CARDIOVASCULAR DISEASE IN COMPANION ANIMALS

CARDIOVASCULAR DISEASE IN COMPANION ANIMALS

Dog, Cat, and Horse

2nd Edition

Wendy A. Ware, John D. Bonagura

with contributions by Brian A. Scansen

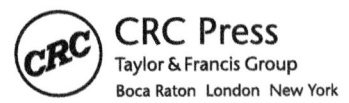

CRC Press is an imprint of the
Taylor & Francis Group, an **informa** business

Second edition published 2022
by CRC Press
6000 Broken Sound Parkway NW, Suite 300, Boca Raton, FL 33487-2742

and by CRC Press
2 Park Square, Milton Park, Abingdon, Oxon, OX14 4RN

© 2022 Taylor & Francis Group, LLC

First edition published by Manson Publishing Ltd 2007, and CRC Press 2011

CRC Press is an imprint of Taylor & Francis Group, LLC

Reasonable efforts have been made to publish reliable data and information, but the author and publisher cannot assume responsibility for the validity of all materials or the consequences of their use. The authors and publishers have attempted to trace the copyright holders of all material reproduced in this publication and apologize to copyright holders if permission to publish in this form has not been obtained. If any copyright material has not been acknowledged please write and let us know so we may rectify in any future reprint.

Except as permitted under U.S. Copyright Law, no part of this book may be reprinted, reproduced, transmitted, or utilized in any form by any electronic, mechanical, or other means, now known or hereafter invented, including photocopying, microfilming, and recording, or in any information storage or retrieval system, without written permission from the publishers.

For permission to photocopy or use material electronically from this work, access www.copyright.com or contact the Copyright Clearance Center, Inc. (CCC), 222 Rosewood Drive, Danvers, MA 01923, 978-750-8400. For works that are not available on CCC please contact mpkbookspermissions@tandf.co.uk

Trademark notice: Product or corporate names may be trademarks or registered trademarks and are used only for identification and explanation without intent to infringe.

ISBN: 978-1-4822-4622-3 (hbk)
ISBN: 978-0-3677-0937-2 (pbk)
ISBN: 978-0-429-18663-9 (ebk)

Typeset in Garamond
by KnowledgeWorks Global Ltd.

Supplementary online media for each chapter can be accessed via book's webpage at https://www.routledge.com/9781482246223.

Look for the Online Media icon:

CONTENTS

Abbreviations xxix

Preface to Cardiovascular Disease in Companion Animals xxxv

About the Authors xxxvii

SECTION I Fundamentals of Clinical Cardiology

1   The Normal Cardiovascular System 3
     General Considerations 3
     The Heart 3
        External Features 3
        Internal Features 6
           Left Heart 6
           Right Heart 8
        Conduction System 9
        Cardiac Electrophysiology 10
           Resting Membrane Potential 11
           Fast-response Action Potential 11
           Slow-response Action Potential 12
        Myocardial Contraction 12
           Electrical–Mechanical Coupling 13
           Myocardial Relaxation 14
        The Heart as a Pump 14
           Cardiac Output 15
           Contractility 15
           Preload 15
           Afterload 16
           Response to Pressure or Volume Loading 16
           Ventricular Function Assessment 17
           Cardiac Cycle and Generation of Heart Sounds 18
           Pressure–Volume Loops 19
        Autonomic Control of the Heart 20
           Effects of Sympathetic Stimulation 20
           Effects of Parasympathetic (Vagal) Stimulation 21

    Cardiac Energy Supply 21
        Coronary Blood Flow 21
  The Circulation 22
    Hemodynamic Concepts 22
        Flow, Pressure, Resistance Relationships 22
        Resistance 22
        Viscosity 23
        Blood Flow Velocity 23
        Laminar and Turbulent Flow 23
    The Vasculature 23
        Arterial System 23
        Arterial Blood Pressure 23
        Microcirculation and Lymphatics 24
        Venous System 25
    Control of the Circulation 25
        Local (Intrinsic) Control 26
        Neurohormonal (Extrinsic) Control 27
        Vascular Receptors 27
        Vascular Reflexes 28
        Hormonal (Humoral) Factors 29
  Cardiovascular Responses to Stress and Exercise 30
  Notes 30
  Suggested Additional Reading and References 31

2 Cardiovascular Examination 33
  General Considerations 33
    Medical History 33
    Clinical Signs of Heart Disease and Failure 33
    Observation of the Patient 35
  Physical Examination 35
    Evaluation of Mucous Membranes 35
    Evaluation of Arterial Pulses 36
    Evaluation of Jugular Veins 36
    Precordial Palpation 37
    Cardiac Auscultation 37
        The Stethoscope 38
        Heart Sounds and Auscultation Technique 38
        Heart Sound Alterations 40
    Respiratory Auscultation 40
        Respiratory Sounds 41
    Evaluation for Abnormal Fluid Accumulation 42
  Suggested Additional Reading and References 42

3 Cardiac Radiography 45
  General Considerations 45
    Radiographic Views 45
    Patient Positioning 46
    Technique Considerations 46
    Systematic Evaluation 46
  The Cardiac Silhouette 46
    The Normal Canine Heart 46
        Vertebral Heart Size 47
    Additional Assessment Methods 50
    The Normal Feline Heart 50
        Vertebral Heart Size 50
    Generalized Cardiomegaly 51

  Small Cardiac Silhouette 52
  Cardiac Chamber Enlargement Patterns 52
   Left Atrium 53
   Left Ventricle 55
   Right Atrium 55
   Right Ventricle 56
Intrathoracic Blood Vessels 58
  Aorta 58
  Main Pulmonary Artery 58
  Lobar Pulmonary Arteries and Veins 58
   Undercirculation Pattern 60
   Overcirculation Pattern 60
   Pulmonary Arteries Larger Than Veins 61
   Pulmonary Veins Larger Than Arteries 61
  Vena Cava 61
The Pulmonary Parenchyma 61
  Pulmonary Patterns 61
  Pulmonary Edema 62
The Pleural Space 64
  Pleural Effusion 64
  Pneumothorax 64
Equine Thoracic Radiography 66
Additional Cardiac Imaging Modalities 67
Suggested Additional Reading and References 67

4   Echocardiography **71**
General Considerations 71
Principles of Echocardiography 72
  Physics and Terminology 72
  Transducer Characteristics 73
  Practical Guidelines and Pitfalls 74
  Image Properties 75
  Image Planes and Display 75
  Image Artifacts 79
   Clinical Utility of Imaging Artifacts 80
The Echocardiographic Examination 80
  Patient Preparation 80
  Sedation 80
  Imaging Technique 81
  Examination Questions and Diagnostic Approach 82
   Pulmonary Imaging and Cavity Effusions 82
   Cardiac Lesions 82
   Cardiac Size and Function 84
Two-dimensional Echocardiography 84
  Standard 2D Echocardiographic Views 84
   Right-sided, Long-axis Image Planes 84
   Clinical Utility of Right-sided, Long-axis Images 85
   Right-sided, Short-axis Image Planes 86
   Clinical Utility of Right-sided, Short-axis Images 86
   Left Apical Images 86
   Clinical Utility of Left Apical Images 88
   Left Cranial Images 88
  Contrast 2D Echocardiography 88
M-mode Echocardiography 88
  Normal M-mode Patterns 90
   Left Ventricle 90

  Mitral Valve 90
  Aortic Valve and Left Atrium 92
  Clinical Utility of the M-mode Exam 92
Cardiac Size and Function Measurement 93
 General Considerations and Pitfalls of Cardiac Chamber Measurement 95
  Methods Used 95
  Measurements in Cats 95
  Other Issues 95
  Identifying Chamber Enlargement 95
Left Atrial Size and Function 103
 Suggested Approach 103
  Atrial Function 103
Left Ventricular Size and Function 104
 Different Approaches 104
 Suggested Approach 105
Right Atrial and Ventricular Size and Function 106
 Suggested Approach 106
Great Vessels 106
Cardiac Chamber Size and Clinical Decision-Making 107
Doppler Echocardiography 107
 Doppler Principles 108
 Overview of Doppler Modalities 112
  Pulsed Wave Doppler Imaging 112
  Color Doppler Imaging 112
  Continuous Wave Doppler Imaging 112
  Tissue Doppler Imaging 112
 Presentation Formats for Doppler Imaging 113
 Doppler Examination—General Approach 113
 Normal Doppler Findings 114
 Semilunar Valves 114
  Left Ventricular Outflow 117
  Right Ventricular Outflow 117
 Atrioventricular Valves 117
  Mitral Valve 118
  Tricuspid Valve 118
 Pulmonary Veins, Left Auricle, and Hepatic Veins 118
  Pulmonary Venous Flow 118
  Atrial Function 119
  Hepatic Veins and Caudal Vena Cava 119
 Tissue Doppler Imaging 119
 Principles of Diagnosis Using Doppler Echocardiography 120
  Abnormal Blood Flow Patterns 120
  Abnormal Blood Flow Velocity 120
 PISA, Vena Contracta, and Jet Area 121
  Proximal Isovelocity Surface Area 121
  Vena Contracta 122
  Jet in the Receiving Chamber 122
 Continuity Relationship and Stenosis 122
 Bernoulli Relationship and Clinical Applications 122
  Valve Stenosis, Gradients, and Pressure Half-time 124
  Valvular Regurgitation 125
  Pulmonary and Systemic Hypertension 126
  Shunts 126
 Doppler Assessment of Ventricular Systolic Function 127
 Doppler Assessment of Ventricular Diastolic Function 127

  Overview and Practical Considerations 127
  Relaxation Abnormality 129
  Pseudonormal Filling 129
  Restrictive Filling 129
 Other Echocardiographic Imaging Applications 129
  Transesophageal Echocardiography 129
  3D Echocardiography 130
  Advanced Image Analysis 130
 Suggested Additional Reading and References 130

5 Electrocardiography **135**
 General Considerations 135
  ECG Lead Systems 136
   Standard Limb Leads 137
   Precordial Leads 138
   Base-Apex Lead 138
  Recording a Standard ECG 138
   Recording a Base-Apex ECG 139
 Approach to ECG Interpretation 139
  Heart Rate 139
  Heart Rhythm 140
   Abnormal Rhythms: Basic Concepts 140
  ECG Measurements 142
 Cardiac Rhythm Assessment 142
  Sinus Rhythm and Variations 142
   Sinus Arrhythmia 143
   Sinus Pause or Arrest 143
  Abnormal Cardiac Rhythms 143
   Supraventricular Premature Complexes 143
   Atrial Tachycardia 145
   Atrial Flutter 145
   Atrial Fibrillation 146
   Atrioventricular Reentrant Tachycardia 147
   Ventricular Premature Complexes 147
   Ventricular Tachycardia 148
   Accelerated Idioventricular Rhythm 149
   Ventricular Parasystole 149
   Isorhythmic Atrioventricular Dissociation 150
   Ventricular Fibrillation 150
   Escape Complexes and Rhythms 150
  Abnormal Cardiac Conduction 151
   Atrioventricular Conduction Disturbances 151
   Intraatrial Conduction Disturbances 153
   Intraventricular Conduction Disturbances 153
   Ventricular Preexcitation 153
 Mean Electrical Axis 155
 Cardiac Chamber Enlargement 156
  Atrial Enlargement Patterns 156
  Ventricular Enlargement Patterns 156
   Right Ventricle 156
   Left Ventricle 156
 Other ECG Abnormalities and Considerations 157
  Small-voltage QRS Complexes 157
  Electrical Alternans 157
  ST-T Abnormalities 157

         The QT Interval... 158
         Effects of Drugs and Electrolyte Abnormalities on the ECG.. 159
            Hyperkalemia.. 160
            Hypokalemia... 161
         Common ECG Artifacts... 161
      Ambulatory ECG... 162
         Holter Monitoring.. 162
         Cardiac Event Recording... 162
         Smartphone and Other Wireless ECG Recording.. 163
         Exercise ECG in Horses... 164
      Suggested Additional Reading and References 165

6   Cardiac Catheterization and Angiocardiography.. 167
      General Considerations 167
      Cardiovascular Catheterization.. 167
         Preparation and Planning 167
         Equipment 168
            Imaging 168
            Hemodynamic Monitoring 169
            Needles, Sheaths, Catheters, and Wires 170
         Patient Preparation 172
         Vascular Access 172
      Angiocardiography... 174
         Nonselective Versus Selective Injection 174
         Equipment and Supplies.. 174
            Power Injector.. 174
            Contrast Agents.. 174
      Common Interventional Procedures 175
         Via Right Heart Catheterization.. 175
            Cardiac Pacing.. 175
            Pulmonary Balloon Valvuloplasty 177
         Via Left Heart Catheterization 179
            Patent Ductus Arteriosus Occlusion 179
            Aortic Balloon Valvuloplasty... 181
         Hybrid Catheterization.. 184
      Suggested Additional Reading and References 184

SECTION II   Clinical Manifestations of Cardiovascular Disease

7   Exercise Intolerance.. 189
      General Considerations 189
      Approach to the Patient with Exercise Intolerance.. 192
      Suggested Additional Reading and References 193

8   Intermittent Collapse and Syncope... 195
      General Considerations 195
         Causes of Syncope 196
      Approach to the Patient with Syncope or Intermittent Collapse 199
      Suggested Additional Reading and References 202

9   Cough.. 203
      General Considerations 203
      Approach to the Coughing Patient 205
      Suggested Additional Reading and References 208

10	**Respiratory Distress**	**211**
	General Considerations	211
	Causes of Respiratory Distress	212
	Hypoxemia	214
	Pulmonary Edema	215
	Pleural Effusion	216
	Pulmonary Thromboembolism	216
	Approach to the Patient with Respiratory Difficulty	217
	Patterns of Breathing	218
	Clinical Examination	219
	Clinical Testing and Management	219
	Suggested Additional Reading and References	221
11	**Murmurs and Abnormal Heart Sounds**	**225**
	General Considerations	225
	Cardiac Murmurs	225
	Murmur Characteristics	226
	Timing	226
	Intensity	226
	Point of Maximal Intensity and Radiation	226
	Shape and Quality	227
	Nonpathologic Murmurs	228
	Dogs	228
	Cats	228
	Horses	228
	Pathologic Systolic Murmurs	228
	Mitral Regurgitation	229
	Tricuspid Regurgitation	229
	Ventricular Outflow Obstructions	230
	Ventricular Septal Defect	230
	Pathologic Diastolic Murmurs	230
	Murmurs in Both Systole and Diastole	231
	Continuous Murmur	231
	To-and-Fro Murmur	231
	Abnormal Transient Sounds	231
	Gallop Sounds	232
	S_3 Gallop	232
	S_4 Gallop	232
	Systolic Clicks and Ejection Sounds	232
	Other Considerations in Cardiac Auscultation	233
	Approach to the Patient with a Murmur or Other Abnormal Heart Sound	233
	Suggested Additional Reading and References	235
12	**Abnormal Heart Rate or Rhythm**	**237**
	General Considerations	237
	Rapid Heart Rate and Arrhythmias	240
	Slow Heart Rate and Arrhythmias	241
	Approach to the Patient With Abnormal Heart Rate or Rhythm	242
	Suggested Additional Reading and References	245
13	**Abnormal Mucous Membrane Color**	**247**
	General Considerations	247
	Pallor	247
	Cyanosis	247
	Methemoglobinemia	249

	Approach to the Patient with Abnormal Mucous Membrane Color	250
	Suggested Additional Reading and References	252
14	**Arterial Pulse Abnormalities**	**253**
	General Considerations	253
	Hypokinetic Pulses	254
	Hyperkinetic Pulses	255
	Pulse Deficits	256
	Other Pulse Abnormalities	256
	Approach to the Patient with an Arterial Pulse Abnormality	257
	Suggested Additional Reading and References	258
15	**Jugular Vein Distension or Pulsation**	**261**
	General Considerations	261
	Approach to the Patient with Jugular Vein Distension or Pulsation	263
	Central Venous Pressure Measurement	264
	Suggested Additional Reading and References	266
16	**Abdominal Distension**	**267**
	General Considerations	267
	Abdominal Effusions	267
	Other Causes of Abdominal Distension	270
	Approach to the Patient with Abdominal Distension	270
	Suggested Additional Reading and References	272
17	**Subcutaneous Edema**	**275**
	General Considerations	275
	Cranial Caval Syndrome	277
	Lymphedema	278
	Myxedema	278
	Approach to the Patient with Subcutaneous Edema	278
	Suggested Additional Reading and References	279
18	**Cardiomegaly**	**281**
	General Considerations	282
	Approach to the Patient with Cardiomegaly	284
	Suggested Additional Reading and References	285
19	**Clinical Laboratory Abnormalities**	**287**
	Routine Laboratory Tests	287
	Complete Blood Count	287
	Serum Biochemistries	289
	Renal Function Tests	289
	Liver and Pancreatic Enzymes	289
	Electrolytes	289
	Proteins	290
	Muscle Enzymes	290
	Urinalysis	290
	Tests for Parasites and Other Infections	290
	Cardiac Biomarkers	290
	Cardiac Troponins	290
	Natriuretic Peptides	291
	Other Tests	293
	Approach to the Patient	293
	Suggested Additional Reading and References	294

SECTION III Heart Failure

20 Heart Failure: Pathophysiology and Patient Assessment 299
  Pathophysiology 300
    General Perspectives 300
    Contractility Failure 300
    Increased Workload 300
    Diastolic Dysfunction 301
    Clinical Associations 301
    Cardiac Responses 302
    Neurohormonal Mechanisms 303
      Sympathetic Nervous System 303
      Baroreceptor Function 305
      Renin–Angiotensin–Aldosterone System 305
      Arginine Vasopressin (Antidiuretic Hormone) 307
      Endothelin 308
      Cytokines and Inflammation 308
      Natriuretic Peptides and Other Endogenous Vasodilatory Substances 308
      Other Factors 310
    Renal Responses 310
    Exercise Capacity 311
      Cardiac Cachexia 312
  Clinical Manifestations of Congestive Heart Failure 312
    Presenting Signs 312
      Cardiogenic Shock 313
    Diagnosis 313
      Laboratory Tests 313
  Assessment of Heart Disease and Heart Failure Severity 313
    Heart Disease/Failure Staging System 313
    Heart Failure Functional Classification Systems 314
  Suggested Additional Reading and References 314

21 Drugs for the Treatment of Heart Failure 317
  Diuretics 317
    Furosemide and Other Loop Diuretics 317
      Torsemide 319
    Spironolactone 319
    Thiazides 320
  Angiotensin Converting Enzyme Inhibitors 320
    Enalapril 322
    Benazepril 322
    Other ACE Inhibitors 322
  Other Vasodilators used in Heart Failure 323
    Hydralazine 323
    Amlodipine 324
    Prazosin 324
    Nitrates 324
  Positive Inotropic Agents 325
    Pimobendan 325
    Digoxin 327
      Digoxin Toxicity 327
      Serum Digoxin Concentration 328
      Management of Digoxin Toxicity 328
    Catecholamines 330
      Dobutamine 330

      Dopamine 330
      Other Phosphodiesterase-3 Inhibitors.. 330
   Other Drugs Used in Heart Failure... 331
      Sildenafil.. 331
      Beta-blockers in Chronic Heart Failure 331
         Carvedilol... 332
         Metoprolol and Atenolol... 332
      Newer Therapies 332
         Angiotensin Receptor Blockade and Natriuretic Peptide Potentiation 332
         Other Strategies 333
   Suggested Additional Reading and References 334

22 Management of Heart Failure **337**
   Considerations for Managing Preclinical Heart Disease.. 337
      Initial Signs of Congestive Heart Failure.. 340
   Acute Decompensated Congestive Heart Failure in Dogs and Cats 340
      Oxygen Supplementation and Ventilation 341
      Diuretic Therapy... 341
      Vasodilator Therapy 344
      Other Therapies for Acute Congestive Heart Failure 346
      Inotropic Support.. 346
      Heart Failure from Diastolic Dysfunction 347
      Monitoring and Initial Follow-up... 348
   Chronic Heart Failure Management in Dogs... 349
      Drug Therapy 350
      Dietary Considerations..351
         Omega-3 Fatty Acids 351
         Other Dietary Supplements..351
         Inappetence 352
      Exercise.. 352
      Long-term Management of Diastolic Dysfunction... 353
      Monitoring and Follow-up Evaluation... 353
      Approach to Refractory CHF 354
   Chronic Heart Failure Management in Cats 356
      Management of Diastolic Dysfunction.. 357
      Dietary and Other Recommendations 357
      Monitoring and Follow-up Evaluation... 357
      Approach to Refractory CHF 358
   Management of Heart Failure in Horses.. 358
      Acute Congestive Heart Failure 358
      Considerations for Ongoing Therapy.. 359
   Suggested Additional Reading and References 359

SECTION IV   Heart Rhythm Disturbances

23 Arrhythmias: Pathophysiology and Clinical Associations.. **363**
   Electrophysiologic Mechanisms 363
      Enhanced and Abnormal Automaticity... 364
      Triggered Activity 365
      Reentry... 365
   Cardiac and Hemodynamic Consequences... 368
      Effects of Heart Rate 368
      Ineffective Atrial Contraction... 368

  Loss of Atrioventricular Synchrony 369
  Ventricular Dyssynchrony 369
 Clinical Causes and Associations of Arrhythmias 369
 Suggested Additional Reading and References 371

24 **Antiarrhythmic Therapies** **373**
 Drug Classification Systems 373
 Antiarrhythmic Drugs 374
  Class I Antiarrhythmic Drugs 374
   Lidocaine 375
   Procainamide 376
   Quinidine 376
   Mexiletine 378
   Phenytoin 378
   Class Ic Agents 378
  Class II Antiarrhythmic Drugs 379
   Propranolol 380
   Atenolol 380
   Metoprolol 380
   Esmolol 381
   Other Beta-blocking Drugs 381
  Class III Antiarrhythmic Drugs 381
   Sotalol 381
   Amiodarone 382
   Other Class III Agents 383
  Class IV Antiarrhythmic Drugs 384
   Diltiazem 384
   Verapamil 385
  Other Drugs with Antiarrhythmic Effects 385
   Digoxin 385
   Ivabradine 385
   Other Agents 386
  Anticholinergic Drugs 386
   Atropine Sulfate and Glycopyrrolate 386
   Atropine Response Test 387
   Other Anticholinergic Agents 387
  Sympathomimetic Drugs 387
   Isoproterenol 387
   Bronchodilator Drugs 387
   Epinephrine 387
  Other Drugs 388
   Phenylephrine 388
   Edrophonium 388
 Vagal Maneuver 388
 Pacing Therapy 388
 Cardioversion and Defibrillation 391
  Cardioversion 391
   Intracardiac Electrical Mapping and Catheter Ablation 392
  Defibrillation 393
 Suggested Additional Reading and References 393

25 **Management of Cardiac Arrhythmias** **397**
 Initial Management Considerations 397
  Patient Assessment 397
  Rhythm Diagnosis 398

Decision to Treat 399
　　　General Supportive Measures.. 400
　Sinus Rhythm Disturbances 401
　　Sinus Tachycardia 401
　　Sinus Bradycardia 401
　　Sinus Node Dysfunction 405
　　　Sick Sinus Syndrome 405
　Atrial Rhythm Disturbances.. 406
　　Atrial Premature Complexes 407
　　Atrial Tachycardia 407
　　　Paroxysmal (Nonsustained) Atrial Tachycardia 407
　　　Sustained Atrial Tachycardia 407
　　Atrial Flutter and Fibrillation 409
　　　Atrial Flutter 409
　　　Atrial Fibrillation 409
　　　Atrial Fibrillation Management in Dogs 411
　　　Atrial Fibrillation Management in Cats 412
　　　Atrial Fibrillation Management in Horses 413
　　Atrial Standstill 416
　Atrioventricular Reentrant (Reciprocating) Tachycardia 417
　AV Junctional Rhythms.. 419
　　Atrioventricular Blocks.. 419
　Ventricular Rhythm Disturbances 422
　　Ventricular Premature Complexes 422
　　Accelerated Idioventricular Rhythm 423
　　Ventricular Tachycardia 424
　　　Nonsustained (Paroxysmal) Ventricular Tachycardia 424
　　　Sustained Ventricular Tachycardia 424
　　Therapy for Ventricular Arrhythmias 424
　　　In-hospital Therapy for Ventricular Arrhythmias.. 424
　　　Chronic Therapy for Ventricular Arrhythmias 426
　　Ventricular Flutter and Fibrillation 428
　　Lethal Arrhythmias and Cardiopulmonary Arrest 428
　Suggested Additional Reading and References 430

SECTION V Cardiovascular Diseases

26　Congenital Cardiac Shunts.. 435
　Congenital Cardiovascular Disease in General 435
　Pathophysiology.. 437
　　Left-to-Right Shunting 437
　　Right-to-Left Shunting 437
　Patent Ductus Arteriosus (Left-to-Right Shunting).. 439
　　Clinical Features 441
　　Diagnostic Tests.. 442
　　Management 444
　　　Transcatheter Ductal Occlusion 446
　　　Surgical Ductal Ligation 447
　　　Changes and Prognosis Following Ductal Closure 448
　Reversed Patent Ductus Arteriosus (Right-to-Left Shunting) 449
　　Clinical Features 450
　　Diagnostic Tests.. 450
　　Management 452

Ventricular Septal Defect (Left-to-Right Shunting)..454
    Clinical Features 456
    Diagnostic Tests...456
    Management 458
Reversed Ventricular Septal Defect (Right-to-Left Shunting)..460
    Clinical Features 460
    Diagnostic Tests...460
    Management 460
Atrial Septal Defects 461
    Clinical Features of Left-to-Right Shunting Atrial Septal Defect..................................462
    Diagnostic Tests in Left-to-Right Shunting Atrial Septal Defect 462
Reversed Atrial Septal Defect (Right-to-Left Shunting)..464
    Clinical Features and Diagnostic tests for Right-to-Left Shunting ASD........................464
    Management of Atrial Septal Defect 465
Patent Foramen Ovale 465
Atrioventricular Septal Defect 466
    Clinical Features 466
    Diagnostic Tests...467
    Management 467
Tetralogy of Fallot..467
    Clinical Features 469
    Diagnostic Tests...470
    Management 471
Suggested Additional Reading and References 472

27 Congenital Valvular Malformations...**477**
Pathophysiology...478
    Ventricular Outflow Obstruction...478
    Semilunar Valve Regurgitation 479
    Atrioventricular Valve Regurgitation 480
    Atrioventricular Valve Stenosis 480
Aortic Stenosis...480
    Clinical Features 481
    Diagnostic Tests...482
    Management 488
        Prognosis...489
Pulmonic Stenosis..490
    Clinical Features 492
    Diagnostic Tests...492
    Management 497
        Prognosis...499
Mitral Dysplasia 500
    Clinical Features 500
    Diagnostic Tests...500
    Management 504
        Prognosis...504
Tricuspid Dysplasia..504
    Clinical Features 505
    Diagnostic Tests...505
    Management 506
        Prognosis...507
Suggested Additional Reading and References 508

28 Other Cardiovascular Malformations **511**
Cor Triatriatum..511

- Cor Triatriatum Dexter ... 511
  - Clinical Features ... 511
  - Diagnostic Tests ... 511
  - Management ... 512
- Cor Triatriatum Sinister ... 512
  - Clinical Features ... 512
  - Diagnostic Tests ... 514
  - Management ... 514
- Endocardial Fibroelastosis ... 515
- Vascular Developmental Considerations ... 515
  - Aortic Arch Embryology and Anatomy ... 515
  - Venous Embryology and Anatomy ... 515
- Vascular Ring Anomalies ... 516
  - Persistent Right Aortic Arch ... 516
  - Other Vascular Ring Anomalies ... 516
    - Double Aortic Arch ... 516
    - Right Ductus Arteriosus ... 516
    - Aberrant (Retroesophageal) Subclavian Arteries ... 517
  - Clinical Features ... 518
  - Diagnostic Tests ... 519
  - Management ... 520
- Other Aortic Arch Anomalies ... 520
  - Truncus Arteriosus Communis ... 520
  - Coarctation of the Aorta ... 521
  - Tubular Hypoplasia of the Aorta ... 521
  - Interruption of the Aorta ... 521
- Other Causes of Aortic Dilation ... 521
  - Aortocardiac and Aortopulmonary Fistulae ... 522
- Arteriovenous and Venovenous Malformations ... 523
  - Arteriovenous Malformations ... 523
  - Portosystemic Vascular Anomalies ... 523
  - Venous Malformations ... 524
    - Persistent Left Cranial Vena Cava ... 524
    - Left Azygous Vein ... 525
    - Anomalies of the Caudal Vena Cava ... 526
    - Venous Aneurysms ... 526
    - Retrocaval Ureter ... 526
- Suggested Additional Reading and References ... 526

29 Degenerative Valvular Disease of the Dog ... 529
- The Normal Mitral Valve ... 529
- Pathophysiology ... 530
  - Valvular Changes ... 531
    - Valve Lesion Severity ... 533
  - Myocardial and Chamber Remodeling ... 534
  - Other Pathophysiologic Changes ... 537
- Clinical Features ... 537
  - Physical Findings ... 538
  - Complicating Factors ... 540
- Diagnostic Tests ... 540
  - Clinical Laboratory Tests ... 540
  - Radiography ... 541
  - Electrocardiography ... 545
  - Echocardiography ... 545

Left Heart Evaluation	546
Right Heart Evaluation	554
Systemic Vascular Function	554
Management	554
Preclinical (Stage B) Degenerative Mitral Valve Disease	554
Stage B1	554
Stage B2	556
Onset of Congestive Heart Failure (Stage C)	558
Mild to Moderate Signs of CHF	559
Severe Signs of CHF	560
Transition to Home Care	560
Monitoring Heart Failure Therapy	561
Strategies for End-Stage or Refractory (Stage D) Heart Failure	561
Mitral Valve Repair and Other Interventions	561
Complications and Comorbid Conditions	561
Pulmonary Hypertension	561
Arrhythmias	562
Ruptured Chordae Tendineae	562
Left Atrial Tears	562
Chronic Respiratory Disease	563
Abnormal Blood Pressure	564
Renal Dysfunction and Other Systemic Problems	564
Prognosis	565
Suggested Additional Reading and References	566

30 Valvular Heart Disease of the Horse 573

Causes of Equine Valvular Disease	573
Pathophysiology of Valvular Regurgitation	574
Clinical Features	578
Cardiac Murmurs	578
Systolic Murmurs	579
Diastolic Murmurs	579
Other Clinical Findings	579
Clinical Outcomes and Overall Risk Assessment	581
Diagnostic Tests	581
Echocardiography in Valvular Heart Disease	581
Mitral Regurgitation	582
Aortic Regurgitation	586
Assessment of Left Heart Chambers	586
Tricuspid Regurgitation	588
Other Diagnostic Tests	588
Management	588
Prognosis	589
Suggested Additional Reading and References	589

31 Infective Endocarditis 591

Predisposing Factors	591
Pathophysiology	592
Cardiac Consequences	593
Systemic Consequences	594
Causative Organisms	594
Clinical Features	596
Physical Findings	596
Diagnostic Tests	597

Blood Cultures..597
　　　Molecular and Serologic Testing..598
　　　Radiography and Electrocardiography...599
　　　Echocardiography..599
　Management...600
　　　Follow-up and Monitoring 603
　　　　Prognosis...604
　　　　Antibiotic Prophylaxis 604
　Suggested Additional Reading and References 604

32　Myocardial Diseases of the Dog..607
　Idiopathic Dilated Cardiomyopathy..607
　　Pathophysiology 608
　　　Clinical Features 610
　　　　Physical Findings 611
　　　Diagnostic Tests in Preclinical (Occult) DCM..612
　　　　Electrocardiography in Preclinical DCM 613
　　　　Echocardiography in Preclinical DCM..614
　　　Diagnostic Tests in Overt DCM...616
　　　　Radiography in Overt DCM..616
　　　　Electrocardiography in Overt DCM..617
　　　　Echocardiography in Overt DCM...620
　　　Management of Preclinical DCM..621
　　　　Prognosis in Preclinical DCM 622
　　　Management of Overt DCM..622
　　　　Prognosis in Overt DCM 624
　Arrhythmogenic Right Ventricular Cardiomyopathy..624
　　　Pathophysiology 625
　　　Clinical Features 626
　　　Diagnostic Tests..627
　　　Management..628
　　　　Prognosis...629
　Hypertrophic Cardiomyopathy...629
　　　Pathophysiology 629
　　　Clinical Features 629
　　　Diagnostic Tests..630
　　　Management..630
　Secondary Myocardial Diseases..630
　　　Tachycardia-Induced Cardiomyopathy...630
　　　Doxorubicin Toxicity...631
　　　Nutritional Deficiencies and Metabolic Abnormalities..632
　　　　Taurine 633
　　　　L-carnitine 634
　　　　Catecholamine-Associated Myocardial Disease 634
　　　　Muscular Dystrophy 635
　　　　Other Conditions 635
　　　Ischemic Heart Disease 636
　Infective Myocarditis...636
　　　Clinical Features and Diagnostic Tests...636
　　　Management..638
　　　Viral Myocarditis...639
　　　Bacterial Myocarditis...639
　　　　Lyme Disease 639
　　　Protozoal Myocarditis..640
　　　　Chagas Disease...640

	Other Protozoal Diseases	641
	Miscellaneous Causes of Myocarditis	641
Noninfective Myocarditis		641
	Traumatic Myocarditis	641
Note		643
Suggested Additional Reading and References		643

33 Myocardial Diseases of the Cat ... 649

- Hypertrophic Cardiomyopathy ... 649
  - Pathophysiology ... 651
    - Cardiac Morphologic Abnormalities ... 652
  - Myocardial Functional and Hemodynamic Abnormalities ... 653
  - Clinical Features ... 656
    - Screening for Hypertrophic Cardiomyopathy ... 656
    - History ... 657
    - Physical Findings - Auscultation ... 657
    - Physical Findings–Congestive Heart Failure ... 659
  - Diagnostic Tests ... 660
    - Laboratory Tests ... 660
    - Radiography ... 661
    - Electrocardiography ... 663
    - Echocardiography ... 664
  - Management ... 671
    - Management of Preclinical HCM ... 671
    - Prognosis in Preclinical HCM ... 672
    - Acute Congestive Heart Failure ... 673
    - Chronic Heart Failure ... 675
    - Other Complications and Prognosis ... 678
- Restrictive Cardiomyopathy ... 678
  - Pathophysiology ... 678
  - Clinical Features ... 679
  - Diagnostic Tests ... 679
  - Management ... 681
    - Prognosis ... 682
- Dilated Cardiomyopathy ... 682
  - Pathophysiology ... 682
  - Clinical Features ... 682
  - Diagnostic Tests ... 683
  - Management ... 685
    - Prognosis ... 686
- Arrhythmogenic Right Ventricular Cardiomyopathy ... 686
  - Pathophysiology ... 686
  - Clinical Features ... 686
  - Diagnostic Tests ... 686
  - Management ... 687
    - Prognosis ... 687
- Cardiomyopathy of "Nonspecific Phenotype" ... 687
  - Clinical Features and Diagnostic Tests ... 687
  - Management ... 687
- Secondary Myocardial Disease ... 688
  - Causes ... 688
    - Pressure Overload ... 688
    - Hyperthyroidism ... 688
    - Miscellaneous Causes ... 689
    - Corticosteroid-Associated Congestive Heart Failure ... 689

Myocarditis 689
    Causes 689
    Pathophysiology 690
    Clinical Features 690
    Diagnostic Tests 691
    Management 691
Suggested Additional Reading and References 691

34 Myocardial Diseases of the Horse **695**
Causes of Equine Myocardial Disease 695
Pathophysiology 696
Specific Myocardial Disorders 697
    Myocardial Toxicity 698
    Myocarditis 698
    Idiopathic Dilated Cardiomyopathy 698
    Tachycardia-Induced Cardiomyopathy 699
    Infiltrative Cardiomyopathy 699
    Ischemic Myocardial Disease 699
    Hypertensive Cardiomyopathy 700
    Myocardial Fibrosis 700
Clinical Features 701
Diagnostic Tests 701
    Laboratory Tests 701
    Electrocardiography 702
    Echocardiography 702
Management 703
    Medical Therapy for Congestive Heart Failure 703
    Prognosis 703
Suggested Additional Reading and References 704

35 Pericardial Diseases and Cardiac Tumors **705**
Congenital Pericardial Malformations 706
    Peritoneopericardial Diaphragmatic Hernia 707
        Pathophysiology 707
        Clinical Features 708
        Diagnostic Tests 708
        Management 708
Acquired Pericardial Effusions 710
    Types of Effusion 710
        Transudative Effusions 710
        Hemorrhagic Effusions 711
        Exudative Effusions 711
        Pericarditis in Horses 712
        Chylous Effusions 712
    Pathophysiology 712
        Cardiac Tamponade 713
    Clinical Features 714
        Physical Findings 715
        Pericarditis in Horses 715
    Diagnostic Tests 716
        Laboratory Tests 716
        Radiography 716
        Electrocardiography 717
        Echocardiography 717
        Other Imaging 722

  Central Venous Pressure and Right Heart Catheterization 722
  Pericardial Fluid Evaluation 722
  Pericarditis in Horses 723
 Management 723
  Pericardiocentesis 724
  Complications of Pericardiocentesis 727
  Management After Pericardiocentesis 728
  Management of Pericardial Effusion in Horses 729
Constrictive Pericardial Disease 730
 Pathophysiology 730
 Clinical Features 730
 Diagnostic Tests 730
 Management 732
Cardiac Tumors 732
 Pathophysiology 733
 Clinical Features 734
  Physical Findings 735
 Diagnostic Tests 735
 Management 740
Suggested Additional Reading and References 742

36 Thromboembolic Disease **745**

Normal Hemostasis 745
 Fibrinolysis 747
 Mechanisms Opposing Thrombosis 747
Pathophysiology 748
 Mechanisms of Pathologic Thrombosis 748
 Thromboembolism and Common Disease Conditions 749
 Systemic Arterial Thromboembolic Disease 750
 Pulmonary Arterial Thromboembolic Disease 753
 Venous Thrombosis 754
Clinical Features 755
 Arterial Thromboembolism 755
  Arterial Thromboembolism in Cats 755
  Arterial Thromboembolism and Thrombosis in Dogs 756
  Coronary Thromboembolism 757
  Pulmonary Thromboembolism 757
  Venous Thrombosis 757
Diagnostic Tests 757
 Laboratory Tests 757
 Radiography 759
 Echocardiography 759
 Other Diagnostic Imaging 761
Management of Thromboembolic Disease 763
 General Therapeutic Principles 763
 Antiplatelet Therapy 764
  Clopidogrel 764
  Aspirin 764
  Other Antiplatelet Drugs 765
 Anticoagulant Therapy 765
  Unfractionated Heparin 765
  Low Molecular Weight Heparin 765
  Newer Anticoagulant Agents 766
 Fibrinolytic Therapy 766
  Tissue Plasminogen Activator 766

	Other Fibrinolytic Agents	767
	Other Considerations	768
	Prognosis	769
	Thromboembolic Disease Prophylaxis	769
	Antiplatelet and Anticoagulant Strategies	769
	Warfarin	770
	Suggested Additional Reading and References	770
37	**Vascular Diseases**	**775**
	Pathophysiology	775
	Arteriovenous Fistula	776
	Clinical Features	776
	Diagnostic Tests	777
	Management	778
	Arteriosclerosis	778
	Atherosclerosis	779
	Intramural Coronary Arteriosclerosis	780
	Medial Hypertrophy of Pulmonary Arteries	780
	Clinical Features of Arteriosclerosis	780
	Vascular Mineralization	780
	Vasculitis (Arteritis)	781
	Thrombosis and Embolism	782
	Thrombotic Diseases	782
	Arterial Embolic Disease	783
	Venous Embolic Disease	783
	Other Vascular Diseases	784
	Suggested Additional Reading and References	786
38	**Systemic Hypertension**	**787**
	Blood Pressure in Normal Animals	787
	Risk for Target Organ Disease	788
	Predisposing Conditions	789
	Pathophysiology	789
	Kidney Disease	790
	Endocrine Disease	791
	Other Associations	792
	Pathologic Effects of Hypertension	793
	Clinical Features	794
	Physical Findings	795
	Blood Pressure Measurement	795
	Direct Measurement	796
	Indirect Measurement	796
	Doppler Method	798
	Oscillometric Method	799
	Other Diagnostic Tests	799
	Laboratory Tests	799
	Radiography and Electrocardiography	800
	Echocardiography	800
	Management	802
	Decision to Treat	802
	Antihypertensive Strategies	803
	Monitoring Therapy	805
	Management of Hypertensive Emergencies	805
	Prognosis	807
	Antihypertensive Agents	807

Angiotensin Converting Enzyme Inhibitors..807
  Angiotensin Receptor Blockers...807
    Telmisartan...807
  Amlodipine..808
  Other Drugs..809
  Suggested Additional Reading and References 810

39 **Pulmonary Hypertension**..**813**
  Pathophysiology..815
    Cor Pulmonale..816
    Pulmonary Arterial Hypertension 817
    Pulmonary Venous Hypertension 819
    Pulmonary Disease and Hypoxia..819
    Pulmonary Thromboembolism 821
    Parasitic Disease...822
    Other Causes of Pulmonary Hypertension...823
  Clinical Features...823
    Physical Findings 824
  Diagnostic Tests 824
    Laboratory Tests 825
    Radiography..825
    Electrocardiography..827
    Echocardiography..827
    Cardiac Catheterization 833
    Other Tests...833
  Management...833
    Phosphodiesterase-5 Inhibitors 834
    Additional Medical Therapy...835
    Other Considerations 836
      Prognosis..836
  Suggested Additional Reading and References 836

40 **Heartworm Disease**..**841**
  Dirofilaria immitis...841
    Heartworm Transmission..841
      Heartworm Life Cycle...841
    Pathophysiology 843
      Dogs..843
      Cats...844
    Clinical Features...846
      Dogs..846
      Cats...846
    Heartworm Testing..846
      Serologic Tests 847
      Detection of Microfilariae 849
    Other Diagnostic Tests...850
      Dogs..850
      Cats...854
    Management of Heartworm Disease in Dogs 856
      Pretreatment Assessment..856
      Initial Doxycycline and Macrocyclic Lactone Therapy..856
      Melarsomine Treatment..858
      Assessing Adulticide Efficacy 859
      Alternatives to Melarsomine Adulticide Therapy..860
      Treatment of Dogs with Complicated Heartworm Disease................................860

    Postadulticide Pulmonary Thromboembolism... 861
    Microfilaricide Therapy... 862
    Caval Syndrome... 863
  Management of Heartworm Disease in Cats... 866
  Heartworm Prevention in Dogs... 867
    Macrocyclic Lactones... 867
    Lack of Efficacy Concerns... 868
    Vector Control... 869
    Minimizing Heartworm Transmission Associated with Relocated Dogs... 869
  Heartworm Prevention in Cats... 870
Angiostrongylus Vasorum... 870
  Pathophysiology... 870
  Clinical Features... 871
    Physical Findings... 871
  Diagnostic Tests... 871
    Laboratory Tests... 871
    Imaging... 872
  Management... 873
  Prognosis... 873
    Prevention... 873
Suggested Additional Reading and References... 873

Summary Drug Table for Dogs... 877
Summary Drug Table for Cats... 889
Summary Drug Table for Horses... 899

Index... 905

ABBREVIATIONS

2D	two-dimensional	**APC**	atrial premature complex
3D	three-dimensional	**A_R**	(Doppler) atrial reversal (wave)
4D	four-dimensional	**AR**	aortic valve regurgitation
5-HT	5-hydroxytryptophan, serotonin	**ARB**	angiotensin receptor blocker
αSMA	alpha-smooth muscle actin	**ARNI**	angiotensin receptor blocker and neprilysin inhibitor
A	late diastolic (atrial kick) mitral or tricuspid inflow (motion or velocity)	**ARVC**	arrhythmogenic right ventricular cardiomyopathy
A-a	alveolar–arterial (O_2 gradient)	**AS**	aortic stenosis
Ab	antibody	**ASD**	atrial septal defect
ABV	aortic balloon valvuloplasty (or BAV, balloon aortic valvuloplasty)	**AST**	aspartate aminotransferase
		AT	(Doppler flow) acceleration time
ACDO	Amplatz® Canine Duct Occluder	**ATE**	arterial thromboembolism
ACE	angiotensin converting enzyme	**ATP**	adenosine triphosphate
Ach	acetylcholine	**ATPase**	adenosine triphosphatase
ACVIM	American College of Veterinary Internal Medicine	**AV**	atrioventricular
		A-V	arteriovenous
ADH	antidiuretic hormone	**AVP**	arginine vasopressin
ADP	adenosine diphosphate	**AVRT**	atrioventricular reciprocating tachycardia
ADPase	adenosine diphosphatase		
AF	atrial fibrillation	**AVSD**	atrioventricular septal defect
Ag	antigen	**BAL**	bronchoalveolar lavage
AHS	American Heartworm Society	**BAPGM**	Bartonella alpha Proteobacteria growth medium
ALD	aldosterone		
ALS	advanced life support	**BAV**	balloon aortic valvuloplasty (or aortic balloon valvuloplasty, ABV)
ALT	alanine aminotransferase		
Ang	angiotensin	**BEG**	"boutique," exotic protein-based or grain-free (diets)
Ang1R	angiotensin-1 receptor(s)		
Ang2R	angiotensin-2 receptor(s)	**BENCH**	
ANP	atrial natriuretic peptide	**(study)**	The effect of benazepril on survival times and clinical signs of dogs with congestive heart failure (BENCH study group, 1999; see Chapter 21 references)
Ao	aorta/aortic		
AoSA	aorto-septal angle		
AoV	distance between the open aortic valve leaflets; maximal aortic orifice diameter		
		BLS	basic life support

BNP	brain natriuretic peptide	DC	direct current
BP	blood pressure	DCM	dilated cardiomyopathy
BPV	balloon pulmonary valvuloplasty (or pulmonary balloon valvuloplasty, PBV)	DCRV	double-chambered right ventricle
		DDD	dual-paced, dual-sensed, dual-response (pacing mode)
BUN	blood urea nitrogen	DELAY (study)	Delay of appearance of symptoms of canine degenerative mitral valve disease treated with spironolactone and benazepril (Borgarelli, 2020; see Chapter 29 references)
Ca^{++}	calcium ion		
cAMP	cyclic adenosine monophosphate		
CATSCAN (study)	Cardiomyopathy prevalence in 780 apparently healthy cats in rehoming centers (Payne, 2015; see Chapter 33 references)		
		DHA	docosahexaenoic acid
		DIC	disseminated intravascular coagulation
CaVC	caudal vena cava/caval		
CB	cutting balloon (catheter)	DISH	discrete interventricular septal hypertrophy
CBC	complete blood count		
CDI	color Doppler imaging (CF Doppler)	DMVD	degenerative mitral valve disease (also called chronic mitral valve disease, CVMD, and myxomatous mitral valve disease, MMVD)
CF	color flow (Doppler)		
cGMP	cyclic guanosine monophosphate		
CK	creatine kinase	DNA	deoxyribonucleic acid
CKCS	Cavalier King Charles Spaniels	dP/dt	change in pressure/time (rate of LV pressure change)
CK-MB	cardiac-specific isoenzyme of CK		
CHD	congenital heart disease	dP/dt_{max}	maximal rate of LV pressure rise during isovolumic contraction
CHF	congestive heart failure		
cm/s	centimeters/second	DSH	domestic shorthair (cat)
CMVD	chronic mitral valve disease (also called degenerative mitral valve disease, DVMD, and myxomatous mitral valve disease, MMVD)	DT	(Doppler flow) deceleration time
		DUST	discrete upper septal thickening
		DV	dorsoventral (position or view)
		E	early diastolic mitral or tricuspid inflow (motion or velocity)
CNP	C-type natriuretic peptide		
CNS	central nervous system	E_a	early diastolic annular tissue velocity (sometimes expressed as E′, e′, or Em)
CO	cardiac output		
CO_2	carbon dioxide		
CPR	cardiopulmonary resuscitation	EADs	early afterdepolarizations
CRI	constant/continuous rate infusion	ECG	electrocardiogram/electrocardiographic
CRT	capillary refill time		
CSA	cross-sectional area	echo	echocardiographic/echocardiography
CT	computed tomography		
CTD	cor triatriatum dexter	ECM	extracellular matrix
cTn	cardiac troponin (also, cTnI and cTnT)	ECVIM	European College of Veterinary Internal Medicine
CURATIVE (guidelines)	Consensus on the Rational Use of Antithrombotics in Veterinary Critical Care (Goggs, 2019; see Chapter 36 references)	EDP	end-diastolic pressure (ventricular)
		EDTA	ethylene diamine tetraacetic acid
		EDV	end-diastolic volume (ventricular)
		EDVI	end-diastolic volume index
		EF	ejection fraction
CV	cardiovascular	EIPH	exercise-induced pulmonary hemorrhage
CVP	central venous pressure		
CvRD	cardiovascular-renal axis disorder	ELISA	enzyme-linked immunosorbent assay
CW	continuous wave (Doppler)		
D5W	5% dextrose in water	eNOS	endothelial nitric oxide synthase
D	diastolic (wave or volume), depending on context	EP	electrophysiologic
		EPA	eicosapentaenoic acid
DADs	delayed afterdepolarizations	Epi	epinephrine

Abbreviation	Definition
EPIC (study)	Effect of pimobendan in dogs with preclinical myxomatous mitral valve disease and cardiomegaly: the EPIC study (Boswood, 2016; see Chapter 29 references)
EPSS	(mitral) E-point to septal separation
EROA	effective regurgitant orifice area
Es, E$_{max}$	slope of the end-systolic pressure-volume relationship
ESVC	European Society for Veterinary Cardiology
ESVI	end-systolic volume index
ET	(Doppler flow) ejection time
ETN	endothelin
f	fibrillation (waves)
FA	fatty acid(s)
FAC	fractional area change
FAST	focused assessment with sonography in trauma
FAT	focal atrial tachycardia
FATCAT (study)	Secondary prevention of cardiogenic arterial thromboembolism in the cat: the double-blind, randomized, positive-controlled feline arterial thromboembolism; Clopidogrel vs. Aspirin trial (Hogan, 2015; see Chapter 36 references)
FDA	(United States) Federal Drug Administration
FDPs	fibrinogen/fibrin degradation products
FIV	feline immunodeficiency virus
Fr	French (diameter size, for catheterization equipment)
FS	fractional shortening
GAGs	glycosaminoglycans
GFR	glomerular filtration rate
GI	gastrointestinal
H$_2$O	water
HARD	heartworm-associated respiratory disease
HCl	hydrochloride
HCM	hypertrophic cardiomyopathy
HFpEF	heart failure with preserved ejection fraction
HFrEF	heart failure with reduced ejection fraction
Hg	mercury (as in mm Hg)
HOCM	hypertrophic obstructive cardiomyopathy
HPB	high-pressure balloon
HR	heart rate
HRV	heart rate variability
HSA	hemangiosarcoma
HT	(systemic) hypertension
HW	heartworm
HWD	heartworm disease
I$_{Ca}$	inward Ca^{++} current
I$_f$	funny current
I$_K$	delayed rectifier K$^+$ current
I$_{Kr}$	rapid component of I$_K$
I$_{Ks}$	slow component of I$_K$
I$_{K1}$	inward rectifier K$^+$ current
I$_{NCX}$	sodium-calcium exchange current
I$_{to}$	transient outward K$^+$ current
ICS	intercostal space
IFA	immunofluorescent antibody
IGF	insulin-like growth factor
IL	interleukin
IM	intramuscular/intramuscularly
IMHA	immune-mediated hemolytic anemia
iNOS	inducible nitric oxide synthase
INR	international normalization ratio
IO	intraosseous
IRIS	International Renal Interest Society
ISACHC	International Small Animal Cardiac Health Council
ISFM	International Society of Feline Medicine
ISI	international sensitivity index (for thromboplastin)
IV	intravenous/intravenously
IVRT	isovolumic (isovolumetric) relaxation time
IVS	interventricular septum/septal
K$^+$	potassium ion
KCl	potassium chloride
kVp	kilovoltage peak
L	cardiac long axis (VHS measurement), or liter, depending on context
L1	first stage larvae
L2	second stage larvae
L3	third stage larvae
L4	fourth stage larvae
L5	immature adult heartworms, or fifth stage larvae
L/R	left/right (echocardiograph inversion switch)
L-to-R	left-to-right (shunt flow direction)
LA	left atrium/atrial
LAA	left atrial appendage
LAFB	left anterior fascicular block
LAO	left anterior oblique (position)
LAu	left auricle (atrial appendage)
LAx	long axis

LBBB	left bundle branch block	**NT-proBNP**	N-terminal probrain (B-type) natriuretic peptide
LD50	lethal dose causing death in 50% of cases	**NYHA**	New York Heart Association
LDH	lactate dehydrogenase	**O₂**	oxygen
LMWH	low molecular weight heparin	**OTN**	over-the-needle (catheter)
LPFB	left posterior fascicular block	**P**	pressure
LRS	lactated Ringer's solution	**P wave**	atrial muscle depolarization waveform
LV	left ventricle/ventricular		
LVID	left ventricular internal dimension	**P-P**	P wave to P wave interval
		ΔP	perfusion pressure
LVIDd	left ventricular internal diameter at end-diastole	**PA**	pulmonary artery/arterial
		PAI-1	plasminogen activator inhibitor type 1
LVIDdN	LVIDd normalized to body weight		
LVIDs	left ventricular internal diameter at end-systole	**PBV**	pulmonary balloon valvuloplasty (or BPV, balloon pulmonary valvuloplasty)
LVOT	left ventricular outflow tract		
MAP	mean arterial pressure	**PCH**	pulmonary capillary hemangiomatosis
MAPSE	mitral annular plane systolic excursion		
		pCO₂	partial pressure of carbon dioxide
mAs	milliamperes x seconds	**PCR**	polymerase chain reaction
MEA	mean electrical axis (on ECG)	**PCV**	packed cell volume
MF	microfilariae	**PCWP**	pulmonary capillary wedge pressure
MHS	manubrium heart score		
MHz	megahertz	**PDA**	patent ductus arteriosus
miRNA	microRNA	**PDE**	phosphodiesterase
mL	milliliter	**PDE-3**	phosphodiesterase-type 3 isoenzyme
mm	millimeter		
mm Hg	millimeters of mercury	**PDE-5**	phosphodiesterase-type 5 isoenzyme
mm/s	millimeters/second		
MMPs	matrix metalloproteinases	**PDK4**	pyruvate dehydrogenase kinase isozyme 4
MMVD	myxomatous mitral valve disease (also: chronic mitral valve disease, CMVD; degenerative mitral valve disease, DVMD)		
		PEA	pulseless electrical activity
		PFO	patent foramen ovale
		PG	pressure gradient
MR	mitral valve regurgitation (insufficiency)	**PH**	pulmonary hypertension
		PICALM	phosphatidylinositol-binding clathrin assembly protein
MRI	magnetic resonance imaging		
MS	mitral valve stenosis	**PISA**	proximal isovelocity surface area
m/s	meters/second	**PLCVC**	persistent left cranial vena cava
mV	millivolts	**PMI**	point of maximal (murmur) intensity
MVD	mitral valve dysplasia		
MYBPC	myosin binding protein C	**PNS**	parasympathetic (cholinergic) nervous system
Na⁺	sodium ion		
NaCl	sodium chloride	**pO₂**	partial pressure of oxygen
NCX-1	sodium-calcium exchanger	**PO**	*per os*, oral/orally
NE	norepinephrine	**POC**	point-of-care
NH	neurohormonal	**PPDH**	peritoneopericardial diaphragmatic hernia
nNOS	neuronal nitric oxide synthase		
NO	nitric oxide	**PR**	pulmonary valve regurgitation
NOS	nitric oxide synthase	**PRAA**	persistent right aortic arch
NPR	natriuretic peptide receptor	**PREDICT (study)**	Prediction of first onset of congestive heart failure in dogs with degenerative mitral valve disease (Reynolds, 2012; see Chapter 29 references)
NSAID	nonsteroidal anti-inflammatory drug		
NT-proANP	N-terminal proatrial (A-type) natriuretic peptide		

PRF	pulse-repetition frequency (of pulsed wave Doppler modalities)	**RMP**	resting membrane potential
		RNA	ribonucleic acid
		RPADI	right pulmonary artery distensibility index
PROTECT (study)	Efficacy of pimobendan in the prevention of congestive heart failure or sudden death in Doberman Pinschers with preclinical dilated cardiomyopathy (Summerfield, 2012; see Chapter 22 references)	**rPDA**	reversed patent ductus arteriosus
		RRR	resting (sleeping) respiratory rate
		rt-PA	recombinant tissue plasminogen activator
		RT-PCR	reverse transcriptase-polymerase chain reaction
		RV	right ventricle/ventricular
PS	pulmonary (pulmonic) stenosis	**RVIDd**	right ventricular internal diameter in diastole
PT	prothrombin time		
PTE	pulmonary thromboembolism	**RVOT**	right ventricular outflow tract
PVC	premature ventricular complex	**rVSD**	reversed ventricular septal defect
PVOD	pulmonary veno-occlusive disease	**RyR2**	cardiac ryanodine receptor
PVR	pulmonary vascular resistance	**S**	cardiac short axis (VHS measurement) or systolic (wave or volume), depending on context
PW	pulsed wave (Doppler)		
Q	flow		
QRS	ventricular muscle depolarization waveform(s)	S_1	first heart sound ("lub")
		S_2	second heart sound ("dub")
QTc	heart rate-corrected QT interval	S_3	third heart sound (ventricular gallop)
QUEST (study)	Effect of pimobendan or benazepril hydrochloride on survival times in dogs with congestive heart failure caused by naturally occurring myxomatous mitral valve disease (Häggström, 2008; see Chapter 21 references)	S_4	fourth heart sound (atrial gallop)
		SA	sinoatrial
		SAM	(mitral) systolic anterior motion
		SAS	subaortic stenosis
		SAx	short axis
		SC	subcutaneous/subcutaneously
R	resistance	**SDMA**	symmetric dimethylarginine assay
R-R	R wave to R wave interval (also, QRS to QRS complex interval)	**SERCA**	sarcoendoplasmic reticulum calcium ATPase
R-to-L	right-to-left (shunt flow direction)	**SI**	sphericity index
RA	right atrium/atrial	**SMOD**	Simpson's method of disks
RAAS	renin-angiotensin-aldosterone system	**SNS**	sympathetic (adrenergic) nervous system
RAO	right anterior oblique (position)	SpO_2	oxygen saturation
RAu	right auricle (atrial appendage)	**spp.**	species
rASD	reversed atrial septal defect	**SR**	sarcoplasmic reticulum
RBBB	right bundle branch block	**SSS**	sick sinus syndrome
RBC	red blood cell	**SV**	stroke volume
RCM	restrictive cardiomyopathy	**SVEP (study)**	Efficacy of enalapril for prevention of congestive heart failure in dogs with myxomatous valve disease and asymptomatic mitral regurgitation (Kvart, 2002; see Chapter 22 references)
RDW	RBC distribution width		
RECOVER	Reassessment Campaign on Veterinary Resuscitation (see Chapter 25 reference citations)		
REVEAL (study)	International collaborative study to assess cardiovascular risk and evaluate long-term health in cats with preclinical hypertrophic cardiomyopathy and apparently healthy cats (Fox, 2018; see Chapter 33 references)	**SVT**	supraventricular tachycardia
		TFPI	tissue factor pathway inhibitor
		T of F	tetralogy of Fallot
		T wave	ventricular muscle repolarization waveform
		TAPSE	tricuspid annular plane systolic excursion

TDI	tissue Doppler imaging		heart failure in dogs chronically treated with enalapril alone for compensated, naturally occurring mitral valve insufficiency. (Atkins, 2007; see Chapter 22 references)
TdP	*torsades de pointes*		
TE	thromboembolism or thromboembolic		
TEE	transesophageal echocardiography/echocardiographic	**VF**	ventricular fibrillation
TFAST	thoracic focused assessment with sonography for trauma	**VHD**	valvular heart disease
		VHS	vertebral heart size (score, scale, sum)
TGF	transforming growth factor		
TICM	tachycardia-induced cardiomyopathy	**VICs**	valve interstitial cells
		VLAS	vertebral left atrial size
TIMPs	tissue inhibitors of MMPs	**Vmax**	maximal (peak) velocity (spectral Doppler)
TNF	tumor necrosis factor		
t-PA	tissue plasminogen activator	**VO$_{2\,max}$**	maximal rate of O$_2$ uptake
TR	tricuspid valve regurgitation	**VPC**	ventricular premature complex
TTE	transthoracic echocardiography	**V/Q**	(pulmonary) ventilation/perfusion
TVD	tricuspid valve dysplasia	**VSD**	ventricular septal defect
UCM	unclassified cardiomyopathy	**VT**	ventricular tachycardia
UFH	unfractionated heparin	**VTI**	velocity-time integral (Doppler echocardiography)
US	ultrasound		
v	vertebrae (as in VHS)	**VVI**	ventricular-paced, ventricular-sensed, inhibited (pacing mode)
V	velocity		
VD	ventrodorsal (position or view)	**VVIR**	ventricular-paced, ventricular-sensed, inhibited, rate modulation (pacing mode)
VDD	ventricular-paced, dual-sensed, dual-response (pacing mode)		
VECs	valve endothelial cells	**WBC**	white blood cell
VETPROOF (study)	Results of the veterinary enalapril trial to prove reduction in onset of	**WPW**	Wolff–Parkinson–White (preexcitation pattern or syndrome)

PREFACE TO *CARDIOVASCULAR DISEASE IN COMPANION ANIMALS*
(2nd edition to *Cardiovascular Disease in Small Animal Medicine*)

Our aim in writing this new and expanded edition was to create a comprehensive yet easily accessible clinical cardiology reference for practicing veterinarians, residents, interns, and veterinary students. Veterinary nurses and others with an interest in the subject might also find it useful. This book reflects the authors' extensive clinical and teaching experience in veterinary cardiology over the past four decades, as well as a review of wide-ranging literature. We have tried to present an overview of cardiovascular medicine in companion animal species that is relevant to veterinarians engaged in canine, feline, and equine clinical practices, and that is well-integrated across chapters, and richly illustrated. We hope this textbook will be helpful and easy to use in your study of cardiology, as well as your day-to-day practice. While the text is focused toward companion animal practitioners, we have included some advanced topics because we believe these provide a useful perspective regarding the current scope of veterinary cardiology.

The extensive use of visual images is a core feature of this book, as it was for the previous edition. Many new images are included, while others have been brought forward from the first edition. The vast majority of clinical images were collected during the course of the authors' practices. We are indebted also to a number of colleagues, who generously allowed us to include their images in various chapters. In addition, some figures originally published elsewhere have been included, with permission, to help illustrate key concepts. We are especially pleased that Dr. Brian A. Scansen agreed to write a new chapter on *Cardiac Catheterization and Angiocardiography* (Chapter 6) for this edition because of his extensive expertise and current developments in this area. Brian also contributed importantly to the chapters on *Other Cardiovascular Malformations* (Chapter 28) and *Thromboembolic Disease* (Chapter 36).

We have organized this text into five main sections. The first, *Fundamentals of Clinical Cardiology* (Chapters 1–6), presents clinically relevant overviews of cardiovascular structure and function; aspects of the cardiovascular examination; and the diagnostic modalities of cardiac radiography, echocardiography, electrocardiography, and cardiac catheterization and angiocardiography. The second section (Chapters 7–19) offers a problem-based approach to various *Clinical Manifestations of Cardiovascular Disease*. Section three (Chapters 20–22) focuses on the clinical syndrome of *Heart Failure*, from its pathophysiology and clinical signs to management strategies. Section four of the book (Chapters 23–25) deals with *Heart Rhythm Disturbances*, including underlying mechanisms and consequences, antiarrhythmic drugs and other therapeutic options, and the management of various arrhythmias. The final and largest section (Chapters 26–40) contains chapters on important congenital and acquired *Cardiovascular Diseases* of dogs, cats, and horses. We have cited some specific references within the text but have not attempted to reference every statement in the book. Many of the original sources we reviewed during our writing are included in the *Suggested Additional Readings and References* list at the end of each chapter. More extensive bibliographies and a collection of supplemental media, are available online for the interested reader. The videos and additional images are especially useful for learning about modalities such as echocardiography.

We have striven for consistency in our use of abbreviations throughout the book. For ease of reference, a list of abbreviations is included. One pitfall inherent to a volume covering such a broad and intertwined subject as cardiovascular disease is the risk of discussing certain concepts repeatedly in different chapters. In an effort to avoid unplanned redundancy and control the overall size of the text, we have chosen to include many cross-references within. We recognize that this can be an annoyance to the reader, but hope that by referencing specific page numbers as much as possible, any inconvenience will be minimized.

This project has been an "adventure" of greater proportions than we originally anticipated. Yet, despite the many challenges along the way, stubborn perseverance as well as a sense of humor allowed us to bring it to conclusion... and remain friends. We want to thank Michael Manson and Jill Northcott of Manson Publishing, for requesting the writing of this second edition and for coordinating its transition while in-process to CRC Press, Taylor and Francis Group. We also are most grateful to Alice Oven, Senior Editor for Veterinary Medicine at CRC Press, Taylor and Francis Group, for her steadfast patience and encouragement throughout the lengthy writing process. In addition, we thank Linda Leggio, Production Editor at Taylor and Francis, and Elizabeth King, Project Manager at KnowledgeWorks Global, for their mighty efforts in shepherding this project into its final form. There are many others who, in various ways, have contributed to our ability to write this book. We want to acknowledge our many colleagues, mentors, patients and their owners, as well as the house officers and thousands of students we have taught over the years. We have learned a huge amount from you all, and hope that what we have written will in turn benefit others. Finally, our sincere thanks and appreciation to our family members and friends who, willingly or not, have supported us through this process. You now can stop asking us if the book is finally finished.

Wendy A. Ware and John D. Bonagura

ABOUT THE AUTHORS

Wendy Ware is *Professor Emerita* of the Departments of Veterinary Clinical Sciences and Biomedical Sciences at the Iowa State University College of Veterinary Medicine. She served as Cardiologist in the ISU Lloyd Veterinary Medical Center for many years and was the first faculty member to hold the Phyllis M. Clark Professorship in Cardiology. Wendy is a Diplomate of the American College of Veterinary Internal Medicine (specialty of Cardiology) and former President of the ACVIM Board of Regents. She also has served as Associate Editor for Cardiology for the Journal of Veterinary Internal Medicine. Dr. Ware authored the textbook *Cardiovascular Disease in Small Animal Medicine*, and subsequently, co-wrote and edited *Self-Assessment Color Review of Small Animal Cardiopulmonary Medicine*, both produced by Manson Publishing. She has authored the "Disorders of the Cardiovascular System" section in Nelson & Couto's *Small Animal Internal Medicine* since its inaugural edition. Her other contributions include numerous journal articles and individual book chapters, as well as many hours of continuing education presentations to veterinarians.

John Bonagura is an Adjunct Professor in the Department of Clinical Sciences at North Carolina State University College of Veterinary Medicine, and *Professor Emeritus* of Veterinary Clinical Sciences at the Ohio State University College of Veterinary Medicine. John is a Diplomate of the American College of Veterinary Internal Medicine (specialties of Cardiology and Internal Medicine) and former President of the specialty of Cardiology. Dr. Bonagura is the long-time Editor of *Kirk's Current Veterinary Therapy*, co-author of a *Colour Atlas of Veterinary Cardiology*, and has written or co-authored over 250 scientific publications, reviews, and book chapters. He has given an extensive number of continuing education presentations to veterinarians around the world. Among his awards are the Ohio State University Distinguished Teacher Award, the Bourgelat International Award of the BSAVA, and the Kirk Lifetime Achievement Award from the ACVIM.

Brian Scansen is an Associate Professor in the Department of Clinical Sciences at the Colorado State University College of Veterinary Medicine and Biomedical Sciences, and Service Head of Cardiology and Cardiac Surgery in the James L Voss Veterinary Teaching Hospital. Brian is a Diplomate of the American College of Veterinary Internal Medicine (specialty of Cardiology) and is fellowship-trained in veterinary interventional radiology. His particular interests include congenital heart disease, interventional cardiology, and cardiac computed tomography.

Section I

Fundamentals of Clinical Cardiology

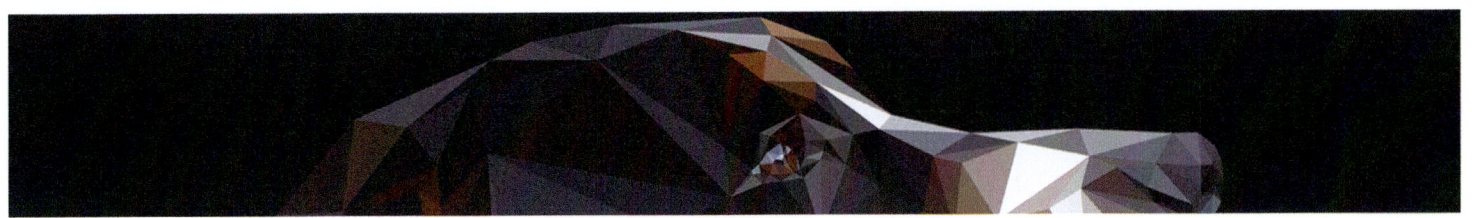

1
THE NORMAL CARDIOVASCULAR SYSTEM

Knowledge of cardiac anatomy and physiology is essential for understanding, diagnosing, and treating diseases of the heart and blood vessels. This chapter offers an overview of normal cardiovascular (CV) structure and function, with some important clinical correlations that illustrate their relevance to clinical practice.

General Considerations

The CV system delivers nutrients and removes metabolic by-products throughout the body. It also supports flow-dependent organ functions such as ventilation and urine formation. The two major component circulations (pulmonary and systemic) are linked in series; therefore, a functional abnormality involving either circulation could negatively affect the other. The coronary circulation originates from the aortic root and returns myocardial venous blood to the heart. The systemic circulation supplies the various organs of the body through a set of parallel circulations. The smaller pulmonary circulation provides oxygen (O_2) and carbon dioxide (CO_2) exchange and contributes to acid-base regulation. **Figure 1.1** schematically illustrates the normal path of blood flow and approximate normal pressures for small animals. Right-sided pressures tend to be higher in large animals, related in part to posture and head position.

Three complementary diagnostic perspectives help provide a conceptual framework for understanding CV system abnormalities: anatomic localization, (patho)physiologic or functional abnormality, and etiologic diagnosis. Each yields insight into a patient's underlying disease process and can inform clinical management decisions. The anatomic localization of disease might involve the cardiac valves (and endocardium), myocardium, pericardium, cardiac impulse formation and conduction system, the respiratory system (with its secondary effects on the heart), or the systemic vasculature. Functional abnormalities could relate to a leaky or stenotic cardiac valve, poor myocardial contractility (systolic dysfunction), impaired cardiac filling (diastolic dysfunction), arrhythmias and their effect on cardiac output (CO), abnormal systemic-pulmonary communications (shunts), congestive heart failure, pulmonary hypertension, systemic hypertension, or cardiogenic shock. In most cases, a combination of physiologic abnormalities is involved. Third, the patient's etiologic diagnosis is important to consider. Specific etiologies might involve degenerative disease, congenital malformation (anomaly), metabolic or endocrine disease, a neoplastic or nutritional disorder, inflammatory disease (infective or parasitic, immune-mediated, idiopathic), ischemia, and iatrogenic injury, toxicity, or trauma. The reader is referred to the chapters on specific diseases and clinical problems in this text as well as the section "Suggested Additional Reading and References" and online bibliography for further details.

The Heart

External Features

The heart is comprised of four chambers, four cardiac valves, two great vessels, and a number of systemic and pulmonary venous attachments. Superficially the chambers are divided by different grooves or sulci. The atria are dorsal to the coronary or atrioventricular (AV) groove that surrounds the heart circumferentially. The paraconal sulcus (groove) on the left craniolateral surface of the heart separates the left ventricle (LV) from the outflow portion of the right ventricle (RV). The subsinuosal sulcus (groove) is located caudally and separates the caudal portions of the RV and the LV. Because the ventricular septum is angled, these grooves only approximate the demarcation of these chambers. As animals age, fat is gradually deposited within these cardiac sulci; this is especially dramatic in horses. In animals with cachexia, the normally white epicardial fat and connective tissue undergo serous atrophy,

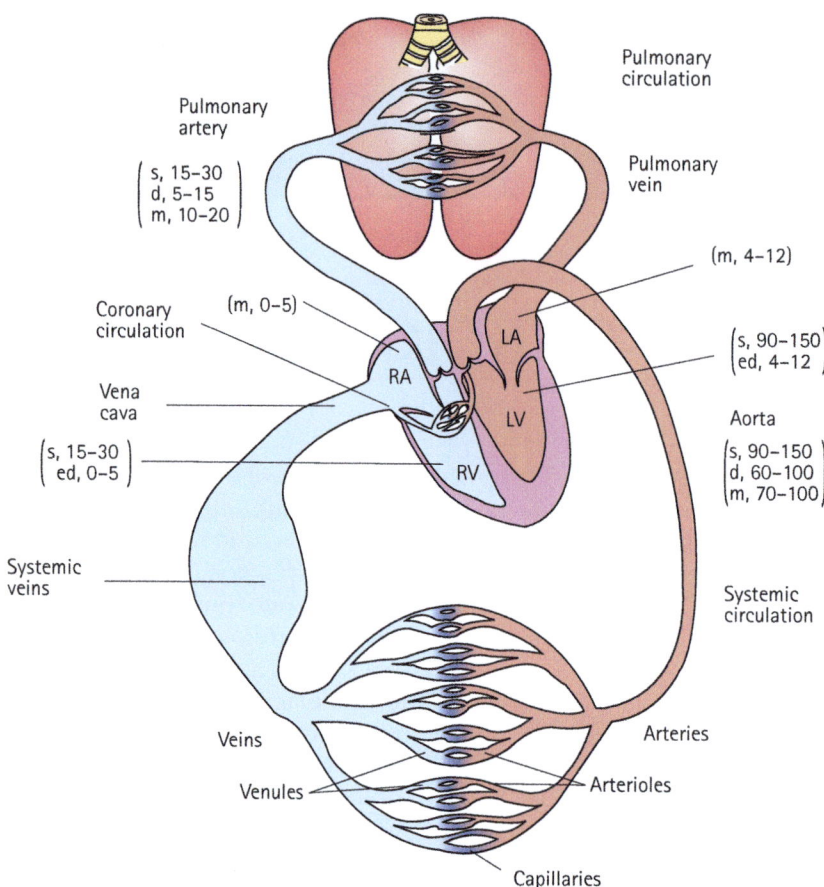

Figure 1.1 Schematic diagram of the cardiovascular system. Examples of normal pressures (mm Hg) in different regions noted in parentheses. d, diastolic; ed, end-diastolic; LA, left atrium; LV, left ventricle; m, mean; RA, right atrium; RV, right ventricle; s, systolic.

taking on a gelatinous appearance at necropsy. Epicardial fat must be distinguished from superficial cardiac lymphatics that appear as white streaks over the cardiac surface. These are seen most prominently in horses.

The pericardium is a double-layered sac that surrounds the heart. It consists of a thin visceral (epicardial) layer of mesothelial cells that is closely adhered to the heart. This lining reflects at the heart base to form the serous lining of the fibrous, parietal pericardium. The latter is contiguous with the mediastinal pleura. A small amount of serous fluid acts as a lubricant between the visceral and parietal pericardial layers. The pericardial space is a common site of disease, which often involves abnormal fluid accumulation and cardiac tumors. See Chapter 35 for more information about pericardial structure and clinical disorders.

The left and right coronary arteries arise from the sinuses of Valsalva, behind the left and right coronary cusps (leaflets) of the aortic valve, respectively. These arteries course over the external surface of the heart before their branches penetrate into the myocardium (**Figure 1.2**). The left coronary artery divides into a circumflex branch that traverses the AV (coronary) groove and a paraconal branch, which descends along the craniolateral sulcus separating the two ventricles.

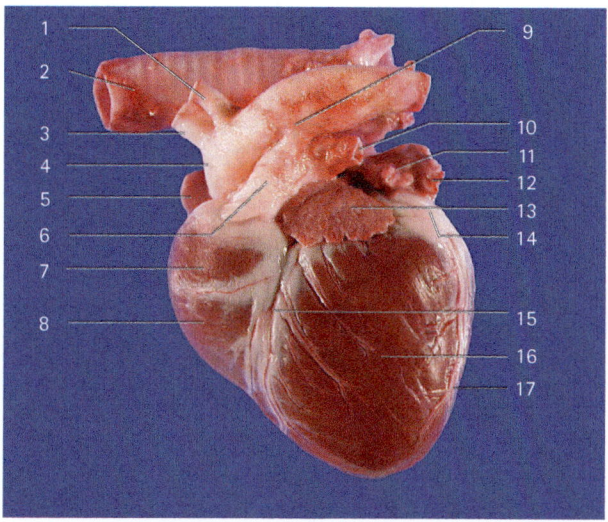

Figure 1.2 Canine heart: External view from the left. 1. L subclavian a., 2. Trachea, 3. Brachiocephalic trunk, 4. Aorta, 5. R auricle, 6. Main pulmonary a. (pulmonary trunk), 7. Conus arteriosus, 8. R ventricle, 9. Ligamentum arteriosum, 10. L pulmonary a., 11. Pulmonary v., 12. L atrium, 13. L auricle, 14. Coronary groove (with circumflex branch of L coronary a.), 15. Cranial (paraconal) interventricular branch of L coronary a., 16. L ventricle, 17. Caudal (subsinuosal) interventricular branch of L coronary a. a., artery; L, left; R, right; v., vein.

The left coronary system is dominant in most dogs, which means the circumflex branch supplies the subsinuosal artery that is distributed to the caudal aspect of the heart. Most cats and horses have a right dominant system, where the subsinuosal artery is derived from the right coronary artery. Coronary artery malformations and myocardial infarctions caused by extramural coronary artery disease occur sporadically in companion animals, however atherosclerotic coronary disease, so common in humans, is rare.

Venous return from the systemic circulation enters the right atrium (RA) through the cranial vena cava, caudal vena cava, and potentially from the azygous vein, which often connects to the cranial vena cava (**Figure 1.3**). Pulmonary venous return enters the dorsal left atrium (LA). There are seven pulmonary veins in most species, although three major pulmonary venous confluences are typically visualized by echocardiography in dogs and cats. Venous anomalies are under-recognized, as suggested by computerized tomography studies in dogs. Some venous admixture occurs normally when systemic bronchial veins, which serve the visceral pleura of the lungs, join the pulmonary veins and mix desaturated with well-oxygenated blood. These venous connections can become clinically relevant in the settings of congestive heart failure, pulmonary hypertension, and cyanotic congenital heart disease. Venous return from the heart muscle is via small coronary veins that eventually drain into the great coronary (cardiac) vein. This vein empties into the coronary sinus, an opening into the RA just ventral to that of the caudal vena cava.

The LV forms the caudoventral aspect of the heart; its point, termed the cardiac apex, normally is located to the left of the midline in dogs, cats, and horses (**Figure 1.2**). The apex is especially prominent and pointed in horses (**Figure 1.4**).

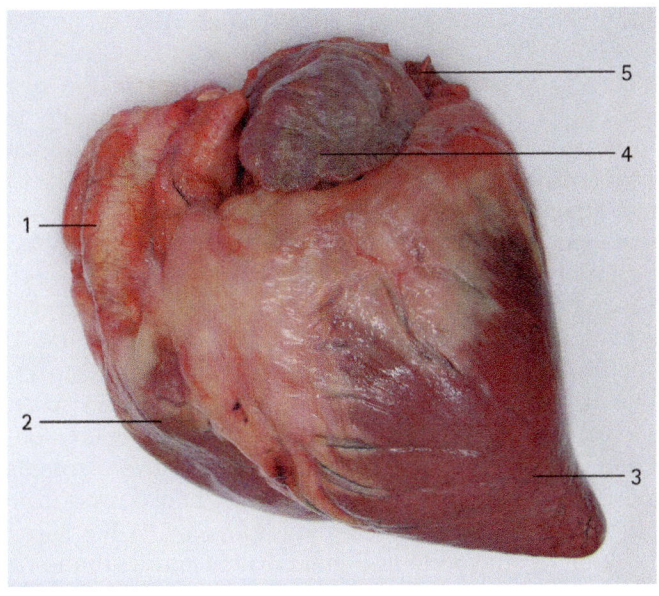

Figure 1.4 Equine heart: External view from the left. 1. Main pulmonary a. (pulmonary trunk), 2. R ventricle (outflow region), 3. L ventricle (note pointed apex), 4. L auricle, 5. L atrium. a., artery; L, left; R, right.

Palpation of the apical (precordial) impulse during physical examination is useful because it provides an important landmark for valve region and murmur localization during cardiac auscultation. The LV is cone-shaped and surrounded on its right, cranial, and left craniodorsal aspects by the RV. The LA straddles the midline dorsocaudal to the LV; its appendage or left auricle (LAu) projects craniolaterally with the blind end (tip) directed toward the pulmonary artery (PA). The LAu can become especially prominent in cats with cardiomyopathy and is the major source of arterial thromboembolism in this species (see Chapters 33 and 36).

The aorta arises from the center of the heart base, cranial to the LA and to the right of the PA. The bulbous sinuses of Valsalva, from which the two coronary arteries originate, join the ascending aorta at the sinotubular junction. The ascending aorta projects cranially and rightward, then smoothly arches dorsally and to the left to join the descending aorta. Because the ascending aorta angles to the right of midline, cardiac murmurs that originate from the LV outflow region (as with subaortic stenosis) often radiate well to the cranial right thorax, as turbulent flow enters the ascending aorta. The definitive aortic arch normally is derived from the left fourth fetal arch. Persistence of the right arch, instead of the left, is the most common cause of a vascular ring anomaly that entraps the esophagus and prevents normal swallowing of solid food in neonates (p. 516). Beyond the aortic arch, the fetal ductus arteriosus extends ventrally and cranially from the descending aorta to connect with the PA, at the origin of its left principal branch. This duct normally closes shortly after birth, leaving just a remnant (*ligamentum arteriosusm*). However, persistent patency of this structure is common in dogs and also occurs in cats and in horses (rarely). Because this vascular connection is

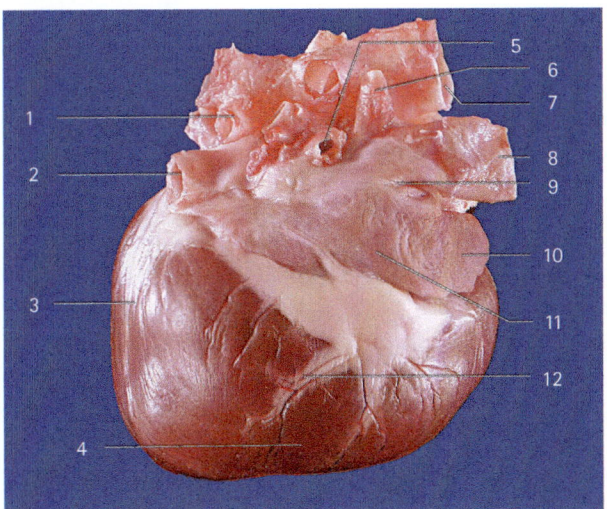

Figure 1.3 Canine heart: External view from the right. 1. Pulmonary v. ostium, 2. Caudal vena cava, 3. Caudal (subsinuosal) interventricular sulcus, 4. R ventricle, 5. R pulmonary a., 6. Azygous v., 7. Trachea, 8. Cranial vena cava, 9. Region of sinoatrial node, 10. R auricle, 11. R atrium, 12. Branches of R coronary a. a., artery; L, left; R, right; v, vein.

extracardiac, the murmur of patent ductus arteriosus is heard best over the PA at the left, craniodorsal heart base (p. 441).

The RA occupies the dorsal right aspect of the heart, above the RV inflow tract; however it expands cranially and caudally to join the two vena cavae. The right atrial appendage or auricle (RAu) is broader-based than the LAu; its tip points cranially and to the left. Additionally, pectinate muscles are not confined to the RAu. The inlet of the RV is to the right of the midline. Heart murmurs caused by tricuspid valve disease are heard best on the right side of the chest. However, the RV traverses the midline cranial to the LV. The RV outflow tract and PA form the left craniodorsal aspect of the heart. Accordingly, while the pulmonary valve is part of the "right heart" it is anatomically located on the left side of the thorax. Murmurs caused by pulmonary valve disease are loudest at the left cranial heart border. When viewed from a left thoracotomy or by echocardiography, the PA lies superficial to (left of) the aorta and immediately cranial to the LAu. It divides into two main branches, the left and the right PAs. The left branch typically extends dorsal to the tracheal carina, and might be evident on lateral thoracic radiographs.

Internal Features

The inner lining of the heart is known as the endocardium (**Figure 1.5**). It consists of three layers. A continuous sheet of endothelial cells covers the internal cardiac surface and is contiguous with the intimal layer of attached arteries and veins. Just below the endothelium lies a thin subendothelial layer of collagen and elastic fibers, with a few smooth muscle cells. The deeper portion of the endocardium (subendocardial layer) consists of connective tissue that often contains specialized cardiomyocytes capable of rapid cardiac conduction (Purkinje cells). The myocardium, with its working contractile cells, lies between the endocardium and pericardium; it forms the bulk of the cardiac wall. In general, the wall thickness of each cardiac chamber reflects the degree of systolic pressure generated within.

The four cardiac valves are thin, flexible fibrous flaps covered with endothelium. Each valve is anchored to a valve annulus, characterized by varying degrees of fibrous ring or tissue organization. These valvular rings, along with connective tissue at the center of the heart (membranous septum and fibrous trigone), form the "fibrous skeleton" of the heart.

Left Heart   The LA includes a smooth-chambered venous cavern (body) that collects venous return and a muscular appendage (LAu), which is of different embryologic origin. Interlacing pectinate muscles produce a raised and irregular internal surface within the auricle. Venous return from the multiple pulmonary veins enters the dorsal LA. Three venous inflows (or ostia) usually are evident in dogs on color Doppler echocardiography and computed tomography (CT). These represent a confluence of pulmonary veins from the right cranial and middle lobes (seen closest to the atrial septum), the left and right caudal and accessory lung lobes, and the two segments of the left cranial lobe (entering craniolateral to the caudal confluence). The left AV (mitral) valve separates the LA from the LV. The atrial septum separates the LA from the RA and includes the flap of the fetal *foramen ovale*, which is a common location for atrial septal defects.

There is a short segment of cardiac septum, between the atrial and ventricular septa, that interconnects all four cardiac chambers; this is termed the AV septum. The septal mitral leaflet inserts more dorsally than the septal tricuspid leaflet into the AV septum and because of this ventrodorsal offset, the left side of the AV septum functions as ventricular septum while the right side is indistinguishable from the atrial septum. Defects in the AV septum are associated with both (primum) atrial and (inlet) ventricular septal defects, as well as malformations of the AV valves (p. 466).

The conical LV connects to the LA at the mitral valve and to the aorta at the aortic valve (**Figures 1.6** and **1.7**). The LV endocardial surface is fairly smooth, with only shallow indentations (*trabeculae carneae*). Thin false tendons (variously called "LV moderator bands" or "LV trabecula") span the distance between the subaortic ventricular septum and papillary muscles, and represent ramifications of the specialized conduction tissues of the left bundle branch. The ventricular mass is formed mostly by a continuum of myocardial fibers arrayed in layers of varying orientation from endocardium to epicardium and base to apex. Between the cardiomyocytes (histologically) are supporting elements that include normal

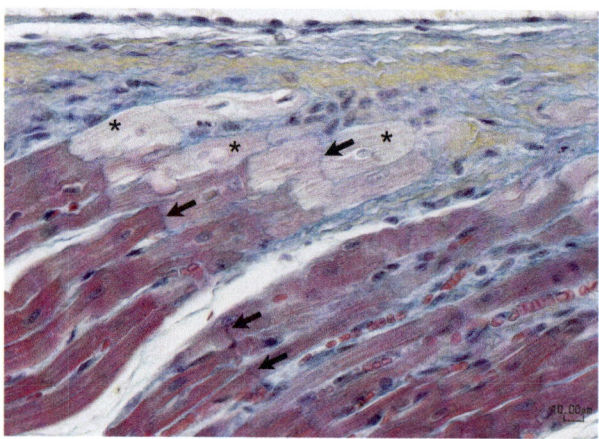

Figure 1.5 Photomicrograph showing endocardial and part of inner myocardial layers from the left ventricle of a dog. The endocardium consists of an endothelial layer (top of image), some subendothelial connective tissue, and a deeper subendocardial layer containing pale-staining Purkinje cells (black asterisks). Purkinje cells (fibers) are modified myocytes with rapid-conduction properties and fewer contractile elements than regular myocytes. Below these conduction fibers is the deeper red myocardium itself (bottom half of image). Purple-staining intercalated disks (black arrows) join the ends of adjacent regular myocytes and Purkinje cells; the centrally located nuclei of these cells also are visible. There is a dense capillary network within the myocardium. Rows of red blood cells within capillaries lie between the myocytes in the lower right portion of this image. Crossman's trichrome stain; 40× magnification. (Image courtesy of Dr. E Uemura.)

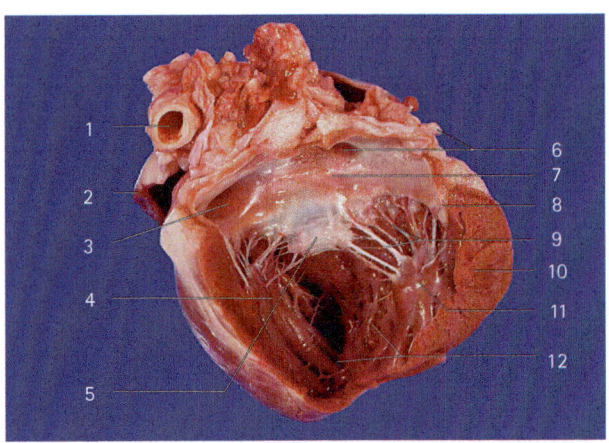

Figure 1.6 Canine heart: Left ventricular inflow tract. 1. Descending aorta, 2. R ventricular wall (cut), 3. L auricle, 4. Ventral (subauricular; anterior) papillary m., 5. Septal (anterior) mitral cusp, 6. Pulmonary v., 7. Interatrial septum, 8. Parietal (posterior) mitral cusp (cut), 9. Chordae tendineae, 10. L ventricular free wall, 11. Dorsal (subatrial; posterior) papillary m., 12. Trabeculae carneae. L, left; m., muscle; R, right; v, vein.

collagen as well as intramural coronary vessels and capillaries (**Figure 1.5**). Disease of the heart muscle is referred to generally as "cardiomyopathy"; several forms are clinically important in companion animals (see Chapters 32–34).

The LV has an inflow region (inlet) and outflow tract (outlet). The ventricle fills during diastole and ejects blood during systole. Myocardial contraction causes longitudinal, radial, and circumferential shortening; this increases intraventricular pressure and functionally narrows the LV, which pushes blood toward the outflow tract and aorta. Rotational movements in opposite directions at the apex and base also cause the LV to twist and untwist during systole and diastole, respectively. These movements are captured by 2D echocardiography and more advanced analysis methods that track myocardial deformation (strain). Both ventricles share and are separated by the interventricular septum (IVS), which extends from the aortic root to the ventricular apex. The subaortic region of the IVS is thinner and contains more fibrous elements than the rest of the (muscular) IVS. The IVS forms an arc along the right-cranial aspect of the circular LV when viewed in cross-section by echocardiography, CT, or magnetic resonance imaging (MRI). The thicknesses of the LV wall and IVS depend on the size of the animal, the systolic pressure load, and LV diastolic volume. LV wall and IVS thicknesses are similar; however, the septum does include both LV and RV components and often is slightly thicker in diastole than the LV free wall when measured by 2D echocardiography. This is especially obvious dorsally in some feline breeds such as Maine Coon cats and Bengals, as well as in normal horses.

The mitral valve, similar to the right AV (tricuspid) valve, is part of an "apparatus" comprised of several different support structures including the chordae tendineae, papillary muscles, valve annulus, and atrial wall (**Figure 1.6**). Disease of any component or geometric changes in the atria or ventricles can lead to valvular dysfunction (usually insufficient closure). Degenerative mitral valve disease is the most important cause of heart disease in the dog (Chapter 29). Abnormal mitral valve function also occurs commonly with cardiomyopathies, congenital malformations, and infection (endocarditis).

The two mitral leaflets are identified by an inconsistent nomenclature. The cranioventral leaflet also is called the anterior, cranial, or septal leaflet. The leaflet closer to the LV free wall, and positioned more caudodorsally, is called the posterior, caudal, parietal, or mural leaflet. Regardless of veterinary nomenclature, clinicians (especially echocardiographers) most often use the human terminology of "anterior" and "posterior" for these mitral components. The anterior mitral leaflet is cranial, contiguous with the caudal aspect of the aortic root, and extends more fully into the lumen of the LV chamber when compared to the posterior leaflet. This mitral-aortic fibrous continuity is an important anatomic feature of cardiac anatomy and is especially useful during echocardiography. The anterior leaflet functionally separates the LV inflow and outflow tracts (**Figure 1.7**), with the former confined by the mitral valve orifice and the latter formed by the anterior leaflet, ventricular septum, aortic valve orifice, and proximal aorta. The posterior mitral leaflet has a wider mural circumference and includes some incomplete scallops, which are especially prominent in horses. The mitral valve is open in diastole and closed during systole to facilitate the one-way movement of blood.

The mitral valve is supported by stout chordae tendineae of varying thicknesses that attach each leaflet to the two large papillary muscles (also identified by human echocardiographic nomenclature). The anterior and posterior papillary muscles arise near the left cranial (septal) and right caudal (mural) aspects of the LV, respectively. Variation in the arrangement of papillary muscles is not uncommon (as is the case in humans) and a smaller "third" papillary muscle often is observed by echocardiography cranial to

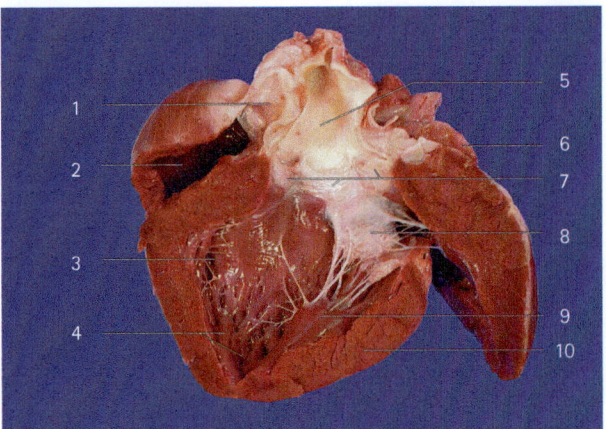

Figure 1.7 Canine heart: Left ventricular outflow tract. 1. Pulmonary trunk, 2. R ventricular outflow region (conus), 3. Interventricular septum, 4. Trabeculae carneae, 5. Ascending aorta, 6. L auricle, 7. Aortic valve cusps, 8. Septal (anterior) mitral cusp, 9. Dorsal (subatrial; posterior) papillary m., 10. L ventricle. L, left; m., muscle; R, right.

the anterior papillary muscle. This structure—perhaps similar to the anterolateral muscle bundle of Moulaert in human hearts—often is misdiagnosed as an anomaly, and it becomes more prominent when there is LV hypertrophy.

Chordae tendineae from both papillary muscles attach to each mitral leaflet. The chordae typically divide into several branches before inserting either at the free edge or onto the ventricular surface of the leaflet. Chordae that support the leaflet's free edge are known as commissural chordae tendineae. Chordae that insert into the leaflet's ventricular surface (sometimes called "mitral valve leaflet chordae") provide major support for the leaflet during systole; they usually are thicker than the commissural chordae. Other classification schemes also have been used for chordae tendineae, including designation of primary chords (attaching to the leaflet edge) and secondary chords (attaching to the ventricular surface of the valve). If one of these collagenous strands ruptures, the severity of valvular regurgitation (insufficiency) that results relates in part to the chord's insertion site and structure. Chapter 29 provides additional details about the normal mitral valve.

The aortic valve has three semilunar leaflets (cusps) and is located centrally within the fibrous cardiac skeleton (**Figure 1.8**). The right and noncoronary cusps of the aortic valve are located dorsally, above the subaortic IVS. The valve normally opens fully during systole. During diastole, the higher aortic pressure holds the leaflets closed to prevent backflow into the LV. Obstruction to LV outflow, most often at the subvalvular level (subaortic stenosis), is a relatively common congenital malformation in dogs. Aortic valve regurgitation (insufficiency) occurs sporadically in dogs, especially with infective endocarditis of this valve. Aortic valve degeneration and insufficiency is quite common in older horses.

Right Heart The RA is relatively large, with a venous cavern that ends blindly in a somewhat more muscular RAu. The auricle has a broad base and the pectinate muscles project from this appendage into the RA proper. The sinoatrial (SA) node is located subepicardially in the cranial RA, near the junction of the cranial vena cava and RAu and opposite the crista terminalis. The SA node artery, which arises from the right coronary artery, supplies blood to the SA node. The AV node is located subendocardially in the ventral right aspect of the interatrial septum, near the septal tricuspid leaflet. Both of these nodes, although microscopic, are critically important to normal impulse formation and cardiac conduction. They are highly influenced by the autonomic nervous system; each node receives extensive sympathetic and parasympathetic innervation. The RA contains three to four venous openings: the cranial and caudal vena cavae; the coronary sinus; and the azygous vein, although this is variable in some animals. The right side of the atrial septum includes the *fossa ovale*, the remnant of the fetal *foramen ovale*; this is the most common location for an atrial septal defect.

The RV lies ventral to the RA. The normal RV free-wall thickness is about 30–40% of the LV free-wall thickness. This reflects the much lower systolic pressure generated here. The inner RV surface has prominent muscular ridges (*trabeculae carneae*; **Figure 1.9**). A muscular band (*septomarginal trabecula*, moderator band), which carries conduction system fibers, extends from the IVS to the RV free wall. It is especially prominent in horses. A cardiomyopathy primarily affecting the RV occurs in some dogs and cats.

The tricuspid (right AV) valve separates the RA and RV. It has two distinct leaflets in dogs and cats. The lateral (parietal) leaflet is larger with incomplete commissures. The smaller

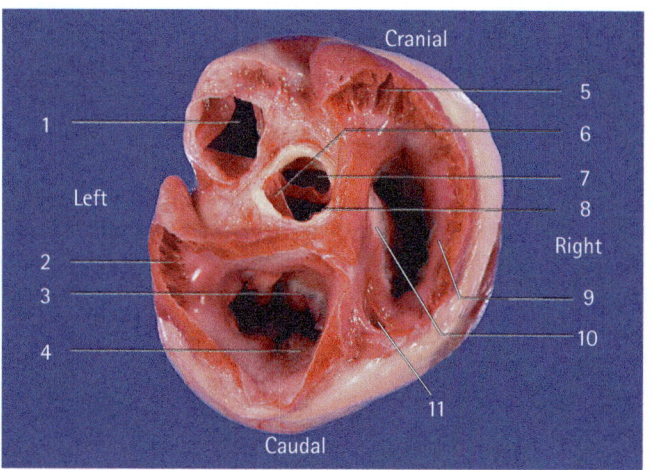

Figure 1.8 Canine heart: Dorsal view showing orientation of cardiac valves. 1. Pulmonary valve, 2. Pectinate mm. in L auricle, 3. Mitral valve: Septal (anterior) leaflet, 4. Mitral valve: Parietal (posterior) leaflet, 5. Pectinate mm. in R auricle, 6. Aortic valve: L cusp, 7. Aortic valve: R cusp, 8. Aortic valve: Noncoronary (septal) cusp, 9. Tricuspid valve: Parietal leaflet, 10. Tricuspid valve: Septal leaflet, 11. Coronary sinus. L, left; mm., muscles; R, right.

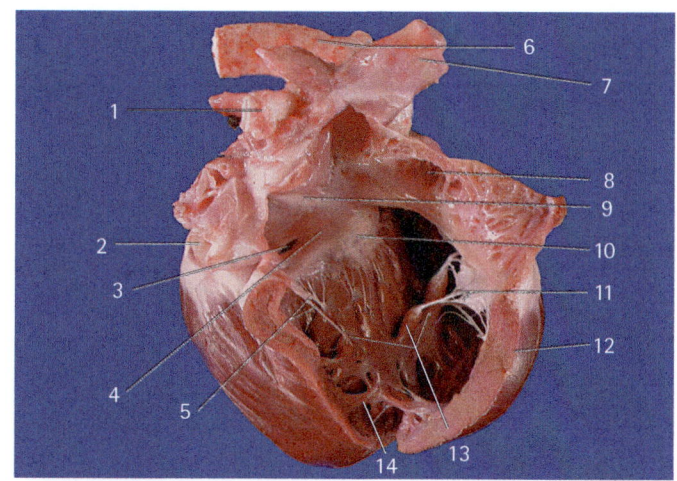

Figure 1.9 Canine heart: Right ventricular inflow tract. 1. R pulmonary a., 2. Caudal vena cava, 3. Coronary sinus, 4. Region of AV node, 5. Chordae tendineae, 6. Aorta, 7. Cranial vena cava, 8. R auricle, 9. Interatrial septum, 10. Septal tricuspid leaflet, 11. Parietal tricuspid leaflet (cut), 12. R ventricular free wall, 13. Papillary mm., 14. Trabeculae carneae. a., artery; AV, atrioventricular; mm., muscles; R, right.

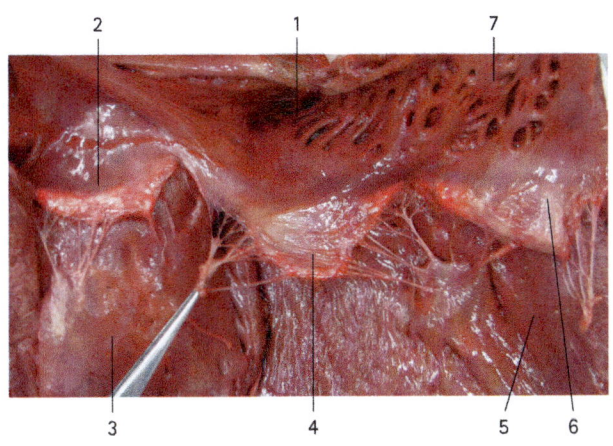

Figure 1.10 Equine heart: Right ventricular inflow tract. 1. R atrium, 2. Septal tricuspid leaflet, 3. Interventricular septum, 4. L tricuspid leaflet, 5. R ventricular free wall with papillary m., 6. R tricuspid leaflet, 7. R auricle. L, left; m., muscle; R, right.

septal (medial) leaflet inserts into the AV septum, slightly ventral to the level of the septal mitral leaflet. In horses, the tricuspid valve includes three complete leaflets (**Figure 1.10**), similar to people. The leaflets are named septal, right (along the lateral wall), and left (closest to the RV outflow tract). Generally, there are three main papillary muscles; however, their number and configuration vary and up to five (with some indistinct) papillary muscles can be present, especially in the RV conus, as evidenced by chordal attachments to the valve.

Functionally, the RV includes an inflow region, trabecular apex, and outflow tract. The muscular supraventricular crest separates the RV inflow and outflow tracts dorsally. Therefore, unlike the mitral and aortic valves, the tricuspid and pulmonic valves are not adjacent or in fibrous continuity with each other. A muscular conus (RV outflow tract) leads to the semilunar pulmonary valve, which is structurally similar but thinner than the aortic valve (**Figure 1.11**). There are no coronary ostia behind pulmonary valve cusps. Congenital malformations as well as acquired abnormalities can affect the right heart's valves.

Conduction System

Electrical activation stimulates cardiac contraction. Specialized myocardial cells ("pacemakers") spontaneously generate action potentials because they possess the property of "automaticity." These action potentials then propagate throughout the heart along an organized electrical conduction system. Electrical impulses normally originate from cells within the SA node, usually from its mid- to cranial region. Impulses then spread into the RA, LA, and via the AV conduction system, into the ventricles (**Figure 1.12**). Specialized fibers (in three internodal pathways) facilitate conduction across the RA, into the LA (via Bachmann's bundle), and to the AV node. After passing through the AV node, the electrical current quickly spreads along the His–Purkinje system into the ventricular myocardium.

The SA node is the normal pacemaker of the heart because the cells here have the fastest intrinsic rate of automaticity (spontaneous diastolic depolarization). This tissue depolarizes spontaneously because of the activity of pacemaker currents that reduce (make less negative) the transmembrane potential until a firing threshold is reached (see section "Slow-Response Action Potential"). This spontaneous depolarization occurs independent of neural control. However, autonomic effects on pacemaker currents can be profound and provide clinically important heart rate (HR) and rhythm regulation. Although primary disease of the SA node occurs sometimes, most sinus rhythm variations result from the effects of the autonomic nervous system, body temperature, endocrine status, or drugs.

The AV node is the electrical "gatekeeper" to the ventricles. Normally, no other pathway allows electrical impulses to pass from the atria to the ventricles. AV nodal cells are small and branching, and like SA nodal cells, depolarize via slow-response action potentials. These factors cause slowed (decremental) conduction across the AV node. This allows time for atrial contraction and final ventricular filling to occur before ventricular activation begins. The AV node has three regions: the dorsal-most atrionodal region, the central nodal region, and the nodal-His region. Spontaneous pacemaker activity normally occurs in the nodal region, although at a slower rate than in the SA node. Therefore, it does not become manifest unless the SA nodal rate becomes abnormally slow. As with the SA node, the conduction of impulses across the AV node is markedly affected by autonomic activity.

Electrical impulses enter a bundle of rapidly conducting (Purkinje) fibers after passing through the AV node. This "bundle of His" (AV bundle) quickly transmits impulses into the left and right bundle branches. The right bundle branch courses subendocardially down the right side of the IVS, crosses the RV within the septomarginal trabecula, and branches distally to activate the RV free wall. RV dilation that

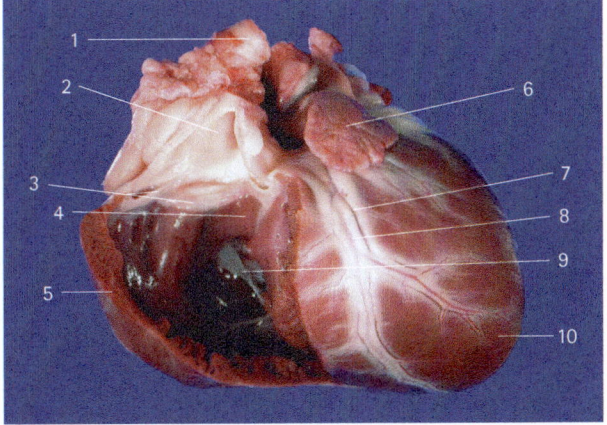

Figure 1.11 Canine heart: Right ventricular outflow tract. 1. Aorta, 2. Main pulmonary a. (pulmonary trunk), 3. Pulmonary valve, 4. Supraventricular crest, 5. R ventricle, 6. L auricle, 7. Great coronary v., 8. Cranial interventricular branch of L coronary a. (in cranial, paraconal, interventricular groove), 9. Tricuspid valve, 10. L ventricle. a., artery; L, left; R, right, v, vein.

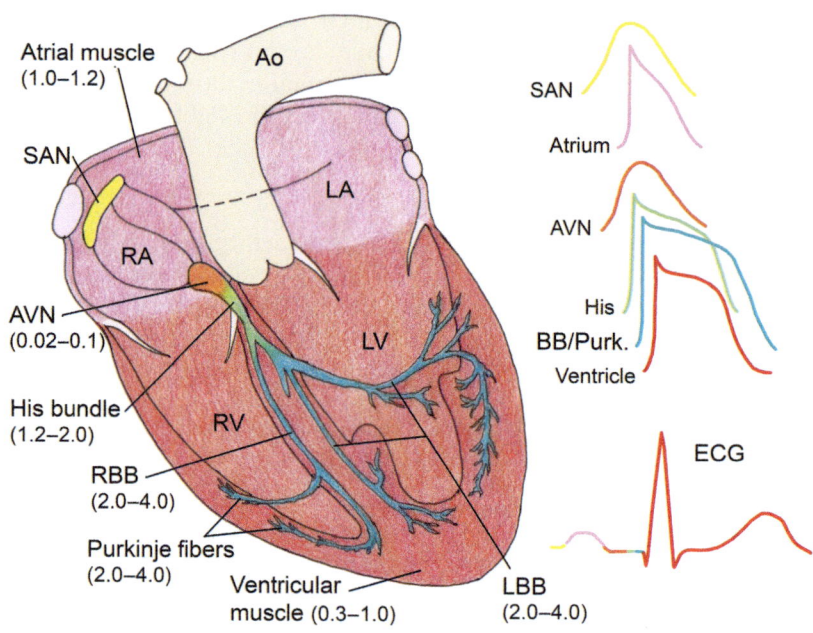

Figure 1.12 Cardiac conduction system. Major components of the conduction system are illustrated on the left, with approximate conduction speed (m/s) in parentheses. On the right, representative action potentials are color-coded to the cardiac conduction system and myocardium. A composite ECG (below) illustrates the electrical activation sequence. Ao, aorta; BB/Purk., bundle branches and Purkinje fibers; AVN, atrioventricular node; ECG, electrocardiogram; LA, left atrium; LBB, left bundle branch (posterior fascicle to the right); LV, left ventricle; RA, right atrium; RBB, right bundle branch; RV, right ventricle; SAN, sinoatrial node.

unduly stretches this muscular strand can damage the conduction fibers within and interrupt conduction to the RV free wall (known as "right bundle branch block"). On the left side of the IVS, the thick left bundle branch divides into a small septal fascicle, a posterior (caudal) fascicle serving the caudoventral aspect of the LV wall, and an anterior fascicle serving the craniolateral LV wall. A branching system of terminal Purkinje fibers transmits electrical impulses from the bundle branches into the ventricular myocardium. In dogs and cats, as in people, these terminal Purkinje fibers penetrate only partially into the myocardium (so-called "Type A" heart). Penetration of the terminal Purkinje fibers is deeper and more extensive throughout the ventricular myocardium in horses, as well as other large mammalian species and birds ("Type B" heart). This allows for more extensive and rapid electrical activation of the ventricles. Failure of electrical impulse transmission from atria to ventricles is referred to as AV block. This can occur at the level of the AV node, His bundle, or bilaterally in the bundle branches.

Cardiac Electrophysiology

Cardiac cells are polarized (more negative on the inside) and undergo depolarization (becoming less negative on the inside) in an organized manner. After depolarization, the cells undergo a process of repolarization. Cardiac action potentials occur in association with changes in cell membrane permeability to sodium (Na^+), potassium (K^+), and calcium (Ca^{++}) ions. Transmembrane movement of these ions depends on the opening and closing of numerous ion-specific channels, with different controls affecting opening and closing kinetics. The specific channels present in a cell membrane depend on the type and location of the cardiac cell. Furthermore, the conductance of different ions can be affected by changes in serum electrolyte concentrations, acid-base balance, autonomic influence, and tissue oxygenation, as well as by the effects of various drugs and cardiac disease states.

The duration of cardiac action potentials is much longer than that of noncardiac tissues. This allows time for myocardial relaxation and refilling between contractions. Cardiac action potentials also differ among types of heart cells, depending on cellular location and function. There are two main types of cardiac action potentials. The "fast-response" action potential is typical of atrial and ventricular muscle cells and Purkinje fibers. Depolarization of these cells must be initiated by current flow from an adjacent cell. Other cardiac cells exhibit the property of automaticity and can depolarize on their own via the "slow-response" (pacemaker) action potential. As mentioned above, this pacemaker action potential is characteristic of SA and AV nodal cells. However, diseased or ischemic myocardial cells sometimes also develop the functional characteristics of a slow-response cell.

In general, ion channels are affected by transmembrane voltage, time constants, ion concentrations, ligands (such as norepinephrine [NE] or other beta-agonists and acetylcholine [Ach]), pH, adenosine, and drugs. Cardiac arrhythmias can result from changes in these various factors. The efficacy of different antiarrhythmic drugs relates to their effect on different ion channels, as well as the arrhythmia's underlying mechanism (see Chapters 23 and 24). For example, a calcium channel blocker such as diltiazem will affect phase 0 depolarization in nodal (slow-response) cells, but is less likely to affect ventricular myocytes or Purkinje cells. Conversely, a sodium channel blocker like lidocaine will have minimal effect on nodal cells, which depend on Ca^{++} entry for their activation.

Resting Membrane Potential The cardiac cell membrane (sarcolemma) maintains a gradient of ions between the intra- and extracellular environment. In normal myocardial cells at rest, the electrical potential difference across the sarcolemma is about −90 mV; inside the cell is negative compared with the outside. This resting membrane potential (RMP) is largely determined by the equilibrium between chemical and electrostatic forces for K^+ (as described by the Nernst equation[1] and the concept of the Gibbs–Donnan equilibrium). The concentration of K^+ inside the cell is much greater than that outside; conversely, extracellular Na^+ and Ca^{++} concentrations far exceed intracellular concentrations. The resting sarcolemma is relatively permeable to K^+, but largely blocks migration of Na^+ and Ca^{++} as well as negatively charged intracellular proteins. K^+ tends to diffuse outward along its concentration gradient through K^+-specific channels despite an opposing electrostatic force attracting the positive ions into the cell. A tiny inward leak of Na^+ also occurs. Normal RMP and ionic concentrations are maintained by the membrane's electrogenic Na^+, K^+-ATPase pump, which moves three Na^+ ions out for every two K^+ ions in. Digoxin is a drug that blocks ("poisons") this pump, which partially relates to the drug's mechanism of action.

Fast-Response Action Potential When a stimulus reduces the membrane potential to a less negative "threshold" level, activation of Na^+-specific membrane channels allows a rapid Na^+ influx that initiates an action potential (phase 0; **Figure 1.13**). A small amount of ionic current moving from adjacent cells across gap junctions often provides this stimulus. Activation (as well as subsequent inactivation) of these channels depends on the level of membrane potential (voltage-dependence), and this inward Na^+ current (I_{Na}) occurs only briefly (time-dependence). Inactivation (closure) of the Na^+ channels produces an effective refractory period. A return toward RMP, as well as time, is necessary for Na^+ channels to recover from inactivation and become responsive to another stimulus. The steepness of the phase 0 upstroke, as well as its amplitude, influences the velocity of impulse conduction along the myocardial membranes. This largely explains the fast conduction velocity in fast-response cells; conversely, nodal (slow-response) cells have a gradual phase 0 slope and relatively slow conduction velocity. If fast-response cells are stimulated when membrane potential is less negative than

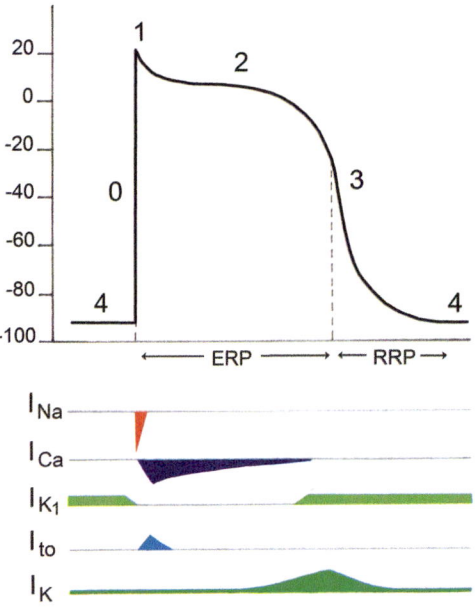

Figure 1.13 Fast-response action potential. Phases of the action potential are indicated, with the timing and direction of some important ion currents shown below; inward currents depicted below the baseline, outward currents, above. I_{Ca} represents the L-type Ca^{++} current, I_{K1} is the inward rectifier (important for maintaining resting membrane potential), and I_K includes the rapid and slow components of the delayed rectifier current (important for repolarization). See section "Fast-Response Action Potential" for further explanation. ERP, effective refractory period; RRP, relative refractory period.

normal RMP, Na^+ channels are partially inactivated and conduction velocity of the resulting action potential (if it even occurs) is slowed. Regions of slowed conduction and unidirectional conduction block predispose to reentrant arrhythmias (p. 365). A number of antiarrhythmic drugs, such as lidocaine and quinidine, block I_{Na}.

The rapid upstroke of the fast-response action potential is followed by a brief partial repolarization (phase 1) caused by a transient outward K^+ current (I_{to}) in some cardiac cells. Voltage-activated membrane Ca^{++} channels (L-type) slowly open during the latter part of phase 0, allowing an inward Ca^{++} current (I_{Ca}), which is responsible for phase 2 (the plateau). The duration of phase 2 is longer in ventricular myocardial cells than those in the atria. The Ca^{++} that enters the myocardial cells during phase 2 induces electrical–mechanical coupling (see section "Electrical–Mechanical Coupling"). As the Ca^{++} channels slowly inactivate, the inward Ca^{++} flux decreases and outward movement of K^+ increases, leading into repolarization (phase 3). Several types of K^+ channels are important in this process, especially the slow (I_{Ks}) and rapid (I_{Kr}) components of the I_K (delayed rectifier) current. The inwardly rectifying K^+ current (I_{K1}) also contributes at the end of the repolarization period and helps maintain RMP (phase 4) as well. Reduced outward K^+ flux during phases 2 and 3, or enhanced inward Ca^{++} flux, can delay repolarization and predispose to serious and potentially fatal arrhythmias.

Some antiarrhythmic drugs block (certain) potassium channels; they can exert both antiarrhythmic and proarrhythmic effects, depending on the situation.

The effective refractory period (from phase 0 until membrane potential reaches about −50 mV during phase 3) is a time when the cell cannot be re-excited. Immediately following is the relative refractory period, when a stronger than normal stimulus might elicit another action potential, although conduction velocity is likely to be slowed because of partial Na$^+$ channel inactivation. Normal excitability is achieved only after full repolarization.

Slow-Response Action Potential Two important properties of the heart are automaticity (the ability to initiate a heartbeat) and rhythmicity (the regularity of this activity). Cells with slow-response action potentials allow the heart to beat spontaneously because, instead of a consistent RMP, they undergo spontaneous diastolic (phase 4) depolarization (**Figure 1.14**). Spontaneous depolarization is characteristic of SA and AV nodal cells. These cells also have a less negative maximum diastolic membrane potential than cells characterized by the fast-response action potential.

The process of spontaneous (phase 4) diastolic depolarization results from the combined effects of: activation of the so-called "funny" current (I_f, carried by inward Na$^+$ and K$^+$ movement, especially at more negative levels of membrane potential and under beta-receptor, sympathetic stimulation); cessation of outward K$^+$ leak; transmembrane Na$^+$–Ca^{++} exchange, and activation of a transient (T-type) Ca^{++} influx. The process of spontaneous depolarization involves the concept of a SA nodal "membrane (or voltage) clock" and a "Ca^{++} clock" that work together to control SA node activation. The slow-response action potential upstroke (phase 0) and also the peak of phase 2 depend on slow (L-type) Ca^{++} channel activation; there is no recognizable phase 1 or plateau. Phase 3 (repolarization) depends on outward K$^+$ currents (I_K). Conduction velocity also is much slower along cells characterized by slow-response action potentials and the refractory period is longer. Consequently, conduction is more easily blocked in these cells.

The SA nodal cells normally have the most rapid intrinsic rate of spontaneous diastolic depolarization. Therefore, they usually reach threshold first and control the heartbeat. If the sinus rate slows or stops, other slow-response fibers lower in the conduction system (so-called "subsidiary pacemakers") can initiate a heartbeat. This is termed "escape" pacemaker activity (also see p. 141) and is a normal cardiac rescue mechanism. Subsidiary pacemakers are located mostly in the His–Purkinje system. Ultimately, the rate at which SA (or other automatic) cells activate the heart depends on the slope of their spontaneous phase 4 depolarization, as well as maximal diastolic potential and threshold potential.

Myocardial Contraction

Cardiac myocytes act as a "functional syncytium," or as if they were a single cellular unit, unlike skeletal muscle. Gap junctions (nexi) within the intercalated disks that separate adjacent myocytes promote cell-to-cell conduction and communication (**Figure 1.15**). Gap junctions, as points of contact

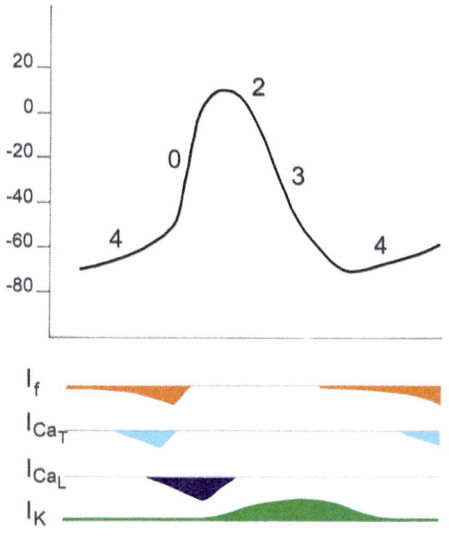

Figure 1.14 Slow-response action potential. Phases of the action potential are indicated, with the timing and direction of some important ion currents shown below; inward currents depicted below the baseline, outward currents, above. See section "Slow-Response Action Potential" for further explanation.

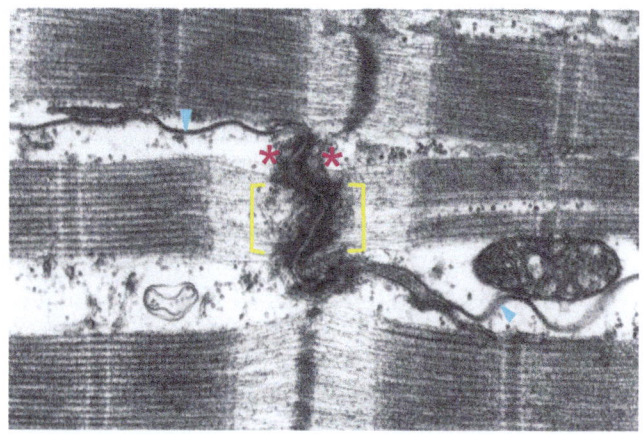

Figure 1.15 Ultrastructure of myocardial intercalated disks. This image is centered on a Z disk (Z line) between two sarcomeres. Gap junctions (light blue arrowheads) allow transfer of chemical signals between adjacent cells. Desmosomes (bright pink asterisks) have filaments that extend into the cytoplasm and are important in attaching adjacent cells together. The fascia adherens (yellow brackets) are located between desmosomes and anchor the actin filaments. (From Frappier BL, Eurell JA (editors). Dellman's Textbook of Veterinary Histology. 6th edition. 2006. p. 90.)

between the intracellular fluid of adjacent cells, facilitate local ionic current flow and action potential propagation. This allows coordinated contraction and relaxation, as if the cardiac muscle cells were a single entity.

At the subcellular level, sarcomeres (demarcated by Z lines or disks) are the basic contractile units within myocytes (**Figure 1.16**). Thin actin filaments attach to the Z lines and interdigitate with thick myosin filaments. Contraction (sarcomere shortening) occurs as these filaments slide along each other by the cycling of cross-bridges (formed by heavy meromyosin heads interacting with sites on the actin filaments). This cycling requires the presence of adenosine triphosphate (ATP) and Ca^{++}. The actin filaments are composed of two helical chains attached to a twisting tropomyosin support molecule. The troponin complexes consist of proteins (troponins I, C, and T), which regulate contraction. They are attached to the tropomyosin backbone of the actin filaments. Troponin I, in conjunction with tropomyosin, inhibits cross-bridge formation during diastole when intracellular free Ca^{++} is low. When Ca^{++} becomes available in systole (see next paragraph), it activates troponin C, which then binds to troponin I. This induces a conformational change that exposes myosin binding sites on the actin strand and subsequently allows interaction between adjacent actin and myosin filaments. Myocardial injury causes leakage of troponin proteins; clinical assays for circulating troponin I and T can provide a sensitive and specific test for cardiac muscle damage.

Electrical–Mechanical Coupling The Ca^{++} influx that occurs during phase 2 of cardiac cell activation triggers the intracellular release of more Ca^{++} from the sarcoplasmic reticulum (SR) via the calcium release (ryanodine; RyR2) receptor (**Figure 1.17**). This process is known as electrical–mechanical or excitation–contraction coupling. It is this increase in free intracellular Ca^{++} from the SR that allows contraction to proceed. The SR is an intracellular network of tubules surrounding the myofibrils that sequesters and releases Ca^{++} (**Figure 1.16**). Invaginations of the cell membrane (T tubule system) facilitate action potential propagation along the cells. Coupling of electrical excitation to mechanical contraction is enhanced by the close proximity of T tubules to parts of the SR. Sympathetic (beta-receptor) activation increases

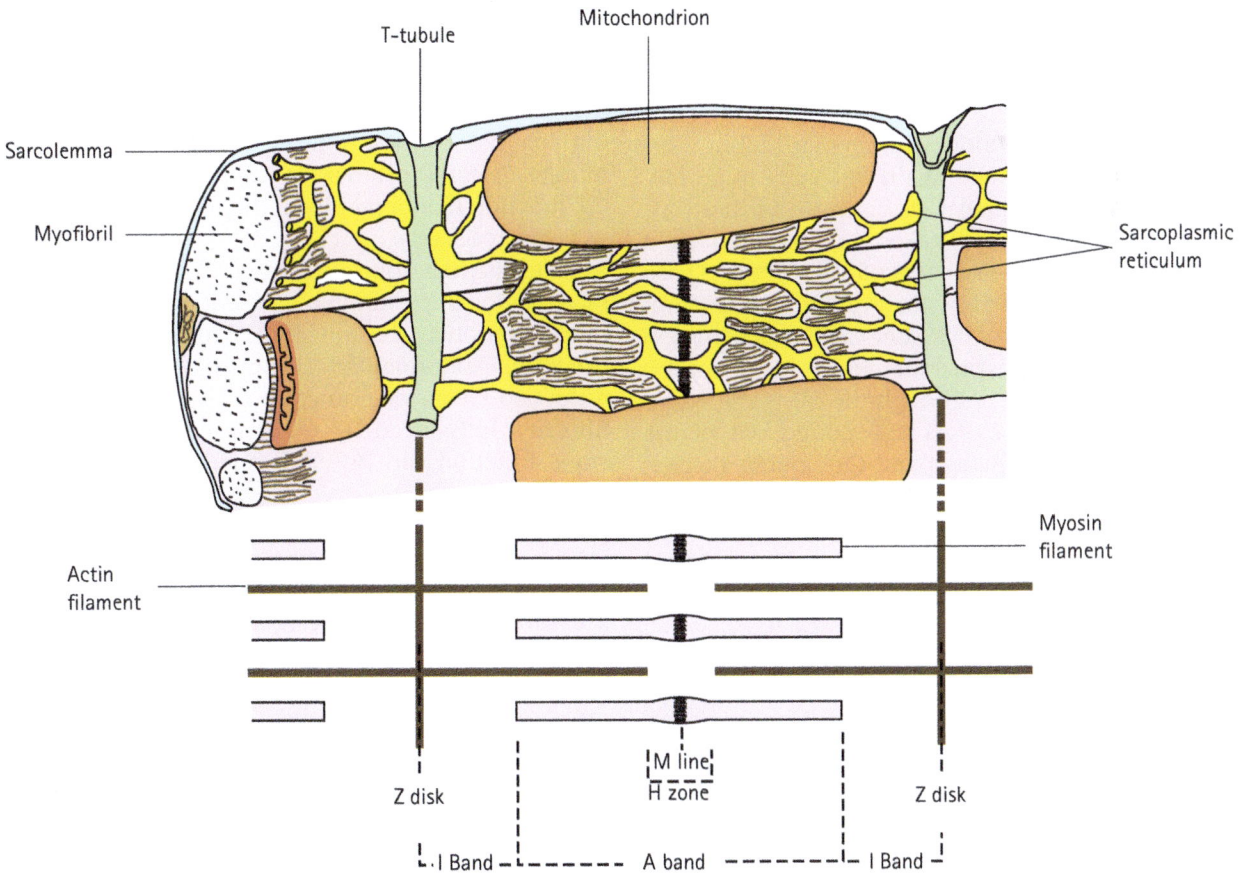

Figure 1.16 Diagram of myocardial cell components involved with excitation and contraction (above) and schematic illustration of the contractile elements (below). Location of isotropic (I) bands and anisotropic (A) band between the Z disks is indicated. See section "Myocardial Contraction" for more information.

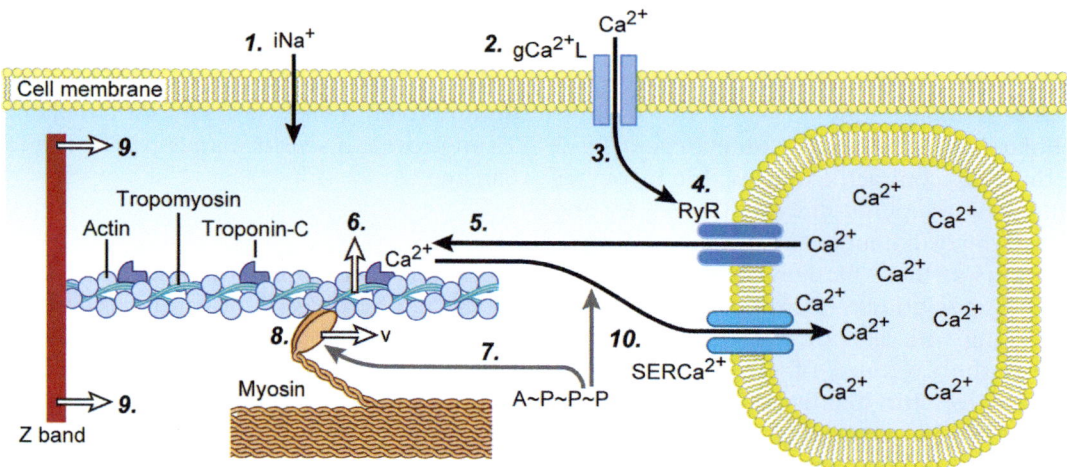

Figure 1.17 Schematic illustration of the excitation–contraction coupling process. 1. Inward Na⁺ current (phase 0) of the fast-response action potential (AP) depolarizes the myocardial cell membrane. 2. Voltage-gated Ca⁺⁺ channels in the membrane open as the membrane depolarizes. 3. A small amount of extracellular Ca⁺⁺ enters through these open channels (during phase 2 of AP). 4. This Ca⁺⁺ activates ryanodine receptors (RyR) and triggers the release of Ca⁺⁺ stored within the (intracellular) sarcoplasmic reticulum (SR). 5. A large amount of Ca⁺⁺ leaves the SR, becoming available to interact with troponin-C. 6. The Ca⁺⁺–troponin-C complex removes the inhibition of troponin-I (not shown), which then allows the heavy meromyosin heads to bind with actin. 7. The hydrolysis of adenosine triphosphate (ATP) releases energy, which fuels the movement of the myosin heads. 8. The myosin heads, bound to actin, now cycle (ratchet) and pull the actin filaments inward. 9. The Z bands move toward each other as the sarcomeres (Z-to-Z distance) shorten during contraction. 10. Energy from ATP hydrolysis also fuels the sarcoendoplasmic reticulum Ca⁺⁺ ATPase (SERCA) Ca⁺⁺ reuptake pump of the SR membrane; this resequesters free intracytoplasmic Ca⁺⁺ into the SR. The rapid drop in free Ca⁺⁺ causes actin–myosin disengagement and myocardial relaxation. (Diagram courtesy of Dr. RL Hamlin.)[8]

SR Ca⁺⁺ release, as well as indirectly promotes Ca⁺⁺ reuptake to facilitate relaxation.

Myocardial Relaxation During cell repolarization, Ca⁺⁺ influx falls off as the membrane again becomes impermeable to Ca⁺⁺. The SR is not stimulated to release further Ca⁺⁺ into the cytosol and now actively takes Ca⁺⁺ back up via a pump called sarcoendoplasmic reticulum Ca⁺⁺ ATPase (SERCA). This pump is regulated by the protein phospholamban. The rapid resequestering of cytosolic Ca⁺⁺ makes this ion unavailable to the contractile apparatus and leads to inhibition of cross-bridge formation. Although the SR is the major site of Ca⁺⁺ reuptake, some Ca⁺⁺ is transported out of the cell via membrane Na/Ca exchange and Ca⁺⁺ pump mechanisms. Mitochondrial uptake of free Ca⁺⁺ becomes important when intracellular Ca⁺⁺ levels are pathologically high. Slowed or incomplete reuptake of Ca⁺⁺ in diastole increases cardiac stiffness and adversely affects filling. Impaired myocardial relaxation can develop acutely with myocardial ischemia; chronically it can contribute to heart failure, especially in cats with hypertrophic cardiomyopathy. Catecholamines accelerate relaxation in normal myocardium by phosphorylating phospholamban and removing its inhibition of SERCA.

The Heart as a Pump

The ventricles fill during diastole and eject during systole. This occurs over 100,000 times each day in a normal canine heart. Cardiac pump function can be described in a number of ways. The stroke volume (SV) is the volume of blood pumped from either ventricle with each heart contraction. The HR is the frequency of cardiac contractions per minute. The CO is the volume of blood pumped from either ventricle over one minute. Systemic arterial blood pressure is another variable of CV function that depends on the interaction between CO and vascular resistance.

The heart's ability to function as a pump is based on interrelationships among the sequence of electrical activation, ventricular diastolic function, and ventricular systolic function. Abnormalities in any of these determinants can reduce CO. Diastolic function is complicated and ventricular filling is influenced by multiple factors. Conceptually, diastolic function can be envisioned as an interaction among ventricular relaxation, venous (filling) pressures, and ventricular compliance (or distensibility). In early diastole, active relaxation of the myocardium (an energy-dependent process) is important for rapidly reducing intraventricular pressure. In addition, the recoil and untwisting of the ventricles greatly affect early ventricular filling. Then the combined effects of blood return from the venous system, atrial pressure, ventricular compliance, the duration of diastole, and atrial contraction strength contribute to the ventricular volume achieved by the end of diastole (also known as preload). Ventricular compliance (defined as change in volume/change in pressure, which is the reciprocal of stiffness) becomes increasingly important as diastole and ventricular filling progress. Venous pressure and venous return to the heart are affected by numerous factors, as summarized later in this chapter (section "Venous System"). The duration of diastole depends on the HR. As HR increases, diastole becomes shorter and atrial contraction contributes a proportionately greater amount to EDV. If atrial contraction is lost (as with atrial fibrillation), serious negative effects on cardiac performance can result, especially at higher HRs.

Systolic function depends on myocardial contractility (inotropy) as well as the loading conditions (preload and afterload) imposed on the ventricular fibers. Abnormal valvular function can negatively affect ventricular function in the setting of heart disease. The synchronization of ventricular filling and contraction also is important and involves at least three different aspects of electromechanical coordination. The first is AV synchrony, which mainly depends on heart rhythm and the timing between atrial and ventricular activation (PR interval on ECG; see section "Cardiac Cycle and Generation of Heart Sounds"). Intraventricular synchrony of contraction relates to the sequence of mechanical activation and relaxation within a ventricular chamber. Interventricular synchrony compares the ejection periods of the left and right ventricles. Synchrony can be altered by arrhythmias, conduction disturbances, and various cardiac diseases.

Cardiac Output CO is calculated as the product of HR and SV. It generally is expressed as liters or mL/minute. Thus CO = HR (beats per minute) × SV (in L or mL per beat). Frequently, CO is indexed to body size (the "cardiac index"). The normal cardiac index for a resting dog is about 3.1–4.7 liters/minute/m^2. Because the right heart and left heart are in series, CO from the RV equals CO from the LV. However, minor variation between ventricles does occur over brief time periods, such as during phases of respiration. Because CO depends on both frequency of contraction and ventricular function, it is considered a global estimate of the heart as a pump. Invasive methods used to estimate CO are based on the Fick principle[2] and include thermodilution, lithium-based indicator techniques, and other methods. These rarely are used in patients. Noninvasive CO estimation can be done with echocardiography, especially Doppler methods (p. 127).

Normal SV is about 55–65% of the ventricular end-diastolic volume (EDV). The blood remaining in the ventricles after ejection is known as the residual, or end-systolic, volume. This ratio of SV/EDV is termed ejection fraction (EF) and is a global estimate of ventricular function. The ventricular SV and EF are related directly to myocardial contractility and ventricular preload, and related inversely to ventricular afterload.

Contractility The term "contractility" refers to the intrinsic strength of contraction at a given preload and afterload. Contractility also is known as inotropic state or inotropy. Contractility primarily depends on the amount of free intracellular Ca^{++} available during systole, although ATP availability and the sensitivity of the contractile proteins to Ca^{++} also are important. Changes in autonomic nervous activity or HR (the Bowditch, also known as the "treppe" or "staircase," effect) can influence contractility in a positive manner. Positive inotropic agents such as catecholamines and digoxin increase peak contractile force and SV by increasing intracellular Ca^{++} availability. Because the ventricle empties to a greater degree, this can reduce ventricular end-systolic volume. Calcium-sensitizing agents (such as pimobendan) increase myocardial contractility without substantially increasing free Ca^{++} concentration. Negative inotropic agents (such as beta-blockers or calcium-channel blockers) impair Ca^{++} entry across L-type channels, reduce available Ca^{++} and depress contractility.

Impaired myocardial contractility is a defining feature of dilated cardiomyopathy. Reduced contractility also can develop from chronic ventricular volume and pressure overloads. With little exception, anesthetic drugs markedly decrease contractile and overall systolic function. Accurate assessment of systolic (contractile) function is challenging in the setting of valvular heart disease, especially in cases of mitral regurgitation.

Preload The concept of preload refers to the degree of diastolic sarcomere stretch just prior to contraction. This is related to ventricular EDV and end-diastolic pressure (EDP). Diastolic sarcomere stretch (to an optimal length) will increase the force of the subsequent contraction by favorably aligning the contractile elements, and increasing Ca^{++} release and affinity. In the intact heart, as EDV (preload) increases, the volume ejected with each contraction increases. This is the Frank–Starling relationship or Starling's law of the heart (sometimes called "heterometric autoregulation"; **Figure 1.18**, left middle). This mechanism is crucial for beat-to-beat adjustments in SV and for balancing the output of the RVs and LVs.

Although preload directly influences ventricular systolic function, ventricular filling and stretch are determined by factors related to diastolic function (see section "The Heart as a Pump"). Ventricular preload is clinically important. Volume depletion (as from vomiting, diarrhea, urinary loss, or hemorrhage) is likely to reduce preload and CO. Prerenal azotemia, impaired perfusion of other organs, and hypotension can result. Myocardial hypertrophy or infiltration with fibrous tissue also impedes filling by increasing myocardial stiffness. External compression of the heart, as with pericardial disease, is another cause of impaired ventricular filling. When ventricular distensibility is reduced, higher filling pressures are required for any given diastolic volume; this is an operative definition of ventricular "diastolic dysfunction." Consequences of impaired ventricular filling are a smaller EDV and increased venous pressure behind the affected ventricle. Perhaps surprisingly, ventricular dilation also can increase end-diastolic ventricular stiffness, as well as preload (**Figure 1.19**). In either situation, excessively

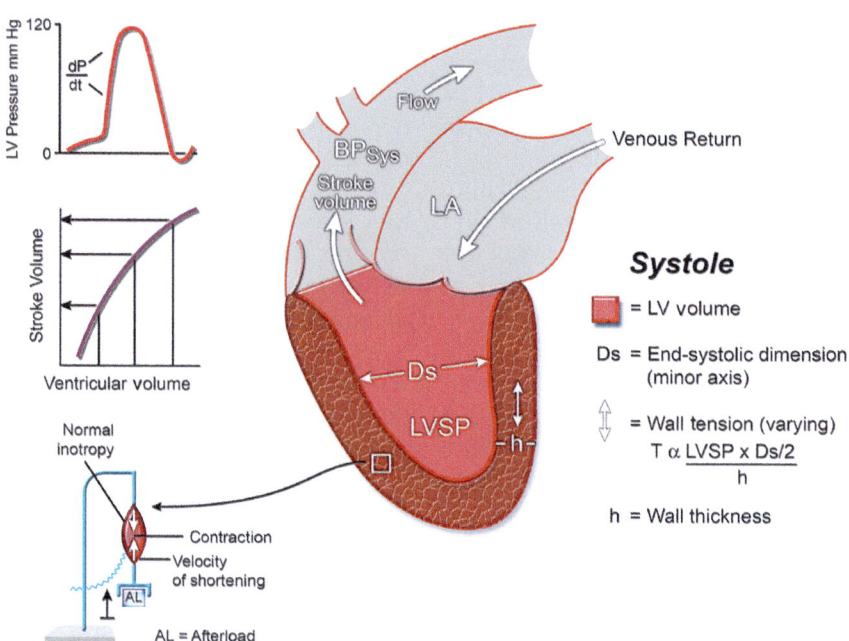

Figure 1.18 Schematic illustration of important concepts of left ventricular (LV) systole; analogous events occur in the right heart. After electrical activation, the LV myocardium contracts and the rapidly developing wall tension increases intraventricular pressure (LVSP, LV systolic pressure), squeezing the blood within the chamber. The upper figure on the left depicts the extremely rapid increase in LVSP. LV wall tension varies throughout systole as pressure increases, blood is ejected from the ventricle, and the ventricular walls thicken during ejection. Maximal wall tension occurs at the instant of aortic valve opening, at which point blood (stroke volume) is ejected into the aorta and systolic blood pressure (BPsys) increases. The wall tension needed to overcome the aortic pressure and arterial impedance is called the "afterload (AL)." This word is based on muscle strip experiments (diagram at lower left) where the AL was literally a weight that had to be lifted and moved by the contracting muscle. Unlike increasing preload, which enhances ventricular function, AL opposes it, reducing the velocity and duration of shortening in the muscle and the stroke volume in the LV. Based on the Laplace relationship (right), the LV wall tension increases with a higher LVSP and with ventricular dilation (Ds/2) but is normalized (reduced) by ventricular hypertrophy that increases wall thickness. This wall thickening explains in part how the LV adapts to systemic hypertension and to aortic stenosis (two disorders that require higher LVSP). The other "loading" condition on the ventricle is preload (also see **Figure 1.19**, diastole). Preload relates the end-diastolic sarcomere stretch (and LV volume) prior to contraction to LV's ability to develop tension and eject a stroke volume. Increasing preload optimizes sarcomere length, which increases the force of contraction and stroke volume (left, middle figure). This is known as the Frank–Starling relationship. Thus, reduced ventricular diastolic volume (such as from dehydration) decreases LV stroke volume, while an increased preload produces a greater stroke volume, even accounting for its effects on afterload. In upper left diagram: dP/dt, change in pressure/change in time (1st derivative of LV pressure).[8]

high ventricular filling pressures promote venous congestion upstream from the affected chamber, leading to edema and cavity effusions.

Afterload Ventricular afterload is a complicated variable. It relates to the contractile force that must be achieved before sarcomeres can shorten and the ventricle ejects blood. Increased afterload has a negative effect on SV. One estimate of afterload is peak wall stress at the instant of aortic valve opening. After ejection has begun, the aorta and vascular system continue to oppose contraction. Impedance is another measure of afterload. Impedance is defined for the LV as the instantaneous change in aortic pressure/aortic flow. Because impedance varies throughout ejection, it cannot be measured practically in patients. From a clinical standpoint, afterload is often equated to arterial blood pressure, however this is an oversimplification. Factors that impede aortic flow, such as elevated blood pressure, (sub)aortic stenosis, reduced arterial compliance, increased vascular resistance, and reflected arterial waves increase impedance afterload. Ventricular wall thickening actually reduces wall stress; whereas, ventricular dilation without sufficient wall hypertrophy increases afterload.

Response to Pressure or Volume Loading A chronic increase in ventricular volume (preload) or systolic pressure generation (afterload) creates greater wall tension (stress) according to the Laplace relationship.[3] Increased wall stress demands greater energy (ATP) and O_2 consumption. As a compensatory response, myocardial hypertrophy develops via an increase in number of sarcomeres. In general, the pattern of hypertrophy depends on the type of overload. Chronic increase in ventricular volume stimulates the formation of new sarcomeres in series, lengthening the myofibers and creating a larger ventricle of normal wall thickness—so-called "eccentric hypertrophy." A classic example is the LV dilation that develops with chronic degenerative (myxomatous) mitral valve disease in the dog (Chapter 29). Diseases

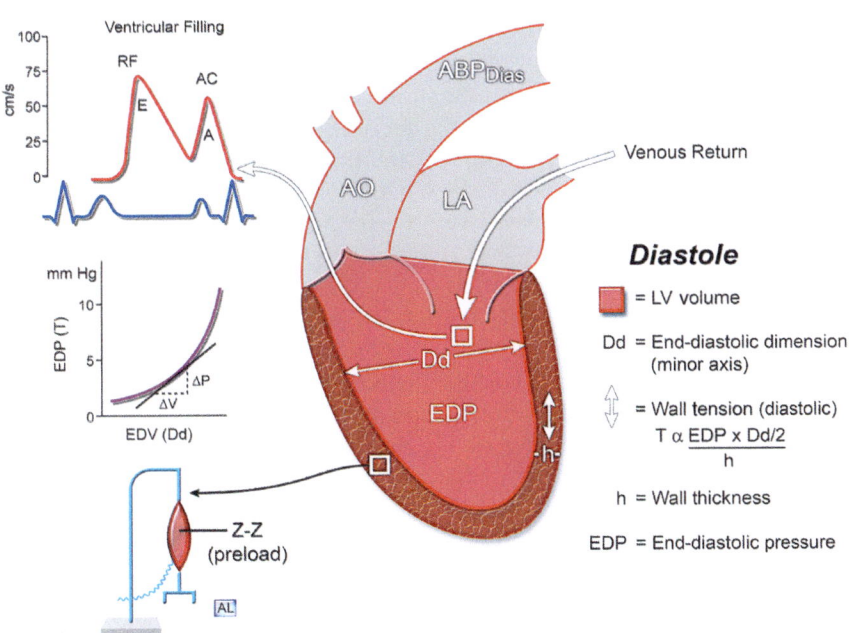

Figure 1.19 Schematic illustration of important concepts of left ventricular (LV) diastole; analogous events occur in the right heart. The volume that distends the ventricle sets the sarcomere length prior to contraction and strongly influences ventricular contractility. This sarcomere length, termed the "preload," is based on muscle strip experiments that prestretched the muscle before stimulation (lower left diagram). The actual end-diastolic ventricular volume (EDV) and diameter (Dd, often measured by echocardiography) depend on the distending effect of end-diastolic pressure (EDP), as well as the stiffness of the muscle and compliance of the ventricular chamber. As venous return increases the LV volume, wall tension develops based on the law of Laplace (right). Tension is directly proportional to the distending pressure and chamber radius (Dd/2) and inversely proportional to wall thickness. The slope of the tangent of the diastolic volume to pressure relationship ($\Delta V/\Delta P$) relates to the compliance of the ventricle and explains in part why severe ventricular dilation is associated with higher filling pressures and risk of pulmonary edema (left, middle figure). As EDV increases, the increasing wall tension resists filling and requires a relatively higher end-diastolic pressure for filling. Furthermore, if a ventricle is stiffer than normal, the diastolic volume–pressure relationship shifts leftward, resulting in less filling at any level of EDP. Diastole is complicated to measure clinically; however, pulsed wave Doppler methods (upper left) can record the two main filling waves of the ventricle. Rapid ventricular filling (RF) in early diastole generates the E wave, while the late diastolic atrial contraction (AC) generates the A wave. The size and contour of these waveforms can reflect changes in diastolic function and ventricular filling pressure.[8]

that demand excessive systolic pressure generation stimulate formation of new sarcomeres in parallel, increasing myofiber diameter and ventricular wall thickness—so-called "concentric hypertrophy." Severe pulmonic or (sub)aortic stenosis provides examples of this (Chapter 27).

Increased myocardial mass could normalize wall stress. However, with progressive cardiac disease, wall stress normalization might not be achieved or sustained despite myocardial hypertrophy. The "cardiomyopathy of overload" is a situation where a chronic workload has led to depressed contractility and systolic heart failure (heart failure with reduced EF). Diastolic heart failure (heart failure with preserved EF) also can develop from chronic workload, especially when the ventricle becomes thick, fibrotic, or ischemic.

Ventricular Function Assessment Overall CV function could be estimated by measuring CO or systemic blood pressure, as noted previously. Ventricular function can be assessed by invasive (catheter-based) or noninvasive methods. Most noninvasive methods used currently are ultrasound-based, including M-mode, 2D and Doppler echocardiography, as well as more sophisticated automated methods. A number of indices can be used to estimate systolic function. Although inotropy is defined in muscle strip experiments by the maximal velocity of fiber shortening (V_{max}), indices of ventricular contractility in the intact heart are imperfect. The slope of the end-systolic pressure–volume relationship (Es, E_{max}, maximal end-systolic elastance) provides a good estimate of contractility, and preload-recruitable stroke work is considered another index of contractile function. Unfortunately, neither are practical to measure in patients. The maximal rate of LV pressure generation during isovolumic contraction (dP/dt_{max}) can be determined invasively from a catheter placed into the LV, and noninvasively in some cases using echocardiography. Although dP/dt_{max} has been considered a gold standard index of LV contractility, it is heavily influenced by preload.

The ventricular EF and the percent reduction in LV diameter or short-axis area from diastole to systole (fractional shortening, FS; and fractional area change, FAC) are common LV function indices measured by echocardiography. These mainly represent global systolic function, as opposed to contractility per se, because these ejection phase indices are especially influenced by loading conditions (preload and afterload), as well as heart rate. Right ventricular function can be estimated echocardiographically by the distance of apical-basilar contraction, area change of the cavity over the cardiac cycle, and by tissue Doppler and special techniques that measure velocity or deformation of the myocardium. Unfortunately, when there is moderate to severe mitral regurgitation, both systolic and diastolic ventricular function indices tend to become hyperdynamic and unreliable related to changes in ventricular load (Chapter 4).

Invasively measured indices of ventricular relaxation include the maximal rate ($-dP/dt_{max}$), and the time constant (tau), of LV pressure decline during isovolumic relaxation. Doppler indices offer noninvasive clues about ventricular filling but are rarely specific for relaxation. The isovolumic relaxation time (IVRT), mitral inflow patterns, and tissue Doppler velocity measurements are in popular use (p. 127).

Cardiac Cycle and Generation of Heart Sounds

Understanding the interrelations among electrical, mechanical, and acoustic events during the cardiac cycle is fundamental to understanding both normal and abnormal cardiac function (**Figure 1.20**). Accurate interpretation of CV examination findings also depends on knowledge of these events. Electrical activation (depolarization) always precedes mechanical activation (contraction).

Atrial electrical activation, indicated by the P wave on ECG, triggers atrial contraction (the "atrial kick"). This provides final ventricular filling (preload) at the end of ventricular diastole. At resting HRs, this represents only 10–20% of the total ventricular EDV. However, at fast HRs, atrial contraction can contribute up to 30% (or more) of the final ventricular volume. Therefore, loss of atrial contraction combined with

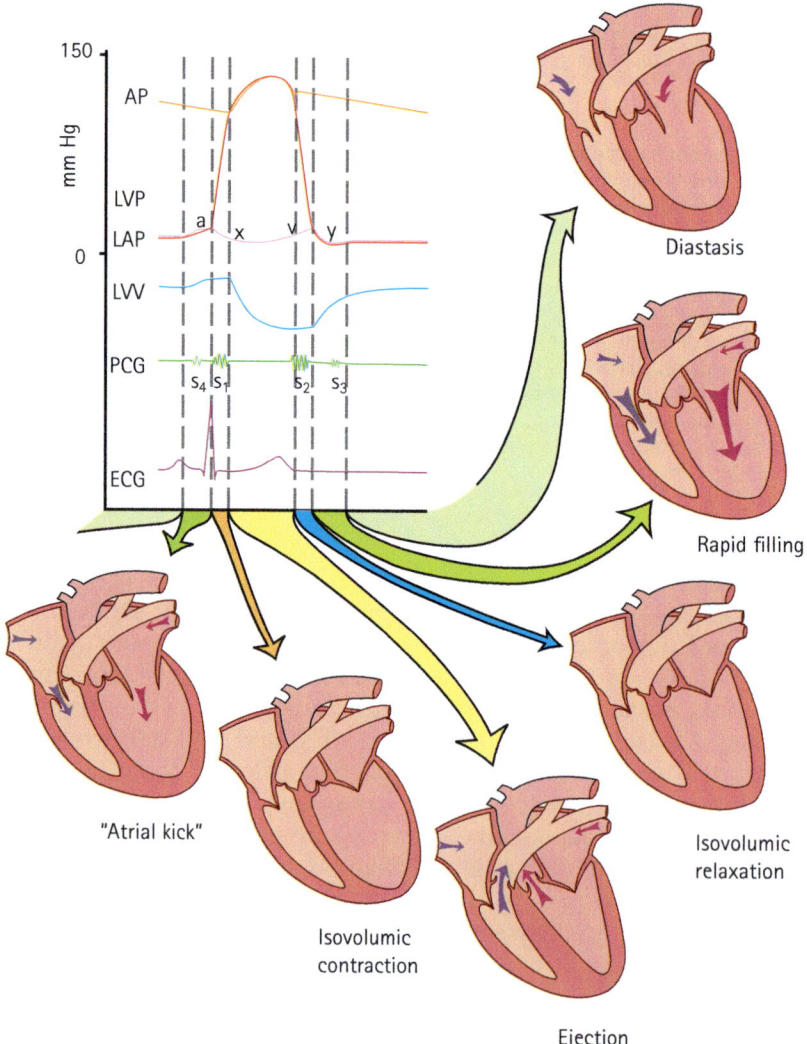

Figure 1.20 Cardiac cycle diagram showing interrelationships among electrical activation; pressures within atrium, ventricle, and associated great vessel; changes in ventricular volume; and heart sounds. Phases of the cardiac cycle are indicated by colored arrows correlating their time of occurrence on the graph with pictoral illustrations of the cardiac events. The timing of the sounds S_3 and S_4 is illustrated, although these sounds are not heard in normal dogs and cats. Similar pressure and volume changes occur in the right heart. (See section "Cardiac Cycle and Generation of Heart Sounds" for explanation of atrial pressure waves.) AP, aortic pressure; ECG, electrocardiogram; LAP, left atrial pressure; LVP, left ventricular pressure; LVV, left ventricular volume; PCG, phonocardiogram.

high HR (as can occur with atrial fibrillation) can markedly impair cardiac filling and output.

Ventricular electrical activation, signaled by the QRS complex on ECG, precedes ventricular contraction (systole). Ventricular pressure is low at the onset of the QRS complex (end-diastole); however, it quickly begins to rise. When ventricular pressure exceeds atrial pressure (also quite low), the AV valves close. Vibrations associated with valve closing and tensing are heard as the first heart sound (S_1, "lub"). From a clinical perspective, this signals the beginning of ventricular systole. Ventricular pressure continues its rapid increase. The brief time from AV valve closure until ventricular pressure rises enough to open the semilunar valves is known as isovolumic (isovolumetric) contraction. After the aortic and pulmonary valves open, ventricular ejection proceeds rapidly as the contracting ventricular walls thicken and shorten. Then the rate of ejection slows as myocardial relaxation begins to occur. These velocity changes can be appreciated on an aortic (or pulmonary) Doppler flow recording.

Ventricular pressure falls quickly as relaxation occurs. When ventricular pressure drops below that in the associated great artery, ejection ceases (after a brief time lag caused by the momentum of blood flow) and the semilunar valves close. Vibrations associated with closing and tensing of these valves create the second heart sound (S_2, "dub"). From a clinical perspective, this signals the end of ventricular systole and the beginning of ventricular diastole. The initial phase of diastole is isovolumic (isovolumetric) relaxation. During this brief period, the ventricular myocardium is actively relaxing and ventricular pressure falls rapidly with no change in volume. When intraventricular pressure drops below that in the atria, the AV valves open and rapid (early) ventricular filling occurs. The greatest increase in ventricular volume occurs during this rapid filling phase, typically to about 80% of final ventricular volume at normal HRs. A slower filling phase (diastasis) follows, although little volume is added here. The duration of diastasis is inversely related to HR. The final phase of ventricular diastole occurs with atrial contraction, as the cycle begins again.

Atrial contraction, at the end of ventricular diastole, produces an increase in atrial pressure called the "a wave." Sometimes a smaller "c wave" also is evident following the "a wave," as ventricular contraction begins (not shown in **Figure 1.20**, see **Figure 1.23**). During initial ventricular ejection, there is a drop in atrial pressure as the atrium relaxes and the AV junction moves downward during ventricular contraction (the "x descent"; **Figure 1.20**). A gradual rise in atrial pressure ("v wave") follows, as blood continues to flow into the atria during ventricular systole. Atrial pressure falls again ("y descent") when the AV valves open in early diastole. Continued filling during diastasis produces a gradual, small rise in atrial (and ventricular) pressures.

Only two heart sounds (S_1 and S_2) are heard in normal dogs and cats. However, two other sounds might become audible with certain myocardial abnormalities. The S_3 (ventricular gallop sound) results from accentuated low-frequency vibrations associated with the end of early (rapid) diastolic filling. The S_3 is most likely to be heard in dogs (or cats) with LV dilation and failure (as from dilated cardiomyopathy with elevated filling pressures). The S_4 (atrial gallop sound) is associated with blood and tissue oscillations at the time of atrial contraction. The S_4 might be heard with an abnormally stiff LV (such as from hypertrophic cardiomyopathy). Normal horses, in contrast to small animals, have an audible S_4, and often an S_3 or ventricular sound, as well. These sounds become more accentuated with myocardial disease, as in small animals. In horses with physiological (or pathological) AV block, an isolated S_4 sound heard during pauses in the rhythm indicates that atrial, but not ventricular, contraction has occurred.

Pressure–Volume Loops The changes in LV pressure and volume that occur during the cardiac cycle can be depicted in a loop without regard to timing; this helps illustrate functional abnormalities. **Figure 1.21** shows a normal pressure–volume loop compared with the changes induced by systolic dysfunction (poor myocardial contractility), diastolic dysfunction (impaired ventricular filling), and chronic volume overload. Such changes underlie

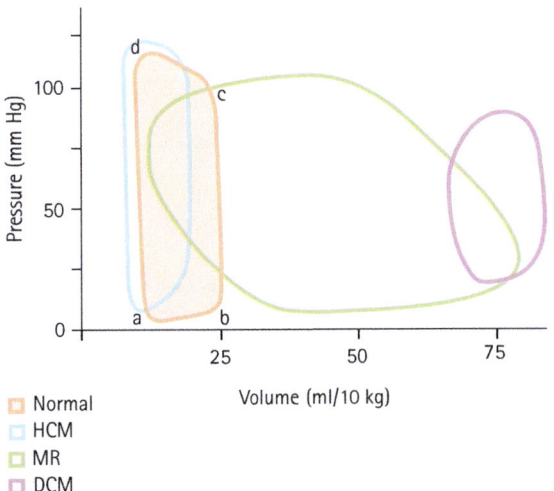

Figure 1.21 The normal left ventricular pressure–volume relationship is illustrated in orange. Ventricular filling occurs from "a" to "b." Mitral valve closure and end-diastolic volume and pressure occur at point "b." From "b" to "c" is isovolumic contraction and from "c" to "d" is ejection. The change in ventricular volume from "c" to "d" represents the stroke volume. Isovolumic relaxation occurs from "d" to "a," where the mitral valve opens. Changes typical of various chronic heart diseases also are depicted. Hypertrophic cardiomyopathy (HCM, blue loop) is associated with increased ventricular stiffness, elevated end-diastolic pressure, and reduced volume. Large end-diastolic and stroke volumes are typical for severe, chronic mitral regurgitation (MR, green loop). There is no true isovolumic contraction because of the MR. Likewise for isovolumic relaxation because MR continues after aortic valve closure; elevated atrial pressure causes rapid inflow shortly thereafter. In dilated cardiomyopathy (DCM, red loop), both end-diastolic and end-systolic volumes are large and stroke volume is small because of the chronically poor contractility and secondary volume retention. Elevated filling pressure develops as ventricular dilation and stiffness increase.

the clinical, radiographic, and echocardiographic findings associated with various heart diseases.

Autonomic Control of the Heart

Although cardiac innervation is not necessary for action potential generation and contraction, parasympathetic and sympathetic nerves play an important role in modulating cardiac activity (**Figure 1.22**). NE released at the sympathetic nerve terminals, and also circulating epinephrine and NE, act as adrenergic agonists. Ach is the neurotransmitter released by parasympathetic neurons. Varying levels of sympathetic and parasympathetic (vagal) "tone" combine to regulate cardiac responses under a wide variety of conditions. Arterial baroreceptor reflexes have a profound influence on efferent autonomic traffic.

Effects of Sympathetic Stimulation Adrenergic receptors are widespread throughout the heart and are mainly of the beta$_1$ subtype. Stimulation of these receptors increases HR (*chronotropy*) and conduction velocity (*dromotropy*), shortens the refractory period, and enhances myocardial contractility (*inotropy*) and relaxation (*lusitropy*). Beta-adrenergic stimulation enhances L-type calcium channel opening, which increases contractility because more Ca^{++} enters the myocytes during depolarization and more Ca^{++} is released from the SR. Beta-receptor stimulation also accelerates myocardial relaxation by reducing troponin's affinity for Ca^{++} and accelerating SR reuptake of Ca^{++} via the phospholamban-SERCA regulatory system. Sympathetic stimulation of the SA node hyperpolarizes these cells, thus activating an inward flux of Na^+ and K^+ (I_f) which causes faster spontaneous diastolic (phase 4)

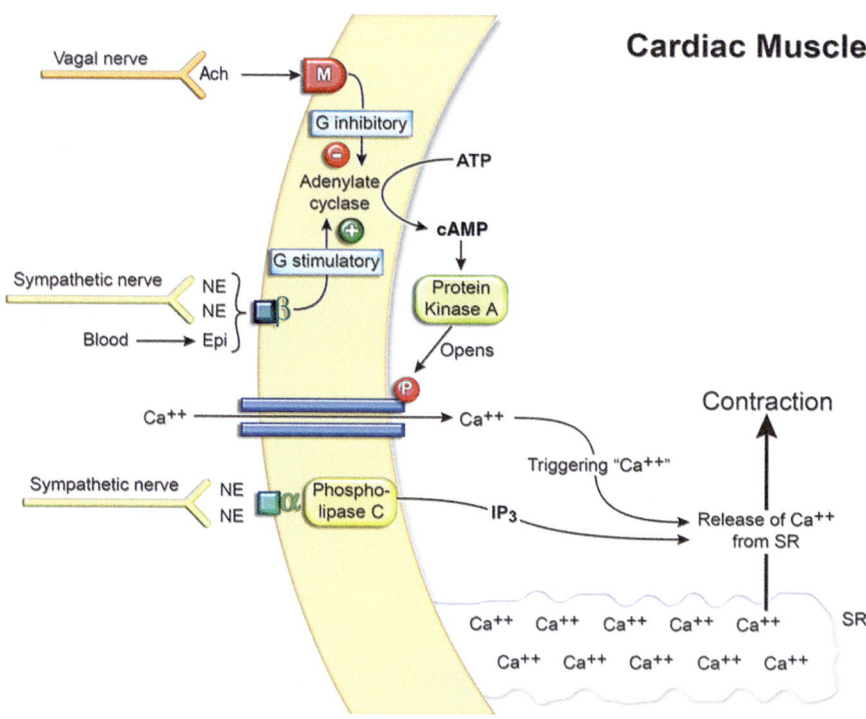

Figure 1.22 Autonomic control in the heart. Most beta-adrenergic receptors in the heart are myocardial beta$_1$ receptors, with some beta$_2$ receptors. There are few alpha-adrenergic receptors in companion animal species. The agonists for beta- and alpha-receptors are norepinephrine (NE, released from sympathetic nerves) and epinephrine (Epi, released by the adrenal medulla). Simply put, the essence of cardiac beta-stimulation is faster, stronger, and quicker. Under sympathetic stimulation of the beta-receptors, the heart beats faster (positive chronotropy), conducts current more rapidly (positive dromotropy), contracts more vigorously (positive inotropy), relaxes faster (positive lusitropy), and becomes more excitable (positive bathmotropy). Beta-receptors link by a stimulatory G protein to the adenylate cyclase system, which generates cyclic adenosine monophosphate (cAMP), as well as other messengers such as protein kinase A. cAMP works via protein kinase A to increase calcium channel opening, which increases Ca^{++} entry across its L-type channel; this increases the strength of contraction. It also acts to phosphorylate the membrane protein phospholamban. This reduces the braking (depressing) effect of phospholamban on the Ca^{++} reuptake pump (SERCA), which in turn increases the rate of Ca^{++} uptake into the sarcoplasmic reticulum (SR) and therefore, relaxation (lusitropic effect).

The alpha-receptors are less prominent in cardiac muscle; some species have little or none. Their main agonist is NE released from sympathetic nerves. The alpha-receptor's signaling system is different; the receptor is coupled to phospholipase C, which generates inositol triphosphate (IP$_3$), a second messenger that increases Ca^{++} release from the SR to create a positive inotropic effect.

Muscarinic (M) receptors are widely distributed in atrial myocardium, the SA node, and the AV node. They are less numerous in ventricular muscle, although some are present. Vagal stimulation releases the agonist, acetylcholine (Ach), from parasympathetic nerves. Ach stimulates the M2 receptor, which is coupled to an inhibitory G protein. This in turn inhibits adenylate cyclase. Thus, vagal stimulation depresses contractile function, especially in the atria where vagal innervation is most prominent.[8]

depolarization. Therefore, these cells reach threshold and generate the next action potential sooner, leading to an increase in heart (sinus) rate. This also decreases beat-to-beat HR variability, in contrast to the influence of vagal activity. Enhanced opening of L-type calcium channels also speeds AV conduction velocity besides facilitating pacemaker activity. Drugs that block beta-receptors antagonize these sympathetic effects.

Effects of Parasympathetic (Vagal) Stimulation Vagal (muscarinic) innervation to the heart is much more prominent in SA and AV nodal tissue and atrial myocardium, compared to the ventricular tissues. Vagal stimulation slows the SA node rate by antagonizing sympathetic activity and by reducing the slope of diastolic depolarization via an Ach-activated outward K^+ current (I_{KAch}). AV conduction also is slowed. Thus, the physiologic control of HR is mediated by the autonomic nervous system mainly by changes in the slope of diastolic (phase 4) depolarization in SA nodal cells. Vagal stimulation also accelerates repolarization; this effect is more pronounced in atrial myocardial cells. Normally, vagal influences predominate at rest.

Periodic variation in the sinus rate is called sinus arrhythmia. This is related to reflex-mediated fluctuations in the degree of vagal tone and usually is associated with the respiratory cycle (respiratory sinus arrhythmia). HR increases with inspiration (as vagal tone diminishes) and decreases during expiration (as vagal tone rises). Sinus arrhythmia can be quite pronounced in resting dogs and horses. Physiological second-degree AV block often occurs in horses during periods of HR slowing, as a further manifestation of increasing vagal tone. Sinus arrhythmia also occurs in resting cats, although the HR variability is more subtle.

Measurement of HR variability can indicate an underlying imbalance in autonomic activity. HR variability decreases in situations of stress, as sympathetic activity increases and vagal influence diminishes. Low HR variability has been associated with reduced survival in various disease conditions. HR variability can be measured over various durations of time and in several ways. These include time-domain indices (which quantify the variability among interbeat intervals), frequency-domain indices (which measure signal energy or power within several frequency bands), and nonlinear measurements of the unpredictability of a time series (for example, with Poincaré plots).

Parasympathetic nerves produce an antisympathetic effect on atrial myocardial cells. Because few ventricular cells receive direct vagal innervation, this effect is less prominent in the ventricular myocardium. However, parasympathetic neurons indirectly affect the myocardium through Ach-mediated activation of muscarinic cholinergic receptors located on sympathetic nerve terminals. This inhibits NE release from these terminals, which weakens the effects of sympathetic activation on ventricular cells.

Cardiac Energy Supply

The heart requires a high level of energy to support contraction, as well as other cellular functions. Myocardial O_2 needs rise when HR, contractility, and wall tension increase, as occurs with sympathetic activation. Ironically, higher HR also reduces the diastolic period when most coronary flow occurs.

Coronary arterioles deliver O_2 to the cells via a dense myocardial capillary network. Regulation of coronary arteriolar tone is tightly coupled to the myocytes' energy status and metabolic vasodilation is the most important control. The myocardium contains many mitochondria, which produce ATP by oxidative phosphorylation; fatty acids are the major source of energy for the heart. Mitochondrial ATP production is impaired when excess intracellular Ca^{++} leads to mitochondrial Ca^{++} overloading.

Coronary Blood Flow Overall, coronary blood flow is proportional to the driving pressure across the coronary circulation and is expressed by the following relationship: (aortic pressure − coronary sinus [or RA] pressure)/coronary vascular resistance. Coronary flow varies throughout the cardiac cycle because of pressure fluctuations within the chambers and ventricular walls. Because the major coronary arteries lie on the external surface of the heart, flow moves in an epicardial-to-endocardial direction. During systole, when intraventricular pressure rises, coronary flow in subendocardial regions diminishes or ceases. It may even reverse direction when intraventricular pressure is abnormally high (as with severe subaortic stenosis). Thus, most coronary flow occurs during diastole. Situations that shorten diastole or impair ventricular relaxation can negatively affect coronary blood flow. For example, when the active phase of myocardial relaxation is slowed, as occurs with ischemia, the early diastolic rise in coronary flow is impaired. At fast HRs, coronary flow (as well as ventricular filling) diminishes because diastole is abbreviated. When myocardial stiffness also is increased, tachycardia further compromises ventricular filling and perfusion.

Because coronary flow moves in the epicardial-to-endocardial direction, the subendocardial myocardium is most susceptible to ischemia when coronary flow is inadequate. At the same time, the subendocardial myocardium also undergoes greater mechanical stress and requires greater O_2 uptake, especially when myocardial energy needs increase (as with high afterload or sympathetic stimulation). A rough estimate of LV myocardial O_2 demand is provided by multiplying HR by arterial BP (as a proxy for afterload); this is known as the "double product." Coronary blood flow that is insufficient for the myocardial demand promotes myocardial ischemia, cell death, and replacement fibrosis. This contributes to the ventricular dysfunction associated with diseases such as hypertrophic cardiomyopathy and severe subaortic stenosis.

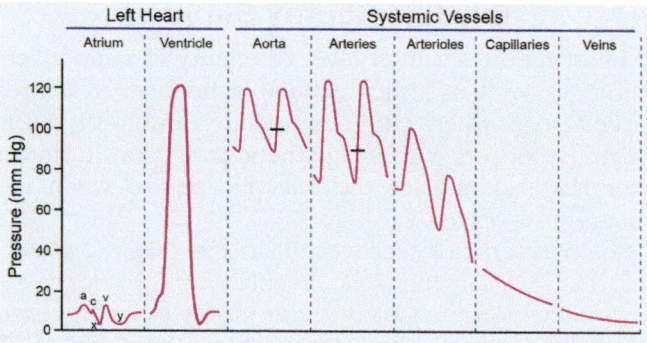

Figure 1.23 Schematic example of normal pressures and waveform contours across the systemic circulation. Left atrial pressure variations occur during the cardiac cycle from atrial contraction ("a wave"), onset of ventricular contraction ("c wave"), atrial relaxation and downward AV junction movement during ventricular systole ("x descent"), continued atrial filling during ventricular systole ("v wave"), and atrial emptying as the AV valves open in early diastole ("y descent"). Two cardiac cycles are shown for aorta, (large) arteries, and arterioles. The horizontal black bars indicate mean pressure, in the aorta and large peripheral arteries. Note that peak systolic pressure in the latter exceeds that in the aorta; this is caused by the effect of reflected pressure waves from the more peripheral smaller and stiffer arteries. Pulsatile arterial pressure waves become damped as blood travels through ever smaller arteries and arterioles. Capillary flow is nonpulsatile, as is venous flow. However, especially when right heart filling pressure is elevated, right atrial pressure waves can reflect backward into the large veins (see Chapter 15).[8]

The Circulation

Total blood volume is about 8–10% of body weight (80–100 ml/kg) in the dog and about 10% of body weight in the horse. The systemic circulation contains about 75% of the total blood volume at any one time, compared with 25% in the pulmonary circulation. Systemic veins act as storage (capacitance) vessels and usually contain about 70–80% of the systemic blood volume. The spleen serves as another important blood reservoir, particularly in the horse and dog. About 11–15% of blood in the systemic circulation is contained within arterial vessels and 5% within the capillary beds. In contrast, blood within the pulmonary circulation is distributed evenly among arterial, capillary, and venous vessels. **Figure 1.23** shows normal pressures and waveform contours across the systemic circulation. Pressure waveforms in the pulmonary circulation are similar; however, mean blood pressure in the pulmonary circulation is about one-seventh of that in the systemic circuit. A complex system of regulatory mechanisms controls systemic perfusion pressure, as well as the distribution of blood flow among body systems according to their changing metabolic needs.

Hemodynamic Concepts

Flow, Pressure, Resistance Relationships Blood flow (volume/unit time) through any part of the circulation depends directly on the driving (perfusion) pressure and inversely on vascular resistance. These fundamental relationships are summarized by the equation: $Q = \Delta P/R$, where Q = blood flow, ΔP = pressure difference across the vessel(s) in question (that is, perfusion pressure), and R = vascular resistance. When referring to the output from either the left or right heart, $Q = CO$.

In the systemic circulation, ΔP is the difference between mean aortic pressure and mean RA pressure; R is total peripheral (systemic vascular) resistance. Sometimes left heart CO is estimated only as mean aortic pressure/R, ignoring mean RA pressure because normally it is quite low. For the pulmonary circulation, ΔP is the difference between mean pulmonary arterial and LA pressures; R is pulmonary vascular resistance. Because the pulmonary and systemic circulations are in series, the output from each ventricle must be balanced over time (left heart CO = right heart CO). Resistance in the normal pulmonary circulation is about one-seventh that in the systemic circulation. This allows lung perfusion to occur at relatively low pressures (**Figure 1.1**). While perfusion P (ΔP) is the force that pushes blood through the vasculature, the term "blood pressure (BP)" refers to the transmural pressure in a vessel, or the distending force/unit area of vessel wall.

Resistance Vascular resistance, or impediment to flow, is an important variable that affects blood flow rate and the distribution of that flow among various vascular beds. The reciprocal of resistance is conductance, a measure of flow for a given pressure difference. Blood vessel radius has the greatest impact on resistance and flow. Poiseuille's law summarizes the effects of vessel dimension, flow velocity, pressure, and viscosity on blood flow.[4] According to the relationships described by this law, resistance is inversely proportional to vessel radius to the fourth power (r^4), and directly proportional to blood viscosity. The exponential effect of vessel radius on resistance has important implications with regard to CV pathophysiology and therapy.

Within the systemic circulation as a whole, the highest vascular resistance is at the level of the arterioles. Widespread arteriolar dilation or constriction can lead to systemic hypotension or hypertension, respectively. For example, in patients with septic shock, hypotension might persist despite fluid volume resuscitation and increased CO because of widespread arteriolar vasodilation caused by metabolic acidosis and continued production of nitric oxide (NO) and other vasodilating factors. Catecholamine and vasopressin therapy might be needed to stimulate arteriolar constriction, increase systemic resistance, and maintain BP.

In the pulmonary circulation, there are three general levels of resistance to flow: pulmonary arterioles, pulmonary capillaries, and LA (essentially, pulmonary venous) pressure. Widespread compression of alveoli can promote increased pulmonary vascular resistance. Left-sided heart failure increases pressure in the LA, which impedes pulmonary flow to the left heart and raises pulmonary venous and capillary pressures. In contrast, RA pressure and systemic capillary pressure or compression do not influence systemic vascular resistance.

Viscosity Viscosity is a measure of resistance to flow. The apparent viscosity of blood is determined mainly by the hematocrit. At higher hematocrit values, there is greater friction between successive layers of blood flowing within vessels, and therefore greater viscosity. A normal hematocrit value provides the best balance between ease of flow and ability to deliver O_2 to the tissues.

Blood Flow Velocity Blood flow velocity at any level of the circulation is related to the total cross-sectional area at that level, as well as to flow rate. For a given flow (or CO), as cross-sectional area decreases, velocity increases; this is known as the continuity relationship. For this reason, a narrowed valve orifice abruptly accelerates blood flow velocity. Conversely, blood flow velocity is slowest in the systemic capillary beds because total capillary cross-sectional area is huge, compared to that of the aorta, where velocity is fastest.

Laminar and Turbulent Flow Blood flowing in smooth, straight vessels tends to form layers (streamlines) that slip over each other; flow is faster toward the center of the vessel, while the outer layers drag along the vessel wall. This laminar flow can easily be disrupted and become turbulent (disorganized). Turbulent flow is characterized by the formation of whorls or "eddy currents." Factors that promote turbulence include high flow velocity (as with ventricular outflow obstruction), low blood viscosity (from anemia), wide vessel diameter, sudden change in vessel diameter or direction, and pulsatile flow. A measure of the tendency for turbulence to occur is described by Reynold's number.[5] Reynold's numbers over a so-called "critical" level (~2,000–2,300) are likely to be associated with an audible murmur. Resistance to blood flow increases when flow is turbulent.

The Vasculature

Arterial System Arteries provide a high-pressure reservoir for the pulsatile CO, as well as a conduit for blood to the body's tissues. The strong elastic walls of the large arteries keep systolic pressure from becoming excessively high. Their recoil maintains pressure during diastole, which drives blood toward the peripheral tissues (**Figure 1.24**). Smaller arteries are less compliant as the proportion of elastin in their walls is less (**Figure 1.25**). Arterioles have more muscular walls, with an increased wall thickness/lumen ratio. As noted above, the greatest increase in systemic vascular resistance occurs at the level of the arterioles, which act as "control valves" to the microcirculation. There is rich sympathetic innervation to the smooth muscle within arteriolar walls, which allows the arterioles control over blood flow distribution to the different tissues according to metabolic needs.

The pulsatile pressure within the great arteries gradually is dampened by the elastic recoil of the arterial walls and the progressively increasing resistance of the arterial tree. Blood flow in the capillary beds is nonpulsatile.

Arterial Blood Pressure Arterial blood pressure is expressed as systolic pressure/diastolic pressure, in mm Hg. "Systolic pressure" is the highest pressure that occurs with each cardiac ejection. In the great arteries, a small pressure deviation (the "incisura" or "dicrotic notch") occurs following the systolic pressure peak; this is associated with semilunar valve closure. "Diastolic pressure" is the lowest arterial pressure, attained just before the next ejection. "Pulse pressure"

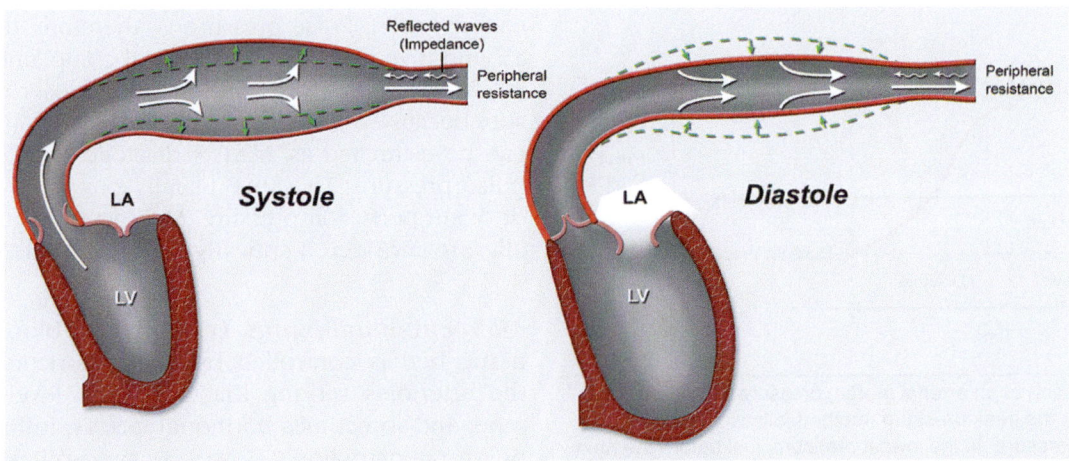

Figure 1.24 The large elastic arteries expand during systole to accept the ejected stroke volume without excessive increase in arterial pressure. During diastole, recoil of their elastic walls maintains arterial pressure, which helps drive blood flow (larger white arrows) through the circulation. LA, left atrium; LV, left ventricle.[8]

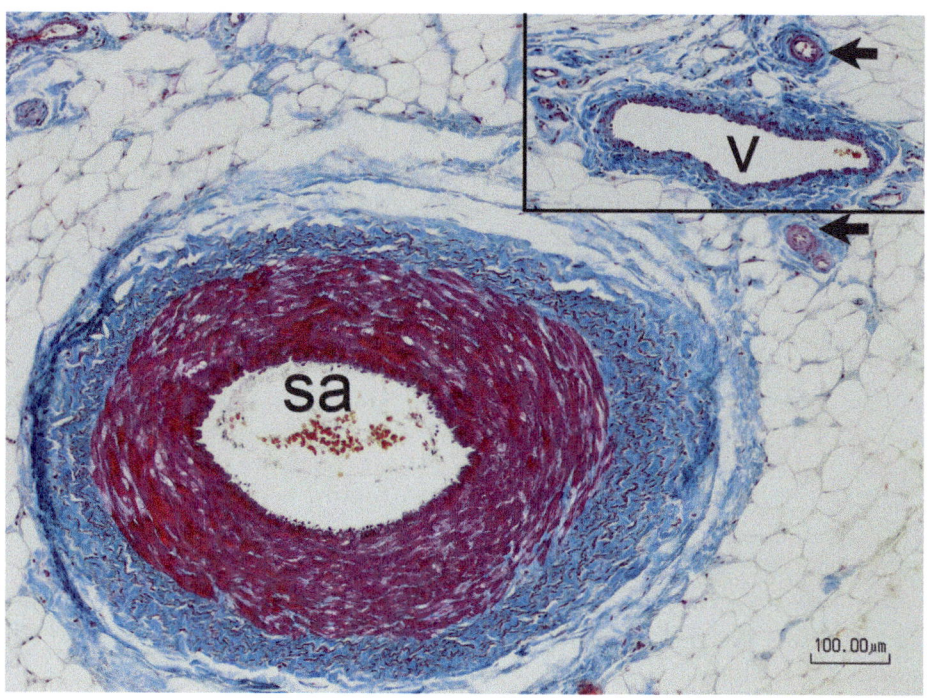

Figure 1.25 Photomicrograph showing cross-section of a small artery (sa). The tunica intima (interna) consists of an endothelial cell layer covering a small amount of subendothelial connective tissue and an inner elastic membrane (which appears plicated as an artifact of fixation). The relatively thick tunica media consists mainly of smooth muscle cells (stained deep pink here), arranged perpendicular to the long axis of the vessel. The outer tunica externa (adventitia) is mostly collagen fibers (blue), with fibroblasts and some wavy elastic fibers (purple) interspersed. The inset shows a smaller vein (v), an arteriole (arrow; two arterioles are indicated in the main image also), and several tiny venules. The walls of veins are quite thin compared to their lumen size (seen partially collapsed here), but do contain a small number of smooth muscle cells. Mallory stain; 10× magnification. (Image courtesy of Dr. E Uemura.)

is the difference between systolic and diastolic arterial pressures (**Figure 1.26**). The pulse pressure is the major determinant of how strong the peripheral arterial pulse feels on palpation. Several factors influence pulse pressure, especially the SV, the compliance of the arterial system, the rapidity of diastolic blood run-off into the peripheral vasculature, and, to a lesser degree, the character of ventricular ejection. When SV increases, the rise in arterial pressure is greater because a larger volume must be accommodated in the arterial tree with each heartbeat. Pulse pressure also is wider at a slow HR because diastolic blood pressure falls lower (there is more time for pressure decline as blood flows from aorta into the periphery) and subsequent SV is greater (there is more time for ventricular filling). When the compliance (distensibility) of the arterial tree is greater, there is less pressure rise with each ejection. Pulse pressure is, therefore, directly related to SV and inversely related to arterial compliance.

Mean arterial pressure (MAP) is closer to diastolic pressure because diastole has a longer duration than systole. MAP can be estimated as: MAP = diastolic arterial pressure + 1/3 pulse pressure. The MAP usually provides the best estimate of organ perfusion pressure. MAP values <60 mm Hg, generally, are considered critically low in patients.

Microcirculation and Lymphatics Blood flow to each tissue bed is controlled by the constriction or dilation of the arterioles serving that bed. The level of sympathetic tone, and sometimes hormonal factors, influence the degree of vasoconstriction. However, precapillary arterioles are influenced greatly by local metabolic (vasodilatory) factors because of their close contact with the tissues they serve. Capillaries, with their single endothelial cell layer, are where

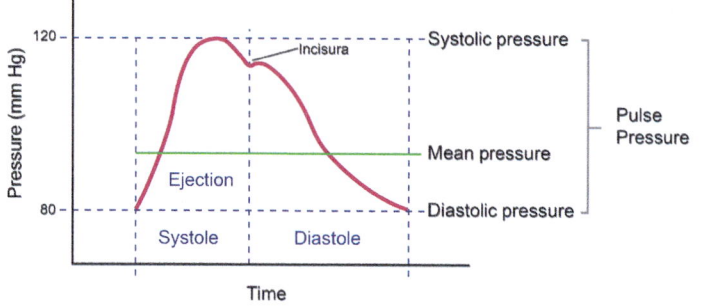

Figure 1.26 Illustration of an arterial (aortic) pressure waveform. "Systolic pressure" is the peak pressure reached following ventricular ejection. "Diastolic pressure" is the lowest pressure, just before the next ejection. The incisura indicates the time of aortic valve closure. The "pulse pressure" is the difference between the systolic and diastolic pressures. "Mean pressure" is often estimated as diastolic pressure + 1/3 of the pulse pressure.[8]

nutrient and waste exchange occur. Fick's Law of Diffusion[6] describes factors that influence the rate of transfer of substances between the capillary and the interstitium surrounding the body's cells. Increases in cell metabolic rate lead to enhanced delivery of O_2 and various nutrients by alterations in all these factors except the diffusion coefficient. This is accomplished via increased capillary recruitment and blood flow, and increased concentration gradients between capillary and interstitium.

Fluid movement across the capillary membrane depends on the relationship between hydrostatic and oncotic pressures in both capillary and interstitium (Starling's forces).[7] This concept is of paramount clinical relevance because it explains the mechanism of edema (or effusion) formation in many diseases. Recent evidence highlights the importance of the tissue interstitium in regulating plasma volume in health and disease, generating cellular signals, and preventing edema. Hydrostatic pressure within capillaries tends to push fluid through the membrane pores into the interstitium, especially at the arteriolar end of the capillary. Plasma proteins are too large to pass through pores in the normal capillary membrane (there is high colloid oncotic pressure within the capillary). Usually, the capillary oncotic pressure tending to hold fluid within the vessel almost balances the outward hydrostatic force (pressure) tending to push fluid into the interstitium, so that there is a small net flow into the interstitium. Most of the filtered fluid is reabsorbed by the venous side of the capillaries; the rest is removed by lymphatics.

Lymph vessels mobilize excess fluid from the interstitial space. Some interstitial proteins also are removed, which reduces net fluid flow out of the capillaries. Lymph fluid from most of the body returns to the cranial vena cava via the thoracic duct; return from the right forelimb, neck, and head is by the right lymphatic duct. The rate of lymph flow increases when interstitial free fluid pressure rises. This can result from increased capillary hydrostatic pressure (as with heart failure, venous obstruction, or overinfusion of IV fluids), decreased plasma colloid oncotic pressure (from severe hypoproteinemia), and increased interstitial protein accumulation (usually from increased capillary permeability, as with inflammatory disorders). Tissue edema develops when the rate of interstitial fluid accumulation exceeds the maximal rate of lymph flow. This is more likely to occur in acute settings, because lymphatic drainage can dramatically increase over time. For example, in dogs, pulmonary edema is likely to develop when mean LA pressure rises rapidly to over 18 mm Hg. However, with chronic progressive LA pressure elevation, values of up to 40 mm Hg might not cause overt pulmonary edema.

Venous System   Veins return blood to the heart; one-way valves help prevent backflow. Because virtually all systemic venous blood eventually reaches the RA (there is a small venous admixture in the lungs and in the heart), systemic venous return essentially equals CO. Mean systemic venous pressure depends on sympathetic tone (venoconstriction) as well as blood volume. Pressure in the RA and adjoining segments of the vena cavae, also known as central venous pressure (CVP), influences pressure in all systemic veins. CVP usually is measured clinically in cm H_2O, although sometimes it is measured in mm Hg (1 mm Hg = 1.36 cm H_2O). In normal dogs and cats, CVP ranges from 0 to 10 cm H_2O, with trends up or down carrying the greatest clinical relevancy.

Systemic veins can expand to store some blood volume, or constrict to return it to the central circulation. Functionally, these are termed unstressed and stressed venous volumes, representing the volumes filling the systemic veins and the volume available to increase venous return to the heart. Fluid therapy can increase both, while venoconstriction is likely to affect the stressed volume and facilitate venous return. The compliance of veins is about 24 times greater than that of arteries, so a large increase in venous volume can occur with little change in pressure or stressed volume. Systemic venous constriction can maintain arterial flow and pressure when up to 20% of the total blood volume is lost. The spleen also acts as an important blood reservoir in the horse and dog; splenic contraction increases the amount of blood in circulation and therefore, venous return to the heart.

Systemic veins are the major blood reservoir for the body. Increasing venous return is associated with both an increase in cardiac output, due to improved preload, and impairment of venous return at RA pressure increases. Eventually, a classic Guytonian equilibrium is achieved between venous return and cardiac output. In contrast to systemic veins, pulmonary venous capacitance is small and increased venous volume can predispose to pulmonary edema.

Normally, no pulsations are seen in veins because pressure pulses are not transmitted forward from the arteries through the capillaries. However, pressure waves can be transmitted backward from the right heart into the large veins, especially when RA pressure is elevated (see section "Cardiac Cycle and Generation of Heart Sounds," and Chapter 15).

Control of the Circulation

Fairly constant arterial blood pressure is needed for normal tissue perfusion. The rapidly acting BP regulatory mechanisms are primarily neural and hormonal in origin. The arterial baroreceptor reflexes are most important. However, long-term arterial BP control depends on blood volume also, which involves renal regulation of sodium and water balance. In addition, a host of local factors influences the degree of vascular constriction or dilation within different regional circulations.

Blood flow regulation in the peripheral circulation depends on three general mechanisms: neural (autonomic) regulation, hormonal factors, and local control systems that include endothelial-derived factors, paracrine controls, and

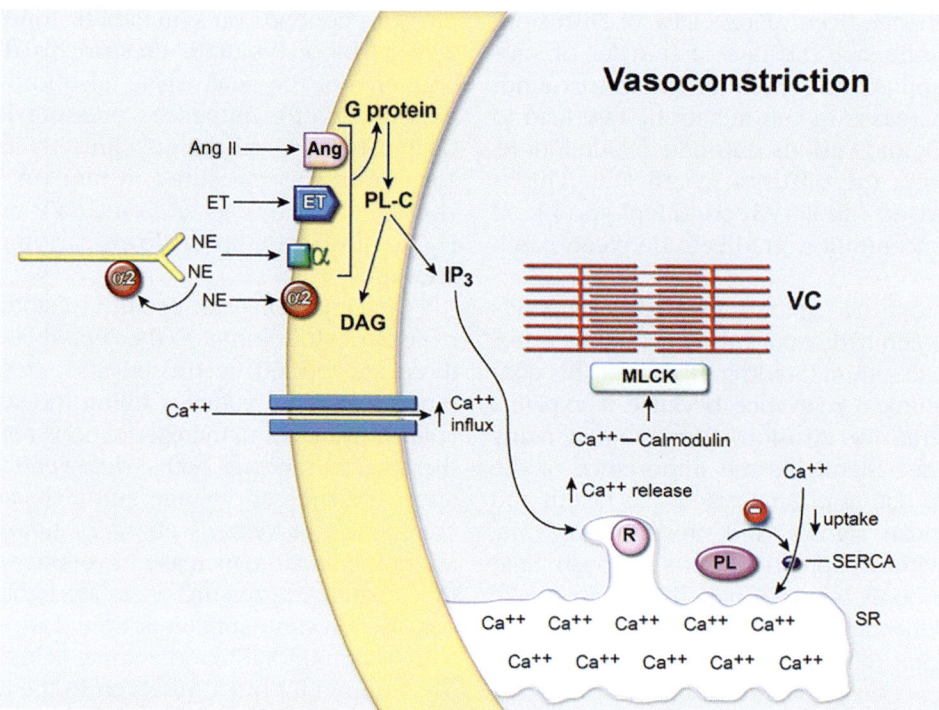

Figure 1.27 Vasoconstriction. Extracellular Ca^{++} enters the vascular smooth muscle (VSM) cell via the long-lasting (L-type) Ca^{++} channels. Various receptors modulate the ion's entry, including alpha-adrenergic receptors (stimulated by norepinephrine, NE), and also receptors for angiotensin (Ang) II and endothelin (ET), as well as vasopressin (not depicted). These receptors interact with the G protein that regulates Ca^{++} entry, via phospholipase-C (PL-C)-mediated formation of the second messenger, inositol triphosphate (IP_3). Ca^{++} entry stimulates the sarcoplasmic reticulum (SR) to release stored Ca^{++} via the calcium release channel (R). Diacyl glycerol (DAG) also is formed, which can increase Ca^{++} sensitivity and enhance vasoconstriction. Ca^{++} released by the SR (and complexed with calmodulin) binds to the enzyme myosin light chain kinase (MLCK). The activated MLCK phosphorylates myosin light chains, allowing these to interact with thin actin filaments of the VSM cell sarcomere. Actin-myosin interaction leads to VSM contraction and vasoconstriction. Unlike cardiac muscle (which quickly contracts and relaxes), VSM maintains a tonic contraction for long periods.[8]

cellular metabolites (**Figures 1.27** and **1.28**). The relative importance of central compared to local control is not uniform across the circulation. For example, neural control predominates in splanchnic tissues, however local metabolic factors are most important in the heart. Ultimately, it is constriction and relaxation of arteriolar smooth muscle that regulates blood flow distribution throughout the body, total peripheral resistance, and BP. Vascular smooth muscle in most tissues is innervated only by sympathetic fibers. A level of partial contraction (vascular "tone") exists that appears to be independent of nervous system control. An increase in sympathetic nerve activity stimulates further contraction, while reduced sympathetic nerve traffic allows dilation.

Vascular smooth muscle contraction is mediated by increased intracellular Ca^{++}, most often via agonist binding to membrane receptor-operated Ca^{++} channels. Intracellular Ca^{++} release from the SR also contributes. Agonists include catecholamines, angiotensin (Ang)II, and vasopressin. Voltage-operated Ca^{++} entry also can stimulate contraction. In contrast to cardiac muscle, where Ca^{++}-troponin interaction (on actin filaments) controls contraction, vascular smooth muscle contraction depends on myosin activation by Ca^{++} complexed to calmodulin and interacting with myosin light chain kinase.

When these regulatory systems are activated acutely, it is generally for correction of abnormal BP. Chronic activation of vasoconstrictor systems occurs in disorders such as heart failure. Chronic activation also is associated with renal sodium retention as well as mechanisms that promote tissue hypertrophy and fibrosis.

Local (Intrinsic) Control Several mechanisms influence blood flow at the local tissue level. A major one is the concentration of vasodilator metabolites produced by the tissue's cells, which adjusts blood flow according to local metabolic needs (metabolic regulation). Examples of local vasodilator substances include K^+, adenosine, CO_2, and metabolic acids including lactic acid. Local vasodilation also occurs from a number of paracrine and inflammatory mediators including NO, prostacyclin (PGI_2), kinins, and histamine. Examples of local vasoconstrictor substances include O_2 (relevant to the treatment of cerebral edema) and the prostaglandin thromboxane A2, which also causes platelet aggregation.

Many arterioles have the intrinsic ability to constrict (or dilate) in response to increased (or decreased) pressure and stretch, so that a steady flow rate is maintained. This is known as autoregulation. Another local mechanism is

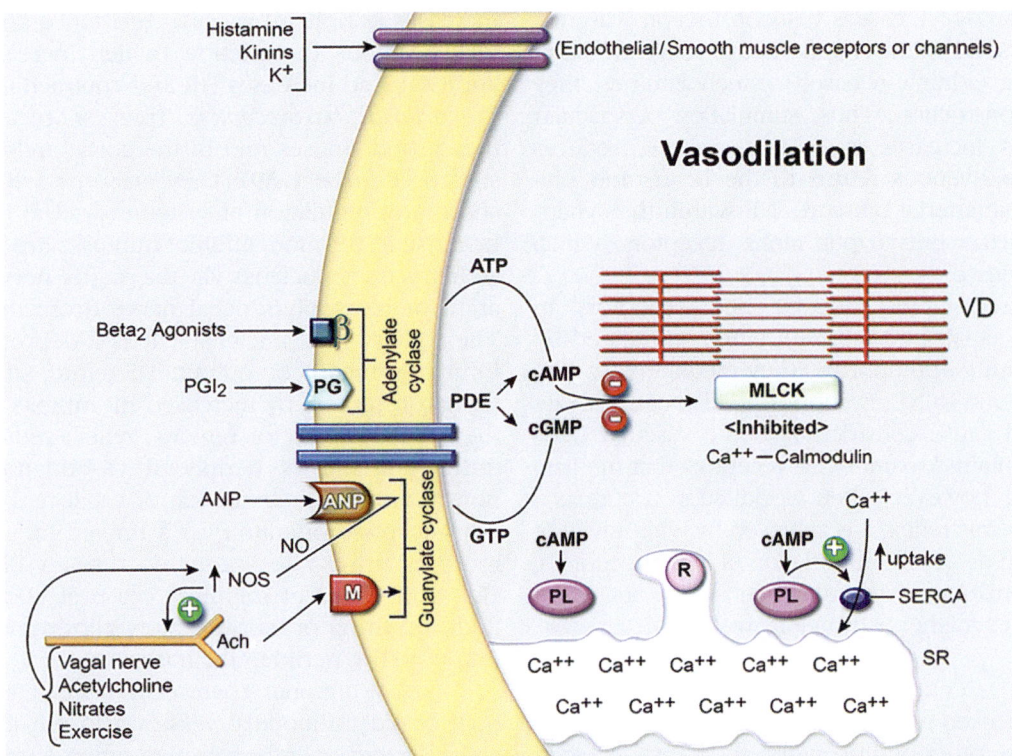

Figure 1.28 Vasodilation occurs mainly by reduction in cytosolic Ca^{++} concentration, which reduces the degree of vascular smooth muscle constriction. Factors or drugs that decrease cytosolic Ca^{++} concentration, or promote increased reuptake into the sarcoplasmic reticulum (SR), reduce tonic constriction and therefore, allow vasodilation. In addition, there are membrane-associated vasodilator systems. These include $beta_2$-adrenergic receptors, and receptors for prostacyclin (PGI_2), A- and B-type natriuretic peptides (ANP, shown), and acetylcholine (Ach; muscarinic receptor, M). These receptors signal through the second messengers cyclic adenosine monophosphate (cAMP) and cyclic guanosine monophosphate (cGMP). Both of these messengers inhibit the Ca^{++}-myosin light chain kinase (MLCK) interaction, leading to vasodilation. Nitric oxide (NO), derived from nerves and endothelial cells via NO synthase (NOS), also signals the guanylate cyclase system to increase intracellular cGMP. NO production is increased by parasympathetic activity, exercise (shear stress in the endothelium), and nitrate drugs. Reuptake of Ca^{++} into the SR is influenced by the sarcoendoplasmic reticulum Ca^{++}-ATPase (SERCA). Increased SERCA activity leads to vasodilation; inhibition promotes continued vasoconstriction. Phospholamban (PL) is a membrane protein that inhibits SERCA. When phospholamban is inhibited (for example, by the action of cAMP), Ca^{++} reuptake leads to vasodilation. Various intracellular phosphodiesterase (PDE) enzymes degrade cAMP and cGMP. PDE-inhibitor drugs (such as pimobendan, which inhibits PDE-3, or sildenafil, which inhibits PDE-5) function as vasodilators.[8]

endothelial-mediated regulation. This can promote vasodilation (as with NO release in response to increased blood flow and shear stress), or vasoconstriction (as when endothelin, ETN-1 is released from injured endothelium). The ETNs are a family of potent vasoconstrictors released from endothelial cells. When produced in increased amounts, they can act as hormones as well as local paracrine factors. ETN A and B are thought to be important in pulmonary disease and pulmonary hypertension.

Neurohormonal (Extrinsic) Control Control of the circulation as a whole, including the regulation of systemic arterial BP within narrow limits, is mediated centrally by the autonomic nervous system. Hormonal (humoral) controls also contribute to some extent, as well as play an important role in blood volume regulation. The sympathetic (adrenergic) nervous system (SNS) activates the CV system (pressor response) via the neurotransmitter NE. Sympathetic innervation extends to the veins (capacitance vessels) as well as arteries and arterioles throughout the body. Capillaries are not innervated. Vascular reflexes, or hormonal stimuli, that activate the central pressor region increase the number of efferent sympathetic impulses. This increases NE release at the vascular nerve terminals and, thus, the degree of vasoconstriction. Sympathetic innervation is greater in the small arteries, arterioles, and veins than in larger arteries. Inhibition of the central pressor region reduces sympathetic efferent traffic and results in vasodilation.

The parasympathetic (cholinergic) nervous system (PNS) has inhibitory effects on the heart. However, parasympathetic activation has minimal effect on total peripheral resistance because the PNS innervates only vasculature in the head and some viscera, not skeletal muscle or skin. Ach is its neurotransmitter.

Vascular Receptors The density and distribution of different receptors within the vasculature varies depending on the organ system and tissue. Postsynaptic $alpha_1$-receptors are most important; stimulation by NE causes vasoconstriction. Vascular wall alpha$_2$-receptors are extrasynaptic and usually are stimulated by circulating (adrenal-released) catecholamines; they also mediate vasoconstriction. Thus, stimulation of vascular alpha$_{(1 \text{ or } 2)}$-receptors increases vascular resistance, reduces compliance, increases venous return to the heart, and ultimately raises systemic arterial pressure. NE within the synaptic clefts also stimulates presynaptic alpha$_2$-receptors, which inhibit further NE release.

There are extrasynaptic vascular beta$_2$-receptors in many tissues (such as skeletal muscle); when stimulated by low levels of circulating epinephrine, they mediate vasodilation. They also respond to NE. Epinephrine also can activate alpha-receptors and cause constriction. Some vascular beds (especially renal) contain dopaminergic receptors that mediate vasodilation. Overall, however, when vasodilation occurs as a function of an autonomic reflex, it is achieved by withdrawal of sympathetic tone and decreased stimulation of alpha-receptors, rather than by stimulation of vascular beta$_2$-receptors. Local vasodilator substances might contribute as well.

Vascular Reflexes Central sympathetic and parasympathetic output is influenced by afferent signals from baroreceptors, chemoreceptors, other brain centers, and skin receptors. Widespread activation of sympathetic vasoconstrictor fibers increases peripheral vascular resistance and arterial BP, stimulates venous constriction (which increases venous return and CO), and increases HR and contractility.

Arterial baroreceptors (pressor receptors), located in the carotid sinuses and in the aortic arch, are stimulated by stretch (**Figure 1.29**). They are especially important in the short-term regulation of systemic arterial BP. When stretched by a rise in BP, more afferent impulses are sent to the medulla (solitary tract nucleus) via the vagus nerve (from the aortic arch) or glossopharyngeal nerve (from the carotid sinuses). The solitary tract nucleus acts as a depressor control, which inhibits sympathetic output. Therefore, stimulation of vascular baroreceptors by increased BP inhibits the central sympathetic vasoconstrictor regions, which reduces efferent nerve traffic and allows peripheral vasodilation and BP reduction. Concurrent stimulation of vagal regions also slows HR. Baroreceptors operate over a limited range of BPs. Maximal receptor firing rates occur at a mean BP of 180–200 mm Hg, while afferent impulses cease at about 50–60 mm Hg. Reduced firing of baroreceptors allows more vasoconstrictor output to the peripheral circulation.

Cardiopulmonary baroreceptors located in the atria, ventricles, and pulmonary vessels also are tonically active and can alter peripheral resistance when stimulated by intracardiac and pulmonary pressures changes. For example, atrial

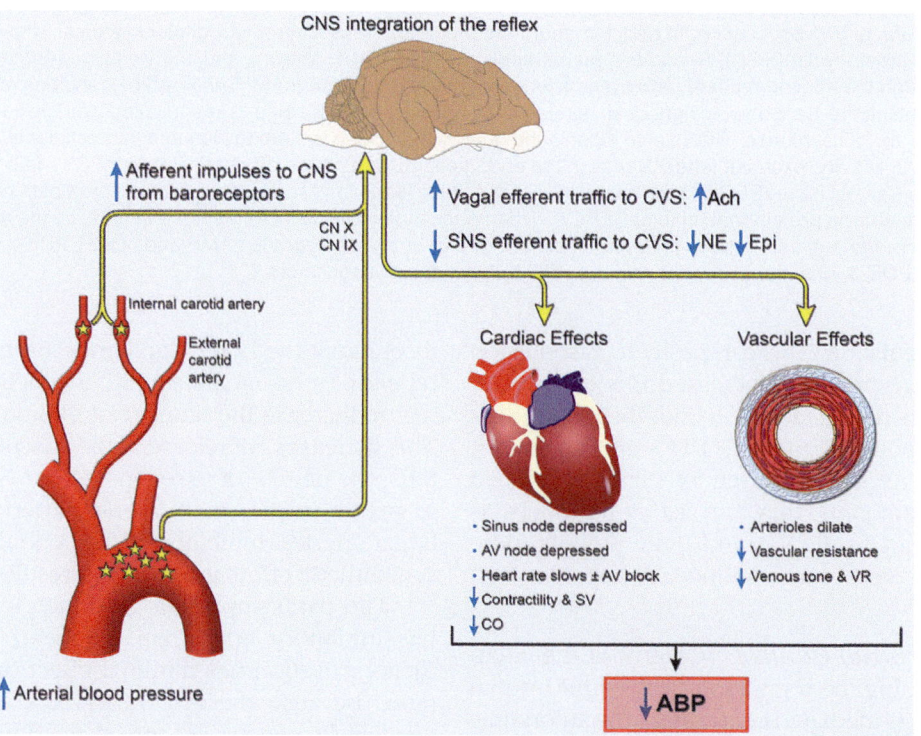

Figure 1.29 Arterial baroreceptor reflex schematic illustration. Stretch (baro-)receptors in the carotid sinuses and aortic arch respond to changes in arterial pressure. Increased arterial pressure (stretch) stimulates an increase in afferent nerve traffic to the brain, which ultimately inhibits efferent sympathetic nerve traffic and enhances vagal traffic to the CVS. The resulting decreases in heart rate, CO, and vasoconstriction lead to reduction in blood pressure. See section "Vascular Reflexes" for further details. ABP, arterial blood pressure; Ach, acetylcholine; AV, atrioventricular; CN, cranial nerve; CNS, central nervous system; CVS, cardiovascular system; Epi, epinephrine; NE, norepinephrine; CO, cardiac output; SNS, sympathetic nervous system; SV, stroke volume; VR, venous resistance.[8]

receptor stretch mediates reduced sympathetic output to the kidneys (increasing renal blood flow and urine output), although it enhances sympathetic output to the sinus node (increasing HR). Cardiopulmonary baroreceptor activation can alter BP reflexively by inhibiting the vasoconstrictor center in the medulla, as well as inhibiting renin (and thus Ang), aldosterone, and antidiuretic hormone release. Changes in the rate of urine output resulting from cardiopulmonary baroreceptor effects are important in blood volume regulation, too. Peripheral chemoreceptors in the area of the aortic arch (aortic bodies) and carotid sinuses (carotid bodies) react to changes in PO_2, PCO_2, and pH of the blood. They mainly are involved with regulating respiration but can influence the medullary vasomotor regions to some degree.

Hormonal (Humoral) Factors Epinephrine and NE also can function as hormones, when released into the circulation by the adrenal gland. This normally is less important in BP control than NE release from sympathetic nerve terminals. Epinephrine in low concentrations dilates resistance vessels (a beta-adrenergic effect) in some tissues (such as skeletal muscle). However, high concentrations of epinephrine induce vasoconstriction (alpha-adrenergic effect). NE mediates vasoconstriction (alpha-adrenergic effect).

The renin-angiotensin-aldosterone system (RAAS) influences vascular smooth muscle tone and blood volume through a complex interplay of effects. The traditional description of the RAAS cascade focuses on the production of AngII via a two-step process (**Figure 1.30**). First, the inactive precursor protein, angiotensinogen, is cleaved by renin into the 10-amino acid peptide AngI, also called AngI(1-10); renin release from the kidney occurs in response to increased sympathetic activation, reduced renal perfusion pressure, hypovolemia, and decreased distal tubular sodium load. Angiotensin converting enzyme (ACE) converts AngI into the active, 8-amino acid peptide, AngII or AngII(1-8). AngII's effects include potent vasoconstriction and reduced sodium and water secretion, through stimulation of aldosterone release from the adrenal cortex and direct renal effects. AngII stimulates thirst and promotes vasopressin release from the pituitary gland, too. Angiotensin type 1 receptors (Ang1Rs) mediate all these AngII effects. Synthesis of RAAS components also can occur at the local tissue level, where the effects of AngII and aldosterone promote myocardial and vascular wall hypertrophy and fibrosis. The entire RAAS cascade does not end with AngII, however. Multiple other enzyme pathways and Ang metabolites have been identified, some of which have counterbalancing vasodilatory and natriuretic effects. Chapter 20 (p. 305) provides some additional information about this "expanded" RAAS in the context of heart failure. Vasopressin (also called antidiuretic hormone) is released from the pituitary gland in response to low arterial BP as well as osmotic stimuli. It has a direct vasoconstrictor effect. It also plays an indirect role in BP regulation by stimulating renal volume retention and thirst.

The natriuretic peptides, atrial or A-type (ANP) and brain or B-type (BNP) natriuretic peptides, are hormones released from the myocardium in response to stretch and, in the case

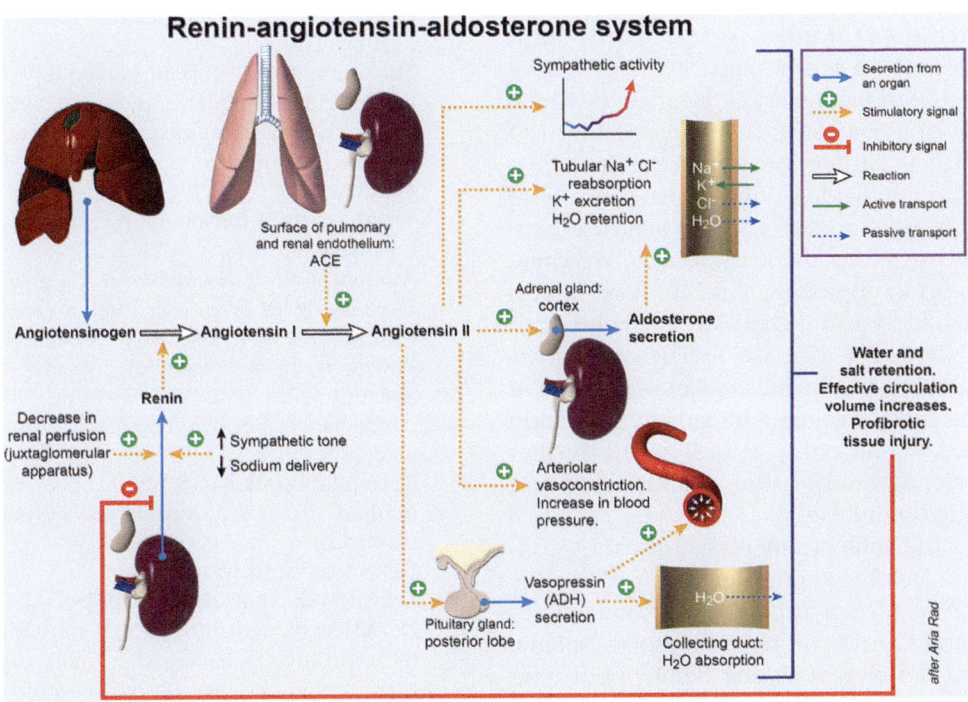

Figure 1.30 Schematic diagram illustrating components and effects of the renin-angiotensin-aldosterone system. ACE, angiotensin converting enzyme; ADH, antidiuretic hormone.[8]

of BNP, potentially from cardiomyocyte hypertrophy and ischemia. These hormones induce diuresis and vasodilation. In essence, they antagonize the effects of AngII at the vascular, renal and tissue levels. See Chapter 20 (p. 308) for more information about natriuretic peptides.

Cardiovascular Responses to Stress and Exercise

The CV system can respond to a variety of stressors. Some of these are physiological, such as exercise and the need for increased gastrointestinal blood flow after eating. Others relate to a sudden fall in arterial pressure and involve acute activation of BP control mechanisms (see section "Control of the Circulation"). Various forms of shock are relevant here, too. Heart failure sometimes disrupts CV homeostasis acutely; however, progressive and chronic neurohormonal compensatory mechanism activation is more common in companion animals (Chapter 20).

Certain structural and functional adaptations are associated with athletic activity and training. This is an expansive subject and CV responses to athletic training can vary with the species, intensity and duration of exercise, environment (temperature and humidity), and past training. Issues related to the equine athlete are discussed more fully in other sources (see section "Suggested Additional Readings and References"). Some general principles of exercise physiology are reviewed here briefly.

Aerobic capacity, or maximal rate of O_2 uptake ($VO_{2\,max}$), is considered an important indicator of athletic ability. The ability to greatly increase CO during exercise is the most important factor in determining aerobic capacity. Horses have the ability to produce a high maximal CO. Heart size (which is a major determinant of SV) and HR determine CO (as CO = SV × HR). Heart size is proportionately larger in racing breeds, and especially in individual elite athletes. Exercise training can increase heart size and a larger ventricle produces a larger SV. HR increases markedly during maximal exercise, for example, up to approximately 240 beats/min in the galloping horse. While SV can increase to a small degree during exercise, it is the great increase in HR that allows CO in the elite equine athlete to increase from ~30 L/min at rest to over 350 L/min during racing. Sympathetic activation also increases myocardial contractility as well as HR, further enhancing CO. Systemic arterial pressure also increases and MAP can reach around 200 mm Hg.

Besides a high CO, the ability to increase arterial O_2 content also is an important factor in supporting maximal aerobic capacity. Arterial O_2 content is a function of blood hemoglobin concentration and O_2 saturation. In the horse, splenic contraction can almost double circulating hemoglobin concentration, compared to resting level. Proportionately, equine spleen size is larger than other species, and racing breeds have larger spleens than nonracing breeds.

Distribution of the CO among various tissues is markedly altered during exercise. For example, blood flow to skeletal muscle at rest is about 10–20% of the total CO; however, it can increase to 80–90% of CO during maximal exercise. Simultaneously, the percentage of CO to the splanchnic and renal circulations might drop from ~50% to ~5%. These shifts result from regional changes in arteriolar resistance and capillary recruitment.

The marked increase in CO during exercise distends the pulmonary vasculature and, although this is a relatively low-resistance and low-pressure system, pulmonary arterial pressure does greatly increase during strenuous exercise. Mean pulmonary arterial pressures of 90–140 mm Hg have been documented in horses during exercise. This likely relates in part to LA pressure elevation during high intensity exercise, which promotes high pulmonary capillary pressure. Combined with marked alveolar pressure fluctuations and other factors, this exercise-induced pulmonary hypertension can lead to alveolar capillary rupture (exercise-induced pulmonary hemorrhage). Besides these CV factors, $VO_{2\,max}$ also depends on the respiratory system's ability to take up O_2 (which can be a limiting factor at maximal exercise), as well as the diffusion of O_2 into skeletal muscle mitochondria and muscle oxidative enzyme capacity.

Notes

1. Nernst equation:
   $E_K = -61.5 \log([K^+]_i/[K^+]_o)$
   E_K, potassium equilibrium potential; $[K^+]_i$, intracellular K^+ concentration; $[K^+]_o$, extracellular K^+ concentration.
2. Fick principle:
   The amount of a substance taken up (or released) by an organ per unit time is equal to the arterial-venous concentration difference of that substance × blood flow.
3. Laplace relationship:
   $\tau = Pr/w$
   τ, wall stress; P, transmural pressure; r, chamber radius; w, wall thickness.
4. Amount of flow in a vessel over a given time:
   Q = velocity of flow ($[\Delta Pr^2]/8\eta l$) × cross-sectional area (πr^2)
   r, vessel radius; η, viscosity; l, vessel length.
   Rewritten, this is Poiseuille's law: $Q = (\Delta Pr^4)/8\eta l$
   Since Q = flow and ΔP = pressure difference, the rest equals conductance. Because resistance is the reciprocal of conductance: $R = 8\eta l/\pi r^4$.
5. Reynold's number = $(\sigma/\eta)VD$
   σ, fluid density; η, viscosity; V, average velocity; D, vessel diameter.
6. Fick's Law of Diffusion:
   Diffusion of a substance = $DA([Sc] - [Si])/\Delta x$
   D, diffusion coefficient for that substance; A, area available for diffusion (this increases when more capillaries are open); [Sc], concentration of the substance within the capillary; [Si], concentration of the substance within the interstitium; Δx, distance over which the substance must travel (this decreases when more capillaries are open).

7. Starling's forces:
$$Q_f = k[(P_c + \pi_i) - (P_i + \pi_p)]$$
Q_f, fluid movement; P_c, capillary hydrostatic pressure; P_i, interstitial fluid hydrostatic pressure; π_I, interstitial fluid oncotic pressure; π_p, plasma oncotic pressure; k, filtration constant for capillary membrane.
8. Computer graphic artwork by **Tim Vojt** BFA, Senior Medical Illustrator, The Ohio State University College of Veterinary Medicine.

Suggested Additional Reading and References

Also See Online Comprehensive Bibliography at: https://www.routledge.com/9781482246223.

Ames MK, Atkins CE, Pitt B. The renin-angiotensin-aldosterone system and its suppression. J Vet Intern Med 2019;33:363–382.

Bacha Jr WJ, Bacha LM. Cardiovascular system. In, Color Atlas of Veterinary Histology. 3rd edition. Wiley-Blackwell, Ames, IA. 2012. pp. 77–88.

Bezuidenhout AJ. Heart and arteries, veins, lymphatic system. In, Evans HE, de Lahunta A (editors). Miller's Anatomy of the Dog. 4th edition. Saunders Elsevier, St. Louis, MO. 2013. pp. 428–562.

Borgarelli M, Tursi M, La Rosa G, et al. Anatomic, histologic, and two-dimensional-echocardiographic evaluation of mitral valve anatomy in dogs. Am J Vet Res 2011;72:1186–1192.

Brown CM, Holmes JR. Haemodynamics in the horse: 1. Pressure pulse contours. Equine Vet J 1978;10:188.

Brown CM, Holmes JR. Haemodynamics in the horse: 2. Intracardiac, pulmonary arterial and aortic pressures. Equine Vet J 1978;10:207.

Coulson A, Lewis N. An Atlas of Interpretive Radiographic Anatomy of the Dog and Cat. 2nd. Blackwell, Oxford, UK. 2008.

Drourr L, Lefbom BK, Rosenthal SL, et al. Measurement of M-mode echocardiographic parameters in healthy adult Maine Coon cats. J Am Vet Med Assoc 2005;226:734–737.

Erickson HH. The cardiovascular system. In, Reece WO (editor). Duke's Physiology of Domestic Animals. 13th edition. Wiley-Blackwell, Ames, IA. 2015. pp. 30–41.

Eurell JA. Muscle. In, Eurell JA, Frappier BL (editors). Dellmann's Textbook of Veterinary Histology. 6th edition. Blackwell, Ames, IA. 2006. pp. 79–90.

Gaudette S, Hughes D, Boller M. The endothelial glycocalyx: structure and function in health and critical illness. J Vet Emerg Crit Care 2020;30:117–134.

Hall JE. The heart. In, Hall JE (editor). Guyton and Hall: Textbook of Medical Physiology. Saunders Elsevier, Philadelphia, PA. 2016.

Hinchcliff KW, Kaneps AJ, Geor RJ (editors). Equine Sports Medicine and Surgery. 2nd edition. Saunders Elsevier, St. Louis, MO. 2014. (ISBN 978 0 7020 4771 8).

Katz AM. Physiology of the Heart. 5th edition. Wolters Kluwer, Philadelphia, PA. 2010.

Lamb AP, Meurs KM, Hamlin RL. Correlation of heart rate to body weight in apparently normal dogs. J Vet Cardiol 2010;12:107–110.

Marlin D, Nankervis K. Cardiovascular responses. In, Equine Exercise Physiology. Blackwell, Oxford, UK. 2002. pp. 113–126.

Navas de Solis C. Cardiovascular response to exercise and training, exercise testing in horses. Vet Clin North Am Equine Pract 2019;35:159–173.

Pappano AJ, Wier WG. The cardiovascular system. In, Koeppen BM, Stanton BA (editors). Berne & Levy Physiology. 7th edition. Elsevier, Philadelphia, PA. 2018. pp. 300–432.

Plendl J. Cardiovascular system. In, Eurell JA, Frappier BL (editors). Dellmann's Textbook of Veterinary Histology. 6th edition. Blackwell, Ames, IA. 2006. pp. 117–133.

Poole DC, Erickson HH. Cardiovascular function and oxygen transport: responses to exercise and training. In, Hinchcliff KW, Geor RJ, Kaneps AJ (editors). Equine Exercise Physiology. Saunders Elsevier, Edinburgh, UK. 2008. pp. 212–245.

Reece WO, Rowe EW. The cardiovascular system. In, Functional Anatomy and Physiology of Domestic Animals. Wiley-Blackwell, Ames, IA. 2018. pp. 220–257.

Shaffer F, Ginsberg JP. An overview of heart rate variability metrics and norms. Front Public Health 2017;5:258.

Shih AC. Cardiac monitoring in horses. Vet Clin North Am Equine Pract 2019;35:205–215.

Singh B. The cardiovascular system. In, Singh B (editor). Dyce, Sack and Wensing's Textbook of Veterinary Anatomy. 5th edition. Elsevier, St. Louis, MO. 2018.

Spiegel R. Stressed vs. unstressed volume and its relevance to critical care practitioners. Clin Exp Emerg Med 2016;31(3):52–54.

Stephenson RB. Cardiovascular physiology. In, Klein BG (editor). Cunningham's Textbook of Veterinary Physiology. 5th edition. Saunders Elsevier, St. Louis, MO. 2013. pp. 158–262.

Watras JM. Cardiac muscle. In, Koeppen BM, Stanton BA (editors). Berne & Levy Physiology. 7th edition. Elsevier, Philadelphia, PA. 2018. pp. 268–279.

Webb AI, Weaver BMQ. Body composition of the horse. Equine Vet J 1979;11:39–47.

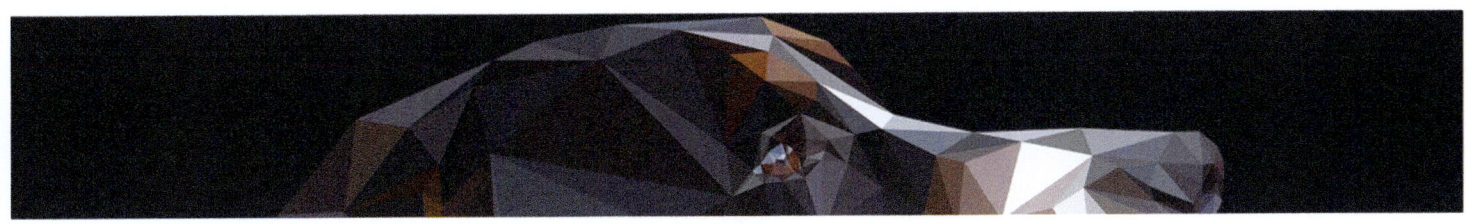

2
CARDIOVASCULAR EXAMINATION

The cardiovascular (CV) examination can be divided arbitrarily into the medical history provided by the caretaker, physical diagnosis focused on CV issues, and diagnostic studies that include imaging, electrocardiography, and clinical laboratory tests. The medical history can reveal evidence of a previously unsuspected heart or vascular abnormality, as well as inform the management of animals with defined CV disease. While there are no specific (pathognomonic) historical signs of heart disease in animals, certain problems raise suspicion for an underlying CV disorder. Taken collectively, the history, physical examination, and appropriate diagnostic studies can exclude or establish the presence of CV disease and define underlying anatomic, pathophysiologic, and etiologic processes. Information obtained from the history and physical examination helps the clinician select and prioritize additional diagnostic studies, with the goals of establishing the diagnosis, staging disease severity, and guiding any indicated therapy.

General Considerations

Medical History

The patient's signalment (species, breed, age, and gender) often is relevant to diagnosis. Experienced clinicians leverage their knowledge of epidemiology within the first minutes of history-taking and physical examination. Some congenital and acquired heart abnormalities are more prevalent in certain species, breeds, or age ranges. Conversely, some disorders are highly uncommon in certain species; for example, degenerative valve disease would be a rare cause of a murmur in cats. Some conditions have a sex predisposition as described in later chapters on specific diseases. Knowing the work or performance expectations for the animal also is important. Strenuous activity imposes a greater burden on the CV system, which could pose a risk to the patient or to a rider. Historical information particularly pertinent in patients with CV disease includes that listed in **Table 2.1**.

Clinical Signs of Heart Disease and Failure

Cardiac disease does not invariably lead to clinical "heart failure." Furthermore, problems seen commonly with cardiac failure can be manifestations of noncardiac disease, as well. Objective signs that are consistent with the presence of heart disease include moderate to loud cardiac murmurs, most persistent heart rhythm disturbances, jugular venous pulsation or distension, and cardiomegaly (see Chapters 11, 12, 15, and 18). The animal's owner or caretaker generally is unaware of these findings until they are discovered during CV examination. Other clinical signs that suggest, but are less specific for, cardiac disease or failure are the usual presenting complaints. These include coughing, abnormal respiratory pattern or effort, exercise intolerance or poor performance, weakness, syncope, abdominal distension, subcutaneous edema, and cyanosis (see Chapters 7–10, 13, 16, and 17). Some animals are presented for nonspecific signs (**Table 2.2**). It is important to note that the "suggestive" signs of heart disease and failure can be manifestations of noncardiac disease as well; none are specific for heart disease.

Most clinical signs caused by heart failure relate to high venous pressure behind the heart (congestive signs) or inadequate blood flow out of the heart (low output signs; also see **Table 20.1**, p. 300). Congestive signs related to right-sided heart failure stem from systemic venous hypertension and resulting increase in systemic capillary hydrostatic pressures. Typical consequences of right-sided congestive heart failure (CHF) are effusions within the serous body cavities as well as subcutaneous edema in horses. In contrast, elevated left ventricular (LV) filling pressure leads to pulmonary venous hypertension, which predisposes to left-sided CHF with its principle consequence of pulmonary edema. Increased

Table 2.1 Information Relevant to the General Medical History[a]

Signalment (Species, Breed, Age, Sex)
- Current client complaint or concern
- Previously established medical diagnoses

Current Medical Therapy
- Medications prescribed currently (or in the past) for the presenting problem
  - Including dispensing size, amount/dosage, and administration frequency and compliance
- Response to therapy (none, partial, or complete)
- Other medications or supplements

Preventive Care
- Vaccination status
- Deworming status
- Parasite prevention (internal, external)
- Heartworm prevention (for dogs and cats)
- Dental care

Diet and Appetite
- Food consumed (type and volume)
- Nutritional supplements
- Appetite (normal, increased, decreased, partial, or complete anorexia)
- Water consumption

Environment
- Where the animal was obtained
- Current geographic location
- Travel history
- Housing (indoors or outdoors)
- Other animals at home (type and health)
- Potential exposure to toxins or contaminated food/water or poisonous plants

Body as a Whole
- Changes in attitude (or interactions with people or other animals)
- Weight gain or loss
- Changes in body condition including muscle mass
- Trembling or shaking

Activity and Exercise
- Recent changes in activity or exercise capacity compared to normal for that animal
- Tiring or fatigue with exercise
- Exertional weakness or collapse

Collapse or Syncope
- Frequency
- Precipitating activity or events
- Obtain full description of episodes

Respiratory System Signs
- Change in rate, depth, or pattern of ventilation
- Respiratory noise
- Respiratory distress
- Coughing
  - What precipitates coughing episodes
  - Character of the cough
  - If sputum is produced or swallowing occurs after coughing

Mucous Membranes (and/or Tongue)
- Pink or blue
- Changes with exercise

Organ System Review
- Digestive: oral cavity or dental issues; vomiting, gagging, or diarrhea; recent bowel movements (if observed)
- Urinary: Changes in urinary habits; color of urine (if observed)
- Dermatologic: Skin or ear lesions or problems; subcutaneous edema
- Musculoskeletal: Joint or bone disorders; lameness or gait abnormalities
- Nervous: History of seizures or possible neurologic problems
- Ophthalmologic: Recent changes in vision; chronic ocular conditions

Allergies/Hypersensitivities—Known or Recurrent Allergies
- Food allergies
- Medication allergies or previous adverse drug events

[a] The clinician should review a full medical history. To increase efficiency and consistency in this, have a trained veterinary nurse/technician complete a "checklist" of specific questions during an initial conversation with the client. The clinician then can further explore any historical issues and patient problems during the subsequent physical examination and client interview.

Table 2.2 Historical Problems Commonly Associated with Cardiovascular Disease[a]

Respiratory Signs (Appearing at Rest or Following Exercise)
- Tachypnea (increased respiratory rate)
- Hyperpnea (increased rate and depth of respiration)
- Coughing
- Respiratory distress (variously called: Dyspnea, shortness of breath, respiratory difficulty, labored breathing)
- Cyanosis (blue tinge to the mucous membranes)

Changes in Exercise Capacity and Mobility
- Exercise intolerance
- Reduced performance in athletic dogs or horses
- Episodic weakness or collapse
- Syncope (fainting) and near-syncope (presyncope)
- Acute paresis (from arterial thromboembolism)

Abnormal Swelling of the Body
- Abdominal distension (ascites)
- Subcutaneous edema (mainly in horses)

Nonspecific Signs
- Listlessness or lethargy
- Decreased interaction with people or other animals
- Poor appetite
- Increased thirst (can occur with incipient congestive heart failure)
- Vomiting (possible sign of heartworm disease in cats or pericardial disease in dogs)
- Hemoglobinuria (with caval syndrome of heartworm disease)
- Regurgitation of solid food after weaning (from a vascular ring anomaly)
- Colic in horses (with *Strongylus vulgaris* infection or from reduced cardiac output)

[a] Note: These signs are not exclusive to cardiovascular disease.

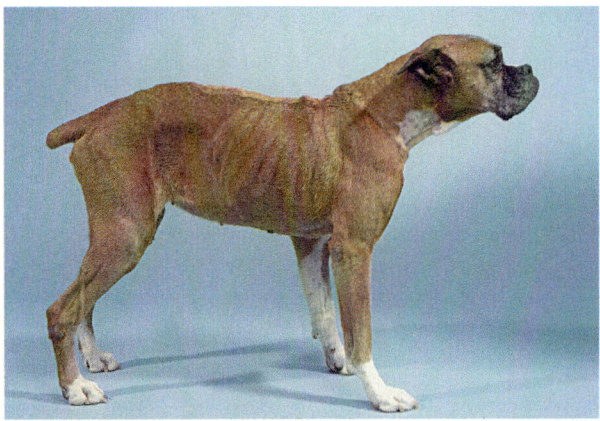

Figure 2.1 Cardiac cachexia is evident in this Boxer with chronic right-sided heart failure. Note the loss of muscle mass dorsally. Ascites caused the abdominal distension.

compromise, and other factors. Chapters 9, 10, 15–17, and 36 provide further information about respiratory signs, abnormal body appearance, and other problems the patient might display. Overall body condition is variable in patients with CV disorders, especially in early disease stages; some animals are thin, while others are obese. However, weight loss is common in advanced CV disease with heart failure, or when underlying infectious or multisystemic disease exists. Dramatic loss of muscle mass and body condition (cardiac cachexia) can occur with chronic heart failure (**Figure 2.1**; also see p. 312; and **Figure 32.4**, p. 611). Animals with congenital disease may have stunted growth.

pulmonary venous pressures also promote the development of pulmonary hypertension, usually of mild to moderate severity (see Chapter 39), as well as varying volumes of pleural effusion that tend to vary across species. Because the circulations are organized in series, and the normal right ventricle is designed for relatively low-pressure work, pulmonary hypertension can lead to signs of right-sided heart failure. This is especially common in animals with chronic left-sided heart failure from degenerative mitral valve disease or a cardiomyopathy. Concurrent tricuspid regurgitation or atrial fibrillation exacerbates right ventricular (RV) dysfunction. Clinical signs of low cardiac output are similar for both LV and RV disease, because output from the left heart is coupled to that from the right.

Physical Examination

A general physical examination should be done in conjunction with the CV examination. Vital signs can initially be noted by a technician, if available, and reassessed during the evaluation. The animal's body weight, temperature, and respiratory and heart rates should be recorded. While attention might be focused on the CV system, other body systems, as well as hydration status, should be systematically evaluated and any abnormalities recorded. An overview of CV examination components is presented in the following text; Chapters 11–17 contain further details and illustrations. In most cases, noninvasive systemic arterial blood pressure measurement also is recommended as part of the initial database (p. 795).

Observation of the Patient

Prior to the actual physical examination, it is important to observe the patient's attitude, posture, conformation and body condition, level of anxiety, and respiratory pattern; the gait is observed before or following examination, as possible. The animal's general appearance depends on the severity of underlying disease, hemodynamic and respiratory

Evaluation of Mucous Membranes

Mucous membrane color and capillary refill time (CRT) provide a crude estimate of the adequacy of peripheral perfusion and tissue oxygenation. Oral membranes usually are assessed, but caudal (preputial or vaginal) membranes also can be evaluated. The ocular conjunctiva can be used if oral membranes are pigmented. When laboratory tests show

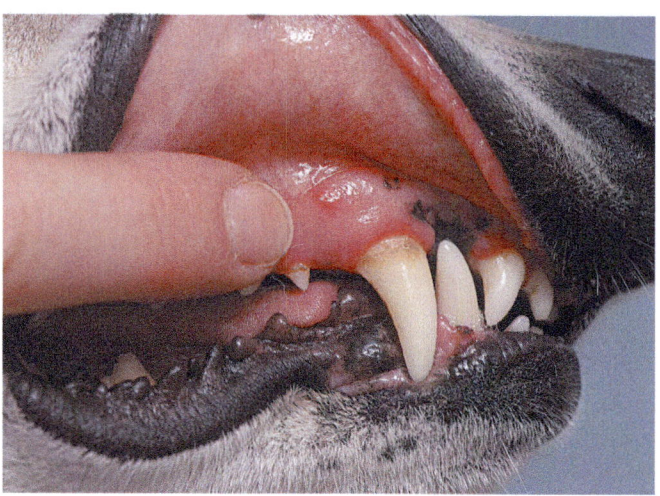

Figure 2.2 Normal pink mucous membrane color. Digital pressure will blanch the membrane and allow determination of CRT.

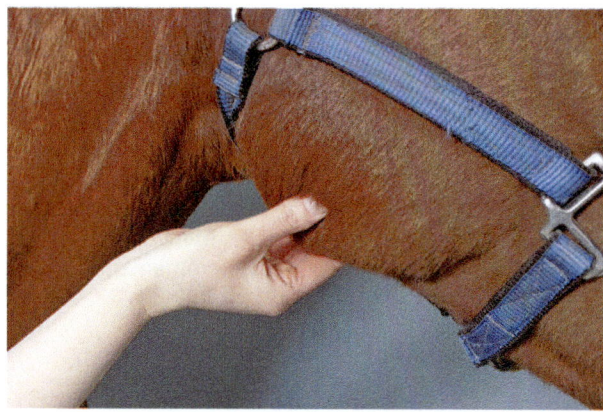

Figure 2.3 Arterial pulse palpation using the facial artery in a horse.

erythrocytosis (polycythemia), caudal mucous membrane color should be compared with that of the oral membranes, regardless of whether a cardiac murmur is detected. This is to screen for differential cyanosis (p. 249), a characteristic finding for reversed patent ductus arteriosus. Cranial and caudal membrane comparison also is relevant for dogs with exertional rear limb weakness, which is another manifestation of this anomaly. Several CV, respiratory, and hematologic abnormalities can alter the normally pink color of the mucous membranes (Chapter 13).

The CRT is assessed by applying digital pressure to blanch the membrane; color should return within 2 seconds (**Figure 2.2**). Dehydration and other causes of decreased cardiac output prolong the CRT because of high peripheral sympathetic tone and vasoconstriction. Thus, mucous membrane pallor can result from either anemia or peripheral vasoconstriction. Anemic animals should have normal CRT unless hypoperfusion also is present, although assessment of CRT is difficult in severely anemic animals because color contrast is lacking.

Evaluation of Arterial Pulses

The strength, regularity, and rate of the peripheral arterial pressure waves are assessed by palpation of the femoral or other peripheral arteries. A facial or digital artery commonly is used in the horse; alternatives include the carotid, great metatarsal, and coccygeal arteries (**Figure 2.3**). Subjective evaluation of pulse strength is based on the difference between systolic and diastolic arterial pressures (the "pulse pressure"; p. 23). When the pulse pressure is wide, the pulse feels strong on palpation. However, the rate of systolic arterial pressure rise is another factor that can influence perceived pulse intensity. For example, LV outflow obstruction (as with aortic stenosis) can cause delayed pressure rise, whereas high sympathetic tone promotes rapid pressure change. It is important to note that systolic and diastolic arterial blood pressures cannot reliably be determined by arterial palpation; these must be measured.

Even normal femoral pulses can be difficult to palpate in cats. The feline pulse usually can be found by gently working a fingertip toward the proximal femur between the dorsomedial thigh muscles, in the area of the femoral triangle (**Figure 2.4**). Excessive digital pressure can obscure the pulse, however.

Normally, there is a pulse for every heartbeat. However, some arrhythmias disrupt this relationship, resulting in fewer arterial pulses than heartbeats. This creates a "pulse deficit." Pulse deficits can be detected by simultaneously palpating the arterial pulse and counting the direct heart rate (obtained by chest wall palpation or auscultation). Whenever a pulse deficit is discovered, only direct methods should be used to assess heart rate. In addition, an electrocardiogram (ECG) should be recorded to define the heart rhythm. See Chapter 14 for further information about arterial pulse abnormalities.

Evaluation of Jugular Veins

Systemic venous and right heart filling pressures are reflected in the jugular veins. When the animal is standing with the head in a normal position and jaw parallel to the floor, these veins should not be distended. Persistent jugular venous

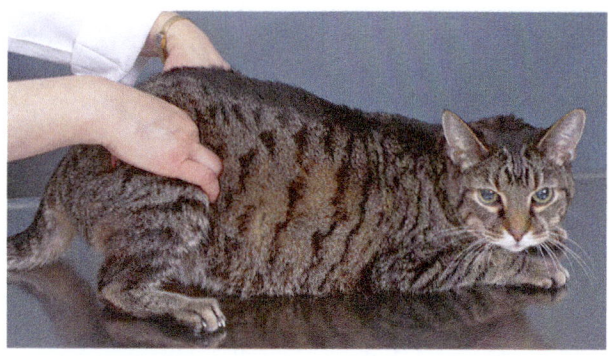

Figure 2.4 Arterial palpation in cats can be challenging. Gently palpate bilaterally for the femoral pulses deep within the femoral triangles.

distension suggests either an increased central venous pressure or obstruction to cranial vena caval flow.

Jugular pulse waves are related to pressure changes accompanying atrial contraction, relaxation, and right heart filling (**Figure 1.20**, p. 18; and Chapter 15). Pulsations extending above the point of the shoulder in a standing animal generally are abnormal. Occasionally, the carotid pulse wave is transmitted through adjacent soft tissues, mimicking a jugular pulse in thin or excited animals. A true jugular pulse can be differentiated from carotid transmission by lightly occluding the jugular vein below the area of the visible pulse. If the pulse disappears, it is a true jugular pulsation; if the pulse continues, it is being transmitted from the carotid artery. In horses, the jugular vein can collapse when atrial pressure falls during the cardiac cycle; the normal refilling of the vein sometimes might be confused with a pathological jugular pulse.

The major reasons for pathological jugular pulses are increased right atrial (RA) pressures from any cause, impaired RV diastolic function with compensation by a vigorous RA contraction (giant "a wave"), moderate to severe tricuspid regurgitation ("v wave" or "c-v wave"), and arrhythmias causing atrioventricular (AV) dissociation (cannon "a wave"). The latter are most common with complete AV block and ventricular tachycardias. Regardless of the cause, the finding of an abnormal jugular pulse should prompt assessment of heart rhythm and the right side of the heart.

The abdominojugular (hepatojugular) reflux (reflex) test sometimes can uncover impaired RV function in small animals, even when jugular distension or pulsations are absent at rest. To conduct this test, have the animal stand quietly with an assistant controlling the head to facilitate jugular vein visualization. Apply pressure to the cranial abdomen for 20–30 seconds (**Figure 2.5**); this pressure will increase systemic venous return for a time. While previously termed the hepatojugular reflux, pressure on the abdomen and not the liver per se is in play. Persistent jugular distension or pulsations during abdominal pressure constitutes a positive (abnormal) test and implies that either RV function is compromised, pulmonary blood flow is reduced, or significant tricuspid regurgitation is present. Normal animals have no change in jugular vein appearance or only transient pulsation.

Precordial Palpation

Normally, the strongest systolic impulse occurs over the area of the left cardiac apex, located at approximately the 5th intercostal space (ICS) near the costochondral junction. To detect the apical impulse, palpate the precordium by placing the palm and fingers of each hand on the corresponding side of the animal's chest wall over the heart. A weaker impulse usually is present on the right hemithorax near the 3rd to 4th ICS. Cardiomegaly, a space-occupying mass, or lung disease can shift or alter the precordial impulse. LV dilation displaces the apex impulse caudoventrally. Ventricular hypertrophy can produce a stronger impulse (precordial heave). A stronger precordial impulse on the right chest wall compared with the left can signal RV hypertrophy, or cardiac displacement into the right hemithorax (as from a mass lesion, lung consolidation or atelectasis, or chest deformity). Reduced intensity of the precordial impulse can be caused by obesity, weak cardiac contractions, pericardial effusion, intrathoracic masses, pleural effusion, or pneumothorax. The precordium also can be percussed in horses for the area of cardiac dullness, with displacement suggesting cardiomegaly. However, percussion is today a rarely taught skill and infrequently used.

The term "precordial thrill" refers to palpable chest wall vibrations caused by an extremely loud cardiac murmur. A thrill feels like a focal "buzzing" sensation. A precordial thrill is usually localized over the area where the murmur is loudest.

Cardiac Auscultation

Heart rate and rhythm, heart sounds, and respiratory sounds are evaluated by thoracic auscultation. The clinician with skill and experience in auscultation can detect many serious heart diseases, especially in conjunction with the patient's signalment, clinical situation, and other physical findings. Auscultation remains an important component of the patient exam. Chapter 11 addresses abnormal heart sounds more extensively.

Heart sounds are sudden intracardiac changes in turbulent blood flow, pressure, and associated vibrations in adjacent tissues during the cardiac cycle (p. 18). Much of this sound is too low in frequency or intensity to be heard. Audible heart sounds are classified as transient sounds (those of short duration) and cardiac murmurs (longer audible vibrations occurring during a normally silent part of the cardiac cycle). Heart murmurs generally are associated with turbulent blood flow, although their generation is more complex. The most important descriptors related to heart murmurs are timing within the cardiac cycle and point of maximal intensity

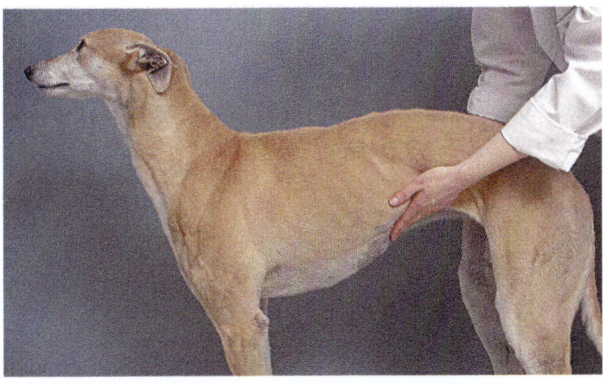

Figure 2.5 Apply pressure to the cranial abdomen to test for abdominojugular reflux. Jugular vein distension that appears while abdominal pressure is applied constitutes a positive (abnormal) test. Normal animals have little to no change in the jugular veins. A normal head and neck position, as shown here, is important when evaluating jugular veins.

over the precordium. These sounds can be further qualified by their pitch (frequency), loudness or intensity ("grade"), duration, and quality (timbre). The latter is affected by the physical characteristics of the vibrating structures and the transmission media. The turbulence associated with audible heart murmurs generally relates to some combination of high velocity flow, flow disturbance related to structural heart disease, or reduced blood viscosity (as with anemia).

The Stethoscope The stethoscope must be used properly to obtain maximal benefit from auscultation. Ideally, the stethoscope should have relatively short double tubing and comfortable but snuggly fitting ear tips. The binaural ear tubes should angle rostrally (toward the examiner's nose) to align with the examiner's ear canals. The traditional stethoscope has a stiff, flat diaphragm and a cuplike bell on the chestpiece, which the operator rotates to select the desired side (**Figure 2.6**). The diaphragm is applied firmly to the chest wall; this allows better transmission of higher frequency sounds, such as normal heart sounds and breath sounds. The bell, applied lightly to the chest to create an air seal, facilitates detection of lower frequency sounds such as S_3 and S_4 (gallop sounds; p. 19 and 232) and some diastolic murmurs. Many stethoscopes contain (single or dual) "tunable diaphragms." These demonstrate an adjustable frequency response, functioning as a diaphragm under firm pressure and a bell when applied lightly. The acoustic response of the tunable diaphragm is further modified by gradually changing the pressure up and down. Stethoscope size is another consideration, as the chestpiece of adult human models can be too large for cats and small dogs. Stethoscopes featuring electronic amplification might be helpful to individuals with a hearing impairment, but in general are not recommended because of the potential for artifacts and distortion. However, there is renewed interest in such devices related in part to an increased trend to telemedicine.

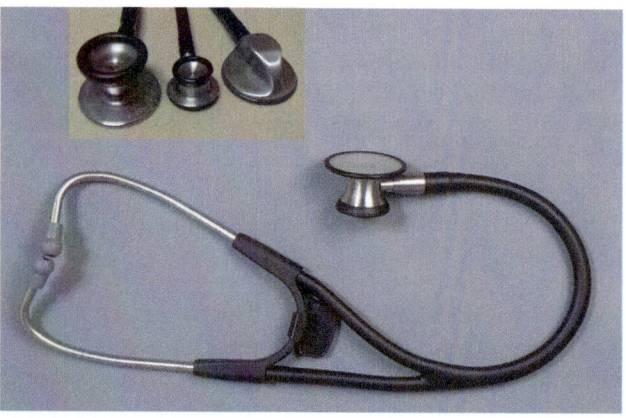

Figure 2.6 Traditional stethoscope with diaphragm and bell. Inset shows (from left to right) bell side of traditional chestpiece, bell of pediatric stethoscope head, and single "tunable" diaphragm chestpiece.

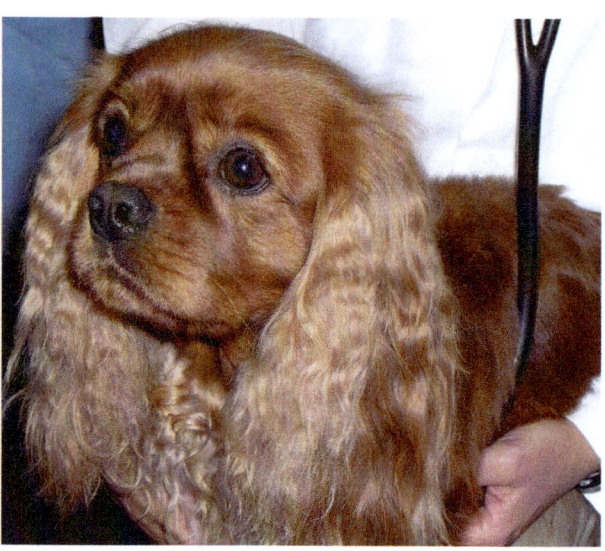

Figure 2.7 Cardiac auscultation is enhanced when the environment is quiet and the patient is calm, breathing quietly, and in a normal standing position (if possible).

Heart Sounds and Auscultation Technique Because many heart sounds are difficult to hear, patient cooperation and a quiet environment are important during auscultation. Ideally, both the animal and examiner are relaxed and calm. If possible, the animal should be standing so that the heart is in its normal position (**Figure 2.7**). Placing a hand under the abdomen can help restrain cats and small dogs. Respiratory sounds can interfere with heart sound assessment and can mimic murmurs, especially when heart and respiratory rates are synchronized. Panting in dogs is discouraged by gently holding the patient's mouth shut. Breath sounds can be decreased further by placing a finger over one or both nostrils for a short time; this often slows the heart rate slightly as well, which can be helpful. Intermittently whistling or having an assistant blow puffs of air at the animal's face also can reduce respiratory rate and artifacts. Purring in cats often can be interrupted by holding a finger over one or both nostrils (**Figure 2.8**), gently compressing the larynx, holding the cat, waving an alcohol-soaked cotton ball near the cat's nose, or turning on a nearby water faucet. Additional artifacts that can interfere with auscultation include other respiratory noises, shivering or muscle twitching, hair rubbing against the stethoscope (mimics pulmonary crackles), gastrointestinal sounds, and extraneous room noises. Pressing too firmly on a small animal's chest could distort the thorax and create abnormal flow patterns and murmurs.

One challenge when learning auscultation relates to precise placement of the chestpiece to detect various abnormalities. The exact orientation of the heart and location of valve areas within the thorax vary with species, breed, chest conformation, and size of the heart. However, the relative location among valve areas is fairly consistent; from cranial to caudal: Pulmonic, aortic, tricuspid (on the right), and mitral (**Figures 2.9** and **2.10**). The authors recommend locating

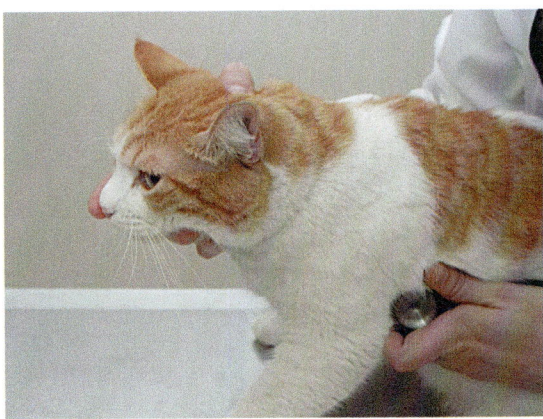

Figure 2.8 Gentle occlusion of one nostril (or briefly, both) during auscultation helps slow respiration, minimize lung sounds in dogs, and interrupt purring in cats.

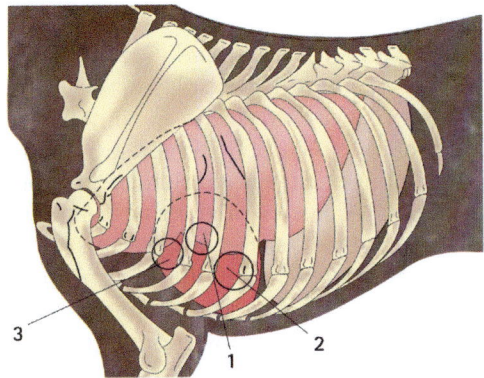

Figure 2.9 Approximate locations of cardiac valve areas on the left hemithorax in the dog. 1, aortic; 2, mitral; 3, pulmonic.

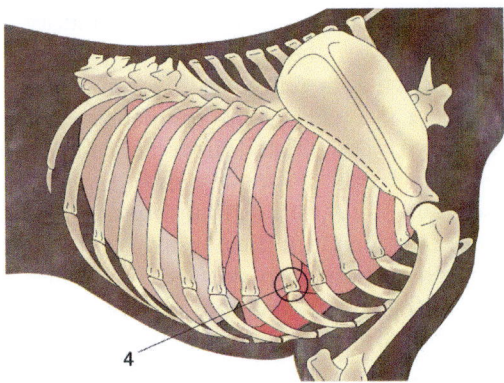

Figure 2.10 Approximate location of the tricuspid valve area on the right hemithorax in the dog. 4, tricuspid.

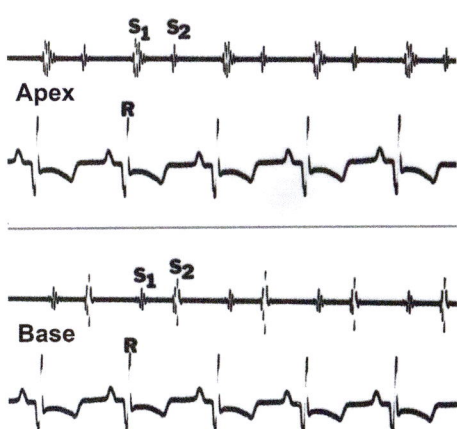

Figure 2.11 Simultaneous phonocardiographic and electrocardiographic recordings showing the timing and relative intensity of the S_1 and S_2 at the cardiac apex (top) compared to the cardiac base (bottom). (Image courtesy of Dr. RL Hamlin.)

is loudest, usually is about one to two ICSs craniodorsal to the mitral valve. Approximately one ICS cranioventral to the aortic valve is the pulmonary valve, over which S_2 splitting or a tympanic pulmonary closure sound would be best detected. Sounds from the tricuspid valve are best heard over the right hemithorax, slightly cranial to the level of the mitral valve. Both sides of the chest should be carefully auscultated in all species, with special focus on the valve areas, as well as the sternal borders and pulmonary artery region, just craniodorsal to the heart. In cats, differentiating the valve areas is challenging because the heart lies more horizontally in the chest compared with dogs and horses. Furthermore, the stethoscope chestpiece often covers more than one valve area simultaneously. The palpable apex beat often is along the sternum in cats. It is important to auscultate along both sides of the sternum, caudally and cranially (**Figure 2.12**). Functional or outflow obstruction murmurs in cats usually are loudest along

the patient's left apical impulse by precordial palpation, and beginning cardiac auscultation at this point. Then from here gradually move the stethoscope's chestpiece over all areas of the precordium. Near or slightly dorsal to this left apical reference point is the mitral valve area, where the S_1 sound is loudest (**Figure 2.11**). The aortic valve area, where the S_2

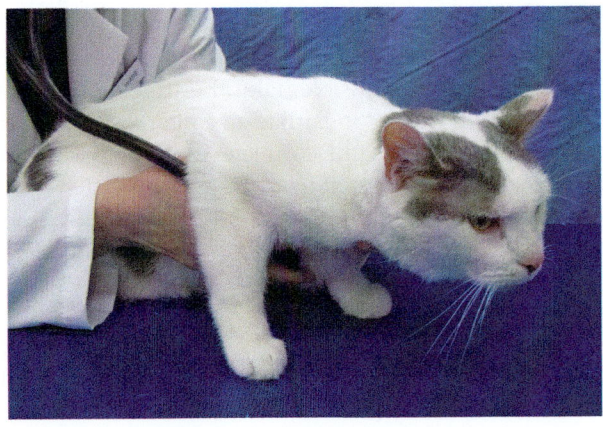

Figure 2.12 It is important to auscultate along both sides of the sternum in cats, because of their more horizontal cardiac orientation. Most abnormal heart sounds are heard best over either the left or right sternal border.

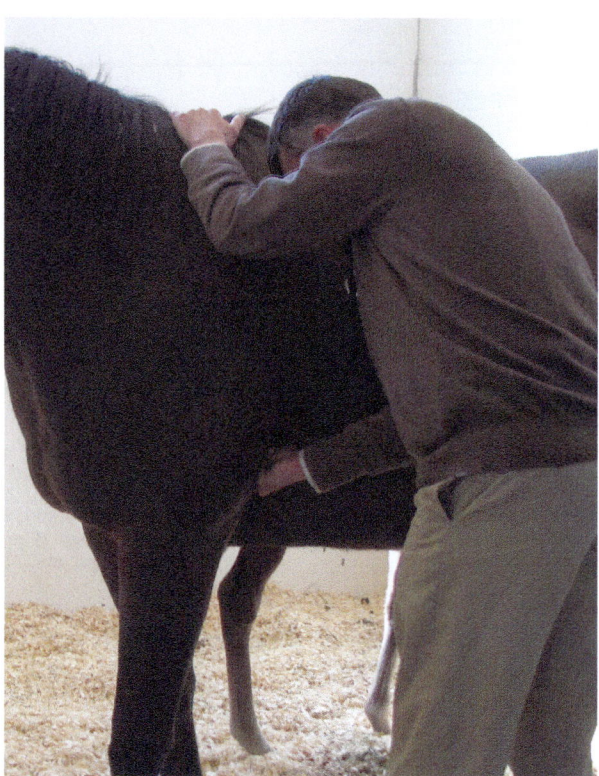

Figure 2.13 In horses, cardiac sounds originating from the heart base typically are heard best with the stethoscope chestpiece pressed into the "armpit," medial to the triceps muscle. A quiet environment is important.

the left or right cranial sternal border, whereas mitral regurgitation murmurs typically are heard best at the caudal sternal border near the apex. In horses, the base of the heart is oriented more craniodorsally (or upright); sounds from the aortic and pulmonic valve regions usually are heard best when the stethoscope chestpiece is pressed into the area between left forelimb and cranial thorax (**Figure 2.13**). Nevertheless, there are exceptions to all these generalizations.

It is important to focus on cardiac sounds separately from respiratory sounds during the process of auscultation. Full assimilation of sounds from both systems simultaneously is unlikely, so whenever possible, take the time to concentrate on each system in turn. For cardiac auscultation, focus on the individual heart sounds and correlate them to the events of the cardiac cycle. The normal heart sounds (S_1 and S_2) provide the framework for timing abnormal sounds, so they must be accurately identified. Usually their paired timing enables this. Also, the precordial impulse occurs just after S_1 (systole) and the arterial pulse between S_1 and S_2. After differentiating the S_1 and S_2, listen for any abnormal sounds in systole and diastole, successively. It is important to understand the events of the cardiac cycle (see **Figure 1.20** and associated text, p. 18) and to identify the timing of extra sounds and murmurs as systolic (between S_1 and S_2) or diastolic (after S_2 until the next S_1). The point of maximal intensity (PMI) on the chest wall of any abnormal sound(s) should be located as well. The PMI generally is identified in terms of a particular valve area, ICS, or location at the left or right cardiac apex or base. In horses, a multiphasic cardiac "murmur" might represent a friction rub associated with pericarditis. See Chapter 11 for further information about murmurs and other abnormal heart sounds.

Heart Sound Alterations Cardiac arrhythmias often cause variation in the intensity, or even absence, of heart sounds. Detecting the influence of sustained or recurrent arrhythmias on the normal heart sounds is relatively straightforward. Abnormal heart rate (slow or fast), noncyclic irregularity of the rhythm, premature or extra sounds, abrupt pauses, marked variation in intensity of sounds, and muddled or split sounds are typical features of heart rhythm disturbances. These abnormalities can be further defined by recording an electrocardiogram.

The appreciation of altered transient heart sounds, however, is a subtlety of auscultation that requires both knowledge and attention to examination detail; it is a more advanced and learned skill. The first (S_1) or second (S_2) heart sounds sometimes are altered in intensity or split (also see **Table 11.2**, p. 231). Loud sounds are common in thin-chested animals and those with high sympathetic tone. Soft or muffled heart sounds can indicate pericardial or pleural effusion; however, a soft S_1 also can be a sign of myocardial failure, as with dilated cardiomyopathy. In some horses with pleuropneumonia, the heart sounds are not muffled but instead transmit more widely over the thorax, presumably through consolidated lung tissue. A split or sloppy-sounding S_1 could be normal, especially in large dogs and horses, or it might result from ventricular premature contractions or an intraventricular conduction delay.

Normal physiologic splitting of S_2 can be heard sometimes in (usually large) dogs and often in horses because of variations in stroke volume through the respiratory cycle; this is most noticeable over the pulmonary valve. During inspiration, increased venous return to the right heart tends to delay pulmonic valve closure in systole, while the greater vascular capacity of the inflated lungs reduces LV filling and accelerates aortic valve closure. During expiration, LV filling increases while RV filling diminishes, producing more synchronous aortic and pulmonic valve closure. Pathologic splitting of S_2 can result from delayed ventricular activation or prolonged RV ejection secondary to ventricular premature beats, right bundle branch block, a ventricular or atrial septal defect, or moderate to severe pulmonary hypertension. The S_3 and especially the S_4 sounds are heard in most normal horses, but almost never in normal dogs and cats.

Respiratory Auscultation

Prior to respiratory auscultation, it is important to note the patient's level of comfort or distress, any sounds audible without a stethoscope, and the pattern of ventilation (p. 218), which sometimes can suggest the nature of airway, pulmonary, or pleural space disease that might exist. Patients with orthopnea, abducted elbows, alar flaring, open mouth breathing, hyperpnea, or other signs of respiratory distress should be provided supplemental O_2 and sedation, as possible, before examination (Chapter 10).

Respiratory auscultation involves consistent placement of the stethoscope diaphragm over multiple dorsal and ventral listening areas, as well as over the larynx and trachea. Patient noncooperation can impede effective auscultation. Abnormal, and sometimes normal, breath sounds might be heard only after inducing the animal to breath more deeply. In small animals, this can be done by closing the mouth and occluding one or both nostrils for a brief time. A rebreathing bag sometimes is tolerated by horses. These maneuvers could reveal abnormal adventitial sounds, such as lung crackles, that were not heard previously during more shallow breathing.

Respiratory Sounds Normal bronchial breathing generates ("vesicular" or "bronchovesicular") sounds related to turbulent air movement through major airways and the related tissue vibrations. These are similar to the sound of wind gently blowing through tree branches. These normal breath sounds are more prominent during inspiration and over the large intrathoracic airways. They might be barely audible over the lung periphery. The intensity of normal breath sounds increases when airflow rate and turbulence are greater (as with panting or excitement). Panting is considered a normal variation of breathing in dogs; a brief pause separates the harsh inspiratory and expiratory component sounds which are heard best over the trachea. It is nearly impossible to assess the lungs in a panting dog because of diffuse upper airway noise transmission.

Bronchial sounds can become harsher or markedly asymmetrical with pulmonary disease (including pneumonia and pulmonary edema) and airway obstruction. Breath sounds also are louder in thin-chested animals because of better sound transmission. Lung consolidation in horses with pleuropneumonia can improve the transmission of heart sounds across the thorax; however, this finding is uncommon in dogs and cats. Lung sounds are muffled or absent over areas of pneumothorax, lung consolidation (or atelectasis), or solid tissue (for example, a mass or diaphragmatic hernia). Large-volume pleural effusion will cause muffled sounds ventrally. In some animals with pleural effusion, breath sounds might be increased dorsally. Breath sounds can be difficult to hear in normal cats, in animals with shallow respirations, and animals with obesity, emphysema, pulmonary hyperinflation, or pleural effusion.

Abnormal ("adventitious") lung sounds are superimposed on normal breath sounds and usually are loudest over the area of disease. Adventitious sounds can be divided into those originating from the upper or lower airways (and pleura). The upper airways extend from the nose to the tracheal carina. Loud respiratory noises generally point to a major airway obstruction or collapse; these frequently are evident even without a stethoscope. "*Stertor*" is the term used for snoring or snorting sounds that occur with pharyngeal or nasopharyngeal obstructive disease. "*Stridor*" is a harsh, (usually) high-pitched, and prolonged inspiratory sound caused by laryngeal or upper tracheal obstruction. Stridor, in most cases, is heard best over the larynx; it suggests narrowing at or near the glottis, as with laryngeal paralysis or a mass lesion. Sounds related to laryngeal obstruction are not inevitably high-pitched, and might be detected as an altered inspiratory sound worsened by exercise. Loud obstructive airway sounds heard during both inspiration and expiration suggest a fixed obstruction in the upper airways. Respiratory clicking or low-pitched "clucking" sounds suggest dynamic pharyngeal or tracheal obstruction. A loud honk is nearly pathognomonic for tracheal collapse in a small breed dog. Noises originating from the upper airways, such as purring, stridor, stertor, and vocalizations, are referred easily to the thorax. Auscultation over the trachea and thoracic inlet helps the clinician differentiate these upper airway sounds from sounds arising lower in the respiratory system.

Abnormal sounds arising from the lower airways include crackles, wheezes, and rhonchi. Their location and the phase of respiration when heard should be noted. *Pulmonary crackles* ("rales") are short, discontinuous, nonmusical sounds of varying intensity. Fine crackles sometimes are described as the sounds of puffed rice cereal when milk is first poured on, a few hairs rolled between your fingers (held near your ear), crumpling cellophane, or soft radio static. Loud crackles are likened to Velcro being pulled apart (and sometimes are called "Velcro rales"). Crackles usually are caused by the sudden popping open of collapsed small airways as airway pressure equalizes. They generally are heard during inspiration and in dependent lung regions. Crackles might occur sometimes when these airways are partially filled with fluid or secretions. Although often associated with pulmonary edema ("wet lungs"), these sounds are equally common with other lung diseases such as pneumonia, bronchitis, and pulmonary fibrosis. Indeed, the loudest crackles usually are associated with primary lung disease rather than pulmonary edema.

Wheezes (sometimes called "sibilant rhonchi") are high-pitched musical or whistling sounds that occur when partial airway obstruction causes audible oscillation of the airway walls. Wheezes usually occur during expiration. Bronchoconstriction, bronchial wall thickening, secretions, lower airway foreign body or mass lesions, and dynamic or external airway compression can cause expiratory wheezes. Common clinical associations include asthma and bronchitis. However, wheezes also can occur with large bronchus collapse or compression related to marked left atrial enlargement, hilar lymphadenopathy, or a pulmonary mass. Rigid tracheal or main bronchus narrowing also could generate inspiratory wheezes. A *rhonchus* is a long, continuous sound of varying pitch and is typical of bronchial disease. Lower-pitched "sonorous rhonchi" suggest fluid or exudate in large airways, such as with severe pneumonia or bronchitis.

Pleural friction rubs typically are inspiratory sounds heard over the thorax and caused by rubbing of inflamed visceral and parietal pleural surfaces. These rubs are more common in horses with pleuropneumonia or pleuritis. Occasionally, they might be heard in small animals, especially when both air and fluid are present within the pleural space. Suspending ventilation briefly can distinguish pleural from pericardial friction rubs, as the latter will continue with ventricular contraction and filling.

Subcutaneous edema might be apparent on visual inspection, as well as by palpation, especially in horses; it is most pronounced in dependent areas because of gravitational effects. Abnormal jugular vein distension or pulsation usually accompanies fluid accumulation caused by right-sided heart failure, unless circulating blood volume is reduced (for example, after diuretic use). Hepatomegaly, with or without splenomegaly, also might be palpable in cats and dogs with right-sided heart failure.

Evaluation for Abnormal Fluid Accumulation

Elevated systemic venous pressure promotes abnormal fluid accumulation within body cavities or (less noticeably in small animals) within the subcutaneous tissue of dependent areas (Chapters 16 and 17). An ultrasound examination can quickly reveal the presence of ascites or pleural effusion. However, palpation and ballottement of the abdomen and percussion of the chest in the standing animal also can help the clinician detect effusions. Abdominal ballottement involves placing the palm of one hand on one side of the abdomen, then sharply tapping the other side of the abdomen with the fingertips of the opposite hand. A fluid wave can be felt against the palm when moderate-to-large volume ascites is present. Chest percussion (**Figure 2.14**) over normal aerated lung causes a resonant drumlike sound. Areas of fluid accumulation or solid tissue produce a dull (hyporesonant) sound. Various percussion techniques can be used, including placing one hand (or one or two fingers) flat on the thorax and sharply tapping the back of this hand (or the top of the fingers) with the fingertips of the opposite hand. Alternately, one can just sharply tap the thorax directly with the fingertips of one hand or use a reflex hammer. Although this technique requires practice, it can help the clinician identify pleural fluid, cardiomegaly, or a large thoracic mass, especially in larger animals.

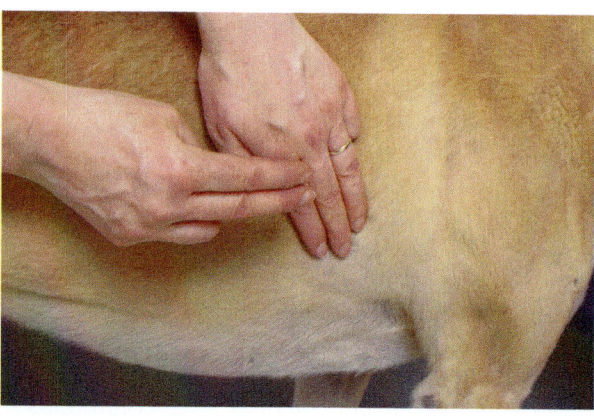

Figure 2.14 Chest percussion using the technique of placing one hand flat on the thorax and sharply tapping it with the fingers of the opposite hand (see section "Evaluation for Abnormal Fluid Accumulation").

Suggested Additional Reading and References

Also See Online Comprehensive Bibliography at: https://www.routledge.com/9781482246223.

Bakos Z, Voros K. Comparative examination of percussional and echocardiographic determination of the cardiac dullness area in healthy horses. Acta Vet Hung 2007;55:277–286.

Blass KA, Schober KE, Bonagura JD, et al. Clinical evaluation of the 3M Littmann Electronic Stethoscope Model 3200 in 150 cats. J Feline Med Surg 2013;15:893–900.

Bonagura JD. Equine heart disease: an overview. Vet Clin North Am Equine Pract 1985;1:267–274.

Bond BR. Fine tuning the history and physical examination: correlations with miscellaneous techniques. Clin Tech Small Anim Pract 2005;20:203–210.

Chizner MA. Cardiac auscultation: rediscovering the lost art. Curr Probl Cardiol 2008;33:326–408.

Conn RD, O'Keefe JH. Cardiac physical diagnosis in the digital age: an important but increasingly neglected skill (from stethoscopes to microchips). Am J Cardiol 2009;104:590–595.

Dickson D, Little CJL, Harris J, et al. Rapid assessment with physical examination in dyspnoeic cats: the RAPID CAT study. J Small Anim Pract 2018;59:75–84.

Ferasin L, Ferasin H, Little CJL. Lack of correlation between canine heart rate and body size in veterinary clinical practice. JSAP 2010;51:412–418.

Gerring EL. Clinical examination of the equine heart. Equine Vet J 1984;16:552–555.

Hardy RM. General physical examination of the canine patient. Vet Clin North Am Small Anim Pract 1981;11:453–467.

Keen JA. Examination of horses with cardiac disease. Vet Clin North Am Equine Pract 2019;35:23–42.

Kvart C, Haggstrom J. Cardiac Auscultation and Phonocardiography in Dogs, Horses and Cats. Uppsala, 2002 (self-published).

Lorello O, Ramseyer A, Burger D, et al. Cardiovascular variables in eventing and endurance horses over a season. J Vet Cardiol 2019;21:67–78.

Mesquita CT, Reis JC, Simoes LS, et al. Digital stethoscope as an innovative tool on the teaching of auscultatory skills. Arq Bras Cardiol 2013;100:187–189.

Paepe D, Verjans G, Duchateau L, et al. Routine health screening: findings in apparently healthy middle-aged and old cats. J Feline Med Surg 2013;15:8–19.

Parent C, King LG, Walker LM, et al. Clinical and clinicopathologic findings in dogs with acute respiratory distress syndrome: 19 cases (1985–1993). J Am Vet Med Assoc 1996;208:1419–1427.

Reef VB. Assessment of the cardiovascular system in horses during prepurchase and insurance examinations. Vet Clin North Am Equine Pract 2019;35:191–204.

Rozanski E, Chan DL. Approach to the patient with respiratory distress. Vet Clin North Am Small Anim Pract 2005;35:307–317.

Schwarzwald CC. Disorders of the cardiovascular system. In, Reed SM, Bayly WM, Sellon DC (editors). Equine Internal Medicine. 4th edition. 2018. Elsevier, St. Louis, MO. pp. 387–541.

Sharp CR, Rozanski EA. Physical examination of the respiratory system. Top Companion Anim Med 2013;28:79–85.

Smith Jr. FWK, Keene BW, Tilley, LP, et al. Rapid Interpretation of Heart and Lung Sounds: A Guide to Cardiac and Respiratory Auscultation in Dogs and Cats. Saunders, Philadelphia, PA. 2006.

Tseng LW, Waddell LS. Approach to the patient in respiratory distress. Clin Tech Small Anim Pract 2000;15:53–62.

Vörös K, Bonnevie A, Reiczigel J. Comparison of conventional and sensor-based electronic stethoscopes in detecting cardiac murmurs of dogs. Tierärztliche Praxis Kleintiere 2012;40:103–111.

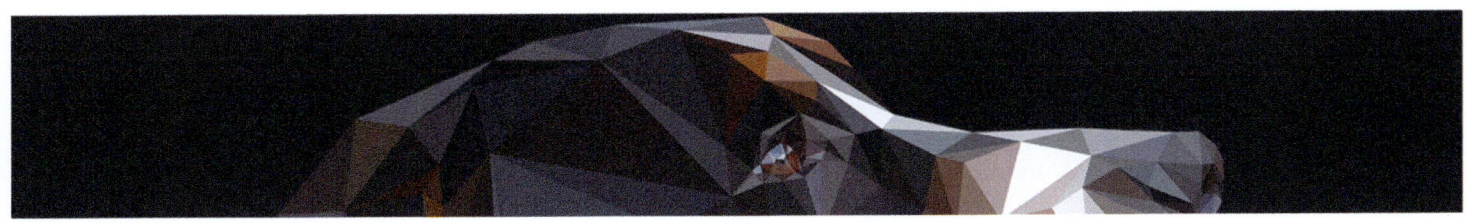

3
CARDIAC RADIOGRAPHY

Good quality thoracic radiographs can provide vital information about overall cardiac size and shape, pulmonary blood vessel size, and possible lung edema or other infiltrates, especially in small animals. Potential abnormalities of the major airways, pleural space, mediastinum, and diaphragm also can be detected. Although computed tomography (CT) and magnetic resonance imaging (MRI) yield higher-resolution images of thoracic structures; in dogs and cats, radiography is the most efficient means for initial evaluation of the thorax as a whole, accepting the increased use of point-of-care (POC) ultrasound. Nevertheless, a major limitation of radiography is that fluid has the same opacity as soft tissue. Consequently, the heart appears as a homogeneous fluid/tissue opacity; internal cardiac structures cannot be discerned and pericardial effusion cannot be readily differentiated from cardiomegaly. Subtle changes in pulmonary interstitial opacity and small pulmonary nodules also can be missed by radiography, but usually are evident with CT imaging. This chapter focuses mainly on cardiac radiography in dogs and cats. Considerations regarding radiographic evaluation of the equine heart and lungs are on p. 66.

General Considerations

Radiographic Views

At least two views should be evaluated: Right or left lateral and dorsoventral (DV) or ventrodorsal (VD). However, a three-view study, with both left and right lateral exposures, is preferred. Slight change in the appearance of the heart and other structures can occur with different patient positions. Especially for studies repeated over time, it is best to be consistent in the views used to evaluate the heart and lungs. However, additional complementary lateral or DV/VD views might yield further relevant information in some cases.

The right lateral view often is preferred for cardiac evaluation in dogs and cats. On left lateral view, in comparison, the heart usually appears slightly rounder with the apex lifted off the sternum, which can mimic mild right ventricular (RV) enlargement. The left atrium (LA) can appear more prominent on the left lateral projection, even when of normal size. Conversely, the left main bronchus is easier to visualize on the left lateral view, and bronchial narrowing is easier to identify.

Lateral recumbency sometimes complicates interpretation of lung opacity. Because the two lung fields are superimposed, overinterpretation of pulmonary opacity can occur, particularly if small pulmonary vessels are mistaken for infiltrate. Lateral recumbency produces some atelectasis in the dependent lung. The better-inflated upper (nondependent) lung fields display greater definition between aerated lung and soft tissue structures on lateral view. Unilateral pulmonary disease can be better delineated using both right and left lateral views. However, it might be overlooked entirely with a single lateral view when infiltrates are present only in the dependent lung (closest to the cassette).

The DV view provides better definition of the hilar area and caudal pulmonary vessels when compared to a VD view. If one uses clarity of vessel margins as an objective sign arguing *against* a diagnosis of pulmonary edema or infiltration, the DV often is more useful and can prevent an erroneous diagnosis of pulmonary edema. Furthermore, a DV position is better tolerated when respiration is compromised. When the patient is in ventral recumbency (for DV view), the ventral diaphragm's slightly cranial orientation tends to push the cardiac apex leftward. However, the heart also has a more upright orientation, which can create a rounder silhouette. Yet consistent DV positioning can be more difficult. Furthermore, even small, as well as moderate, pleural effusions can efface the cardiac border on DV view. When the VD view is used, the heart appears more elongated, with a more rounded cranial right aspect. The VD view often is technically easier to obtain in terms of patient positioning. The VD view might be better for detecting some lung lesions, especially in the accessory lobe. Furthermore, small-volume pleural effusion will appear within the lung fissures and costophrenic angles but is unlikely to obscure the cardiac silhouette.

Patient Positioning

Proper (not obliquely tilted) patient positioning is important for accurate assessment of the cardiac shape and size, as well as the pulmonary parenchyma. Conscious sedation can assist positioning and also relieve stress associated with the procedure, for both patient and technicians. In some jurisdictions, sedation becomes a de facto legal requirement for routine veterinary radiography, because personnel cannot remain near the imaging field during exposures.

The forelimbs should be pulled forward so the cranial thorax is well visualized. For DV/VD views, the sternum, vertebral bodies, and dorsal spinous processes should be superimposed so that the ribs appear symmetrical and the spine straight. External foreign matter on the body wall (such as dirt, water, alcohol or ultrasound gel) should be removed. For a lateral view the sternum and spine should be equidistant to the cassette so that the ribs are aligned parallel with each other. Chest rotation, with the sternum lower than the spine, increases the apparent size of the LA and heart base.

In the horse, standing lateral horizontal beam radiographs are all that can be obtained, except in some small foals or miniature horses that can be placed in lateral and VD positions, similar to small animals. Four lateral views usually are necessary to evaluate the entire thorax in the standing adult horse: Cranioventral, craniodorsal, caudoventral, caudodorsal.

Technique Considerations

High kilovoltage peak (kVp) and low milliamperes × seconds (mAs) radiographic technique generally is recommended, especially for analog film systems. This technique produces a long scale of contrast (many shades of gray) which provides better resolution among soft tissue structures. The shortest exposure time possible should be used to minimize respiratory motion. With modern digital systems it can be challenging to obtain consistent exposures over time due to automated settings, so this should be considered when assessing pulmonary parenchyma. If the ribs and spine appear darker on comparison films, it is likely that the exposure was different. Radiographic exposure ideally is made at the time of peak inspiration to give the best contrast between pulmonary air and soft tissue opacity. On expiration, lung opacity is greater, the heart is relatively larger, the diaphragm may overlap the caudal heart border, and pulmonary vessels are poorly delineated. Each of these imaging consequences can lead to errors of radiographic interpretation, including a false-positive diagnosis of "pulmonary edema." Conversely, intentional expiratory exposures are useful for identifying dynamic intrathoracic airway collapse.

Systematic Evaluation

The images should be examined systematically. This includes noting which views were taken and assessing the technique and whether images are digital or analog, the patient's body morphology and positioning, presence of artifacts, and phase of respiration during exposure. Obesity will increase the radiographic opacity of the lungs, and can reduce lung expansion; mediastinal or pericardial fat deposits can mimic mass lesions or cardiomegaly. The enhanced contrast resolution capability and postprocessing options of digital radiography systems make these factors somewhat less problematic compared with analog film systems.

All visible structures should be evaluated. Using a systematic approach helps the clinician avoid overlooking unexpected abnormalities. Any observations made must be integrated with the patient's clinical signs and an understanding of anatomy and physiology.

The Cardiac Silhouette

The Normal Canine Heart

Breed differences in chest conformation influence the radiographic appearance of the heart. In dogs with rounded or barrel-shaped chests, the cardiac silhouette has greater sternal contact and a more horizontal orientation on the lateral view (**Figure 3.1**). On DV/VD views, the heart has an oval to rounded shape; this can mimic right heart enlargement, especially if there is increased mediastinal or pericardial fat. Narrow-chested and deep-chested dogs have an upright and elongated appearance to the heart on lateral view (**Figure 3.2**). On DV/VD views, the heart looks relatively small and, in some cases, appears almost circular. Because of the variation in chest conformation, as well as the influences of respiration, positioning, and cardiac cycle (larger during diastole) on the apparent size of the

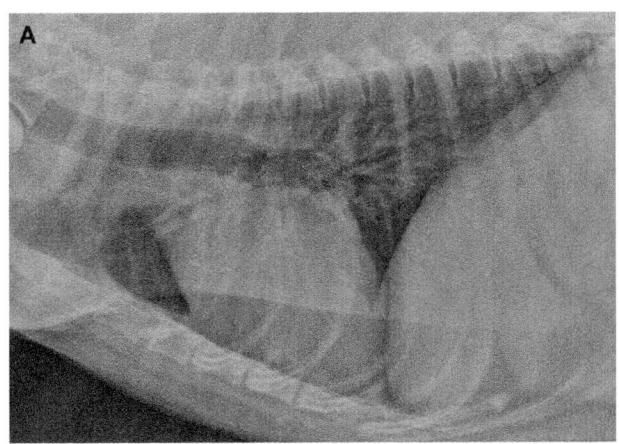
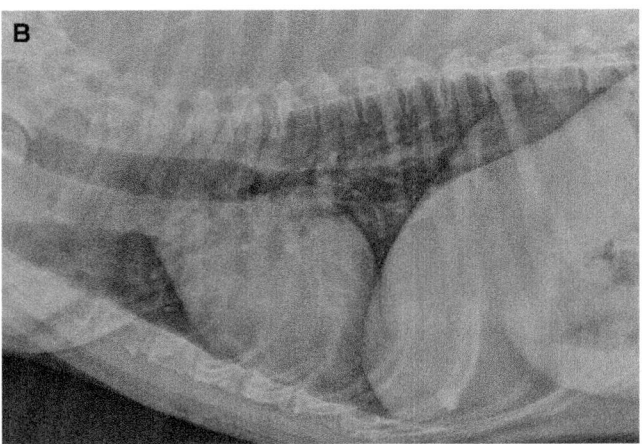
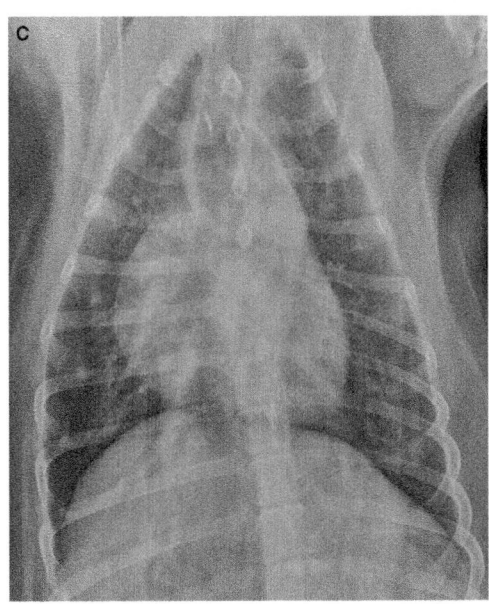

Figure 3.1 Right (A) and left (B) lateral and DV (C) views from a normal 9-year-old spayed female Basset Hound show the wider cardiac silhouette common in breeds with a rounded, barrel-shaped chest.

heart, mild cardiomegaly can be difficult if not impossible to identify radiographically. Occasionally, the cardiac apex is displaced into the right hemithorax on DV/VD views. If there are no other abnormal signs, this might be a normal variation. The cardiac shadow in puppies normally appears slightly large relative to the thoracic size, compared with adult dogs. The thymus may obscure the cranial heart border.

Various methods have been used to assess cardiac size, although chest conformation and cardiac position can influence results. Comparisons to vertebral length are widely used for assessing generalized cardiomegaly (vertebral heart size, VHS) and also, especially in dogs with degenerative (myxomatous) mitral valve disease (DMVD), left atrial size (vertebral left atrial size, VLAS). Additional methods (described in the following paragraphs) have included comparisons of cardiac radiographic dimensions to manubrium length, calculation of cardiac sphericity, and others.

Vertebral Heart Size There is good correlation between body length and heart size, although breed, chest conformation, and vertebral malformation present confounding influences, minimizing the value of a "one size fits all"

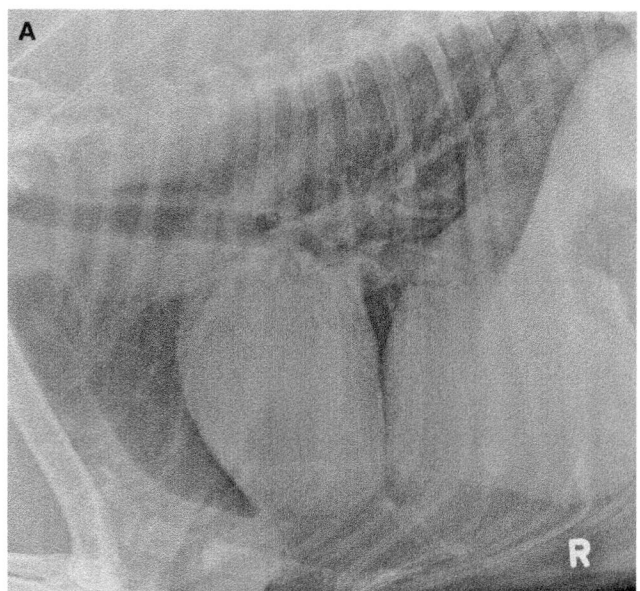
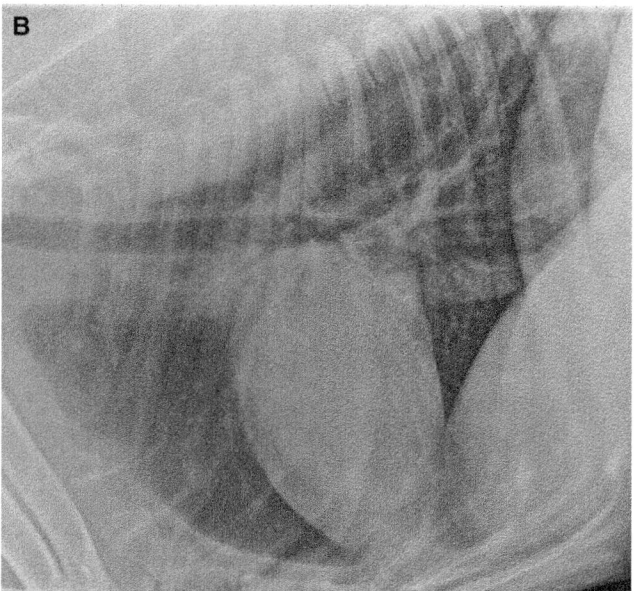
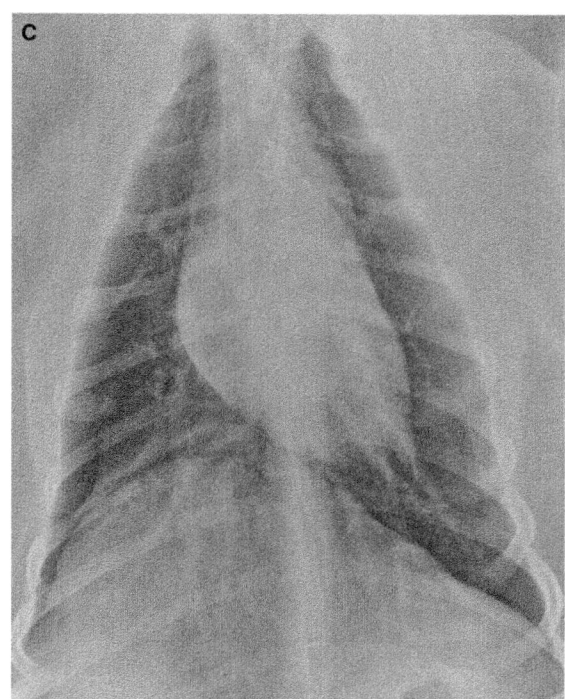

Figure 3.2 Right (A) and left (B) lateral and DV (C) views from a normal 6-year-old neutered male Doberman Pinscher. Note the elongated, upright orientation (A and B) and small DV profile (C) common in breeds with a deep, narrow chest.

approach to this form of cardiac quantitation; **Table 3.1** illustrates this issue. Despite these minor limitations, the VHS (also known as the vertebral heart score, scale, or sum), is widely used to identify and quantify cardiomegaly in dogs and cats (Buchanan, 1995). VHS measurements are obtained using a lateral view (**Figure 3.3**) in dogs. There are differences between values obtained from left versus right lateral radiographs; accordingly, the same view should be used for serial examinations within a patient. In general, the VHS is slightly greater in right lateral compared to left lateral projection (Greco, 2008). The cardiac long axis (L) is measured from the ventral border of the origin of the left mainstem bronchus to the most ventral aspect of the cardiac apex. The short axis (S) is measured perpendicular to L within the central third of

Table 3.1 Vertebral Heart Size and Canine Breed Variations

Dog Breed	VHS Range (mean ± 2 SD[a])	Reference
Composite—various breeds together	8.7–10.7	Buchanan, 1995
Composite—various large breeds	9.7–10.5	Marin, 2007
Mixed breed (16.25 ± 4 kg)	9.1–10.2	Bodh, 2016
Australian Cattle Dog	9.5–11.5 (R lat); 9.3–11.3 (L lat)	Luciani, 2019
Beagle	9.4–11.3	Kraetschmer, 2008
Boston Terrier[d]	8.9–14.5	Jepsen-Grant, 2013
Boxer	10.0–13.2	Lamb, 2001
Boxer	~11–11.5[b]	Pinto, 2002
Bulldog[d]	10.3–15.1	Jepsen-Grant, 2013
Cavalier King Charles Spaniel	9.6–11.6	Lamb, 2001
Cavalier King Charles Spaniel	9.8–11.8	Hansson, 2005
Chihuahua	8–11.0	Puccinelli, 2020
Cocker Spaniel	~11[b]	Pinto, 2002
Dachshund	8.7–10.7	Jepsen-Grant, 2013
Dachshund	10.3 (9.25–11.55; R lat); 10.1 (8.7–11.3; L lat)[c]	Birks, 2017
Doberman Pinscher	8.8–11.2	Lamb, 2001
Doberman Pinscher	~10.2[b]	Pinto, 2002
German Shepherd	8.1–11.3	Lamb, 2001
Greyhound	10.3–10.7	Marin, 2007
Indian Spitz	9.8–10.5	Bodh, 2016
Labrador Retriever	9.6–12	Lamb, 2001
Labrador Retriever	9.8–10.8	Bodh, 2016
Lhasa Apso[e]	8.0–11.2	Jepsen-Grant, 2013
Norwich Terrier	9.4–11.8	Taylor, 2020
Pomeranian	8.7–12.3	Jepsen-Grant, 2013
Poodle	9.1–11.1	Ana, 2004
Pug	8.9–12.5	Jepsen-Grant, 2013
Shih Tzu	8.3–10.7	Jepsen-Grant, 2013
Turkish Shepherd	8.4–11.0	Gulanber, 2005
Whippet (racing line)	10.3–12.2	Bavegems, 2005
Whippet (show line)	9.3–12	Bavegems, 2005
Yorkshire Terrier	8.7–10.7	Lamb, 2001
Yorkshire Terrier	8.7–11.1	Jepsen-Grant, 2013

[a] The use of 2 standard deviations is generally valid for large data sets encompassing >100 subjects. Accordingly, the "reference ranges" shown above are likely too narrow considering the sample sizes of most studies are relatively small.
[b] No standard deviation reported.
[c] Reported as median (range), n = 51.
[d] Anomalous thoracic vertebrae are associated with increase in VHS.
[e] VHS influenced by body condition score.
Abbreviations: R lat, right lateral view; L lat, left lateral view.

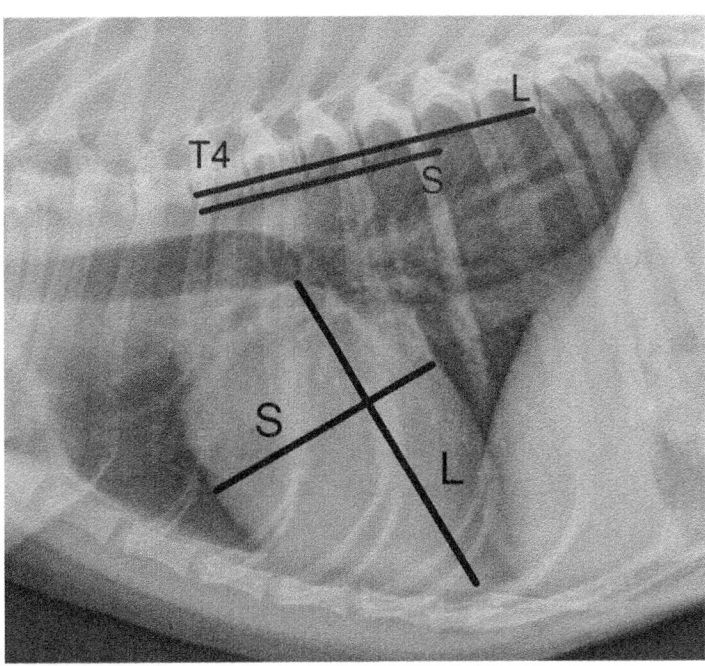

Figure 3.3 Lateral radiograph from a 4-year-old mixed-breed dog demonstrating the method for measuring vertebral heart size (VHS). In this example, L = 5.9v, S = 4.2v; therefore, the VHS = 10.1v, which is normal. L, long-axis heart dimension; S, short-axis heart dimension; T4, 4th thoracic vertebra; v, vertebrae.

the cardiac silhouette, where the cardiac width is greatest. Both L and S are compared with the thoracic spine, beginning at the cranial edge of T4; each length is estimated to the nearest 0.1 vertebra. The sum of measurements L and S is the VHS. A VHS between 8.5 and 10.5 vertebrae (v) is considered normal for most breeds, although there is substantial variation among breeds (**Table 3.1**). For example, in dogs with a short thorax like the Miniature Schnauzer, an upper limit of 11v is considered normal, whereas an upper limit of 9.5v reportedly is normal in dogs with a long thorax, such as Dachshunds. Normal puppies also have a VHS within the reference range for adult dogs. Whenever possible, the clinician should seek online references for current reports on breed-associated normal values as these are constantly updated. The cardiac cycle can have a minor, yet potentially significant, effect on the measured VHS. Using fluoroscopic frames obtained during peak inspiration, measured VHS increased by a mean of 0.36v from end-systole to end-diastole in a group of healthy dogs (Brown, 2020). When LA enlargement is marked, measurement of the L dimension from apex to the ventral aspect of the elevated left main bronchus (rather than the carina) has been suggested in order to reflect this extension of cardiac size. Unfortunately, most breed-specific studies of VHS consist of relatively small sample sizes (<100 dogs) and the method used by others to suggest the "normal" range in those studies (+/−2 standard deviations) is insufficient, underestimating the normal prediction limits. This should be kept in mind, especially when contemplating a therapy based on VHS alone.

In most cases, serial changes in VHS are more meaningful, accepting that absolute values exceeding 12–12.6 vertebral bodies are abnormal for the vast majority of breeds. A number of studies (Boswood, 2020; Lord, 2011) have indicated that the most rapid increase, estimated by a VHS "velocity" in vertebral bodies per month, occurs near the onset of congestive heart failure (CHF). This change, along with increases in the sleeping respiratory rate, represents a practical method for the detection of pulmonary edema. A general rate of change in VHS that suggests CHF is impending or present, used by the authors, is 0.1 vertebral bodies/month. Because there can be substantial interobserver variability in VHS measurement (Hansson, 2005), the same clinician should measure serial radiographs of the same lateral view.

A vertebral scoring system (VLAS) to estimate LA size was described for dogs with DMVD, where a VLAS ≥2.3v suggested LA enlargement; control dogs had a median VLAS of 2.1v (interquartile range, 1.8–2.3; Malcolm, 2018). A right or left lateral image can be used for this. The VLAS is fairly well correlated with echocardiographic LA to aortic root ratios. Another study in normal dogs reported a median VLAS of 1.9v (reference interval, 1.4–2.2v), with no effect of body weight, sex, and age (Vezzosi, 2020). See p. 542 and **Figure 29.12** for VLAS measurement method. In evaluating dogs with DMVD, various cut-offs have been proposed to indicate a dog is likely to fulfill EPIC-study criteria for initiating therapy with pimobendan (to delay CHF). In one study, a VLAS >2.6 was proposed as optimal (Mikawa, 2020) and in another, VLAS >2.5 was optimal, although values >3.0 were most specific (Stepien, 2020). As a general guideline, the authors suggest that a VLAS of 2.8 or more indicates at least moderate left atrial dilation in a dog.

Additional Assessment Methods

Manubrium heart scores (MHSs) are obtained by measuring the lengths of the manubrium and the cardiac short- and long-axes in mm on a right lateral view. Various ratios that can be used include the cardiac short axis to manubrium (short-MHS), long axis to manubrium (long-MHS), and sum of short and long axes to manubrium (overall-MHS). Additional short- and long-axis measurements can be obtained from the VD view and similar ratios constructed; however, the ratios using measurements from the VD view are greater than those derived from lateral view (Mostafa, 2017).

A radiographic cardiac sphericity index can be calculated using right lateral view. A more spherical silhouette can suggest right-sided cardiomegaly (or pericardial effusion). The ratios of long-axis:short-axis (Guglielmini, 2012) and short-axis:long-axis (Mostafa, 2020) have both been described. The latter study, involving a modest number of dogs, reported that for large breed dogs, a cardiac sphericity index >78% and a short-MHS ≥2.2 suggested right heart disease; for small breed dogs, these values were 83% and ≥2.5, respectively. The same study reported that left heart disease was likely in large breed dogs that had a combination of short-MHS ≥2.2, long-MHS >2.8, and overall-MHS >5.0; for small breed dogs, the respective cut-off values were ≥2.5, ≥3.0, and ≥5.5.

Other methods include the following. On lateral view, the normal cardiac apex-to-base length is less than or equal to 2/3 of the distance from apex to spine, as measured along a line aligned with the long axis of the heart. The cardiac width, measured parallel to the orientation of the trachea, is usually 2.5–3.5 intercostal spaces (ICSs). On DV view, the cardiac long axis usually is about 5 ICSs, from rib 3 through 8. The widest cardiac dimension is less than or equal to ½ to 2/3 the width of the thoracic cavity at the same level.

The Normal Feline Heart

The feline heart generally is aligned more parallel to the sternum on lateral view than that of dogs (**Figure 3.4**). This more horizontal orientation is accentuated in older cats. On DV/VD view, the cardiac apex usually is on the midline or only slightly leftward compared to dogs. Radiographic positioning, as well as patient resistance to restraint, can influence the relative size, shape, and position of the heart and trachea. These influences are greater in cats than in dogs because of greater thoracic flexibility. The normal feline heart is less than or up to 2 intercostal spaces wide and less than 70% of the height of the thorax on the lateral view, although some variation exists. On DV/VD views, the heart usually is no more than 1/2 (up to 2/3) the width of the thorax. Cardiac cycle phase has only a small influence on heart size and shape; however, the effect is greater on DV view compared with VD. In kittens, as in puppies, the relative size of the heart compared to the thorax is larger than in adults because of a smaller lung volume.

Vertebral Heart Size The VHS also is useful in cats (**Figure 3.5**). Normal VHS range on lateral view in cats is reported as 6.7–8.1v, with a mean of 7.5v. A VHS over 8.0v on lateral view raises suspicion for heart disease. However, especially in cats with respiratory distress, a VHS over 9.3v is highly specific for cardiac disease (Sleeper, 2013).

Cardiac measurement from a DV/VD view is more consistent in cats than in dogs and can be clinically useful. The mean short-axis cardiac dimension taken from a DV/VD view, compared with the thoracic spine beginning at the cranial edge of T4 on lateral view, is 3.4–3.5v, with a normal upper limit of 4 vertebrae.

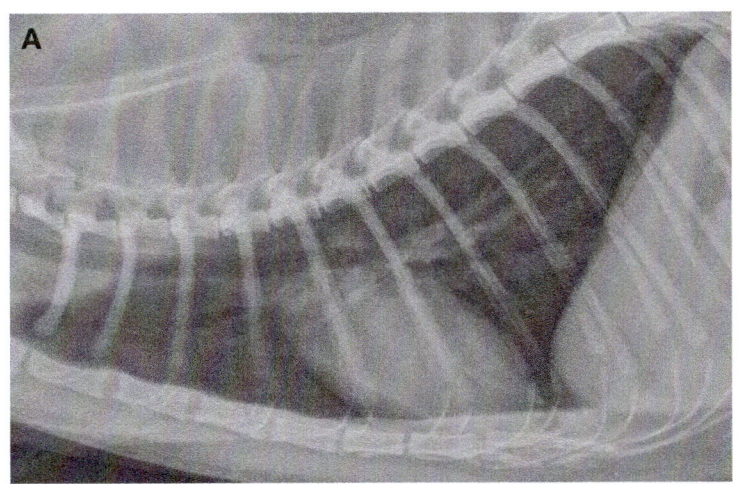
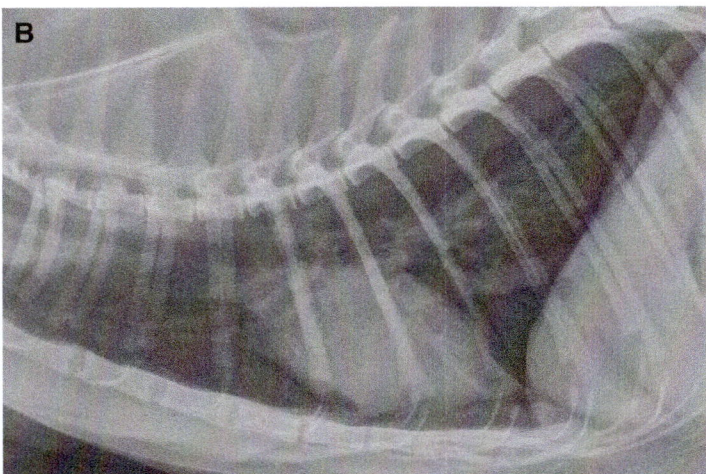
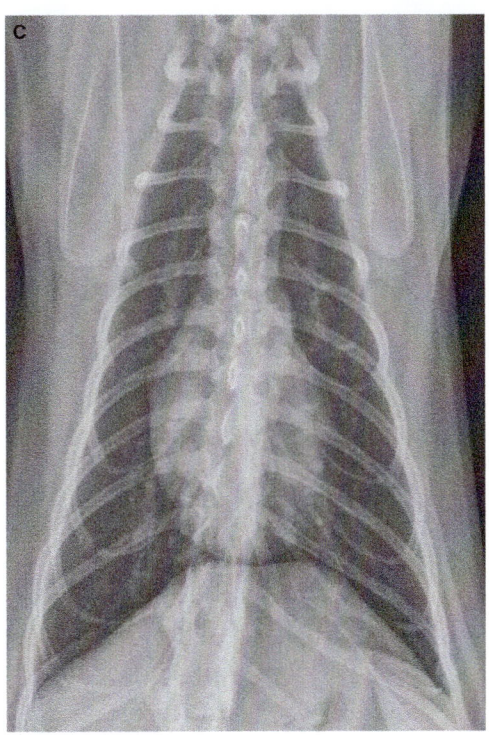

Figure 3.4 Right (A) and left (B) lateral and DV (C) views from a normal, 8-year-old spayed female domestic longhair cat.

A modified VHS scoring system to assess LA size on lateral view has been described for cats (LA-VHS), although measurement precision appears problematic. The LA-VHS is obtained by plotting the cardiac long-axis dimension (as for standard VHS measurement), then drawing a line perpendicular to this (and dorsal to the caudal vena cava [CaVC]) which extends to the caudal LA border. The length of this perpendicular line across the LA is compared with the thoracic spine beginning at the cranial edge of T4. LA-VHS values in normal cats were reported as a median of 1.0v (range 0.72–1.30v; Schober, 2007) and mean of 0.87v (± 0.21v; Guglielmini, 2014).

Generalized Cardiomegaly

Generalized cardiomegaly can result from enlargement of all four, or combinations of several, chambers. Fluid accumulation within the pericardial sac also increases cardiac silhouette size, generally with an increase in roundness or sphericity.

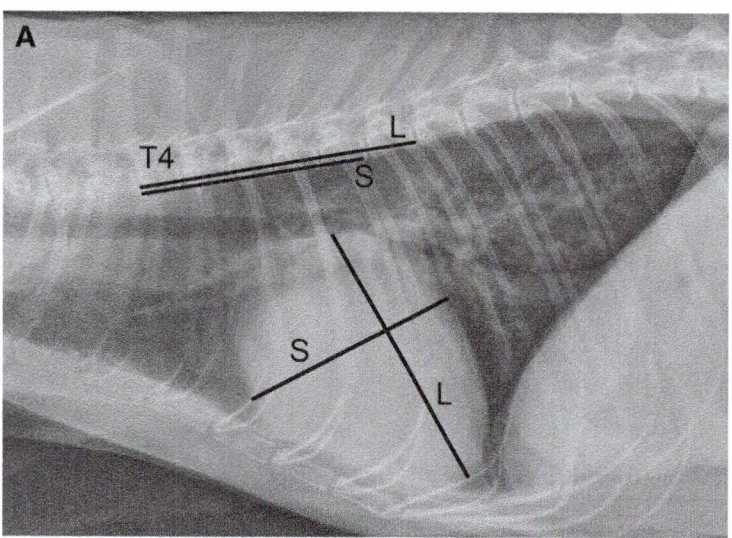
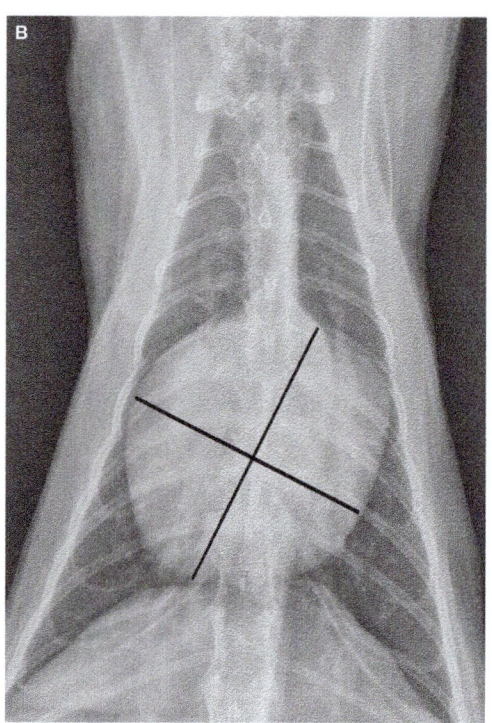

Figure 3.5 Right lateral (A) radiograph demonstrating vertebral heart size (VHS) measurement in an 11-year-old domestic shorthair cat with hypertrophic cardiomyopathy. The VHS of 10.9v was spuriously large because of pericardial effusion (secondary to congestive heart failure). Short-axis VHS measurement on DV view (B) was 4.9v (see p. 50).

In addition, the heart could appear relatively enlarged if the lungs are underinflated. When abnormal cardiac size or shape is suspected radiographically, it is important to ask if other supportive or commonly associated findings also are evident on physical examination and other test findings. The contours of different chambers usually are visible when the heart itself is enlarged, although marked RV and RA dilation can create a rounded cardiac silhouette (**Figure 3.6**). Fluid, fat (**Figure 3.7**), or viscera within the pericardial sac tends to obliterate specific chamber contours and can cause a globoid heart shadow (Chapter 35). Differentiation of fat from fluid opacity is easier with a lateral view. Common differential diagnoses for various cardiac enlargement patterns are listed in **Table 3.2**. Specific patterns are discussed in the following text.

Small Cardiac Silhouette

An abnormally small heart shadow (microcardia) results from poor venous return (as with severe hypovolemia). The cardiac apex is more pointed and might be elevated from the sternum on lateral view (**Figure 3.8**). The heart looks small on both lateral and DV/VD views. Other findings with hypovolemia include small pulmonary vessels and a thin CaVC. Sometimes, thoracic overexpansion with gas trapping can cause the heart to artifactually appear small, mimicking microcardia.

Cardiac Chamber Enlargement Patterns

Most diseases that cause cardiac dilation or hypertrophy affect at least two chambers; rarely is there isolated enlargement of one chamber. For example, mitral insufficiency leads to both LV and LA enlargement; pulmonic stenosis causes RV enlargement, a main pulmonary artery bulge, and, often, RA dilation. Even if only one side of the heart is enlarged, the cardiac silhouette can appear generally increased because different chambers are superimposed radiographically. Nevertheless, recognition of specific chamber and great vessel enlargement patterns can be helpful in diagnosis and in staging of disease. The orientation of normal cardiac chambers and major vessels is shown in **Figures 3.9** and **3.10**. Typical enlargement patterns are illustrated in **Figure 3.11**. Regions of an imaginary clock face superimposed on the cardiac silhouette often are used to describe areas of enlargement, especially on

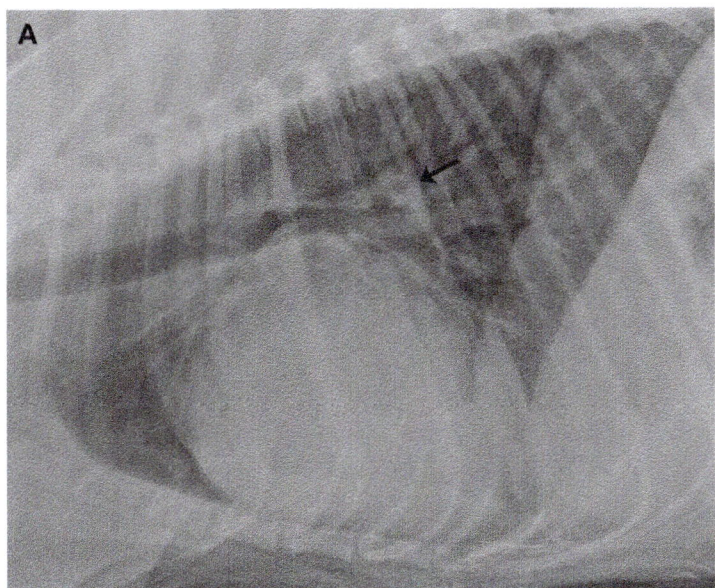
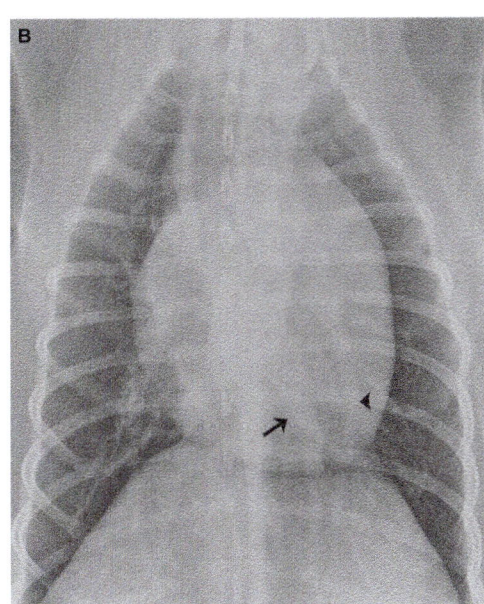

Figure 3.6 Right lateral (A) and DV (B) views from a 7-year-old male neutered Golden Retriever with dilated cardiomyopathy and moderate mitral regurgitation. There is generalized cardiomegaly (VHS ~12.8v), with left atrial prominence (A; arrow). Although pulmonary edema is absent, the left caudal pulmonary vein (B; arrow) is slightly larger than its accompanying artery (arrowhead), indicating venous congestion.

DV/VD views. Specific cardiac chamber enlargement sometimes occurs even when the overall VHS is normal. For example, RV enlargement in some dogs with pulmonary hypertension or pulmonic stenosis changes the cardiac shape without increasing the VHS (**Figure 27.26A**, p. 493).

Left Atrium The LA is the most dorsocaudal chamber of the heart, although its appendage extends cranially to the left (**Figure 3.9**; see also **Figure 1.8**, p. 8). On lateral view, the LA bulges dorsally and caudally as it enlarges, while the left and possibly right mainstem bronchi are pushed dorsally

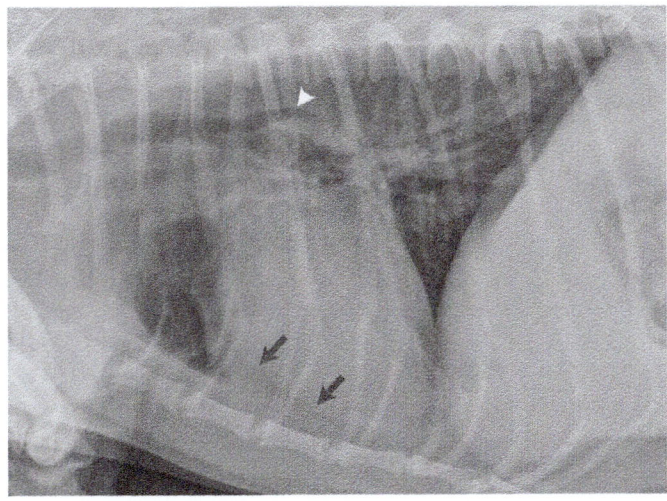

Figure 3.7 Fat accumulation in the pericardium can mimic cardiomegaly. However, in this radiograph from an obese 7-year-old male Shih Tzu, the demarcation between fat and soft tissue (heart) opacity (gray arrows) is evident. VHS is ~9.1v. The small amount of gas in the esophagus (white arrowhead) is an incidental finding.

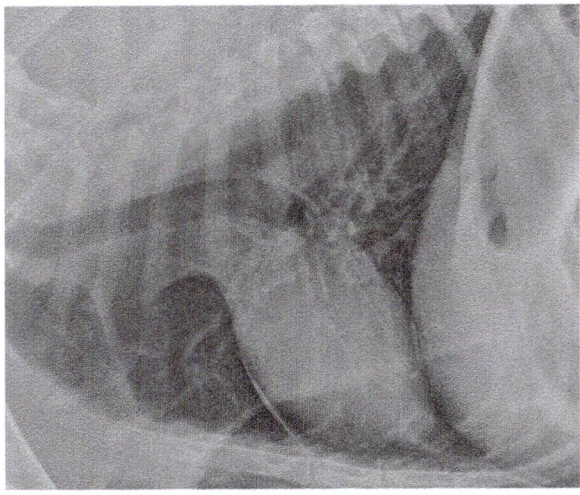

Figure 3.8 An abnormally small cardiac silhouette (microcardia) is present in this 8-year-old female Great Dane with severe gastric dilatation and volvulus. Note the separation of the cardiac apex from the sternum, as well as the collapsed caudal vena cava and small pulmonary vessels.

Table 3.2 Causes for Radiographic Cardiomegaly

Generalized Enlargement of the Cardiac Shadow
- Dilated cardiomyopathy
- Mitral and tricuspid valve insufficiency
- Pericardial effusion
- Intrapericardial mass or peritoneopericardial diaphragmatic hernia
- Ventricular or atrial septal defect
- Tricuspid valve dysplasia
- Patent ductus arteriosus
- Systemic hypertension
- "Athletic" heart
- Hyperthyroidism
- Acromegaly
- Large arteriovenous fistula
- Chronic (moderate to severe) anemia
- Intracardiac mass
- Intrapericardial fat—(could mimic cardiomegaly)

Left Atrial Enlargement
- Mild mitral valve insufficiency
- Hypertrophic cardiomyopathy
- Early dilated cardiomyopathy, especially Doberman Pinschers
- (Sub)aortic stenosis

Left Atrial and Ventricular Enlargement
- Mitral valve insufficiency
- Dilated cardiomyopathy
- Hypertrophic cardiomyopathy
- Ventricular septal defect
- Patent ductus arteriosus
- (Sub)aortic stenosis
- Aortic valve insufficiency
- Systemic hypertension
- "Athletic" heart
- Hyperthyroidism
- Mass lesion involving left heart
- Acromegaly

Right Atrial and Ventricular Enlargement
- Tricuspid valve insufficiency
- Atrial septal defect
- Pulmonic stenosis
- Heartworm disease
- Tetralogy of Fallot
- Other reversed-shunting congenital defects
- Other causes of pulmonary hypertension
- Mass lesion involving right heart

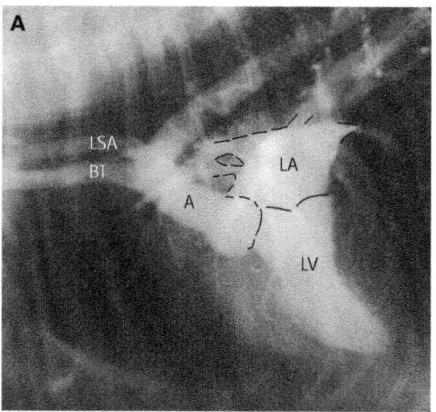

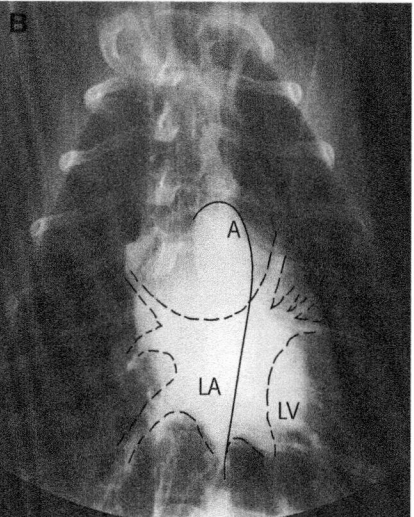

Figure 3.9 Lateral (A) and DV (B) views from a nonselective venogram (levo phase) in a normal 4-year-old dog show pulmonary venous inflow, left cardiac chambers, and aorta. A, aorta; BT, brachiocephalic trunk; LA, left atrium; LSA, left subclavian artery; LV, left ventricle.

(**Figure 3.12**; see also Figures **29.10–29.12**, p. 543). Left mainstem bronchus compression (or collapse) is common with severe LA enlargement (**Figure 3.13**; see also **Figure 29.11B**, p. 543), especially during expiration. In cats, the caudal heart border is normally quite straight on a lateral view; LA enlargement causes subtle to sometimes marked convexity of the dorsocaudal heart border, with elevation of the mainstem bronchi (**Figure 3.14**). However, echocardiography is a much more sensitive tool for identifying mild to moderate LA enlargement than radiography, especially in cats.

On DV/VD views, the mainstem bronchi are pushed laterally and curve slightly around a markedly enlarged LA (see Figure **29.10B**, p. 543); this sometimes is referred to as the "bowed-legged cowboy" sign, although it is an inconsistent feature of LA dilation. Left auricular enlargement causes a bulge in the 2 to 3 o'clock position of the cardiac silhouette in cats and dogs. LA enlargement increases the opacity of the caudal heartbase. Massive enlargement sometimes appears as a large, rounded soft tissue mass summated between the carina and the caudal border of the heart (**Figure 3.12**). In cats, left auricular enlargement that widens the left-cranial aspect of the heart, combined with apex shifting to the midline, produces a "valentine"-shaped silhouette (**Figure 3.14**).

The extent of LA enlargement depends not only on the pressure or volume load imposed, but also on its duration. For example, mitral regurgitation (MR) of slowly increasing severity can result in massive LA enlargement without

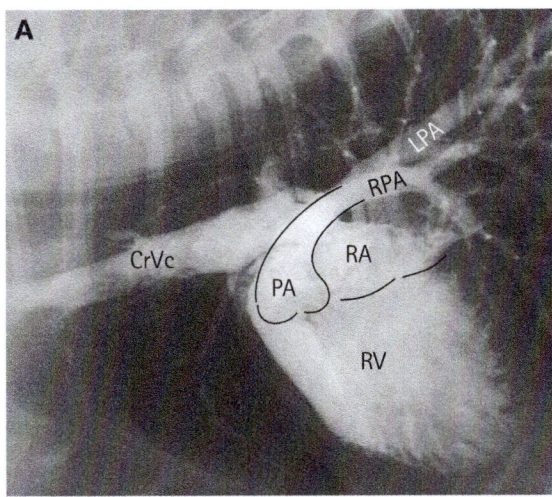 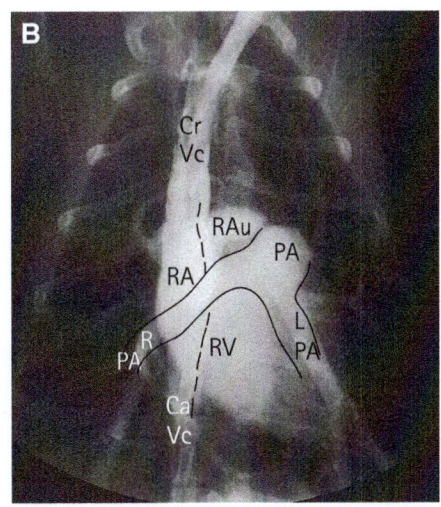

Figure 3.10 Lateral (A) and DV (B) views from a nonselective venogram (dextro phase) in a normal 4-year-old dog highlight the cranial vena cava, right cardiac chambers, and pulmonary arterial tree. CaVc, caudal vena cava; CrVc, cranial vena cava; LPA, left pulmonary artery; PA, main pulmonary artery; RA, right atrium; RAu, right auricle; RPA, right pulmonary artery; RV, right ventricle.

pulmonary edema, if there is sufficient time for chamber dilation to occur at relatively low pressures. Conversely, rupture of chordae tendineae causes acute valvular regurgitation and when LA pressure rises quickly, pulmonary edema can develop with little radiographic evidence of enlargement.

Left Ventricle LV enlargement is manifested on a lateral view by a taller or longer heart with dorsal displacement of the tracheal bifurcation (carina) and CaVC. The intrathoracic trachea appears closer and more parallel to the spine (**Figure 3.12**). The caudal heart border becomes convex, with the apex still against the sternum. Marked LV dilation also can create the appearance of generalized cardiomegaly. On DV/VD view, the heart usually appears elongated, with rounding and enlargement in the 2 o'clock to 5 or 6 o'clock area. Cats with hypertrophic cardiomyopathy (Chapter 33) often maintain a pointed appearance to the cardiac apex, which might shift to the left or more often toward the midline or right. Concurrent atrial enlargement can produce the classic "valentine"-shaped silhouette (**Figure 3.14B**). Other affected cats show apex rounding and more generalized cardiomegaly.

Right Atrium On lateral view, RA and auricular enlargement might cause widening of the cardiac silhouette and a bulge at the cranial border of the heart. Sometimes, the trachea is elevated over the cranial portion of the heart, but then courses ventrally. On DV/VD views, the cardiac silhouette bulges in the 9 to 11 o'clock position. Because the RA

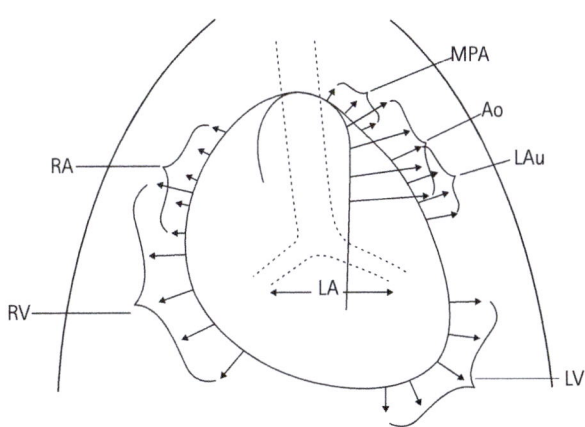 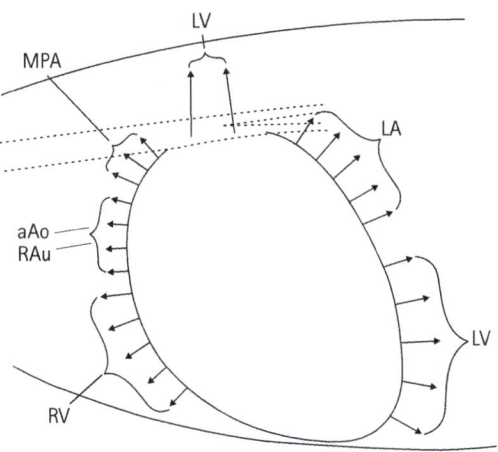

Figure 3.11 Diagrams illustrating common enlargement patterns of the heart chambers and great vessels on DV (left) and lateral (right) radiographic views. aAo, ascending aorta; Ao, aorta (descending); LA, left atrium; LAu, left auricle; LV, left ventricle; MPA, main pulmonary artery; RA, right atrium; RAu, right auricle; RV, right ventricle.

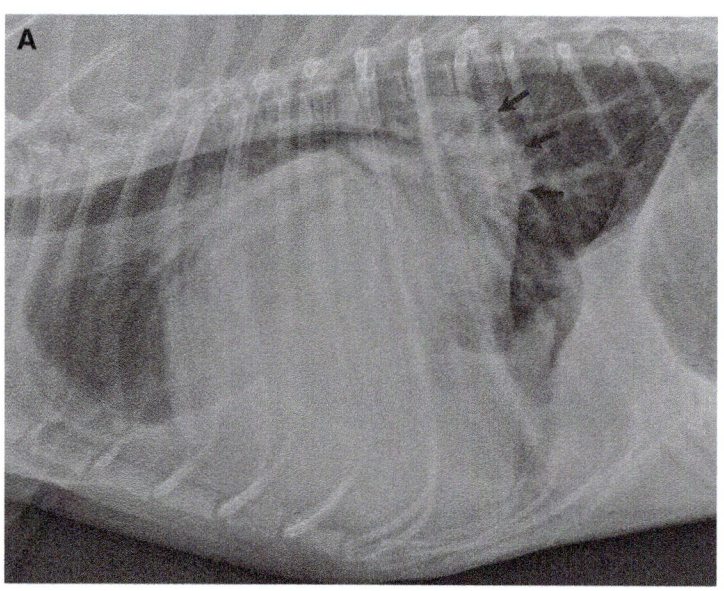
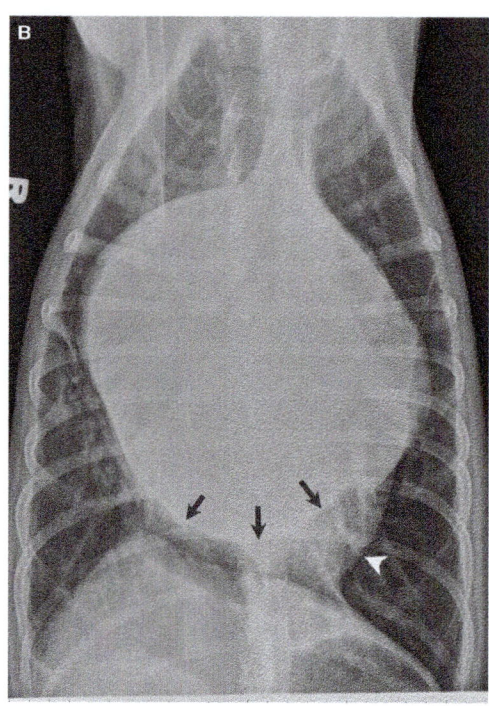

Figure 3.12 Left ventricular (LV) and massive left atrial (LA) enlargement (arrows) is present in this 5-year-old female mixed-breed dog with mitral valve dysplasia and severe valvular regurgitation. (A) The LA enlargement creates a prominent dorsocaudal bulge (arrows) on right lateral view. LV enlargement elongates the heart, elevates the carina dorsally, aligns the trachea parallel to the spine, and raises the cranial aspect of the caudal vena cava where it joins the heart. On DV view (B), prominent left auricular distension is evident in the 3 o'clock region. The main bronchi are pushed laterally, although not easily seen in this image. The left atrium appears summated over the LV, although its caudal border (small arrows) is distinct from the ventricular apex (white arrowhead).

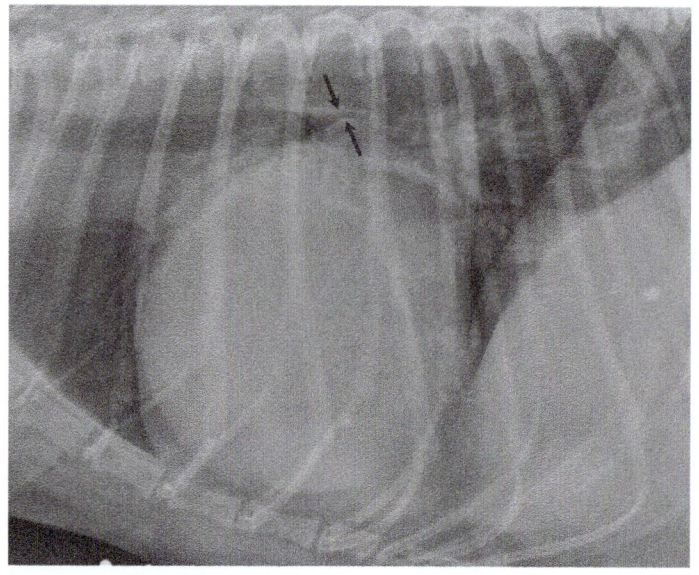

Figure 3.13 Marked left atrial enlargement and left mainstem bronchus compression (arrows) are present in this 10-year-old male neutered mixed-breed dog with advanced degenerative mitral valve disease and increased cough frequency. There is no radiographic evidence for pulmonary edema. Left lateral thoracic radiograph.

is largely superimposed on the RV, differentiation from RV enlargement is difficult. However, concurrent enlargement of both chambers is common.

Right Ventricle RV enlargement (dilation or hypertrophy) usually causes increased widening and convexity of the cranioventral heart border on lateral view (**Figure 3.15**). The trachea over the cranial heart border sometimes appears elevated. However, the VHS is not always increased, especially with RV concentric hypertrophy. With marked RV enlargement and relatively normal left heart size, the apex becomes elevated from the sternum, especially on the right lateral view (**Figure 27.27A**, p. 493; and **Figures 39.6A** and **39.9A**, p. 822 and 826). The carina and CaVC also are elevated dorsally. Because of breed variation in chest conformation, the degree of sternal contact of the cardiac silhouette is not a reliable sign of RV enlargement. The heart on DV/VD view can take on a reverse-D configuration if left-sided enlargement is absent (**Figure 27.28B**, p. 494; and **Figures 39.6B** and **39.9B**, p. 822 and 826). The apex can shift leftward, while the right cardiac border bulges rightward, causing widening and rounding of the 6 to 9 o'clock area.

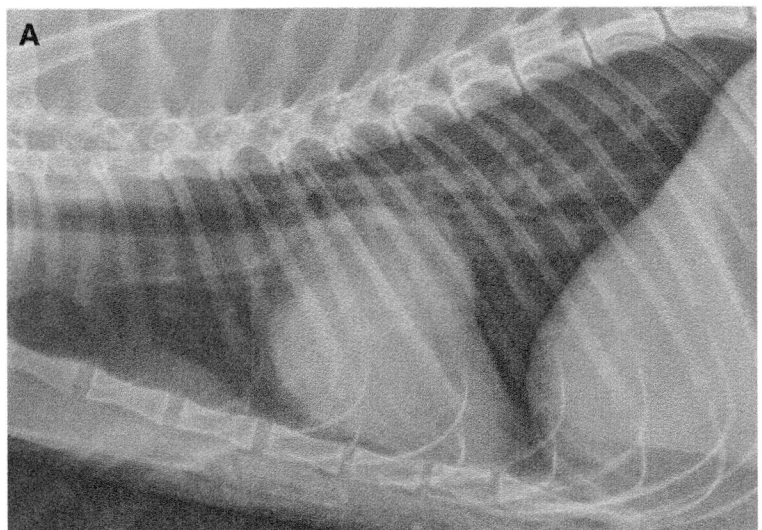
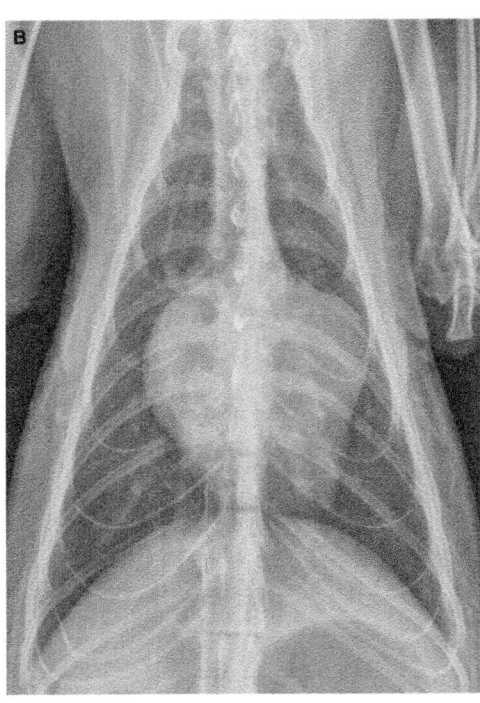

Figure 3.14 This 3-year-old neutered male domestic shorthair cat with end-stage hypertrophic cardiomyopathy has severe left atrial enlargement. Note the mild convexity of the dorsocaudal cardiac border and tracheal elevation on right lateral view (A), and the widened cranial heart borders on DV view (B). The left ventricular apex point is fairly well-maintained, creating a so-called "valentine"-shaped heart silhouette.

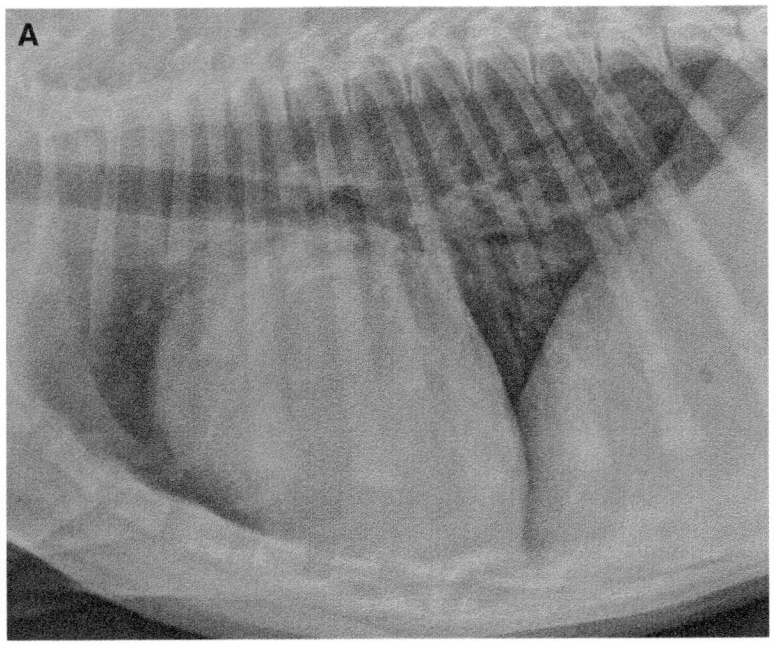
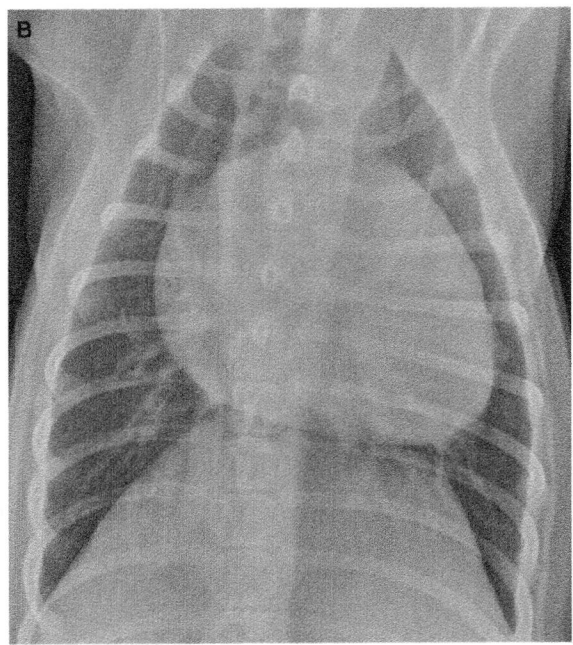

Figure 3.15 Right ventricular and atrial enlargement resulted from tricuspid valve dysplasia in this 6-month-old male Bouvier des Flandres. (A) The cardiac silhouette is widened cranially on right lateral view. (B) On DV view, the right cardiac border bulges prominently and the apex is shifted leftward.

Intrathoracic Blood Vessels

Aorta

The aorta and main pulmonary artery both tend to dilate in response to chronic arterial hypertension or increased turbulence, as with poststenotic dilation (**Table 3.3**). Subaortic stenosis (p. 480) produces dilation of the ascending aorta. However, this can be difficult to see on lateral view because of this structure's location within the mediastinum. Widening and increased opacity of the dorsocranial heart shadow often is observed. On DV/VD view, there might be mediastinal widening just cranial to the heart. Turbulence induced by a patent ductus arteriosus causes localized dilation of the descending aorta just caudal to the aortic arch. This "ductus bump" is seen on DV/VD view at the 2 to 3 o'clock area (**Figure 26.1B**, p. 437). Idiopathic aortic dilatation is common also, especially in cats and in canine breeds with high subaortic stenosis prevalence. This could represent a primary aortopathy, as seen in the Leonberger dog.

The aortic arch in cats often is more prominent than in dogs on lateral view. Older cats especially can have a wavy, undulating appearance to the thoracic aorta (**Figure 3.16**). On DV/VD view, the aortic arch can look large, with a prominent knob at the junction of the aortic arch and descending aorta (**Figure 3.16**). Arterial blood pressure should be checked, although not all these cats are hypertensive. On DV/VD view in both dogs and cats, it is easier to identify the thoracic aorta near the diaphragm; from there, follow it cranially to assess its contour.

Main Pulmonary Artery

Main pulmonary artery dilation appears on lateral radiograph as a bulge at the cranial heart base, superimposed over the trachea. On DV/VD view in the dog, main pulmonary trunk enlargement causes a bulge in the 1 to 2 o'clock position (**Figure 27.27B**, p. 493; also **Figures 39.6B** and **39.8B**, p. 822 and 826). Valvular pulmonic stenosis, pulmonary hypertension, and left-to-right shunts are the usual causes (Chapters 27, 39, and 40). In the cat, the main pulmonary trunk's position is slightly more medial and it usually is obscured within the mediastinum.

Lobar Pulmonary Arteries and Veins

The paired lobar arteries and veins should be the same size as each other; although on the left (but not the right) lateral projection, the cranial lobar pulmonary vein sometimes appears slightly larger than the artery even in normal dogs. Four pulmonary vascular patterns are commonly described (see the following sections and **Table 3.3**). The size and appearance of the pulmonary vasculature can provide important clinical information. The cranial lobar vessels are best evaluated on lateral view. Vessels in the nondependent ("up"-side) lung are

Table 3.3 Causes of Abnormal Intrathoracic Vessel Size[a]

Aorta

- Aortic root and ascending aorta dilation
  - Subaortic stenosis (poststenotic dilation)
  - Systemic hypertension
  - Aortopathy / Idiopathic dilation
- Aortic arch
  - Systemic hypertension
  - Aging change in some geriatric cats
  - Aortopathy / Idiopathic dilation
- Proximal descending aorta dilation
  - Patent ductus arteriosus

Main Pulmonary Artery Dilation

- Pulmonic valve stenosis (poststenotic dilation)
- Pulmonary hypertension (heartworm disease and other causes)
- Overcirculation (left-to-right cardiac shunts; large arteriovenous fistula)

Lobar Pulmonary Vessels

- Smaller than normal (undercirculation)
  - Severe dehydration and hypovolemia
  - Right ventricular inflow obstruction
  - Tetralogy of Fallot
  - Severe pulmonic stenosis
  - Severe cardiac tamponade
  - Right-sided congestive heart failure
  - Pulmonary overinflation or overexposed radiographic images can cause pulmonary vessels to appear small
- Larger than normal (overcirculation)
  - Left-to-right cardiac shunts (atrial and ventricular septal defects, patent ductus arteriosus)
  - Overhydration
  - Large arteriovenous fistula
  - Other hyperdynamic state
  - Acute left-sided congestive heart failure with pulmonary hypertension, especially cats
- Lobar arteries larger than veins
  - Pulmonary arterial hypertension (heartworm disease and other causes)
- Lobar veins larger than arteries
  - Pulmonary venous hypertension (left-sided congestive heart failure; rarely, obstruction to left heart inflow)

Caudal Vena Cava

- Larger than normal
  - Increased intracaval pressure (right-sided congestive heart failure, cardiac tamponade, constrictive pericardial disease, cor triatriatum dexter, other obstruction to right heart inflow)
- Smaller than normal
  - Hypovolemia
  - Poor venous return
  - Pulmonary overinflation
  - Sometimes secondary to expiratory phase of ventilation

[a] See text for vascular size assessment methods.

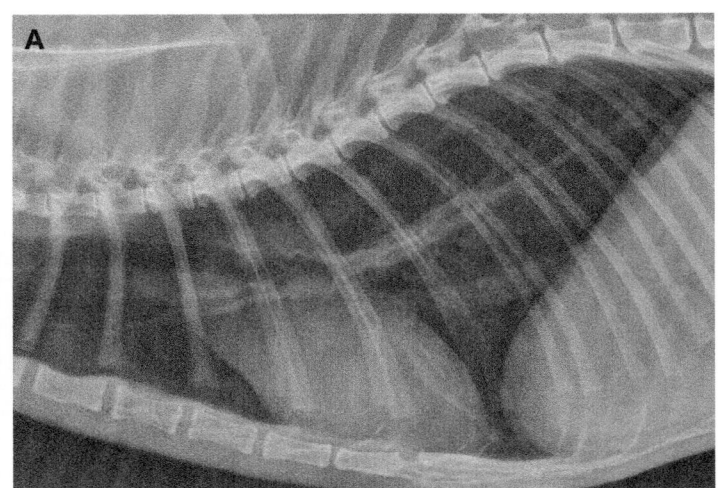
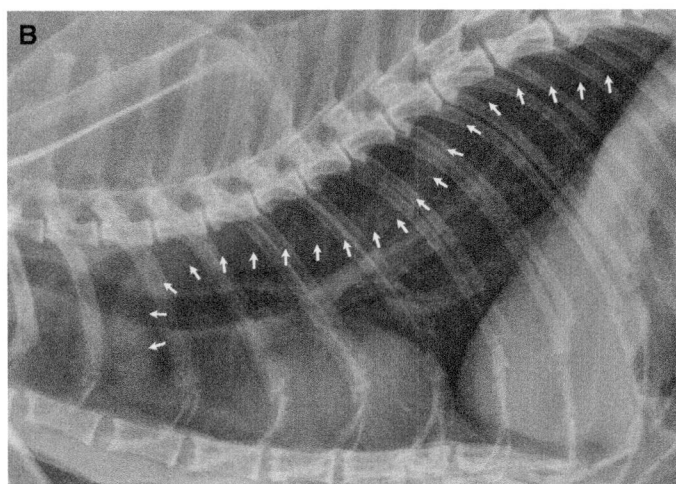
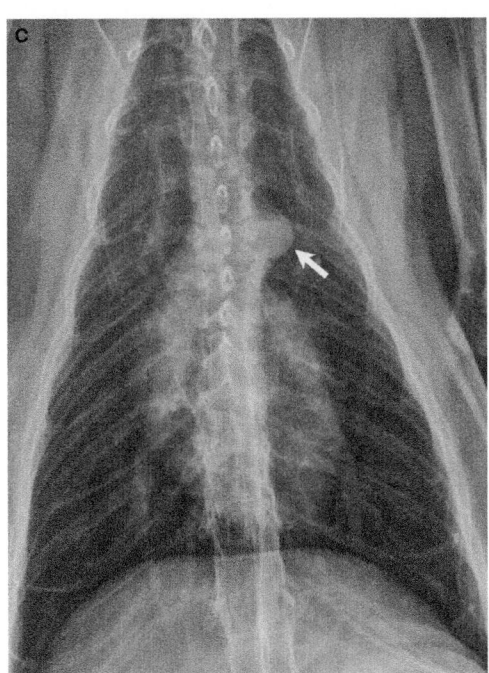

Figure 3.16 A prominent aortic arch and wavy, or redundant, thoracic aorta can be seen on the lateral views (A) from a 13-year-old neutered male domestic longhair cat, and especially (B) from a 17-year-old spayed female Birman cat with chronic renal disease. Small arrows delineate the ventral border of the thoracic aorta. Both cats had systemic arterial hypertension. The heart often is more horizontally oriented in geriatric cats; this is particularly notable in the Birman (B). (C) The large aortic arch can create a knoblike appearance (arrow) on DV view, as seen in a 13-year-old spayed female domestic shorthair with hyperthyroidism and hypertension.

usually clearest and larger than in the dependent lung. The right cranial lobar vessels are easiest to see on left lateral view; with right lateral positioning, these vessels might be superimposed on the left cranial lobar vessels. On both lateral views, the left cranial lobar vessels often are more obscure because of their more dorsal location (where mediastinal tissue is thicker) and superimposition with other vessels.

The pulmonary arteries are dorsal to the accompanying veins and bronchi. The right pulmonary artery passes ventral to the carina and appears end-on as a round/oval opacity. The width of the cranial lobar vessels is measured where the vessels cross the 4th rib in dogs, or at the cranial heart border (4th–5th rib) in cats. These vessels normally are no wider than 0.5–1 times the diameter of the proximal 1/3 of the 4th rib.

In normal cats, the vessel-to-rib ratio usually ranges between 0.6 and 0.8.

The caudal lobar vessels are easier to see on DV, rather than VD view. This is because they are somewhat magnified, have less adjacent lung atelectasis, and are more perpendicular to the primary X-ray beam, with minimal distortion. Caudal lobar arteries originate cranial to the tracheal bifurcation and lie lateral to their accompanying bronchi and veins. Caudal lobar veins enter the heart caudal to the tracheal bifurcation. Caudal lobar vessels are measured where they cross the 9th rib in dogs, and 9th or 10th rib in cats. Normal vessels generally are 1/2 to 1 times the width of the rib where they cross. However, the diameter of the right caudal pulmonary artery and vein slightly exceed that of the 9th rib, in about 2/3 of healthy dogs (Oui, 2014). In cats, pulmonary arteries are considered enlarged if their width exceeds 1.5 times that of the 9th rib (at the cross point). Pulmonary vessels should taper as they extend distally. The relation of pulmonary lobar arteries and veins to each other might be easier to remember with the phrase "veins are central and ventral," that is, on DV/VD and lateral views, respectively.

Undercirculation Pattern Pulmonary undercirculation is characterized by narrowed pulmonary arteries and veins, along with increased lung field lucency (**Figure 3.17A**). Severe dehydration, hypovolemia, obstruction to RV inflow, right-sided congestive heart failure (CHF), and tetralogy of Fallot can cause this pattern. Some animals with pulmonic stenosis appear to have pulmonary undercirculation, as do many dogs with cardiac tamponade. Pulmonary overinflation and overexposure of radiographs also minimize the appearance of pulmonary vessels.

Overcirculation Pattern An overcirculation pattern occurs when the lungs are hyperperfused (**Figure 3.17B**). Left-to-right cardiac shunts, overhydration, and other hyperdynamic

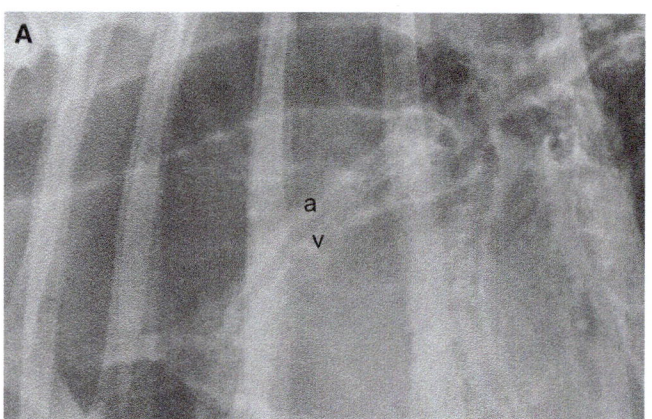
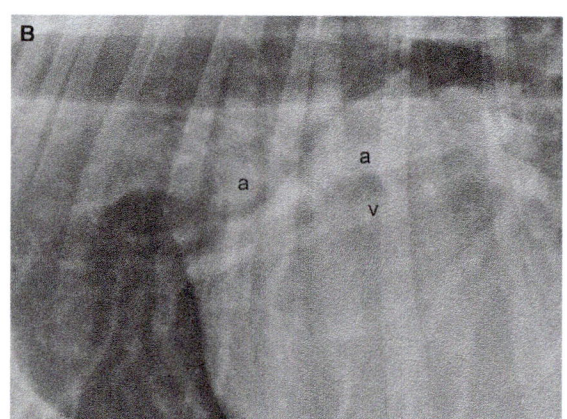
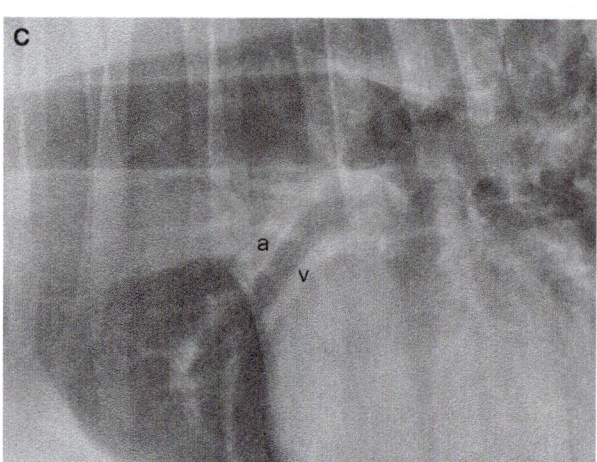
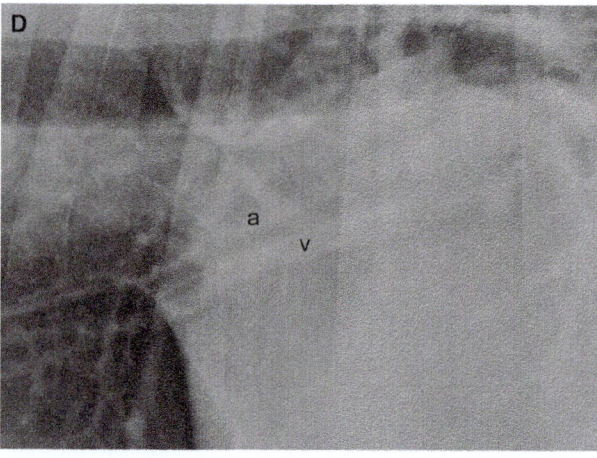

Figure 3.17 Pulmonary vascular patterns. (A) Pulmonary undercirculation (arteries and veins both are small) in a 15-year-old female Cocker Spaniel with multisystemic disease and severe dehydration. (B) Pulmonary overcirculation (arteries and veins both are large) in a 7-month-old female English Springer Spaniel with patent ductus arteriosus. (C) Enlarged pulmonary arteries in a 9-year-old neutered male, mixed-breed dog with pulmonary hypertension from severe heartworm disease. (D) Distended pulmonary veins caused by left-sided congestive heart failure in a 9-year-old male German Shepherd with long-standing mitral regurgitation. a, artery; v, vein.

states can cause this. Pulmonary arteries and veins are both large. The increased pulmonary perfusion also causes a generally increased lung opacity ("haziness"), although careful scrutiny will show that the vessels are just distended, not obscured. Some deep-chested, large-breed dogs (such as German Shepherds) seem to have prominent yet normal pulmonary vascular markings.

Pulmonary Arteries Larger Than Veins Pulmonary arteries that are wider than their accompanying veins indicate pulmonary arterial hypertension (**Figure 3.17C**). The dilated pulmonary arteries can become tortuous and blunted, with poorly visualized terminal portions. Heartworm disease is a common cause (Chapter 40); patchy to diffuse interstitial pulmonary infiltrates also are commonly seen with heartworm disease.

Pulmonary Veins Larger Than Arteries Prominent pulmonary veins are a sign of venous congestion, usually from left-sided CHF. On both left and right lateral views, the cranial lobar veins are larger and denser than their accompanying arteries and may sag ventrally (**Figure 3.17D**). Dilated and sometimes tortuous pulmonary veins might be evident adjoining the dorsocaudal aspect of an enlarged LA in dogs and cats with chronic pulmonary venous hypertension. However, pulmonary venous distension is not always seen in patients with left-sided heart failure, especially after diuretic therapy, and as noted above a small discrepancy in cranial venous and arterial diameter might be seen normally on the left lateral view of the dog. Cats with acute cardiogenic pulmonary edema often have enlargement of both pulmonary veins and arteries.

Vena Cava

The cranial vena cava normally forms the straight ventral border of the cranial mediastinum, although it is not visible as a separate structure. The CaVC, on lateral view, normally angles cranioventrally from diaphragm to heart. Enlargement of either ventricle pushes the CaVC–cardiac juncture dorsally and creates a more horizontal CaVC orientation.

The diameter of the CaVC is approximately that of the descending thoracic aorta, although its size varies with respiration. Persistent widening of the CaVC suggests increased intracaval pressure. This can occur with RV failure (including from severe outflow obstruction or pulmonary hypertension), cardiac tamponade, pericardial constriction, or other obstruction to right heart inflow (**Figure 3.18**). Based on a study in dogs with right-sided heart disease, the following ratios between CaVC diameter and other thoracic structures indicate abnormal CaVC distension (Lehmkuhl, 1997):

- CaVC/aortic diameter (at the same intercostal space as CaVC measurement) >1.5
- CaVC/length of the thoracic vertebra directly above the tracheal bifurcation >1.3
- CaVC/width of right 4th rib (just ventral to the spine) >3.5

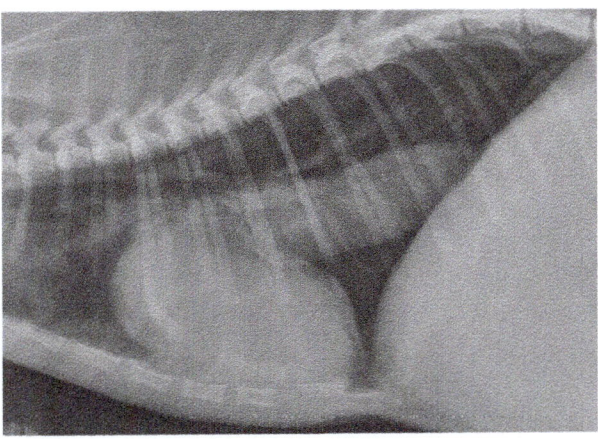

Figure 3.18 Massive caudal vena caval distension and right heart enlargement in a 4-month-old female Maine Coon cat with tetralogy of Fallot. The pulmonary stenosis and consequent right ventricular hypertrophy were severe. Right atrial dilation also was severe. Tricuspid regurgitation was minimal in this case.

A thin or rapidly tapering vena cava can be associated with hypovolemia, poor venous return, or pulmonary overinflation, and sometimes it is normal, related to the phase of ventilation (see **Figure 3.8**).

The Pulmonary Parenchyma

Pulmonary Patterns

Increased pulmonary opacity has been categorized into bronchial, vascular, alveolar, and diffuse or nodular interstitial patterns. In reality most patterns are mixed. For example, pulmonary edema might cause interstitial perivascular and peribronchial infiltrates as well as air bronchograms (alveolar pattern). Abnormal parenchymal infiltrates are easier to visualize in nondependent lung regions because the greater pulmonary inflation there provides better contrast within the air-filled lung (for example, the right lung lobes on left lateral view, or accessory lobe on VD view). The distribution of these patterns within different lung regions, and whether they are focal or diffusely disseminated, can have diagnostic significance. For example, infiltrates caused by cardiogenic pulmonary edema in dogs generally have a perihilar distribution, while those from bacterial pneumonia typically are located cranioventrally.

Bronchial patterns highlight the walls of the larger airways. Prominent bronchial markings can occur from aging changes or bronchial mineralization. Bronchial wall thickening also results from accumulation of cellular infiltrate or edema. Thick end-on bronchi have been described as "donuts" or "ring shadows"; when viewed from the side, the thickened parallel walls have been called "tramlines." Abnormally dilated bronchi (bronchiectasis) can result from chronic severe airway disease. Pulmonary vascular patterns are described in the section "Lobar Pulmonary Arteries and

Veins". Pulmonary overcirculation causes a vascular pattern of increased lung opacity.

Interstitial opacities can be unstructured, nodular, or miliary (like millet seeds). A diffuse or unstructured increase in interstitial opacity can occur with early or resolving pulmonary edema or some cellular infiltrates (such as diffuse lymphoma or interstitial pneumonias). However, mild diffuse opacity or haziness often is related to nonpathologic causes such as aging, fat accumulation, expiration, or underexposed images. Obesity tends to reduce maximal lung expansion, which also contributes to increased pulmonary opacity. However, if the increased lung opacity has blurred or obscured the edges of the pulmonary vessels and the increased opacity is evident on DV/VD view, in addition to a lateral projection, it is not just an artifact. Nodular interstitial opacities of different size are typical of metastatic lung disease or granulomatous inflammation. Additional rule-outs include end-on vessels (that should become smaller toward the lung periphery), osteomas, and external causes (including nipples, ticks).

Alveolar patterns occur when terminal air spaces fill with fluid. The intense fluid opacity obscures the tissue margins of adjacent structures (such as the heart, vessels, and diaphragm), producing the silhouette sign. Air bronchograms become visible as the severity of alveolar infiltration progresses. These are branching lucent lines caused by air-filled bronchi surrounded by fluid opacity. A lobar sign is also common, where the edge of a lobe with increased opacity creates a sharp margin against an adjacent, normally aerated lobe.

The distribution of an alveolar pattern can be patchy throughout several lung lobes, or localized to certain regions or an individual lobe. Edema, infectious and inflammatory debris, hemorrhage, and water (from near drowning) can cause this pattern. In addition, lung lobe torsion, with consolidation or collapse of the lung from gas reabsorption, can lead to a lobar sign, as can a primary lung tumor. The right middle lobe is especially prone to reabsorption atelectasis and reduced volume.

Decreased lung opacity can occur with pulmonary hyperinflation (as with feline asthma and emphysema), bronchiectasis, image overexposure, or as a normal variation. Overly lucent lungs can be mistaken for pneumothorax.

Pulmonary Edema

Pulmonary edema is an increase in lung water and solute. It accumulates initially in the interstitium around vessels and bronchi, causing radiographically ill-defined vessels and thickened bronchial walls. As the edema worsens, areas of fluffy or mottled fluid opacity progressively become more confluent. The lung pattern can be unstructured interstitial or alveolar as described previously. The distribution of these pulmonary infiltrates often helps characterize their cause. Cardiogenic pulmonary edema in dogs typically is located in dorsal and perihilar areas, and is often bilaterally symmetric; however, some dogs with cardiogenic edema have an asymmetric or concurrent ventral distribution of opacities (**Figures 3.19–3.21**).

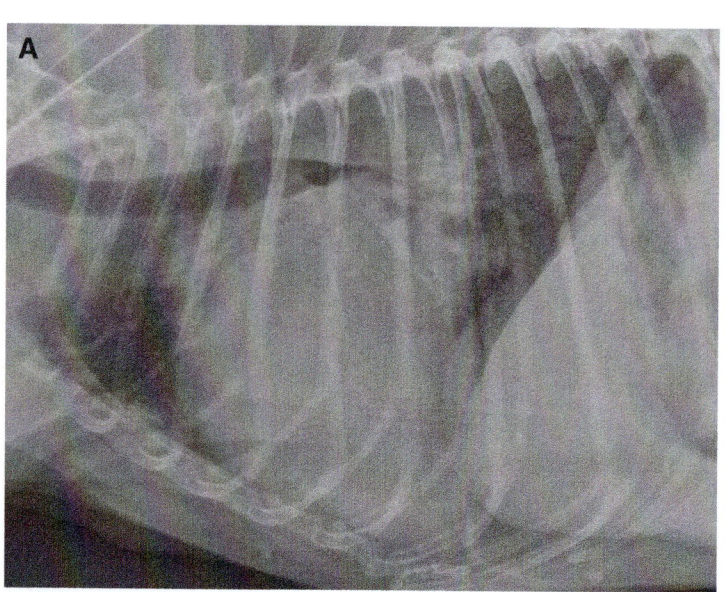
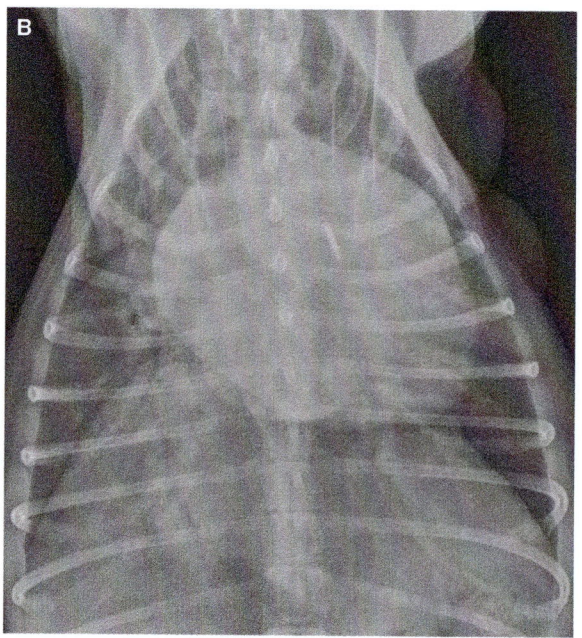

Figure 3.19 Mild cardiogenic pulmonary edema secondary to degenerative mitral valve disease in an 11-year-old female Minature Schnauzer. The typical dorsohilar distribution is evident on right lateral view (A), although the DV projection (B) shows that the infiltrate is worse in the right and caudal lung regions.

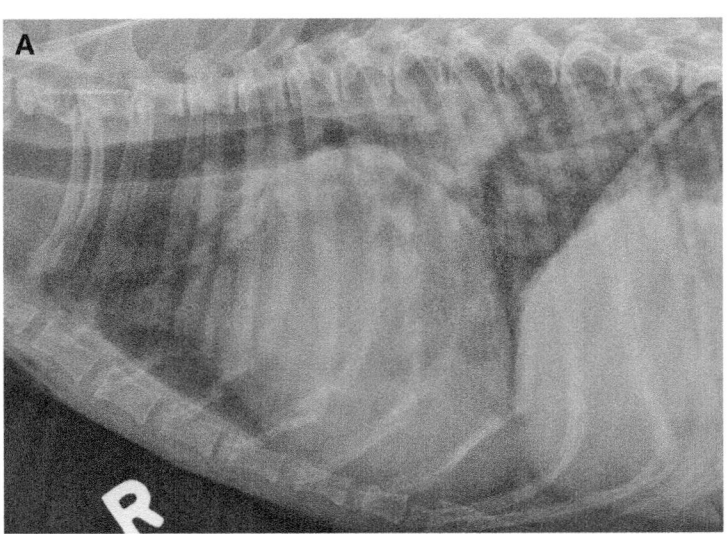
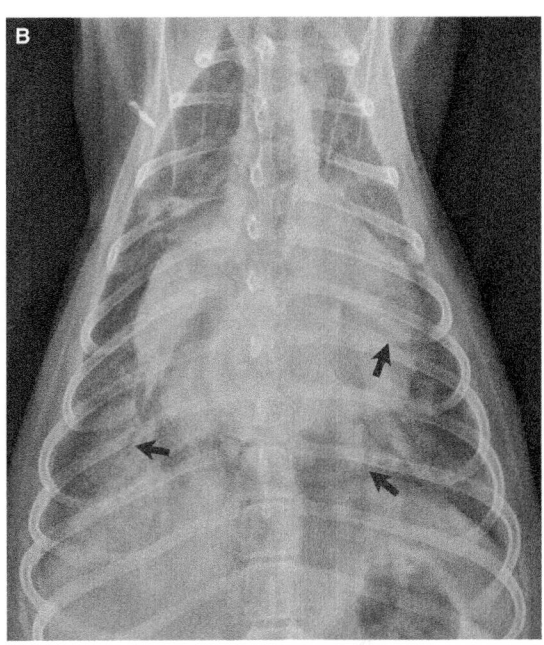

Figure 3.20 More widespread, patchy pulmonary edema in a 12-year-old female Havanese with degenerative mitral valve disease. (A) Infiltrates extend into the cranial lung (right lateral view). (B) DV view shows air bronchograms (arrows) in the caudal lung regions.

An asymmetric pulmonary edema pattern is observed in some dogs with MR and acute CHF (often worse on the right). This could relate to an eccentric MR jet (Diana, 2009); nevertheless, many jets are directed eccentrically toward the left pulmonary veins and not all produce asymmetric pulmonary edema, in the authors' experience.

Cats with cardiogenic edema can have widely varying patterns of pulmonary opacities. These often consist of unstructured interstitial opacities with an uneven and patchy distribution that can extend throughout the lung fields or be concentrated in the middle zones (**Figure 3.22**). The opacities could involve peribronchial and perivascular areas, as

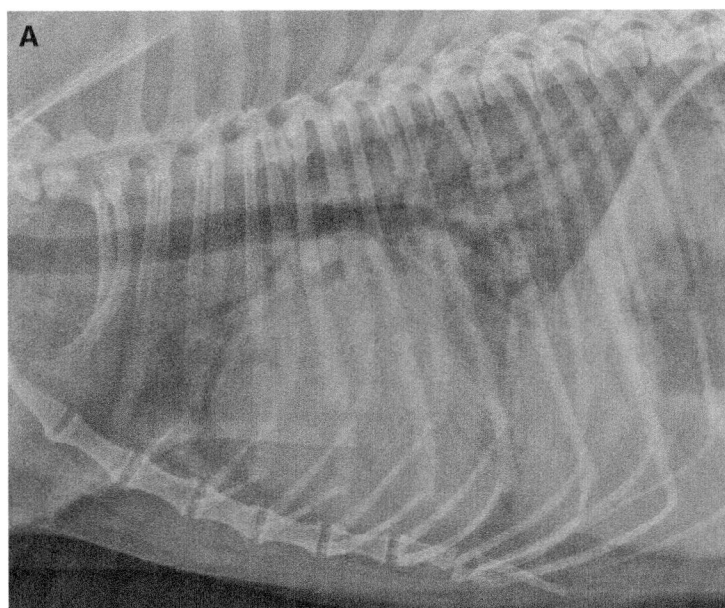
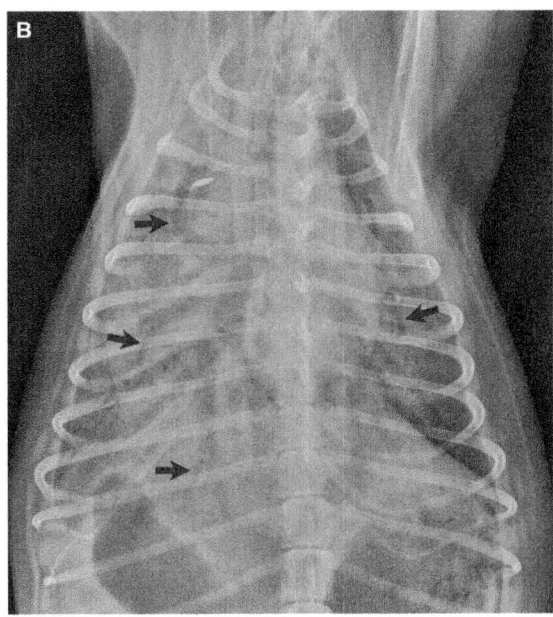

Figure 3.21 Severe pulmonary edema in a 10-year-old spayed female Cavalier King Charles Spaniel with progressive respiratory distress. Widespread air bronchograms are present throughout the lung fields in both lateral (A) and DV (B; arrows) views. The alveolar pattern is particularly severe on the right (B).

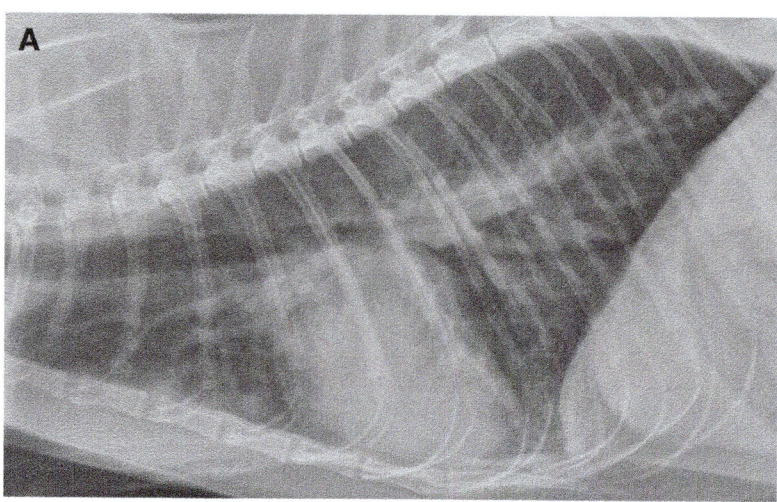
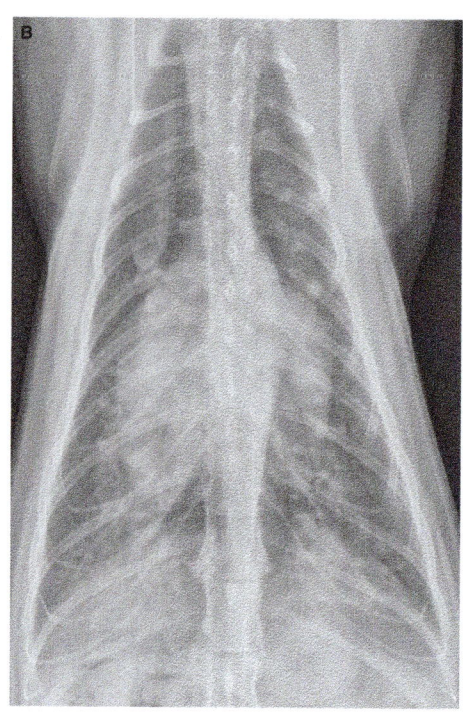

Figure 3.22 Recurrent pulmonary edema in a 7-year-old male neutered domestic shorthair cat with hypertrophic cardiomyopathy and marked left atrial enlargement (A). The vertebral heart score is ~9.4v. There is a diffuse, slightly patchy pulmonary bronchointerstitial pattern. The pulmonary vessels are enlarged, especially caudally (B), although the pulmonary infiltrate partially obscures them.

well as progress to an alveolar pattern with worsening edema. Cardiogenic edema usually is accompanied by cardiomegaly, with or without vascular distension (involving either pulmonary arteries, veins, or both).

Other classic patterns of pulmonary infiltrate distribution have been described. Noncardiogenic pulmonary edema tends to be bilateral and dorsocaudal. Infiltrates from bacterial pneumonia usually gravitate to cranioventral regions. Lung lobe atelectasis or torsion tends to be lobar or regional and accompanied by a mediastinal shift.

The Pleural Space

Pleural Effusion

As free pleural fluid accumulates between lung lobes, wedge-shaped areas of soft tissue or fluid opacity that "point" toward the center of the chest become visible. On a lateral view, ventral opacity (fluid) separates the lungs from the sternum. A scalloped appearance often is seen at the fluid/lung interface on this projection. On DV/VD view, this opacity separates the lung lobes from each other and the chest wall and blunts the normally sharp costophrenic angles (**Figures 3.23** and **3.24**). The cardiac silhouette is better visualized on a VD view because the fluid collects at the dorsal aspect of the thorax; however, this position may exacerbate respiratory distress. Large-volume pleural effusion causes partial lung collapse, rounding of lobar borders, and silhouetting of the cardiac and mediastinal shadows. Pleural fluid and reduced lung expansion hinder recognition of pulmonary parenchymal infiltrates. Other findings that often accompany cardiogenic pleural effusion include a wide CaVC, cardiomegaly, hepatomegaly, and abdominal effusion.

Some conditions can mimic small-volume pleural effusion. Pleural fibrosis in old dogs accentuates pleural fissure lines, although the peripheral areas do not look thicker or wedge-shaped, as with effusion. Fat within the caudal mediastinum, between caudally located lung lobes, or lining the chest wall also can mimic pleural effusion.

Pneumothorax

The lateral view is more sensitive for detecting a small volume of free air in the pleural space. The lung border appears separated from the diaphragm and dorsal thoracic wall; the heart shifts toward the dependent lung and looks elevated from the sternum. On DV/VD view, the lungs retract from the chest wall; a DV view more readily reveals free air,

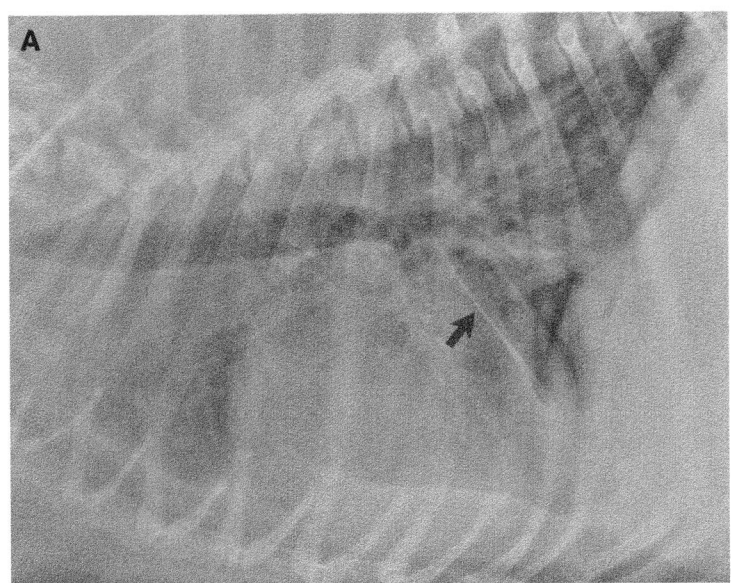
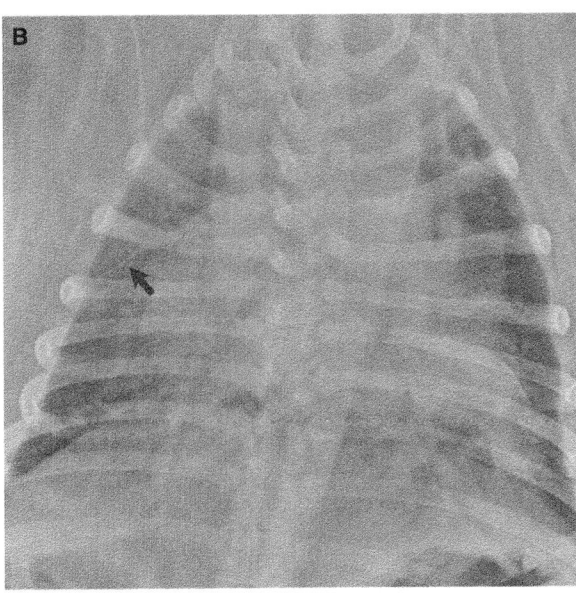

Figure 3.23 Pleural fissure lines (arrows) on both lateral (A) and DV (B) radiographs indicate mild pleural effusion in a 6-year-old neutered male Bulldog with severe pulmonary disease, moderate pulmonary hypertension, and cor pulmonale. A diffuse, patchy increase in pulmonary opacity is worse in the left caudal region.

which rises to the widest (dorsal) part of the thorax. With larger amounts of free air, the relatively collapsed lungs appear more opaque.

Pneumothorax sometimes is misdiagnosed on a lateral view when the heart appears to be separated from the sternum, as with hypovolemia (microcardia), very narrow deep-chested conformation, lung hyperinflation, left lateral recumbency, or causes of a mediastimal shift. On DV/VD view, skinfolds sometimes are mistaken for pneumothorax. Regions where free air is suspected should be inspected carefully; subtle markings from vessels or bronchi indicate aerated lung is present.

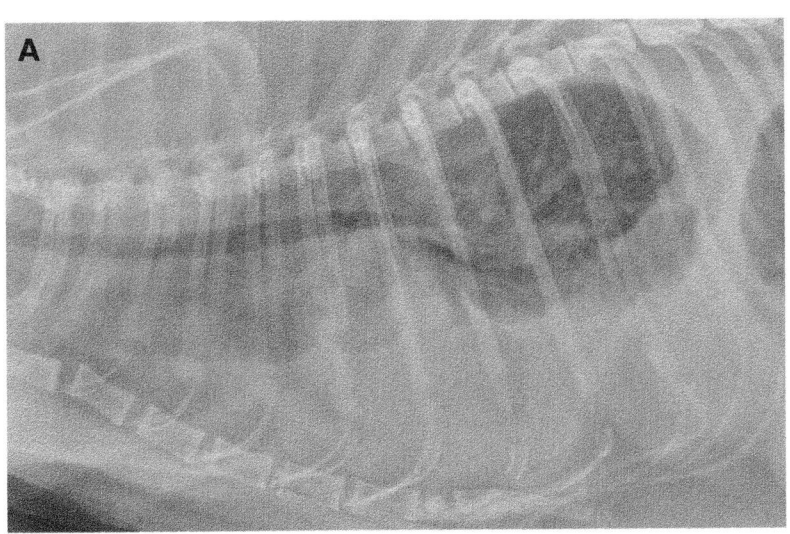
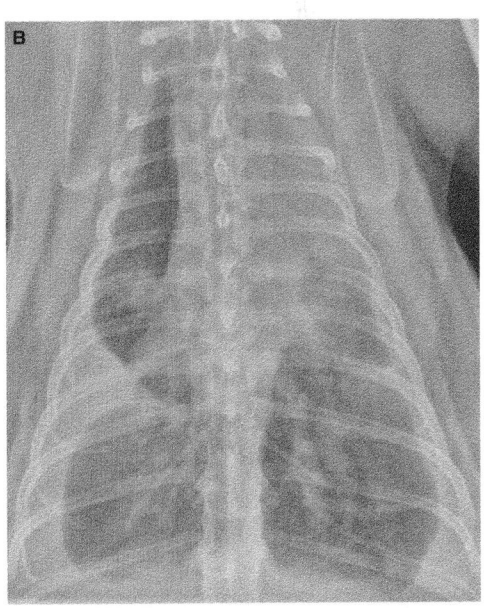

Figure 3.24 Lateral (A) and DV (B) radiographs show marked pleural effusion in an 11-year-old neutered male cat with hypertrophic cardiomyopathy and chronic congestive heart failure. The cat was presented for respiratory distress. The left caudal pulmonary lobar vessels are distended (B) and concurrent pulmonary edema is likely. Pulmonary edema alone originally developed 2 1/2 years earlier; initial onset of pleural effusion occurred a year later.

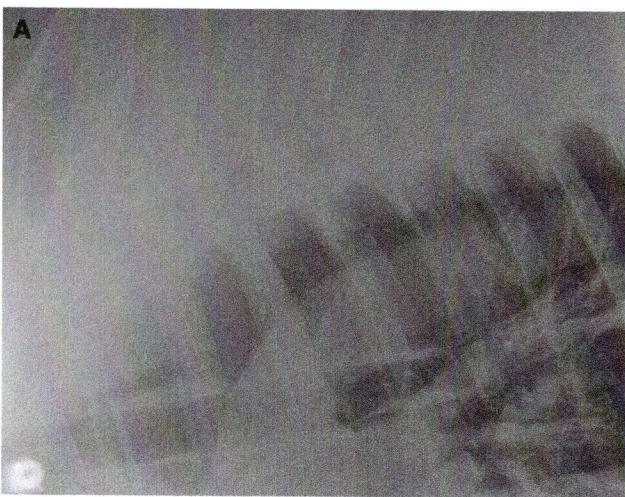 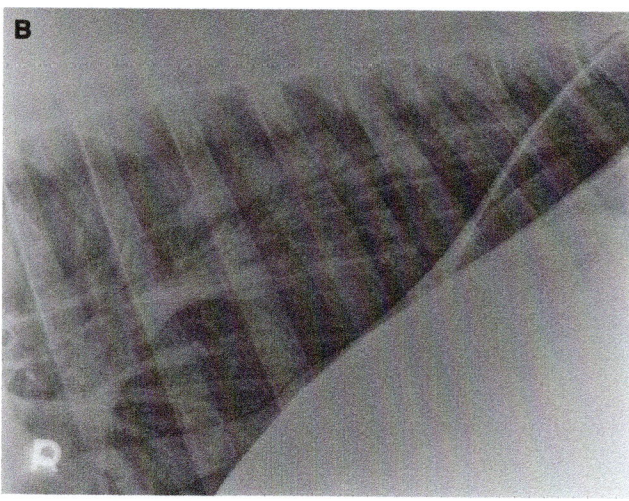

Figure 3.25 Craniodorsal (A) and caudodorsal (B) radiographs from a normal 3-year-old Quarter horse gelding. The dorsal heart border, cranial aorta, and caudal trachea are well delineated in (A). The caudal aspect of the left atrium, caudal vena cava, and caudal lung regions are visible in (B); the diaphragm occupies the lower right aspect of the image.

Equine Thoracic Radiography

Thoracic radiography of the mature equine thorax can be performed in "segments" using lateral projections. In general, the equipment needed to expose thoracic radiographs in the horse is found at larger equine centers and referral hospitals. When performed, four lateral images usually are obtained (cranioventral, craniodorsal, caudoventral, and caudodorsal). Despite the possibilities of radiography, cardiomegaly is far easier to recognize using ultrasound in this species. Images of the dorsocaudal lung fields can be instructive in terms of identifying pulmonary infiltration (compare **Figures 3.25** and **3.26**) and pleural effusion. However, edema must be distinguished from more common interstitial pneumonias or other inflammatory pulmonary diseases. Moreover, thoracic ultrasound can be used effectively to identify intrapulmonary densities (lung rockets, pulmonary consolidation) and is more sensitive for finding small pleural effusions. One specific use of radiography is for additional guidance during placement of the radiopaque electrode catheters used in transvenous cardioversion of atrial fibrillation (p. 392). Overall, thoracic radiography plays a minor role in the recognition of heart disease and failure in horses.

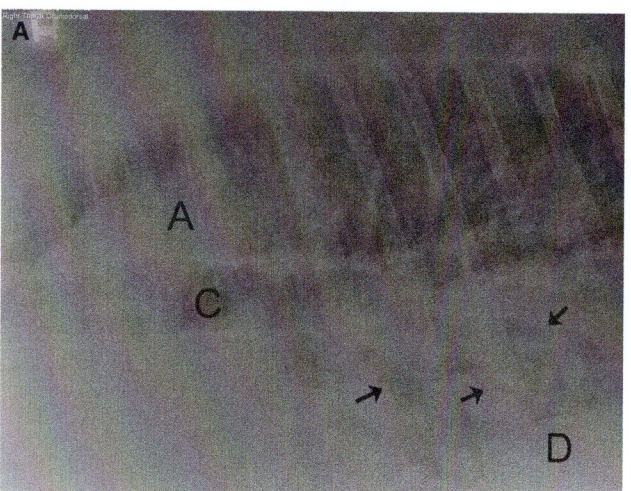 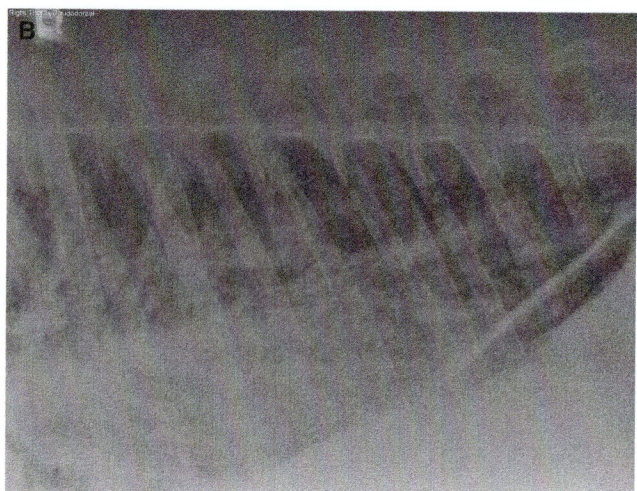

Figure 3.26 Craniodorsal (A) and caudodorsal (B) radiographs from a 10-year-old Paint mare with congestive heart failure and severe pulmonary edema. Pulmonary opacity is greatest in the hilar and central lung regions, but also extends to the periphery. The caudal cardiac border and vascular margins are obscured. Air bronchograms (arrows) are evident in (A). A, cranial descending aorta; C, carina; D, diaphragm.

Additional Cardiac Imaging Modalities

CT imaging can allow better differentiation of specific tissue densities within the thorax and detect subtle changes in the size, shape, or position of structures (**Figure 3.27**). CT is more sensitive than plain thoracic radiography for identifying pulmonary nodules, bronchiectasis, and interstitial lung diseases, such as fibrosis (Armbrust, 2012; Johnson, 2005). CT angiography, with volume rendering, can provide a three-dimensional view of the cardiac and pulmonary vasculature. This is useful for identifying and defining congenital CV lesions, especially those involving the great vessels (**Figures 28.12**, **28.13**, and **28.18**, p 517, 518, and 520), and also thromboembolic disease (**Figure 36.6**, p. 753). Optimal image resolution requires ECG gating and a period of breath-holding. The need for anesthesia or deep sedation and use of potentially toxic contrast agent and ionizing radiation are limitations.

MRI allows detailed views of soft tissue, especially the heart and great vessels, as well as some surrounding structures without employing ionizing radiation. Both CT and MRI yield excellent spatial resolution, although MRI provides better temporal resolution than CT. Temporal resolution, for both modes, can be improved by reconstructing single images from multiple cardiac cycles; however, sinus arrhythmia and extrasystoles can cause erroneous data reconstruction. Besides the need for anesthesia, MRI (and CT) involves greater expense than other current imaging modalities. They also are more time-intensive and have limited availability.

Both CT and MRI could provide better estimation of cardiac volumes and ejection fraction using the Simpson method compared to one- or two-dimensional echocardiography, which require geometric assumptions to calculate volume. CT might overestimate LV diastolic volume; however, for systolic volume, stroke volume, and ejection fraction there appears to be no difference between CT and MRI modalities (Sieslack, 2013). Although myocardial function assessments can be done with MRI, there are additional challenges, especially related to heart rate, veterinary patient size, and costs and availability of this technology for cardiac studies.

Nuclear imaging studies also can aid in evaluating CV shunts, and myocardial function or perfusion. The most commonly used radiopharmaceutical is ^{99m}technetium (pertechnetate). First-pass radionuclide angiocardiography can be used to identify and estimate the severity of shunts within the heart or proximal great vessels. The compound ^{99m}technetium-macroaggregated albumin is used in animals suspected to have a right-to-left shunt. These larger particles normally are trapped in the lung; however, a right-to-left shunting defect allows radioactivity to be detected in other parts of the body. ECG-gated equilibrium radionucleotide angiocardiography can assess ventricular volume changes through the cardiac cycle and allow estimation of ejection fraction. However, complicating factors include heart rate variation from sinus arrhythmia and the superimposition of RV and LV radioactivity. Nuclear imaging studies also can be used to screen for areas of myocardial ischemia or scarring. These studies use different radiopharmaceuticals (such as ^{201}Thallium, ^{82}rubidium, or others) and alternate imaging techniques (such as single photon emission CT or positron emission tomography), rather than the traditional gamma camera.

Suggested Additional Reading and References

Also See Online Comprehensive Bibliography at: https://www.routledge.com/9781482246223.

Armbrust LJ, Biller DS, Bamford A, et al. Comparison of three-view thoracic radiography and computed tomography for detection of pulmonary nodules in dogs with neoplasia. J Am Vet Med Assoc 2012;240:1088–1094.

Bavegems V, Van Caelenberg A, Duchateau L, et al. Vertebral heart size ranges specific for whippets. Vet Radiol Ultrasound 2005;46:400–403.

Benigni L, Morgan N, Lamb CR. Radiographic appearance of cardiogenic pulmonary oedema in 23 cats. J Small Anim Pract 2009;50:9–14.

Birks R, Fine DM, Leach SB, et al. Breed-specific vertebral heart scale for the Dachshund. J Am Anim Hosp Assoc 2017;53:73–79.

Bodh D, Hoque M, Saxena AC, et al. Vertebral scale system to measure heart size in thoracic radiographs of Indian Spitz, Labrador Retriever and Mongrel dogs. Vet World 2016;9:371–376.

Boswood A, Gordon SG, Haggstrom J, et al. Temporal changes in clinical and radiographic variables in dogs with preclinical myxomatous mitral valve disease: the EPIC study. J Vet Intern Med 2020;34:1108–1118.

Bouyssou S, Specchi S, Desquilbet L, et al. Radiographic appearance of presumed noncardiogenic pulmonary edema and correlation with the underlying cause in dogs and cats. Vet Radiol & Ultrasound 2017;58:259–265.

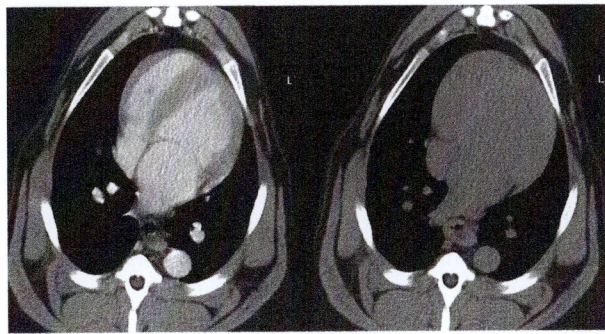

Figure 3.27 Transverse thoracic CT images from a normal dog (dorsal recumbency) at the level of the heart. Image on the left is after IV contrast injection and delineates the four cardiac chambers. Left ventricle and atrium are to the right in each image. L, left.

Brown CS, Johnson LR, Visser LC, et al. Comparison of fluoroscopic cardiovascular measurements from healthy dogs obtained at end-diastole and end-systole. J Vet Cardiol 2020;29:1–10.

Buchanan JW. Vertebral scale system to measure heart size in radiographs. Vet Clin North Am Small Anim Pract 2000;30:379–393.

Buchanan JW, Bucheler J. Vertebral scale system to measure canine heart size in radiographs. J Am Vet Med Assoc 1995;206:194–199.

Carolina ABC. Radiographic evaluation of the cardiac silhouette in clinically normal poodles through the vertebral heart size (VHS) method. Braz J Vet Res Anim Sci 2004;41:261–266.

Coulson A, Lewis ND. An Atlas of Interpretive Radiographic Anatomy of the Dog and Cat. Blackwell Science, Oxford, UK. 2002.

Daniel GB, Berry CR (editors). Textbook of Veterinary Nuclear Medicine. American College of Veterinary Radiology, Harrisburg, PA. 2006.

De Rycke LM, Gielen IM, Simoens PJ, et al. Computed tomography and cross-sectional anatomy of the thorax in clinically normal dogs. Am J Vet Res 2005;66:512–524.

Diana A, Guglielmini C, Pivetta M, et al. Radiographic features of cardiogenic pulmonary edema in dogs with mitral regurgitation: 61 cases (1998–2007). J Am Vet Med Assoc 2009;235:1058–1063.

Duler L, LeBlanc NL, Cooley S, et al. Interreader agreement of radiographic left atrial enlargement in dogs and comparison to echocardiographic left atrial assessment. J Vet Cardiol 2018;20:319–329.

Drost WT. Transitioning to digital radiography. J Vet Emerg Crit Care 2011;21:137–143.

Farrow CS, Green R, Shively M. Radiology of the Cat. Mosby, St. Louis, MO. 1994. pp. 46–130.

Greco A, Meomartino L, Raiano V, et al. Effect of left vs. right recumbency on the vertebral heart score in normal dogs. Vet Radiol Ultrasound 2008;49:454–455.

Guglielmini C, Baron Toaldo M, Poser H, et al. Diagnostic accuracy of the vertebral heart score and other radiographic indices in the detection of cardiac enlargement in cats with different cardiac disorders. J Feline Med Surg 2014;16:812–825.

Guglielmini C, Baron Toaldo M, Quinci M, et al. Sensitivity, specificity, and interobserver variability of survey thoracic radiography for the detection of heart base masses in dogs. J Am Vet Med Assoc 2016;248:1391–1398.

Guglielmini C, Diana A. Thoracic radiography in the cat: identification of cardiomegaly and congestive heart failure. J Vet Cardiol 2015;17:S87–S101.

Guglielmini C, Diana A, Santarelli G, et al. Accuracy of radiographic vertebral heart score and sphericity index in the detection of pericardial effusion in dogs. J Am Vet Med Assoc 2012;241:1048–1055.

Gulanber EG, Gonenci R, Kaya U, et al. Vertebral scale system to measure heart size in thoracic radiographs of Turkish Shepherd (Kangal) dogs. Turk J Vet Anim Sci 2005;29:723–726.

Hansson K, Haggstrom J, Kvart C, et al. Interobserver variability of vertebral heart size measurements in dogs with normal and enlarged hearts. Vet Radiol Ultrasound 2005;46:122–130.

Hayward NJ, Baines SJ, Baines EA, et al. The radiographic appearance of the pulmonary vasculature in the cat. Vet Radiol Ultrasound 2004;45:501–504.

Jepsen-Grant K, Pollard RE, Johnson LR. Vertebral heart scores in eight dog breeds. Vet Radiol Ultrasound 2013;54:3–8.

Johnson VS, Corcoran BM, Wotton PR, et al. Thoracic high-resolution computed tomographic findings in dogs with canine idiopathic pulmonary fibrosis. J Small Anim Pract 2005;46:381–388.

Keyserling CL, Buriko Y, Lyons BM, et al. Evaluation of thoracic radiographs as a screening test for dogs and cats admitted to a tertiary-care veterinary hospital for noncardiopulmonary disease. Vet Radiol Ultrasound 2017;58:503–511.

Kraetschmer S, Ludwig K, Meneses F, et al. Vertebral heart scale in the beagle dog. J Small Anim Pract 2008;49:240–243.

Lamb CR, Nelson JR. Diagnostic accuracy of tests based on radiologic measurements of dogs and cats: a systematic review. Vet Radiol Ultrasound 2015;56: 231–244.

Lamb CR, Wikeley H, Boswood A, et al. Use of breed-specific ranges for the vertebral heart scale as an aid to the radiographic diagnosis of cardiac disease in dogs. Vet Rec 2001;148: 707–711.

Lehmkuhl LB, Bonagura JD, Biller DS, et al. Radiographic evaluation of caudal vena cava size in dogs. Vet Radiol Ultrasound 1997;38:94–100.

Lisciandro GR, Fulton RM, Fosgate GT, et al. Frequency and number of B-lines using a regionally based lung ultrasound examination in cats with radiographically normal lungs compared to cats with left-sided congestive heart failure. J Vet Emerg Crit Care 2017;27:499–505.

Litster AL, Buchanan JW. Radiographic and echocardiographic measurement of the heart in obese cats. Vet Radiol Ultrasound 2000;41:320–325.

Lord PF, Hansson K, Carnabuci C, et al. Radiographic heart size and its rate of increase as tests for onset of congestive heart failure in Cavalier King Charles Spaniels with mitral valve regurgitation. J Vet Intern Med 2011;25:1312–1319. Erratum in: J Vet Intern Med. 2012;26:223.

Luciani MG, Withoeft JA, Mondardo Cardoso Pissetti H, et al. Vertebral heart size in healthy Australian cattle dog. Anat Histol Embryol 2019;48:264–267.

MacDonald KA, Kittleson MD, Garcia-Nolen T, et al. Tissue Doppler imaging and gradient echo cardiac magnetic resonance imaging in normal cats and cats with hypertrophic cardiomyopathy. J Vet Intern Med 2006;20:627–634.

Malcolm EL, Visser LC, Phillips KL, et al. Diagnostic value of vertebral left atrial size as determined from thoracic radiographs for assessment of left atrial size in dogs with myxomatous mitral valve disease. J Am Vet Med Assoc 2018;253: 1038–1045.

Marin LM, Brown J, McBrien C, et al. Vertebral heart size in retired racing Greyhounds. Vet Radiol Ultrasound 2007;48:332–334.

Mikawa S, Nagakawa M, Ogi H, et al. Use of vertebral left atrial size for staging of dogs with myxomatous valve disease. J Vet Cardiol 2020;30:92–99.

Morandi F, Daniel GB, Gompf RE, et al. Diagnosis of congenital cardiac right-to-left shunts with 99mTc-macroaggregated albumin. Vet Radiol Ultrasound 2004;45:97–102.

Mostafa AA, Berry CR. Radiographic assessment of the cardiac silhouette in clinically normal large- and small-breed dogs. Am J Vet Res 2017;78:168–177.

Mostafa AA, Peper KE, Berry CR. Use of cardiac sphericity index and manubrium heart scores to assess radiographic cardiac silhouettes in large- and small-breed dogs with and without cardiac disease. J Am Vet Med Assoc 2020;256:288–896.

O'Brien RT. Thoracic Radiography for the Small Animal Practitioner. Teton NewMedia, Jackson, WY. 2001.

Olive J, Javard R, Specchi S, et al. Effect of cardiac and respiratory cycles on vertebral heart score measured on fluoroscopic images of healthy dogs. J Am Vet Med Assoc 2015;246:1091–1097.

Oui H, Oh J, Keh S, et al. Measurements of the pulmonary vasculature on thoracic radiographs in healthy dogs compared to dogs with mitral regurgitation. Vet Radiol Ultrasound 2015;56:251–256.

Oura TJ, Young AN, Keene BW, et al. A valentine-shaped cardiac silhouette in feline thoracic radiographs is primarily due to left atrial enlargement. Vet Radiol Ultrasound 2015;56:245–250.

Pinto AC, Iwasaki M. Radiographic methods in the cardiac evaluation in dogs. Veterinaria Noticias. Univ Fed Uberlandia Brazil 2002;8:67–75.

Puccinelli C, Citi S, Vezzosi T, et al. A radiographic study of breed-specific vertebral heart score and vertebral left atrial size in Chihuahuas. Vet Radiol Ultrasound 2020.

Sanchez X, Prandi D, Badiella L, et al. A new method of computing the vertebral heart scale by means of direct standardisation. J Small Anim Pract 2012;53:641–645.

Schober KE, Maerz I, Ludewig E, et al. Diagnostic accuracy of electrocardiography and thoracic radiography in the assessment of left atrial size in cats: comparison with transthoracic 2-dimensional echocardiography. J Vet Intern Med 2007;21:709–718.

Schober KE, Wetli E, Drost WT. Radiographic and echocardiographic assessment of left atrial size in 100 cats with acute left-sided congestive heart failure. Vet Radiol Ultrasound 2014;55:359–367.

Scollan KF, Bottorff B, Stieger-Vanegas S, et al. Use of multidetector computed tomography in the assessment of dogs with pericardial effusion. J Vet Intern Med 2015;29:79–87.

Sieslack AK, Dziallas P, Nolte I, et al. Comparative assessment of left ventricular function variables determined via cardiac computed tomography and cardiac magnetic resonance imaging in dogs. Am J Vet Res 2013;74:990–998.

Sleeper MM, Buchanan JW. Vertebral scale system to measure heart size in growing puppies. J Am Vet Med Assoc 2001;219:57–59.

Sleeper MM, Roland R, Drobatz KJ. Use of vertebral heart scale for differentiation of cardiac and noncardiac causes of respiratory distress in cats: 67 cases (2002–2003). J Am Vet Med Assoc 2013; 242:366–371.

Stepien RL, Rak MB, Blume LM. Use of radiographic measurements to diagnose stage B2 preclinical myxomatous mitral valve disease in dogs. J Am Vet Med Assoc 2020;256:1129–1136.

Taylor CJ, Simon BT, Stanley BJ, et al. Norwich Terriers possess a greater vertebral heart scale than the canine reference value. Vet Radiol Ultrasound 2020;61:10–15.

Thrall DE (editor). Textbook of Veterinary Diagnostic Radiology. 6th edition. Elsevier, St. Louis, MO. 2013.

Toal RL, Losonsky JM, Coulter DB, et al. Influence of cardiac cycle on the radiographic appearance of the feline heart. Vet Radiol 1985;26:63–69.

Vezzosi T, Mannucci T, Pistoresi A, et al. Assessment of lung ultrasound B-lines in dogs with different stages of chronic valvular heart disease. J Vet Intern Med 2017;31:700–704.

Vezzosi T, Puccinelli C, Tognetti R, et al. Radiographic vertebral left atrial size: A reference interval study in healthy adult dogs. Vet Radiol Ultrasound 2020;61:507–511.

Ward JL, Lisciandro GR, Keene BW, et al. Accuracy of point-of-care lung ultrasonography for the diagnosis of cardiogenic pulmonary edema in dogs and cats with acute dyspnea. J Am Vet Med Assoc 2017;250:666–675.

Winter MD, Giglio RF, Berry CR, et al. Associations between "valentine" heart shape, atrial enlargement and cardiomyopathy in cats. J Feline Med Surg 2015;17:447–452.

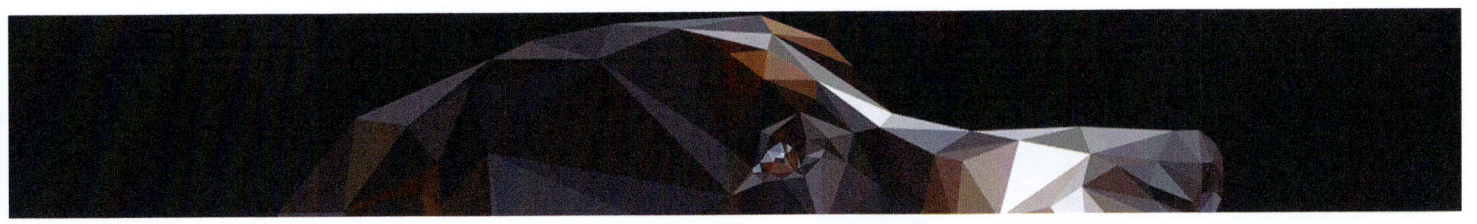

4
ECHOCARDIOGRAPHY

Cardiac ultrasound (US), or echocardiography, is the noninvasive gold standard for assessing heart disease. Echocardiographic (echo) examination offers the best available balance between convenience, availability, cost-effectiveness, and diagnostic yield. Cardiac US delineates both the morphology and function of the heart, along with the appearance of contiguous great arteries and venous entries. Pleural and pericardial effusions, mass lesions within or around the heart, and most serious congenital and acquired diseases of cardiac valves, myocardium, and great arteries are readily visualized by US imaging. When Doppler echo studies are included, the velocity patterns of normal and abnormal blood flow can be tracked. Complementary Doppler modalities deliver quantitative estimates of heart function, intracardiac pressures, and blood flow.

General Considerations

Three imaging modalities currently predominate in veterinary medicine: Two-dimensional (2D) grayscale cardiac imaging, the motion or M-mode study, and various forms of Doppler echocardiography. The foundation for most echo examinations is 2D imaging, also known as brightness or B-mode imaging. This modality generates the many adjacent lines of US that compose the 2D image frame. These images are updated rapidly (at rates of 30–120 per second with modern equipment) to create "real-time" cardiac motion, which is subsequently stored in digital video loops for subjective and quantitative analysis. Both M-mode and Doppler studies are guided by the anatomic template provided by 2D imaging. These echo modalities are complementary. Three- and four-dimensional (3D and 4D) echo imaging with various analyses based on artificial intelligence algorithms also are available, but are expensive and rarely used in routine practice. We consider such advanced methods only briefly in this chapter.

A transthoracic, "parasternal" (intercostal) approach is used for nearly all canine, feline, and equine echo studies (**Figures 4.1** and **4.2**). Limited subcostal imaging windows also are used for small animals. Specialized, endoscope-mounted transducers are available for transesophageal imaging. Transesophageal echocardiography (TEE) requires general anesthesia and mainly is used to guide interventional catheterization procedures.

As with any diagnostic test, the echocardiogram should be interpreted within the context of the patient's history, cardiovascular (CV) examination findings, and other imaging and laboratory test results. The principles of echo examination and interpretation are similar across species. Three critical elements affect the usefulness of echocardiography:

- Technical proficiency in performing the study
- The examiner's understanding of CV anatomy, disease, and pathologic physiology
- The availability of US equipment appropriate for the patient under study

For example, it is nearly impossible to image a cat effectively using a transducer optimal for a large dog. It follows that point-of-care (POC) US systems with a single transducer are limited in the range of patient sizes that can be evaluated effectively. Conversely, a US system equipped with several carefully selected transducers can provide optimal imaging for patients of wide-ranging size. Operators should scale their echo examinations to their level of training, experience, and knowledge. As with any advanced technique, echo methods and interpretation are learned in stages, to minimize missed or erroneous diagnoses (Bonagura, 2020). Complicated cardiac cases, particularly those involving congenital disease, and patients with special imaging requirements are best referred to a specialist with the US imaging system and training sufficient to deliver a complete diagnosis and assessment. Similarly, asymptomatic patients with heart disease often are

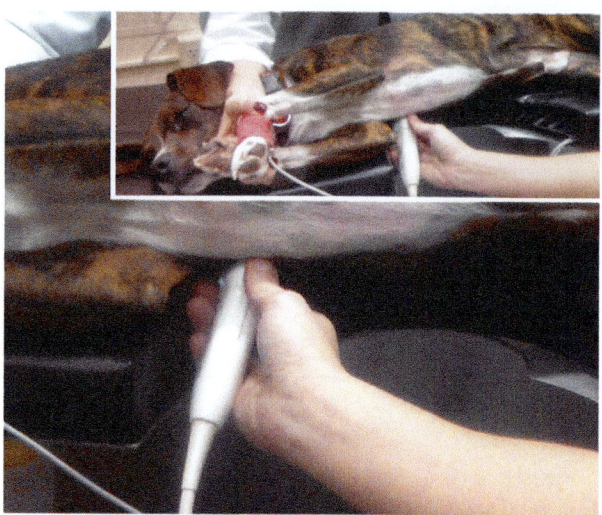

Figure 4.1 Recording a transthoracic echocardiogram in a dog using a cutout table. This method is widely used for dogs and cats. How the operator orients the transducer's index marker—under the thumb or index finger—determines the left/right orientation of the image. The console's electronic invert button should be used as needed to display the image conventionally (generally, cranial structures to the viewer's right side).

more challenging to evaluate than those with overt signs, such as congestive heart failure (CHF).

This chapter offers an introduction to transthoracic echocardiography (TTE) appropriate for general small animal and equine practices. More information related to US physics, technology, noncardiac imaging, and advanced image analysis can be found in section "Suggested Additional Readings and References." The chapter begins with an overview of principles, definitions, and technical issues. A general approach to diagnosis by echocardiography follows. Last, the individual echo modalities of importance to most veterinary practitioners are presented. Typical examples of normal imaging patterns are described, and useful reference values (when available) are provided for each modality. Some illustrative examples of their use in identifying and quantifying cardiac diseases also are given. Additional echo images and videos related to specific congenital and acquired diseases are included in the associated chapters and in the online repository.

Principles of Echocardiography

Physics and Terminology

Echocardiography uses pulsed, high-frequency sound waves, typically within the 2.0–13 megahertz (MHz) frequency bands (1 MHz = 1,000,000 cycles/second). Sound waves at these frequencies are inaudible and behave according to the laws of optics. As such, the US beam is transmitted, reflected, refracted, and absorbed, similar to visible light energy. Ultrasound is emitted in pulses when the transducer crystals are electrically shocked, or activated, to vibrate. When US encounters a tissue interface of different acoustic density, a small amount is reflected or "echoed" back to the transducer, while the balance continues to propagate through the far-field tissues. This US signal is progressively attenuated the deeper it travels away from the transducer face; greater signal loss occurs with higher-frequency transducers. Returning echoes deform the crystals, creating signals processed relative to time and space. The instant of US pulse emission, the timing of returned acoustic signals, and the average velocity of US propagation through tissues (~1,540 meters/second, or m/s) all are known; consequently, the spatial orientation of reflective interfaces or targets within the sound field can be determined.

The interaction between US and tissue depends in part on the characteristics of the reflective tissue interface. For example, a strong mirror like or specular reflector (such as the pericardium) returns a larger proportion of transmitted US back to the transducer. Such reflectors also generate prominent artifacts, including mirror images (discussed below). Specular reflectors, such as the tissue-blood interface within the heart and blood vessels, also tend to be visualized best when the incidence angle between the ultrasound beam and the target is 90 degrees. Right-sided parasternal long-axis views usually provide better images of the cardiac chambers because the US beam is oriented perpendicular to many structures; that is, they are imaged in axial resolution. Conversely, apical transducer placement orients the chamber walls roughly parallel to the US beam, leveraging the lateral resolution of the imaging system. Having the US beam parallel to blood flow is essential for accurate Doppler echocardiography; however, it produces 2D images of lower overall quality. Tissue reflectors that are irregular in shape create random scatterings of

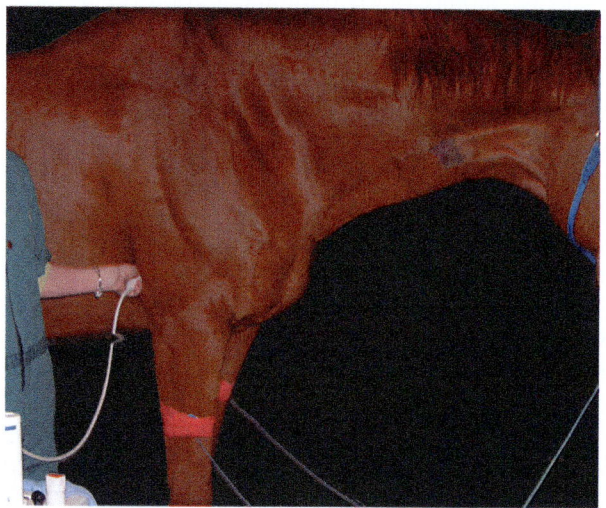

Figure 4.2 Recording a transthoracic echocardiogram in a standing horse. Notice the operator is resting the hand holding the transducer on the olecranon. Slightly advancing the animal's forelimb will facilitate transducer placement. The echo system has been moved away to show the hand position; typically, the operator would face in the same direction as the horse, with the system opposite the horse's shoulder. This method also can be used for giant-breed dogs; some examiners use this position routinely.

US; only that which returns to the transducer (backscatter) is processed. The resulting images tend to have various shades of gray relating to the transducer frequency and backscatter processing, which is controlled in part by the operator. Red blood cells (RBCs) scatter US in all directions and represent very weak reflectors. This explains why the blood pool is relatively devoid of echoes and specialized signal processing is needed to capture blood flow in Doppler echocardiography. Most automated imaging controls optimize the image to create an echo-free blood pool; this processing is useful, unless there is a specific desire to identify spontaneous or saline echocontrast within the chambers. Additionally, during color Doppler imaging, processing that minimizes grayscale within the chambers helps ensure that screen pixels can prioritize blood flow information.

Modern cardiac US systems emit numerous adjacent US lines from the transducer face and blend the returning echoes to compose a wedged-shaped, 2D image of grayscale dots or screen pixels. This extremely thin, planar image of the heart reveals both the relative position and intensity of the reflectors within the sound field. The echo image is calibrated in centimeters and measurements typically are made in cm or mm (as seen in the scales in the 2D and M-mode images of **Figure 4.3**). By repeatedly updating static images or frames over time, a 2D image of the beating heart is visualized in real-time (see supplemental media). Alternatively, a single line of echoes from moving US targets, graphed over time, is used to generate the M-mode image. The operator can make adjustments of the transducer and console controls to optimize the image plane and image quality.

Transducer Characteristics

A US transducer is a handheld instrument containing numerous crystal elements connected electrically to the echocardiograph system. Transducers convert one form of energy to another, and in the case of US, exhibit the property of piezoelectricity. This means that as transducer elements are shocked into vibration, they emit pulses of US from the transducer face; then, the returning US deforms the crystals, sending electrical signals back to the system. Thus, transducers function as both transmitters and receivers of US, although different elements might be involved with each task. Most modern transducers contain hundreds of crystal elements. Electronic activation and steering of this array in phase creates a wedge-shaped US beam, that when unfocused, widens as it leaves the transducer face. This beam is assumed to have a finite planar (x, y) sector shape, although there is also a width (z-axis) to the beam, from which some imaging artifacts can arise. There are both near and far fields within the sound beam. These are roughly delineated by an operator-controlled focal zone, where the beam narrows before it diverges into the far field. Unlike abdominal or vascular imaging, cardiac imaging uses only one focal zone to maintain temporal resolution. The positioning of the focal zone markedly influences the overall image resolution and the generation of far-field imaging artifacts.

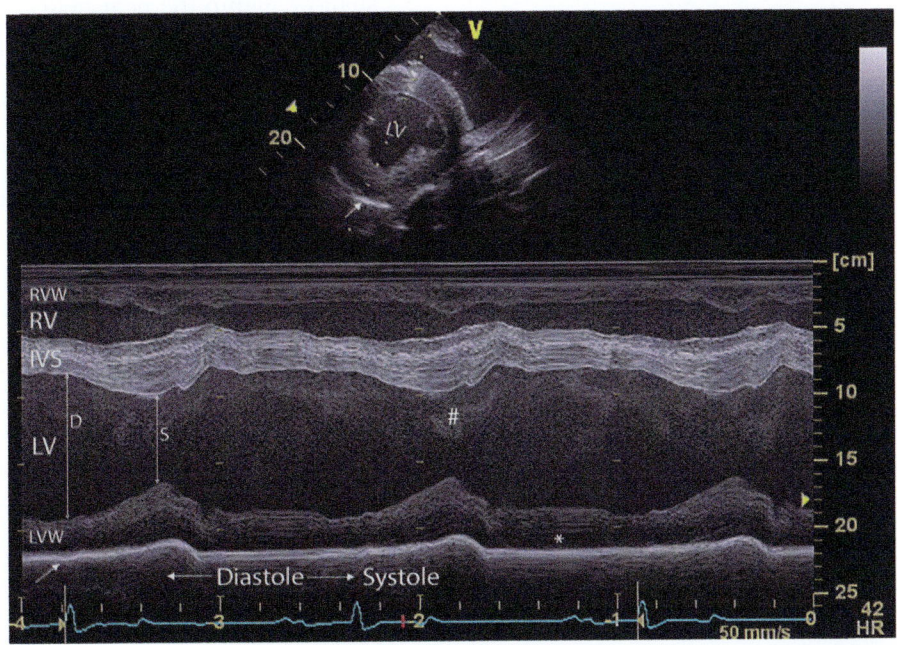

Figure 4.3 Duplex 2D (short-axis; top) and M-mode (bottom) echocardiographic image from a horse. Note calibration marks indicating the distance from the transducer face (in cm). This standard M-mode image was obtained across the ventricles and shows the right ventricular wall (RVW), right ventricular cavity (RV), interventricular septum (IVS), left ventricular cavity (LV), and left ventricular posterior wall (LVW). The bright reflection of the pericardium is evident (arrows). Note the changes over the cardiac cycle in LV diameter (D, diastole; S, systole) and in cardiac wall thicknesses. The LV fractional shortening is calculated as (D-S)/D and reported as a fraction or percentage. Spontaneous echocontrast (#)—a common finding in the horse—is present within the LV cavity. Differences in grayscale within the LV wall (*) can be confused with a pericardial effusion.

There is an important trade-off between image clarity (resolution) and US penetration based on transducer frequency. Higher-frequency US waves produce better resolution of small structures; however, these shorter wavelengths demonstrate less penetrating ability because more energy is absorbed and scattered by the tissue reflectors. Conversely, a transducer producing lower-frequency US offers greater depth of penetration but less resolution of adjacent structures. Typically, the highest frequency transducer that allows adequate penetration is selected for 2D and M-mode imaging.

One engineering solution to the penetration–resolution problem involves the use of harmonic (octave) imaging. A lower (fundamental) frequency of US is emitted within a relatively narrow frequency band, but only the octave frequency of returning US (generated by the tissues) is processed. For example, a transducer might emit at a fundamental frequency of 2.5 MHz, but the system processes images only from tissue vibrations in the 5 MHz band. The clinical utility of harmonic imaging depends on the US system and patient size. It is more useful in larger dogs and in horses, which are imaged at greater depths. Harmonic imaging is less valuable for cats and toy-breed dogs. Downsides to harmonic imaging include a significant reduction in frame rate and the potential for returning echoes to be "thicker," as is seen sometimes with cardiac valves. This situation can be identified by turning octaves "off" and converting back to fundamental frequency imaging.

Doppler imaging uses the opposite approach to transducer frequency. Lower frequency crystal elements within a transducer array are activated for greater sensitivity in detecting the direction and velocity of blood flow. The operator usually can adjust both 2D and Doppler frequencies independently in the system software or console. Learning to properly preset these controls is one key to obtaining high-quality echo images.

Optimal transducer frequencies for small animals range from approximately 2.5 to 5.0/5.0 to 10.0 MHz (fundamental/harmonic) for dogs and 8 to 13 MHz for cats. A lower-frequency transducer often is needed for optimal color flow and spectral Doppler imaging. For example, it might be appropriate to image a small dog or cat at 12 MHz and then drop down to a 7–9 MHz transducer for better Doppler sensitivity. Horses usually are imaged with transducers in the 1.5–4 MHz range; harmonic imaging often is useful, because their physiologic bradycardia permits quality imaging at lower frame rates. Although a typical transducer array consists of hundreds of elements with different frequency characteristics, most transducers work best near their central or "nominal" frequency. Accordingly, despite the purported frequency ranges advertised by vendors, adequately imaging patients of widely disparate body sizes using a single echo transducer is not feasible.

Practical Guidelines and Pitfalls

The heart is unique because of its rapidly changing motion over time. This presents a challenge for practitioners using a US system designed for imaging multiple body regions. Transducers used for superficial tissues, such as linear transducers, and imaging presets designed for static tissues such as those in the abdomen, are inappropriate for echocardiography. Practically, the most frequent trade-offs are between *image resolution and tissue penetration*, and between *overall image quality and temporal (time) resolution*. The latter is indicated by the frame rate/second during an examination. Some of the more important issues are outlined below.

Aside from system and equipment limitations, such as limited transducer availability, improper operator adjustments of the US system console often lead to inferior image quality. Some common adjustment errors are listed here:

- Using noncardiac presets
- Imaging with a 2D sector that is too wide or deep, leading to suboptimal frame rates; for example, <30 frames/second or <20/second for color imaging in dogs, and <60 frames/second or <30/second for color imaging in cats
- Scanning at frame rates that are excessively high (which degrades image quality)
- Setting image "quality" controls at the highest values (which increases line density but markedly reduces frame rate)
- Using excessive pixel averaging and persistence (which blurs the image)
- Using more than one transducer focal zone (another cause for slow frame rates)
- Using a transducer focal zone placement that is too shallow within the near field
- Failing to optimize the transmit power, the return gain, and the reject controls
- Not experimenting with various grayscale image options (such as image compression and grayscale maps or curves)
- Using harmonic imaging at shallow imaging depths of field

"Out of the box" imaging presets rarely are sufficient for optimal veterinary imaging; accomplished examiners learn how to adjust the console and create their own presets. Some of the technical details of setting up an echo system can be found in standard textbooks (Bonagura, 2020). For an initial setup, operators should:

- Select a depth of field just beyond the distal pericardium
- Modify the sector width to achieve frame rates of 30–60/second in dogs (for grayscale imaging)
- Move a single focal zone to just within the greatest depth of field
- Set gain, image "quality," and grayscale postprocessing and compression settings "to the middle"

Adjusting one single control at a time will often yield substantial differences. Most US systems incorporate automated gain and image processing controls; these are a good starting point before making further adjustments. Doppler settings require a more advanced understanding of control settings. Some of these controls are discussed below (see section "Doppler Echocardiography").

Image Properties

Certain terminology is used to describe US images. These are relative terms and the ultrasonic appearance of tissues is strongly influenced by transducer frequency, operator settings on the console, and the postprocessing of returned backscatter. Tissues that strongly reflect US are called "hyperechoic" or of greater "echogenicity." This is observed normally with the pericardium and valves, but might also be observed within pathologic regions of myocardial fibrosis or myocarditis. Poorly reflecting tissues are "hypoechoic," whereas targets such as fluid that do not reflect US are labeled "anechoic" or "sonolucent." Combinations of these patterns are "heterogeneous" or "mixed echoic," as observed in normal myocardial walls and with cardiac tumors. Closely located reflectors of different acoustic densities are common. One example is in the far field of right parasternal images, where the posterior papillary muscle and subendocardium appear more hyperechoic while the adjacent myocardium of the left ventricular (LV) wall seems nearly anechoic. This finding can prompt a misdiagnosis of pericardial effusion, especially in horses.

The strength of received echoes, along with image processing, determines the grayscale appearance of 2D images. The operator can adjust many of the factors controlling the image, while others depend on the character of the tissues and orientation of the beam. Highly reflective tissue boundaries, with a greater mismatch in acoustic impedance, produce stronger signals. Thus, signals of cardiac valves, aortic walls, endocardium, and parietal pericardium tend to be especially "bright" or hyperechoic. Practically, many of the highest-quality images will be obtained using long- and short-axis views from the right thorax and employing axial resolution. The opposite situation applies to Doppler imaging, where a US beam parallel to the direction of the moving blood or tissue targets provides optimal signal strength and the most accurate quantitation of flow velocity.

Ultrasound beam energy decreases as distance from the transducer increases because of beam divergence and the absorption, scatter, and reflection of soundwave energy. These factors reduce the intensity of echoes returning from deeper structures. Therefore, adjustments in the echo console's controls, such as time-gain compensation, are needed to optimize the signals. Highly reflective interfaces, such as bone/tissue or air/tissue, create artifacts that prevent visualization of deeper soft-tissue interfaces. However, tissue deep to a sonolucent near field can appear hyperechoic because more US energy reaches it; this is known as "acoustic enhancement" or through-transmission. Through-transmission of the US beam might be blocked by a strongly hyperechoic object, such as a rib, which casts an acoustic (dark) shadow in the far field. An air/fluid interface can create strong near-field reverberation artifacts that extend across the far field. These are both impediments and of diagnostic value (see section "Clinical Utility of Imaging Artifacts").

Image Planes and Display

Grayscale, real-time (updated) 2D imaging is the most important modality currently used for cardiologic evaluation in veterinary medicine. A well-conducted 2D examination is fundamental both to basic and advanced imaging studies. However, the examiner must understand the 3D structure of the heart and the need to acquire images from multiple and orthogonal 2D tomographic planes. These views are described as long-axis, short-axis, apical, and angled (**Figures 4.4–4.13**). Additionally transducer placements at the subcostal or subxiphoid positions are useful for evaluating the caudal vena cava (CaVC) and hepatic veins, and aligning Doppler images to the LV outflow tract in dogs. In distinction to (human) medicine, and because of the different thoracic conformation of our canine, feline and equine patients, most veterinary long- and short-axis images are obtained from right-sided, intercostal transducer positions. These views place the right atrium (RA) or ventricle in the near field (closest to the transducer), image most of the chamber walls using axial resolution, and can extend from cardiac

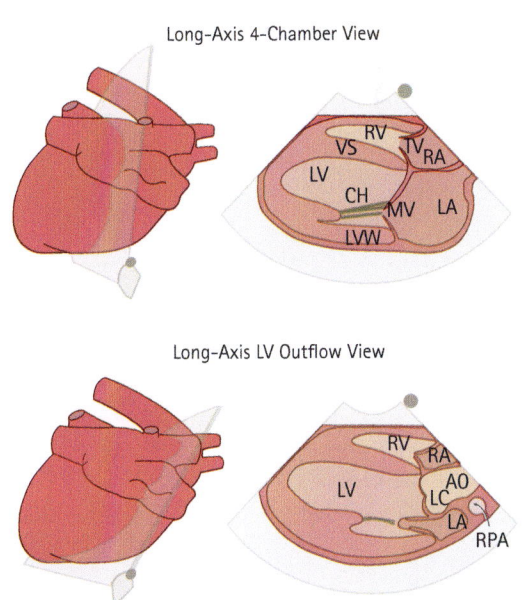

Figure 4.4 Drawings of right parasternal (intercostal) long-axis views optimized for the LV inlet (top) and the LV outlet (bottom). Ao, aorta; CH, chordae tendineae; LA, left atrium; LC, left coronary cusp of aortic valve; LV, left ventricle; LVW, left ventricular wall; MV, mitral valve; PA, pulmonary artery (trunk); RA, right atrium; RPA, right pulmonary artery; RV, right ventricle; TV, tricuspid valve; VS, (inter)ventricular septum. (From Thomas WP et al. Recommendations for standards in transthoracic two-dimensional echocardiography in the dog and cat. J Vet Intern Med 1993;7:247–252.)

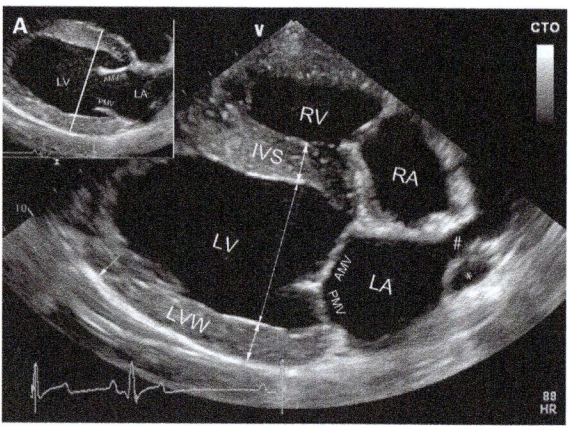
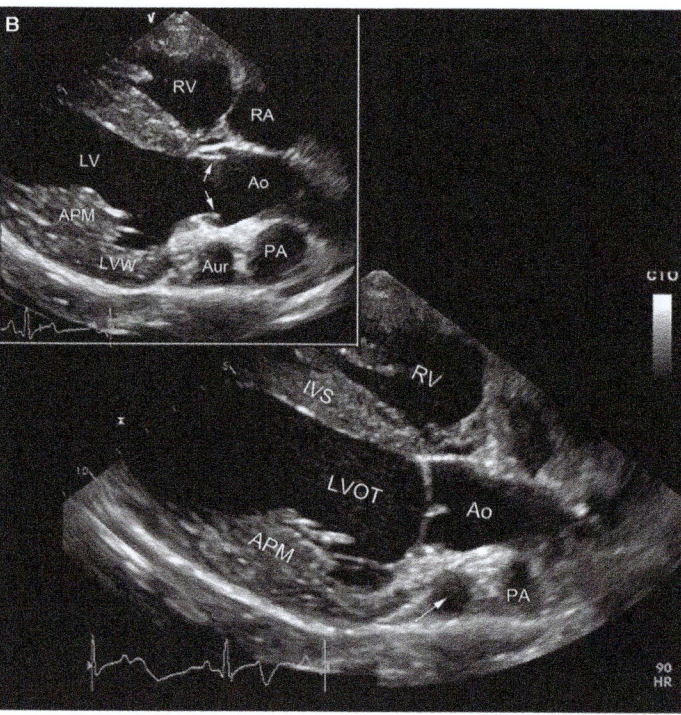

Figure 4.5 Long-axis images from a dog optimized for the LV inlet (A) and LV outflow tract (B). Compare these to **Figure 4.4**. (A) Double-headed arrows indicate wall and chamber dimensions. Single-headed arrow indicates the reflection of the pericardium. The right pulmonary vein (#) and artery (*) are adjacent (dorsal) to the LA. Inset shows the LV during diastole with a line crossing the chordal level. (B) Single arrow points to a portion of the left atrial appendage. Main image obtained during diastole. The inset, during systole, shows the opened aortic valve leaflets (arrows). AMV, anterior mitral valve leaflet; APM, anterior papillary muscle; Aur, (left) auricle; IVS, interventricular septum; LVOT, left ventricular outflow tract; PA, (right) pulmonary artery; PMV, posterior mitral valve leaflet. Other abbreviations as in **Figure 4.4**.

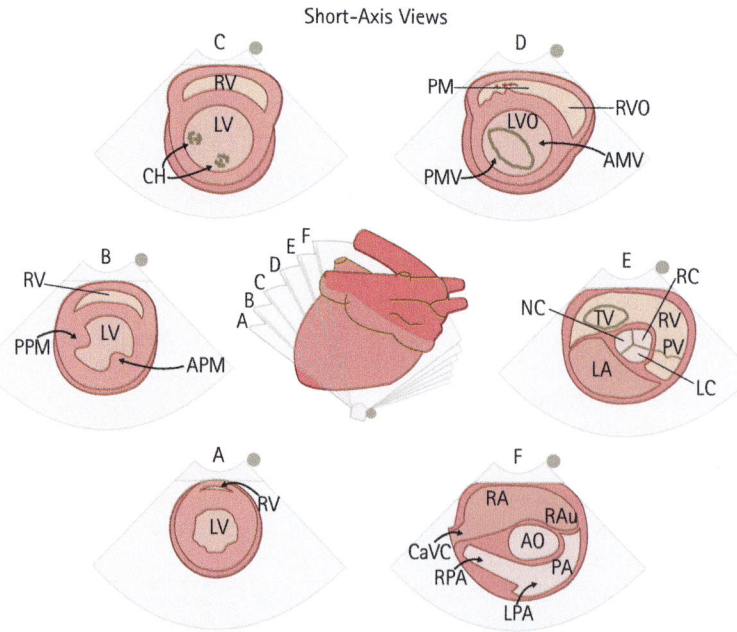

Figure 4.6 Drawings of right parasternal (intercostal) short-axis views recorded at right angles to the long-axis images shown in **Figure 4.4**. Progressive dorsal angulation (A to F) demonstrates different tomographic planes. AMV, anterior mitral valve leaflet; APM, anterior papillary muscle; CaVC, caudal vena cava; LPA, left pulmonary artery; LVO, left ventricular outflow tract; NC and RC, noncoronary and right coronary cusps of aortic valve; PA, pulmonary artery; PM, papillary muscles; PMV, posterior mitral valve leaflet; PPM, posterior papillary muscle; PV, pulmonary valve; RAu, right auricle; RVO, right ventricular outflow tract. Other abbreviations as in **Figure 4.4**. (From Thomas WP, et al. Recommendations for standards in transthoracic two-dimensional echocardiography in the dog and cat. J Vet Intern Med 1993;7:247–252.)

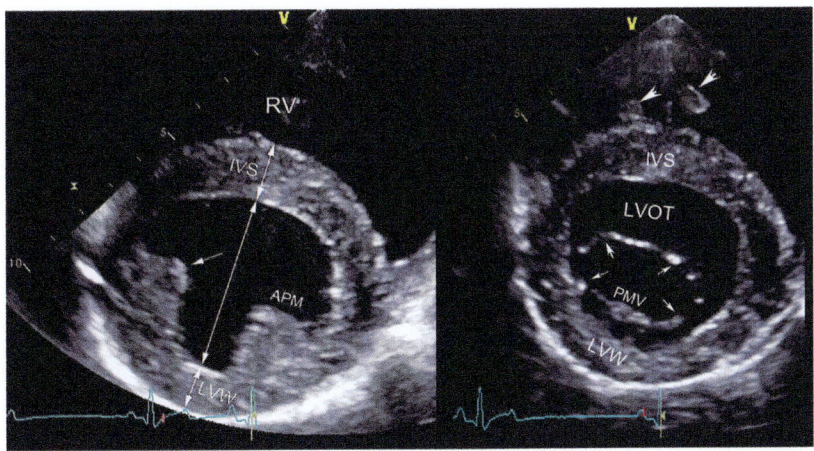

Figure 4.7 Short-axis images from a dog obtained at the levels of the papillary muscles and mitral valve. Compare these to **Figure 4.6**, planes B and D. The left panel shows the "high" papillary muscle level, with a chordal attachment at the posterior papillary muscle (arrow); double-headed arrow lines show diastolic measurements for the interventricular ventricular septum (IVS), LV cavity, and LV wall. The right panel shows the two leaflets of the mitral valve open in diastole (small arrows) in this so-called "fish-mouth" view of the valve. Two papillary muscles in the RV are evident in cross-section (arrowheads). Abbreviations as in **Figures 4.4–4.6**.

base to apex. Short-axis images are collected by rotating the transducer about 90 degrees from the long-axis views and sweeping the sector from apex to base. Apical views generally are recorded from the left caudoventral intercostal spaces. These are "long-axis" images of the heart; however, the near field displays the apical regions of the left and right ventricles. Angled images are usually hybrid, showing some structures in long and others in short axis.

Conventions of imaging dictate that cranial and dorsal structures should be oriented toward the observer's right side (although regrettably, this standard often is ignored in veterinary examinations). Thus, atria and great vessels are displayed on the right side of the viewing screen. Most examiners place the reference notch of the transducer—which corresponds to the vendor icon on the 2D image—under either their thumb or their forefinger; either approach generates an image flipped 180 degrees from the other. Regardless of how the transducer is held and rotated, the electronic left/right (L/R) inversion switch on the echo system should be activated to achieve the standard orientation of cranial structures and great vessels to the right side of the display. Exceptions to this guideline are used for left apical four- and five-chamber images, in which the left ventricle is displayed to the viewer's right.

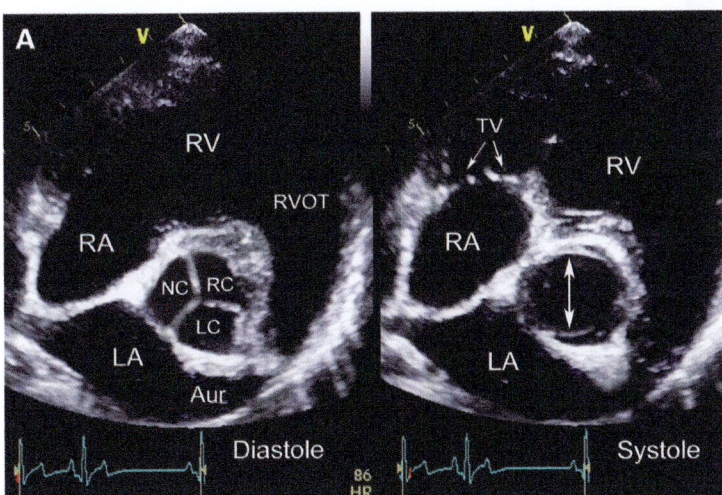
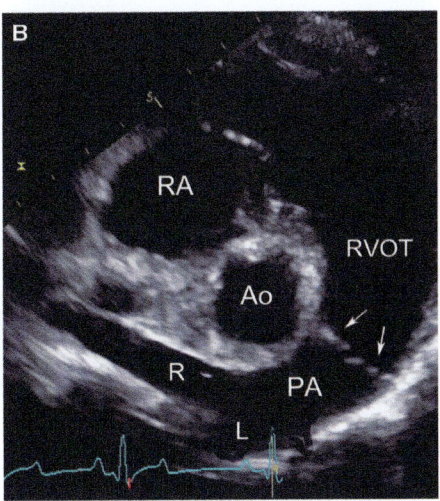

Figure 4.8 Short-axis images from a dog obtained at the levels of the aorta/left atrium (A) and the pulmonary artery (B). Compare these to **Figure 4.6** planes E and F. (A) Images show structures in diastole (left) and systole (right; aortic valve open, double-headed arrow). (B) Image (in diastole) is optimized to show the bifurcation of the pulmonary artery. The pulmonary valve is closed (arrows). RVOT, right ventricular outflow tract; other abbreviations as in **Figures 4.4–4.6**.

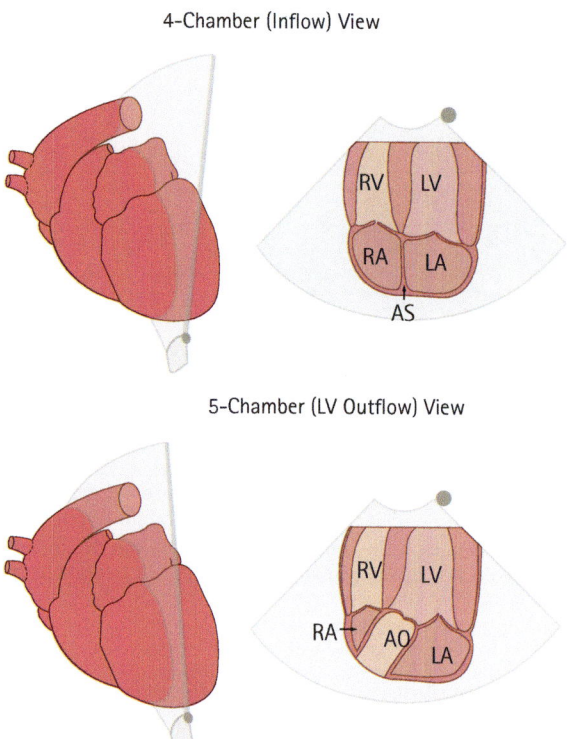

Figure 4.9 Drawings of apical (left caudal) images displayed with the left ventricle (LV) and left atrium (LA) by convention to the viewer's right. AS, atrial septum; other abbreviations as in **Figure 4.4**. (From Thomas WP, et al. Recommendations for standards in transthoracic two-dimensional echocardiography in the dog and cat. J Vet Intern Med 1993;7:247–252.)

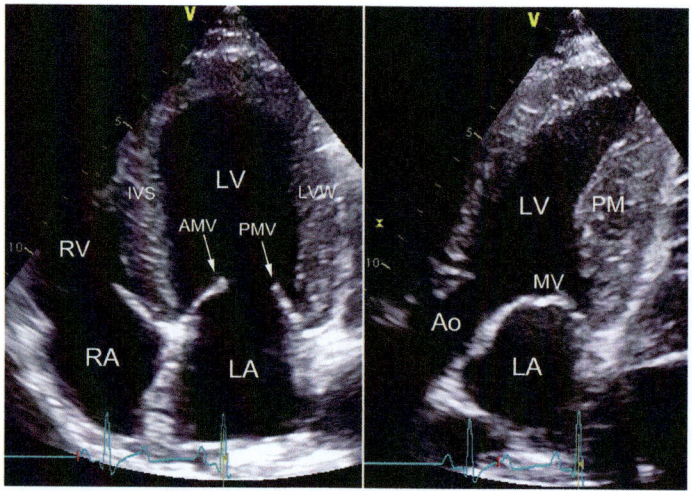

Figure 4.10 Left apical four-chamber (left) and three-chamber (right) images from a dog. The three-chamber image is rotated about 90 degrees from the four-chamber view, with additional cranial and dorsal angulation of the ultrasound beam. By convention, the LV is displayed to the viewer's right in the apical four-chamber image. The apical three-chamber image also is termed an apical long-axis; it is optimally displayed with the aorta to the viewer's right side. Abbreviations as in **Figures 4.4–4.6**.

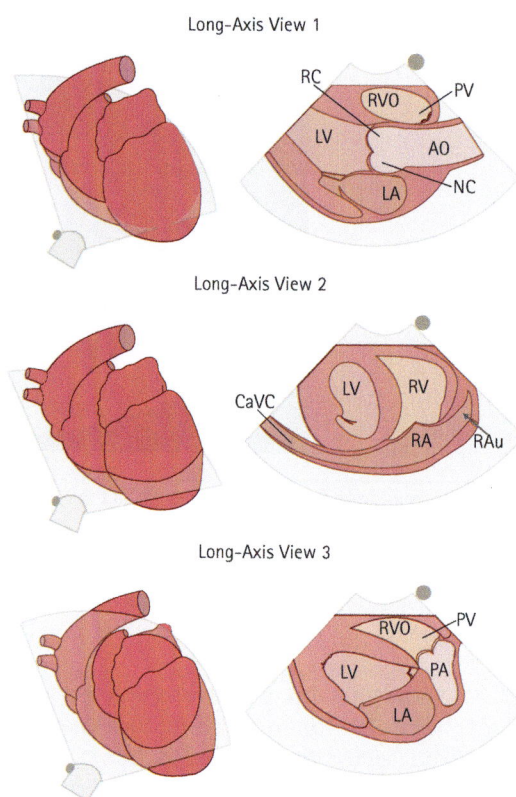

Figure 4.11 Drawings showing long-axis and hybrid images from the left cranial parasternal transducer position. The transducer is held with the sector marker oriented toward the patient's nose and the beam parallel to the long axis of the aorta (view 1). Pushing the transducer's cable end away from the operator (view 2) will reveal the right auricle (RAu); this view is used to see tumors of the right atrium and its auricle. The caudal vena cava sometimes is visualized, as well. Pulling the transducer cable upward, through view 1 and orienting the beam dorsally, will reveal the RV outflow tract (RVO), pulmonary valve, and pulmonary artery (view 3). Subtle variations in angulation will cause modifications of this view. Examples of these image planes are found in the chapters on cardiac diseases. Other abbreviations as in **Figures 4.4–4.6**. (From Thomas WP, et al. Recommendations for standards in transthoracic two-dimensional echocardiography in the dog and cat. J Vet Intern Med 1993;7:247–252.)

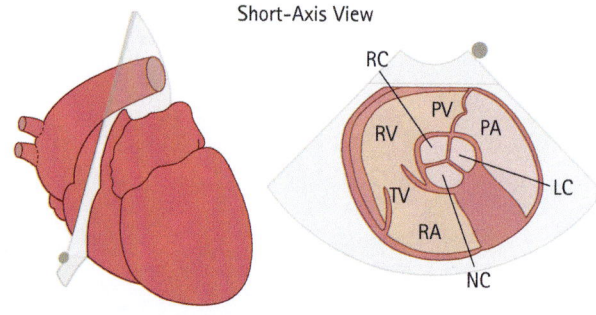

Figure 4.12 Drawing of the left cranial image short-axis view showing the RV inlet and outlet with the aorta in the center in short axis. Notice the pulmonary valve is closer to the transducer when imaged from the left side. Abbreviations as in **Figure 4.6**. (From Thomas WP, et al. Recommendations for standards in transthoracic two-dimensional echocardiography in the dog and cat. J Vet Intern Med 1993;7:247–252.)

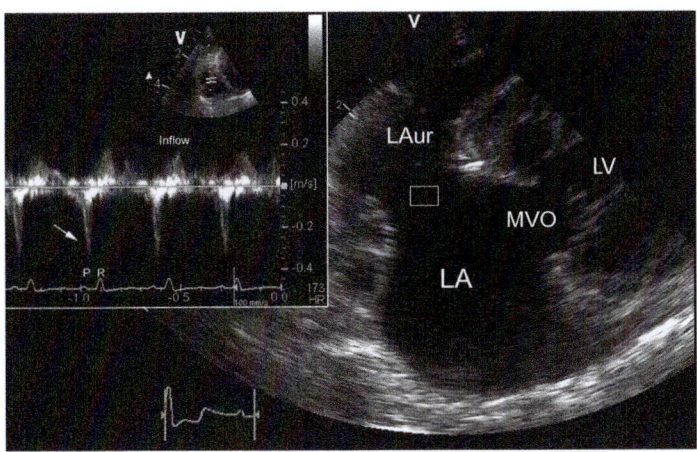

Figure 4.13 Left cranial images optimized for the left atrial appendage (LAur) in a cat. This image is especially important when screening for thrombi. In this case, the tip of the auricle is free of thrombus. The mitral orifice (MVO) also is evident between the body of the left atrium (LA) and left ventricle (LV). The inset shows a recording of RBC velocities using pulsed wave Doppler with the sample volume placed just into the LAur; active atrial emptying velocity shown (arrow).

Image Artifacts

Artifacts are common during US examinations (Feldman, 2009). Some of these cause little confusion, as when mirror image artifacts appear in the far field. However, other artifacts can mimic lesions. Because phased array transducer systems create both a primary beam and lateral secondary beams (side lobes), a common artifact is created by the joining of returning vibrations from side lobes into the primary US beam path (**Figure 4.14**). These usually are curved or arced in appearance. A beam width artifact is similar, in that a structure along the z-axis of the imaging beam is displayed within the sector of the x-y plane. This also is more common in the far field, where the US beam progressively widens. Such displacements are problematic when they are projected into an otherwise anechoic cardiac chamber, because they can be mistaken for either the left atrial wall, a cardiac mass or thrombus, a valve or mural vegetation, or spontaneous echocontrast. Conversely, echo image "dropout" often occurs in an area of relative tissue thinning, such as the *fossa ovalis* in the interatrial septum. This area of echo dropout sometimes is confused as a septal defect, especially during color Doppler imaging. Therefore, it is important to visualize a suspected mass, thrombus, or septal defect in multiple imaging planes; if that can be done, the lesion is likely to be real.

Some artifacts are associated with multiple acoustic signals. Reverberation artifacts develop when two strong reflectors create a zone where US waves echo between them, before returning to the receiving crystals of the transducer face. In cardiac imaging, a single strong reflector and part of the transducer face can function as paired reflectors to create repetitions of the strong reflector. Reverberations also are common when the parietal pleural-lung interface is encountered during thoracic scanning. Reverberation (or repetition) artifacts of this type are recognized by two or more, *equidistant*, hyperechoic, but progressively attenuated images of the strong reflector at increasing depths of field. Comet tail artifact is another form of reverberation, but is associated with two closely spaced reflectors within the sound field. In this situation, the reverberations occur internal to the reflectors, and once returned to the transducer, blend into a single vertical echo artifact that attenuates in the far field. Reverberation artifacts with diagnostic value for pulmonary disease are discussed in the next section.

Mirror image artifacts are created when the US beam strikes a strong (far-field) reflector, reverberates off the "back edge" of another strong reflector, and then returns from the far-field reflector to the transducer. This artifact often is observed deep to the pericardium, or lateral to the right ventricular outflow tract (RVOT) and pulmonary trunk, when imaging from the right side. The artifact extends in the opposite direction from the "mirror" of the strong reflector, and can occur with 2D, M-mode, or color Doppler imaging. Some of these artifacts can be minimized simply by selecting an appropriate depth of field for the patient. Narrowing the sector width can crop mirror image artifacts at the sector edges.

Artifacts and poor image quality also can result from inadequate skin–transducer contact, insufficient use of US gel, trapping of air within the hair coat, and selection of a transducer that is the wrong shape (such as linear) or too low in frequency for the intended imaging targets. Individual patient characteristics also affect the quality of images obtained. Images often are poor in animals with barrel-shaped chest conformation, a sternal deformity, obesity, or of uncooperative temperament during the exam. Lung artifact and rib interference can prevent good visualization of the entire heart. Additionally, even a rapid heart rate can substantially degrade the quality of an image.

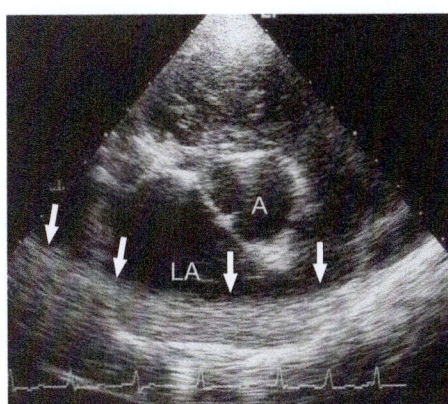

Figure 4.14 A band of false echoes, secondary to a side lobe artifact (arrows), is evident within the enlarged left atrium (LA) of a dog. The simultaneous ECG at bottom shows atrial fibrillation. A, aorta. Right parasternal short-axis view.

Clinical Utility of Imaging Artifacts Although artifacts pose a hindrance to image acquisition and interpretation, there are some clinical uses (Feldman, 2009). One is the "ring-down" artifact, a form of reverberation, associated with the trapping of gas within fluid. This occurs with pulmonary edema or lung infiltration. These artifacts appear as relatively narrow, echogenic to hyperechoic vertical streaks, devoid of repetitive linear patterns and less attenuating than classical reverberation artifacts. During thoracic (lung) US imaging, pulmonary ring-down artifacts (also called B-lines and lung rockets) typically originate from the linear, hyperechoic near-field pleural-pulmonary echo interface (or A-line) before extending into the far field (see **Figure 33.11**, p. 665). B-lines move laterally on the imaging screen with ventilation. The generation of this artifact relates to the dynamics of US interacting with trapped gas, which functions as a US oscillator and continuous generator of secondary sound waves. Multiple ring-down artifacts can coalesce and these are likely to indicate true lung pathology (as opposed to single or isolated streaks that sometimes occur in normal animals). B-lines often are confused with attenuating comet tail reverberations (caused by calcific or fibrotic reflectors). Ring-down artifacts frequently are observed in left-sided CHF, but they are more generally a marker for interstitial and alveolar lung diseases, including pulmonary fibrosis, noncardiogenic lung edema, and pneumonia.

The Echocardiographic Examination

Patient Preparation

The small animal is gently restrained in lateral recumbency (**Figure 4.1**); better-quality images usually are obtained when the heart is imaged "underneath," from the recumbent side. A table or platform with an edge cut-out is useful, as this allows the echocardiographer to position and manipulate the transducer from the animal's dependent side. The assistant should gently pull the lower elbow cranially to improve examiner access, as opposed to tugging on the limbs or holding the feet, which are poorly tolerated by cats and might incite certain dogs. Placing a soft Elizabethan collar on a cat or a soft muzzle on a potentially fractious dog helps protect the operator and assistants. Some cats prefer hiding their heads under a towel or blanket, and if available, one from the cat's carrier or a towel previously sprayed with a pheromone is used. Large animals are imaged as they stand in an examination area, box, or stocks. Some examiners also evaluate dogs in this way, although the authors prefer a recumbent canine patient, especially for detailed examinations. When examining a horse the operator should stand or sit in the same direction as the patient and face the console controls. The examiner and US system are then moved to the patient's opposite side, if required to complete the study. A focused examination of the heart and thorax is appropriate for patients in respiratory distress; the canine patient can stand while being gently restrained, and the cat in distress is encouraged to rest in sternal recumbency at the edge of the examining table (to provide transducer access). Supplemental oxygen should be supplied as accepted and mild sedation is indicated to reduce stress in these patients.

Attention to the room conditions and patient preparation can ease workflow and save time and stress. A quiet environment often is key for a successful examination; this includes minimizing loud speech, silencing the audio channel of spectral Doppler, and preventing sudden noise interruptions. The hair over the transducer placement site should be clipped to improve skin contact and image clarity. Although some patients are not shaved for cosmetic reasons (or for focused echo or lung US exam in a dyspneic patient), most examinations are improved in quality by first clipping the hair. When clipping is not possible, initially wetting the skin with isopropyl alcohol will improve transducer contact and reduce artifacts caused by air trapping; however, this chemical can damage some transducer faces. Furthermore, alcohol alone does not provide optimal acoustic impedance for coupling the skin to the transducer. US gel always should be applied to produce a consistent, air-free coupling between skin and transducer. Clipping and using copious gel also reduces the pressure needed to maintain transducer contact. Efficiency is improved, as well; continual repositioning of the transducer to find a "window" and the associated excessive transducer pressure create patient discomfort. Failing to follow these simple guidelines can eventually prompt the need for sedation, which might otherwise have been avoided if a quiet environment, clipping, gel, and a light touch (with more patience) had been employed. Yet, having said this, tranquilization or sedation is needed in a substantial number of cases to protect all involved or to obtain a technically sufficient study.

Sedation

Most dogs and cats do not require chemical restraint; however, if the patient will not lie or stand quietly for the examination with physical restraint, light sedation usually is effective. Heavier sedation is needed for fractious patients, squirmy young animals, or for prolonged studies. Although highly effective as a sedative, dexmedetomidine is avoided in dogs and cats because of its deleterious effects on heart rate, afterload, and cardiac function. In horses, although xylazine (typically 200 mg IV for an adult horse) and detomidine are often used if sedation is required, even in this species it is recommended to first obtain basic images and quantify ventricular size and function, prior to sedation (or after its effects have largely diminished).

Nearly every dog becomes adequately sedated for an echocardiogram when an appropriate combination of drugs is used. Buprenorphine (0.005–0.01 mg/kg) or butorphanol (0.2–0.25 mg/kg), mixed in the same syringe with acepromazine (0.025–0.03 mg/kg) and administered IM or IV, works well for dogs and has minimal effect on echo measurements. The concern for using acepromazine at these low doses in otherwise healthy dogs is overstated, and its sedation benefit used in combination with an opioid is underappreciated. Nevertheless, when acepromazine is to be avoided, a higher dose of butorphanol is often more effective (consider 0.3 mg/kg IM, up to 0.5 mg/kg IM for especially challenging dogs). For recheck examinations, trazodone (2–5 mg/kg PO) administered prior to leaving the home will reduce anxiety and promote sedation in some dogs. Reduce the dose of acepromazine by ~50% if it is to be administered concurrently with trazodone.

Sedation of cats is more problematic and can require a "staged" approach, depending on the response to a lower-intensity regimen. Butorphanol (0.2–0.25 mg/kg IM) mixed with acepromazine (0.1 mg/kg IM) followed by 20–30 minutes of rest in the carrier—along with gentle handling—is often sufficient to quiet a cat for the examination. Acepromazine is well tolerated at this dose in asymptomatic cats, but is avoided in those that are hypothermic or hypotensive. The dose is reduced by 50% if given IV. Unfortunately, some cats require more intense levels of sedation. The aforementioned dose of butorphanol and acepromazine can be followed with ketamine (2 mg/kg IV) for a short period of immobilization, although this regimen can increase heart rate undesirably. Ketamine administration also has been shown to increase the measured thickness of the interventricular septum (IVS) and LV wall, and to decrease LV diastolic dimension. A better alternative is to add alfaxalone (1–2 mg/kg IM) should acepromazine-butorphanol prove insufficient. Alternatively, if the need for heavy sedation is anticipated, a combination of butorphanol (0.2 mg/kg, IM) and alfaxalone (1.5–2 mg/kg IM), mixed in the same syringe, can be used initially (Thibault, 2015). When recheck examinations are planned, oral gabapentin (100 mg PO for most cats, 2h prior to the echocardiogram) might provide some anxiolytic benefit.

Imaging Technique

The right and left parasternal transducer positions are used most often. Subxiphoid positioning is helpful for specific situations in small animals, such as obtaining maximal aortic flow velocity (in dogs) or evaluating size and collapsibility of the CaVC. Dorsal intercostal and subcostal positions also provide a window to the CaVC and hepatic veins, and occasionally to the heart and great vessels. Ideally, a simultaneous ECG recording is made during the echo study. Images with patient name, identification number, and date should be stored on digital media for subsequent analysis and measurement. Even in the POC setting, best practices include storing labeled images for subsequent review.

For small animals, most operators begin the examination with the patient right side down, facing the same direction as the operator, and commence imaging through a table cutout. The transducer is held in the right hand and the imaging console is adjusted with the left. The guidelines offered here are based on this starting position; obviously, the hands can assume opposite roles if the examiner and the imaging system are positioned at the opposite end of the exam table. After imaging from the right side, the small animal patient is "turned and flipped" to a left side down position, facing in the opposite direction from the operator. Some operators prefer to image a standing patient, and a small minority examine the patient in recumbency with the spine positioned toward the operator.

The sector reference edge (seen on the screen as a vendor icon) is held under the thumb or index finger; the operator should employ the electronic L/R inversion switch as needed to maintain image display conventions. Otherwise, the RVOT and pulmonary trunk might be displayed, incorrectly, to the viewer's left side. The transducer footprint, with copious gel, is placed firmly but gently over the precordial impulse at the right thorax to begin. The transducer position is adjusted to locate an "acoustic window" that allows clear visualization of the heart or great vessels. The initial degree of transducer rotation depends on whether long- or short-axis images will be obtained. For long-axis, the reference edge should be rotated about 40 degrees clockwise (from the perspective of looking down the transducer cable). Minor adjustments to the patient's forelimb or torso position might be required. Transducer placement and adjustment are done in a similar manner when imaging from the left precordium, or other appropriate site. Initial placement for left-sided images is at the edge of the sternum, where the most caudoventral apical impulse is palpable. The initial transducer rotation is minimal (10–20 degrees clockwise with a craniodorsal tilt).

The usual right-sided acoustic window for a horse is just above the olecranon; the operator faces forward (with transducer in left hand) and can rest the edge of the left palm on top of the patient's elbow. The reference sector notch should be placed straight up and the transducer initially tilted cranially to see the main pulmonary artery and then slowly directed caudally to an inflow image of the left heart. The starting point on the left side is slightly caudal to the elbow on the left, again with the sector reference pointed dorsally (and transducer in right hand). The electronic L/R inversion switch might be needed to maintain proper image orientation, depending on the preset.

The four essential transducer movements are: placement, rotation, pointing or tilting, and fine-plane angulation, in order of extreme to most discrete adjustments of the US beam. With training and experience, standardized images can be acquired quickly, provided the operator uses appropriate veterinary presets and is skilled at adjusting the instrumentation console. The techniques involved cannot be fully learned from a textbook, but essential elements include knowledge, training, practice, experience, and follow-up assessment of skills and echo diagnoses (Bonagura, 2020). Without a systematic approach, examinations are likely to be inefficient, incomplete, or nondiagnostic for appropriate patient care.

The extent of the examination should address pertinent clinical questions and might range from a focused echocardiogram to an extensive cardiac evaluation of congenital heart disease. The basic echo examination includes the standard long- and short-axis 2D images from the right parasternal position (**Figures 4.4–4.8**), along with important cardiac measurements obtained from carefully timed 2D frames. This is where most beginning sonographers start. With more experience, complementary M-mode examinations are recorded; these are especially useful for fast frame rates or timing of flow events with color Doppler imaging. Left apical or caudal (in small animals and foals) and left cranial images are more challenging to obtain; however, they are essential for spectral Doppler studies and when a cardiac mass lesion is suspected. Off-angle or hybrid views might also be needed to further evaluate specific lesions or visualize the lobar pulmonary arteries. When the veterinarian decides to invest sufficient capital and time to obtain Doppler evaluations of transvalvular flow and flow disturbances, multiple right- and left-sided imaging positions will be required. A complete examination can become time-consuming, as functionally, some studies represent a noninvasive cardiac catheterization. There is a point where referral to a cardiologist is the best option to ensure quality of patient care, as well as practicality.

Most general practitioners with an interest in learning echocardiography should therefore focus on 2D and selective M-mode imaging, while considering the associated costs, training, and range of noncardiac disorders they are likely to evaluate with US. Doppler examinations mainly are used to identify the sources of audible murmurs, estimate intracardiac pressures, and assess diastolic heart function; these are all advanced techniques and require increasingly expensive hardware. Modifications of "FAST" scans (for Focused Assessment with Sonography in Trauma) are useful for evaluating the thorax and abdomen more generally and for detecting cavity effusions and pulmonary edema associated with CHF. In cases of respiratory distress, the finding of a small to normal left atrial size usually is sufficient to rule out left-sided CHF. Additional, noncardiac (lung) US of the thorax is instructive, as mentioned in section "Clinical Utility of Imaging Artifacts" and described more fully by the medical BLUE and the VetBLUE® imaging protocols (see Lichtenstein, 2015; Lisciandro, 2014).

Examination Questions and Diagnostic Approach

Table 4.1 summarizes key issues in echocardiography relevant to general clinical practice and, while not comprehensive, it outlines questions that should be addressed during a complete echo examination. For the current discussion, application of Doppler imaging presumes an advanced level of training and experience. Imaging of cardiac chambers and lesions by 3D or TEE are not considered. The general questions posed in **Table 4.1** are approached using a systematic evaluation of extracardiac serous cavities (pericardial, pleural, and peritoneal spaces); the lung parenchyma in patients with respiratory signs; each individual cardiac chamber and heart valve; the pulmonary and systemic venous entries; and the great vessels along with their proximal branches, when evident.

Pulmonary Imaging and Cavity Effusions Noncardiac imaging in patients with heart disease should focus on the presence or absence of cavity effusions and, in patients with respiratory signs, the identification of artifacts originating from pulmonary disease. When there is pneumonia associated with pleural effusion, thoracic imaging might reveal a hepatized appearance to the lung with reverberations stemming from mobile or static, air-filled bronchi within the lung. Moving gas patterns in a lung without loss of volume is more suggestive of pneumonia or of pulmonary neoplasia; whereas static bronchial gas reverberations in a lung showing reduced volume is more typical of pulmonary atelectasis, with residual gas in bronchi. The latter is commonly observed in chronic right-sided or biventricular CHF. Identification of intrapulmonary fluid in the form of B-lines requires some experience, but is suggestive of left-sided CHF, as described previously (p. 80; see also **Figure 33.11**, p. 665).

Serous cavity effusions might be obvious or require identification from multiple imaging planes; the right parasternal short- and long-axis views are used for initial screening for pleural and pericardial effusions. Pleural effusion is a potential sign of CHF; however, this fluid often is caused by other thoracic disease, including neoplasia, lymphatic disorders, and infections. When pleural effusion is identified, any concurrent pericardial and peritoneal effusions should be noted. The finding of tricavitary effusions suggests CHF caused by right heart disease or cardiac tamponade. Pleural effusion, in the absence of pericardial fluid or overt cardiac disease, points to a noncardiac cause; especially in older animals, mediastinal or pulmonary mass lesions should be sought. Subxiphoid (subcostal) transducer placement can reveal ascites near the diaphragm, caudal pleural and pericardial effusions, and CaVC size (and its respiratory variation). A CaVC of normal- to small-diameter, and which varies with respiration, argues against a diagnosis of right-sided CHF. Small-volume ascites sometimes is evident in the caudal abdomen near the bladder.

Cardiac Lesions Specific cardiac lesions in companion animal species relate to congenital and acquired disease of the pericardium, myocardial walls, heart valves, and the blood vessels connecting to the heart or great arteries. These lesions are manifested as *morphologic* or *motion* abnormalities in these structures and are visualized by 2D or M-mode echo imaging across the affected area. Shunts, outflow tract stenosis, or valvular incompetency might be strongly suspected from combining auscultation with 2D echo findings; however,

Table 4.1 Echocardiographic Exam: Suggested Systematic Approach and Outcomes

From 2D and M-mode Imaging

Consideration	Key Questions
Congestive heart failure	• Is there pleural effusion? • Is there ascites? • Is evidence for pulmonary edema ("B-lines") or infiltration present? • Is there atrial dilation or evidence of gross cardiac disease?

Pericardium	• Is pericardial effusion present?
	  • If yes, what is the volume and appearance?
	  • Is there evidence of cardiac tamponade?
	• Is a cardiac or heart base mass evident?

Cardiac chambers and cardiomegaly	• Are the four cardiac chambers identified?
	• Are there normal ventricular connections to inlet and outlet valves?
	• Are the chambers of normal proportions to each other?
	• Is the ventricular septum normally rounded, or flattened?
	• Are any myocardial morphologic lesions or defects present?
	• Do the ventricular wall thicknesses and chamber volumes (areas) appear normal?
	  • Are measurements of ventricular chamber size and wall thicknesses normal for the species, body weight, and breed?[a]
	• Do LA and RA chamber volumes (areas) appear normal?
	  • Are measurements of atrial chamber size normal for the species, body weight, and breed?[a]

Ventricular systolic function[b]	• Does ventricular wall motion appear normal across visualized segments?
	  • Is LV short-axis fractional area change >40%?
	  • Does the mitral valve annulus move vigorously toward the apex?
	• Is interventricular septal motion normal in systole and diastole?
	• What is the subjective assessment of LV EF?
	  • What are the calculated values for LV systolic function (FS, fractional area change, Simpson's EF)?[a]
	• What is the subjective assessment of RV systolic function?
	  • What are the measured or calculated values of RV systolic function (TAPSE, fractional area change)?[a]
	• Is the cardiac rhythm normal?

Great vessels	• Are the outflow tracts and great vessels arranged normally? • Any abnormalities or dilation seen in the aorta or pulmonary trunk and branch pulmonary arteries? • Are there intraluminal abnormalities (such as heartworms, thrombus, mass)?

From 2D, M-mode, and Doppler Imaging

Consideration	Key Questions

Cardiac valves	• Are the mitral and tricuspid valves normal, in terms of:
	  • Morphology and thickness of the leaflets/cusps?
	  • Support apparatus: chordal attachments and papillary muscles?
	  • Motion?
	  • Is there stenosis (from motion and Doppler studies)?
	  • Is there regurgitation (from Doppler studies)?
	• Are the aortic and pulmonary valves normal, in terms of:
	  • Morphology, number, symmetry, and thickness of the leaflets/cusps?
	  • Motion?
	  • Is there stenosis (from motion and Doppler studies)?
	  • Is there regurgitation (from Doppler studies)?

Diastolic ventricular function; atrial function and filling pressures[a, b]	• Is LV diastolic function normal? • Are LA size and function normal? • Are pulmonary venous entries and flow patterns normal? • Are LV filling pressure estimates normal? • Is RV diastolic function normal? • Is there evidence for elevated RA pressure (dilated coronary sinus or vena cava)?
Arterial hypertension	Is there 2D or Doppler evidence for pulmonary hypertension? Is there 2D or Doppler evidence for systemic hypertension?

Overall Assessment

What is the nature, severity, clinical significance, and prognosis of the cardiac findings?
Is therapy potentially indicated?[c]

[a] Some of these measurements and calculations usually are done "offline," after the examination has concluded.
[b] The following assessments are more advanced and require integration of 2D imaging, pulsed wave and continuous wave Doppler flow, and pulsed wave tissue Doppler imaging. In addition, advanced (referral or investigational) methods, such as myocardial strain imaging, might have a role for more sensitive assessment of cardiac systolic and diastolic function.
[c] Therapy should be guided only by a veterinarian completely familiar with the patient and all related medical issues. Direction of treatment presumes a patient–client–veterinarian relationship.

Abbreviations: EF, ejection fraction; FS, fractional shortening; LA, left atrial; LV, left ventricular; RA, right atrial; RV, right ventricular; TAPSE, tricuspid annular plane systolic excursion.

color and continuous wave Doppler studies are needed to confirm and fully quantify the severity of blood flow disturbances. Numerous examples of these are included throughout this book.

Cardiac Size and Function Cardiomegaly, dilation of the great vessels, ventricular wall motion, and systolic ventricular function are evaluated both subjectively and by specific measurements and calculations, described later. Chamber enlargement or wall thickening can develop from compensatory hypertrophy associated with a shunt or valvular lesion, or as the essential component of a primary cardiomyopathy. With experience, examiners can learn to "eyeball" normal systolic function of the ventricles. However, only moderate to severe depression of ventricular function is evident using subjective analysis.

Atrial enlargement is an important marker of (hemodynamically and) clinically important cardiac disease. Atrial dilation accompanies shunts (from increased venous return), atrioventricular (AV) valve disease (from regurgitation or stenosis of the valve), diastolic or systolic ventricular dysfunction (as in cardiomyopathies), or heart failure in general (from cardiac dysfunction and increased venous pressures). Subjective analysis can identify moderate to severe atrial chamber enlargement, although measurements should be obtained also. Atrial function is measured by 2D, M-mode, or Doppler techniques and has prognostic value in some diseases, especially the feline cardiomyopathies.

Enlargement of the aorta or pulmonary trunk usually stems from one of four causes: systemic or pulmonary hypertension (PH), left-to-right shunting, outflow-tract stenosis ("poststenotic dilation"), or as an idiopathic (often genetically predisposed) dilation.

Most measurements focus on chamber size and ventricular systolic function. However, some disorders are characterized mainly by diastolic dysfunction, at least initially. Assessments of diastolic heart function are intertwined with estimations of ventricular filling pressures. These are complicated assessments, but some basics are considered below under Doppler echocardiography. Estimations of venous and atrial ("filling") pressures are pertinent to predicting the likelihood that a patient has, or is likely to experience, CHF. Although dilation of the atria (or venous connections) indirectly suggests elevated pressure, when this dilation develops gradually, mean atrial pressure might actually be close to normal. A more complete analysis requires advanced Doppler flow and tissue imaging (Schober, 2015).

Two-Dimensional Echocardiography

Two-dimensional echocardiography projects a wedge-shaped image onto the viewing screen and updates the image frame (typically at 1/30th of a second or faster) to create a smooth, real-time image of cardiac structure and motion. This modality is used for identifying cardiac anatomy and quantifying cardiac chamber size and function. The 2D echo examination also is the platform that guides other modalities, including M-mode and Doppler imaging. Because of the planar nature of the 2D exam, suspected lesions should be scanned from multiple acoustic windows to further verify and delineate abnormalities. Focal heart lesions, such as a ventricular septal defect (VSD), valvar vegetation, or segmental myocardial hypertrophy, are confirmed by using complementary 2D image planes.

In addition to the artifacts discussed previously, there are other pitfalls. One is using an off-angle imaging plane that truncates chambers or artificially "thickens" the myocardial walls. For example, in companion animals, images showing the greatest LV length often are obtained from the right parasternal long-axis view; in contrast, LV length frequently is truncated on left apical images. Another issue is insufficient temporal resolution, which can be a problem at high heart rates in dogs and even normal heart rates in cats. When the acquisition frame rate is too slow, the number of truly end-diastolic images available for measurement is limited; this increases the risk of erroneously measuring "diastolic" wall thickness during systole. Temporal resolution is a substantial problem with 2D color Doppler imaging, because longer processing time is needed for Doppler shifts to be collected and overlaid on the 2D grayscale image. Slow 2D color Doppler frame rates commonly lead to the misdiagnosis of mitral or tricuspid valvular regurgitation.

Standard 2D Echocardiographic Views

Common 2D image planes are designated as right-sided or left-sided (based on transducer placement) and as long-axis, short-axis, or apical (caudal sternal) images, as noted previously. Various hybrid or angled image views also might be employed. Most standard views are similar among dogs, cats and horses, with only minor differences across species and breeds. The majority of images are obtained from the right parasternal (intercostal) positions (directly over the heart and close to the sternum). Some 2D images are named for the number of chambers captured. Thus, images are subclassified by the transducer position, the tomographic plane, and chambers imaged.

Right-sided, Long-axis Image Planes These sagittal views (**Figures 4.4** and **4.5**) are obtained with the transducer at the right thorax and with the imaging plane parallel to the long-axis of the heart. The right atrium and ventricle are nearest the transducer in these planes. The left heart chambers are in the far field. When visualized, the aorta arises from roughly the center of the heart, between the dorsal IVS and anterior leaflet of the mitral valve.

Right parasternal long-axis images in dogs and horses usually are optimized for the left atrium (LA), mitral valve and LV inflow tract, or for the LV outflow tract (LVOT) and ascending aorta. Switching between these views typically is done with a

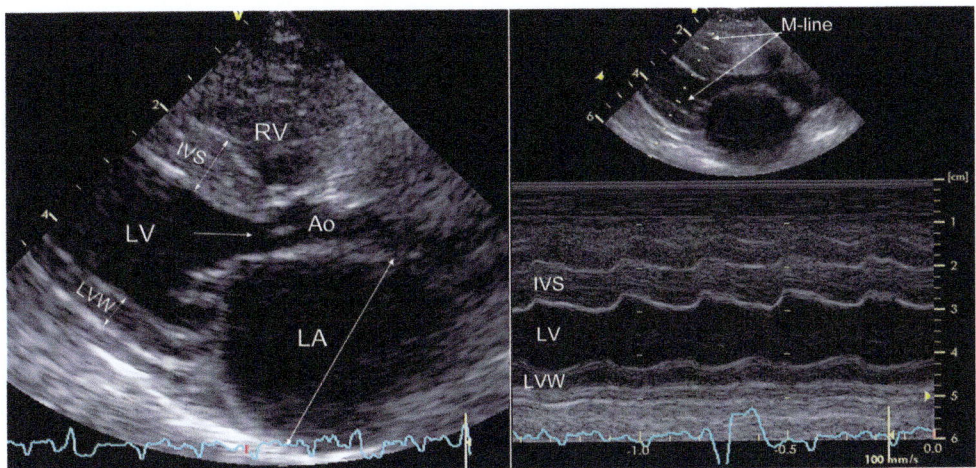

Figure 4.15 The left panel shows a right parasternal, 2D long-axis left ventricular (LV) inflow-outflow tract image, recorded in a cat with end-stage hypertrophic cardiomyopathy and severe left atrial dilation (midchamber diameter is ~27 mm at the line indicated). There is residual interventricular septal hypertrophy, but the LV wall is normal in thickness. The LV outflow tract is indicated (arrow) in this typical feline view. The right panel shows an M-mode image generated from the M-line (cursor) position shown on the small 2D image above. This case has reduced LV systolic function, characterized by decreased fractional shortening. Other abbreviations as in **Figures 4.4** and **4.5**.

simple clockwise rotation of the transducer (from the perspective of looking down the transducer cable). The dorsal portion of the LA might need to be "cut off" to completely visualize the ventricle from apex to base. In cats, the long-axis image of the left heart is more similar to that in humans, with good visualization of most of the LV chamber and a good portion of the LA and LVOT (**Figure 4.15**). However, the operator also can exclude the aorta and place the RA, atrial septum, and LA in the imaging field. This provides a standard four-chamber image, showing the widest feline left atrial diameter and allowing a long-axis measurement of the LA (**Figure 4.16**).

Placing the transducer more ventrally and angulating dorsally in dogs and horses creates a "tipped" long-axis image with a LV inflow-outflow tract view, although the size of the LA and ventricle are not maximal with this orientation. This maneuver highlights a general imaging tip for 2D studies: When the transducer is placed ventrally and angled dorsally, the IVS and parallel structures will appear more vertically oriented on the screen; whereas, when the transducer is placed more dorsally and perpendicular to the chest wall, the septum and other structures will appear more horizontal on the screen.

Clinical Utility of Right-Sided, Long-Axis Images The fundamental long-axis views, along with minor modifications of these, permit visualization of the mitral, aortic, and tricuspid valves; LV cavity; cardiac septa; and the RV inflow tract. Long-axis images are effective for diagnosing the majority of common congenital and acquired heart diseases. Clear exceptions are disorders of the RVOT, pulmonary valve, and the pulmonary trunk, which require different planes.

The LV inflow tract view optimized for the mitral valve is most commonly used to assess congenital and acquired lesions of this valve, as well as enlargement of the right heart and atrial septal defects. The modified, long-axis LV inflow-outflow tract view can demonstrate dynamic LVOT obstruction and eccentric jets of mitral regurgitation (MR). The optimized LVOT view is used to identify hypertrophy of the dorsal IVS, membranous VSDs, subvalvular aortic stenosis, aortic valve lesions, and disorders of the proximal aorta, such as idiopathic dilation. Left heart cavity and LV wall measurements are made from long-axis images, including ratios of the LA to the aorta (see p. 103). An optimized image of the LA that excludes the aorta also shows the entry of right pulmonary veins and adjacent origin of the right pulmonary

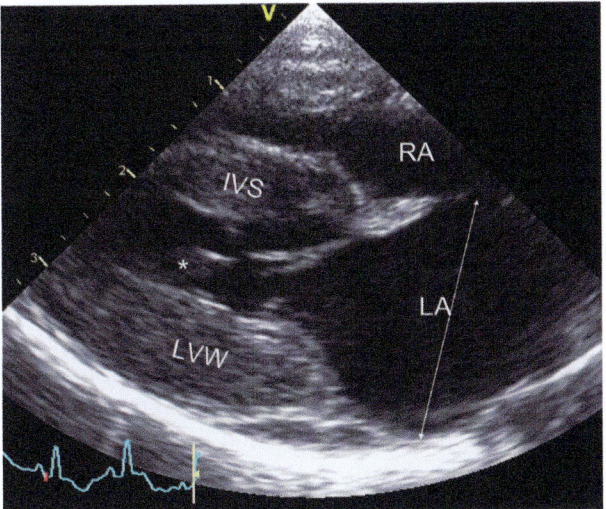

Figure 4.16 A left ventricular (LV) inflow tract (four-chamber) image from the right parasternal position, recorded in another cat with hypertrophic cardiomyopathy. The interventricular septum (IVS) and LV free wall (LVW) are thickened. The left atrium (LA), measured at end-systole, is enlarged. A papillary muscle (*) is evident. RA, right atrium.

artery (in cross-section; **Figure 4.5A**). Increased pressure in the LA often dilates the pulmonary vein relative to the artery, whereas the opposite finding occurs with PH. Accordingly, the ratio of the vein to artery increasingly is being used for assessment of pulmonary pressure dynamics when Doppler studies cannot be obtained (Visser, 2017).

LV systolic function is commonly underestimated when inspecting long-axis views because the focus is on changes in ventricular septal to LV wall distance, while apical to basilar shortening is less obvious. However, focusing on movement of the apical region and mitral annulus is useful for evaluating longitudinal systolic LV function, especially in larger dogs where it is relatively more important. Again, the greatest LV length often is obtained from parasternal right-sided images, as compared to left apical transducer placement. As such, tracings of LV internal area and length at end-diastole and end-systole from the right side are often used to estimate LV volumes and global LV ejection fraction (EF), similar to the approach used in apical views (see section "Left Ventricular Size and Function").

Images of the RA and ventricle are visualized in the near field when viewed from right parasternal long-axis planes. However, right heart anatomy is complicated and the chambers are incompletely visualized, with only the inflow tract and tricuspid valve leaflets seen. When compared to left apical images, the RV chamber is foreshortened in the sagittal plane, exhibiting a triangular appearance. Both RV and right atrial chambers increase in size as the transducer is placed more dorsally on the thorax (until lung tissue obscures the image). These imaging issues lend inaccuracies to right heart chamber measurements. Some clinicians do attempt to measure the right ventricle below the tricuspid valve, and subjective assessments are possible. The RV free-wall thickness usually is <50% of the LV (posterior) wall thickness. Adjusting the transducer focal zone closer to the transducer, or selecting a higher-frequency transducer, optimizes the resolution of these near-field structures.

Right-Sided, Short-Axis Image Planes A series of transverse (axial) views are obtained initially, or following acquisition of long-axis images, depending on the examiner's preference. These tomographic planes are obtained with the transducer at roughly 90 degrees perpendicular to the long-axis views (**Figures 4.6–4.8**). Transverse imaging at the levels of the left apex, LV papillary muscles, and mitral valve (the "fish mouth" view) reveals a circular-appearing left ventricle and crescent-shaped right ventricle in normal animals. The posterior (caudodorsal) papillary muscle usually is closer to the transducer and the anterior (cranioventral) papillary muscle farther away (the opposite of humans), although cardiac rotation or shifting can modify this, especially in cats. The posterior (caudal or mural) mitral leaflet is closest to the LV free wall.

When the transducer is angled further dorsally from the mitral valve, and rotated slightly clockwise (as you look down the cable to the transducer), the aorta (Ao) appears in cross-section. The aortic root is located between the IVS and anterior (cranial or septal) mitral valve leaflet, roughly in the middle of the image. In this plane, the LA and its appendage are observed in the far field. If the image is properly oriented, the auricular tip points toward the right side of the imaging screen. The aortic cusps are identified as right (closest to transducer), left (nearest the LA) and noncoronary (straddling the atrial septum). The coronary artery ostia can be seen with careful angulation, especially in the horse where a dominant right coronary artery is readily visible. This view also is used commonly to measure the LA and aortic root size in all species.

With further cranial and dorsal angulation from the Ao-LA image plane, the left auricle disappears and the pulmonary trunk and its main branches are revealed in a long-axis orientation, to the right side of the image. This is a hybrid view, as the aorta persists in short-axis (**Figures 4.6** and **4.8B**). Although the right heart structures are truncated in short-axis planes, both the tricuspid and pulmonary valves can be assessed because the crescent-shaped right ventricle wraps around the more circular left ventricle. The general appearance of the right heart is a "U" with portions of the tricuspid leaflets and inflow tract separated from the RVOT and pulmonary valve by muscle of the supraventricular crest.

Clinical Utility of Right-Sided, Short-Axis Images In addition to providing anatomic detail from ventral to dorsal, the right-sided, short-axis image planes are used frequently for cardiac size quantitation, especially for LV and RV wall thicknesses and chamber dimensions. The LV minor axis is visualized, and the dimension between the IVS and LV free wall (between the two papillary muscles) is one measure of overall LV chamber size (LV internal diameter; **Figure 4.7**). Most examiners guide M-mode studies from short-axis images (see section "M-mode Echocardiography"); however, identical measurements can be made using the electronic calipers on a frozen 2D image. This is a more accurate approach when the M-line is off-angle or if there is segmental wall thickening, as is common with feline cardiomyopathies. Dorsal short-axis planes allow quantitation of the LA, aorta and the pulmonary trunk (**Figure 4.17**).

Left Apical Images The left apical, four-chamber view and its many variations allow visualization of the LV inflow and outflow tracts, three valves, the proximal aorta, CaVC entry into the RA, and relative chamber proportions. This image is displayed against convention; that is, the more caudal left heart chambers are displayed toward the viewer's right side. A common technical pitfall is failure to place the transducer face sufficiently caudal and ventral, at the sternal edge. The heart should appear nearly vertical, as if suspended from its apex, when this view is properly recorded. The apical four-chamber view is the springboard for other apical images. Unfortunately, apical images have limitations, including that (1) the LV length often is truncated in dogs; (2) the view is limited or unavailable in mature horses (although more possible in foals); and (3) it often is extremely difficult to align a Doppler cursor parallel to aortic flow in cats. Using the dog as the example, modifications of transducer rotation and

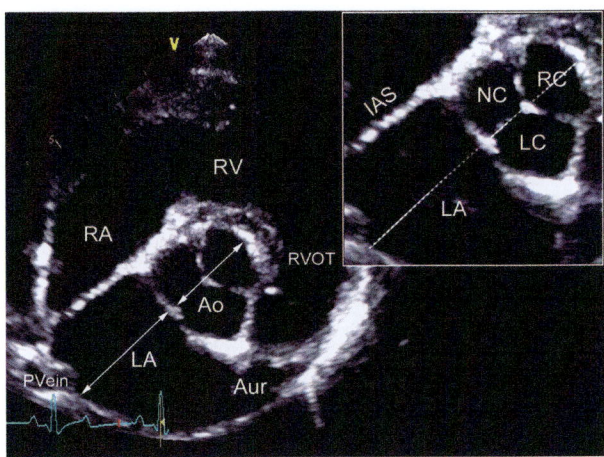

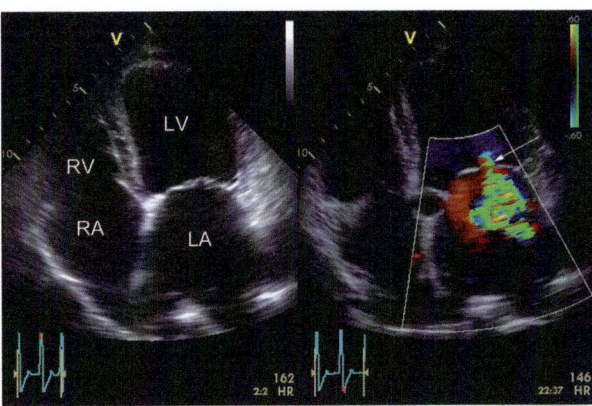

Figure 4.17 Short-axis method for measuring the left atrium (LA) relative to the aorta. The image is frozen in early diastole once the aortic valve closes. A line that bisects the aorta, drawn along the commissure of the left and noncoronary cusps (inset), is continued across the LA. The dimensions of the LA and Ao, measured along this line, are used to generate the so-called "Swedish" LA/Ao ratio for assessing left atrial size. IAS, interatrial septum; PVein, pulmonary vein. Other abbreviations as in **Figure 4.6**.

angulation from the "home base" of the apical four-chamber image can yield the following useful images:

- Apical five-chamber view (a slight cranial tilt will reveal the proximal aorta)
- Apical three-chamber view, also called an apical long-axis (obtained by rotating the transducer ~90 degrees clockwise with steep craniodorsal angulation, then activating the L/R invert to display the aorta to the right)

Figure 4.18 Apical four-chamber images from a dog with dilated cardiomyopathy and mitral regurgitation. The color Doppler image (right) shows a relatively central jet of valvular regurgitation. Turbulence encoding shows the regurgitant jet area in green. Abbreviations as in **Figure 4.4**.

- Apical two-chamber view showing the LA and ventricle (obtained by rotating the transducer counter-clockwise about 120 degrees from the four-chamber view and tilting slightly ventrally)

Some of these images are shown in **Figures 4.9**, **4.10**, and **4.18**.

Optimized views of the right heart can be obtained by modifying the apical four-chamber view. Rotating the transducer clockwise from the four-chamber view, while pushing the cable end away from the examiner, brings the image plane ventral to the LA to reveal the terminal CaVC in long axis as it enters the RA. Moving the transducer one intercostal space cranially from the left apical four-chamber view and angulating caudally yields an optimized view of the RV inlet (**Figure 4.19**).

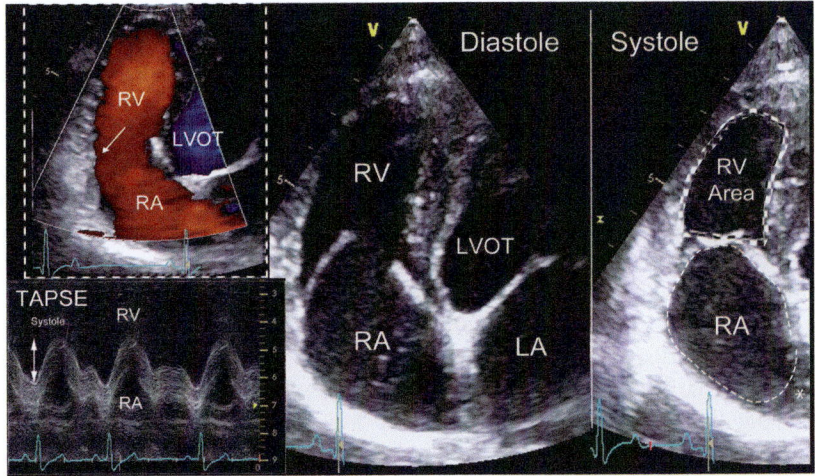

Figure 4.19 Modified left apical image optimized for the right ventricle from a dog (center panel). The longitudinal anatomy and function of the right ventricle (RV) can be evaluated in this view. The fractional area change of the RV is calculated by tracing the inflow area in diastole and systole (right panel). The right atrial area also can be traced, but is more complicated because the venous entry of the caudal vena cava (*, right panel) creates an indistinct border between the two. The lower left inset shows an M-mode recording for Tricuspid Annular Plane Systolic Excursion (TAPSE) measurement. This is generated by aligning the M-mode cursor along the lateral wall of the RV to record basilar to apical movements of the tricuspid annulus (from diastole to systole, arrow). The color Doppler image (upper left panel) shows low-velocity flow from RA to RV during diastole (coded red, toward the transducer); the arrow indicates the tricuspid annulus.

Clinical Utility of Left Apical Images In addition to providing opportunities to visualize the AV valves, and inflow and outflow tracts, the apical four-chamber view provides subjective comparison of right and left sides of the heart (provided the center of the US beam passes to the anatomical left of the IVS). The LV area can be traced in systole and end-diastole (see below), as for the right parasternal long-axis view, to estimate LV volumes and systolic function, including EF. However, in most dogs and horses, the chamber is likely to be slightly truncated in this view. The apical imaging planes are used to evaluate blood flow across the mitral and tricuspid valves and often are the best ways to demonstrate valvular regurgitation or congenital stenosis. Advanced methods of tissue Doppler imaging (TDI) are applied using these views, too. The right ventricle imaged by the modified apical view is probably the best image for evaluating the tricuspid valve and RV function (**Figure 4.19**). However, the RVOT cannot be viewed from this plane.

Left Cranial Images Cranial long-axis, short-axis, and hybrid views are obtained from left cranial transducer positions. These more advanced images allow further evaluation of the outflow tracts, great vessels, right auricle, left atrial appendage, and IVS (**Figures 4.11–4.13**). Although these are not required for most routine diagnoses, they can be crucial in some cases. Other chapters contain examples of their value in delineating congenital heart disease, cardiac masses or thrombi, and diseases of the great arteries.

Contrast 2D Echocardiography

Contrast echocardiography or "bubble study" is a technique used mainly with 2D imaging. A substance that alters the sonographic characteristics of the blood pool is injected rapidly either into a peripheral vein or (uncommonly) selectively into a cardiac chamber. These solutions or suspensions alter the acoustic properties of the blood by creating microcavitations ("microbubbles") or releasing gases that function as powerful reflectors of US. Agitated saline solution (sometimes mixed with some of the patient's blood) is used most often as an echocontrast agent in veterinary practice. There also are commercially available solutions of microspheres licensed for human use that contain perfluorocarbon gas, which is released when US disrupts the containing shell. The main differences are that injection of agitated saline into a peripheral vein opacifies only the right heart chambers, unless there is a right-to-left shunt (**Figure 4.20**). Saline microbubbles do not pass through the pulmonary capillaries. Thus, unless arteriovenous (A-V) shunts have been opened (from disease or atelectasis) the bubbles from agitated saline do not traverse the lung. In contrast, commercially available echocontrast agents do pass through the pulmonary circulation and can be used to outline left heart endocardial borders or a cardiac mass or thrombus.

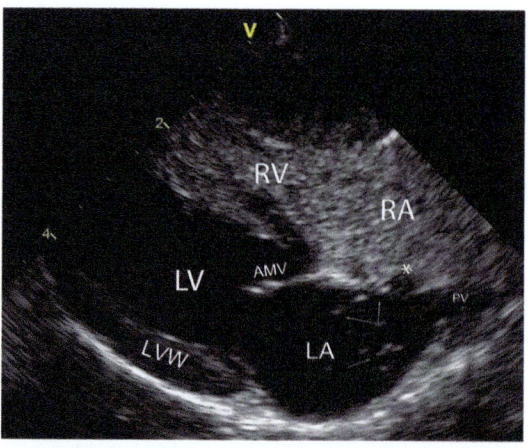

Figure 4.20 Saline contrast echo "bubble" study in a dog with a patent foramen ovale and pulmonary stenosis. A bolus of sterile, agitated saline solution was rapidly injected IV, creating bright bubbles that opacify the lumen of the right atrium (RA) and ventricle (RV). A small number of these echodense "microbubbles" have entered the left atrium (LA, arrows) from the region of the fossa ovalis (*) because the right heart pressures are elevated. AMV, anterior mitral valve leaflet; LVW, left ventricular wall; PV, pulmonary vein. Right parasternal four-chamber view.

Although color Doppler echocardiography generally has replaced the use of contrast echocardiography in dogs and cats, this technique is still helpful for identifying a right-to-left shunting atrial septal defect, patent foramen ovale, or patent ductus arteriosus (PDA). In the latter case, the agitated saline microbubbles are identified flowing within the abdominal aorta (**Figure 26.26**, p. 453).

M-mode Echocardiography

M-mode echocardiography was the original cardiac US modality. It still has utility in veterinary practice because of its rapid sampling rates (about 1000/second), excellent temporal (time) resolution, compatibility with color Doppler imaging, and often higher-resolution borders of wall segments and ventricular chambers. Unlike 2D imaging, which employs an array of crystals, the M-mode study is generated from activation of a single US crystal within the array. Using the 2D image as an anatomical template, the M-mode US beam is guided by the operator across structures of interest using a track ball and M-line (cursor line). The result is a graphical, "one-dimensional" view of imaging targets displayed relative to their depth from the transducer.

M-mode stands for "motion" mode. The images obtained are reflections from the various tissue interfaces traversed by the US beam as they move toward and away from the static transducer during the cardiac cycle (**Figures 4.21** and **4.22**). The M-mode image "graph" is created by sweeping the instantaneous images horizontally, across time, on the x-axis. The M-mode study should be recorded with a simultaneous ECG to show precise timing within the cardiac cycle.

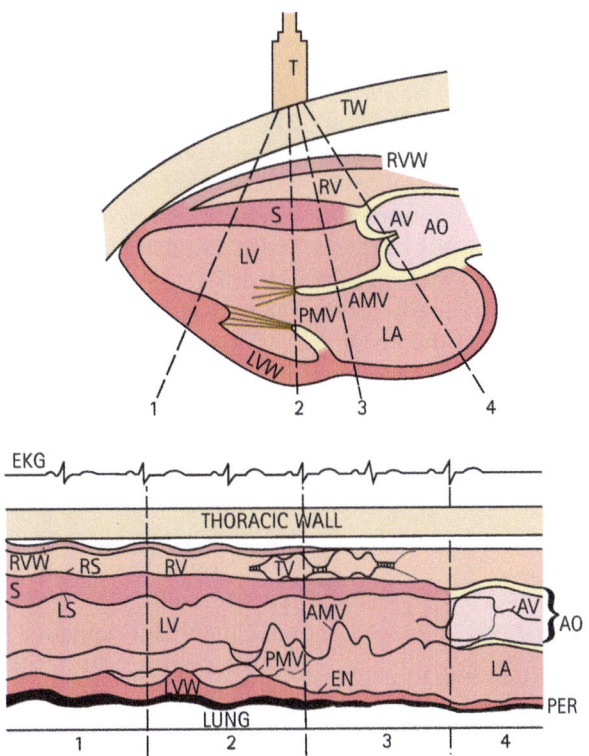

Figure 4.21 Schematic diagram illustrating how various tissue interfaces crossed by the one-dimensional M-line cursor (upper panel) are displayed across time in M-mode imaging (lower panel). The M-line typically is directed from ventricular to chordal/high papillary to mitral to aortic levels. Although the long-axis view is shown here to depict different levels from apex to base, short-axis views often are used in practice to guide cursor placement. AMV, anterior mitral valve leaflet; Ao, aorta; AV, aortic valve; EN, endocardium; IVS, interventricular septum; LA, left atrium; LS, left edge of septum; LV, left ventricle; LVW, left ventricular wall; PER, pericardium; PMV, posterior mitral valve leaflet; RS, right edge of septum; RV, right ventricle; RVW, right ventricular wall; S, interventricular septum; T, transducer; TV, tricuspid valve; TW, thoracic wall.

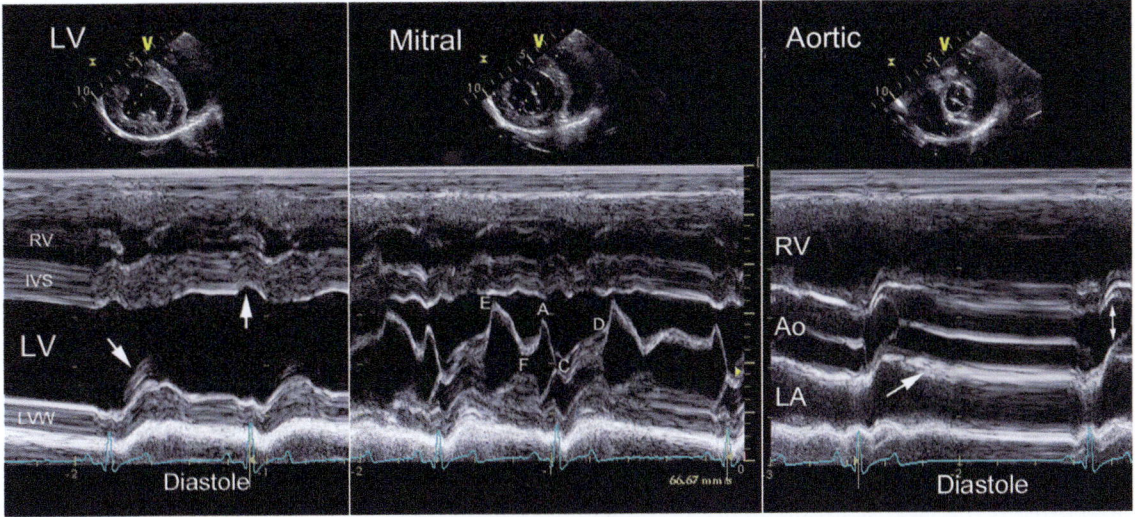

Figure 4.22 M-mode images from a dog obtained at the ventricular (left), mitral (center), and aortic (right) levels. Compare these to **Figure 4.21**. Note M-line orientation in the small 2D images above. (Left panel) During systole, some papillary muscle echos (down-pointing arrow) might be captured near the LVW. Atrial contraction causes brief upward motion (up-arrow) of the IVS. (Center panel) Letters identify mitral leaflet motion. For example, the E-point represents maximal opening in early diastole (during rapid ventricular filling) and the A-point follows atrial contraction; see text for further descriptions. Cardiac cycle length also influences the motion of the leaflets. (Right panel) During diastole, echoes from the closed aortic leaflets appear midway between the parallel aortic wall echoes (posterior wall indicated by larger arrow). During systole, the aortic leaflets separate (double-headed arrow at right); two leaflets are visible in this recording, although often only one is evident. In the dog and horse, because the M-line crosses the junction of the LA and its appendage (see associated 2D image), M-mode significantly underestimates left atrial size. However, in most cats, M-mode does capture left atrial size fairly well. Abbreviations as in **Figure 4.21**.

Although measurements of some cardiac dimensions and motion might be more accurately assessed from M-mode tracings, difficulties are encountered in placing the M-line consistently along standardized paths. Optimal visualization and consistency of measurement are achieved only when the images are recorded in axial resolution (reflectors are perpendicular to the US beam). Consistent placement of the line relative to internal structures and image planes is critical, and too often ignored. Other limitations include translational motion and rotation of the beating heart such that the cursor does not actually remain within the same targets over the cardiac cycle. For example, it is common for the cursor to cross the edge of the papillary muscle as the heart rotates, thereby spuriously increasing apparent LV wall thickness. Furthermore, when there is regional or asymmetrical ventricular hypertrophy, wall thickness measurements obtained by M-mode might not be representative.

Normal M-mode Patterns

The usual M-mode examination includes three image planes:

- The ventricular level, transecting the left ventricle at the chordae tendineae or "high" papillary muscle plane
- The mitral valve level
- The aortic root/left atrial level

The examiner must understand the normal M-mode patterns of cardiac motion in these three planes in order to properly acquire and interpret the images. Typical examples are shown in **Figures 4.15**, **4.21**, and **4.22**). Other than LV size measurements, analysis of the M-mode study is largely subjective. Common M-mode features of various cardiac diseases are addressed in the related chapters and summarized in **Table 4.2**.

Left Ventricle When the papillary muscles are excluded, the left ventricle is roughly bullet-shaped, with a longitudinal or major axis (length) and two perpendicular minor axes. The M-mode study follows the wall motion of this chamber across the minor axis extending from the dorsal IVS to the LV posterior wall between the dorsal edges of the two papillary muscles. Because the papillary muscles provide a clear reference target for the M-line, the short-axis view often is used to obtain the M-mode study. However, a source of potential error is the lack of strong anatomic reference within the IVS; this could lead to an oblique angulation of the US beam, with consequent overestimation of LV chamber size. A good practice is to verify that the beam is relatively perpendicular to the IVS and LV free wall in long-axis view prior to switching to a short-axis view. Placing the cursor too dorsally on the IVS will artificially reduce LV systolic function measures, because such cursor positioning can approach the so-called "hinge point" between septal myocardium and the fibrous aortic root, which moves in the opposite direction during systole.

Once the mitral valve opens in early diastole, the IVS and LV posterior wall quickly move away from each other as the rapid ventricular filling phase occurs (p. 19). A small early diastolic "dip" is observed in the IVS motion, reflecting different rates of ventricular filling and overall cardiac motion. Changes associated with the respiratory cycle cause the RV chamber to fill relatively more during inspiration, which moves the IVS away from the transducer; this reflects both increased right heart filling and translational motion with ventilation. Additional small movements in both walls are observed after atrial contraction and during the QRS complex, related to isovolumetric (isovolumic) contraction. Immediately after the QRS complex is inscribed, the aortic valve opens and ejection begins. This is characterized by progressive thickening of the ventricular walls and movement of the IVS and LV wall toward each other (inward), with a slight timing offset of about 40 ms in maximal excursions. The maximal upward excursion (or apogee) of the LV wall coincides with aortic valve closure. The thickening and excursion of the LV wall from end-diastole to its apogee is a useful estimate of systolic function. This LV wall "amplitude" normally exceeds that of the IVS. When ventricular septal amplitude exceeds that of the LV wall in dogs, there is either significant LV volume overload or impaired segmental LV systolic function.

Mitral Valve The M-mode study at the mitral valve level tracks the opening and closing movements of both leaflets but focuses more on the anterior leaflet, closest to the IVS. Normal motion (**Figure 4.22**, center) is characterized by an early diastolic opening (E-point) that briefly brings the tip of the anterior mitral leaflet close to the IVS. The posterior (caudal) leaflet moves in the opposite direction. Posterior leaflet motion often is easier to visualize in patients with LV dilation. Following the E-point is a period of reduced LV filling (diastasis) with partial valve closure (F); this motion is lost when there is tachycardia. After the P wave of the ECG, atrial contraction reopens the mitral valve (A-point). At the onset of ventricular systole, the two mitral leaflets are brought to apposition (C). During systole the closed valve targets move toward the septum in a manner that parallels the LV wall. Once end-systole (D) is reached, the leaflets separate again with rapid ventricular filling (E), completing the cardiac cycle.

The distance between the opening E-point of the anterior leaflet and IVS is referred to as the "E-point to septal separation" (EPSS). In the absence of left-sided valvular disease, this distance is inversely related to LV EF. The EPSS in dogs normally is less than 7 mm, even in large breeds and typically is zero in many small breeds. The C-point typically occurs during the QRS complex, but it can be delayed in the setting of increased LV end-diastolic pressure. This can create a so-called "B-shoulder" or bump between the A-point and C-point of mitral valve excursion. Other abnormalities in

Table 4.2 M-mode Echocardiography—Some Diagnostic Clues

Structure	Finding	Interpretation	Comment
Left ventricle	Increased chamber diameter	Volume overload; DCM Athletic heart	Secondary to left-to-right shunts (PDA, VSD), mitral or aortic regurgitation, or primary or secondary DCM phenotype
Left ventricle	Reduced wall excursions	LV systolic dysfunction	Abnormal septal motion (including paradoxical motion and dyssynchrony) can falsely decrease systolic function measurements
Left ventricle	Increased end-diastolic wall thickness	Left ventricular hypertrophy; pseudohypertrophy	Usually results from ventricular outflow tract obstruction, hypertension, or HCM; pseudohypertrophy is artifact of dehydration or other cause of poor LV filling
IVS	Dyssynchronous motion relative to the LV wall	Myocardial disease; conduction disorder	Can occur in otherwise normal hearts; reduces value of fractional shortening
IVS	Flattened motion during the cardiac cycle	RV pressure overload	Septal and RV wall thicknesses are also increased usually
IVS	Paradoxical motion	RV volume overload	Septum moves toward RV in systole; RV chamber is dilated
IVS	Exuberant septal motion	LV volume overload	Septal excursion > LV wall excursion
Mitral valve	Increased EPSS	Dilated left ventricle with impaired systolic function (in most cases—see comment)	Increased distance between anterior mitral leaflet E-(opening) point and IVS. Also r/o mitral stenosis or aortic regurgitation
Mitral valve	Systolic fluttering	Possible chordal tear	Usually accompanies a musical murmur of mitral regurgitation
Mitral valve	Diastolic fluttering	Aortic regurgitation jet striking the anterior leaflet	Might have fluttering of the IVS if multiple jets of aortic regurgitation
Mitral valve	Concordant leaflet motion	Mitral stenosis; valve fusion	Posterior leaflet does not fully separate and move in opposite direction to anterior leaflet in diastole
Mitral valve	Chaotic leaflet motion	Flail mitral leaflet	Major chordal rupture, usually caused by degenerative (myxomatous) disease or endocarditis
Mitral valve	Systolic anterior motion	Dynamic LV outflow tract obstruction	Anterior leaflet strikes septum in mid-to-late systole; common in HOCM and occasionally with subaortic stenosis or mitral dysplasia
Mitral valve	Premature closure	Aortic regurgitation with elevated LV diastolic pressure	Also, r/o closure caused by a short cardiac cycle, as with atrial fibrillation or VPC
Mitral valve	Delayed closure after the QRS complex ("B-shoulder")	Increased LA and LV diastolic pressures	Typical of DCM with congestive heart failure
Aortic root	Decreased amplitude of motion	Reduced CO	Common with DCM
Aortic valve	"Boxcars" appearance	Possible reduced CO or dilated aortic root	In animals, it is unusual to clearly visualize two wide-open leaflets in systole
Aortic valve	Systolic leaflet fluttering	Increased ejection velocity	Common in subaortic stenosis and HOCM, but can be a normal finding in many animals, including those with functional ejection murmurs
Aortic valve	Midsystolic closure	Dynamic LV outflow tract obstruction	Valve partially closes then reopens; common in HOCM
Aortic valve	Diastolic fluttering	Aortic regurgitation	From primary aortic valve disease or aortic root dilation
Aortic valve	Inadequate leaflet separation	Valvular aortic stenosis; poor stroke volume	Eccentric closure line suggests stenosis with bicuspid or otherwise abnormal aortic valve; or r/o causes of low CO

Abbreviations: CO, cardiac output; DCM, dilated cardiomyopathy; EPSS, E-point septal separation; H(O)CM, hypertrophic (obstructive) cardiomyopathy; IVS, interventricular septum; LA, left atrial; LV, left ventricular; PDA, patent ductus arteriosus; r/o, rule out; RV, right ventricular; VPC, ventricular premature complex/contraction; VSD, ventricular septal defect.

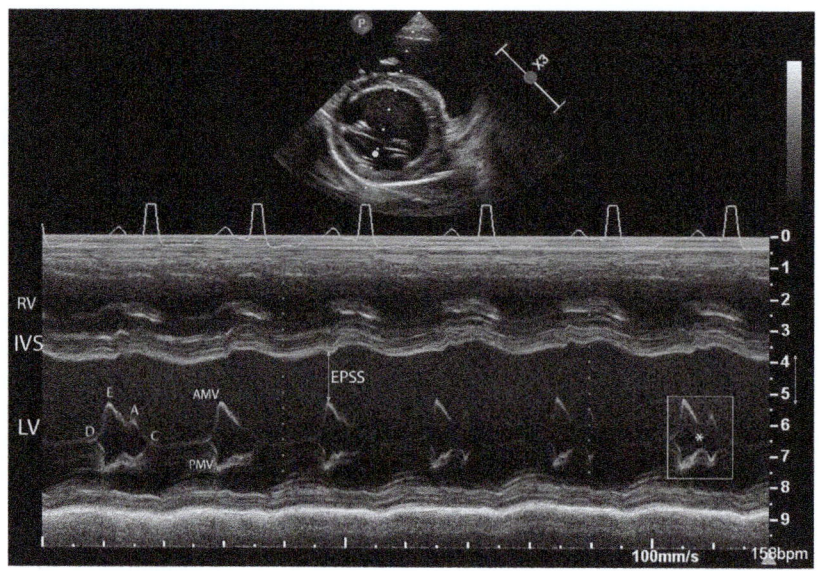

Figure 4.23 Duplex 2D and M-mode images at the mitral valve level in a French Bulldog with dilated cardiomyopathy. The value of M-mode study is still evident inasmuch as it shows the LV is dilated, the overall systolic shortening is reduced, and the E-point to septal separation (EPSS) is increased at >10 mm, indicating reduced LV ejection fraction. The two mitral leaflets create a "double-diamond" appearance (*) with approximately equal excursions of the posterior (PMV) and anterior (AMV) leaflets. Other abbreviations as in **Figures 4.21** and **4.22**.

mitral motion are summarized in **Table 4.2** and illustrated in **Figure 4.23**.

Aortic Valve and Left Atrium The M-mode cursor bisects the circular aortic root at the valve level. In dogs and in horses, it crosses two leaflets and the junction of left atrial body and appendage. Because the M-line does not transect the full extent of the LA in this view, the M-mode examination should not be used to measure left atrial size in these species. In cats, although M-mode echocardiography usually better reflects left atrial size, maximal chamber diameter is not imaged consistently. However, fractional shortening of the LA (the percentage change in diameter from filling to emptying) can be measured using the M-mode cursor in cats.

The proximal aorta moves toward the transducer during systole; overall, aortic root amplitude correlates generally with stroke volume. Aortic valve opening and closing movements can be tracked during the M-mode examination, but this one-dimensional ("ice pick") view limits the diagnostic information available. In most healthy animals, only one aortic leaflet will be seen well throughout the cardiac cycle, although the opening distance between two leaflets usually is evident during systole. Generally, lesions of the aortic valve are better identified with 2D or 3D imaging.

Despite these limitations, the high-frequency sampling of this modality permits capture of rapid valvular movements such as high-frequency systolic fluttering of the leaflets during rapid ejection or partial midsystolic valve closure and reopening correlating to the onset of dynamic LV obstruction, such as with hypertrophic cardiomyopathy (HCM) or some cases of subaortic stenosis (**Figure 27.12**, p. 485). Diastolic fluttering of the aortic valve and of the aortic root (and anterior mitral leaflet on mitral level images) might be seen in cases with aortic regurgitation (AR; **Table 4.2**; also see **Figures 30.13**, p. 583, and **31.11**, p. 601).

Clinical Utility of the M-mode Exam For many clinicians, the M-mode examination is mostly of historical interest and largely has been replaced by capture and measurement of digital 2D images at high frame rates. However, this modality still has utility in veterinary practice, because diseases can change cardiac motion or the position of imaging targets within the imaging field. For example, in normal hearts, a properly recorded image at the ventricular level provides a rapid and reasonable representation of LV wall thickness and chamber size. If subjective evaluation reveals no regional wall abnormalities, a normal M-mode study of the ventricle can confirm this with objective measures. M-mode imaging can verify normal, low, or hyperdynamic LV systolic function, again assuming there are no regional wall motion disturbances. Analysis of interventricular septal motion also offers insight regarding ventricular chamber volumes and pressures. Abnormal pressures or high-velocity blood flow jets can alter the motion of the cardiac valves, as is often seen best with M-mode (see **Figures 26.32B**, p. 459, and **33.20B**, p. 670).

The M-mode study can be combined with color Doppler imaging to generate an accurate spatial map of flow disturbances across the cursor line. This is especially valuable for timing of flow events (**Figures 4.24** and **4.25**). For example, brief backflow signals that occur as the valves close often are misinterpreted as clinically significant valvular regurgitation during 2D color Doppler imaging. Color M-mode can

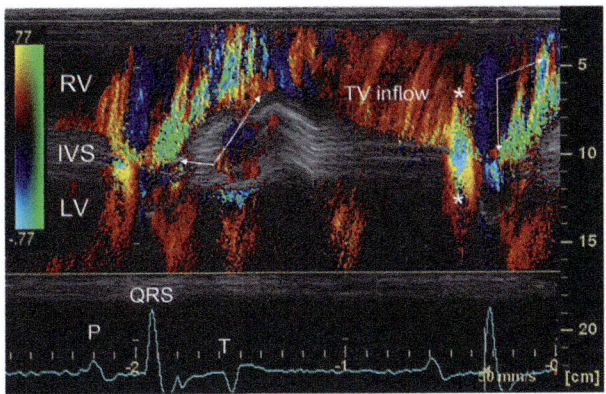

qualitative and quantitative insights into a variety of heart diseases. Many of the most common diagnostic clues are outlined in **Table 4.2**.

Cardiac Size and Function Measurement

Enlargement of cardiac chambers and great vessels can indicate the type of heart disease present, as well as its severity (**Table 4.3**). Some disorders, such as the cardiomyopathies, are fundamentally characterized by changes in cardiac chamber size and function. The progression of chronic valvular disease is reflected in changes of cardiac measurements. The severity of a cardiac shunt is reflected by enlargements in chambers carrying the extra volume. As a noninvasive imaging modality, echocardiography has become the foremost method for quantifying heart size and function.

Figure 4.24 Color M-mode showing the timing (x-axis and ECG) and spatial orientation (y-axis) of flow across a ventricular septal defect. Close up of the ventricular septum (IVS) shows a turbulent (mosaic/green) systolic flow pattern (arrows) crossing the septum into the right ventricle (RV). During diastole, low velocity transtricuspid (TV) flow enters the RV (encoded in darker red). There is also presystolic left-to-right shunting after the atrial contraction (*). LV, left ventricle.

The number of measurements and calculations that can be generated using echocardiography is nearly endless. Busy clinicians should focus on those with the greatest clinical impact. Measurements are made with digital calipers, often within a programmed software routine (**Figures 4.3, 4.5, 4.7, and 4.15–4.17**). Although there are dedicated workstations and web hosting sites for making cardiac measurements, the majority are done on the echo system at the time of examination. Left heart measurements in companion animals have traditionally be obtained from M-mode studies, but can be more readily learned by measuring frozen

faithfully define the duration of these signals with greater time resolution than conventional color flow mapping, and with less need for signal processing compared to spectral Doppler studies.

Although valvular thickening and valvar lesions, such as vegetations or thrombi, can be seen using the M-mode exam, these changes are best visualized by 2D (or 3D) imaging. However, targeting the ventricular chambers and the rapidly moving valvular structures within the M-line offers both

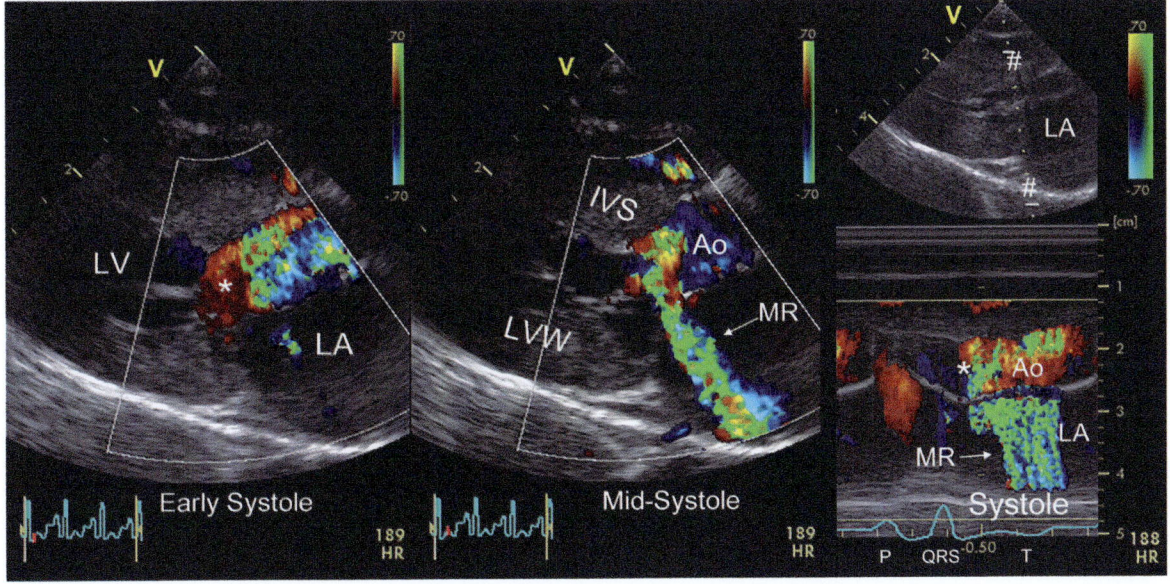

Figure 4.25 Long-axis images of the feline left ventricular inflow and outflow tracts recorded in early-systole (left panel) and midsystole (center panel), from a cat with hypertrophic cardiomyopathy, systolic anterior motion of the mitral valve, and dynamic left ventricular outflow tract (LVOT) obstruction. Color Doppler imaging has been activated. There is a mid-late systolic jet of mitral regurgitation (MR, arrows). The right panel shows a color M-mode recording from the same cat; the M-line (between the # in 2D image above) crosses the LVOT and the mitral orifice. Note the timing of the turbulence in the 2D and M-mode recordings: turbulent flow begins in the aorta (*) before the prominent eccentric jet of MR develops. The color M-mode clearly shows that the MR does not begin until midsystole. Other abbreviations as in **Figure 4.4**.

Table 4.3 Causes of Cardiac Chamber and Great Vessel Enlargement

Enlarged Structure	Differential Diagnoses
Left atrium	Left-to-right shunt (PDA, VSD)
	Mitral valve disease (regurgitation or stenosis)
	Cardiomyopathy (any form)
	Left heart failure (any cause)
Left ventricle—eccentric hypertrophy or dilation	Left-to-right shunt (PDA, VSD)
	Mitral valve disease (regurgitation or stenosis)
	Cardiomyopathy (dilated, end-stage of other cardiomyopathy phenotypes)
	Chronic aortic regurgitation
	Left heart failure (any cause)
Left ventricle—concentric hypertrophy or wall thickening	Aortic stenosis (any type/localization)
	Hypertrophic cardiomyopathy
	Systemic hypertension
	Myocarditis
	Transient myocardial thickening of cats
	Infiltration (neoplastic, inflammatory)
Aorta	Subaortic/aortic stenosis (poststenotic dilation)
	Dynamic LV outflow tract obstruction
	Idiopathic aortoannular ectasia
	Systemic hypertension
	Genetic aortopathy (as in Leonberger dogs)
Right atrium and right ventricle	ASD; anomalous pulmonary vein drainage
	Tricuspid valve disease (regurgitation or stenosis)
	Some cardiomyopathies, including advanced ARVC and silent atrium
	Pulmonic stenosis (concentric RV hypertrophy)
	Pulmonary hypertension (mixed or concentric RV hypertrophy)
	Right heart failure (any cause)
Pulmonary artery	Pulmonic stenosis (poststenotic dilation)
	Left-to-right shunt (ASD, VSD, PDA)
	Pulmonary hypertension (any cause; lobar PA dilation also)

Abbreviations: ARVC, arrhythmogenic right ventricular cardiomyopathy; ASD, atrial septal defect; LV, left ventricular; PA, pulmonary artery; PDA, patent ductus arteriosus; RV, right ventricular; VSD, ventricular septal defect.

2D images, as long as true end-diastolic and end-systolic frames are selected. Measurement of the LA should always be done using 2D (or 3D) methods; similarly, quantitation of right atrial, RV, and pulmonary arterial size is accomplished mainly with 2D imaging.

The timing of measurements is important. End-diastolic measurements are obtained between the onset of the QRS complex and peak of the R wave. The timing for ventricular systolic measurements is more subjective, but typically occurs just after the end of the T wave. When using 2D imaging for ventricular measurements, the frame immediately prior to mitral valve opening is selected. For M-mode studies of the left ventricle, systolic measurements are obtained at the maximal (greatest) excursion of the ventricular walls (either the septal nadir or apogee of the LV posterior wall), or at the point when the ventricular lumen is smallest. Atrial measurements are greatest just prior to AV valve opening (end-systole). However, there are some notable exceptions to these guidelines, as indicated below.

The same images used to assess heart enlargement also are relevant for measuring heart function. There are dozens of different approaches, but practically, 2D and M-mode studies are used for routine cardiac work. The fundamental global assessment of LV or RV function is the EF, which is simply the ventricular stroke volume (volume ejected) divided by the end-diastolic volume (the volume at the end of ventricular filling). Arithmetically, $EF = (D-S)/D$, where D is the end-diastolic volume, S represents the end-systolic volume, and D-S is the stroke volume. Frequently, surrogates for EF are used in veterinary practice. If diastolic and systolic areas are used, the function index is called "fractional area change." This is done most often using short-axis images of the left ventricle, left apical images of the right ventricle, or the left apical four-chamber and two-chamber images for the LA (recognizing that the atria fill as the ventricles empty). When volumes in the EF formula are replaced with linear dimensions (as with M-mode study of the left ventricle), the functional index is termed "fractional shortening" (FS; **Figure 4.3**). Normal values differ depending on whether volumes, areas, or dimensions are used; however, the concept of the EF formula is the same.

Another approach to measuring ventricular function involves tracking longitudinal movement at the lateral AV valve annulus from a left apical transducer position. For the right ventricle, this is called "tricuspid annular plane systolic excursion" (TAPSE; **Figure 4.19**). For the left ventricle and mitral annulus, the abbreviation is MAPSE. These are relatively simple to perform using M-mode echocardiography. They are repeatable provided the cursor is aligned well with annular motion, that is, the angle of incidence between cursor and longitudinal shortening is small. Although often underutilized, these approaches can be especially useful in cases where systolic function, as measured by FS, is borderline.

It also is possible to measure segmental cardiac function. These function tests potentially are more sensitive for detecting preclinical disease; however, they require advanced technologies and have not been standardized for animals.

Examples include TDI (p. 119) and myocardial speckle-tracking (p. 130) to determine segmental deformation or strain. Currently, few clinical (and no therapeutic) decisions are based only on segmental myocardial analysis.

Diastolic ventricular function should not be overlooked in terms of importance to certain diseases such as HCM and aortic stenosis. Diastolic assessment is largely the province of Doppler echocardiography. These are more advanced techniques. They are discussed briefly at the end of this introductory chapter.

General Considerations and Pitfalls of Cardiac Chamber Measurement

Methods Used Three different methods are used by cardiologists for measuring a ventricular wall or cardiac chamber. This has created issues of standardization. The most common approach involves the "leading edge to leading edge" method, which incorporates one endocardial border into the measurement (or one near-field wall in the case of the aorta or pulmonary artery). The second approach involves measuring at the blood–tissue interface (inner edge approach), which essentially incorporates two endocardial borders into a wall measurement and none into a luminal diameter. A third approach, used for the left ventricle, employs the trailing edge for the IVS, inner edge for the LV chamber at the blood–tissue interface, and the leading edge for the posterior LV wall (Bonagura, 2020).

Measurements in Cats Special comment is relevant regarding ventricular wall thickness measurement in cats. Most published studies in cats have used M-mode imaging with a leading edge method of measurement such that one endocardial border is included. These results might not be identical to those obtained using 2D measurements and a tissue–blood interface approach. While inclusion of one or two endocardial border thicknesses might seem trivial, in cats this decision could change the diagnosis from "normal" to "hypertrophied"; this is an issue that is currently unresolved. Some practical suggestions are provided later in this section. The frame- or sampling rate of imaging also influences measurement accuracy in cats because rapid heart rates make it more difficult to freeze a true end-diastolic image, and in fact, also increase relative wall thicknesses (Sugimoto, 2017). Frame-by-frame analysis is crucial in asymptomatic cats to avoid overdiagnosis of HCM. Ventricular septal measurements are especially prone to overinterpretation. Many large cats have a slightly thicker IVS and LV free wall; this is more prominent in some breeds, such as Bengal cats. In some cats, a prominent false tendon exits the dorsal IVS and tracks along its LV surface before extending toward the papillary muscles. The insertion point of this conduction bundle within the septum is normally thicker, and should not be included in IVS measurements. There are other roadblocks to accurate LV assessment in cats. For example, the posterior papillary muscle extends quite dorsally in long-axis views; this muscle commonly is captured by the M-mode cursor, inappropriately increasing apparent LV wall thickness. Additionally, dehydration and diuretic therapy reduce LV chamber volume, which leads to a pseudohypertrophy of the ventricular walls.

Other Issues Quantitation of LV lumen size in horses and in dogs is hampered by imprecise placement of the M-mode cursor. Additionally, there is a subaortic "divot" observed in these species; this can measure nearly 1 cm in the horse. When using the short axis for LV measurement in the horse, it is common to select a plane that is too ventral, which underestimates chamber size. In both horses and in dogs, the opposite error occurs when the measurement extends obliquely from between the papillary muscles across and into the septal "divot," which overestimates LV size. One potential check is to compare measurements from both short- and long-axis planes when assessing LV diameter. Marked differences in diastolic values should prompt reconsideration of the image plane(s) used.

Experienced examiners are relatively proficient at subjectively recognizing what might be considered moderate to severe cardiomegaly. However, most examiners cannot identify mild chamber enlargement or wall thickening without completing specified measurements and reviewing slow motion video loops. Changes over time are relatively reliable for detecting progressive heart enlargement, especially when the repeated measurement exceeds the normal variability for that measurement (typically 5–15% for echo variables). Changes in echo measurements are especially valuable for monitoring progressive LV volume overload caused by chronic mitral or aortic valvular disease in dogs and horses, and left atrial chamber size in cats with cardiomyopathy.

Identifying Chamber Enlargement Five general approaches might be considered for assessing cardiac chamber enlargement. The first is "subjective," based on clinician experience and the size relationships among chambers; with experience, moderate to severe enlargement can be identified subjectively. The second involves detecting progressive heart enlargement over time, assuming the changes are beyond physiological and day-to-day variation. As noted above, these generally need to be greater than 5–10% from the prior examination, depending on the measured or calculated echo variable. The third method involves calculation of various "ratios." For example, normal diastolic RV wall thickness should be <50% (and is usually 35–40%) of LV wall thickness, assuming good near-field resolution and exclusion of the epi/pericardial thickness. There are a number of useful indices relating the left and right heart

Table 4.4 Left Atrial and Left Ventricular to Aortic Ratios Obtained from Normal Dogs

LA/Ao Short-Axis Ratios and Prediction Intervals	Method; Number; Reference; Comments
1.42 (median) 1.14, 1.65 (lower, upper prediction limits)	Maximal diastolic; n = 122; Visser, 2019; short-axis aorta
0.97, 1.76 (lower, upper prediction intervals)	Maximal diastolic; n = 233; Rishniw, 2019; short-axis aorta
0.75, 1.65 (lower, upper prediction intervals)	Minimal diastolic; n = 233; Rishniw, 2019; short-axis aorta
LA/AoV Long-Axis Ratios and Prediction Intervals	**Method; Number; Reference**
2.24 (median); 1.88, 2.57 (lower, upper prediction limits)	Long-axis AoV; n = 122; Visser, 2019
LV/AoV 2D Ratios and Prediction Intervals	**Method; Number; Reference**
2.29 (median); 1.79, 2.59 (lower, upper prediction limits)	Long-axis AoV; n = 122; Visser, 2019
2.32 (median); 1.80, 2.89 (lower, upper prediction limits)	Short-axis AoV; n = 122; Visser, 2019
LA/Ao (Long-Short Axis) Ratio	**Method; Number; Reference**
1.33, 2.17 (lower, upper prediction limits)	Long-axis LA, short-axis aorta; n = 233; Rishniw, 2019
Left Ventricular Wall Thickness by Aortic Weight Ratios	**Method; Reference; Comments**
4.14, 8.15 (lower, upper prediction limits)	2-D aortic valve systolic diameter; Strohm, 2018[a] See footnote[a] for formula
2.96, 5.82 (lower, upper prediction intervals)	Using M-mode aortic diastolic diameter; modified Brown, 2003[b] See footnote[b] for formula

[a] Weighted ratio can be calculated using this equation: **0.5677 *Body weight in kg$^{1/3}$**; from Strohm, 2018.

[b] Weighted ratio can be calculated using this equation: **0.795 * Body weight in kg$^{1/3}$**; from Brown, 2003. The weight-based constant is larger because M-mode measurements of the aorta include a sinus of Valsalva and are larger than those obtained between opened aortic valve leaflets.

Examples: If the LV wall in diastole measures 11 mm in a 10 kg dog, the aortic weighted LV diastolic wall thickness (using the Strohm constant of 0.5677 determined from 2D aortic diameter) is as follows: **LVWd/wAo = (11 mm/[0.5677] * [10$^{.333}$])** = 11 mm/(0.5677 * 2.15) = 11/1.221 = **9.01**, an aortic weighted value that exceeds the upper prediction limit of 8.15 shown in the table. This weighted aortic ratio represents a thickened LV wall. Using the Brown constant of 0.795 (derived from M-mode echocardiograms of diastolic aortic size), the aortic weighted ratio would equal **LVWd/wAo = (11 mm/[0.795] * [10$^{.333}$])** = 11/1.711 = **6.43**, a value that exceeds the upper prediction limit of 5.82. Note that while constants from different studies were used, the upper prediction limits were calculated from a single multibreed study of 80 healthy dogs (Strohm, 2018) using the robust CLSI method for prediction limits (with 90% confidence limits around the highest values). Both Brown and Strohm weight-based aortic constants identified LV wall hypertrophy or thickening in this case example.

Abbreviations: Ao, aorta; AoV, distance between opened aortic valve leaflets (maximal aortic orifice diameter); LA, left atrium.

chambers to the aorta (**Table 4.4**). However, aortic-based ratios are not interchangeable, and the precise imaging planes and timing of the cardiac measurements must be reported. In the authors' experience, some of these ratios are useful for identifying even mild cardiomegaly.

A fourth approach to chamber quantitation involves "allometric scaling" to body size. This mainly is done in dogs and to a limited degree in horses, but it is also relevant to cats (**Tables 4.5** and **4.6**). For example, in dogs a normalized diastolic LV and systolic LA dimension, based on allometric scaling, should not exceed about 1.65 (see tables). In warmblood horses (**Table 4.7**), the LV diameter normalized to a bodyweight (Wt) of 500 kg can be estimated as Diameter (500) = Measured diameter/Wt$^{1/3}$ × 500$^{1/3}$. More details are needed regarding this type of scaling in all species. Unfortunately, many of the published prediction ranges tend to be specific, but quite insensitive, for cardiomegaly.

Finally, identifying cardiomegaly using breed-specific normal values can be considered when suitable reference studies are available. A number of these have been published and some are summarized in **Tables 4.7–4.10**. Uniformly accepted guidelines for cardiac size measurement are lacking and some studies are single-center with small sample sizes; thus, the values for common echo measurements shown in the tables should be regarded as approximate. Weight, breed, age, and exercise training affect measured echo variables.

In an attempt to keep recommendations for quantifying chamber size as practical as possible, only a limited number of methods and reference data are presented. These undoubtedly reflect the perspectives of the authors and there is considerable controversy regarding optimal approaches. The reader is referred to the figures for examples of these measurements, and to the tables for reference ranges.

Table 4.5 Canine Echocardiographic Left Atrial and Ventricular Dimensions—Allometric Scaling

Allometric Scaling to Weight (kg)	Left Atrium—2D (long-axis)[1] End-Systolic Measurement (cm)		Left Ventricle—2D and M-mode Diastolic Dimensions (cm)[1,2]							
Weight	Predicted LA diameter[a]	Upper prediction interval	Predicted LV diameter (2D, long-axis)[1]	LV upper prediction interval (2D, long-axis)[1]	Predicted LV diameter (2D, short-axis)[1]	LV upper prediction interval (2D, short-axis)[1]	Predicted LV diameter M-mode (short-axis)[1]	LV upper prediction interval (M-mode)[1]	Predicted LV diameter (M-mode)[2]	LVEDDN 1.7[b] (M-mode)[2]
1	1.00	1.60	1.00	1.60	1.00	1.70	1.00	1.67	1.00	1.70
2	1.24	1.98	1.24	1.99	1.24	2.12	1.23	2.05	1.23	2.08
3	1.40	2.25	1.42	2.26	1.42	2.41	1.39	2.32	1.38	2.35
4	1.53	2.46	1.55	2.48	1.55	2.63	1.51	2.53	1.50	2.56
5	1.64	2.63	1.66	2.66	1.66	2.83	1.62	2.70	1.61	2.73
6	1.74	2.78	1.76	2.82	1.76	2.99	1.71	2.85	1.69	2.88
7	1.82	2.92	1.85	2.96	1.85	3.14	1.79	2.99	1.77	3.01
8	1.90	3.04	1.93	3.09	1.93	3.28	1.86	3.11	1.84	3.13
9	1.97	3.15	2.00	3.20	2.00	3.40	1.93	3.22	1.91	3.24
10	2.04	3.26	2.07	3.31	2.07	3.52	1.99	3.32	1.97	3.35
11	2.10	3.36	2.13	3.41	2.13	3.63	2.05	3.42	2.02	3.44
12	2.16	3.45	2.19	3.51	2.19	3.73	2.10	3.51	2.08	3.53
13	2.21	3.53	2.25	3.60	2.25	3.82	2.15	3.60	2.13	3.61
14	2.26	3.62	2.30	3.68	2.30	3.91	2.20	3.68	2.17	3.69
15	2.31	3.69	2.35	3.76	2.35	4.00	2.25	3.75	2.22	3.77
16	2.36	3.77	2.40	3.84	2.40	4.08	2.29	3.83	2.26	3.84
17	2.40	3.84	2.45	3.92	2.45	4.16	2.33	3.90	2.30	3.91
18	2.44	3.91	2.49	3.99	2.49	4.24	2.37	3.96	2.34	3.98
19	2.48	3.97	2.54	4.06	2.54	4.31	2.41	4.03	2.38	4.04
20	2.52	4.04	2.58	4.12	2.58	4.38	2.45	4.09	2.41	4.10
21	2.56	4.10	2.62	4.19	2.62	4.45	2.49	4.15	2.45	4.16
22	2.60	4.16	2.66	4.25	2.66	4.51	2.52	4.21	2.48	4.22
23	2.63	4.22	2.69	4.31	2.69	4.58	2.55	4.26	2.51	4.27
24	2.67	4.27	2.73	4.37	2.73	4.64	2.59	4.32	2.55	4.33
25	2.70	4.33	2.77	4.42	2.77	4.70	2.62	4.37	2.58	4.38
26	2.74	4.38	2.80	4.48	2.80	4.76	2.65	4.42	2.61	4.43
27	2.77	4.43	2.83	4.53	2.83	4.82	2.68	4.47	2.64	4.48
28	2.80	4.48	2.87	4.59	2.87	4.87	2.71	4.52	2.66	4.53
29	2.83	4.53	2.90	4.64	2.90	4.93	2.74	4.57	2.69	4.58
30	2.86	4.58	2.93	4.69	2.93	4.98	2.76	4.62	2.72	4.62
31	2.89	4.62	2.96	4.74	2.96	5.03	2.79	4.66	2.74	4.67
32	2.92	4.67	2.99	4.78	2.99	5.08	2.82	4.71	2.77	4.71
33	2.95	4.71	3.02	4.83	3.02	5.13	2.84	4.75	2.80	4.75
34	2.97	4.76	3.05	4.88	3.05	5.18	2.87	4.79	2.82	4.79
35	3.00	4.80	3.08	4.92	3.08	5.23	2.90	4.83	2.84	4.84
36	3.03	4.84	3.10	4.96	3.10	5.28	2.92	4.88	2.87	4.88
37	3.05	4.88	3.13	5.01	3.13	5.32	2.94	4.92	2.89	4.91
38	3.08	4.92	3.16	5.05	3.16	5.37	2.97	4.96	2.91	4.95
39	3.10	4.96	3.18	5.09	3.18	5.41	2.99	4.99	2.94	4.99
40	3.13	5.00	3.21	5.13	3.21	5.45	3.01	5.03	2.96	5.03

[a] Other exponents have been generated from different studies but are generally similar for long axis measurements of the left atrium at end systole shown here. In a study by Marchesotti, 2019, Normalized LA = (in cm)/weight (in kg)$^{0.324}$, where the median was 1.29 (converted to cm from the original reported mm) and the 95% prediction interval was 0.97–1.72, similar to the Visser study limits of 0.65–1.65 based on their equation, Normalized LA = LA (cm)/weight (kg)$^{0.309}$. In a multicenter study by Rishniw, 2019, the LA exponent was a nearly identical 0.31 with an upper prediction interval for the normalized long axis LA of 1.64–1.79.
For LVID diastolic, the normalized value was calculated from Visser[1] (2019) as Normalized LVIDD = LV (cm)/weight$^{(x\ or\ y)}$, where x = 0.316 for 2D imaging and y = 0.299 for M-mode imaging. The exponent for the study of Cornell[2], 2004 is 0.294. The upper (97.5%) limit for predictive values in that study were larger (Normalized LVID in diastole × 1.85) and somewhat less sensitive to LV enlargement when compared to the Visser (2019) upper limits. Note: (Visser) limit is similar to the Normalized LVIDD × 1.7 calculated from the Cornell (2004) data and commonly used to identify "clinically significant" LV dilation. A recent study (published during printing of this text), based on >6,000 non-sighthound dogs, showed exponents of 0.322 for LVIDd & 0.346 for LVIDs (Esser, 2020).
[b] Criterion used in EPIC clinical trial of myxomatous mitral valve disease in dogs; see Boswood (2016). The allometric scaling was from Cornell (2004).

Abbreviations: LA, left atrium; LV, left ventricle; LVEDDN, normalized left ventricular end-diastolic dimension.

Table 4.6 Feline Echocardiographic Measurements—Allometric Scaling

M-mode Data from 19,866 Cats[1]				2D Measurement Data from 150 Cats[2]							
Weight (kg)	IVSd (mm)	LVIDd (mm)	LVWd (mm)	Weight range (kg) (number)	LAD-LAx (mm)	IVSd-LAx (mm)	IVSd-SAx (mm)	LVIDd-LAx (mm)	LVIDd-SAx (mm)	LVWd-LAx (mm)	LVWd-SAx (mm)
1.5	3.1 (4.0)	11.9 (15.0)	2.9 (3.8)								
2	3.3 (4.3)	12.8 (16.0)	3.1 (4.1)								
2.5	3.4 (4.5)	13.6 (17.0)	3.2 (4.4)	<3 (n = 24)	13.37 (13.98)	4.34 (4.52)	4.44 (4.64)	13.07 (13.75)	12.72 (13.52)	3.63 (3.89)	3.96 (4.18)
3	3.5 (4.7)	14.2 (17.8)	3.4 (4.5)	>3 to ≤4 (n = 49)	14.09 (14.49)	4.55 (4.67)	4.67 (4.81)	13.87 (14.33)	13.68 (14.22)	3.94 (4.12)	4.21 (4.37)
3.5	3.7 (4.9)	14.8 (18.5)	3.6 (4.7)								
4	3.8 (4.9)	15.4 (19.2)	3.7 (4.8)	>4 to ≤5 (n = 38)	14.65 (14.93)	4.71 (4.81)	4.86 (4.96)	14.50 (14.82)	14.41 (14.79)	4.19 (4.33)	4.41 (4.53)
4.5	3.9 (5.1)	15.8 (19.8)	3.8 (5.0)								
5	3.9 (5.2)	16.3 (20.3)	3.9 (5.1)	>5 to ≤6 (n = 25)	15.20 (15.48)	4.87 (4.97)	5.04 (5.14)	15.13 (15.45)	14.63 (15.79)	4.44 (4.58)	4.62 (4.74)
5.5	4.0 (5.3)	16.7 (20.9)	4.0 (5.3)								
6	4.1 (5.4)	17.1 (21.4)	4.1 (5.4)	>6 to ≤7 (n = 9)	15.64 (15.85)	4.99 (5.07)	5.19 (5.29)	15.63 (15.87)	15.82 (16.12)	4.64 (4.74)	4.78 (4.88)
7	4.2 (5.6)	17.8 (22.2)	4.3 (5.6)	>7 (n = 5)	16.12 (16.28)	5.13 (5.21)	5.35 (5.43)	16.18 (16.36)	16.51 (16.73)	4.66 (4.94)	4.85 (5.05)
8	4.3 (5.8)	18.4 (23.0)	4.4 (5.8)								
9	4.4 (5.9)	19.0 (23.7)	4.5 (5.9)								
10	4.5 (6.0)	19.5 (24.4)	4.6 (6.1)								

[1] M-mode data from Haggstrom, et al (2016); shown as predicted value (upper prediction interval) for each body weight.
[2] 2D data from Schober, et al (2018); shown as mean (upper reference limit). Both studies are based on allometric scaling of the data.

Abbreviations: IVSd, diastolic interventricular septal thickness (mm); LAD, maximal left atrial dimension (long axis); LAx, long-axis image plane; LVIDd, diastolic left ventricular dimension, LVWd, diastolic left ventricular wall thickness; SAx, short-axis image plane.
Data from the studies of Haggstrom, et al (2016)[1] and from Schober, et al (2018)[2]; see References for citations.

Table 4.7 Equine Echocardiographic Measurements[a]

Echo Variable	Study (reference)					
	Gunther-Harrington, 2018	Young, 2005	DeCloedt, 2020	Huesler, 2016	Zucca, 2018	Buhl, 2005
Number	30	358	29	31	30	
Breed	Thoroughbred	National Hunt/TB	Warmblood	Warmblood	Standardbred	Standardbred Various
Age (Years)	3.8 (0.9)	>2	8 (4)	12 (4)	3.8 (1.6)	
Weight (kg)	—	461.5 (3.6[b])	566 (48)	574 (58)	435 (36)	441 (43)–481 (36)
LA (2D) Lax	13.0 (0.7) 11.8–14.7[c]			11.9 (0.7) 10.2–13.5[c]	11.5 (0.5) 10.4–12.4[c]	
LA (2D) SAx	10.9 (0.7) 9.8–12.2[c]					
Aorta (2D)	7.5 (0.6) 6.6–8.6[c,d]			7.6 (0.5) 6.3–9.0[c]	7.79 (0.46) 6.84–8.94	
Aorta (M-mode)	7.5 (0.6) 6.6–8.6[c,d]					
Aorta 2D Normalized (500)						
IVSd	3.3 (0.4) 2.7–4.0[c]	2.62 (0.003[b])				
IVSd Normalized (500)				3.0 (0.3) 2.2–3.9[c]	3.10 (0.41) 2.23–38.3	
LVIDd	12.1 (1.0) 10.5–13.7[c]	12.96 (0.11[b])	11.1 (9.9–13.5)		11.6 (1.28) 8.74–13.6[c]	10.87 (0.86) first exam 12.16 (0.8) last exam
LVIDd normalized (500)				11.1 (0.9) 8.9–13.3[c]		
LVIDs	6.9 (1.1) 5.0–8.7[c]	7.93 (0.12[b])	6.4 (4.6–8.1)			
LVS Normalized (500)						
LVFWd	2.8 (0.3) 2.2–3.4[c]	2.27 (0.002[b])	—	2.5 (0.3) 1.8–3.3[c]	2.55 (0.36) 1.90–3.19	2.19 (0.18) first exam 2.43 (0.17) last exam
LVWd Normalized (500)						
LV Fractional Shortening %	42.2 (7.6) 30.8–58.0[c]		43 (6)		35.2 (3.9) 31–46	

Note: Normalized (500) dimensions indicate the measurement was allometrically scaled to a warmblood breed weighing 500 kg.
[a] All measurement values are in centimeters unless otherwise noted and data are reported as a mean (SD) or mean (SEM[b]) or as a median (lower–upper values).
[c] Indicates a range is a calculated reference interval.
[d] Method not stated.

Abbreviations: IVSd, interventricular septal thickness end-diastole; LA, left atrium; LVIDd, left ventricular internal dimension end-diastole; LVIDs, left ventricular internal dimension end-systole; LVWd, left ventricular free-wall thickness end-diastole; TB, thoroughbred.

Table 4.8 Canine Breed-Specific M-mode Measurements

Breed[a] (Reference)	n	Weight (kg)	LVIDd (mm)	LVIDs (mm)	IVSd (mm)	LVWd (mm)	LV FS (%)
Miniature Poodle (Morrison, 1992)	20	3[b] (1.4–9.0)	20 (16–28)	10 (8–16)	—	5 (4–6)	47 (35–57)
Italian Greyhound (della Torre, 2000)	20	5 ± 2	22.2	—	6.4	7.1	42.7
Cavalier King Charles Spaniel (Misbach, 2014)	134	8.7 (6.0–14.5)	[21.4–41.1]	[10.9–24.6]	[4.8–8.8]	[4.9–8.5]	—
Beagle (Crippa, 1992)	50	8.9 ± 1.5 (5.5–12)	26.3 19.9–33.1	15.7 8.9–22.5	6.7 4.5–8.9	8.2 4.4–12	40 22–58
Beagle (Hanton, 2005)	108	12.5 ± 2.0	31.2 26.6–35.8	20.4 15–25.8	7.7 5.5–9.9	6.5 4.3–8.7	34.8 24–45.2
West Highland White Terrier (Baade, 1999)	24	10.3 ± 0.9	28.8 17.4–40.2	20 12.6–27.4	6.9 4.1–10.7	6.4 4–8.8	35 21–49
English Cocker Spaniel (Gooding, 1986)	12	12.2 ± 2.25	33.8 27.2–40.4	22.2 16.6–27.8	–	7.9 5.7–10.1	34.3 25.3–43.3
Mudi (Voros, 2009)	28	12.8 ± 5.1	33.6 28–39.2	21.4 17.2–25.6	8.4 6.4–10.4	9.2 8.0–11.4	36.3 27.1–45.5
Whippet (Bavegems, 2007)	105	13.2 ± 2.1	37.3 27.9–44.8	26.9 19.8–34.1	9.4 7.0–11.8	8.8 6.6–10.9	27.7 17.4–38.1
Whippet (della Torre, 2000)	20	15 ± 2	35.9	–	8.6	9.0	32.2
Corgi (Morrison, 1992)	20	15 (8–19)	32 (28–40)	19 (12–23)	–	8 (6–10)	44 (33–57)
Border Collie (Jacobson, 2013)	20	19 (15–29)	34.5 26.5–42.5	25.6 19.2–32	8.61 5.6–11.6	8.79 4.45–13.1	25.6 17.5–33.7
Pointer (Sisson, 1991)	16	19.2 ± 2.8	31.2 34.4–44	25.3 20.5–30.1	6.9 4.7–10.1	7.1 5.7–8.5	35.5 27.5–43.5
Afghan (Morrison, 1992)	20	23 (17–36)	42 (33–52)	28 (20–37)	–	9 (7–11)	33 (24–48)
Alaskan Sled Dog (Stepien, 1998)	77	23.4 ± 3.1	43.8 36.8–50.8	34.0 25.8–42.2	8.9 5.3–12.5	8.8 6.2–11.4	23 9–37
Hungarian Vizsla (Voros, 2009)	45	24.5 ± 4.2	42.9 33.1–52.7	26.7 18.1–35.3	10.6 7.8–13.4	11.1 7.9–14.3	38.6 28.4–48.8
English Bull Terrier (O'Leary, 2003)	14	– (18–30.2)	38 32–44	13 9–17	10 6–14	10 8–12	32.5 24–41
Labrador Retriever (Gugjoo, 2014)	24	23.7 (18–30)	38.39 29.4–45.3	23.90 14.5–36.8	9.20 5.6–12.5	8.86 6.8–11.3	37.7 18.75–49.66
Greyhound (Page, 1993)	16	26.6 ± 3.5	44.1 28.1–50.1	32.5 25.5–39.5	10.6 7.2–14	12.1 8.7–15.5	25.3 12.7–37.9
Greyhound (della Torre, 2000)	20	27 ± 3	42.7	–	11.9	12.9	24.6
Hungarian Greyhound (Voros, 2009)	22	27.8 ± 4.0	45.3 39.3–51.3	28.9 21.3–36.5	11.8 8.4–15.2	12.3 9.3–15.3	36.8 24.2–49.4
Boxer (Herrtage, 1994)	30	28 ± 7.1	40 30–50	26.8	9 5–13	10 6–14	33 17–49
Greyhound (Snyder, 1995)	11	29.1 ± 3.7	46.9 40.7–53.1	33.3 28.1–38.5	13.4 10–16.8	11.6 8.2–15	28.8 20.4–37.2
Golden Retriever (Morrison, 1992)	20	32 (23–41)	45 (37–51)	27 (1.8–3.5)	–	10 (8–12)	39 (27–55)
German Shepherd (Muzzi, 2006)	60	30.2 ± 3.98	41.7 31.7–51.7	31 20.8–41.2	9.6 8.7–10.5	8.8 6.6–11	28.6 15.2–41.7
German Shepherd (Kayar, 2006)	50	M: 34.3; F: 35.1 (28–40)	49.5 40.1–58.9	34.3 27.6–41.5	9.75 6.87–12.6	9.5 7.1–12	31.4 24.6–38.2

Table 4.8 Canine Breed-Specific M-mode Measurements (Continued)

Breed[a] (Reference)	n	Weight (kg)	LVIDd (mm)	LVIDs (mm)	IVSd (mm)	LVWd (mm)	LV FS (%)
German Shepherd (de Oliveira, 2014)	23	M:34.9 ± 3.7	40.8 32.9–48.6	28.1 22–34.1	10 7.1–12.9	9.8 7.5–12.1	–
Doberman Pinscher (O'Sullivan, 2007)	23	–	40.1 34.7–45.5	31.4 25.9–36.9	–	8 5.6–10.4	21.7 14.4–29
Doberman pinscher (Calvert, 1986)	21	36	46.8 38.5–55.1	30.8 24.2–37.4	9.6 8.4–10.8	10.6 8.4–10.8	34.2 30.6–37.8
Estrela mountain dog (Lobo, 2008)	74	46.9 ± 8.8	F:48.9 38.9–58.9 M:51.8 44.0–59.6	33.0 24.2–41.8	11.0 9.0–14	11.2 8–14.4	34.4 23–45.9
Spanish mastiff (Bayon, 1994)	12	52.4 ± 3.3	47.7 44.9–50.5	29 26.8–31.2	10.8 9–10.6	10.7 8.9–10.5	39
Newfoundland (Koch, 1996)	27	61 47–61.5	50 44–60	35.5 29–44	11.5 7–15	10 8–13	30 22–37
Great Dane (Koch, 1996)	15	62 52–75	53 44–59	31.5 34–45	14.5 12–16	12.5 10–16	25 18–36
Irish wolfhound (Vollmar, 1999)	262	65.0 ± 8.75	53.2 45.2–61.2	35.4 29.8–41	9.3 5.7–12.9	9.8 6.6–13	34 25–43
Irish wolfhound (Koch, 1996)	20	68.5 50–80	50 46–59	36 33–45	12 9–14.5	10 9–13	28 20–34

Notes: Neither the range of reported values nor the interval of 2 standard deviations in either direction from the mean should be construed as normal reference ranges. At best, these provide a rough approximation of the normal variation within a breed and might represent too conservative or a too liberal a "range of normal," depending on the sample size and the distribution of the values. Additionally, methods of measurement can influence the data.

[a] Breeds listed in order of smallest to largest body weight in the study samples.

[b] All single values represent mean values or median values. Variability around central tendency is indicated variously as ±1SD; the interval encompassing ±2SD from the mean (and shown in the table in this format: xx.x–yy.y); as the range of reported values (noted in parentheses); or as a reference range suggested by the study authors [noted in brackets].

Abbreviations: F, female; IVSd, interventricular septal thickness in diastole; LV FS, Left ventricular fractional shortening (SF%); LVIDd, Left ventricular diameter in diastole; LVIDs, left ventricular diameter in systole; LVWd, left ventricular free-wall thickness in diastole; M, male; n, number of dogs.

Table 4.9 Normal Feline M-mode Echocardiographic Measurements: Multibreed Studies

M-mode Variable	Study (Reference)						
	Sisson, 1991 n = 78[a]	Moise, 1986 n = 11	Jacobs, 1985 n = 30	Fox, 1985 n = 30[b]	Smith, 2013 n = 24[a]	Mottet, 2012 n = 30[a]	Petric, 2012 n = 50[a]
Left Atrium (S)	11.7 ± 1.7	12.1 ± 1.8	12.0 ± 1.4	10.3 ± 1.4		11.0 [10.6–11.5]	
Aorta (D)	9.5 ± 1.4	9.5 ± 1.5	9.5 ± 1.1	9.4 ± 1.1		9.3 [9.1–9.5]	
Left Atrium (S): Aorta (D)	1.25 ± 0.18	1.29 ± 0.23	1.30 ± 0.17	1.10 ± 0.18		1.17 [1.13–1.21]	
Left Ventricular Diameter (D)	15.0 ± 2.0	15.1 ± 2.1	15.9 ± 1.9	14.0 ± 1.3	13.4 ± 0.2	15.0 [14.2–16.7]	13 (8.8–18.9)
Left Ventricular Diameter (S)	7.2 ± 1.5	6.9 ± 2.2	8.0 ± 1.4	8.1 ± 1.6		7.8 [7.2–8.4]	7.4 (4.0–11.4)
LV Fractional Shortening	52.1 ± 7.1	55.0 ± 10.2	49.8 ± 5.3	42.7 ± 8.1	46 ± 12	47.8 [45.5–50.0]	46 (32–68)
Interventricular Septum (D)	4.2 ± 0.7	5.0 ± 0.7	3.1 ± 0.4	3.6 ± 0.8	3.5 ± 0.8	4.0 [3.7–4.3]	4.1 (2.7–5.7)
Left Ventricular Wall (D)	4.1 ± 0.7	4.6 ± 0.5	3.3 ± 0.6	3.5 ± 0.8	3.9 ± 0.6	4.2 [3.9–4.5]	4.1 (2.3–5.7)

Note: All linear measurements tabulated in millimeters and expressed as mean ±SD, median (range), or mean [95% confidence interval]. See text for specific suggestions for assessing left atrial and ventricular size.

[a] Body weights: Sisson: 4.7 ± 1.2 kg; Smith: 4.3 ± 0.7; Mottet: 3.97 (3.6–4.3); Petric: 5.1 (2.2–8.0).

[b] Cats sedated with ketamine; heart rate mean (±SD): 255/min (±36).

Abbreviations: D, end-diastole; S, end-systole.

Table 4.10 Normal Feline M-mode and 2D Echocardiographic Measurements: Single Breed studies

M-mode Variable	Gundler, 2008 MCC	Drourr, 2005 Male MCC	Drourr, 2005 Female MCC	Chetboul, 2005 MCC	Granstrom, 2011 British Shorthair	Chetboul, 2012 Sphynx	Mottet, 2012 Sphynx	Kayar, 2014 Turkish Van	Scansen, 2015 Bengals
	n = 42	n = 46	n = 59	n = 23	n = 282	n = 53	n = 72–89	n = 40	n = 66
Left Atrium (S)	11.6 ± 2.0	14.4 ± 1.4	13.2 ± 1.6		9.5 (6.7–14.4)[a]		12.1 [11.7– 12.4]	9.4 [6.6–12.4]	13.3 {10.9–15.8}[a] 14.9 {12.1–17.5}
Aorta (D)	8.9 ± 1.6	11.7 ± 1.2	10.8 ± 1.1		8.7 (6.1–11.5)[a]		9.7 [9.5–10.0]	8.2 [7.9–8.6]	9.1 {7.8–10.5}[a]
Left Atrium/Ao	1.3 ± 0.3	1.24 ± 0.15	1.23 ± 0.16	1.0 ± 0.2	1.1 (0.9–1.4)[a]	0.9 ± 0.14	1.24 [1.21–1.28]	1.14 [1.0–1.3]	1.5 {1.1–2.0}[a] 1.5 {1.2–1.8}[b]
Left Ventricular Diameter (D)	14.8 ± 2.5	19.4 ± 1.8	17.9 ± 2.2	16.9 ± 1.8	15.0 (11.0–21.2)	15.2 ± 1.6	16.3 [15.9–16.7]	14.8 [14.2–15.4]	16.0 {12.6–19.2}
Left Ventricular Diameter (S)	8.7 ± 2.4	9.5 ± 1.8	8.5 ± 1.9	9.1 ± 1.5	7.4 (0.5–12.1)	7.2 ± 1.5	8.1 [7.6–8.5]	7.6 [4.6–11.0]	8.7 {5.4–12.0}
LV Fractional Shortening	41.8 ± 9.9	51.1 ± 7.6	52.4 ± 7.8	47 ± 6.0	50 (29–95.8)	53 ± 7.0	50.7 [48.5–52.8]	48.4 [45.7–51.1]	45 {26.7–61.9}
Interventricular Septum (D)	4.3 ± 1.2	4.2 ± 0.6	3.8 ± 0.7	4.7 ± 0.7	3.8 (2.6–5.2)	4.4 ± 0.4	4 [3.8–4.2]	3.7 [3.5–3.8]	4.8 {3.7–6.1}
Left Ventricular Wall (D)	4.1 ± 0.8	4.4 ± 0.6	4.1 ± 0.6	4.6 ± 0.6	3.8 (2.6–5.0)	4.2 ± 0.6	4.1 [4.0–4.3]	3.66 [3.4–3.9]	4.6 3.4–5.8}
Body Weight (kg)	4.9 ± 1.3	6.47 ± 0.92	4.86 ± 1.17	5.0 ± 1.0	4.1 (2.2–8.3)	3.76 ± 1.09	3.62 [3.5–3.8]	Females: 3.41 kg Males: 4.16 kg	4.4 ± 1.1

Notes:
1. All linear measurements in millimeters and expressed as mean ±SD; median (range) or mean [95% confidence interval of the mean], or mean {95% prediction intervals}.
2. All measurements derived from M-mode studies unless indicated otherwise.
3. See text for specific suggestions for assessing left atrial and ventricular size.
4. Significantly larger LV internal diameters are found in male versus female Maine Coon cats and Van cats for some variables.
5. A relatively weak but statistically significant relationship is identified between body weight and some echocardiographic variables.
[a] Left atrial and aortic diameters and ratio calculated from short-axis 2D images using method of Hansson (Vet Radiol Ultrasound 2002;43:568–575).
[b] Left atrial dimensions calculated from long-axis 2D images.

Abbreviations: D, end-diastole; MCC, Maine Coon cats; S, end-systole; Ao, aorta; LV, left ventricular.

Left Atrial Size and Function

Left atrial dilation (dilatation) develops from increased pressure or volume in the LA, as occurs with left-to-right shunting, primary mitral valve disease, secondary or functional MR (because of abnormal annular and subvalvular support), cardiomyopathies, and significant LV systolic or diastolic dysfunction. High cardiac output states, including hyperthyroidism and anemia, also can induce left atrial dilation, perhaps from volume retention. The LA also dilates in response to primary atrial myocardial disease, chronic bradyarrhythmias, or persistent tachyarrhythmias with secondary LV dysfunction. When heart disease is chronic, the magnitude of enlargement relates to the hemodynamic burden and prognosis of the underlying lesion, where a LA of normal size portends a more favorable short-term prognosis. Notable exceptions are peracute causes of heart failure, such as MR from ruptured chordae tendineae or infective endocarditis. In these cases, left atrial dilation might be minimal and if atrial distensibility is low, CHF can be severe. Typically, left atrial size is increased in patients with left-sided CHF; however, the LA might appear relatively normal after diuretic therapy has contracted the plasma volume, especially in cats.

The quantitation of left atrial size or volume is perhaps the most important of all echo measurements. Most simple methods for measuring the LA (linear measures, ratios of LA to Ao) are surrogates for atrial volume estimates. One pitfall is the influence of asymmetrical chamber remodeling, if incorporated in the measurement path. This can affect the strength of correlation of an atrial diameter to the actual atrial volume. For example, in dogs with chronic mitral valve disease, markedly dilated pulmonary venous entries (**Figure 4.18**) can artificially inflate atrial chamber size. A pulmonary vein often is near the path of the short-axis plane measurement (**Figure 4.17**). In the long-axis view, remodeling often leads to displacement of the atrial septum toward the RA (**Figure 4.16**); this increases the midchamber diameter of the LA. Sometimes the LA will appear enlarged in one plane, but not the other; this might represent actual differences in how the chamber enlarges with different diseases.

Using the principles of measurement discussed earlier, left atrial size can be quantified by absolute values (for breed or species, as in cats), scaling measurements allometrically, constructing ratios of LA to Ao size (Rishniw, 2019); and observing changes on serial examinations. Volumetric approaches using single 2D and 3D imaging have been reported (Höllmer, 2013). Maximal atrial volume occurs just after the end of the T wave on the ECG and more precisely, immediately before mitral valve opening as visualized by 2D imaging. While many measurements of the LA are obtained at end-systole, this is not always the case. In some methods—notably, the short-axis approach—the size of the LA might be determined in early diastole, or at its minimal value at end-diastole. This emphasizes that various LA/Ao ratios are not interchangeable.

Suggested Approach A suggested approach from right parasternal images:

- Measure the end-systolic dimension of the LA in the four-chamber plane (**Figure 4.5A**) and the maximal opening distance between the aortic valve leaflets (AoV) in the LVOT long-axis plane (**Figure 4.5B**); Long-axis LA diameter in normal cats is <15 to 16 mm (**Table 4.6**). For dogs normalize LA diameter as: nLAD=LA(cm)/bodyweight (kg)$^{0.31}$ where normal is <1.7. Normal long-axis LA/AoV is <2.6 in most dogs.
- Measure early diastolic left atrial and aortic dimensions in the short-axis plane (**Figure 4.17**); construct LA/Ao ratios. Normal short-axis LA/Ao is <1.5-1.6 (cats) and <1.6-1.7 (dogs).
- Optionally, in dogs and cats, trace LA area at end-systole and at the R wave (end-diastole) to estimate atrial areas and fractional area change (**Figure 4.26**)

Applying suitable formulas also permits the estimation of left atrial volumes and atrial EF from these area traces, as discussed later for the left ventricle. The left atrial area also can be traced in short-axis plane; this is done most often in horses. Approximate reference values are shown in **Tables 4.5–4.10**.

Atrial Function Decreased atrial function is an under-recognized feature of cardiac disease. It reduces cardiac output, predisposes to atrial thrombosis in cats, and probably relates to the likelihood of atrial arrhythmias, such as atrial fibrillation. The atrial cycle includes three functions:

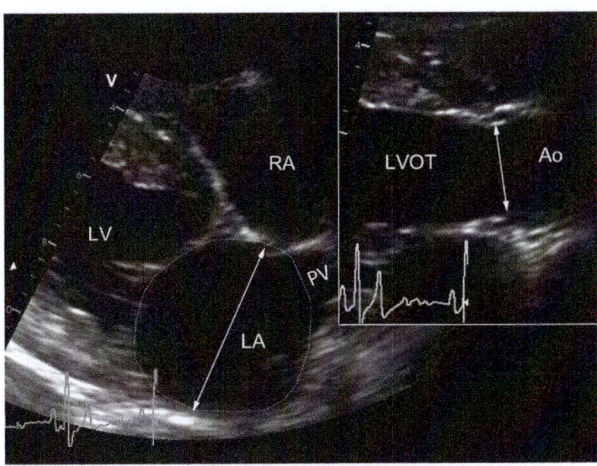

Figure 4.26 Long-axis measurements of the left atrium (LA) and aorta. Maximal end-systolic diameter, maximal distance between opened aortic valve leaflets (AoV, inset), and a tracing of the end-systolic area of the LA are shown. Maximal linear dimension can be compared to normal values for body size and by creating a ratio of LA/AoV (normally <2.65 in dogs), similar to the short-axis approach shown in **Figure 4.17**. However, normal values depend on the approach taken and are not interchangeable. Tracing atrial area at minimal and maximal values allows for estimation of the LA's global function.

(1) as a "reservoir" during ventricular systole, while the mitral valve is closed and the atrium fills; (2) as a "conduit" during early diastole to middiastole, as the open mitral valve serves as a passageway between atrium and ventricle; and (3) as a "pump," when active atrial contraction follows the P wave of the ECG. Atrial function indices use measurements obtained during one or more of these phasic changes of atrial physiology. Atrial function also is influenced by ventricular diastolic function, venous pressures filling the chamber, and the presence of any MR. Although atrial function is not routinely quantified in animals, it can provide useful information. In cats, decreased left atrial function correlates to the likelihood of severe CHF and risk for blood flow stagnation and atrial thrombosis. In horses, failure to recover atrial function after conversion from atrial fibrillation to sinus rhythm indicates a greater risk for reversion. Measuring the fractional area change or FS of left atrial diameter is a simple approach to assessing function of the LA, although more data are needed before specific values can be used for prognostication. The authors routinely measure left atrial appendage function using pulsed wave (PW) Doppler echo imaging (p. 119) in cats with cardiomyopathy.

Left Ventricular Size and Function

The diseased left ventricle can undergo several morphologic adaptations, including simple dilation, dilation with a normal wall thickness (eccentric hypertrophy), wall thickening at the expense of the ventricular lumen (concentric hypertrophy), and concentric hypertrophy with chamber dilation (mixed hypertrophy). Another form of ventricular remodeling observed in human hypertensive and aged patients is a concentric remodeling where LV mass is normal but wall thicknesses are increased; this is not currently reported in dogs or cats.

Certain cardiac diseases are associated with these patterns of ventricular enlargement. Simple dilation occurs in the worst cases of dilated cardiomyopathy (DCM) or fulminating myocarditis. Eccentric hypertrophy is typical of volume overload (valvular regurgitation and left-to-right shunts) and compensated DCM. Concentric hypertrophy most often is associated with aortic stenosis, HCM, systemic hypertension, and some cases of hyperthyroidism and obesity. Mixed hypertrophy is observed in combined aortic stenosis and insufficiency, and with aortic stenosis or HCM complicated by myocardial failure. Wall thickening also can develop secondary to myocardial inflammation and edema caused by myocarditis or with so-called transient myocardial thickening in cats (p. 688). Ideally, these different forms of hypertrophy would be quantified by estimation of LV volume and mass; however, this is rarely done in veterinary practice. Although measurements of LV wall thickness are especially relevant to certain conditions, such as aortic stenosis, systemic hypertension, or relative wall thickness in DCM, this issue is most acute in cats more prone HCM.

Different Approaches

Linear, area, and volumetric methods can be used to analyze LV chamber size and function. Traditionally, veterinarians have focused on linear measurements from the M-mode exam or from frozen 2D images. As with the LA, such measurements are surrogates for ventricular volume, which represents a better standard for identifying cardiomegaly (and estimating LV EF). This assumes that LV volumes are accurately estimated and scaled to body size. Some of the volumetric approaches used for echo examinations in people are readily applicable to veterinary patients. The recommended approach is the method of discs, often referred to as Simpson's method (**Figure 4.27**). Calculation of LV volumes requires tracing the LV area and measuring the chamber length in diastole and systole. This can be done from the right parasternal long-axis view (if the LV apex is included) or from the left apical four-chamber view (as in **Figure 4.27**; although the LV often is truncated in this view). All echo systems have software that permits ventricular volume calculation by this method. Unfortunately, estimating ventricular volumes from the M-mode echocardiogram using variations of the cube-based formulas leads to overestimation of LV size as the chamber dilates. While linear measurements still are useful, relying on derivations of volume from the M-mode exam is discouraged, except for normal hearts.

Ventricular hypertrophy refers to an increase in ventricular mass, not simply to an increase in wall thickness. As such, a dilated left ventricle with normal wall thickness represents an eccentrically hypertrophied chamber.

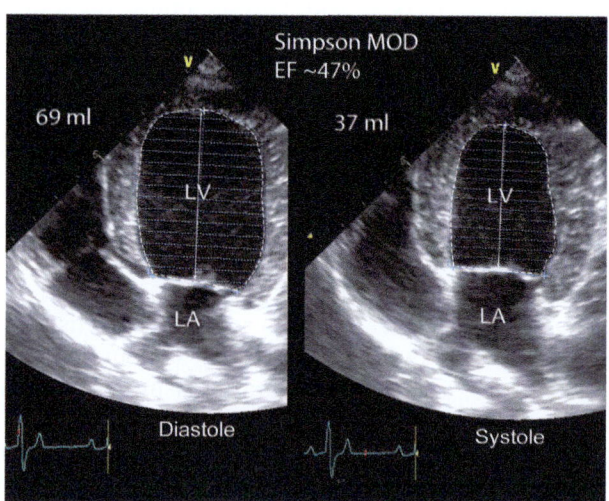

Figure 4.27 Left apical four-chamber images from a dog taken at end-diastole (left) and end-systole (right). The original area-length traces have been enhanced. The (Simpson's) method of discs is used to estimate ventricular volumes and ejection fraction (EF); these are calculated by the echo system software. The EF is calculated as (End-diastolic volume − End-systolic volume)/End-diastolic volume. Additionally, ventricular volume indices in systole and diastole can be derived by dividing the volume by body surface area. These volumes can be used to identify chamber dilation and reduced systolic function of the left ventricle (LV). LA, left atrium.

With concentric hypertrophy, cardiac mass is increased but characterized mainly by wall thickening with a normal to reduced luminal size. Although it is possible to estimate overall ventricular mass by combining various wall and area measurements, linear determinations of wall thicknesses currently represent a more practical approach in our patients. Multiple measurements of the same wall segments should be averaged to reduce the influence of measurement errors.

Sometimes there is a tendency to perform serial echocardiograms to "follow heart size"; however, follow-up echo studies should focus on more pertinent issues than just overall size. One example is to focus on left atrial size and function in cats, as well as the presence of any "smoke" (spontaneous echocontrast) or thrombosis in the feline LA. Another, more advanced evaluation involves Doppler estimates of ventricular filling and pulmonary arterial pressures (see the Doppler Echocardiography section). A common use of serial echo exams in dogs with asymptomatic mitral valve disease involves monitoring LV and atrial size to determine when to initiate treatment aimed at delaying CHF (p. 546). Last, in dogs with apparent diet-induced or tachycardia-induced DCM, improvement in LV size and function on follow-up examinations might indicate a reason to discontinue therapy.

Suggested Approach   From right parasternal images:

- Measure LV end-diastolic and end-systolic dimensions and FS from short-axis plane, including guided M-mode echo exam (**Figures 4.3** and **4.22**). In dogs use allometric scaling to normalize the LVIDd as: nLVIDd=LVID(cm)/bodyweight (kg)$^{0.31}$. Normal is <1.65-1.7.
- Repeat the LV diastolic measurements in the right parasternal long-axis plane as a check against poor cursor placement (**Figure 4.5**). In cat compare to Table.
- In dogs, construct LV/Ao ratios (similar to the LA/AoV for long axis), A normal long-axis LV/AoV is <2.6. Normalized LVIDd = (cm)/bodyweight (kg)$^{0.31}$. Normal is <1.65.
- Estimate LV systolic and diastolic volumes and EF using Simpson's method of discs from right parasternal long-axis (or apical four-chamber images, or both) if LV FS is low or the LV is dilated.
- Optionally, trace the LV diastolic and systolic areas in short-axis to calculate fractional area change (**Figure 4.28**); normal is >35% to 40%. Perform MAPSE to measure longitudinal shortening.

Ventricular internal dimensions or volumes can be compared to reference standards when available. A generally accepted approach is one of calculating the "normalized" LV dimensions based on allometric scaling (**Table 4.5**). Optionally, compare measured or calculated values to breed-specific references when available (**Table 4.8**). Many, but not all, of these approaches are applicable to horses (**Table 4.7**).

In cats, both M-mode and 2D measurements of the LV and atrial chambers and LV walls should be made with consideration of previously discussed pitfalls. Measurements should be compared to a reference (**Tables 4.6, 4.9,** and **4.10**). Additionally, a narrative of any hypertrophy should be included in the echo report, because the pattern of thickening can influence the overall prognosis. As noted by Häggström (2015), "there is a problem in differentiating mild disease from a normal phenotype, and the margin for error is small." Many cardiologists select a wall measurement of between 5.5 and

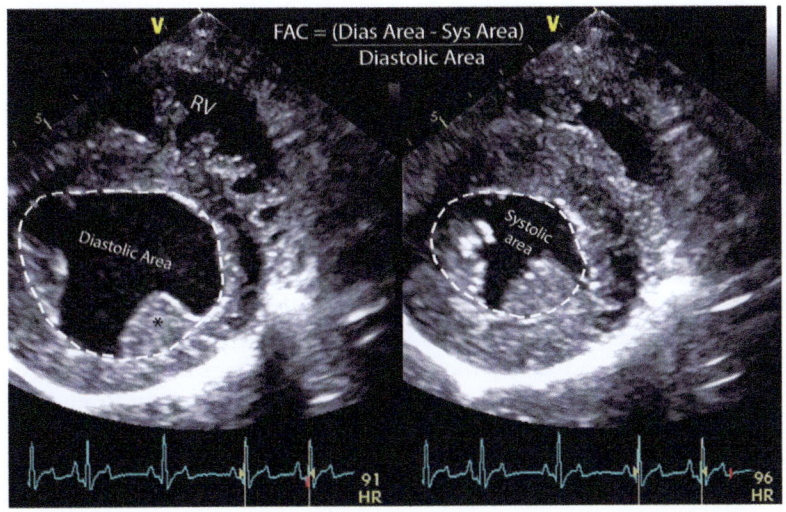

Figure 4.28 Short-axis fractional area change (FAC). Shortening in multiple minor dimensions is evident. The image is from the papillary muscle level and the left ventricular (LV) short axis area is measured by tracing through the endocardial border–papillary muscle interface. The FAC is the same formula as for shortening fraction, but uses areas instead of linear measurements. This method is most valuable when there is dyssynchrony between the ventricular septum and LV free wall on M-mode study. One issue with this approach, as shown here, is the difficulty in obtaining perfectly symmetrical papillary muscle and circular LV shapes in both phases of the cardiac cycle. *, anterior papillary muscle.

5.9 mm as the upper limit of normal for diastolic thicknesses in the "average" cat. However, not all cardiologists agree and some contend that an upper limit of normal is closer to 5 mm. Additionally, body size is relevant; some normal, heavy cats and specific breeds can have predicted LV diastolic wall thicknesses approaching 6 mm (Häggström, 2016). As a general guideline, the authors use a diastolic thickness of or exceeding 5.5 mm as a relatively sensitive cut-off for LV hypertrophy, and a value of 6 mm or greater as specific for LV hypertrophy in cats of average size. LV wall thickness in many healthy cats is less than 5 mm. Nevertheless, there can be significant heterogeneity in wall thickness related to the segment measured and breed.

Right Atrial and Ventricular Size and Function

Compared to the left side, the right atrial and ventricular cavities are more complex geometrically, and the limited acoustic windows available to image these chambers make the right heart challenging to measure. The right ventricle includes an inlet, an apical portion, and an outlet; it projects from right to left, caudal to cranial, and ventral to dorsal. This anatomy is relevant to quantifying RV chamber size and function. The RV cavity is difficult to assess subjectively or measure consistently because it appears as a rapidly tapering triangle when viewed from the right parasternal long-axis view or a crescent adjacent to the LV or aorta when viewed in the short-axis planes (**Figures 4.4–4.8**). The internal references needed to direct cursor placements for right heart measurements using M-mode are neither necessarily static nor consistent in the setting of heart disease. Defining mild RV enlargement is especially challenging.

The size of the RA from the right parasternal windows changes, depending on how dorsally one places or angulates the transducer. A good acoustic window can lead to overestimation of this chamber's size. The left apical four-chamber view is probably better for subjective identification of moderate to severe right atrial enlargement, because both atria are relatively circular in this plane. The LA normally appears slightly larger than the RA when the two atria are viewed side-by-side. This comparison presumes that the center of the US beam falls to the anatomic left side of the ventricular septum.

There are a number of useful studies now published that provide some normative data for RV and atrial measurements and RV function (Visser, 2017), as well as studies related to the diagnosis of PH (see below). However, each carries some limitations based on available imaging planes or comorbidities. For example, the presence of right-sided CHF will further augment chamber diameters because of elevated filling pressures. The traced right atrial area can be indexed to body surface area or aortic diameter; this measure is obtained from a modified left apical image, optimized for the right heart (**Figure 4.19**). With regard to identifying RV hypertrophy, the diastolic RV wall thickness can be measured with a higher-frequency transducer from the right parasternal windows. Diastolic RV thickness should be <50% of the diastolic LV wall measurement if pericardial echoes are excluded; typically, the RV wall is about 1/3 as thick as the left.

Suggested Approach A suggested approach to measuring right heart size and function in dogs is as follows:

- Subjectively compare the right and left heart chambers in the parasternal short-axis and left apical four-chamber views (**Figures 4.6** and **4.10**, left)
- Record RV longitudinal shortening (TAPSE) and optionally, RV diastolic and systolic areas to calculate fractional area change (**Figure 4.19**)
- Compute a ratio of right atrial traced area to aortic dimension (Vezzosi, 2018)

More advanced analysis involves TDI (p. 119) of the longitudinal contraction velocity (S) or myocardial strain analysis of the lateral RV wall. When assessments of RV function are made, these are obtained from the modified apical view optimized for the right heart (**Figure 4.19**). Last, the coronary sinus and CaVC (as well as the hepatic veins) can be subjectively assessed or measured for normal changes during ventilation. Subjective dilation or minimal respiratory variation in these vessels suggests increased right atrial pressure or volume overload.

Great Vessels

Cardiomegaly might be accompanied by dilation of the aorta or the pulmonary trunk. Pulmonary trunk dilation usually is associated with three major abnormalities: left-to-right shunts, PH (including that caused by dirofilariasis and left heart disease), and pulmonic stenosis. Idiopathic dilation is encountered infrequently. The differential diagnoses for aortic dilation are somewhat more extensive and include: (sub)aortic stenosis, PDA, malformations of the conotruncal tissues (tetralogy of Fallot, pulmonary atresia, truncus arteriosus), systemic hypertension, idiopathic or breed-related aortopathy, and hypertrophic obstructive cardiomyopathy. Middle-aged to older cats also can develop idiopathic dilation, sometimes with tortuosity of the aorta. Idiopathic aortic dilation is identified regularly in dogs, too. This could be a differential diagnosis when radiography suggests a craniodorsal heart base mass. Familial aneurysm of the aorta is reported in Leonberger dogs. Breeds prone to subaortic stenosis, including Golden Retrievers, Rottweilers, and Newfoundland dogs, sometimes have isolated aortopathy characterized by mild to marked dilation of the ascending aorta that often extends into the arch. These dogs can have an otherwise normal LVOT.

Dilation of a great vessel often is evident from subjective evaluation. Many examiners perform a subjective assessment and compare the aorta in cross-section to the pulmonary artery in long-axis (**Figure 4.8**, right; also see **Figures 39.6C**, p. 822 and **39.12D**, p. 829). As a guideline, the normal pulmonary trunk, just distal to the pulmonic valve, appears no wider than the short-axis aorta at the same level. Assuming normal aortic dimensions, this rule of thumb can be used to identify a dilated or attenuated pulmonary artery. It is possible to measure the aorta and compare it to reference values (that mostly have been generated by M-mode studies), but this is not commonly done. Importantly, dimensions across the aortic sinuses are significantly wider than those measured between the attachment (hinge) points of the aortic valve, the opened valve leaflets, or the sinotubular junction.

Measurements of the right branch of the main pulmonary artery also have proven useful, especially in patients with PH (Visser, 2017). In these cases, the normal diastolic to systolic variation in pulmonary artery diameter, or its distensibility, is reduced. This can be measured simply with M-mode or 2D calipers as the diameter change from diastole to systole divided by the maximal (systolic) diameter. This measurement is made from right-sided, short-axis images optimized for branching of the pulmonary arteries (**Figure 39.17**, p. 832). It is important to optimize the image for maximal right pulmonary artery size throughout the cardiac cycle, to minimize translational motion artifact. In addition, it is instructive to compare the diameters of the right pulmonary vein and adjacent pulmonary artery from a right parasternal long-axis image, optimized for the LV inflow tract (**Figure 4.5A**). In patients with chronic left atrial pressure elevation or severe MR, the pulmonary vein tends to be larger than the artery. In contrast, with pulmonary arterial hypertension caused by increased pulmonary vascular resistance, the opposite finding occurs.

Cardiac Chamber Size and Clinical Decision-Making

The number of measurements and calculations that can be obtained by echo exam is huge and choosing the most important ones can be overwhelming. The selection of highest-priority measurements for a patient is informed by the clinical epidemiology of heart disease within the particular species and the individual's differential diagnosis. For example, measuring systolic function in a heart that is swinging within a pericardial effusion is of little value until the effusion is drained. Similarly, systolic function indices in primary mitral valve disease of small-breed dogs has limited clinical utility. In contrast, identifying reduced LV systolic function is the *sine qua non* for diagnosing the DCM phenotype. Sometimes, measurements fundamentally define the cardiac disease, as with idiopathic aortopathy or feline HCM. In congenital heart disease, cardiac chamber measurements also are useful for guiding prognosis and catheter or surgical intervention. For instance, LV dilation with PDA or a severely hypertrophied RV wall with pulmonary stenosis would argue for catheter-based or surgical intervention, with recognition that a comprehensive approach is needed when deciding on therapy for cardiac malformations. Evaluation of a dog or cat with an arrhythmia often includes echocardiography, along with the consideration of genetic risk for cardiomyopathy and laboratory tests (such as a cardiac troponin) to identify active myocardial injury. Last, considering perhaps 50% (or more) of feline cardiac murmurs are functional (physiological), a normal echo exam essentially rules out HCM or a congenital malformation as the underlying cause.

The most common diseases diagnosed by veterinarians in clinical practice are chronic degenerative (myxomatous) mitral valve disease (DMVD) in dogs and HCM in cats. For dogs with chronic MR caused by DMVD, the decision to intervene with preemptive therapy to delay or prevent CHF (with pimobendan, ± an ACE inhibitor) is based largely on accurate measurement of left heart dimensions and the degree of remodeling (see Chapter 29). Echo exams done in most healthy cats are prompted because of a cardiac murmur. After excluding known causes of LV thickening, such as systemic hypertension and hyperthyroidism, the LV wall and left atrial measurements will largely determine if a cat is diagnosed with a functional heart murmur (and treated normally) or labeled with a diagnosis of HCM (followed by a lifetime of client worry, patient stress, and all the attendant costs of reevaluations). Moderate to severe left atrial dilation in cats presents both a guarded prognosis for life and a high risk for CHF or thromboembolism. Accordingly, antiplatelet therapy such as clopidogrel or a Factor Xa inhibitor (apixaban or rivaroxaban) generally will be indicated.

Finally, finding that cardiac chambers and great vessels are normal in size also is valuable for clinical assessment and client reassurance. For example, in a mature Golden Retriever or Boxer dog with a soft to moderate ejection murmur and equivocal diagnosis of subaortic stenosis, normal cardiac measurements realistically can allow the dog to exercise at will, avoid treatment, and after perhaps a single recheck, forego further echo examinations. In mature dogs with a soft to moderate murmur of MR, identifying normal chamber sizes offers a favorable prognosis for the upcoming year, informs us that neither therapy nor intense home monitoring of respiratory rate are needed, and realistically allows that dog to be treated as usual.

Doppler Echocardiography

Doppler echocardiography is an US modality that detects the direction and velocity of moving blood flow and tissues in relation to the stationary US transducer. All Doppler examinations are based on the detection of a *frequency difference* ("shift") between that of the emitted US and that of echoes returning from *moving* reflectors, typically from moving RBCs. Echoes reflected from blood flow (or tissue) moving away from the transducer return at lower frequencies; those reflected from targets moving toward the transducer echo back at higher frequencies. Clinical applications of Doppler imaging relate to the detection of blood flow, including abnormal direction, velocity, and turbulence, within the flow profile. Accordingly, Doppler examinations can confirm the presence of shunts, valvular regurgitation, and valvular stenosis, as well as other flow obstructions. More advanced Doppler studies can quantify global and regional ventricular function, atrial function, and estimate intravascular pressures. The assessment of diastolic heart function and cardiac filling pressures is based mainly on Doppler modalities.

Doppler Principles

Doppler studies are based on the principle that when US waves are reflected back from a moving object to a stationary receiver, a change in US wavelength occurs. When the source of the reflected US travels toward the transducer, the returning wavelength is shorter than that emitted. Conversely, when the reflecting source moves away from the transducer, the returning wavelength will be longer, correlating to a lower frequency. This is akin to the increase and subsequent decrease in the pitch of a racing car engine as it speeds toward and then away from a stationary observer.

In the typical Doppler examination, blood cells are the moving reflectors of US. In the specially processed Doppler mode of TDI (tissue Doppler imaging) the myocardial wall is the target. Compared to the nominal transducer frequencies of 1–12 MHz, Doppler shifts are relatively small (measured in kilohertz) and fall within the audible range. As such, spectral Doppler instruments include an audio channel that allows the operator to hear the Doppler shifts. These sounds are helpful for optimizing Doppler studies, but they also can frighten animals; so, practically, the audio volume is turned off, monitored with headphones, or set at the minimal volume.

The Doppler equation, as rewritten for velocity, indicates two important points. The first is that Doppler shifts are directly proportional to the *velocity* of moving blood or tissue. The second is that the *angle of incidence* between the US beam and the direction of blood movement affects the velocity estimate. As such:

$$V = F_d(C)/2F_o \cos \Theta$$

where (V) is the velocity of flow (or tissue), expressed in meters or centimeters/second (m/second or cm/second); F_d is the frequency shift; F_o the initial emitted frequency; C the velocity of US in tissue; and Θ the intercept angle between the US beam and path of the reflector. The emitted or carrier frequency (F_o) is known, and the average velocity of US in tissue (1540 m/second) and factor of 2 (which corrects for the "return trip") are constants. Importantly, in cardiac Doppler the US beam must travel nearly parallel to the direction of target movement to accurately record the velocity; when the incident angle Θ is 0 or 180 degrees, the cosine function equals plus or minus 1 and therefore, does not contribute to the velocity calculation. Moving targets usually change direction and velocity during the cardiac cycle. So, at any given time point, the speed of the targets (in m/second or cm/second), the intercept angle, and the direction of movement relative to the transducer determine the magnitude and sign (+ or –) of the Doppler frequency shifts.

Doppler signal processing ultimately yields four variables analyzed by the examiner: *direction, velocity, variance* (instantaneous differences in direction and velocities), and **time** within the cardiac cycle. Variance generally relates to turbulence within a small region of interest, termed a sample volume. Doppler information is displayed either in color-coded format, called "color Doppler" (**Figures 4.18, 4.24, 4.25, and 4.29**), or in a graphical display, called "spectral Doppler" echocardiography (**Figures 4.30–4.35**).

Detailed discussion of Doppler physics and instrumentation are beyond the scope of this textbook, but are critical issues for clinicians who plan to perform these studies (for more information, see Armstrong, 2010). One technical point related to the angle between US beam and direction of target motion merits extra consideration, because it affects our interpretation of Doppler shifts. If US returns from reflectors that are moving at right angles to the emitted US beam, no Doppler shift is recorded (because the cosine of 90 degrees = 0). Furthermore,

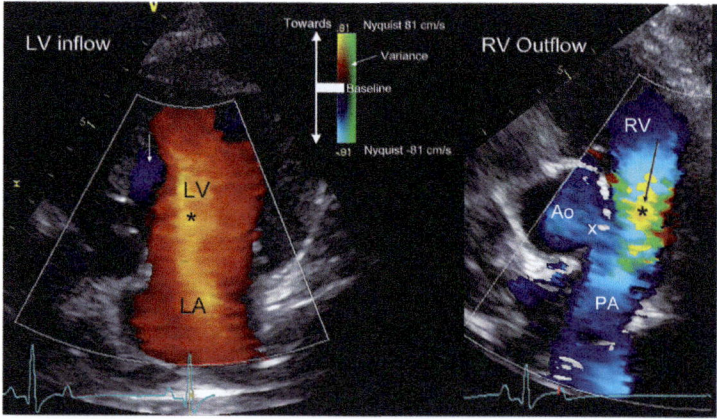

Figure 4.29 Color Doppler imaging at the inflow tract of left ventricle (LV) and outflow tract of right ventricle (RV) in a normal dog. Flow toward the transducer is coded in shades of red, and away in shades of blue. If no Doppler shifts are detected the encoding is black (zero baseline). Using an enhanced map, the slower-velocity cells (or those interrogated at a greater angle of incidence) are coded in darker shades (left panel, arrow), whereas those moving faster are brighter (*) or create a normal signal alias. When velocities exceed the (base-line adjusted) Nyquist limits, the color reverses and can be identified as an alias surrounded by the fastest moving flow coded in the opposite direction (see right panel *). Color bleeding (x, right panel) is a common artifact. There is no aorticopulmonary window in this case, but simply an instrument prioritization of the pixels for color-coding instead of grayscale; thus, the aortic wall is not seen.

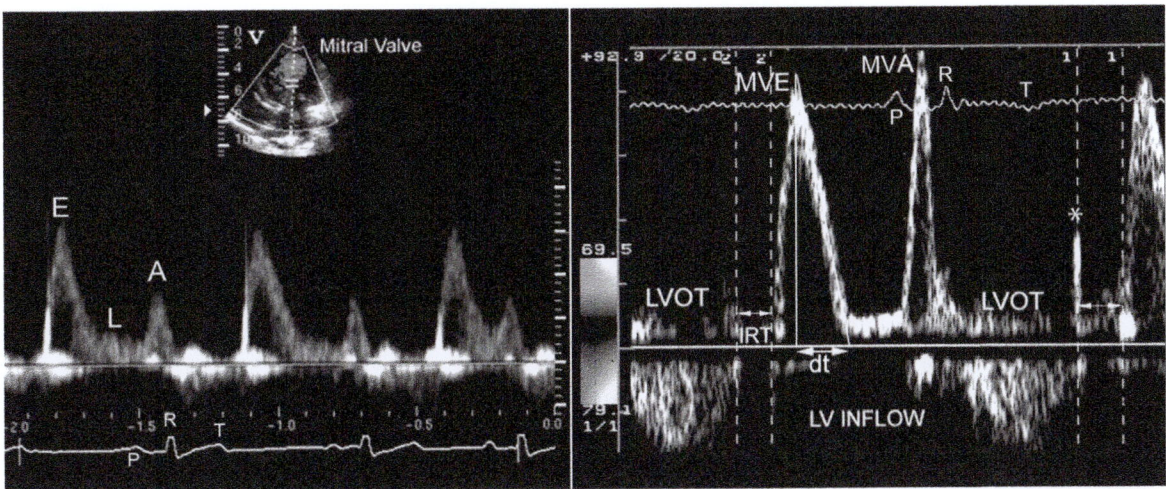

Figure 4.30 Pulsed wave Doppler recordings of transmitral flow. The left panel shows early diastolic filling (E), middiastolic (L), and atrial contraction (A) waves. The right panel shows isovolumetric relaxation time (IRT) measurement using the left ventricular outflow tract (LVOT) flow signal and aortic valve closure noise (*), and the mitral deceleration time (dt) measurement. MVA, mitral valve A wave; MVE, mitral valve E wave.

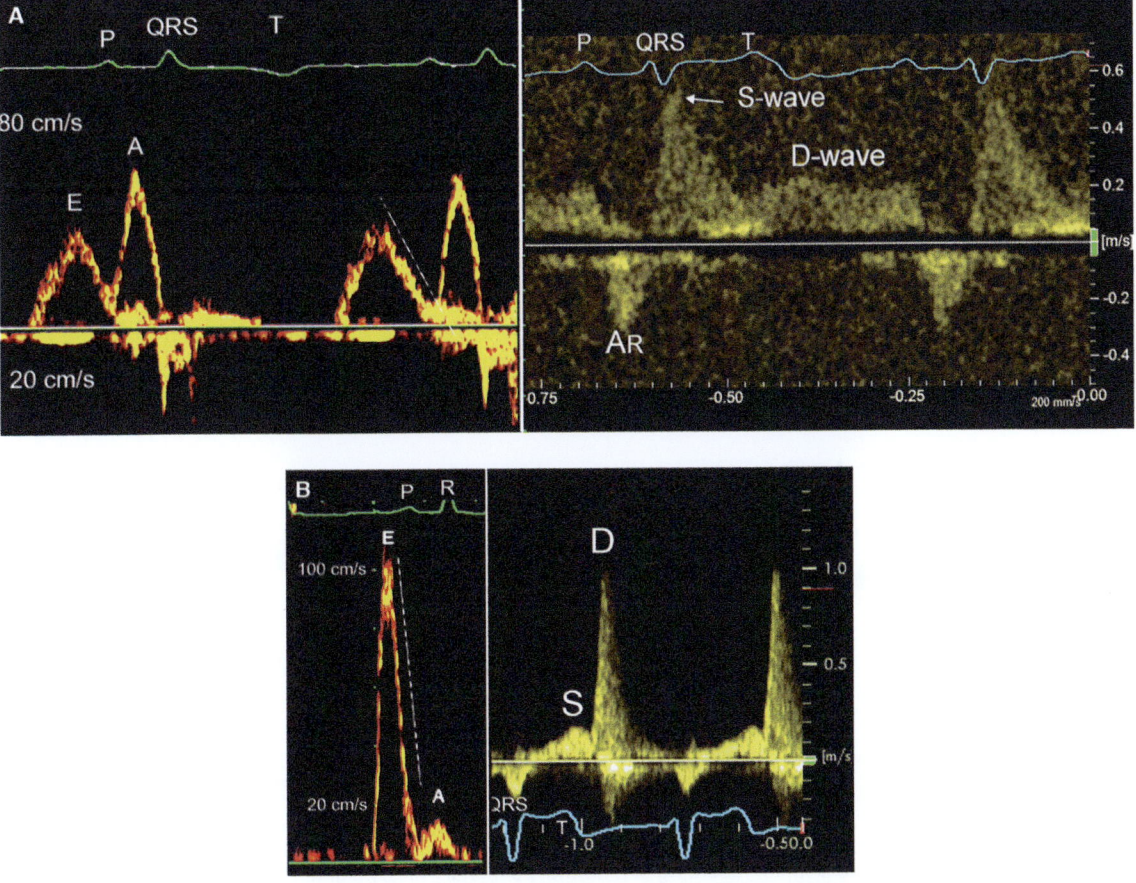

Figure 4.31 Assessment of diastolic function. (A) Transmitral inflow showing a relaxation abnormality with prolonged deceleration time and E/A reversal in a healthy old cat (left panel). Comparable pulmonary venous flow (right panel) but in a cat with hypertrophic cardiomyopathy; normally the S and D waves are more similar in velocity, but impaired relaxation has reduced the D wave and vigorous atrial contraction has led to a prominent atrial reversal (AR) wave. (B) Restrictive transmitral filling pattern in a cat with end-stage cardiomyopathy and congestive heart failure (CHF). The transmitral E wave (left panel) is high-velocity, with abbreviated deceleration time; the A wave is small, indicating reduced atrial function and elevated end-diastolic ventricular pressure. A restrictive pulmonary venous flow pattern in a cat (right panel). Note the small S and high-velocity D wave; compare this to the right panel in (A). Restrictive filling patterns indicate a high risk for CHF.

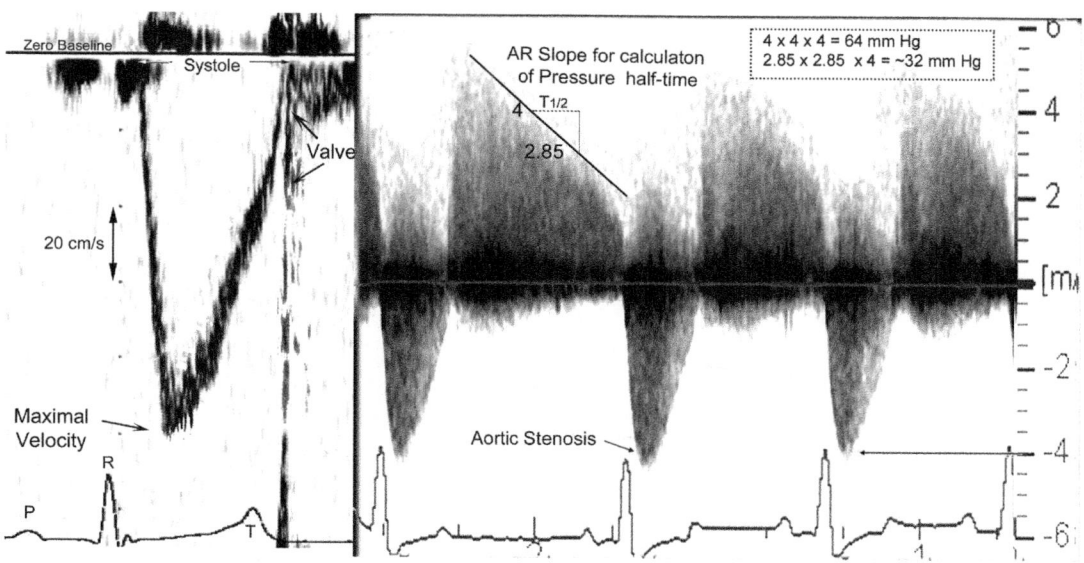

Figure 4.32 Pulsed wave Doppler recording from the ascending aorta in a normal dog (left) and continuous wave Doppler recording of aortic stenosis and regurgitation in a dog with infective endocarditis (right). The normal aortic profile shows rapid acceleration (compare to normal pulmonary flow signal in **Figure 4.33**), with some normal spectral dispersion during deceleration. Aortic valve closure results in valve noise ("valve"), a useful timing clue. The dog with aortic stenosis has an increased ejection velocity (about 4 m/s, corresponding to a pressure gradient of ~64 mm Hg). The profile of the aortic regurgitation (AR) spectrum is that of a steep decline in velocity. The "pressure half-time" is the duration in ms needed for the estimated pressure to decrease by 50% based on the simplified Bernoulli equation; shorter values indicate more severe regurgitation. The time between 4 m/s (64 mm Hg) and ~2.85 m/s (~32 mm Hg) is the pressure half-time in this case. This same principle can be applied to stenotic inflow valves.

because the cosine function is nonlinear, any returning signals associated with incidence angles exceeding 22 degrees significantly underestimate true velocity. Accordingly, cardiology examinations must be performed so that the orientation of the US beam is as parallel to blood flow (or tissue movements) as possible. This depends completely on the examiner, requiring appreciation for both normal flow and the eccentric paths of pathologic flow observed with shunts, regurgitant jets, and flow across stenoses. Although subjective angle correction can be done on the console, and often is used in peripheral vascular imaging, this procedure *never* is used for cardiac Doppler interrogation. Motion in the third plane of flow is unknown and the path of abnormal flow usually diverts from the confines of normal 2D anatomy. In spectral Doppler studies, the optimal angle is determined by carefully inspecting the images and by listening to the Doppler shifts in the audio channel.

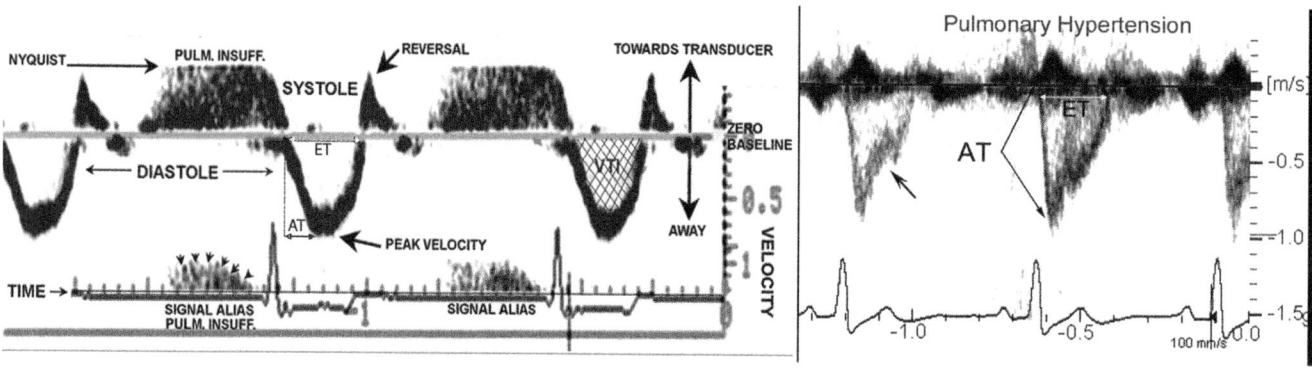

Figure 4.33 Left panel contains a pulsed wave Doppler recording of a normal pulmonary artery signal. This recording illustrates many of the principles of spectral Doppler including the triangular ejection profile, with acceleration time (AT) and ejection time (ET) indicated; the zero baseline shifted upward to record the outflow signal; the diastolic spectral dispersion (turbulence) caused by physiologic pulmonary insufficiency (insuff.), and the aliasing of this signal because of the baseline shift; and the velocity-time integral (VTI) or "stroke distance." The stroke distance fundamentally is the area under the ejection curve; when multiplied by pulmonary cross-sectional area, it provides an estimate of right ventricular stroke volume. Nyquist = the aliasing velocity. The right panel depicts how marked pulmonary hypertension (PH) can alter the morphology of the pulmonary flow profile. Faster outflow acceleration relates to increased arterial stiffness, creating a profile more like that of the aorta. While the AT shortens, the ET prolongs, which decreases the AT/ET ratio. The recording also shows a notch (arrow) during deceleration. PH-induced alterations in pulmonary vascular impedance and abnormally strong reflection waves are thought to underlie the brief decline in systolic velocity.

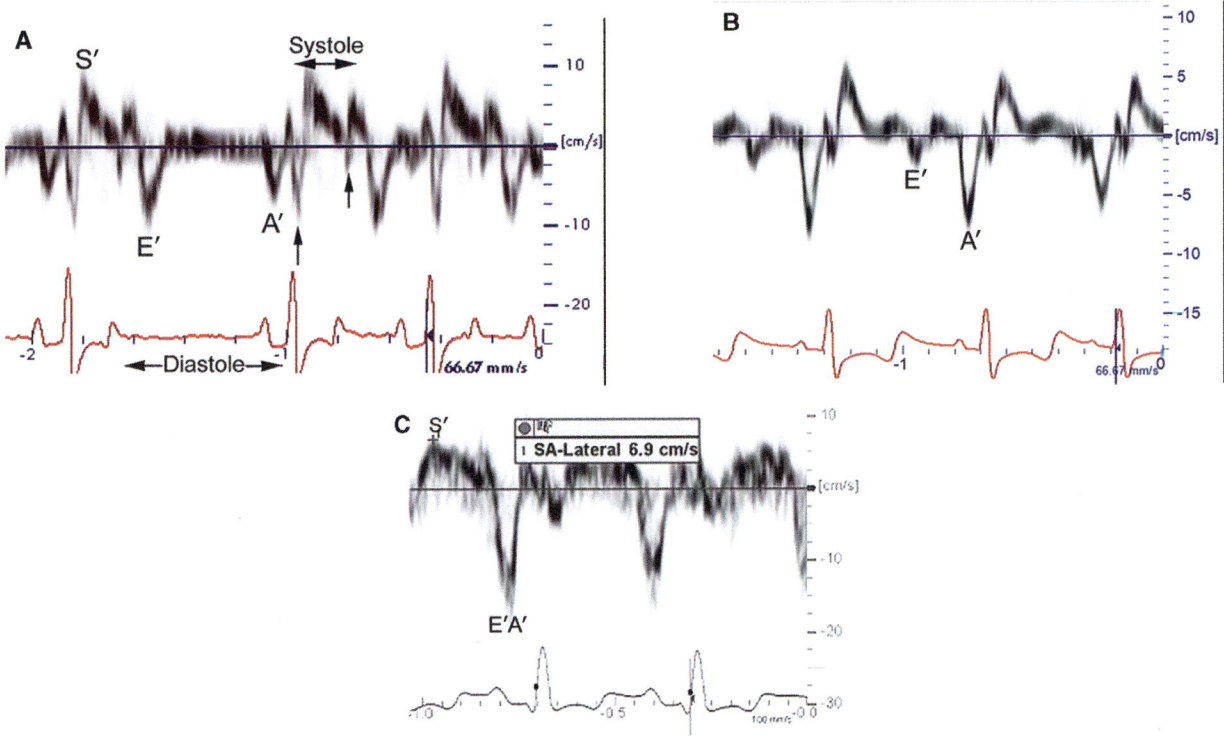

Figure 4.34 Tissue Doppler imaging in three dogs. (A) Tissue velocities associated with early diastolic recoil (E′) and atrial contraction (A′) in a normal dog, recorded from the lateral left ventricular (LV) wall near the mitral annulus. Velocities related to isovolumetric contraction (before the QRS) and relaxation (after the T wave) are indicated (arrows). The systolic wave (S′) also is shown. Absolute tissue velocity depends on the site of recording, patient size, and ventricular preload. Waveforms also are altered by disease. (B) Relaxation abnormality of the right ventricular (RV) wall in a dog with pulmonary stenosis and RV hypertrophy. Note the reversal of E′ and A′ wave velocities, indicating slowed early relaxation and shifting of filling to later in diastole. (C) Reduced S′ wave velocity in a giant-breed dog with dilated cardiomyopathy; normally, S′ recorded from the lateral LV wall would be >12 cm/sec.

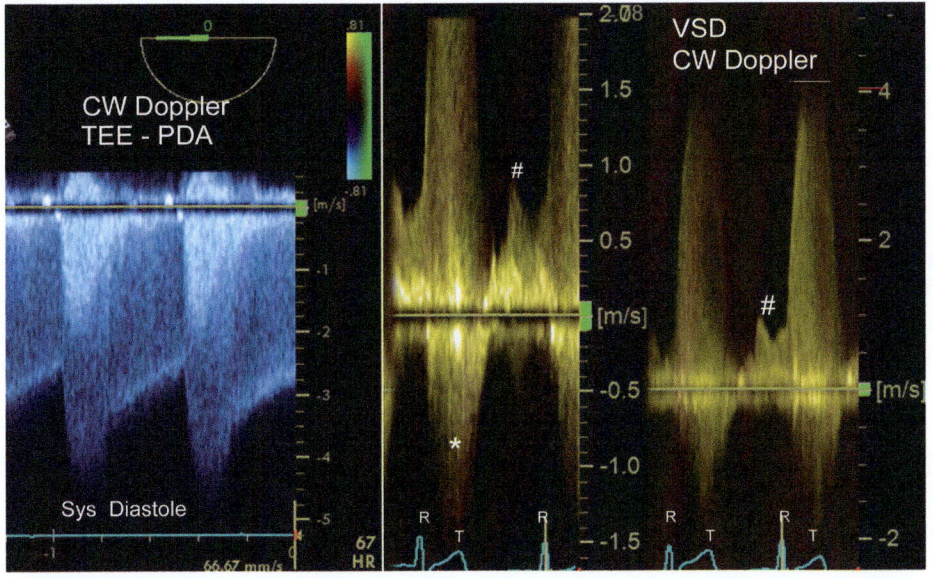

Figure 4.35 The left panel shows a continuous wave (CW) Doppler recording made during transesophageal echocardiography (TEE) in a puppy with patent ductus arteriosus (PDA). Continuous high-velocity flow is evident, although the velocities are attenuated by the hypotension of general anesthesia. Sys, systole. The right panel shows both high-pulse repetition frequency (PRF) pulsed wave Doppler (to the left) and CW Doppler imaging (to the right) in an English Bulldog puppy with a ventricular septal defect (VSD). Even with high-PRF Doppler, the VSD shunt velocity is too fast to accurately interrogate the flow, resulting in a signal alias (*). After switching to CW Doppler, a peak velocity of just over 4 m/s is recorded. Systemic blood pressure should be measured at the same time, because sedation or young age often is associated with relatively low systolic blood pressure. In this case, the VSD was small and restrictive. Low-velocity diastolic shunting, or more likely, transtricuspid inflow, is evident during diastole (#).

Overview of Doppler Modalities

Standard Doppler modalities include color (or color flow) Doppler imaging (CDI; CF Doppler) and the spectral Doppler modalities of pulsed wave (PW) Doppler, continuous wave (CW) Doppler, and tissue Doppler imaging (TDI). The spectral Doppler outputs display a velocity scale above and below a zero velocity baseline, reflective of the Doppler frequency shifts (**Figures 4.30–4.35**). In CDI, a directional flow-velocity map tracks targets moving toward and away from the transducer in shades of red and blue, respectively (**Figure 4.29**). The various Doppler modalities, with the exception of CW Doppler, are based on emission of short pulses of US (similar to a strobe light), followed by longer periods during which the transducer "listens" for returning Doppler shifts. These acquisition periods limit the maximum number of US pulses transmitted across the imaging field. The number of pulses per second is the "pulse-repetition frequency" (PRF). The maximal flow velocities that can be faithfully recorded are displayed at the two extremes of the velocity scale (the Nyquist limits; equal to 1/2 PRF). When faster flow velocities (exceeding the Nyquist velocity) return to the transducer, the displayed US signal is "wrapped" around the zero velocity baseline, thereby contaminating the velocity signal in the opposite direction (**Figures 4.24, 4.29, 4.30,** and **4.33**). This flow—displayed falsely in the opposite direction—is a *"signal alias."* Signal aliasing is common, even with normal blood flow, and it must be recognized to interpret CDI and PW Doppler images.

Pulsed Wave Doppler Imaging The PW Doppler exam records Doppler shifts within a discrete operator-controlled area known as the sample volume (typically encompassing a width of 1–4 mm). Therefore, the source of returning "flow" information is known. PW Doppler uses a single sample volume that the operator steers within a 2D image. A hybrid modality termed high pulse-repetition frequency Doppler uses multiple sample volumes, which increase the PRF and Nyquist limits, roughly doubling these values for each additional sample volume. However, as more sample volumes are applied, the source of the returning signals becomes less certain, lending "range ambiguity" to the spectrum. Practically, when there is signal aliasing in PW Doppler, most operators switch to CW Doppler.

Color Doppler Imaging The CDI examination, also called color flow mapping, is a sophisticated form of PW Doppler. This modality uses dozens of sample volumes arranged in contiguous scan lines emanating spokelike from the transducer. Lines of Doppler shifts are rapidly processed within an operator adjustable *region of interest* that is overlaid on the 2D image. Instantaneous mean velocity within each sample volume is displayed over the cardiac cycle. CDI can reveal both normal and abnormal blood flow patterns. Most systems code blood flow moving away from the transducer as blue and flow toward as red (Blue Away, Red Toward, or "BART"). Zero velocity is indicated by black, meaning either no flow or that flow direction is perpendicular to the US beam angle of incidence. Variation in velocity of flow usually is displayed with enhanced color maps, where intensities of color hue indicate relative velocities (**Figure 4.29**). These maps enhance the visibility of the fastest-moving normal flow, as well as abnormal jets associated with lesions. Signal aliasing is displayed as an abrupt reversal or "wrap around" of color. Additionally, multiple velocities and directions of blood flow (turbulence) can be captured within a region of interest at any point in the cardiac cycle. System algorithms attempt to depict turbulent flow as mosaics of color or by encoding sample volumes using variance maps that usually add yellow or green to the edge of the red/blue display. Importantly, both signal aliasing and variance mapping can occur even with normal flow in CDI, because Nyquist limits generally are low and variance coding is strongly influenced by instrument settings. While these colorations direct the attention of the operator, they do not necessarily indicate an abnormal flow pattern.

In addition to signal aliasing, another inherent limitation to color flow Doppler is the challenge of maintaining temporal resolution, because of the relatively long processing time needed to compose a 2D color Doppler frame. An underused modality, termed color M-mode echocardiography, uses just one line of color-coded Doppler and overlays this onto a traditional grayscale M-mode study (**Figures 4.24** and **4.25**). The result is a rapidly sampled map of blood flow crossing this single line. Color M-mode has great utility for timing of flow events and avoiding problems with temporal resolution.

Continuous Wave Doppler Imaging The CW Doppler examination differs from PW Doppler by activating one crystal that constantly emits US while another crystal constantly samples the returning Doppler frequency shifts. Consequently, CW Doppler is not limited by PRF and can accurately record and display velocities exceeding 6 m/second without signal aliasing. Accurate velocity depiction assumes the operator maintains the angle of incidence close to zero. High velocities are typical of regurgitant and stenotic flow patterns and most left-to-right cardiac shunts, such as VSD and PDA. As reflected US is sampled down a line directed across the entire imaging field, all returning Doppler shifts superimpose. Thus, there always is range ambiguity related to the source of the returning signals and the velocity spectrum is inherently "turbulent," showing multiple velocities within the spectral display envelope. Practically, the operator uses CDI and PW Doppler to identify locations of turbulence and high-velocity flow, and then quantifies the maximal velocities using CW Doppler.

Tissue Doppler Imaging TDI usually is displayed in the same graphical format as for PW Doppler, but TDI is characterized by intense, low-velocity signals reflected from the moving myocardium (**Figure 4.34**). For example, while normal aortic flow is greater than 100 cm/second (1 m/second), TDI recordings usually fall within the 5–20 cm/second range. In usual PW and CW Doppler, the US system is set to accentuate echoes from RBCs (which are weak reflectors) while filtering out the "noise" of stronger, low-velocity signals reflected from valves and myocardial walls. Tissue velocity imaging requires special instrumentation that includes turning off low-velocity (wall or clutter) filters. TDI mainly is used for estimating ventricular filling pressures and assessing ventricular systolic and diastolic function, as discussed below.

Presentation Formats for Doppler Imaging

Spectral Doppler modalities graphically display the direction (relative to the transducer's position) and velocity of blood flow and tissue movements (**Figures 4.30–4.35**). The x-axis displays time, as marked by the electrocardiogram. The y-axis depicts the Doppler shifts as positive or negative velocities, relative to a zero velocity baseline. The operator can adjust the baseline to prioritize velocities in the positive (shift baseline "down") or negative (shift baseline "up") direction relative to the transducer. The y-axis indicates both the direction and velocity estimates of the moving targets. Properly adjusted spectral Doppler recordings of blood flow present a subtle grayscale spectrum, with its intensity linked to the relative number (or bins) of RBCs traveling within a velocity range. This grayscale is especially evident in CW Doppler, as the cursor records all Doppler shifts along the interrogating beam.

Normal blood flow travels within a narrow velocity spectrum. The densest compression of grayscale is found just inside the maximal velocity envelope and is termed the "modal" velocity. In contrast, abnormal flow often is turbulent and demonstrates a broader range of velocities, termed "spectral dispersion." Pathologic flow often is faster than normal and can create a signal alias in PW Doppler and CDI images. In these situations, maximal velocities can be quantified accurately only by using CW Doppler.

CDI, as noted previously, overlays a region of interest on a 2D image. The color map serves the same function as the graphical display except that only direction and relative velocity of flow are depicted. Time is shown by the updating of successive imaging frames or by combining CDI with M-mode imaging to create a graphical output (color M-mode). The operator can adjust the size and location of the color region of interest and modify the velocity scale by altering the PRF of the system. Higher PRF increases the Nyquist limit in each direction but filters out lower-frequency Doppler shifts, which produces less color flow mapping. Other console controls, including low-velocity filtering and adjusting color "quality" (which affects the packet size of US pulses) also affect the velocity scale. As with spectral Doppler, the zero baseline can be adjusted in CDI, but this is done only in special circumstances, such as for proximal isovelocity surface area (PISA) analysis (p. 121).

Doppler Examination—General Approach

A Doppler examination should include images from both right and left sides of the thorax and, at minimum, capture and quantify CDI and PW Doppler images of the inflow and outflow tracts. The examiner steers the PW sample volume and color region of interest with a trackball, then captures spectral Doppler and CDI loop recordings of blood flow. Grayscale 2D imaging guides the acquisition of these recordings.

In *normal* dogs and cats, all blood flow velocity spectra can be obtained from the left thorax using: left apical images (for mitral and aortic valves), a modified left apical image optimized for the tricuspid valve, and one of the left cranial positions aligned to RV outflow and pulmonary artery. The pulmonary artery also can be interrogated from the right thorax using cranial short-axis images; however, the vessel tends to curve away from optimal US beam alignment. Both right- and left-sided short-axis images of the aorta can offer reasonable alignment to a good portion of tricuspid transvalvular flow. For aortic blood flow in dogs, the highest velocity usually is recorded from the subcostal (subxiphoid) position. However, in the absence of LVOT obstruction, recording aortic velocity from the left apical five- or three-chamber image usually is sufficient for practical purposes. Subcostal (subxiphoid) windows always should be used when measuring LVOT velocity in dogs with (and with suspected) aortic stenosis or elevated LVOT velocities. Unfortunately, subcostal imaging offers no clear advantage for aortic flow alignment in cats.

In addition to "screening" the ventricular inlets and outlets by CDI and PW Doppler, additional evaluations of blood flow patterns often are necessary for individual patients. These are based on clinical suspicions, as well as any morphologic lesions identified during 2D imaging. For example, in cats with left atrial dilation, assessment of left auricular filling and emptying should be done using PW Doppler interrogation (**Figure 4.13**).

Complementary imaging planes are needed in animals with cardiac disease, beyond those used to map normal flow. For example, right parasternal long- and short-axis images often are best for aligning to a VSD, and a right parasternal long-axis image might optimally record an eccentric jet of MR, AR, or tricuspid regurgitation (TR). Modified short-axis views from the left thorax are best for visualizing the shunt of a PDA. Consequently, CDI is activated to evaluate the mitral, tricuspid, and aortic valves using both left and right parasternal long- and short-axis image planes. Other views are obtained based on findings during the active examination.

Accurate timing of flow events is a critical aspect of Doppler imaging. M-mode and spectral Doppler modalities accurately depict time during the cardiac cycle. However, timing of flow events can be confusing with CDI, especially when watching real time image motion. Two common errors in CDI are (1) mistaking a "flash" of blue in the LA for a jet of MR, when the signal is simply low-velocity, presystolic backflow of blood from a closing valve; and (2) mistaking color "bleeding" for a shunt (**Figure 4.29**, right). Digital loops should be captured and reviewed in slow motion or frame-by-frame to match flow events with time in the cardiac cycle. The ECG assists in determining this timing; a marker or cursor superimposed on the ECG delineates the period encompassed by the 2D image frame. Mechanical systole usually begins during the latter half of the QRS complex and ends just after inscription of the T wave. LV ejection begins after the QRS is fully inscribed (**Figure 4.32**, left). The ECG interval between the end of the P wave and onset of the QRS complex delineates the period of events related to atrial contraction. The exact point where atrial events begin and conclude, relative to ECG complexes, is influenced by the PR interval, heart rate, and LV end-diastolic pressure. Cardiac and valve motion on the 2D image, adjacent blood flow events, and spectral Doppler and color M-mode recordings also inform the timing assessment.

Finally, a technically proficient Doppler examination requires appropriate transducer selection, adjustment of the Doppler console controls, imaging skill, and appreciation of normal variation. Knowledge of cardiac diseases, ability to alter the examination based on contemporaneous findings, and appreciation of technical and interpretation errors also are critical. The imaging goals for spectral recordings are the delineation of a clean envelope and a clear peak, with distribution that reflects the number of RBCs contributing to the different velocity bins. Suboptimal technique or instrument settings can produce misleading diagnoses or disease severity assessment.

Normal Doppler Findings

The movement of blood depends on the development of a pressure gradient within the heart and circulation. Blood flow observations should be evaluated within the context of the cardiac cycle. For routine analysis, this can be divided into five arbitrary phases:

- Early diastole (from isovolumetric relaxation through rapid ventricular filling)
- Mid-diastole (diastasis)
- Atrial contraction (end-diastole or presystole)
- Early systole (from isovolumetric contraction to the peak velocity of ejection)
- Late systole

Corresponding events in the great vessels, atria, and connecting large veins also are targets for analysis, as described below. Understanding the normal events is pivotal to appreciating Doppler studies of blood flow and tissue movements; these are reviewed in Chapter 1 (p. 19). Timing of events also is important. High frame rates are needed for discrete timing of flow events when only 2D grayscale or CDI are used.

For the left side of the heart, relatively small instantaneous pressure gradients—called "impulse gradients"—drive blood across the cardiac valves. Although differences in peak systolic pressures in the left ventricle and aorta are negligible, a small impulse gradient is generated by the rise in LV pressure preceding that in the aorta. Similarly, small differences in left atrial and LV diastolic pressures are sufficient to propel blood across the wide mitral valve orifice. Corresponding but smaller impulse gradients are recorded in the right side of the heart. Together these generate the normal PW Doppler velocities recorded within the inflow and outflow tracts of the ventricles. Some of the reported normal values obtained with PW Doppler (without angle correction) in healthy dogs and cats are listed in **Table 4.11**.

Normal, or laminar, blood flow as captured by PW Doppler is characterized by a relatively compact modal velocity spectrum with less intense (fainter) velocity variations clustered to either side. In contrast, CDI uses a much larger region of interest, which contains a larger range of velocities and often maps flow moving in different directions. The fastest-moving red cells are characterized in PW Doppler by the edge of the velocity envelope, and in CDI by the brightest non-aliasing shades of color (if enhanced maps are used).

As discussed above, a Doppler signal alias is a common feature of PW Doppler and can be normal, or it can be an indicator of pathologic flow. An alias is recognized in PW Doppler by a velocity spectrum that "wraps" around the display and appears at the top or bottom (but on the opposite side of the zero baseline) so that flow seemingly originates from the opposite direction. When signal aliasing develops in spectral PW Doppler, most examiners shift the spectral baseline up or down to increase the Nyquist limit in the direction of recorded flow. However, if this maneuver cannot prevent aliasing, then CW Doppler should be activated to accurately record the maximal velocity. High PRF Doppler echocardiography also can be used, but this is done less commonly. Signal aliasing also occurs within normal flow patterns with CDI.

Semilunar Valves

Normal blood flow in the RVOT and LVOT is characterized by velocity spectra with roughly triangular profiles and a relatively high-pitched, whistling sound in the system's audio channel (**Figures 4.32** and **4.33**). The area under these triangular curves, known as the "velocity-time integral," (VTI), relates directly to ventricular stroke volume. Both maximal and mean ejection velocities are relevant to assessing cardiac function and disease. The "maximal instantaneous velocity" is the highest velocity recorded at the edge of the envelope, assuming the image has not been bloomed by overgaining or too much transmit power. The "mean ejection velocity" is the sum of the instantaneous velocities measured during systole divided by the systolic ejection time. Practically, these velocities are measured using calibrated electronic screen calipers that permit tracing of the outer edge of the modal velocity-time envelope. Outflow tract velocities and VTI increase with higher ventricular stroke volume. This commonly is observed with sympathetic or pharmacologic stimulation of

Table 4.11 Pulsed Wave Doppler Variables in Healthy Dogs and Cats[a]

Doppler Variable	Suggested Canine Reference[b]	Study (Reference)								
Species (number) ⇨	Composite of studies	Gaber, 1991 Dogs, n = 28	Yuill, 1991 Dogs, n = 20	Brown, 1991 Dogs, n = 28	Bonagura, 1998 Dogs, n = 15	Schober, 2001[e] & 1998[f] Dogs, n = 92[e] n = 14[e]	Petric, 2012 Cats, n = 31 to 53	Disatian, 2008 Cats, n = 87	Chetboul, 2006 Cats, n = 100[g]	Santilli, 1998 Cats, n = 20
Aorta	1.7 m/s (PW) <2.0 m/s (CW) Uncertain: 2.0–2.4 m/s[c]	1.189 ± 0.178 m/s	1.181 ± 0.108 m/s	1.06 ± 0.21 m/s	1.154 ± 0.153 m/s		1.04 m/s (0.77–1.40 m/s)		1.10 ± 0.2 m/s	
Pulmonary artery	<1.4 m/s	0.998 ± 0.153 m/s	0.981 ± 0.094 0.955 ± 0.103 Right side (top) Left side	0.84 ± 0.17 m/s	1.06 ± 0.138 m/s 1.068 ± 0.102 m/s Right, Left		0.96 m/s (0.65–1.21 m/s)		0.9 ± 0.2 m/s	
Mitral E wave[d]	<1.05 m/s	0.75 ± 0.118 m/s	0.862 ± 0.095 m/s		0.739 ± 0.089 m/s	Means: 0.69–0.77 m/s 0.52, 0.93 m/s 10, 90 percentiles[e]	0.68 m/s (0.48–1.01 m/s)	0.7 ± 0.14 m/s	0.7 ± 0.1 m/s	0.67 ± 0.13 m/s
Mitral A wave	MVE > MVA; Decreases with age	0.538 ± 0.087 m/s			0.459 ± 0.106 m/s	Means: 0.48–0.57 m/s[f] 0.52, 0.93 m/s 10, 90 percentiles[e]	0.56 m/s (0.38–0.73 m/s)	0.65 ± 0.14 m/s Ratio of E/A: 1.1 ± 0.2	0.5 ± 0.1 m/s Ratio of E/A: 1.5 ± 0.3	0.59 ± 0.14 m/s Ratio of E/A: 1.19 ± 0.3
Tricuspid E-wave	<0.90 m/s	0.562 ± 0.161 m/s	0.689 ± 0.084 m/s		0.597 ± 0.088 m/s					
Tricuspid A wave	TVE wave > TVA				0.454 ± 0.068 m/s					
Pulmonary venous flow diastolic wave	S < D typical S:D <1.4					Means: 0.5–0.57 m/s[f] 0.36, 0.82 m/s 10, 90 percentiles		0.47 ± 0.1 m/s		0.44 ± 0.09 m/s
Pulmonary venous flow systolic wave	S < D typical S:D <1.4					Means: 0.34–0.45 m/s[f] 0.24, 0.7 m/s 10, 90 percentiles for all age groups		0.48 ± 0.14 m/s		0.39 ± 0.12 m/s

(Continued)

Table 4.11 Pulsed Wave Doppler Variables in Healthy Dogs and Cats[a] *(Continued)*

Doppler Variable	Suggested Canine Reference[b]	Study (Reference)							
		Gaber, 1991	Yuill, 1991	Brown, 1991	Bonagura, 1998	Schober, 2001 & 1998	Petric, 2012	Disatian, 2008	Chetboul, 2006	Santilli, 1998
Pulmonary venous flow reversal (A_R) wave (velocity)	A_R < 0.9 m/s Duration A_R < MVA					Means: 0.21–0.24 m/s[f] 0.15, 0.3 m/s 10, 90 percentiles[e]		0.23 ± 0.06 m/s		
Pulmonary vein A_R (duration)	>30 ms					Means 67–70 ms[f] 53, 103 10 90 percentiles[e]		52.9 ± 13.5 ms		
Isovolumetric relaxation time[d]	<65 ms					60 ms ± 20[g] Means: 43–47 ms[f] 31, 65 ms 10, 90 percentiles[e]	58 ms (35–84 ms)	46.2 ± 7.6 ms	43 ± 9 ms (all cats) 50 ± 11 ms DSH 55 ± 11 ms MCC	55.4 ± 13 ms
Mitral deceleration time[d]						Means: 67–80 ms[f] 49, 110 ms 10, 90 percentiles	68 ms (49–113 ms)			59.9 ± 14 ms

Note: All velocity values are expressed in meters per second (m/s); all time values are expressed in milliseconds (ms).

[a] Values reported are mean ± 1SD or as a median (range); Doppler data reported have *not* been angle-corrected.

[b] For small studies with normal distribution, a suggested normal range is the mean ± 2.5 to 3SD. For samples >120, 2SD are appropriate. Reference limits for dogs suggested by the authors are indicated in this column and are subject to refinement with future studies. For feline reference values, the reader is referred to the three studies presented in the table.

[c] The upper limit defining peak aortic velocities is controversial. Peak aortic velocities using pulsed wave (PW) Doppler recorded from the left apex typically are <1.70 m/s in dogs without cardiac murmurs; continuous wave (CW) Doppler increases the signal to noise and records slightly higher peak velocities, with values <2.0 m/s suggested as normal. The velocity range between 2.0 and 2.4 m/s often is associated with an ejection murmur and, in the absence of any 2D imaging lesions, is considered ambiguous or equivocal for aortic stenosis. In normal dogs, slightly higher maximal velocities usually are recorded from the subxiphoid (subcostal) position using CW Doppler. See references for further details.

[d] Mitral valve (MV) E-velocity and MVE:MVA normally decrease with increasing age; mitral valve deceleration time and isovolumetric relaxation time normally prolong with increasing age.

[e] Study of the mitral valve involved dogs of varying age groups—the data quoted in ranges are the range of four sets of means for 84 of the healthy study dogs, divided into four arbitrary age groups of n = 30 (<2 years of age), n = 30 (≥2 to <4 years of age), n = 13 (≥4 to <6 years of age), and n = 11 (≥6 to <10 years of age).

[f] Study of 14 dogs for which pulmonary venous flow patterns are reported (Schober, 1998)

[g] 50 of 100 cats were Maine Coon cats

Abbreviations: MCC, Maine Coon cats; DSH, domestic shorthair cats.

contractility, volume expansion that increases ventricular preload, and during slower heart rates and situations of reduced diastolic blood pressure. The presence of any obstructing lesion in the outflow tracts also increases velocity and VTI; however, this is caused by abnormal ventricular systolic pressure and does not correlate with an increased stroke volume, as discussed below. Anesthetics and sedatives often depress outflow tract velocities. Variation in VTI also is observed during ventilation. Furthermore, the examiner must be aware of the influence of cardiac translation, the motion that occurs when the heart moves back-and-forth across the cursor and sample volume. Translation is caused by contraction and filling and by thoracic movements that attend ventilation.

Doppler color-coding of blood flow across the normal ventricular outflow tracts depends in part on the transducer location. Generally, apical or subcostal images are used for the LVOT, in which case the flow will move away from the transducer and be coded in shades of blue, according to the relative velocities within the region of interest. Again, signal aliasing is common and can be normal. Here, an alias in CDI is recognized as an abrupt change in color (to red) within a zone encoded bright blue. In contrast to apical images, when the LVOT is assessed from a right-parasternal transducer position, the aorta is nearly perpendicular to the US beam. As such, flow velocities are underestimated and normal flow is more difficult to detect. However, pathologic blood flow, being faster, can be highlighted in these long-axis views. When there is aortic dilation, the LVOT flow might be encoded red, especially if a right-craniodorsal transducer position is used. Nearly all transducer positions used to evaluate the RVOT will demonstrate flow with blue encoding. Signal aliasing within the zone of fastest moving pulmonary artery flow appears as a red core surrounded by blue as the Nyquist limit (for that direction) is exceeded.

Left Ventricular Outflow The velocity of the normal LVOT spectrum increases as the PW Doppler sample volume is moved from the subaortic vestibule into the ascending aorta. Normally there is rapid velocity acceleration, with a thin acceleration envelope and relatively sharp peak (**Figure 4.32**). The deceleration limb of the aortic spectrum is approximately twice the thickness. Valve opening and closure noise might be sampled as well and these assist in timing of flow events. The velocity peaks just distal to the valve, and in healthy resting dogs is usually <1.7 m/second; however, velocities can approach or slightly exceed 2 m/second. Outflow tract velocity profiles in normal cats are similar to those of dogs, although peak velocities are lower. It is difficult to align the cursor with aortic blood flow in cats, and velocities typically are underestimated.

The upper limit of normal for LVOT ejection velocity still is debated. Canine breeds with smaller aortic dimensions relative to LV size, such as Boxer dogs and Bull Terriers, often have a mildly accelerated ejection velocity that is considered either normal variation or mild aortic stenosis, depending on one's perspective. The most common reason for *physiologic* increase in LVOT velocity is increased stroke volume, as observed in dogs with bradycardia caused by complete AV block or in excited dogs, from increased sympathetic stimulation. No velocity cut-off is both sensitive and specific for delineating normal outflow from mild aortic stenosis. However, as resting maximal LVOT velocities approach 2.5 m/second, the liability for having LVOT obstruction certainly is greater (see Chapter 27).

The normal aortic valve does not leak. However, brief perivalvular AR of uncertain clinical significance sometimes is seen in healthy young dogs and cats. Holodiastolic AR is regarded with suspicion, though. Heavy sedation, especially with alpha-2 agonist agents, also can induce AR. In older animals, trivial to mild AR, silent to auscultation, often is observed in dogs and horses with valvular degeneration and in cats with aortic root dilation.

Right Ventricular Outflow When compared to the aorta, the pulmonary artery velocity profile is slower to accelerate, more rounded at the peak, and slightly lower in maximum velocity (usually <1.4 m/second). Furthermore, physiologic pulmonary regurgitation (PR) of low velocity (<2.2 m/second) is both normal and common in all species (**Figure 4.33**, left).

Physiologic reasons for increased RVOT velocity are similar to those noted above for the LVOT. In healthy cats, high ejection velocities sometimes develop from increased sympathetic tone and dynamic obstruction within the RV infundibulum. This creates a mid-to-late-systolic blood flow acceleration characterized by a dagger-shaped profile, with a concave acceleration limb typical of other dynamic obstructions (**Figure 33.21**, p. 671). It has been suggested that iatrogenic RVOT obstruction can be induced by excessive thoracic pressure with the transducer. Hypovolemia also predisposes to dynamic RVOT obstruction.

Normally, the acceleration of RBCs ejected into the low resistance pulmonary circulation is characterized by a gradual upstroke or "acceleration time," (AT). However, especially in animals with PH (associated with increased pre-capillary vascular resistance), the ratio of AT to "ejection time," (ET) becomes smaller (**Figure 4.33**, right); this is discussed further in Chapter 39. The change in pulmonary flow profile can be explained by the increased resistance and vascular impedance within the pulmonary circuit, which morphs the RVOT ejection profile into one more resembling that of the LVOT.

Atrioventricular Valves

Ventricular filling is measured with a sample volume placed near the tips of the opened mitral or tricuspid valve. Normal diastolic blood flow has two peaks, an early rapid filling wave (E wave) and a lower velocity presystolic wave due to atrial contraction (A wave). The audio signals are multiphasic with two distinct sounds. During slower heart rates in dogs and horses, a low-velocity signal of mid-diastolic filling can be recorded during ventricular diastasis. This also can be pathological if atrial pressures are increased. Normal values for transmitral and transtricuspid PW Doppler imaging are shown in **Table 4.11**.

Filling patterns in the ventricles are affected by AV pressure gradients that are influenced by numerous factors, including: myocardial relaxation and ventricular untwisting; ventricular chamber distensibility; heart rate; venous pressures; ventricular afterload; ventilation; pericardial constraint; ventricular interdependence; and the presence of any cardiac lesions, especially mitral or tricuspid valve disease or left-to-right shunts. Even in healthy animals, the transmitral flow velocities depend greatly on heart rate and ventricular filling pressures. These multiple determinants complicate the assessment of ventricular diastolic function, as is described later (see section "Doppler Assessment of Ventricular Diastolic Function", p. 127).

Mitral Valve The typical appearance of transmitral flow recorded at the tips of the opened valve is an "M-shaped" waveform, consisting of two triangular peaks. The first velocity peak (the E wave) represents early diastolic ventricular filling. The second velocity peak (or A wave) is caused by atrial contraction (A; **Figure 4.30**). The first (E) relates to blood being sucked into the ventricle during the rapid ventricular filling phase, and the second (A), to the pumping of blood into the ventricle. LV filling initially is rapid, usually achieving a maximum inflow velocity of about 75–80 cm/second (0.75–0.8 m/second) in dogs. The mitral velocity spectral profile is relatively "tight" around the modal velocity. With increased transmitral flow, the E wave velocity becomes higher and spectral dispersion increases. Following the E wave peak there is a rapid deceleration of LV inflow. In healthy hearts, enhanced sympathetic tone physiologically abbreviates this "deceleration time" (DT) by promoting vigorous diastolic relaxation and ventricular suction. This reduction in mitral DT must be distinguished from DT shortening caused by high left atrial pressures operating on a stiff left ventricle. At slow heart rates, during ventricular diastasis, mitral inflow velocities are low and can be masked by excessive baseline (low-velocity) filtering. Atrial contraction (A wave) peak velocity averages about 50–60 cm/second (0.5–0.6 m/second) in dogs. In healthy animals and at normal heart rates, the A wave is smaller and briefer than the corresponding E wave.

The normal mitral inflow (filling) velocity relationship is E wave > A wave. LV diastolic dysfunction and increased filling pressures cause abnormalities of this relationship. As discussed below this analysis actually is complicated. The E wave often exceeds 1 m/second when there is a high cardiac output, as with anemia, or when fusion of the E and A waves occurs during tachycardia. This is especially common and problematic in cats. Completely fused E and A waves should not be analyzed. Preload directly affects the E wave and A wave velocities. For example, volume overload increases the filling velocities, while dehydration and diuretic therapy decrease them. The E/A ratio decreases in healthy dogs and cats as they age, reflecting slower ventricular relaxation and greater dependence on atrial contraction. A technical error also can alter the ratio; moving the sample volume closer to the LA causes the A wave velocity to increase.

During systole, a general concept of interpretation is that the mitral valve does not normally leak. However, it actually is common to see tiny jets of MR in dogs, horses, and humans, including in some younger animals. These regurgitant jets are silent to cardiac auscultation. However, they pose a problem during assessment of young animals for breeding soundness, or horses with impaired exercise capacity. Additionally, as dogs and horses mature, small jets of mitral regurgitation are commonly observed related to valvular thickening and degenerative valve disease. These will be evident before any murmur is detected and are of no immediate clinical concern. It is less common to find MR in the absence of cardiac pathology in cats. However, as noted above, a frequent mistake with CDI is misinterpreting valve closure backflow for pathological MR. Many such cats are labeled as having heart disease, when in fact they simply have a functional or physiological heart murmur.

Tricuspid Valve The tricuspid valve recording is qualitatively similar to that of the mitral valve, with some important differences. Peak inlet velocities are lower than for the left heart (**Table 4.11**); this relates to the larger tricuspid orifice circumference, as well as difficulty obtaining fully apical images of the RV inflow tract. There often is greater spectral dispersion of the inlet signal, which might indicate difficulties in aligning to inflow in all planes. A dispersed, positive low-velocity systolic wave also is recorded in many studies; this can be confusing if a simultaneous ECG is not recorded. Small jets of physiologic TR are common in all species; such TR is evident in over 50% of cases examined from multiple acoustic windows. This is especially problematic in cats with a functional heart murmur loudest over the right thorax, as the clinical significance of the tricuspid regurgitant flow can be ambiguous.

Pulmonary Veins, Left Auricle, and Hepatic Veins

Doppler studies can be used to interrogate the velocity patterns in the pulmonary veins, CaVC and hepatic veins, as well as in the left atrial appendage. These are more advanced studies, but they can provide valuable information regarding diastolic heart function and cardiac filling pressures. Increased pressures are a common element of heart failure.

Pulmonary Venous Flow Pulmonary venous velocities have been measured from healthy dogs and cats under a variety of conditions using both TTE and TEE. Pressure gradients between the pulmonary venous system and LA drive flow across the pulmonary venous ostia. These pressure gradients reflect the diastolic and systolic functions of the left ventricle and mitral valve, as well as plasma volume status. Ventricular diastolic dysfunction or mitral valve disease can markedly influence the appearance of the pulmonary venous waveforms. Pulmonary venous flow profiles are polyphasic and reflect the three major functions of the LA over the cardiac cycle. From the apical position, two positive waves (S, D) and one negative or atrial reversal wave (A_R) are recorded within the atrial connection of the pulmonary veins (**Figure 4.31**). Analysis of these waveforms relates mainly to the assessment of LV filling pressures and diastolic left heart function.

At the conclusion of atrial contraction, one or two forward S waves are registered. The first begins just before the QRS complex and probably relates to suction created by atrial relaxation. This usually blends into the second S wave, which follows the QRS complex and occurs while the LA functions as a *reservoir* for venous return (during ventricular systole). The genesis of this second S wave is the negative pressure created within the LA by descent of the mitral annulus during ventricular contraction and the RV pressure pulse pushing venous return through the lungs. The S wave becomes smaller relative to the D wave in the setting of LV failure and elevated left atrial pressure, which impedes venous return while the mitral valve is closed. Severe MR often contaminates the S wave when the regurgitant jet extends into a pulmonary vein.

During proto-diastole, another forward flow wave is recorded as the LA functions as a *conduit* (or passageway) for venous return. This D wave is explained by the pulmonary vein-to-LV gradient that is exposed at mitral valve opening. The pulmonary vein D wave occurs as the transmitral E wave records early LV filling. Accordingly, conditions that increase the transmitral E wave velocity, especially high cardiac output or increased pulmonary venous pressure, also augment the pulmonary venous D wave.

In late diastole, after the P wave on ECG, the LA functions to *pump* blood into the ventricle. This causes the transmitral A wave while simultaneously generating the pulmonary venous A_R wave. The A_R wave reflects backward movement of blood into the pulmonary veins during atrial contraction and LV filling. The ratio of mitral A wave duration to A_R duration is about 1.2–1.5 in healthy dogs. This ratio decreases with reduced LV distensibility and increased end-diastolic pressures.

Atrial Function   The reservoir, conduit, and pump functions of the atria can be evaluated using echocardiographic and Doppler methods. This often is done in cats with a large LA. The evaluation includes measurements of left atrial size, pulmonary venous flow, and various assessments of left atrial function. Left atrial EF can be estimated by tracing the 2D area of the LA after filling and emptying, or by calculating atrial fractional shortening from M-mode-derived measurements.

Another approach to assessing the LA involves recording the filling and emptying velocities at the mouth of the left auricle using PW Doppler. In healthy cats, two or three waveforms are identified (Schober, 2015). One consideration is to focus on the active contraction of the appendage; this left auricular ejection velocity normally exceeds 25 cm/second in cats (**Figure 4.13**). As a general guideline, peak auricular velocities between 20 and 25 cm/second are suspicious for impaired left atrial function; those <20 cm/second usually are associated with significant atrial disease, increased risk of blood stasis characterized by echogenic "smoke," and an overall higher risk for arterial thromboembolism. As a practical outcome, the recommendation for antithrombotic prophylaxis often is based on the combined assessment of left atrial size, auricular contraction, and the pertinent medical history. Advanced "black box" technologies, such as speckle-strain analysis also can be applied to the LA, as for the ventricle; however, these are beyond the scope of this chapter.

Hepatic Veins and Caudal Vena Cava   Right atrial filling pressures can be estimated by combining 2D and M-mode imaging of the CaVC over the respiratory cycle, observing CDI flow patterns in the hepatic veins, and recording PW Doppler velocities in the hepatic veins, although the latter evaluation requires better definition. In normal animals, CaVC diameter varies as thoracic pressure increases and decreases with ventilation. The hepatic venous velocity profile, as recorded by PW Doppler imaging, is similar to that seen in the pulmonary veins, with S, D, and A_R waves. The first two waves are antegrade (toward the RA) while the A_R wave is retrograde.

Internal dimension measurements of the CaVC by 2D or M-mode imaging can provide an index of collapsibility. With increased right atrial pressures, the CaVC and hepatic veins usually appear distended on 2D imaging, while collapsibility over the respiratory cycle decreases. This must be distinguished from translational motion affecting the US beam path. Higher systemic venous pressures also cause the D wave of the hepatic venous flow to increase, while the S wave decreases because pressure in the RA is higher. Strong retrograde A_R waves also might be present.

Tissue Doppler Imaging

Myocardial motion and velocity can be recorded using TDI. A PW Doppler sample volume is placed within the myocardium, typically adjacent to the mitral or tricuspid annulus (**Figure 4.34**). Using the various left apical transducer positions, the three most common recording sites are at the lateral and septal LV walls at the mitral annulus, and the lateral RV wall with the sample volume near the tricuspid annulus. These TDI profiles appear as low-velocity, mirror images of transmitral and transtricuspid blood flow patterns. Early diastolic recoil of the ventricle results in a negative tissue velocity called E′ or e′ ("E-prime" or "E_a" for the annulus). Late diastolic recoil following atrial contraction produces a negative, lower-velocity tissue waveform, a′ or A_a. A single positive wave (s′) is evident during systole, coinciding with ventricular ejection and apical displacement of the annulus. Additionally, rapid oscillations are observed coincident with isovolumetric relaxation and isovolumetric contraction. Peak myocardial velocities in dogs are low, usually <20 cm/second, and as previously discussed, the instrumentation settings must be optimized to record these signals. Tissue velocities vary by species (lower in cats), body weight (in dogs), and methodology (single sample PW Doppler versus segmental analysis using tissue-based color Doppler or speckle tracking, which averages a larger segment of tissue). The examiner must be mindful of the angle of interrogation (incidence) of the US beam to the moving targets. For example, it is challenging to align to apical-basilar movements in horses and the lateral wall of dogs and cats poses more technical challenges than the IVS. Similar to transmitral flow, the normal E' is greater than A'. Myocardial annular velocities are used in the assessment of left and right ventricular diastolic function, filling pressures, and evaluation of segmental systolic function as discussed below.

Principles of Diagnosis Using Doppler Echocardiography

The most important uses of Doppler imaging are confirmation of normal blood flow velocities across the cardiac valves, detection of abnormal flow patterns caused by valve disease and shunts, recognition of PH, and quantitation of valvular heart diseases. Additionally, Doppler studies are integral to ventricular diastolic function assessment and right heart evaluation.

Abnormal Blood Flow Patterns PW Doppler originally was used to screen for abnormal blood flow patterns. The typical finding was the contamination of an expected inflow or outflow tract signal with a turbulent or high-velocity jet. Additionally, the examiner would search for turbulent flow signals in the *receiving chamber* adjacent to an imaged lesion, such as a VSD or abnormal mitral valve. Today that role has been assumed by CDI, although the principles of evaluation are the same. The advantage of CDI is the ability to screen relatively large regions for valvular regurgitation, stenosis, shunting, and other flow disturbances. Small shunts and regurgitant flow patterns, muscular VSDs, and flow disturbances caused by subtle lesions are better visualized with this modality. The color flow study also guides placement of the PW Doppler sample volume and steerable CW Doppler cursor across normal and suspicious areas of flow, thus streamlining the examination. Analysis of cardiac color Doppler images is mainly subjective; this mode provides only semi-quantitative estimates of velocity. Because larger regions of interest are examined, the angle of incidence between US beam(s) and blood flow is variable, although this is less of a concern than with spectral studies where tight alignment to blood flow is a priority.

Clinical questions should be considered when performing a Doppler examination. For example, in a patient without a cardiac murmur, an extensive Doppler evaluation is unnecessary unless required to assess ventricular function or filling pressures. Routine color flow mapping of the ventricular inlets and outlets combined with PW Doppler recordings of their velocity spectra should suffice. Conversely, when a cardiac murmur is present, a more comprehensive examination is necessary and should be informed by the physical examination findings. The examiner must integrate the 2D (or 3D) images with the Doppler findings. For example, in a dog with a left apical systolic murmur and thickened or prolapsing mitral valve leaflets, at least three or four complementary image planes should be used to search for (and assess the extent of) MR by CDI. In a cat or horse with a systolic murmur, a cause should be sought with CDI using multiple planes before rendering a diagnosis of "functional" or "physiological" murmur. Frequently, only one imaging plane will provide the diagnosis or offer the optimal alignment to blood flow for further quantitation using CW Doppler. A similar but more detailed approach is needed for evaluating congenital malformations of the heart. For instance, a common CDI mistake is to misdiagnose venous return from the CaVC as an atrial septal defect. Interrogation of the atrial septum from multiple planes likely will avoid this error.

Spectral Doppler and color M-mode imaging are complementary to CDI. Whether normal or abnormal flow is detected, the precise timing and maximal velocity of that flow should be determined. MR, for example, might not be holosystolic, but this is difficult to assess with only 2D color Doppler imaging. In the rapidly beating heart of a cat or excited dog, it is especially important to time color flow events. This can be done using a spectral Doppler mode or by meticulously placing the M-mode cursor through the flow pattern of interest. A graphic color M-mode display offers spatial and time resolution of flow events across the M-line. With some practice and study, this technique can be an invaluable part of the flow assessment.

Abnormal Blood Flow Velocity High blood flow velocities can arise in several ways. One is simply from the normal pressure differences in the circulation that are exposed by a shunt or an incompetent heart valve. Another involves systemic hypertension or PH superimposed on an insufficient semilunar heart valve. A third involves the increased (ventricular or atrial) pressure needed to accelerate blood across a stenotic valve or region. These abnormal flow patterns are depicted by turbulence or variance displays in CDI and PW Doppler; they are further quantified with CW Doppler and the application of physical laws. Especially pertinent to veterinary medicine are the continuity equation and the Bernoulli relationship, discussed below.

In the setting of cardiac pathology, the assessment of a high-velocity flow profile recorded by CW Doppler offers both diagnostic and quantitative information about the type and severity of disease (**Figure 4.35**). Examples include aortic stenosis, pulmonic stenosis, dynamic LVOT obstruction (from hypertrophic cardiomyopathy), mitral and tricuspid valvular stenosis, VSD, regurgitation across any of the heart valves, and PDA. This dynamic is driven by a pressure gradient that moves the blood from higher- to lower-pressure sides of the lesion at velocities typically ranging from 2.5 to 7 m/second.

PISA, Vena Contracta, and Jet Area

A relationship between lesion size, pressures, and RBC velocity characterizes flow across stenotic lesions, incompetent valves, and shunts. The majority of these lesions involve a *restrictive orifice*, which means that pressures do not equilibrate across the two sides of the lesion despite the presence of a communication. For instance, with mild mitral or tricuspid valvular regurgitation, systolic ventricular pressures are normal and atrial pressures increase only minimally because the *regurgitant orifice* is small enough to restrict flow across the valve. If this was not the case, and the lesion was *unrestrictive*, pressures would equilibrate from ventricle to atrium (leading to uncontrollable CHF). In practice, there are variations that range from highly restrictive to nonrestrictive lesions; the latter occurs with large septal defects, where the two ventricles function as a common chamber with matching pressures. The instantaneous pressure difference or *gradient* measured across the lesion also determines the velocity at which blood moves from higher-pressure source, through the lesion, and into the lower pressure sink or *receiving chamber*. The flow pattern across a lesion often is characterized by three components (**Figure 4.36**):

- A proximal region of flow convergence, characterized by isovelocity shells of RBCs
- A narrowed vena contracta of flow crossing the orifice
- A jet of turbulent blood flow into the receiving chamber

Each of these components can be used in the diagnosis and analysis of cardiac lesions.

Proximal Isovelocity Surface Area The pattern of blood flow approaching a valve lesion, stenosis, or a shunt is observed best using CDI. The common disorder of MR can be used as an example. Proximal to the regurgitant orifice, RBCs converge toward the lesion in accelerating isovelocity shells. The blood essentially is pushed across the regurgitant valve by the higher pressure on the ventricular side. In idealized flow models, these isovelocity shells are hemispherical in shape. If the operator slowly shifts the color map baseline down to create a 20–40 cm/second aliasing limit, one

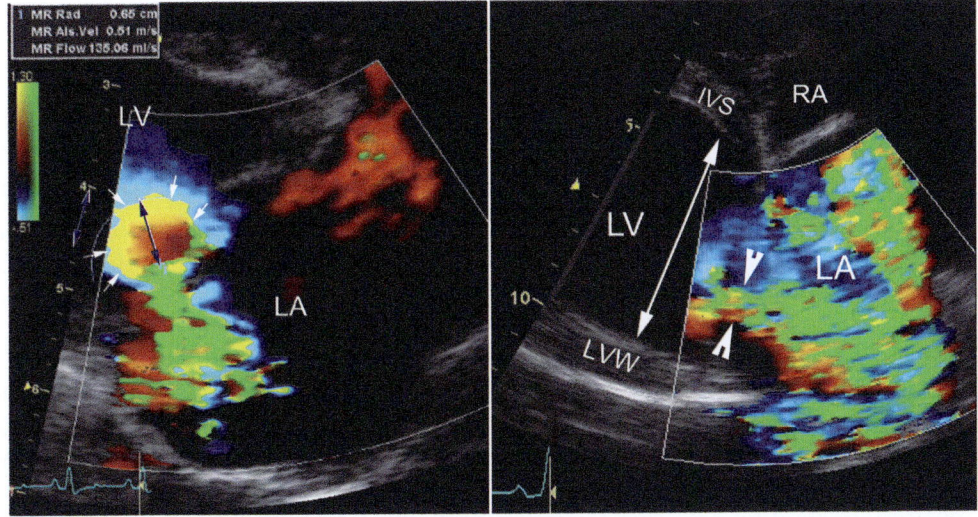

Figure 4.36 Color Doppler imaging of mitral regurgitation (MR) in two dogs. The left panel shows the flow pattern into a regurgitant orifice. Flow moving from left ventricle (LV) into the left atrium (LA) accelerates (from dark blue to cyan), then aliases (to yellow and dark red), then becomes a "jet" (green) within the regurgitant orifice. Note the roughly circular appearance of the signal alias (white arrows) at 51 cm/second (see color bar). This "ball on a jet" is the proximal isovelocity surface area (PISA), which ideally is formed as a hemisphere but often appears this way. The distance to the regurgitant orifice (double-headed arrow) is the radius of the proximal isovelocity shell. The regurgitant flow rate and regurgitant orifice area can be estimated using calculation software. PISA patterns often are seen with regurgitant and stenotic valves and across left-to-right shunts. The right panel contains a close up image of a *vena contracta* (arrowheads) in a dog with MR from dilated cardiomyopathy. Note the flow encoding below (red) and above (blue) the regurgitant jet, indicating the image is at about right angles to the *vena contracta*. In general, for any given body size, the larger the *vena contracta* the more severe the MR; however, there are a number of confounding limitations, such as the presence of multiple jets or an asymmetrical regurgitant orifice. Color bleeding or mirror image artifact causes turbulence to appear outside the LA at the bottom of the right image.

of these isovelocity shells might be captured as a signal alias called a *proximal isovelocity surface area (PISA)*. The speed of this velocity shell is known, based on the Nyquist aliasing velocity, and the distance from the center of the PISA to the regurgitant orifice can be measured. This distance represents the radius of the hemisphere. In general, at a set aliasing velocity, the farther the PISA from the regurgitant orifice the greater the volume of regurgitant flow. Conversely, a small or indeterminate PISA radius suggests only mild regurgitation. The PISA aliasing velocity and the radius to the orifice are incorporated, along with the VTI of the MR jet (determined from CW Doppler), into a hydraulic formula that calculates regurgitant flow rate and effective regurgitant orifice area (EROA). Such calculations are advanced and usually performed by software in the echo system. Because veterinary patients vary greatly in size, the calculation of an EROA probably is of less practical value unless it is indexed to body size. However, this PISA principle is important and the approach will be more relevant once surgical valvular repair becomes more common. The same principle can be applied to evaluate flow across a septal defect or regurgitant tricuspid or aortic valve.

Vena Contracta As the isovelocity shells of blood enter the (regurgitant) orifice, they form into a high-velocity *jet* that functionally narrows immediately past the regurgitant orifice. This is termed the "vena contracta"; it might be observed by zooming the CDI image and (ideally) imaging perpendicular to this part of the high-velocity jet (**Figures 4.18** and **4.36**, right). The diameter of the *vena contracta* relates to the size of the EROA, with recognition that the geometry might not be symmetric and multiple jets can be present. A small *vena contracta* (such as 1–2 mm wide in a small-breed dog with MR) indicates milder regurgitation; whereas, a larger *vena contracta* width (5–6 mm) is compatible with severe MR. Again these values must somehow be scaled to body size.

Jet in the Receiving Chamber As the regurgitant jet exits the orifice and *vena contracta*, it enters the receiving chamber as turbulent blood flow. This often is referred to as a "jet" or "turbulence" and in patients with MR, is observed within the LA using CDI (**Figures 4.18** and **4.25**). This is the most obvious way of diagnosing valvular regurgitation and the most commonly used (and misused) method for assessing severity by CDI. Some operators will calculate a jet area in relation to the area of the atrium. However, there are problems with this approach. For example, centrally oriented jets tend to spray, entraining RBCs that are already in the atrium into the "turbulence"; conversely, eccentric jets that hug the atrial wall create a smaller jet area-to-atrial area, but can represent severe MR. Jet area is greatly affected by instrument settings and transducer selection. The echocardiographer should evaluate multiple planes when using this approach. Realistically, standards for grading severity of regurgitation based on jet area have not been established yet in veterinary medicine. The clinician is advised to combine results from CDI with measurements of ventricular and atrial size (as previously discussed). When standard console settings are used for CDI, central jets that extend less than halfway into the atrium are likely to indicate mild regurgitation. Jets that extend to the dorsal atrial wall or enter the pulmonary venous ostia are more likely to indicate severe MR. Nevertheless, multiple factors can affect this extension, including jet direction and systolic blood pressure, which is the driving force for the regurgitant jet. The severity of regurgitation also will affect the CW spectrum, as discussed below.

Continuity Relationship and Stenosis

The continuity relationship states that the product of flow velocity × cross-sectional area along a single path is a constant (p. 23). When the cross-sectional area (CSA) along the path of blood flow decreases abruptly, RBCs progressively accelerate and converge across the region proximal to the stenosis. This principle is straightforward when dealing with stenotic valves or outflow tracts. It also is relevant to regurgitant valve orifices and to restrictive shunts, though less often used here. If the proximal CSA is measured by 2D imaging, the velocity (V) in the proximal area by PW Doppler, and the stenotic jet velocity by CW Doppler, then a functional CSA of the lesion can be estimated as follows: $CSA_{Stenotic} = (CSA_{Proximal} \times V_{Proximal})/Velocity_{Stenotic}$, assuming the same volume of blood crosses both normal and stenotic zones.

Bernoulli Relationship and Clinical Applications

The continuity relationship emphasizes the interaction between flow velocity and orifice area, while the Bernoulli relationship relates flow velocity (measured by CW Doppler through a shunt, stenosis, or incompetent valve) to the instantaneous pressure difference (gradient) across the lesion (**Table 4.12**). Knowledge of the pressure gradient across a lesion can assist with clinical assessment and prognosis. Details of the full Bernoulli relationship are beyond the scope of this chapter (Weyman, 1994). However, the simplified Bernoulli equation is used in daily practice. Instantaneous pressure gradient (in mm Hg) is calculated from the product of $4V^2$ (where maximal velocity, V, is measured in m/second). For example, in a case of aortic stenosis, a peak ejection velocity of 4.5 m/second would correspond to a maximal pressure gradient of 81 mm Hg ($4 \times 4.5 \times 4.5 = 81$).

The maximal instantaneous pressure gradient is obtained by placing the measurement cursor at the highest velocity point of the spectral envelope and allowing the system to apply the simplified Bernoulli equation to the measurement. Determination of the mean pressure gradient requires tracing

Table 4.12 Clinical Applications of the Simplified Bernoulli Equation[a]

Pulmonic Stenosis (PS)
- Record the peak velocity profile in m/s across the stenosis.
- Use the simplified Bernoulli equation (PG = $4V^2$) to determine the maximum instantaneous PG across the RVOT.
- RV systolic pressure = Peak gradient + 20 to 25 mm Hg (where 20 to 25 mm Hg is an estimate of PA systolic pressure, based on catheterization experience).
- Verify RV systolic pressure if there is a TR jet available (see the section "Pulmonary Hypertension").
- If a dynamic subvalvular component is identified, also calculate the peak end-systolic dynamic obstruction PG.
- If there is an increase in the proximal velocity (V_1) before the fixed obstruction that peaks in midsystole, recalculate the distal valvular obstruction using both the PA velocity (V_2) and the proximal velocity, as peak gradient = $4(V_2 - V_1)^2$.
- Trace the outer envelope of the PA VTI to determine the mean PG.
- Mean gradient is usually ≈ 55–60% of the peak instantaneous gradient.

Aortic Stenosis (AS, Subaortic Stenosis)
- Record the maximal velocity profile in m/s across the stenosis.
- Use the simplified Bernoulli equation (PG = $4V^2$) to determine the maximum instantaneous PG across the LVOT, where V is maximal velocity (m/s).
- Measure noninvasive systemic arterial blood pressure.
- Maximal LV systolic pressure = Systolic arterial blood pressure + Maximal instantaneous PG.
- Trace the outer envelope of the aortic VTI to determine the mean PG across the LVOT.
- Mean gradient is usually ≈ 55–60% of the peak instantaneous gradient.

Pulmonary Hypertension (PH)
- Measure the peak velocity of TR, if present.
- Abnormal TR velocity is >2.6 m/s; >3.0 m/s typically is used to indicate PH in the absence of any outflow stenosis.
- High-velocity TR correlates to elevated RV systolic pressure.
- Peak systolic pressure in the PA equals peak RV systolic pressure.
- Peak PA pressure equals the calculated RV-to-RA instantaneous PG plus RA pressure (usually zero, unless there is CHF).
- To estimate mean and diastolic PA pressures, record the maximal velocity of any pulmonary insufficiency and calculate the PA pressure in early and late diastole, respectively, using the simplified Bernoulli equation. The PA diastolic pressure = RV diastolic pressure + Doppler-derived PA to RV diastolic PG (in the absence of CHF, RV diastolic pressure is assumed to be zero, or is estimated by inspection of the jugular veins, caudal vena cava collapsibility, or from CVP measurement).

Ventricular Septal Defect (VSD)
- Determine the peak velocity across the aortic valve. If aortic velocity is <2 m/s, assume LV systolic pressure = the systemic arterial systolic pressure (measured simultaneously by noninvasive means). If aortic velocity is >2 m/s, calculate the gradient; see the section "Aortic Stenosis".
- Measure the peak velocity across the VSD. Assuming close parallel alignment with flow, one can use the simplified Bernoulli equation to estimate the peak instantaneous LV-to-RV PG.
- RV systolic pressure = Systolic arterial blood pressure − the PG between left and right ventricles.
- Interpretation is difficult if there is concurrent RV outflow obstruction or subaortic stenosis, or if the angle of Doppler interrogation is >20°.

Patent Ductus Arteriosus (PDA)
- Use the simplified Bernoulli equation to estimate the peak aortic-to-PA PG and PA systolic pressure.
- PA systolic pressure = Systolic arterial blood pressure − the PG between the aorta and PA.
- The peak aortic-to-PA systolic gradient should be approximately 80–100 mm Hg in normotensive animals with left-to-right shunting PDA.
- Poor alignment with flow, or a long narrow ductus might produce a lower PG despite normal PA pressures.
- Markedly decreased shunt gradients, <20–30 mm Hg, suggest moderate to severe PH.

Mitral or Tricuspid Valve Stenosis
- Estimate the transvalvular diastolic gradients using the modified Bernoulli equation.
- Trace the diastolic envelope to measure both maximal diastolic and mean diastolic PGs.
- Also calculate the pressure half-time, the time (in seconds) required for the instantaneous PG to decrease by 50%, as calculated from the Bernoulli equation (see text).
- Results can be altered by a high heart rate (which shortens diastolic flow time), increased transvalvular flow (from a concurrent shunt, AV valvular regurgitation), or high cardiac output states (increased sympathetic activity, fever, or anemia).

Aortic Regurgitation and Pulmonary Regurgitation
- Estimate the transvalvular early and end-diastolic gradients from the modified Bernoulli equation.
- Trace the diastolic envelope to measure both maximal diastolic and mean diastolic PGs.
- Calculate the pressure half-time, the time (in seconds) required for the instantaneous PG to decrease by 50%.

[a] Simplified Bernoulli equation: Pressure gradient = 4 × Maximal Velocity^2.

Abbreviations: AV, atrioventricular; CHF, congestive heart failure; CVP, central venous pressure; LV, left ventricle; LVOT, left ventricular outflow tract; PA, pulmonary artery; PG, pressure gradient; PH, pulmonary hypertension; RA, right atrial; RV, right ventricular; RVOT, right ventricular outflow tract; TR, tricuspid regurgitation; VTI, Doppler velocity-time integral.

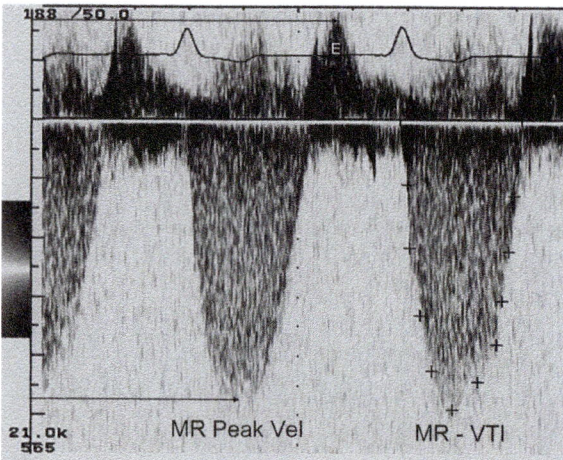

Figure 4.37 Continuous wave Doppler recording from a dog with severe mitral regurgitation (MR). The transmitral inflow E wave is high-velocity (about 1.7 m/s; normal is <1 m/s), indicating high end-systolic left atrial pressure. The MR jet's maximal velocity is <5 m/s (~4.7 m/s). Using the simplified Bernoulli relationship (4×4.7^2), the systolic difference between left ventricular (LV) and atrial (LA) pressures is ~88 mm Hg (normal is ~120 mm Hg). Assuming good alignment with regurgitant flow, this indicates either systemic hypotension, high LA pressure, or both. Looking at both the diastolic and systolic flow profiles, the findings are compatible with severe MR. This is supported by the velocity-time integral (VTI) tracing (at right), which shows a somewhat early peak to the MR jet, indicating LA pressure is rapidly increasing. The VTI can be used to estimate the mean velocity of the MR flow pattern and therefore, the mean pressure gradient during that phase of the cardiac cycle.

the outline of the outer modal envelope of the velocity spectrum (**Figures 4.37** and **4.38**). The echo system calculates the mean gradient from the VTI. Conceptually, the mean gradient can be thought of as the sum of an infinite number of instantaneous gradients measured over the period of interest

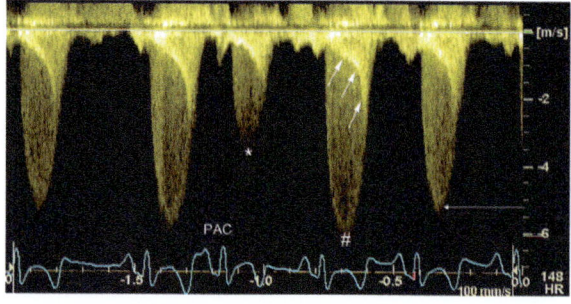

Figure 4.38 Continuous wave Doppler recording from a dog with fixed and dynamic pulmonary stenosis. The congenital obstructive lesion has led to a peak velocity across the valve of just over 5 m/s, which translates to an instantaneous maximal pressure gradient of about 100 mm Hg ($4 \times 5^2 = 100$). A late-peaking dynamic obstruction also is evident (arrows), superimposed on the flow profile of the fixed obstruction; note the "dagger-shape" of this profile, which is typical of dynamic obstructions. A premature atrial complex (PAC) illustrates the effect of stroke volume. The premature beat's smaller stroke volume produces reduced outflow velocity (*) and pressure gradient. The beat that follows typically is stronger (post-extrasystolic potentiation) and has a larger stroke volume, increasing the maximal velocity (#).

(systole or diastole) and then divided by the number of measurements taken.

There are substantial risks for both under- and over-estimating pressure gradients using the Bernoulli equation and, therefore, misclassifying the severity of heart disease. The maximal instantaneous pressure gradient recorded by CW Doppler will be underestimated unless the US beam angle of incidence is close to 0 degrees or 180 degrees. Velocity estimates of pressure gradient will be significantly underestimated at intercept angles exceeding 22 degrees. The greatest risks for overestimation involve: application of angle correction (which should never be done in the heart), expansion of the velocity spectrum caused by excessive transmit power, selecting a carrier (transducer) frequency that is too low, over-gaining the receiver Doppler shifts, or selecting inappropriate compression and grayscale processing.

In some ways, the continuity equation approach is more valid for evaluating the severity of certain lesions compared to the pressure difference approach. Pressure gradients depend heavily on the amount of *flow* crossing the lesion (**Figure 4.38**). When stroke volume increases (as with anemia, high sympathetic tone, or after successful balloon valvuloplasty of a stenotic valve), the gradient across the lesion also increases. If ventricular stroke volume is diminished (as from heart failure or cardiodepressive drugs), the opposite occurs. Thus, estimation of stenosis severity based solely on pressure gradient can be erroneous, because this method discounts the effect of blood flow. The continuity relationship method intuitively seems preferable and it has been used to estimate LVOT stenosis severity in dogs. However, limitations to this approach include the need to measure the CSA and velocity in the proximal zone, as well as to consider the vast range of patient sizes encountered in veterinary practice. For example, the clinical significance of a stenotic orifice area of 0.44 cm² would be quite different in a miniature compared to a standard poodle.

Despite these limitations, most veterinarians focus on pressure gradients and widely employ the simplified Bernoulli equation. However, this assessment should always be tempered by consideration of the flow. Besides the identification and quantification of stenotic lesions, other applications of the simplified Bernoulli equation include diagnosis of systemic hypertension or PH, assessment of shunt severity, and further evaluation of valvular regurgitation severity. These are considered below.

Valve Stenosis, Gradients, and Pressure Half-Time The concept of identifying valvular or subvalvular stenosis by CW Doppler and determining its severity using the Bernoulli and continuity relationships have been summarized in the previous sections. It is commonly accepted that trivial to mild stenosis is a controversial diagnosis when based only on a maximal velocity. However, the assessment of moderate to severe aortic and pulmonic stenosis is well established. Usually the proximal blood flow velocity (V_1) is ignored and either maximal (peak) velocity (V_2) or the mean velocity are measured. In cases of stenoses in series, as with combined subvalvular and valvular stenoses, both V_1 and V_2 need to be considered, and appropriate reference texts should be consulted. Both maximal and mean pressure gradients should be determined in outflow tract stenosis, to minimize the effect of overgaining the return signal. Because the maximal velocity is squared to determine the gradient, even small errors can cause clinical miscalculation related to severity assessment. Experience indicates that mean systolic gradients in the outflow tracts are approximately 55–60% of the maximal instantaneous gradient. So, the specific gradient used must be indicated.

Obstruction to right or left ventricular inflow also can be assessed using the simplified Bernoulli relationship. When there is stenosis associated with AV valvular malformation, congenital supravalvular ring, or a tumor, the pressures in the atrium and veins behind the obstruction increase. The consequence is a faster inflow velocity than would be expected. Because increased E wave velocity also can be seen in CHF, additional imaging features should be considered before making the diagnosis of mitral or tricuspid stenosis. Obviously, assessment of the 2D anatomy is critically important, too.

Another derivation of the Bernoulli equation is the "pressure half-time"; this is applied in cases of inflow tract stenosis or when assessing the severity of aortic regurgitation. The pressure half-time is defined as the *time* in milliseconds needed for the transvalvular, diastolic pressure gradient to decrease by 50%. Normally the mitral (and tricuspid) E wave is quickly inscribed and its velocity rapidly declines. Conceptually, small increases in pressure half-time occur when the ventricle relaxes slowly due to disease; this is visualized as a prolonged E wave deceleration time. In the case of anatomic mitral or tricuspid stenosis, the inflow velocity decay is markedly prolonged; it appears as a flattened slope between the E and A waves and it can be quantified by determining the pressure half-time (**Figure 4.39**). Fundamentally, a prolonged pressure half-time indicates that more time is needed to reduce the pressure gradient between the atrium and ventricle. In humans, this time duration can be included in calculations that estimate mitral valve orifice area. Although this approach has been applied to dogs and cats, there are few supportive data and in most cases, the subjective appearance of a prolonged pressure half-time indicates the presence of stenosis.

When pressure half-time measurements are applied to the assessment of aortic and pulmonary regurgitation, the question is essentially, how rapidly does the pressure gradient decline? In severe aortic or pulmonary regurgitation (**Figure 4.32**, right), the pressure half-time is short because of rapidly rising ventricular and declining arterial pressures. In contrast, with mild semilunar valve regurgitation, the arterial to ventricular pressure gradient is maintained and the pressure half-time is long (that is, its slope is shallow).

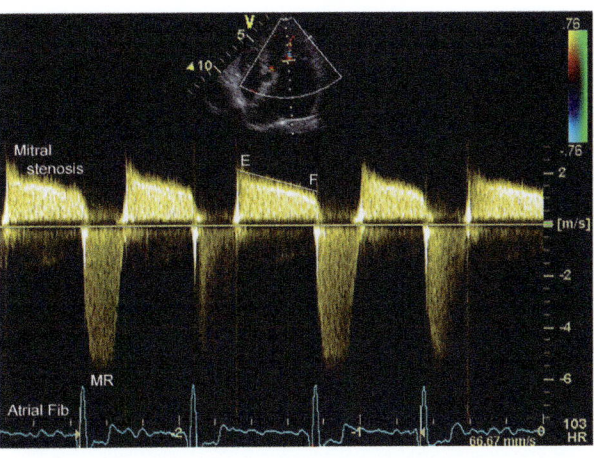

Figure 4.39 Prolonged pressure half-time in a dog with mitral stenosis, and regurgitation (MR), caused by valve dysplasia. The cardiac rhythm is atrial fibrillation (note the lack of an A wave in the transmitral profile). The E to F slope is extremely shallow, indicating maintenance of a pressure gradient across the stenotic mitral valve throughout diastole. Early-diastolic transmitral velocity (E) is nearly twice normal because of high left atrial pressure. Also note the high-velocity MR jet.

When there is mitral or tricuspid valve stenosis, the inflow pattern changes in several ways. Besides a prolonged pressure half-time, the E wave velocity is increased, reflecting higher mean atrial pressure and a higher diastolic pressure gradient as the valve opens. A common compensation for inflow tract stenosis is atrial hypertrophy, such that atrial contraction generates a higher than normal A wave velocity also. Frequently, this velocity exceeds that of the E wave. However the A wave will be lost if atrial fibrillation supervenes.

Valvular Regurgitation The concept of valvular regurgitation is discussed above in terms of the PISA, the vena contracta, and the receiving chamber jet area. Additional information usually can be obtained by looking at the contour and density of the CW Doppler image. When using "standard" instrument settings and transducers, a weak or poorly defined VTI suggests less severe regurgitation. The appearance of a triangular and lower-velocity CW profile is compatible with severe MR or TR. In terms of the simplified Bernoulli equation, this can be explained by the more rapid rise in atrial pressure that occurs with severe AV valvular regurgitation, which reduces the transvalvular pressure gradient and the corresponding velocity. In contrast, when atrial pressure is lower, the regurgitant jet tends to have a more rounded and central systolic peak. The influence of systolic arterial blood pressure also must be considered, because this will dictate LV systolic pressure and influence measured MR velocity.

As discussed below, peak MR or TR velocity correlates to the pressure within the respective ventricle. Assuming a normal atrial pressure, increased regurgitant velocity relates to either hypertension on that side of the circulation or an outflow obstruction, such as subaortic or pulmonic stenosis. This can be another method for checking the severity of an outflow tract stenosis and the corresponding intraventricular systolic pressure in patients with congenital heart disease.

When MR or TR is severe, or in the setting of CHF, the early ventricular filling wave also will increase in velocity. Assessing left atrial pressure is challenging in this case, because the E wave will be most affected by the pressure in the atrium at the end of (ventricular) systole. Although atrial pressure can be high throughout the cardiac cycle, as in CHF, with AV valve regurgitation the increase also can be confined to end-systole, as seen in the v wave of the atrial pressure curve (**Figure 15.3**, p. 263). When atrial pressure elevation only occurs in the latter part of systole, the likelihood of CHF is lower, although the E wave velocity will be increased. Nevertheless, in the setting of MR (or TR), a normal mitral (or tricuspid) inflow velocity argues against severe regurgitation or impending CHF. A high-velocity E wave and lower-velocity regurgitant MR jet implies severe valvular disease (**Figure 4.37**).

Diastolic regurgitation across the aortic and the pulmonary valves can be assessed in a manner similar to that previously discussed for the AV valves. Additionally, as discussed above, the pressure half-time can be applied. With moderate to severe aortic or pulmonary valve regurgitation, the pressure within the receiving chamber (ventricle) increases more rapidly; this reduces the diastolic pressure difference between great vessel and ventricle, resulting in a corresponding decline in regurgitant velocity. As a result, the measured pressure half-time is shorter, and subjectively appears as a steep velocity slope (**Figure 4.32**).

Pulmonary and Systemic Hypertension Doppler echocardiography is the principal method by which PH is identified noninvasively. Although there are 2D imaging features that correspond to this diagnosis (including dilation of the main and branch pulmonary arteries), estimation of pulmonary artery pressures using the Bernoulli relationship can demonstrate the presence and estimate the severity of PH. This method is based on detecting either a higher than normal velocity of TR (in the absence of intraventricular or pulmonary valvular stenosis, or a large VSD) or (in the absence of measurable TR) of pulmonary regurgitation; the right atrial pressure also must be considered. In patients with normal pulmonary arterial and RV systolic pressures, TR velocity usually is less than 2.6 m/second, and definitely less than 3 m/second. These cut-off values are slightly higher in standing horses. The concept is that as pulmonary artery systolic pressure increases, so too must RV systolic pressure, and if there is TR, blood will be forced into the RA at a higher velocity. For example, if right atrial pressure is ignored, a peak TR velocity of 3 m/second will correlate to an estimated systolic RV (and pulmonary arterial) pressure of 36 mm Hg, which is the calculated pressure gradient; this corresponds with mild PH. A 4 m/second peak TR velocity (calculated gradient of 64 mm Hg) would relate to moderate to severe PH, with systolic pressure exceeding 60 mm Hg. In patients with CHF, the elevated right atrial pressure must be considered and added to the calculated TR pressure gradient. One approach is to add 10 mm Hg when there is CHF. For horses, the value of 20 mm Hg might be more appropriate. Thus for the preceding example, the patient's systolic pulmonary artery pressure would be closer to 70–80 mm Hg. Central venous pressure could be measured and used as proxy for right atrial pressure.

Diastolic velocity across a regurgitant pulmonary valve also can be used to identify PH. The regurgitant velocity in early diastole can estimate mean pulmonary artery pressure, although further data are needed regarding this. The pressure half-time also is relevant, because severe pulmonary regurgitation often results in a steep slope and shortened pressure half-time.

Other methods for assessing PH by Doppler include measuring the ratio of the RV outflow AT divided by the ET. As pulmonary vascular resistance rises and becomes more like that in the systemic arteries, RV outflow acceleration becomes more abrupt and ET becomes relatively prolonged. Values of this AT/ET ratio predicting PH depend largely on whether the cause is pre-capillary, as with heartworm disease, or post-capillary secondary to left-sided heart failure. In general, the most severe alterations in AT/ET will be seen in cases of pre-capillary PH. This can include the appearance of a notch during flow deceleration, presumably from abnormal pulmonary arterial wave propagation characteristics (downstream impedance mismatch) with prominent reflection waves, which abruptly reduce systolic velocity (**Figure 4.33**, right).

Although indirect systemic blood pressure measurement usually is preferred, systemic hypertension also might be uncovered by applying the Bernoulli equation to a mitral or aortic valve regurgitant jet. In normotensive patients with MR, the maximal velocity usually is less than 6 m/second. If the MR peak velocity exceeds 6.3–6.4 m/second, systemic hypertension should be suspected. Complementary findings, such as LV concentric hypertrophy or aortic dilation, can help support a diagnosis of systemic hypertension. In general, however, the relationship between intracardiac estimates of systemic blood pressure and peripheral noninvasive measurements has not been strong, so this method cannot be entirely relied upon. Failure to obtain optimal alignment with the regurgitant jet also will reduce the estimated LV pressure.

Shunts Finally, the Bernoulli equation often is applied to cardiac shunts (**Figure 4.35**). The CW Doppler exam is the standard for documenting the high-velocity flow across a shunt. As a general principle, the systemic-to-pulmonary pressure gradient reflects (inversely) the size of a shunt. For example, in a left-to-right shunting PDA or VSD the corresponding pressure gradient should be approximately 100 mm Hg, as shown in **Table 4.12**. This gradient corresponds to a maximum velocity of 5 m/second through the defect. If systemic arterial pressure is depressed because of sedation, the corresponding left-to-right shunting velocity also will be lower. Restrictive shunts maintain a near normal pressure difference on each side of the circulation, so for PDA and VSD, the velocity will approximate 5 m/second assuming good alignment to flow. Conversely, because the pressure difference across a large or unrestricted shunt is smaller, peak velocity will be lower. As an example, a 3 m/second shunt velocity in a dog with a VSD (assuming optimal alignment with shunt flow) suggests a large defect with reduced pressure differential between the ventricles, which implies some degree of PH or RVOT obstruction. This should be confirmed by 2D imaging and ensuring that the maximum velocity has been faithfully recorded. Because pressures in the RA and LA are low, the pressure gradient across an isolated atrial septal defect typically is small.

Doppler Assessment of Ventricular Systolic Function

Doppler imaging has a minor role in the assessment of ventricular systolic function. The TDI recording of ventricular annular S' waves is used most commonly today. Although a variety of systolic time indices can be derived from the ventricular outflow profile, measurements such as pre-ejection period and ejection time rarely are used in practice. Various combined indices of cardiac function such as the Tei index of myocardial performance also are used infrequently; while not discussed further here, more details can be found in the section "Suggested Additional Reading and References."

Ventricular stroke volume (SV), cardiac output (CO), and shunt fractions can be estimated using PW Doppler methods. After measuring the diameter (d; in cm) across the location of the PW Doppler sample volume, CSA is determined as $\pi(d/2)^2$. The volume of flow is directly proportional to the area under the velocity (cm/second) - time (s) integral or VTI (this area is called "stroke distance," with units in cm). Multiplying the VTI (cm) by the CSA (in cm^2) yields a calculated SV. It is most accurate to determine this at the aortic valve, although the pulmonary trunk could be used as well. SV multiplied by heart rate provides a rough estimate of CO. When estimating shunt fractions, multiple volumetric calculations are needed to determine systemic versus pulmonary blood flow. Overall, such volumetric calculations are performed infrequently in routine clinical practice and we probably underestimate the information provided, especially variables such as forward SV in dogs with MR.

Doppler Assessment of Ventricular Diastolic Function

Diastole extends from the time of aortic valve closure to mitral valve closure. Active myocardial relaxation begins even before ejection is complete, and this initiates a complicated process that allows the AV valves to open and normal ventricles to fill under low venous pressures during both rest and exercise. Abnormal ventricular diastolic function leads to elevation in filling pressures. Severe diastolic dysfunction is considered a negative prognostic finding. Pericardial diseases characteristically cause abnormal filling, but diastolic function abnormalities also occur with, and can complicate, myocardial diseases and conditions associated with ventricular volume or pressure overloads. As with tests of systolic function, the assessment of diastolic function is confounded by moderate to severe MR in the setting of preserved or hyperdynamic ventricular systolic function. **Table 4.13** summarizes some echo indices of ventricular diastolic function, relative to the severity of diastolic dysfunction.

Overview and Practical Considerations   Diastolic function is complicated. No single index incorporates all the determinants of ventricular filling. Some relevant factors include active myocardial relaxation, ventricular fiber restoring forces (recoil and untwisting), myocardial stiffness, chamber compliance, pericardial restraint, ventricular interaction, and atrial contractility. Additional influences include ventricular loading, inotropy, heart rate, and coronary blood flow. The interplay among these factors is complex.

The most important concept underlying echo methods of diastolic filling assessment is that most indices measure the *combined effects* of diastolic heart function and ventricular filling pressures. Filling pressures for the left heart relate to mean pressure in the LA (the average atrial pressure over the cardiac cycle, which is strongly influenced by pulmonary venous pressure) and to LV end-diastolic pressure, which is affected by LV compliance and the strength of atrial contraction.

Transient increases in atrial pressure during a vigorous atrial contraction can compensate for impaired ventricular relaxation and recoil, as long as the instantaneous heart rate is not so fast that it abbreviates diastole. Conversely, chronic elevation in mean left atrial pressure usually relates to severe LV functional impairment, including decreased chamber compliance or distensibility and neurohormonal-renal compensations leading to volume retention. The identification of high pulmonary venous pressures during the diastolic assessment often indicates a need for drug (diuretic, inodilator) therapy to prevent or treat CHF. Conversely, mild diastolic dysfunction associated with lower mean left atrial pressure implies a more favorable short-term prognosis (or indicates that previous therapy for CHF has been successful). Of importance to veterinarians is the point that ventricular diastolic function can appear normal, or even hyperdynamic, when there is moderate to severe volume overload with relatively well-preserved ventricular systolic function. This limits the value of diastolic assessment in most small-breed dogs with chronic MR. The most commonly used LV diastolic function assessments are the analysis of transmitral inflow velocity patterns and TDI of LV wall motion. Normal patterns of transmitral and pulmonary venous flow, and of LV wall TDI, are described above. Diastolic dysfunction usually is classified into three (or four) broad categories, which are summarized below and in **Table 4.13**, and illustrated **Figures 4.30, 4.31,** and **4.34**).

Table 4.13 Ventricular Diastolic Function and Filling Pressures

Functional Designation		Estimates of Left Ventricular Diastolic Function and Ventricular Filling								
		LA Size	**Mitral: E, A**	**TDI: e', a'**	**IVRT**	**Mitral: DT**	**E/e'**	**E/IVRT**	**PVF: S, D**	**PVF: A_R**
Normal	Normal diastolic function	Normal	E > A	e' > a'	Normal	Normal	Normal	Normal	S < D (dog) S ≈ D (cat)	Duration MVA > A_R
Grade 1 dysfunction	Relaxation abnormality	Normal to ↑	E < A	e' < a'	↑	↑	N to ↓	N to ↓	S > D	Duration MVA > A_R ↑ A_R velocity
Grade 2 dysfunction	Pseudonormal filling	↑	E > A	e' < a'	Normalizes	Normalizes	N to ↑	N to ↑	Variable	Duration MVA: A_R variable; ↑ A_R velocity
Grade 3 dysfunction	Restrictive filling: reversible	↑↑	E ≫ A	↓e', ↓a'	↓	↓	↑	↑	S < D	Duration MVA < A_R
Grade 4 dysfunction	Restrictive filling: irreversible	↑↑	E ≫ A	↓e', ↓a'	↓	↓	↑	↑	S < D	Duration MVA < A_R

Notes:

1. The patterns shown here are general findings; it is uncommon for each variable to change in the manner shown exactly in this table.
2. Diastolic function is very difficult to assess in primary mitral regurgitation (see text). Higher end-systolic LA pressure develops because of the regurgitant volume and this has a disproportionate influence on early diastolic filling. Additionally, both systolic and early diastolic motion tend to increase in primary mitral valve disease. Compared to cardiomyopathies, much higher ratios of mitral E wave to TDI e′ and mitral E wave to IVRT are needed before increased filling pressures can be identified.
3. Sinus tachycardia can lead to fusion of E and A waves and uninterpretable patterns; atrial fibrillation eliminates the A wave and short cardiac cycles can reduce mitral DT.

Abbreviations: IVRT, isovolumetric relaxation time; LA, left atrial; Mitral: DT, mitral valve deceleration time; Mitral: E A, transmitral filling velocities in early diastole (E) and after atrial contraction (A); MVA, transmitral A wave (duration); N, normal; PVF: A_R, pulmonary venous flow atrial reversal wave; PVF: D S, pulmonary venous flow diastolic (D) & systolic (S) waves; TDI e′ a′, tissue Doppler imaging longitudinal tissue velocity in early diastole (e′) and after atrial contraction (a′); ↓, decreased; ↑, increased; ↑↑, moderate to severe LA enlargement. Normal means within reference range for species.

Relaxation Abnormality Evidence of *delayed ventricular relaxation* is probably the most common finding of diastolic dysfunction. It can be identified even in healthy dogs and cats as an aging change. When delayed relaxation is evident the following are observed:

- Isovolumetric (isovolumic) relaxation time (IVRT) is prolonged
- Mitral E wave amplitude is reduced, with E<A
- Mitral E wave deceleration time is prolonged
- Early diastolic recoil in the LV wall is diminished, with a lower tissue velocity e′ wave and decreased e′/a′
- The pulmonary venous flow D wave decreases relative to the S wave

As long as heart rate is normal, impaired early filling is compensated for by shifting ventricular filling fractions to late diastole. This is evident as increased amplitudes of the transmitral A wave, tissue Doppler annular a′ wave, and pulmonary venous A_R wave. Collectively, these findings are typical of *Grade 1 diastolic dysfunction*. This rarely is associated with CHF unless fluid therapy, protracted tachycardia, or acute volume overload cause increased filling pressures. The most obvious changes during real-time examination are E wave to A wave reversal in both the PW Doppler transmitral and TDI recordings. The reduced transmitral E wave velocity indicates that filling pressures are not high and therefore, the likelihood of CHF is relatively low at this stage.

Pseudonormal Filling Diastolic function abnormalities are less apparent once mean venous and atrial pressures increase. Higher ventricular filling pressures mask Doppler findings of impaired relaxation because the mitral valve opens sooner under higher pressure and the LA empties more readily. This compensation produces what is termed pseudonormal filling, which normalizes the mitral E/A ratio, mitral deceleration time, and IVRT. However, the early diastolic recoil measured with TDI does not normalize and TDI demonstrates that e′<a′. The pulmonary venous flow is characterized by an S wave that still exceeds the D wave and in some cases, the duration of the pulmonary venous A_R wave will exceed that of the transmitral A wave. Collectively, these findings define *Grade 2 diastolic dysfunction* and indicate the patient is at higher risk for CHF. Thoracic radiographs should be obtained in these cases and home respiratory rate monitoring implemented. The potential for lowering venous pressures with drug therapy (angiotensin converting enzyme inhibitor, low-dose diuretic, dietary sodium restriction, pimobendan) should at least be considered.

Restrictive Filling Progressive ventricular disease usually is associated with a loss of ventricular distensibility. This is a more severe form of diastolic dysfunction, which can be overcome only by increased venous pressures. Although such pressure increase can partially mitigate the resistance to cardiac filling, capillary pressures also increase, which predisposes to pulmonary edema, pleural effusion, or both. Myocardial relaxation and ventricular distensibility both are impaired at this stage, and most ventricular filling is limited to early diastole. The result is the so-called *restrictive filling pattern* evident in the transmitral flow pattern; this is considered *Grade 3 diastolic dysfunction*.

Typical Doppler findings include a high-velocity E wave, shortened deceleration time, and attenuated A wave, so that E≫A. The precise E/A ratios defining this stage have not been sufficiently defined for dogs and cats. Often, the diminutive A wave is filtered out by the low-velocity (wall) filter setting. The changes in the E wave are caused by the combination of initial filling under high left atrial pressure and increased ventricular stiffness, which causes the AV pressure gradient to quickly approach zero, thus stopping further ventricular inflow (**Figure 4.31B**). The small A wave is explained by the reduced left atrial-to-LV end-diastolic pressure difference, and possibly by concurrent atrial myocardial failure. In most cases of cardiomyopathy, the early diastolic tissue recoil (e′) is not normalized by high filling pressures. Thus, with restricted filling, mitral E/A and mitral E/e′ ratios are greatly increased.

The IVRT actually *shortens* in restrictive filling because high venous pressures initiate earlier filling. This is characterized by an increase in the E/IVRT ratio in both dogs and in cats. Complementary changes are observed in the pulmonary venous flow profile. This is characterized by a small systolic filling (S)wave (related to high pressure and reduced compliance in the LA), a pronounced D wave (from high pulmonary venous pressure, paralleling the tall transmitral E wave), and sometimes, a prolonged A_R wave (as pulmonary veins offer less resistance to flow than the noncompliant left ventricle). These changes might be reversed by cardiac drug therapy that includes diuretic(s), an angiotensin converting enzyme inhibitor, and often, pimobendan. If filling patterns then return to a Grade 2 (pseudonormal) pattern, this is evidence of therapeutic success; however, if the diastolic abnormalities do not improve, *Grade 4 diastolic dysfunction* is said to be present.

Other Echocardiographic Imaging Applications

Transesophageal Echocardiography

Cardiac structures can be imaged through the esophageal wall with specialized transducers mounted on a flexible, steerable endoscope tip. TEE can provide clearer images of some cardiac structures (especially those at or above the AV junction) compared with TTE because interference from the chest wall and lung is avoided. TEE can be especially helpful for defining

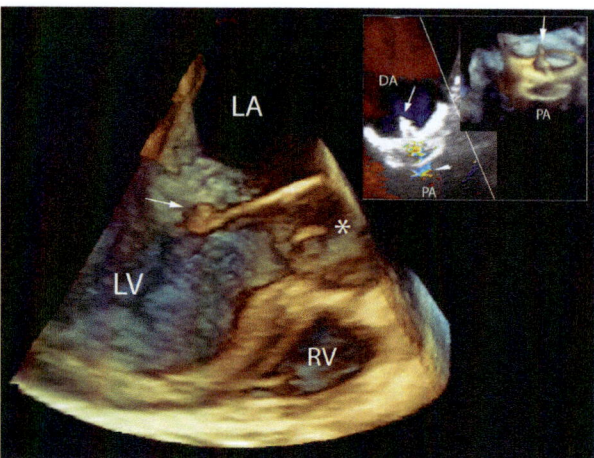
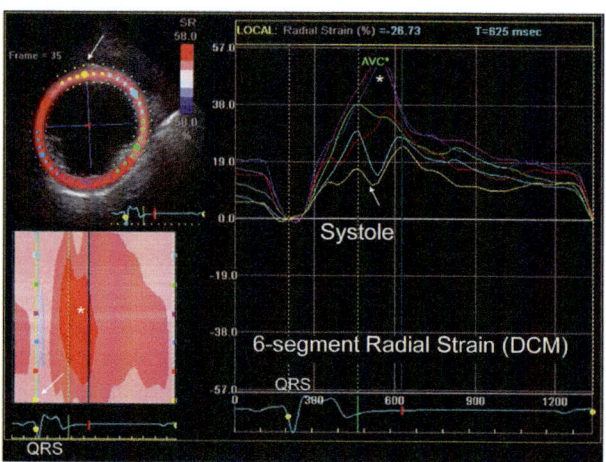

Figure 4.40 Three-dimensional echocardiography in a dog with patent ductus arteriosus. The dilated left ventricle (LV), mitral valve (arrow) and aorta (*) are shown. The inset images show 2D (color flow, left) and 3D (right) close-ups of an Amplatz canine ductal occluder. The device is positioned within the ductus and has been released from the retaining cable. The two occluding discs and the cable screw connector on the aortic side of the device (arrow) are evident. DA, descending aorta; LA, left atrium; PA, pulmonary artery; RV, right ventricle.

Figure 4.41 Radial strain recorded across the left ventricle in a dog with preclinical dilated cardiomyopathy. The colored lines relate to the six arbitrary short axis segments selected by the (human) algorithm. Note that the yellow segment (three arrows) is the least deforming in both the curves (at right) and in the color panel (at lower left); these both track radial strain over the cardiac cycle. Conversely, the segments coded in purple and blue exhibit the greatest strain (*). The marked disparity across the segments is abnormal and typical of myocardial disease or conduction disturbance. Normal segmental radial strain is >40% in dogs.

some congenital malformations, identifying atrial thrombi or tumors, evaluating valves for endocarditis lesions, and guiding cardiac interventional procedures (**Figure 26.16**, p. 446; and **Figure 4.40**, inset). The need for general anesthesia, or heavy sedation, and the expense of the endoscopic transducers are the main disadvantages of TEE. The interested reader should consult the references (including Bonagura & Luis Fuentes, 2020, and others) for more detail on TEE and other advanced echocardiographic imaging applications.

3D Echocardiography

The development of various methods for obtaining 3D reconstruction or real-time (4D) imaging of the heart and other structures represents an advanced application of echocardiography (**Figure 4.40**). Although still confined to a small number of referral centers, its availability is becoming more widespread. Limitations of 3D echocardiography currently are based on three factors: cost, technology (most transducers are too large for small animals or employ image processing speeds that are too slow for horses, as well as smaller animals), and a lack of demonstrated clinical value over other available modalities. Current technology requires several cardiac cycles in order to acquire sufficient data for quality 3D real-time or reconstruction. Regardless, this modality has been used for diagnostic evaluation, procedural planning, and quantitation of chamber size in dogs and horses. Once these limitations are addressed, 3D imaging is likely to become a clinical standard. 3D echocardiography allows anatomic and blood flow abnormalities to be viewed from any angle by rotating or bisecting the image. The greatest clinical potential for 3D imaging relates to morphologic evaluation prior to cardiac surgical procedures.

Advanced Image Analysis

An increasing number of advanced image processing methods are available for anatomic and functional assessments of the heart and valves. Representing a form of artificial intelligence, these applications usually are vendor specific and represent unnecessary expenses for a veterinary practice. Some of these applications can rapidly measure ventricular volumes along with global and segmental function. There are methods for quantifying ventricular dyssynchrony and outlining the sequence of cardiac activation. There certainly is hope that these indices could be more sensitive measures of cardiac function, but few veterinary studies have been validated against gold standards or by longitudinal studies that show an impact on clinical decision making. One of the most common uses is determination of myocardial strain (deformation) using a methodology of tissue speckle tracking (**Figure 4.41**). There is a substantial research literature about these "black box" methods in veterinary medicine; however, their limited current use (and high expense) precludes further discussion here.

Suggested Additional Reading and References

Also See Online Comprehensive Bibliography at: https:// www.routledge.com/9781482246223.

Armstrong WF, Ryan T. Feigenbaum's Echocardiography. 7th edition. Wolters Kluwer Health/Lippincott Williams & Wilkins, Philadelphia, PA. 2010.

Baade H, Schober K, Oechtering G. Echokardiographische Normwerte bei West Highland White Terriern und Boxern unter besonderer Beruecksichtigung der Rechtsherzfunktion. Proceedings of the 7th Annual Congress of the German Society of Veterinary Internal Medicine and Laboratory Diagnostics. 1999.

Bavegems V, Duchateau L, Sys SU, et al. Echocardiographic reference values in whippets. Vet Radiol Ultrasound 2007;48:230–238.

Bayon A, Fernandez del Palacio MJ, Montes AM, et al. M-mode echocardiography study in growing Spanish mastiffs. J Small Anim Pract 1994;35:473–479.

Bonagura JD, Luis Fuentes V. Echocardiography. In, Mattoon J, Nyland T (editors). Small Animal Diagnostic Ultrasound. 4th edition. Saunders Elsevier, St. Louis, MO. 2020.

Bonagura JD, Miller MW, Darke PG. Doppler echocardiography. I. Pulsed-wave and continuous-wave examinations. Vet Clin North America Small Anim Pract 1998;28:1325–1359.

Boon J. Veterinary Echocardiography. 2nd edition. Wiley, Ames, IA. 2011.

Boswood A, Häggström J, Gordon SG, et al. Effect of pimobendan in dogs with preclinical myxomatous mitral valve disease and cardiomegaly: the EPIC study—a randomized clinical trial. J Vet Intern Med 2016;30:1765–1779.

Brown DJ, Knight DH, King RR. Use of pulsed-wave Doppler echocardiography to determine aortic and pulmonary velocity and flow variables in clinically normal dogs. Am J Vet Res 1991;52:543–550.

Brown DJ, Rush JE, MacGregor J, et al. M-mode echocardiographic ratio indices in normal dogs, cats, and horses: a novel quantitative method. J Vet Intern Med 2003;17:653–662.

Buhl R, Ersbøll AK, Eriksen L, et al. Changes over time in echocardiographic measurements in young Standardbred racehorses undergoing training and racing and association with racing performance. J Am Vet Med Assoc 2005;226(11):1881–1887. Notes: Racing Standardbreds followed over time—data are from the initial and the last examinations.

Calvert CA, Brown J. Use of M-mode echocardiography in the diagnosis of congestive cardiomyopathy in Doberman Pinschers. J Am Vet Med Assoc 1986;189:293–237.

Chetboul V, Bussadori C, DeMadron E (DeMadron E, editor). Clinical Echocardiography of the Dog and Cat. Elsevier, St. Louis, MO. 2016.

Chetboul V, Petit A, Gouni V, et al. Prospective echocardiographic and tissue Doppler screening of a large sphynx cat population: reference ranges, heart disease prevalence and genetic aspects. J Vet Cardiol 2012;14:497–509.

Chetboul V, Sampedrano CC, Tissier R, et al. Quantitative assessment of velocities of the annulus of the left atrioventricular valve and left ventricular free wall in healthy cats by use of two-dimensional color tissue Doppler imaging. Am J Vet Res 2006;67:250–258.

Chetboul V, Sampedrano CC, Tissier R, et al. Reference range values of regional left ventricular myocardial velocities and time intervals assessed by tissue Doppler imaging in young nonsedated Maine Coon cats. Am J Vet Res 2005;66:1936–1942.

Chetboul V, Taton C. Encyclopedie Animee D'Imagerie Cardiovasculaire Ultrsonore Du Chien Et Du Chat. Elsevier Masson, Issy-les-Moulineaux, France. 2018.

Chetboul V, Tissier R. Echocardiographic assessment of canine degenerative mitral valve disease. J Vet Cardiol 2012;14(1):127–148.

Cornell CC, Kittleson MD, Della Torre P, et al. Allometric scaling of M-mode cardiac measurements in normal adult dogs. J Vet Intern Med 2004;18:311–321.

Crippa L, Ferro E, Melloni E, et al. Echocardiographic parameters and indices in the normal beagle dog. Lab Anim 1992;26:190–195.

de Oliveira VM, Chamas PP, Goldfeder GT, et al. Comparative study of 4 echocardiographic methods of left ventricular measurement in German Shepherd dogs. J Vet Cardiol 2014;16:1–8.

Decloedt A, Ven S, De Clercq D, et al. Assessment of left ventricular function in horses with aortic regurgitation by 2D speckle tracking. BMC Vet Res 2020;16(1):93. Notes: Data from control horses.

della Torre PK, Kirby AC, Church DB, et al. Echocardiographic measurements in greyhounds, whippets and Italian greyhounds—dogs with a similar conformation but different size. Aust Vet J 2000;78:49–55.

Disatian S, Bright JM, Boon J. Association of age and heart rate with pulsed-wave Doppler measurements in healthy, nonsedated cats. J Vet Intern Med 2008;22:351–356.

Drourr L, Lefbom BK, Rosenthal SL, et al. Measurement of M-mode echocardiographic parameters in healthy adult Maine Coon cats. J Am Vet Med Assoc 2005;226:734–737.

Esser LC, Borkovec M, Bauer A, et al. Left ventricular M-mode prediction intervals in 7651 dogs: Population-wide and selected breed-specific values. J Vet Intern Med. 2020;34:2242-2252.

Feldman MK, Katyal S, Blackwood MS. US artifacts. Radiographics 2009;29(4):1179–1189.

Fox PR, Bond BR, Peterson ME. Echocardiographic reference values in healthy cats sedated with ketamine hydrochloride. Am J Vet Res 1985;46:1479–1484.

Gaber C. Doppler echocardiography. Probl Vet Med 1991;3:479–499.

Goldberg SJ, Allen HD, Marx GR, et al. Doppler echocardiography. 2nd edition. Lea & Febiger, Philadelphia, PA. 1988.

Gooding JP, Robinson WF, Mews GC. Echocardiographic assessment of left ventricular dimensions in clinically normal English Cocker Spaniels. Am J Vet Res 1986;47:296–300.

Granstrom S, Godiksen MT, Christiansen M, et al. Prevalence of hypertrophic cardiomyopathy in a cohort of British shorthair cats in Denmark. J Vet Intern Med 2011;25:866–871.

Gugjoo MB, Hoque M, Saxena AC, et al. Reference values of M-mode echocardiographic parameters and indices in conscious Labrador Retriever dogs. Iran J Vet Res 2014;15(4):341–346.

Gundler S, Tidholm A, Haggstrom J. Prevalence of myocardial hypertrophy in a population of asymptomatic Swedish Maine Coon cats. Acta Vet Scand 2008;50:22.

Gunther-Harrington CT, Arthur R, Estell K, et al. Prospective pre- and post-race evaluation of biochemical, electrophysiologic, and echocardiographic indices in 30 racing thoroughbred horses that received furosemide. BMC Vet Res 2018;14(1):18. Notes: Racing Thoroughbred horses.

Häggström J, Andersson ÅO, Falk T, et al. Effect of body weight on echocardiographic measurements in 19,866 pure-bred cats with or without heart disease. J Vet Intern Med 2016;30(5):1601–1611.

Häggström J, Luis Fuentes V, Wess G. Screening for hypertrophic cardiomyopathy in cats. J Vet Cardiol 2015;17(Suppl 1):S134–S149.

Hanton G, Gautier M, Bonnet P, et al. Effect of milrinone on echocardiographic parameters after single dose in Beagle dogs and relationship with drug-induced cardiotoxicity. Toxicol Lett 2005;155:307–317.

Hatle L, Angelsen B. Doppler Ultrasound in Cardiology: Physical Principles and Clnical Applications. 2nd edition. Lea & Febiger, Philadelphia, PA. 1985.

Herrtage ME. Echocardiographic measurements in the normal Boxer (abstract). Proceedings of the 4th European Society of Veterinary Internal Medicine Congress. 1994. p. 172.

Höllmer M, Willesen JL, Tolver A, et al. Left atrial volume and phasic function in clinically healthy dogs of 12 different breeds. Vet J 2013;197(3):639–645.

Huesler IM, Mitchell KJ, Schwarzwald CC. Echocardiographic assessment of left atrial size and function in warmblood horses: reference intervals, allometric scaling, and agreement of different echocardiographic variables. J Vet Intern Med 2016;30(4):1241–1252. Warmblood horses; 12 (4) years old; 574 (58) kg.

Jacobs G, Knight DH. M-mode echocardiographic measurements in nonanesthetized healthy cats: effects of body weight, heart rate, and other variables. Am J Vet Res 1985;46:1705–1711.

Jacobson JH, Boon JA, Bright JM. An echocardiographic study of healthy Border Collies with normal reference ranges for the breed. J Vet Cardiol 2013;15:123–130.

Kayar A, Gonul R, Or ME, et al. M-mode echocardiographic parameters and indices in the normal German shepherd dog. Vet Radiol Ultrasound 2006;47:482–486.

Kayar A, Ozkan C, Iskefli O, et al. Measurement of M-mode echocardiographic parameters in healthy adult van cats. Jpn J Vet Res 2014;62:5–15.

Kisslo J, Adams DB, Belkin RN. Doppler Color Flow Imaging. Churchill Livingstone, New York, NY. 1988.

Koch J, Pedersen HD, Jensen AL, et al. M-mode echocardiographic diagnosis of dilated cardiomyopathy in giant breed dogs. Zentralbl Veterinarmed A 1996;43:297–304.

Lichtenstein DA. Recent advances in chest medicine: BLUE-protocol and FALLS-protocol: two applications of lung ultrasound in the critically ill patients. Chest 2015;147(6):1659–1670.

Lisciandro GR1, Fosgate GT, Fulton RM. Frequency and number of ultrasound lung rockets (B-lines) using a regionally based lung ultrasound examination named vet BLUE (veterinary bedside lung ultrasound exam) in dogs with radiographically normal lung findings. Vet Radiol Ultrasound 2014;55(3):315–322.

Lobo L, Canada N, Bussadori C, et al. Transthoracic echocardiography in Estrela Mountain Dogs: reference values for the breed. Vet J 2008;177:250–259.

Marchesotti F, Vezzosi T, Tognetti, R, et al. Left atrial anteroposterior diameter in dogs: reference interval, allometric scaling, and agreement with the left atrial-to-aortic root ratio. Vet Med Sci 2019;81(11):1655–1662.

Misbach C, Lefebvre HP, Concordet D, et al. Echocardiography and conventional Doppler examination in clinically healthy adult Cavalier King Charles Spaniels: effect of body weight, age, and gender, and establishment of reference intervals. J Vet Cardiol 2014;16:91–100.

Moise NS, Dietze AE. Echocardiographic, electrocardiographic, and radiographic detection of cardiomegaly in hyperthyroid cats. Am J Vet Res 1986;47:1487–1494.

Morrison SA, Moise NS, Scarlett J, et al. Effect of breed and body weight on echocardiographic values in four breeds of dogs of differing somatotype. J Vet Intern Med 1992;6:220–224.

Mottet E, Amberger C, Doherr MG, et al. Echocardiographic parameters in healthy young adult Sphynx cats. Schweizer Archiv fur Tierheilkunde 2012;154:75–80.

Muzzi RA, Muzzi LA, de Araujo RB, et al. Echocardiographic indices in normal German Shepherd dogs. J Vet Sci 2006;7:193–198.

Nanda NC. Comprehensive Textbook of Echocardiography. Jaypee Brothers Medical Publishers, New Delhi, India. 2013.

O'Leary CA, Mackay BM, Taplin RH, et al. Echocardiographic parameters in 14 healthy English Bull Terriers. Aust Vet J 2003;81:535–542.

O'sullivan ML, O'Grady MR, Minors SL. Assessment of diastolic function by Doppler echocardiography in normal Doberman Pinschers and Doberman Pinschers with dilated cardiomyopathy. J Vet Intern Med 2007;21:81–91.

Oh JK, Seward JB, Tajik AJ. The Echo Manual. 3rd edition. Lippincott Williams & Wilkins, Philadelphia, PA. 2007.

Orvalho JS. Real-time three-dimensional echocardiography: from diagnosis to intervention. Vet Clin North Am Small Anim Pract 2017;47(5):1005–1019.

Otto CM. Textbook of Clinical Echocardiography. 5th edition. Saunders Elsevier, Philadelphia, PA. 2013.

Oyama MA. Advances in echocardiography. Vet Clin North Am Small Anim Pract 2004;34(5):1083–1104.

Page A, Edmunds G, Atwell RB. Echocardiographic values in the greyhound. Aust Vet J 1993;70:361–364.

Petric AD, Rishniw M, Thomas WP. Two-dimensionally-guided M-mode and pulsed wave Doppler echocardiographic evaluation of the ventricles of apparently healthy cats. J Vet Cardiol 2012;14:423–430.

Ribas T, Bublot I, Junot S, et al. Effects of intramuscular sedation with alfaxalone and butorphanol on echocardiographic measurements in healthy cats. J Feline Med Surg 2015;17(6):530–536.

Rishniw M, Caivano D, Dickson D, et al. Two-dimensional echocardiographic left-atrial-to-aortic ratio in healthy adult dogs: a reexamination of reference intervals. J Vet Cardiol 2019;26:29–38.

Santilli RA, Bussadori C. Doppler echocardiographic study of left ventricular diastole in non-anaesthetized healthy cats. Vet J 1998;156:203–215.

Scansen BA, Morgan KL. Reference intervals and allometric scaling of echocardiographic measurements in Bengal cats. J Vet Cardiol 2015;17(Suppl 1):S282–295.

Schober KE, Chetboul V. Echocardiographic evaluation of left ventricular diastolic function in cats: Hemodynamic determinants and pattern recognition. J Vet Cardiol 2015;17(Suppl 1):S102–S133.

Schober KE, Fuentes VL. Effects of age, body weight, and heart rate on transmitral and pulmonary venous flow in clinically normal dogs. Am J Vet Res 2001;62:1447–1454.

Schober KE, Fuentes VL, McEwan JD, et al. Pulmonary venous flow characteristics as assessed by transthoracic pulsed Doppler echocardiography in normal dogs. Vet Radiol Ultrasound 1998;39:33–41.

Schober K, Savino S, Yildiz V. Reference intervals and allometric scaling of two-dimensional echocardiographic measurements in 150 healthy cats. J Vet Med Sci 2017 Nov;79(11):1764–1771. Predicted allometrically scaled values, with upper 95% confidence interval.

Sisson DD, Knight DH, Helinski C, et al. Plasma taurine concentrations and M-mode echocardiographic measures in healthy cats and in cats with dilated cardiomyopathy. J Vet Intern Med 1991;5:232–238.

Sisson D, Schaeffer D. Changes in linear dimensions of the heart, relative to body weight, as measured by M-mode echocardiography in growing dogs. Am J Vet Res 1991;52:1591–6.

Smith DN, Schober KE. Effects of vagal maneuvers on heart rate and Doppler variables of left ventricular filling in healthy cats. J Vet Cardiol 2013;15:33–40.

Snyder PS, Sato AE, Atkins CE. A comparison of echocardiographic indices of the nonracing, healthy greyhound to reference values from other breeds. Vet Radiol Ultrasound 1995;36:387–392.

Stepien RL, Hinchcliff KW, Constable PD, et al. Effect of endurance training on cardiac morphology in Alaskan Sled dogs. J Appl Physiol 1998;85:1368–1375.

Strohm LE, Visser LC, Chapel EH, et al. Two-dimensional, long-axis echocardiographic ratios for assessment of left atrial and ventricular size in dogs. J Vet Cardiol. 2018;20:330–342.

Sugimoto K, Fujii Y, Ogura Y, et al. Influence of alterations in heart rate on left ventricular echocardiographic measurements in healthy cats. J Feline Med Surg 2017;19(8):841–845.

Vezzosi T, Domenech O, Iacona M, et al. Echocardiographic evaluation of the right atrial area index in dogs with pulmonary hypertension. J Vet Intern Med 2018;32(1):42–47.

Visser LC. Right ventricular function: imaging techniques. Vet Clin North Am Small Anim Pract 2017;47(5):989–1003.

Visser LC, Ciccozzi MM, Sintov DJ, et al. Echocardiographic quantitation of left heart size and function in 122 healthy dogs: a prospective study proposing reference intervals and assessing repeatability. J Vet Intern Med 2019;33:1909–1920.

Vollmar AC. Echocardiographic measurements in the Irish wolfhound: reference values for the breed. J Am Anim Hosp Assoc 1999;35:271–277.

Voros K, Hetyey C, Reiczigel J, et al. M-mode and two-dimensional echocardiographic reference values for three Hungarian dog breeds: Hungarian Vizsla, Mudi and Hungarian Greyhound. Acta Vet Hung 2009;57:217–227.

Wess G, Domenech O, Dukes-McEwan J, et al. European Society of Veterinary Cardiology screening guidelines for dilated cardiomyopathy in Doberman Pinschers. J Vet Cardiol 2017;19(5):405–415.

Weyman AE. Principles and Practice of Echocardiography. 2nd edition. Lea & Febiger, Philadelphia, PA. 1994.

Young LE, Rogers K, Wood JL. Left ventricular size and systolic function in Thoroughbred racehorses and their relationships to race performance. J Appl Physiol (1985) 2005;99(4):1278–1285. Notes: A number of racing types were studied (flat/sprinters and National Hunt horses of different ages); values tabulated are from the National Hunt horses unadjusted for weight.

Yuill CD, O'Grady MR. Doppler-derived velocity of blood flow across the cardiac valves in the normal dog. Can J Vet Res 1991;55:185–192.

Zucca E, Ferrucci F, Croci C, et al. Echocardiographic measurements of cardiac dimensions in normal Standardbred racehorses. J Vet Cardiol 2008;10(1):45–51. Note: Trained Standardbred horses.

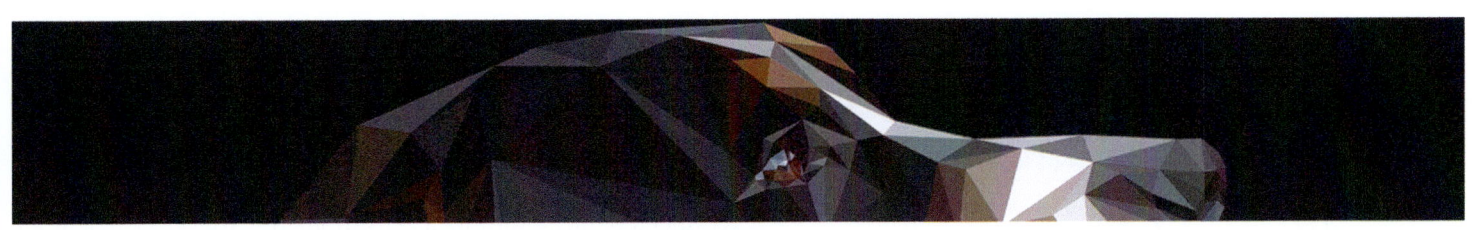

5
ELECTROCARDIOGRAPHY

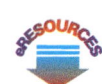

The electrocardiogram (ECG or EKG, from the German *elektrokardiogramm*) records the electrical activity (depolarization and repolarization) of cardiac muscle from the body surface. It provides information on heart rate (HR), rhythm, and intracardiac conduction. ECG findings might also suggest the presence of specific chamber enlargement, myocardial disease, ischemia, pericardial disease, certain electrolyte imbalances, and some drug toxicities. However, the ECG does not record cardiac mechanical activity; therefore, the ECG by itself cannot be used to assess the strength (or even presence) of cardiac contractions, diagnose congestive heart failure, or predict whether the patient will survive anesthesia or a surgical procedure. This chapter provides guidelines for ECG acquisition, interpretation, and ambulatory monitoring. ECG features typical of specific diseases are discussed more fully in the chapters describing those conditions. Approaches to managing abnormal cardiac rhythms are found in Chapters 24 and 25. For other means of evaluating cardiac electrical activity, such as intracardiac recording, high-resolution (signal averaged) ECG, and HR variability analysis, the reader is referred to other sources (see section "Suggested Additional Readings and References" and the online bibliography).

General Considerations

The normal cardiac rhythm originates in the sinoatrial (SA) node and follows the cardiac conduction pathway illustrated in **Figure 1.12** (p. 10). The ECG waveforms, P-QRS-T (**Figure 5.1**), are generated as the heart muscle is depolarized and then repolarized (p. 10). **Table 5.1** summarizes the events underlying ECG waveforms and time intervals. The P wave represents the depolarization of both atria; the small atrial repolarization (T_a) wave that follows is not usually visible unless the subsequent QRS complex is delayed or absent. The P wave in horses often appears notched, or bifid. The equine P wave configuration often changes from notched to single-peaked during excitement or exercise, and with a more prominent T_a wave, as sympathetic tone increases (and vagal influence wanes). A negative-positive P wave also can occur in normal horses at rest.

The QRS complex as a whole represents electrical activation of ventricular muscle, regardless of whether individual Q, R, or S components are present or not. When referring to time intervals between successive QRS complexes, the shorthand term "R-R interval" is often used. Regarding specific nomenclature for describing QRS morphology, lowercase letters are often used to describe a deflection of low voltage (q, r, or s) while uppercase (capital) letters are used for comparatively high-voltage deflections (Q, R, or S). For example, the QRS complex illustrated in **Figure 5.1** could be more specifically described as a qR wave (there is no s wave in lead II for this dog); nevertheless, this waveform results from ventricular myocardial depolarization and therefore is still considered a "QRS complex." The configuration of the QRS complex depends on the lead recorded, as well as the ventricular activation pattern in that animal. There is some normal variation from animal to animal within species and marked differences in ventricular activation patterns between dogs and cats (Type A, or I, activation) and horses (Type B, or IIA, activation, related to more complete ventricular penetration of Purkinje fibers).

The ST segment and T wave correspond to ventricular repolarization, a process that is more variable in animals than in humans in terms of the spread of current and T wave morphologies. For example, negative/positive or diphasic T-waves are normal in animals. During exercise, healthy horses can exhibit some deviation of the ST segment and increased T wave amplitude, compared to their baseline. However, especially in small animals, marked changes in ST segment or T wave morphology over time generally are considered abnormal. Because the repolarization process depends on depolarization, whenever a QRS complex is abnormal, the subsequent ST-T-wave will usually be affected. Such "secondary ST-T changes" should not be over-interpreted.

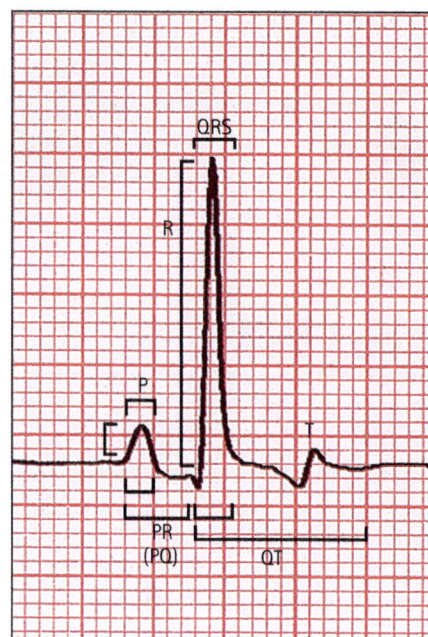

Figure 5.1 Lead II ECG complex from a dog; 50 mm/s, 1 cm = 1 mV. P-QRS-T waveforms and intervals are indicated. Each small box is 0.02 second in duration (x-axis) and 0.1 mV in amplitude (y-axis).

ECG Lead Systems

The ECG system consists of a current source (the heart) that generates a varying, instantaneous electrical field over a volume conductor (the thorax). This field, measured in potential difference, is detected by recording electrodes that are connected physically to a galvanometer (the ECG machine) with lead cables. The ECG system electronically connects individual electrodes to generate various electrocardiographic leads. The ECG system displays the interaction between leads and the depolarization and repolarization processes of the heart in the form a graphical tracing. The ECG is printed or displayed with time on the horizontal (x-) axis; the direction of current flow (polarity) and potential difference across electrodes (in millivolts) are depicted on the vertical (y-) axis.

Several standard leads are used to evaluate cardiac electrical activity (**Table 5.2**). The leads are created by the placement of the electrodes and their electronic connection by the ECG machine. Both bipolar and unipolar ECG leads are used

Table 5.1 Normal ECG Waveforms

Waveform	Description
P wave	Atrial muscle activation (depolarization) wave; normally is positive in leads II and aVF. Measure from beginning to end of waveform.
PR interval	Also called PQ interval. Includes duration of atrial muscle activation, and conduction over the AV node, bundle of His, and Purkinje fibers. Measure from onset of P wave to onset of QRS complex.
QRS complex	Ventricular muscle activation wave; by definition, Q is the first negative deflection (if present), R is the first positive deflection, and S is the negative deflection after the R wave. Measure from beginning to end of entire waveform.
J point	Junction point between end of QRS complex and onset of ST-T.
ST segment	Represents the period between ventricular depolarization and repolarization (correlates with phase 2 of the action potential).
T wave	Ventricular muscle repolarization wave.
QT interval	Total time of ventricular depolarization and repolarization. Measure from onset of QRS complex through end of T wave.

Table 5.2 ECG Lead Systems

Standard Bipolar Limb Leads
- I — RA (−) compared with LA (+)
- II — RA (−) compared with LL (+)
- III — LA (−) compared with LL (+)

Augmented Unipolar Limb Leads
- aVR — RA (+) compared with average of LA and LL (−)
- aVL — LA (+) compared with average of RA and LL (−)
- aVF — LL (+) compared with average of RA and LA (−)

Unipolar Chest Leads[a]
- V_1, rV_2 (CV_5RL) — 5th right ICS near sternum
- V_2 (CV6LL) — 6th left ICS near sternum
- V_3 — 6th left ICS, equidistant between V_2 and V_4
- V_4 (CV6LU) — 6th left ICS near costochondral junction
- V_5 and V_6 — Spaced as for V_3 to V_4, continuing dorsally in 6th left ICS
- V_{10} — Over dorsal spinous process of 7th thoracic vertebra

Orthogonal Leads
- X — Lead I (right to left) in the frontal plane
- Y — Lead aVF (cranial to caudal) in the midsagittal plane
- Z — Lead V_{10} (ventral to dorsal) in the transverse plane

[a] Compared to Wilson's central terminal
Abbreviations: ICS, intercostal space; LA, left arm; LL, left leg; RA, right arm.

clinically. Bipolar leads (I, II, and III) record the electrical potential differences between two electrodes on the body surface. Unipolar leads employ a recording (positive) electrode on the body surface and compare that potential to a negative pole or zero reference formed by "Wilson's central terminal." The axis for these leads is from the positive electrode to the center of the heart. Unipolar chest leads (such as V_3, located near the left apex) and augmented unipolar limb leads can be recorded.

Leads exist within planes, and these are designated in ECG analysis as frontal (corresponding to the cranial-caudal, right-left plane of a ventrodorsal radiograph), sagittal (corresponding to the cranial-caudal, ventro-dorsal plane of a lateral radiograph), and transverse or horizontal (encompassing the right-to-left and ventral-to-dorsal plane orthogonal to the other two). A lead's orientation with respect to the heart is called the "lead axis." A lead records waves of cardiac depolarization and repolarization aligned parallel to its axis. If the direction of myocardial activation parallels the lead axis, a relatively large deflection is recorded. As the angle between the lead axis and the direction of the activation increases (up to 90 degrees), the ECG deflection in that lead progressively decreases. The ECG deflection becomes miniscule to nonexistent (isoelectric) when the activation wave is oriented perpendicular to the lead axis. Each lead also is considered to have a positive and a negative pole. A positive ECG deflection is recorded if the activation wave moves toward the positive electrode of that lead. If the wave of depolarization travels away from the positive pole, a negative deflection is recorded in that lead. The opposite concept occurs with ventricular repolarization such that repolarization moving toward the positive electrode generates a negative deflection in that lead.

Standard Limb Leads For standard limb leads, electrodes are placed on the forelimbs and left rear limb with a ground electrode traditionally put at the right rear limb (see section "Recording a Standard ECG"). The standard limb lead system records cardiac electrical activity within the frontal plane (as depicted by a DV or VD radiograph). Left-to-right and cranial-to-caudal activation and repolarization currents are recorded in this plane. **Figures 5.2** and **5.3** illustrate the six standard frontal leads superimposed on the torso (hexaxial lead system) and representative recordings from a normal dog. The standard bipolar limb leads (I, II, and III) record electrical potential differences between two electrodes on the body surface. The positive electrode is at the left forelimb (or LA) for lead I (with right forelimb negative), and at the left rear limb (LF) for lead II (with right forelimb negative) and lead III (with left forelimb negative). The lead axis for bipolar leads is oriented between the two electrodes.

The unipolar limb leads generate small surface voltages; these are augmented electronically by comparing the positive electrode of the lead to the averaged potential of the other two limb electrodes (a process that enhances the overall

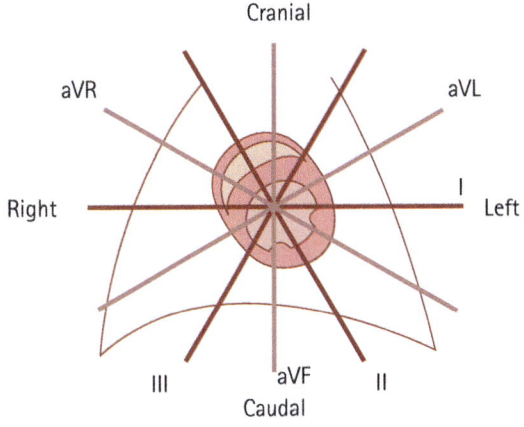

Figure 5.2 Diagram illustrating the orientation of the six standard limb leads with respect to the heart in the frontal plane. The outline of the thorax surrounds the cardiac ventricles. All leads are labeled at their positive pole. (See section "Standard Limb Leads" and **Table 5.2**.)

voltage). Although the lead axis for augmented limb leads is still directed through the center of the heart, the methodology increases the voltage by about 50%. Augmented limb leads are named for the lead's positive (surface) electrode; for example, the positive pole of lead aVF is located at the left rear limb ("foot"). In ECG theory, limbs are simply extensions of the torso, such that for standard limb leads, the lead axis system is shown within "Einthoven's triangle", delimited by two forelimb electrodes at the axilla and the left rear limb electrode situated (hypothetically) near the umbilicus.

Lead I records electrical boundaries (or interfaces between polarized and depolarized myocardium) moving in the right-to-left (or left-to-right) direction and lead aVF records cranial-to-caudal boundaries. Thus, these leads are "orthogonal" (at right angle to each other) and help to define—along with chest lead V_{10}—the frontal, sagittal, and transverse (horizontal) planes of ECG analysis. Leads II, III, aVR, and aVL record boundaries moving in any direction within the frontal plane, except those perpendicular to the lead axis. The predominant atrial and ventricular depolarization boundaries move right-to-left and cranial-to-caudal, making leads II and aVF the most commonly used leads for recording heart rhythm in dogs and cats.

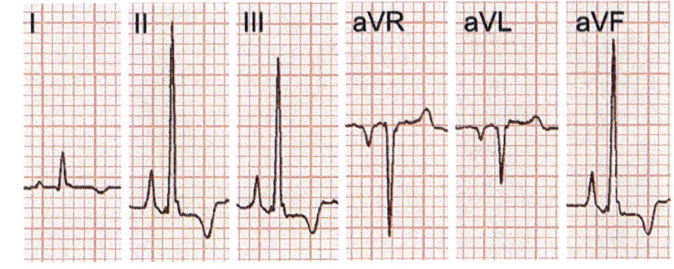

Figure 5.3 ECG complexes from a normal dog. 25 mm/s, 1 cm = 1 mV.

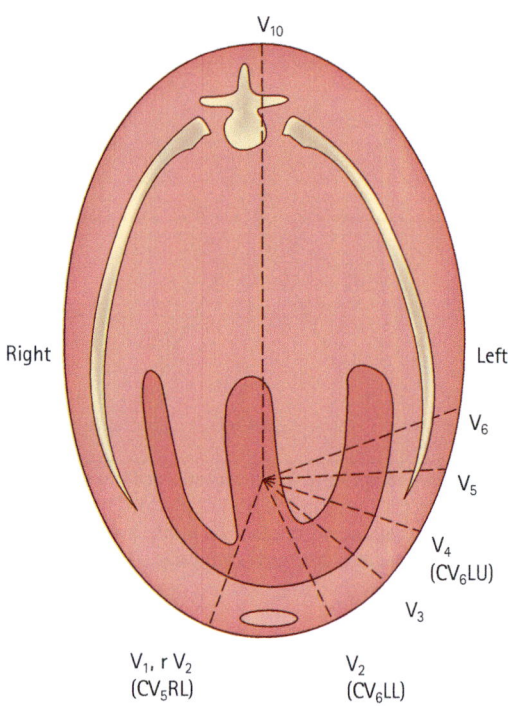

Figure 5.4 Diagram illustrating the orientation of selected chest leads with respect to the heart in the transverse plane. The cardiac ventricles, ribs, and thoracic vertebra are indicated within the outline of the thorax. (Also see **Table 5.2**.)

Precordial Leads Unipolar chest (precordial) leads "view" the heart from various vantage points along the transverse plane (**Figure 5.4**). When lead V_{10} is combined with leads I and aVF, an orthogonal lead system is generated that views the heart in three perpendicular planes (**Table 5.2**).

Base-Apex Lead The so-called "base-apex" lead is used most often to record the HR and rhythm in standing horses. The positive electrode is located at the left apex and the negative electrode at the right jugular furrow. This lead records cardiac electrical activity across three planes simultaneously and is oriented from the positive electrode (located left, caudal, and ventral) to the negative electrode (located to the right, cranial and dorsal). During normal sinus rhythm, the base-apex lead produces positive (above baseline) P waves that often are notched (bifid), especially in relaxed horses. The QRS complexes are mostly negative (below baseline) in this lead, with either an rS or QS pattern (**Figure 5.5**). The T waves can be negative, positive, or biphasic and can flip from negative to positive as HR increases above 40–50 beats/minute. Recording instructions are below.

Recording a Standard ECG

The standard resting ECG in small animals is recorded with the patient placed in right lateral recumbency on a nonconducting surface. The forelimbs are held parallel to each

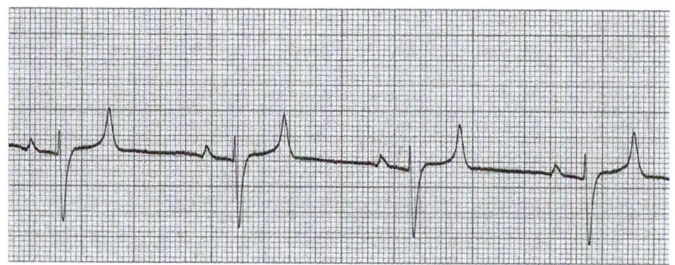

Figure 5.5 Base-apex lead ECG showing normal sinus rhythm in a 15-year-old Arabian mare. Note that the P waves are positive and the QRS complexes are mostly negative (with small R waves and large S waves). Although not seen on this recording, the P waves in normal resting horses often have a notched appearance. Positive T waves, as seen in this case, are common; other normal horses might have biphasic T waves in this lead. 25 mm/s, 0.5 cm = 1 mV.

other and perpendicular to the torso (**Figure 5.6**). Other body positions can alter the recorded waveform amplitudes and affect the calculated mean electrical axis (MEA). However, if information about HR and rhythm only is needed, almost any recording position is fine. The animal is held gently in position to minimize movement artifacts. A relaxed and quiet animal yields a better-quality recording. Intermittently holding a dog's mouth shut to discourage panting or placing a hand on the chest of a trembling animal might be helpful.

Forelimb electrodes usually are placed at or slightly below the elbows, not touching the chest wall or each other. Hind limb electrodes are placed at the stifles or hocks. The electrodes labeled LA and RA stand for the left and right arms in humans (forelimbs for animals); electrodes labeled LF and RF designate placement at the left foot and right foot (rear limbs), respectively. Although the precise location of limb electrodes should be less important than lateral positioning of the torso and maintaining proximal forelimbs at right angles to the spine, placement of electrodes too

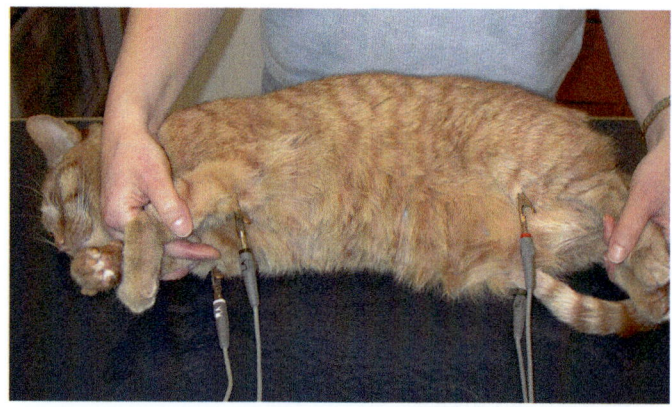

Figure 5.6 Normal patient positioning for routine ECG recording in cats and dogs. Note that the proximal limbs are perpendicular to the trunk and the electrodes are not touching each other or the trunk. The cat is lying on a nonconducting pad.

proximal on the limb can change the ECG in some patients. ECG contact paste or (less ideally) alcohol is used to ensure good skin contact when using alligator clip or plate electrodes. Alternative techniques could include alligator clip electrodes attached to the haircoat, with ultrasound gel used to provide contact between skin and hair, or use of pre-gelled electrode pads adhered to the patient's footpads or shaved skin (Ferasin, 2006). Communication between two electrodes via a bridge of paste or alcohol, or by physical contact, should be avoided.

A good ECG recording has a clean baseline, with minimal artifact from patient movement or electrical interference. The ECG complexes should be centered and totally contained within the background grid so that neither the top nor bottom of the QRS complex is truncated ("clipped"). If the complexes are too large to fit entirely within the lead's grid, the calibration should be changed from standard (1 cm = 1 mV) to half-standard (0.5 cm = 1 mV). To measure waveform amplitude, the calibration used for recording each lead must be known. A calibration square wave (1 mV amplitude) should be inscribed, or the calibration otherwise indicated, during the recording. The paper or sweep speed and lead(s) recorded also must be identified. Frequently, little attention is paid to somatic muscle filters, but activation of these can result in substantial diminution of overall QRS voltages. Standard recording includes 0.67–150 Hz, but filtering at upper cutoff values of 40 Hz might be needed to reduce baseline noise such as muscle tremor. Underfiltering can lead to ringing (small sign-wave) artifacts, especially in the ST segment. This is not an issue for rhythm diagnosis, but is relevant to analysis of chamber size. The interested reader can find more information in the Clinical Guidelines from the Society of Cardiological Science and Technology (SCST, 2017).

Recording a Base-Apex ECG A base-apex ECG can be obtained in the standing horse by attaching the RA (negative) electrode at the right jugular furrow and the LA (positive) electrode to the chest wall over the left apex and setting the ECG machine to record "lead I" (**Figure 5.7**). To reduce electrical artifacts and provide grounding, the RL (ground) electrode usually is attached at the left jugular furrow or withers and the LL electrode anywhere distant to the active (right and left forelimb) electrodes, although these other electrodes sometimes can be left unattached.

Approach to ECG Interpretation

A consistent approach to ECG interpretation is recommended. First, determine if the tracing is of adequate technical quality (all complexes within the grid, minimal artifact) and the patient, date, paper speed, lead(s) used, and calibration are identified. Then the HR, heart rhythm, and MEA (in

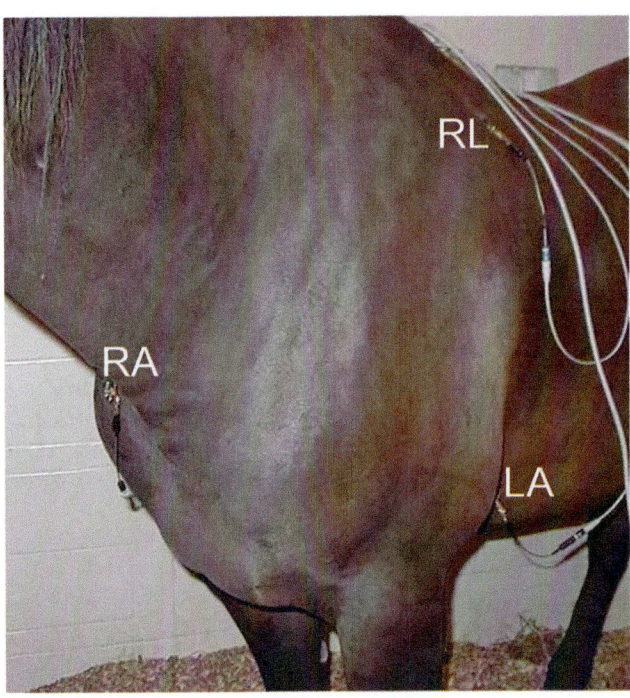

Figure 5.7 Electrode placement for the base-apex lead; the ECG machine is set to record lead I (see section "Recording a Base-apex ECG"). LA, left arm (forelimb); RA, right arm (forelimb); RL, right leg (rear limb; ground electrode).

dogs and cats, if multiple frontal leads have been recorded) are determined. Finally, the individual waveforms are measured (see **Table 5.3**).

Heart Rate

The HR is the number of complexes (or beats) per minute. This can be calculated by counting the QRS complexes within a 3- or 6-second period and then multiplying by 20 or 10, respectively. Some ECG machines inscribe 1-second marks on the recording. Some one-channel recorders might use paper with small vertical hash marks at the top margin that can be used to calculate time elapsed (for example, at 25 mm/s 3 seconds elapse between two marks; at 50 mm/s, 1.5 seconds). If the heart rhythm is regular, the following method is useful for determining the instantaneous HR: Count the number of large, 5 mm boxes delimited by two consecutive R waves at a recording speed of 25 mm/s. For one large box, the instantaneous rate is 300/minute; this proceeds as follows: for 2 boxes (150/minute), three boxes (100/minute), four boxes (75/minute) and five boxes (60/minute). If the paper speed is 50 mm/s the estimated heart rate is doubled. Another approach is dividing 3,000 by the number of small boxes between consecutive R wave to R wave (R-R) intervals (with the recording at 50 mm/s). However, because variation in HR is quite common, especially in dogs and horses, these methods are limited. Therefore, estimating the average HR over several

Table 5.3 Guide for ECG Interpretation

1. Identify the patient, lead(s), paper/sweep speed, calibration, and any artifacts.
2. Determine the heart (ventricular) rate.
   - Is it normal, or too slow or fast for the species? (See **Table 5.4**.)
3. Identify if the rhythm is regular (R-R intervals evenly spaced) or irregular.
   - If irregular, search for any recurring patterns.
4. Identify P waves and QRS-T complexes, and the relationship between these waveforms (PR [PQ] interval and QRS to subsequent P).
5. Is sinus rhythm present (with or without other abnormalities)?
6. Are all P waves followed by a QRS and all QRS complexes preceded by a P wave?
   - Evaluate the morphology and consistency of the P waves, QRS complexes, and ST-T segments.
   - Is an intermittent AV conduction disturbance present?
   - Is a consistent temporal relationship between P waves and QRS complexes totally lacking, with a slow and regular QRS occurrence (implying complete AV block with ventricular escape rhythm)?
7. If premature (early) complexes are present, do their QRS waveforms look the same as the sinus QRS complexes for that patient, implying atrial or junctional (supraventricular) origin? Or are they wide and of different morphology than sinus complexes, implying a ventricular origin or, possibly, abnormal (aberrant) ventricular conduction of a supraventricular complex (as with a bundle branch block pattern)?
8. Are premature QRS complexes preceded by an abnormal P wave (suggesting atrial origin)?
9. Are there baseline undulations instead of clear and consistent P waves, with an irregular (+/-rapid) QRS occurrence (compatible with atrial fibrillation)?
10. Are there long pauses in the underlying rhythm before an abnormal complex occurs (escape complex or rhythm)? Are these escape complexes of ventricular or supraventricular origin (based on QRS morphology)?
11. During sinus rhythm, measure the waveform amplitudes and durations (see **Table 5.4**).
    - Consider conduction intervals across the atria (P wave duration), AV conduction system (PR interval), ventricles (QRS duration), and overall repolarization time (QT interval, in light of the heart rate).
    - Are all (sinus) waveform measurements within normal limits for the species, or is there a pattern consistent with chamber enlargement or slowed conduction?
    - Assess the ST-T segment for repolarization abnormalities; as possible, determine if ST-T changes are primary or secondary (to abnormal QRS complex morphology).
12. For sinus (or supraventricular ectopic) QRS complexes, estimate the mean electrical axis (MEA) in the frontal plane, if multiple limb leads are available; see **Figure 5.52** and p. 155.
    The orientation of the terminal electrical activity of the ventricle (last 50% of QRS complex).
    Is the QRS morphology typical for a particular bundle branch or fascicular block, or does it suggest other intraventricular conduction disturbance?

seconds is often more accurate and practical than calculating an instantaneous HR. **Table 5.4** lists normal HR ranges for sinus rhythms in dogs, cats, and horses.

Heart Rhythm

Heart rhythm refers to the cardiac electrical activation process. It is designated by terms that describe the origin, and sometimes the conduction pattern, of electrical impulses through the heart. For example, the term "sinus rhythm" indicates that the impulses arise from the normal pacemaker cells within the sinus node; without further description, it is implied that normal conduction follows. To assess the heart rhythm, first estimate the ventricular rate and scan the ECG recording for irregularities and identify the individual waveforms. Determine the presence and pattern of P waves, QRS complexes, and T waves. Then evaluate the relationship between P and QRS-T waveforms. Calipers are useful for assessing waveform regularity and interrelationships. Common rhythm abnormalities are described below.

Abnormal Rhythms: Basic Concepts The general term "bradycardia" describes a heart rhythm that is slow, without identifying its site of origin. Conversely, a "tachycardia" is a heart rhythm with an HR faster than normal. For example, sinus bradycardia and sinus tachycardia are rhythms that originate in the sinus node, but have an HR that is slower or faster, respectively, than normal for the species at rest.

Depolarizations originating from outside the sinus node (ectopic complexes) are abnormal and cause an arrhythmia (or "dysrhythmia"). Ectopic complexes are described by their general site of origin and their timing (**Figures 5.8** and **5.9**). The configuration of the ECG waveforms is used to surmise whether the ectopic complexes are likely of supraventricular (atrial, atrioventricular [AV] junctional) or ventricular

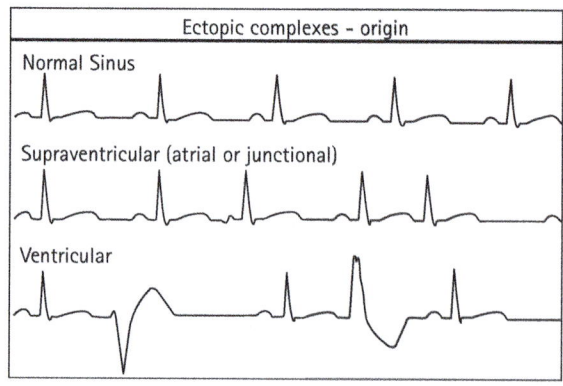

Figure 5.8 Diagram illustrating the concept of supraventricular versus ventricular origin of ectopic complexes. Impulses arising from atrial tissue or the AV junctional region typically have essentially the same QRS configuration as the patient's sinus-origin complexes, because intraventricular conduction follows the normal pathway. From Ware WA. Diagnostic tests for the cardiovascular system. (In, Nelson RW, Couto CG (editors). Small Animal Internal Medicine. 6th edition. Elsevier, St Louis, MO. 2019. p. 41.)

Table 5.4 ECG Reference Ranges

ECG Variable	Dog	Cat	Horse
Heart rate	60 to 160 beats/min, adults; up to 220 beats/min in young puppies	(120) 140 to 240 beats/min	28 to 44; to 100 beats/min in foals[b]
Mean electrical axis (frontal plane)	+40 to +100 degrees	0 to +160 degrees	Variable
Measurements (lead II)			
P wave duration (maximum)	0.04 sec; to 0.05 sec in large/giant breeds	0.035 to 0.04 sec	0.16 sec
P wave height (maximum)	0.4 mV	0.2 mV	Variable (0.25 to possibly 0.5 mV)[c]
PR interval	0.06 to 0.13 sec; up to 0.14 sec in giant breeds	0.05 to 0.09 sec	0.16 to 0.32 sec (small breeds) or 0.20 to 0.50 sec (large breeds)
QRS complex duration (maximum)	0.05 sec (small breeds) to 0.06 sec (large breeds)	0.04 sec	0.12 sec (small breeds) or 0.14 sec (large breeds)
R wave height (maximum)	2.5 mV (small breeds) to 3 mV (large breeds)[a]	0.9 mV, any lead; <1.2 mV QRS total excursion, any lead	2.2 or 2.3 mV[c]
ST segment deviation	<0.2 mV depression; <0.15 mV elevation	< 0.1 mV deviation	Unclear; variable deviation can occur during exercise
T wave	Usually <25% of R wave height; can be positive, negative, or biphasic	Maximum 0.3 mV; can be positive (most common), negative, or biphasic	Variable
QT interval duration	0.15 to 0.25 (to 0.27) sec; varies inversely with HR	0.12 to 0.18 (range 0.07 to 0.2) sec; varies inversely with HR	0.32 to 0.56 sec (small breeds) or 0.36 to 0.60 sec (large breeds); varies inversely with HR
Chest leads			
V_1, rV_2	Positive T wave	R wave 1.0 mV maximum	
V_{2-3}	S wave 0.8 mV maximum; R wave 2.5 mV maximum[a]		
V_{4-6}	S wave 0.7 mV maximum; R wave 3 mV maximum[a]		
V_{10}	Negative QRS; negative T wave	R/Q <1.0; negative T wave	

Note: Each small box on the standard ECG grid is 0.02 second wide at 50 mm/s paper or sweep speed, 0.04 second wide at 25 mm/s, and 0.1 mV high at a calibration of 1 cm = 1 mV.

[a] May be greater in young (under 2 years old), thin, deep-chested dogs.
[b] Some sources report up to ~50 beats/minute for adults and ~140 beats/minute for foals.
[c] However, the base-apex lead is recorded more commonly than lead II in horses.

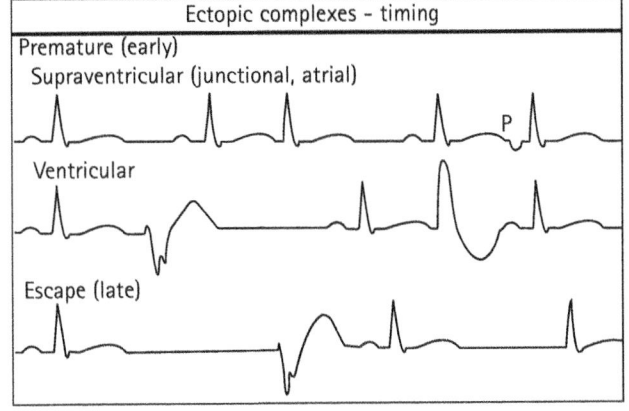

Figure 5.9 Concept of premature vs late (escape) timing for supraventricular & ventricular origin ectopic complexes. (From Ware WA. Diagnostic tests for the cardiovascular system. In, Nelson RW, Couto CG (editors). Small Animal Internal Medicine. 6th edition. Elsevier, St Louis, MO. 2019. p. 41.)

origin. Supraventricular origin impulses usually are conducted through the ventricles via the normal conduction pathway; therefore, these QRS complexes typically assume a morphology similar to that animal's sinus complexes. The configuration of complexes of ventricular origin reflects their abnormal origin (and usually slower) pattern of conduction across the ventricles. Additionally, when depolarization is abnormal, repolarization will appear differently when compared to normally generated and conducted complexes. The concept of timing refers to whether the ectopic complex occurred earlier than the next expected sinus impulse ("premature") or after a longer pause ("late" or "escape"). Escape complexes represent activation of a latent, subsidiary pacemaker (p. 12). The relative prematurity of ectopic complexes is also relevant to ECG assessment. For example, very early ventricular ectopic complexes that encroach on the prior T wave have "R-on-T" timing, whereas, premature complexes that occur just before the next normal P wave appears are termed "late diastolic."

Premature ectopic complexes can occur singly, in couplets, or in multiples; three or more in sequence comprise an episode or a "run" of tachycardia. Episodes of tachycardia can be brief (nonsustained or "paroxysmal") or prolonged (sustained). Ectopy can develop with a haphazard distribution or in recognizable patterns. For example, when a premature complex follows each normal QRS, a bigeminal pattern exists. The origin of the premature complexes determines whether the rhythm is further described as "atrial" or "ventricular" bigeminy. When abnormal complexes arise every third beat, the pattern of trigeminy is evident.

The concept of myocardial fibrillation refers to rapid and chaotic electrical activation. Multiple small reentrant circuits or waves of activation cause uncoordinated depolarization of the affected chambers. Because the subsequent mechanical activation also is disorganized, no effective contraction occurs in those chambers.

Abnormal delay or failure of conduction through the AV node or infranodal conduction pathways is another relatively common cause of arrhythmias. These are often associated with a slowed HR. Because AV nodal conduction velocity normally is relatively slow, AV conduction failure can arise from conditions or drugs that enhance vagal tone, drugs that affect calcium entry, or diseases that further impair AV conduction. "Physiologic" AV block occurs when a supraventricular tachyarrhythmia, such as atrial fibrillation (AF) or atrial tachycardia, stimulates the AV node at a rate faster than it normally can conduct. Drugs that slow AV conduction are used therapeutically to enhance physiologic AV block. It should be emphasized that transient AV block can be normal in some dogs with high resting vagal tone and is normal in standing horses, serving as a mechanism to lower arterial blood pressure. These blocks should abate with sympathetic stimulation.

ECG Measurements

Estimation of MEA is described below (p. 155). Although HR and rhythm can be assessed using any lead, waveforms and intervals generally are measured using lead II (**Figure 5.1**), or the base-apex lead in horses. Waveform amplitudes are recorded in millivolts (mV) and durations in seconds. Each measurement should include only one thickness of the inscribed (pen) line. At a paper speed of 25 mm/s, each small (1 mm) box on the ECG grid is 0.04 seconds in duration from left to right. At a paper speed of 50 mm/s, each small box equals 0.02 seconds. At standard calibration, a deflection of the pen up or down 10 small boxes (1 cm) equals 1 mV. Limb lead voltages tend to be much smaller in cats compared to dogs. The size of QRS complexes in horses can be quite variable, likely related to the pattern of ventricular activation in this species. **Table 5.4** contains normal ECG reference ranges for cats, dogs, and horses. While measurements for most normal animals fall within these ranges, measurements for some subpopulations or breeds can lie outside. As previously noted, manual frequency filters that reduce baseline artifact are available on many ECG machines. Activating these filters can markedly attenuate ECG waveforms; the accompanying reduction of QRS amplitude could complicate the assessment of ECG chamber enlargement.

Cardiac Rhythm Assessment

Cardiac arrhythmias are disorders of impulse formation, conduction, or both. Heart rhythm disturbances can vary in seriousness from mere ECG curiosity to life-threatening electrical irregularity. The hemodynamic consequences might be tolerated, or induce clinical signs of hypotension. The underlying cellular mechanisms are complicated, and frequently beyond our ability to delineate in the clinical setting. Chapter 23 addresses basic mechanisms, hemodynamic consequences, and clinical associations of cardiac arrhythmias. Chapters 24 and 25 describe arrhythmia management strategies. This section focuses on criteria for recognizing common cardiac arrhythmias.

Sinus Rhythm and Variations

Sinus rhythm is the heart's normal rhythm; it is manifested by the P-QRS-T waveforms described previously when HR is normal for the species (**Figures 5.1**, **5.10**, and **5.11**). The P waves are positive in the caudal leads (II and aVF); sometimes biphasic, negative-to-positive P wave deflections might occur, but not the opposite configuration (that is, positive to negative). Horses often have a notch in the P wave, especially at slower heart rates (higher vagal tone). Sinus PR (or "PQ") intervals are consistent, although minor variation can occur with fluctuations in vagal tone, especially in horses. The QRS-to-QRS (R-R) intervals occur regularly, with less than 10% variation in timing in regular ("normal") sinus rhythm. The T waves can be either positive or negative in normal animals but should be consistent for a given individual (although changes can occur in exercising horses). T waves often are biphasic in dogs and horses. Sinus arrhythmia (described below) is a common and

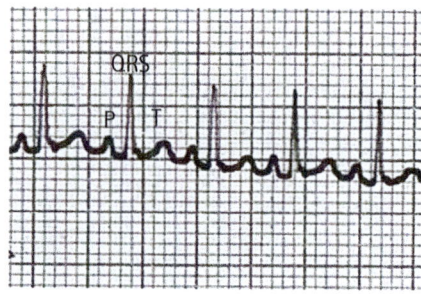

Figure 5.10 Normal sinus rhythm in a cat. The QRS voltage is within normal limits for cats and smaller than is typical for dogs. Lead II, 25 mm/s, 1 cm = 1 mV.

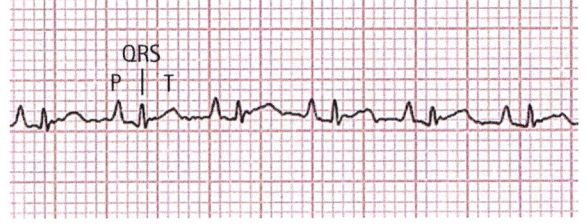

Figure 5.11 Sinus rhythm a cat. Normal cats can have tiny QRS complexes. Lead II, 25 mm/s, 1 cm = 1 mV.

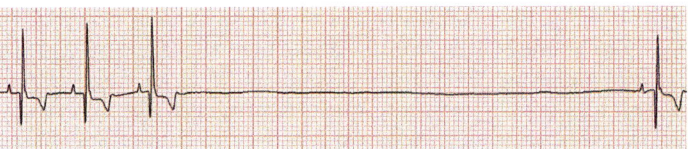

Figure 5.13 Episode of sinus arrest (~4-second duration) with resumption of sinus rhythm in an older American Cocker Spaniel with pulmonary carcinoma and hypertension. Lead II, 25 mm/s, 0.5 cm = 1 mV.

normal variation. Abnormal sinus HRs (sinus tachycardia or bradycardia) usually stem from altered autonomic tone associated with various clinical conditions, drugs, or less often, by structural heart disease or heart failure (**Table 12.1**, p. 238).

Sinus tachycardia typically is a regular rhythm, usually demonstrating only subtle variation in QRS-to-QRS intervals. The mechanism underlying this rhythm is increased sympathetic tone, and an underlying cause for this should be sought. Extremely rapid sinus tachycardia (for example, ≥240/minute in dogs) can cause T wave–P wave fusion and complicate the rhythm diagnosis. Sinus bradycardia can have regular or irregular QRS-to-QRS intervals, depending on the etiology. Escape complexes sometimes occur with sinus bradycardia. Normal sinus-origin QRS complexes are narrow and upright in leads II and aVF; however, an intraventricular conduction disturbance (or ventricular enlargement) can change this appearance (see p. 153).

Sinus Arrhythmia This normal rhythm variation is characterized by a cyclic slowing and speeding of the sinus rate. It is usually, but not always, associated with respiration (**Figure 5.12**). With respiratory sinus arrhythmia, the sinus rate increases during inspiration and decreases with expiration as vagal tone fluctuates through the respiratory cycle. The term "wandering pacemaker" refers to a cyclic change in P wave configuration, which can accompany sinus arrhythmia and is related to a shift in pacemaker location within the relatively extensive tissues constituting the SA node. Increased vagal tone can shift the pacemaker location to the more ventrocaudal aspect of the SA node, away from its usual mid- to cranial nodal site. The P waves (in lead II) become taller and spiked during inspiration (as vagal tone diminishes) and flatter in expiration (as vagal tone increases). This is considered

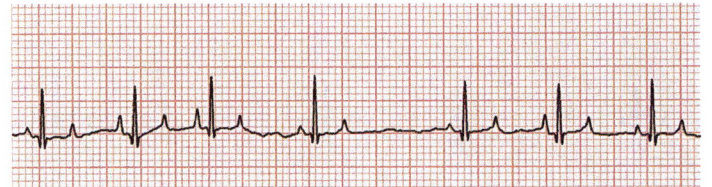

Figure 5.12 Normal sinus arrhythmia with wandering pacemaker in an English Cocker Spaniel with pneumonia and chronic bronchitis. The QRS complexes are abnormally small. Lead II, 25 mm/s, 1 cm = 1 mV.

a normal variation and is especially common in dogs. Sinus arrhythmia is present often in horses and dogs; it can be especially prominent in brachycephalic breeds. It also occurs in resting cats, although it is not usually seen in the clinic in this species. Exaggerated sinus arrhythmia is associated with chronic pulmonary disease in some animals.

Sinus Pause or Arrest Long pauses during sinus arrhythmia can occur from (normal or pathological) increases in vagal tone, or might be an early sign of sinus node dysfunction. Many drugs also depress sinus node function, leading to sinus bradycardia or arrest. A pause in sinus activity lasting at least twice the duration of the patient's usual QRS-to-QRS interval usually is considered "sinus arrest" (**Figure 5.13**). Either an escape complex or resumption of sinus activity can follow. Long pauses in the sinus rhythm (usually >5-6 sec in dogs) can cause weakness or syncope. Sinus arrest cannot be differentiated with certainty from SA block on the surface ECG, although pauses that are a multiple of the normal cycle length are suggestive of the latter rhythm. Sinus arrest is a major feature of the sick sinus syndrome (p. 405 and **Figure 25.3**; also **Figure 12.6**, p. 241).

SA block occurs when sinus impulse conduction to the atrial myocardium fails. This abnormality could exist if the P wave to P wave (P-P) interval on either side of a long pause is exactly 2 to 3 times the normal P-P interval. However, because sinus arrhythmia is so common, this is challenging to diagnose with certainty. SA block with Wenckebach periodicity is a variant that can be identified with more certainty; it is characterized by a progressively decreasing P-P interval followed by a relatively long pause.

Sinus node reentry is an arrhythmia characterized by two consecutive P-QRS-T complexes with identical P waves. The second P wave closely follows the preceding T wave by a fixed interval (coupling). However, sinus arrhythmia occurring as paired complexes, or some cases of atrial bigeminy arising from the craniodorsal right atrium, can mimic sinus node reentry.

Abnormal Cardiac Rhythms

Supraventricular Premature Complexes These rhythm disturbances originate above the ventricles (and usually above the AV node), typically in the atrial tissues or less often, the AV junction (**Figures 5.14** and **5.15**). Because their conduction into and through the ventricles occurs via the normal conduction pathway, their QRS configuration is normal, unless an intraventricular conduction disturbance or ventricular enlargement pattern is concurrently present. Premature complexes that arise within the atria (outside the SA node) usually are preceded by an abnormal positive, negative, or biphasic P wave designated as a P´ wave (pronounced "P-prime"; see **Figure 5.14**, and also **Figure 25.3**, p. 405). Sometimes, the tissues below the atria are incompletely repolarized, resulting in slow conduction of the premature P´ wave. This will be manifest as a prolonged P´-to-QRS interval (a form of physiological AV block) or even a transient QRS widening or bundle branch block pattern. If an ectopic P´ wave occurs before the AV node has sufficiently repolarized, the impulse might not be conducted into the ventricles at all, resulting in a nonconducted APC (**Figure 5.16**). This is another example of physiologic AV block, in the setting of a supraventricular tachyarrhythmia. Junctional complexes typically are not preceded by a P´ wave; however, retrograde conduction backward into the atria can cause a negative P´ wave after, superimposed on, or even preceding the resulting QRS complex.

The more general term "supraventricular" is used if it is unclear whether the origin of the ectopic complex(es) or tachyarrhythmia is atrial or junctional (**Figures 5.17** and **5.18**).

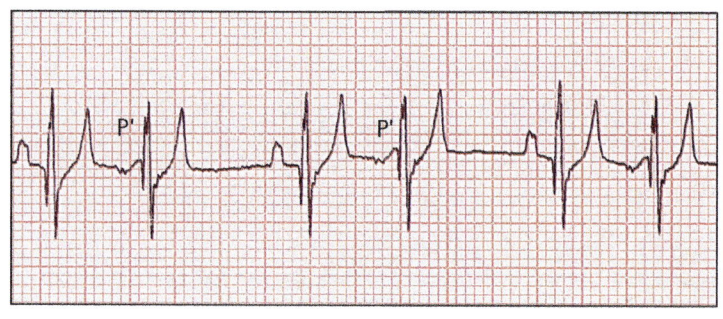

Figure 5.14 Atrial bigeminy in a 6-year-old female Irish Wolfhound several days after surgery for gastric dilatation-volvulus. Note the notched negative P´ waves. Lead II, 25 mm/s, 1 cm = 1 mV.

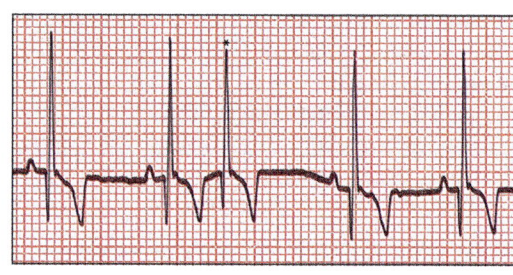

Figure 5.15 Junctional premature complex (*) in an older male Doberman Pinscher. Lead II, 25 mm/s, 1 cm = 1 mV.

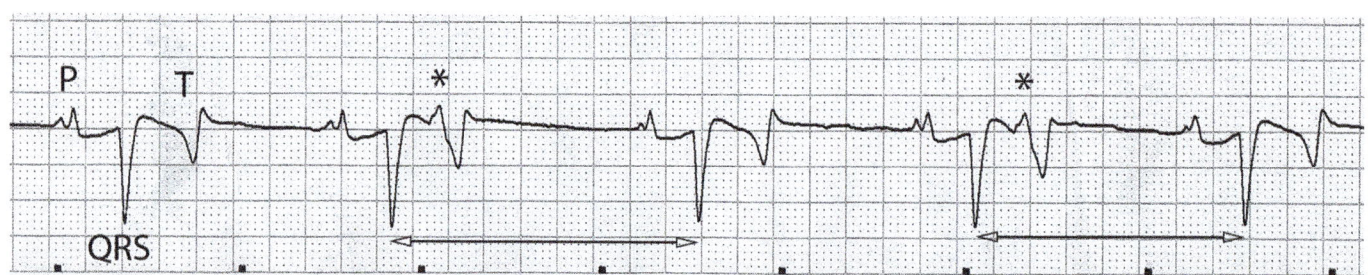

Figure 5.16 ECG from a horse with nonconducted atrial premature complexes (APCs). The normal bifid P waves (P), negative QRS complexes, and biphasic T waves (T) of the equine base-apex lead are present for all cycles. However, the T waves of two sinus complexes are deformed by premature atrial complexes (*) that are blocked in the AV node and therefore not transmitted into the ventricles. The first APC likely penetrated the sinoatrial node and reset the cycle length, leading to a longer R-R interval surrounding the APC (horizontal arrow on left); this did not occur with the second APC. However, note that the length of the left arrow is less than two normal cycle lengths. Base-apex lead; 25 mm/s.

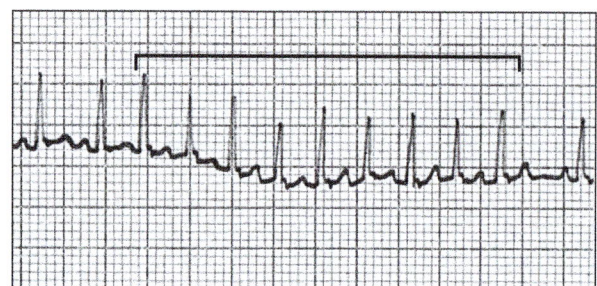

Figure 5.17 Paroxysm of supraventricular tachycardia (bracket) in a geriatric Siamese cat. Lead II, 25 mm/s, 1 cm = 1 mV.

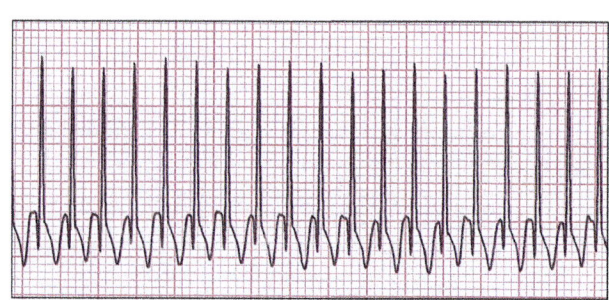

Figure 5.18 Sustained supraventricular (likely AV reentrant) tachycardia at 360 beats/min in a Labrador Retriever puppy with mitral & tricuspid valve dysplasia. Lead II, 25 mm/s, 1 cm = 1 mV.

Clinically, it is important to distinguish whether the arrhythmia involves atrial myocardium (supraventricular) or originates below it (junctional/ventricular). Supraventricular premature beats usually penetrate and depolarize the sinus node. This resets the sinus rhythm, creating a so-called "noncompensatory" (or less-than-compensatory) pause. In other words, if the underlying sinus rhythm is regular, the interval between the QRS complex preceding and following the premature complex is less than two normal R-R intervals (**Figure 5.19**). Premature atrial complexes can be associated with more advanced atrial arrhythmias, including atrial tachycardia, atrial flutter, and AF.

A sustained AV junctional-origin (idionodal) rhythm can cause AV dissociation if it does not simultaneously depolarize the atria. AV dissociation occurs when atrial (sinus) activation and ventricular activation are not directly related; junctional premature activity can cause the AV conduction system to be refractory when a normal sinus impulse reaches it. Thus, it is a matter of timing, rather than impaired AV conduction, per se. An accelerated idionodal rhythm usually becomes overdrive suppressed when the sinus rate increases, similar to what happens with an accelerated idioventricular rhythm (see below). However, there can be various forms of apparent synchronization where the two rhythms independently become stable relative to each other, or P waves can migrate around the junctional QRS complexes without capturing the ventricles. Junctional rhythms cause a normal-looking, narrow QRS complex, unless there is aberrant intraventricular conduction (see below).

Atrial Tachycardia Atrial tachycardia originates from an abnormal atrial focus; it can occur as a paroxysmal or sustained tachycardia. The diagnosis of focal atrial tachycardia (FAT) can be challenging. First, the repetitive atrial impulses can occur over a range of rates (in dogs typically >200/minute and sometimes approaching 360/minute; this overlaps with the atrial cycle lengths observed with atrial flutter). Second, ectopic P′ waves often are hidden within the QRS-T complexes. Third, in dogs, FAT frequently originates near the crista terminalis of the right atrium; this generates P′ waves

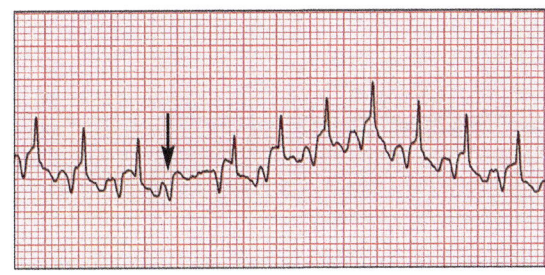

Figure 5.20 Atrial tachycardia at a rate of 200 beats/minute in an 11-year-old Yorkshire Terrier. Note the negative P′ waves, one of which is not conducted (arrow). Lead II, 25 mm/s, 1 cm = 1 mV.

of similar morphology to those arising from the sinus node (Santilli, 2010).

At slower atrial discharge rates, FAT induces a regular (QRS) rhythm, but if the atrial rate exceeds the AV node's ability to conduct every impulse, physiologic AV block occurs that can lead to irregular QRS intervals (**Figure 5.20**). A consistent ratio of atrial to ventricular activation (such as 2:1 or 3:1 AV conduction) preserves the regularity of this arrhythmia; however, a diagnostic clue is a sudden doubling or halving of the ventricular rate suggesting an abrupt change in AV conduction. If atrial tachycardia is accompanied by delayed intraventricular conduction or bundle branch block, it can be difficult to differentiate this rhythm from ventricular tachycardia (**Figure 5.21**). Electrical alternans (p. 157) can occur, especially during the onset of the tachycardia, due to variable intraventricular conduction. This finding is rare in sinus tachycardia but often observed in pathologic supraventricular tachycardias.

Atrial Flutter Atrial flutter—also called macro-entrant atrial tachycardia—results from a single circuit wave of electrical activation that regularly cycles through the atrial myocardium. Classic atrial flutter mainly involves circuits in the right atrium and develops in association with right atrial dilation. The circuit moves counter-clockwise using the vena cavae as anatomic obstacles to sustain the reentrant loop. Flutter cycle lengths easily can exceed 300/minute in small animals and approach 250/minute in horses. The ventricular response rate

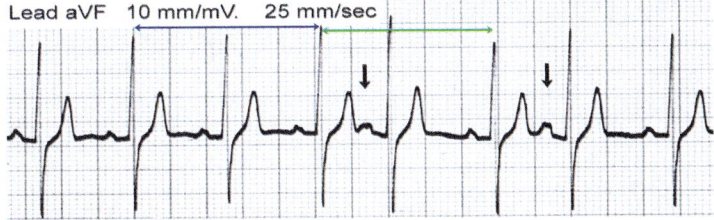

Figure 5.19 Atrial premature complexes (APCs; arrows) with a background of normal sinus rhythm in a dog. Blue line over the 2nd-4th QRS complexes shows normal time for 3 sinus beats (2 full cycle lengths). The shorter green line illustrates an APC-induced "noncompensatory" pause; i.e., the distance from the QRS before the APC to that after it is <2 normal cycle lengths. Lead aVF, 25 mm/s, 1 cm = 1 mV.

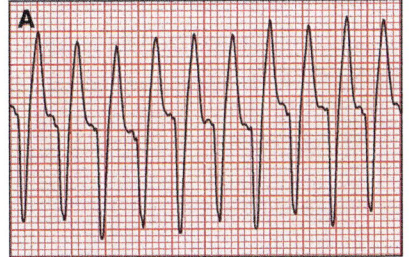 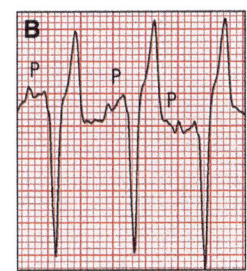

Figure 5.21 (A) Wide-complex supraventicular tachycardia in a male Irish Wolfhound with preexisting right bundle branch block is easily mistaken for ventricular-origin tachycardia. (B) Sinus rhythm in the same dog. Both ECGs Lead II, 25 mm/s, 0.5 cm = 1 mV.

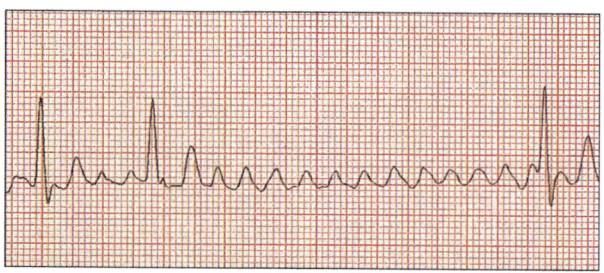

Figure 5.22 Atrial flutter recorded in an older German Shorthair Pointer with heart failure. Note the "sawtooth" flutter waves at a rate of about 330/minute. Lead II, 50 mm/s, 1 cm = 1 mV.

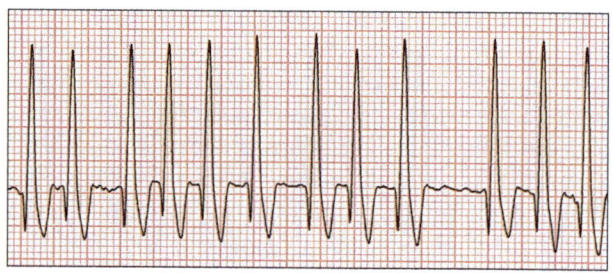

Figure 5.24 Atrial fibrillation with an uncontrolled ventricular rate of 220/minute in a 4-year-old male Labrador Retriever with dilated cardiomyopathy. Note the irregular R-R intervals and small fibrillation ("f") waves in the baseline. Lead II, 25 mm/s, 0.5 cm = 1 mV.

to atrial flutter (that is, the HR) depends on AV conduction and this response can be irregular or regular. "Sawtooth" flutter waves in the baseline (without an isoelectric shelf between the waves) represent recurrent atrial activation and can be seen between the QRS complexes (**Figures 5.22** and **5.23**). However, atypical forms of atrial flutter also occur and can resemble ectopic atrial tachycardias. Atrial flutter is a relatively unstable rhythm in small animals. It often degenerates into AF, although it sometimes converts to sinus rhythm. Atrial flutter also is a common transitional arrhythmia in horses undergoing quinidine conversion of AF. Atrial enlargement is a common underlying factor in small animals. However, atrial flutter can occur without overt disease in horses, giant-breed dogs, and dogs with other conduction disorders.

Atrial Fibrillation Atrial electrical activation in AF is rapid and chaotic because of multiple, small reentrant circuits. About 350–400 impulses per minute are typical of horses and this rate exceeds 500/minute in dogs and cats. The AV node is bombarded by many chaotic electrical impulses, however some die out within the AV node and do not reach the ventricles. Ultimately, it is the AV conduction velocity and recovery time that determine the (ventricular) HR. No P waves are evident because uniform atrial depolarization is lacking. The ECG baseline usually shows irregular undulations known as fibrillation (f) waves (**Figures 5.24–5.26**). These vary from fine, imperceptible f waves (as in most cats) to large baseline undulations (typical of horses and some dogs). Because

organized electrical activity is absent, effective atrial contractions also are lacking. The loss of the atrial kick can reduce ventricular filling and cardiac output (p. 18), especially during stress, exercise, anesthesia, or in congestive heart failure. AF causes an irregular heart rhythm, usually with a rapid rate (related to increased sympathetic tone). HR in patients with AF should be monitored using an ECG because counting the HR by auscultation can be highly inaccurate. The QRS complexes usually are normal in configuration, although minor variation in QRS complex voltage is common; this can be pronounced in cats (**Figure 5.25**). Moreover, an underlying intraventricular conduction disturbance (see below), such as an intermittent or sustained bundle branch block, can coexist. Sometimes during AF, an isolated wide QRS complex follows

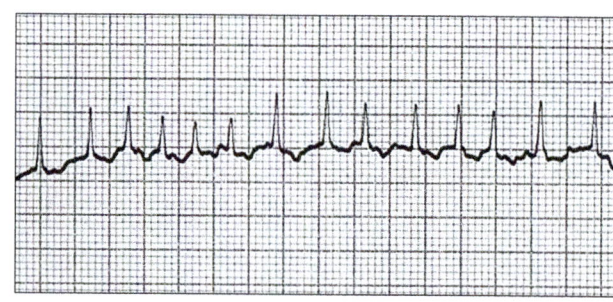

Figure 5.25 Atrial fibrillation in a cat with cardiomyopathy and marked left atrial enlargement. Besides the irregular QRS timing, there is some variation in QRS size as well. Lead II, 25 mm/s, 1 cm = 1 mV.

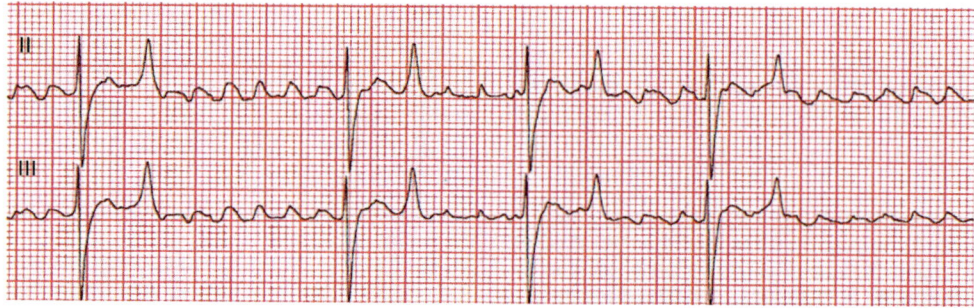

Figure 5.23 Atrial flutter in a horse. Note the regular flutter waves, especially after the 1st and 4th complexes. Simultaneous leads II and III, 25 mm/s.

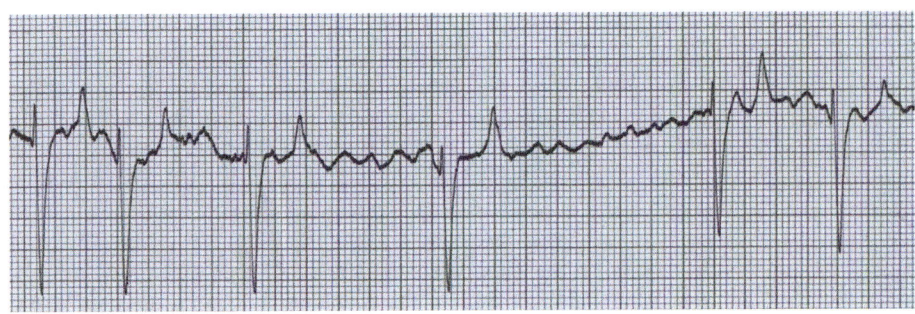

Figure 5.26 Atrial fibrillation in a 12-year-old Thoroughbred with severe mitral regurgitation. The heart rate is mildly increased at ~60 beats/minute. Base-apex lead, 25 mm/s, 1 cm = 1 mV.

a short R-R interval which was preceded by a long R-R interval. Although a VPC is one possible cause, the wide QRS actually might be an aberrantly conducted supraventricular impulse. This is known as Ashman's phenomenon (or phase 3 aberrancy); it occurs when ventricular activation begins before the intraventricular conduction system has fully recovered from the prior activation. Horses with AF often develop widened QRS complexes during exercise. This could result from aberrant ventricular conduction at fast HRs, although ventricular ectopy also must be ruled out.

AF and other recurrent or persistent atrial arrhythmias tend to be a consequence of severe atrial disease and enlargement, especially in dogs and cats (Chapter 23). AF often is preceded by another atrial tachyarrhythmia. Sometimes, AF occurs spontaneously, particularly in giant-breed dogs and horses, without evidence of underlying heart disease ("lone AF"). The HR (ventricular response rate) generally is normal in these animals (see p. 409).

Atrioventricular Reentrant Tachycardia A particular form of supraventricular tachycardia (SVT) involves a reentrant pathway incorporating the atrial muscle, AV node, ventricular muscle, and an accessory atrioventricular electrical pathway within a circuit loop (Chapter 23 and **Figure 23.4A**, p. 367; and **Figure 25.10**, p. 418). These tachyarrhythmias variously are termed AV reentrant tachycardia, AV nodal reentrant tachycardia, and the more general reciprocating SVT. This potentially can occur with functional longitudinal dissociation within the AV node into slow- and fast-conducting fibers, or more likely through incorporation of an accessory (muscular) AV pathway that forms a bypass around the AV node. The usual AV reciprocating SVT involves an "orthodromic" tachycardia circuit, where the impulse descends the AV node, activates the ventricular muscle (producing a narrow QRS complex), but then ascends the accessory AV pathway to enter the atrial muscle (producing a retrograde P'-wave), and reenters the proximal AV node. Subtle electrical alternans is commonly observed, especially at the onset of a paroxysmal AV tachycardia. There also are other variants, including antidromic conduction with wide-QRS tachycardia. A premature atrial or ventricular impulse can initiate the reentrant tachycardia by inducing conduction along just one limb of the two AV circuits (see section "Ventricular Preexcitation" for additional information).

Ventricular Premature Complexes Ventricular premature complexes (VPCs or PVCs) originate below the AV node, usually distal to the bundle of His. Conduction of these ectopic impulses across the ventricular myocardium can be quite abnormal and slow compared to supraventricular impulse conduction via the normal, rapidly conducting His-Purkinje system. Consequently, the QRS-T complexes produced by ventricular ectopic impulses typically are wider and of different morphology compared to that animal's normal sinus QRS complexes (**Figures 5.27–5.31**). The shape and duration of ventricular ectopic QRS complexes depends on their site of origin, as well as intraventricular conduction characteristics. Although VPCs do conduct at least partially retrograde (backward) into the AV conduction system, they usually do not enter into the atria. Therefore, the sinus node activation process continues undisturbed; the P wave immediately following the VPC typically is blocked within the AV conduction system.

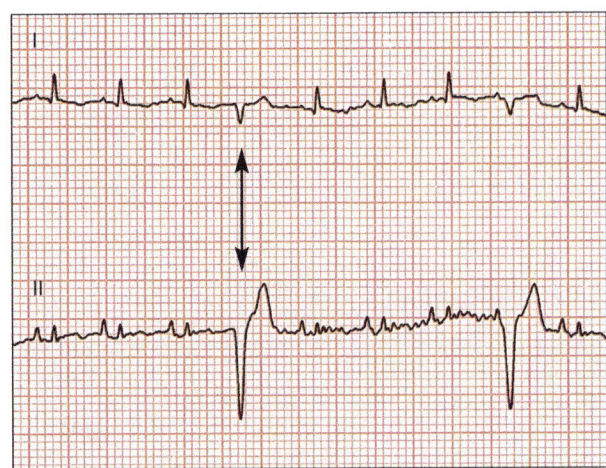

Figure 5.27 Intermittent ventricular premature complexes (arrow) in a 15-year-old male cat with hypertrophic cardiomyopathy. Baseline muscle tremor artifact also is present in lead II (right half of tracing). Leads I and II, 25 mm/s, 1 cm = 1 mV.

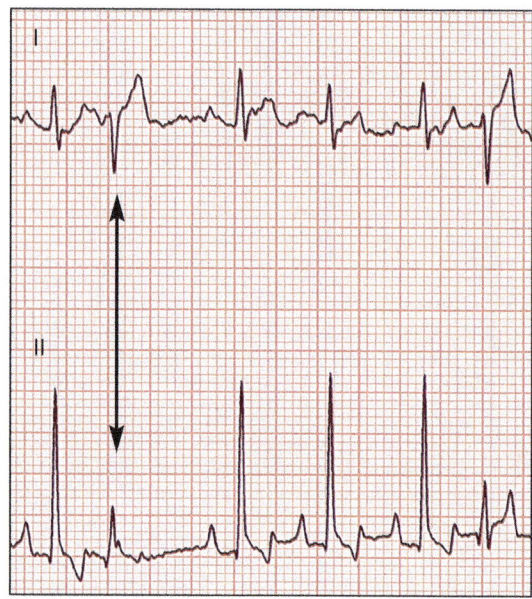

Figure 5.28 Intermittent ventricular premature complexes (arrow) in a young female Great Dane with exercise intolerance. The voltage of ventricular-origin ectopic complexes is not always larger than that of normal sinus QRS complexes, as seen here. Leads I and II, 25 mm/s, 1 cm = 1 mV.

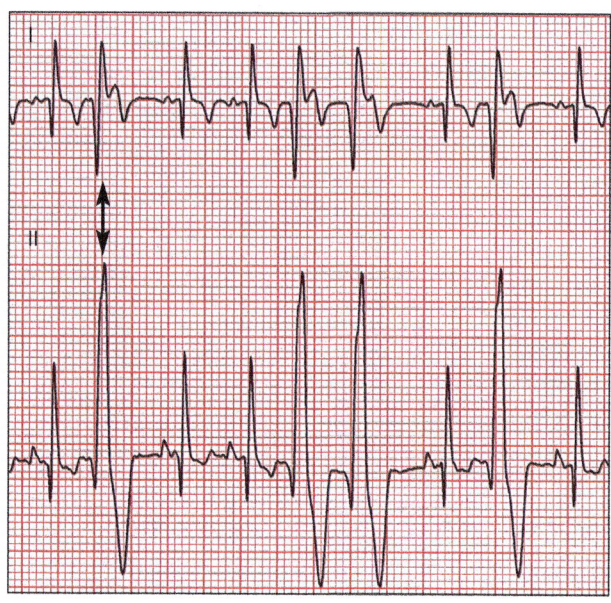

Figure 5.30 Two single (arrow) and a couplet of monomorphic ventricular premature complexes in a 4-year-old female Boxer with arrhythmogenic right ventricular cardiomyopathy. The upright (positive) configuration of the ectopic complexes in lead II is typical for this disease. Leads I and II, 25 mm/s, 1 cm = 1 mV.

This generates a pause after the VPC that is termed "fully compensatory," so that the R-R interval of the two normal complexes surrounding the VPC measure twice the normal R-R interval (assuming an underlying regular sinus rhythm). Careful scrutiny of the ECG can reveal a blocked P wave in the ST segment or T wave of the VPC. Sometimes, the sinus impulse immediately following a VPC is conducted, although partial (concealed) retrograde conduction of the VPC into the AV node prolongs the PR interval (**Figure 5.31**). This is typical of "interpolated" VPCs, which occur between two sinus complexes without a compensatory pause, and typically at slower sinus rates. When VPC configuration is consistent, the complexes are described as "uniform" or "monomorphic." When VPCs in an individual have differing ECG configurations, they are said to be "multiform" or "polymorphic." Multiform VPCs (or polymorphic ventricular tachycardia) could indicate greater electrical instability.

Ventricular Tachycardia Three or more sequential VPCs constitute the rhythm of ventricular tachycardia (**Figures 5.32–5.35**). Typically, the tachycardia rate exceeds the underlying sinus rate and the ectopic QRS intervals are regular. Nonconducted sinus P waves might be seen superimposed on or between the ventricular complexes. Successful conduction of a sinus P wave into the ventricles, uninterrupted by another VPC, is known as a "capture beat." If the normal ventricular activation sequence is interrupted by another VPC, a "fusion" complex can result. The configuration of a fusion complex represents a melding of the normal QRS and that of the VPC. Fusion complexes are preceded by a P wave with shortened PR interval. They often are observed at the onset or end of a paroxysm of ventricular tachycardia. Identification of P waves, whether conducted or not, or fusion complexes

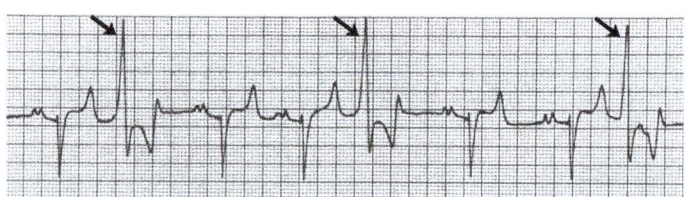

Figure 5.29 Single, monomorphic ventricular premature complexes (VPCs; arrows) in a horse. The background sinus complexes have a normal P-QRS-T configuration. A nonconducted P wave is obscured by each VPC, although one is evident in the ST segment of the VPC on the right. Base-apex lead, 25 mm/s.

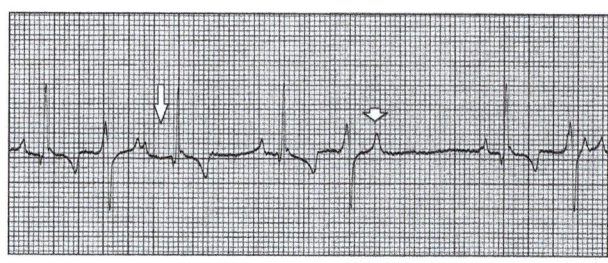

Figure 5.31 The ventricular premature complexes (VPCs) in this older, asymptomatic dog caused concealed retrograde AV nodal conduction, as evidenced by the prolonged PR interval after the first VPC (arrow) and conduction block after the P wave coinciding with the second VPC's T wave (arrowhead). Lead II, 50 mm/s, 1 cm = 1 mV.

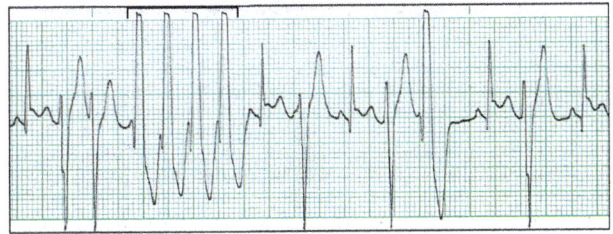

Figure 5.32 Multiform ventricular premature complexes (VPCs) in a young Golden Retriever with intracardiac rhabdomyosarcoma and syncope. A brief paroxysm of ventricular tachycardia (positive QRS polarity; bracket), one couplet (negative QRS polarity), and several single VPCs are present in this short recording. Lead II, 25 mm/s, 1 cm = 1 mV.

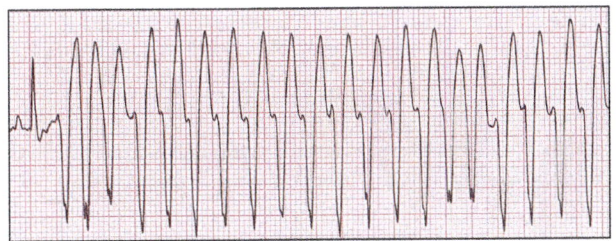

Figure 5.33 A rapid, slightly irregular ventricular tachycardia (at ~280 beats/minute) in a 9-year-old female Dalmatian with dilated cardiomyopathy and episodic weakness. Lead II, 25 mm/s, 1 cm = 1 mV.

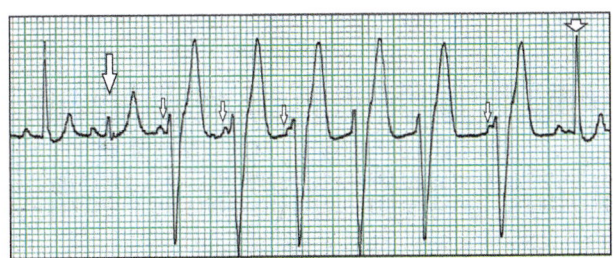

Figure 5.34 A fusion complex (large arrow) occurred at the onset of ventricular tachycardia (or accelerated idioventricular rhythm; ~140 beats/min) in a dog. The ventricular rhythm slows, & the sinus complex that follows (thick arrowhead) is known as a "capture beat." Nonconducted sinus P waves are evident (small arrows). Lead II, 25 mm/s, 1 cm = 1 mV.

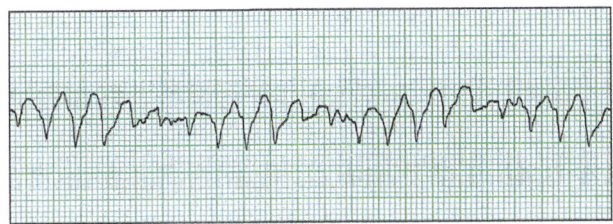

Figure 5.35 Polymorphic ventricular tachycardia (torsades de pointes) in an 11-year-old Siamese cat with dilated cardiomyopathy. QT interval prolongation was evident during a preceding period of sinus rhythm. Note that the configuration of the complexes changes progressively over time, as if the QRS orientation were rotating around the baseline. Lead II, 25 mm/s, 1 cm = 1 mV.

(**Figure 5.34**) helps the clinician differentiate ventricular tachycardia from SVT with abnormal intraventricular conduction.

Polymorphic ventricular tachycardia has QRS complexes that vary in size, polarity, and often, rate. Sometimes, the QRS configuration appears to rotate around the isoelectric baseline (**Figure 5.35**). Torsades de pointes is a specific form of such polymorphic ventricular tachycardia that is associated with QT interval prolongation (see also **Figure 23.3**, p. 366, and p. 365).

Accelerated Idioventricular Rhythm   Also called idioventricular tachycardia and "slow" ventricular tachycardia, this rhythm occurs at a rate of about 70–100 (up to ~150) beats/minute in the dog, perhaps somewhat faster in the cat, and at about 60–90 beats/minute in the horse. Because the rate is slower and close to the sinus rate, it often is considered less serious. In animals with accelerated idioventricular rhythm, the ventricular-origin or fusion complexes typically appear when the sinus rate slows (including in the longer cycles of sinus arrhythmia) and disappear as the sinus rate increases (because the ventricular focus becomes overdrive suppressed; **Figure 5.36**). Accelerated idioventricular rhythm occurs commonly in dogs recovering from motor vehicle or other trauma (p. 641). In all species, accelerated idioventricular rhythms are associated with anesthesia, catecholamine use, gastrointestinal disease, and abnormal electrolyte or acid-base imbalances. This arrhythmia usually causes no deleterious effects and usually resolves with time or correction of the underlying condition. Nevertheless, deterioration to ventricular tachycardia is possible, so monitoring is warranted.

Ventricular Parasystole   This uncommon rhythm disturbance also is caused by a focus of automatic cells. However, in the situation of parasystole, the automatic focus is surrounded by ischemic or otherwise injured cardiac cells which isolate the parasystolic focus and protect it from depolarization when the surrounding myocardium becomes depolarized during sinus (or other) rhythm. This phenomenon is known as "entrance block," where normal depolarizing waves cannot penetrate into the parasystolic focus; thus, these automatic cells are not overdrive suppressed by a faster rhythm. However, spontaneous action potentials can exit the

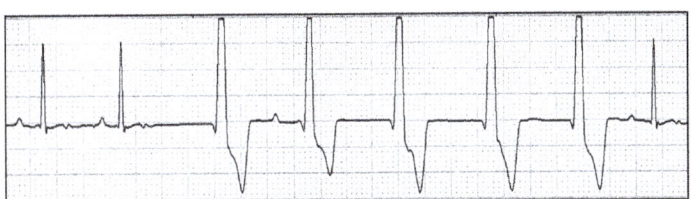

Figure 5.36 An accelerated idioventricular rhythm emerged when the sinus rate slowed in a dog that was hit by a car 1 day ago. This uniform ventricular rhythm (at ~80 beats/min) caused no instability and resolved spontaneously. Lead II, at 25 mm/s, 0.5 cm = 1 mV.

parasystolic focus and will activate the surrounding myocardium when it is not refractory. The ECG characteristics of ventricular parasystole include VPCs with varying coupling intervals to the preceding sinus QRS complexes, intervals of time between the VPCs that are multiples of a common denominator, and intermittent fusion complexes. Parasystole is an uncommon rhythm that can be relatively benign.

Isorhythmic Atrioventricular Dissociation Isorhythmic AV dissociation refers to the situation where independent atrial (sinus, usually) and ventricular pacemakers discharge and activate their respective chambers at almost equal rates for a fairly prolonged time. The timing of the two pacemakers can suggest that the two rhythms are synchronized. Rhythms that can produce isorhythmic AV dissociation include an accelerated idioventricular (or idionodal) rhythm, complete AV block with ventricular escape rhythm, ventricular pacing, ventricular tachycardia, and focal junctional tachycardia. Two patterns of isorhythmic AV dissociation have been described. The most common is Type I synchronization, in which there is a periodic but slight variation in timing between P waves and QRS complexes; the P waves appear to march into and out of the regularly spaced QRS complexes (**Figure 5.37**). In type II synchronization, the timing between P waves and QRS complexes is relatively fixed. If the P-to-QRS timing is short, type II synchronization could create the appearance of ventricular preexcitation; however, with isorhythmic AV dissociation atrial depolarization does not cause ventricular depolarization because the two rhythms are independent. Labrador Retrievers seem predisposed to focal junctional tachycardia. Electrophysiologic study in a small number of cases determined that ventricular activation originated from a His bundle focus (Perego, 2012). Isorhythmic AV dissociation sometimes is seen in horses or other species during inhalation anesthesia. Depending on the timing between atrial and ventricular activation, the contribution of atrial contraction to ventricular filling could be reduced or absent. However, if the overall HR is fairly normal the hemodynamic effect of isorhythmic AV dissociation is likely to be minimal.

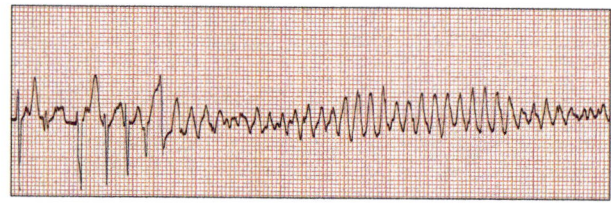

Figure 5.38 Irregular ventricular ectopic activity (left) degenerated into coarse ventricular fibrillation toward the center of this ECG strip in a dog under anesthesia. Lead II at 25 mm/s, 0.5 cm = 1 mV.

Ventricular Fibrillation This lethal rhythm is characterized by multiple waves of chaotic reentrant electrical activity within the ventricles (**Figure 5.38**). Consequently, as in the atria during AF, there is no coordinated mechanical activity and the ventricles cannot function as a pump. Ventricular fibrillation (VF) can be "coarse," with larger ECG baseline oscillations, or "fine."

Ventricular flutter appears as rapid sine-wave activity on the ECG (**Figure 5.39**). This severe, unstable arrhythmia sometimes precedes VF. Ventricular asystole is the absence of ventricular electrical (and mechanical) activity.

Escape Complexes and Rhythms Escape complexes represent the spontaneous discharge of subsidiary cardiac pacemakers (p. 12). These occur after a pause in the dominant (usually sinus) rhythm. If sinus rhythm with normal AV conduction does not resume, the escape focus will continue to discharge, and after a brief period of "warm-up," become manifest at its own intrinsic rate. Once established, escape rhythms usually are regular in timing. However, escape activity is suppressed by faster pacemaker activity, whether of normal (sinus) or abnormal (ectopic) origin. For example, VPCs or a paroxysmal SVT can (overdrive) suppress an escape rhythm. Escape complexes and escape rhythms constitute a protective mechanism. Therefore, it is important to recognize escape activity and not use antiarrhythmic drugs, which potentially can suppress this "back-up" pacemaker activity. An escape rhythm constitutes a "secondary" diagnosis associated

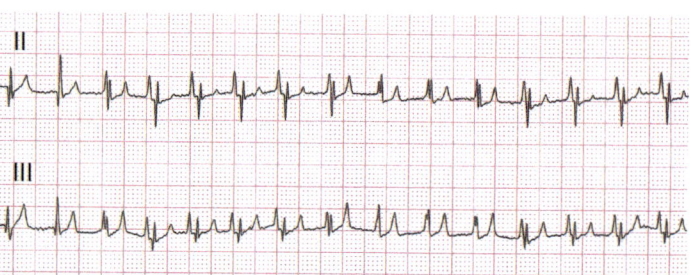

Figure 5.37 Isorhythmic AV dissociation in an older Shih Tzu with pulmonary hypertension and respiratory distress. Sinus P waves appear to move in and out of the QRS complexes, which arise from an idionodal or idioventricular focus. The P waves are abnormally tall, consistent with P pulmonale. Leads II & III, 25 mm/s, 1 cm = 1 mV.

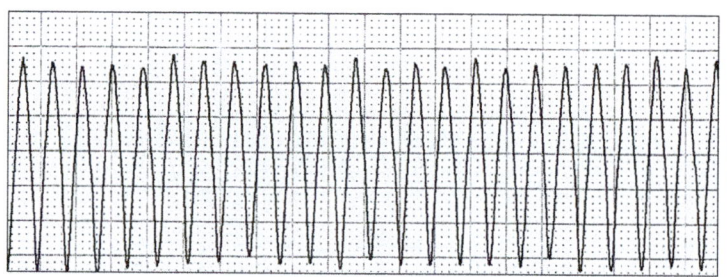

Figure 5.39 Ventricular flutter in a 7-year-old Great Pyrenees with dilated cardiomyopathy. The fairly uniform sine-wave appearance makes the differentiation between QRS complexes and T waves unclear. Ventricular fibrillation occurred soon after this recording; resuscitation was unsuccessful. Lead II, 25 mm/s, 1 cm = 1 mV.

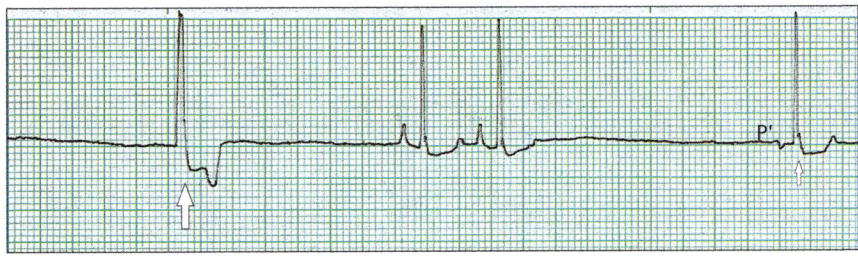

Figure 5.40 Ventricular (large arrow) and atrial (small arrow) escape complexes interrupt periods of sinus arrest in a 9-year-old female Miniature Schnauzer with sick sinus syndrome. Note the small ectopic P′ wave prior to the atrial escape complex. Lead II at 25 mm/s, 1 cm = 1 mV.

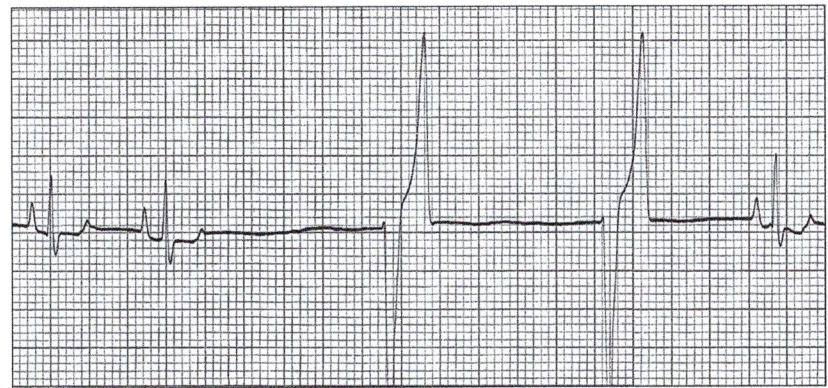

Figure 5.41 A ventricular escape rhythm began after sinus arrest occurred in a 12-year-old male Scottish Terrier with heart failure and syncope. Lead II at 25 mm/s, 1 cm = 1 mV.

with sinus bradycardia, sinus arrest, atrial standstill, and high-grade AV block. A terminal escape rhythm also commonly occurs prior to death, with the QRS complexes becoming progressively wider and slower in frequency.

Escape activity can originate from automatic cells in the atria, the AV junction, or the ventricles (**Figures 5.40** and **5.41**); the site of origin determines the width and morphology of the QRS complexes. In general, the more distal the site of an escape pacemaker, the wider the QRS-T complex. Ventricular escape rhythms (also called idioventricular rhythms) develop at approximately 20–40/minute in dogs, 15–25/minute in horses, and remarkably, at rates of 70–130 (or more)/minute in cats. Junctional escape rhythms generally occur at 40–60 beats/minute in dogs. These HR ranges are generalizations; the rate of an escape rhythm can be altered by metabolic factors, catecholamines, site of origin, and drug effects.

Abnormal Cardiac Conduction

Atrioventricular Conduction Disturbances Impaired AV conduction results in delayed or blocked transmission of atrial electrical activity (P waves) into the ventricles. Causes of abnormal AV conduction include excessive vagal tone, drugs (such as digoxin, xylazine, dexmedetomidine, diltiazem, beta-blockers, and anesthetic agents), and organic disease of the AV node or infranodal conduction system (His bundle and bundle branches). AV block also is called "heart block." Three "degrees" of AV conduction block severity are described. First-degree AV block means that conduction time from atria to ventricles is abnormally prolonged, although all atrial depolarizations ultimately are conducted (**Figure 5.42**).

Second-degree AV block is characterized by intermittent AV conduction; some P waves are not followed by a QRS complex. Second-degree heart block can be further classified in several ways. Mobitz type I (Wenckebach) block is characterized by progressive prolongation of the PR interval before a nonconducted P wave occurs. Typically, the conducted

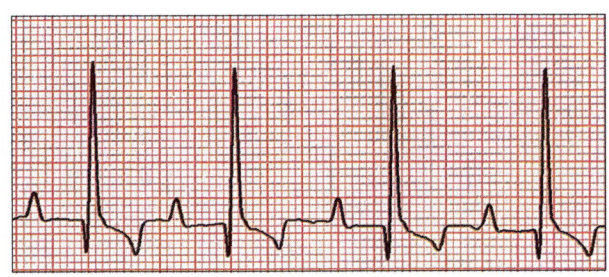

Figure 5.42 Sinus rhythm with first-degree AV block in a 13-year-old female American Cocker Spaniel being treated with digoxin. The PR interval is 0.16 second. Lead II at 50 mm/s, 1 cm = 1 mV.

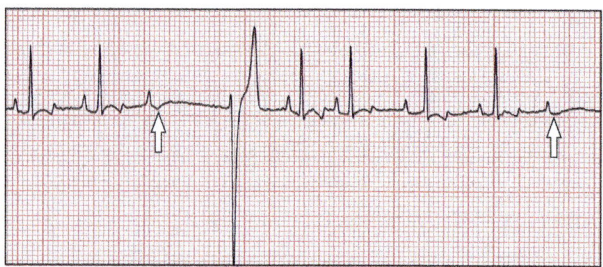

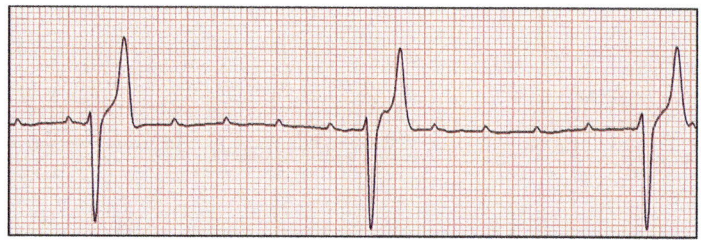

Figure 5.43 Sinus arrhythmia with second-degree AV block in a 12-year-old female West Highland White Terrier with chronic pulmonary disease. Note that T_a waves (arrows; p. 135) are evident following the blocked P waves because they are not obscured by QRS complexes. A ventricular escape complex occurred after the first blocked P wave. Lead II at 25 mm/s, 1 cm = 1 mV.

Figure 5.45 Third-degree (complete) AV block with a ventricular escape rhythm in an older male Weimaraner. Sinus P waves are unrelated to the ventricular escape complexes. Lead II, 25 mm/s, 0.5 cm = 1 mV.

impulses have a normal (narrow) QRS duration. Type I second-degree AV block often is associated with high vagal tone, drugs, or disorders within the AV node itself (**Figure 5.43**). Resting horses commonly have Mobitz type I AV block with occasional "dropped" (nonconducted) P waves; (**Figure 5.44**); this is a normal expression of vagal tone that also helps regulate systemic blood pressure. Mobitz type II second-degree AV block is characterized by uniform PR intervals preceding the blocked impulses. This is associated more often with disease lower in the AV conduction system (bundle of His or major bundle branches); in some cases, the QRS complex is widened also, indicating more diffuse conduction system disease. Some consider 2:1 AV block (where every other P wave is conducted) as a form of type II AV block. "High-grade" second-degree AV block, which indicates a P:QRS ratio of 3:1 (or higher), is another typical variant of type II AV block.

Additional subclassification of second-degree AV block is based on the duration of the QRS complexes following conducted P waves. Type A second-degree AV block is characterized by a narrow QRS configuration, which more likely indicates the block is within or near the AV node. In contrast, type B second-degree AV block is characterized by widened or abnormal QRS complexes, suggesting more diffuse disease within the infranodal or intraventricular conduction systems. As noted above, type B is more often encountered with Mobitz type II block. Junctional (nodal) or ventricular escape complexes commonly occur during second-degree AV block, particularly during longer pauses between ventricular activations.

Third-degree or complete AV block is present when no sinus (or supraventricular) electrical impulses are conducted into the ventricles. P waves often indicate a concurrent regular sinus rhythm or sinus arrhythmia. However, these P waves are not temporally related to the QRS complexes, which result from a (usually) regular ventricular escape rhythm (**Figures 5.45** and **5.46**). The duration and configuration of the ventricular escape complexes depends on their site of origin. A ventricular escape rhythm is necessary for survival in patients with complete AV block.

The ECG differentiation of second-degree from third-degree AV block sometimes might be confusing. In most cases, second-degree AV block causes an irregular ventricular rhythm; if escape complexes appear intermittently, they generally are of different configuration than the patient's normal

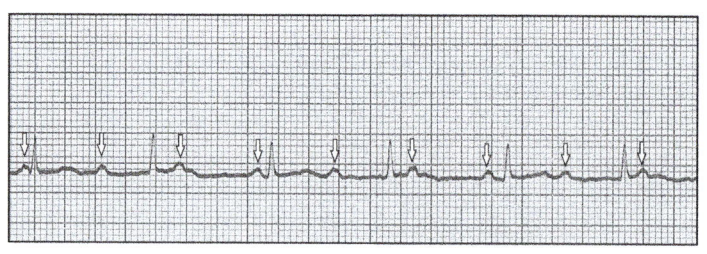

Figure 5.46 Complete AV block with ventricular escape rhythm in a cat with cardiomyopathy. The ventricular rate (~150 beats/min) is higher than the usual escape rate in cats. Sinus P waves indicated by arrows. Lead II, 50 mm/s, 1 cm = 1 mV. (ECG courtesy of Dr J Tyler.)

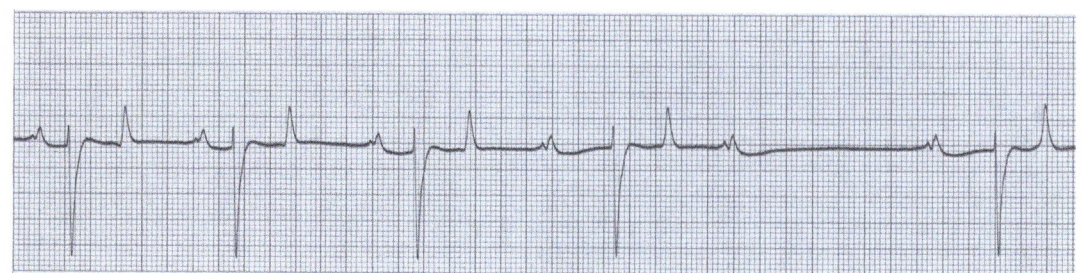

Figure 5.44 Mobitz type I (Wenckebach) second-degree AV block in a normal 12-year-old Thoroughbred. Note the gradual PR interval prolongation prior to the nonconducted P wave, as well as the normal bifid P wave morphology. Base-apex lead, 25 mm/s.

sinus QRS complexes. The P-to-QRS interval in patients with second-degree block is fairly consistent, although some variation occurs with Mobitz type I block (see above). In contrast, there are no consistent P-to-QRS intervals with third-degree AV block; usually there is a regular, slow ventricular escape rhythm with uniform QRS complex appearance. However, in some cases with third-degree AV block, ventricular premature complexes or shifts in the escape focus might cause rhythm irregularities and variation in QRS appearance. Additionally, ventriculophasic sinus arrhythmia is commonly observed with higher grades of AV block, such that the P-P intervals surrounding a QRS complex are shorter than those not encompassing a ventricular complex.

Intraatrial Conduction Disturbances Several abnormalities of intraatrial conduction can occur. Conduction failure between the SA node and the surrounding atrial muscle is called SA block. This cannot reliably be differentiated from sinus arrest on the ECG, although the interval between P waves should be a multiple of the normal P-P interval in classic SA block. Prolonged sinus arrest or SA block can lead to an atrial, junctional, or ventricular escape rhythm.

Atrial standstill indicates a loss of normal atrial electrical and mechanical functions. Regardless of sinus node activity, the atrial muscle cannot respond to electrical stimulation. Atrial standstill occurs with moderate to severe hyperkalemia, which interferes with myocardial cell depolarization (p. 160); this is reversible with treatment of the electrolyte disturbance. Persistent atrial standstill is caused by myocardial disease, typically with fibrous tissue replacement. P waves are characteristically absent, although sometimes diminutive, but ineffective, atrial deflections from remaining islands of atrial muscle might be evident. A junctional or ventricular escape rhythm develops to maintain some cardiac output (**Figure 25.9**, p. 416).

Intraventricular Conduction Disturbances Slowed or blocked impulse transmission within any of the major bundle branches causes an intraventricular conduction disturbance (aberrant conduction). Electrical activation of any ventricular muscle served by the diseased conduction bundle must originate in adjacent myocardium; the spread of this depolarization is both late and slow. This causes QRS widening, as well as a shift in the orientation (axis) of the terminal QRS toward the region of delayed activation (**Table 5.5** and **Figures 5.47–5.49**). The right bundle branch or the septal, anterior, and posterior fascicles of the left bundle branch can be affected singly or in various combinations. A block in all branches causes third-degree (complete) heart block. Right bundle branch block (RBBB) can occur in otherwise normal dogs and cats, or from conduction tissue degeneration, right ventricular (RV) disease, or distension. Left bundle branch block (LBBB) usually is related to clinically relevant left ventricular (LV) myocardial or conduction disease. The left anterior fascicular

Table 5.5 Ventricular Chamber Enlargement[a] and Conduction Abnormality Patterns in Dogs and Cats

Normal
- Normal mean electrical axis
- No S wave in lead I
- R wave is taller in lead II than in lead I
- In lead CV_6LL, R wave is larger than S wave

Right Ventricular Enlargement
- Right axis deviation
- S wave is present in lead I
- S wave in lead V_2 (CV_6LL) & V_3 >R wave (or >0.8 mV, dogs); rSr' in V_1 (CV_5RL)
- QS ("W"-shaped QRS) in lead V_{10}
- Positive T wave in lead V_{10} (in most breeds)
- Prominent S wave in leads II, aVF ± III

Right Bundle Branch Block (RBBB)
- As for right ventricular enlargement, with terminal QRS prolongation (and broad S wave if complete RBBB)

Left Ventricular (Concentric) Hypertrophy
- Left axis deviation
- R wave in lead I is taller than R wave in leads II and aVF
- qR complex but no S wave in leads I and aVL
- Progressively deeper S-waves in leads II, aVF and III

Left Anterior Fascicular Block (LAFB)[b]
- As for left ventricular hypertrophy, possibly with wider QRS

Left Ventricular Dilation (Eccentric Hypertrophy)
- Normal frontal axis
- R wave is taller than normal in leads II, aVF, and CV_6LL
- Widened QRS; ST segment might be slurred and displaced, and T wave might be enlarged

Left Bundle Branch Block (LBBB)
- Normal frontal axis
- Very wide and sloppy QRS
- Small Q wave might be present in leads II, III, and aVF (incomplete LBBB, or left posterior fascicular block)

---
[a] Not all patients with ventricular dilation or hypertrophy manifest the "typical" ECG ventricular enlargement criteria.
[b] Criteria uncertain in dogs.

block (LAFB) pattern is common with LV hypertrophy, as in cats with hypertrophic cardiomyopathy (**Figure 33.10**, p. 664). Intraventricular conduction disturbances that do not clearly fit the above patterns also can occur and can cause an unusual or widened QRS configuration.

Ventricular Preexcitation Accessory conduction pathways are anomalous bundles of myocardial fibers that extend from atrium to ventricle, perforating the insulation of the fibrous rings and bypassing the normal AV conduction system. Affected animals usually have a single accessory pathway, although some have multiple anomalous pathways. Several types of preexcitation and accessory pathways have been described, mainly in dogs; right-sided atrial to ventricular connections are most common (Santilli, 2007). Other

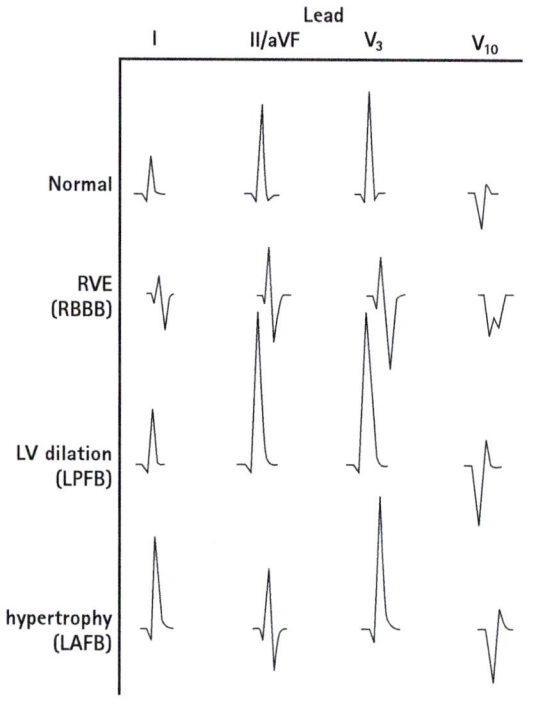

Figure 5.47 Typical QRS configurations resulting from ventricular enlargement or conduction delay in selected leads. LAFB, left anterior fascicular block; LPFB, left posterior fascicular block; LV, left ventricular; RBBB, right bundle branch block; RVE, right ventricular enlargement.

accessory pathways might be identified near or within the AV node or bundle of His. Preexcitation occasionally is identified in cats and horses, as well. A short PR interval is the most characteristic feature of ventricular preexcitation.

Early activation (preexcitation) of part of the ventricular myocardium occurs when atrial-to-ventricular (antegrade) conduction occurs over the accessory conduction pathway, bypassing the slowly conducting AV node. In the classical Wolff–Parkinson–White (WPW) preexcitation pattern, early depolarization of ventricular myocardial fibers (distant to the normal site of initial activation) not only shortens the PR interval, it also widens the initial portion of the QRS complex.

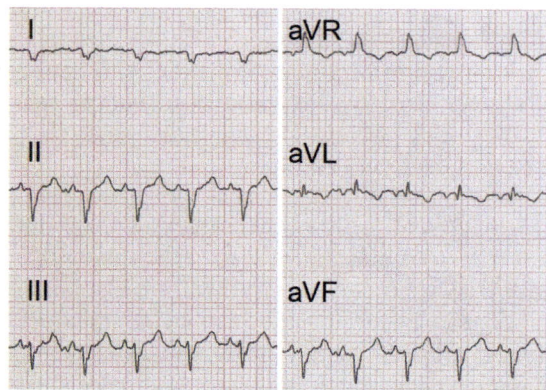

Figure 5.48 Sinus rhythm with a right bundle branch block (RBBB) pattern in a Manx cat with restrictive cardiomyopathy, but no evidence for right ventricular enlargement. Leads as marked; 25 mm/s, 1 cm = 1 mV.

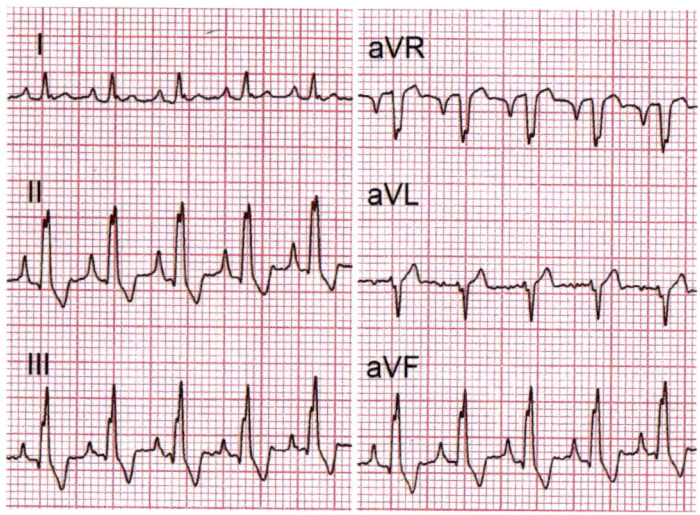

Figure 5.49 Sinus rhythm with a left bundle branch block (LBBB) pattern in a female Dalmatian with dilated cardiomyopathy. The QRS complexes are unusually small. Leads as marked; 25 mm/s, 1 cm = 1 mV.

This widened and slurred QRS onset is called a "delta wave" (**Figure 5.50**); occasionally, a discrete wave within the PR segment might represent a delta wave. Depolarization of the remaining (non-preexcited) ventricular myocardium follows via the AV node and His-Purkinje system. Therefore, the resulting QRS is a type of fusion complex. Because this ventricular activation process is abnormal, the QRS complexes and their T waves in patients with preexcitation often are larger than normal. Other types of accessory pathways can connect the atria or dorsal areas of the AV node directly to the bundle of His or proximal bundle branches. These cause a short PR interval without a delta wave and the QRS is more normal in morphology.

Animals with an accessory pathway can have consistent or intermittent preexcitation during sinus rhythm (**Figure 5.51**). However, an accessory pathway can be "concealed" (not evident on ECG). Animals with one or more concealed accessory pathways show no evidence of preexcitation during sinus rhythm because antegrade conduction over the accessory

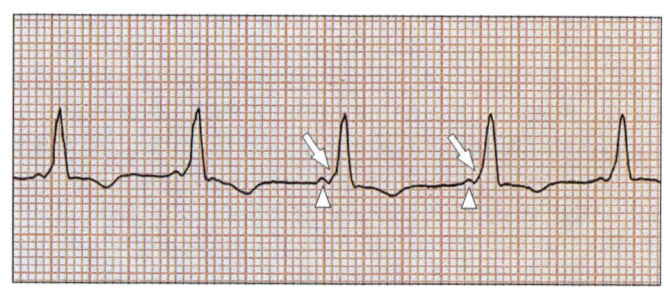

Figure 5.50 Sinus rhythm with ventricular preexcitation in a 4-month-old kitten with occasional syncope (AV reciprocating tachycardia was suspected but not documented). Small P waves (arrowheads) are followed by delta waves (arrows), indicating early ventricular activation from an extranodal accessory pathway. Lead V_6, 50 mm/s, 1 cm = 1 mV.

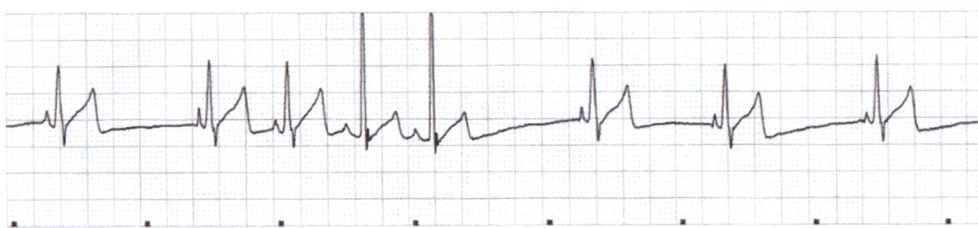

Figure 5.51 Intermittent ventricular preexcitation was identified during general anesthesia in a horse. This ECG segment shows that antegrade conduction occurred over the abnormal bypass tract (note the shortened PR interval) in all but the 4th and 5th complexes from the left. Monitor lead, 25 mm/s. (ECG courtesy of Dr. D Riedesel.)

pathway does not occur. Yet the accessory path might permit retrograde (ventricular-to-atrial) conduction, as discussed previously for AV reentrant tachycardia. In dogs, it appears that unidirectional retrograde conduction is more common than bidirectional conduction (Santilli, 2007). The danger with an accessory pathway is not ventricular preexcitation itself, but the potential for a rapid "AV reciprocating tachycardia," which is a reentrant SVT using the accessory pathway and AV node. Usually, the tachycardia's impulses travel into the ventricles through the AV node (antegrade or "orthodromic" conduction) and then back to the atria via the accessory pathway. This creates normal-appearing, narrow QRS complexes during the tachycardia (**Figure 25.10**, p. 418), unless an intraventricular conduction disturbance also is present. Retrograde P′ waves buried in the ST segment (RP′) usually are present. Less often, the direction of the reentrant circuit is reversed ("antidromic" AV reciprocating tachycardia); this creates a wide-QRS tachycardia that must be distinguished from ventricular tachycardia. Incessant or very-rapid AV reciprocating tachycardias can cause weakness, syncope, congestive heart failure (secondary to tachycardia-induced cardiomyopathy), and death. The presence of the WPW pattern on ECG in conjunction with a rapid AV reciprocating tachycardia causing clinical signs characterizes the WPW syndrome and points to the mechanism of the SVT. Development of AF in a patient with ventricular preexcitation potentially can lead to VF via rapid conduction of fibrillation waves down the accessory pathway. This is rare but should be considered when a wide-QRS tachycardia is irregular in cycle length.

Mean Electrical Axis

The MEA describes the average direction of the ventricular depolarization process in the frontal (cranial-caudal and left-right) plane, unless another orientation is specified. It represents the summation of the various instantaneous vectors that occur throughout ventricular muscle depolarization and that create the QRS complex. Especially in dogs and cats, estimation of the MEA helps the clinician identify major intraventricular conduction disturbances, as well as some ventricular enlargement patterns, because these shift the average direction (axis) of ventricular activation. Body position and cardiac orientation within the thorax can influence the MEA. For dogs and cats, positioning in standard right lateral recumbency during ECG recording is recommended. The MEA in most normal dogs and cats (and horses) is oriented caudally and leftward, near the positive side of lead II or aVF. Cats have greater variability in MEA than dogs (**Figure 5.52**). Sometimes, an animal without apparent heart disease will have a MEA outside the normal range. A left shift has been reported in some healthy Doberman Pinschers, too (Carnabuci, 2019). Nevertheless, an MEA outside the normal range usually signals an underlying abnormality.

The simplest approaches to estimating the MEA in the frontal plane involve inspection of all six limb leads (but not the chest or base-apex leads). By convention, the reference positions of these leads are defined by degrees (from 0 to ±180 degrees) around a circle (**Figure 5.52**). The positive pole (electrode) of most leads lies on the "positive" side of the circle; however, it is important to note that the positive pole of leads aVR and aVL lie within the "negative" quadrants of the circle. When estimating the MEA, consider only the QRS complexes (not P or T waves) that occur during sinus rhythm. A number of methods, including computerized ECG analysis and analysis of just two limb leads, can be used to estimate the MEA, but the following two approaches are most commonly used in veterinary practice. These methods are approximate, but clinically useful.

- Find the lead (I, II, III, aVR, aVL, or aVF) with the largest R wave (note that the R wave is by definition a positive deflection), or the greatest net positive area under the QRS. The positive electrode of this lead shows the approximate MEA.
- Find the lead (I, II, III, aVR, aVL, or aVF) with the most isoelectric QRS complexes (where the positive and negative deflections or areas are about equal). Then identify the lead perpendicular to this lead on the hexaxial lead diagram (**Figure 5.2** or **Figure 5.52**). If the patient's QRS complex configuration in this perpendicular lead is mostly positive, the MEA is toward the positive pole of this lead. If the QRS in the perpendicular lead is mostly negative, the MEA is oriented toward the negative pole. If all leads appear isoelectric, the frontal axis is indeterminate.

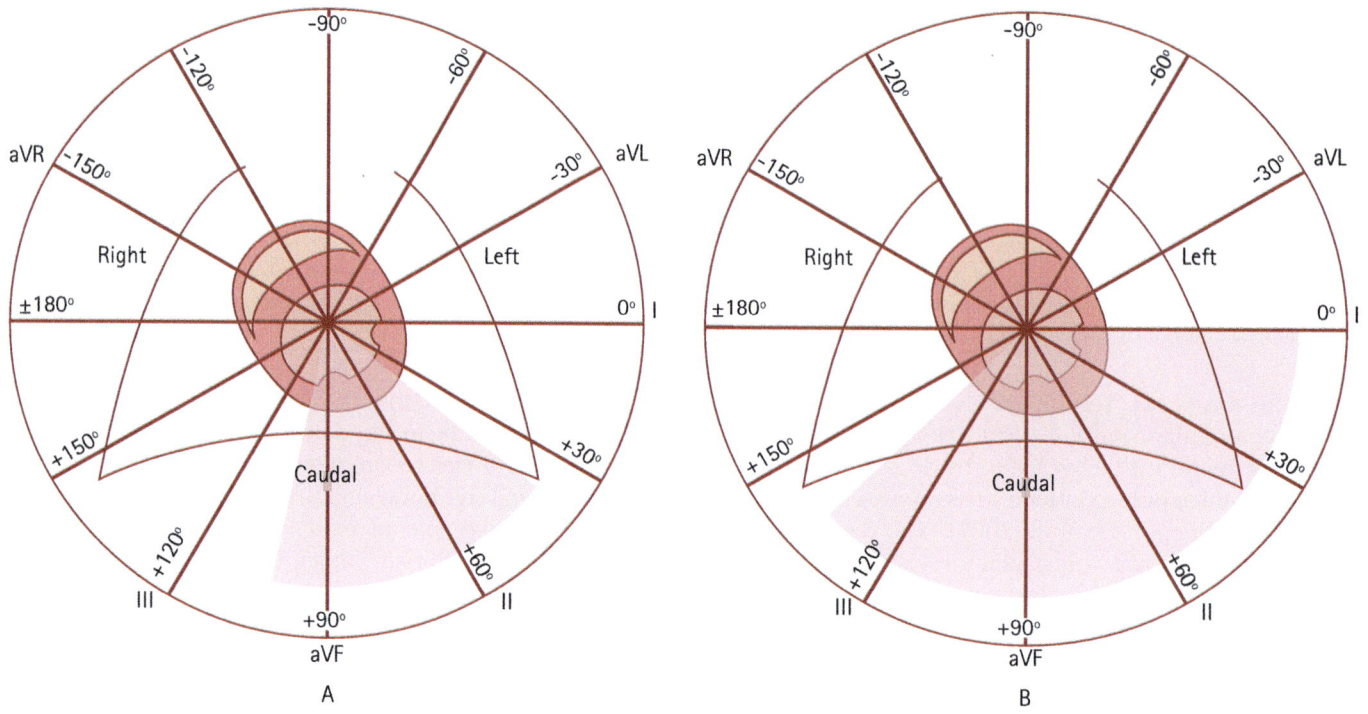

Figure 5.52 Diagram illustrating frontal plane leads and the normal mean electrical axis (MEA) ranges for dogs (A) and cats (B). Conventional (positive and negative) degree locations around the circle are indicated for all leads. Each lead is labeled at its positive pole.

Cardiac Chamber Enlargement

Certain changes in ECG waveform patterns can suggest enlargement or conduction disturbance related to a particular cardiac chamber (**Table 5.5**). However, cardiac enlargement often occurs without these ECG changes. Thus, ECG analysis for cardiomegaly is relatively insensitive and sometimes nonspecific.

Atrial Enlargement Patterns

Left atrial (LA) enlargement commonly prolongs the P wave duration; this pattern also is known as "P mitrale." Sometimes, the P wave is notched as well as wide. Slowed intraatrial conduction and moderate to severe right atrial (RA) dilation also can cause wide and notched P waves. In horses, notched P waves are normal as long as the P wave duration is within reference range. RA enlargement might be manifest by tall, spiked P waves (also called "P pulmonale"). This is also nonspecific and LA dilation can sometimes increase the P wave amplitude, especially in cats. Atrial enlargement can magnify the usually obscured atrial repolarization (T_a) wave, too. The T_a wave appears as a brief baseline shift in the opposite direction of the P wave (**Figure 5.43**).

Ventricular Enlargement Patterns

Normal QRS voltages in the limb leads usually are under 2.5 mV in dogs and infrequently exceed 0.7 mV in healthy cats. Frontal plane QRS voltages in horses are generally between those of normal dogs and cats.

Right Ventricle Right axis deviation and an S wave in lead I are strong criteria for RV enlargement. Other ECG changes often can be found as well (**Figure 5.47**). Three or more of the criteria listed in **Table 5.5** generally accompany marked RV enlargement. Mild RV enlargement usually is not evident on the ECG because the forces of LV activation normally are so dominant. It is important to note that the RBBB pattern can mimic or accompany RV enlargement.

Left Ventricle LV dilation and eccentric hypertrophy (p. 16) often increase R wave voltage in the caudal limb leads (II and aVF) and might widen the QRS complex. A complete LBBB or left posterior fascicular block (LPFB) pattern can mimic or accompany LV dilation. LV concentric hypertrophy is inconsistently associated with left axis deviation (LAFB pattern). **Table 5.5** and **Figures 5.47–5.49** summarize ECG patterns typical for ventricular enlargement or conduction delay. Common clinical associations are listed in **Table 5.6**.

Table 5.6 Some Clinical Associations of ECG Enlargement Patterns

Left Atrial Enlargement
- Mitral insufficiency (acquired or congenital)
- Cardiomyopathies
- Patent ductus arteriosus
- (Sub)aortic stenosis
- Ventricular septal defect

Right Atrial Enlargement
- Tricuspid insufficiency (acquired or congenital)
- Chronic respiratory disease ± pulmonary hypertension
- Atrial septal defect
- Pulmonic stenosis

Left Ventricular Enlargement (Dilation)
- Mitral insufficiency
- Dilated ± other cardiomyopathies
- Aortic insufficiency
- Patent ductus arteriosus
- Ventricular septal defect
- Subaortic stenosis

Left Ventricular Enlargement (Hypertrophy)
- Hypertrophic cardiomyopathy
- Subaortic stenosis

Right Ventricular Enlargement
- Pulmonic stenosis
- Tetralogy of Fallot
- Tricuspid insufficiency (acquired or congenital)
- Severe pulmonary hypertension (including heartworm disease)

Other ECG Abnormalities and Considerations

Small-Voltage QRS Complexes

In dogs, small-voltage QRS complexes in the limb leads can accompany pleural or pericardial effusions, obesity, intrathoracic mass lesions, hypovolemia, and hypothyroidism. However, small-voltage complexes occasionally are seen in dogs without identifiable abnormalities and are common in some breeds, such as the Boxer and the English bulldog. Small-voltage QRS complexes are normal in cats.

Electrical Alternans

Every-other-beat alteration in QRS complex size is known as electrical alternans. Most often, electrical alternans during sinus rhythm is associated with a large-volume pericardial effusion. The effusion allows the heart to swing back and forth inside the pericardium, altering its orientation within the thorax on alternating beats (p. 717 and **Figures 35.21** and **35.22** p. 719). Rapid, regular SVT (as opposed to sinus tachycardia) can also cause subtle electrical alternans, especially at the onset of the arrhythmia.

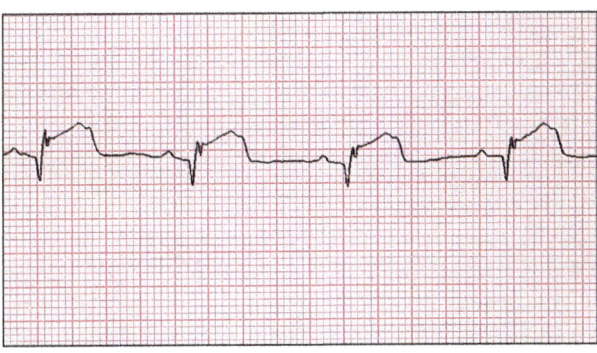

Figure 5.53 Sinus rhythm with ST segment elevation in a 2-year-old Pomeranian with severe valvular pulmonic stenosis. Ischemia of the markedly hypertrophied right ventricular wall was the suspected cause for the ST segment deviation. Lead II, 50 mm/s, 1 cm = 1 mV.

ST-T Abnormalities

The ST segment extends from the end of the QRS complex (also called the J point) to the onset of the T wave. It represents the time between ventricular depolarization and the onset of repolarization. However, in companion animals, the ST segment slopes into the T wave without a clear demarcation because repolarization begins immediately after depolarization. ST segment abnormalities can be primary (caused by abnormalities of the repolarization process) or secondary to abnormalities of ventricular depolarization. Deviation of the ST segment from the isoelectric baseline (**Figures 5.53** and **5.54**) and changes in its duration can occur. Elevation (>0.15 mV in dogs or >0.1 mV in cats) or depression (>0.2 mV in dogs or >0.1 mV in cats) of the J point and ST segment in leads I, II, or aVF can be caused by ischemia or other myocardial injury. For example, pericarditis can be a cause of ST segment elevation (**Figure 35.23**, p. 719). Secondary ST segment deviation could stem from ventricular hypertrophy, aberrant conduction, and some drugs (including digoxin). Prominent T_a waves associated with atrial enlargement or tachycardia can

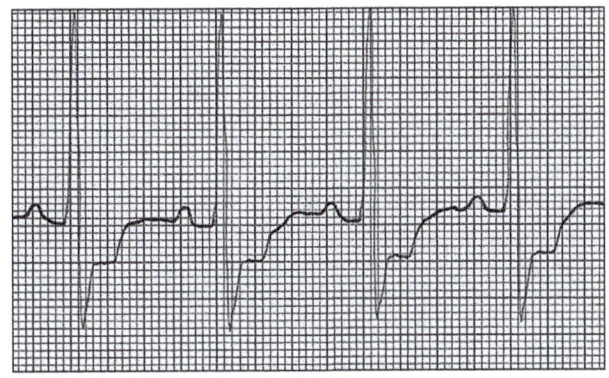

Figure 5.54 Sinus rhythm with ST segment depression in a 5-month-old Newfoundland puppy with severe subaortic stenosis and presumed left ventricular ischemia. Lead II, 50 mm/s, 1 cm = 1 mV.

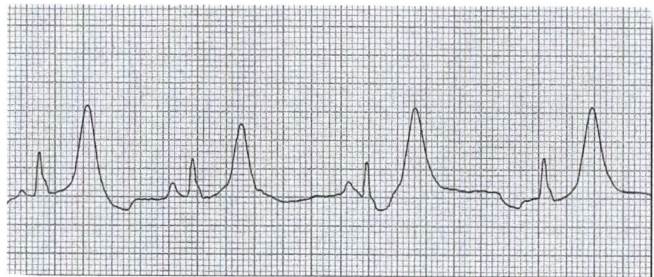

Figure 5.55 Sinus rhythm with very large T waves in a 12-year-old Yorkshire Terrier. Hypoxia secondary to airway disease was suspected, based on the history of cough, dyspnea, and absence of a cardiac murmur. Lead II, 50 mm/s, 1 cm = 1 mV.

Table 5.7 Some Causes of ST Segment, T Wave, and QT Abnormalities

Depressed J Point/ST Segment
- Myocardial ischemia
- Myocardial infarction/injury (subendocardial)
- Hyperkalemia or hypokalemia
- Cardiac trauma
- Secondary change (ventricular hypertrophy, aberrant conduction, VPCs)
- Digoxin ("sagging" appearance)
- Pseudodepression (caused by prominent T_a wave)

Elevated J Point/ST Segment
- Pericarditis
- Left ventricular subepicardial injury
- Myocardial infarction (transmural)
- Myocardial hypoxia
- Secondary change (ventricular hypertrophy, aberrant conduction, VPCs)
- Digoxin toxicity

Prolonged QT Interval
- Many drugs have the potential to slow repolarization by affecting the I_{Kr} or I_{Na} current (including antiarrhythmic agents such as quinidine, procainamide, sotalol, amiodarone, flecainide, disopyramide, dofetilide, ibutilide; antimicrobials such as erythromycin, azithromycin, clarithromycin, ciprofloxacin, levofloxacin, fluconazole; antipsychotics such as chlorpromazine, haloperidol, droperidol, thioridazone; and cisapride, domperidone, methadone, propofol, sevoflurane, chloroquine, and others)
- Hypocalcemia
- Hypokalemia
- Ethylene glycol poisoning
- Secondary to prolonged QRS
- Cardiomyopathies
- Some infectious and inflammatory conditions (including tick toxicity)
- Hypothermia
- Central nervous system abnormalities (including subarachnoid hemorrhage)
- Other acquired causes of cardiac ion channelopathy
- Inherited cardiac ion channel mutation (congenital long QT syndrome; rare)

Shortened QT Interval
- Hypercalcemia
- Hyperkalemia
- Digitalis toxicity
- Inherited short QT syndrome; reported in people but not animals yet

Large T Waves
- Myocardial hypoxia
- Ventricular enlargement
- Intraventricular conduction abnormalities
- Hyperkalemia (some cases)
- Metabolic or respiratory diseases
- Normal variation

Tented T Waves
- Hyperkalemia

Abbreviation: VPC, ventricular premature complex.

mimic ST segment depression (pseudodepression). In heavily exercising horses, ST segment deviation and increased T wave amplitude are common and considered physiologic alterations. These changes likely represent some imbalance of myocardial oxygen demand and delivery.

The T wave, representing ventricular muscle repolarization, can be positive, negative, or biphasic in normal companion animals. Differences in size, shape, or polarity from previous recordings in an individual animal might be clinically relevant, but this requires more definition. Primary abnormalities of the T wave are related to factors that affect repolarization; these can include hyperkalemia, hypercalcemia, hypoxia, and hypothermia (**Figure 5.55**). Secondary changes are related to abnormalities of ventricular depolarization, including cardiac enlargement patterns, bundle branch block or other intraventricular conduction disturbance, and VPCs. Secondary ST-T changes tend to be of opposite polarity to the main QRS deflection. **Table 5.7** lists some causes of ST-T abnormalities. T wave alternans indicates beat-to-beat variability in repolarization. Although seemingly uncommon in companion animals, it might be evident on the surface ECG or could be virtually undetectable without specialized ECG analysis (microvolt alternans). T wave alternans is a risk factor for sudden arrhythmic death in people.

The QT Interval

The QT interval represents the total time of ventricular depolarization and repolarization. This interval varies inversely with average HR, largely reflecting underlying cardiac autonomic influences. The QT interval is shorter at faster HRs, although the relationship is not linear. Besides autonomic tone, various drugs and other factors influence the QT interval duration (**Table 5.7**). Variations in the QT interval also have been reported in different breeds of athletic horses and there is much variability among individuals, as well (Pedersen, 2016). Abnormally prolonged QT duration and heterogeneous repolarization predispose to potentially fatal ventricular arrhythmias. Acquired causes of QT prolongation include a number of drugs, some toxins, electrolyte

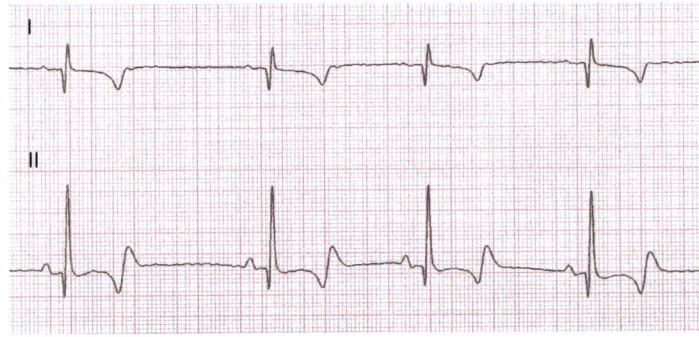

Figure 5.56 Resting ECG from a 9-month-old male English Springer Spaniel with inherited QT prolongation. The heart rate (HR) is 60 beats/min and QT interval is ~0.36 sec. When this dog's HR rose to 110 beats/min, the QT interval decreased to 0.27 sec, with QTc ~0.31 sec. The QTc of normal related dogs at the same HR was 0.23-0.25 sec. QTc, corrected QT interval (VandeWater formula). Leads I and II, 50 mm/s, 1 cm = 1 mV.

Table 5.8 Effects of Electrolyte Abnormalities and Selected Drugs[a] on the ECG

Hyperkalemia (Figures 5.57–5.59)
- Peaked (tented), ± large T waves
- QT interval abbreviation
- Flat or absent P waves
- Widened QRS
- ST segment depression
- Slowed HR

Hypokalemia
- ST segment depression
- Small, biphasic (or variably enlarged) T waves
- QT interval prolongation
- Tachyarrhythmias
- Widened QRS or P wave
- ± AV block

Hypercalcemia
- Few effects
- Abbreviated QT interval
- Prolonged conduction
- Tachyarrhythmias

Hypocalcemia
- Prolonged QT interval
- Tachyarrhythmias
- ± T wave alternans

Digoxin
- PR prolongation
- Sinus bradycardia or arrest
- Second- (or third-) degree AV block
- Accelerated junctional rhythm
- Ventricular premature complexes
- Ventricular tachycardia
- Paroxysmal atrial tachycardia with block
- Atrial fibrillation with slow ventricular rate

Quinidine/Procainamide
- Atropine-like effects
- QT prolongation
- AV block
- Ventricular tachyarrhythmias
- QRS widening
- Sinus arrest

Lidocaine
- AV block
- Ventricular tachycardia
- Sinus arrest

Beta-Blockers
- Sinus bradycardia
- PR prolongation
- AV block

Barbiturates/Thiobarbiturates
- Ventricular bigeminy

Halothane/Methoxyflurane
- Sinus bradycardia
- Ventricular arrhythmias (increased sensitivity to catecholamines, especially halothane)

Alpha$_2$-Blockers (Xylazine, Medetomidine, Dexmedetomidine)
- Sinus bradycardia
- Sinus arrest/sinoatrial block
- AV block
- ±Ventricular tachyarrhythmias (especially with concurrent halothane, epinephrine)

[a] Adverse or toxic effects; also see **Table 5.7** for partial list of other drugs that can affect repolarization.

disturbances, cardiomyopathies, subarachnoid hemorrhage, infectious and inflammatory lesions including tick (*Ixodes holocyclus*) toxicity, and other conditions that alter cardiac ion channel function. Inherited QT prolongation (long QT syndrome) is common in people, but only recently was reported in one family of dogs with sudden death (**Figure 5.56**, also p. 365 and **Figure 23.3**; Ware, 2015).

Equations to predict expected QT duration based on HR (corrected QT interval, QTc) have been derived for normal dogs and cats, as well as people. Nevertheless, these efforts to define more clearly the QT interval–HR relationship all have limitations with regard to accuracy and also their ability to identify arrhythmia risk. With regular sinus rhythm, the QTc can be calculated using the R-R interval from the preceding beat (that is, the instantaneous HR). In contrast, marked variability in R-R intervals occurs with respiratory sinus arrhythmia. However, an R-R interval derived from the average HR can be used in QTc calculations because QT duration remains essentially unchanged during respiratory sinus arrhythmia. Newer methods of dynamic beat-to-beat QT to R-R analysis appear to be better for assessing arrhythmia vulnerability, however they are not as simple to perform as QTc calculations (see section "Suggested Additional Reading and References" and the online bibliography).

Effects of Drugs and Electrolyte Abnormalities on the ECG

Digoxin, antiarrhythmic agents, and anesthetic drugs often alter heart rhythm and conduction either by their direct electrophysiologic effects or by affecting autonomic tone (see Chapters 23 and 24). **Table 5.8** summarizes some common ECG manifestations of such drug effects. Abnormalities of potassium homeostasis have marked and complex influences on cardiac electrophysiology and, consequently, on the ECG. Noticeable ECG changes caused by other electrolyte disturbances occur infrequently (**Table 5.8**). Hypomagnesemia has no reported effects on the ECG; however, it can predispose to digoxin toxicity and arrhythmias, as well as exaggerate the effects of hypocalcemia.

Hyperkalemia Mild hyperkalemia actually can have an antiarrhythmic effect by reducing automaticity and enhancing repolarization speed and uniformity. However, rapid or severe increases in serum potassium concentration can cause arrhythmias. This mainly relates to reduced (less negative) resting membrane potential, which inactivates sodium channels and opens potassium channels; these changes in turn lead to slowed conduction velocity and shortened refractory period, respectively. Several ECG changes can occur as serum potassium concentration rises, although these can be inconsistent in ill animals (**Figures 5.57–5.59**). Experimentally, as serum K$^+$ rises to near 6 mmol/l (6 mEq/l), an early ECG change is a narrowed and peaked ("tented") T wave, where the waveform's down stroke mirrors the upstroke. The characteristic tented T wave appearance can be more apparent in some leads than in others, and the area under the T wave (that is, the wave's voltage) can be large or small.

SA nodal cells are relatively resistant to the effects of hyperkalemia. Nevertheless, the sinus rate slows with worsening hyperkalemia, especially in dogs and horses (sinus rate can be normal in cats). Atrial muscle excitability diminishes and P waves tend to flatten as serum K$^+$ approaches 7 mmol/l (7 mEq/l); this tissue becomes inexcitable and P waves disappear above ~8 mmol/l (8 mEq/l). Despite progressive unresponsiveness of the atrial myocardium, specialized fibers can transmit sinus impulses to the AV node. This is known as a "sinoventricular" rhythm (sinus origin but without P waves); it can mimic atrial standstill.

Progressive QRS widening, caused by slowing of intraventricular conduction, also occurs as serum K$^+$ rises above 6 mmol/l (6 mEq/l). With severe hyperkalemia (>10 mmol/L [>10 mEq/L]), reentry or afterdepolarizations can lead to ventricular tachycardia or fibrillation and asystole. Hypocalcemia, hyponatremia, and acidosis accentuate the ECG changes caused by hyperkalemia, whereas hypercalcemia and hypernatremia tend to counteract them.

Therapy for life-threatening hyperkalemia is aimed at promoting intracellular translocation of potassium, antagonizing the membrane effects of potassium, and removing the underlying cause. There is no prospective study delineating the most effective and safe therapy and various methods have their proponents. Therapeutic options for severe hyperkalemia include: 10% calcium gluconate (50–100 mg/kg; or 0.5–1.5 ml/kg, slow IV bolus over 10–30 minutes); regular insulin (0.25–0.5 U/kg IV) given with glucose (2 g/U insulin, diluted to a 10% solution); terbutaline sulfate (4–8 mcg/kg, SC); or sodium bicarbonate (1–2 mEq/kg, slow IV bolus over 5–10 minutes). For horses, insulin-glucose therapy doses of 0.1 U regular insulin/kg body weight with 0.5–1 g glucose (or dextrose)/kg IV infused over 15 minutes have been recommended. The sodium bicarbonate therapy option usually is reserved for refractory cases because it can provoke hypocalcemia (in some cats with urethral obstruction), hyperphosphatemia, and possibly also paradoxical cerebrospinal fluid acidosis. When infusing calcium salts, the ECG should be monitored; if sudden HR slowing, QT interval prolongation, or VPCs develop, the calcium

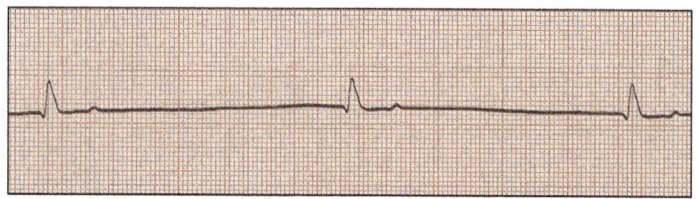

Figure 5.57 Marked hyperkalemia (serum K$^+$,10.5 mEq/L) in a dog with hypoadrenocorticism caused bradycardia, loss of P waves, peaked (tented) but tiny T waves, and delayed ventricular activation. Lead II, 50 mm/s, 1 cm = 1 mV.

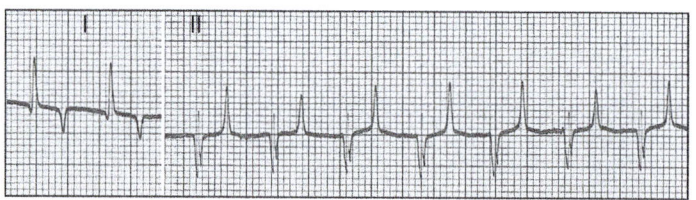

Figure 5.58 Leads I & II from a male cat with urethral obstruction. Serum K$^+$ was 10.2 mEq/L. Calibration 2 cm = 1mV, 25 mm/s.

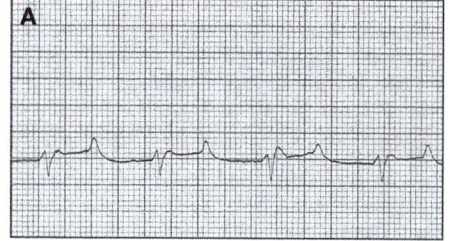
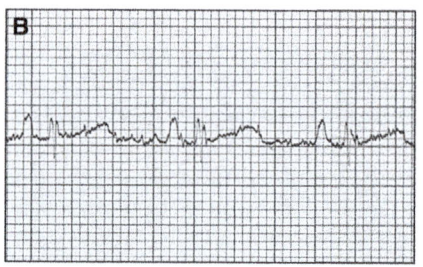

Figure 5.59 (A) ECG from a male cat with urethral obstruction (serum K$^+$ not available). (B) Eight hours post-treatment in the same cat, sinus rhythm and normal P waves are evident; the QRS complexes and T waves also appear normal. Some muscle tremor artifact is present in this strip. Lead II, 50 mm/s, 1 cm = 1 mV.

administration should be discontinued because these can indicate hypercalcemia.

Hypokalemia Hypokalemia could increase spontaneous automaticity of cardiac cells, as well as nonuniformly slow repolarization and conduction. These effects predispose to supraventricular and ventricular arrhythmias. Hypokalemia can cause progressive ST segment depression, reduced (or increased) T wave amplitude, QT interval prolongation, and the appearance of U waves (a low-voltage wave following the T wave that usually is not evident; it might indicate delayed Purkinje fiber or other myocardial cell repolarization). Severe hypokalemia also can increase QRS and P wave amplitudes and durations, as well as lead to bradycardia, AV block, and cardiac arrest. Hypokalemia exacerbates digoxin toxicity and reduces the effectiveness of class I antiarrhythmic agents (Chapter 24). Hypernatremia and alkalosis worsen the effects of hypokalemia on the heart. Concurrent magnesium deficiency might exacerbate the effects of and interfere with correction of hypokalemia.

Common ECG Artifacts

Artifacts complicate ECG interpretation and can mimic arrhythmias. Some common ECG artifacts are illustrated (**Figures 5.60–5.65**). Electrical interference can be minimized or eliminated by properly grounding the ECG machine. Turning off other electrical equipment or lights on the same circuit, placing the animal on an electrically insulated pad, or having a different person restrain the animal might help also. ECG artifacts sometimes are confused with arrhythmias. However, artifacts do not disturb the underlying cardiac rhythm. In contrast, ectopic complexes often disrupt the underlying rhythm and they are followed by a T wave. Determining whether the ECG deflection in question changes the underlying rhythm and also is followed by a T wave usually allows the clinician to differentiate between intermittent artifacts and arrhythmias. Recording more than one lead simultaneously for comparison is helpful, as well.

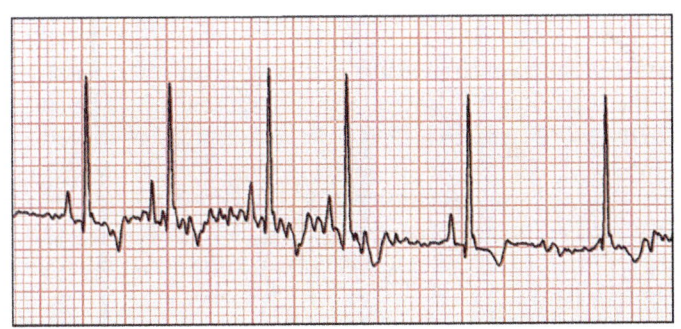

Figure 5.60 Intermittent muscle tremor (shiver) artifact in a dog with sinus arrhythmia and wandering pacemaker. Lead II, 25 mm/s, 1 cm = 1 mV.

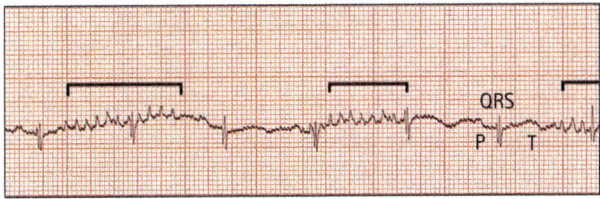

Figure 5.61 Sinus rhythm with purr artifact (brackets) and mild 60-Hz interference (seen best superimposed on P and T waves and baseline segments in between) from a cat with cardiomyopathy. Lead II, 50 mm/s, 1 cm = 1 mV.

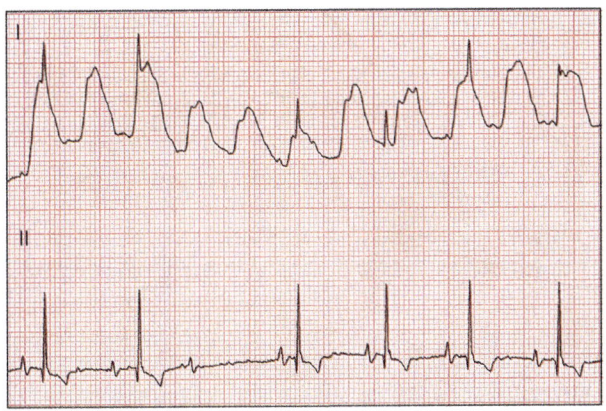

Figure 5.62 Simultaneous leads I and II ECG recording from a dog. Left limb movement caused by the dog's panting obscures the rhythm in lead I; however, lead II clearly shows sinus arrhythmia with one nonconducted P wave (Mobitz I, Wenckebach, second-degree AV block). 25 mm/s, 1 cm = 1 mV.

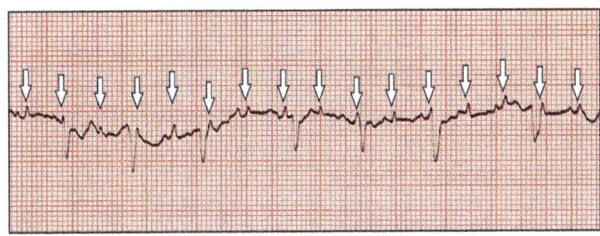

Figure 5.63 ECG from a 9-year-old cat with hypertrophic cardiomyopathy, moderate pericardial effusion, and multiple myeloma. The large negative deflections could be mistaken for ventricular ectopic complexes; however, closer inspection reveals no accompanying T waves and no disruption of the underlying sinus rhythm. The negative deflections occurred when the cat moved its leg. Arrows indicate sinus QRS complexes. Lead III, 25 m/s, 1 cm = 1 mV.

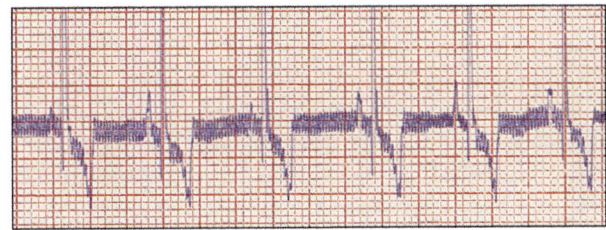

Figure 5.64 Sixty-Hz (electrical) interference is evident in the baseline of this lead aVF ECG from a dog with sinus rhythm. 25 mm/s, 1 cm = 1 mV.

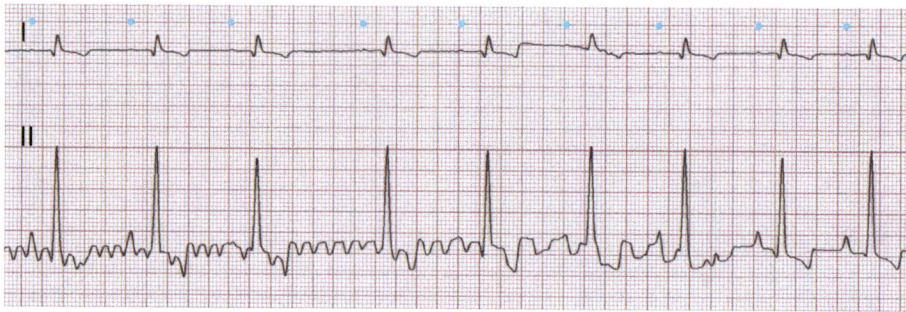

Figure 5.65 Prominent baseline artifact in lead II (bottom) in the first part of this ECG strip from a dog could be mistaken for atrial flutter. However, lead I shows no artifact and sinus P waves (indicated by blue dots) are present throughout. 50 mm/s, 1 cm = 1 mV.

Ambulatory ECG

Holter Monitoring

Holter monitoring provides a continuous recording of cardiac electrical activity during normal daily activities, exercise, and sleep. Intermittent cardiac arrhythmias can be detected and quantified, and cardiac causes of syncope or episodic weakness can be identified (Chapter 8). Holter monitoring also is used to assess efficacy of antiarrhythmic drug therapy, and to screen for arrhythmias associated with cardiomyopathy or other diseases. Measures of heart rate variability during periods of sinus rhythm can be derived from Holter recordings, as well. Time-domain, Frequency-domain, and Poincaré plot analyses provide information on underlying sympathetic and vagal influence. See section "Suggested Additional Reading and References" and the online bibliography for more information about heart rate variability assessment. The Holter monitor is a small battery-powered recorder worn by the patient, typically for 24 hours. Two or three ECG channels are recorded from modified chest leads. During the recording period, the animal's activities should be noted in a patient diary for later correlation with simultaneous ECG events. An event button on the Holter recorder can be pressed if syncope or other episode is witnessed. Newer devices are single, flat electrode patches that have a low profile and require less bandaging.

The digitized Holter recording is analyzed using computer algorithms that classify the recorded complexes. Because fully automated computer analysis can result in significant misclassification of QRS complexes and artifacts from veterinary patient recordings, review and editing by a trained Holter technician experienced with veterinary recordings are important for accurate analysis. A summary report, with selected and enlarged portions of the recording incorporated, is produced for examination by the clinician. In addition, a full disclosure report of the entire recording should be visually scanned and compared with the selected ECG strips, as well as with the times of clinical signs or activities noted in the patient diary (**Figure 5.66**; see section "Suggested Additional Reading and References" and the online bibliography for more information). Holter monitoring equipment and analysis are available through commercial Holter scanning services, university veterinary teaching hospitals, and cardiology specialty practices.

Normal animals can experience wide variation in HR throughout the day. Maximum sinus rates up to 300 beats/minute have been recorded in some dogs during excitement or strenuous activity. Episodes of bradycardia (<50 beats/minute) are common, especially during quiet periods and sleep; HRs of 20–30 beats/minute (or even lower) have been recorded in normal dogs. Sinus arrhythmia, sinus pauses (sometimes for over 5 seconds), and occasional second-degree AV block also can occur in normal dogs, especially at times when the mean HR is low. In normal cats, HRs also vary widely over 24 hours (from below 70 to over 290 beats/minute). While regular sinus rhythm often predominates in normal cats, sinus arrhythmia is evident at slower HRs. VPCs occur only sporadically in normal dogs and cats, although a slight increase in prevalence is likely with age. There is considerable debate regarding the number of VPCs considered "normal" for a dog or a specific breed in 24 hours.

Cardiac Event Recording

External cardiac event monitors are small loop recorders that can store brief periods of a single modified chest lead ECG within their microprocessor's memory. They can be worn for longer time periods than Holter monitors; however, they cannot store prolonged, continuous ECG activity as the Holter recorder can. Event recorders are used most often to discern whether episodic weakness or syncope is caused by a cardiac arrhythmia (Chapter 8). When an episode is observed, the owner must activate the recorder, which then stores the ECG from a predetermined time frame (usually from 45 seconds before activation to 15 seconds after). The stored recordings are sent via telephone to a receiving station for downloading and analysis.

Implantable loop recorders provide a means of monitoring heart rhythm for several months, without the skin irritation, mobility limitations, and artifact from lead wire or electrode movement that can be problematic with external

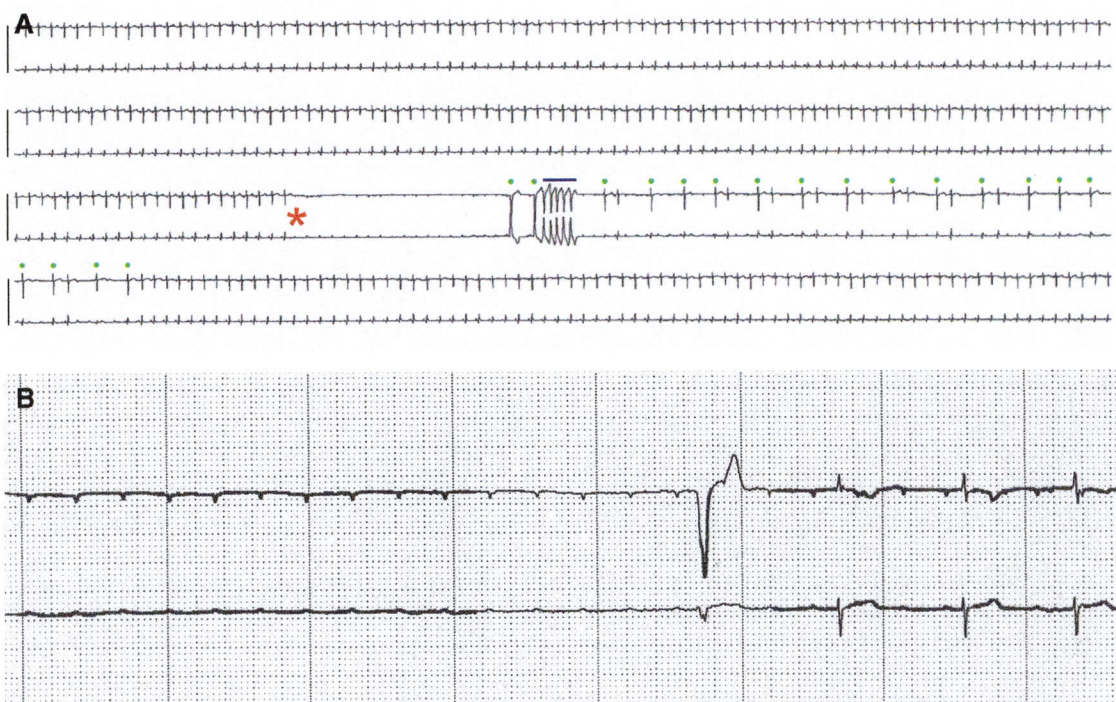

Figure 5.66 (A) Portion of a two-channel, full-disclosure Holter recording from a 14-year-old domestic shorthair cat with syncope. The segment shown was recorded a couple minutes before midnight. Vertical black bars on the left indicate the paired, simultaneously recorded ECG channels. The first two sets of lines show that the cat was in sinus rhythm. On the third pair of lines, AV conduction abruptly ceases (red asterisk) although regular P waves continue. About 6 seconds later, two ventricular escape complexes appear (first two green dots), followed by a brief paroxysm of ventricular tachycardia (blue bar). Additional ventricular escape complexes (green dots) follow, although intermittent AV conduction also occurs (unmarked QRS complexes). On the bottom line, four ventricular escape complexes occur before normal AV conduction resumes. (B) A brief segment of the same Holter recording, from a different time of day, again shows complete (third-degree) AV block. Only P waves are present initially until a ventricular escape complex appears. The last three QRS complexes shown represent a different ventricular escape focus.

ambulatory ECG monitoring. The small (~2 × 5 cm) device is surgically implanted subcutaneously on the left chest, overlying and aligned with the axis of the heart; sedation and local anesthesia often are adequate for implantation, although some animals might require general anesthesia. Newer devices are much smaller (somewhat larger than a microchip), and are implanted using a loader under conscious sedation with a local block and only a small stab incision in the skin. These devices can be used for ECG monitoring for 2–3 years. The ECG, recorded from two electrodes on the casing of the device, is held in a temporary memory buffer, similar to external event recorders, until manual or automatic activation triggers storage of an ECG segment into more permanent, but still limited, memory. A compatible pacemaker programmer is needed to set parameters for activation and the duration of ECG saved before and after activation (within available limits); the programmer also is used to download recorded ECG segments for evaluation. Automatic activation is triggered by "bradycardia," "tachycardia," and "asystole," according to preset determinants for rate and number of detected heartbeats. A dedicated external activator device can be used to manually activate the ECG save function whenever syncope or another event is observed. Manual, compared to automatic, activation appears to be much more effective for identifying arrhythmias associated with syncope in animals.

Smartphone and Other Wireless ECG Recordings

A small handheld ECG recording device (Kardia Mobile, AliveCor Inc., Mountain View, CA; or AliveCor Veterinary Heart Monitor) connected by Bluetooth to a smartphone with the correlated app allows brief, intermittent ECG rhythm recordings to be obtained quickly, either in-clinic or by the animal's owner at home or in the field. A pdf file of the recording can be sent via email to the clinician. The device is positioned directly on the patient's left chest, aligned with the heart, after parting the haircoat and wetting the electrode sites with alcohol (**Figure 12.8**, p. 244). Some clinicians also have obtained good recordings by fastening a lead wire to each electrode plate and connecting to the patient with alligator clip electrodes. HR and cardiac rhythm diagnosis obtained from smartphone ECG recordings correlate closely with standard 6-lead ECG recordings in most cases. Smartphone ECG recording also can be useful for arrhythmia screening in horses. In this species, recording from both sides of the thorax has been recommended because P wave definition appears to be better from the right thorax, while the diagnostic quality of QRS and QT intervals is likely to be better from the left thorax (Corradini, 2020). Poor electrode contact and patient movement can impair waveform recognition and create artifacts during smartphone ECG recording. When an arrhythmia is suspected but not clearly defined or the nature of the underlying rhythm is in doubt, it is important to obtain a standard (or other ambulatory) ECG recording to verify the rhythm.

In-hospital ECG telemetry, where available, is another method for continuous or intermittent rhythm monitoring within a limited distance. Wireless ECG patch monitoring systems also have been developed for use in people; these either store ECG data for later analysis or perform real-time analysis and transmission. One system described recently in dogs and cats uses two precordial electrodes with an attached battery-powered electronic sensor, which communicates with an android smart device via Bluetooth technology (Brloznik, 2019). Because the ECG data are stored on the android device, continuous Bluetooth coupling is necessary. Although excessive motion artifact during strenuous activity is problematic, continuous ECG monitoring for several days is possible.

Exercise ECG in Horses

ECG recordings made during and immediately following exercise can provide important information about heart rate and rhythm in horses used for athletic work. This is particularly relevant for animals with persistent AF that cannot be converted to sinus rhythm, or that have a history of transient AF, intermittent premature beats, reduced exercise performance, episodic weakness, or abnormal cardiac structure. An exercise ECG also would be prudent during prepurchase evaluation when a pathologic murmur or unexpected arrhythmia is discovered. Besides documenting the peak HR achieved and the effects of exercise on cardiac rhythm, exercise testing can reveal change in murmurs heard during examination at rest, as well as rhythm abnormalities that occur during postexercise recovery. Additionally, pre- and postexercise echocardiography, if available, could demonstrate an exercise-induced change in cardiac function. Pre- and postexercise measurement of cardiac troponin I might be useful in some cases. Nevertheless, although exercise ECG testing can alert the clinician to potentially serious cardiac rhythm disturbances, it is important to note that the overall sensitivity, specificity, and reliability of such testing for predicting serious future arrhythmias and identifying underlying heart disease are not fully characterized. In addition, exercise ECG testing is not appropriate for some horses, including those with congestive heart failure, severe valvular disease complicated by AF, complex ventricular tachyarrhythmias, markedly reduced ventricular contractile function, or pulmonary hypertension.

Exercise ECG testing can be done using a high-speed treadmill, at a racetrack, or during other field exercise. The ECG is usually recorded by telemetry, Holter monitor, or potentially with a standard ECG machine (during treadmill exercise). An exercise ECG, in contrast to use of an HR monitor alone, can reveal the occurrence of specific arrhythmias in addition to HR changes. Lunging exercise provides a lower-intensity workout, although that might provide some useful information. However, an exercise intensity similar to or greater than what is required for the horse's normal or desired work is usually better, especially when the animal's performance suffers only during peak effort. For horses with a history (or increased risk) of collapse, a high-speed treadmill should be used for testing, to avoid injury to a rider. Providing an additional sudden and unexpected sympathetic stimulation can be useful because it could uncover an inappropriately rapid HR, abnormal intracardiac conduction, and sympathetic-induced arrhythmias.

HR acceleration occurs as exercise begins; the HR should stabilize at a level appropriate for the work intensity. An unexpectedly high HR could indicate underlying disease involving the cardiac, pulmonary or musculoskeletal systems, or it might instead indicate an inadequate level of fitness. General guidelines for normal horses exercising on level ground include HR ranges of 70–140 beats/minute at the trot, 120–160 beats/minute at the canter, 150–180 beats/minute at a gallop, and >180 beats/minute at a hard gallop (Schwarzwald, 2018). Exercise on an incline increases these HR ranges. Maximum HR reached is usually between 210 and 240 beats/minute, although young horses might exceed this. As HR increases, the conduction intervals shorten and marked ST-T wave alterations commonly develop. Various arrhythmias can occur during exercise. While occasional premature complexes might not be concerning, the development of AF or an ectopic tachycardia is abnormal. Such arrhythmias could underlie reduced performance during high-intensity exercise. Ventricular tachyarrhythmias induced by exercise could cause collapse or even sudden death. Sudden-onset AF has caused collapse in sporadic cases, also. QRS widening during exercise and ventricular tachyarrhythmias with R-on-T timing could indicate underlying myocardial disease and electrical instability. Those findings appear to be more common in horses with a history of AF. The risk for sudden death might be higher in horses with AF and exercise-induced ventricular tachyarrhythmias.

Upon stopping exercise, the HR usually falls below 100 beats/minute within about 5 minutes. Following a period of sustained maximal exercise intensity, complete recovery to normal resting HR could take up to an hour. Multiple factors can influence the rate of HR recovery, including environmental temperature and humidity, as well as the animal's fitness level, temperament, and underlying cardiac health. Various arrhythmias could occur in the immediate postexercise period. Sinus arrhythmia, along with first- or second-degree AV block, usually is related to changes in vagal tone and likely not of clinical concern. The clinical relevance of isolated premature complexes that occur only in the postexercise period is unclear. However, the development of AF, supraventricular tachycardia, or ventricular tachycardia at any time during exercise testing is abnormal.

Suggested Additional Reading and References

Also See Online Comprehensive Bibliography at: https://www.routledge.com/9781482246223.

Blake RR, Shaw DJ, Culshaw GJ, et al. Poincare plots as a measure of heart rate variability in healthy dogs. J Vet Cardiol 2018;20:20–32.

Brložnik M, Likar Š, Krvavica A, et al. Wireless body sensor for electrocardiographic monitoring in dogs and cats. J Small Anim Pract 2019;60:223–230.

Carnabuci C, Tognetti R, Vezzosi T, et al. Left shift of the ventricular mean electrical axis in healthy Doberman Pinschers. J Vet Med Sci 2019;81:620–625.

Coleman MG, Robson MC. Evaluation of six-lead electrocardiograms obtained from dogs in a sitting position or sternal recumbency. Am J Vet Res 2005;66:233–237.

Corradini I, Fernandez-Ruiz A, Barba M, et al. Stall-side screening potential of a smartphone electrocardiogram recorded over both sides of the thorax in horses. J Vet Intern Med 2020.

Côté E, Richter K, Charuvastra E. Event-based cardiac monitoring in small animal practice. Compend Contin Educ Pract Vet 1999;21:1025–1033.

Couroucé-Malblanc A, van Erck-Westergren E. Exercise testing in the field. In, Hinchcliff KW, Kaneps AJ, Geor RJ (editors). Equine Sports Medicine and Surgery. Saunders Elsevier, Edinburgh. 2014.

Decloedt A, de Clercq D, van der Vekens N, et al. Noninvasive determination of atrial fibrillation cycle length by atrial colour tissue Doppler imaging in horses. Equine Vet J 2014;46:174–179.

DeProspero DJ, Adin DB. Visual representations of canine cardiac arrhythmias with Lorenz (Poincare) plots. Am J Vet Res 2020;81:720–731.

Durando M. Exercise and stress testing. In, Marr CM (editor). Cardiology of the Horse. Saunders Elsevier, Edinburgh. 2010.

Epstein V. Relationship between potassium administration, hyperkalaemia and the electrocardiogram: an experimental study. Equine Vet J 1984;16:453–456.

Ferasin L, Amodio A, Murray JK. Validation of 2 techniques for electrocardiographic recording in dogs and cats. J Vet Intern Med 2006;20:873–876.

Flethoj M, Kanters JK, Haugaard MM, et al. Changes in heart rate, arrhythmia frequency, and cardiac biomarker values in horses during recovery after a long-distance endurance ride. J Am Vet Med Assoc 2016;248:1034–1042.

Fossa AA, Zhou M. Assessing QT prolongation and electrocardiography restitution using a beat-to-beat method. Cardiol J 2010;17:230–243.

Frick L, Schwarzwald CC, Mitchell KJ. The use of heart rate variability analysis to detect arrhythmias in horses undergoing a standard treadmill exercise test. J Vet Intern Med 2019;33:212–224.

Gattland L, Holmes JR. ECG recording at rest and during exercise in the horse. Equine Vet Educ 1990;2:28.

Hall LW, Dunn JK, Delaney M, et al. Ambulatory electrocardiography in dogs. Vet Rec 1991;129:213–216.

Hanas S, Tidholm A, Egenvall A, et al. Twenty-four-hour Holter monitoring of unsedated healthy cats in the home environment. J Vet Cardiol 2009;11:17–22.

Harvey AM, Faena M, Darke PG, et al. Effect of body position on feline electrocardiographic recordings. J Vet Intern Med 2005;19:533–536.

Hiraga A, Sugano S. History of research in Japan on electrocardiography in the racehorse. J Equine Sci 2015;26:1–13.

Holmes JR. Electrocardiography in the diagnosis of common cardiac arrythmias in the horse. Equine Vet Educ 1990;2:24.

Kraus MS, Gelzer AR, Rishniw M. Detection of heart rate and rhythm with a smartphone-based electrocardiograph versus a reference standard electrocardiograph in dogs and cats. J Am Vet Med Assoc 2016;249:189–194.

Lamb AP, Meurs KM, Hamlin RL. Correlation of heart rate to body weight in apparently normal dogs. J Vet Cardiol 2010;12:107–110.

Lee PM, Brown RHT. Establishing 24-hour Holter reference intervals for clinically healthy puppies. Res Vet Sci 2019;125:253–255.

MacKie BA, Stepien RL, Kellihan HB. Retrospective analysis of an implantable loop recorder for evaluation of syncope, collapse, or intermittent weakness in 23 dogs (2004–2008). J Vet Cardiol 2010;12:25–33.

Meurs KM, Spier AW, Wright NA, et al. Use of ambulatory electrocardiography for detection of ventricular premature complexes in healthy dogs. J Am Vet Med Assoc 2001;218:1291–1292.

Mitchell KJ. Equine electrocardiography. Vet Clin North Am Equine Pract 2019;35:65–83.

Navas de Solis C. Cardiovascular response to exercise and training, exercise testing in horses. Vet Clin North Am Equine Pract 2019;35:159–173.

Oyama MA, Kraus MS, Gelzer AR. Rapid Review of ECG Interpretation in Small Animal Practice. CRC Press, Boca Raton, FL. 2014.

Pedersen PJ, Karlsson M, Flethoj M, et al. Differences in the electrocardiographic QT interval of various breeds of athletic horses during rest and exercise. J Vet Cardiol 2016;18:255–264.

Perego M, Ramera L, Santilli RA. Isorhythmic atrioventricular dissociation in Labrador retrievers. J Vet Intern Med 2012;26:320–325.

Petrie JP. Practical application of Holter monitoring in dogs and cats. Clin Tech Small Anim Pract 2005;20:173–181.

Physick-Sheard PW, McGurrin MK. Ventricular arrhythmias during race recovery in Standardbred racehorses and associations with autonomic activity. J Vet Intern Med 2010;24:1158.

Reef VB, Bonagura J, Buhl R, et al. Recommendations for management of equine athletes with cardiovascular abnormalities. J Vet Intern Med 2014;28:749–761.

Rishniw M, Porciello F, Erb HN, et al. Effect of body position on the 6-lead ECG of dogs. J Vet Intern Med 2002;16:69–73.

Ryan N, Marr CM, McGladdery AJ. Survey of cardiac arrhythmias during submaximal and maximal exercise in Thoroughbred racehorses. Equine Vet J 2005;37:265–268.

Santilli RA, Ferasin L, Voghera SG, et al. Evaluation of the diagnostic value of an implantable loop recorder in dogs with unexplained syncope. J Am Vet Med Assoc 2010;236:78–82.

Santilli RA, Perego M, Crosara S, et al. Utility of 12-lead electrocardiogram for differentiating paroxysmal supraventricular tachycardias in dogs. J Vet Intern Med 2008;22:915–923.

Santilli RA, Perego M, Perini A, et al. Electrophysiologic characteristics and topographic distribution of focal atrial tachycardias in dogs. J Vet Intern Med 2010;24:539–545.

Santilli RA, Spadacini G, Moretti P, et al. Anatomic distribution and electrophysiologic properties of accessory atrioventricular pathways in dogs. J Am Vet Med Assoc 2007;231:393–398.

Schwarzwald CC. Disorders of the cardiovascular system. In, Reed SM, Bayly WM, Sellon DC (editors). Equine Internal Medicine. 4th edition. Elsevier, St. Louis, MO. 2018. pp. 387–541.

Schwarzwald CC, Kedo M, Birkmann K, et al. Relationship of heart rate and electrocardiographic time intervals to body mass in horses and ponies. J Vet Cardiol 2012;14:343–350.

SCST, Clinical Guidelines by Consensus: Recording a standard 12-lead electrocardiogram. Review date June 2017. https://www.bmj.com/sites/default/files/response_attachments/2016/09/CAC_SCST_Recording_a_12-lead_ECG_final_version_2014_CS2v2.0.pdf

Shaffer F, Ginsberg JP. An overview of heart rate variability metrics and norms. Front Public Health 2017;5:258.

Tag TL, Day TK. Electrocardiographic assessment of hyperkalemia in dogs and cats. J Vet Emerg Crit Care 2004;18:61–67.

Verheyen T, Decloedt A, van der Vekens N, et al. Ventricular response during lungeing exercise in horses with lone atrial fibrillation. Equine Vet J 2013;45:309–314.

Vezzosi T, Buralli C, Marchesotti F, et al. Diagnostic accuracy of a smartphone electrocardiograph in dogs: comparison with standard 6-lead electrocardiography. Vet J 2016;216:33–37.

Vezzosi T, Tognetti R, Buralli C, et al. Home monitoring of heart rate and heart rhythm with a smartphone-based ECG in dogs. Vet Rec 2019;184:96.

Vezzosi T, Vitale V, Sgorbini M, et al. Two methods for 24-hour Holter monitoring in horses: evaluation of recording performance at rest and during exercise. J Equine Vet Sci 2019;79:127–130.

Vibe-Petersen G, Nielsen K. Electrocardiography in the horse. (A report of findings in 138 horses.) Nord Vet Med 1980;32:105–121.

Ware WA. Twenty-four-hour ambulatory electrocardiography in normal cats. J Vet Intern Med 1999;13:175–180.

Ware WA, Reina-Doreste Y, Stern JA, et al. Sudden death associated with QT interval prolongation and KCNQ1 Gene mutation in a family of English springer spaniels. J Vet Intern Med 2015;29:561–568.

Wright KN, Connor CE, Irvin HM, et al. Atrioventricular accessory pathways in 89 dogs: clinical features and outcome after radiofrequency catheter ablation. J Vet Intern Med 2018;32:1517–1529.

Zucca E, Ferrucci F, Di Fabio V, et al. The use of electrocardiographic recording with Holter monitoring during treadmill exercise to evaluate cardiac arrhythmias in racehorses. Vet Res Commun 2003;27(Suppl 1):811–814.

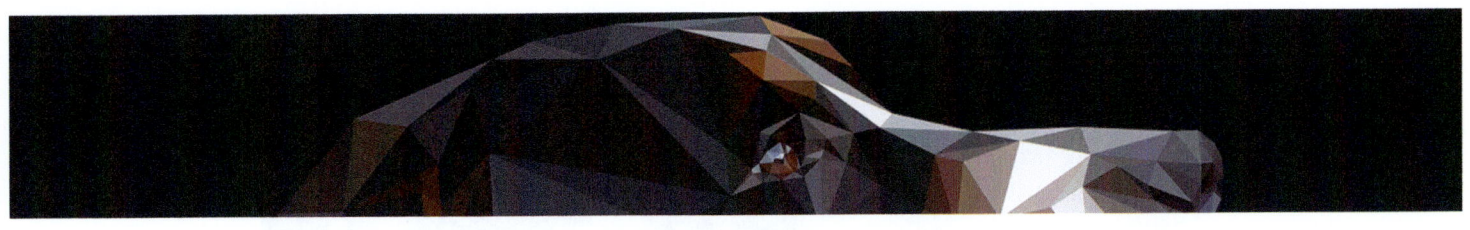

6

CARDIAC CATHETERIZATION AND ANGIOCARDIOGRAPHY

Contributed by Brian A. Scansen

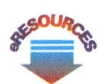

General Considerations

Cardiac catheterization involves the insertion of sheaths, catheters, guide wires, and devices into the cardiovascular (CV) system to directly measure pressures and evaluate flow (hemodynamics), sample oxygen content or saturation (oximetry), or selectively inject contrast agents to outline and characterize vascular and cardiac structures (angiocardiography). Catheterization of most organ systems was performed by the Egyptians, Greeks, and Romans and is by no means a modern invention. It was not until the evolution of radiography, from a novelty in the late 1800s to a diagnostic subspecialty by the early twentieth century, that the two techniques of catheterization and radiographic imaging were combined in order to visualize the gastrointestinal, renal, and CV systems in animals and people. Until the 1980s, angiocardiography and cardiac catheterization were done solely for diagnostic purposes; this remained the gold standard for characterizing CV disease until the advent of echocardiography, especially Doppler modalities. Today, purely diagnostic catheterizations are performed rarely because noninvasive tests such as echocardiography, computed tomography (CT), and magnetic resonance imaging (MRI) can provide a rapid and accurate diagnosis in most cases.

Interventional cardiology represents an additional step in the evolution of radiography and catheterization. Interventional cardiology is the subspecialty of CV medicine that affects a therapeutic outcome through minimally invasive catheterization of peripheral blood vessels or body orifices, while guided by imaging. Examples include balloon dilation of stenotic valves or other lesions; coil, particle, or device occlusion of anomalous vessels or diseased vascular beds; stent implantation for narrowed or obstructed lumens; biopsy or extraction of tumors or foreign material; drainage or infusion catheter placement for medicinal or nutritional support; and others.

Catheterization studies within the heart and vasculature require detailed knowledge of the equipment used and the technical skills of catheterization, as well as a thorough understanding of thoracic and CV anatomy. Additional skills and anatomic knowledge are required to effectively plan an intervention, select appropriate equipment, verify that the intervention is being done at the correct site during the procedure, and troubleshoot unexpected findings or complications. This chapter provides an overview of catheterization techniques and a framework for interpretating hemodynamic and angiocardiographic studies discussed in subsequent chapters.

Cardiovascular Catheterization

Preparation and Planning

The catheterization laboratory should provide a sterile environment for interventional procedures, along with storage space for related supplies (including various catheters, wires, and devices). Equipment needed for cardiac catheterization procedures also includes high-quality fluoroscopic imaging (optimally with rotational capability or biplane features), a portable ultrasound machine (for vascular access and transesophageal echocardiography, TEE), a power injector (for rapid delivery of iodinated contrast), anesthetic and hemodynamic monitoring equipment (including for intravascular pressure recording), an adequate number of monitors (for

Cardiovascular Disease in Companion Animals

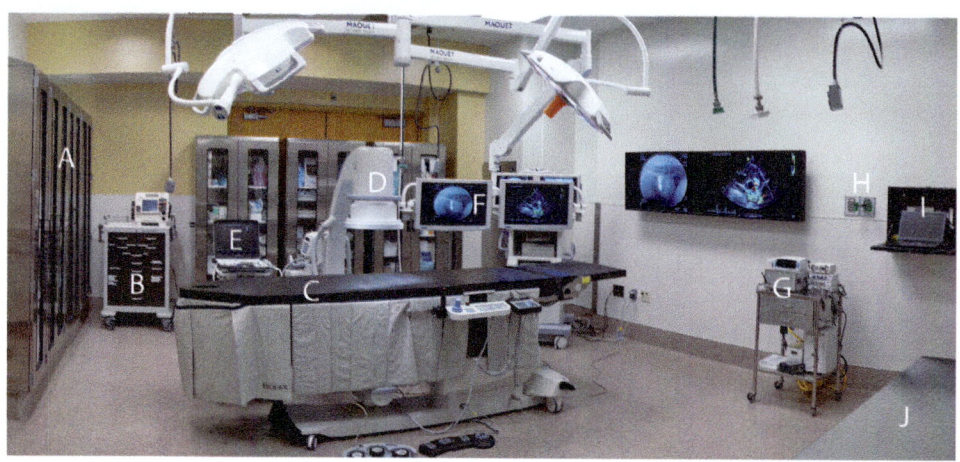

Figure 6.1 A catheterization laboratory ideally would contain: (A) adequate storage space for catheters, wires, and devices; (B) a crash cart with defibrillator and emergency medications; (C) a radiolucent table; (D) a fluoroscopic C-arm; (E) a transesophageal echocardiography system; (F) moveable monitors that can be positioned within view of the operator; (G) hemodynamic recording equipment; (H) an oxygen source for anesthetic equipment; (I) a computer terminal for charting and access to the electronic record and archived patient images; and (J) a table for laying out sterile equipment and supplies. Not shown is a power injector, for controlled and rapid injections of contrast.

visualizing live images and hemodynamic parameters), and a crash cart with a cardioverter-defibrillator and supplies for emergency intervention (**Figure 6.1**).

Properly trained personnel are as important in the catheterization laboratory as the technical equipment. Interventional procedures typically are performed by veterinary specialists with advanced training. The operator should have thorough understanding of the disease process that the intervention is targeting, the imaging modality being used, and the equipment and techniques required for successful intervention. A veterinary technician should be designated to oversee organization, inventory, and maintenance of the catheterization suite and its equipment. This person should be available during all catheterization procedures to prepare the patient and equipment, aid in hemodynamic recording and image review or measurement, and efficiently provide the operator with catheters, devices, and other supplies as needed throughout the intervention. The catheterization technician should be familiar with all commonly used equipment and, ideally, could be a resource to help troubleshoot options if a case requires alternative approaches. Separate from the catheterization technician, it is important to have a skilled anesthetist proficient in CV diseases of animals who can maintain patient stability and comfort throughout the procedure and recovery process.

Prior to any procedure, a complete diagnostic and therapeutic plan should be devised, taking into consideration the expected findings and equipment likely to be needed based upon pre-catheterization imaging studies. All potential complications should be anticipated, with an emergent strategy identified for each possible obstacle. This plan should be reviewed with all members of the team, especially the secondary operator, catheterization technician, and anesthetist. The client should be informed of the potential risks of the procedure, as well as the expected outcome, and consent obtained.

Equipment

Imaging Most catheterization procedures require fluoroscopic guidance. Desirable features of the fluoroscopic system include digital archiving, high resolution imaging (optimally a 1024 × 1024 or 2048 × 2048 matrix), sufficient energy generation to penetrate the thorax and abdomen of a large dog, ability to display and record fast frame rates (25–30 frames per second or higher), and capability for electronic magnification, digital subtraction and road-mapping. Fluoroscopic systems can be portable (requiring only a standard electrical outlet), or large fixed systems with separate power supply. Higher-quality imaging and advanced capabilities are available on the fixed systems, albeit at higher cost. Fluoroscopes employ either an analog image intensifier or a digital flat panel detector to generate the image. Advantages of flat panel detectors over image-intensifiers include lack of geometric distortion, a uniform response across the field-of-view, and a smaller size of the detector which improves access to the patient. Most veterinary fluoroscopic systems in use today are image intensifier-based systems; however, flat panel detector technology is available in some academic and tertiary care centers. Many human catheterization laboratories employ biplane fluoroscopic systems that provide real-time imaging of two orthogonal views to improve anatomic guidance. New generation fluoroscopic systems also can perform rotational angiography to circumferentially record a single injection from all angles and create a three-dimensional reconstruction of the anatomy, allowing selection of the optimal angle to guide intervention. Finally, some systems have the capability of importing anatomic landmarks from cross-sectional imaging

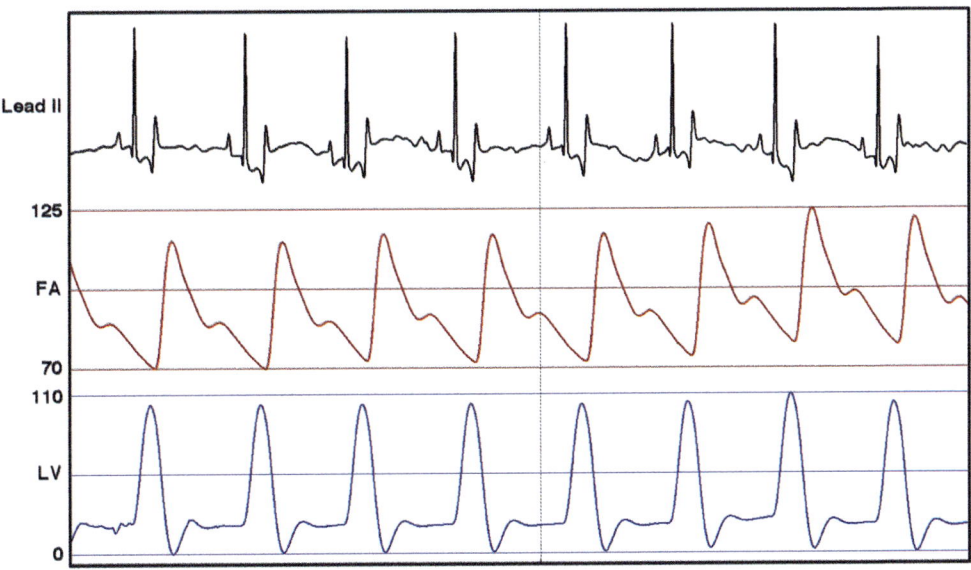

Figure 6.2 Simultaneous lead II electrocardiogram (top tracing), and pressures recorded from the femoral artery (FA; middle tracing) and left ventricle (LV; bottom tracing) in a normal dog. Pressure scale (mm Hg) is on the left (middle and bottom tracings). Note the normal dicrotic notch (incisura) in the FA pressure wave. The LV pressure falls to near zero in diastole.

studies (CT or MRI) or real-time echocardiographic imaging onto the live two-dimensional fluoroscopic image to improve guidance during the intervention.

Ultrasound capability, with both vascular and TEE probes, is desired in the catheterization laboratory. Ultrasound guidance during percutaneous vascular access can be useful and minimizes complications of vascular catheterization. TEE aids in catheter and device placement within the heart or adjacent great vessels, and in monitoring an intervention's success in real-time.

Hemodynamic Monitoring Changes in intracardiac hemodynamics guide many cardiac interventions, including the pressure gradient across a stenosis or alterations in ventricular function. The ability to monitor intravascular and intracardiac pressures, as well as cardiac rhythm, is important during cardiac catheterization and intervention (**Figures 6.2** and **6.3**). This could be as simple as an anesthetic monitor or as complex as a dedicated hemodynamic computer station.

The availability of blood gas analysis also is important for some cases, in which oxygen saturation or content

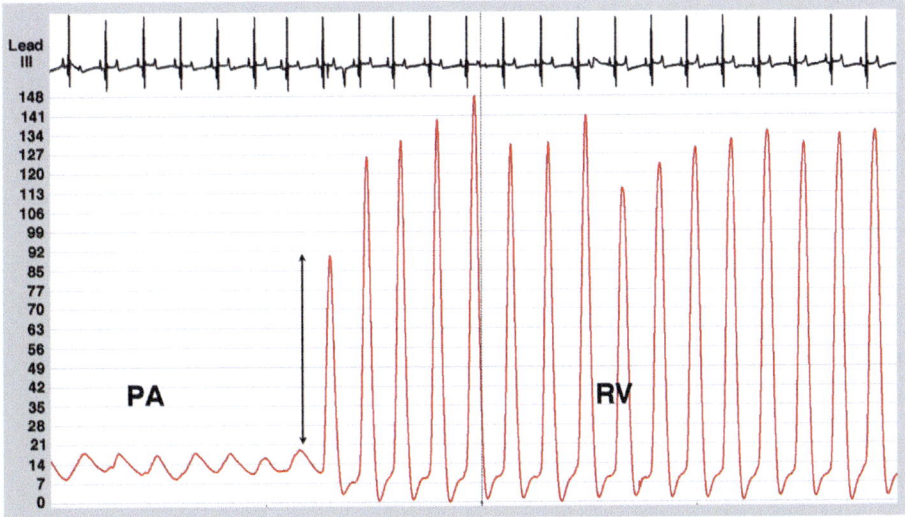

Figure 6.3 Pressure recording with simultaneous lead III electrocardiogram during pullback (of the catheter tip) from pulmonary artery (PA) to right ventricle (RV) in a dog with severe pulmonary valve stenosis. Note the dramatic increase in systolic pressure as the catheter tip crosses the valve (double-headed arrow) into the RV. Pressure scale (mm Hg) on left.

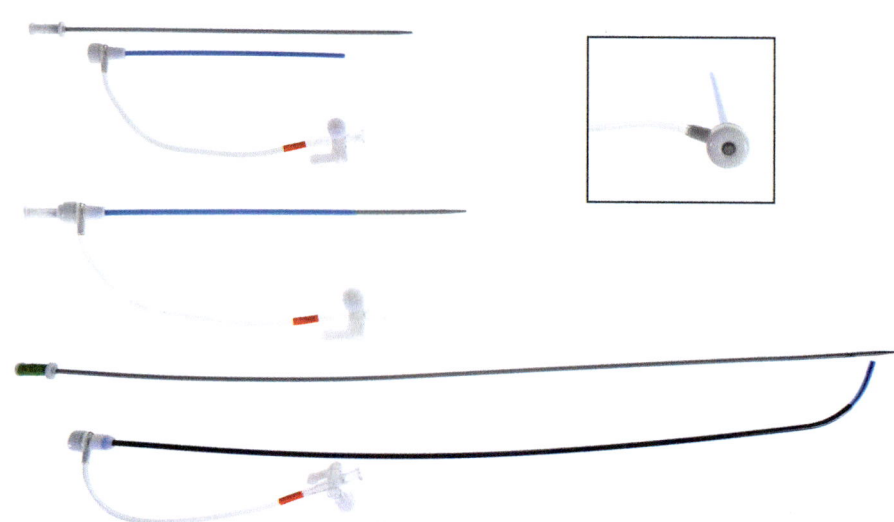

Figure 6.4 Examples of introducer sheaths for vascular access. From top to bottom: A 7-Fr by 13 cm dilator and sheath with side port, the same 7-Fr 13 cm sheath with the dilator in place, and a 7-Fr by 45 cm Ansel dilator and sheath with an angled tip and side port. Inset in upper right corner shows the hemostatic valve at the back of most vascular access sheaths.

measurements are needed for oximetry runs. Although used less commonly now in veterinary medicine, oximetry can reveal an abnormal, localized increase (step-up) or decrease (step-down) in oxygen saturation caused by intracardiac shunting.

Needles, Sheaths, Catheters, and Wires Access to the peripheral vessel during catheterization is gained by placing an introducer sheath, through which catheters, wires, or devices can be safely advanced (**Figure 6.4**). The sheath typically is inserted over a wire, which was directed into the vessel lumen through an access needle or over-the-needle (OTN) catheter (**Figure 6.5**). Sheaths have an inner dilator, which tapers to a known wire diameter; this allows for a smooth transition from wire, to dilator, to outer sheath diameter. Traditionally, 18-gauge or 19-gauge access needles were used in combination with wires of 0.035 in. or 0.038 in. diameter to achieve access. Wires of 0.035 in. diameter can be passed through most 18-gauge OTN catheters. However, whether using an access needle or an OTN catheter, the operator should verify that the desired wire passes easily before gaining access to the vessel or organ. The needle or OTN catheter is placed into the vessel using palpation or ultrasound guidance; placement is verified by a "flash" of blood. When the access needle is within the vessel lumen, a guide wire is advanced to provide a scaffold over which the introducer sheath can be directed. In small animals, vascular access through a microintroducer, a 4-French (Fr) or 5-Fr sheath that tapers to a 0.018 in. guide wire, is a preferred strategy because this allows a smaller gauge access needle (typically 21-gauge or 22-gauge) to be used and causes less trauma to the target vessel. Once a microintroducer is in place, a larger-diameter guide wire can be advanced into the vessel lumen through the microintroducer, which then is exchanged for a conventional introducer sheath of the desired size. A sheath can be short or long, of variable shape depending on the desired procedure, and typically has a hemostatic valve and side port (**Figure 6.4**). The size of an introducer sheath is given by its internal diameter (for example, an 8-Fr sheath has an inner diameter of 8-Fr), in contrast to catheter sizing.

Catheters are long, thin, radiopaque tubes of variable shape and size that allow the operator to access different

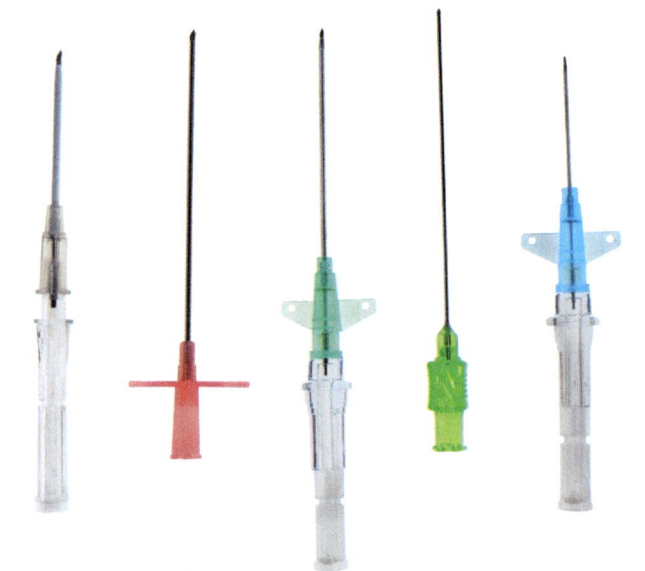

Figure 6.5 Examples of needles and catheters used for percutaneous vascular access. From left to right: 16-gauge over-the-needle (OTN) catheter, 18-gauge arterial access needle, 18-gauge OTN catheter, 21-gauge arterial access needle, and 22-gauge OTN catheter.

body structures under fluoroscopic guidance (**Figure 6.6**). They have a standard luer adaptor on one end for connection to syringes and other medical devices. Although dozens of catheter shapes are available, for a variety of image-guided procedures, most catheterization laboratories stock a limited selection of frequently used shapes and sizes. Examples include catheters with an angled tip of ~45 degrees (Berenstein and multipurpose catheters), a reverse-curve catheter (Chung, left Judkins, and Rösch inferior mesenteric catheters), a double-curve catheter (Cobra and right Judkins catheters), flow-directed catheters with an inflatable balloon on the end (balloon wedge-pressure and Swan-Ganz catheters), and angiographic catheters (Berman and pigtail catheters). Most veterinary procedures are performed through 4-Fr or 5-Fr catheters, although larger-bore catheters up to 8-Fr might be desired for angiographic studies to allow more rapid contrast material administration. Catheters that are smaller than 3-Fr are termed microcatheters; they are highly flexible, which allows access to tortuous or small vessels. While larger catheter sizes generally are stiffer, which improves "pushability" and torque control, this varies by catheter design, material, and manufacturer. Some catheters have a hydrophilic coating to provide a slippery, atraumatic surface when advanced into the body. Catheter size is determined by the outer diameter of the catheter, in contrast to the sizing system for introducer sheaths. That is, a 5-Fr catheter fits through a 5-Fr sheath because the inner diameter of the sheath and outer diameter of the catheter are equivalent. In practice, a sheath one size larger than the desired catheter size allows for greater technical ease. Specialized catheters include balloon dilation catheters.

Catheter advancement into a vessel or other body structure is performed over a guide wire in almost all circumstances because manipulating a guide wire to the desired site for imaging or intervention is easier and safer than direct catheter advancement. After the guide wire has been positioned, the hollow catheter can be advanced over the wire to the target location, using the wire as a "guide." Like catheters, guide wires of variable shape, diameter, stiffness, taper, and composition are available (**Figure 6.7**). Standard guide wires generally are 0.035 in. diameter and 150 or 180 cm long; microwires are those with a diameter of 0.018 in. or less. Exchange-length guide wires are 260 cm or longer; these allow the removal of one catheter and replacement with another catheter over the same wire without losing the position of the guide wire in the body. Traditional guide wires have a stainless steel core of variable stiffness within a stainless steel spring coil, the entirety of which is coated in polytetrafluoroethylene (Teflon); additional heparin coatings commonly are used to reduce thrombogenicity. Newer generations of guide wires have a nitinol core, which is a super elastic alloy that provides good torque control, with greater flexibility and maneuverability compared to stainless steel. Hydrophilic guide wires commonly are employed because their coating is slippery when wet. Hydrophilic guide wires create less friction when inserted into the body, reducing the force required to advance the guide wire and allowing atraumatic catheterization when the anatomy is tortuous. The end, or tip, of a guide wire is preformed by the manufacturer into various shapes that facilitate catheterization, including straight, angled, complex curvature, and J-tipped. Other guide wires have a tip that

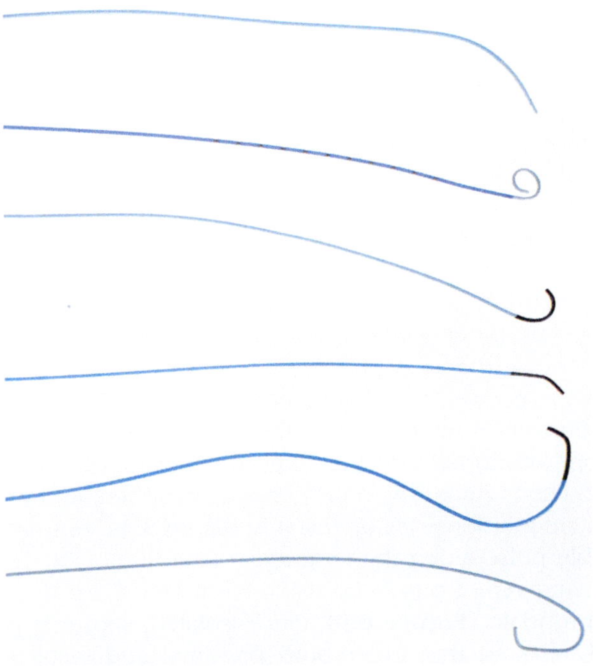

Figure 6.6 Examples of catheter shapes and sizes used during interventional procedures. From top to bottom: 6-Fr NIH, 5-Fr marker pigtail, 5-Fr RIM, 4-Fr Kempe, 5-Fr Cobra hydrophilic and 4-Fr left Judkins catheters. Fr, French (size); NIH, National Institutes of Health; RIM, Rösch inferior mesenteric.

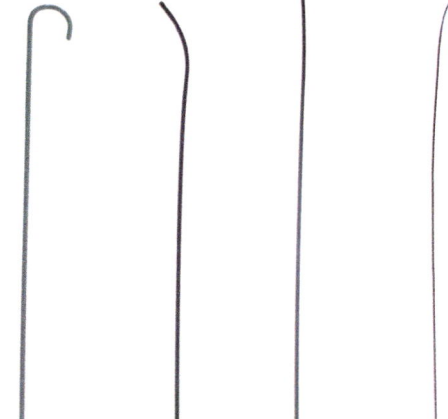

Figure 6.7 Examples of guide wire shapes and diameters used during cardiac catheterization procedures. From left to right: 0.038 in. Teflon-coated stainless steel wire with 3 mm J-tip, 0.035 in. hydrophilic guide wire with angled tip, 0.032 in. hydrophilic guide wire with straight tip, and 0.014 in. stainless steel guide wire with angled tip.

can be manipulated at the time of catheterization into the desired shape. Guide wires with a 45-degree angulation commonly are used to enter ("select") specific vascular branches. J-tipped guide wires are used to provide an atraumatic tip within a vessel lumen or to avoid selection of vascular branch points during advancement. The tip of a guide wire also has a variable taper, meaning the portion of the wire that is floppy prior to reaching the stiff core; many wires have a short taper of 1–3 cm, while others are made with a 10 cm or longer taper. Greater flexibility at the tip can facilitate access of tortuous anatomy; the wire's stiff core is needed to provide a sufficient scaffold over which to advance a catheter. Core stiffness can vary from standard to super-stiff or even ultra-stiff, with varying indications for each representing a compromise between stability for advancement of catheters or devices and stress on the structure catheterized.

When passing catheters into the heart, it always is preferable to cross cardiac valves in the antegrade direction, with a flow-directed (balloon-tipped) catheter or one with a J-tip or pigtail. Potentially, advancing an end-hole catheter across the valve could perforate a valve leaflet, ensnare chordae tendineae, or otherwise damage the valve apparatus. However, a balloon-tipped or pigtail catheter will preferentially enter the true valve orifice and minimize trauma to the valve.

Patient Preparation

Most contrast studies and CV interventional procedures are performed with the animal under general anesthesia and positioned in right or left lateral recumbency. Lateral positioning allows the operator to monitor dorsal-ventral and cranial-caudal motion of catheters and wires as they are advanced into the thorax. Although less common than lateral imaging for cardiac intervention, the ventrodorsal (VD) projection allows visualization of left-to-right laterality and the cranial-caudal position of catheters introduced into the thorax; however, the dorsal-ventral localization of catheters or wires is not possible. Several additional imaging planes could be used to highlight and optimize the imaging of cardiac structures. Variations from the traditional lateral or VD projection typically are identified by an angle, which refers to the position of the radiographic detector in relation to the animal's thorax in a VD position. Commonly used oblique projections in human medicine include the right and left anterior obliques (RAO and LAO, respectively) with variable cranial or caudal angulation. Typically, the image intensifier is rotated a variable number of degrees to the animal's right (RAO) or left (LAO); 10 to 30 degrees of cranial or caudal angulation also might be employed. Altering the angle of the C-arm can elongate structures (such as the left ventricular, LV, outflow tract in subaortic stenosis, SAS) or provide a more directly perpendicular visualization plane during device deployment (for example, of the atrial septum during closure of an atrial septal defect). These viewing angles have not been standardized in veterinary medicine. In practice, adjusting the angle of the C-arm is most useful for optimizing the angiographic imaging plane in order to make a specific measurement (for example, to better visualize the minimal ductal diameter of a patent ductus arteriosus, PDA) or to compensate for suboptimal patient positioning on the table.

Vascular Access

Venous access for interventional procedures typically is achieved percutaneously using the external jugular vein or femoral vein in dogs and cats (**Figure 6.8**). The skin over the vein is clipped, scrubbed, and draped in a sterile fashion. A 1–2 mm skin incision is made over the site of needle access with a #11 blade and an access needle or OTN catheter is advanced through the skin incision into the vein. Ultrasound can be useful to guide needle access, although palpation of the vein often is sufficient. For the femoral vein, the puncture is made 2–3 mm caudomedial to the palpable arterial pulse because the femoral vein lies medial to the femoral artery and nerve (**Figure 6.9**). The vein should bleed back through the needle hub, confirming position within the vessel lumen; if necessary, negative pressure with a syringe applied to the needle hub confirms back-bleeding. Once luminal positioning is confirmed, a guide wire is advanced through the needle into the vessel lumen. Pressure is placed on the vein as the access needle or catheter is removed and wire position maintained. An introducer sheath then is advanced into the vein over the wire and sutured in place to the proximate skin. In general, a 0.035 in. guide wire is used through an 18-gauge OTN catheter for access in large dogs; an 0.018 in. guide wire through a 22-gauge OTN catheter is used to place a microintroducer in small dogs and cats.

Arterial access is similar to that described for venous access, with a few additional considerations. Percutaneous femoral arterial access could be performed, and in people is the standard of care, with manual compression and reduced mobility prescribed after sheath removal to allow hemostasis of the arteriotomy. However, manual compression was found to provide insufficient hemostasis in dogs following percutaneous arterial access. Therefore, most arterial interventions are done following surgical exposure of the femoral artery. The inguinal region is clipped, scrubbed, and draped. A 3–4 cm incision is made distal to the inguinal ring over the palpable pulse along the long axis of the limb. The femoral artery and vein are isolated using blunt and sharp dissection as appropriate (**Figure 6.9**). Once isolated, suture is passed loosely around the artery both proximal and distal to the site of puncture; then an access needle or OTN catheter is advanced into the artery as described above for venous access. Because intravascular pressure is much greater in the artery than a vein, back-bleeding can be substantial once access is achieved. Rapid exchange, as well as pressure over the access

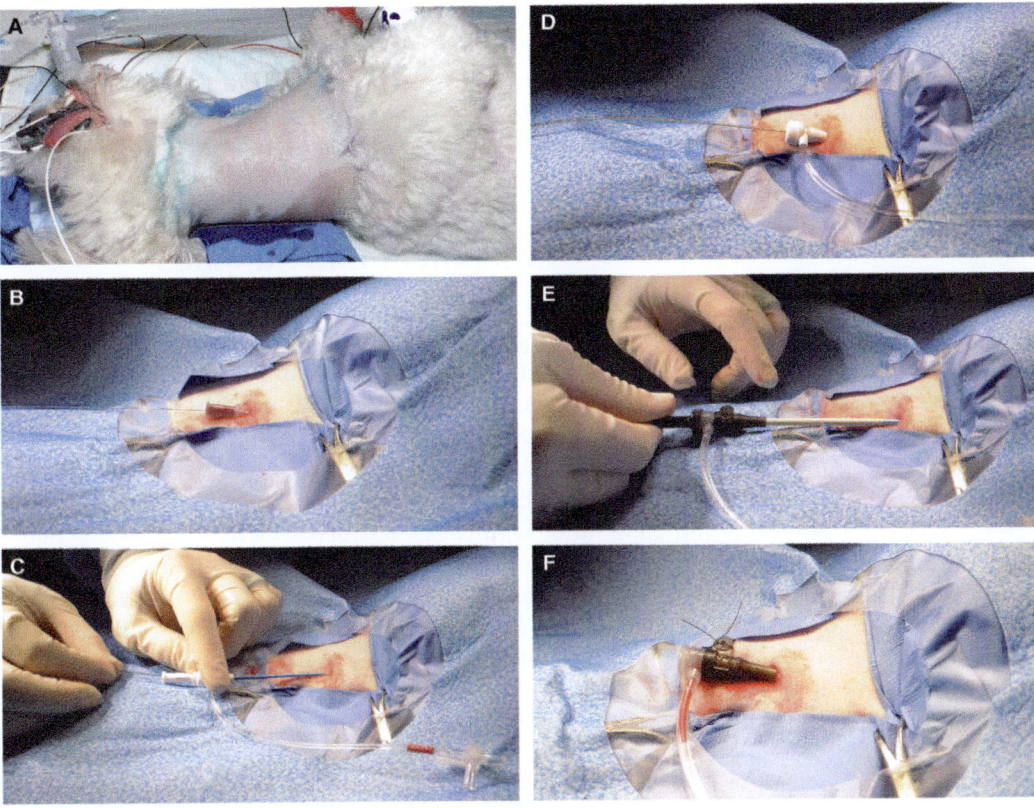

Figure 6.8 Percutaneous venous access to the canine external jugular vein. (A) The neck has been shaved and surgically scrubbed. (B) After the site was draped and a 2 mm skin incision made, a 22-gauge catheter and then a 0.018 in. guide wire are directed into the vessel lumen. (C) After the catheter is removed, a 4-Fr microintroducer is advanced over the guide wire. (D) After the 0.018 in. wire is removed, a 0.035 in. guide wire is advanced through the microintroducer to provide a stronger scaffold for the introducer sheath. (E) The microintroducer has been removed and the introducer sheath (9-Fr, in this case) is advanced over the guide wire. (F) The introducer sheath is sutured to the adjacent skin of the neck and the procedure can proceed. The use of a microintroducer is optional, but preferred in small dogs or cats to limit damage to the vessel.

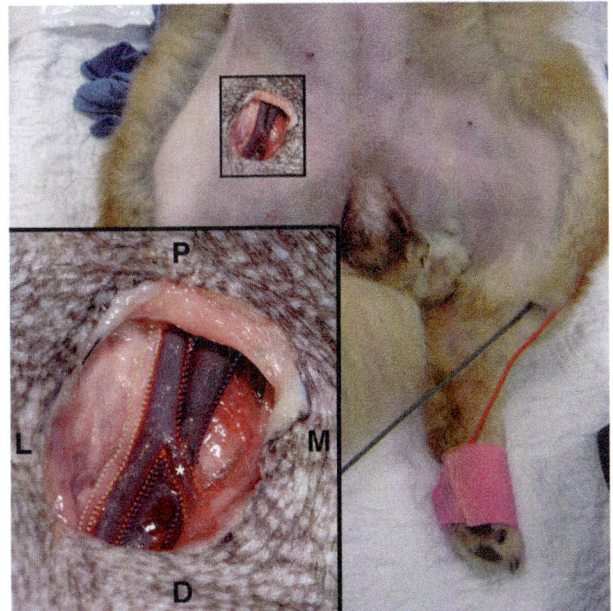

Figure 6.9 Preparation for femoral arterial or venous catheterization. The dog is in dorsal recumbency for surgical cut-down to the femoral triangle; the small inset indicates this anatomic location. The larger inset image shows the right femoral vasculature (canine cadaver dissection). The femoral nerve (outlined in yellow) is craniolateral to the femoral artery (outlined in red), which is craniolateral to the femoral vein (outlined in blue). The white asterisk indicates the proximal caudal femoral artery branch. D, distal; L, lateral; M, medial; P, proximal.

site during wire manipulation and introducer sheath placement, are required to minimize blood loss.

A similar approach is used for carotid arterial access, although the surgical approach is deeper than for femoral arterial access. Carotid arterial access is achieved through a lateral incision in the neck, dorsal to the jugular vein. The artery also can be approached from the ventral neck, with an incision lateral to the trachea. The carotid artery is found with the vagosympathetic trunk at the dorsolateral border of the trachea; the vagus nerve should be gently and bluntly dissected from the carotid artery prior to vascular access. Following the catheterization procedure, the femoral or carotid artery either is ligated above and below the access site or surgically repaired. Cats and dogs have sufficient collateral flow to allow ligation of either the common femoral artery or the carotid artery, though this limits ability to re-intervene and is, in the author's opinion, suboptimal for a procedure meant to be minimally invasive. The author has published successful use of a vascular closure device in a coagulopathic dog following percutaneous femoral arterial access (Scansen, 2017). This is a common strategy in human medicine to minimize complications from manual compression after percutaneous arterial access. Several devices are available that can provide effective hemostasis while maintaining arterial patency and vessel preservation. They could help avoid a surgical approach to the artery, thereby reducing pain or discomfort during recovery. However, their use in veterinary medicine remains to be more fully tested.

Angiocardiography

Because heart rates in dogs and cats are fairly rapid, opacification of CV structures following contrast injection occurs and disappears quickly. Frame-by-frame review of a digitally recorded angiographic image series ("run") is needed to examine the anatomy and perform measurements. Fast imaging frame rates are important during contrast injection to avoid "missing" a lesion in a high-flow organ such as the heart or great vessels. Digital subtraction angiography is a technique where a fluoroscopic image of the animal's anatomic structures (ribs, spine, solid organs) is stored prior to contrast agent administration and then digitally "subtracted" from the images in the remainder of the cine run (**Figure 6.10**). This enhances visualization of the radiographic contrast in finer detail by removing overlying anatomy that might obscure the structure of interest. Road-mapping is similar in that a previously recorded angiogram can be overlaid onto a live fluoroscopic image; guide wires or catheters then can be directed toward structures of interest without requiring additional contrast administration. Road-mapping and digital subtraction angiography are used mainly in vascular rather than cardiac interventions, because the beating heart prevents maintenance of the mask throughout the cine run or superimposed on live fluoroscopy. Nevertheless, digital subtraction angiography still can be useful for evaluating the great vessels, coronary anatomy, or pulmonary and aortic branch arteries.

Nonselective versus Selective Injection

Most angiograms are acquired using selective injection into the chamber or structure of interest. Nonselective angiography refers to contrast injection into a peripheral vein; image acquisition must be appropriately timed (by waiting until contrast reaches the desired anatomic site) in order to observe flow in the targeted area of the circulatory system. Selective angiography allows the operator to see precisely the area of interest and deliver more concentrated contrast agent to visualize the target site optimally. Nonselective studies can cause the lesion to be obscured or misinterpreted when superimposed structures are opacified simultaneously.

Equipment and Supplies

Power Injector   Hand injection generally does not achieve a sufficiently tight bolus of contrast material to optimally opacify a cardiac chamber in medium- and large-sized dogs. Automated power injectors allow the operator to program the volume, flow rate, and pressure of an injection to maximize opacification of the desired heart or great vessel locations within 1–2 cardiac cycles. It is important to use angiographic catheters and high-pressure tubing when a power injector is used. The preferred angiographic catheter is one with the largest diameter possible for the task, of the shortest feasible length, and with multiple side holes and a closed or tapered tip—all to maximize flow and minimize tissue trauma. A Berman or pigtail catheter generally is a good choice. Conversely, a catheter with only an end-hole is a poor choice for angiographic studies, particularly within the heart, because the full force of the injection is directed through the single end-hole and catheter recoil is likely. Additionally, if the end-hole is against a vessel wall or the endocardium, high-pressure injection could cause tissue damage.

Contrast Agents   Contrast agents used for angiocardiography are almost exclusively iodine-based particles (carbon dioxide gas rarely is used as a negative contrast agent). Iodine has a relatively high atomic weight, which equates to radiodensity; the degree of opacity with this agent is directly proportional to the total amount of iodine in the image. Second-generation contrast agents (developed in the 1970s) are nonionic monomers,

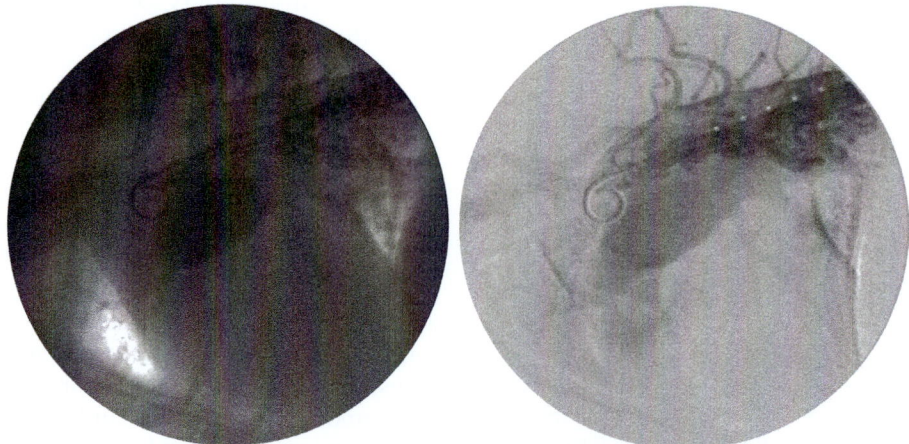

Figure 6.10   Angiographic images from a dog with aortopulmonary malformation showing the effect of digital subtraction. Left: conventional fluoroscopic imaging; bony structures can obscure intravascular contrast in standard fluoroscopic images. Right: same image after using digital subtraction, which provides better detail of the vasculature by masking all structures in the image prior to contrast injection.

which attach an amide group to an iodinated benzoic ring and prevent dissociation in solution. These agents cause many fewer adverse reactions than early-generation agents. They are termed low-osmolar agents because the particles do not dissociate once in solution. These agents still have an osmolality two to three times that of the blood (550–850 mOsm/kg). Iohexol is a second-generation contrast agent that is used commonly in veterinary medicine. Iodixanol is a third-generation agent; it is an iso-osmolar dimer made by combining two non-ionic tri-iodinated benzoic rings together. This arrangement does not dissociate in solution, has an iodine:particle ratio of 6:1, and has the same osmolality of blood (290 mOsm/kg). Although no studies are available in veterinary medicine, a meta-analysis of human patients at risk for contrast-induced nephropathy found a lower risk of adverse reaction for iodixanol compared to iohexol (Solomon, 2005).

The the contrast agent's viscosity also is important because this affects flow rate during injection. Warming the contrast can decrease viscosity and allow for a more rapid injection rate. Iodinated contrast agents are available in variable concentrations; highly concentrated solutions require smaller volumes for comparable degrees of radioopacity. Adverse contrast reactions appear to be rare in animals. Both the agent used and the total amount of contrast injected probably are important contributors to this risk. However, no prospective studies are available and recommendations vary widely. In general, the authors attempt to keep the cumulative contrast dose used for a CV procedure to < 720 mg iodine/kg, although some animals have received as much as 2,400 mg iodine/kg without apparent adverse effects. More conservative doses and concurrent pre- and post-catheterization fluid diuresis are advisable for animals with renal impairment.

Common Interventional Procedures

Via Right Heart Catheterization

Cardiac Pacing Permanent transvenous cardiac pacing has been done in dogs since the 1970s (Musselman, 1976). The primary indication for cardiac pacing in small animals is a symptomatic bradycardia (see Chapters 24 and 25). Temporary transvenous pacing is reserved for situations where the animal is not clinically stable enough for general anesthesia, for animals that might require short-term pacing (such as with intoxications), and when it is unclear whether a patient's bradycardia has contributed substantially to end-organ dysfunction (renal, hepatic, or cardiac). In the latter situation, temporary pacing can answer the question of whether heart rate normalization will improve the organ dysfunction.

Permanent pacemaker implantation in dogs is performed with the animal in left lateral recumbency and the right side of the neck exposed. Sterile technique is essential. Perioperative antibiotics often are given at the time of temporary pacemaker implantation, although there is no definitive evidence to support their use. The skin of the neck from ventral midline to dorsal midline is clipped and the skin aseptically scrubbed and draped. A 4–5 cm incision is made over the proximal right external jugular vein and the vein is isolated by blunt dissection. Suture or vessel loops are placed proximal and distal to the planned site of venous access to control the vein and limit hemorrhage. Tenotomy scissors, or a #11 blade, are used to create a 2–3 mm incision in the lateral wall of the jugular vein. Through this venous incision, a pacing lead of appropriate length is inserted with the aid of a vein pick, and advanced under fluoroscopic guidance to the right ventricular (RV) apex. Once positioned in the RV apex, a temporary pulse (pacing) generator is attached, to control the rhythm until the permanent pulse generator is connected. When using a bipolar pacing system, the sterile permanent pulse generator could be used here instead of an external temporary generator as long as sterility is maintained.

Pacing lead tips come in two varieties—passive or active fixation (**Figure 6.11**). Passive fixation leads have small polyurethane tines, which (ideally) become ensnared within the trabeculations of the right ventricle and then promote fibrosis with the surrounding tissue, and eventual rigid adherence. Active fixation leads have a small metallic screw at the tip, which penetrates into the RV myocardium when turned in a clockwise manner. To protect the vasculature and tricuspid valve during lead advancement and positioning, the screw tip is either retracted inside a housing at the lead tip or enclosed in a mannitol cap. Once the mannitol coating is in contact with blood it begins to dissolve, allowing 3 to 10 minutes to maneuver the lead into an appropriate and safe position before the sharp screw is exposed.

Positioning of the lead tip can be troublesome. In the authors' experience, the most stable pacing position is at the RV apex, which is seen as the most ventral and caudal aspect of the cardiac silhouette on a lateral projection and on midline

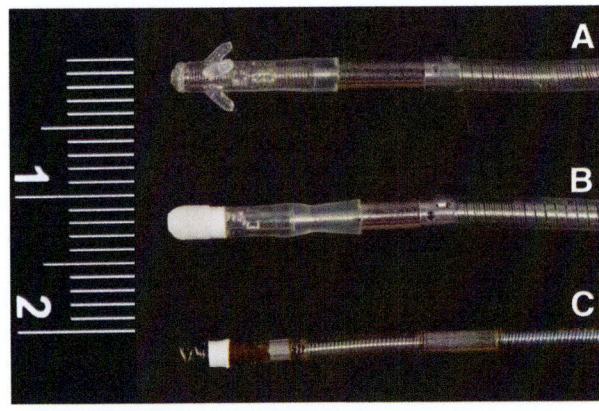

Figure 6.11 Various pacing lead tips. (A) Passive fixation leads have small polyurethane tines. Active fixation leads (B, C) are screwed into the myocardium. Some forms of active fixation leads have a mannitol-coated cap (B) which dissolves during placement within the animal to expose the screw tip (C).

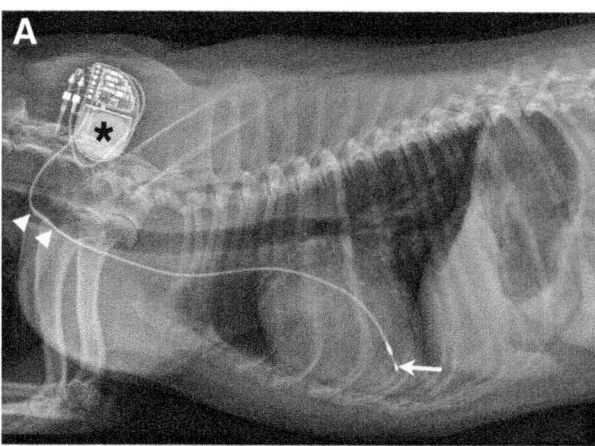
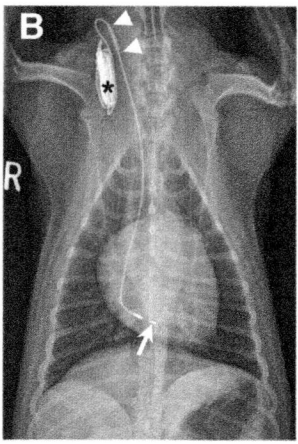

Figure 6.12 Lateral (A) and ventrodorsal (B) thoracic radiographs from a 5-year-old Beagle with a permanent transvenous pacing system implanted. The pulse generator (asterisk) is in the dorsal neck; the lead tip (arrow) is at the right ventricular apex. The sewing sleeve (visible as a subtle opacity between the arrowheads) encircles the lead at the jugular venous access site.

with a slight deflection toward the left chest wall on a VD projection (**Figure 6.12**). Depending on the animal's body habitus, as well as the degree and type of cardiac chamber enlargement, these landmarks might not be consistent. Use of variably shaped stylets can aid in proper lead positioning. Chronic pacing of the RV apex has been associated with progressive myocardial dysfunction in humans. Although lead placement has been tried at the RV septum or LV free wall (within a coronary vein) in dogs to avoid the complications of apical pacing (Estrada, 2015), this is not commonly done in clinical practice.

After the lead appears to be in a stable position, the patient's head and neck are carefully brought through a normal range of motion under fluoroscopic visualization in order to confirm minimal movement of the lead tip within the RV. A second incision, at roughly 5 cm dorsal to the jugular incision and equidistant between the point of the shoulder and the base of the right ear, is then made in a dorsoventral direction. Blunt and sharp dissections are used to find the superficial muscle of the neck that is deep to the subcutaneous adipose tissue. This muscle is incised and a pocket created below of just sufficient size to contain the permanent pulse generator. A tunnel then is made using hemostats from this pocket to the jugular incision and the pacing lead is brought up with a gentle bend into the pocket. The permanent generator is connected to the pacing lead, any excess lead length is coiled carefully under the generator to avoid kinking, and the unit is placed within the pocket. All incisions are closed routinely in three layers. The neck is bandaged to protect the incisions and provide mild compression to minimize serous fluid accumulation within the generator pocket; the neck bandage generally is left in place for approximately 3 days postoperatively.

Temporary transvenous pacing requires a vein capable of accepting a 5-Fr or 6-Fr vascular sheath. In dogs, this typically is either the external jugular or lateral saphenous vein; in cats, the jugular vein is used almost exclusively. If the jugular vein is used, the left external jugular vein should be chosen, in order to reserve the right jugular vein for permanent pacemaker implantation. Rarely, the presence of a (congenital) persistent left cranial vena cava complicates pacing lead placement via the left jugular vein, although it still is possible in most cases. All supplies required for temporary pacing should be assembled first, to limit the duration of sedation in these often-unstable animals. Although temporary pacing can be performed without fluoroscopic guidance, the ability to visualize proper placement of the lead and troubleshoot any difficulties during lead passage makes fluoroscopic visualization strongly advisable in all but the most desperate of circumstances. Once the operator is prepared, the patient is given local analgesia, in combination with a minimal degree of sedation or injectable anesthesia just sufficient to minimize motion, so that the pacing lead can be safely and efficiently placed. Inhalation anesthetics and cardiodepressant medications should be avoided. An anticholinergic could be given, but this seldom is effective for normalizing the rhythm.

Temporary pacing leads used in animals are available with or without a balloon at the tip of the lead. The balloon-tipped lead can facilitate passage into the RV because the balloon is carried by the blood flow. The non-balloon-tipped lead has a smaller outer diameter and is useful for small patients. Most balloon-tipped leads require a 6-Fr vascular sheath, while the non-balloon-tipped leads often will pass through a 5-Fr sheath. Lead wires with a curved tip, or used with a curved stylet, can be easier to pass into the RV. When a balloon-tipped pacing catheter is used, the introducer sheath might need to be one Fr size larger than the pacing catheter.

A variety of methods can be used to gain venous access for the temporary pacing lead. Some temporary pacing kits come with a presized over-the-needle catheter through which the lead can be advanced. The modified Seldinger technique also can be used to place a standard introducer or a (4-Fr) microintroducer, which can facilitate guide wire placement for the standard introducer in cases with challenging venous access. After the introducer sheath has been advanced into the vein, it is sutured to the skin to avoid backward migration. The temporary pacing lead often is inserted through a sterile (60 cm) sleeve (to facilitate lead repositioning later without compromising sterility) before it is advanced through the introducer sheath and its tip directed into the RV apex, under fluoroscopic guidance. The external electrode wires of the pacing lead then are connected to a temporary pulse generator, and pacing is commenced. The sterile sleeve is attached to the introducer sheath.

Complications associated with pacing include lead dislodgement, arrhythmias during implantation, seroma formation at the pulse generator site, infection of a pacing system component, and programming difficulties. Major complications have reportedly occurred in 13% to 33% of patients. Most dogs (well over 70%) are alive at 1 year after pacemaker implantation; mean survival time reportedly is between 2 and 3 years.

Pulmonary Balloon Valvuloplasty Pulmonary valve stenosis (PS) is a common congenital heart defect of dogs. It is variably reported as the third most common (in North America) to most common (in Europe) canine congenital heart defect (p. 490). Without therapy, dogs with severe valvular PS are at increased risk for exercise intolerance, syncope, sudden cardiac death, congestive heart failure, and in some cases, cyanosis from a right-to-left shunt. Pulmonary balloon valvuloplasty (PBV; or balloon pulmonary valvuloplasty, BPV) was first performed in a dog in 1980 (Buchanan, 2002). Clinical cardiologists now do this procedure routinely for dogs and some cats with a severe pressure gradient or clinical signs associated with PS. Morbidity and mortality generally are low with this procedure and there is evidence that PBV can improve clinical signs and survival.

Prior to intervention, pulmonary valve morphology should be characterized as best as possible and required balloon size(s) estimated. Transthoracic echocardiography with Doppler is the current standard method for evaluating pulmonary valve morphology, annular size, and stenosis severity. Severely dysplastic valves (those with redundant tissue, annular hypoplasia, or a subvalvular fibrous ring) are less likely to respond as well to PBV and clients should be so advised. Nevertheless, because it is difficult to quantify the degree of valvular fusion by echocardiography alone and cases with valve dysplasia still could respond at least partially to PBV, the procedure generally is recommended for severe PS. The author also has attempted stent implantation into the RV outflow tract and across the annulus of such dogs with fair improvement in clinical signs and pressure gradient (Scansen, 2014).

Continuous wave spectral Doppler is used to estimate the pressure gradient across the stenotic valve area (p. 122). Color flow Doppler imaging is used to optimize alignment parallel to the direction of the turbulent jet. Most cardiologists consider the stenosis mild at a gradient of 10–49 mm Hg, moderate at 50–79 mm Hg, and severe when the gradient is 80 mm Hg or greater. The decision to pursue PBV is influenced by the pressure gradient, with greater benefit more likely in cases with severe stenosis. As with all Doppler estimates, the velocity measured depends not only on the valve orifice size, but also on the transvalvular flow and ventricular systolic function at the time of measurement. Changes in sympathetic tone, intravascular volume status, or intrinsic ventricular contractility can alter the measured velocity.

Many balloon dilation catheters are commercially available; they vary in profile, material, size, and maximal pressure tolerance. The ideal balloon for PBV is made of a noncompliant material (so that it will only expand to its stated size), is of a low profile (meaning that it folds tightly over the shaft to form a small diameter for introduction into the vasculature), and is on a flexible shaft that will accommodate an appropriately sized guide wire and provide good tracking and pushability when advanced into the heart. Because some of the above characteristics are contradictory to one another, the choice of balloon dilation catheter represents a trade-off among characteristics, which all should be considered in the context of the individual patient's size and anatomy. Factors that influence the selection of a balloon dilation catheter include the size of introducer needed to access the animal's vasculature (the maximal introducer size that can be placed is limited in small dogs and cats); the size and angulation of the patient's RV lumen (a small, severely hypertrophied heart cannot tolerate a stiff guide wire or inflexible catheter shaft); and the valve anatomy (which will influence the desired balloon's diameter, length, nominal pressure and burst pressure). A higher maximal pressure increases the radial force that the balloon can apply to a stenotic valve; however, higher-pressure balloons typically are stiffer and have a larger profile, which requires a larger introducer. Within the same line of balloon dilation catheters, the larger the balloon diameter, the lower its maximal burst pressure. As such, extremely large balloons typically have the lowest maximal pressure; this supports the recommendation to utilize a double balloon technique in dogs with a pulmonary valve diameter exceeding 20 mm. Some veterinarians re-sterilize and reuse balloon dilation catheters; however, this practice is not recommended for several reasons. The re-sterilization process could alter the nominal and burst pressures of the balloon, it is challenging to re-constrain the balloon catheter to the same low profile as when new, and there is a theoretical risk of pyrogen reaction to proteins that remain on the re-sterilized balloon. Current balloon dilation catheters are made for one-time use only and their cost is affordable for most clients who pursue PBV. As such, new equipment is preferred for each animal, although a selection of re-sterilized balloons might be kept for charitable cases.

The PBV procedure is performed transvenously, either via the external jugular vein or femoral vein. The jugular vein is preferred in small dogs because, as a larger vessel than the femoral vein, it can accommodate a larger introducer sheath. The femoral vein typically is chosen when an arterial study is to be done concurrently, given the close proximity of femoral artery and vein. Percutaneous access via an appropriately sized introducer is achieved with the animal in lateral (for jugular vein) or dorsal (for femoral vein) recumbency. The vascular sheath selected should be at least one French size larger than that required by the anticipated balloon dilation catheter. After the right heart is catheterized, intracardiac pressures are measured to evaluate the starting RV pressure and RV-to-pulmonary artery gradient.

After the right heart and pulmonary artery pressures have been obtained, right ventriculography is performed using an appropriate angiographic catheter (typically a Berman catheter); then, pulmonary annulus diameter is measured to help determine the balloon size needed (**Figure 6.13**). Angiographic and echocardiographic measurements of pulmonary annulus diameter are compared and a catheter chosen with balloon diameter of approximately 1.3 to 1.5 times the pulmonary annulus diameter.

A (balloon-tipped) pulmonary wedge pressure catheter is positioned across the pulmonary valve and into a distal pulmonary artery branch. The left pulmonary artery (the dorsal pulmonary artery branch when viewed from a lateral image) is preferred because it provides a smoother and more secure path for balloon dilation catheter advancement, compared to the right pulmonary artery. Next, a J-tipped exchange length guide wire (typically greater than 180 cm length) is advanced through the wedge pressure catheter and into the distal pulmonary artery branch. The J-tip is preferred because it is less traumatic to the artery. The diameter and stiffness of the guide wire chosen depends on patient size and the stiffness of the balloon dilation catheter to be used. Guide wires of 0.035 in. diameter in a standard stiffness or super-stiffness are preferred for PBV. However, in small dogs or those with severe RV hypertrophy, the super-stiff guide wires place too much pressure on the tricuspid valve and the RV endocardium, particularly when they are advanced from a jugular venous approach. Conversely, for larger dogs, standard stiffness guide wires are overly flexible and do not maintain the balloon in proper position during inflation; therefore, super-stiff guide wires are preferred for large dogs or inflexible balloon dilation catheters. For very small dogs (or cats), the chosen balloon dilation catheter might not accept a 0.035 in. guide wire. In such instances, a 0.018 in. or 0.025 in. guide wire can be used, but these wires provide even less stability during advancement and inflation of the balloon dilation catheter so stiffer varieties should be selected.

To prepare the balloon catheter for insertion, first the protective plastic sheath around the balloon is removed. A three-way stopcock is attached to the balloon catheter port; a pressure inflation device is connected to one port and a 12 mL Luer-Lock syringe attached to the other port. Within the inflation device, a mixture of iodinated contrast and saline (from 1:1 to 1:3, contrast to saline) is drawn up and 3–4 mL of a similar mixture is drawn into the syringe. For larger balloons, a lesser proportion of contrast to saline should be used because the rate of balloon deflation depends partially on the viscosity of the fluid used for inflation; contrast is necessary to visualize inflation, but its viscosity causes a slower deflation rate. The balloon dilation catheter then is purged of air using the three-way stopcock and the syringe. The central lumen of the balloon dilation catheter is flushed to remove air and the catheter is slowly advanced over the guide wire to a position spanning the pulmonary valve annulus. A projected reference image of the RV angiogram can aid in achieving proper balloon positioning; platinum marker bands on the balloon dilation catheter allow the operator to center the balloon within the annulus, or site of stenosis.

Rapid balloon inflation is then done using live fluoroscopy in order to visualize the development of a balloon "waist" at the stenotic site and to allow adjustment (retraction or advancement) of the catheter if its position changes (**Figure 6.14**). The pressure generated by the inflation device should be monitored and increased to the balloon's nominal pressure. Exceeding this nominal pressure (the pressure at which the balloon reaches its advertised diameter) can be done if the stenotic waist persists; however, the balloon's burst pressure should not be exceeded. Once the desired pressure is reached, or if the balloon migrates from the site of stenosis, the balloon is rapidly deflated. The duration of balloon

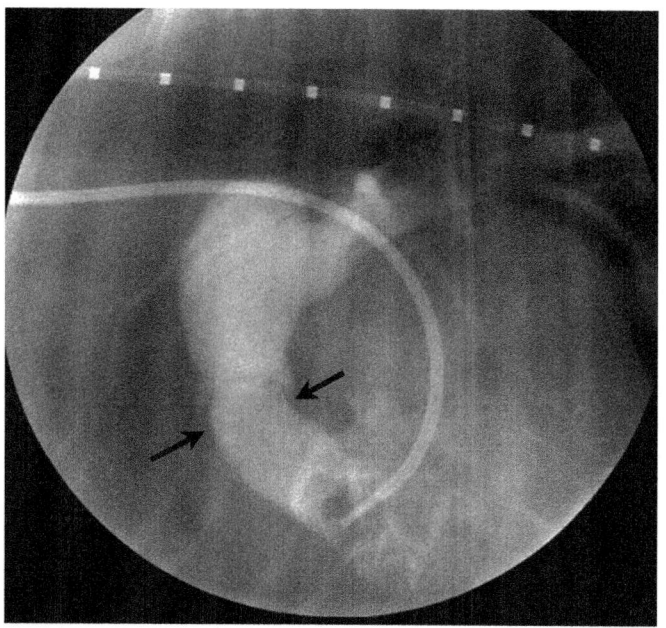

Figure 6.13 Right ventricular (RV) angiocardiogram from a 2-year-old Shih Tzu with pulmonary valve stenosis. Note the fused and doming valve (arrows) in this systolic frame, as well as poststenotic dilation of the main pulmonary artery. RV hypertrophy also is evident. A calibrated marker catheter is within the esophagus.

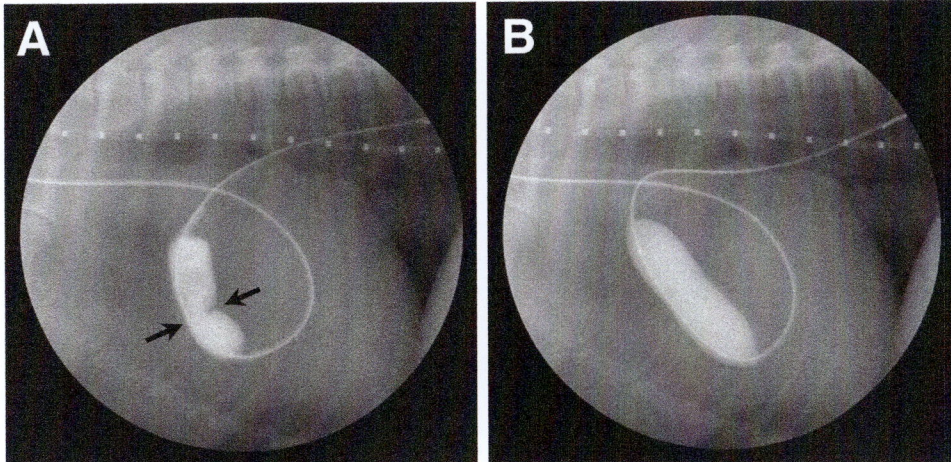

Figure 6.14 Fluoroscopic images during balloon pulmonary valvuloplasty in the dog of Figure 6.13. (A) The balloon dilation catheter has been advanced over a guide wire so that the balloon straddles the stenotic valve. As the balloon is rapidly inflated, a stenotic waist (indentation; arrows) appears at the pulmonary annulus. (B) Increasing pressure within the balloon tears the stenotic valve, causing the waist to disappear.

inflation should not exceed 5–6 seconds. A precipitous drop in systemic arterial pressure is expected, with rapid recovery within the following 5–10 seconds. The desired outcome with PBV is disappearance of the stenotic waist and the lack of a recurrent waist on subsequent re-inflations. Typically, 2–4 inflations are performed to confirm the waist was engaged and resolved. RV pressure and pressure gradient across the pulmonary valve are measured again; if the result is satisfactory, all equipment is removed. After the vascular sheath is removed, hemostasis is achieved with a purse-string suture around the access site and 5 minutes of applied pressure. If the jugular vein was used for access, a neck bandage is placed to keep the site clean as the animal recovers. The prognosis for PBV generally is good if significant reduction in pressure gradient can be achieved.

The coronary artery anatomy is of particular importance in brachycephalic dogs with PS. Anomalous coronary arterial circulations, characterized by either a single right coronary ostium (**Figures 27.22** and **27.23**, p. 490 and 491) or single left coronary ostium, have been identified in English Bulldogs and Boxers (Buchanan, 2001; Visser, 2013). In such cases, the coronary artery that lacks a patent ostium arises from the contralateral coronary artery and passes adjacent and cranial to the pulmonary valve annulus. Evaluation of coronary anatomy in brachycephalic dogs with PS should include imaging of the coronary ostia, either by aortic angiography during catheterization or cross-sectional imaging such as CT angiography prior to intervention. Performing PBV with a standard-size balloon (balloon:annulus ratio of 1.2 to 1.5) in a dog with a coronary artery anomaly could result in coronary artery avulsion, other damage, and death. PBV has been attempted in such cases using a more conservative balloon:annulus ratio of 0.9 to 1.0, with some reduction in stenosis severity observed (Fonfara, 2010). The long-term benefit of conservative ballooning in these dogs remains uncertain.

Via Left Heart Catheterization

Patent Ductus Arteriosus Occlusion PDA is a common congenital heart defect in dogs; it is the most common defect in some surveys. PDA also occurs occasionally in cats. Without therapy, the prognosis generally is poor. Therefore, closure of the ductus either by surgical ligation or interventional occlusion is recommended as soon as possible.

Transcatheter therapy for PDA was first reported in dogs in 1994 (Miller, 1994). In the initial decade of transcatheter PDA therapy, transarterial or transvenous coil delivery was the predominant method used for ductal closure. Thereafter, human implants of variable design were tried for PDA occlusion in dogs and in 2007 a device designed and optimized for canine anatomy came on the market (Nguyenba, 2007). The canine-specific device, the Amplatz® Canine Duct Occluder (ACDO), now is the preferred transcatheter device for PDA occlusion in dogs because of its excellent safety and efficacy record and ease of deployment. There remain a subset of small dogs (and cats), however, in which vascular access of sufficient size to deliver an ACDO is not possible; in these small dogs, coils remain a useful technique to achieve ductal closure. A nitinol device for small canine PDA has been evaluated with good results, but is not yet commercially available (Stauthammer, 2015).

The technique for nearly all cases of transcatheter PDA occlusion begins with the animal in dorsal recumbency and access to the femoral triangle (typically the right side is chosen). Dorsal recumbency is used for ease of access and catheter advancement from the groin; once access is achieved, the animal or fluoroscope can be turned to visualize the procedure from a lateral imaging plane. For the ACDO and transarterial coil delivery, the femoral artery is isolated by surgical cut-down and a combination of blunt and sharp dissection (**Figure 6.9**). Although percutaneous access might be feasible for femoral arterial access, postoperative hemorrhage is a greater concern. A long sheath with dilator is placed into the artery and advanced over a guide wire to the aortic isthmus; the guide wire and dilator then are removed. Angiography is performed through the long sheath to delineate ductal anatomy and minimal ductal diameter; this provides adequate clarity in most dogs (**Figure 6.15A**). If sufficient contrast flow cannot be achieved through the sheath, a pigtail catheter is advanced through the vascular sheath and a power injection made into the ascending aorta; however, this rarely is necessary. Measurement of the minimal ductal diameter at the pulmonary ostium is made from the angiographic image and compared to TEE measurements of minimal ductal diameter.

An appropriately sized ACDO is chosen, with a central waist that is 1.5–2.0 times the minimal ductal diameter. The hydrophilic guide wire and sheath dilator then are replaced within the vascular sheath and directed across the PDA into the pulmonary trunk under fluoroscopic guidance, taking care to not engage the pulmonary valve with the stiff dilator or sheath. The dilator and guide wire are removed again and the device is prepared for implantation. The ACDO set screw should be tested by removing the device and screwing it back onto the delivery cable. The device must screw on and off easily or it should not be implanted in the animal. When tightening, the device should be turned until it stops (fully tight) and then turned back a half turn; it should not be overtightened. While on the delivery cable, the ACDO is vigorously flushed and purged of all air bubbles by extruding and reconstraining the device under saline. The ACDO then is advanced into the long sheath and passed out into the pulmonary trunk, taking care to extrude only the pulmonary artery disc. The entire system (sheath, delivery cable) then is withdrawn slightly until the open pulmonary artery disc engages with the pulmonary ostium of the PDA (**Figure 6.15B**). Slight tension is placed on the system to ensure the disc is flush with the PDA–pulmonary artery junction. This tension is maintained as the sheath is slowly retracted over the delivery cable to expand the ductal disc within the PDA ampulla (**Figure 6.15C**). After the ductal disc has been deployed, a slight forward advancement of the delivery cable often is needed to allow the device to regain its cupped shape.

The position of the ACDO device on the fluoroscopic image should be compared to the prior angiogram to confirm it is in the correct location of the PDA. Gentle pushing and pulling on the delivery cable helps confirm that the device is seated appropriately; however, even an optimally positioned

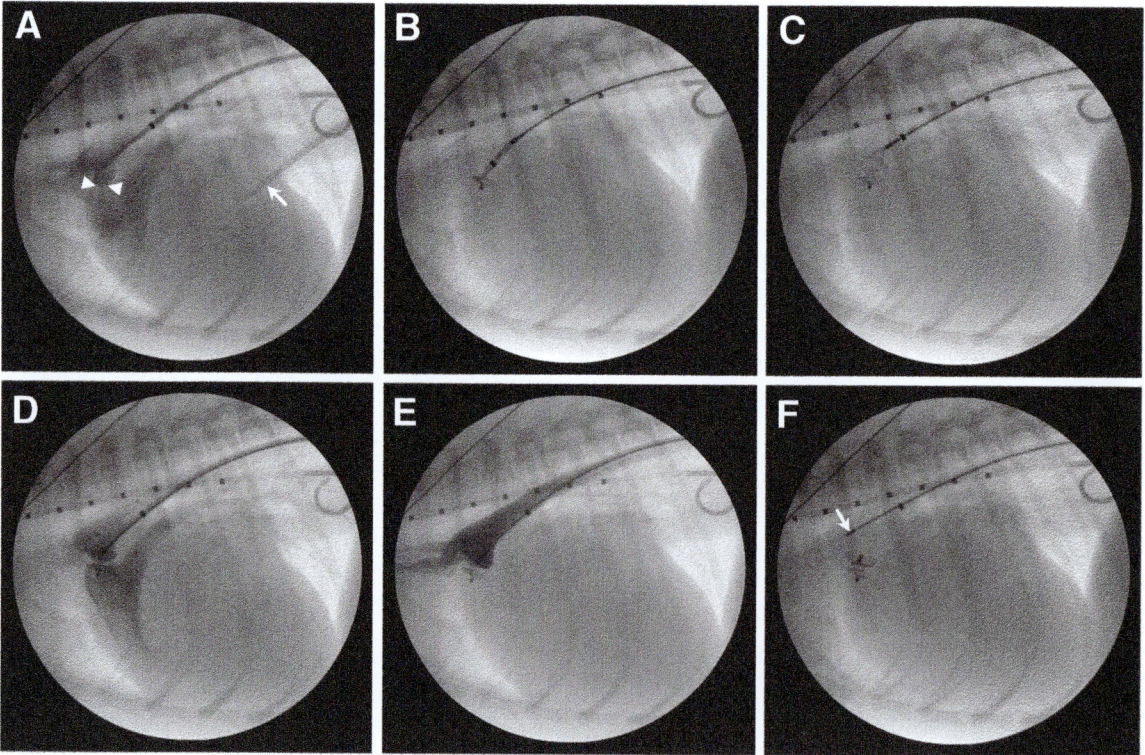

Figure 6.15 Transcatheter closure of patent ductus arteriosus in a Cavalier King Charles Spaniel by Amplatz Canine Duct Occluder (ACDO); this dog also has pulmonary valve stenosis. (A) A long vascular sheath is advanced into the thoracic aorta and angiography used to define the ductal location, anatomy, and minimal ductal diameter (between arrowheads). Another catheter (arrow), not used for ACDO placement, is in the right atrium. (B) The pulmonary disc is deployed within the pulmonary trunk, then brought back against the pulmonary ostium. (C) The ductal disc is partially deployed within the ductal ampulla. (D) Angiography immediately after ACDO deployment shows moderate flow through the center of the device. (E) Contrast injection at 10 minutes postdeployment shows complete ductal closure. (F) Counterclockwise rotation of the delivery cable releases the device from the cable screw (arrow).

device can be pushed or pulled out of the PDA if too great a force is exerted. The authors typically wait 5 minutes after deployment and then perform an angiogram through the long vascular sheath to confirm ductal closure. If a small amount of central flow still is observed, it will likely close without further intervention (**Figure 6.15D** and **E**). However, if there is contrast flow cranial or caudal to the waist, around the device, the device has been improperly positioned and should be re-deployed. In lieu of repeated angiogram(s), TEE with color flow Doppler can be used to observe the ductus and ACDO for persistent flow. If placement is satisfactory, the ACDO device is released using counterclockwise rotation of the delivery cable, either with the supplied pin or a hemostat; then the cable and sheath are removed (**Figure 6.15F**). The femoral access site is repaired or ligated, and the skin closed. The animal should be kept sedated and quiet overnight; echocardiography is performed the next day to confirm ductal closure.

The procedure for transarterial coil delivery is comparable to that described for ACDO deployment, except a 4-Fr or 5-Fr catheter is used for vascular access, either alone or through an introducer sheath. Most cases that undergo transarterial coil delivery have insufficient vascular size for an ACDO, so the catheter is placed directly into the vessel (rather than through a sheath) with a hemostatic valve or Tuohy-Borst adaptor placed on the catheter hub to control hemorrhage. Angiography is done as described for an ACDO, although through the catheter rather than a sheath. Coil selection also is based on the minimal ductal diameter, with a coil loop diameter twice the minimal angiographic ductal diameter chosen. Typically, 0.038 in. or 0.035 in. coils are used for small dogs. The catheter tip is positioned in the ductus and its position verified by hand contrast injections. The coil is advanced carefully through the catheter to the ductal ampulla. If detachable coils are used, they are mounted on the delivery cable and advanced through the catheter to the ductus. The catheter is retracted to expose the coil and, once positioning is appropriate, the coil is released by counterclockwise rotation of the delivery cable. If nondetachable coils are used, they are advanced through the catheter using a straight-tipped guide wire of the same thickness as the coil. The drawback to nondetachable coils is that repositioning or retraction into the catheter is not possible; therefore, confirmation of appropriate coil size and deployment location are paramount to success. Transarterial coil delivery is used most often for dogs (or cats) of small size (typically 2.0–3.5 kg) and with narrow pulmonary ostia, because these cases appear most amenable to coil occlusion. There are reports of smaller coils being deployed in even smaller dogs (1–2 kg), either from a carotid or femoral arterial approach. If the animal is smaller than 2.5 kg, the authors typically recommend surgical ligation.

Transvenous coil delivery also is possible in small dogs or cats via retrograde cannulation of the ductus. This technique allows for easier vascular access in small animals because the jugular or femoral vein is larger and more pliable than the femoral artery. Percutaneous access might be used for transvenous coil delivery. Catheterization of the PDA from venous access requires placement of an end-hole catheter into the pulmonary trunk, and then advancing it over a straight-tipped flexible guide wire that has been advanced across the ductus to the descending aorta. The delivery is comparable to that described for transarterial coil delivery. However the detachable coil system is preferred to allow the coil to be exposed in the descending aorta, then withdrawn into the ductal ampulla, followed by the delivery cable being retracted slightly into the pulmonary trunk so that a small segment of coil spans the ductal ostium prior to release (**Figure 6.16**).

The prognosis after transcatheter PDA occlusion is quite good, with perioperative survival rates of 90–100% and median survival of greater than 11.5 years. Factors reported to have a negative effect on survival time include the presence of clinical signs, concurrent congenital heart disease, large breed, older age, increased weight, and severe mitral regurgitation documented within 24 hours of ductal closure (Saunders, 2014).

Aortic Balloon Valvuloplasty SAS is a common congenital defect of large-breed dogs; valvular aortic stenosis rarely is encountered (p. 480). Interventional therapy for SAS remains controversial. One prospective case-control study showed no survival benefit for aortic balloon valvuloplasty (ABV; or, balloon aortic valvuloplasty, BAV) compared to medical therapy (atenolol) alone (Meurs, 2005). New developments in interventional treatment options, including cutting balloon (CB) followed by high-pressure balloon (HPB) valvuloplasty, have been tried in dogs with SAS with reasonable short- and mid-term results (Kleman, 2013; Schmidt, 2010). An HPB can withstand inflation pressure of greater than 8 atmospheres. Long-term results with this strategy remain unknown, however, and comparison to medical therapy or the natural history of the disease has not yet been made. Whether the long-term prognosis for dogs with severe SAS is improved by the combined CB and HPB procedure remains to be seen. An interim analysis of 28 dogs that underwent this procedure found that peak systolic pressure gradient decreased from a mean of 143 mm Hg to 78 mm Hg at 1 day postprocedure, 84 mm Hg at 1 month, 89 mm Hg at 3 months, 92 mm Hg at 6 months, and 116 mm Hg at 12 months post-ABV (Kleman, 2013). Six dogs died after the combined ABV, including three dogs euthanized for progressive myocardial failure, one euthanized for syncope, and two dogs with sudden death. Although this procedure can reduce peak pressure gradient to some degree and exercise capacity might be improved, randomized prospective study is required to assess overall benefit. The reduction in pressure gradient achieved is typically to the high moderate range (70–80 mm Hg), which means considerable obstruction persists. Because the procedure is costly, involves arrhythmic and anesthetic risks, and is of uncertain benefit, the authors currently reserve this procedure for cases that

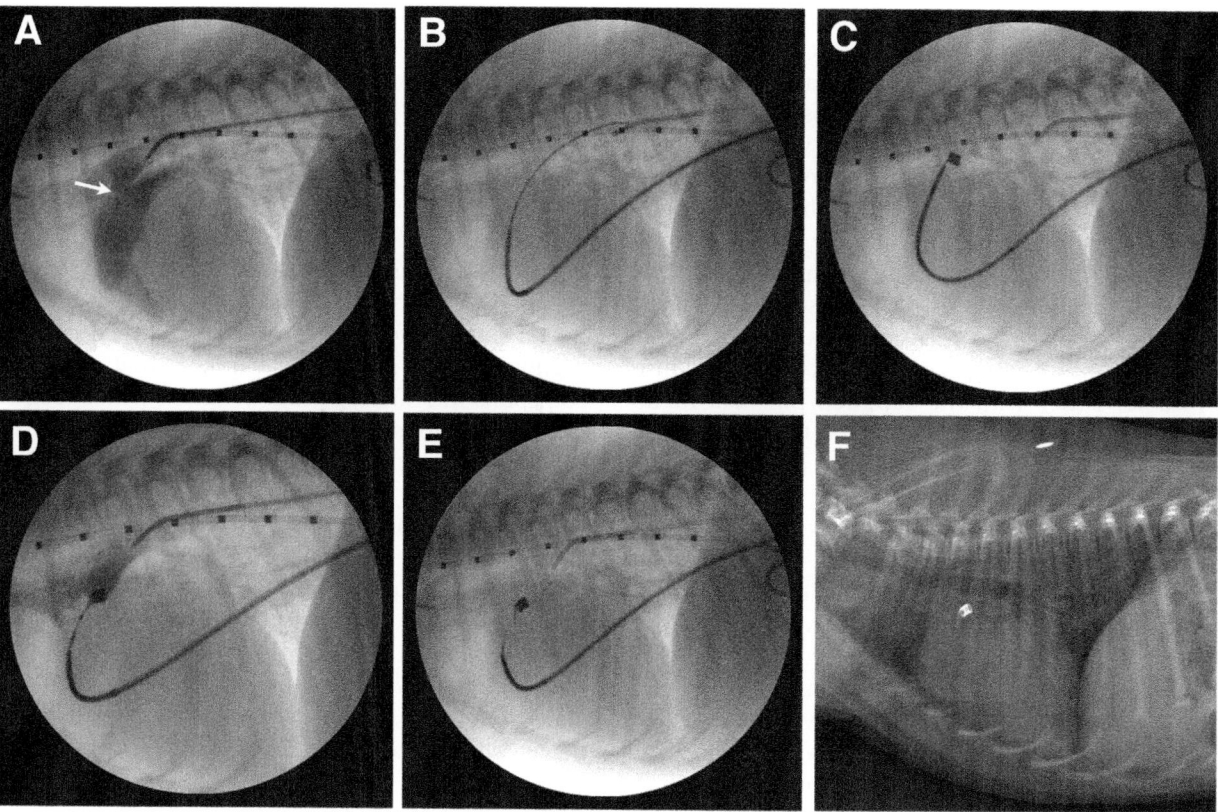

Figure 6.16 Transvenous coil deployment in a small dog with patent ductus arteriosus. (A) Aortography highlights the ductal anatomy, location of the pulmonary ostium (arrow), and minimal ductal diameter. (B) Right heart catheterization directs a guide wire from the pulmonary artery, retrograde across the ductus and into the descending aorta. (C) The detachable coil is delivered to the aorta, extruded within the ductal ampulla, and pulled back toward the pulmonary ostium. (D) One coil loop is brought across the ostium and into the pulmonary trunk; repeat aortography shows near complete ductal occlusion in this case. (E) The coil is detached from the delivery cable once appropriate positioning and angiography are complete. (F) Postoperative radiograph shows final coil position.

display clinical signs (syncope, weakness, congestive heart failure) or that are at high risk for clinical signs based on the severity of the stenosis (for example, >150 mm Hg instantaneous pressure gradient) and cardiac remodeling.

The approach for ABV typically is via a carotid artery cutdown. The dog is positioned in dorsal or lateral recumbency; the ventral and lateral neck (either right or left) is clipped, prepped, and draped. A 3–4 cm incision is made along the lateral border of the trachea and blunt and sharp dissection used to expose the common carotid artery, which is carefully separated from the vagosympathetic trunk. Suture or vessel loops are passed around the carotid artery, cranial and caudal to the proposed access site, to stabilize the vessel during access. Arterial puncture is performed with an 18-gauge over-the-needle catheter or arterial access needle, then a vascular sheath of 1 to 2 French sizes larger than required by the desired HPB balloon catheter is advanced into the vessel. A marker pigtail catheter is advanced into the left ventricle after aortic pressure has been measured; LV pressure is measured to quantify the gradient across the SAS. It can be challenging to pass the catheter across the aortic valve in these dogs because aortic valve excursion is limited by reduced forward flow. Rarely, the pigtail catheter will advance alone through the valve orifice. Alternatively, a guide wire with a long floppy tip can be used to *gently* probe the aortic orifice; with repeated attempts it will cross in most cases and the pigtail angiographic catheter can then be advanced over the guide wire into the left ventricle. Left ventriculography is performed to delineate the site of subaortic obstruction, as well as to assess LV size and function, presence of mitral regurgitation, coronary arterial anatomy, and any other concurrent defects (**Figure 6.17A**).

Following the contrast study, a 0.018 in. guide wire that has been preshaped to create a (single to) double loop (or 360 to 720-degree curve) at the end is inserted through the angiographic catheter; the loop allows the guide wire to seat within the LV apex without injuring or perforating it. Once this guide wire is in position, the angiographic catheter is removed. Then the CB catheter is advanced over the preplaced guide wire to the level of the subaortic ridge and the balloon is inflated rapidly, then deflated (**Figure 6.17B**). Selection of CB size is based upon the minimal stenotic diameter of the LV outflow tract, with a roughly 1:1 balloon-to-stenosis diameter chosen. The largest CB diameter currently available

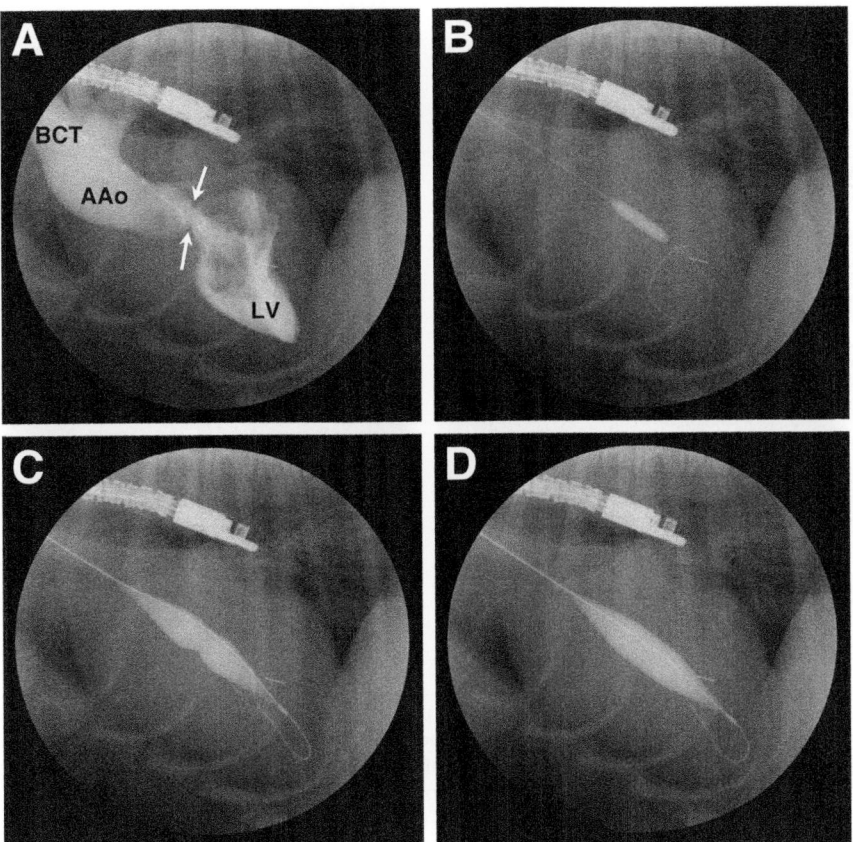

Figure 6.17 Left ventriculography (A) and balloon aortic valvuloplasty in a Golden Retriever dog with subaortic stenosis. The left ventricle (LV) is concentrically hypertrophied, the left ventricular outflow tract is narrowed with a discrete ridge (between arrows), and there is poststenotic dilation of the ascending aorta (AAo) and brachycephalic trunk (BCT). (B) A cutting balloon dilation catheter is advanced across the subaortic ridge, then inflated to score the fibrous lesion. (C) After the cutting balloon catheter is withdrawn, a high-pressure balloon dilation catheter is positioned across the lesion and the balloon rapidly inflated. The stenotic subaortic lesion creates a central indentation (waist) in the balloon. (D) With higher balloon pressure, the subaortic ring is torn and the waist abolished. A transesophageal echocardiography probe is at the top in all images.

commercially is 8 mm; this is large enough to engage the subaortic ridge in most dogs with SAS. After two to three inflation cycles, the CB is fully deflated and this catheter is withdrawn, leaving the guide wire in place. The pigtail catheter is reinserted over the 0.018 in. guide wire, then the wire is exchanged for an ultrastiff 0.035 in. guide wire with a long floppy tip. The end of the 0.035 in.guide wire also is preshaped with a (single to) double loop and positioned in the LV apex. HPB catheter sizing is based on the true aortic valve annulus diameter; a ratio of 0.9–1:1, HPB diameter-to-aortic valve annulus diameter is used. The HPB catheter is advanced over the 0.035 in. guide wire so that the HPB straddles the subaortic lesion; then the balloon is inflated rapidly, and then deflated. Transvenous RV burst pacing at 200-240 beats/min during HPB inflation can aid accurate balloon positioning by limiting LV forward stroke volume. As with PBV, successful inflation involves a stenotic waist that disappears with increased balloon pressure and does not recur on subsequent inflations (**Figure 6.17C** and **D**). After 2-3 inflations across the outflow tract, the HPB catheter is removed. LV and aortic pressures are remeasured to compare the change in gradient from preoperative level. A contrast injection at the aortic root usually is done to assess aortic valve insufficiency. Once satisfactory results are achieved, all equipment is withdrawn. The carotid access site is allowed to bleed temporarily prior to repair so that any thrombus around the introducer sheath exits the carotid opening before it is closed. The carotid artery is repaired with 5-0 or 6-0 monofilament suture, the surgical incision is closed in three layers, and the neck is bandaged routinely. Cardiac rhythm monitoring and administration of analgesia, sedation, and prophylactic antibiotics are employed during recovery.

A similar approach to ABV can be pursued for dogs with valvular aortic stenosis; however, the CB is not used. Rather, standard balloon dilation catheters are utilized as described for PBV, because these dogs have fusion of the aortic valve leaflets and do not require scoring and high pressure tearing of the fibrous tissue typical for SAS. As described previously for the HPB, the ratio of conventional balloon diameter-to-aortic valve annulus in the setting of valvular aortic stenosis is also 0.9–1:1. This is to limit the risk of postoperative aortic insufficiency.

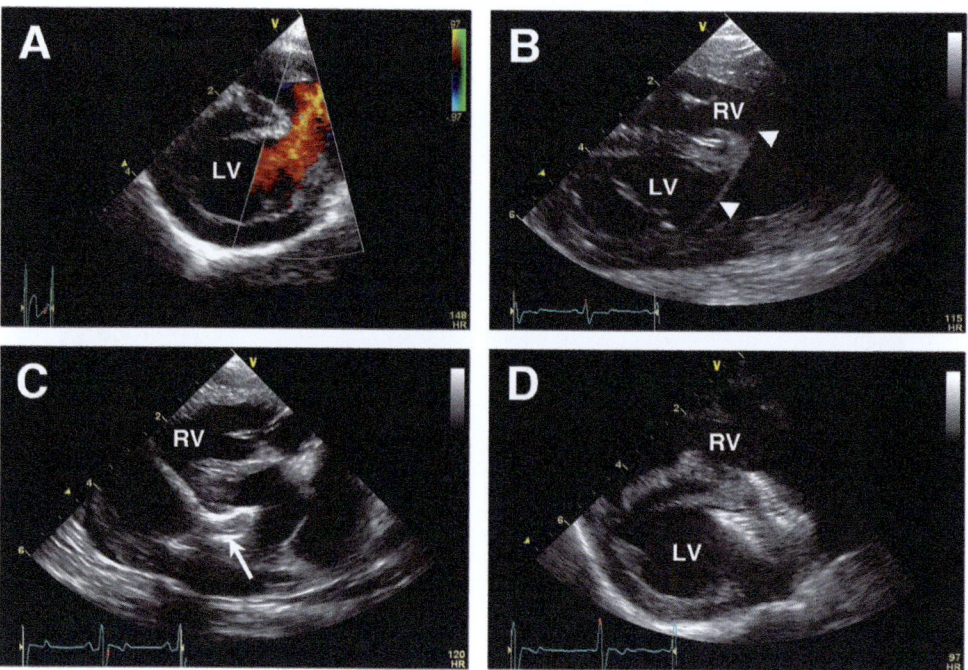

Figure 6.18 Hybrid perventricular ventricular septal defect (VSD) closure using an Amplatzer™ muscular ventricular septal occluder in a Cavalier King Charles Spaniel with a large muscular VSD. (A) The defect is visible as a large anechoic space in the interventricular septum on transthoracic echocardiography (short-axis view); color flow Doppler indicates left-to-right shunting (coded red). (B) A right lateral thoracotomy was done to access the heart for hybrid intervention; this epicardial echocardiographic image shows a guide wire (arrowheads) traversing the right ventricular (RV) free wall and crossing the VSD into the left ventricle (LV). (C) The sheath is placed across the VSD and the distal retention disc (arrow) deployed within the LV (long-axis view). (D) Postoperative transthoracic echocardiogram illustrates the device in place and appropriately spanning the interventricular septum (short-axis view).

Hybrid Catheterization

A hybrid procedure is one that utilizes a surgical approach combined with image-guided intervention. As an example of hybrid catheterization, a device used to close a ventricular septal defect (VSD) could be delivered directly through the RV wall with echocardiographic guidance, rather than by a transvascular approach. This is known as perventricular VSD occlusion. The strategy can be effective for animals that are too small for transvascular device delivery. Some transcatheter devices require delivery systems of 9-Fr or larger, which can be too large for vascular access in small dogs or cats. In such cases, a right lateral thoracotomy can be done to expose the RV free wall of the beating heart. A purse-string suture is placed around the proposed access site prior to myocardial puncture to control hemorrhage. Then a vascular access needle is inserted directly across the RV free wall, guided by echocardiography; a guide wire is placed through the access needle so that the desired delivery system can be advanced (**Figure 6.18**). Echocardiographic and fluoroscopic guidance facilitate placement, as with transcatheter delivery of the same device. Such a hybrid approach not only can overcome the challenge of vascular access in a small dog, it can allow for a more direct path to the defect, which makes device deployment more straightforward than a conventional, percutaneous approach. The hybrid approach also can be used for transatrial occlusion of an atrial septal defect. The more invasive nature of this technique and potential for increased morbidity are drawbacks. Other veterinary uses for hybrid catheterization could include the delivery of balloon dilation catheters directly through the left atrium for treatment of mitral stenosis or cor triatriatum sinister. Future options for mitral valve repair or replacement also are likely to use a hybrid approach given the complexities of left heart access and the large delivery systems required of these techniques.

Suggested Additional Reading and References

Also See Online Comprehensive Bibliography at: https://www.routledge.com/9781482246223.

Achen SE, Miller MW, Gordon SG, et al. Transarterial ductal occlusion with the Amplatzer vascular plug in 31 dogs. J Vet Intern Med 2008;22:1348–1352.

Akerstrom F, Pachon M, Puchol A, et al. Chronic right ventricular apical pacing: adverse effects and current therapeutic strategies to minimize them. Int J Cardiol 2014;173:351–360.

Blossom JE, Bright JM, Griffiths LG. Transvenous occlusion of patent ductus arteriosus in 56 consecutive dogs. J Vet Cardiol 2010;12:75–84.

Buchanan JW. Causes and prevalence of cardiovascular diseases. In, Kirk RW, Bonagura JD (editors). Current Veterinary Therapy XI: Small Animal Practice. WB Saunders Co., Philadelphia, PA. 1992. pp. 647–654.

Buchanan JW. Pathogenesis of single right coronary artery and pulmonic stenosis in English Bulldogs. J Vet Intern Med 2001;15:101–104.

Buchanan JW. Pulmonic stenosis caused by single coronary artery in dogs: four cases (1965–1984). J Am Vet Med Assoc 1990;196:115–120.

Buchanan JW, Anderson JH, White RI. The 1st balloon valvuloplasty: an historical note. J Vet Intern Med 2002;16:116–117.

Buchanan JW, Patterson DF. Selective angiography and angiocardiography in dogs with congenital cardiovascular disease. J Am Vet Radiol Soc 1965;6:21–39.

Estrada AH. Cardiac pacing. In, Weisse C, Berent A (editors). Veterinary Image-Guided Interventions. Wiley-Blackwell, Ames, IA. 2015.

Eyster GE, Eyster JT, Cords GB, et al. Patent ductus arteriosus in the dog: characteristics of occurrence and results of surgery in one hundred consecutive cases. J Am Vet Med Assoc 1976;168:435–438.

Fonfara S, Martinez Pereira Y, Swift S, et al. Balloon valvuloplasty for treatment of pulmonic stenosis in English Bulldogs with an aberrant coronary artery. J Vet Intern Med 2010;24:354–359.

Francis AJ, Johnson MJ, Culshaw GC, et al. Outcome in 55 dogs with pulmonic stenosis that did not undergo balloon valvuloplasty or surgery. J Small Anim Pract 2011;52:282–288.

Gordon SG, Nelson DA, Achen SE, et al. Open heart closure of an atrial septal defect by use of an atrial septal occluder in a dog. J Am Vet Med Assoc 2010;236:434–439.

Gordon SG, Saunders AB, Achen SE, et al. Transarterial ductal occlusion using the Amplatz® canine duct occluder in 40 dogs. J Vet Cardiol 2010;12:85–92.

Grifka RG, Miller MW, Frischmeyer KJ, et al. Transcatheter occlusion of a patent ductus arteriosus in a Newfoundland puppy using the Gianturco-Grifka vascular occlusion device. J Vet Intern Med 1996;10:42–44.

Hamlin RL. Angiocardiography for the clinical diagnosis of congenital heart disease in small animals. J Am Vet Med Assoc 1959;135:112–116.

Hildebrandt N, Stertmann WA, Wehner M, et al. Dual chamber pacemaker implantation in dogs with atrioventricular block. J Vet Intern Med 2009;23:31–38.

Hogan DF, Green HW III, Gordon S, et al. Transarterial coil embolization of patent ductus arteriosus in small dogs with 0.025-inch vascular occlusion coils: 10 cases. J Vet Intern Med 2004;18:325–329.

Hogan DF, Green HW, Sanders RA. Transcatheter closure of patent ductus arteriosus in a dog with a peripheral vascular occlusion device. J Vet Cardiol 2006;8:139–143.

Johnson MS, Martin M, Edwards D, et al. Pulmonic stenosis in dogs: balloon dilation improves clinical outcome. J Vet Intern Med 2004;18:656–662.

Johnson MS, Martin MW, Henley W. Results of pacemaker implantation in 104 dogs. J Small Anim Pract 2007;48:4–11.

Johnson V. Diagnostic imaging: reflecting on the past and looking to the future. Vet Rec 2013;172:546–551.

Kittleson M, Thomas W, Loyer C, et al. Single coronary artery (type R2A). J Vet Intern Med 1992;6:250–251.

Kleman ME, Estrada AH, Maisenbacher HW III, et al. How to perform combined cutting balloon and high pressure balloon valvuloplasty for dogs with subaortic stenosis. J Vet Cardiol 2012;14:351–361.

Kleman ME, Estrada AH, Tschosik ML, et al. An update on combined cutting balloon and high pressure balloon valvuloplasty for dogs with severe subaortic stenosis. J Vet Intern Med 2013;27:632–633.

Lehmkuhl LB, Bonagura JD, Jones DE, et al. Comparison of catheterization and Doppler-derived pressure gradients in a canine model of subaortic stenosis. J Am Soc Echocardiogr 1995;8:611–620.

Locatelli C, Spalla I, Domenech O, et al. Pulmonic stenosis in dogs: survival and risk factors in a retrospective cohort of patients. J Small Anim Pract 2013;54:445–452.

Meurs KM, Lehmkuhl LB, Bonagura JD. Survival times in dogs with severe subvalvular aortic stenosis treated with balloon valvuloplasty or atenolol. J Am Vet Med Assoc 2005;227:420–424.

Miller MW, Stepien RL, Meurs KM, et al. Echocardiographic assessment of patent ductus arteriosus (PDA) after occlusion. Proceedings of the 12th ACVIM Forum. 1994. p. 305.

Miller SJ, Thomas WP. Coil embolization of patent ductus arteriosus via the carotid artery in seven dogs. J Vet Cardiol 2009;11:129–136.

Musselman EE, Rouse GP, Parker AJ. Permanent pacemaker implantation with transvenous electrode placement in a dog with complete atrioventricular heart block, congestive heart failure and Stokes-Adams syndrome. J Small Anim Pract 1976;17:149–162.

Nguyenba TP, Tobias AH. The Amplatz canine duct occluder: a novel device for patent ductus arteriosus occlusion. J Vet Cardiol 2007;9:109–117.

Nguyenba TP, Tobias AH. Minimally invasive per-catheter patent ductus arteriosus occlusion in dogs using a prototype duct occluder. J Vet Intern Med 2008;22:129–134.

Oliveira P, Domenech O, Silva J, et al. Retrospective review of congenital heart disease in 976 dogs. J Vet Intern Med 2011;25:477–483.

Orton EC. Transcatheter mitral valve implantation (TMVI) for dogs. Proceedings of the 30th Annual ACVIM Veterinary Medical Forum. 2012. pp. 185–187.

Oyama MA, Sisson DD, Lehmkuhl LB. Practices and outcome of artificial cardiac pacing in 154 dogs. J Vet Intern Med 2001;15:229–239.

Pollard RE, Pascoe PJ. Severe reaction to intravenous administration of an ionic iodinated contrast agent in two anesthetized dogs. J Am Vet Med Assoc 2008;233:274–278.

Ristic J, Marin C, Baines E, et al. Congenital pulmonic stenosis a retrospective study of 24 cases seen between 1990–1999. J Vet Cardiol 2001;3:13–19.

Saunders AB, Carlson JA, Nelson DA, et al. Hybrid technique for ventricular septal defect closure in a dog using an Amplatzer® duct occluder II. J Vet Cardiol 2013;15:217–224.

Saunders AB, Gordon SG, Boggess MM, et al. Long-term outcome in dogs with patent ductus arteriosus: 520 cases (1994–2009). J Vet Intern Med 2014;28:401–410.

Scansen BA, Cober RE, Bonagura JD. Congenital heart disease In, Bonagura JD, Twedt DC (editors). Kirk's Current Veterinary Therapy XV. 15th edition. Saunders, St. Louis. 2014. pp. 756–761.

Scansen BA, Hokanson CM, Friedenberg SG, et al. Use of a vascular closure device during percutaneous arterial access in a dog with impaired hemostasis. J Vet Emerg Crit Care 2017;27(4):465–471.

Scansen BA, Kent AM, Cheatham SL, et al. Stenting of the right ventricular outflow tract in 2 dogs for palliation of dysplastic pulmonary valve stenosis and right-to-left intracardiac shunting defects. J Vet Cardiol 2014;16:205–214.

Schmidt M, Estrada A, Maisenbacher HW, et al. Combined cutting balloon and high pressure balloon angioplasty in dogs with severe subaortic stenosis is effective at mid-term follow-up. Cath Cardiovas Interv 2010;76:1.

Schneider M, Hildebrandt N. Transvenous embolization of the patent ductus arteriosus with detachable coils in 2 cats. J Vet Intern Med 2003;17:349–353.

Schneider M, Hildebrandt N, Schweigl T, et al. Transvenous embolization of small patent ductus arteriosus with single detachable coils in dogs. J Vet Intern Med 2001;15:222–228.

Schranz D, Michel-Behnke I. Advances in interventional and hybrid therapy in neonatal congenital heart disease. Semin Fetal Neonatal Med 2013;18:311–321.

Seibert JA. Flat-panel detectors: how much better are they? Pediatr Radiol 2006;36:173–181.

Singh MK, Kittleson MD, Kass PH, et al. Occlusion devices and approaches in canine patent ductus arteriosus: comparison of outcomes. J Vet Intern Med 2012;26:85–92.

Sisson D. Use of a self-expanding occluding stent for nonsurgical closure of patent ductus arteriosus in dogs. J Am Vet Med Assoc 2003;223:999–1005.

Sisson D, Thomas WP, Woodfield J, et al. Permanent transvenous pacemaker implantation in forty dogs. J Vet Intern Med 1991;5:322–331.

Smith PJ, Martin MW. Transcatheter embolisation of patent ductus arteriosus using an Amplatzer vascular plug in six dogs. J Small Anim Pract 2007;48:80–86.

Solomon R. The role of osmolality in the incidence of contrast-induced nephropathy: a systematic review of angiographic contrast media in high risk patients. Kidney Int 2005;68: 2256–2263.

Stauthammer CD, Olson J, Leeder D, et al. Patent ductus arteriosus occlusion in small dogs utilizing a low profile Amplatz® canine duct occluder prototype. J Vet Cardiol 2015;17: 203–209.

Stauthammer CD, Tobias AH, Leeder DB, et al. Structural and functional cardiovascular changes and their consequences following interventional patent ductus arteriosus occlusion in dogs: 24 cases (2000–2006). J Am Vet Med Assoc 2013;242:1722–1726.

Stern DJ, Gunasekaran T, Sanders RA. Periprocedural vascular access complications associated with percutaneous femoral arterial access using the modified Seldinger's technique in dogs during cardiac catheterization: a single-center experience. J Vet Cardiol 2020;32:28–32.

Stern JA, Tou SP, Barker PC, et al. Hybrid cutting balloon dilatation for treatment of cor triatriatum sinister in a cat. J Vet Cardiol 2013;15:205–210.

Stokhof AA, Sreeram N, Wolvekamp WT. Transcatheter closure of patent ductus arteriosus using occluding spring coils. J Vet Intern Med 2000;14:452–455.

Tashjian RJ, Albanese NM. A technique of canine angiocardiography with the interpretation of a normal left lateral angiocardiogram. J Am Vet Med Assoc 1960;136:359–365.

Trehiou-Sechi E, Behr L, Chetboul V, et al. Echoguided closed commissurotomy for mitral valve stenosis in a dog. J Vet Cardiol 2011;13:219–225.

Vance A, Nelson M, Hofmeister EH. Adverse reactions following administration of an ionic iodinated contrast media in anesthetized dogs. J Am Anim Hosp Assoc 2012;48: 172–175.

Visser LC, Scansen BA, Schober KE. Single left coronary ostium and an anomalous prepulmonic right coronary artery in 2 dogs with congenital pulmonary valve stenosis. J Vet Cardiol 2013;15:161–169.

Weisse C, Berent A (editors). Veterinary Image-Guided Interventions. Wiley Blackwell, Ames, IA. 2015.

Wess G, Thomas WP, Berger DM, et al. Applications, complications, and outcomes of transvenous pacemaker implantation in 105 dogs (1997–2002). J Vet Intern Med 2006;20:877–884.

Section II

Clinical Manifestations of Cardiovascular Disease

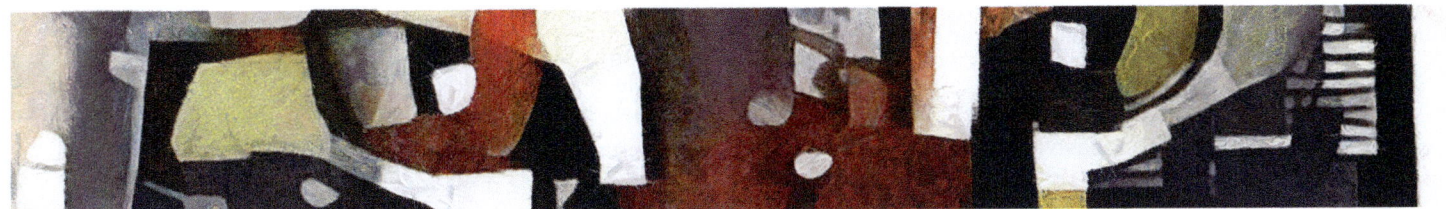

7

EXERCISE INTOLERANCE

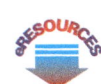

Exercise intolerance, as a clinical sign, can have variable meaning depending on the observer's perspective. It does not, by itself, imply loss of consciousness. The use and expected performance level of the animal influence how easily exercise intolerance is perceived. While mild compromise is likely to be detected quickly in racing animals, exercise ability might become profoundly impaired before it is noticed in relatively inactive house pets. To some owners, exercise intolerance could mean a decreased interest in play, lethargy, or weakness. Whatever the client's definition of exercise intolerance, the observation indicates that the animal is unable to sustain activity for as long or as fast as it previously could or should be able to do. Cardiovascular (CV) disease, as well as abnormalities in many other body systems, can underlie exercise intolerance (**Figure 7.1**). Other clinical signs often accompany exercise intolerance, including heavy breathing, cough, generalized weakness, or collapse.

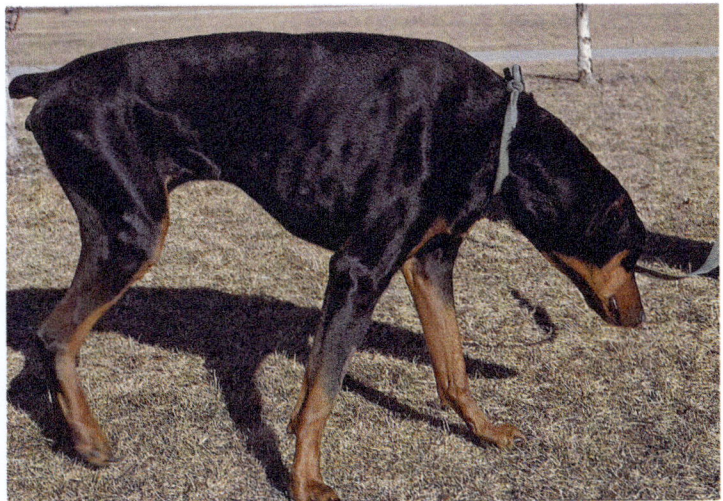

Figure 7.1 This dog tired easily and was unable to sustain previously normal levels of exercise. Dilated cardiomyopathy was diagnosed.

General Considerations

Several mechanisms, alone or in combination, can interfere with the animal's ability to sustain an optimal activity level. These could involve a number of body systems (**Table 7.1**). In general, factors that can impair exercise ability include

Table 7.1 Some Causes of Exercise Intolerance

Cardiovascular
- Impaired forward cardiac output
  - Arrhythmias (tachy- or brady-arrhythmias)
  - Poor myocardial contractility
  - Advanced valvular insufficiency of any cause
  - Cardiac tamponade
  - Constrictive pericardial disease
  - Congenital or acquired ventricular outflow or inflow obstructive lesion
  - Moderate to severe pulmonary hypertension
  - Other causes
- Pulmonary venous congestion or CHF (especially with impaired oxygenation):
  - Congenital CV shunts
  - Congenital or acquired mitral or aortic valve disease (insufficiency or stenosis)
  - Hypertrophic myocardial disease
  - Overt pulmonary edema
  - Post-capillary pulmonary hypertension
  - Overt pleural effusion
  - Large-volume ascites
- Right-to-left shunt leading to poor muscle oxygenation
- Systemic hypotension:
  - Heart failure
  - Hypovolemia
  - Drug effect or other causes of reduced vascular tone

(Continued)

Cardiovascular Disease in Companion Animals 189

Table 7.1 Some Causes of Exercise Intolerance *(Continued)*

- Systemic hypertension
- Vascular disease:
  - Arterial thromboembolic disease (pulmonary or systemic)
  - Thrombophlebitis or systemic venous thrombosis
  - Aortoiliac thrombosis
  - Arteriovenous fistula
  - Aortic root rupture (aortocardiac fistula)
- Combinations of the above

Respiratory
- Infiltrative lung disease
  - Infectious
  - Inflammatory
  - Neoplastic
- Pleural space disease
  - Effusion of any kind
  - Pneumothorax
  - Diaphragmatic hernia
- Pulmonary vascular disease
  - Heartworm disease
  - Other causes of pulmonary hypertension
  - Pulmonary thromboembolism
- Airway obstruction
  - Laryngeal paralysis
  - Tracheal or bronchial collapse
  - Airway compression
  - Foreign body or mass lesion
- Bronchitis
  - Infectious
  - Inflammatory or allergic
- Pharyngeal mass, infection, or inflammation
- Mediastinal mass or infection

Musculoskeletal
- Muscle strain
- Myositis
- Stress fracture
- Tendonitis
- Degenerative joint disease
- Infectious or inflammatory arthritis or osteitis
- Other causes of muscle, bone, or joint pain
- Loss of condition (disuse atrophy, cachexia, geriatric sarcopenia)
- Overexertion/overtraining

Neurologic
- Spinal cord injury
  - Trauma
  - Infection or inflammation
  - Vascular accident
- Intracranial disease
  - Trauma
  - Infection or inflammation
  - Vascular accident
  - Toxin
- Peripheral nerve disease
  - Trauma
  - Infection or inflammation
  - Vascular accident
  - Toxin
- Myasthenia gravis

Dehydration and Hypovolemia

Anemia
- Acute or chronic blood loss
- Hemolysis
- Associated with chronic disease

Metabolic or Endocrine Disease
- Hyper- or hypoadrenocorticism
- Hypothyroidism
- Diabetes mellitus
- Hyper- or hypoparathyroidism
- Pheochromocytoma
- Marked electrolyte imbalance
  - Hypo- or hypercalcemia
  - Hypo- or hyperkalemia
  - Hypo- or hypernatremia
  - Hypomagnesemia
  - Hypoglycemia
- Renal failure
- Pancreatitis
- Hepatopathy
- Nutritional deficiency (from poor diet or impaired absorption/metabolism)
- Cachexia
- Marked acidosis or alkalosis

Inflammatory Disease
- Systemic or local infection or fever
- Immune-mediated disease
- Neoplastic disease and cachexia

Pain

Obesity

Marked Ascites

Impaired Vision

Drug Effects
- Glucocorticoids
- Antihypertensives
- Anticonvulsants
- Sedatives
- Antihistamines
- Others

Abbreviations: CHF, congestive heart failure; CV, cardiovascular.

insufficient capacity to increase muscle perfusion, inadequate oxygen delivery to tissues, damaged musculoskeletal structural components (muscle, bone, tendon, joint tissues, etc.), metabolic or endocrine derangements, localized or systemic inflammation, neurologic deficits, pain, and other abnormalities.

Although the focus of this text is the CV system, other body systems also must be considered in the individual patient. Many animals with cardiac disease concurrently have other abnormalities that could contribute to reduced exercise ability. For example, inadequate oxygen delivery to working muscle might occur from impaired pulmonary gas exchange (from an underlying lung disease or airway obstruction), or from reduced blood oxygen carrying capacity (as with anemia), as well as from factors that reduce muscle perfusion. Limitations on skeletal muscle perfusion during exercise could be caused not only by reduced forward cardiac output (CO) from heart disease, but also by dehydration or impaired muscle vasodilatory capacity, perhaps related to hormonal factors, vessel wall edema, or deconditioning.

Cardiac disease often limits exercise capacity when the heart is unable to increase forward CO sufficiently. **Table 7.1** outlines common CV pathophysiologic causes; specific etiologies are numerous. Even when underlying cardiac structure and contractility are normal, arrhythmias inhibit maximal exercise performance. In addition, they exacerbate the negative effects of other underlying cardiac, as well as noncardiac, abnormalities on CO (**Figure 7.2**). Besides limitations on maximum CO from underlying heart disease, animals with congestive heart failure (CHF) also can have impaired pulmonary function related to edema, pulmonary hypertension, or pleural effusion. Reduced diastolic function (for example, from severe myocardial hypertrophy or scarring) even without overt CHF can limit CO and also promote pulmonary vascular congestion and shortness of breath with exercise. In some cases, there might be cardiac pain associated with ischemia (angina) that could negatively affect exercise ability, too.

Abnormal peripheral circulation contributes to inadequate skeletal muscle perfusion and fatigue during exercise. For example, there is an impaired vasodilatory response in animals with heart failure. Increased sympathetic tone, angiotensin II (both circulating and locally produced), and vasopressin are some factors that can contribute to impaired skeletal muscle vasodilatory capacity. In other cases, partial peripheral vascular obstruction caused by thromboemboli or vascular disease (see Chapters 36 and 37) limits exercise ability. Cramping pain and weakness in the affected leg(s) that progressively worsens with activity (intermittent claudication) is typical of inadequate or obstructed peripheral blood flow. These are typical features of aortoiliac thrombosis in dogs, cats, and horses. A weak or absent arterial pulse, coolness, pallor, pain, lack of sweating and venous return (horses), muscle contracture, or even paresis might be evident in the pelvic limbs. Another classic example is the reversed patent ductus arteriosus where desaturated blood is preferentially shunted to the descending aorta, the caudal limbs. Affected dogs become weaker in the pelvic limbs with progressive exercise as oxygen demand outstrips delivery. These patients recover after a short rest, thereby mimicking the clinical findings of myasthenia gravis.

Animals with advanced heart failure can exhibit weakness at rest or with minimal exercise. Causes include low blood pressure (BP), arrhythmias, reduced muscle mass (cardiac cachexia), or electrolyte disturbances (especially hypokalemia). Low BP could relate to poor forward CO because of underlying heart disease and the effects of vasodilatory or diuretic drugs. Hypotensive patients also might be somewhat hypothermic.

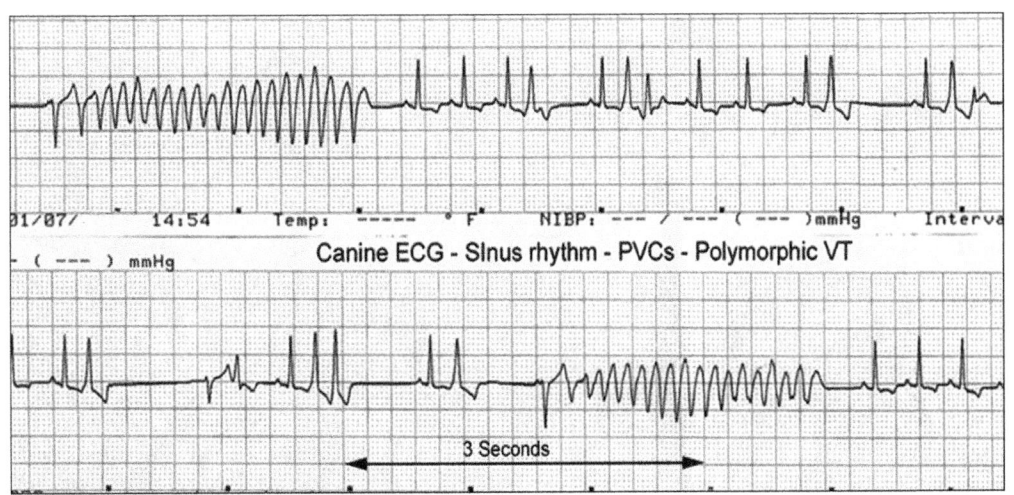

Figure 7.2 Intermittent tachy- or brady-arrhythmias can impair exercise ability and potentially cause collapse. Intermittent ventricular premature complexes and brief paroxysms of polymorphic ventricular tachycardia were identified in this dog.

Approach to the Patient with Exercise Intolerance

Because exercise intolerance is such a nonspecific sign, it is important to take a broad view, especially during initial patient evaluation (**Figure 7.3**). A detailed history and careful examination often provide information that helps focus further diagnostic testing. Questions relating to the time course and progression of the exercise intolerance, recent changes in observed behavior or physical status, and medications administered are important. A thorough physical examination is essential. Evidence for disease in all body systems, not just the CV, respiratory, and musculoskeletal systems, should be noted. A pain response or swelling detected on palpation of limbs, joints, local muscle groups, or spinal regions could indicate local disease or trauma, or it might be a manifestation of more widespread infectious, inflammatory, or neoplastic disease. An increased respiratory rate could indicate primary pulmonary disease or CHF, or it might signal pain, fever, anemia, or other abnormality. Respiratory pattern, especially with activity, might provide clues (p. 218). For example, increased inspiratory effort, especially when accompanied by stridor or hoarseness, could indicate laryngeal paralysis or mass lesion. An endocrinopathy, such as hypothyroidism or hyperadrenocorticism, might be accompanied by alopecia or other skin lesions evident on physical exam.

A routine laboratory database is recommended as part of the initial workup, including CBC, biochemical profile,

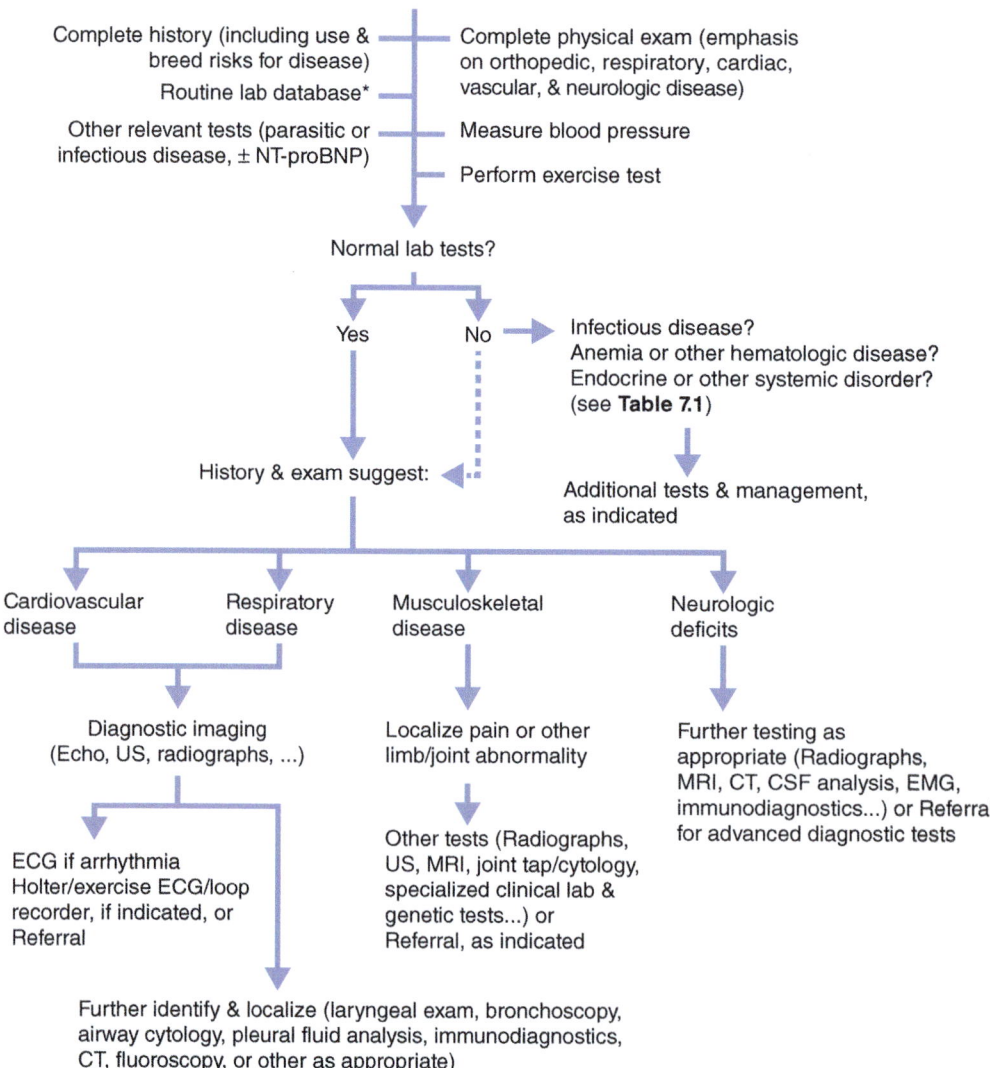

Figure 7.3 Approach to the patient with exercise intolerance. These general guidelines focus on the dog, but aspects apply to horses & cats too. *Includes CBC, biochemical profile, urinalysis, and for Labrador Retrievers, genetic testing for centronuclear myopathy. CSF, cerebral spinal fluid; CT, computed tomography; ECG, electrocardiography; echo, echocardiography; EMG, electromyography; MRI, magnetic resonance imaging; NT-proBNP, N-terminal probrain natriuretic peptide; US, ultrasonography.

urinalysis, heartworm testing (for dogs and cats), and arterial BP measurement. Depending on the individual situation, thoracic and abdominal radiographs, as well as additional cardiac, respiratory, neurologic, endocrine, or orthopedic assessments, might be indicated. Ambulatory electrocardiography could uncover contributory arrhythmias, especially during exercise.

If heart disease is suspected to underlie or contribute to exercise intolerance, the specific cardiac etiology and its severity should be defined as best as possible. Information obtained from general physical and CV-focused examinations (Chapter 2), thoracic radiography (Chapter 3), and echocardiography (Chapter 4) are helpful for this. Results of ambulatory or resting electrocardiography (Chapter 5) also can contribute importantly.

Exercise testing is critical in horses and focused on both horse and rider safety, as well as performance. The typical exam begins with assessment of orthopedic soundness and identification of neurologic deficits and then proceeds to the cardiorespiratory evaluation. Respiratory noise or endoscopic evidence of upper airway obstruction during exercise (as with laryngeal or soft palate abnormalities), endoscopic or bronchoalveolar lavage evidence of exercise-induced pulmonary hemorrhage, and identification of exercise-associated arrhythmias are key elements of the evaluation.

Optimal management for the patient with exercise intolerance depends on accurate identification of contributing factors and whether these can be treated effectively. Recognition that multiple abnormalities could underlie any individual patient's impaired exercise ability is important. For example, a dog with advanced degenerative mitral valve disease also might have chronic airway disease or collapse, degenerative joint disease, and obesity—each of which can cause exercise intolerance by itself. In most cases, some degree of exercise restriction is advisable, at least temporarily if not for the long term.

Suggested Additional Reading and References

Also See Online Comprehensive Bibliography at: https://www.routledge.com/9781482246223.

Aleman M. A review of equine muscle disorders. Neuromuscul Disord 2008;18:277–287.

Barnett L, Martin MW, Todd J, et al. A retrospective study of 153 cases of undiagnosed collapse, syncope or exercise intolerance: the outcomes. J Small Anim Pract 2011;52:26–31.

Beard W. Upper respiratory causes of exercise intolerance. Vet Clin North Am Equine Pract 1996;12:435–455.

Bohanon TC, Beard WL, Robertson JT. Laryngeal hemiplegia in draft horses. A review of 27 cases. Vet Surg 1990;19:456–459.

Brown K, Stefanovski D, Davidson E. Prevalence of adverse events and their effect on completion of high speed treadmill exercise tests at a single institution (2000–2015). Equine Vet J 2020;52:232–237.

Buhl R, Carstensen H, Hesselkilde EZ, et al. Effect of induced chronic atrial fibrillation on exercise performance in Standardbred trotters. J Vet Intern Med 2018;32:1410–1419.

Campbell FE. Cardiac effects of pulmonary disease. Vet Clin North Am Small Anim Pract 2007;37:949–962.

Cerda-Gonzalez S, Talarico L, Todhunter R. Noninvasive assessment of neuromuscular disease in dogs: use of the 6-minute walk test to assess submaximal exercise tolerance in dogs with centronuclear myopathy. J Vet Intern Med 2016;30:808–812.

Chesen AB, Whitfield-Cargile C. Update on diseases and treatment of the pharynx. Vet Clin North Am Equine Pract 2015;31:1–11.

Davenport-Goodall CL, Parente EJ. Disorders of the larynx. Vet Clin North Am Equine Pract 2003;19:169–187.

Dean PW. Upper airway obstruction in performance horses. Differential diagnoses and treatment. Vet Clin North Am Equine Pract 1991;7:123–148.

Durando MM. Cardiovascular causes of poor performance and exercise intolerance and assessment of safety in the equine athlete. Vet Clin North Am Equine Pract 2019;35:175–190.

Flaminio MJ, Gaughan EM, Gillespie JR. Exercise intolerance in endurance horses. Vet Clin North Am Equine Pract 1996;12:565–580.

Fogarty U, Buckley T. Bronchoalveolar lavage findings in horses with exercise intolerance. Equine Vet J 1991;23:434–437.

Foreman JH. Metabolic causes of equine exercise intolerance. Vet Clin North Am Equine Pract 1996;12:537–554.

Fraipont A, Van Erck E, Ramery E, et al. Subclinical diseases underlying poor performance in endurance horses: diagnostic methods and predictive tests. Vet Rec 2011;169:154.

Gaughan EM. Skeletal origins of exercise intolerance in horses. Vet Clin North Am Equine Pract 1996;12:517–535.

Hinchcliff KW, Kaneps AJ, Geor RJ. Equine Sports Medicine and Surgery. 2nd edition. Saunders Elsevier, Edinburgh. 2014.

Hoffman AM, Mazan MR, Ellenberg S. Association between bronchoalveolar lavage cytologic features and airway reactivity in horses with a history of exercise intolerance. Am J Vet Res 1998;59:176–181.

Kobluk CN, Gross GM. Exercise intolerance and poor performance in western performance and sprint horses. Vet Clin North Am Equine Pract 1996;12:581–606.

Lilich JD, Gaughan EM. Diagnostic approach to exercise intolerance in racehorses. Vet Clin North Am Equine Pract 1996;12:555–564.

Lilja-Maula L, Lappalainen AK, Hyytiainen HK, et al. Comparison of submaximal exercise test results and severity of brachycephalic obstructive airway syndrome in English bulldogs. Vet J 2017;219:22–26.

Little WC, Kitzman DW, Cheng CP. Diastolic dysfunction as a cause of exercise intolerance. Heart Fail Rev 2000;5:301–306.

Martin BB, Davidson EJ, Durando MM, et al. Clinical exercise testing: overview of causes of poor performance. In, Hinchcliff KW, Kaneps AJ, Geor RJ (editors). Equine Sports Medicine and Surgery. Saunders Elsevier, Edinburgh. 2004.

Martin BB Jr., Reef VB, Parente EJ, et al. Causes of poor performance of horses during training, racing, or showing: 348 cases (1992–1996). J Am Vet Med Assoc 2000;216:554–558.

Maxie MG, Physick-Sheard PW. Aortic-iliac thrombosis in horses. Vet Pathol 1985;22:238–249.

Mitten LA. Cardiovascular causes of exercise intolerance. Vet Clin North Am Equine Pract 1996;12:473–494.

Moore BR. Lower respiratory tract disease. Vet Clin North Am Equine Pract 1996;12:457–472.

Morris E. Application of clinical exercise testing for identification of respiratory fitness and disease in the equine athlete. Vet Clin North Am Equine Pract 1991;7:383–401.

Morris EA, Seeherman HJ. Clinical evaluation of poor performance in the racehorse: the results of 275 evaluations. Equine Vet J 1991;23:169–174.

Navas de Solis C. Cardiovascular response to exercise and training, exercise testing in horses. Vet Clin North Am Equine Pract 2019;35:159–173.

Navas de Solis C. Exercising arrhythmias and sudden cardiac death in horses: review of the literature and comparative aspects. Equine Vet J 2016;48:406–413.

Nogueira RB, Palacio MJ, Lopez JT, et al. Alterations in the large peripheral circulation in dogs with heart failure. Vet J 2011;188:101–104.

Nollet H, Deprez P. Hereditary skeletal muscle diseases in the horse. A review. Vet Q 2005;27:65–75.

Parente EJ. Testing methods for exercise intolerance in horses. Vet Clin North Am Equine Pract 1996;12:421–433.

Rossmeisl JH, Duncan RB, Inzana KD, et al. Longitudinal study of the effects of chronic hypothyroidism on skeletal muscle in dogs. Am J Vet Res 2009;70:879–889.

Rovira S, Munoz A, Benito M. Hematologic and biochemical changes during canine agility competitions. Vet Clin Pathol 2007;36:30–35.

Valberg SJ. Muscular causes of exercise intolerance in horses. Vet Clin North Am Equine Pract 1996;12:495–515.

Wall L, Mohr A, Ripoli FL, et al. Clinical use of submaximal treadmill exercise testing and assessments of cardiac biomarkers NT-proBNP and cTnI in dogs with presymptomatic mitral regurgitation. PLoS One 2018;13:e0199023.

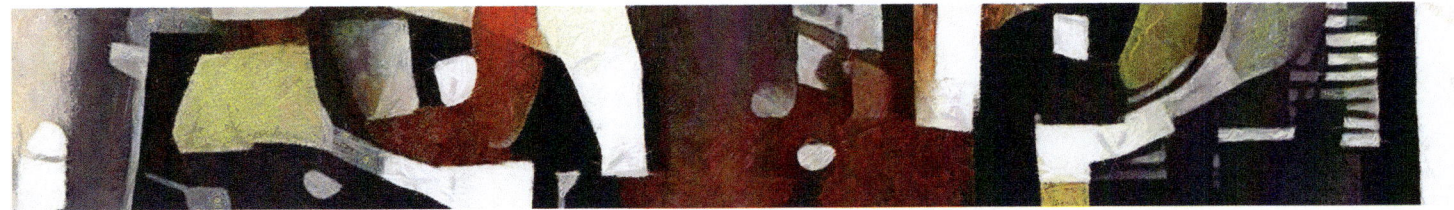

8

INTERMITTENT COLLAPSE AND SYNCOPE

Syncope is a sudden, transient loss of consciousness (sometimes called a "blackout" in people), as well as loss of postural tone (collapse). Syncope results from an abrupt decrease in cerebral perfusion or essential substrate delivery. It can be difficult to differentiate syncope from seizure activity or, sometimes, episodes of transient weakness (collapse without unconsciousness). Likewise, identifying the specific underlying cause of a collapse or syncopal event in an individual can be challenging. In many cases, the specific proximate cause remains undefined.

General Considerations

Syncope is often associated with sudden exertion or excitement. During a syncopal event, the animal usually collapses into lateral recumbency (**Figure 8.1**). However, this is variable; sometimes, collapsing on the sternum or even "going over backwards" might be observed. Limb stiffening, opisthotonic posture, micturition, and vocalization are common. However, facial fits, persistent tonic and clonic motion, defecation, a prodromal aura, (postictal) dementia, and neurologic deficits typically are not associated with cardiovascular (CV) syncope. Nevertheless, profound hypotension or asystole can cause hypoxic "convulsive syncope," with seizure-like activity or twitching. Convulsive syncopal episodes are preceded by loss of muscle tone. Conversely, seizure activity caused by underlying neurologic disease usually is preceded by atypical limb or facial movement or staring spells before postural tone is lost. Presyncope ("grayout" or near-syncope) might appear as mental dullness with transient wobbliness or weakness, especially in the hindlimbs. Presyncope can occur when reduction in brain perfusion, or substrate delivery, is not severe enough to cause unconsciousness.

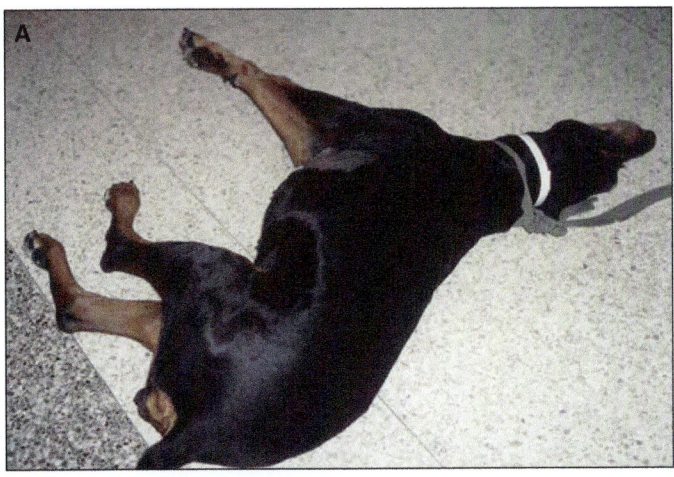
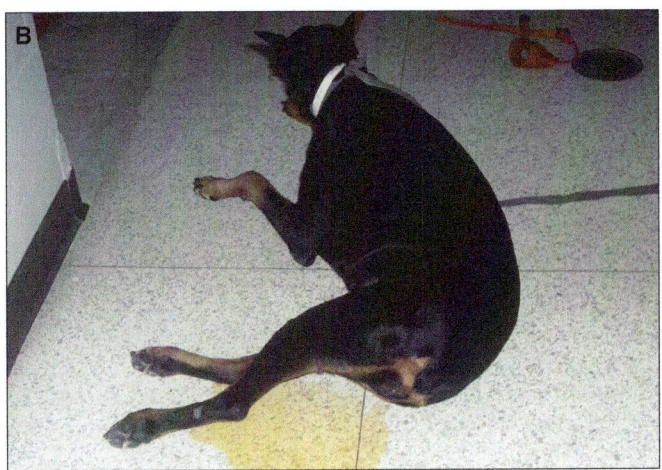

Figure 8.1 Syncope in a female Doberman Pinscher with paroxysmal ventricular tachycardia. (A) Sudden collapse into lateral recumbency was followed immediately by extension and stiffening of the forelimbs and neck. (B) The dog lost bladder control, but regained consciousness within about a minute. (A) From Ware WA. The cardiovascular examination. (In, Nelson RW, Couto CG (editors). Small Animal Internal Medicine. 6th edition. 2019. Elsevier, St. Louis. p. 2.)

Causes of Syncope

Many diseases can be associated with syncope (**Table 8.1**). Mechanisms underlying syncope usually involve either acutely reduced cardiac output (CO; often related to arrhythmias or severe structural heart disease), ventricular outflow obstruction, hypoxia or hypoglycemia with normal cerebral blood flow, or a combination of bradycardia and decreased vascular resistance related to neurocardiogenic reflexes. A fall in CO or vascular resistance reduces mean arterial pressure and, consequently, cerebral perfusion. Syncope occurs when cerebral blood flow falls below a critical level; this is about 30–50% of normal in people, although it might differ for quadripeds. Reduced cerebral blood flow also can result from cerebrovascular or other intracranial disease. Some cases of syncope might involve multiple mechanisms. For example, syncope associated with subaortic stenosis (p. 480) could relate to left ventricular (LV) outflow obstruction, arrhythmias, and also neurocardiogenic reflex mechanisms.

Table 8.1 Potential Causes of Syncope[a]

Cardiovascular
- Arrhythmias (see Chapters 5, 12, and 25)
  - Tachyarrhythmias
    - Ventricular tachyarrhythmias (tachycardia, flutter, fibrillation)
    - Supraventricular (atrial or AV junctional) tachyarrhythmias
    - Atrial fibrillation
  - Bradyarrhythmias
    - Sinus node dysfunction (sinus arrest, sick sinus syndrome)
    - Atrial standstill
    - High-grade second- or third-degree AV block
    - Reflex-mediated bradycardia
    - ?Sleep apnea in brachycephalic breeds
- Impaired cardiac output
  - Myocardial failure (see Chapters 32–34)
    - Dilated cardiomyopathy
    - Myocarditis
    - Myocardial ischemia or infarction (rare)
  - Severe valvular insufficiency (see Chapters 27, 29–31)
  - Cardiac rupture (with tamponade)
- Impaired cardiac filling
  - Hypertrophic cardiomyopathy (see Chapter 33)
  - Restrictive cardiomyopathy (see Chapter 33)
  - Cardiac tamponade (see Chapter 35)
  - Constrictive pericarditis (see Chapter 35)
  - Intracardiac tumor (see Chapter 35)
- Ventricular outflow or inflow obstructions
  - (Sub)aortic or pulmonic stenosis (see Chapter 27)
  - Hypertrophic obstructive cardiomyopathy (see Chapter 33)
  - Mitral or tricuspid stenosis (see Chapter 27)
  - Intracardiac tumor or thrombus
- Pulmonary vascular disease
  - Pulmonary hypertension (including heartworm disease; see Chapters 39 and 40)
  - Pulmonary thromboembolism (see Chapters 36 and 39)
- Congestive heart failure of any cause
- Cyanotic heart disease (right-to-left shunts; see Chapter 26)
  - Tetralogy of Fallot
  - Eisenmenger's physiology ("reversed" ASD, VSD, or PDA)
- Vascular disease
  - Aortic, pulmonary artery, or other large artery rupture
  - Cerebrovascular disease; hemorrhage or thromboembolism
  - Other acute hemorrhage (external or internal)
  - Acute pulmonary or systemic thromboembolism

Noncardiac
- Neurologic
  - Cerebrovascular disease (including from severe hypothyroidism in dogs)
  - Thrombotic (feline cardiomyopathy) or hemorrhagic (systemic hypertension) stroke
  - Brain tumor
  - Seizures
  - Narcolepsy/cataplexy
- Metabolic and hematologic
  - Anemia (hemolysis, blood loss, bone marrow suppression)
  - Hemoglobin abnormalities
  - Hypoadrenocorticism
  - Hypoglycemia (insulinoma, other neoplasia, insulin overdose, idiopathic [puppies, toy breeds], sepsis, liver failure)
- Diseases causing hypoxemia (primary respiratory or pleural space disease, right-to-left shunts)
- Cardiovascular active drugs (often from overdosing)
  - Calcium channel blockers
  - Beta-adrenergic blockers
  - Alpha-adrenergic blockers

Reflex
- Neurocardiogenic (vasovagal)
- Situational
  - Cough
  - Micturition, defecation
- Carotid sinus hypersensitivity
- Primary and secondary autonomic failure syndromes (reported in people)

[a] Many of these causes can lead to sudden death, also.
Abbreviations: ASD, atrial septal defect; AV, atrioventricular; PDA, patent ductus arteriosus; VSD, ventricular septal defect.

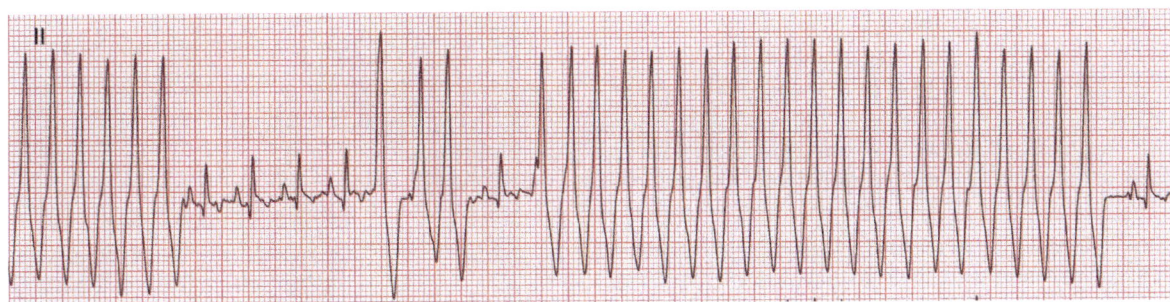

Figure 8.2 ECG from a 6-year-old male Boxer with a history of syncope. Paroxysms of rapid ventricular tachycardia (at ~300 beats/minute) interrupt the background sinus rhythm. The upright (positive) configuration of the ectopic QRS complexes is typical for arrhythmogenic right ventricular cardiomyopathy, the underlying diagnosis. Lead II; 25 mm/s; 1 cm = 1 mV.

Syncope often is associated with excitement or exertion, when the demand for CO and oxygenation is increased. Cardiac arrhythmias, as well as organic heart disease, commonly are involved. Underlying functional or structural heart abnormalities exacerbate the negative effect of arrhythmias on CO. Even when the heart rhythm is normal, diseases that reduce myocardial contractility, impair filling, or obstruct ventricular outflow can prevent adequate rise in CO to meet increased demand during activity or excitement. This group of causes includes pulmonary arterial hypertension due to heartworm disease, severe pulmonary disease, or idiopathic pulmonary vascular disease. Tachyarrhythmias, such as paroxysmal ventricular or supraventricular tachycardias and atrial fibrillation (Chapters 5 and 12), can markedly reduce CO by compromising ventricular filling and stroke volume (**Figure 8.2**). Recall the relationship: CO = Heart rate (HR) × Stroke volume. Bradyarrhythmias, such as complete atrioventricular (AV) block or sinus arrest, can profoundly reduce HR and, therefore, CO (**Figures 8.3** and **8.4**). Even sinus bradycardia, which normally is well tolerated, can induce syncope in the setting of exertion or when there is reflex vasodilation. Sudden death also can result from various arrhythmias associated with syncope.

In animals with normal CO, insufficient cerebral oxygen delivery can result from impaired blood oxygenation, as occurs

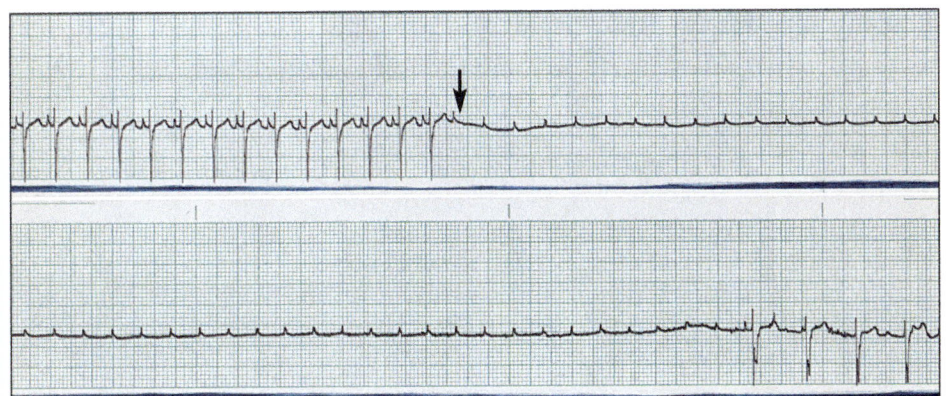

Figure 8.3 Continuous lead II ECG strip recorded from an 18-year-old spayed female domestic shorthair cat with syncope. Sinus rhythm is present at the top left, although the QRS complexes show a right bundle branch block pattern. Conduction failure then occurs (arrow) in the left bundle branch and/or AV node, causing third-degree (complete) AV block. Sinus P waves continue during the ventricular asystole that follows (~12 seconds duration); syncope occurred during this time (Figure 8.4). Finally, a ventricular escape rhythm appears (bottom right). 25 mm/s; 1 cm = 1 mV.

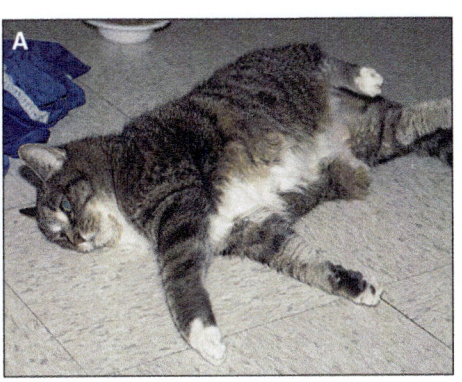
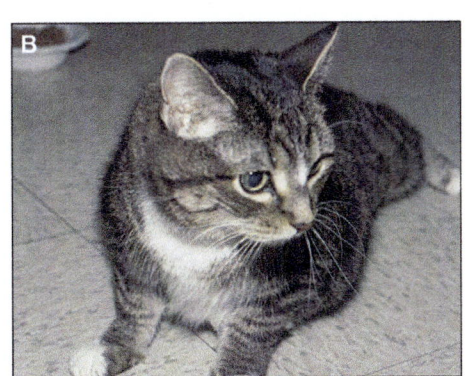

Figure 8.4 (A) After a few seconds of unsteadiness, syncope occurred during ventricular asystole in the cat of Figure 8.3. The limbs stiffened, but twitched briefly. (B) After several seconds, the cat regained consciousness and righted herself, then walked away normally.

with right-to-left shunts, anemia, or severe pulmonary disease (**Figure 8.5**). Hypoglycemia also can precipitate syncope, especially with exertion, although weakness and seizures are more common manifestations. Diseases that increase intracranial pressure can impair blood flow to the brain by reducing cerebral perfusion pressure and compressing intracranial vessels. Recall the relationship: Blood flow = Perfusion pressure/Vascular resistance; in the brain, Perfusion pressure = Mean arterial pressure–Intracranial pressure. Cerebrovascular disease (including stroke) can critically reduce cerebral blood flow either by vascular obstruction or rupture.

Neurocardiogenic or reflex (previously called vasovagal) syncope is thought to occur in some cases (**Figure 8.6**), although this mechanism is probably under-recognized in companion animals. Neurocardiogenic reflex mechanisms commonly underlie syncope in people, where upright posture increases susceptibility to gravitational effects on the circulation and orthostatic hypotension, and sympathetic surges stimulate myocardial c-fibers that trigger an inappropriate

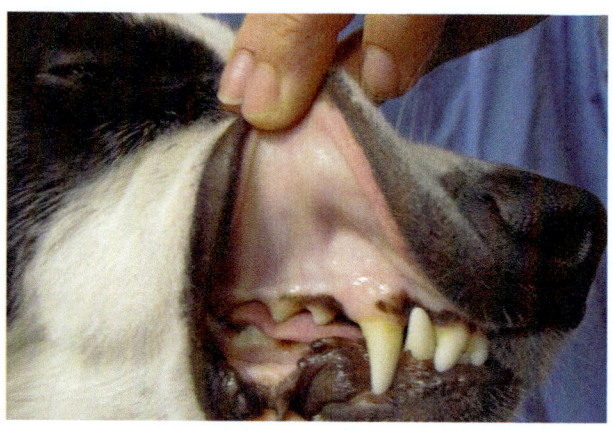

Figure 8.5 This young Border Collie was referred for cardiac evaluation because of exercise intolerance, collapse episodes, tachycardia, and a soft systolic murmur. Her heart rhythm was sinus tachycardia. She had a hematocrit of 8%; cardiac structure and function were normal.

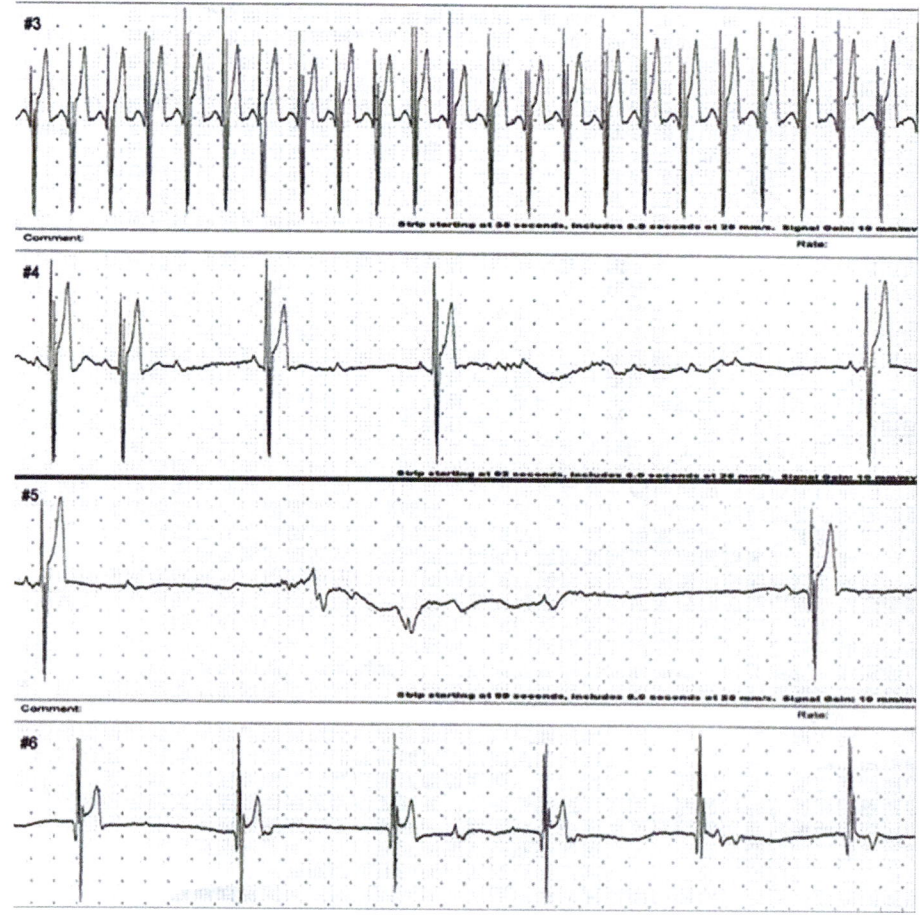

Figure 8.6 ECG event monitor recording from a young dog with excitement-induced syncope. The progression of heart rate and rhythm changes is consistent with reflex-mediated syncope. Sinus tachycardia is recorded in the top strip. Shortly thereafter, the heart rate slows markedly and sinus arrhythmia with intermittent second-degree AV block develops (second strip). This progresses rapidly to high-grade second-degree AV block; syncope occurred during the period of ventricular asystole (third strip). Finally, escape complexes appear (bottom strip); their relatively narrow QRS duration suggests a high-ventricular or junctional origin. The last two complexes on the right are slightly different in configuration, suggesting an alternate escape focus.

and exaggerated baroreceptor reflex. These are characterized by vagally induced bradycardias (sinus bradycardia, sinus arrest, and AV blocks) and concurrent peripheral vasodilation, which is difficult to document in animals. Quadrupedal posture makes this less likely in companion animals, although it does seem that sudden excitement might precipitate this in dogs. Holter monitor recordings in a small series of dogs with suspected neutrally mediated syncope revealed progressive sinus bradycardia and sinus arrest, often with an unstable ventricular escape rhythm, leading to the collapse; transient (or sometimes, persistent) atrial fibrillation (AF) then developed (Porteiro Vazquez, 2016). Inappropriate parasympathetic stimulation was thought to have impaired pacemaker cell function and then provoked acute AF in these cases. Syncope that occurs during sudden bradycardia after a burst of sinus tachycardia also has been observed regularly in dogs, especially small-breed dogs with advanced AV valve disease; excitement often precipitates such an episode. In some cases, younger dogs without apparent cardiac disease are affected. Doberman Pinschers and Boxers can experience a similar syndrome (Domingues, 2020). Whether and to what degree vasodilation occurs in these dogs is unknown because of the difficulty in documenting blood pressure (BP) during the syncopal episode. It is suspected that an acute sympathetic surge induced by excitement or exercise provokes a similar reflex vagal response to vasovagal syncope in people, which then results in bradycardia as well as hypotension. Activation of ventricular mechanoreceptors by forceful contractions, especially when ventricular filling is reduced, could play a role. The resulting surge in afferent neural traffic is thought to mimic that associated with hypertension, stimulating a paradoxical brainstem response of sympathetic withdrawal and vagal activation. Syncope in dogs with pheochromocytoma might represent a neurocardiogenic response to surges in sympathetic activity. It is also possible that neurocardiogenic mechanisms could be involved in animals with anemia and syncope.

Arrhythmic causes of syncope can occur during sleep such that a loss of consciousness might not be observed, but might result in seizure-like activity, opisthotonus, urination, or sudden death. Airway obstruction and sleep apnea are associated with arrhythmias in people. This has been reported in dogs and the authors have observed protracted sinus arrest and asystole in dogs during sleep on ambulatory ECG recordings (including Cavalier King Charles Spaniels with upper airway obstruction).

Syncope precipitated by coughing (cough syncope, "cough-drop") is a form of situational syncope (**Table 8.1**) that occurs more often in dogs with brachycephalic conformation, underlying airway disease or collapse, or with chronic mitral regurgitation and marked left atrial (LA) enlargement. Coughing transiently increases intrathoracic pressure (which reduces venous return to the heart) and intracranial pressure (which reduces cerebral perfusion pressure). The fall in CO and cerebral perfusion pressure can reduce cerebral blood flow below the level needed to maintain consciousness. Coughing also can reflexly stimulate vagally mediated bradycardia and vasodilation, which can contribute to hypotension and syncope.

The true incidence of syncope in dogs and cats is unknown. A survey of the Purdue Veterinary Medical Database over a 10-year period done by one of the authors (Ware, 2002) indicated that syncope had occurred in an estimated 0.15% of dogs and 0.03% of cats. While syncope might be underreported, this low prevalence in dogs and cats compared with people (estimated as high as 30–50%) suggests that neurocardiogenic syncope caused by orthostatic hypotension, is rare in quadrupeds. Syncope occurs more frequently in older animals. It is associated most often with cardiac disease and, to a lesser extent, other disease processes. According to the database survey noted earlier, about two-thirds of the dogs with syncope had cardiac disease, with or without an arrhythmia. Less frequently, respiratory diseases, anemia, or various other metabolic, neoplastic, or neurologic conditions were diagnosed concurrently in these dogs with syncope. Similarly, about two-thirds of cats with syncope were noted to have myocardial disease, with or without an arrhythmia. In a case series of dogs with syncope of undiagnosed cause, resolution or clinical improvement occurred with time in over half; a minority experienced clinical deterioration or death (Barnett, 2011).

Episodic weakness, without loss of consciousness, also can result from the mechanisms outlined for syncope in this chapter and **Table 8.1**. Additional considerations for sudden weakness especially with activity include myopathies, joint or spinal pain, pulmonary hypertension, and airway obstruction. Exercise-induced weakness with collapse of the rear limbs in particular might signal a reversed patent ductus arteriosus (p. 449), degenerative myelopathy, or myasthenia gravis.

Approach to the Patient with Syncope or Intermittent Collapse

The clinical history and physical examination often give clues to the underlying cause of episodic collapse (**Figure 8.7**). Detailed description of the episodes themselves, as well as preceding events, prodromal signs, and the animal's mentation and behavior after the event, can be helpful in differentiating CV syncope from seizure activity or other causes of collapse. Other information to be collected includes the number and frequency of previous events, whether the patient has had signs of cardiopulmonary or other systemic disease, what medications the animal is taking, and whether there has been collapse or sudden death in related animals. Video recordings of events obtained by clients can be especially useful if the full episode is recorded. For example, in canine narcolepsy/cataplexy, there is often an initial stimulus related to feeding and the dog often appears to just fall asleep. Owner

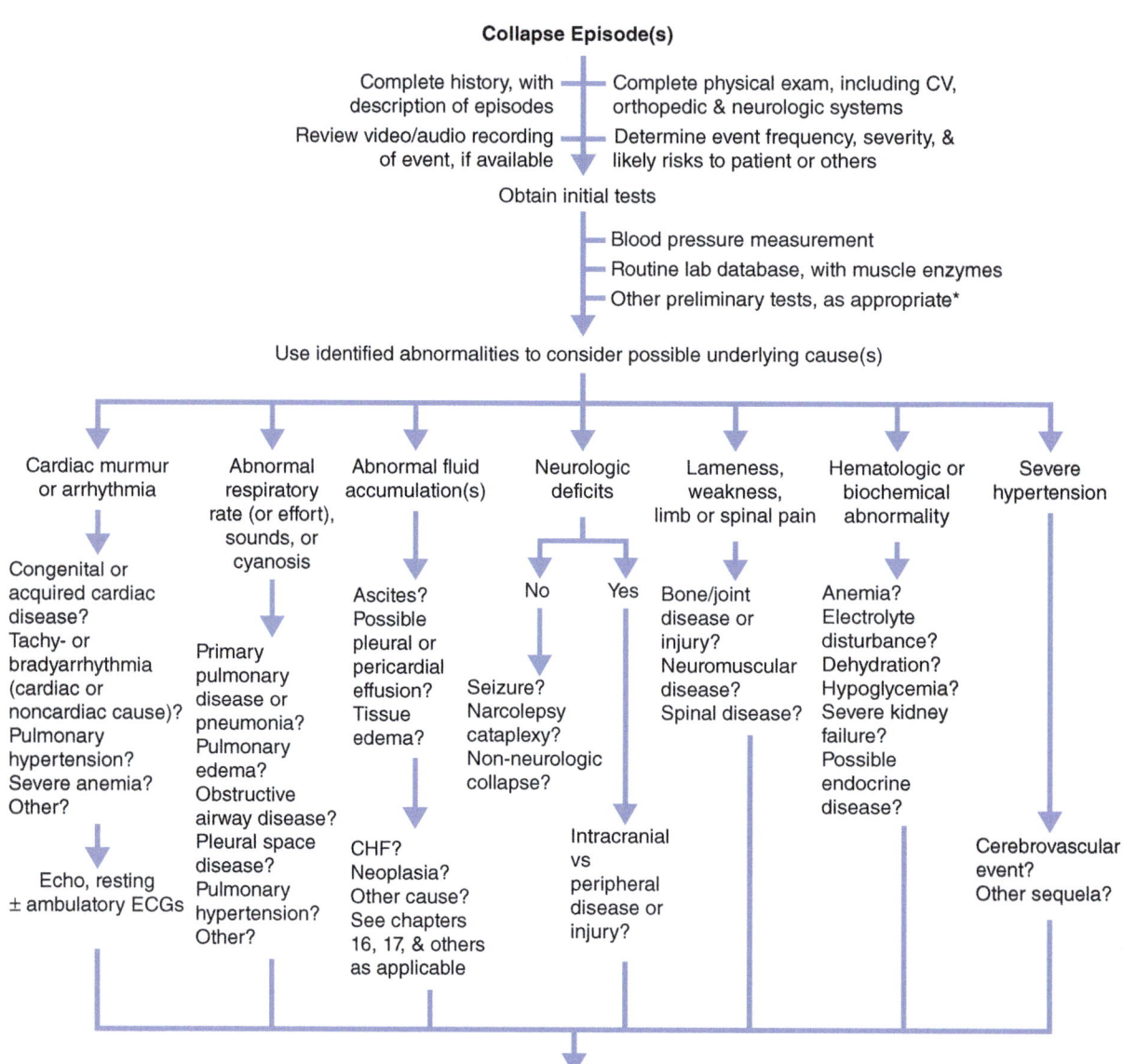

Figure 8.7 Approach to the patient with intermittent collapse. These are general guidelines; exceptions can occur. *This could include tests for heartworm or other parasitic disease, screening ultrasound exam, radiographs, etc. CNS, central nervous system; CHF, congestive heart failure; CV, cardiovascular; ECG, electrocardiogram; Echo, echocardiogram.

descriptions of witnessed events are critical to the diagnosis, and these can be confirmed or possibly recharacterized after viewing videos. The physical examination should evaluate all body systems thoroughly, with particular focus on the CV (Chapter 2), nervous, and respiratory systems.

A routine database of complete blood count (CBC), biochemical profile, urinalysis, heartworm test, and arterial BP measurement should be done. Although these tests often are normal, contributory underlying disease might be revealed. Endocrine tests (such as for adrenal or thyroid function) could be useful in some cases. A baseline electrocardiogram (ECG) is recommended; although when auscultation findings are normal, the resting ECG is usually nondiagnostic but could suggest underlying cardiac enlargement, conduction abnormality, or arrhythmia that might contribute to syncope. Thoracic radiographs are taken to evaluate the lungs, pleural space, mediastinum and pulmonary vasculature, as well as the cardiac size and shape. Suspicion for an underlying cardiac cause for syncope usually is generated by the combination of history, physical examination, the ECG, and thoracic radiographs. Echocardiography can confirm the presence and severity of cardiac structural or functional abnormalities that could lead to syncope or increase risk for arrhythmias.

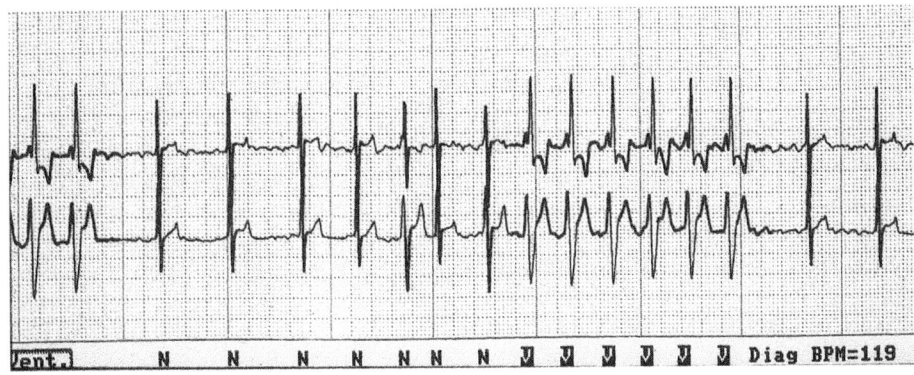

Figure 8.8 Brief segment from a 24-hour Holter recording in a dog with compensated heart failure and atrial fibrillation, with well-controlled ventricular rate in the clinic. Although the dog's medical status appeared stable, recent syncopal episodes prompted the Holter monitoring. Paroxysmal ventricular tachycardia was documented, as shown here; no ventricular ectopy had been evident during clinic visits. Ventricular antiarrhythmic therapy was instituted and no further syncope was reported.

Ambulatory ECG monitoring (Holter or external event monitor, or implantable loop recorder) can help identify or exclude cardiac arrhythmias as a cause for syncope (**Figure 8.8**) The reported diagnostic yield, both positive and negative results, has ranged from 42% to 85%. Event monitors usually are worn for a 1–2-week period and have a higher diagnostic yield than Holter monitoring, especially in animals with structural heart disease. Implantable loop recorders provide a longer monitoring time, which can improve diagnostic yield, and now include small recorders implantable under sedation and local anesthesia (p. 162). A syncopal episode must occur during monitoring to make a definitive diagnosis.

Not all arrhythmias cause hemodynamic compromise sufficient to induce syncope or collapse. While brady- or tachyarrhythmias might underlie the syncopal event, a cardiac arrhythmia can be excluded as the precipitating cause in many other cases, when collapse occurs during normal HR and rhythm. Holter monitoring (over one to seven days) is most likely to be diagnostic in animals that have multiple syncopal episodes over a short period of time, although the historical frequency of syncope does not predict likelihood of an event during Holter monitoring. Nevertheless, Holter monitoring is useful for quantifying the type and severity of arrhythmias, identifying arrhythmias in asymptomatic patients, and assessing antiarrhythmic drug efficacy. Because continuous loop event monitors (external or implantable) allow a longer monitoring period than traditional Holter monitors, they are optimal for patients with infrequent symptoms. These digital loop recorders monitor heart rhythm continuously; when activated, the ECG from a brief period prior to and following activation is saved into memory. The disadvantages of external event monitors are that they do not record potentially significant arrhythmias unless activated, and internal recorders must be programmed to collect appropriate ECG data from animals. Neither will quantify the frequency of arrhythmias.

When neurologic signs are present, an electroencephalogram (EEG), computed tomography (CT) or magnetic resonance imaging of the head, or other neurologic testing could be helpful. However, without a typical seizure history (such as tonic/clonic movement, postictal confusion) or abnormal neurologic examination, the diagnostic yield of these tests is likely to be low. Likewise, specific tests for musculoskeletal or neuromuscular abnormalities could be useful in some individuals.

Therapy is aimed at managing underlying disease(s) and avoiding precipitating factors, such as exertion or environmental stressors, as far as possible. This might include instituting or adjusting medications for heart failure (Chapter 22) or hypertension (Chapters 38 and 39), correcting anemia, or treating respiratory or metabolic diseases. When an arrhythmia appears to be the proximate cause, antiarrhythmic drug therapy or pacing is used as appropriate (Chapter 25). However, pacing is unlikely to modulate hypotension caused by neurocardiogenic syncope if the predominant mechanism is peripheral vasodilation. However, in cases of a sudden fall in heart rate, there are special pacing algorithms that can be activated to mitigate clinical signs.

Several medical strategies have been tried to manage suspected neurocardiogenic (reflex-mediated) syncope; however, none of these are backed by clinical trial evidence. Beta-blockers could be tried as a means to blunt the initiating sympathetically induced tachycardia and vigorous ventricular contraction, although exacerbation of bradycardia and suppression of escape activity can be a concern, and this treatment often backfires. Other strategies that have been effective anecdotally include a methylxanthine drug (such as theophylline or aminophylline), starting with a low dose and titrating up to effect, or low-dose digoxin in animals with chronic AV valve disease. In younger dogs without overt cardiac disease, salting the food to maintain plasma volume and even sodium retaining drugs such as fludrocortisone have been tried. In patients with proven sinus arrest but without other findings of sick sinus syndrome, the anticholinergic drug hyoscyamine has been used with variable clinical response (see Chapter 25).

Suggested Additional Reading and References

Also See Online Comprehensive Bibliography at: https://www.routledge.com/9781482246223.

Barnett L, Martin MW, Todd J, et al. A retrospective study of 153 cases of undiagnosed collapse, syncope or exercise intolerance: the outcomes. J Small Anim Pract 2011;52:26–31.

Basso C, Fox PR, Meurs KM, et al. Arrhythmogenic right ventricular cardiomyopathy causing sudden cardiac death in boxer dogs: a new animal model of human disease. Circulation 2004;109:1180–1185.

Bharati S, Cantor GH, Leach JB III, et al. The conduction system in sudden death in Alaskan sled dogs during the Iditarod race and/or during training. Pacing Clin Electrophysiol 1997;20:654–663.

Bright JM, Cali JV. Clinical usefulness of cardiac event recording in dogs and cats examined because of syncope, episodic collapse, or intermittent weakness: 60 cases (1997–1999). J Am Vet Med Assoc 2000;216:1110–1114.

Calvert CA, Brown J. Influence of antiarrhythmia therapy on survival times of 19 clinically healthy Doberman pinschers with dilated cardiomyopathy that experienced syncope, ventricular tachycardia, and sudden death (1985–1998). J Am Anim Hosp Assoc 2004;40:24–28.

de Solis CN, Althaus F, Basieux N, et al. Sudden death in sport and riding horses during and immediately after exercise: a case series. Equine Vet J 2018;50:644–648.

Domingues M, Brookes VJ, Oliveira P, et al. Heart rhythm during episodes of collapse in boxers with frequent or complex ventricular ectopy. J Small Anim Pract 2020;61:127–136.

Durando MM. Cardiovascular causes of poor performance and exercise intolerance and assessment of safety in the equine athlete. Vet Clin North Am Equine Pract 2019;35:175–190.

Dutton E, Dukes-McEwan J, Cripps PJ. Serum cardiac troponin I in canine syncope and seizures. J Vet Cardiol 2017;19:1–13.

Ferasin L. Recurrent syncope associated with paroxysmal supraventricular tachycardia in a Devon Rex cat diagnosed by implantable loop recorder. J Feline Med Surg 2009;11:149–152.

Fukushima R, Araie T, Itou N, et al. Canine case of swallowing syncope that improved after pacemaker implantation. J Vet Med Sci 2018;80:460–464.

Hyun C, Filippich LJ. Molecular genetics of sudden cardiac death in small animals—a review. Vet J 2006;171:39–50.

Kiryu K, Machida N, Kashida Y, et al. Pathologic and electrocardiographic findings in sudden cardiac death in racehorses. J Vet Med Sci 1999;61:921–928.

Lyle CH, Blissitt KJ, Kennedy RN, et al. Risk factors for race-associated sudden death in Thoroughbred racehorses in the UK (2000–2007). Equine Vet J 2012;44:459–465.

Lyle CH, Turley G, Blissitt KJ, et al. Retrospective evaluation of episodic collapse in the horse in a referred population: 25 cases (1995–2009). J Vet Intern Med 2010;24:1498–1502.

MacKie BA, Stepien RL, Kellihan HB. Retrospective analysis of an implantable loop recorder for evaluation of syncope, collapse, or intermittent weakness in 23 dogs (2004–2008). J Vet Cardiol 2010;12:25–33.

Meurs KM, Stern JA, Reina-Doreste Y, et al. Natural history of arrhythmogenic right ventricular cardiomyopathy in the boxer dog: a prospective study. J Vet Intern Med 2014;28:1214–1220.

Meurs KM, Weidman JA, Rosenthal SL, et al. Ventricular arrhythmias in Rhodesian Ridgebacks with a family history of sudden death and results of a pedigree analysis for potential inheritance patterns. J Am Vet Med Assoc 2016;248:1135–1138.

Miller RH, Lehmkuhl LB, Bonagura JD, et al. Retrospective analysis of the clinical utility of ambulatory electrocardiographic (Holter) recordings in syncopal dogs: 44 cases (1991–1995). J Vet Intern Med 1999;13:111–122.

Navas de Solis C. Exercising arrhythmias and sudden cardiac death in horses: review of the literature and comparative aspects. Equine Vet J 2016;48:406–413.

Obreztchikova MN, Sosunov EA, Anyukhovsky EP, et al. Heterogeneous ventricular repolarization provides a substrate for arrhythmias in a German shepherd model of spontaneous arrhythmic death. Circulation 2003;108:1389–1394.

Ohad DG, Lenchner I, Bdolah-Abram T, et al. A loud right-apical systolic murmur is associated with the diagnosis of secondary pulmonary arterial hypertension: retrospective analysis of data from 201 consecutive client-owned dogs (2006–2007). Vet J 2013;198:690–695.

Payne JR, Borgeat K, Brodbelt DC, et al. Risk factors associated with sudden death vs. congestive heart failure or arterial thromboembolism in cats with hypertrophic cardiomyopathy. J Vet Cardiol 2015;17(Suppl 1):S318–S328.

Perego M, Porteiro Vazquez DM, Ramera L, et al. Heart rhythm characterisation during unexplained transient loss of consciousness in dogs. Vet J 2020;263:105523.

Phan A, Yates GD, Nimmo J, et al. Syncope associated with swallowing in two British Bulldogs with unilateral carotid body tumours. Aust Vet J 2013;91:47–51.

Porteiro Vazquez DM, Perego M, Santos L, et al. Paroxysmal atrial fibrillation in seven dogs with presumed neurally-mediated syncope. J Vet Cardiol 2016;18:1–9.

Rasmussen CE, Falk T, Domanjko Petric A, et al. Holter monitoring of small breed dogs with advanced myxomatous mitral valve disease with and without a history of syncope. J Vet Intern Med 2014;28:363–370.

Santilli RA, Ferasin L, Voghera SG, et al. Evaluation of the diagnostic value of an implantable loop recorder in dogs with unexplained syncope. J Am Vet Med Assoc 2010;236:78–82.

Thomason JD, Kraus MS, Surdyk KK, et al. Bradycardia-associated syncope in 7 Boxers with ventricular tachycardia (2002–2005). J Vet Intern Med 2008;22:931–936.

Ward JL, DeFrancesco TC, Tou SP, et al. Outcome and survival in canine sick sinus syndrome and sinus node dysfunction: 93 cases (2002–2014). J Vet Cardiol 2016;18:199–212.

Ware WA. Causes and diagnosis of syncope. Proceedings of the 26th Annual Waltham/OSU Symposium. Columbus, OH. 2002.

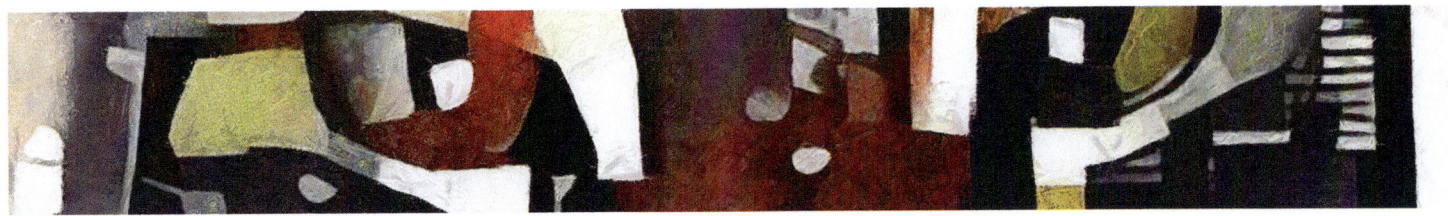

9
COUGH

The cough reflex is a protective mechanism that helps clear the airways of secretions and foreign substances. Mechanical or chemical stimulation activates rapid and slowly adapting receptors and C-fiber receptors in the larynx, trachea, carina, and bronchi to initiate the cough reflex. Other potential sites for stimulating cough include the pericardial and pleural surfaces, the diaphragm, and even the stomach. Afferent impulses from the airway receptors travel mainly through the vagus nerves to the medulla, which triggers a sequence of events. An initial inspiration is followed by closure of the glottis. Then, forceful contraction of the expiratory muscles sharply raises intrathoracic pressure. Finally, the epiglottis and vocal folds suddenly open widely, allowing air to explode out of the lungs and carry irritant material toward the pharynx. The strong lung compression narrows the airways, further increasing airflow velocity. Coughing can occur voluntarily also. Persistent coughing often is a sign of disease.

General Considerations

The cough reflex can be stimulated by the presence of foreign matter, accumulated secretions or fluid within the airways, airway collapse or compression, and the effects of inhaled irritants or inflammatory mediators (**Table 9.1** and **Figures 9.1–9.3**), although mechanisms triggering cough in some disorders are incompletely understood. Occasionally, coughing occurs in animals with disease of the pleural, pericardial, diaphragmatic, mediastinal, or nasal tissues; it is unclear if airway receptor stimulation is somehow involved in these cases. Cough receptors appear to be absent in the pulmonary alveoli and interstitium. Stimulation of the cough reflex is thought not to arise from those regions.

A cough is termed "productive" when secretions (of mucus, edema fluid, exudate, or blood) are brought up from the lung or airways. This feature might not be noticed by the owner because animals usually do not expectorate these secretions. The cough might have a moist sound. Swallowing motions generally follow a productive cough. In some cases, retching or expectoration occurs. Conditions that stimulate a productive cough include bronchopneumonia, chronic bronchitis, bronchiectasis, pulmonary edema, and hemoptysis. Postnasal drip from nasal or nasopharyngeal disease can also lead to coughing, including expectoration of foamy secretions.

A "nonproductive" or "dry" cough often is described as honking, or a "goose-honk" sound. Minimal secretions are involved. Conditions that usually induce a dry cough include tracheal or bronchial collapse, tracheobronchial irritation, mainstem bronchus compression (as from hilar lymphadenopathy or perhaps massive left atrial, LA, enlargement), and allergic pulmonary disease including asthma (**Figure 9.4**). A nonproductive cough also can be associated with heartworm disease (HWD). The importance of gastroesophageal reflux in animals as a cause of nocturnal or daily coughing is unresolved.

Hemoptysis is the coughing up of bloody foam or secretions. Although uncommon, it most often is associated with HWD, pulmonary hypertension, pulmonary embolism, or pulmonary neoplasia. Hemoptysis can also occur from a foreign body, mycotic infection, severe left-sided congestive heart failure (CHF) including from mitral stenosis, coagulopathy, lung lobe torsion, and rarely, pulmonary neoplasia.

Coughing often has been considered a common sign of cardiogenic pulmonary edema, especially in dogs with degenerative (myxomatous) mitral valve disease (DMVD). However, it appears that radiographic evidence for pulmonary edema is inconsistently associated with coughing in many dogs with DMVD. Coughing in these cases is often associated with radiographically abnormal airway patterns, as well as LA enlargement (Ferasin, 2013), suggesting airway disease or left bronchial compression as causes. The association between LA enlargement and cough in dogs with DMVD also has been questioned, although this point is controversial.

Table 9.1 Common Causes of Coughing

Airway Disease/Irritation
- Pharyngitis and tonsillitis
- Postnasal drip
- Laryngitis and laryngeal paresis
- Tracheobronchitis
- Collapsing trachea or mainstem bronchus
- Mainstem bronchus compression by enlarged left atrium or hilar lymphadenopathy
- Airway foreign body
- Airway mass lesion
- Canine chronic bronchitis, bronchiectasis
- Feline bronchial disease
- Equine asthma/bronchitis
- Allergic bronchitis
- *Oslerus osleri* infection (dog)
- Esophageal dysfunction

Pulmonary Disease
- Edema (not usually associated with cough in cats):
  - Cardiogenic (high pulmonary venous pressure)
  - Noncardiogenic (as with increased capillary permeability, neurogenic edema, hypoproteinemia)
- Pneumonia:
  - Bacterial
  - Aspiration
  - Viral
  - Fungal (including *Blastomyces dermatitidis, Histoplasma capsulatum, Coccidioides immitis,* and *Cryptococcus neoformans* [dog and cat])
  - Protozoal (including *Toxoplasma gondii* [cat]; *Pneumocystis carinii* [dog])
- Eosinophilic pulmonary disease

Neoplasia
- Primary
- Metastatic

Parasites
- Heartworms (*Dirofilaria immitis* [dog and cat]; *Angiostrongylus vasorum* [dog])
- Lungworms (including *Paragonimus kellicotti* and *Capillaria aerophila,* [dog and cat]; *Aelurostrongylus abstrusus* [cat]; *Crenosoma vulpis* [dog])
- Larval migration (*Toxocara canis* and other intestinal parasites)

Other
- Pleural, pericardial, diaphragmatic, mediastinal, and nasal diseases
- Gastroesophageal reflux disease
- Enalapril or other angiotensin converting enzyme inhibitors (p. 320)

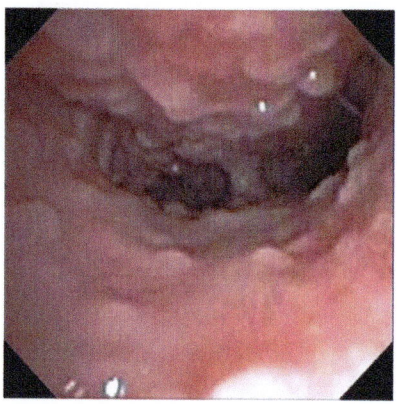

Figure 9.1 Bronchoscopy image at the carina from a 12-year-old Miniature Pinscher with chronic bronchitis shows mucosal edema, inflammation, and polypoid mucosal proliferation (nodules) secondary chronic inflammation. Cytologic exam showed intense inflammation (neutrophils and eosinophils) with no organisms evident. (Image courtesy of Dr. J Morrison.)

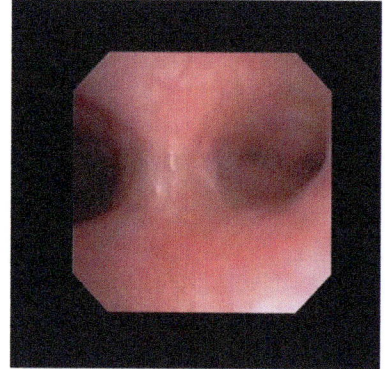

Figure 9.2 Collapse of the left mainstem bronchus (on right side of image), presumably with some compression by the enlarged left atrium, contributed to persistent coughing in an 11-year-old Cavalier King Charles Spaniel mix with degenerative mitral valve disease and compensated, stage C heart failure. Bronchomalacia from chronic bronchitis is a common comorbidity in such cases.

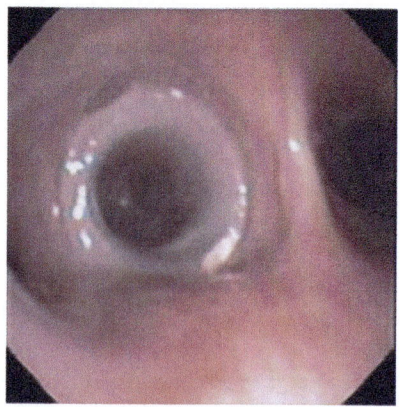

Figure 9.3 Bronchoscopic image from a 1-year-old spayed Bichon Frise with a persistent, nonproductive cough of 5 weeks duration and recent onset of collapse episodes. Marked bradycardia and cyanosis occurred during several collapse episodes. A whitish circular foreign body (FB) is visible in the right middle lobar bronchus. The freely moveable FB was extracted; it was a plastic, cone-shaped tip from a tube of caulk. Presumably, the FB would slip out of the bronchial orifice during coughing fits and obstruct airflow in the trachea, leading to the observed collapse, cyanosis, and bradycardia. (Image courtesy of Drs. J Clemans and K Deitz.)

Clearly, many dogs with DMVD have concurrent bronchitis and bronchomalacia with associated airway collapse (Singh, 2012). However, radiographic features of left bronchial compression are commonly observed in advanced DMVD, especially on left lateral radiographs of dogs with severe mitral regurgitation. Furthermore, coughing does occur in larger

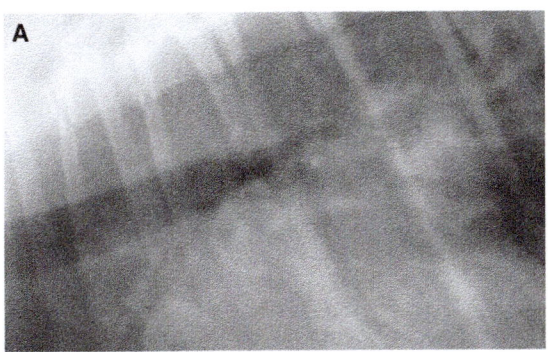
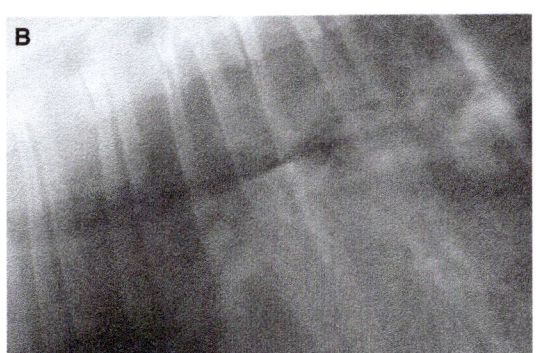
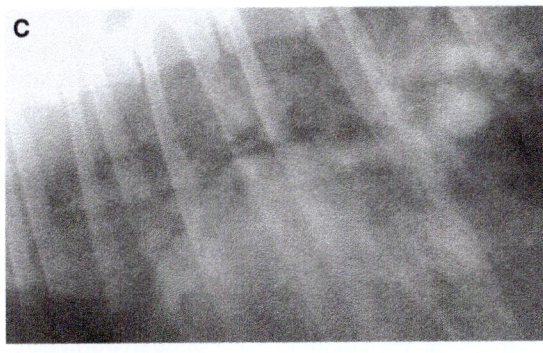

Figure 9.4 (A) Fluoroscopic image taken during inspiration in a 9-year-old female Bolognese dog with chronic mitral regurgitation and cough with excitement. Note the left atrial enlargement and some main bronchus compression. (B) In early expiration, the airways narrow further. (C) Complete expiratory airway collapse follows shortly.

breed dogs and in some horses with cardiogenic pulmonary edema. Cats infrequently cough with CHF although some will, especially with fulminant pulmonary edema. A useful caveat is that cough without resting or sleeping tachypnea is an *unlikely* sign of left-sided CHF. In patients with a normal sleeping respiratory rate (<25/minute) or with only mild left atrial dilation, underlying airway disease is likely to be the major contributor to coughing. Lastly, coughing in cardiac patients might also be explained by clearing of pooled secretions following sleep or the triggering of some poorly defined reflex related to elevated left atrial pressure.

Coughing in cats often is associated with reactive airway disease, bronchitis, HWD (Chapter 40), or lungworms (**Table 9.1**). Pharyngeal irritation, nasopharyngeal polyp, drainage of nasal/pharyngeal secretions into the larynx and trachea, and hairballs also can cause coughing, as well as gagging sounds, in cats. Because cough receptors are lacking in alveolar regions, lung parenchymal disease usually does not stimulate the cough reflex. As noted, cats with CHF generally do not cough. Nevertheless, an occasional cat with cardiogenic pulmonary edema or pleural effusion does have a history that includes coughing. Pleuritis in cats, such as that secondary to chronic chylothorax, can stimulate coughing.

In horses also, coughing can be a sign of airway inflammation, either infectious or noninfectious. Cough is a common sign of recurrent airway obstruction (asthma) in horses; mucoid nasal discharge also is common in affected animals. Some coughing, either at rest or during exercise, has been reported in up to about half of racehorses (Thoroughbreds, Standardbreds, barrel racing horses), although coughing could be more common in nonracing sport horses (Leguillette, 2016). Exercise-induced pulmonary hemorrhage or variable airway inflammation could underlie this. Nevertheless, horses with CHF and pulmonary edema do sometimes manifest coughing, in addition to increased respiratory rate and effort.

Approach to the Coughing Patient

It is important to differentiate coughing from gagging or retching, or from other sounds the patient might make. Gagging or retching often is associated with upper gastrointestinal (GI) or pharyngeal disease, although animals frequently retch at the end of a coughing episode. Expectorated mucous or foam that is bile-tinged indicates vomitus rather than respiratory secretions. Expectorated blood or bloody foam should be presumed to originate in the lungs until proven otherwise.

Coughing associated with CHF can occur either at rest or during exercise, but is worse with activity. Dogs with pulmonary edema can develop nocturnal dyspnea and cough at night. The cough might sound productive and be associated with retching and expectoration of fluid, especially if alveolar

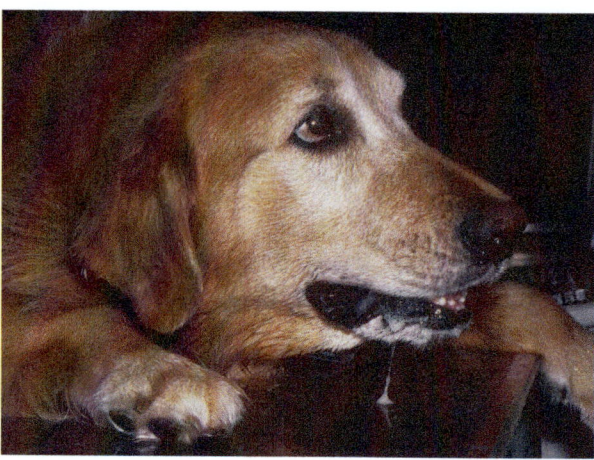

Figure 9.5 A 9-year-old male Golden Retriever with no prior health issues developed a soft cough, which progressed over several days to respiratory distress. The dog had severe cardiogenic pulmonary edema caused by dilated cardiomyopathy.

Table 9.2 An Approach to the Coughing Patient

Determine If the Animal Is Truly Coughing
- History, observation, video recordings with sound, physical examination.
  - Rule out vomiting, gagging/retching, reversed sneeze, and so on.

Consider Evidence for Pulmonary Parenchymal Involvement or Other Concurrent Disease
- Signalment, history, physical examination, systemic signs, and other findings (see text).
- Rule out a primary airway cause or cardiopulmonary compromise.
- Is respiratory rate, character or effort abnormal?
- What is the sleeping respiratory rate?
- Is exercise tolerance reduced?
- Any physical or laboratory evidence for a generalized or systemic disease process?

Evaluate Thoracic Radiographs (see Figure 9.6).
Select Other Diagnostic Tests as Appropriate (see text)
- Consider all findings.

Treat Based on Underlying Etiology
- For cardiogenic pulmonary edema, see Chapter 22 and other chapter(s) on specific cardiovascular diseases.
- For heartworm disease, see Chapter 40.
- For disease complicated by pulmonary hypertension, see Chapter 39.
- For primary airway, pulmonary parenchymal, and other noncardiac disease, consult appropriate reference sources.
- For persistent nonproductive cough, consider adjunctive antitussive therapy

edema is present (**Figure 9.5**). However, this is not specific because the common conditions of chronic bronchitis with bronchomalacia (and airway collapse) sometimes induce a similar cough as respiratory secretions can pool, especially during sleep. Fulminant pulmonary edema can lead to pink-red froth flowing from the mouth and nares, as well as dyspnea. Loud, brassy or honking coughing in dogs is more typical of major airway irritation or collapse (tracheal collapse, left mainstem bronchus compression; **Figures 9.2** and **9.4**). Soft coughing is more typical of small airway or lung parenchymal disease, including edema. Either type of cough is compatible with cardiovascular disease.

An initial determination must be made as to whether airway irritation, left-sided CHF, or primary pulmonary disease is most likely responsible for the coughing (**Table 9.2** and **Figure 9.6**). This guides more specific testing and initial therapy. The patient's signalment and history can help suggest whether conditions such as infectious disease, acute reactive airway disease, chronic airway disease or collapse, CHF, or HWD are more likely in that individual. Diseases that involve the pulmonary parenchyma and interfere with normal lung function, including pulmonary edema, often cause reduced exercise tolerance, as well as increased resting respiratory rate and effort. Sometimes, the cough interferes with sleep at night; this is classic but not pathognomonic for left-sided CHF. Cough can become worse with activity, especially in patients with CHF, collapsing trachea, inflammatory airway disease, HWD, and other lung diseases. Primary airway disease usually is associated with normal resting respiratory rate and activity level, unless airway obstruction is present, although excitement, activity, and pulling against a collar or leash can provoke the cough. A major airway obstruction, such as laryngeal paresis, is typically associated with audible noise during ventilation. As previously noted, a productive cough in the early morning or after resting can occur as airway secretions accumulated during sleep are cleared. Some diseases cause signs of both airway and lung parenchymal disease, including chronic bronchitis with secondary infection, neoplasia, and parasitic diseases.

The physical examination can provide etiologic clues. The patient's demeanor and character of respirations (Chapter 10) might help in localizing the disease process. Palpation of the cervical trachea could stimulate a cough in animals with collapsing trachea; however, this maneuver also can provoke a cough when the trachea is irritated from another cause of chronic cough. Abnormal lung or heart sounds heard on auscultation might, or might not, indicate the main clinical abnormality. For example, a coughing dog with a murmur of mitral regurgitation (MR) and pulmonary crackles might have left-sided CHF; however, the pulmonary crackles could instead be a manifestation of underlying chronic lung disease, with incidental MR. Alternatively, the cough could be secondary to chronic bronchitis, collapsing trachea, or mainstem bronchus compression from marked LA enlargement, rather than pulmonary edema.

Thoracic radiographs are an important diagnostic tool, especially in small animals. They should be evaluated for the presence and pattern of any pulmonary infiltrates, cardiomegaly (including specific chamber enlargement criteria;

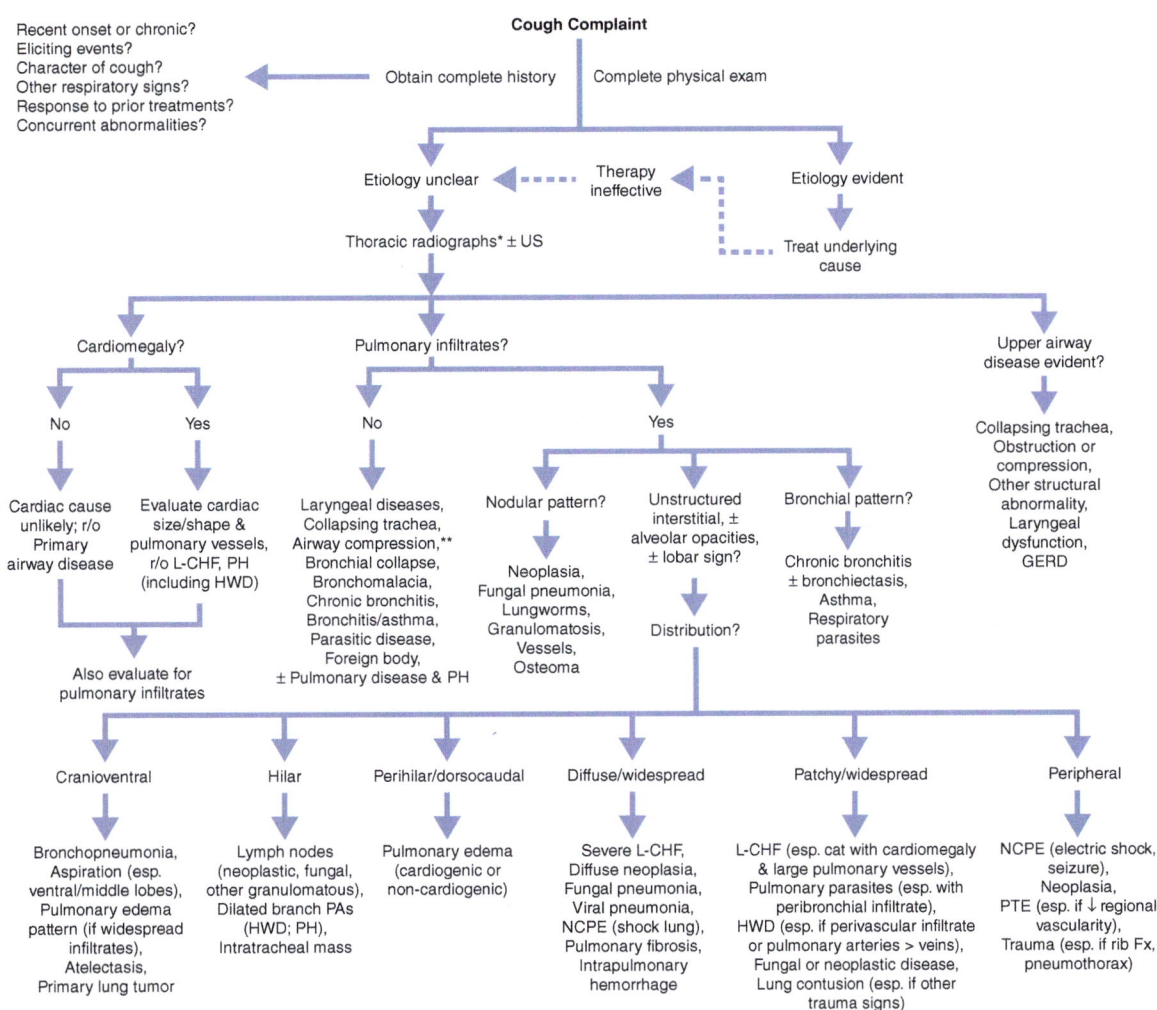

Figure 9.6 Approach to the patient with cough. These are general guidelines; exceptions can occur. Diseases listed below are rule-outs to consider. *Also note evidence for pleural effusion or air, & abnormalities of other structures (see **Tables 10.2 & 10.3**, p. 213). **Hilar lymphadenopathy, lung tumor, dilated esophagus. Fx, fracture; L-CHF, left-sided congestive heart failure; GERD, gastroesophageal reflux disease; HWD, heartworm disease; NCPE, noncardiogenic pulmonary edema; PAs, pulmonary arteries; PH, pulmonary hypertension; PTE, pulmonary thromboembolism; r/o, rule out; US, ultrasonography.

Chapter 3), evidence of large airway disease, and pleural space or vascular abnormalities. Diagnosis of dynamic airway collapse might require fluoroscopy, comparison of inspiratory and expiratory exposures, or bronchoscopy. If pulmonary edema is suspected based on the appearance and distribution of pulmonary infiltrates, especially with concurrent cardiomegaly, a diuretic trial and further cardiac assessment are indicated. If the animal already is being treated for heart failure of known cause, intensification of therapy is warranted.

If radiography must be delayed for any reason, point-of-care lung ultrasound could be a useful and rapid screening test in some animals. Especially in dogs presented for cough, lung ultrasound helps differentiate those likely to have underlying pulmonary edema, or another parenchymal abnormality, from those with primary airway disease. The criteria of ≥10 total B-lines and ≥2 sites strongly positive for B-lines were both 92% sensitive and 94% specific for cardiogenic pulmonary edema, in one study (Ward, 2019).

Other diagnostic tests are indicated if the cause of coughing is unclear. The choice of these depends on the patient's signalment, history, physical examination, and radiographic findings. Such tests might include a complete blood count, serum biochemical profile, airway washings (tracheal wash or bronchoalveolar lavage), heartworm tests, fungal serology, fecal tests, bronchoscopy, lung biopsy, and computerized tomography of the thorax, among other tests.

Treatment for the coughing patient should be directed at the underlying disease process whenever possible. An accurate diagnosis is obviously important; for example, it makes no sense to prescribe a cough suppressant or antibiotic for a dog coughing from left-sided CHF. Guidelines for managing heart failure can be found in Chapter 22, as well as in chapters on specific heart diseases. HWD is discussed in Chapter 40. The reader is urged to consult other sources for current treatment recommendations for primary respiratory and airway diseases.

Table 9.3 Antitussive Therapy

Cough Suppressants (for Dogs Only)	
Butorphanol	Dog: 0.5–1 mg/kg PO q6–12h
Hydrocodone bitartrate	Dog: 0.25 mg/kg PO q6–12h[b]
Dextromethorphan	Dog: 1–2 mg/kg PO q6–8h
Bronchodilators[a]	
Aminophylline	Dog: 11 mg/kg PO q8h
	Cat: 5 mg/kg PO q12h
Theophylline (long-acting)	Dog: 10 mg/kg PO q12h
	Cat: 20-25 mg/kg PO q24-48 h (in evening)
Oxtriphylline elixir	Dog: 14 mg/kg PO q8h
	Cat: none
Terbutaline	Dog: 1.25–5 mg/dog PO q8–12h
	Cat: 1/8–1/4 of 2.5 mg tablet/cat PO q12h

[a] May be useful if bronchospasm is provoking cough.
[b] Lower initial doses often are increased over time as tolerance develops.

Antitussive therapy can be useful in selected cases. However, a productive cough generally is not suppressed because it helps clear the airways. Underlying airway inflammation should be addressed prior to resorting to chronic antitussive drug therapy, as this will not address the etiology or damage caused by chronic inflammation. For persistent coughing that is not associated with infection or pulmonary edema, antitussive therapy can provide some relief to both patient and owner (**Table 9.3**). Such situations include dynamic large airway collapse and mainstem bronchus compression associated with marked LA enlargement when pulmonary edema is absent.

Suggested Additional Reading and References

Also See Online Comprehensive Bibliography at: https://www.routledge.com/9781482246223.

Bedenice D, Mazan MR, Hoffman AM. Association between cough and cytology of bronchoalveolar lavage fluid and pulmonary function in horses diagnosed with inflammatory airway disease. J Vet Intern Med 2008;22:1022–1028.

Bosshard S, Gerber V. Evaluation of coughing and nasal discharge as early indicators for an increased risk to develop equine recurrent airway obstruction (RAO). J Vet Intern Med 2014;28:618–623.

Canning BJ. Afferent nerves regulating the cough reflex: mechanisms and mediators of cough in disease. Otolaryngol Clin North Am 2010;43:15–25.

Christley RM, Hodgson DR, Rose RJ, et al. Coughing in Thoroughbred racehorses: risk factors and tracheal endoscopic and cytological findings. Vet Rec 2001;148:99–104.

DeFrancesco TC, Rush JE, Rozanski EA, et al. Prospective clinical evaluation of an ELISA B-type natriuretic peptide assay in the diagnosis of congestive heart failure in dogs presenting with cough or dyspnea. J Vet Intern Med 2007;21:243–250.

Drobatz KJ, Saunders HM, Pugh CR, et al. Noncardiogenic pulmonary edema in dogs and cats: 26 cases (1987–1993). J Am Vet Med Assoc 1995;206:1732–1736.

Egenvall A, Hansson K, Sateri H, et al. Pulmonary oedema in Swedish hunting dogs. J Small Anim Pract 2003;44:209–217.

Ferasin L, Crews L, Biller DS, et al. Risk factors for coughing in dogs with naturally acquired myxomatous mitral valve disease. J Vet Intern Med 2013;27:286–292.

Guglielmini C, Diana A, Pietra M, et al. Use of the vertebral heart score in coughing dogs with chronic degenerative mitral valve disease. J Vet Med Sci 2009;71:9–13.

Hawkins EC, Clay LD, Bradley JM, et al. Demographic and historical findings including exposure to environmental tobacco smoke, in dogs with chronic cough. J Vet Intern Med 2010;24: 825–831.

Hawkins EC, Rogala AR, Large EE, et al. Cellular composition of bronchial brushings obtained from healthy dogs and dogs with chronic cough and cytologic composition of bronchoalveolar lavage fluid obtained from dogs with chronic cough. Am J Vet Res 2006;67:160–167.

Johnson LR. Laryngeal structure and function in dogs with cough. J Am Vet Med Assoc 2016;249:195–201.

Johnson LR, Pollard RE. Tracheal collapse and bronchomalacia in dogs: 58 cases (7/2001–1/2008). J Vet Intern Med 2010;24:298–305.

Kittleson MD, Kienle RD. Small Animal Cardiovascular Medicine. Mosby, London, UK. 1998. pp. 36–46.

Lara JP, Dawid-Milner MS, Gonzalez-Baron S. Effects of bronchoconstriction on the cough reflex in the cat. Rev Esp Fisiol 1993;49:235–240.

Leguillette R, Steinmann M, Bond SL, et al. Tracheobronchoscopic assessment of exercise-induced pulmonary hemorrhage and airway inflammation in barrel racing horses. J Vet Intern Med 2016;30:1327–1332.

Macready DM, Johnson LR, Pollard RE. Fluoroscopic and radiographic evaluation of tracheal collapse in dogs: 62 cases (2001–2006). J Am Vet Med Assoc 2007;230:1870–1876.

Marr CM. Cardiac and respiratory disease in aged horses. Vet Clin North Am Equine Pract 2016;32:283–300.

Prandota J. Furosemide: progress in understanding its diuretic, anti-inflammatory, and bronchodilating mechanism of action, and use in the treatment of respiratory tract diseases. Am J Ther 2002;9:317–328.

Rettmer H, Hoffman AM, Lanz S, et al. Owner-reported coughing and nasal discharge are associated with clinical findings, arterial oxygen tension, mucus score and bronchoprovocation in horses with recurrent airway obstruction in a field setting. Equine Vet J 2015;47:291–295.

Rose RJ, Hodgson DR. Protocols for common presenting complaints. In, Rose RJ, Hodgson DR. Manual of Equine Practice. WB Saunders Co., Philadelphia, PA. 2000. pp. 31–32.

Schober KE, Hart TM, Stern JA, et al. Detection of congestive heart failure in dogs by Doppler echocardiography. J Vet Intern Med 2010;24:1358–1368.

Singh MK, Johnson LR, Kittleson MD, et al. Bronchomalacia in dogs with myxomatous mitral valve degeneration. J Vet Intern Med 2012;26:312–319.

Sudo T, Hayashi F, Nishino T. Responses of tracheobronchial receptors to inhaled furosemide in anesthetized rats. Am J Respir Crit Care Med 2000;162:971–975.

Ward JL, Lisciandro GR, Ware WA, et al. Lung ultrasonography findings in dogs with various underlying causes of cough. J Am Vet Med Assoc 2019;255:574–583.

Widdicombe JG. A brief overview of the mechanisms of cough. In, Chung KF, Widdicombe J, Boushey HA. Cough: Causes, Mechanisms and Therapy. Blackwell, Oxford, UK. 2003. pp. 17–23.

Yamaya Y, Suzuki K, Watari T, et al. Bronchoalveolar lavage fluid and serum canine surfactant protein A concentrations in dogs with chronic cough by bronchial and interstitial lung diseases. J Vet Med Sci 2014;76:593–596.

Zhu BY, Johnson LR, Vernau W. Tracheobronchial brush cytology and bronchoalveolar lavage in dogs and cats with chronic cough: 45 cases (2012–2014). J Vet Intern Med 2015;29:526–532.

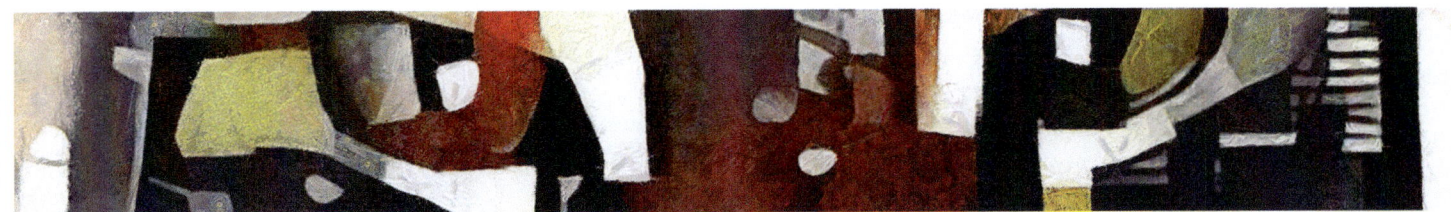

10
RESPIRATORY DISTRESS

Normal respiration is characterized by quiet, active inspiration followed by passive expiration. Both phases are smooth and symmetrical. The breath is initiated by medullary neurons, however neural control of breathing also involves other brainstem centers, cervical vertebral segments, and the cerebral cortex. This allows involuntary rhythmic breathing, as well as involuntary nonrhythmic control (as during swallowing) and voluntary control. The diaphragm is the main inspiratory muscle. During contraction the diaphragmatic dome moves caudally, enlarging the thorax and creating the negative intrathoracic pressure that pulls air into the lungs. The external intercostal muscles also help by moving the ribs cranially and outward during inspiration. Contraction of abductor muscles in the nares, pharynx, and larynx maximizes upper airway diameter to facilitate airflow during inspiration. During passive exhalation, elastic recoil of the lung and chest wall moves air out. Abdominal and internal intercostal muscles also are used for expiration; their contraction decreases thoracic size, thereby increasing intrathoracic pressure and forcing air out of the lungs.

General Considerations

The breathing rate is influenced by numerous factors such as exercise, ambient temperature, excitement, digestive tract filling, pregnancy and other causes of abdominal enlargement, and many diseases. Normal dogs and cats have resting (sleeping) respiratory rates of between 16 and 25 breaths/minute; a guideline of <30 breaths/minute often is used clinically. Resting respiratory rates in adult horses generally range between 8 and 16 breaths/minute.

Pulmonary, pleural space, and airway diseases can influence the pattern of breathing and associated breath sounds. The nasal cavity and upper airways offer the greatest resistance to normal inspiration. However, abnormally high inspiratory resistances often are encountered in brachycephalic breeds of dogs and cats; a prolonged inspiratory phase of breathing is a typical compensation. Lung stiffness can be altered by pulmonary capillary congestion, lung edema, or interstitial fibrosis; more rapid but shallow breathing occurs in compensation. Resistance to exhalation generally is low, but it increases with narrowing of a principle bronchus (as with left bronchial compression) or as a consequence of diffuse bronchial disease with bronchomalacia.

Animals with respiratory difficulty usually have an increased effort and rate of breathing, among other signs (**Table 10.1**). Several descriptive terms are used:

- "Tachypnea" is an increase in respiratory rate. This term typically is not used to describe panting as a means of heat dissipation in dogs, which is normal. However, excessive panting or rapid shallow breathing can occur from respiratory compromise. Panting in cats often is a sign of respiratory compromise, although it can occur with stress and hyperthermia, too.
- "Hyperpnea" is increased depth (and rate) of breathing.
- "Dyspnea," as used in human medicine, is the awareness of difficulty in breathing, breathlessness, or the sensation of air hunger. A number of mechanisms are thought to underlie this; systemic chemoreceptors and vagal C-fibers, present throughout the respiratory tract, appear to be the main peripheral sensors. In veterinary use, the term is synonymous with labored breathing or respiratory distress.
- "Orthopnea" refers to respiratory distress so severe that it causes the animal to assume a certain upright posture and resist other body positions. Dogs with orthopnea stand or sit with elbows abducted, which allows full rib expansion, and neck extended. They resist being positioned in lateral or dorsal recumbency (**Figures 10.1** and **10.2**). Cats often crouch in a sternal or squatting position with elbows abducted and neck extended; open-mouth breathing usually

Table 10.1 Signs of Hypoxemia

Restlessness and anxiety
↑ Respiratory rate
↑ Respiratory effort
Extended head and neck
Assuming a posture to optimize airflow and ventilation
Orthopnea
Pale grayish or cyanotic mucous membranes (unless marked anemia)
± Arrhythmias or tachycardia (less often, bradycardia)
± Syncope

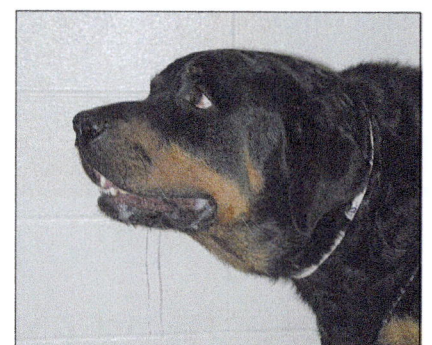

Figure 10.2 Orthopnea in a 4-year-old Rottweiler with severe bacterial pneumonia. Note the head and neck extension, anxious expression, and drooling saliva.

is a sign of severe respiratory distress (**Figures 10.3** and **10.4**). Horses with orthopnea also stand with elbows abducted, neck extended, and nostrils flared prominently (**Figure 10.5**).

- "Paradoxical" breathing occurs when the abdomen moves in the opposite direction to the ribcage. It often is a sign of chronic respiratory disease or impending respiratory failure and can occur with a variety of disorders.

Animals with severe dyspnea are reluctant to eat, drink, or even swallow saliva. Some patients exhibit greater respiratory effort during inspiration or during expiration. Both phases are equally labored in others. The localization and pathophysiology of the underlying disease process influence the pattern as well as the rate of breathing (see section "Patterns of Breathing").

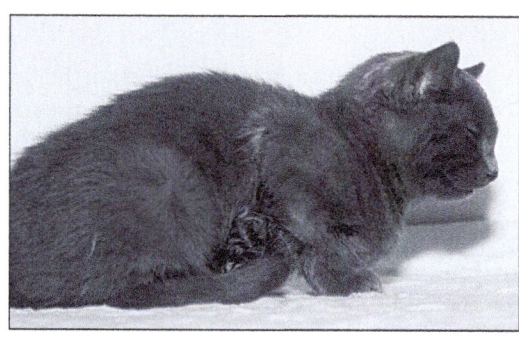

Figure 10.3 The crouched position of this 4-month-old kitten with hypoxemia from tetralogy of Fallot is typical for cats with orthopnea. Subtle open-mouth breathing is apparent.

Causes of Respiratory Distress

The underlying causes of respiratory difficulty most often involve either respiratory system disease, at any level from external nares to pulmonary alveoli to pleural space, or cardiovascular (CV) dysfunction. The most common CV causes for respiratory distress are pulmonary edema or pleural effusion from congestive heart failure (CHF), congenital right-to-left shunts, heartworm disease, and pulmonary thromboembolism (PTE). Other diverse causes also interfere with respiration, such as impaired blood oxygen-carrying capacity, pleural space disease, and disruption of thoracic cage integrity or respiratory muscle function (**Table 10.2**). Hyperthermia

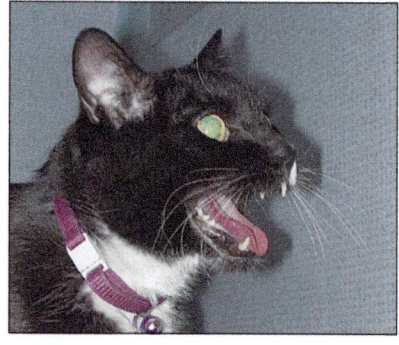

Figure 10.4 Severe respiratory distress with open-mouth breathing in a 10-year-old cat with fulminant pulmonary edema caused by restrictive cardiomyopathy.

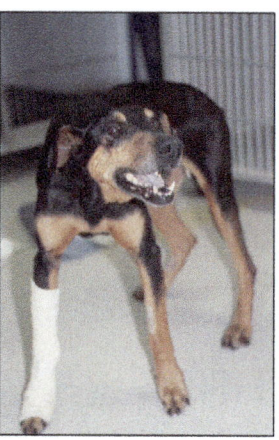

Figure 10.1 Respiratory distress in a 9-year-old male Doberman Pinscher with metastatic bronchoalveolar carcinoma, pulmonary thrombosis, and PaO_2 of 47 mm Hg. Note the wide-based stance, with head and neck extension (typical of orthopnea) and cyanotic tongue.

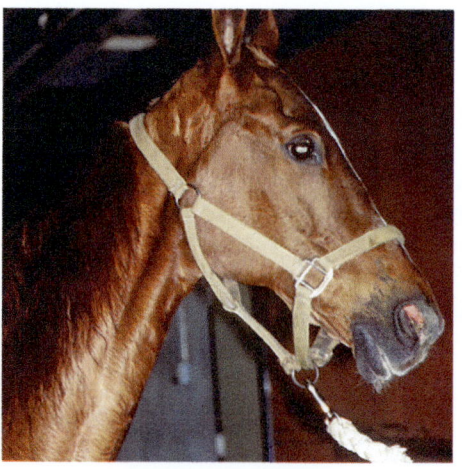

Figure 10.5 Note the widely flared nostrils (as well as marked jugular vein distension) in this 18-year-old American Saddlebred gelding with biventricular congestive heart failure (CHF) caused by dilated cardiomyopathy. Sweating might be observed in some horses with CHF.

Table 10.2 Causes of Respiratory Difficulty, Tachypnea, and Distress

Nasal Cavity and Nasopharynx
- Nasopharyngeal polyp
- Rhinitis/sinusitis
- Fungal infection (including cryptococcosis, aspergillosis)
- Neoplasia (including lymphoma, carcinomas, mast cell tumor, fibrosarcoma)
- Other mass lesion (including cyst, abscess)
- Foreign body
- Nasopharyngeal stenosis
- Brachycephalic airway abnormalities (stenotic nares, elongated soft palate)

Larynx
- Unilateral or bilateral paralysis
- Neoplasia (including lymphoma, squamous cell carcinoma, adenocarcinoma)
- Granulomatous laryngitis
- Abscess
- Other mass lesion (including cyst)
- Edema or laryngospasm
- Foreign body
- Trauma (hemorrhage, fractured cartilage, subcutaneous emphysema)
- Brachycephalic airway abnormalities (everted laryngeal saccules, laryngeal malformation)

Trachea
- Collapse
- Foreign body
- Tracheal mass or parasitic granuloma
- Tracheal compression (mediastinal, esophageal)
- Trauma
- Brachycephalic airway abnormalities (hypoplastic trachea)

Bronchi
- Collapse (bronchomalacia)
- Compression (left atrium, hilar lymph nodes, pulmonary mass lesions)
- Chronic bronchitis/bronchiectasis (accumulation of secretions or exudate)
- Bronchospasm (including asthma, inhaled irritant)

Pulmonary Parenchyma
- Edema—cardiogenic (left-sided CHF), causes include:
  - Dilated cardiomyopathy (Chapters 32–34)
  - Acquired mitral or aortic valve disease (Chapters 29–31)
  - Feline myocardial diseases (Chapter 33)
  - Certain congenital heart defects (Chapters 26–28)
- Edema—noncardiogenic, causes include:
  - Acute upper airway obstruction
  - Neurogenic (seizures, electrocution)
  - Hypervolemia
  - Smoke inhalation
  - Near drowning
  - Sepsis
  - Severe hypoproteinemia
  - Rapid lung expansion
- Pneumonia (including bacterial, fungal, aspiration, viral, protozoal)
- Hemorrhage (including coagulopathy, foreign body, neoplasia, and extreme exercise in horses)
- Fibrosis (including from certain drugs, viral or other infections, dusts, and organic allergens)
- Parasites (including *Aelurostrongylus* species, *Paragonimus* species)
- Pulmonary thromboemboli (Chapters 36 and 39)
- Heartworm disease (Chapter 40)
- Neoplasia (primary or metastatic)
- Trauma (including pulmonary contusion, traumatic cysts/bullae)

Pleural Space[a]
- Pleural effusion: Modified Transudate—cardiogenic (CHF), causes include:
  - Dilated cardiomyopathy (Chapters 32–34)
  - Acquired tricuspid valve disease (rare as isolated cause; Chapters 29–31)
  - Feline myocardial diseases (Chapter 33)
  - Pericardial diseases (Chapter 35)
  - Heartworm disease (Chapter 40)
  - Certain congenital heart defects (Chapters 26–28)
- Pleural effusion: Transudate/modified transudate—noncardiogenic, causes include:
  - Neoplasia (including lymphoma, mesothelioma, thymoma, and metastatic diseases; varying degrees of hemorrhage are relatively common)
  - Diaphragmatic hernia
  - Lung lobe torsion (can be hemorrhagic)
  - Severe hypoproteinemia
- Pleural effusion: Nonseptic exudate, causes include:
  - Feline infectious peritonitis
  - Neoplasia
  - Chronic lung lobe torsion or diaphragmatic hernia
  - Chronic chylothorax
- Pleural effusion: Chylothorax, causes include:
  - Severe right-sided CHF
    - Feline myocardial diseases (Chapter 33)
    - Congenital right heart disease
    - Pericardial diseases, including constriction
  - Mediastinal lymphoma
  - Trauma
  - Lymphangiectasia
  - Congenital lymphatic malformation
  - Heartworm disease (Chapter 40)
  - Cranial vena cava thrombosis (Chapter 36)
- Pyothorax (septic exudate; including bite wound, systemic infection, migrating foreign body)
- Hemothorax or hemorrhagic effusions (including trauma, coagulopathy, neoplasia, lung lobe torsion)
- Fungal infection
- Pneumothorax (including trauma, iatrogenic, *Paragonimus* infection, ruptured congenital bullae)

Diaphragm/Thoracic Cavity
- Diaphragmatic hernia, including traumatic, congenital peritoneopericardial (Chapter 35)
- Primary or metastatic neoplasia (including cranial mediastinal masses)
- Massive pericardial effusion (Chapter 35)

Chest Wall
- Neuromuscular disease
- Trauma (including rib fractures, flail segment, muscle tears)
- Congenital pectus excavatum and other thoracic anomalies

Other Causes
- Marked abdominal enlargement (from ascites, gastric dilatation/volvulus, etc.)
- Neurologic disease (including coma, brainstem or high cervical injury)
- Drug-induced respiratory depression (from sedative or anesthetic agents)
- ↓ O_2-carrying capacity (from anemia, carbon monoxide toxicity or smoke inhalation, methemoglobinemia)
- Metabolic acidosis, some drug reactions (e.g. opioids in cats), pain, shock, sepsis[b]

---

[a] Typical effusions are indicated, however, there is considerable variation and overlap related to causes and chronicity. This list is not exhaustive.
[b] Some causes of tachypnea involve altered central control of ventilation or sympathetic responses to injury or pain.
Abbreviations: CHF, congestive heart failure; O_2, oxygen.

and metabolic diseases, as well as some toxicoses, can cause apparent "dyspnea" by affecting thermoregulation, blood pH, oxygen (O_2) transport or delivery, or through stimulation of the central nervous system.

Inadequate partial pressure of oxygen (hypoxemia) or excessive carbon dioxide (CO_2; hypercarbia, hypercapnia) leads to respiratory distress. Ventilation normally is regulated reflexly in response to changes in the partial pressure of arterial carbon dioxide ($PaCO_2$), sensed by central and peripheral chemoreceptors. Central chemoreceptors (in the medulla) are highly sensitive to changes in cerebral spinal fluid pH, which is inversely related to $PaCO_2$. Small changes in alveolar pCO_2 affect ventilation. Hypoxia also affects the central respiratory center directly. Peripheral chemoreceptors in the carotid bodies, located near the bifurcation of the common carotid arteries, and to a lesser extent the aortic bodies, respond more to low partial pressure of arterial O_2 (PaO_2) and reflexly stimulate ventilation. However, these chemoreceptors also respond to elevated $PaCO_2$, decreased pH, low perfusion rate, and increased temperature to raise the rate and depth of ventilation.

Besides chemoreceptor-mediated reflex effects on ventilation, other mechanisms influence ventilatory rate and depth. Dyspnea associated with pulmonary vascular congestion or thromboembolism (as well as the ventilatory response to exercise) could be mediated through C-fiber (nonmyelinated nerve) endings associated with the bronchial and pulmonary microcirculation (J-receptors). Primary central nervous system (CNS) disease occasionally causes abnormal regulation of respiratory rate or rhythm.

Hypoxemia

Several abnormalities lead to hypoxemia, a decrease in arterial oxygen tension (**Table 10.3**). These usually involve either alveolar hypoventilation, pulmonary ventilation/perfusion (V/Q) mismatch with venous admixture (shunt), anatomic right-to-left shunt, or a combination of these factors. Impaired alveolar gas diffusion or low O_2 content of inspired air are other potential causes of hypoxemia. In addition, tissue hypoxia can result from reduced blood O_2-carrying capacity (as with anemia or hemoglobinopathy), even with normal PaO_2, because they reduce blood O_2 content.

Table 10.3 Causes of Hypoxemia & Decreased Oxygen Content

Alveolar hypoventilation
Ventilation/perfusion (V/Q) mismatch
Shunt (intrapulmonary or right-to-left cardiac)
↓ Inspired O_2 concentration (F_iO_2)
Diffusion impairment
Abnormal hemoglobin (reduced oxygen carrying capacity)

Abbreviation: F_iO_2, fraction of inspired oxygen.

When ventilation of pulmonary alveolar units is inadequate, insufficient O_2 is available for absorption into alveolar capillaries and CO_2 is retained. Alveolar hypoventilation can occur from pleural space disease, multiple rib fractures with or without flail chest, respiratory muscle dysfunction or fatigue, severe upper airway obstruction, markedly increased small airway resistance, CNS disease with abnormal neural control of respiration, chest compression (such as from an overly tight bandage), or decreased lung elasticity (as with severe pulmonary fibrosis). Hypoventilation also can occur from the respiratory depressant effects of drugs used for sedation or anesthesia, as well as the use of an excessively large breathing circuit during inhalation anesthesia, which functionally increases anatomic "dead space."

V/Q mismatch occurs with relative overperfusion of poorly or nonventilated lung regions or by ventilation of poorly perfused regions. Pulmonary arterioles normally constrict in response to low O_2 levels. Such vasoconstriction shifts blood flow from poorly ventilated regions preferentially toward well-ventilated areas, which minimizes V/Q mismatch. Accumulation of alveolar fluid or exudate and bronchoconstriction, as well as the degree of hypoxic vasoconstriction, impact the balance of ventilation to perfusion. Inflammatory mediators associated with pneumonia or other lung disease could interfere with hypoxic vasoconstriction and contribute to greater V/Q abnormality. V/Q mismatch occurs with pulmonary edema, pulmonary interstitial disease and fibrosis, airway obstruction with partial lung collapse, and lung collapse (atelectasis) related to pleural space disease, diaphragmatic hernia, and multiple rib fractures.

When alveoli collapse or fill with fluid or exudate, gas exchange ceases in those units. Deoxygenated blood flowing through adjacent pulmonary capillaries functionally creates an area of arteriovenous (A-V) shunt or "venous admixture." Alveolar flooding from severe pulmonary edema and pulmonary consolidation from pneumonia are common causes of functional intrapulmonary A-V shunt. True anatomic shunts, such as a pulmonary A-V fistula or right-to-left shunting intracardiac malformation or reversed patent ductus arteriosus (PDA), also cause hypoxemia.

Diffusion impairment occurs when alveolar capillary wall thickening prevents rapid equilibration between capillary blood and alveolar gas. It is thought to be an uncommon cause of hypoxemia in companion animals.

Hypoxemia causes visible cyanosis when the concentration of desaturated hemoglobin exceeds 5 g/dl (Chapter 13). Oral mucous membranes appear grayish ("muddy") or bluish (cyanotic). In animals with a normal packed cell volume (PCV), cyanosis usually indicates severe hypoxemia (PaO_2 <45–50 mm Hg). Animals with erythrocytosis (polycythemia) could appear cyanotic with less severe hypoxemia by virtue of their greater hemoglobin content. Anemic animals can be severely hypoxemic without cyanosis. Hypoxemia and cyanosis are difficult to detect with carbon monoxide toxicity or methemoglobinemia because mucous membrane color is altered; even with a normal PaO_2, total blood O_2 content is reduced. "Central" cyanosis is associated with generalized hypoxemia; "peripheral" cyanosis refers to local hemoglobin desaturation caused by poor peripheral circulation (as with arterial thromboembolism).

Pulmonary Edema

Pulmonary edema, excess accumulation of pulmonary extravascular water, occurs when capillary transudation or exudation exceeds pulmonary lymphatic drainage capacity. An imbalance in Starling's forces usually underlies pulmonary edema formation (**Figure 10.6**; also see p. 25). The most common mechanism is increased pulmonary capillary hydrostatic pressure, which results from high pulmonary venous pressure (as with left-sided CHF), hypervolemia, or pulmonary overcirculation that overwhelms the left heart (as with left-to-right shunting cardiac defects). This is also termed "high-pressure" pulmonary edema, and tends to have relatively low protein content. Another mechanism is increased capillary permeability, which occurs with diseases that directly or indirectly injure the capillary membrane. This "low-pressure" leakage of albumin and other large molecules into the alveoli and surrounding interstitium causes edema fluid with protein content similar to plasma. These distinctions are not absolute, as large increases in pulmonary capillary pressure (such as to 30–50 mm Hg) also can create gaps in the membrane ("stress failure") which allow protein and even red blood cell (RBC) leakage, as in exercise induced pulmonary hemorrhage of horses. Low plasma osmotic pressure from severe hypoalbuminemia (as with ≤10 g/l, ≤1 g/dl) promotes fluid transudation out of the capillaries. Moderate hypoalbuminemia magnifies the tendency for edema formation from other mechanisms. Pulmonary lymphatic obstruction or high lymphatic pressure secondary to elevated systemic venous pressure also will promote pulmonary edema formation. Neurogenic pulmonary edema is thought to result from a surge in circulating epinephrine or a neural response that causes acute constriction of pulmonary venous sphincters and high pulmonary venous pressure. Pulmonary edema also can develop with rapid reexpansion of collapsed lung tissue, probably from increased capillary permeability; however, this is rarely noted clinically in animals. High-altitude pulmonary edema, of unclear mechanism, also is recognized.

Overt pulmonary edema presumably is preceded by a prodromal stage, where increased lymph flow maintains a normal amount of extravascular fluid. With chronicity, lymphatic drainage of the lung can dramatically increase, allowing for compensation for left-sided heart disease. However, acute elevations in pulmonary capillary hydrostatic pressure or permeability are less well-tolerated. Peracute increases in hydrostatic pressure can lead to edema with hemorrhage and is recognized as blood-tinged froth. The progression of pulmonary edema severity has been described in four stages:

- *Stage 1 (increased interstitial fluid).* Distended lymphatics are seen around adjacent bronchi and pulmonary arteries. Gas exchange is well-preserved and physical signs are minimal, although mild dyspnea might occur with exercise.
- *Stage 2.* Interstitial edema accumulates along portions of alveolar septa and between adjacent alveoli, sometimes described as "crescentic filling" of alveoli. Increased respiratory effort might be noted at rest.
- *Stage 3 (alveolar flooding).* "Quantal" alveolar flooding develops, where some units are totally fluid-filled and others are clear or show only crescentic filling, especially in dependent lung regions. Blood flow past flooded alveoli creates venous admixture (shunt), which eventually leads to hypoxemia and increased alveolar–arterial (A-a) O_2 gradient. Pulmonary crackles are heard on inspiration, especially in dependent regions.
- *Stage 4.* Froth now enters the airways (**Figure 10.7**; also see **Figure 9.5**, p. 206) and effectively stops gas exchange.

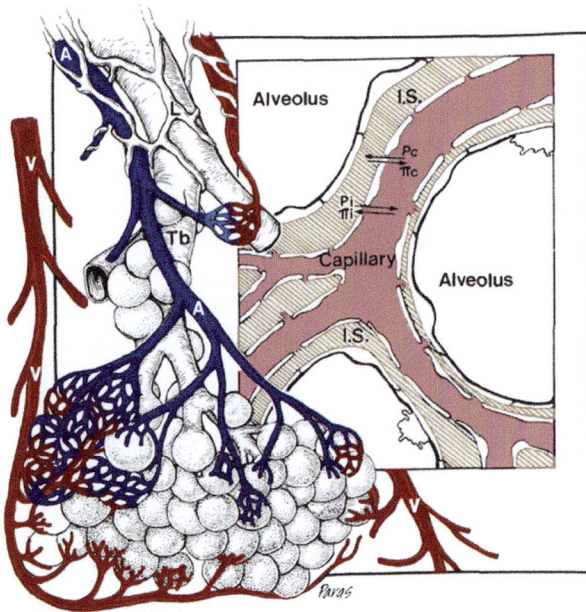

Figure 10.6 Schematic of a respiratory unit. Small arterioles branch into capillary networks, which surround the alveoli. The enlargement (inset) indicates Starling's forces, which control fluid movement into or out of the capillary. P_c, capillary hydrostatic pressure; π_c, capillary colloid osmotic pressure; P_i, interstitial hydrostatic pressure; π_i, interstitial colloid osmotic pressure; A, arteriole; V, venule; L, lymphatic vessel; Tb, terminal bronchiole; I.S., interstitial space. (Modified from Ware WA, Bonagura JB. Pulmonary Edema. In, Fox PR, Sisson D, Moise NS (editors). Canine and Feline Cardiology. Saunders, Philadelphia. 1999. p. 252.)

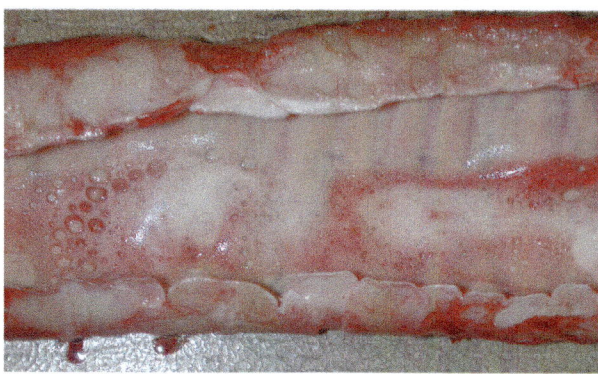

Figure 10.7 Postmortem image showing foamy pulmonary edema fluid within the trachea of a Quarterhorse gelding. The horse died of acute congestive heart failure following rupture of a major mitral chorda tendineae.

Pleural Effusion

The pleural surfaces include mechanisms for both systemic and pulmonary venous drainage. Normal pleural fluid is an ultrafiltrate derived from systemic capillaries along the thoracic wall. Lymphatic stoma within the parietal pleural surface normally absorb excess pleural fluid. Many cardiac and a large number of noncardiac diseases cause pleural fluid accumulation. As with tissue edema formation, effusion generally results from an imbalance of Starling's forces: Increased systemic capillary hydrostatic pressure or permeability, reduced lymphatic drainage, or low capillary oncotic pressure. Elevated right heart filling pressure increases systemic venous and capillary pressures, causing greater transudation into the pleural space, as well as the peritoneal and sometimes pericardial spaces. This can occur with any disease that raises right heart filling pressure, including primary right heart diseases, pericardial diseases, obstructive intracardiac mass lesions, and severe pulmonary hypertension. It also can occur with conditions that obstruct venous inflow to the heart, such as cranial vena cava thrombosis. Pleural effusion can also develop from predominately left-sided heart failure, as often observed in cats and horses. This likely stems from increased lymph formation at the visceral pleural surface (as these capillaries eventually drain into pulmonary veins) along with secondary right heart dysfunction. Additionally, third spacing of fluid accumulation that occurs in CHF might be a relevant factor.

Fluid appearance, protein concentration, and cell content typify different effusions (**Table 10.4**). The pleural fluid's character depends on the underlying mechanism. A modified transudate is typical for cardiac causes, although chronic cardiogenic pleural effusion can become chylous, especially in cats. Because the mediastinum typically is fenestrated in dogs, cats, and horses, pleural effusion usually is bilateral, with possible exceptions of some proteinaceous effusions and pyothorax. The volume of fluid, as well as how rapidly it accumulates, influences the degree of respiratory compromise. Chronic effusions can lead to pleural reactions and fibrosis, which further impairs expansion of the lungs.

Pulmonary Thromboembolism

PTE usually causes tachypnea or respiratory distress and its onset often is rapid. The extent of vascular obstruction, along with any concurrent pulmonary parenchymal disease, influences the severity of respiratory signs. Hypoxia develops mainly from complicated changes in V/Q matching within the lung, although secondary hemorrhage, edema and bronchoconstriction can contribute. The extent of vascular obstruction also influences overall pulmonary vascular resistance; large or extensive PTE could cause severe pulmonary hypertension, poor left ventricular filling and cardiac output, and signs of right heart failure (Chapter 39). Conditions that predispose to systemic venous thrombus formation (for example, by causing venous stasis, endothelial damage, or hypercoagulability; Chapter 36), as well as heartworm disease (Chapter 40) and other conditions, can promote PTE development. Besides

Table 10.4 Pleural Effusions

Type	Appearance	Protein	Nucleated Cells	Predominant Cells	Common Causes
Pure transudate	Clear	<30 g/L (<3 g/dL)	<1,000/microL	M, L, mesothel.	↓ capillary oncotic P (hypoalbuminemia)
Modified transudate	Slightly turbid; amber/pinkish	up to 35 g/L (<3.5 g/dL)	to 5,000/microL	M, L, mesothel., PMN	↑ capillary hydrostatic P (R-CHF, ↓ lymph drainage)
Exudate	Turbid to opaque; amber, pink, or white	>30 g/L (>3 g/dL)	>5,000/microL	PMN, M, L, E (degenerate PMN +/− bacteria if septic)	↑ capillary permeability (septic or nonseptic inflammation)
Hemorrhage	Red-tinged to frank blood	Similar to peripheral blood	Variable	RBC, PMN, M	Vascular disruption (trauma, inflammation, coagulopathy)
Chyle	Turbid to milky white or pink	Variable	~5,000–10,000/microL	Mature L, M, PMN	↓ lymphatic drainage (lymphatic obstruction or rupture, lymphangiectasia, ↑ systemic venous P)

Abbreviations: E, eosinophils; L, lymphocytes; M, macrophages; mesothel., mesothelial cells; P, pressure; PMN, neutrophils; R-CHF, right-sided congestive heart failure; RBC, red blood cells.

tachypnea and respiratory distress, increased lung sounds, a systolic murmur, and hepatosplenomegaly also might be evident with PTE. Chest pain and hemoptysis are common signs in people with PTE, but not easily recognized in animals.

Approach to the Patient with Respiratory Difficulty

The severity of the animal's respiratory compromise as well as surrounding circumstances influence the clinician's approach. Care must be taken not to increase patient distress. Brief observation before the patient is handled, with or without a cursory physical examination (including pulse rate and chest auscultation), might be all that is possible initially. A severely dyspneic animal should be given supplemental O_2 immediately. A point-of-care thoracic/lung ultrasound exam (p. 80) with the patient in sternal recumbency often can be done simultaneously and can help direct initial therapy. A complete physical examination and other testing are delayed until the patient is more stable (**Figure 10.8**). Various methods for O_2 administration are described. Although a commercial temperature-controlled O_2 cage is ideal, other methods include O_2 administered into a plexiglass anesthetic induction box (for small patients), by nasal cannula (at 50–100 ml O_2/kg/min with humidification), or flow-by (at ~2–5 L O_2/min) via face mask or just holding the O_2 delivery tubing near the patient's nose or mouth (**Figures 10.9** and **10.10**). Whatever the method, it is important to avoid increasing patient stress and overheating. While 100% O_2 usually is given initially, concentrations

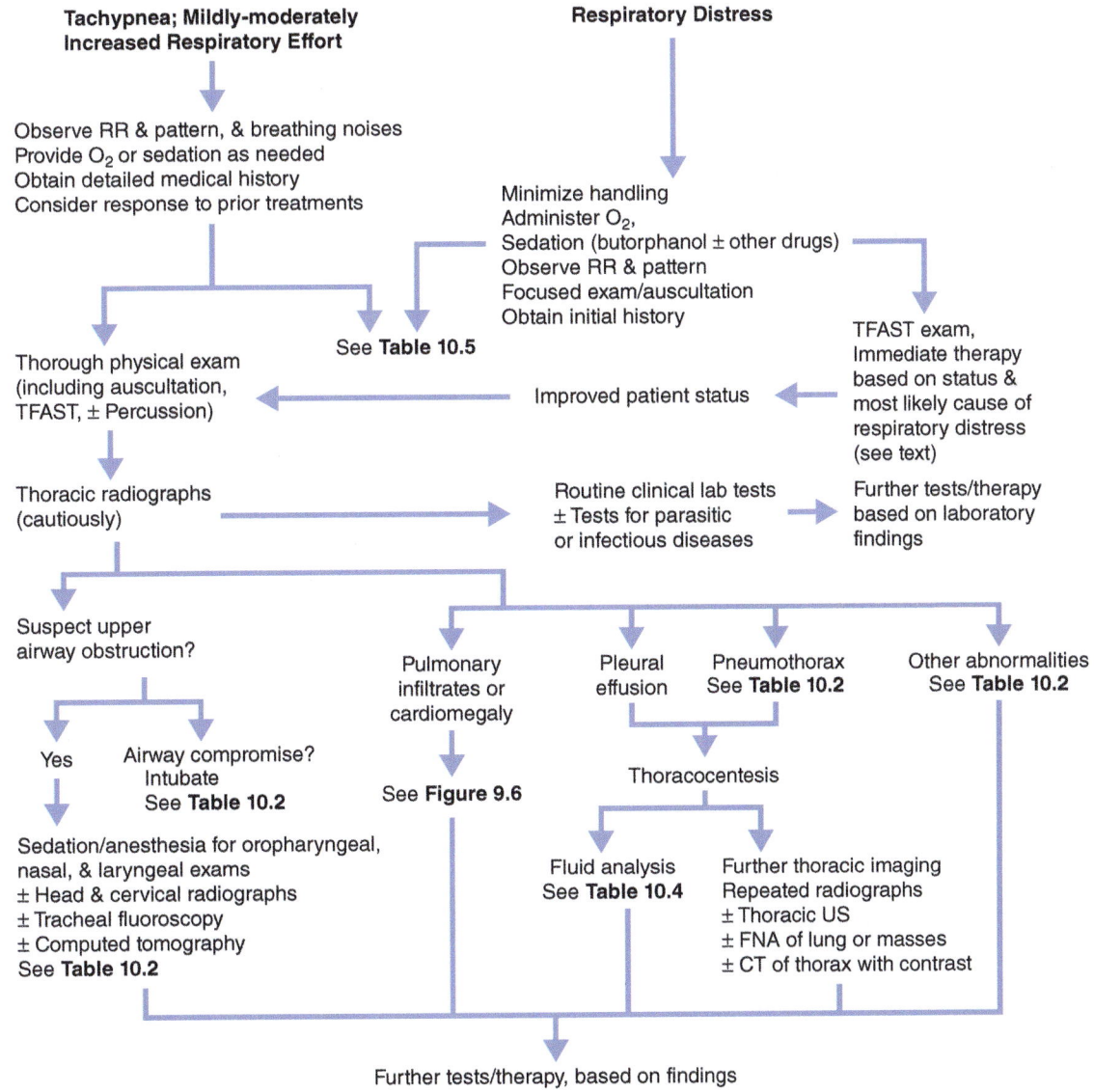

Figure 10.8 Approach to the patient with increased respiratory effort or respiratory distress. These are general guidelines; exceptions can occur. CT, computed tomography; FNA, fine needle aspirate; RR, respiratory rate; TFAST, thoracic focused assessment with sonography for trauma (used here to include rapid/focused echocardiogram); US, ultrasonography.

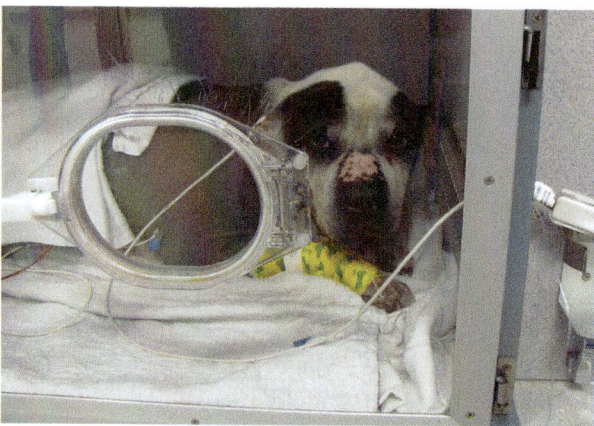

Figure 10.9 A commercial temperature- and humidity-controlled O_2 cage is practical for providing supplemental O_2 in small animals.

exceeding 50-60% should not be administered for more than 12 hours unless absolutely required. A nasal cannula is useful for more long-term O_2 administration. As long as undue patient stress can be avoided, placing an IV catheter as soon as possible allows for initial blood tests (such as PCV, blood smear, and total protein, blood urea nitrogen and glucose concentrations) and provides access for emergency drugs and fluids.

Observation of the patient's rate and character of respirations, including whether inspiration or expiration is more labored (**Table 10.5** and section "Patterns of Breathing"), attitude and level of alertness, mucous membrane color, general body condition, and evidence of trauma or other external abnormalities can be done with minimal or no physical contact. Most dyspneic animals have respiratory rates

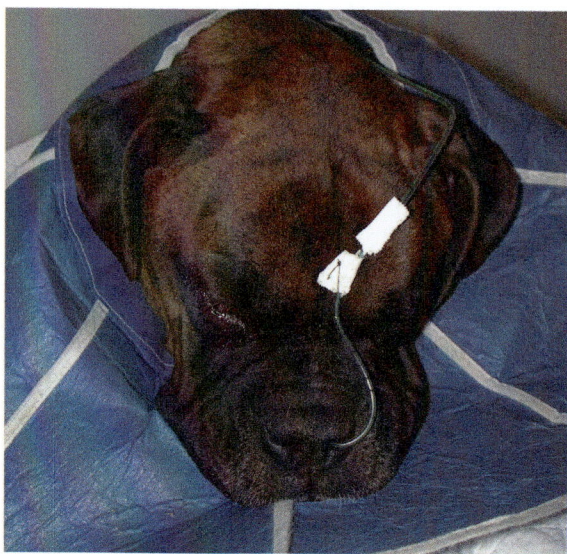

Figure 10.10 Humidified O_2 being administered by nasal cannula in a Boxer with heart failure. The tube is held in place by sutures in the skin near the nares (or bridge of the nose), as well as on the forehead (using adhesive tape "wings"). A soft Elizabethan collar helped protect the tube placement in this dog.

Table 10.5 Respiratory Signs by Disease Localization[a]

Nasal Cavity and Nasopharynx
- Stertor
- Open-mouth breathing
- Nasal discharge
- Cough
- Gagging or retching
- Reversed sneezing (nasopharynx)

Larynx
- Stridor or altered inspiratory pitch
- Inspiratory difficulty
- Cough
- Change in voice or bark

Trachea
- Inspiratory difficulty or noise (cervical trachea)
- Expiratory difficulty or noise (intrathoracic trachea)
- Mixed inspiratory and expiratory difficulty (especially with fixed obstruction)
- Cough

Lower Airways/Bronchi
- Expiratory difficulty
- Cough
- Wheezes

Pulmonary Parenchyma
- Tachypnea
- Mixed inspiratory and expiratory difficulty
- Pulmonary crackles (especially toward end of inspiration)
- Areas of ↑ or ↓ breath sounds

Pleural Space/Thoracic Cavity
- Tachypnea, or slower labored breathing
- Hyperpnea (marked distress)
- Areas of muffled breath sounds, especially ventrally
- Areas of hypo- or hyperresonance on percussion

Chest Wall/Other
- ↓ Chest wall excursion
- Abnormal chest wall appearance or motion

[a] Cyanosis can occur with any disease causing >50 g/L (>5 g/dL) of desaturated hemoglobin.

>50–60 breaths/minute. Rates often are slower with airway obstruction or a large volume of pleural effusion.

Overly stressed and anxious animals can benefit from sedation (for example, 0.1–0.2 mg/kg butorphanol tartrate, IV in dogs and cats; or 0.025–0.1 mg/kg acepromazine maleate, IV or IM; use the lower range in the dog). A complete medical history should be obtained as soon as possible.

Patterns of Breathing

The patient's respiratory rate and character can provide clues to the underlying disease process. Reduced lung compliance produces a "restrictive" breathing pattern, characterized by tachypnea with more rapid and shallow breaths. This breathing pattern minimizes the work of ventilating stiffer lungs.

Both phases of respiration could appear labored, especially when there is bronchial involvement. Pulmonary congestion, with or without edema, as well as interstitial or infiltrative lung diseases, including pulmonary fibrosis, produce this pattern. Such diseases reduce the surface area available for gas exchange, as well as decrease pulmonary compliance. Pulmonary crackles (p. 41) often are heard on inspiration; these can be especially loud with fibrosis. Partial lung collapse from pleural fluid accumulation or other pleural space abnormalities also decreases lung compliance and causes tachypnea. However, large-volume pleural effusion often causes progression to hyperpnea, with more labored inspiration and pronounced abdominal effort.

An "obstructive" breathing pattern is associated with airway narrowing. Slower, deeper breathing reduces frictional resistance and the work of breathing. However, the breathing rate can be normal or increased with peripheral airway obstruction or from the effects of irritant receptors in the airways. The location of narrowing determines which phase of respiration is more labored and (often) prolonged. Expiratory difficulty is characteristic of lower airway obstruction, such as with bronchial narrowing (bronchospasm, secretions, thickened walls) and intrathoracic tracheal or mainstem bronchial compression or collapse. Wheezing might be heard during exhalation. Air-trapping in peripheral lung regions is common with obstructive bronchial disease. Some animals with chronic lower airway obstruction have an expiratory heave or grunt.

Inspiratory difficulty, with slow or labored inspiration, generally is associated with upper airway obstruction, including nasal disease, laryngeal or pharyngeal obstruction, intratracheal mass lesions, and cervical tracheal collapse. Abnormal inspiratory sounds might be apparent without a stethoscope, especially stridor or stertor (p. 41). A fixed obstruction can prolong both inspiration and expiration, and cause a noise during each phase.

Tachypnea and hyperpnea are not always related to hypoxemia or abnormalities of pulmonary mechanics. Hypercarbia and acidosis cause hyperpnea as an attempt to blow off CO_2. This could be interpreted as dyspnea. Moreover, thermoregulation and behavioral responses to respiratory distress can modify the rate or depth of breathing. CNS injury (as from infection, neoplasia, vascular accident, or trauma) can produce an abnormal rate or character of ventilation.

Clinical Examination

Initial therapy, in addition to supplemental O_2, sometimes is warranted before complete examination or diagnostic tests can be done safely. However, an expedient observation of the patient and ventilatory pattern, efficient thoracic auscultation, and a focused thoracic and cardiac ultrasound exam can help the clinician quickly identify large-volume pleural effusion, lung infiltrates, left atrial enlargement, pericardial effusion, or other abnormalities. These exams often allow differentiation of cardiac from noncardiac causes of respiratory distress. Depending on the clinician's judgment as to the likely cause, initial therapy might include furosemide, pimobendan, and a vasodilator (for suspected pulmonary edema; Chapter 22); bronchodilators (for suspected bronchospasm, plus corticosteroid for noninfectious inflammatory causes); thoracocentesis (for suspected pleural effusion or pneumothorax); or sedation/anesthesia for pharyngeal/laryngeal inspection and intubation, or for emergency tracheostomy for upper airway obstruction. Ventilatory support might be needed in some cases. (See section "Suggested Additional Readings and References" and the online bibliography for further information on these techniques.)

A complete physical examination should be done as soon as is safely possible (see Chapters 2 and 11–17 for further details on aspects of CV examination). Besides the respiratory abnormalities, signs of other organ system disease might be apparent, such as a cardiac murmur, gallop sound, or arrhythmia; neurologic deficits; ocular abnormality; a palpable mass; organomegaly; or evidence for abnormal fluid accumulation. Careful pulmonary auscultation is important and could help in localizing the disease process. Pulmonary crackles might indicate the presence of pulmonary edema; however, it is important to remember that they instead could signal lung diseases such as pneumonia, bronchitis, and pulmonary fibrosis. Loud crackles are more likely to be associated with primary lung disease rather than pulmonary edema. Chest percussion (p. 42) might reveal areas of increased (air) or decreased (fluid/solid tissue) thoracic resonance. Body temperature elevation can occur from increased respiratory effort and anxiety, as well as from infectious, inflammatory, or neoplastic disease. Reduced chest compressibility in cats could indicate a cranial mediastinal mass or large pleural effusion; however, geriatric cats normally have reduced chest compliance.

Clinical Testing and Management

Thoracic radiographs are obtained as soon as the animal's breathing has stabilized. The DV, rather than the VD, view usually is less stressful for patients with respiratory difficulty. Both left and right lateral views are helpful, especially if unilateral disease is suspected. Radiographs of the upper cervical and nasopharyngeal regions might be useful if signs suggest upper airway disease, although direct visual examination is also needed. Pleural fluid or air of more than minimal volume should be removed by thoracocentesis to improve ventilation before additional testing is done. Thoracic radiographs taken again after full lung expansion usually yield more diagnostic information.

Additional diagnostic testing is guided by patient history, observation, physical abnormalities, and radiographic or point-of-care ultrasound findings. This might include direct nasopharyngeal or laryngeal examination, complete blood count (CBC), serum biochemistries, pleural fluid analysis, echocardiography (Chapter 4), electrocardiography (Chapter 5), pulse oximetry or arterial blood gas analysis, capnography, fungal or heartworm serologic tests, lymph node aspirates, coagulation profile, fecal tests, bronchoscopy, bronchoalveolar lavage, pulmonary fine needle aspiration or biopsy, computed tomography (CT) scan, thoracoscopy, pulmonary function testing, and pulmonary or ventilation scintigraphy.

Pulse oximetry is a useful noninvasive means of estimating hemoglobin saturation (SpO_2) and monitoring the animal's response to O_2 administration, although it will not differentiate PaO_2 gradations above 100 mm Hg. For example, in a patient with normal lung function breathing 100% O_2, PaO_2 is 500 mm Hg yet hemoglobin saturation is still 100%. Pulse oximetry also does not indicate if hypoventilation (hypercarbia) is the cause of hypoxemia. The technique can be inaccurate, especially in patients that are poorly perfused, moving, deeply pigmented, or that have thick fur. Although **Table 10.6** includes approximate correlation of selected SpO_2 values with PaO_2 based on the normal hemoglobin dissociation curve, it must be remembered that SpO_2 is not sensitive enough to replace PaO_2 in many clinical patients. In a study including over 1,000 dogs on mechanical ventilation, as well as a cohort of normal dogs breathing room air, an SpO_2 of 95% was less than 78% sensitive for predicting hypoxemia (PaO_2 <80 mm Hg; Farrell, 2019).

Arterial blood gas analysis will allow differentiation of alveolar hypoventilation from other causes of hypoxemia (**Table 10.6**), verify the need for O_2 supplementation, and monitor its effectiveness; however, the stress of arterial puncture and availability of rapid analysis capability must be considered (**Table 10.7**). Venous partial pressure of O_2 (PvO_2) does not reflect pulmonary function, although it can provide a rough estimate of whether tissue oxygenation is adequate. When obtained from a central vein, PvO_2 <30 mm Hg suggests either decreased O_2 delivery to the tissues or an increased O_2 consumption. Venous PCO_2 ($PvCO_2$) usually is 3–6 mm Hg higher than $PaCO_2$; this can provide an estimate of ventilatory status.

Calculation of the A-a O_2 gradient can help in disease assessment (**Table 10.6**). In the normal lung, the partial pressure of O_2 in the alveolus (PAO_2) should approximately be equal to that in the pulmonary capillary and, therefore, in arterial blood (PaO_2). Higher than normal gradients occur with V/Q mismatch, shunt, and impaired gas diffusion. The ratio of PaO_2 to the fraction of inspired O_2 (F_iO_2) also provides a rough estimate of lung function (**Table 10.6**). Unexplained respiratory distress with a high A-a gradient should generate suspicion for acute PTE.

Specific therapy depends on the etiology and pathophysiology involved, as well as the species. However, general principles apply to all cases: Remove or minimize any airway obstruction, promote full lung expansion by removing pleural air or fluid, improve oxygenation using supplemental O_2, and reduce patient anxiety. In some cases, high-flow nasal oxygen administration or assisted ventilation might be necessary (see section "Suggested Additional

Table 10.6 Assessment of Hypoxemia

Pulse Oximetry

Approximate correlation of hemoglobin saturation (SpO_2) with PaO_2:

SpO_2 (%)	PaO_2 (mm Hg)
99–100	>100
96	80
91	60

Arterial Blood Gas Analysis

Normal values (room air):
- PaO_2 = 85–100 mm Hg
- $PaCO_2$ = 35–45 mm Hg
- pH = 7.35–7.45
- HCO_3 = 21–27 mmol/L

O_2 supplementation recommended if PaO_2 < 60(–80) mm Hg (or SpO_2 <92%), or if signs of hypoxemia are evident. O_2 supplementation is of minimal help when hypoventilation (unless assisted ventilation is provided), pleural space disease, or anatomic shunt is the cause of hypoxemia.

Assisted ventilation recommended if $PaCO_2$ is persistently > 45 mm Hg after O_2 supplementation (indicates alveolar hypoventilation), and airway obstructive or anesthesia-related causes are excluded.

Alveolar-arterial (A-a) O_2 Gradient

A-a gradient = PAO_2–PaO_2
- PAO_2 = F_iO_2 (P_B–P_{H2O})–$PaCO_2$/R

A-a Gradient (mm Hg; on room air at sea level) = (150–[$PaCO_2$/0.8])–PaO_2
- <10–15 is normal
- >15 indicates compromised ability of lung to oxygenate blood
- >30 indicates severely impaired gas exchange

↑ A-a gradient occurs with V/Q mismatch, shunt, diffusion impairment.

Hypoxemia with normal A-a gradient is associated with hypoventilation (hypercapnia) or ↓ inspired O_2 concentration.

PaO_2:F_iO_2 Ratio

Allows quick estimation of oxygenation, but is less accurate than A-a gradient because $PaCO_2$ is not considered.

PaO_2:F_iO_2 Ratio and Lung Function
- 500 is normal
- 300–500 indicates mild disease
- 200–300 indicates moderate disease
- <200 indicates severe disease

F_iO_2(%) × 5 = Approximate PaO_2 (assuming normal lung function in animal at sea level)

F_iO_2(%)	PaO_2 (mm Hg)
0.2 (room air)	100
1.0 (100% O_2)	500

Abbreviations: F_iO_2, fraction of inspired O_2; PAO_2, partial pressure of O_2 in alveolar air; PaO_2, partial pressure of O_2 in arterial blood; $PaCO_2$, partial pressure of CO_2 in arterial blood; P_B, barometric pressure; P_{H2O}, partial pressure of water; R, respiratory quotient (assumed to be 0.8 for fasting animal).

Table 10.7 Arterial Blood Sample Acquisition

Supplies
- 25-gauge needle; 3-cc syringe; heparin (1,000 U/mL); rubber blood tube stopper or cork; clippers; surgical scrub solution; and alcohol.

Preparation
- Attach the needle to the syringe. Heparinize both by drawing heparin into the syringe and then expelling it back into its bottle, leaving heparin only in the needle hub.
- Choose the arterial puncture site: The femoral artery is used most often, but the dorsal pedal artery is an alternative, especially if there is difficulty accessing the femoral artery or if restraint in lateral recumbency would exacerbate respiratory distress.
- At least one assistant will be needed to help with restraint and positioning.

Femoral Artery Puncture
- Position the animal in lateral recumbency. Extend the lower hindlimb and abduct and flex the upper hindlimb to expose the inguinal area. Lift the prepuce or caudal mammary tissue if necessary to gain adequate access to the femoral artery in the inguinal region.
- Clip hair from the puncture site and surgically scrub the area. Palpate for the arterial pulse, then position the artery between the tips of the first two fingers of the free hand.
- Position the prepared needle/syringe at a 60- to 90-degree angle to the skin. Hold the syringe at the plunger end so that it is possible to pull back on the plunger without having to reposition the hand (and risk moving the syringe and needle).
- Slowly insert the needle through the skin into the artery (between the fingertips) while watching for a flash of bright red blood in the needle hub. It may help to apply a tiny amount of pull on the plunger after the needle penetrates the skin.
- Aspirate 1.0–1.5 ml of blood. Withdraw the needle and immediately apply direct pressure to the puncture site for at least 5 minutes.
- Immediately after withdrawing the needle, hold the syringe/needle upright to expel all air bubbles, then insert the needle into the rubber stopper or cork. Place on ice for transport to the lab.

Dorsal Pedal Artery Puncture
- Position animal with the hindlimbs to one side in sternal (or lateral) recumbency. Extend and stabilize the lower hindlimb. Palpate for the arterial pulse along the dorsal and proximal metatarsal area (slightly medial to midline) to locate the puncture site.
- Clip hair from the puncture site and surgically scrub the area. Proceed as for femoral artery puncture, except hold the syringe at a 15- to 30-degree angle to the skin (more parallel).

Reading and References" and the online bibliography for additional recommendations and details). Guidelines for managing patients with heart failure are in Chapters 20–22 and in chapters on specific cardiac diseases. Other appropriate sources should be consulted for further information on diagnosis and management of the many noncardiac diseases that cause respiratory difficulty.

Suggested Additional Reading and References

Also See Online Comprehensive Bibliography at: https://www.routledge.com/9781482246223.

Balakrishnan A, Drobatz KJ, Silverstein DC. Retrospective evaluation of the prevalence, risk factors, management, outcome, and necropsy findings of acute lung injury and acute respiratory distress syndrome in dogs and cats: 29 cases (2011–2013). J Vet Emerg Crit Care 2017;27:662–673.

Benavides K, Rozanski E, Anastasio JD, et al. The effect of inhaled heliox on peak flow rates in normal and brachycephalic dogs. J Vet Intern Med 2019;33:208–211.

Boiron L, Hopper K, Borchers A. Risk factors, characteristics, and outcomes of acute respiratory distress syndrome in dogs and cats: 54 cases. J Vet Emerg Crit Care 2019;29:173–179.

Campbell VL. Respiratory complications in critical illness of small animals. Vet Clin North Am Small Anim Pract 2011;41:709–716.

Ceccherini G, Lippi I, Citi S, et al. Continuous positive airway pressure (CPAP) provision with a pediatric helmet for treatment of hypoxemic acute respiratory failure in dogs. J Vet Emerg Crit Care 2020;30:41–49.

Connolly DJ, Brodbelt DC, Copeland H, et al. Assessment of the diagnostic accuracy of circulating cardiac troponin I concentration to distinguish between cats with cardiac and non-cardiac causes of respiratory distress. J Vet Cardiol 2009;11:71–78.

Connolly DJ, Soares Magalhaes RJ, Fuentes VL, et al. Assessment of the diagnostic accuracy of circulating natriuretic peptide concentrations to distinguish between cats with cardiac and non-cardiac causes of respiratory distress. J Vet Cardiol 2009;11(Suppl 1):S41–S50.

Corona TM, Aumann M. Ventilator waveform interpretation in mechanically ventilated small animals. J Vet Emerg Crit Care 2011;21:496–514.

DeClue AE, Cohn LA. Acute respiratory distress syndrome in dogs and cats: a review of clinical findings and pathophysiology. J Vet Emerg Crit Care 2007;17:340–347.

Drobatz KJ, Saunders HM, Pugh CR, et al. Noncardiogenic pulmonary edema in dogs and cats: 26 cases (1987–1993). J Am Vet Med Assoc 1995;206:1732–1736.

Dunkel B, Dolente B, Boston RC. Acute lung injury/acute respiratory distress syndrome in 15 foals. Equine Vet J 2005;37:435–440.

Edwards TH, Erickson Coleman A, Brainard BM, et al. Outcome of positive-pressure ventilation in dogs and cats with congestive heart failure: 16 cases (1992–2012). J Vet Emerg Crit Care 2014;24:586–593.

Epstein S. Pulse oximetry. In, Ettinger SJ, Feldman EC, Côté E (editors). Textbook of Veterinary Internal Medicine. 8th edition. Elsevier, St. Louis, MO. 2017. pp. 374–376.

Farrell KS, Hopper K, Cagle LA, et al. Evaluation of pulse oximetry as a surrogate for PaO2 in awake dogs breathing room air and anesthetized dogs on mechanical ventilation. J Vet Emerg Crit Care 2019;29:622–629.

Forrester SD, Moon ML, Jacobson JD. Diagnostic evaluation of dogs and cats with respiratory distress. Compend Cont Educ Pract Vet 2001;23:56–68.

Fox PR, Oyama MA, Hezzell MJ, et al. Relationship of plasma N-terminal pro-brain natriuretic peptide concentrations to heart failure classification and cause of respiratory distress in dogs using a 2nd generation ELISA assay. J Vet Intern Med 2015;29:171–179.

Greensmith TD, Cortellini S. Successful treatment of canine acute respiratory distress syndrome secondary to inhalant toxin exposure. J Vet Emerg Crit Care 2018;28:469–475.

Haskins SC. Hypoxemia. In, Silverstein DC, Hopper K (editors). Small Animal Critical Care Medicine. 2nd edition. Saunders Elsevier, St. Louis, MO. 2015. pp 81–86.

Hezzell MJ, Ostroski C, Oyama MA, et al. Investigation of focused cardiac ultrasound in the emergency room for differentiation of respiratory and cardiac causes of respiratory distress in dogs. J Vet Emerg Crit Care 2020;30:159–164.

Hopper K. Basic and advanced mechanical ventilation. In, Silverstein DC, Hopper K (editors). Small Animal Critical Care Medicine. 2nd edition. Saunders Elsevier, St. Louis, MO. 2015. pp. 161–174.

Hopper K. Discontinuing mechanical ventilation. In, Silverstein DC, Hopper K (editors). Small Animal Critical Care Medicine. 2nd edition. Saunders Elsevier, St. Louis, MO. 2015. pp. 190–194.

Jagodich TA, Bersenas AME, Bateman SW, et al. High-flow nasal cannula oxygen therapy in acute hypoxemic respiratory failure in 22 dogs requiring oxygen support escalation. J Vet Emerg Crit Care 2020;30:364–375.

Janson CO, Hezzell MJ, Oyama MA, et al. Focused cardiac ultrasound and point-of-care NT-proBNP assay in the emergency room for differentiation of cardiac and noncardiac causes of respiratory distress in cats. J Vet Emerg Crit Care 2020;30:376–383.

Johns SM, Nelson OL, Gay JM. Left atrial function in cats with left-sided cardiac disease and pleural effusion or pulmonary edema. J Vet Intern Med 2012;26:1134–1139.

Johnson LR, Vernau W. Bronchoscopic findings in 48 cats with spontaneous lower respiratory tract disease (2002-2009). J Vet Intern Med 2011;25:236–243.

Keir I, Daly J, Haggerty J, et al. Retrospective evaluation of the effect of high flow oxygen therapy delivered by nasal cannula on PaO2 in dogs with moderate-to-severe hypoxemia. J Vet Emerg Crit Care 2016;26:598–602.

Lisciandro GR, Fosgate GT, Fulton RM. Frequency and number of ultrasound lung rockets (B-lines) using a regionally based lung ultrasound examination named vet BLUE (veterinary bedside lung ultrasound exam) in dogs with radiographically normal lung findings. Vet Radiol Ultrasound 2014;55:315–322.

Lisciandro GR, Fulton RM, Fosgate GT, et al. Frequency and number of B-lines using a regionally based lung ultrasound examination in cats with radiographically normal lungs compared to cats with left-sided congestive heart failure. J Vet Emerg Crit Care 2017;27:499–505.

Mason DE, Ainsworth DM, Robertson JT. Respiratory emergencies in the adult horse. Vet Clin North Am Equine Pract 1994;10:685–702.

Mazzaferro EM. Oxygen therapy. In, Silverstein DC, Hopper K (editors). Small Animal Critical Care Medicine. 2nd edition. Saunders Elsevier, St. Louis, MO. 2015. pp. 77–80.

Mueller ER. Suggested strategies for ventilatory management of veterinary patients with acute respiratory distress syndrome. J Vet Emerg Crit Care 2001;11:191–198.

Palmer JE. Neonatal foal resuscitation. Vet Clin North Am Equine Pract 2007;23:159–182.

Pouzot-Nevoret C, Hocine L, Negre J, et al. Prospective pilot study for evaluation of high-flow oxygen therapy in dyspnoeic dogs: the HOT-DOG study. J Small Anim Pract 2019;60:656–662.

Powell LL. Causes of respiratory failure. Vet Clin North Am Small Anim Pract 2002;32:1049–1058.

Prosek R, Sisson DD, Oyama MA, et al. Distinguishing cardiac and noncardiac dyspnea in 48 dogs using plasma atrial natriuretic factor, B-type natriuretic factor, endothelin, and cardiac troponin-I. J Vet Intern Med 2007;21:238–242.

Rademacher N, Pariaut R, Pate J, et al. Transthoracic lung ultrasound in normal dogs and dogs with cardiogenic pulmonary edema: a pilot study. Vet Radiol Ultrasound 2014;55:447–452.

Rozanski E, Chan DL. Approach to the patient with respiratory distress. Vet Clin North Am Small Anim Pract 2005;35:307–317.

Rozanski EA. Oxygenation and ventilation. Vet Clin North Am Small Anim Pract 2015;45:931–940.

Sauvé V, Drobatz KJ, Shokek AB, et al. Clinical course, diagnostic findings and necropsy diagnosis in dyspneic cats with primary pulmonary parenchymal disease: 15 cats (1996–2002). J Vet Emerg Crit Care 2005;15:38–47.

Sharp CR, Rozanski EA. Physical examination of the respiratory system. Top Companion Anim Med 2013;28:79–85.

Sigrist NE, Adamik KN, Doherr MG, et al. Evaluation of respiratory parameters at presentation as clinical indicators of the respiratory localization in dogs and cats with respiratory distress. J Vet Emerg Crit Care 2011;21:13–23.

Sleeper MM, Roland R, Drobatz KJ. Use of the vertebral heart scale for differentiation of cardiac and noncardiac causes of respiratory distress in cats: 67 cases (2002–2003). J Am Vet Med Assoc 2013;242:366–371.

Smith KF, Quinn RL, Rahilly LJ. Biomarkers for differentiation of causes of respiratory distress in dogs and cats: part 1–cardiac diseases and pulmonary hypertension. J Vet Emerg Crit Care 2015;25:311–329.

Sumner C, Rozanski E. Management of respiratory emergencies in small animals. Vet Clin North Am Small Anim Pract 2013;43:799–815.

Wang RL, Xu K, Yu KL, et al. Effects of dynamic ventilatory factors on ventilator-induced lung injury in acute respiratory distress syndrome dogs. World J Emerg Med 2012;3:287–293.

Ward JL, Lisciandro GR, Keene BW, et al. Accuracy of point-of-care lung ultrasonography for the diagnosis of cardiogenic pulmonary edema in dogs and cats with acute dyspnea. J Am Vet Med Assoc 2017;250:666–675.

Webster RA, Mills PC, Morton JM. Indications, durations and outcomes of mechanical ventilation in dogs and cats with tick paralysis caused by ixodes holocyclus: 61 cases (2008–2011). Aust Vet J 2013;91:233–239.

Wilkins PA, Palmer JE. Mechanical ventilation in foals with botulism: 9 cases (1989–2002). J Vet Intern Med 2003;17:708–712.

Wilkins PA, Seahorn T. Acute respiratory distress syndrome. Vet Clin North Am Equine Pract 2004;20:253–273.

Wilson DV, Schott II HC, Robinson NE, et al. Response to nasopharyngeal oxygen administration in horses with lung disease. Equine Vet J 2006;38:219–223.

Zocchi L. Physiology and pathophysiology of pleural fluid turnover. Eur Respir J 2002 Dec;20(6):1545–1558. doi: 10.1183/09031936.02.00062102. PMID: 12503717.

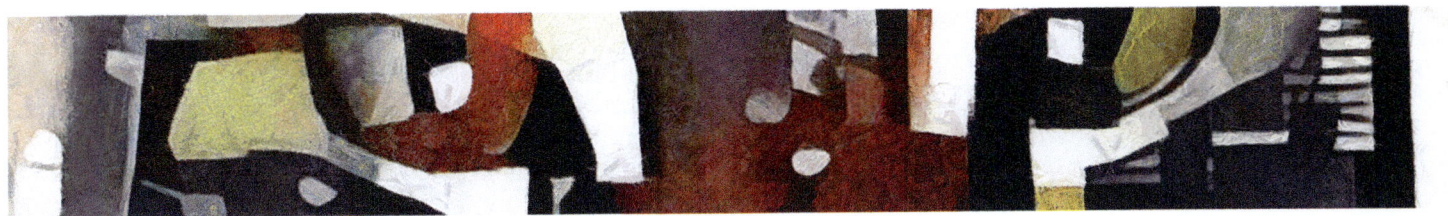

11
MURMURS AND ABNORMAL HEART SOUNDS

Heart sounds are caused by audible vibrations of cardiohemic tissues. Normal heart sounds are the first sound (S_1), timed with closure and tensing of the atrioventricular (AV) valves and associated structures at the onset of systole, and the second sound (S_2), associated with closure of the aortic and pulmonic valves following ejection (p. 18, and **Figure 1.20**). These are the only transient heart sounds heard in normal dogs and cats. In contrast, in addition to S_1 and S_2, the atrial or fourth sound (S_4) and the ventricular or third sound (S_3) are normal heart sounds in horses (see section "Gallop Sounds" and p. 19). Proficiency in recognizing abnormal heart sounds and their origin is not easily achieved; however, this is a skill that can provide important clinical insight. In animals with abnormal heart sounds or a cardiac murmur, it is especially important to understand the cardiac cycle events associated with these sounds and to identify their timing relative to systole (between S_1 and S_2) and diastole (from S_2 until the next S_1).

General Considerations

Identifying an abnormal heart sound as "systolic" or "diastolic" is critical to understanding its origin. Besides the paired onomatopoeic "lub-dub" associated with S_1 and S_2 during sinus rhythm, palpation can help the clinician differentiate these sounds (and, therefore, the timing of systole). The precordial impulse occurs just after S_1, peaking at the opening of the aortic valve, and the arterial pulse is palpable between S_1 and S_2. Additionally, subtle changes in the relative intensity of the two sounds occur as the stethoscope chestpiece is moved toward or away from the source of each sound.

Many sounds generated by the heart are too low in frequency and intensity to be audible, even with the stethoscope. Any hearing impairment adds further limitation. Low-frequency sounds, such as the gallop sounds, must be of greater intensity (loudness) than higher pitched sounds to be heard. When relatively loud sounds also are present (such as a loud murmur or environmental noise), the examiner might not consciously hear any softer sounds because of the phenomenon of "masking." Therefore, efforts to optimize conditions for auscultation are important. These include using a good quality stethoscope with proper technique, listening in a quiet environment, and examining a calm patient that is breathing quietly and standing in a normal position, whenever possible (p. 38).

Cardiac Murmurs

Murmurs are defined as audible vibrations of prolonged duration occurring during a normally silent period of the cardiac cycle. Murmurs are associated with turbulent blood flow, although the precise source of sound generation is likely more complicated, involving periodic fluctuations within the wake of the high-velocity flow stream. Although many cardiac murmurs are pathologic (organic), other murmurs are nonpathologic or "functional," occurring when the heart is structurally normal.

Hemodynamically, most organic and functional murmurs are associated with higher than normal blood flow velocity. Additional associations in the genesis of cardiac murmurs include reduced blood viscosity (anemia), and blood flow into a large or dilated vessel. Interestingly, velocity, viscosity, and diameter are also the determinants of turbulent flow based on Reynold's critical number (p. 23). Sympathetic nervous system activation (as with stress, exercise, fever, anemia, and hyperthyroidism) can increase ejection velocity across normal ventricular outflow tracts, initiate or enhance dynamic ventricular outflow obstruction, and increase intracardiac and intravascular pressures. Adrenergic drive is a common cause of functional murmurs and it accentuates many pathologic murmurs (such as from aortic or pulmonic stenosis, and mitral or aortic regurgitation). Increased transvalvular flow volume related to cardiac shunts also augments transvalvular flow velocity; this can initiate or accentuate a murmur across a normal or stenotic valve. Lastly, harmonic oscillations within the heart or great vessels can produce musical or vibratory murmurs; these can be functional ("innocent") or pathologic in origin. Specific examples of these mechanisms of murmur generation are discussed below.

Pathologic causes of murmurs usually relate to valvular insufficiency, narrowing (stenosis) of valves or surrounding regions, or shunts. Nonpathologic (functional) murmurs can result from physiologic alterations or robust blood flow; these common murmurs are invariably systolic in dogs and cats, and usually of lower intensity (see section "Nonpathologic Murmurs"). Especially when a soft to moderate-intensity murmur is heard, it can be difficult to discern whether structural cardiac disease is the underlying cause or not. For example, in a large survey of apparently healthy cats of all ages, about 40% of the cats had a systolic murmur; yet, a large percentage of these were determined to be functional (Payne, 2015). Older cats are more likely to have a murmur (up to 60% of cats ≥9 years old) and, while these animals are more likely to have underlying cardiomyopathy, functional murmurs still are relatively common (Chapter 33). In certain breeds of dog, including Boxers and Bull Terriers, a soft to moderate ejection murmur is frequently heard at the left heart base in otherwise healthy dogs. This murmur might be functional or due to mild subaortic stenosis (SAS), which is common in these breeds; often the echocardiographic results are ambiguous. Functional, as well as pathologic, murmurs are common in horses, as well; their timing within the cardiac cycle can be systolic or diastolic. The patient's history, physical findings, and results of echocardiography or other clinical tests help the clinician identify a murmur's underlying cause, although the cause of some murmurs remains ambiguous.

Murmur Characteristics

Timing Cardiac murmurs can be described by their timing within the cardiac cycle (systolic or diastolic, or portions thereof; **Figure 11.1**), intensity (grade), point of maximal intensity (PMI) on the precordium, pattern of radiation over the chest wall, quality (timbre), and pitch. Systolic murmurs can occur in early (protosystolic), middle (mesosystolic), or late (telesystolic) systole, or throughout systole (holosystolic or pansystolic). Diastolic murmurs generally occur in early diastole (protodiastolic) or throughout diastole (holodiastolic). Occasionally, a murmur is heard at the very end of diastole (just before the next S_1); this timing is termed presystolic. Continuous murmurs, such as that of patent ductus arteriosus (PDA), begin in systole and extend without interruption through S_2 into all or part of diastole. To-and-fro murmurs are combinations of systolic and diastolic murmurs with a brief pause at the time of S_2; an example is aortic stenosis and insufficiency.

Intensity The intensity (loudness) of a murmur generally is graded on a 1–6 scale (**Table 11.1**), although some clinicians use a 1–5 scale. While the six-grade system has been established for decades in medicine, alternative approaches have been suggested (Rishniw, 2018; Caivano, 2018). For example, a simpler four-level grading scheme might be useful, at least for dogs with degenerative (myxomatous) mitral valve disease (DMVD) or ventricular outflow obstruction (pulmonic or aortic stenosis), where louder murmurs generally indicate more severe disease. However, confounding issues include a considerable overlapping in murmur grades in terms of the severity of disease (readily evident if one examines raw data of these studies), and the fact that murmur intensity does not always reflect the severity of underlying cardiac disease. Part of the ongoing confusion in grading murmurs in the authors' view stems from a lack of commonly accepted descriptions used to delineate the various grades. As shown in **Table 11.1**, and based on extensive teaching experience, grades 3 and 4 tend to be the most confused, but even beginners can appreciate the differences among the other murmur grades. Furthermore, many factors can influence murmur intensity, including the patient's level of myocardial contractility, red cell mass (viscosity), pressure gradient across a septal defect or other abnormal cardiovascular (CV) communication, and chest conformation or obesity. No grading system is ideal, and sometimes a grade 4 murmur in a thin patient will sound subjectively louder than a grade 5 in an obese one, where a thrill is palpable. These differences are related largely to extracardiac factors. The examiner's experience, stethoscope quality, and hearing acuity, as well as the selection and use of the chestpiece also have influence.

Point of Maximal Intensity and Radiation The PMI of a murmur usually is indicated by the hemithorax (right or left) and intercostal space or valve area where it is located, or by the terms apex or base. The base generally refers to the aortic and pulmonary valve areas and the precordium overlying the great arteries. Loud murmurs radiate to other areas over the chest wall. The areas to which a murmur radiates often are characteristic of the source and the potential to project sound across solid structures (such as the apex). Murmurs characteristically radiate in the direction of abnormal blood flow, as sound is often generated downstream from the anatomical

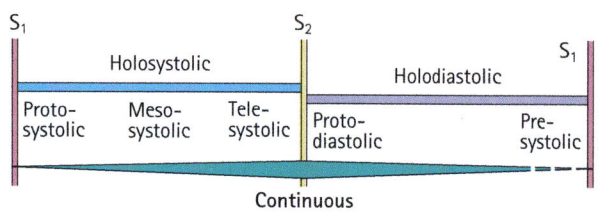

Figure 11.1 The timing of murmurs in relation to the normal heart sounds.

Table 11.1 Murmur Intensity Grading

Commonly Used Six-Grade System[a]

Grade	Murmur Intensity
1	Very soft, localized murmur; heard only over its site of origin after listening intently in quiet surroundings
2	Soft murmur, yet heard easily over its site of origin and confined to a single valve area or auscultatory location
3	Moderate intensity murmur; radiates to more than one precordial area
4	Loud murmur, but without a (consistent) precordial thrill; radiates widely and usually can be heard over most precordial regions
5	Loud murmur accompanied by a palpable precordial thrill; radiates widely and usually can be heard well over all precordial regions
6	Very loud murmur accompanied by a precordial thrill and also can be heard with the stethoscope lifted slightly away from the chest (over its site of origin); radiates widely and usually can be heard well over all precordial regions

A Proposed Four-Level Grading System[b]

Descriptive Grade	Comparable Six-Grade System Designation	Definition
Soft	1/6 and 2/6	Murmur is softer than the heart sounds (S_1 and S_2), which can be heard easily
Moderate	3/6	Murmur intensity is equal to that of S_1 and S_2, which still can be heard easily
Loud	4/6	Murmur is louder than S_1 and S_2. One or both heart sounds could be masked by the murmur, or are distinctly softer than it
Palpable	5/6 and 6/6	Murmur is accompanied by a palpable thrill, regardless of its perceived loudness on auscultation

[a] Roman, rather than Arabic, numerals often are used also. This is based on the original murmur grading system proposed by Levine and modified mainly by the addition of the precordial thrill to distinguish grades 5 and 6 from other murmur grades (Alpert, 1990).
[b] Rishniw (2018), Caivano (2018); p. 226.

source of the murmur. Thus, the entire thorax, thoracic inlet, and carotid artery areas should be auscultated.

Shape and Quality   A murmur can be described by its phonocardiographic shape, which arises from the hemodynamic forces that generate it. **Figure 11.2** depicts the typical (if somewhat stereotypical) configurations of various murmurs. The holosystolic or plateau-shaped murmur begins at the time of S_1 and is of uniform intensity throughout systole. Loud murmurs of this type might prevent distinction of S_1 and S_2 from the murmur. AV valve insufficiency and interventricular septal defects commonly cause a holosystolic murmur because the abnormal turbulent flow occurs throughout ventricular systole, beginning before the opening and ending after closure of the semilunar valves. A crescendo-decrescendo or diamond-shaped murmur starts softly, builds intensity and then diminishes; the S_1 and S_2 usually can be identified before and after the murmur, respectively. This murmur type also is called an ejection murmur because it occurs during blood ejection. The most common causes are rapid, normal ejection into the aorta or pulmonary artery (functional or physiological ejection murmurs) and ventricular outflow obstruction caused by stenosis. The time of peak flow determines the peak intensity of the murmur. Generally, cases of severe stenosis are louder and peak later in systole, often blending into the second heart sound. Conversely, functional murmurs and those caused by mild outflow tract obstruction usually peak in early to mid-systole. A decrescendo murmur tapers from its initial intensity over time; it can occur in systole or diastole, usually from valvular regurgitation. Functional protodiastolic murmurs in horses also are decrescendo in shape. A crescendo murmur does the opposite, abruptly increasing in loudness before stopping. The best example is mitral valve prolapse leading to late systolic mitral regurgitation (MR) in the horse.

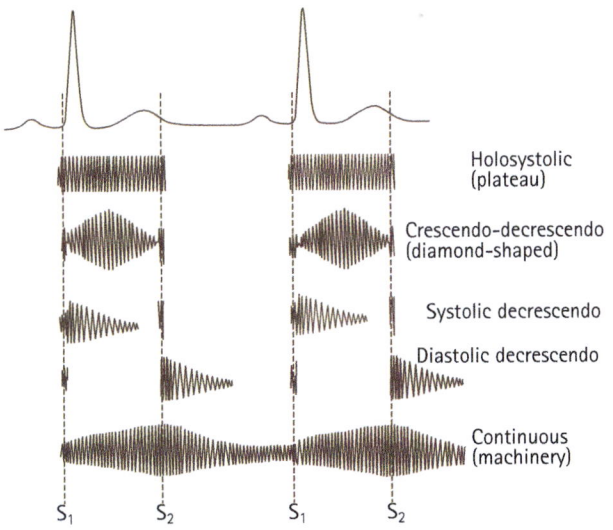

Figure 11.2 Depiction of the (phonocardiographic) configuration and timing of various cardiac murmurs. (From Ware WA. The cardiovascular examination. In Nelson RW, Couto CG (editors). Small Animal Internal Medicine. 6th edition. Elsevier, St Louis, MO. 2019. p. 10.)

The pitch and quality (timbre) of a murmur relate to its various frequency components. Murmurs usually are of higher frequency than transient sounds. "Noisy" or "harsh" murmurs contain mixed frequencies; the vast majority of murmurs have this characteristic. "Musical" and vibratory murmurs essentially comprise a fundamental frequency with its overtones. Mitral and aortic valve regurgitation sometimes have a musical component to their audible spectrum.

Nonpathologic Murmurs

Functional (nonpathologic) murmurs tend to be systolic and heard best at the left heart base, over the aortic and pulmonic valves and great vessels. Functional murmurs result from some physiological alteration in the absence of a structural cardiac abnormality. They sometimes are called physiologic murmurs, especially when a physiological explanation can be invoked. Causes of high sympathetic tone frequently underlie these murmurs, including anxiety, pain, colic, exercise, low blood pressure, and administration of sympathomimetic drugs. High output states (also related to sympathetic activation) increase blood flow velocities; these include moderate to severe anemia, fever, hyperthyroidism, and peripheral arteriovenous (A-V) fistulae. Other causes include hypoproteinemia, an athletic heart, and extreme bradycardia. All these conditions can increase blood flow velocity. Functional murmurs can change with exercise or excitement; some become louder, others softer, and some only appear with exercise or excitement. This also is true for functional diastolic murmurs in horses (see section "Horses").

Innocent murmurs (such as those heard in some puppies, kittens, and foals) occur without identifiable physiologic cause or structural cardiac disease. In one survey, the prevalence of innocent murmurs in mixed-breed dogs was 0.1%; in mixed-breed cats, it was 0.16% or even up to 0.2% when dynamic left or right ventricular (LV or RV) outflow obstruction was included (Schrope, 2015). This study showed a slight male predominance for both species. However, there is certainly a much higher incidence of innocent murmurs in many purebred dogs examined by specialists. For example, in one report, 36% of 227 Cairn Terrier puppies examined had innocent heart murmurs detected (van Staveren, 2019). The authors would suggest similar results in many other breeds, including those prone to SAS.

Dogs Innocent and physiologic murmurs are heard best at the left base and are systolic in timing. They usually are of soft, or occasionally moderate, intensity and have a crescendo-decrescendo (ejection-type) configuration, with S_1 and S_2 clearly evident. Innocent puppy murmurs become softer with time and generally disappear by about 4–6 months of age. Functional ejection murmurs are common in many large breed dogs, including those with a high prevalence of SAS, as well as some at low risk (Greyhounds). Based on Doppler echocardiographic studies, these ejection murmurs arise from the LV outflow tract in association with rapid ejection of blood into the ascending aorta. These murmurs can persist well past maturity. They are indistinguishable from those caused by trivial or mild aortic stenosis, and their origin can be confusing even after detailed echocardiography. Although these functional murmurs pose no apparent health risk to the dog, they do create challenges when evaluating potential candidates for breeding.

Cats Functional murmurs in cats are systolic in timing and usually heard best at the cranial left (or right) sternal border, so it is important to listen in these ventral locations. Common physiologic causes include hyperthyroidism, anemia, and high sympathetic tone (from excitement and other causes). Some cats with aortic dilation (perhaps from systemic hypertension) have an audible murmur. Dehydration or hypovolemia can promote dynamic ventricular outflow obstruction and murmur development. Likewise, a murmur might occur with dynamic mid-ventricular obstruction associated with LV hypertrophy of any cause, including hyperthyroidism or hypertension, especially when sympathetic tone is high. Dynamic RV outflow obstruction is another cause of functional ejection murmurs, especially in stressed cats. Furthermore, it is possible to induce an iatrogenic RV outflow murmur in some cats by applying excessive pressure to the chest wall during auscultation. Functional (as well as pathological) murmurs in cats often change in intensity over time or with excitement and heart rate.

Horses Nonpathologic murmurs in horses usually are systolic in timing, associated with normal ventricular ejection, of soft to moderate intensity, and peak in early to mid-systole, as described earlier. However, soft diastolic murmurs are heard in some normal horses too. These can occur in association with early ventricular filling (between the S_2 and S_3 sounds) or with atrial systole (a presystolic murmur, between the S_4 and S_1 sounds). Functional diastolic murmurs might be heard over the ventricular area on either side of the thorax; they can vary in intensity with changes in excitement, exercise, and even normal heart rate variation. Some protodiastolic murmurs are musical, vibratory, or squeaky in nature. Importantly, these murmurs are short in contrast to the holodiastolic murmur of aortic regurgitation. In foals, innocent systolic flow murmurs are common. In addition, newborns can have a continuous murmur from persistent flow in the ductus arteriosus during the first few days after birth, until the ductus closes.

Pathologic Systolic Murmurs

Systolic murmurs commonly are either holosystolic (plateau-shaped) or mid-systolic (crescendo-decrescendo or ejection) in configuration. It can be difficult to differentiate between these types of murmurs, especially for the inexperienced listener. However, establishing that a murmur occurs in systole (rather than diastole), determining its PMI, and grading its intensity are the most important steps toward diagnosis. The typical location of various murmurs over different areas of the chest wall is shown in **Figure 11.3**. In general, pathologic murmurs tend to be louder over the left thorax with the exceptions of tricuspid regurgitation and most (membranous) ventricular septal defect murmurs, which are louder on the right.

Mitral Regurgitation The murmur of MR (mitral insufficiency) is heard best in the area of the mitral valve and projects well to the palpable left apex. MR murmurs can radiate both dorsally and to the right hemithorax. In cats, MR murmurs are heard best along the caudal sternal border, near the palpable apex beat, although this is a generalization. Malfunction or malformation of any part of the mitral apparatus can lead to valve insufficiency. Thus, causes of MR include DMVD, infective endocarditis, congenital malformation (dysplasia) of the valve or its supporting structures (chordae, papillary muscles), chordal rupture, and diseases causing LV dilation or hypertrophy. MR murmurs radiate well dorsally and often to the left base and right chest wall.

Characteristically, MR causes a holosystolic, mixed frequency or harsh murmur, often characterized as "blowing" in quality. However, the murmur might be heard in early systole (protosystolic) and taper into a decrescendo configuration, either with mild MR, where the leakage ceases in late systole, or with sudden and severe valve insufficiency, as the atrial-to-ventricular pressure gradient diminishes. In horses, the MR murmur often has a crescendo configuration, peaking in late systole; this is likely from valve prolapse. In cats with dynamic LV outflow tract obstruction, the systolic anterior motion of the mitral valve can cause a mid-to-late systolic murmur that often diminishes or disappears with beta-adrenergic blockade. Occasionally, MR murmurs have a musical or "whoop-like" quality.

The intensity of a MR murmur caused by DMVD is related largely to the severity of valve leakage, up to a point. In particular, soft murmurs (grade 1–2/6) are associated with mild disease and minimal cardiac remodeling. Moderate to loud murmurs indicate more severe disease, but with substantial overlapping of severity. Also, with advancing DMVD, the S_1 tends to become progressively louder; this is thought to result from increasing LV dilation combined with well-maintained ventricular systolic function. However, murmur loudness does not necessarily correlate with disease severity when MR is associated with other etiologies, such as dilated cardiomyopathy. Increased arterial pressure can increase the intensity of a MR murmur of any cause, while hypotension can diminish it. MR associated with mitral systolic anterior motion (SAM) from dynamic LV outflow obstruction varies with the degree of obstruction and sympathetic tone.

Tricuspid Regurgitation The murmur of TR is loudest at the right apex and over the tricuspid valve area and tends to radiate dorsally. A noticeably different pitch or quality from a concurrent MR murmur, a right precordial thrill, jugular pulsations, or signs of right-sided heart failure can help differentiate TR from radiation of a MR murmur to the right chest wall. Causes of TR include degenerative (myxomatous) valve disease, infective endocarditis (rare in companion animals and uncommon in horses), and congenital malformations (dysplasia). Diseases that induce RV hypertrophy or dilation can also cause TR, such as pulmonary hypertension (including heartworm caval syndrome, where worms are found within the tricuspid valve orifice). TR murmurs often are softer than MR murmurs, except when severe pulmonary hypertension is present. Septal leaflet prolapse is common in degenerative tricuspid valve disease and results in an eccentric jet directed laterally, directly at the thoracic wall. This situation can create a loud murmur, including a precordial thrill, even when the overall regurgitation volume is mild to moderate.

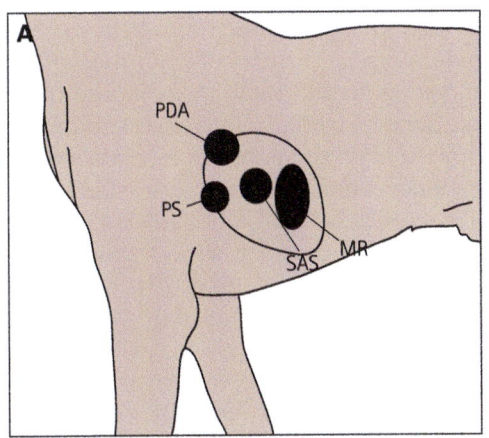 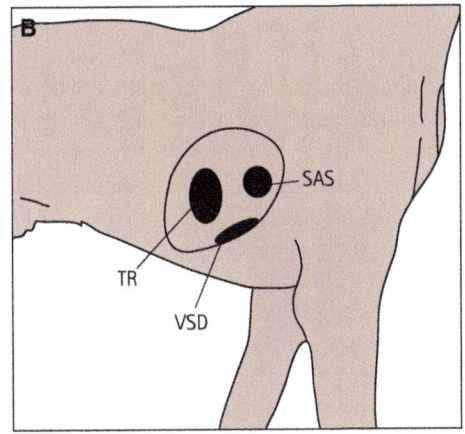

Figure 11.3 Typical areas of maximal intensity for common congenital and acquired murmurs on the left (A) and right (B) chest walls. MR, mitral valve regurgitation; PDA, patent ductus arteriosus; PS, pulmonic stenosis; SAS, subaortic stenosis; TR, tricuspid valve regurgitation; VSD, ventricular septal defect.

Ventricular Outflow Obstructions Murmurs caused by ventricular outflow obstruction are crescendo-decrescendo in shape and most often are heard at the left base. These can be caused either by a fixed subvalvular, valvular, or supravalvular narrowing or a dynamic muscular or mitral valvular obstruction. These murmurs become louder as stroke volume or contractile strength increases, as occurs with exercise, increased sympathetic tone, increased venous return, and following a premature beat.

The murmur of SAS is heard well at the lower left base and radiates prominently up the ascending aorta (that curves toward the right) to the right cardiac base. With extreme poststenotic dilation of the aorta, the murmur of SAS can be loudest on the right side. The murmur of SAS also radiates craniodorsally on the left side and up the carotid arteries. Loud SAS murmurs occasionally can be heard on top of the skull (calvarium). However, detection of an ejection-type "murmur" (or bruit) that is isolated to the thoracic inlet should not be misdiagnosed as SAS. This vibration usually is derived from partial compression of the carotid artery, either by the stethoscope or from the patient's neck position. Another point of confusion can be distinguishing the murmur of severe SAS from mitral regurgitation. This is challenging because the mitral valve area and subaortic vestibule are in anatomic continuity, severe SAS causes a late peaking murmur that can obscure S_2, there can be concurrent MR in dogs with SAS, and the subaortic murmur sometimes radiates ventrally toward the left apex. (In these cases, late-rising, hypokinetic arterial pulses strongly suggest LV outflow tract obstruction). Infrequently, concurrent aortic regurgitation (AR) is severe enough to cause a diastolic murmur (see section "To-and-Fro Murmur"). Finally, although valvular and supravalvular aortic stenoses are uncommon, their murmurs can be loudest over the right cranial thorax because the high-velocity jet radiates directly into the ascending aorta.

Dynamic LV outflow and mid-ventricular obstructions are most common in feline hypertrophic cardiomyopathy and especially those cats with systolic anterior motion of the mitral valve. In this species, the associated murmur is heard best at the cranial sternal borders, although this is variable and can be confused by concurrent MR, which tends to be louder more apically. Dynamic LV mid-ventricular or outflow tract obstructions also can occur in cats and dogs with other disorders. These include: Concentric LV hypertrophy from SAS, systemic hypertension, or other causes; profound LV volume depletion; mitral valve dysplasia, especially when associated with systolic anterior motion of the valve; and severe concentric RV hypertrophy, such as that caused by pulmonic stenosis (and that alters LV geometry).

The systolic murmur of pulmonic stenosis (PS) is heard best cranially at the left base, originating at the pulmonary valve more ventrally and radiating dorsally into the main pulmonary artery, which is located "high" on the left base. Because these structures are close to the thoracic wall, murmurs of PS frequently are loud and practically always loudest on the left side. "Relative" PS occurs when flow through the valve is greatly increased, even though the valve itself is structurally normal. Causes include a large left-to-right shunting atrial or ventricular septal defect, VSD. In addition, valvular PS sometimes is associated with an early systolic ejection click, indicating a fused but mobile valve, or with a tricuspid regurgitation (TR) murmur, due to ventricular or right atrial remodeling or concurrent tricuspid valve malformation.

Ventricular Septal Defect VSD also will cause a harsh, blowing-type holosystolic murmur, although some midsystolic peaking commonly is seen on a phonocardiogram. The PMI usually is located at the right sternal border (for perimembranous defects), reflecting the direction of the intracardiac shunt. Less commonly, when the VSD is located in the RV outlet region (subarterial VSD), the murmur is louder over the left, dorsal heart base. A large VSD could cause a murmur of relative PS as well. Prolapse of part of the aortic valve into the defect might cause an audible AR murmur. The intensity of a VSD murmur often is inversely correlated to the size of the defect; for example, a small defect typically causes a loud murmur because a high pressure gradient is maintained across the ventricular septum. As such, prognosis should never be based on auscultation alone.

Pathologic Diastolic Murmurs

Diastolic murmurs are relatively uncommon in dogs and cats. In small animals, AR caused by bacterial endocarditis is the most likely etiology, although congenital valve malformations, aortic leaflet prolapse associated with a VSD, or AR secondary to SAS do occur. Degenerative aortic valve disease is common, but rarely severe enough to generate an audible murmur. Aortopathy with aortic root dilation is very common in cats (and less so in dogs) related to systemic hypertension or advancing age. Aortic regurgitation is a common Doppler finding in aortic root dilation, although a diastolic murmur associated with this regurgitation is infrequently audible.

In contrast, degenerative aortic valve disease is common in older horses. The diastolic murmur of AR begins at the time of S_2 and is heard best at the left base over the aortic valve; it often radiates to the right base. The murmur of AR is decrescendo in configuration and extends a variable time into diastole, depending on the pressure difference between aorta and LV. In most cases, AR is holodiastolic, and there frequently is some presystolic accentuation following the atrial contraction (Chapter 30). The genesis of that accentuation is unresolved. At normal heart rates, the murmur is particularly long, and in cases of physiologic AV block, exceptionally so. Some AR murmurs in horses exhibit a musical quality, with descriptions of "cooing," "buzzing," and "like a dive-bomber plane" often reported. The differential diagnosis of degenerative AR in the horse includes infective endocarditis, noninfective valvulitis, and malalignment VSD with aortic root prolapse (causing the diastolic component in the murmur complex).

Clinically relevant pulmonary valve regurgitation (PR) is rare, although an audible murmur would be more likely in the face of severe pulmonary hypertension with pulmonary artery dilation. In referral practices, it is common to detect a decrescendo murmur of pulmonary regurgitation following successful balloon valvuloplasty of PS. Some canine cases of congenital PS also have an audible murmur of PR, especially if the pulmonary trunk is severely dilated. Lastly, a soft, low diastolic rumble is described in humans with congenital mitral or tricuspid stenosis. However, these are rare lesions in animals, cause faint murmurs that require patient cooperation to hear, and are almost never heard in dogs, cats, and horses.

Murmurs in Both Systole and Diastole

Continuous Murmur Continuous (machinery) murmurs begin in systole and extend through S_2 into diastole, indicating that a significant pressure gradient exists continuously between two connecting locations. Murmurs of this type become shorter and less intense in the setting of pulmonary hypertension, which reduces the pressure differential and diminishes the shunt velocity. PDA is the classic cause of a continuous murmur in dogs and cats. A rare cause is aortopulmonary window, where a defect in the arterial wall connects the ascending aorta and main pulmonary artery. Pulmonary hypertension is common with this defect, and can cause the murmur to be only systolic or even absent. Ruptured sinus of Valsalva aneurysm (aortocardiac fistula) and rupture of the aorta into the pulmonary artery (both most common in horses) are other potential causes of continuous murmurs. Central A-V shunts (arteriovenous malformations) and peripheral A-V fistulae might be associated with a thoracic or locally audible continuous murmur (bruit), respectively. To-and-fro murmurs are not considered continuous, while the combined murmurs of ventricular septal defect (systolic) and aortic regurgitation (diastolic) can be readily mistaken as continuous.

PDA is by far the most common cause of a continuous murmur in veterinary practice. At slow heart rates, this murmur might become inaudible toward the end of diastole, as the pressure gradient diminishes. The PDA murmur is loudest high at the left base above the pulmonic valve area (over the main pulmonary artery). This murmur tends to radiate cranially, ventrally, and to the right. The systolic component usually is louder and heard well all over the chest, whereas the diastolic component is more localized to the left base, in many cases. If only the cardiac apical area is auscultated, the diastolic component (and the correct diagnosis) could be missed. Concurrent MR associated with LV dilation is common, and also can create a systolic murmur at this location. The clinician can better appreciate the timing by slowly advancing the stethoscope from apex to base and back, listening for lengthening of the murmur at the base. For practical purposes, the finding of a continuous murmur rules out a "reversed" PDA (p. 449). Identifying the murmur of PDA in cats is more challenging because of their higher heart rate and greater risk of developing progressive pulmonary hypertension. In this species, the murmur might be described as a "long" systolic murmur (but in realty one that spans into diastole).

To-and-Fro Murmur Continuous murmurs can be confused with concurrent systolic ejection and diastolic decrescendo murmurs. However, with these so-called "to-and-fro" murmurs, the ejection murmur component tapers in late systole, allowing the S_2 to be heard as a distinct sound. The most common cause of to-and-fro murmurs is the combination of SAS and AR. Sometimes, to-and-fro murmurs are heard in dogs with PS and PR, especially after balloon valvuloplasty.

Abnormal Transient Sounds

Transient sounds are vibrations of brief duration. They occur with abrupt changes in blood flow and pressure. Normal transient sounds are the S_1 and S_2. Changes in the intensity, or splitting, of the S_1 or S_2 sound sometimes indicate underlying pathology (**Table 11.2**). Split sounds result from asynchronous closure of the left and right heart valves. Systolic clicks can be nonejection or related to ejection. Diastolic transient (also called "gallop") sounds normally are not heard in dogs and cats. In normal horses, however, an audible S_4 sound is common. The S_3 is softly audible in many horses, as well.

Table 11.2 Altered Intensity of Heart Sounds

Loud S_1
- Thin chest wall
- High sympathetic tone
- Tachycardia
- Systemic arterial hypertension
- Shortened PR intervals[a]

Loud, Snapping S_2
- Pulmonary hypertension (from heartworm disease, primary pulmonary disease, congenital shunt with Eisenmenger's physiology, left heart failure, and other causes)

Muffled Sounds (Especially S_1)
- Pericardial effusion
- Obesity
- Diaphragmatic hernia
- Dilated cardiomyopathy (myocardial failure)
- Hypovolemia/poor ventricular filling
- +/-Pleural effusion

[a] An intermittently louder S_1 could occur with ventricular premature beats, as the timing between atrial and ventricular contraction changes. Additionally, the S_2 can vary in intensity or be absent, depending on the prematurity of the ventricular ectopic beats (and degree of ventricular filling).

Gallop Sounds

The S_3 and S_4 heart sounds occur during diastole (Figure 1.20, p. 18). As noted in Chapter 1, the two major features of diastole are the rapid filling phase where blood is actively sucked into the ventricle, and the atrial contraction phase where blood is pumped into the ventricle. These filling events are driven by small pressure gradients and occur against the backdrop of ventricular compliance or stiffness. Both filling pressures and compliance frequently are altered in disease. Gallop sounds relate to these phases of diastole.

These transient sounds are lower in frequency and usually softer than the S_1 and S_2, and thus are harder to hear. Because they are of lower frequency, gallop sounds generally are heard best with the bell of the stethoscope (or with only light pressure applied to a single-sided tunable chestpiece). When the S_3 or S_4 is audible, the heart can mimic the sounds of a galloping horse, hence the term "gallop rhythm." However, this term can be confusing because the presence or absence of an audible S_3 or S_4 has nothing to do with the heart's electrical rhythm. At very fast heart rates, differentiation of S_3 from S_4 is difficult. If both sounds are present, they might be superimposed (called a summation gallop).

Audible gallop sounds in dogs and cats, or loud gallop sounds in horses, generally indicate ventricular diastolic dysfunction. Congestive heart failure (CHF) and increased left atrial pressure intensify the gallop sounds. A gallop sound might be the only auscultatory abnormality in some cases of cardiomyopathy or hypertensive heart disease.

S_3 Gallop The S_3, also known as an S_3 gallop or ventricular gallop, is associated with low frequency vibrations during the rapid ventricular filling phase. This is a normal sound in trained horses and related to vigorous suction of blood into a compliant ventricle, which then vibrates near the end of rapid filling. However, an audible S_3 in a dog or cat (or a loud S_3 in a horse) usually indicates CHF in the setting of ventricular dilation or hypertrophy with reduced chamber compliance. Greater ventricular stiffness is compensated by increasing venous and atrial filling pressures; these lead to high-velocity ventricular filling that terminates abruptly as ventricular stiffness supervenes. The Doppler correlate to this sound is the restrictive mitral filling pattern (see Chapter 4). This extra sound can be fairly prominent or quite subtle. It is heard best over the cardiac apex and might be the only auscultable abnormality in cardiomyopathies, especially dilated cardiomyopathy. An S_3 gallop is probably overlooked in dogs and horses with severe MR and CHF; it might be detected as a soft "thud" at the conclusion of the holosystolic murmur, where it can be misinterpreted as an S_2. The ventricular gallop can diminish in intensity or abate with successful therapy of CHF and reduction of venous pressures.

S_4 Gallop The S_4 gallop, also called an atrial or presystolic gallop, is associated with low frequency vibrations induced by blood flow into the ventricles during atrial contraction. An audible S_4 in dogs and cats can occur with abnormal ventricular relaxation and increased ventricular stiffness so long as atrial function is preserved. LV hypertrophy, as with hypertrophic cardiomyopathy, hyperthyroidism, or systemic hypertension, and myocardial ischemia are typical underlying causes. A transient S_4 gallop sometimes is heard in older stressed or anemic cats and could represent aging changes in ventricular relaxation. It can be combined with an S_3 as a summation gallop in CHF. As atrial function deteriorates from progressive left atrial dilation, this gallop becomes unreliable as a signal of diastolic dysfunction.

The S_4 occurs immediately before the first sound in normal horses, creating what has been termed a "pseudosplit" S_1. This relationship (timing) will vary with the P-R interval of the ECG. Horses with second-degree AV block typically have an audible, isolated S_4 (without accompanying S_1 and S_2) associated with the nonconducted atrial activation. The presence of atrial fibrillation causes the S_4 sound to disappear, because coordinated atrial contractions are lost. A pitfall is confusing a split first heart sound for a closely timed S_4-S_1; the loss of the atrial sound will be confirmed if attention is paid to the erratic rhythm, which tends to be nonpatterned in atrial fibrillation. The atrial sound also is inconsistent or lost with junctional or ventricular arrhythmias, as well as in the setting of severe hyperkalemia. Abnormally increased ventricular stiffness is likely to enhance S_4 intensity.

Systolic Clicks and Ejection Sounds

Other brief abnormal sounds sometimes are audible. Systolic clicks are classified as ejection or nonejection. The most common are single to multiple, high frequency mid- to late-systolic sounds heard best over the mitral valve or tricuspid valve areas (see **Figure 29.7**, p. 539). These sounds can occur with degenerative valvular disease, mitral or tricuspid valve prolapse, congenital mitral dysplasia, and potentially from hypertrophic cardiomyopathy, although this requires verification. These clicks are thought to result from abrupt tension or checking of a redundant valve or abnormal chordae tendineae. A concurrent murmur of valvular insufficiency might be present. In dogs with DMVD, a mitral or tricuspid click sometimes is heard before the typical MR murmur develops.

Ejection clicks are less common. An early systolic, high-pitched ejection sound at the left base sometimes is heard in animals with valvular PS associated with mobile but fused pulmonary valve leaflets, as well as from conditions that cause dilation of a great artery, such as pulmonary hypertension. These sounds are thought to arise either from the sudden checking of a fused pulmonic valve or the rapid filling of a dilated vessel during ejection.

Other Considerations in Cardiac Auscultation

Several factors influence the intensity of the normal heart sounds, including body habitus and level of excitement (**Table 11.2**, and p. 231). An auscultatory finding highly suggestive of severe pulmonary hypertension (Chapter 39) is a loud, snapping S_2 sound, which can also be split (see next paragraph). Rhythm disturbances that cause an abbreviated PR interval, so that ventricular contraction begins while the AV valves are still wide open, generate a louder S_1 as do contractions associated with increased LV pressure generation (as with high sympathetic tone or systemic hypertension). Conversely, factors that increase the distance between the heart and stethoscope, or that reduce contractile strength, will soften or muffle the heart sounds; these include pericardial effusion, obesity, hypovolemia, and dilated cardiomyopathy (**Table 11.2**). Arrhythmias cause variability in the intensity, as well as the regularity, of the heart sounds.

Physiologic splitting of S_2 (p. 40) is most noticeable in horses, and sometimes large-breed dogs, and is associated with delayed closure of the pulmonic relative to the aortic component of that sound. Pathologic splitting of the heart sounds occurs with asynchronous ventricular contraction or abnormally prolonged ejection from one ventricle compared to the other. Splitting is challenging to identify and is more appreciated when the delay occurs within the right ventricle as the pulmonary component of S_2 normally occurs last. Common causes of split heart sounds include ventricular premature contractions, bundle branch blocks, severe pulmonary hypertension (split S_2), and septal defects (split S_2). Fixed splitting of the S_2 (with little or no respiratory variation) is a characteristic auscultatory finding of large atrial septal defects. Split sounds can be distinct as in pulmonary hypertension where the pulmonary component of S_2 also is tympanic, or sound less crisp or "muddled" as the two components prolong the first or second sound. This feature can sometimes distinguish supraventricular from ventricular tachycardias, where sounds are normal or split, respectively.

Pericardial diseases can cause several abnormal auscultatory findings. The most common finding is muffled heart sounds, usually associated with large-volume pericardial effusion, but occasionally with constrictive pericardial disease (Chapter 35). Rarely, constrictive pericardial disease causes an audible pericardial knock. This early diastolic sound results from sudden checking of ventricular filling by the restrictive pericardium (similar to a ventricular gallop). Pericardial friction rubs can accompany pericarditis (p. 715). These are heard more often in large animal species and only rarely in dogs with pericarditis. Pericardial friction rubs can occur as triple sounds (in mid-systole and mid- and late-diastole), although sometimes only a double or single rub sound is heard.

Several cardiac conditions might cause no cardiac murmur, or perhaps only a subtle murmur or other abnormal sound. This can be the case in animals with dilated, hypertrophic, or restrictive cardiomyopathy (Chapters 32–34). Pericardial disease or effusion does not cause a murmur, although the animal might have a concurrent abnormality that does, such as DMVD or an intracardiac tumor. Congenital CV shunts with concurrent severe pulmonary hypertension might be associated with no or only a soft systolic murmur. This occurs when pulmonary and systemic pressures are fairly equivalent ("balanced"), causing minimal to no flow across the shunt. This also occurs in animals with a congenital shunt and more severe pulmonary hypertension, where hypoxemia from chronic right-to-left shunting has stimulated development of erythrocytosis. The consequent increase in blood viscosity, especially in the setting of equilibration of pressures across the shunt, can reduce blood flow turbulence to an inaudible level (p. 23).

Approach to the Patient with a Murmur or Other Abnormal Heart Sound

When a murmur or other abnormal heart sound is discovered on physical exam, it is important to characterize the sound(s) as best as possible and to pay careful attention to other aspects of the CV exam. This is especially urgent for patients with historical or clinical signs that might be caused by cardiac disease. Yet these observations also are important when a murmur or abnormal sound is discovered incidentally in an animal with no clinical signs. Findings from the CV exam, in addition to auscultation (Chapter 2), help the clinician decide whether a murmur (or other sound) is likely to be pathological, as well as clinically relevant (Côté, 2015). While not all murmurs indicate underlying cardiac structural abnormality, many do. Likewise, some abnormal transient sounds indicate early or well-compensated disease (such as mitral clicks in DMVD or sometimes, atrial gallops in hypertrophic cardiomyopathy); whereas, others (such as a ventricular gallop) might indicate a life-threatening situation.

Identifying the anatomic origin of the abnormal sound is an important initial step. For murmurs, this generally relates to the PMI (**Figure 11.4**). The next step is to determine the likely underlying etiology of the abnormal sound. For example, is the animal's murmur caused by a structural abnormality (congenital, degenerative, or infective disease) or perhaps a physiologic change (such as fever, anemia, hyperthyroidism, or other)? The patient's species, breed, and sex might generate a higher degree of suspicion for certain cardiac diseases where an associated increase in prevalence is known. For example, DMVD in Cavalier King Charles Spaniels and other small breeds, dilated cardiomyopathy in Doberman Pinschers, or hypertrophic cardiomyopathy in Maine Coon cats.

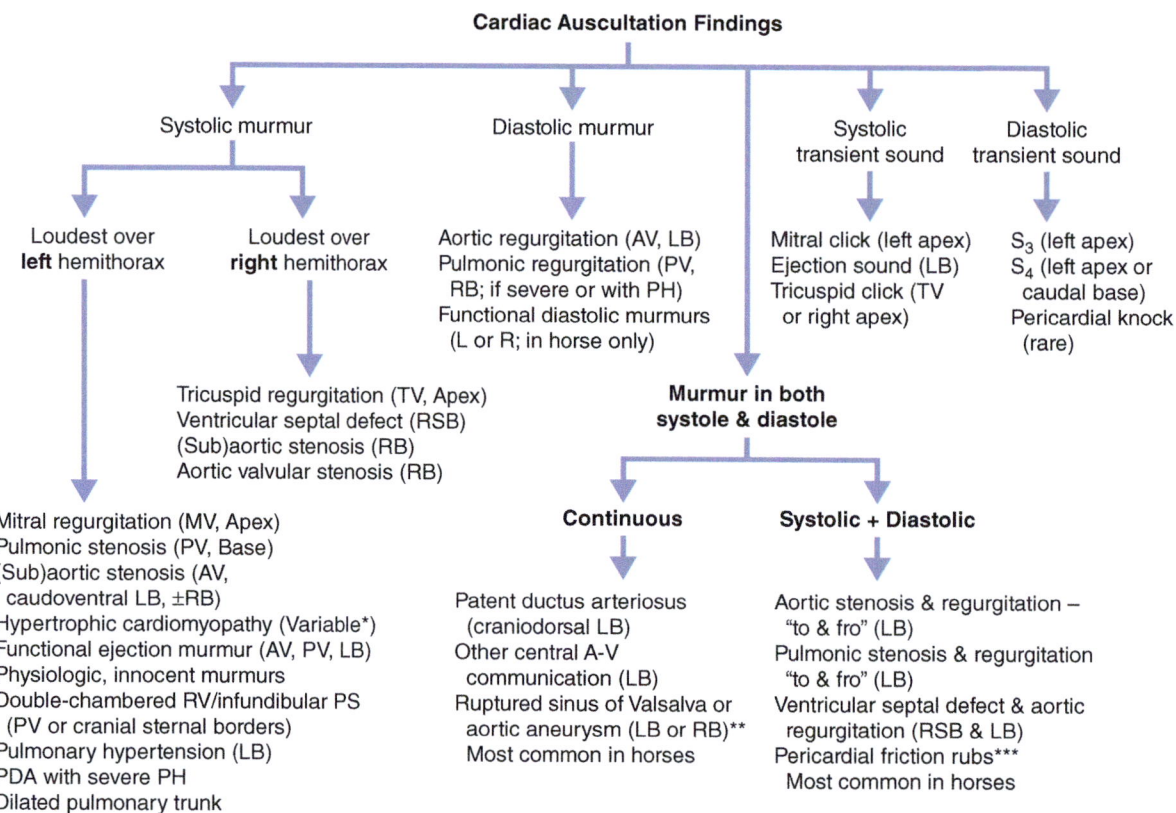

Figure 11.4 Approach to the patient with abnormal cardiac auscultation findings, with lists of diagnostic considerations; exceptions can occur. Usual point of maximal intensity (PMI) noted in parentheses. *Murmur can be from mitral systolic anterior motion, mitral regurgitation, left midventricular obstruction, or dynamic RV outflow obstruction. PMI can be caudal (apical) or cranial sternal border, & louder on left or right. **PMI depends on site (into right heart vs pulmonary artery). ***Can be mistaken for a murmur. A-V, arteriovenous; AV, aortic valve; LA, left apex; LB, left base; MV, mitral valve; PDA, patent ductus arteriosus; PH, pulmonary hypertension; PV, pulmonary valve; RB, right base; RSB, right sternal border; RV, right ventricular; TV, tricuspid valve.

The presence and severity of any adverse hemodynamic or clinical consequences, such as cardiac chamber dilation or hypertrophy, edema or effusions, myocardial dysfunction, and arrhythmias inform additional diagnostic testing and therapeutic strategies.

The clinical approach to the patient could vary depending on: (1) Whether potentially related clinical signs are present or not; (2) the timing, PMI, or intensity (loudness) of a murmur that was heard; (3) the characteristics and timing of an identified transient sound; (4) the type of alteration heard in a normal heart sound (S_1 or S_2, and in horses, also S_3 or S_4); (5) the signalment and intended use of the animal; and (6) whether there are other patient concerns, such as an upcoming surgical procedure or other known stressors. **Table 11.3** summarizes pertinent observations and considerations that can help the clinician decide if additional cardiac diagnostic testing (especially echocardiography) is indicated immediately, could be delayed for a time, or might even be unnecessary.

Echocardiography (Chapter 4), particularly when done by a veterinary cardiologist, provides the most detailed and specific clinical information about the structure and function of the heart and proximal vessels. Echocardiography is currently the best screening tool for cardiomyopathy in cats, although the quantitative NT-proBNP test can help in gauging the relative risk of feline heart disease and is a practical first step before referral. This biomarker and an echocardiogram also are indicated in large breed dogs with a murmur of MR. Unlike older small breed dogs with MR, which typically have reasonably normal LV function, MR in large breed dogs could indicate dilated cardiomyopathy, more rapid LV function deterioration even with degenerative valve disease, congenital mitral valve malformation (dysplasia), or infective endocarditis.

Other clinical tests can complement echocardiographic findings, and sometimes are useful for initial screening. Thoracic radiographs (Chapter 3) can reveal overt cardiomegaly or abnormal cardiac contours, as well as pulmonary infiltrates, intrathoracic vascular patterns, mediastinal abnormalities, and pleural space disease. However, radiographs are not adequately sensitive to reliably detect or differentiate mild congenital diseases or acquired valvular or myocardial diseases prior to the development of cardiomegaly. Nonetheless, serial radiographic screening can

Table 11.3 Additional Cardiac Diagnostic Testing[a] Is Recommended for Patients with a Murmur or Other Abnormal Heart Sound When:

- Clinical or historical signs consistent with CV disease are present
- Other abnormal findings are present on CV exam, such as:
  - Jugular vein pulsation or distension
  - Hyper- or hypokinetic arterial pulses
  - Abnormal mucous membrane color or refill time
  - Displaced or otherwise abnormal maximal precordial impulse
  - Abnormal heart rate or rhythm
- The animal possibly will be used for breeding
- The animal is intended (or being used) for service, performance, or athletic work (such as law enforcement or military, search and rescue, guide or other support work; hunting or field trial, and racing)
- The animal is to undergo an anesthetic or surgical procedure, or other stressor (such as shipping or other travel)
- The animal has a close relative with congenital cardiac disease
- A systolic murmur is heard and:
  - The PMI is the left base and intensity is loud (grade 3/6 or higher)
  - The PMI is the left apex (± both S_1 and S_2 are obscured) and especially if a large breed dog
  - The PMI is on the right hemithorax
  - The murmur radiates up the carotid arteries
  - The PMI is at the left base, intensity is soft (grade 1-2/6), animal is asymptomatic, and the clinician is unclear if the cause is structural heart disease or not
- A continuous murmur is heard (of any intensity)
  - Except if in a <4-day-old foal (re-examine in a couple days)
- A diastolic murmur is heard (of any intensity) in a dog or cat
  - (Soft, brief diastolic functional murmurs can occur in horses)
- An abnormal transient sound is heard:
  - An S_3 or S_4 in a dog or cat
  - An especially loud S_3 or S_4 in a horse
  - A split S_2 sound (except physiologic splitting, typically in horses)
  - Marked alteration in S_1 or S_2 intensity
- The owner requests further cardiac evaluation

[a] Echocardiography especially; see text.

be useful in some situations, particularly for adult small breed dogs with a systolic murmur loudest at the left apex, where MR caused by DMVD is most likely. In these dogs, the finding of a normal cardiac size and shape generally indicates that the condition is not yet of clinical importance, although it should be re-assessed over time. Circulating NT-proBNP concentrations (p. 291) often are elevated in animals with cardiomegaly and advanced cardiac disease; however, in milder disease there can be much overlap with normal. Breed specific differences in normal range exist as well. Furthermore, NT-proBNP elevation can occur with some noncardiac conditions, such as renal disease. Electrocardiography (Chapter 5) can help the clinician identify an arrhythmia heard on auscultation. An electrocardiogram (ECG) also might reveal an abnormal mean electrical axis or other cardiac chamber enlargement criteria; however, this can be inconsistent and echocardiography is more sensitive for identifying chamber dilation and hypertrophy. See chapters on specific diseases for further information and patient management guidelines.

Suggested Additional Reading and References

Also See Online Comprehensive Bibliography at: https://www.routledge.com/9781482246223.

Alpert MA. Systolic murmurs. In, Walker HK, Hall WD, Hurst JW (ed). The History, Physical, and Laboratory Examinations. Butterworths, Boston. 1990. Chapter 26. (https://www.ncbi.nlm.nih.gov/books/NBK345/).

Bavegems VC, Duchateau L, Polis IE, et al. Detection of innocent systolic murmurs by auscultation and their relation to hematologic and echocardiographic findings in clinically normal Whippets. J Am Vet Med Assoc 2011;238:468–471.

Blass KA, Schober KE, Bonagura JD, et al. Clinical evaluation of the 3M Littmann Electronic Stethoscope Model 3200 in 150 cats. J Feline Med Surg 2013;15:893–900.

Blissitt K. Auscultation. In, Marr CM, Bowen IM (editors). Cardiology of the Horse. 2nd edition. Saunders Elsevier, Edinburgh. 2010. pp. 91–104.

Caivano D, Dickson D, Martin M, et al. Murmur intensity in adult dogs with pulmonic and subaortic stenosis reflects disease severity. J Small Anim Pract 2018;59:161–166.

Côté E, Edwards NJ, Ettinger SJ, et al. Management of incidentally detected heart murmurs in dogs and cats. J Vet Cardiol 2015;17:245–261.

Côté E, Manning AM, Emerson D, et al. Assessment of the prevalence of heart murmurs in overtly healthy cats. J Am Vet Med Assoc 2004;225:384–388.

Detweiler DK, Patterson DF. Abnormal heart sounds and murmurs of the dog. J Small Anim Pract 1967;8:193–205.

Dirven MJ, Cornelissen JM, Barendse MA, et al. Cause of heart murmurs in 57 apparently healthy cats. Tijdschr Diergeneeskd 2010;135:840–847.

Drut A, Ribas T, Floch F, et al. Prevalence of physiological heart murmurs in a population of 95 healthy young adult dogs. J Small Anim Pract 2015;56:112–118.

Fabrizio F, Baumwart R, Iazbik MC, et al. Left basilar systolic murmur in retired racing greyhounds. J Vet Intern Med 2006;20:78–82.

Ferasin L, Ferasin H, Kilkenny E. Heart murmurs in apparently healthy cats caused by iatrogenic dynamic right ventricular outflow tract obstruction. J Vet Intern Med 2020;34:1102–1107.

Fielding CL, Meier CA, Balch OK, et al. Risk factors for the elimination of endurance horses from competition. J Am Vet Med Assoc 2011;239:493–498.

Hanifin C. Cardiac auscultation 101: a basic science approach to heart murmurs. JAAPA 2010;23:44–48.

Hassdenteufel E, Kresken JG, Henrich E, et al. NT-proBNP as a diagnostic marker in dogs with dyspnea and in asymptomatic dogs with heart murmur. Tierarztl Prax Ausg K Kleintiere Heimtiere 2012;40:171–179.

Hoglund K, Ahlstrom CH, Haggstrom J, et al. Time-frequency and complexity analyses for differentiation of physiologic murmurs from heart murmurs caused by aortic stenosis in Boxers. Am J Vet Res 2007;68:962–969.

Hoglund K, Haggstrom J, Bussadori C, et al. A prospective study of systolic ejection murmurs and left ventricular outflow tract in Boxers. J Small Anim Pract 2011;52:11–17.

Keen JA. Examination of horses with cardiac disease. Vet Clin North Am Equine Pract 2019;35:23–42.

Kriz NG, Hodgson DR, Rose RJ. Prevalence and clinical importance of heart murmurs in racehorses. J Am Vet Med Assoc 2000;216:1441–1445.

Ljungvall I, Rishniw M, Porciello F, et al. Murmur intensity in small-breed dogs with myxomatous mitral valve disease reflects disease severity. J Small Anim Pract 2014;55:545–550.

Marinus SM, van Engelen H, Szatmari V. N-terminal pro-B-type natriuretic peptide and phonocardiography in differentiating innocent cardiac murmurs from congenital cardiac anomalies in asymptomatic puppies. J Vet Intern Med 2017;31:661–667.

Nakamura RK, Rishniw M, King MK, et al. Prevalence of echocardiographic evidence of cardiac disease in apparently healthy cats with murmurs. J Feline Med Surg 2011;13:266–271.

Naylor JM, Wolker RE, Pharr JW. An assessment of the terminology used by diplomates and students to describe the character of equine mitral and aortic valve regurgitant murmurs: correlations with the physical properties of the sounds. J Vet Intern Med 2003;17:332–336.

Ohad DG, Lenchner I, Bdolah-Abram T, et al. A loud right-apical systolic murmur is associated with the diagnosis of secondary pulmonary arterial hypertension: retrospective analysis of data from 201 consecutive client-owned dogs (2006-2007). Vet J 2013;198:690–695.

Patterson DF, Detweiler DK, Glendenning SA. Heart sounds and murmurs of the normal horse. Ann N Y Acad Sci 1965;127:242–305.

Payne JR, Brodbelt DC, Luis Fuentes V. Cardiomyopathy prevalence in 780 apparently healthy cats in rehoming centres (the CatScan study). J Vet Cardiol 2015;17(Suppl 1):S244–257.

Pyle RL. Interpreting low-intensity cardiac murmurs in dogs predisposed to subaortic stenosis. J Am Anim Hosp Assoc 2000;36:379–382.

Reef VB. Assessment of the cardiovascular system in horses during prepurchase and insurance examinations. Vet Clin North Am Equine Pract 2019;35:191–204.

Rishniw M. Murmur grading in humans and animals: past and present. J Vet Cardiol 2018;20:223–233.

Rishniw M, Thomas WP. Dynamic right ventricular outflow obstruction: a new cause of systolic murmurs in cats. J Vet Intern Med 2002;16:547–552.

Schrope DP. Prevalence of congenital heart disease in 76,301 mixed-breed dogs and 57,025 mixed-breed cats. J Vet Cardiol 2015;17:192–202.

Serfass P, Chetboul V, Sampedrano CC, et al. Retrospective study of 942 small-sized dogs: prevalence of left apical systolic heart murmur and left-sided heart failure, critical effects of breed and sex. J Vet Cardiol 2006;8:11–18.

Stepien RL, Kellihan HB, Luis Fuentes V. Prevalence and diagnostic characteristics of non-clinical mitral regurgitation murmurs in North American Whippets. J Vet Cardiol 2017;19:317–324.

Szatmari V, van Leeuwen MW, Teske E. Innocent cardiac murmur in puppies: prevalence, correlation with hematocrit, and auscultation characteristics. J Vet Intern Med 2015;29:1524–1528.

van Staveren MDB, Szatmári V. Age when presumptive innocent cardiac murmurs spontaneously disappear in clinically healthy Cairn terrier puppies. Vet J 2019;248:25–27.

Voros K, Bonnevie A, Reiczigel J. Comparison of conventional and sensor-based electronic stethoscopes in detecting cardiac murmurs of dogs. Tierarztl Prax Ausg K Kleintiere Heimtiere 2012;40:103–111.

Young LE, Rogers K, Wood JL. Heart murmurs and valvular regurgitation in thoroughbred racehorses: epidemiology and associations with athletic performance. J Vet Intern Med 2008;22:418–426.

Zucca E, Ferrucci F, Stancari G, et al. The prevalence of cardiac murmurs among standardbred racehorses presented with poor performance. J Vet Med Sci 2010;72:781–785.

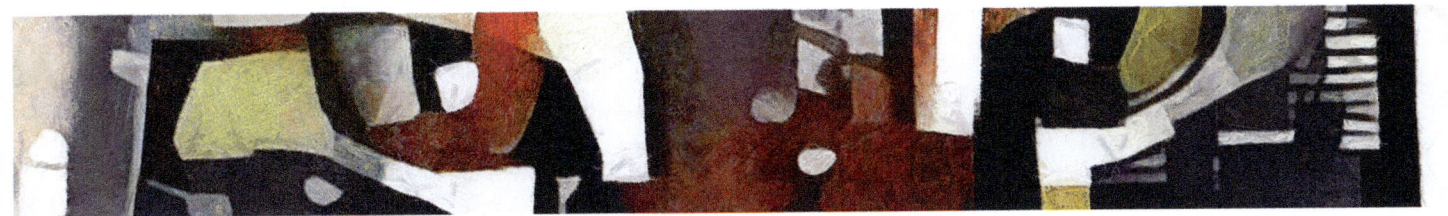

12
ABNORMAL HEART RATE OR RHYTHM

An unexpected heart rate (HR) or abnormal cardiac rhythm might be encountered during auscultation or while palpating the arterial pulse or precordium in a patient. An owner also might have noticed an unusual heart rate or rhythm in the animal at home. This clinical problem can pertain to heartbeats originating from an ectopic focus (that is, from somewhere outside the sinus node), to abnormal intracardiac conduction, or even to heart rhythms of normal (sinus) origin but inappropriate or unexpected HR for the clinical context. Fundamental questions in affected patients relate to whether the cardiac rhythm is arising from the sinus node (or not), whether nonsinus rhythm disturbances are superimposed on or replacing an otherwise normal sinus rhythm, and whether any clinical effects of the disturbance(s) are evident.

It can be helpful to first identify if the patient's HR is unexpectedly rapid (therefore, some kind of tachycardia) or unexpectedly slow (a bradycardia), and then decide if the rhythm is regular or irregular. Such categorization will suggest certain rhythm diagnoses that typically manifest those characteristics (**Tables 12.1** and **12.2** and text that follows). Approximate normal HR ranges (per minute) during clinical examination are 60–160 for dogs, 140–240 for cats, and 28–44 for mature horses. Higher rates can occur in young or excited animals. Conversely, when evaluated by ambulatory monitoring, most healthy dogs have sinus arrhythmia with an average HR of about 70–85 beats/minute over 24 hours of recording. No substantive correlation between HR and body weight is apparent in healthy dogs (Lamb, 2020). Especially during sleep, sinus bradycardia, transient second-degree atrioventricular (AV) block, and wandering atrial pacemaker are common manifestations of high vagal tone. The daily average HR in cats typically is 150–170 beats/minute on 24-hour Holter recordings, although significant variation in average HR occurs among cats. At home, monitored cats often exhibit periods of sinus arrhythmia, although this usually gives way to regular sinus rhythm in the clinic. Horses usually have high resting vagal tone. As documented on ambulatory electrocardiographic recordings, a prominent sinus arrhythmia or bradycardia, often with intermittent second-degree AV block or periods of sinus arrest, are typical in horses at rest. However, sudden stimuli can provoke periods of sinus tachycardia. Healthy animals might have a few non-sinus (ectopic) heartbeats, too, especially as they age. Although the "normal" cut-off for number of ectopic complexes is controversial, it often is considered to be less than 10 atrial or ventricular premature complexes in a 24-hour period. The presence of escape complexes during sinus pauses in a sleeping animal is considered normal variation.

General Considerations

Cardiac arrhythmias occur for many reasons. Some arrhythmias are of no clinical consequence. Others cause hypotension, weakness, syncope, or sudden death, especially in animals with underlying disease (Chapter 25). The presence of an arrhythmia might be suspected from the animal's history, or identified on physical examination. An accurate ECG diagnosis is important (Chapter 5 and Table 5.3, p. 140); therefore, it is crucial to obtain a representative ECG recording. The clinical situation and whether the arrhythmia causes relevant hemodynamic disturbance also are important. Adequate assessment might require ambulatory ECG monitoring.

The sinus node is influenced by a number of autonomic and metabolic factors, and it participates in multiple CV and respiratory reflexes. For example, changes in body temperature, circulating thyroid concentration, and serum potassium concentration directly affect sinus nodal discharge. The major factors that normally control sinus node rate are sympathetic and vagal neural activity, as well as circulating catecholamines; conditions outside the heart greatly influence these factors. Sinus tachycardia reflects increased sympathetic tone associated with underlying physiologic or pathologic conditions, or drug-induced vagal blockade, or beta-adrenergic stimulation (**Table 12.1**). Abnormally slow sinus rhythms might

Table 12.1 Causes of Sinus Bradycardia and Tachycardia

Sinus Bradycardia
- Cardiovascular causes
  - Cardiac arrest (before or after)
  - Cardiogenic shock (cats)
  - Sinus node disease (dogs)
  - Cardiac drugs (beta-blockers, calcium channel-blockers, digoxin, amiodarone; IV lidocaine in cats)
- Increased vagal tone (any cause)
  - Physiologic variation (athletic dog; sleeping)
  - Increased intracranial pressure (Cushing's reflex)
  - Brainstem lesions
  - Ocular pressure
  - Carotid sinus pressure
  - Vasovagal reactions (reflex mediated, neurocardiogenic)
  - Other causes (including lower airway, pharyngeal, or gastrointestinal obstruction)
- Metabolic and endocrine diseases
  - Hypothermia
  - Hypothyroidism
  - Hypoxemia/hypoxia
  - Severe metabolic disease (such as uremia, hyperkalemia)
- Tranquilizers (acepromazine) and sedatives (dexmedetomidine, alpha-2 agonists, anesthetic agents)
- Miscellaneous drugs or preservatives (often idiosyncratic reactions)

Sinus Tachycardia
- Increased sympathetic tone (general causes)
  - Exercise
  - Excitement
  - Anxiety or fear
  - Pain
  - Infection and sepsis
  - Colic (horses, multifactorial)
- Reflex-mediated sinus tachycardia
  - Heart failure
  - Shock
  - Hypovolemia
  - Hypotension
- Metabolic and endocrine diseases
  - Hyperthermia/fever
  - Hyperthyroidism
  - Anemia
- Hypoxia (secondary to ventilatory responses)
- Drugs (including anticholinergics, sympathomimetics)
- Toxicities (including chocolate, hexachlorophene)
- Electric shock

Table 12.2 Differential Diagnoses for Common Heart Rate and Rhythm Disturbances

Rapid, Regular Rhythms[a]
- Sinus tachycardia
- Sustained supraventricular tachycardia with regular AV conduction (atrial, AV reciprocating, or junctional)
- Sustained ventricular tachycardia (can be irregular)
- Sinoventricular rhythm (atrial standstill) in cats with hyperkalemia

Rapid, Irregular Rhythms
- Atrial or supraventricular premature contractions
- Paroxysmal atrial or supraventricular tachycardia
- Focal atrial tachycardia or macro-reentry atrial tachycardia (flutter) with variable AV conduction
- Atrial fibrillation
- Ventricular premature contractions
- Paroxysmal ventricular tachycardia

Slow, Regular Rhythms[a]
- Sinus bradycardia (can be irregular with sinus arrhythmia when vagally mediated)
- Complete (third degree) AV block with stable ventricular escape rhythm
- Sinoventricular rhythm from hyperkalemia (can be irregular; in cats, heart rate can be normal)
- Atrial standstill with regular junctional or ventricular escape rhythm

Slow, Irregular Rhythms
- Sinus bradycardia with sinus arrhythmia (sinus bradyarrhythmia)
- Sinoatrial block
- Sinus arrest
- Sick sinus syndrome (sometimes also with paroxysmal supraventricular tachycardia and premature beats, so-called bradycardia–tachycardia syndrome)
- Sinoventricular rhythm from hyperkalemia (can be regular or irregular)
- second-degree AV block
- Complete (third-degree) AV block with unstable or variable escape rhythms
- Persistent atrial standstill with unstable escape rhythms

[a] Some regular rhythms are characterized by variable intensity or split heart sounds (see text).

indicate high vagal tone (usually from noncardiac conditions) or primary sinus node disease (**Table 12.1**; also see **Figures 5.12** and **5.13**, p. 143; and p. 405). Sinus arrhythmia, with its recurring fluctuation in rate and P wave morphology (p. 143), is a normal rhythm variation that is common in dogs (over a month old) and in horses. Sinus arrhythmia usually reverts to a regular sinus rhythm as sympathetic influence increases and vagal tone diminishes; for example, this typically occurs at HRs above 150 beats/minute in dogs and 50 beats/minute in horses. Chronic pulmonary disease often is associated with pronounced respiratory sinus arrhythmia. Cats in the clinic setting, in contrast to dogs, rarely manifest sinus arrhythmia; therefore, when this rhythm variation is identified in a cat, it might indicate pathology. Nevertheless, resting cats normally do manifest some degree of sinus arrhythmia at home. A slow sinus rhythm or arrhythmia can be a normal finding, especially in athletic dogs and horses. Horses and dogs also can experience sinoatrial block, which is difficult to distinguish from sinus arrhythmia or sinus node dysfunction, but is physiologic in some animals.

Multiple factors underlie the development of cardiac rhythm disturbances. In general, underlying mechanisms can be categorized as disorders of impulse formation, disorders of impulse conduction, or combinations of both (p. 363). These general mechanisms can underlie either rapid or slow rhythm disturbances. For example, abnormal impulse formation could cause an ectopic tachycardia originating from cells that do not normally demonstrate automaticity. Ectopic rhythms also can develop in the ventricle when normally suppressed Purkinje cells develop faster spontaneous activity and compete with the sinus node discharge. Abnormal impulse conduction can cause profound bradycardia when conduction through the AV node fails, or it can underlie a tachycardia via a re-entrant mechanism (**Figure 25.10A**, p. 418). It is often difficult to identify the specific electrophysiologic mechanism underlying a particular arrhythmia. Furthermore, intraventricular conduction disturbances can confuse the clinician during ECG interpretation, even when the basic rhythm is sinus and the conduction disturbance does not substantially limit cardiac function (**Figures 12.1–12.4**).

The clinical context is important when assessing the significance of a rhythm disturbance. Some arrhythmias can be especially dangerous in animals undergoing general anesthesia, as well as those that are critically ill or in shock, or with structural heart disease. For example, severe electrolyte disturbances, especially involving serum potassium, can promote the development of dangerous arrhythmias (**Figure 12.5**). Some diseases are associated with higher risk for sudden arrhythmic death, in particular, dilated cardiomyopathy (especially in Doberman Pinschers) and arrhythmogenic (right ventricular) cardiomyopathy in Boxers (Chapter 32; see also **Figures 5.30** and **5.33**, p. 148, 149). Diseases that cause marked myocardial concentric hypertrophy, with consequent subendocardial ischemia and fibrosis, such as subaortic stenosis (Chapter 27) and feline hypertrophic cardiomyopathy (Chapter 33) also are associated with a higher rate of sudden death. An inherited disorder of cardiac autonomic maturation, with ventricular tachyarrhythmias

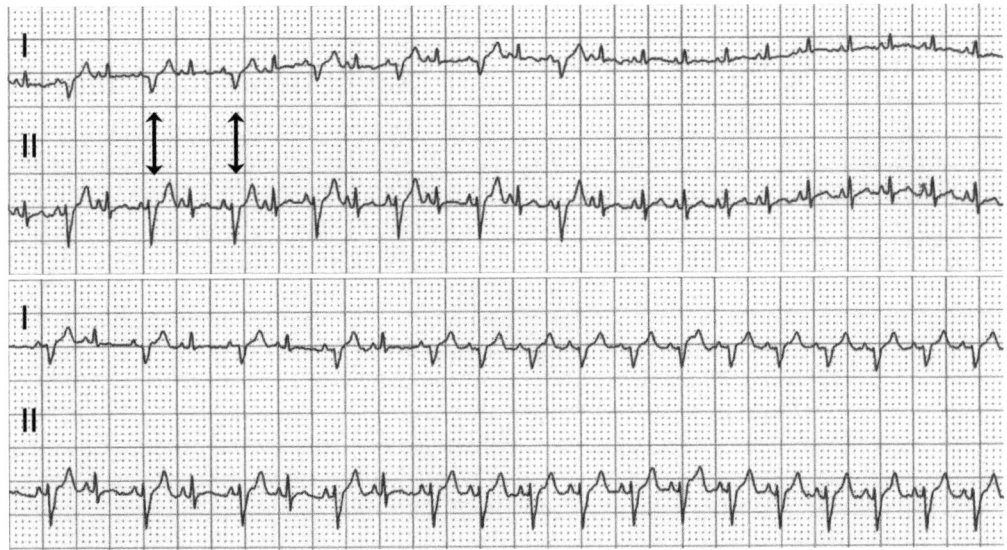

Figure 12.1 Simultaneous lead I & II ECG strips from a cat with sinus rhythm and intermittent right bundle branch block (RBBB). The abnormally conducted QRS complexes (arrows) might be mistaken for ventricular premature complexes; however, note that each is preceded by a P wave at the same PR interval as the normally conducted sinus QRS complexes. The top strip initially shows RBBB in every other QRS complex, followed by all normally conducted complexes. The bottom strip begins with RBBB in every other complex, but then all the rest of the complexes are conducted with RBBB. The cat had mild interventricular septal hypertrophy, without right ventricular enlargement. 25 mm/s, 1 cm = 1 mV.

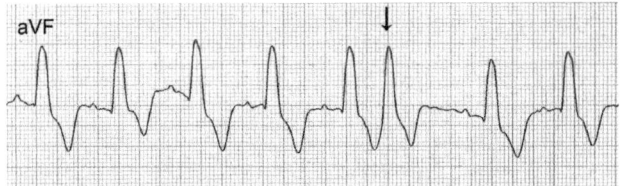

Figure 12.2 ECG from a Boston Terrier with chronic mitral regurgitation and irregular heart rhythm shows sinus rhythm (note consistent P waves & PR intervals), with 1 premature complex (arrow). Yet with the abnormal QRS morphology (from a left bundle branch block) this might be mistaken for ventricular ectopy. Note that the premature QRS complex looks the same as the sinus QRS, indicating supraventricular origin (& same manner of intraventricular conduction). Lead aVF, 50 mm/s, 1 cm = 1 mV.

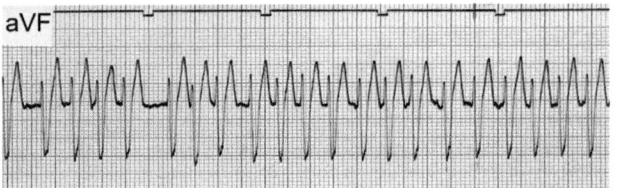

Figure 12.3 ECG from an older female German Shepherd with lethargy, ascites, recent onset of soft cough, and rapid irregular heartbeat. The heart rate is ~240 beats/min. Because the QRS complexes appear so wide and abnormal, the rhythm might be mistaken for ventricular tachycardia; however, the lack of visible P waves (especially during longer intervals) and irregular QRS timing are most consistent with atrial fibrillation. Right bundle branch block caused the abnormal QRS morphology. Lead aVF, 25 mm/s, 1 cm = 1 mV.

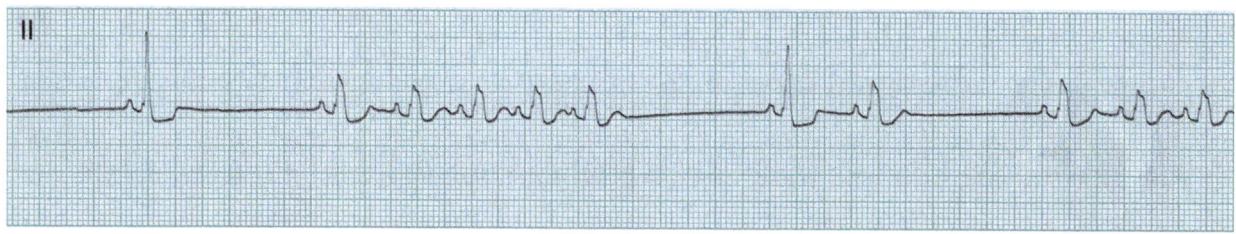

Figure 12.4 This ECG was recorded from a 12-year-old Weimaraner with an irregular rhythm following surgery for gastric dilatation-volvulus. Many of the QRS complexes are wide and abnormal; however, they all are preceded by a normal P wave and consistent PR interval. The rhythm is sinus arrhythmia, with an intermittent (rate-dependent) left bundle branch block (LBBB). The time needed for repolarization within the left bundle is abnormally prolonged in this dog, to the extent that conduction fails in this part of the intraventricular conduction system when the heart rate becomes faster than the recovery time of the left bundle branch. No antiarrhythmic therapy is indicated at this time because the cardiac rhythm is normal. LBBB often is a sign of clinically significant, and possibly progressive, underlying myocardial disease. If conduction were to fail in the right bundle branch, too, complete AV block would result. An echocardiogram and periodic ECG monitoring are advised. Lead II, 25 mm/s.

predisposing to sudden death, occurs in some young German Shepherd Dogs. Similarly, ventricular arrhythmias that sometimes cause sudden death have been recognized in young Rhodesian Ridgebacks, and Leonberger dogs (Chapter 23).

Conversely, isolated ventricular premature complexes (VPCs) and accelerated idioventricular rhythms that occur commonly after thoracic trauma in previously healthy animals generally are benign and resolve without therapy (**Figure 5.36**, p. 149 and p. 641). Healthy older animals might have occasional premature complexes and in most cases, these are well tolerated; although when such rhythms occur in horses, they require further assessment during exercise. VPCs are uncommon in healthy young animals. Arrhythmias that compromise cardiac output, arterial blood pressure, and coronary perfusion promote myocardial ischemia, cardiac pump function deterioration, and sometimes, sudden death (**Figures 5.38** and **5.39**, p. 150). These arrhythmias typically are either very rapid (sustained ventricular or supraventricular tachyarrhythmias), very slow (such as advanced AV block with a slow or unstable ventricular escape rhythm), or associated with serious systemic disease (such as hypoadrenocorticism). Sustained rapid tachycardia of either supraventricular or ventricular origin reduces cardiac output acutely, and within several weeks leads to myocardial dysfunction (tachycardia-induced cardiomyopathy) and congestive heart failure (CHF; also see p. 630).

Rapid Heart Rate and Arrhythmias

An abnormally or unexpectedly rapid HR for the clinical context could be caused by sinus tachycardia or an ectopic or reentrant tachyarrhythmia. Sinus tachycardia is a rhythm with regular P to P and QRS to QRS (R-R) intervals. Sustained tachycardias that originate in either atrial or AV junctional tissues (supraventricular) or from a ventricular focus also tend to have regular QRS intervals once they become established. Rapid irregular rhythms can result from: intermittent premature ectopic beats or (paroxysmal) tachycardias that interrupt the underlying sinus rhythm, atrial fibrillation (AF), or a focal atrial tachycardia or macroreentrant atrial tachycardia (atrial flutter) with variable (physiologic) AV block. Characteristics that help the clinician differentiate among these rhythms on the ECG are described in Chapter 5. AF was the most common arrhythmia identified (in almost 34% of cases), followed by ventricular arrhythmias (in 28%) and supraventricular

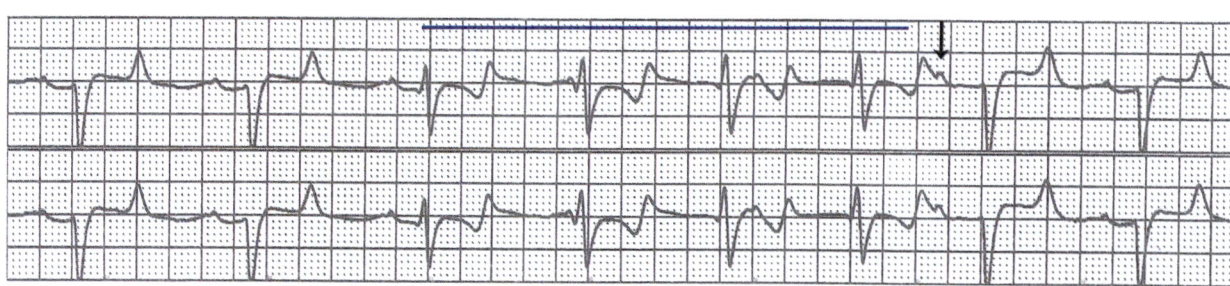

Figure 12.5 Base-apex lead ECG (recorded simultaneously in 2 channels) in a horse with a slightly irregular and rapid heart rate. Sinus rhythm is present, as indicated by the first two complexes. However, a run of ventricular-origin complexes interrupts this (blue bar; note differing QRS and T wave morphology and lack of relationship with the P waves). The last two complexes on the right are sinus in origin. The P wave (arrow) following the last ventricular premature complex (VPC) was conducted with first-degree AV block. The VPC had caused partial (retrograde) depolarization of the AV node, which had not recovered fully by the time this P wave reached it, causing delayed AV conduction. The horse had multiple biochemical abnormalities, including pronounced hypokalemia and hypomagnesemia, which can predispose to serious ventricular tachyarrhythmias; hyponatremia and markedly elevated creatine kinase, aspartate aminotransferase and bilirubin also were evident. 25 mm/s.

arrhythmias (in 24%), in a large European survey of dogs referred for cardiac examination (Noszczk-Nowak, 2017).

AF in cats and dogs occurs most often when there is marked atrial enlargement (**Figures 5.24** and **5.25**, p. 146; also see p. 409). Clinical heart failure is common in affected animals, especially when the ventricular response rate is uncontrolled (high). A rapid, as well as irregular, ventricular activation rate allows little time for ventricular filling. The loss of effective atrial contraction during AF further compromises stroke volume. The contribution of the "atrial kick" to ventricular filling is especially important at faster HRs. Consequently, cardiac output can decrease considerably when AF develops, especially if myocardial function is poor. However, as in horses, AF with a slow ventricular response rate can be an incidental finding, especially in large breed dogs without other evidence of heart disease (lone AF; p. 611; and p. 410). Some of these dogs later develop myocardial dysfunction. Likewise, AF is a common arrhythmia in horses (p. 409).

Ventricular tachyarrhythmias can occur with disorders that affect cardiac tissue directly or indirectly through neurohormonal effects. Central nervous system (CNS) disease can cause ventricular or supraventricular arrhythmias via abnormal neural effects on the heart (brain–heart syndrome). Supraventricular tachyarrhythmias can arise from atrial or junctional tissues through various mechanisms. Heart diseases commonly associated with supraventricular tachyarrhythmias include degenerative mitral or tricuspid valve regurgitation, dilated cardiomyopathy, congenital malformations, and hypertrophic or restrictive cardiomyopathy in cats.

Slow Heart Rate and Arrhythmias

An inappropriately slow HR could result from excessive vagal tone, sinus node disease, atrial myopathy, conduction block in the AV node or the bundle of His, or another abnormality (such as hyperkalemia or hypothermia). Most animals with bradycardia have irregular R-R intervals. The mechanism could be excessive, but variable, vagal tone (as with sinus bradyarrhythmia), intermittent sinus arrest (as with the "sick sinus syndrome," SSS), inconsistent AV conduction (second-degree AV block), or hyperkalemia (with a slow sinoventricular rhythm). A regular, slow heart rhythm might result from regular sinus bradycardia; however, it more often is caused by an ectopic escape rhythm that arises because complete (third-degree) AV block, sinus arrest, or atrial standstill has occurred. See Chapter 5 for the ECG manifestations of these and other rhythm disturbances. AV blocks and sinus pauses were common rhythm disturbances (in nearly 23% and 28% of cases, respectively) reported in a large survey of dogs referred for cardiac examination (Noszczk-Nowak, 2017). The SSS (p. 405) is characterized by sudden episodes of weakness and syncope (with or without convulsive activity; Stokes–Adams seizures) caused by periods of bradycardia or asystole). Some affected dogs also have paroxysmal supraventricular tachyarrhythmias, prompting the name "bradycardia–tachycardia syndrome" (**Figure 12.6**). Older female Miniature Schnauzers and West Highland White Terriers are clearly predisposed, but SSS occurs in males and dogs of other (mostly smaller) breeds also. ECG abnormalities often are pronounced

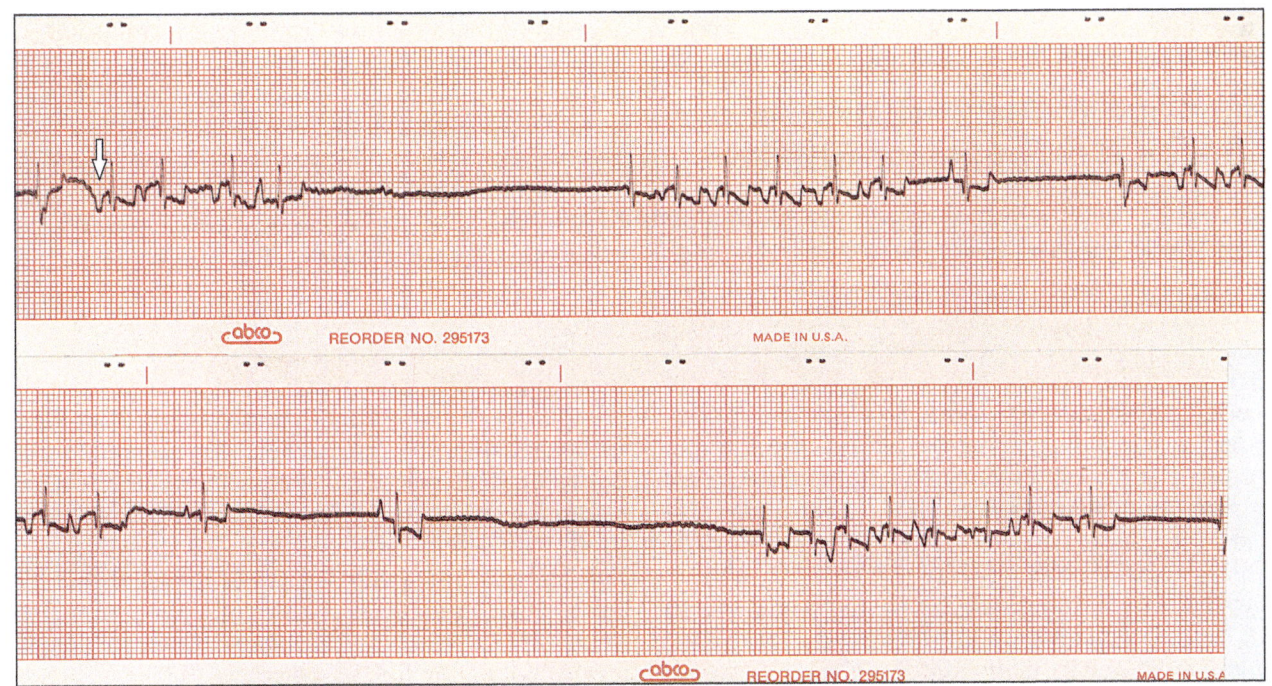

Figure 12.6 Continuous lead II ECG from an older female Miniature Schnauzer with sick sinus syndrome and paroxysmal atrial tachycardia (bradycardia–tachycardia syndrome). The dog had experienced multiple episodes of syncope. An escape complex is seen at the top left, followed by 3 atrial premature complexes (note negative P′ waves; arrow) and a sinus complex. A period of sinus arrest is interrupted by a junctional escape complex, then another paroxysm of atrial tachycardia, followed by a single sinus complex. The rest of the ECG shows similar rhythm variations. 25 mm/s, 1 cm = 1 mV.

in dogs with long-standing SSS. Yet the resting ECG might be normal in other dogs. Ambulatory Holter ECG, implantable loop recorder, or prolonged visual ECG monitoring can help establish the diagnosis.

Diseases associated with abnormal AV conduction have included infective endocarditis (of the aortic valve), hypertrophic cardiomyopathy, infiltrative myocardial diseases, and myocarditis. Idiopathic AV block (presumably from senile degeneration of the AV tissues) is most common, especially in middle-aged to older dogs of many breeds; however, congenital third-degree AV block also has occurred. Symptomatic AV block is less common in cats and is rare in horses. When it does occur in cats, a diagnosis of seizure disorder often is incorrectly assumed because AV block can be intermittent in this species. Complete AV block with a stable, and surprisingly rapid escape rhythm (between 90 and 130 beats/minute), is regularly encountered in older cats without detectable organic heart disease. Sporadic feline cases have been associated with various myocardial or other structural heart diseases.

Hyperkalemia (p. 160 and **Figures 5.57–5.59A**) should be ruled out when P waves are absent or unclear and the HR is somewhat slow (although sinoventricular rhythms in cats can occur at normal to fast rates). Persistent atrial standstill is another arrhythmia characterized by lack of effective atrial electrical activity (no P waves and a flat baseline) in which a junctional or ventricular escape rhythm controls the heart (p. 416). This is most common in dogs. Transient atrial standstill or persistent sinus arrest, of uncertain pathogenesis, occurs in some cats with cardiogenic shock and is reversible with effective medical management of heart failure.

Approach to the Patient with Abnormal Heart Rate or Rhythm

Cardiac arrhythmias in an individual animal can occur quite inconsistently. Their development is influenced by drug therapy, prevailing autonomic tone, baroreceptor reflexes, and variations in HR, as well as underlying disease. Many clinical abnormalities have been associated with cardiac arrhythmias (**Table 23.1**, p. 370). A history that includes episodic weakness, syncope (Chapter 8), or worsening of previously compensated CHF raises suspicion that the patient could have a serious cardiac arrhythmia, even when HR and rhythm are normal on initial evaluation (**Figure 12.7**). Patients with syncope—especially cats and horses—frequently are misdiagnosed with a seizure disorder.

The physical examination might reveal an excessively fast or slow HR, with or without abnormal irregularity. **Table 12.2** lists common arrhythmias, grouped according to a clinical description of the heartbeat. Normal sinus arrhythmia, with its regularly recurring variation in HR, is common in dogs and horses. However, because sinus arrhythmia is rare in cats during clinical exam, any irregularity in heart rhythm is an indication to obtain an ECG in this species. Arterial pulses of variable timing or intensity or pulse deficits might be detected during examination. Likewise, the heart sounds might vary in intensity as well as regularity. In cats with ventricular premature beats, the pause after the premature beat could be easier to detect than the abnormal beat itself. Atrial premature beats in horses might not be conducted to the ventricles and thus, might be detected as an extra atrial sound (S_4) followed by a pause (absent S_1 and S_2), or more likely by the sudden unexpected gap in the rhythm.

Rapidly conducting atrial arrhythmias (such as AF) and premature contractions of any origin often cause pulse deficits. VPCs can cause audible splitting of the heart sounds because of asynchronous ventricular activation. Ventricular and supraventricular tachycardias and AF cause more severe hemodynamic compromise than do isolated premature contractions. Frequent premature contractions, as well as paroxysmal tachycardia, can compromise ventricular filling, especially if underlying heart disease exists. Low cardiac output and hypotension can cause weakness, lethargy, pallor, slow capillary refill time, exercise intolerance, syncope, dyspnea, prerenal azotemia, worsening rhythm disturbances, and, sometimes, altered mentation, seizure activity, and sudden death.

An ECG is essential for differentiating abnormal rhythms and sometimes, for identifying sinus arrhythmia as well. While a routine (resting) ECG documents arrhythmias present during the recording period, it provides only a glimpse of the cardiac rhythms occurring over the course of a day. Because arrhythmias can have marked variation in frequency and severity over time, potentially critical arrhythmias easily can be missed. For this reason, Holter or event monitoring or other forms of extended ECG acquisition, such as implantable loop recorders, are useful in assessing the severity and frequency of arrhythmias, and for monitoring treatment efficacy. Brief ECG recordings obtained by the owner using a smart phone-compatible hand-held recorder (p. 163 and **Figures 12.8** and **12.9**) and emailed to the clinician can help identify persistent cardiac arrhythmias and document HRs when the patient is at home.

Although differentiation of sustained supraventricular tachycardia from sinus tachycardia sometimes is difficult, it is important. Antiarrhythmic drug therapy is indicated for the former (Chapter 25). In patients with sinus tachycardia, alleviation of the underlying cause and administration of IV fluids to reverse hypotension (in animals without edema) should allow sympathetic tone and sinus rate to decrease. A vagal maneuver (p. 388) might help the clinician differentiate these types of tachycardias. Supraventricular tachycardia often causes HRs exceeding 300 beats/minute in dogs and cats; however, it is rare for the sinus rate to be this rapid. Usually, the QRS configuration is normal (narrow and upright in lead II). Yet a concurrent intraventricular conduction disturbance can make a supraventricular tachycardia look like ventricular tachycardia on ECG (**Figures 5.47–5.49**, p. 154).

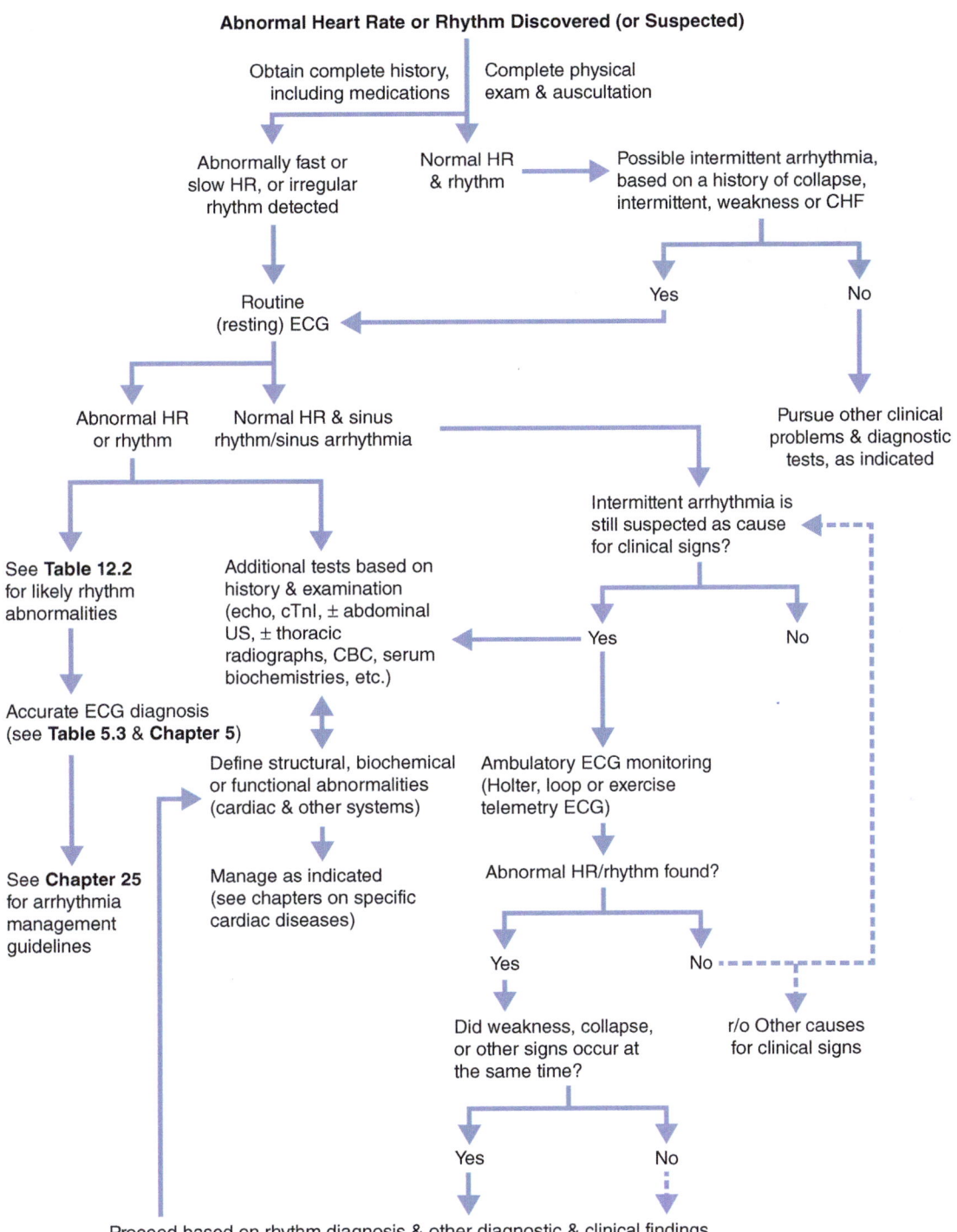

Figure 12.7 Approach to the patient with abnormal heart rate or rhythm. These are general guidelines; exceptions can occur. CBC, complete blood count; CHF, congestive heart failure; cTnI, cardiac troponin I; ECG, electrocardiogram; echo, echocardiogram; HR, heart rate; r/o, rule out; US, ultrasonography.

In most cases of sinus bradycardia, the HR increases in response to exercise, or atropine administration, and no clinical signs are apparent. Symptomatic dogs usually have a HR slower than 50 beats/minute, or pronounced underlying disease. Because sinus bradycardia or bradyarrhythmia is quite rare in cats, a search for underlying cardiac or systemic disease (such as hyperkalemia) is warranted in any cat with a slow HR. In cats with hypotension, hypothermia, and bradycardia, a diagnosis of cardiogenic shock (or shock from another cause) should be on top-of-the-list. High-grade second-degree AV block (many blocked P waves) and complete (third-degree) heart block usually produce signs of low cardiac output (lethargy, exercise intolerance, weakness, or syncope). In dogs, these signs become severe when the HR is consistently below 40 beats/minute

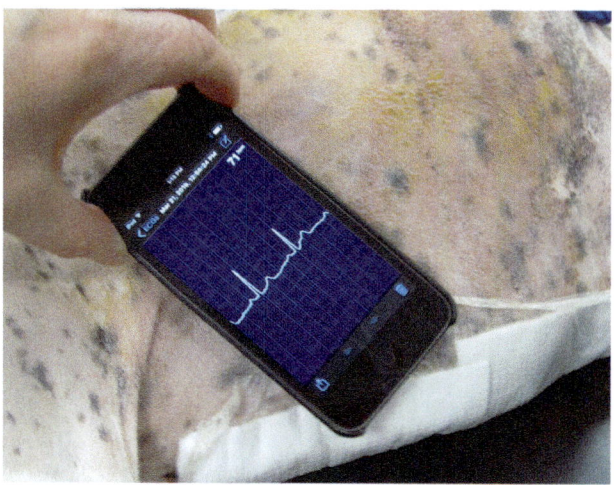

Figure 12.8 Recording an ECG using an AliveCor (Kardia®) device and smart phone app. The device (attached to the back of the phone or an iPod, or in close proximity) is held against the chestwall overlying the heart. Shaving is not necessary; parting the fur then wetting with alcohol generally provides adequate contact.

or when superimposed on valvular or myocardial disease. CHF can be a consequence of chronic bradycardia, especially when other cardiac disease is present.

An atropine challenge test (p. 387) is used in animals with persistent bradycardia or AV block to determine the degree of vagal influence on the arrhythmia. The normal response is an increase in HR of 150%, or to over 130–150 beats/minute (in dogs), or return of AV conduction. Dogs with sick sinus syndrome generally have a subnormal response. Animals with third-degree AV block rarely regain normal conduction, although the P wave (sinus) rate typically increases.

Some rhythm abnormalities do not require therapy, whereas others demand immediate aggressive treatment (Chapter 25). Close patient monitoring is especially important in animals with more serious arrhythmias. Treatment decisions are based on consideration of the origin (supraventricular or ventricular), timing (premature or escape), frequency, and complexity of the rhythm disturbance, as well as the clinical context. Arrhythmias generally considered benign include infrequent premature beats and occasional blocked P waves. Post-traumatic accelerated idioventricular rhythm or slow, monomorphic ventricular tachycardia in animals with otherwise normal cardiac function usually disappears after a few

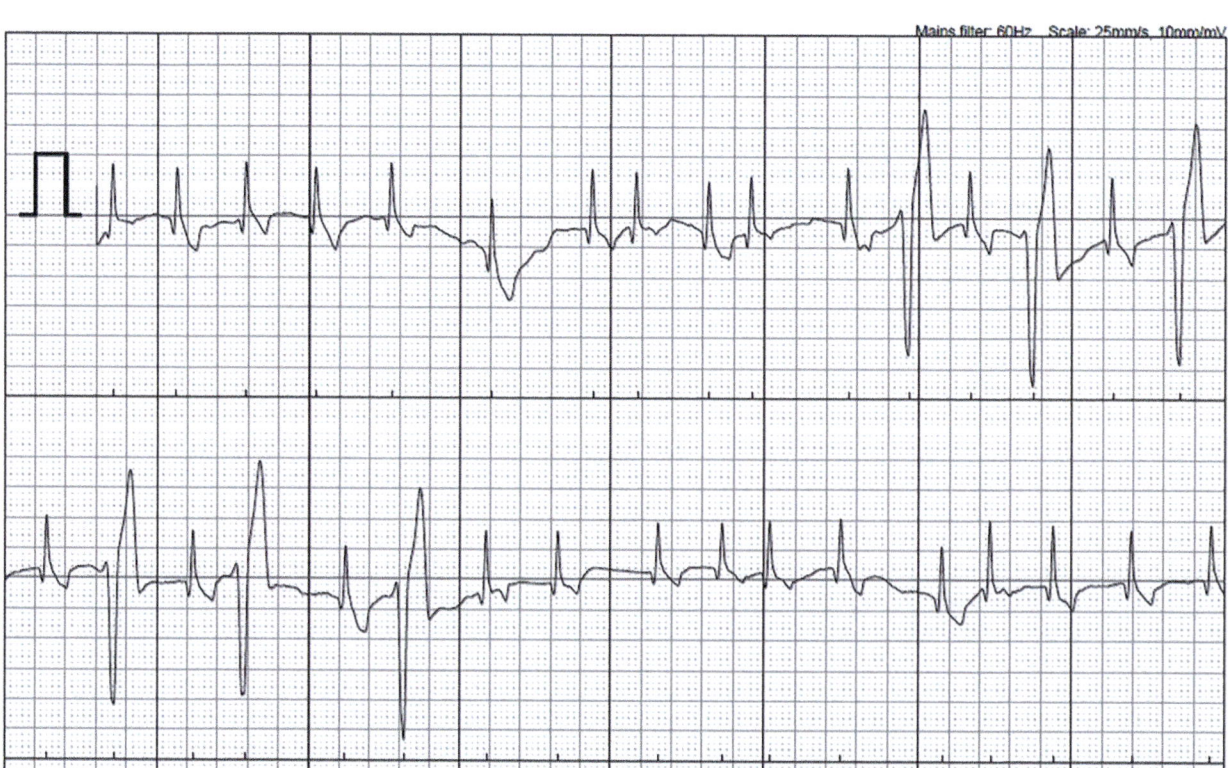

Figure 12.9 Example of a smartphone ECG recording from a dog with atrial fibrillation and intermittent ventricular premature complexes. Good skin contact and minimal patient movement are important optimize the recordings.

days without antiarrhythmic therapy. Correction of underlying electrolyte or acid-base imbalances, hypoxia, abnormal hormone concentrations (such as thyroid), or discontinuing certain drugs can be important for arrhythmia control.

Suggested Additional Reading and References

Also See Online Comprehensive Bibliography at: https://www.routledge.com/9781482246223.

Buhl R, Meldgaard C, Barbesgaard L. Cardiac arrhythmias in clinically healthy showjumping horses. Equine Vet J 2010;42(Suppl 38):196–201.

Côté E. Feline arrhythmias: an update. Vet Clin North Am Small Anim Pract 2010;40:643–650.

Durando MM. Cardiovascular causes of poor performance and exercise intolerance and assessment of safety in the equine athlete. Vet Clin North Am Equine Pract 2019;35:175–190.

Eggensperger BH, Schwarzwald CC. Influence of 2nd-degree AV blocks, ECG recording length, and recording time on heart rate variability analyses in horses. J Vet Cardiol 2017;19:160–174.

Flethoj M, Kanters JK, Haugaard MM, et al. Changes in heart rate, arrhythmia frequency, and cardiac biomarker values in horses during recovery after a long-distance endurance ride. J Am Vet Med Assoc 2016;248:1034–1042.

Jackson BL, Lehmkuhl LB, Adin DB. Heart rate and arrhythmia frequency of normal cats compared to cats with asymptomatic hypertrophic cardiomyopathy. J Vet Cardiol 2014;16(4):215–225.

Kraus MS, Gelzer AR, Rishniw M. Detection of heart rate and rhythm with a smartphone-based electrocardiograph versus a reference standard electrocardiograph in dogs and cats. J Am Vet Med Assoc 2016;249:189–194.

Lamb AP, Meurs KM, Hamlin RL. Correlation of heart rate to body weight in apparently normal dogs. J Vet Cardiol 2010;12:107–110.

Meurs KM, Weidman JA, Rosenthal SL, et al. Ventricular arrhythmias in Rhodesian Ridgebacks with a family history of sudden death and results of a pedigree analysis for potential inheritance patterns. J Am Vet Med Assoc 2016;248:1135–1138.

Moise NS. Inherited arrhythmias in the dog: potential experimental models of cardiac disease. Cardiovasc Res 1999;44:37–46.

Morgan RA, Raftery AG, Cripps P, et al. The prevalence and nature of cardiac arrhythmias in horses following general anaesthesia and surgery. Acta Vet Scand 2011;53:62.

Motskula PF, Linney C, Palermo V, et al. Prognostic value of 24-hour ambulatory ECG (Holter) monitoring in Boxer dogs. J Vet Intern Med 2013;27(4):904–912.

Nakao S, Hirakawa A, Fukushima R, et al. The anatomical basis of bradycardia-tachycardia syndrome in elderly dogs with chronic degenerative valvular disease. J Comp Pathol 2012;146:175–182.

Noszczyk-Nowak A, Michalek M, Kaluza E, et al. Prevalence of arrhythmias in dogs examined between 2008 and 2014. J Vet Res 2017;61:103–110.

Petrie JP. Practical application of Holter monitoring in dogs and cats. Clin Tech Small Anim Pract 2005;20(3):173–181.

Physick-Sheard PW. Seek and ye shall find: cardiac arrhythmias in the horse. Equine Vet J 2013;45:270–272.

Rasmussen CE, Falk T, Domanjko Petric A, et al. Holter monitoring of small breed dogs with advanced myxomatous mitral valve disease with and without a history of syncope. J Vet Intern Med 2014;28(2):363–370.

Reef VB. Assessment of the cardiovascular system in horses during prepurchase and insurance examinations. Vet Clin North Am Equine Pract 2019;35:191–204.

Reef VB, Bonagura J, Buhl R, et al. Recommendations for management of equine athletes with cardiovascular abnormalities. J Vet Intern Med 2014;28:749–761.

Slack J, Boston RC, Soma LR, et al. Occurrence of cardiac arrhythmias in Standardbred racehorses. Equine Vet J 2015;47:398–404.

Taggart P, Critchley H, Lambiase PD. Heart-brain interactions in cardiac arrhythmia. Heart 2011;97:698–708.

Trachsel DS, Bitschnau C, Waldern N, et al. Observer agreement for detection of cardiac arrhythmias on telemetric ECG recordings obtained at rest, during and after exercise in 10 warmblood horses. Equine Vet J 2010;42(Suppl 38):208–215.

Ulloa HM, Houston BJ, Altrogge DM. Arrhythmia prevalence during ambulatory electrocardiographic monitoring of beagles. Am J Vet Res 1995;56:275–281.

Vezzosi T, Buralli C, Marchesotti F, et al. Diagnostic accuracy of a smartphone electrocardiograph in dogs: comparison with standard 6-lead electrocardiography. Vet J 2016;216:33–37.

Vezzosi T, Tognetti R, Buralli C, et al. Home monitoring of heart rate and heart rhythm with a smartphone-based ECG in dogs. Vet Rec 2019;184:96.

Wess G, Schulze A, Geraghty N, et al. Ability of a 5-minute electrocardiography (ECG) for predicting arrhythmias in Doberman Pinschers with cardiomyopathy in comparison with a 24-hour ambulatory ECG. J Vet Intern Med 2010;24:367–371.

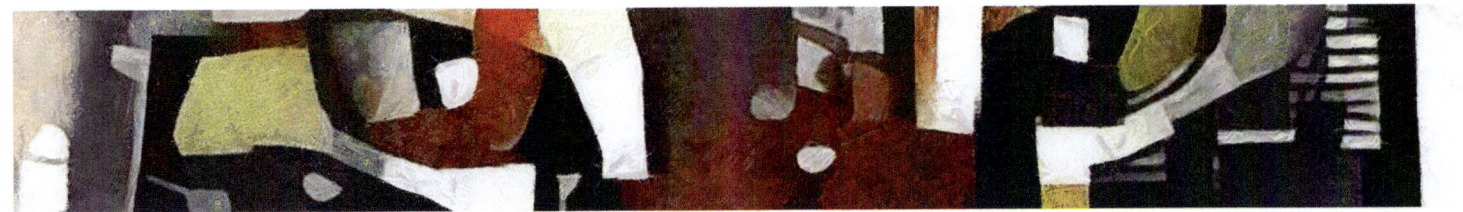

13
ABNORMAL MUCOUS MEMBRANE COLOR

The mucous membranes can provide insight into the adequacy of blood flow to peripheral tissues, as well as information about the circulating blood. Usually, the most important factors influencing membrane color are the degree of peripheral perfusion (tissue blood flow) and the concentration of oxygenated hemoglobin in the blood. Because hemoglobin normally is contained within red blood cells (RBCs), the total amount of hemoglobin is directly correlated with RBC count and packed cell volume (PCV). Additionally, the hemoglobin saturation with oxygen depends on the partial pressure of oxygen in the plasma along with the hemoglobin-oxygen dissociation curve. That relationship can be altered by factors such as pH, combination with other chemical species, or potentially from mutations in hemoglobin affinity for oxygen.

General Considerations

A number of abnormalities alter the normally pink mucous membrane color (**Table 13.1**). Anemia causes mucous membranes to appear pale pink to almost white, depending on its severity (**Figures 13.1** and **13.2**). The mucous membranes of animals with a high PCV or pronounced peripheral vasodilation might appear deep- or brick-red ("injected") in color (**Figure 13.3**), unless hypoxemia causes them to appear cyanotic (**Figures 13.4** and **13.5**, and section "Cyanosis"). In some animals, the presence of other pigments (such as bilirubin) or abnormal forms of hemoglobin (methemoglobin, carboxyhemoglobin) can discolor the blood and membranes. Excess bilirubin accumulation imparts a yellowish color to the plasma and tissues, known as icterus or jaundice. Underlying causes include hepatobiliary disease with bile stasis, and hemolysis (**Figure 40.21**, p. 864). A high concentration of methemoglobin (see section "Methemoglobinemia") interferes with tissue oxygenation and causes the membranes to appear bluish-brown. Carboxyhemoglobin is a complex of carbon monoxide and hemoglobin; carbon monoxide binds much more tightly than oxygen, which prevents normal oxygen delivery to the tissues. In high concentrations (carbon monoxide poisoning), the mucous membranes can appear bright "cherry red," despite poor tissue oxygenation.

Pallor

Pallor refers to abnormal paleness of a tissue. It is generally related to either anemia or reduced tissue perfusion, and in some cases, both. Poor peripheral tissue perfusion results from sympathetically mediated vasoconstriction associated with reduced cardiac output and hypotension, such as in hypovolemic shock, severe dehydration, heart failure, cardiac tamponade, or massive pulmonary embolism. Severe pain also can activate sympathetic vasoconstriction. Reduced peripheral perfusion prolongs capillary refill time (CRT) and causes mucous membrane pallor. In contrast, animals with anemia but normal cardiac output have a normal (1–2 seconds) CRT. However, in animals with profound anemia, the mucous membranes can be so pale that CRT cannot be determined.

Cyanosis

Cyanosis is a bluish discoloration of the tissues; in animals, it is most readily detected in nonpigmented, mucous membranes. Cyanosis occurs when the amount of deoxygenated (reduced) hemoglobin is increased. Multiple disease processes lead to the development of cyanosis, which generally becomes visible only when the concentration of desaturated hemoglobin exceeds 50 g/L (>5 g/dL). Animals with a normal hemoglobin concentration between 100 and 200 g/L (10–20 g/dL, varying with species and age) do not become visibly cyanotic unless hemoglobin oxygen saturation drops below 80%. However, chronic hypoxemia stimulates renal erythropoietin release, increases RBC production, and increases total hemoglobin concentration. Erythrocytosis (sometimes called

Cardiovascular Disease in Companion Animals 247

Table 13.1 Abnormal Mucous Membrane Color

Pale Mucous Membranes
- Anemia
- Poor cardiac output (vasoconstriction)
  - Hypovolemia, severe dehydration
  - Heart failure
  - Cardiac tamponade
  - Sustained tachy- or bradyarrhythmia
  - Intra- or extracardiac blood flow obstruction
  - Massive pulmonary embolism
- Severe pain or other causes of high sympathetic tone & peripheral vasoconstriction

Injected, Brick-Red (or Plethoric) Membranes
- Erythrocytosis (polycythemia)
- Sepsis
- Excitement
- Other causes of peripheral vasodilation, including drugs

Cyanotic Mucous Membranes[a, b]
- Right-to-left shunting congenital cardiac defect
  - Tetralogy of Fallot/Pulmonary atresia
  - Shunt (patent foramen ovale, atrial or ventricular septal defect) with pulmonary hypertension, pulmonic stenosis, or tricuspid valve disease
  - Other complex congenital heart defects
- Airway obstruction
  - Laryngeal paralysis
  - Tracheal collapse
  - Tracheal or bronchial mass or foreign body
- Pulmonary parenchymal disease
  - Pulmonary edema—cardiogenic or noncardiogenic
  - Pneumonias
  - Neoplasia
  - Chronic obstructive airway disease
  - Asthma
  - Pulmonary fibrosis
  - Pulmonary contusion and hemorrhage
  - Other severe lung disease (inflammatory, infectious)
- Pulmonary thromboembolism
- Hypoventilation
  - Pleural effusion (also causes atelectasis)
  - Pneumothorax (also causes atelectasis)
  - Thoracic deformities
  - Diaphragmatic hernia
  - Respiratory muscle fatigue
  - Myopathy
  - Drug overdose (opioids, narcotics)
  - Respiratory center depression from any cause

Differential Cyanosis
- Reversed patent ductus arteriosus[c]

Bluish-Brown Membranes
- Methemoglobinemia
  - Congenital forms
  - Acquired forms (toxicoses)

Bright, Cherry-Red Membranes
- Carboxyhemoglobinemia

Icteric Mucous Membranes
- Hemolysis
- Hepatobiliary disease
- Biliary obstruction

[a] 50 g/L (5 g/dL) desaturated hemoglobin needed for visible cyanosis, therefore, anemic animals might not appear cyanotic.
[b] Peripheral cyanosis uncommonly affects mucous membrane color; causes include arterial thromboembolism, cold exposure, and other causes of local vasoconstriction or blood flow obstruction.
[c] Normally oxygenated blood to head and forelimbs; desaturated blood to more caudal parts of body.

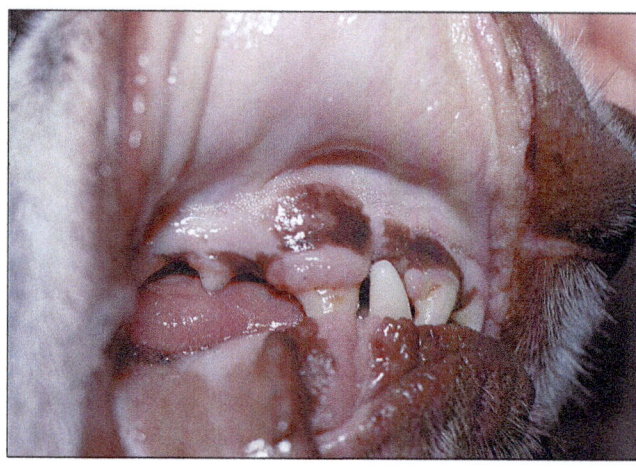

Figure 13.1 Pale mucous membranes can result from high sympathetic tone or anemia; capillary refill time is slowed in the former and usually normal in the latter.

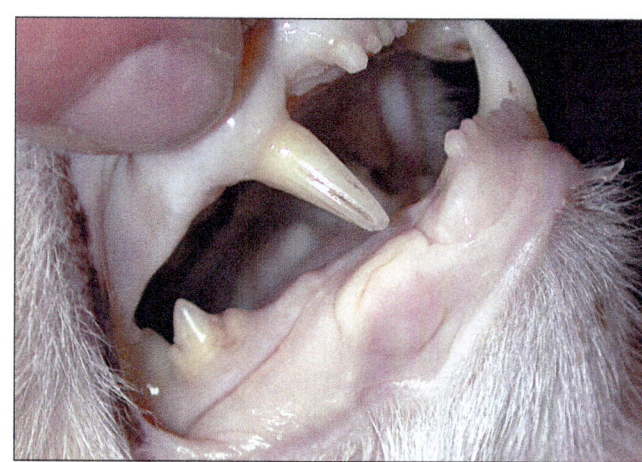

Figure 13.2 Severe anemia, as in this cat, may preclude adequate assessment of capillary refill time.

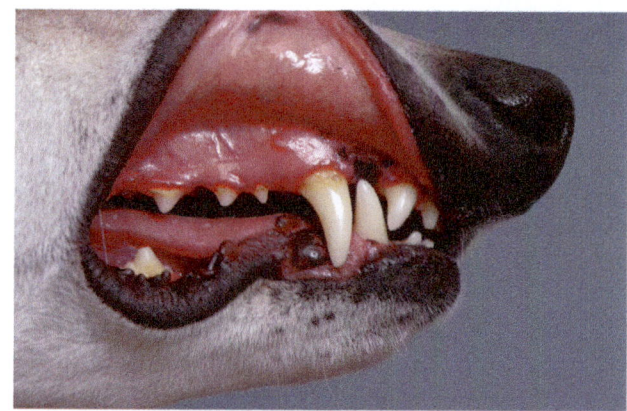

Figure 13.3 Erythrocytosis can increase the intensity of mucous membrane color, causing the membranes to appear deep red. This sometimes is referred to as "injected" or plethoric mucous membranes.

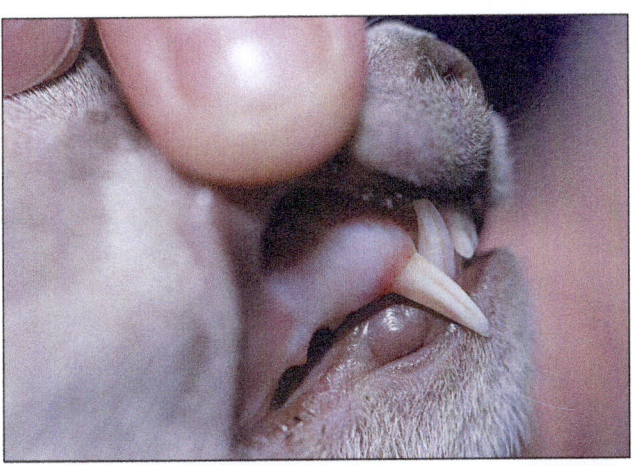

Figure 13.4 The gums have a purplish tint this cyanotic cat with a right-to-left shunting ventricular septal defect and pulmonary hypertension. The young cat had a history of exercise intolerance and fainting. Packed cell volume was almost 70%.

polycythemia) allows cyanosis to be detectable at less severe degrees of hypoxemia, because concentrations of deoxygenated hemoglobin over 50 g/L are easier to achieve. Severely anemic animals, on the other hand, rarely show cyanosis even with profound hypoxemia; with their low hemoglobin levels, the concentration of reduced hemoglobin rarely exceeds that necessary for cyanosis to become manifest.

Cyanosis commonly is categorized as central or peripheral. Central cyanosis usually occurs from serious respiratory disease (with severely impaired gas exchange) or a right-to-left cardiovascular shunt (**Figures 13.4** and **13.5**). These conditions cause systemic arterial hypoxemia. A bluish or "muddy" tinge to the oral mucous membranes, tongue, and caudal membranes is seen. Respiratory causes include marked ventilation-perfusion mismatch that occurs with pulmonary infiltrative diseases or edema, severe hypoventilation from pleural space disease or reduced respiratory drive, and airway obstruction. Anatomic (congenital) cardiac or extracardiac right-to-left shunts cause cyanosis because deoxygenated venous blood flows into the systemic circulation rather than passing through the lungs. In addition to the abnormal venous-to-systemic communication itself (such as a ventricular septal defect or patent ductus arteriosus, PDA), the pathology also involves either pulmonic stenosis (as with tetralogy of Fallot) or severe pulmonary hypertension (see Chapter 26). Atrial shunting in these cases can be across a true atrial septal defect or patent foramen ovale.

Differential cyanosis refers to cyanotic caudal membranes with pink cranial membranes. This is a classic finding with "reversed" PDA. The differential cyanosis occurs because of the anatomical location of the ductus, downstream from the brachiocephalic and left subclavian arteries which perfuse the cranial body. When ductal flow is reversed, deoxygenated blood from the pulmonary artery enters into the descending aorta to perfuse the caudal part of the body (p. 450; and **Figure 26.19**).

Peripheral cyanosis is associated with extremely poor peripheral perfusion and locally desaturated hemoglobin; high tissue oxygen extraction can contribute. Arterial thromboembolism, marked peripheral vasoconstriction, and hypothermia are the most common causes of peripheral cyanosis. Cool, cyanotic footpads or nailbeds in affected limbs are the usual manifestations (**Figures 36.12**, **36.13**, and **36.24**, p. 755, 757 and 769). Occasionally, blood flow obstruction in a limb is caused by a mass lesion or external constriction (as from an excessively tight bandage). Concurrent venous and lymphatic obstruction also causes edema as well as cyanosis of the affected tissue. Protracted ischemia to a limb leads to rhabdomyolysis and tissue necrosis within hours, that might become visible days later (Chapter 37).

Methemoglobinemia

Methemoglobinemia is another cause of cyanotic or dark mucous membranes; the blood appears brownish-blue in color (**Figure 13.6**). Methemoglobin is a product of hemoglobin oxidation, where iron in the heme groups is in the ferric (Fe^{3+}) rather than the normal ferrous (Fe^{2+}) state. This changes oxygen affinity. Methemoglobin itself has impaired ability to bind oxygen. However, within the same tetrameric hemoglobin unit, the binding of oxygen to methemoglobin increases oxygen affinity at other heme sites that still are in the ferrous state. Therefore, affected RBCs have reduced ability to release O_2, which causes a leftward shift in the oxygen-hemoglobin dissociation curve. Consequently, increased methemoglobin concentration can lead to tissue hypoxia. Normally, only low concentrations of methemoglobin are present because methemoglobin reductase enzyme systems in the RBCs rapidly reduce it back to hemoglobin. Ingestion of certain oxidizing drugs or chemicals can

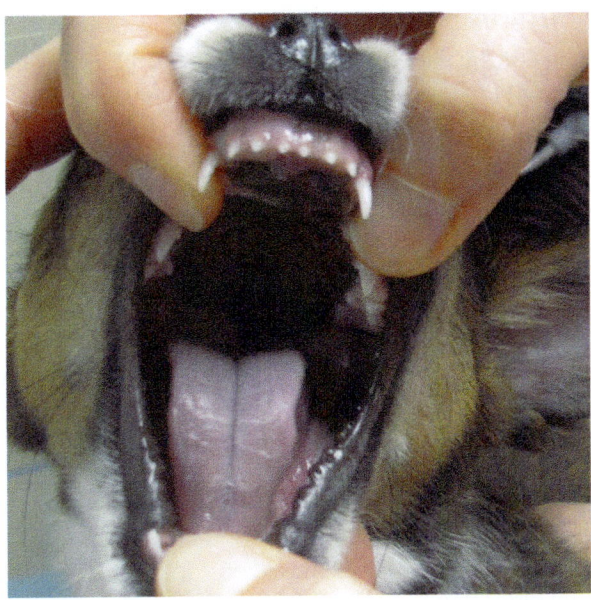

Figure 13.5 The tongue appears bluish-purple in this cyanotic puppy with tetralogy of Fallot, and other cardiac malformations. His packed cell volume was 62%.

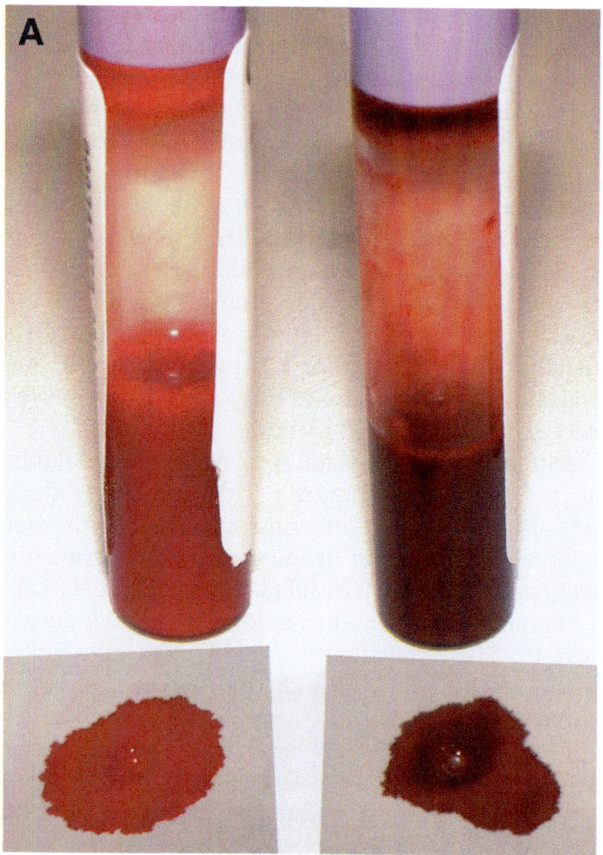 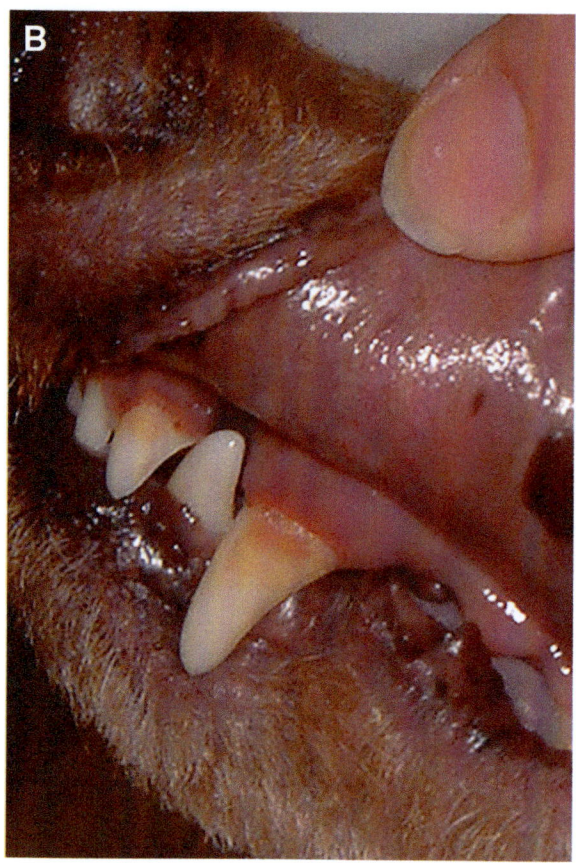

Figure 13.6 (A) Comparison of two blood samples after exposure to oxygen. The sample on the left is from a normal dog. The tube and blood spot on the right are from a young dog with methemoglobinemia, caused by congenital deficiency of methemoglobin reductase. Methemoglobinemia imparts a dark bluish to brownish color to the blood. (B) A slight brownish-blue tinge also is apparent in the mucous membranes of the affected dog. Methemoglobin (oxidized hemoglobin) cannot bind oxygen normally, yet increases oxygen affinity at nonoxidized heme sites. Unlike most cases of cyanosis, caused by low oxygen availability, methemoglobinemia shifts the oxygen-hemoglobin dissociation curve to the left, reducing oxygen release to tissues. (A) Slides courtesy of Dr Kelly Wang.

increase methemoglobin formation to levels that greatly exceed endogenous enzyme capacity, allowing methemoglobin concentration to rise. Acquired methemoglobinemia can occur after ingestion of acetaminophen (especially in cats), garlic, benzocaine and other local anesthetics, sulfonamides and certain other antibiotics, nitrates, nitroglycerin, nitroprusside, and other agents. Congenital forms of methemoglobinemia caused by methemoglobin reductase (or another) deficiency have been recognized in people, dogs, and cats. Red blood cell flavin adenine dinucleotide deficiency and red maple toxicosis are reported to cause congenital and acquired cases of methemoglobinemia in horses, respectively.

Clinical signs can include shortness of breath, lethargy, tachypnea, arrhythmias, hypertension (p. 792), altered mentation, seizures, and coma. Headache also is reported in people. With increasing concentrations of methemoglobin, signs become more severe and can lead to death. A mismatch between hemoglobin oxygen saturation (reduced) and arterial PO_2 (normal) are typical. Lactic acidosis and Heinz body anemia might be detected in some cases. Definitive diagnosis can be obtained with specialized blood gas analysis that includes the partial pressure of detectable methemoglobin. Treatment involves administration of supplemental O_2 (including high-flow and hyperbaric) and methylene blue to reduce oxidized hemoglobin to the ferrous state. However, this chemical can cause adverse effects including Heinz body anemia and, potentially, cardiotoxicity.

Approach to the Patient with Abnormal Mucous Membrane Color

As with other clinical problems, a complete history and physical examination are important (**Figure 13.7**). Any abnormality of mucous membrane color, as well as the patient's CRT (see p. 36), should be noted. Hydration status, heart rate (HR) and rhythm, and other examination details could provide important clues that help direct further testing. An increased HR is common in animals with pallor from either anemia or poor perfusion, but also from other causes of high sympathetic tone.

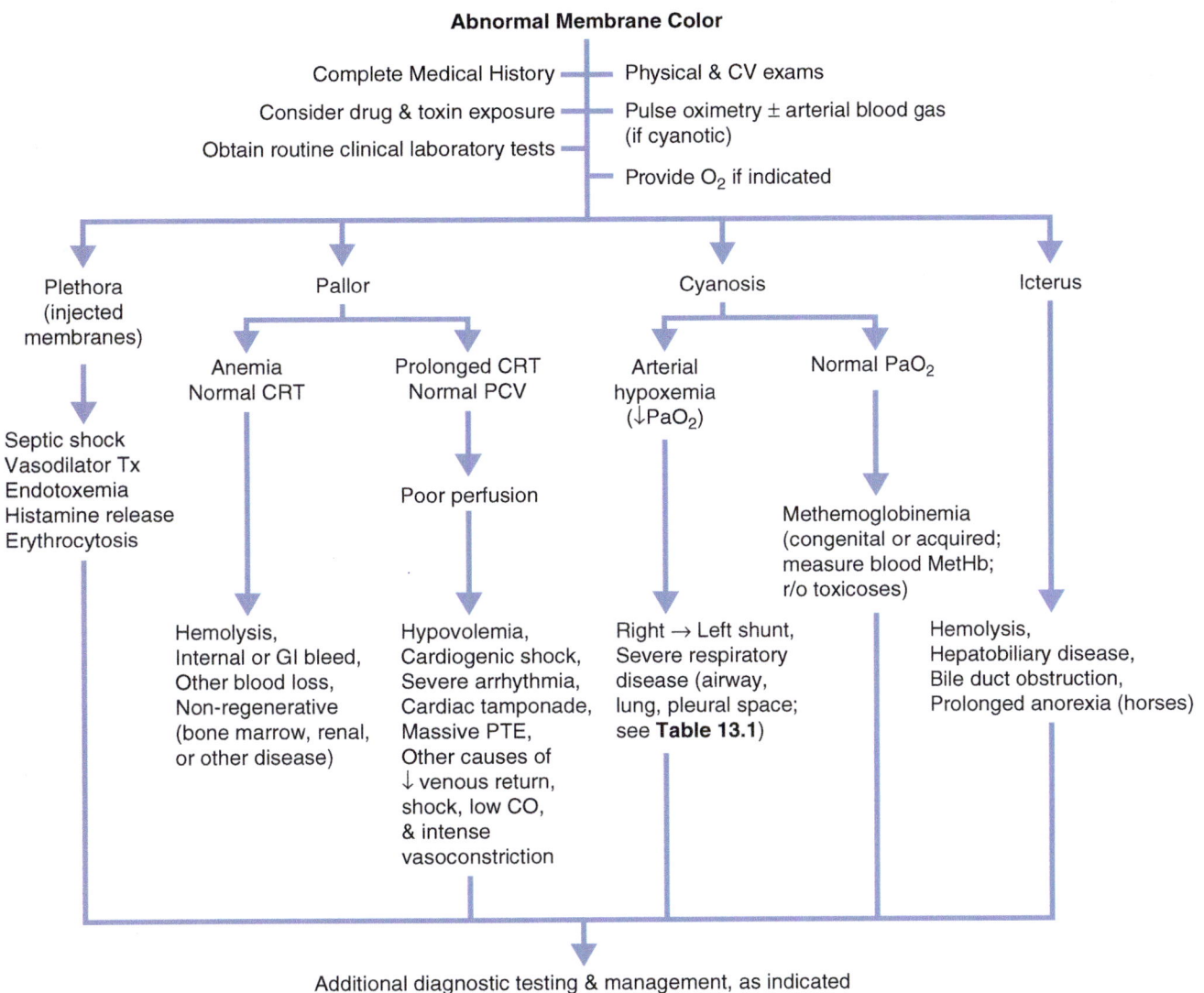

Figure 13.7 Approach to the patient with abnormal mucous membrane color. These are general guidelines & diagnostic considerations; exceptions can occur. CO, cardiac output; CRT, capillary refill time; CV, cardiovascular; GI, gastrointestinal; MetHb, methemoglobin; PCV, packed cell volume; PTE, pulmonary thromboembolism; Tx, therapy.

A yellowish cast to the membranes (icterus, jaundice) should prompt evaluation for hemolysis and hepatobiliary disease. Petechiae in the mucous membranes suggest a platelet disorder.

Especially in animals with a history of rear limb weakness or fatigue, the caudal mucous membrane color (vaginal or preputial) should be examined and compared with oral or other cranial mucous membrane color to determine whether differential cyanosis is present. Differential cyanosis (caudal cyanosis with normal oral membrane color) is a classic finding in reversed PDA. If the color comparison is ambiguous at rest, a period of exercise will accentuate the caudal cyanosis in animals with reversed PDA.

Animals with respiratory distress should be given supplemental oxygen as soon as possible. However, cyanosis caused by an anatomic or large intra-pulmonary right-to-left shunt or from methemoglobinemia are unlikely to respond to conventional oxygen therapy, nor is that from hypoventilation, without ventilatory assistance. A complete blood count (CBC) is indicated in animals with abnormal mucous membrane color, and a blood smear should be inspected for RBC abnormalities. If the PCV (hematocrit) is low, it should be determined whether the anemia is regenerative or nonregenerative (or if recent acute hemorrhage could have occurred). A serum chemistry panel and urinalysis also are part of an initial database. Cyanotic membranes should prompt an assessment of respiratory function as well as a search for a possible right-to-left shunt, or methemoglobinemia. Other tests that might be indicated include radiographs, blood gas analysis and pulse oximetry, slide-agglutination or Coombs' testing, coagulation tests, echocardiography (with saline contrast, p. 88), abdominal ultrasonography, electrocardiogram (ECG), blood pressure, bone marrow analysis, fecal tests, among others.

Suggested Additional Reading and References

Also See Online Comprehensive Bibliography at: https://www.routledge.com/9781482246223.

George LW, Divers TJ, Mahaffey EA, et al. Heinz body anemia and methemoglobinemia in ponies given red maple (*Acer rubrum* L.) leaves. Vet Pathol 1982;19:521–533.

Giger U. Anemia. In, Silverstein DC, Hopper K (editors). Small Animal Critical Care Medicine. 2nd edition. Elsevier-Saunders, St. Louis, MO. 2015. pp. 575–580.

Hall TL, Magdesian KG, Kittleson MD. Congenital cardiac defects in neonatal foals: 18 cases (1992–2007). J Vet Intern Med 2010;24:206–212.

Harvey JW, Stockham SL, Scott MA, et al. Methemoglobinemia and eccentrocytosis in equine erythrocyte flavin adenine dinucleotide deficiency. Vet Pathol 2003;40:632–642.

Jaffey JA, Harmon MR, Villani NA, et al. Long-term treatment with methylene blue in a dog with hereditary methemoglobinemia caused by cytochrome b5 reductase deficiency. J Vet Intern Med 2017;31:1860–1865.

Koster LS, Kirberger RM. A syndrome of severe idiopathic pulmonary parenchymal disease with pulmonary hypertension in Pekingese. Vet Med 2016;7:19–31.

Ohad DG. Pallor. In, Ettinger SJ, Feldman EC, Cote E (editors). Textbook of Veterinary Internal Medicine. 8th edition. Elsevier, St. Louis, MO. 2017. pp. 206–208.

Packer RM, Tivers MS. Strategies for the management and prevention of conformation-related respiratory disorders in brachycephalic dogs. Vet Med 2015;6:219–232.

Rahilly LJ, Mandell DC. Methemoglobinemia. In, Silverstein DC, Hopper K (editors). Small Animal Critical Care Medicine. 2nd edition. Elsevier-Saunders, St. Louis, MO. 2015. pp. 580–585.

Rissi DR, Brown CA. Diagnostic features in 10 naturally occurring cases of acute fatal canine leptospirosis. J Vet Diagn Invest 2014;26:799–804.

Rolim VM, Casagrande RA, Wouters AT, et al. Myocarditis caused by feline immunodeficiency virus in five cats with hypertrophic cardiomyopathy. J Comp Pathol 2016;154:3–8.

Tidholm A. Cyanosis. In, Ettinger SJ, Feldman EC, Cote E (editors). Textbook of Veterinary Internal Medicine. 8th edition. Elsevier, St. Louis, MO. 2017. pp. 210–213.

Tritschler C, Mizukami K, Raj K, et al. Increased erythrocytic osmotic fragility in anemic domestic shorthair and purebred cats. J Feline Med Surg 2016;18:462–470.

Vasiliadou E, Karakitsou V, Kazakos G, et al. Hereditary methemoglobinemia in a cyanotic cat presented for ovariohysterectomy. Can Vet J 2019;60:502–506.

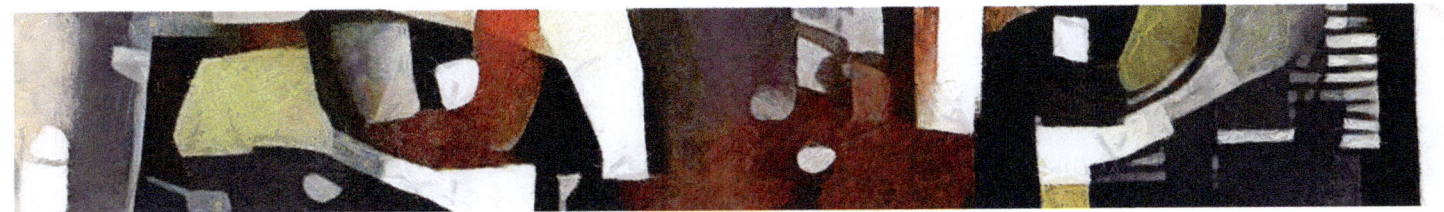

14
ARTERIAL PULSE ABNORMALITIES

The normal arterial pulse exhibits a rapid rise and gradual decline. The arterial pulse upstroke and maximal pressure depend mainly on ventricular systolic function, the compliance of the arterial system, and the previous diastolic blood pressure (BP). Arterial compliance relates to aortic distensibility (the opposite of stiffness) and peripheral arterial resistance. The decline in the arterial pressure is affected largely by heart rate (HR) and factors affecting the diastolic "run-off" of blood, such as peripheral vasodilation or cardiovascular lesions. Thus, changes in HR and rhythm, the degree of cardiac filling, ventricular contractile strength, and vascular function influence the contour of the arterial pulse waves. How strong the peripheral arterial pulse feels on digital palpation relates largely to the "pulse pressure," which is defined as the difference between systolic and diastolic arterial pressures (discussed in more detail below; also see p. 23). As the pulse pressure widens (that is, the difference between systolic and diastolic arterial pressures becomes greater), the arterial pulse feels stronger on palpation. Conversely, as the pulse pressure narrows (difference becomes smaller), the pulse feels weaker. The rate of pressure rise and fall, representing the anacrotic and diacrotic limbs of the recorded arterial pressure waveform, also affect the palpable pulse.

Beyond these cardiac and vascular determinants, there are other considerations during physical diagnosis. For instance, the femoral arterial pulse strength will feel weaker in an obese, compared to a thin, animal even when pulse pressures are comparable. In cats, femoral arterial pulses sometimes are hard to find even with normal body habitus; gentle palpation using a fingertip over the proximal femur at the femoral triangle usually reveals the arterial pulse (p. 36). However, excessive digital pressure can obstruct flow and prevent detection of the pulse. Localized vascular disease or inflammation can result in regional narrowing or dilation of blood vessels. These changes usually are asymmetric and might be most evident in the distal arterial bed.

The arterial pulse generally is palpated in the femoral artery of dogs and cats and the facial artery of the horse. However palpation at alternative sites, such as over the canine metatarsal or equine digital arteries, can be instructive. Physiologically, the prevailing arterial BP does alter aortic compliance and conceivably pulse pressure because higher BP distends the aorta more and renders it less distensible during ventricular ejection. However, practically, the perceived arterial pulse strength on palpation cannot be used to estimate arterial BP. There is no reliable correlation between pulse strength on palpation and systolic (or mean) BP. One exception might be severely hypotensive patients with peripheral vasoconstriction, where more distal pulses can become imperceptible. For example, in a canine study, the loss of the metatarsal pulse was associated with systemic hypotension (Ateca, 2018). However, the opposite situation also might occur if there is peripheral vasodilation, as with sepsis, where a prominent peripheral pulse might be detected even in the setting of lowered BP.

General Considerations

The arterial pulse wave is influenced by the effects of ventricular stroke volume (SV), ejection velocity, arterial compliance, and vascular resistance. Variations in pulse pressure, and therefore perceived arterial pulse strength, relate directly to the input function affected mainly by SV. One determinant of SV is the degree of ventricular filling (preload). Ventricular filling is influenced in turn by the efficiency of the myocardial relaxation process, compliance of the ventricular myocardium, volume of venous return, duration of ventricular diastole, and atrial contraction. SV also

Cardiovascular Disease in Companion Animals 253

is affected by myocardial contractility (direct relationship), as well as by arterial pressure and other factors opposing ejection (afterload; inverse relationship). Conditions that slow left ventricular (LV) ejection and the normally rapid rise in systolic arterial pressure will diminish perceived arterial pulse strength at any given pulse pressure (see section "Hypokinetic Pulses").

Vascular compliance is complicated, but one determinant is aortic input impedance. The aorta is an elastic artery that distends to "store" part of the ventricular SV during ejection and subsequently recoils during diastole to deliver that volume into the arterial system. Increases in aortic stiffness reduce compliance, causing a higher systolic but lower diastolic BP. Thus, a widened pulse pressure might occur in the setting of an aortopathy. This pathophysiology is probably under-recognized in veterinary medicine, but potentially is encountered in a number of disorders (**Table 14.1**). Additionally, the summation of retrograde pulse waves, reflected from the muscular (and potentially stiffer) peripheral arteries, upon the forward pulsatile flow also can influence pulse contour. Overall these vascular changes are likely important but challenging to measure in clinical settings.

HR is another major determinant of pulse pressure and BP. In addition to increasing diastolic ventricular filling time, a slower HR permits a greater decline in diastolic arterial BP and presumably ventricular afterload. Thus, the pulse pressure in patients with a bradycardia often is widened. Mild variation in pulse strength normally accompanies even small fluctuations in the HR, as observed with sinus arrhythmia in dogs or physiologic AV block in horses (**Figure 14.1**). While these physiologic determinants can be enumerated, their interactions and impact on the arterial pulse are complex. Consider subaortic stenosis, where obstruction to outflow (reducing the rate of pressure rise and increasing afterload) competes with the concurrent aortopathy (that reduces arterial distensibility). Nevertheless, some generalizations are possible and **Table 14.1** lists some causes of abnormal arterial pulse strength.

Hypokinetic Pulses

Hypokinetic pulses feel weaker than normal. Most often this occurs when the pulse pressure is narrow, although vascular disease or thrombosis also can affect pulse strength in regional vascular beds (**Table 14.1**; also see Chapters 36 and 37). Situations that diminish the difference between systolic and diastolic arterial pressures usually involve a decrease in SV. Substantial increases in HR from any cause shorten ventricular filling time and therefore might reduce SV. This not only includes sinus tachycardia (associated with heart failure, hypovolemia, or other causes of high sympathetic tone), but also supraventricular and ventricular tachycardias. The latter arrhythmia is also affected by the loss of atrioventricular

Table 14.1 Arterial Pulse Abnormalities and Associations

Hypokinetic (Weak) Pulses
- Reduced ventricular preload
  - Hypovolemia/volume contraction
  - Dehydration
  - Shock (hypovolemic, hemorrhagic, obstructive, cardiogenic)
  - Obstructed venous return (gastric dilation)
  - Hypoadrenocorticism
  - Tachycardia (diminished ventricular filing time)
- Cardiac disease
  - (Sub)aortic stenosis (*pulsus parvus et tardus*)
  - Dilated cardiomyopathy
  - Congestive heart failure (variable)
  - Cardiac tamponade
  - ± Pulmonic stenosis (from ventricular interdependence)

Hyperkinetic (Strong) Pulses
- Sympathetic stimulation (excitement, exercise, etc.)
- Bradycardia
- Hyperthyroidism
- Fever/sepsis
- Anemia
- Laminitis (digital pulse, in horses)

Extremely Hyperkinetic (Bounding) Pulses
- Patent ductus arteriosus ("waterhammer pulse")
- Severe aortic regurgitation ("Corrigan's pulse")
- Other large arteriovenous fistula
- Profound bradycardia (complete AV block)

Variable Pulses
- Pronounced sinus arrhythmia, or sinus rhythm with variable 2nd degree AV block

Irregular Pulse Rate and Strength, Often with Pulse Deficits
- Atrial fibrillation
- Ventricular premature complexes or other irregular tachyarrhythmias

Asymmetrical Pulses, from Right to Left Side
- Arterial thromboembolic disease
- Aorto-iliac disease in dogs and horses (also hypokinetic)
- Other cause of partial to complete arterial vascular obstruction

Alternating Weaker Then Stronger Pulses, Every Other Beat
- Ventricular or atrial bigeminy
- *Pulsus alternans* (associated with severe myocardial failure or volume depletion)

Weaker Pulse during Inspiration
- Cardiac tamponade (*pulsus paradoxus*)
- Marked inspiratory efforts (distress)

Other pulse abnormalities, such as a bifid (bisferiens) pulse, is rarely detectable by palpation.
Abbreviation: AV, atrioventricular.

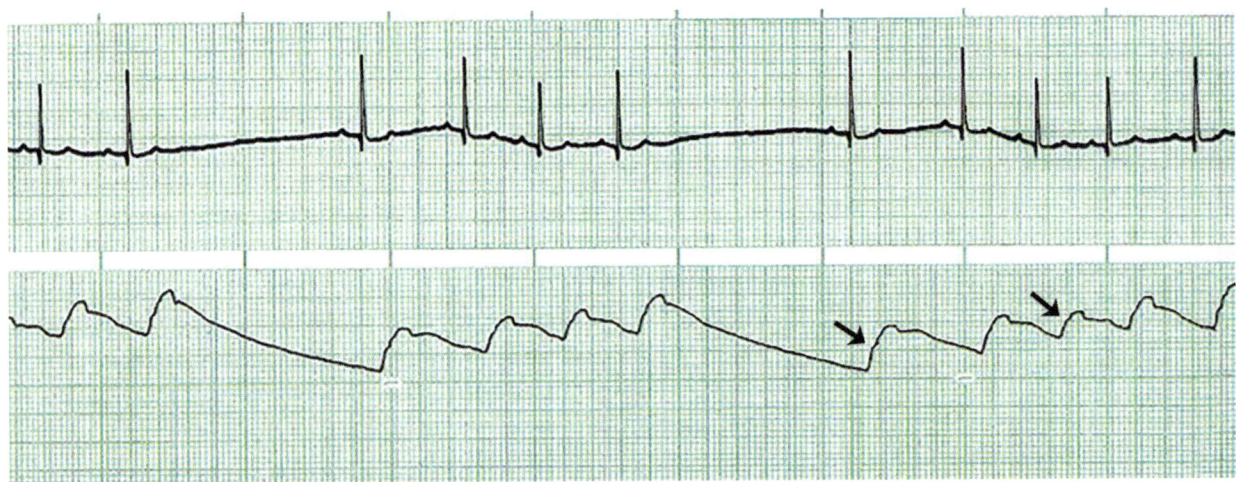

Figure 14.1 Simultaneous lead II ECG (top) and arterial pressure tracing (bottom) from a normal dog with sinus arrhythmia. The varying time intervals between heartbeats affects the width of the pulse pressure (compare the two cycles indicated by arrows), as well as the absolute systolic and diastolic pressures. (Original recording courtesy of Dr. W Reece.)

and ventricular synchrony. Poor venous return to the heart, as occurs with dehydration, hemorrhagic shock, gastric dilation, and pericardial effusion also will reduce SV. Loss of atrial contraction (as with atrial fibrillation) has a negative effect on ventricular end diastolic volume and SV, especially at faster HRs. Although some animals with hypokinetic pulses also might be hypotensive, most have normal BP because of reflex changes in vascular resistance and HR that become activated to maintain arterial pressure.

The pulse also will feel weaker than normal if the rise to maximum systolic arterial pressure is slow and prolonged, as occurs with LV outflow obstruction. Severe subaortic stenosis (SAS) is the most common cause of this. The weak-feeling, or "small and delayed," pulse is known as *pulsus parvus et tardus*. Conversely, the pulse often is normal in case of dynamic LV outflow obstruction (as with feline hypertrophic obstructive cardiomyopathy), because the obstruction occurs in mid- to late systole, after much of the SV has been ejected.

Hyperkinetic Pulses

Stronger than normal (hyperkinetic) pulses occur in a number of conditions. The increase can range from subtle to extreme. The most common cause is a widened pulse pressure, either from an increase in systolic pressure, a greater fall in diastolic pressure (as occurs with rapid blood "run-off" from central arteries to the periphery), or both. Abnormally increased aortic stiffness also increases pulse pressure because normal systolic pressure-dampening distensibility is lost. Marked bradycardia increases pulse strength because prolonged periods of diastole allow arterial pressure to decline more before the next heartbeat. A larger SV results from the longer ventricular filling time and potentially from reduced ventricular afterload. Therefore, the difference between diastolic arterial pressure and the systolic pressure generated by the next ejection is large. High sympathetic tone can increase perceived pulse strength as stronger ventricular contraction, and enhanced SV, produces a rapid rise in arterial pressure during LV ejection. Additionally, "hyperkinetic states" such as fever, hyperthyroidism, anemia, and exercise, as well as use of vasodilator drugs, can increase palpable pulse strength because peripheral vasodilation allows faster flow ("run-off") into the peripheral circulation and more rapid decline in diastolic pressure. These conditions also activate the sympathetic nervous system, which increases ventricular contractility. In cases of regional disease, such as a limb infection or equine laminitis, the more central arterial pulse might feel normal while the local or digital pulse palpates as hyperdynamic.

Exceptionally strong or "bounding" pulses are associated with a large SV and rapid fall (drop-off) in diastolic pressure. The classic cause is the "waterhammer pulse" of a large patent ductus arteriosus (PDA), where much of the SV from LV ejection flows through the ductus into the pulmonary artery; consequently, there is a steep diastolic decline in aortic pressure, along with a mild to moderate increase in systolic pressure related to increased SV (**Figure 26.9**, p. 442). Another important cause of markedly hyperkinetic pulses is severe aortic regurgitation; in this situation, SV also is increased and a large, rapid backflow of blood from aorta to LV causes diastolic arterial pressure to fall steeply. Similar to PDA, other large arterio-venous fistulae also can cause markedly hyperkinetic pulses, because of the rapid blood run-off from arterial to venous vessels. Older adjectives that have been used to describe bounding arterial pulses include "water-hammer," "Corrigan's," "cannonball," or "BB shot" pulses.

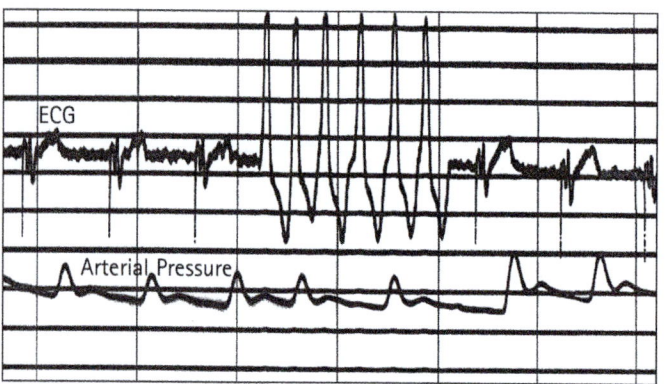

Figure 14.2 Pulse deficits associated with ventricular tachycardia (VT) are shown in this recording from a Bulldog with third-degree AV block and permanent transvenous pacemaker. The ECG (top) shows the paced ventricular rhythm, which is interrupted by paroxysmal VT. An arterial pressure wave follows each paced QRS complex (bottom); but, only two of the six ventricular premature activations result in an arterial pulse wave.

Pulse Deficits

A pulse deficit occurs when there are fewer arterial pulses than cardiac contractions. Various arrhythmias induce pulse deficits by causing the heart to beat before adequate ventricular filling has occurred. Consequently, minimal or even no blood is ejected for those beats and a palpable pulse is absent. Premature beats, atrial fibrillation and ventricular tachyarrhythmias are common causes of pulse deficits (**Figures 14.2** and **14.3**; also **Figure 32.5**, p. 611). To screen for pulse deficits, the arterial pulse rate should be evaluated simultaneously with the direct HR, which is obtained by auscultation or chest wall palpation of the apical impulse. It is important to remember that when the animal has an arrhythmia which causes pulse deficits, the palpated pulse rate will not accurately reflect the animal's true HR. Instead, a direct HR (by auscultation or chest palpation), or preferably an ECG recording, should be used to determine the HR.

Other Pulse Abnormalities

Sometimes, alternately weak then strong arterial pulsations occur. Most often this is caused by a normal heartbeat alternating with a premature beat (bigeminy). The premature beat produces a reduced SV and weaker pulse, while the SV and pulse associated with the following (normal) beat are augmented (this is known as postextrasystolic potentiation). Second-degree atrioventricular (AV) block, which is especially common in resting horses, is another potential cause for variable pulse intensity; however, this does not typically produce every-other-beat variability (**Figure 14.4**). Even marked sinus arrhythmia can cause noticeable variation in arterial pulse strength associated with variations in SV (**Figure 14.1**).

Rarely, beat-to-beat variability in pulse strength occurs despite a regular rhythm; this is known as *pulsus alternans* or Traube's pulse (**Figure 14.5**). The development of pulsus alternans is thought to be related to cyclic changes in myocardial intracellular calcium handling. It can occur with severe myocardial failure, high afterload states, or tachycardia with marked hypovolemia or vasodilation. LV (and systemic arterial) pulsus alternans has been observed in some dogs with

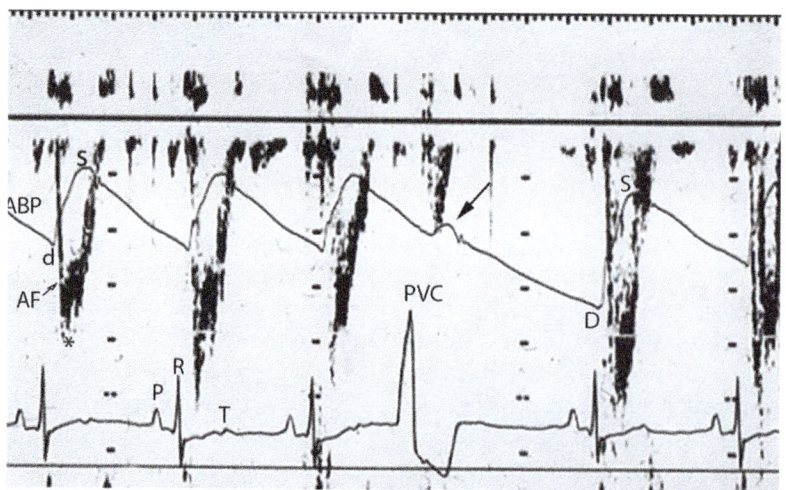

Figure 14.3 Pulsed wave Doppler flow in the aorta (AF), aortic blood pressure (ABP), and ECG (at bottom) from a dog with pulse deficit caused by a premature ventricular complex (PVC). In the first cardiac cycle (*), notice the difference between systolic (s) and diastolic (d) arterial pressures (that is, the pulse pressure), as well as the AF velocity. The PVC causes marked reduction in the associated AF signal and pulse pressure (arrow); this would lead to absence of a palpable arterial pulse (deficit). Note the fall in arterial diastolic pressure and characteristic postextrasystolic potentiation of the pulse pressure (S/D) and AF velocity in the beat following the PVC.

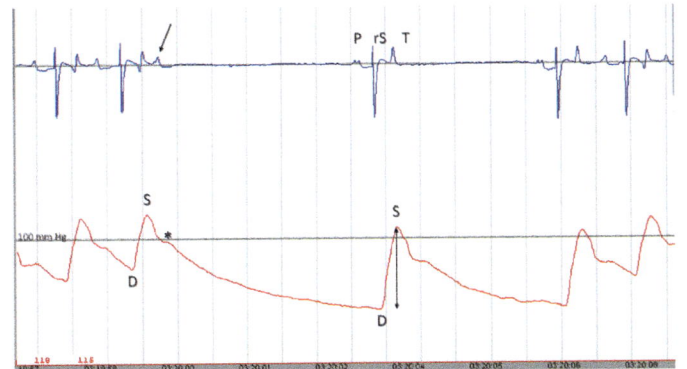

Figure 14.4 Simultaneous ECG (top) and aortic pressure pulse (bottom) from a standing horse with physiologic second-degree AV block (arrow; top). After the blocked P wave, arterial blood pressure (BP) gradually falls to a low diastolic pressure (D). Compare that to the prior waveforms where BP progressively increases with each cardiac cycle. Following the block, the pulse pressure is widened (double-sided arrow) corresponding to a hyperkinetic pulse. Compare that to the pulse pressures in other cycles. S, systolic pressure; *, dicrotic wave caused by reflected pressure waves, a normal finding.

Cardiac tamponade produces an exaggerated decline in systolic arterial pressure (and pulse pressure) during inspiration. This is known as *pulsus paradoxus*. Weaker arterial pulses during inspiration sometimes are clinically detectable in such cases (p. 714, and **Figure 35.15**).

Asymmetrical or absent pulses are another cause for concern. The lack of pulse or a weaker pulse on one side of the body might indicate thromboembolism or other vascular abnormality such as aorto-iliac disease. Absent or asymmetric femoral arterial pulses were found in 6.5% of over 900 Cavalier King Charles Spaniels examined, in one report (Buchanan, 1997). Rare causes of altered pulses might include compression under a mass lesion or deformity, localized arteriovenous fistula, or an obstructive lesion in the aorta, such as a coarctation, which could lead to stronger cranial versus caudal arterial pulsations.

dilated cardiomyopathy, hypovolemia, or under halothane anesthesia. Severe aortic stenosis and hypertension are other potential associations reported in people. Biventricular pulsus alternans has been seen in a dog with severe pulmonic stenosis and concurrent dehydration, sepsis, and tachycardia. Right ventricular (or likely, biventricular) pulsus alternans also has been reported in people with high right ventricular afterload (severe pulmonary hypertension, critical pulmonic stenosis, or massive pulmonary thromboembolism) and right ventricular failure. In situations where systemic arterial pulsus alternans is present, concurrent alternans in right ventricular outflow is likely as well, given the interdependence between right and left ventricles.

Approach to the Patient with an Arterial Pulse Abnormality

A careful patient history and complete physical examination should be obtained, as for animals with other physical abnormalities. It is important to assess arterial pulse rate, regularity, and strength on palpation. Approximate normal HRs per minute in the clinic are 60–160 for dogs, 140–240 for cats, and 28–44 for adult horses. Determine whether pulse deficits are present by simultaneously palpating the arterial pulse and ausculting the heart (or palpating the precordial impulse, if clearly discernable). In dogs and cats, simultaneous palpation of left and right femoral pulses allows assessment of pulse symmetry. This is especially relevant in animals with weakness or lameness in one or both rear limbs. In horses, a rectal examination or ultrasound might be needed to detect aorto-iliac disease or thrombosis. In cases where a pulse cannot be confirmed by palpation, the clinician should attempt to identify arterial flow by clipping the hair and placing a Doppler crystal (one used for noninvasive BP measurement) over that artery, in hope of detecting pulsatile arterial flow in the audio channel.

Pulse abnormalities should be interpreted within the context of the species, body condition, and other physical findings (**Figure 14.6**). Depending on the individual patient situation, further diagnostic testing might include a routine laboratory database (hemogram, serum chemistries, urinalysis), electrocardiogram (ECG), echocardiogram, radiographs, thyroid or other endocrine testing, BP measurement, bacterial cultures, and coagulation tests. Aortic or peripheral vascular diseases (Chapter 37) might require other imaging modalities, including duplex Doppler imaging (B-mode with simultaneous color or pulsed-wave Doppler) using cutaneous, abdominal, or rectal acoustic windows. Traditional radiographic and computed tomographic contrast angiography might be required to detect deeper or central lesions responsible for abnormal arterial pulsations.

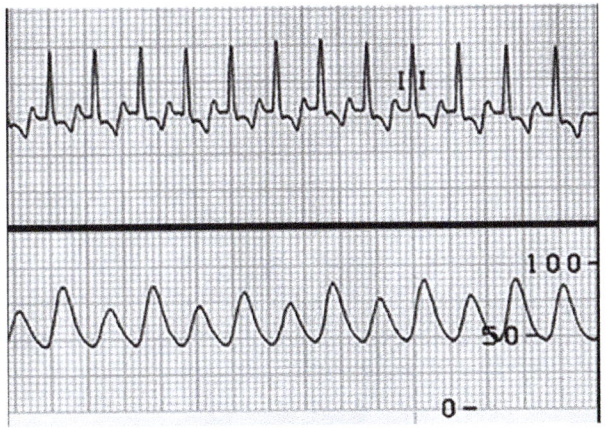

Figure 14.5 Sinus tachycardia with pulsus alternans recorded in a dog with myocardial failure during cardiac catheterization. Note alternating peak systolic arterial pressures (bottom; pressure scale on right). Lead II ECG on top. (Original recording courtesy of Dr. MW Miller.)

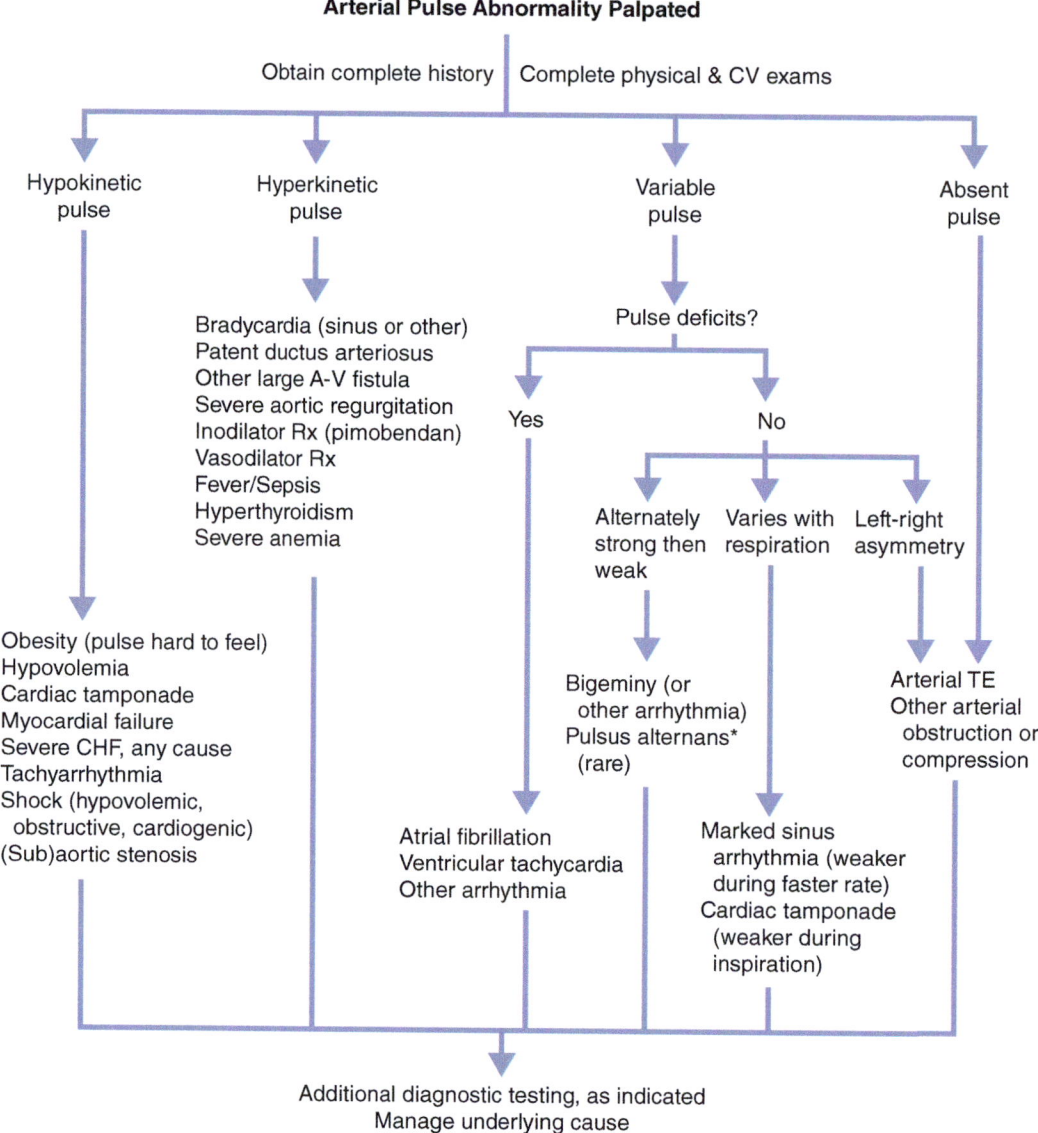

Figure 14.6 Approach to the patient with an arterial pulse abnormality. Common differential diagnoses are listed; other etiologies can occur. A-V, arteriovenous; CHF, congestive heart failure; CV, cardiovascular; Rx, therapy; TE, thromboembolism. *See text p. 256.

Suggested Additional Reading and References

Also See Online Comprehensive Bibliography at: https://www.routledge.com/9781482246223.

Ateca LB, Reineke EL, Drobatz KJ. Evaluation of the relationship between peripheral pulse palpation and Doppler systolic blood pressure in dogs presenting to an emergency service. J Vet Emerg Crit Care 2018;28:226–231.

Boegli J, Schwarzwald CC, Mitchell KJ. Diagnostic value of noninvasive pulse pressure measurements in Warmblood horses with aortic regurgitation. J Vet Intern Med 2019;33:1446–1455.

Buchanan JW, Beardow AW, Sammarco CD. Femoral artery occlusion in Cavalier King Charles Spaniels. J Am Vet Med Assoc 1997;211:872–874.

Conti AA. Nineteenth century "Traube's pulse" and current "Cardiac alternans": significant features in the history of cardiology. La Clinica terapeutica 2012;163:e71–72.

Edwards P, Cohen GI. Both diastolic and systolic function alternate in pulsus alternans: a case report and review. J Am Soc Echocardiogr 2003;16:695–697.

Fitchett DH, Sniderman AD. Inspiratory reduction in left heart filling as a mechanism of pulsus paradoxus in cardiac tamponade. Can J Cardiol 1990;6:348–354.

Freeman GL, Widman LE, Campbell JM, et al. An evaluation of pulsus alternans in closed-chest dogs. Am J Physiol 1992;262: H278–284.

Kahn JH, Starling MR, Supiano MA. Transient dobutamine-mediated pulsus alternans. Can J Cardiol 2001;17:203–205.

Ko JC, Fox SM, Mandsager RE. Effects of preemptive atropine administration on incidence of medetomidine-induced bradycardia in dogs. J Am Vet Med Assoc 2001; 218:52–58.

Moneva-Jordan A, Luis Fuentes V, Corcoran BM, et al. Pulsus alternans in English cocker spaniels with dilated cardiomyopathy. J Small Anim Pract 2007;48:258–263.

Perk G, Tunick PA, Kronzon I. Systolic and diastolic pulsus alternans in severe heart failure. J Am Soc Echocardiogr 2007;20(905):e905–907.

Reef VB, Spencer P. Echocardiographic evaluation of equine aortic insufficiency. Am J Vet Res 1987;48:904–909.

Shaw SP, Rush JE. Canine pericardial effusion: diagnosis, treatment, and prognosis. Compend Contin Educ Vet 2007;29:405–411.

Sisson D, Thomas WP. Endocarditis of the aortic valve in the dog. J Am Vet Med Assoc 1984;184:570–577.

Ware WA, Cheney AB, Murphy S. Biventricular Pulsus Alternans in a Dog with Pulmonic Stenosis and Sepsis. CASE 2021. https://doi.org/10.1016/j.case.2020.12.004

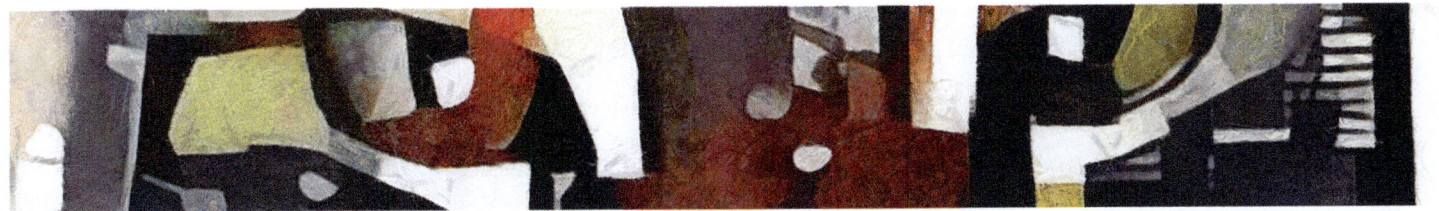

15
JUGULAR VEIN DISTENSION OR PULSATION

Jugular veins distend when pressure within rises. The jugular veins normally are not distended when the animal is standing with its head in a normal erect position and with jaw parallel to the floor. Because of the effects of gravity, jugular veins normally distend when the head is lowered below the level of the right atrium (RA), which is approximately at the point of the shoulder. Likewise, other superficial veins distend or collapse in relation to their gravitational position relative to the heart, as well as the level of venous tone and skin tautness.

Persistent jugular vein distension (when the head is erect) most often is associated with right-sided or biventricular congestive heart failure (CHF; **Figure 15.1**; also **Figure 10.5**, p. 212), including pericardial diseases. Occasionally, lesions that obstruct venous flow from the external jugular veins to the heart are responsible. These include intravascular obstruction within the cranial vena cava or RA (including tricuspid valve stenosis), bilateral jugular thrombosis (including catheter or pacing lead thrombosis), cranial caval compression from a mediastinal mass, and (rarely) obstruction by a cranial lung lobe tumor (**Table 15.1** and **Figure 15.2**). Iatrogenic plasma volume overload can lead to systemic venous distension with subcutaneous edema or pleural effusion. This condition is under-recognized in animals receiving sodium-replete fluids in hospital or in home settings.

Fluctuations in atrial pressure occur during the cardiac cycle related to atrial contraction (a wave), filling (v wave), and emptying (y descent) as well as suction created by ventricular contraction (x' descent) (**Figure 1.20**, p. 18 and related text). Right atrial pressure fluctuations reflect backward into the great veins and sometimes are visible as pulsations in the jugular veins. In the standing normal animal, with head erect, mild jugular pulsations often are noticed at the thoracic inlet up to the point of the shoulder. However, jugular pulsations normally do not extend higher than one third to one half of the distance up the neck from the thoracic inlet, above the point of the shoulder. Jugular pulsations visible higher on the neck indicate increased amplitude of pressure waves in the RA and often, increased mean right atrial pressure. Sometimes, tissue motion caused by pulsation of the underlying carotid arteries mimics jugular pulsations; this should be ruled out (see p. 37). Carotid pulse transmission is more likely to be visible in thin or excited animals. Additionally, prominent collapse of the jugular veins during ventricular contraction (x' descent) or after tricuspid valve opening (y descent) can be confused with a pathologic jugular pulse after the vein refills with blood; this is seen mainly in horses.

General Considerations

Right heart filling pressure and, therefore, central venous pressure (CVP) directly influence the degree of jugular (and other systemic) venous filling. As long as there is no obstructive lesion between the jugular veins and the RA, the appearance of the jugular veins provides an indication of right heart filling pressure. Functionally, CVP is coupled with cardiac output. Conditions that decrease cardiac output can lead to a rise in CVP. Intrathoracic pressure fluctuations during the respiratory cycle also influence CVP. During inspiration, there is a decrease in CVP, which tends to collapse the jugular veins; however, during this time there also is increased venous return and cardiac filling, so any visible pulsations are amplified. Venous distension secondary to elevated pressure in the RA often is accompanied by visible pulsations. Jugular vein distension without pulsation occurs with diseases that restrict or obstruct blood flow through the cranial vena cava or proximal jugular veins, as well as with an obstruction to venous inflow within the RA. Jugular pulsations also might be minimal with impaired right atrial filling (as with cardiac tamponade) or contractility failure (as from dilated cardiomyopathy with atrial fibrillation).

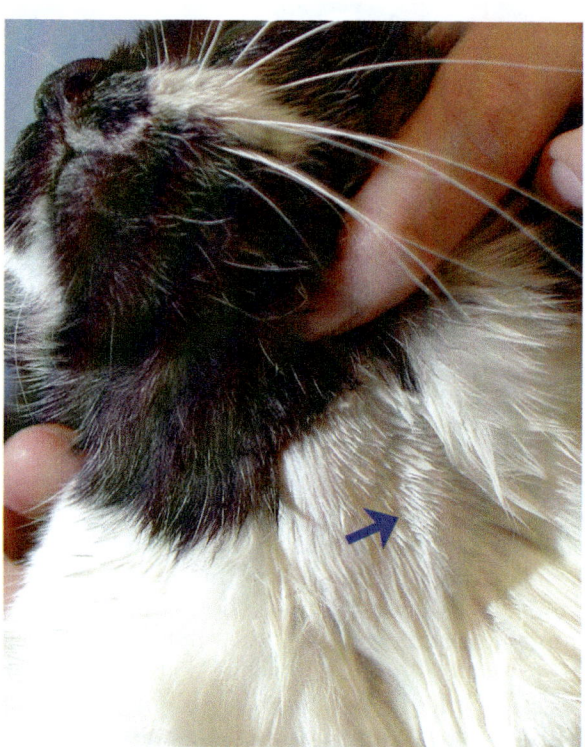

Figure 15.1 Right-sided congestive heart failure secondary to tricuspid valve dysplasia caused prominent jugular vein distension (arrow) in this cat.

Table 15.1 Causes of Jugular Vein Distension/Pulsation

Distension (Obstructed Venous Return)
- Cranial vena caval or bilateral jugular vein thrombosis
- Cranial mediastinal mass (or pulmonary mass) causing external compression
- Cranial right atrial mass obstructing venous return (often with pleural effusion)[a]

Distension (with Elevated Mean Right Atrial Pressure or Right-Sided CHF)
- Tricuspid valve disease (from dysplasia with or without stenosis, degeneration, endocarditis)
- Functional tricuspid regurgitation (from cardiomyopathy or pulmonary hypertension)
- Pulmonary stenosis (valvular, supravalvular, heart base tumor obstructing branch pulmonary arteries)
- Right ventricular cardiomyopathy
- Dilated cardiomyopathy (often complicated by atrial fibrillation)
- Pericardial effusion with cardiac tamponade
- Pulmonary hypertension from any cause (including heartworm disease)
- Volume overload/hypervolemia (iatrogenic, anemia with fluid retention)

Pulsation (with or without Jugular Venous Distension)
- Right ventricular hypertrophy from any cause with increased myocardial stiffness (giant a wave)
- Tricuspid regurgitation from any cause (prominent v wave, also see above list)
- Congenital tricuspid valve stenosis (giant a wave)
- Pulmonic stenosis (giant a wave)
- Complex congenital heart disease (such as tetralogy of Fallot, double-outlet right ventricle)
- Pulmonary hypertension from any cause (including heartworm disease, giant a- or v wave)
- Arrhythmia causing AV dissociation (cannon a wave)
  - Junctional tachycardia
  - Complete (third-degree) AV block
  - Ventricular premature contractions
  - Ventricular tachycardia
- Marked bradycardia
- Pericardial effusion with tamponade
- Constrictive pericarditis
- Hypervolemia

[a] Caudal right atrial obstruction will result in ascites.
Abbreviations: AV, atrioventricular; CHF, congestive heart failure.

As noted above, jugular pulse waves are related to right atrial contraction, filling, and emptying over the cardiac cycle. Atrial pressure waves are more likely to reflect backward a greater distance, and be visible higher on the jugular veins, when mean pressure in the RA is elevated or positive pressure fluctuations are accentuated. For example, tricuspid valve insufficiency can produce a visible jugular pulse after the first heart sound (S_1), as blood regurgitates into the RA during ventricular contraction. The v wave on the atrial pressure tracing becomes magnified and the pressure wave reflects toward the jugular veins (**Figure 15.3**); this is accentuated if CVP also is elevated from heart failure. With severe tricuspid insufficiency, the c and v waves fuse and the x descent is lost (causing "giant cv waves"). In contrast, pathologic jugular pulsations that originate during vigorous right atrial contraction (just prior to the S_1), stem from diseases that increase right ventricular (RV) stiffness and restrict early diastolic (rapid) filling of the ventricle. Ventricular filling then shifts increasingly to the atrial contraction. Examples include RV hypertrophy from any cause, as well as constrictive pericardial disease. The accentuated pressure waves reflect backward as "giant a waves" (**Figure 15.4**).

Cardiac arrhythmias that cause dissociation of atrial and ventricular contractions can produce intermittent, bounding jugular pulse waves. These so-called "cannon a waves" occur when the atria happen to contract against closed atrioventricular (AV) valves, causing retrograde blood flow toward the venae cavae and jugular veins (**Figure 15.5**). Complete (third-degree) AV block with a ventricular escape rhythm and ventricular tachycardia are the most common causes. Identifying cannon a waves in a patient with a regular tachycardia can help to distinguish a ventricular from a supraventricular tachycardia.

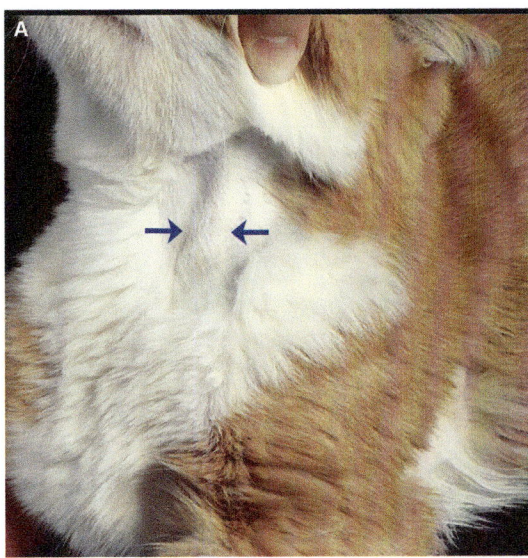
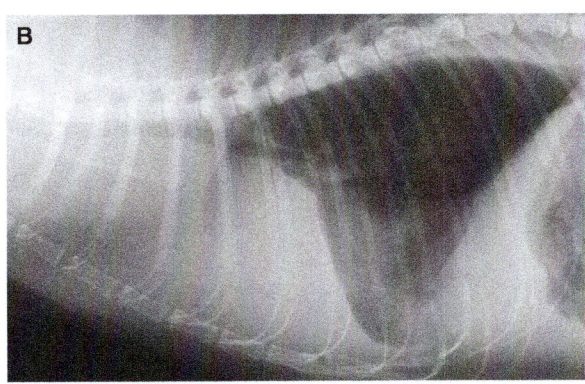

Figure 15.2 Marked jugular vein distension (A; arrows) in a 5-year-old cat with anorexia, lethargy, and respiratory difficulty. The cat also had subcutaneous edema along the ventral jaw, thoracic inlet and forelimbs. (B) Lateral thoracic radiograph from this cat shows soft-tissue/fluid opacity in the cranial mediastinum, which obscures the cardiac silhouette. The caudal displacement of cranial lung lobes and dorsal displacement of the trachea are consistent with a cranial mediastinal mass, which in this case was mediastinal lymphoma. A moderate volume of pleural effusion also is evident. Cranial vena caval compression by the mass led to the jugular distension and cranial body edema (so-called cranial caval syndrome).

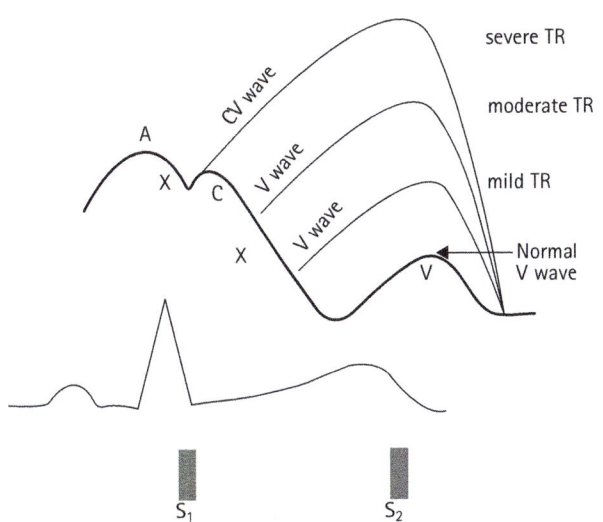

Figure 15.3 Diagram of how the severity of tricuspid regurgitation (TR) affects the jugular pulse wave, timed against ECG waveforms and heart sounds. The bold line indicates the normal jugular venous (right atrial) pressure waveforms. Atrial contraction causes the "a wave" (A). The "x descent" (X) begins with atrial relaxation and descent of the atrial floor at the onset of ventricular contraction. A small "c wave" (C) occurs during ventricular contraction, at the time of the carotid pulse; (the continuation of the x descent often is called the "x' wave"). Continued atrial filling during ventricular systole creates the "v wave" (V). The y descent (not labeled) follows the v wave, as atrial pressure falls after the tricuspid valve opens and ventricular filling begins. Worsening TR severity progressively minimizes the x descent and increases v wave magnitude; severe TR creates a large, combined "cv wave." (From Braunwald E, Perloff JK. Physical examination of the heart and circulation. In, Braunwald E, Zipes DP, Libby P (editors). Heart Diseases: A Textbook of Cardiovascular Medicine, 6th edition. WB Saunders, Philadelphia, PA. 2001. p. 49.)

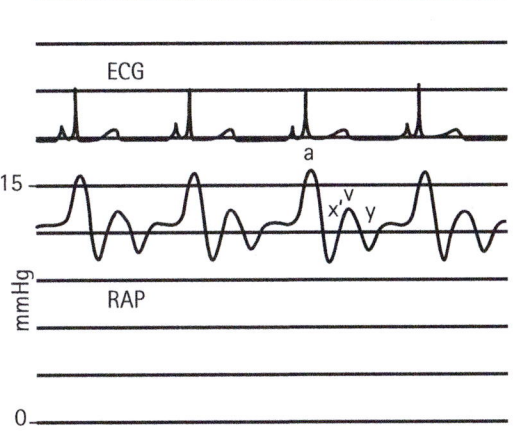

Figure 15.4 Right atrial pressure (RAP) recording from a 5-year-old male Bulldog with pulmonic stenosis and right-sided congestive heart failure (CHF). Jugular distension and pulsation were evident clinically. Overall RAP is elevated (mean ~13 mm Hg) secondary to the CHF. The "a wave" is especially prominent (peak >15 mm Hg), consistent with increased stiffness of the hypertrophied right ventricle.

Approach to the Patient with Jugular Vein Distension or Pulsation

The presence of a jugular vein abnormality offers a window into right atrial pressures and a valuable clue to the underlying disease process. Unfortunately, jugular vein examination often is overlooked, or insufficiently evaluated in longer-haired animals. The patient should be in a normal upright posture, with horizontal head position, for this evaluation. The skin should

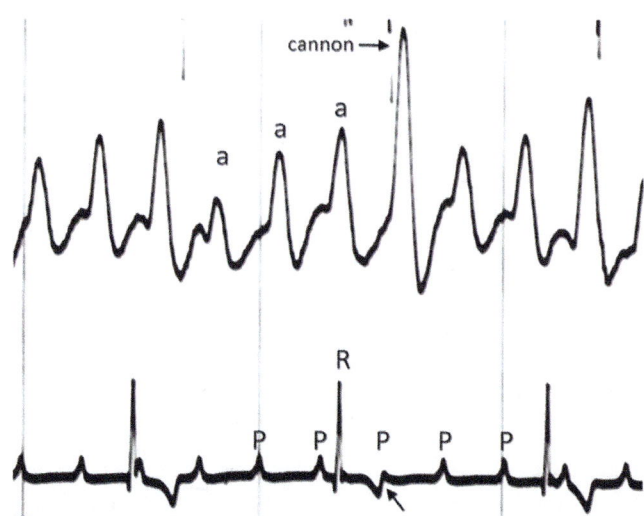

Figure 15.5 Right atrial (RA) pressure (top) and simultaneous ECG (bottom) recording showing "cannon a wave" in a dog with complete atrioventricular (AV) block. Multiple nonconducted P waves (P; bottom tracing) are evident, along with junctional or ventricular escape complexes (R). The atrial contractions that follow the P waves create isolated "a waves" (a) in the RA pressure tracing. By coincidence, one P wave (arrow; bottom) and its associated atrial contraction occur at the end of a ventricular contraction. Atrial contraction against the closed tricuspid valve markedly increases RA pressure, producing a "cannon a wave" (arrow; top). (Recording courtesy of Dr. Robert L Hamlin.)

not be stretched taut and the right jugular vein should be evaluated preferentially. The jugular veins should fill then empty quickly after release of manual compression at the thoracic inlet. The clinician should check for abnormal distension and/or pulsation, and if present, determine whether both veins are equally involved. Especially in anxious or thin animals, it is important to differentiate pulse waves arising from the carotid arteries from true jugular pulsations (see p. 37), or vigorous jugular venous collapse with refilling. A careful history and complete physical examination can provide evidence of heart disease or other potential underlying cause (**Figure 15.6**).

The abdominojugular (hepatojugular) reflux test is a provocative maneuver that can magnify jugular distension and pulsation in small animals with equivocal findings. A positive test most often suggests RV hypertrophy, impaired filling, or tricuspid regurgitation. (See p. 37 for a description of the technique and **Figure 2.5**.)

Abnormal distension of other superficial, ventrally located veins also can occur with right-sided CHF, volume overload, or a central obstruction to venous return. Local or regional venous distension, with or without tissue edema, can be caused by an arteriovenous fistula, thrombophlebitis, or venous thrombosis. Of course, other causes of subcutaneous edema, such as vasculitis, lymphangitis, lymphangiosarcoma, or hypoproteinemia, should be considered if the regional veins are not distended.

Central Venous Pressure Measurement

Measurement of CVP is useful to verify high systemic venous pressure or to monitor right heart filling pressure during fluid therapy in certain patients. The CVP normally is low. Ranges of 5–10 cm H_2O (~3.7–7.4 mm Hg) for normal dogs and standing horses, and 2–5 cm H_2O (~1.5–3.7 mm Hg) for normal cats, have been reported. CVP fluctuations that parallel intrapleural pressure changes occur during respiration.

Intravascular volume, venous compliance, cardiac function, and intrapleural pressure all influence CVP. Diseases that cause right-sided CHF or pericardial restriction to cardiac filling also increase CVP. CVP measurement might help the clinician differentiate these conditions from other causes of pleural or peritoneal effusion. However, a large volume (for example, >20 ml/kg body weight) of pleural effusion can increase intrapleural pressure and compress the heart to the point where cardiac filling is impaired. This can raise CVP even in the absence of cardiac disease. Therefore, in patients with moderate- to large-volume pleural effusion, CVP should be measured after thoracocentesis. Sometimes CVP is used to monitor critical patients receiving large-volume fluid infusions. However, the CVP is not an accurate reflection of left heart filling pressure and as such, is not reliable for detecting the onset (or monitoring treatment) of cardiogenic pulmonary edema. There probably are better methods for assessing volume status, including careful serial study of jugular veins and point-of-care ultrasound examination of the caudal vena cava for size and diameter changes during ventilation.

To measure CVP, a large bore jugular catheter that extends into the RA, or close to it within the cranial vena cava, is placed aseptically. Alternatively, a peripherally inserted central catheter that extends into the vena cava near to the RA can be used. The location of the catheter tip should be verified by radiography, or possibly by ultrasound. The patient

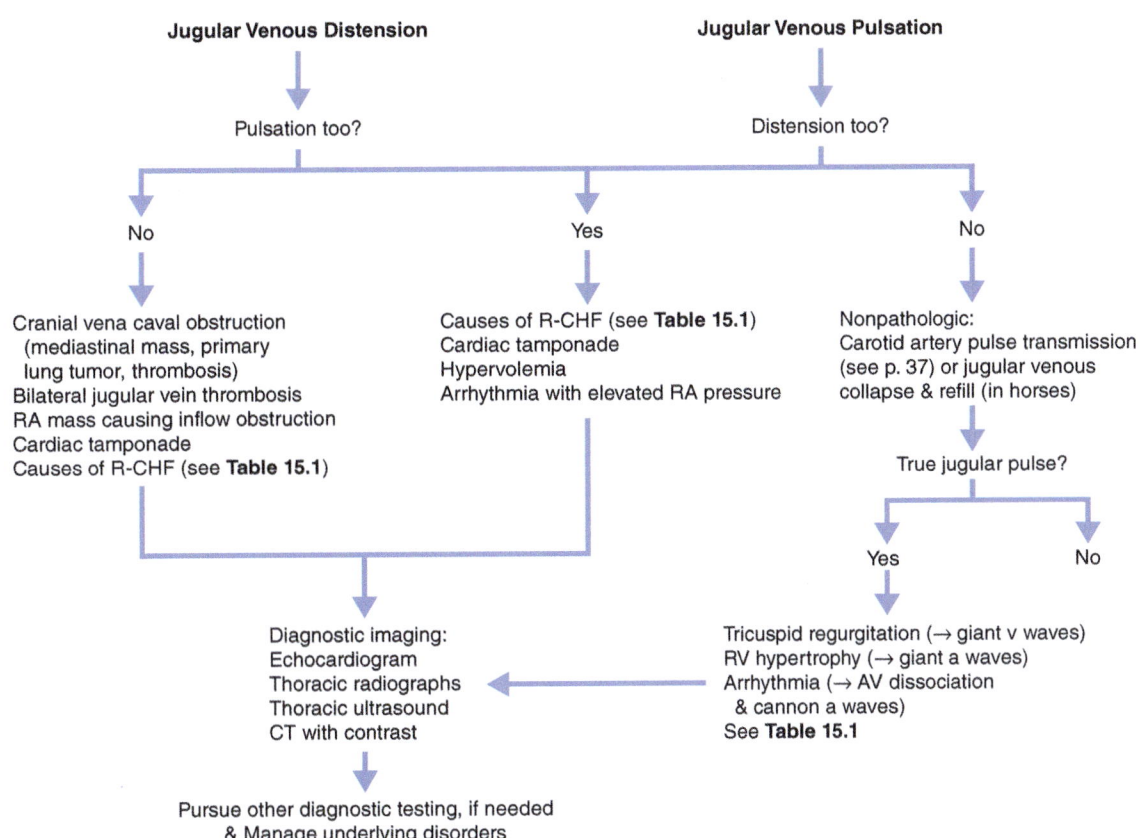

Figure 15.6 Approach to the patient with jugular venous distension or pulsation. These are general guidelines & diagnostic considerations; exceptions could occur. AV, atrioventricular; CT, computed tomography; RA, right atrial; R-CHF, right-sided congestive heart failure; RV, right ventricular.

is placed in lateral or sternal recumbency and the catheter is connected via extension tubing and a three-way stopcock to either a fluid-filled pressure transducer system or a fluid administration set and water manometer. If using the former, position the pressure transducer at the horizontal level of the patient's RA and calibrate zero baseline to atmospheric pressure. Then turn the stopcock off to air and record the patient's CVP (in mm Hg). If using the water manometer system, attach a sterile water manometer tube to the stopcock and position it vertically, with the stopcock (representing 0 cm H_2O) located at the same horizontal level as the patient's RA (**Figure 15.7**). Then turn the stopcock off to the animal, allowing the manometer to fill with sterile crystalloid fluid; finally, turn the stopcock off to the fluid reservoir to allow the fluid column in the manometer to equilibrate with the animal's CVP. Small fluctuations of the fluid meniscus within the manometer occur with the heartbeat; slightly larger movement is associated with respiration. Marked change in the height of the fluid column associated with the heartbeat suggests either severe tricuspid regurgitation or that the catheter tip is within the right ventricle. Repeated measurements will be more consistent when taken with the animal and pressure transducer or manometer in the same position and during the expiratory phase of respiration.

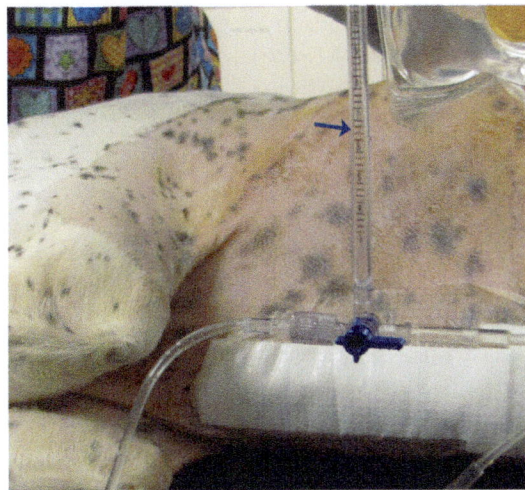

Figure 15.7 Central venous pressure (CVP) measurement using a sterile water manometer, in a dog with a jugular venous catheter that extends into the cranial vena cava. Extension tubing (to the left) connects the jugular catheter to a three-way stopcock. The manometer is inserted (vertically) into the side port of the stopcock and the fluid administration line is connected to the right. The stopcock is suspended at the (horizontal) level of the dog's right atrium, as the zero reference point. First, the stopcock is briefly turned "off" to the dog, so that fluid almost fills the manometer. Next, the stopcock is turned "off" to the fluid line (shown); this allows the fluid level within the manometer to equilibrate with the patient's CVP. This dog's CVP is normal at slightly under 7 cm H_2O (blue arrow).

Suggested Additional Reading and References

Also See Online Comprehensive Bibliography at: https://www.routledge.com/9781482246223.

Byars TD, Dainis CM, Seltzer KL, et al. Cranial thoracic masses in the horse: a sequel to pleuropneumonia. Equine Vet J 1991;23:22–24.

Chow RS, Kass PH, Haskins SC. Evaluation of peripheral and central venous pressure in awake dogs and cats. Am J Vet Res 2006;67:1987–1991.

Conn RD, O'Keefe JH. Cardiac physical diagnosis in the digital age: an important but increasingly neglected skill (from stethoscopes to microchips). Am J Cardiol 2009;104:590–595.

Davis JL, Gardner SY, Schwabenton B, et al. Congestive heart failure in horses: 14 cases (1984-2001). J Am Vet Med Assoc 2002;220:1512–1515.

Drozdzynska MJ, Chang YM, Stanzani G, et al. Evaluation of the dynamic predictors of fluid responsiveness in dogs receiving goal-directed fluid therapy. Vet Anaesth Analg 2018;45:22–30.

Gookin JL, Atkins CE. Evaluation of the effect of pleural effusion on central venous pressure in cats. J Vet Intern Med 1999;13:561–563.

Hall MF. Jugular catheterization and central venous pressure measurement. In, Ettinger SJ, Feldman EC, Cote E (editors). Textbook of Veterinary Internal Medicine. 8th edition. Elsevier, St. Louis, MO. 2017. pp. 303–305.

Hutchinson KM, Shaw SP. A review of Central venous pressure and its reliability as a hemodynamic monitoring tool in veterinary medicine. Top Companion Anim Med 2016;31:109–121.

Machon RG, Raffe MR, Robinson EP. Central venous pressure measurements in the caudal vena cava of sedated cats. J Vet Emerg Crit Care 1995;5:121–129.

Magdesian KG, Fielding CL, Rhodes DM, et al. Changes in central venous pressure and blood lactate concentration in response to acute blood loss in horses. J Am Vet Med Assoc 2006;229:1458–1462.

Mulz JM, Kraus MS, Thompson M, et al. Cranial vena caval syndrome secondary to central venous obstruction associated with a pacemaker lead in a dog. J Vet Cardiol 2010;12:217–223.

Nelson NC, Drost WT, Lerche P, et al. Noninvasive estimation of central venous pressure in anesthetized dogs by measurement of hepatic venous blood flow velocity and abdominal venous diameter. Vet Radiol Ultrasound 2010;51:313–323.

Nolen-Walston RD, Norton JL, Navas de Solis C, et al. The effects of hypohydration on central venous pressure and splenic volume in adult horses. J Vet Intern Med 2011;25:570–574.

Norton JL, Nolen-Walston RD, Underwood C, et al. Repeatability, reproducibility, and effect of head position on central venous pressure measurement in standing adult horses. J Vet Intern Med 2011;25:575–578.

Norton JL, Nolen-Walston RD, Underwood C, et al. Comparison of water manometry to 2 commercial electronic pressure monitors for central venous pressure measurement in horses. J Vet Intern Med 2011;25:303–306.

Palmer KG, King LG, Van Winkle TJ. Clinical manifestations and associated disease syndromes in dogs with cranial vena cava thrombosis: 17 cases (1989–1996). J Am Vet Med Assoc 1998;213:220–224.

Singh A, Brisson BA. Chylothorax associated with thrombosis of the cranial vena cava. Can Vet J 2010;51:847–852.

Tam K, Rezende M, Boscan P. Correlation between jugular and central venous pressures in laterally recumbent horses. Vet Anaesth Analg 2011;38:580–583.

Valverde A, Gianotti G, Rioja-Garcia E, et al. Effects of high-volume, rapid-fluid therapy on cardiovascular function and hematological values during isoflurane-induced hypotension in healthy dogs. Can J Vet Res 2012;76:99–108.

Wilsterman S, Hackett ES, Rao S, et al. A technique for central venous pressure measurement in normal horses. J Vet Emerg Crit Care 2009;19:241–246.

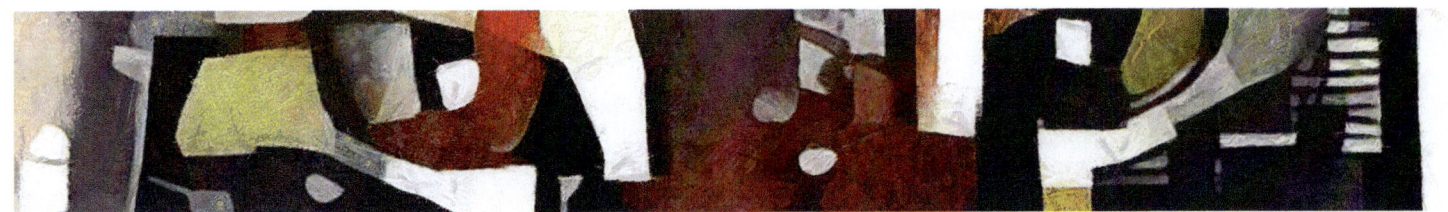

16
ABDOMINAL DISTENSION

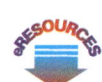

Abdominal distension usually is a sign of an underlying disease process, unless caused by pregnancy or obesity. The abdomen can become distended because of marked intra-abdominal organ enlargement, a large mass lesion, or the accumulation of fat or free peritoneal fluid (**Table 16.1**). A serous membrane of mesothelial cells lines the peritoneal cavity (as the parietal layer) and extends to cover the abdominal organs and the associated vasculature and connective tissue (as the visceral layer). This membrane allows transudation and absorption of fluid, and it can serve a protective function (for example, by walling-off an area of infection). The space between the parietal and visceral peritoneal layers normally contains a small amount of serous fluid. Several disease processes cause excessive abdominal fluid (effusion) to accumulate.

General Considerations

As a manifestation of cardiovascular disease, abdominal fluid accumulation (ascites) is caused by right-sided or biventricular congestive heart failure (CHF) or impaired venous inflow to the right heart (**Figure 16.1**). When associated with heart disease, the fluid is classified cytologically as a transudate, modified transudate, or rarely, chyle (see **Table 10.4**, p. 216, for fluid classification guidelines). In contrast, exudative abdominal effusions, either septic or nonseptic, are characteristic of an inflammatory process involving all or part of the peritoneal cavity (peritonitis). Hemorrhage within the peritoneal space is referred to as a hemoabdomen. Urine collection within the peritoneal space (uroabdomen) is uncommon and most often arises from a rupture of the urinary bladder. The presence of free air in the peritoneal space (pneumoperitoneum), aside from postoperative situations, is a sign of potentially life-threatening bowel devitalization or perforation.

Regardless of the cause, abdominal enlargement tends to push the diaphragm cranially and it can interfere with respiration; compression of abdominal organs, such as the kidneys, could impair their function. Massive abdominal distension, as with large-volume ascites, can cause respiratory distress. Abdominal enlargement can be associated with pain, especially during acute distension of the peritoneal space or stomach. Inflammation of the peritoneum or other intra-abdominal structures is likely to cause pain and systemic signs of disease. Disorders associated with uroabdomen, bile peritonitis, intestinal leakage, or free abdominal air can rapidly progress to systemic signs of critical illness.

Abdominal Effusions

Peritoneal effusion usually results from an imbalance of Starling's forces (Chapter 1), similar to the formation of pleural effusion. An increase in systemic venous or portal hydrostatic pressures is a major cause. Increased capillary endothelial permeability (from inflammation or other vascular disruption) or low capillary colloid oncotic pressure (from severe hypoalbuminemia) are other mechanisms affecting transcapillary fluid movement. Obstruction in the lymphatic drainage system also promotes peritoneal effusion accumulation.

Ascites caused by high venous and (consequently) capillary hydrostatic pressures is categorized according to the location of the pathology. "Posthepatic" or "postsinusoidal" ascites occurs when blood flow is restricted or obstructed between the hepatic veins and the right ventricle. Excessive fluid (hepatic lymph) formation occurs, derived mainly from ultrafiltration across the hepatic capillaries (sinusoids), and the fluid percolates across the liver capsule. If the rate of formation exceeds the lymphatic capacity to drain the peritoneal space, ascites will develop. This fluid typically is a modified transudate related to the "leaky" walls of the sinusoids and associated high protein content. Total protein concentration associated with posthepatic obstruction generally falls

Table 16.1 Causes of Abdominal Distension

Free Peritoneal Fluid
- Transudate
  - Hypoalbuminemia (as from glomerulopathy/nephrotic syndrome, protein-losing enteropathy, intestinal malabsorption or maldigestion, heavy parasitism, liver failure, starvation)
- Modified transudate
  - Right-sided or biventricular CHF
    - Pulmonary stenosis (congenital and acquired, including obstructions of pulmonary artery)
    - Double-chambered right ventricle (intracavitary obstruction)
    - Tricuspid valve insufficiency or tricuspid valve stenosis
    - Dilated cardiomyopathy
    - Pericardial disease (effusion with tamponade, or constrictive)
    - Pulmonary hypertension, including heartworm disease
    - Intracardiac tumor
    - Tachycardia- or bradycardia-induced heart failure
  - Caudal vena caval or right atrial inflow obstruction (Budd–Chiari pathophysiology)
    - Caval thrombus, fibrosis, or neoplastic invasion (pheochromocytoma)
    - External compression of vena cava (tumor, trauma, diaphragmatic hernia)
    - Cor triatriatum dexter
  - Hepatic vein obstruction or thrombosis
    - Hepatic cirrhosis
    - Other causes of portal hypertension
    - Neoplasia (liver, lymphoma, other)
    - Carcinomatosis
    - Mesothelioma
- Chyle
  - Traumatic rupture of major lymph channel
  - Neoplastic obstruction of lymphatics (lymphoma involving lymph channels, other neoplasia)
  - Intestinal lymphangiectasia
  - Intestinal obstruction with rupture of lymphatics
  - Thoracic duct ligation/obstruction
  - Right-sided or biventricular CHF (uncommon; see modified transudate, above)
- Hemorrhage
  - Hemangiosarcoma or other neoplasm (spleen, other sites)
  - Coagulopathy or anticoagulant toxicity
  - Trauma
- Nonseptic exudate
  - Gall bladder or bile duct tear/bile peritonitis
  - Pancreatitis
  - Neoplasia
  - Parasitic peritonitis (as from *Mesocestoides* species)
  - Feline infectious peritonitis (coronavirus)
  - Steatitis (cats)
- Septic exudate
  - Perforated bowel
  - Devitalized intestinal wall (as with ischemia, intussusception, thrombosis)
  - Pyometra/uterine rupture
  - Other septic peritonitis (including *Actinomyces* or *Nocardia* species infection)
- Uroabdomen (ruptured bladder or urethra)

Organ or Soft Tissue Enlargement
- Gastric distention
  - Gastric dilatation +/− volvulus
  - Aerophagia
  - Pyloric obstruction
- Intestinal distension
  - Ileus
  - Intestinal obstruction
  - Obstipation/megacolon
- Hepatomegaly
  - Venous congestion (right-sided or biventricular CHF, caudal caval obstruction)
  - Neoplastic infiltration
  - Hyperadrenocorticism
  - Hepatic lipidosis
- Splenomegaly
  - Venous congestion (including from torsion)
  - Neoplastic infiltration
  - Infection (as from *Rickettsia* and mycoplasma species)
  - Immune-mediated disease
- Fat
- Pregnancy
- Pyometra
- Renomegaly
  - Ureteral obstruction
  - Neoplastic infiltration
  - Cyst
- Tumor (of spleen, liver, lymph nodes, intestine, ovary, retained testicle, or other organ)
- Chronic urinary bladder distension
  - Urethral obstruction
  - Neurologic dysfunction

Marked Abdominal Muscle Weakness
- Hyperadrenocorticism

Abbreviations: CHF, congestive heart failure.

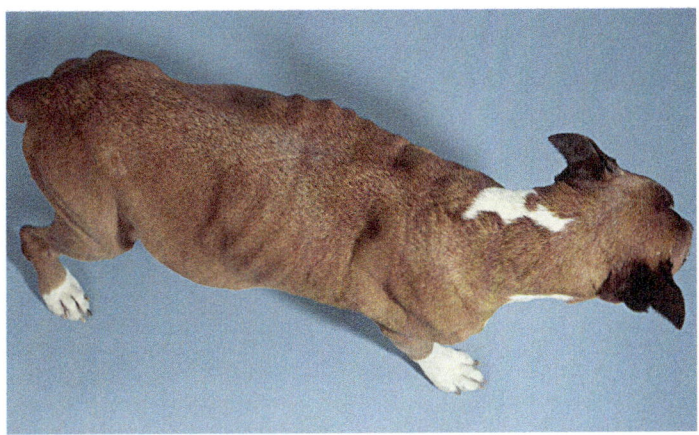

Figure 16.1 Photo of an older male Boxer with ascites secondary to cardiac tamponade, caused by an aortic body tumor. Cachexia is evident from the loss of muscle around ribs and iliac crests.

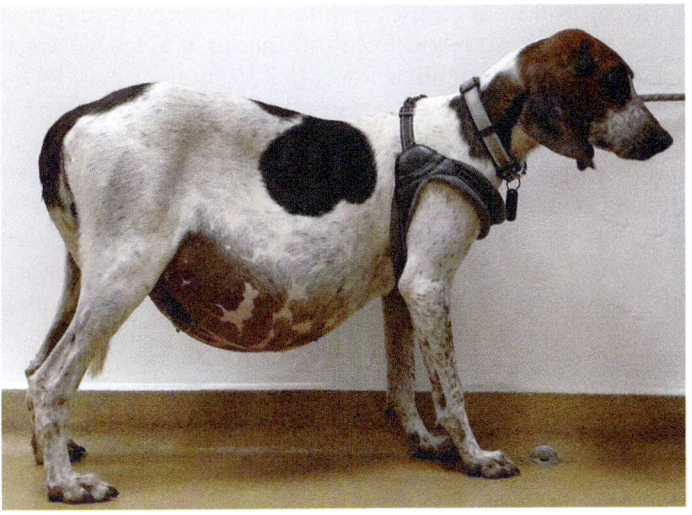

Figure 16.3 This hound dog developed massive ascites secondary to an obstructive lesion in the caudal vena cava.

between 3.0 and 4.0 g/dL, but occasionally exceeds 4 g/dL. This fluid also can be tinged with blood.

Posthepatic ascites usually is secondary to CHF, cardiac tamponade, or constrictive pericarditis (**Figure 16.2**). Uncommon causes include caudal vena caval (CaVC) or hepatic venous obstruction from thrombus, tumor infiltration, trauma, diaphragmatic hernia, or idiopathic fibrous narrowing of the caudal vena cava (**Figure 16.3**; and **Figures 36.19** and **36.20**, p. 762). Intracardiac causes include obstructive intracardiac tumors (Chapter 35), or right atrial (RA) inflow obstruction from congenital tricuspid valve stenosis or cor triatriatum dexter (see Chapters 27 and 28, respectively; and **Figure 28.1**, p. 512). The term "Budd–Chiari-like syndrome or pathophysiology" has been used to describe postsinusoidal portal hypertension and ascites that result from CaVC or RA inflow obstructions.

Dogs are more likely to develop ascites as a manifestation of CHF than cats or horses. Yet heart failure-induced ascites can occur in cats, especially those with dilated, restrictive, or arrhythmogenic right ventricular forms of cardiomyopathy, with congenital malformations involving the right heart, or with pericardial disease. Small amounts of ascites or abdominal fluid collection in horses might be evident only on ultrasound examination of the abdomen. In horses, subcutaneous (ventral) edema is expected as well. When ascites is secondary to CHF, jugular vein distension and pulsation usually are evident because central venous pressure (CVP) is high. However, the jugular veins will appear normal when the inflow obstruction is localized to the caudal right atrium or caudal vena cava. In addition, jugular distension and pulsation can be masked by diuretic therapy, even in patients with residual ascites, although a positive abdominojugular (hepatojugular) reflex often persists. Hepatomegaly also develops from passive venous congestion caused by right heart failure, or RA or CaVC obstruction. Abdominal ultrasound will demonstrate hepatic venous distension and CaVC dilation, with decreased respiratory variation in its diameter.

So-called "hepatic" ascites, caused by primary liver disease, usually is a transudate or modified transudate. The mechanism largely involves portal hypertension, and relates to disease within the portal veins or within the hepatic sinusoids, although other mechanisms might be involved especially with hepatic cirrhosis. "Prehepatic" ascites develops

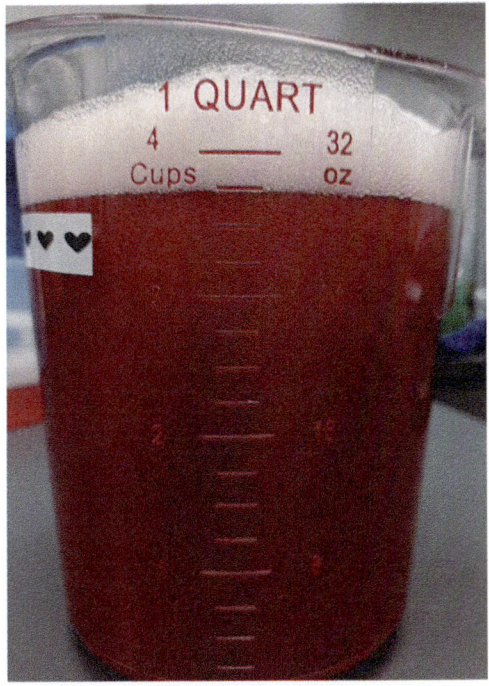

Figure 16.2 A large volume of serosanguinous, modified transudate drained from the abdomen of a dog with right-sided congestive heart failure secondary to pulmonary hypertension.

when blood flow is restricted at the level of the portal vein; excess fluid transudation from the intestinal serosa leads to ascites. This fluid usually is lower in protein than that of posthepatic ascites. Prehepatic causes of ascites are relatively uncommon because collateral portosystemic shunting often develops as portal pressure rises, thus reducing portal hypertension. Complications of surgery are another cause.

Effusions classified as pure transudates are most common with severe hypoalbuminemia. Protein-losing glomerulopathy and enteropathy are likely causes. Chylous abdominal effusion contains intestinal lymph with high lipid content and is comparably rare. Causes of lymphatic disruption and leakage include neoplasia, trauma, infection, and potentially, severe right-sided CHF. Neoplastic infiltration of the abdominal serosa can produce a modified transudate or an exudate related to inflammation and capillary obstruction. Increased capillary permeability as well as inflammatory cell recruitment occur from the effects of inflammatory mediators. Nonseptic exudates also are caused by the presence of bile or urine in the abdominal cavity. Traumatic rupture of the gallbladder or a biliary duct leads to bile peritonitis. A tear in the bladder or ureter results in uroabdomen. Feline infectious peritonitis is an important cause of nonseptic, exudative abdominal effusion in cats. Septic exudates usually are caused by bacterial infection. Sources can include intestinal perforation or devitalization, extension from infection or abscess in adjacent tissues, surgical contamination or wound dehiscence, and injury related to abdominal trauma (blunt or sharp). Bleeding into the peritoneal cavity (hemoabdomen) occurs from trauma, coagulopathy (including rodenticide toxicity), or neoplastic invasion, especially with hemangiosarcoma of the spleen, liver, or other abdominal organs.

During the formation of peritoneal effusion from any cause, fluid is redistributed out of the vascular space into the peritoneal cavity. The reduction in effective plasma volume stimulates compensatory mechanisms (such as the renin–angiotensin–aldosterone system and antidiuretic hormone release) to expand total body water and sodium (p. 29).

Other Causes of Abdominal Distension

Marked organomegaly can cause abdominal distension. Pregnancy must considered in the intact female. Excessive fat accumulation is responsible for abdominal enlargement in some individuals. Chronic venous congestion will enlarge the liver (as with chronic CHF or CaVC obstruction). Splenomegaly is more variable in CHF and uncommonly causes overt abdominal distension. However, congestion from splenic torsion, splenitis, immune mediated diseases, and neoplastic infiltration can be dramatic in some patients. The stomach or intestines can distend greatly with gas or fluid. Examples include aerophagia (usually secondary to respiratory distress), as well as gastric dilatation with or without volvulus, ileus, or bowel obstruction. Obstipation, especially in cats with megacolon, can enlarge the abdomen. Similarly, urinary bladder dilation from chronic urethral obstruction or neurologic dysfunction, or renomegaly secondary to ureteral obstruction, might underlie abdominal distension. Abdominal distension in animals with hyperadrenocorticism is associated with abdominal wall muscle weakness as well as hepatomegaly and often, obesity. Diffuse or localized neoplastic infiltration also causes generalized organ enlargement. Common examples are hemangiosarcoma of the spleen or liver, lymphoma, or primary liver cancers. Discrete mass lesions could be neoplastic or inflammatory in nature.

Abdominal enlargement often progresses slowly and might be interpreted by the owner simply as weight gain. Exceptions include traumatic intra-abdominal hemorrhage, ruptured bladder, or gastric dilatation with or without volvulus. Decreased activity, exercise intolerance, reduced appetite, and increased respiratory rate often accompany abdominal distension of any cause as ventilation becomes restricted by cranial displacement of the diaphragm. Moreover, some disorders associated with ascites also lead to pleural effusion, pulmonary congestion, or pericardial effusion, which also can impact ventilation.

Approach to the Patient with Abdominal Distension

A complete history and a careful physical examination may reveal the likely cause, especially if signs of heart disease or other abnormalities (such as jugular venous distension) are found. Initial diagnostic questions relate to whether the distension is caused by peritoneal fluid accumulation, organomegaly, a mass lesion, or a combination (**Figure 16.4**). Pregnancy should be ruled out in the intact female.

Organomegaly, larger mass lesions, and free peritoneal fluid usually can be detected by abdominal palpation. Small amounts of fluid tend to make the intestines feel slippery as they pass under the examiner's fingers during palpation. A larger volume of ascites will cause a fluid wave during abdominal ballottement (p. 42). A "quick-look" or focused assessment with sonography in trauma (FAST) ultrasound scan also can help rapidly identify abdominal effusion (**Figure 16.5**).

Animals with ascites caused by heart failure generally have concurrent jugular vein distension (usually with pulsation), unless vascular volume has been reduced by diuretic therapy. A murmur, gallop sound, or arrhythmia also is common. Muffled heart sounds are typical of a large pericardial effusion or concurrent pleural effusion. Abdominal tenderness usually is evident with peritonitis and sometimes is present with noninflammatory causes of ascites. Poor body condition (cachexia) is common with chronic heart failure (**Figure 16.1**; also **Figure 2.1**, p. 35), neoplasia, and diseases that cause hypoalbuminemia.

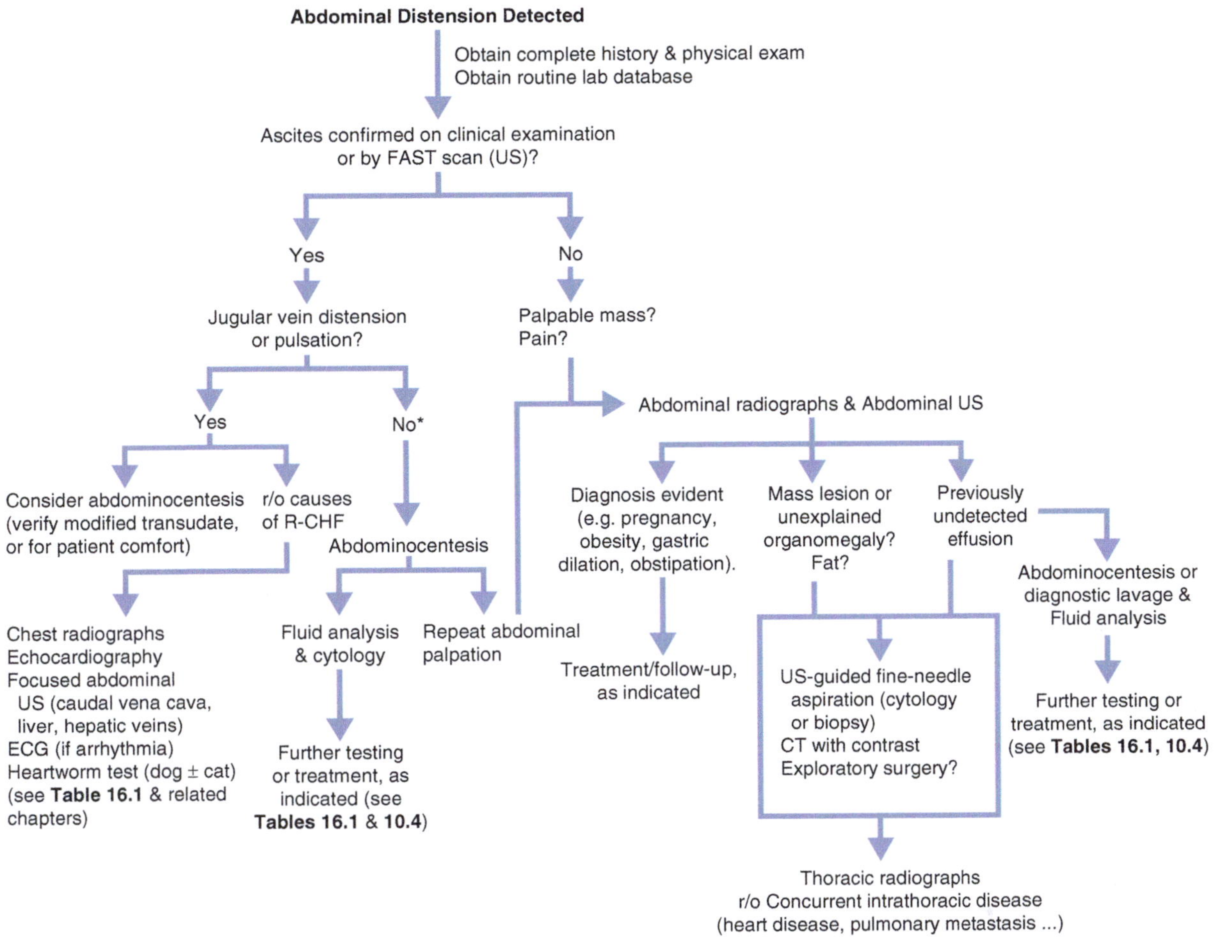

Figure 16.4 Approach to the patient with abdominal distension. These are general guidelines; exceptions can occur. *Jugular distension might not be evident following diuretic therapy or other causes of reduced circulating volume, or if there is isolated caudal vena caval obstruction. R-CHF still should be considered if another etiology of ascites is not evident. CT, computed tomography; ECG, electrocardiogram; FAST, focused assessment with sonography in trauma; R-CHF, right-sided (or biventricular) congestive heart failure; r/o, rule out; US, ultrasound.

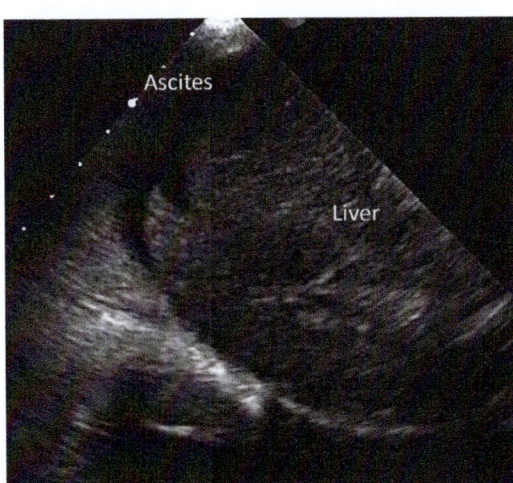

Figure 16.5 Abdominal ultrasound image from a 10-year-old Boxer with a history of collapse episodes. Physical examination had revealed abdominal enlargement, with a slight fluid wave on ballottement. Ascites is visible as the echolucent area adjacent to the liver.

Abdominal radiographs are useful for delineating organomegaly and mass lesions; however, free peritoneal fluid produces a hazy, "ground glass" appearance that obscures serosal margins. Abdominocentesis prior to radiography is recommended in cases with moderate- to large-volume peritoneal effusions to improve radiographic visualization. Nevertheless, gas-filled bowel loops, displacement of other organs by a large mass lesion, or free abdominal gas associated with peritonitis still can be appreciated. A sample of fluid obtained during abdominocentesis should be saved in sterile serum (clot) and EDTA tubes for biochemical and cytologic analysis and culture, if indicated.

Abdominal ultrasonography has largely supplanted radiography for assessment of the peritoneal space, architecture of normal organs and abnormal structures, and assessment of venous drainage and other blood vessels. Changes in echogenicity, shape or size of specific organs, mass lesions, vascular abnormalities, and small volumes of peritoneal effusion can be detected. Ultrasound-guided needle biopsy or aspiration can be performed.

Diagnostic testing in patients with ascites or abdominal organomegaly also should include complete blood count, serum biochemical profile, and urinalysis. Depending on the initial results, further diagnostic evaluation might be indicated. In most patients with ascites, thoracic radiographs and echocardiography are warranted. Additional studies that could be helpful include electrocardiography, heartworm testing, coagulation tests, endocrine tests (such as for hyperadrenocorticism), or computed tomography. Surgical exploration might be necessary in some cases; however, it is important to rule out a cardiac cause for ascites first.

Specific therapy for abdominal effusions is based on the underlying diagnosis. For patients with ascites, diuretic therapy might or might not be helpful, so it is important to identify the underlying cause. Therapy for heart failure is outlined in Chapters 21 and 22; (also see other chapters in this text relevant to specific cardiac diseases). Obstruction to CaVC flow sometimes is amenable to surgical or interventional catheterization procedures (stenting). Abdominocentesis is an important treatment for tense ascites, despite the potential loss of protein. Recent studies have emphasized the negative effects of compression and of high splanchnic venous pressures on renal function. With chronic CHF, or other situations of chronic abdominal fluid accumulation, periodic removal of enough fluid to relieve patient discomfort and improve ventilation is helpful because large-volume ascites can impede respiration.

Suggested Additional Reading and References

Also See Online Comprehensive Bibliography at: https://www.routledge.com/9781482246223.

Bissett SA, Lamb M, Ward CR. Hyponatremia and hyperkalemia associated with peritoneal effusion in four cats. J Am Vet Med Assoc 2001;218:1590–1592, 1580.

Bohn AA. Analysis of canine peritoneal fluid analysis. Vet Clin North Am Small Anim Pract 2017;47:123–133.

Bonczynski JJ, Ludwig LL, Barton LJ, et al. Comparison of peritoneal fluid and peripheral blood pH, bicarbonate, glucose, and lactate concentration as a diagnostic tool for septic peritonitis in dogs and cats. Vet Surg 2003;32:161–166.

Brudvig JM, Swenson CL. Total nucleated cell and leukocyte differential counts in canine pleural and peritoneal fluid and equine synovial fluid samples: comparison of automated and manual methods. Vet Clin Pathol 2015;44:570–579.

Connally HE. Cytology and fluid analysis of the acute abdomen. Clin Tech Small Anim Pract 2003;18:39–44.

Culp WT, Zeldis TE, Reese MS, et al. Primary bacterial peritonitis in dogs and cats: 24 cases (1990–2006). J Am Vet Med Assoc 2009;234:906–913.

Fossum TW, Hay WH, Boothe HW, et al. Chylous ascites in three dogs. J Am Vet Med Assoc 1992;200:70–76.

Glinska-Suchocka K, Slawuta P, Jankowski M, et al. An analysis of pH, pO2 and pCO2 in the peritoneal fluid of dogs with ascites of various etiologies. Pol J Vet Sci 2016;19:141–145.

Gores BR, Berg J, Carpenter JL, et al. Chylous ascites in cats: nine cases (1978–1993). J Am Vet Med Assoc 1994;205:1161–1164.

Hoehne SN, Milovancev M, Hyde AJ, et al. Placement of a caudal vena cava stent for treatment of Budd-Chiari-like syndrome in a 4-month-old Ragdoll cat. J Am Vet Med Assoc 2014;245:414–418.

James FE, Knowles GW, Mansfield CS, et al. Ascites due to pre-sinusoidal portal hypertension in dogs: a retrospective analysis of 17 cases. Aust Vet J 2008;86:180–186.

Jang M, Choi S, Lee I, et al. Computed tomographic features of intra-abdominal hypertension in three dogs. J Vet Emerg Crit Care 2019;29(2):185–189.

Koenig A, Verlander LL. Usefulness of whole blood, plasma, peritoneal fluid, and peritoneal fluid supernatant glucose concentrations obtained by a veterinary point-of-care glucometer to identify septic peritonitis in dogs with peritoneal effusion. J Am Vet Med Assoc 2015;247:1027–1032.

Kull PA, Hess RS, Craig LE, et al. Clinical, clinicopathologic, radiographic, and ultrasonographic characteristics of intestinal lymphangiectasia in dogs: 17 cases (1996–1998). J Am Vet Med Assoc 2001;219:197–202.

Levin GM, Bonczynski JJ, Ludwig LL, et al. Lactate as a diagnostic test for septic peritoneal effusions in dogs and cats. J Am Anim Hosp Assoc 2004;40:364–371.

McLaren PJ, Jocelyn NA. What is your diagnosis? Peritoneal effusion in a 10-year-old horse. Vet Clin Pathol 2016;45:723–724.

Pelosi A, Prinsen JK, Eyster GE, et al. Caudal vena cava kinking in dogs with ascites. Vet Radiol Ultrasound 2012;53:233–235.

Raffan E, McCallum A, Scase TJ, et al. Ascites is a negative prognostic indicator in chronic hepatitis in dogs. J Vet Intern Med 2009;23:63–66.

Salgado BS, Monteiro LN, Grandi F, et al. What is your diagnosis? Ascites fluid from a dog with abdominal distension. Vet Clin Pathol 2012;41:605–606.

Schlicksup MD, Weisse CW, Berent AC, et al. Use of endovascular stents in three dogs with Budd-Chiari syndrome. J Am Vet Med Assoc 2009;235:544–550.

Slawuta P, Glinska-Suchocka K. An attempt to use the peritoneal cavity fluid in the diagnostics of acid-base balance disorders in dogs. Pol J Vet Sci 2013;16:469–475.

Stafford JR, Bartges JW. A clinical review of pathophysiology, diagnosis, and treatment of uroabdomen in the dog and cat. J Vet Emerg Crit Care (San Antonio) 2013;23:216–229.

Steyn PF, Wittum TE. Radiographic, epidemiologic, and clinical aspects of simultaneous pleural and peritoneal effusions in dogs and cats: 48 cases (1982–1991). J Am Vet Med Assoc 1993;202:307–312.

Thomovsky EJ, Johnson PA, Moore GE. Diagnostic accuracy of a urine reagent strip to identify bacterial peritonitis in dogs with ascites. Vet J 2014;202:640–642.

Venzin C, Kook P, Jenni S, et al. Symptomatic treatment of ascites with a peritoneo-vesical automated fluid shunt system in a dog. J Small Anim Pract 2012;53:126–131.

Walters JM. Abdominal paracentesis and diagnostic peritoneal lavage. Clin Tech Small Anim Pract 2003;18:32–38.

Weeden AL, Cherry NA, Breitschwerdt EB, et al. Bartonella henselae in canine cavitary effusions: prevalence, identification, and clinical associations. Vet Clin Pathol 2017;46:326–330.

Wong RW, Gonsalves MN, Huber ML, et al. Erythrocyte and biochemical abnormalities as diagnostic markers in dogs with hemangiosarcoma related hemoabdomen. Vet Surg 2015;44:852–857.

Wright KN, Gompf RE, DeNovo RC Jr. Peritoneal effusion in cats: 65 cases (1981–1997). J Am Vet Med Assoc 1999;214:375–381.

Zoia A, Augusto M, Drigo M, et al. Evaluation of hemostatic and fibrinolytic markers in dogs with ascites attributable to right-sided congestive heart failure. J Am Vet Med Assoc 2012;241:1336–1343.

Zoia A, Drigo M, Simioni P, et al. Association between ascites and primary hyperfibrinolysis: a cohort study in 210 dogs. Vet J 2017;223:12–20.

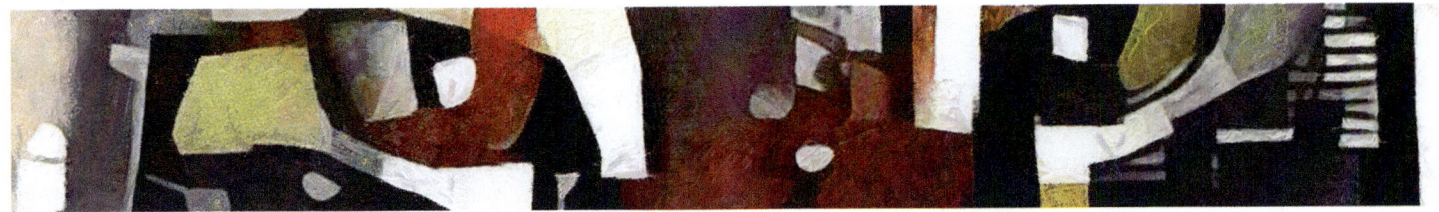

17
SUBCUTANEOUS EDEMA

The interstitium forms the junction between the microcirculation and the tissues. It is an underappreciated component contributing to regulation of metabolism, regional blood flow, and overall fluid balance. Subcutaneous edema is an abnormal increase in the amount of interstitial fluid within the superficial tissues. The relationship between hydrostatic and oncotic pressures across the capillary membrane (Starling's forces; p. 25) defines the general movement of fluid between the interstitial space and the vascular compartment. Fluid filtration into the interstitium is greater on the arterial side of the capillary because intravascular hydrostatic pressure is higher than on the venous side. However, there is greater reabsorption at the venous side, related to oncotic as well as lower hydrostatic pressure effects. This, combined with lymphatic uptake of interstitial fluid, normally maintains a slightly negative interstitial pressure with minimal interstitial fluid.

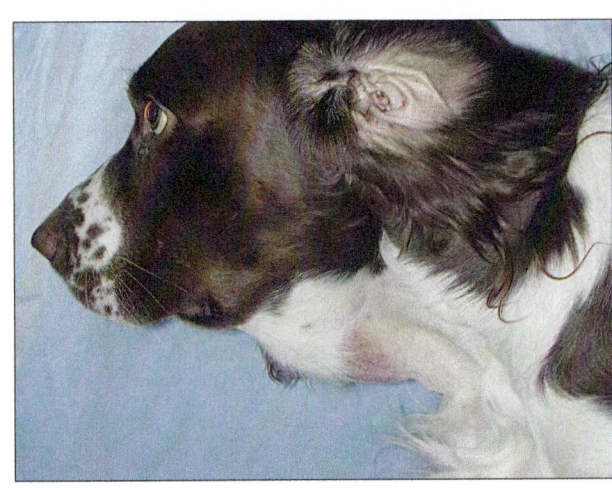

Figure 17.1 Submandibular edema in a 2-year-old male English Springer Spaniel with vasculitis.

General Considerations

Tissue edema develops when the balance of Starling's forces or lymphatic function becomes disrupted. This can occur with increased capillary hydrostatic pressure; low capillary oncotic pressure, mainly from hypoalbuminemia; increased capillary permeability, as with inflammation; or lymphatic obstruction. The effects of gravity cause tissue edema to migrate toward dependent areas of the body, especially where the skin is relatively loose. Subcutaneous edema might be noticeable only along the ventral trunk, under the mandible, or in the lower limbs (**Figures 17.1** and **17.2**). For example, "stocking up" of the distal limb in standing horses is a generally benign form of subcutaneous edema that resolves with exercise. When not associated with inflammatory lesions or secondary infection, edema causes nonpainful swelling. Firm digital pressure applied to edematous superficial tissue leaves behind an indentation, as interstitial fluid in the tissue below is

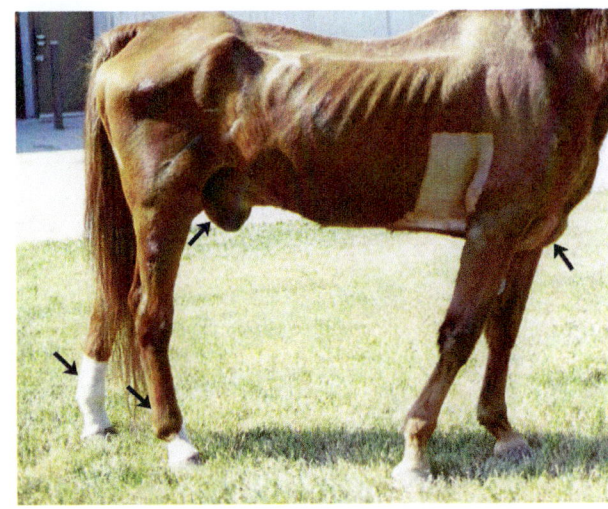

Figure 17.2 Subcutaneous edema gravitated to the ventral thorax, prepuce and distal rear limbs (arrows) in this horse with congestive heart failure and severe cachexia.

Cardiovascular Disease in Companion Animals

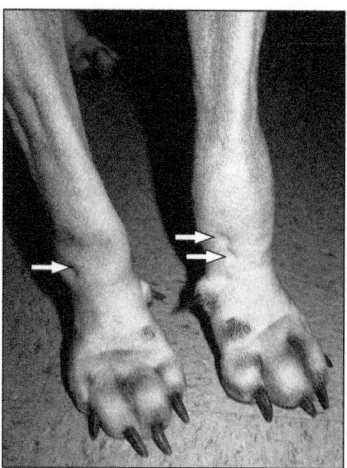

Figure 17.3 Pitting edema in the distal forelimbs of a Great Dane with congestive heart failure from atrioventricular valve insufficiency and myocardial failure. Arrows point to indentations created by digital pressure.

displaced; this is known as "pitting edema" (**Figure 17.3**). The finger-shaped depression persists until interstitial fluid seeps back into the area. Although lymphedema typically is not painful, secondary infections can occur, and tissue edema can be so severe as to stretch the skin painfully. Furthermore, chronic venous or lymphatic obstruction can lead to stasis dermatitis with accompanying skin ulcers, papules, weeping, and other cutaneous findings.

In dogs and cats, subcutaneous edema typically is associated with regional lymphatic or venous obstruction, profound hypoalbuminemia, vasculitis, or localized tissue injury (**Figure 17.4** and **Table 17.1**). Subcutaneous edema caused by high capillary hydrostatic pressure in these two species is more likely to occur from localized venous obstruction or compression (as from thrombosis, compression, or a mass lesion), rather than heart failure. Subcutaneous edema is an uncommon sign of congestive heart failure (CHF) in dogs and cats; increased capillary hydrostatic pressure secondary to high cardiac filling pressure most often causes either pulmonary edema (from left heart failure) or body cavity effusion (from right heart or biventricular failure) in these species. As a practical point, in a dog without ascites or profound hypoproteinemia, CHF is highly unlikely to underlie subcutaneous edema, and when it does occur, the distal rear limbs usually are affected. In contrast, subcutaneous (ventral) edema is a common manifestation of CHF in horses (**Figure 17.2**); the main alternative consideration in this species is vasculitis (as with purpura hemorrhagica). A less common cause of tissue edema is a peripheral arteriovenous (A-V) fistula. Increased local venous (and capillary) pressure related to high flow

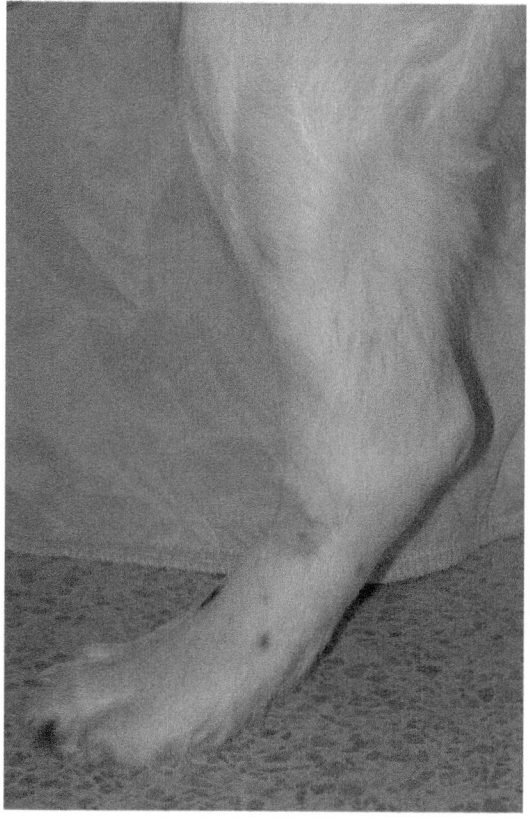 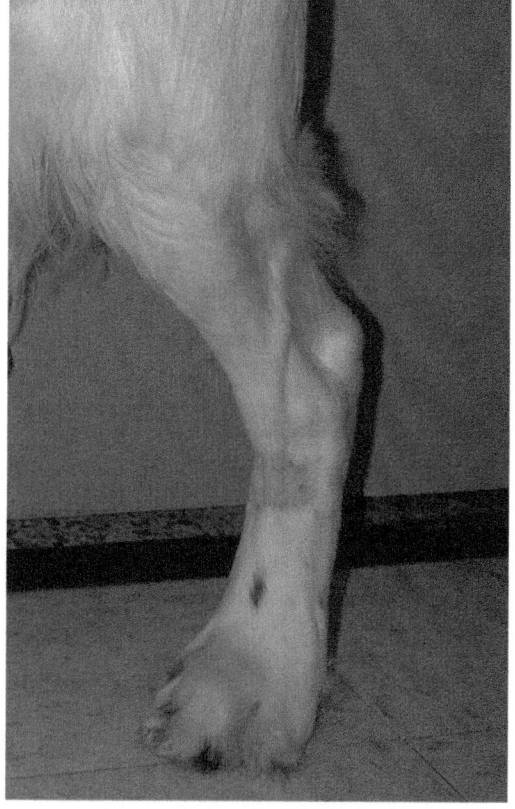

Figure 17.4 (A) Subcutaneous edema secondary to vasculitis is present in the rear limb of a dog. The edema was widespread ventrally along the trunk and other limbs. (B) About a week later, the edema has resolved following treatment.

Table 17.1 Causes of Subcutaneous Edema

Low Capillary Oncotic Pressure
- Hypoalbuminemia, including:
  - Protein-losing glomerulopathy (nephrotic syndrome)
  - Protein-losing enteropathy
  - Intestinal malabsorption or maldigestion
  - Parasites
  - Reduced hepatic production
  - Starvation
  - Exudative skin lesions

High Capillary Hydrostatic Pressure
- Venous thrombosis
- Venous varicosities
- Tissue compression or constriction (as from a mass lesion, rubber band, or tight bandage)
- Right-sided or biventricular CHF (see **Table 16.1**, p. 268, for some causes)
- A-V fistula
- Overhydration (IV fluid administration)

Lymphatic Disease Causing Leakage or Reduced Uptake of Lymph
- Congenital lymphatic dysplasia
- Lymphatic obstruction, including:
  - Lymphoma
  - Other neoplasm causing lymphatic infiltration or compression
- Lymphangitis (bacterial, fungal, Sporotrichosis)
- Trauma

Increased Capillary Permeability
- Vasculitis, including:
  - Immune-mediated (diseases such as purpura hemorrhagica in horses)
  - Infectious (Rickettsia, Ehrlichia, infectious canine hepatitis, Equine viral arteritis, Streptococcus, African Horse Sickness, and many other infectious diseases)
  - Drug-induced
- Thrombophlebitis
- Local tissue infection or inflammation
- Anaphylaxis, including:
  - Secondary to spider bite or insect sting
  - Drug reaction

Abbreviations: A-V, arteriovenous; CHF, congestive heart failure.

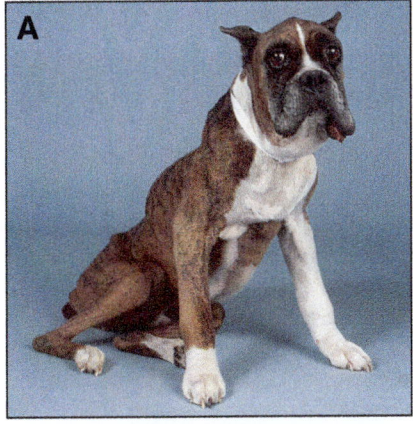

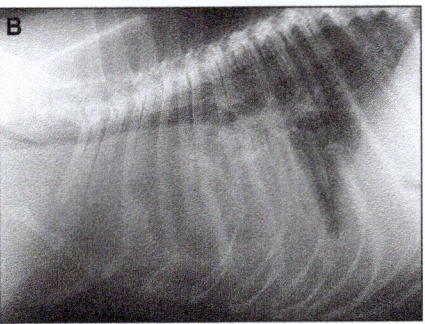

Figure 17.5 Cranial caval syndrome in a 7-year-old male Boxer with cranial mediastinal lymphoma. (A) The head, neck, and forelimbs are swollen with subcutaneous edema; however, muscle wasting is evident in the caudal body. (B) Lateral thoracic radiograph from this dog shows the increased soft tissue opacity cranial to the heart and dorsal tracheal displacement caused by the tumor; mild pleural effusion also is present.

rate and direct connections between arteries and veins can produce subcutaneous edema in patients with an A-V fistula (p. 776). Venous dilation and tortuosity occur as well. Neoplastic obstruction of venous and lymphatic return within the pelvic canal can cause bilaterally symmetric edema of the hind limbs.

Cranial Caval Syndrome

Cranial vena caval compression caused by a cranial mediastinal mass or cranial caval thrombosis can lead to the cranial caval syndrome (**Figures 17.5** and **17.6**; also see **Figure 15.2**, p. 263). Impaired lymphatic drainage is often involved as well because most lymphatics ultimately drain into the cranial vena cava. The cranial caval syndrome is characterized by bilaterally symmetric subcutaneous edema of the head, neck, cranial thorax, and forelimbs. Pleural effusion also is anticipated and the fluid might be chylous, depending on the location of the obstruction. Cranial mediastinal lymphoma and thymoma are the most common neoplastic causes of cranial caval syndrome. Occasionally, a primary lung tumor or large abscess is responsible. Caval thrombosis has been associated with diseases that induce a hypercoagulable state (such as immune-mediated thrombocytopenia or hemolytic anemia, sepsis, nephrotic syndrome, and some cancers), often in conjunction with a central venous catheter or pacemaker lead.

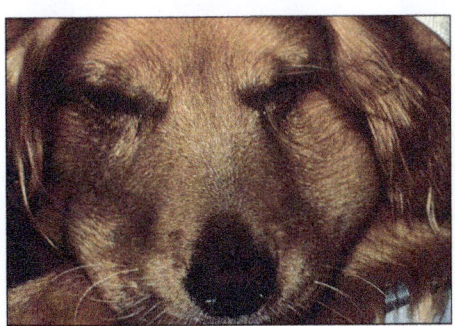

Figure 17.6 Cranial vena caval thrombosis caused marked facial edema in this Golden Retriever. (Image courtesy of Dr. CJ Baldwin.)

Lymphedema

Lymphedema specifically refers to interstitial fluid accumulation secondary to obstructed or leaky lymphatic vessels. Lymphedema fluid tends to have higher protein content (2–5 g/dL), which promotes further interstitial fluid accumulation. Lymphedema can develop with lymph node obstruction, major lymphatic duct leakage, abnormal lymphatic wall function, inadequate number of lymphatic vessels, ineffective fluid uptake by lymph capillaries, or lymphatic overload. Primary lymphedema involves an underlying dysplasia or disease of the lymph vessels or related lymph nodes. This can result from thoracic duct or cisterna chyli hypoplasia, peripheral lymphatic aplasia or malformation, insufficient numbers or development of lymph nodes, or from lymph node or lymphatic fibrosis. Edema caused by lymphatic system malformation often involves the rear limbs; it can be persistent or sometimes, transient. Severe cases can involve widespread lymphedema. The edema usually is bilateral, although it can be asymmetric in severity (**Figure 17.7**). It might develop shortly after birth or later in life.

Secondary lymphedema is more common than primary lymphedema. It occurs when a disease process originating elsewhere damages the lymphatic system. Causes include neoplastic invasion, trauma, infections (lymphangitis) including streptococcus and sporotrichosis, surgery, parasitic invasion, and radiation therapy. Concurrent venous obstruction exacerbates edema formation. Gravitational effects contribute to lymphatic vessel distention, reduction in lymph flow, and greater edema accumulation in ventral regions. The distribution and severity of secondary lymphedema depend on the location and extent of lymphatic obstruction. For example, intrapelvic lymphatic obstruction generally causes bilateral rear limb edema, whereas disease in the popliteal node region can produce localized distal limb edema. A cranial mediastinal mass can cause edema in the entire cranioventral aspect of the body (see section "Cranial Caval Syndrome").

Myxedema

Myxedema is a rare manifestation of morbid hypothyroidism. It is characterized by non-pitting thickening of the skin, especially the forehead, eyelids, and cheeks. Tissue swelling in this condition involves hyaluronic acid deposition in the dermis, rather than subcutaneous edema. In humans, it leads to pericardial effusion but this complication in dogs is poorly established.

Approach to the Patient with Subcutaneous Edema

The history and physical examination could provide important clues to the cause of subcutaneous edema. The distribution of the edema, whether localized to one limb or region or generalized throughout the body, should be noted (**Figure 17.8**). Nonpainful and cool pitting edema usually relates to a mechanism involving either high capillary hydrostatic pressure, hypoalbuminemia, or lymphatic and venous obstruction. Painful swelling that is warmer than surrounding tissue more likely is caused by increased capillary permeability from inflammation or infection. Warm swelling also is reported with A-V fistulae, and there might be a continuous murmur (bruit) over the area if the fistula is large. Other clinical signs help guide diagnostic test selection. In horses, where subcutaneous edema is a common sign of CHF, the jugular veins should be inspected carefully for distension, and a basic echocardiogram and cranial thoracic ultrasound examination should be obtained. A tentative diagnosis of congenital lymphatic dysplasia is reasonable in puppies with bilateral, nonpainful pelvic limb edema accompanied by small to absent popliteal lymph nodes. In primary lymphatic disorders, there will sometimes be concurrent pleural effusion evident by radiography or ultrasound examination.

A routine laboratory database (hemogram, serum biochemical profile, and urinalysis) will reveal hypoalbuminemia, evidence for inflammation, and other abnormal parameters. Thoracic and abdominal radiographs help identify additional areas of fluid accumulation, mass lesions, and organomegaly. Further testing that might be useful can include regional lymph node aspirates or biopsy, skin biopsy, ultrasonography of affected areas and related drainage (venous and lymphatic) vessels, echocardiography, various serologic tests for infectious agents (such as ELISA testing for antibodies to *S. equi*

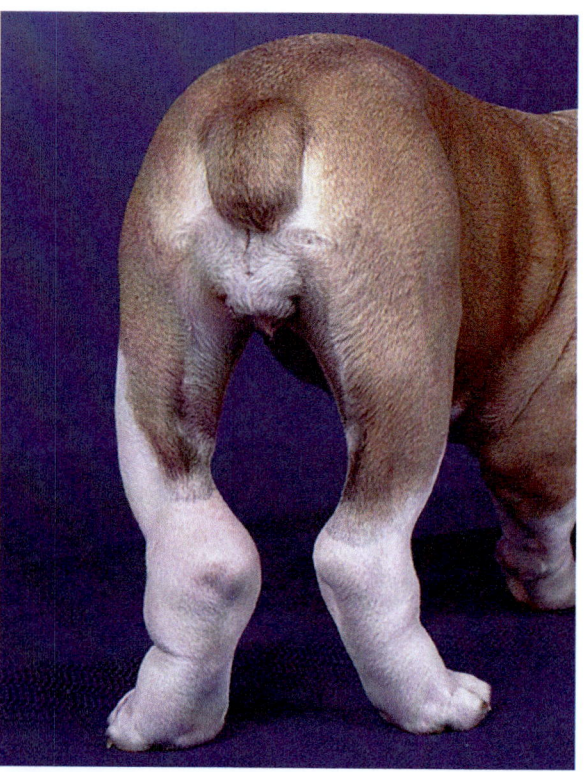

Figure 17.7 Congenital lymphedema in a young Bulldog. Both rear limbs are affected, although edema is more severe in the left rear.

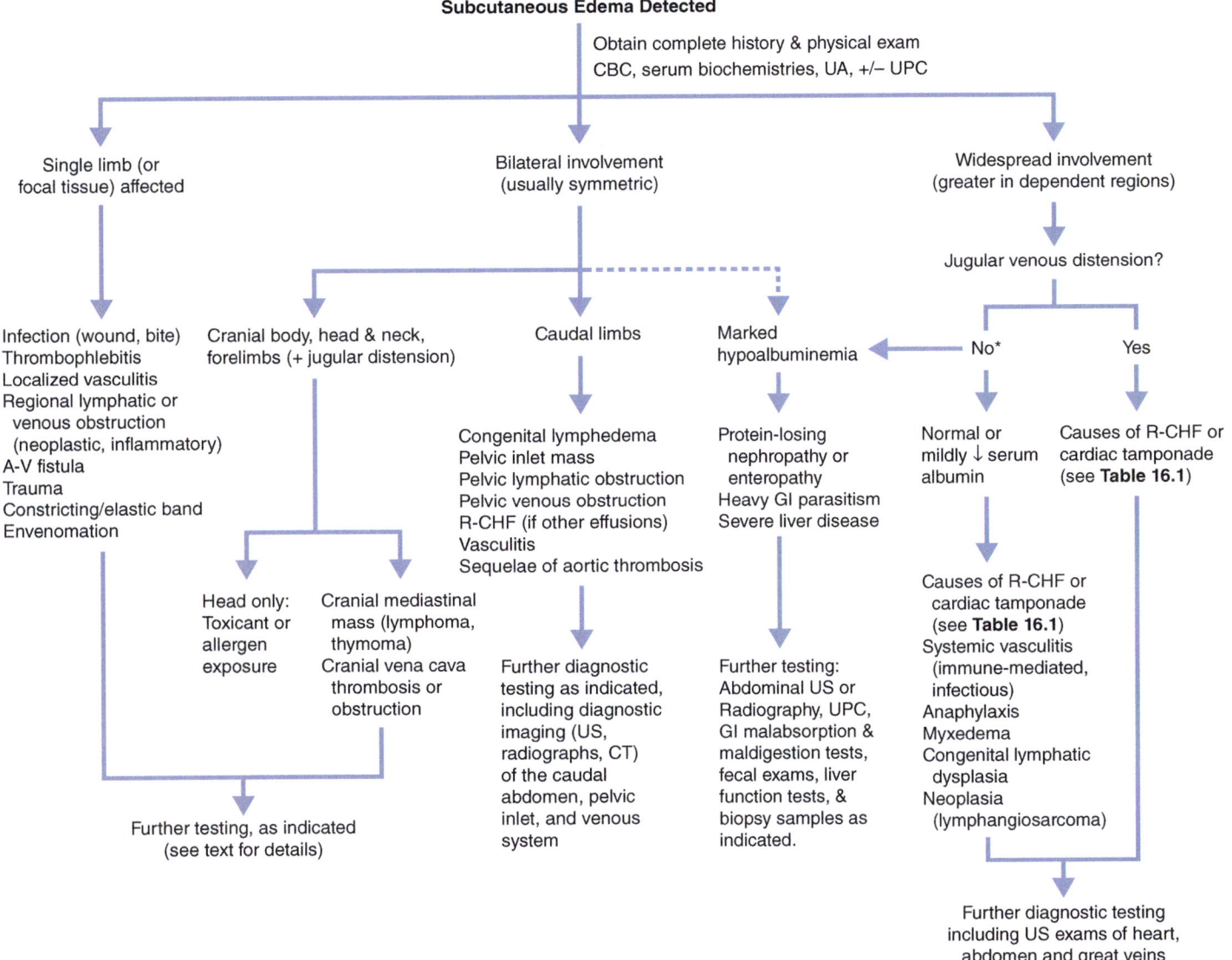

Figure 17.8 Approach to the patient with subcutaneous edema. These are general guidelines and diagnostic considerations; exceptions can occur.
* Jugular distension might not be evident following diuretic therapy or other causes of reduced circulating volume. A-V, arteriovenous; CBC, complete blood count; CT, computed tomography; GI, gastrointestinal; R-CHF, right-sided or biventricular congestive heart failure; r/o, rule out; UA, urinalysis: UPC, urine protein/creatinine ratio; US, ultrasound.

M-like protein), angiography, lymphatic scintigraphy, and other advanced imaging techniques. Although some patients might benefit from diuretic use, management depends on establishing and treating the underlying cause.

Suggested Additional Reading and References

Also See Online Comprehensive Bibliography at: https://www.routledge.com/9781482246223.

Arthur JJ, Kleiter MM, Thrall DE, et al. Characterization of normal tissue complications in 51 dogs undergoing definitive pelvic region irradiation. Vet Radiol Ultrasound 2008;49:85–89.

Basile RC, Rivera GG, Del Rio LA, et al. Anaphylactoid reaction caused by sodium ceftriaxone in two horses experimentally infected by *Borrelia burgdorferi*. BMC Vet Res 2015;11:197.

Bellah JR, Stiff ME, Russell RG. Thymoma in the dog: two case reports and review of 20 additional cases. J Am Vet Med Assoc 1983;183:306–311.

Bouayad H, Feeney DA, Lipowitz AJ, et al. Peripheral acquired arteriovenous fistula: a report of four cases and literature review. J Am Anim Hosp Assoc 1986; 23:205–211.

Bourke CA, Hunt E, Watson R. Fescue-associated oedema of horses grazing on endophyte-inoculated tall fescue grass (*Festuca arundinacea*) pastures. Aust Vet J 2009;87:492–498.

de Keyser K, Janssens S, Buys N. Chronic progressive lymphoedema in draught horses. Equine Vet J 2015;47:260–266.

Fossum TW, King LA, Miller MW, et al. Lymphedema. Clinical signs, diagnosis, and treatment. J Vet Intern Med 1992a;6:312–319.

Fossum TW, Miller MW. Lymphedema. Etiopathogenesis. J Vet Intern Med 1992b;6:283–293.

Leighton RL, Suter PF. Primary lymphedema of the hindlimb in the dog. J Am Vet Med Assoc 1979;175:369–374.

Meyer J, Delay J, Bienzle D. Clinical, laboratory, and histopathologic features of equine lymphoma. Vet Pathol 2006;43:914–924.

Morris DD. Cutaneous vasculitis in horses: 19 cases (1978–1985). J Am Vet Med Assoc 1987;191:460–464.

Murray JD, O'sullivan ML, Hawkes KC. Cranial vena caval thrombosis associated with endocardial pacing leads in three dogs. J Am Anim Hosp Assoc 2010;46:186–192.

Palmer KG, King LG, Van Winkle TJ. Clinical manifestations and associated disease syndromes in dogs with cranial vena cava thrombosis: 17 cases (1989–1996). J Am Vet Med Assoc 1998;213:220–224.

Scansen BA, Bonagura JD. Venous and lymphatic disorders. In, Ettinger SJ, Feldman EC, Cote E (editors). Textbook of Veterinary Internal Medicine. 8th edition. Saunders, St. Louis, MO. 2017. pp. 1349–1360.

Van De Wiele CM, Hogan DF, Green HW 3rd, et al. Cranial vena caval syndrome secondary to transvenous pacemaker implantation in two dogs. J Vet Cardiol 2008;10:155–161.

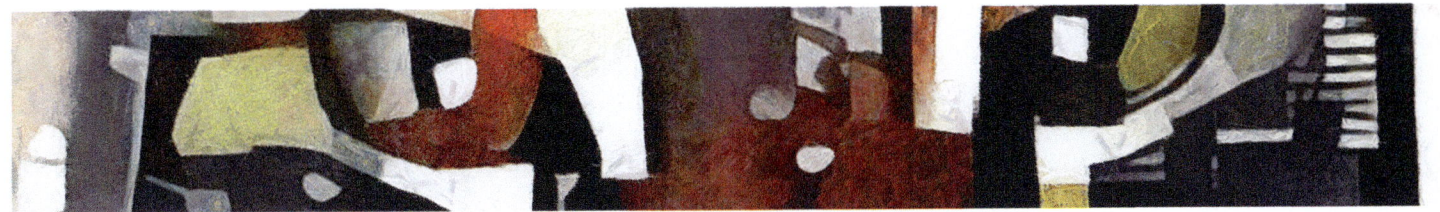

18
CARDIOMEGALY

The term cardiomegaly indicates enlargement of the heart as might be visualized through echocardiography or at the autopsy table. In addition, the term typically is applied to a radiographically large cardiac silhouette; this is most pertinent to evaluation of dogs and cats. Apparent (radiographic) cardiomegaly can occur when fluid or a mass lesion distends the pericardium (**Figure 18.1**). Excessive intrapericardial or mediastinal fat also can mimic the appearance of cardiomegaly (**Figure 18.2**), especially if the cardiac border is not clearly discernable from the adjacent fat density. Likewise, a soft-tissue mass adjacent to the heart might cause the appearance of cardiomegaly (**Figure 18.3**). Clearly, it is important to differentiate true cardiomegaly from factors that mimic it. Additionally, the clinician should focus on the shape of the radiographic cardiac silhouette and the specific chamber enlargement patterns that occur (see Chapter 3).

This chapter provides a general framework for understanding cardiomegaly and in particular, potential changes that might be seen by thoracic radiography or with ultrasound imaging of the heart. It should be recognized that cardiac remodeling in cardiomyopathy or in response to increased work is just one part of perceived cardiomegaly. Dilation of the proximal great vessels and the large veins that enter the heart (venae cavae, pulmonary veins) also can influence the radiographic or ultrasonographic appearance of cardiac shape. Furthermore, the plasma volume and venous filling pressures can increase the filling and size of the heart. For example, moderate to severe dehydration and reduced preload lead to both radiographic "microcardia" and echocardiographic "pseudohypertrophy" of the ventricular walls. These changes are erased by effective fluid therapy. Conversely, renal fluid retention in heart failure, facilitated

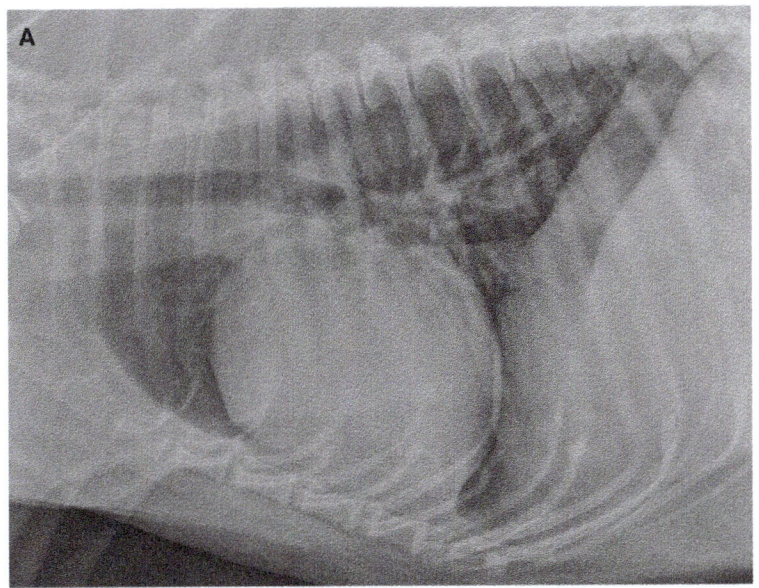
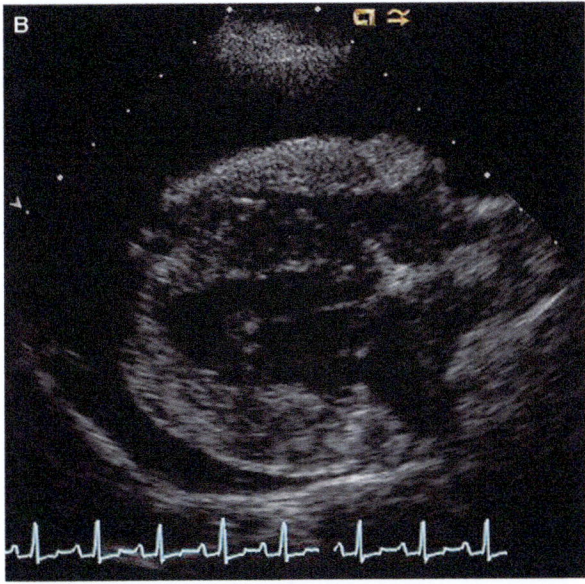

Figure 18.1 (A) Lateral radiograph shows prominent cardiomegaly in a 13-year-old mixed-breed dog referred for lethargy. Dilated cardiomyopathy was suspected; however, the echocardiogram (B) showed pericardial effusion with cardiac tamponade and a small right auricular mass.

Cardiovascular Disease in Companion Animals 281

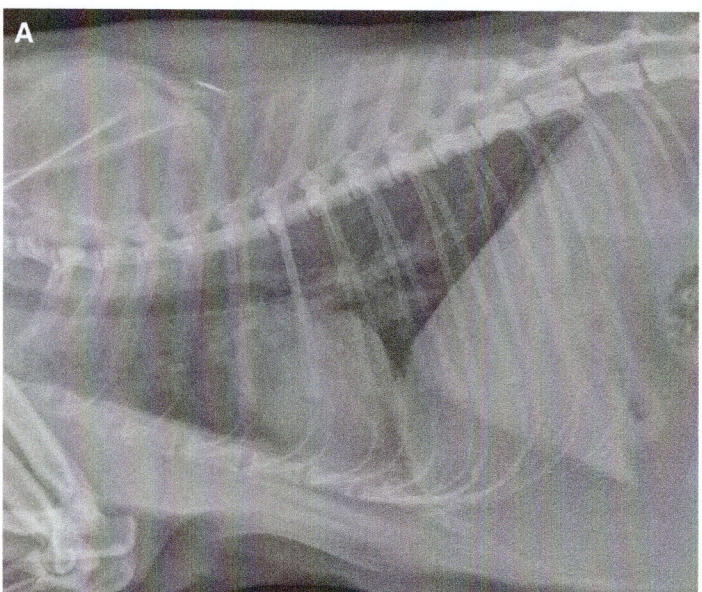
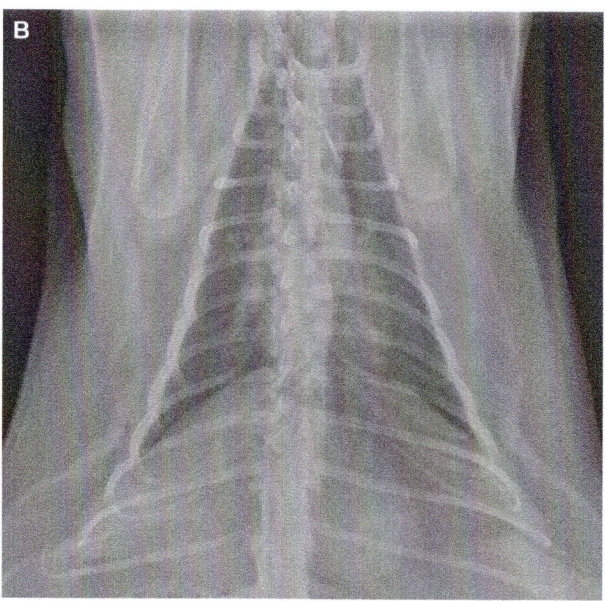

Figure 18.2 A 3-year-old Domestic Shorthair cat with decreased appetite and intermittent vomiting was referred because of a positive (point-of-care) heartworm (HW) antigen test and suspected cardiomegaly. The cardiac silhouette might appear large on lateral (A) and dorsoventral (B) radiographs, but the cat's obesity contributes to this. Echocardiography showed normal cardiac chamber size and wall thickness, with no evidence for HW disease. Clinical signs had resolved within the week, and subsequent HW antigen and antibody tests were negative.

by renin-angiotensin-aldosterone system (RAAS) activation, increases atrial and ventricular volumes and thereby the degree of cardiomegaly. One becomes quite aware of this venous pressure influence after initiating diuresis and pimobendan therapy in acute congestive heart failure (CHF); cardiac size can markedly decrease in less than 24 hours. Intermittent or chronic plasma volume retention also occurs and can gradually lead to changes in heart chamber size as higher venous pressures increase cardiac filling.

General Considerations

A spectrum of pathophysiologic and morphologic changes can underlie "cardiomegaly." The cardiac enlargement process can be generalized to all chambers or involve only the left or right heart chambers, or even a single chamber, depending on the location and type of underlying lesion(s). Furthermore, the proximal great arteries and, less often, the veins can contribute to "bulges" or changes in the shape of the heart and the

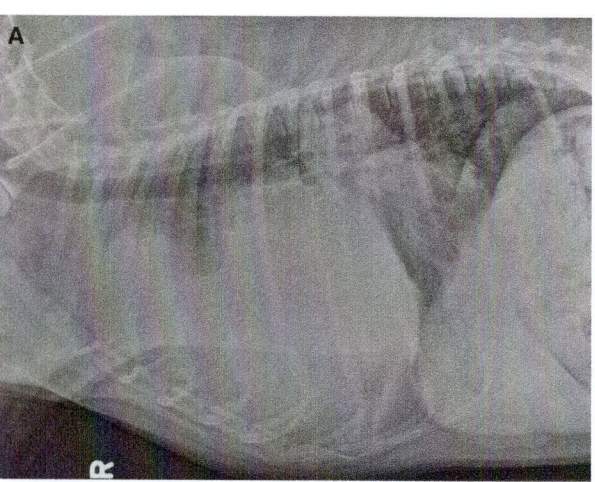
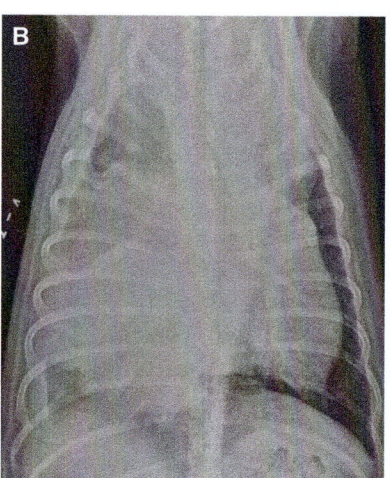
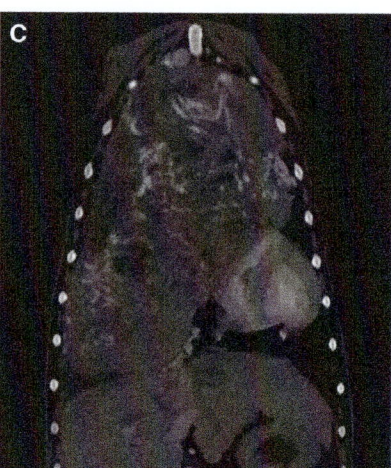

Figure 18.3 A 6-year-old female hound-mix with a 4-week history of coughing, wheezing, reduced appetite, and weight loss was referred for suspected cardiomegaly and dilated cardiomyopathy. Lateral (A) and ventrodorsal (B) radiographs indicate an expansive soft-tissue mass lesion adjacent to the heart, which is displaced leftward (B). Thoracic computed tomography (C) provides better definition of the mass' extent and cardiac displacement. The mass was an undifferentiated carcinoma.

resultant radiographic silhouette. Although certain anticipated patterns of enlargement are associated with specific cardiac diseases, at best these are generalizations. For example, some dogs with dilated cardiomyopathy have radiographic and echocardiographic evidence of mainly left ventricular (LV) and left atrial (LA) dilation; however, other cases show enlargement/dilation of all four chambers. Similarly, right ventricular (RV) and right atrial (RA) enlargement variably occur in degenerative valvular heart disease of dogs and horses, but it becomes more likely with concurrent tricuspid valve regurgitation, pulmonary hypertension, and atrial fibrillation. In view of species and breed differences in chest conformation, the radiographic appearance of heart disease in dogs and cats can range from characteristic to confusing. The following paragraphs summarize some concepts about the development of cardiomegaly in specific disorders.

The type of cardiac chamber enlargement often indicates an adaptive response to chronically increased volume work, as with valvular insufficiency and left-to-right shunts (Chapters 26 and 29–31), or to systolic pressure overload, as with ventricular outflow obstruction or arterial hypertension (Chapters 27 and 38–40). Valvular regurgitation and left-to-right shunts induce an eccentric (dilated) pattern of cardiac hypertrophy. With mitral or tricuspid insufficiency, the chambers on either side of the affected valve enlarge progressively as they alternatively receive and return the additional (regurgitant) volume. Typically, the volume overload and resultant cardiomegaly increase gradually unless an acute event supervenes, such rupture of valve chordae tendineae or the onset of atrial fibrillation. With semilunar valve regurgitation, the receiving chamber undergoes eccentric hypertrophy while the proximal great vessel often dilates as well. Aortic or pulmonary artery dilation in this setting relates to either the underlying arterial disease (such as an aortopathy or pulmonary hypertension) or the expanded ventricular stroke volume. With left-to-right shunts (patent ductus arteriosus, rupture of the aorta into the pulmonary artery, and atrial and ventricular septal defects), the chambers and blood vessels carrying the extra (shunt) volume enlarge. In contrast, right-to-left shunts remodel differently, mostly in relation to the pressure overload of concurrent pulmonary stenosis or severe pulmonary hypertension. In general, pressure overloads cause concentric or mixed hypertrophy, with increased wall thickening, in the ventricle performing the increased work (p. 16). The adjacent atrium often is enlarged in cases of ventricular pressure overload, even when the atrioventricular (AV) valve is competent. This likely stems from ventricular diastolic or systolic dysfunction secondary to the chronic workload and ventricular remodeling, and often portends a future complicated by CHF.

Primary (genetic and idiopathic) cardiomyopathies and myocardial diseases that occur secondary to other disorders are associated with cardiomegaly. The main finding in dilated cardiomyopathy is chamber dilation with eccentric hypertrophy (Chapters 32–34). This also is the usual pattern in infective myocarditis, nutritional cardiomyopathies (taurine deficiency in cats and dogs; legume-rich diets in dogs); toxicoses (doxorubicin, cobalt), and tachycardia-induced cardiomyopathies. However, there are exceptions. For example, severe acute myocarditis and infiltrative myocardial diseases can develop thickened ventricular walls and reduced ejection fraction. Some feline cardiomyopathies, especially end-stage hypertrophic cardiomyopathy and restrictive cardiomyopathy, are most notable for cardiomegaly associated with left or bi-atrial dilation. Right ventricular cardiomyopathies lead mainly to RV and RA dilation, with inconsistent changes in the left heart. In comparison, concentric ventricular hypertrophy or thickening is typical with hypertrophic cardiomyopathy (Chapter 33) and systemic hypertension. These conditions must be distinguished from the physiologic hypertrophy of the athletic heart, especially in horses and some working dogs. Endocrinopathies also can be associated with cardiomyopathy and cardiomegaly, particularly thyrotoxicosis, excess growth hormone production (in cats), and feline diabetes mellitus (**Figures 18.4** and **18.5**; also see p. 688).

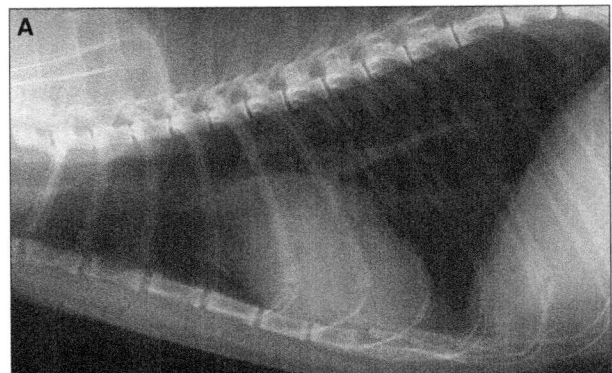
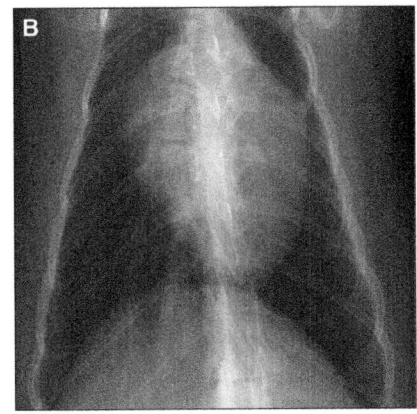

Figure 18.4 Lateral (A) and dorsoventral (B) radiographs from a 14-year-old cat with chronic hyperthyroidism (T_4 >244 nmol/L; 19 mcg/dL) indicate generalized cardiomegaly (vertebral heart size, 8.6v).

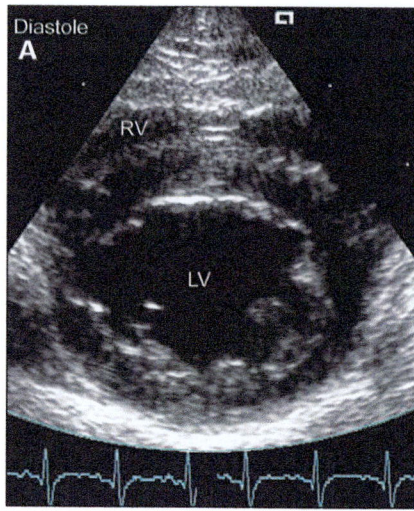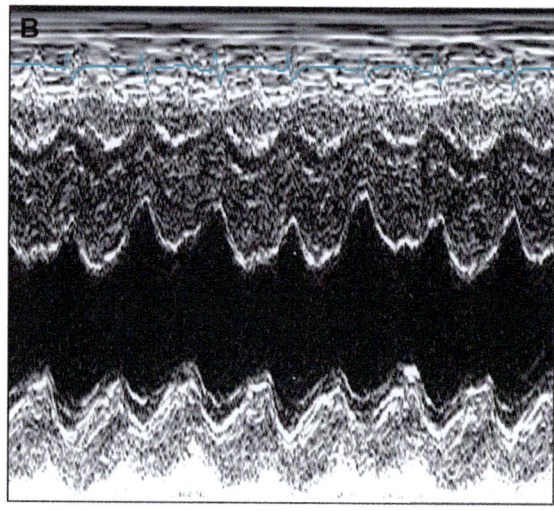

Figure 18.5 (A) Short-axis two-dimensional echocardiographic image, in diastole, and (B) M-mode image at the ventricular level from the cat of **Figure 18.4**. Left ventricular diastolic dimension is increased at 18.4 mm. The vigorous motion of free wall and septum (B) is consistent with a high output state. Left ventricular wall (3.9 mm) and septal (4.2 mm) diastolic thicknesses are normal. Blood pressure in this case was normal. LV, left ventricle; RV, right ventricle.

A cardiac mass lesion can enlarge or distort the heart by its physical presence, or by obstructing blood flow and causing secondary dilation or hypertrophy. Chronic and profound bradycardia, such as from complete (third-degree) AV block, leads to ventricular enlargement as increases in preload and stroke volume become the prime determinants of cardiac output (p. 15). Cardiac enlargement also can develop with chronic anemia; reduced blood viscosity and peripheral vasodilation lead to a high cardiac output state and plasma volume retention. A large arteriovenous (A-V) fistula also produces cardiomegaly; flow through the fistula reduces total peripheral resistance and, along with compensatory volume expansion, increases venous return and cardiac output.

Approach to the Patient with Cardiomegaly

Physical examination findings sometimes suggest the presence of cardiomegaly. Indeed, most patients with clinical signs of CHF, jugular venous distension, or a loud heart murmur are likely to show evidence for cardiomegaly. Caudal displacement of the palpable precordial impulse, or an increase in the area of percussive cardiac dullness (in horses), might be detected when there is left-sided or generalized cardiomegaly. A more prominent right precordial impulse can signal right ventricular hypertrophy (Chapter 2). Likewise, in animals with marked cardiomegaly, a shift from the expected location of cardiac sounds might be discovered during auscultation. However, a mass lesion within the thorax that pushes the heart from its normal position also can displace the precordial impulse and location of heart sounds. Additionally, cardiac enlargement might be suggested by QRS complex enlargement criteria on an electrocardiogram (p. 153 and **Table 5.5**). Of course, imaging techniques should be used to further define suspected cardiomegaly.

When cardiomegaly is suspected, other abnormalities that mimic it must be excluded (such as intrapericardial fluid or fat). Determination of which chamber(s) are enlarged helps the clinician identify the underlying disease process. Thoracic radiographs, echocardiography, and other imaging techniques can provide this information. It is important to discern whether the affected chamber(s) is (are) dilated or increased in wall thickness, or both, and whether other related abnormalities exist. The decision to institute specific therapy in a patient with cardiomegaly must be based on an understanding of the underlying cause, its severity, and the related pathophysiology. **Figure 18.6** outlines an approach for evaluating the patient with cardiomegaly. **Table 3.2** (p. 54) lists some causes of a radiographically enlarged cardiac silhouette.

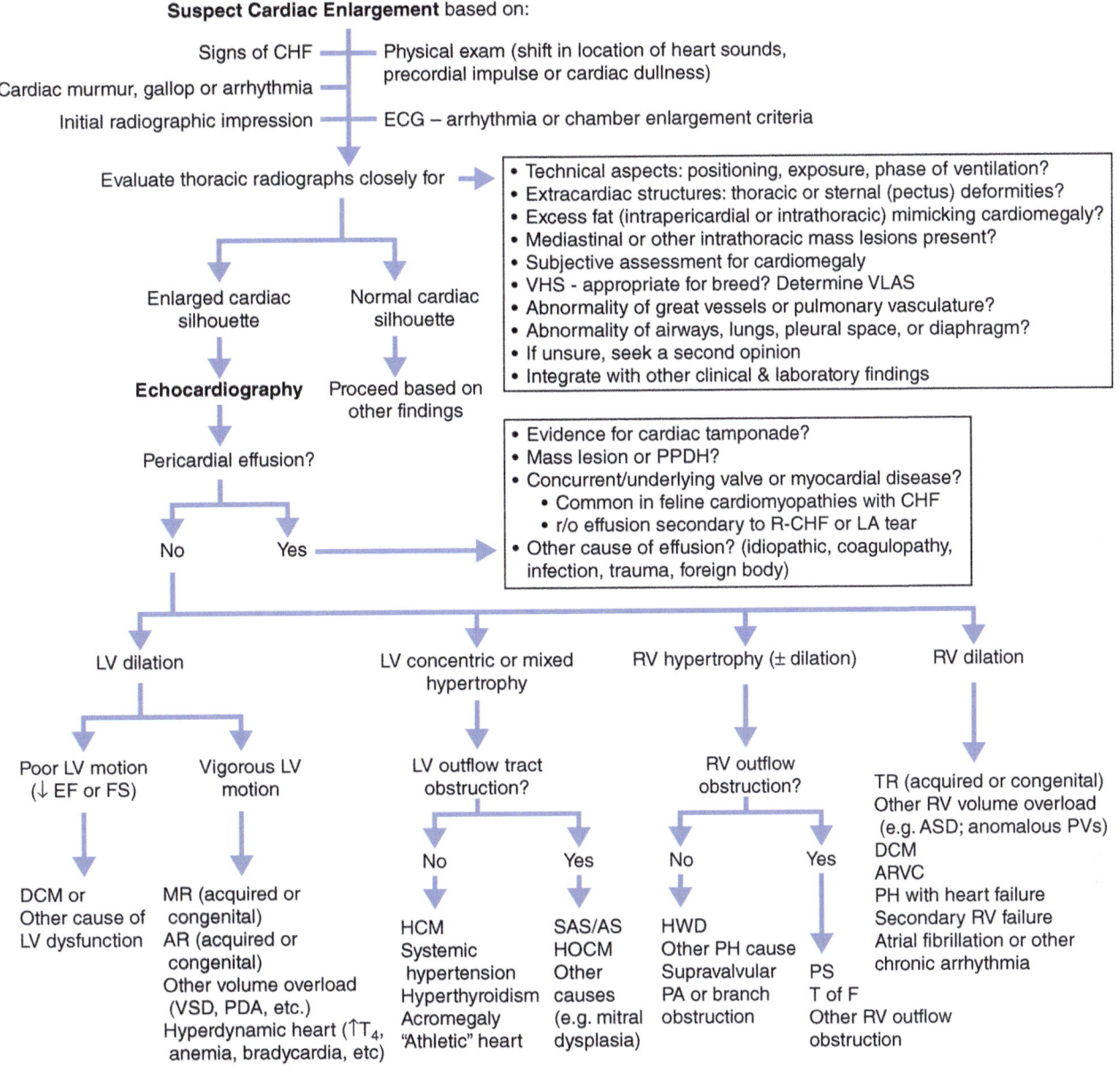

Figure 18.6 Approach to the patient with suspected cardiomegaly. These are general guidelines and diagnostic considerations; exceptions can occur. AR, aortic regurgitation; ARVC, arrhythmogenic right ventricular cardiomyopathy; ASD, atrial septal defect; CHF, congestive heart failure; DCM, dilated cardiomyopathy; ECG, electrocardiogram; EF, ejection fraction; FS, fractional shortening; HCM, hypertrophic cardiomyopathy; HOCM, hypertrophic obstructive cardiomyopathy; HWD, heartworm disease; LA, left atrial; LV, left ventricular; MR, mitral regurgitation; PA, pulmonary arterial; PDA, patent ductus arteriosus; PH, pulmonary hypertension; PPDH, peritoneopericardial diaphragmatic hernia; PS, pulmonic stenosis; PVs, pulmonary veins; r/o, rule out; R-CHF, right-sided (or biventricular) congestive heart failure; RV, right ventricular; SAS/AS, subaortic or aortic valve stenosis; ↑T$_4$, hyperthyroidism; T of F, tetralogy of Fallot; TR, tricuspid regurgitation; VHS, vertebral heart size; VLAS, vertebral left atrial size; VSD, ventricular septal defect.

Suggested Additional Reading and References

Also See Online Comprehensive Bibliography at: https://www.routledge.com/9781482246223.

Guglielmini C, Diana A. Thoracic radiography in the cat: identification of cardiomegaly and congestive heart failure. J Vet Cardiol 2015;17(Suppl 1):S87–101.

Litster AL, Buchanan JW. Vertebral scale system to measure heart size in radiographs of cats. J Am Vet Med Assoc 2000;216:210–214.

Litster AL, Buchanan JW. Radiographic and echocardiographic measurement of the heart in obese cats. Vet Radiol Ultrasound 2000;41:320–325.

Marin LM, Brown J, McBrien C, et al. Vertebral heart size in retired racing Greyhounds. Vet Radiol Ultrasound 2007;48:332–334.

Nakayama H, Nakayama T, Hamlin RL. Correlation of cardiac enlargement as assessed by vertebral heart size and echocardiographic and electrocardiographic findings in dogs with evolving cardiomegaly due to rapid ventricular pacing. J Vet Intern Med 2001;15:217–221.

Oura TJ, Young AN, Keene BW, et al. A valentine-shaped cardiac silhouette in feline thoracic radiographs is primarily due to left atrial enlargement. Vet Radiol Ultrasound 2015;56:245–250.

Rugh KS, Garner HE, Sprouse RF, et al. Left ventricular hypertrophy in chronically hypertensive ponies. Lab Anim Sci 1987;37:335–338.

Sleeper MM, Roland R, Drobatz KJ. Use of the vertebral heart scale for differentiation of cardiac and noncardiac causes of respiratory distress in cats: 67 cases (2002–2003). J Am Vet Med Assoc 2013;242:366–371.

Strohm LE, Visser LC, Chapel EH, et al. Two-dimensional, long-axis echocardiographic ratios for assessment of left atrial and ventricular size in dogs. J Vet Cardiol 2018;20:330–342.

Tominaga Y, Miyagawa Y, Toda N, et al. The diagnostic significance of the plasma N-terminal pro-B-type natriuretic peptide concentration in asymptomatic cats with cardiac enlargement. J Vet Med Sci 2011;73:971–975.

Wilson HE, Jasani S, Wagner TB, et al. Signs of left heart volume overload in severely anaemic cats. J Feline Med Surg 2010;12:904–909.

Yoon Y, Hwang T, Lee H. Prediction of radiographic abnormalities by the use of bag-of-features and convolutional neural networks. Vet J 2018;237:43–48.

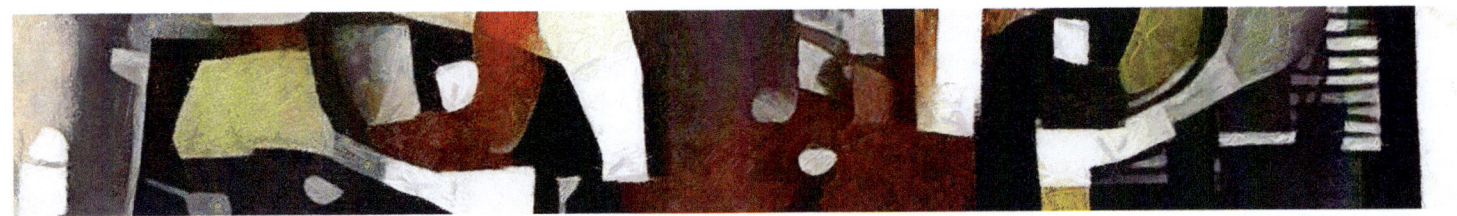

19
CLINICAL LABORATORY ABNORMALITIES

Routine clinical laboratory test results often are nonspecific in animals with cardiovascular (CV) disease. However, sometimes abnormalities reveal evidence of low cardiac output or systemic venous congestion, such as azotemia and mild elevations in liver enzymes, or concurrent noncardiac disease that might influence CV function. Other abnormalities might occur as well, including in patients receiving medical therapy for congestive heart failure (CHF). Multisystemic disease is especially common in older cardiac patients, so general metabolic screening is particularly advisable in this population. Cardiac biomarkers, including troponin and natriuretic peptides, can be useful when screening for cardiac disease or injury. Their utility for guiding therapy and estimating prognosis continues to be explored. In the future, additional biomarkers might be used clinically to help manage animals with CV disease and CHF. Other tests that could be important for individual cases include those for parasitic infection, endocrine abnormalities, and blood taurine concentration, as well as blood cultures and monitoring of therapeutic drug concentrations. Some aspects of the clinical laboratory examination relevant to the CV system are mentioned below and summarized in **Table 19.1**. However, an exhaustive review of all laboratory abnormalities is beyond the scope of this text.

Routine Laboratory Tests

Complete Blood Count

A complete blood count (CBC) might reflect a number of abnormalities associated with various CV diseases. Most abnormalities are secondary, while others could contribute to CV disease. Mild anemia can develop in dogs with chronic CHF. Neurohormonal activation and volume expansion, with impaired ability to excrete free water, are thought to be factors in this. In dogs with advanced CHF, caused by degenerative (myxomatous) mitral valve disease (DMVD), the presence of anemia was identified as a negative prognostic indicator (Yu, 2016).

The hemogram and associated blood smear can reveal a number of abnormalities relevant to CV disease. In particular, anemia lowers blood oxygen-carrying capacity, as well as blood viscosity (p. 23). Moderate to severe anemia, and related to the rapidity of its onset, leads to peripheral vasodilation and sympathetic nervous system activation; consequences include high cardiac output, probable renin-angiotensin-aldosterone system (RAAS) activation, sodium retention, and eventually, cardiomegaly. Circulatory overload, and sometimes CHF, can develop in severe cases. This is most common in cats with marked reductions in hemoglobin. Signs of exercise intolerance, collapse, or even syncope, along with resting tachypnea and sinus tachycardia, are common. The combination of sympathetic activation and reduced blood viscosity produces increased ejection velocities and can cause an audible murmur in the absence of structural cardiac disease. Anemia also can increase the intensity of a previously identified cardiac murmur. Furthermore, moderate anemia can negatively affect previously compensated heart disease. For example, older cats with stable complete heart block can later develop CHF with pleural effusion as anemia progresses.

Erythrocytosis (sometimes referred to as polycythemia) is an increase in circulating red blood cell (RBC) mass. Erythrocytosis can be primary or secondary. Physiologically appropriate secondary erythrocytosis occurs in response to the increased erythropoietin production induced by chronic hypoxemia. Often, this is caused by a congenital right-to-left shunt, such as from Eisenmenger's pathophysiology with a (reversed) patent ductus arteriosus, ventricular septal defect, or atrial septal defect; from pulmonic stenosis or tricuspid valve malformations with a patent foramen ovale; or from complex defects such as tetralogy of Fallot (**Figure 19.1**; also see Chapter 26) and double-outlet right ventricle. Chronic tissue hypoxia associated with pulmonary disease, high altitudes, or carboxyhemoglobinemia also can produce an increase in

Table 19.1 Routine Clinical Laboratory Abnormalities Associated with Cardiovascular Diseases

Complete Blood Count (Hemogram)
- Anemia
- Erythrocytosis (polycythemia)
- Leukocytosis/leukopenia
- Thrombocytopenia
- Hemoglobinemia
- Microfilaria or other parasites (appearing on slide)

Serum Biochemical Abnormalities
- Azotemia
- Elevated liver enzymes (ALT, alkaline phosphatase)
- Hyperkalemia
- Hypokalemia
- Hypomagnesemia
- Hypochloremia
- Increased bicarbonate
- Hyponatremia
- Hypoproteinemia
- Elevated cardiac & skeletal muscle enzymes (creatine kinase, serum AST, serum LDH)

Urinalysis
- Proteinuria
- Hematuria
- Hemoglobinuria
- Pyuria

Cardiac Biomarkers
- Increased NT-proBNP (or C-BNP)
- Increased cTnI

Others (see text and chapters on specific diseases)

Abbreviations: ALT, alanine aminotransferase; AST, Aspartate transaminase; BNP, B-type or brain natriuretic peptide; cTnI, cardiac troponin I; LDH, Lactate dehydrogenase.

might occur in some dogs. Deep red (injected) or cyanotic mucous membranes typically are seen on exam (p. 247).

The RBC distribution width (RDW) is a measure of anisocytosis. RDW is influenced by various CV diseases and, in people, has been shown to have prognostic value. Initial studies in dogs and cats have shown increased RDW in dogs with severe pulmonary hypertension and in cats with CHF. However, an association between RDW and CHF in dogs with degenerative valvular disease has not been identified. The relationship between increased RDW and prognosis is unclear in animals, although progressive increase over time might be a negative prognostic indicator.

Abnormalities of the leukogram in animals with CV disease generally are related to systemic disease. Nevertheless, some animals with acute CHF have mild leukocytosis, which could be associated with high sympathetic tone and epinephrine release or increased proinflammatory cytokines. Studies in dogs have shown increased total leukocyte and neutrophil, and reduced lymphocyte, counts in CHF. Additionally, mean serum C-reactive protein concentration appears to be higher in dogs with decompensated CHF compared to preclinical heart disease and healthy dog groups (Domanjko, 2018). Although dogs with CHF often have values within normal range for these variables, the numbers of neutrophils, band neutrophils, and monocytes were shown to be higher than in dogs without cardiac disease (Hamilton-Elliott, 2018). Neutrophilia, with or without monocytosis, often accompanies infective endocarditis. Eosinophilia (**Figure 19.2**), basophilia, and monocytosis might be seen with heartworm disease (HWD, Chapter 40) and other parasitic conditions, among other causes.

RBC mass. Clinical signs associated with marked erythrocytosis, such as a packed cell volume over 70%, can invoke neurologic abnormalities, including behavioral change or seizures, and exercise intolerance. Anecdotally, paroxysmal sneezing

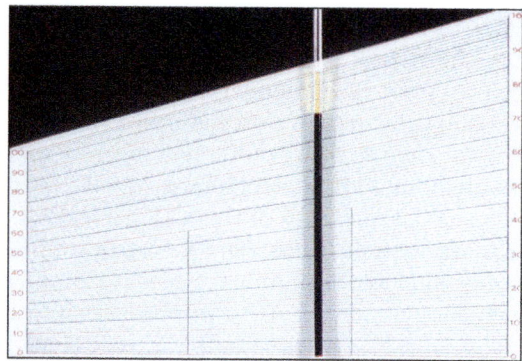

Figure 19.1 Severe erythrocytosis, with a hematocrit of 84%, developed in a 3-year-old Lhasa Apso with tetralogy of Fallot.

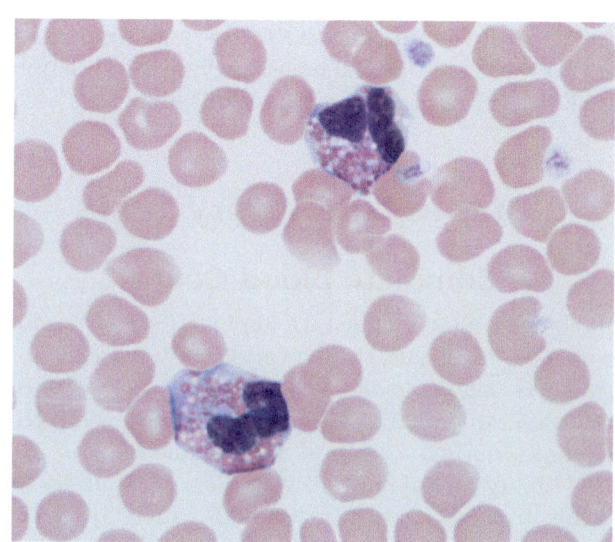

Figure 19.2 Two eosinophils are present in this canine blood smear (Wright-Giemsa stain). Eosinophilia could accompany heartworm disease, other parasitic infections, and hypersensitivity reactions, among other causes. (Image courtesy of Dr. A Viall.)

Mild thrombocytopenia occurs in some cats with heart disease. However, mildly increased platelet counts also have been found in dogs with CHF. Cavalier King Charles Spaniels, with or without DMVD disease, can manifest an autosomal recessive, inherited macrothrombocytopenia. Excluding this breed, however, a difference in mean platelet numbers has not been identified in dogs with DMVD compared to normal dogs. Nonetheless, platelet sensitivity could be enhanced in dogs with DMVD. Increased platelet activation has been shown in cats with hypertrophic cardiomyopathy. Thrombocytopenia and thrombocytosis both have been associated with thromboembolic disease. Mild thrombocytopenia is more common with HWD. An increase in platelet reactivity also occurs in HWD, as well as other causes of pulmonary thromboembolism. Thombocytopenia can develop with endocarditis and systemic infection or sepsis. Marked thrombocytopenia from disseminated intravascular coagulation (DIC) sometimes occurs in animals with CV disease, particularly those with heartworm caval syndrome or endocarditis with sepsis.

Serum Biochemistries

The serum biochemical profile is normal in many animals with CV disease. However, those with low cardiac output (as with dilated cardiomyopathy, DCM) or on chronic CHF medications commonly develop prerenal azotemia, mild electrolyte abnormalities, and sometimes, mild anemia. Primary renal disease and the effects of drug therapy contribute to biochemical abnormalities. Systemic arterial hypertension can exacerbate kidney disease. Embolic renal injury is common with endocarditis and with feline cardiomyopathy. HWD has been associated with glomerular injury and glomerulonephritis.

Renal Function Tests It is important to monitor blood urea nitrogen (BUN) and serum creatinine concentrations in animals with CHF because commonly used therapies can impair renal perfusion. For example, diuretic-induced plasma volume contraction and vasodilator-induced hypotension or renal vasodilation could provoke azotemia and lead to renal failure. In addition, many CV drugs are excreted by renal mechanisms (including enalapril, atenolol, and digoxin) and older animals are especially likely to have underlying renal dysfunction. Chronic kidney disease is prevalent in older dogs and cats with cardiac disease. The development and treatment of CHF can exacerbate kidney disease by reducing renal perfusion, increasing systemic venous congestion, and potentially, by effects of neuroendocrine activation (cardio-renal syndrome; Martinelli, 2016). Concurrent intrinsic renal disease should be strongly suspected when initial, modest dosages of diuretics or angiotensin converting enzyme (ACE) inhibitors lead to moderate or severe azotemia. Furthermore, underlying renal disease often leads to systemic hypertension in cats and dogs (Chapter 38), which further complicates the management of cardiac disease and accelerates renal function deterioration. Serum symmetric dimethylarginine (SDMA) concentration measurement provides an indicator of glomerular filtration rate (GFR) and can help identify early renal dysfunction. SDMA concentration has a linear inverse relationship with GFR. Progressive increases in mean SDMA concentration correlated with the severity of heart failure functional classification in a study of dogs with DMVD (Choi, 2017).

Three specific situations of azotemia merit consideration. First, after intensive diuresis for acute CHF, mild azotemia (as well decreases in serum chloride and potassium) should be expected. These often improve once the patient is stable, drinking and eating. Second, acute renal failure, including serum creatinine concentrations >4 mg/dL, is encountered occasionally with volume depletion and initiation of ACE inhibitor therapy. These patients are highly dependent on angiotensin II for maintaining GFR; the azotemia often is improved by stopping the "-pril" drug and providing judicious fluid volume expansion with 0.45% saline (and potassium chloride supplementation). Third, there often is a disconnection between elevations of serum BUN and creatinine during chronic medical therapy for CHF. This might relate to reduced skeletal muscle generation of creatinine from cardiac cachexia, a higher back-diffusion of urea nitrogen into the blood, or some other factors. Regardless of cause, the BUN often is a better marker of renal perfusion than creatinine in patients undergoing chronic treatment for CHF.

Liver and Pancreatic Enzymes Liver enzymes can become elevated in heart failure from passive venous congestion, organ hypoperfusion, or possibly from the effects of cardiac or other medications. Because some drugs depend on the liver for biotransformation, metabolism, or excretion, alterations in liver function can affect their action and disposition. Chronic CHF with hepatic congestion potentially could lead to hepatic cirrhosis, although this seems uncommon. Elevation of canine pancreatic-specific lipase concentration was identified in dogs with advanced DMVD, suggesting pancreatic injury also occurs in these cases. Pancreatic lipase concentration correlated closely with left atrial-to-aortic diameter ratio, as well as CHF severity, in these dogs (Han, 2015). A clinical observation in cats is that some with cardiogenic shock also develop signs related to splanchnic hypoperfusion, including pancreatitis.

Electrolytes Diuretic therapy used to treat heart failure or systemic hypertension can cause sodium, potassium, and chloride loss. Loop diuretics such as furosemide and torsemide inhibit the 2-chloride transporter and can lead to hypokalemic, hypochloremic, metabolic alkalosis with mild elevation in serum bicarbonate (although a mixed metabolic acidosis/alkalosis also is common and bicarbonate is often normal). Mild to moderate hypochloremia is the most common electrolyte disturbance seen during chronic CHF therapy and it generally is ignored. Practically, a normal serum chloride in advanced CHF suggests insufficient dosing, diuretic resistance, or an issue with drug absorption or client compliance.

Serum potassium, sodium, calcium, and magnesium ion concentrations are critical for maintaining normal membrane potentials and contractility of heart cells. Hypokalemia and hypomagnesemia predispose to arrhythmias and digoxin toxicity. Diuretic therapy can decrease serum potassium and magnesium ion concentrations. Conversely, hyperkalemia can provoke dramatic and lethal arrhythmias (p. 160). Hyperkalemia occasionally occurs in animals with profound myocardial failure or bradycardia, as a consequence of poor renal perfusion. Hyperkalemia also can occur when an ACE inhibitor is administered with spironolactone, although it is usually mild, and therefore ignored. Occasionally on initial presentation, a patient with severe myocardial failure might have hyperkalemia, hyponatremia, and azotemia that mimics hypoadrenocorticism. The combination of hyponatremia and hypoproteinemia can develop with severe chronic heart failure of any cause and is associated with (sodium-free) water retention. This is a negative prognostic sign indicating a situation where RAAS and vasopressin activation is needed to maintain arterial blood pressure. Hypocalcemia and severe hypophosphatemia can reduce myocardial contractility, but these usually are signs of other metabolic or endocrine diseases.

Proteins Total serum protein concentration can be depressed in severe CHF. Mild pan-hypoproteinemia is relatively common in severe right-sided CHF, in particular. Mechanisms could include: dilution from excessive secretion of vasopressin (antidiuretic hormone), protein loss through the kidney or gut because of venous congestion, inadequate hepatic synthesis because of abnormal hepatic circulatory dynamics, anorexia, and cardiac cachexia. The beta and gamma fractions of serum proteins could increase with endocarditis or chronic dirofilariasis.

Muscle Enzymes Myocardial cell injury or necrosis causes leakage of enzymes and regulatory proteins (troponins) into the plasma. Nonspecific markers of cardiac injury, such as creatine kinase (CK), aspartate aminotransferase (AST), lactate dehydrogenase (LDH), and myoglobin, become elevated after severe myocardial necrosis. However, these also can increase with liver or skeletal muscle injury and other conditions. Myocardial isoenzyme activity or another specific cardiac biomarker (such as cardiac troponin I, cTnI; see section "Cardiac Biomarkers") must be measured to prove that the source of abnormal values is the heart. The more cardiac-specific isoenzyme of CK (CK-MB) occurs mainly in the myocardial cytosol and its synthesis increases after cardiac injury. Nevertheless, CK-MB is relatively nonspecific in that it, too, is produced by skeletal muscle and other tissues. Furthermore, CK-MB is not well-conserved among species, so human assays are not recommended. Skeletal muscle ischemia, as occurs with aortic embolism, produces marked elevations of CK and AST, (and often a muscle isoenzyme of alanine aminotransferase, ALT, normally associated with the liver). Generally, in thromboembolic muscle injury, the serum AST will be higher than the serum ALT; the opposite is typical of liver disease.

Urinalysis

In animals with azotemia, the measurement of urine specific gravity prior to administration of any diuretic helps in differentiating prerenal from renal azotemia. However, this is not the case once diuretic therapy has begun. Elevated urine protein concentration and protein:creatinine ratio can be secondary to a glomerulopathy associated with systemic hypertension, HWD or endocarditis, as well as with other causes of renal disease. Hemoglobinuria could be a sign of the hemolysis and DIC that occur with heartworm postcaval syndrome. Urine culture and sensitivity testing might be useful in animals with suspected endocarditis, especially if pyuria is evident.

Tests for Parasites and Other Infections

Serologic tests for circulating heartworm antigen assist in the diagnosis of HWD. Tests for *Dirofilaria immitis* microfilariae also are positive in some canine cases, although rarely so in cats. Heartworm antibody tests are helpful in cats to indicate exposure to the parasite. See Chapter 40 for more information on heartworm testing and laboratory abnormalities associated with HWD.

Fecal flotation and Baermann tests and cytologic examination of airway washings can allow identification of *Angiostrongylus vasorum* larvae and other parasites in endemic areas (p. 871). Other respiratory parasites also might be identified.

Tests for other organisms that can affect the heart, and other body systems, are indicated in some cases. These could include cytological exam of blood smears for various protozoan agents, immunologic tests, or molecular techniques. These infectious agents can cause myocarditis or endocarditis. Serologic testing is available for antibodies to *Trypanosoma cruzi*, the protozoan parasite causing Chagas disease (p. 640). Other immunodiagnostic tests are available to recognize certain rickettsial and bacterial infections, including from *Borrelia* species (associated with Lyme carditis), *Bartonella* species (which can cause myocarditis or endocarditis), Leishmaniasis, and toxoplasmosis, which (rarely) can cause clinical myocarditis in cats.

Cardiac Biomarkers

Cardiac Troponins

The troponins are regulatory proteins attached to actin filaments within myocardial cells (see p. 13). Circulating concentrations of cardiac troponin (cTn) proteins normally are very low. Although normal or only mildly increased levels do not exclude the possibility of cardiac disease, elevations in cardiac troponins (cTnI and cTnT) provide a specific indicator of myocardial cell injury and leakage across the sarcolemma. This cannot differentiate the underlying cause, however. Serum cTn concentrations (especially cTnI) increase with myocardial damage caused by ischemia, inflammation, trauma, toxicosis, or necrosis (also see chapters on specific diseases). These increase relatively rapidly in patients with severe injury. Because the half-life of these biomarkers is short (a couple of hours in the dog), circulating concentrations also can decrease rapidly. Persistent elevation implies continued release. Cardiac troponins often are elevated with chronic heart diseases, although usually to a lesser extent than with acute and severe injury. These "trickle elevations" are thought to reflect ongoing myocardial remodeling and disease. Animals with mild cardiac disease often have normal cTnI concentration, especially with less sensitive assays.

Serum cTnI is a more sensitive marker than cTnT; both have been studied in dogs, cats, and horses. Comparatively higher concentrations of cTnI are found in patients with CHF. Variable cTn elevation occurs with different cardiac diseases and there is overlap with control animals in the absence of CHF. Minimal cTn elevation can occur after strenuous exercise or with diseases where secondary cardiac injury might occur. Increased cTn concentrations have been found in dogs with gastric dilatation/volvulus, with higher concentrations occurring in affected dogs that have more severe arrhythmias. Mildly increased cTn concentrations also can occur with renal dysfunction, blunt trauma, hypertrophic cardiomyopathy and hyperthyroidism (in cats), as well as with systemic infectious and inflammatory diseases. In addition, there seems to be some breed variation in normal cTn concentration. For example, normal Greyhound and Boxer dogs appear to have higher cTn concentrations than other dog breeds. Mild cTn elevation could occur in older animals as well. Studies are ongoing to assess how cTnI can best be used in the diagnosis, management, and prognosis of cardiac disease in companion animals.

Troponin proteins are highly conserved across species, so human assays for cTnI and cTnT can be used. Standard (older) tests for cTnI have a lower limit of detection of about 0.02 ng/mL which might not be adequately sensitive to detect elevations in mild-to-moderate cardiac disease (such as with DMVD in dogs). The upper detection limit is about 40 ng/mL. A high-sensitivity cTnI test designed for humans (with detection range of 0.006–50 ng/mL) has been validated in dogs and cats (ADVIA Centaur TnI-Ultra assay[a]; Siemens Medical Solutions). Mild elevations in dogs with varying severity of DMVD have been documented with high-sensitivity cTnI testing. Similarly, high-sensitivity cTnI testing can identify cats likely to have cardiomyopathy with good sensitivity and specificity, although echocardiography still is recommended for confirmation.

Natriuretic Peptides

The B-type or brain natriuretic peptide (BNP), and to some extent, A-type or atrial natriuretic peptide (ANP), are useful in assessing the presence and potentially the prognosis of heart disease and CHF. In clinical practice, these serve more as functional markers of cardiac disease rather than of a specific pathology. Natriuretic peptides are synthesized and released in response to ventricular strain and hypertrophy, increased vascular volume, hypoxia, ischemia, and tachycardia. Physiologically, these peptides antagonize the RAAS, functioning as natriuretic, vasodilator, and antifibrotic hormones. The nitrogen-terminal fragments (NT-proBNP and NT-proANP) of the respective prohormones remain in circulation longer and reach higher plasma concentrations than the active (C-terminal fragment) molecules; therefore, they are measured most often.

NT-proBNP (and C-BNP) concentrations increase in various cardiac diseases (see chapters on specific diseases). These increases correlate with disease severity, as assessed by radiography and echocardiography, and can provide a surrogate estimate of left atrial pressure. However, certain non-cardiac abnormalities also are associated with increased circulating BNP concentrations, including renal dysfunction, pulmonary hypertension, and hyperthyroidism (in cats). Clearance of natriuretic peptides is partly via the kidney; consequently, serum concentrations could be markedly elevated in patients with severe renal disease.

The structure of proBNP and its fragments is different among dogs, cats, and people, so species-specific assays are required. Careful attention to sample collection and handling instructions is important. NT-proBNP assays for dogs and cats (CardioPet proBNP-Canine and CardioPet proBNP-Feline; IDEXX Labs) and a C-BNP assay for dogs (Cardio-BNP; Antech Diagnostics) are currently available in different countries. BNP tests cannot reliably differentiate among etiologies of heart disease in an individual. It is important to interpret results in the context of patient history, physical examination, and other clinical tests. In populations where a low prevalence of cardiac disease is expected, there is greater likelihood that an elevated result could be a false positive. Additionally, there are marked differences in normal values in canine breeds that are not reflected in the reference laboratory "limits" of normal (Sjöstrand, 2014). Ventricular stretch, as in chronic mitral valve disease, can markedly increase BNP concentrations even when CHF is not present. Thus, the elevation in natriuretic peptides should be viewed as helping to establish "risk," but CHF cannot be diagnosed by BNP testing alone.

Despite these limitations, one potential use is to help differentiate heart failure from other causes of respiratory distress or respiratory signs in cases where other diagnostic tests yield ambiguous results. Plasma NT-proBNP concentrations >1,400–1,600 pmol/L in dogs, or >270 pmol/L in cats, with respiratory signs are supportive for CHF as the cause for dyspnea. Conversely, NT-proBNP concentrations <800 pmol/L in dogs, or <270 pmol/L in cats, suggest a non-cardiac cause for the respiratory distress. The feline point-of-care (POC) NT-proBNP test (SNAP Feline proBNP test; Idexx Laboratories) is most useful for helping rule-out (as opposed to diagnosing) CHF in cats presented with dyspnea of unknown cause because it tends to become positive in the 100–200 pmol/L range (**Figure 19.3**). As an alternative to blood, pleural effusion fluid (diluted 1:1 with saline to increase specificity) can be used for this test; this can be especially useful in patients with respiratory distress. Other potential uses for NT-proBNP concentration testing include assessment of cardiac disease severity and possibly, prognosis. For example, one study found cats that had a larger percentage decrease in NT-proBNP after initial CHF treatment had longer mean survival time, compared to cats with active CHF at recheck (Pierce, 2017). Unfortunately, these reference laboratory test values require time for blood collection, transport, processing, and reporting, none of which is afforded the clinician facing a patient with respiratory distress. Thus, the practical value of these tests is lower, but would improve with faster reporting of reference laboratory results or development of other POC tests that become "positive" at higher values of NT-proBNP.

This biomarker actually is most helpful in cats with preclinical cardiac disease. The NT-proBNP test is highly useful for identifying cats with subclinical cardiomyopathy, especially in cases with a cardiac murmur, arrhythmia, gallop sound, radiographic cardiomegaly, or with close relatives that have been diagnosed with cardiomyopathy. The POC test becomes positive in the 100–150 pmol/L range; NT-proBNP concentrations exceeding 1,000 pmol/L occasionally are encountered in asymptomatic cats. These elevations suggest structural cardiac disease is present, and are an indication for further diagnostic testing by echocardiography, and sometimes, radiography or other tests. However, use of the NT-proBNP test for screening the general feline population or as a breeding soundness test in young healthy cats is not recommended presently, as more false positive results will occur. Male cats appear to have somewhat higher NT-proBNP concentrations than females.

Plasma NT-proBNP might be helpful in identifying Doberman Pincher dogs with occult DCM, although it does not replace an echocardiogram or Holter monitoring. Elevated NT-proBNP concentrations were found in asymptomatic Dobermans with reduced left ventricular systolic function, with or without arrhythmias. In two studies evaluating dogs with a high prevalence of DCM, a cut-off value of >550 pmol/L was found to be 78.6% sensitive and 90.4% specific; a value of >457 pmol/L, 70% sensitive, and a value exceeding 900 pmol/L was 94% specific (Wess, 2011a; Singletary, 2012a). It should be noted that these analyses used a previous analytical method and these values are clearly normal for dogs of most other breeds. Furthermore, accuracy was poor in Dobermans with occult DCM that only had arrhythmias. In Dobermans over 4 years of age, especially if positive for a mutation associated with DCM, NT-proBNP screening could be reasonable if echocardiography and Holter monitoring are not immediately available. However, dogs with elevated concentrations should be further evaluated by echocardiography and Holter monitoring (or at least a 3–5-minute in-hospital ECG recording). NT-proBNP testing is not helpful in Boxers with

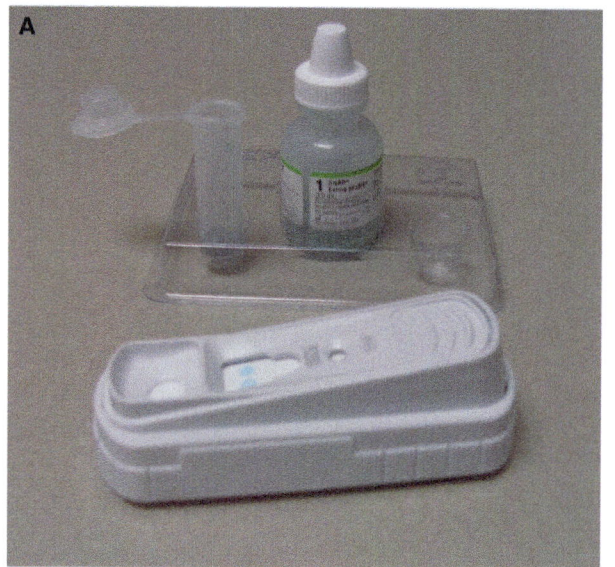 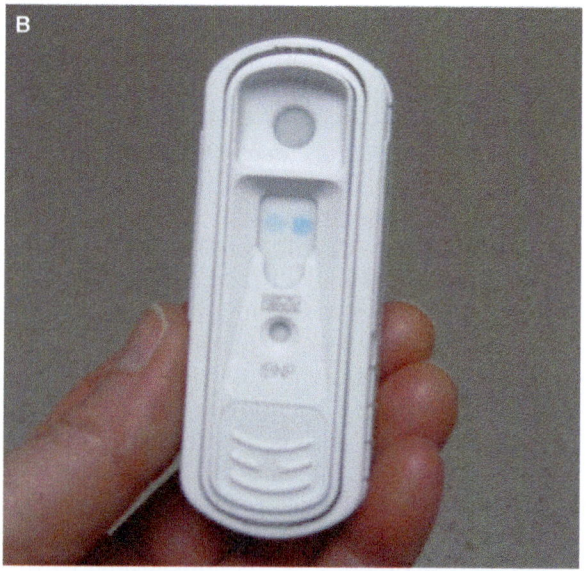

Figure 19.3 Point-of-care feline proBNP test. (A) Blood sample from a 3-year-old cat with respiratory distress is mixed with reagent prior to pouring onto the test device's sample well. (B) The completed test shows a darker blue spot from the patient's sample (on the right), compared to reference (left), indicating a positive (elevated NT-proBNP) result. The cat had hypertrophic obstructive cardiomyopathy with congestive heart failure. (SNAP Feline proBNP Test; Idexx Laboratories.)

arrhythmogenic right ventricular cardiomyopathy (ARVC); no significant difference has been found between affected and clinically normal Boxers. It is not known if NT-proBNP testing would be useful for identifying occult DCM in other breeds.

In dogs with DMVD, NT-proBNP monitoring can help predict stage B2 disease and incipient CHF, and therefore, the need for closer home monitoring (for example, by counting resting respiratory rate often) and more frequent reevaluation visits. A plasma NT-proBNP concentration >1,500 pmol/L was found to indicate increased risk for CHF onset within 3–6 months; other predictors included radiographic vertebral heart score (VHS) >12v and a diastolic left ventricular internal dimension to aortic root ratio (LVID:Ao) >3.0, with greater risk when more than one of these factors was present (Reynolds, 2012). Yet, thoracic radiography still is the gold standard for diagnosis of CHF (pulmonary edema), and NT-proBNP values exceeding 2,500 pmol/L are routinely encountered in dogs with advanced but otherwise compensated DVMD. Nevertheless, high circulating concentrations of natriuretic peptides are associated with overt CHF, disease severity, and worse prognosis in dogs with DMVD, especially when concentrations remain high after therapy has been instituted.

Other biomarkers are being explored. The endothelin (ETN) system is activated in dogs and cats with CHF, as well as those with pulmonary hypertension, so assays for circulating ETN-1 concentration could have future utility. Because ETN is involved in multiple pathologic processes, such assays would not be cardiac specific. Circulating tumor necrosis factor might also be a useful marker of cardiac disease progression, although it, too, is not cardiac specific.

Other Tests

Endocrine testing might be indicated in certain cases. For example, serum thyroxin concentration is relevant in the diagnosis of hyperthyroid heart disease in older cats (>6 years of age), when tachycardia, arrhythmia, murmur, myocardial hypertrophy, weight loss, or palpable thyroid nodule is identified. Dogs with hypothyroidism might exhibit reduced myocardial contractility; severely hypothyroid dogs could develop atherosclerosis. Excessive thyroxine supplementation in dogs can lead to CV signs of increased sympathomimetic activity, ectopy, and to ventricular hypertrophy. Perhaps more importantly, dogs with CHF receiving appropriate thyroid supplementation should have concentrations regularly evaluated and maintained in the low- to mid-normal range considering thyroid hormone increases the demand for cardiac output. Growth hormone excess and diabetes mellitus (persistent hyperglycemia) are associated with cardiomyopathy in cats; unfortunately, there are no readily available assays for growth hormone in this species although circulating insulin-like growth factor-1 can be measured in some reference laboratories to diagnose hypersomatotropism. Diabetic cats should probably be screened for cardiac disease.

Plasma or preferentially, whole blood taurine concentration (or both) should be measured in cats and some dogs with DCM, because low levels could underlie myocardial dysfunction (p. 682 and p. 633). However, taurine concentrations are normal in most dogs with apparent legume-rich ("grain-free") dietary-related cardiomyopathy. Therapeutic drug monitoring is important in certain cases. For example, measuring serum concentrations of digoxin is important in cases where this drug is employed. A (trough) concentration between 0.8 and 1.2 ng/mL, obtained 8–12 hours post-pill, usually is associated with a therapeutic, nontoxic dosage of digoxin in dogs and in horses. Values exceeding 2 ng/mL are more likely to be associated with toxicosis. Assays for some antiarrhythmic and other drugs are available and obtaining plasma concentrations could be helpful in patient management, but rarely are done.

Cytologic and biochemical examination of body cavity fluids can provide important clinical information in many cases; see **Table 10.4**, p. 216 (pleural effusion descriptions), and also p. 710 (pericardial effusions) for further information. Assessment of hypoxemia is described in **Table 10.6** (p. 220).

Coagulation and D-dimer tests can be useful in cases of suspected coagulopathy, thromboembolism, and DIC. An increase in D-dimers occurs in dogs with severe HWD, after heartworm adulticide treatment, and also with other causes of thromboembolism. In dogs with thromboembolic disease, D-dimer concentrations >1,000 ng/mL are highly sensitive in predicting thromboembolism and concentrations >2,000 ng/mL are almost entirely specific. Conversely, low values are helpful for excluding thromboembolism, as in cases of idiopathic pulmonary hypertension.

Blood cultures are important in animals suspected of infective (bacterial) endocarditis. Multiple positive cultures usually are diagnostic for bacteremia. However, as noted previously, specialized immunodiagnostic tests will be necessary for some infectious agents. See Chapter 31 for further details.

Approach to the Patient

The laboratory tests indicated for a particular patient depend on the specific clinical situation and patient characteristics. Even the "routine" laboratory database of CBC, serum chemistry panel and urinalysis, which is recommended and appropriate for many cases, is not necessarily indicated for all patients with heart disease. For example, the biochemical profile and urinalysis would be noncontributory in most cases of asymptomatic congenital heart disease. The use of biomarkers such as cTn and NT-proBNP is evolving. For example, cTn would be an appropriate test in a patient with unexplained arrhythmias, especially in an atypical breed for genetic cardiomyopathy. The POC NT-proBNP test is practical for screening young cats with murmurs prior to spay/neuter; a "negative" test is supportive of a functional murmur, or at least only mild heart disease. Conversely, considering the expense of referral for echocardiography, the reference laboratory quantitation of

NT-proBNP is recommended for mature cats with a cardiac murmur because this can assist with establishing relative risk for structural heart disease.

The importance of considering the animal's signalment, history, and complete physical examination findings cannot be overemphasized when deciding which laboratory tests to obtain. Test interpretation and subsequent therapy to address abnormal findings obviously are intertwined with the specific clinical situation, as well. Many patients with CV disease have concurrent abnormalities involving other body systems, which must be considered when developing diagnostic and therapeutic plans. Because detailed exploration of such other conditions is beyond the scope of this text, the reader is urged to consult other references as appropriate.

Suggested Additional Reading and References

Also See Online Comprehensive Bibliography at: https://www.routledge.com/9781482246223.

Aona BD, Rush JE, Rozanski EA, et al. Evaluation of echocardiography and cardiac biomarker concentrations in dogs with gastric dilatation volvulus. J Vet Emerg Crit Care 2017;27:631–637.

Borgeat K, Connolly DJ, Luis Fuentes V. Cardiac biomarkers in cats. J Vet Cardiol 2015;17(Suppl 1):S74–86.

Borgeat K, Niessen SJM, Wilkie L, et al. Time spent with cats is never wasted: Lessons learned from feline acromegalic cardiomyopathy, a naturally occurring animal model of the human disease. PLoS One 2018;13:e0194342.

Boswood A. Biomarkers in cardiovascular disease: beyond natriuretic peptides. J Vet Cardiol 2009;11(Suppl 1):S23–32.

Choi BS, Moon H, Suh SI, et al. Evaluation of serum symmetric dimethylarginine in dogs with heartworm infection. Can J Vet Res 2017;81:228–230.

Domanjko Petric A, Lukman T, Verk B, et al. Systemic inflammation in dogs with advanced-stage heart failure. Acta Vet Scand 2018;60:20.

Farabaugh AE, Freeman LM, Rush JE, et al. Lymphocyte subpopulations and hematologic variables in dogs with congestive heart failure. J Vet Intern Med 2004;18:505–509.

Flethoj M, Kanters JK, Haugaard MM, et al. Changes in heart rate, arrhythmia frequency, and cardiac biomarker values in horses during recovery after a long-distance endurance ride. J Am Vet Med Assoc 2016;248:1034–1042.

Fox PR, Oyama MA, Hezzell MJ, et al. Relationship of plasma N-terminal pro-brain natriuretic peptide concentrations to heart failure classification and cause of respiratory distress in dogs using a 2nd generation ELISA assay. J Vet Intern Med 2015;29:171–179.

Guglielmini C, Poser H, Pria AD, et al. Red blood cell distribution width in dogs with chronic degenerative valvular disease. J Am Vet Med Assoc 2013;243:858–862.

Gunther-Harrington CT, Arthur R, Estell K, et al. Prospective pre- and post-race evaluation of biochemical, electrophysiologic, and echocardiographic indices in 30 racing thoroughbred horses that received furosemide. BMC Vet Res 2018;14:18.

Hamilton-Elliott J, Ambrose E, Christley R, et al. White blood cell differentials in dogs with congestive heart failure (CHF) in comparison to those in dogs without cardiac disease. J Small Anim Pract 2018;59:364–372.

Han D, Choi R, Hyun C. Canine pancreatic-specific lipase concentrations in dogs with heart failure and chronic mitral valvular insufficiency. J Vet Intern Med 2015;29:180–183.

Harris AN, Beatty SS, Estrada AH, et al. Investigation of an N-terminal prohormone of brain natriuretic peptide Point-of-care ELISA in clinically Normal cats and cats with cardiac disease. J Vet Intern Med 2017;31:994–999.

Heishima Y, Hori Y, Nakamura K, et al. Diagnostic accuracy of plasma atrial natriuretic peptide concentrations in cats with and without cardiomyopathies. J Vet Cardiol 2018;20:234–243.

Herndon WE, Rishniw M, Schrope D, et al. Assessment of plasma cardiac troponin I concentration as a means to differentiate cardiac and noncardiac causes of dyspnea in cats. J Am Vet Med Assoc 2008;233:1261–1264.

Hertzsch S, Roos A, Wess G. Evaluation of a sensitive cardiac troponin I assay as a screening test for the diagnosis of hypertrophic cardiomyopathy in cats. J Vet Intern Med 2019;33:1242–1250.

Hezzell MJ, Block CL, Laughlin DS, et al. Effect of prespecified therapy escalation on plasma NT-proBNP concentrations in dogs with stable congestive heart failure due to myxomatous mitral valve disease. J Vet Intern Med 2018;32:1509–1516.

Hezzell MJ, Rush JE, Humm K, et al. Differentiation of cardiac from noncardiac pleural effusions in cats using second-generation quantitative and point-of-care NT-proBNP measurements. J Vet Intern Med 2016;30:536–542.

Hori Y, Iguchi M, Heishima Y, et al. Diagnostic utility of cardiac troponin I in cats with hypertrophic cardiomyopathy. J Vet Intern Med 2018;32:922–929.

Hori Y, Iguchi M, Hirakawa A, et al. Evaluation of atrial natriuretic peptide and cardiac troponin I concentrations for assessment of disease severity in dogs with naturally occurring mitral valve disease. J Am Vet Med Assoc 2020;256:340–348.

Humm K, Hezzell M, Sargent J, et al. Differentiating between feline pleural effusions of cardiac and non-cardiac origin using pleural fluid NT-proBNP concentrations. J Small Anim Pract 2013;54:656–661.

Keen JA. Examination of horses with cardiac disease. Vet Clin North Am Equine Pract 2019;35:23–42.

Kluser L, Maier ET, Wess G. Evaluation of a high-sensitivity cardiac troponin I assay compared to a first-generation cardiac troponin I assay in Doberman Pinschers with and without dilated cardiomyopathy. J Vet Intern Med 2019;33:54–63.

Kraus MS, Jesty SA, Gelzer AR, et al. Measurement of plasma cardiac troponin I concentration by use of a point-of-care analyzer in clinically normal horses and horses with experimentally induced cardiac disease. Am J Vet Res 2010;71:55–59.

Leroux AA, Al Haidar A, Remy B, et al. Atrial natriuretic peptide as an indicator of the severity of valvular regurgitation and heart failure in horses. J Equine Vet Sci. 2014;34:1226.

Ljungvall I, Hoglund K, Tidholm A, et al. Cardiac troponin I is associated with severity of myxomatous mitral valve disease, age, and C-reactive protein in dogs. J Vet Intern Med 2010;24:153–159.

Martinelli E, Locatelli C, Bassis S, et al. Preliminary investigation of cardiovascular-renal disorders in dogs with chronic mitral valve disease. J Vet Intern Med 2016;30:1612–1618.

Mazzotta E, Guglielmini C, Menciotti G, et al. Red blood cell distribution width, hematology, and serum biochemistry in dogs with echocardiographically estimated precapillary and postcapillary pulmonary arterial hypertension. J Vet Intern Med 2016;30:1806–1815.

Nath LC, Anderson GA, Hinchcliff KW, et al. Serum cardiac troponin I concentrations in horses with cardiac disease. Aust Vet J 2012;90:351–357.

Nelson OL, Andreasen C. The utility of plasma D-dimer to identify thromboembolic disease in dogs. J Vet Intern Med 2003;17:830–834.

Oyama MA. Using cardiac biomarkers in veterinary practice. Clin Lab Med 2015;35:555–566.

Pierce KV, Rush JE, Freeman LM, et al. Association between survival time and changes in NT-proBNP in cats treated for congestive heart failure. J Vet Intern Med 2017;31:678–684.

Polizopoulou ZS, Koutinas CK, Dasopoulou A, et al. Serial analysis of serum cardiac troponin I changes and correlation with clinical findings in 46 dogs with mitral valve disease. Vet Clin Pathol 2014;43:218–225.

Reynolds CA, Brown DC, Rush JE, et al. Prediction of first onset of congestive heart failure in dogs with degenerative mitral valve disease: the PREDICT cohort study. J Vet Cardiol 2012;14:193–202.

Roderick KV, Abelson AL, Nielsen L, et al. Evaluation of red blood cell distribution width as a prognostic indicator in cats with acquired heart disease, with and without congestive heart failure. J Feline Med Surg 2017;19:648–656.

Rossi TM, Pyle WG, Maxie MG, et al. Troponin assays in the assessment of the equine myocardium. Equine Vet J 2014;46:270–275.

Ruaux C, Scollan K, Suchodolski JS, et al. Biologic variability in NT-proBNP and cardiac troponin-I in healthy dogs and dogs with mitral valve degeneration. Vet Clin Pathol 2015;44:420–430.

Shields E, Seiden-Long I, Massie S, et al. 24-hour kinetics of cardiac troponin-T using a "high-sensitivity" assay in thoroughbred chuckwagon racing geldings after race and associated clinical sampling guidelines. J Vet Intern Med 2018;32:433–440.

Singletary GE, Morris NA, Lynne O'sullivan M, et al. Prospective evaluation of NT-proBNP assay to detect occult dilated cardiomyopathy and predict survival in Doberman Pinschers. J Vet Intern Med 2012a;26:1330–1336.

Singletary GE, Rush JE, Fox PR, et al. Effect of NT-pro-BNP assay on accuracy and confidence of general practitioners in diagnosing heart failure or respiratory disease in cats with respiratory signs. J Vet Intern Med 2012b;26:542–546.

Sjöstrand K, Wess G, Ljungvall I, et al. Breed differences in natriuretic peptides in healthy dogs. J Vet Intern Med 2014;28:451–457.

Slack J, Boston RC, Soma L, et al. Cardiac troponin I in racing standardbreds. J Vet Intern Med 2012;26:1202–1208.

Smith KF, Quinn RL, Rahilly IJ. Biomarkers for differentiation of causes of respiratory distress in dogs and cats: part 1–Cardiac diseases and pulmonary hypertension. J Vet Emerg Crit Care 2015;25:311–329.

Stanzani G, Cowlam R, English K, et al. Evaluation of red blood cell distribution width in cats with hypertrophic cardiomyopathy. J Vet Cardiol 2015;17(Suppl 1):S233–243.

Swann JW, Sudunagunta S, Covey HL, et al. Evaluation of red cell distribution width in dogs with pulmonary hypertension. J Vet Cardiol 2014;16:227–235.

Tablin F, Schumacher T, Pombo M, et al. Platelet activation in cats with hypertrophic cardiomyopathy. J Vet Intern Med 2014;28:411–418.

Tanaka R, Yamane Y. Platelet aggregation in dogs with mitral valve regurgitation. Am J Vet Res 2000;61:1248–1251.

Trachsel DS, Schwarzwald CC, Bitschnau C, et al. Atrial natriuretic peptide and cardiac troponin I concentrations in healthy warmblood horses and in warmblood horses with mitral regurgitation at rest and after exercise. J Vet Cardiol 2013;15:105–121.

Van Der Vekens N, Decloedt A, Ven S, et al. Cardiac troponin I as compared to troponin T for the detection of myocardial damage in horses. J Vet Intern Med 2015;29:348–354.

Wess G, Butz V, Mahling M, et al. Evaluation of N-terminal pro-B-type natriuretic peptide as a diagnostic marker of various stages of cardiomyopathy in Doberman Pinschers. Am J Vet Res 2011a;72:642–649.

Wess G, Domenech O, Dukes-McEwan J, et al. European Society of Veterinary Cardiology screening guidelines for dilated cardiomyopathy in Doberman Pinschers. J Vet Cardiol 2017;19:405-415.

Wess G, Daisenberger P, Mahling M, et al. Utility of measuring plasma N-terminal pro-brain natriuretic peptide in detecting hypertrophic cardiomyopathy and differentiating grades of severity in cats. Vet Clin Pathol 2011b;40:237–244.

Winter RL, Saunders AB, Gordon SG, et al. Biologic variability of N-terminal pro-brain natriuretic peptide in healthy dogs and dogs with myxomatous mitral valve disease. J Vet Cardiol 2017;19:124–131.

Winter RL, Saunders AB, Gordon SG, et al. Analytical validation and clinical evaluation of a commercially available high-sensitivity immunoassay for the measurement of troponin I in humans for use in dogs. J Vet Cardiol 2014;16:81–89.

Wolf J, Gerlach N, Weber K, et al. The diagnostic relevance of NT-proBNP and proANP 31-67 measurements in staging of myxomatous mitral valve disease in dogs. Vet Clin Pathol 2013;42:196–206.

Wurtinger G, Henrich E, Hildebrandt N, et al. Assessment of a bedside test for N-terminal pro B-type natriuretic peptide (NT-proBNP) to differentiate cardiac from non-cardiac causes of pleural effusion in cats. BMC Vet Res 2017;13:394.

Yu IB, Huang HP. Prevalence and prognosis of Anemia in dogs with degenerative mitral valve disease. Biomed Res Int 2016;2016:4727054.

Section III

Heart Failure

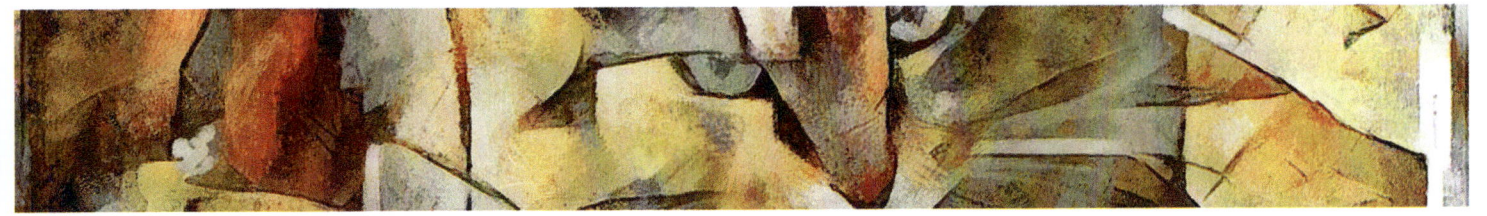

20
HEART FAILURE
Pathophysiology and Patient Assessment

Heart failure often is defined as the state where the heart cannot supply adequate blood flow to meet tissue metabolic demands, or only can do so when cardiac filling pressures are elevated. Heart failure involves abnormalities of systolic (contractile, pumping) or diastolic (filling) function, or both. These abnormalities initially develop without evidence of excess fluid accumulation (congestion) or obvious decline in exercise capacity. Multiple cardiac and systemic "compensatory" mechanisms are activated to sustain cardiac output, systemic arterial blood pressure, and tissue perfusion pressure. Paradigms of heart failure have over time focused on (1) changes in the heart as a pump; (2) the role of the kidneys in compensation and development of the congestive state; (3) neural and hormonal activations; and (4) intracellular and molecular responses to the failing heart. Regardless of the "compensation," these mechanisms are viewed as maladaptive over time because they contribute to progressive cardiovascular (CV) and renal dysfunction, and promote the fluid accumulation which characterizes congestive heart failure (CHF).

As observed in our patients, the end result of heart failure involves signs of low cardiac output or poor tissue perfusion and signs related to congestion, manifested as tissue edema and/or accumulation of effusions within serous body cavities. **Table 20.1** lists common signs associated with heart failure. Diseases that mainly affect the left heart lead to "left-sided" congestive signs. However, while so-called "right-sided" CHF signs are typical manifestations of right heart disease, they also can develop in some animals with left heart (or biventricular) disease.

CHF is not a specific diagnosis, but rather a complex pathophysiologic state and clinical syndrome. It involves an injury stimulus, altered heart and vascular function, and associated structural changes (remodeling) within the heart, the vasculature, and other organs. This remodeling becomes maladaptive and results from (over)expression of compensatory neurohormonal (NH) and other responses to reduced cardiac output and arterial underfilling. In most situations, heart failure is a progressive process. Underlying the state of heart failure are three related cardiac diagnoses: Anatomic/morphologic, etiologic, and pathophysiologic, with the last considered in the following section.

Both the location and the type of lesion are pertinent to the development of cardiac dysfunction and heart failure. Most cases of heart failure stem from congenital or acquired diseases of these structures: (1) Cardiac valves and endocardium (valvular heart diseases); (2) atrial and ventricular myocardium (cardiomyopathies); (3) pericardium (pericardial diseases/pericardial effusions); (4) impulse-forming and conduction system (cardiac arrhythmias); and (5) blood vessels (vascular diseases, including functional disorders like hypertension). The vascular system can be subdivided into the coronary circulation, the systemic circulation (including the aorta), and the pulmonary circulation (including the pulmonary trunk). Many heart diseases are "named" by the type of disorder and one of these five anatomic locations. Examples of these *anatomic diagnoses* include "infective valvular endocarditis", "hypertrophic cardiomyopathy", and "pulmonary arterial hypertension". These tissues can undergo limited responses to injury as defined by the *morphologic* cardiac diagnosis. This is represented by the gross or histopathologic lesion(s) a pathologist might describe. Common lesions include malformation or growth disturbances, disruption (trauma or tearing), hypertrophy, atrophy, apoptosis, degeneration, inflammation (septic or sterile), hemorrhage, infiltration, necrosis, fibrosis, and neoplasia. Blood vessels might be narrowed from vasculitis, degenerative change, smooth muscle hypertrophy, or lipid deposition. Blood vessels also can be occluded by thrombus, embolized material, or neoplasms. Clinicians can suspect or visualize many CV lesions based on physical diagnosis, selected laboratory tests, and noninvasive imaging, especially echocardiography. However,

Cardiovascular Disease in Companion Animals 299

Table 20.1 Clinical Signs of Heart Failure

Low Cardiac Output Signs
- Tiring
- Exertional weakness
- Syncope
- Prerenal azotemia
- Cool extremities (from poor peripheral circulation)
- Pallor and prolonged capillary refill time
- Cardiac arrhythmias

Congestive Signs—"Left-Sided" (from High LV Filling Pressure)
- Pulmonary congestion and edema (tachypnea, increased respiratory effort, orthopnea, cough, pulmonary crackles, tiring, hemoptysis, cyanosis)
- Pleural effusion (in cats and horses)
- Secondary "right-sided" heart failure signs
- Cardiac arrhythmias

Congestive Signs—"Right-Sided" (from High RV Filling Pressure)
- Systemic venous congestion (high central venous pressure, jugular vein distension)
- Hepatic, renal, ± splenic congestion
- Pleural effusion (increased respiratory effort, tiring, orthopnea, cyanosis)
- Ascites (tiring, increased respiratory effort)
- Small pericardial effusion
- Subcutaneous edema (rare in small animals; common in horses)
- Cardiac arrhythmias

Abbreviations: LV, left ventricular; RV, right ventricular.

lesions underlying heart failure might only be confirmed after postmortem examination, or once specialized tests, such as genetic or biochemical markers of disease, are identified.

The *etiologic diagnosis* is the cause of the initiating cardiac injury. This could relate to (1) cardiac malformations; (2) genetic mutations that might present as congenital or acquired disease; (3) degenerative processes; (4) nutritional deficiency (or excess); (5) metabolic and endocrine disorders; (6) toxicities (both natural and drug or chemical-induced); (7) inflammation, from infection or immune-mediated disease; (8) ischemia; (9) thrombosis; and (10) functional dysregulation of the heart or blood vessels (including systemic and pulmonary hypertension, PH). The pathologic basis for some cardiac disorders is unknown (idiopathic), while some others are iatrogenic. The initiating stimulus could occur years before clinical evidence of heart failure appears. Ultimately, maladaptive responses lead to further CV functional impairment and with heart failure, promote renal salt retention, volume expansion, and congestive signs. The development of CHF, therefore, entails an initiating (and often undetected) cardiac injury; a phase of compensation, yet with clinically silent disease progression; and finally, the onset of clinical CHF signs. For most veterinary patients, heart disease is identified only late in this process. From a functional standpoint, heart failure reduces exercise capacity and causes secondary pulmonary dysfunction, as well as metabolic abnormalities that arise from impaired organ perfusion and congestion.

Pathophysiology

General Perspectives

Cardiac lesions create pathophysiologic abnormalities that might eventually lead to the clinical signs of CHF. These are summarized in subsequent paragraphs. The four fundamental pathophysiologic abnormalities of heart failure have been summarized as (1) contractility failure; (2) hemodynamic overload; (3) diastolic heart failure; and (4) arrhythmia. Hemodynamic overloads are divided into those where excessive ventricular volume is pumped during systole (volume overload) or where ventricular pumping occurs at higher than normal systolic pressure (pressure overload). This simple pathophysiologic grouping emphasizes the major hemodynamic mechanisms responsible for CHF, accepting that functional disorders can occur simultaneously, as observed with advanced dilated cardiomyopathy. As such, it offers a useful construct when assessing and managing the individual patient.

Contractility Failure

Contractility or myocardial failure is characterized by a depressed inotropic state and ventricular systolic dysfunction. Over time, the affected ventricle progressively dilates under the influence of increasing filling pressures. Unlike a primary volume overload with secondary ventricular dilation, such as from chronic mitral valve regurgitation, the ventricular stroke volume is not increased. The general appearance of the affected ventricle by echocardiography has the key abnormalities of ventricular chamber dilation with reduced ejection fraction. There can be reduced wall thickness (to luminal ratio) or eccentric hypertrophy (ventricular dilation with a normal wall thickness and increased myocardial mass). "Functional" atrioventricular (AV) valve insufficiency commonly develops as a consequence of progressive ventricular (and valve annulus) dilation, even without concurrent valvular disease. Dilated cardiomyopathy (DCM) is the most notable cause of myocardial failure in animals (Chapters 32–34). Other causes of myocardial failure include persistent, rapid tachycardia (as from sustained supraventricular or ventricular tachycardias); some nutritional or metabolic deficiencies; and cardiac muscle inflammation, infection, or infarction.

Increased Workload

Volume overload heart failure usually is caused either by an incompetent (leaky) valve or an abnormal systemic-to-pulmonary shunt, or sometimes both. A chronic high-output state (such as hyperthyroidism or severe anemia) also can underlie this. The usual appearance of the ventricle affected by volume overload is that of eccentric hypertrophy with normal to increased ejection fraction. Myocardial contractility often is maintained near normal levels for quite some time as the affected chambers progressively dilate, although secondary deterioration of myocardial contractility can occur eventually. Chronic degenerative (myxomatous) mitral valve disease (DMVD), tricuspid regurgitation from degeneration or congenital malformation, and less often, valvular endocarditis (Chapters 29–31) and some congenital shunts and malformations (Chapters 26 and 27, p. 480), are the usual causes of volume overload CHF.

Pressure overload heart failure can develop when the affected ventricle must generate greater than normal systolic pressure in order to eject blood. This occurs with ventricular outflow obstructions or persistently high systemic or pulmonary vascular resistance. An excessive systolic pressure load stimulates myocardial hypertrophy (see "Cardiac Responses" and p. 16). The general appearance of the affected ventricle is that of concentric hypertrophy (reduced chamber size with increased wall thickness and increased myocardial mass), along with normal to increased ejection fraction. Concentric hypertrophy impairs myocardial relaxation and increases ventricular wall stiffness, causing diastolic dysfunction. The pathologic hypertrophy is not accompanied by normal coronary ingrowth, which creates higher risk for myocardial ischemia or infarctions. With a chronic, severe pressure overload, myocardial contractility eventually declines, and secondary chamber dilation can occur. Common causes of ventricular pressure overload include stenosis of the pulmonic or (sub)aortic valve regions (Chapter 27), PH (Chapters 39 and 40), and systemic hypertension (Chapter 38). Pulmonic stenosis and PH associated with congenital heart disease cause concentric right ventricular hypertrophy. In contrast, acquired PH (such as occurs with canine heartworm disease) results in a mixed pattern of hypertrophy, with increased wall thickness and ventricular dilation.

Diastolic Dysfunction

Diastolic dysfunction means that ventricular filling cannot be maintained with normal venous and atrial pressures. This usually occurs from some combination of impaired myocardial relaxation during early- to mid-diastolic filling and reduced ventricular compliance, caused by increased muscle or chamber stiffness in mid- to late diastole. Impaired active relaxation is a common feature of myocardial disease and hypertrophy; it also occurs with myocardial ischemia. Increased stiffness occurs with myocardial hypertrophy, fibrosis, or extreme chamber dilation. External cardiac compression, caused by pericardial effusion (tamponade) or pericardial constraint (constrictive pericarditis), also induces diastolic dysfunction.

Mild (Grade I) diastolic dysfunction is present when active myocardial relaxation is impaired; this change accompanies normal aging, as well. A vigorous atrial contraction can compensate for a relaxation abnormality by briefly increasing atrial filling pressure at end-diastole. In isolation, Grade I dysfunction is not associated with CHF. Moderate diastolic dysfunction (Grade II) is associated with both impaired relaxation and increasing chamber stiffness. The usual compensations are through atrial contraction and fluid retention, which increase mean venous and atrial pressures. This can advance to severe (Grade III) diastolic dysfunction, where ventricular filling can occur only during early diastole, at which time the chamber restricts further active, passive and atrial contributions to filling; this predisposes to CHF. Conditions that shorten diastole, and thereby reduce ventricular filling and coronary perfusion, worsen diastolic dysfunction. Sinus tachycardia (as with exercise), loss of atrial contraction (from atrial fibrillation, AF), erratic cardiac cycles (from AF or premature beats), and loss of AV synchronization (as with ventricular tachycardias) all can exacerbate diastolic dysfunction (also see p. 127).

Diseases characterized by impaired or restricted ventricular filling include hypertrophic and restrictive forms of cardiomyopathy (Chapters 33 and 32, p. 629), pericardial diseases (Chapter 35), and concentric hypertrophy caused by pressure overloads. Consequences of abnormal ventricular wall stiffness or external restriction to venous inflow include elevated ventricular filling pressure and smaller diastolic volume. Even with preserved contractility, reduction in preload can lead to diminished cardiac output, high venous pressures, and CHF. Although contractility initially might be normal in most cases, progressive deterioration can occur. Additional comorbidities could include valvular dysfunction and increased arterial pressures. Relatively uncommon causes of impaired ventricular filling include congenital AV valve stenosis, cor triatriatum, and intracardiac mass lesions.

Clinical Associations

The features of left- and right-sided CHF frequently overlap, as noted previously (**Table 20.1**). Because of the interdependence between right and left ventricles, a disease that initially might involve only one side of the heart will eventually influence the other. For example, dogs with left-sided CHF caused by chronic mitral valve regurgitation might eventually develop congestive signs typical for right heart disease too as a consequence of secondary (postcapillary) PH, or with the onset of AF secondary to left atrial dilation. Furthermore, because capillaries in the visceral (as opposed to parietal) pleura drain into pulmonary veins, persistently high pulmonary venous pressure can promote the accumulation of pleural effusion as well as pulmonary edema; this mechanism is thought to be particularly relevant in cats with cardiomyopathy and horses with chronic heart failure. As another example of ventricular interdependence, pericardial diseases or marked right ventricular dilation shift the interventricular septum leftward as the right ventricle fills; this consequently reduces left heart filling. Ultimately, poor output from either ventricle compromises (filling and) output from the other, because cardiac output from both ventricles must be balanced.

In general, diseases of the mitral and aortic valves will cause signs of left-sided CHF, while those of the tricuspid and pulmonary valves will cause right-sided CHF. Cardiomyopathies usually produce left-sided or biventricular CHF. Pericardial diseases and PH are characterized by signs of right-sided CHF. Congenital left-to-right shunts can cause left-sided (patent ductus arteriosus, PDA; ventricular septal defect, VSD), right-sided (atrial septal defect, ASD), or biventricular CHF (PDA with PH in cats; some cases of VSD, especially in cats and horses; and AV septal defects with AV regurgitation). High output states such as thyrotoxicosis and anemia, as well as chronic tachyarrhythmias, cause biventricular CHF, often with prominent pleural effusion. Chronic bradycardia can cause left- or right-sided failure. In dogs with CHF, large-volume fluid retention most often accumulates within the peritoneal space, although pleural effusion can occur too. In cats and horses, fluid retention within the pleural space is typically most prominent; this often occurs even in the setting of left-sided heart disease. Horses with biventricular or right-side CHF also will have subcutaneous edema. AF and PH are two key factors that can lead to biventricular CHF, even when superimposed on mainly left-heart disease.

Cardiac Responses

Changes in ventricular and atrial size, mass, shape, and stiffness that occur in response to the various mechanical, biochemical, and molecular signals induced by an underlying cardiac injury or stress constitute cardiac remodeling (**Figure 20.1**). Such changes include myocardial cell hypertrophy, apoptosis, excessive interstitial matrix formation, fibrosis, and destruction of normal collagen binding between individual myocytes. The latter, resulting from effects of myocardial collagenases or matrix metalloproteinases, can contribute to dilation or distortion of the ventricle because of slippage between adjacent myocytes. Stimuli for cardiac remodeling include mechanical forces (such as increased wall stress from volume or pressure overload) and also the effects of various neurohormones (see section "Neurohormonal Mechanisms") and proinflammatory cytokines.

Other biochemical abnormalities related to cellular energy production, intracellular Ca^{++} fluxes, protein synthesis, and catecholamine metabolism can contribute; these have been variably identified in different models of heart failure and in clinical patients. Abnormal intracellular Ca^{++} handling and reduced stores in the sarcoplasmic reticulum could relate to decreased activity of the main Ca^{++} reuptake pump (the sarcoendoplasmic reticulum calcium transport ATPase or SERCA), as well as alterations in membrane Na–Ca exchanger and ryanodine receptor functioning. These changes can delay both the rate of systolic rise in myocyte cytosolic Ca^{++} concentration and diastolic Ca^{++} removal; such delays impair systolic and diastolic myocardial function, respectively. Abnormal myofibrillar ATPase activity, troponin regulation, and shifts in contractile element isoform also can reduce contractile function. Myocyte hypertrophy and reactive fibrosis increase total cardiac mass by eccentric and, in some cases, concentric patterns of hypertrophy. Ventricular hypertrophy can increase chamber stiffness, impair relaxation, and cause filling pressures to increase. These abnormalities of diastolic function also can contribute to systolic failure. Furthermore, concentric hypertrophy of the ventricular wall can lead to a relative decrease in myocardial capillary density. This increases the risk for ischemia and impaired mitochondrial ATP production, especially when intraventricular pressures are abnormally increased. Additionally, ventricular remodeling and abnormal intracellular Ca^{++} cycling can promote the development of arrhythmias. For example, slowed diastolic Ca^{++} reuptake within myocytes can facilitate abnormal membrane afterdepolarizations and triggered activity (p. 365). Local membrane conduction abnormalities induced by disease or remodeling can promote reentrant arrhythmias. Either mechanism of arrhythmogenesis could further impair cardiac mechanical function or lead to sudden death.

Myocardial ischemia and necrosis cause acute and sometimes dramatic release of cardiac troponin (cTn) proteins into the circulation. Increases in circulating cTn proteins also can occur with chronic heart diseases, especially as severity worsens. Examples include DMVD, DCM, heartworm disease, PH and pericardial diseases in dogs; cardiomyopathy in cats; and some cases of CHF in horses. Elevated cTn in these conditions presumably reflects ongoing myocardial damage caused by the underlying disease and cardiac remodeling processes. Increased cTnI is associated with myocardial fibrosis and the severity of myocardial arteriosclerosis in dogs with DMVD.

The Frank–Starling relationship (p. 15) describes the observation that an increase in ventricular filling (preload) induces greater contractile force and stroke volume during the next contraction. This beat-to-beat adjustment in cardiac response balances the output of both ventricles and enhances overall cardiac output when there is an acute increase in venous return or hemodynamic load. In the short-term, the

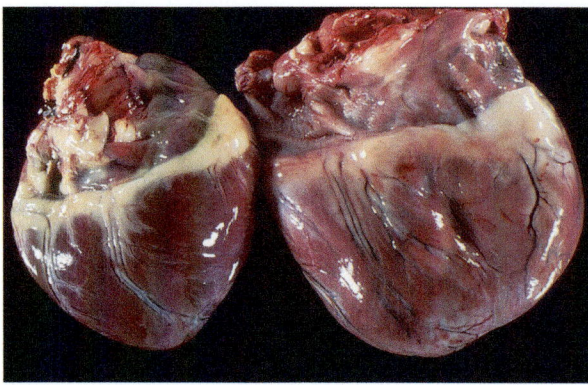

Figure 20.1 The enlarged and rounded heart from a Doberman Pinchser with dilated cardiomyopathy (right) shows the effects of cardiac remodeling. The normal heart from a dog of similar body size (left) is shown for comparison. (Image courtesy of Dr. W Morrison.)

Frank–Starling effect helps normalize cardiac output under conditions of increased pressure or volume loading; however, these conditions also increase cardiac wall stress and myocardial oxygen consumption.

Ventricular wall stress is related directly to ventricular pressure and internal dimensions, and inversely to wall thickness (Laplace's law; p. 16). Compensatory myocardial hypertrophy reduces wall stress and lessens the importance of the Frank–Starling mechanism in chronic heart failure. The pattern of hypertrophy which develops depends on the underlying cardiac disease process. Chronic volume loading increases diastolic wall stress and promotes "eccentric" hypertrophy, where myocardial fiber elongation and chamber dilation occur as new sarcomeres are laid down in series. Reduction in the extracellular collagen matrix and intercellular support structure also occurs in dogs with chronic volume overloading caused by mitral valve insufficiency. Conversely, a chronic increase in systolic pressure load stimulates "concentric" hypertrophy, where myocardial fibers and ventricular walls thicken as contractile units are added in parallel. Abnormal pressure and volume loads both impair cardiac performance over time. Volume loads are better tolerated because myocardial oxygen demand is not as severe; however, decompensation and myocardial failure eventually develop. In primary myocardial diseases, initial loading conditions typically are normal; however, the intrinsic myocardial defects eventually lead to the characteristic dilation or hypertrophy observed. Secondary alterations in preload and afterload also contribute.

High systolic pressure generation increases myocardial oxygen demand; yet, concentric hypertrophy tends to be associated with a relative reduction in the density of capillaries and mitochondria which can predispose to ischemia. Chronic myocardial hypoxia and ischemia stimulate further fibrosis and dysfunction. Impaired active relaxation in early diastole (p. 14) contributes to increased ventricular stiffness and diastolic dysfunction. Another cause of diastolic dysfunction is the external constraint to ventricular filling that occurs with pericardial diseases (Chapter 35). The diastolic impairment also can contribute to systolic dysfunction, not only because of associated reductions in ventricular preload, but additionally because cardiac wall compression compromises myocardial perfusion. In the end, clinical heart failure of various etiologies can be viewed as a state of decompensated hypertrophy, in which ventricular function progressively deteriorates as both contractility and relaxation become more abnormal.

Neurohormonal Mechanisms

NH responses contribute to cardiac remodeling and also have more far-reaching effects. Although these mechanisms support the circulation in situations of acute hypotension and hypovolemia, their chronic activation accelerates further deterioration of cardiac function. The clinical syndrome of CHF is largely the consequence of excessive NH activation over time. Major NH changes in heart failure include increased sympathetic nervous tone, attenuated vagal tone, renin–angiotensin–aldosterone system (RAAS) activation, and increased release of arginine vasopressin (AVP), also known as antidiuretic hormone (ADH). Increased production of endothelin (ETN) and proinflammatory cytokines, as well as altered expression of the counteracting vasodilatory and natriuretic factors, contribute to the complex interplay among these NH mechanisms and their consequences. The various NH mechanisms work independently and in concert. Eventually, the increased vascular volume (through renal Na^+ and water retention and increased thirst), vasoconstriction, and proinflammatory and profibrotic responses that characterize CHF predominate as the counterbalancing natriuretic and vasodilatory mechanisms are overwhelmed (**Figure 20.2**). Although increased lymphatic flow does help moderate the effect of rising venous pressures on capillary fluid dynamics, excessive volume retention eventually results in tissue edema and effusions. Systemic vasoconstriction, mediated by G protein (Gq)-linked vascular smooth muscle receptor activation, redistributes blood flow away from less "vital" organs and increases cardiac workload. This can reduce forward cardiac output, as well as exacerbate cardiac valvular regurgitation. Chronic vasoconstrictive stimulation by these multiple NH mediators also triggers processes that lead to vascular smooth muscle hypertrophy and extracellular matrix remodeling.

The extent to which different NH mechanisms are activated varies with the severity and etiology of heart failure. However, in general, their intensity increases as failure worsens. NH activation initially is selective and regional; generalized systemic activation is a late occurrence. For example, increased cardiac and renal sympathetic activity and natriuretic peptide release occur initially in association with asymptomatic left ventricular (LV) dysfunction. This precedes congestive signs. While the initial stimulus for NH activation is unclear, it is thought that stimulation of low-pressure cardiac receptors, ventricular dilation, and early cardiac remodeling increase sympathetic afferent activity which then initiates the NH activation process. This is in contrast to the concept of low cardiac output or reduced effective circulating blood volume as initiating activators. Nevertheless, reduced cardiac output and arterial baroreceptor unloading eventually lead to systemic NH activation.

Sympathetic Nervous System The effects of sympathetic nervous system (SNS) stimulation (including increased contractility, heart rate, and venous return) can maintain or even increase cardiac output initially. However, over time these SNS effects become detrimental by increasing afterload stress and myocardial oxygen requirements, contributing to cellular damage and myocardial fibrosis, and enhancing the potential for cardiac arrhythmias. Diminished heart rate variability is another manifestation of high sympathetic, and decreased

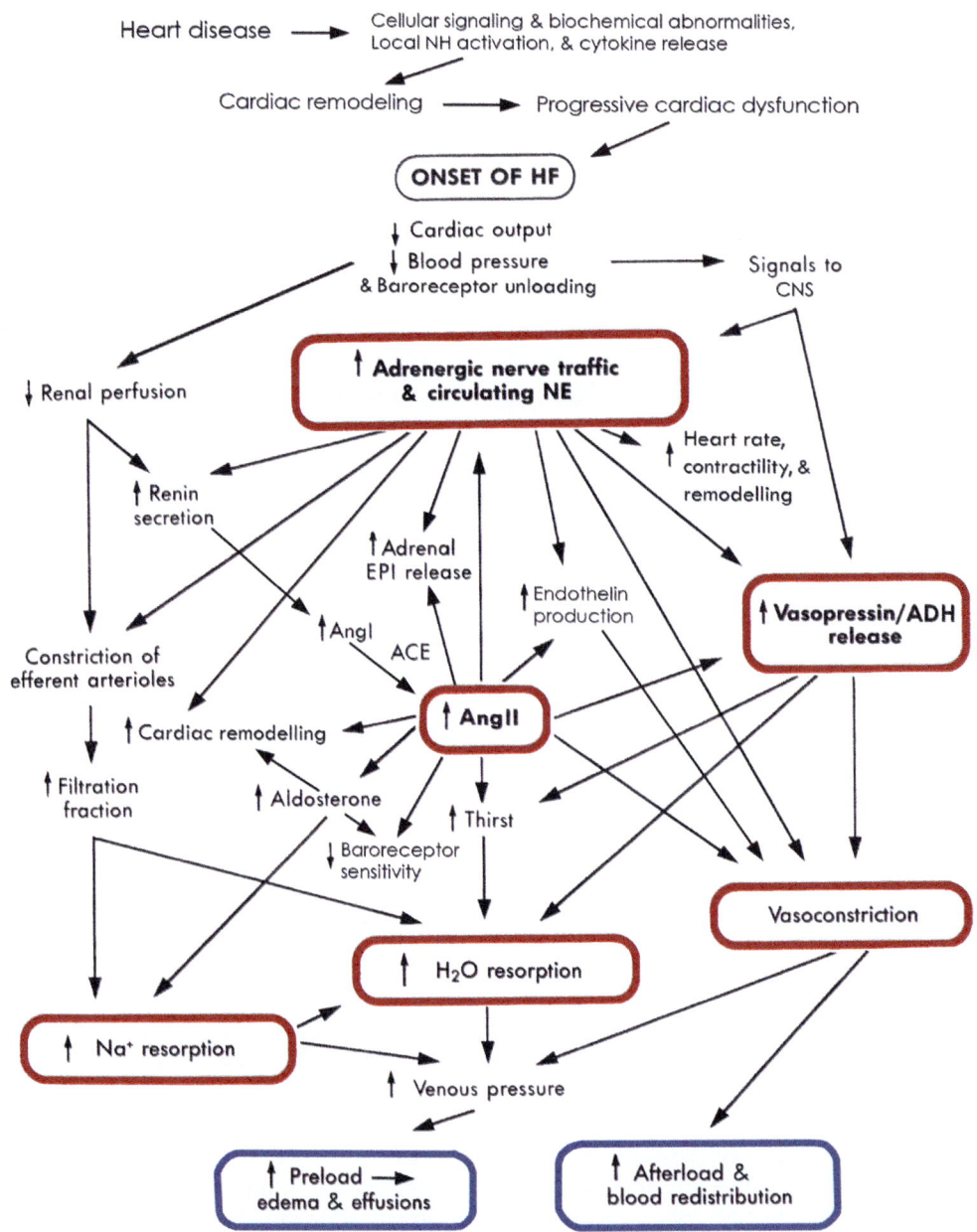

Figure 20.2 Diagram depicting some major neurohormonal interactions and effects during heart failure. ACE, angiotensin-converting enzyme; ADH, antidiuretic hormone; Ang, angiotensin; CNS, central nervous system; EPI, epinephrine; HF, heart failure; NE, norepinephrine; NH, neurohormonal.

parasympathetic, tone. Reduced heart rate variability is known to occur in dogs and other animals with CHF, as well as with other conditions where sympathetic activity is increased.

Norepinephrine (NE) promotes arrhythmias by increasing automaticity, among other electrophysiologic effects. Via $beta_1$-receptor activation, NE increases cyclic adenosine monophosphate (cAMP) production and intracellular Ca^{++} concentrations. Prolonged and excessive exposure contributes to calcium overload and cell necrosis. NE also can stimulate maladaptive myocyte hypertrophy and increase oxidative stress, which can promote apoptosis. The peripheral vasoconstrictive effect of NE and its renal effects to promote volume retention contribute to increased ventricular size and pressure; this also raises myocardial oxygen demand. Increased NE release from sympathetic nerve terminals promotes NE spillover into the circulation, even as cardiac NE stores are depleted. Catecholamine release from the adrenal medulla also can contribute. Elevated circulating NE concentrations are seen in heart failure. Several studies have documented increased NE and epinephrine concentrations in dogs and cats with heart failure, compared to normal animals. Some have shown correlations between increased circulating catecholamine levels and CHF severity and worse prognosis.

Continued exposure to sympathetic stimulation reduces cardiac sensitivity to catecholamines; this occurs via decreased myocardial beta$_1$-receptor density (downregulation), uncoupling of beta$_2$-receptors from the G-regulatory protein complex, and other changes in cellular signaling. However, myocardial beta$_1$-receptor downregulation might help protect the myocardium against the cardiotoxic and arrhythmogenic effects of catecholamines. Beta-blocking drugs can reverse beta$_1$-receptor downregulation but could worsen heart failure. Cardiac beta$_2$- and alpha$_1$-receptors are thought to contribute to myocardial remodeling and arrhythmogenesis, too; however, they do not undergo downregulation. Horses in heart failure appear to have increased beta$_2$-receptor expression rather than beta$_1$-receptor downregulation. The cardiac beta$_3$-receptor subtype could promote deterioration in myocardial function through a negative inotropic effect.

Baroreceptor Function Normal feedback regulation of the sympathetic nervous and hormonal systems depends on arterial and atrial baroreceptor function (p. 28). However, baroreceptor responsiveness becomes blunted in chronic heart failure. Increased sympathetic stimulation and the effects of angiotensin (Ang)II and aldosterone (ALD) contribute to baroreceptor desensitization. This desensitization in turn contributes to sustained sympathetic and hormonal activation, as well as attenuated inhibitory vagal effects. Attenuated baroreflex control of renal sympathetic nerve activity appears to occur even earlier than systemic arterial baroreceptor desensitization in animals with LV dysfunction. Yet baroreceptor dysfunction can improve with heart failure therapy, increased myocardial contractility, decreased cardiac loading conditions, or inhibition of AngII and possibly ALD. Digoxin, and potentially mineralocorticoid receptor blockers (spironolactone), enhance baroreceptor sensitivity toward normal.

Renin–Angiotensin–Aldosterone System The RAAS has far-reaching and complex effects, both systemically and locally. Its chronic activation contributes to the progression of CV, and renal, disease. Systemic RAAS activation follows SNS activation, and in general, coincides with onset of CHF signs. Local tissue activation appears to begin earlier. However, the underlying cardiac disease could influence the time course of systemic RAAS activation. For example, increased plasma renin activity and ALD are not found in all patients with CHF. Conversely, such increases can occur in dogs with only mitral valve prolapse rather than mitral regurgitation per se. Nonetheless, systemic RAAS activation occurs in CHF caused by DCM and probably in advanced failure of other causes, too. Diuretic therapy is known to activate the RAAS, also.

Systemic RAAS activation involves the release of renin from the renal juxtaglomerular apparatus in response to several stimuli, including renal beta$_1$-adrenergic stimulation, low perfusion pressure, and reduced Na$^+$ delivery to the macula densa of the distal renal tubule. Stringent dietary salt restriction, diuretic or vasodilator therapy, dehydration, and even strenuous exercise also promote renin release. Renin converts the precursor peptide angiotensinogen (a globular glycoprotein formed in the liver) to the decapeptide AngI, also notated as AngI(1-10) or Ang1-10 (**Figure 20.3**; also see **Figure 1.30**, p. 29). Angiotensin-converting enzyme (ACE), produced in

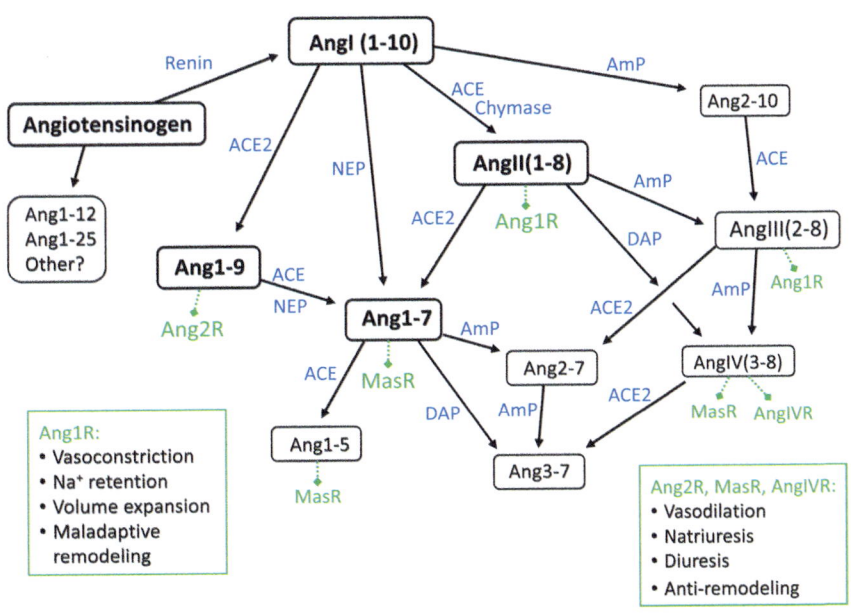

Figure 20.3 Schematic of expanded renin–angiotensin cascade and major effects mediated by various receptors. The different angiotensin molecules are identified by an Arabic number suffix, which denotes amino acid sequence (derived from parent molecule). Other endopeptidase, carboxypeptidase, or aminopeptidase enzymes also can catalyze certain conversions. Additional metabolites not depicted. ACE, angiotensin converting enzyme; AmP, aminopeptidase; Ang, angiotensin; DAP, aspartyl aminopeptidase; NEP, neutral endopeptidase; R, receptor. (Adapted from Larouche-Lebel, 2019)

endothelial cells of the lung and elsewhere, then converts the inactive AngI into the active octapeptide AngII, also notated as AngII(1-8) or Ang1-8. ACE also degrades certain vasodilator kinins, including bradykinin. AngII can be further cleaved to AngIII, or AngIII(2-8), which has similar although less potent actions than AngII. Other enzymes can generate AngII from its inactive precursor, including chymase and other proteases; these are thought to have greater importance at the local tissue level.

AngII exerts diverse effects, both systemically and locally. The majority of AngII effects are mediated by angiotensin type-1 receptors (Ang1R), which are located in the heart, vasculature, kidneys, liver, pituitary gland, and adrenal gland. Ang2R also exist, although AngII has little interaction with these; Ang2R effects largely counteract those of Ang1R. AngII (via Ang1R) is a potent vasoconstrictor. It also causes Na^+ and water retention by a direct effect on the proximal tubule and by stimulating ALD release from the adrenal cortex. Although AngII vasoconstriction affects both afferent and efferent arterioles in renal glormeruli, its effect on efferent arterioles is most pronounced and can maintain glomerular filtration pressure even in the setting of reduced renal blood flow (thereby increasing the filtration fraction). Additional effects of AngII include increased thirst and salt appetite, enhanced neuronal NE synthesis and release, blockade of neuronal NE reuptake, enhanced AVP (ADH) release, and increased adrenal epinephrine secretion. AngII also inhibits renin release as a negative feedback effect. Increased circulating AngII and ALD concentrations have been associated with worse prognosis in people.

Local production of AngII (and ALD) occurs in the heart, blood vessels, adrenal glands, kidney, and other tissues. Tissue chymase is more important than ACE in the production of active AngII within the myocardium and extracellular matrix. Chymase can be released from mast cells, as well as cardiac fibroblasts and vascular endothelial cells during tissue remodeling. A pro-renin pathway also can be involved in local Ang production. AngII produced locally exerts its effects on CV structure and function via G protein (Gq) signaling and several mitogen-activated protein kinases. This local activity promotes tissue remodeling, including hypertrophy, inflammation, and fibrosis, as well as enhanced sympathetic effects. ALD also contributes to this maladaptive remodeling. Local RAAS activation affects the kidney and other tissues, as well. Local vasoconstriction, increased ETN expression, reduced nitric oxide (NO) synthesis, and other effects contribute to vascular endothelial dysfunction. Proinflammatory effects include regulation of cytokine and chemokine expression which ultimately promotes increases in blood pressure, oxidative stress, inflammatory cell infiltration, and fibrosis. Renin–Ang system components also are important in the brain; AngII and AngIII function via Ang1R to increase thirst, AVP release, SNS activity, and blood pressure, and to impair baroreceptor function. Elevated AngII concentrations also might promote development of the skeletal muscle wasting seen with cardiac cachexia.

Additional Ang metabolites and pathways have been identified, which expands the traditional concept of the renin-Ang cascade and its effects (**Figure 20.3**). Some metabolites, including Ang1-7 and Ang1-9, have effects that oppose those of AngII. The enzyme ACE2 (a homologue of ACE) can convert AngII into the heptapeptide, Ang1-7, which has cardioprotective effects mediated by the so-called Mas receptor (MasR). These include vasodilation, stimulation of natriuretic peptide release and NO synthesis, and anti-fibrotic effects. In addition, AngI can be converted (directly and indirectly) into Ang1-7 by several enzymes, including the neutral endopeptidase, neprilysin. Ang1-9 is another cardioprotective metabolite, which is cleaved from AngI by the action of ACE2; Ang1-9 exerts its effects via the Ang2R. Ang2R activation promotes vasodilatory, anti-fibrotic, anti-inflammatory, and other beneficial effects. These pathways become more active when levels of AngI and AngII increase, as occurs in heart failure, especially when an ACE inhibitor or angiotensin receptor blocker (ARB) is used. ACE2 is expressed within the CV system, kidney, lungs, brain, and other locations. Its activity does not appear to be affected by ACE inhibitors. Significant increases in circulating concentrations of AngI, Ang1-7, and Ang1-9 have been documented in dogs with CHF caused by DMVD and on ACE inhibitor therapy, compared to dogs with stage B2 disease that were not receiving an ACE inhibitor, and especially compared to healthy dogs (**Figure 20.4**; Larouche-Lebel, 2019). Similarly, ARB administration to cats with cardiomyopathy appears to increase Ang1-7 production. The benefits of using an ACE inhibitor or ARB in CHF, therefore, could relate not only to reduced production of AngII and degradation of bradykinin, but also to increased production of Ang1-7 and Ang1-9 (and certain other Ang metabolites). In conjunction with this, ACE2-mediated generation of cardioprotective Ang can decrease the availability of AngII and its substrate, AngI.

Circadian variation occurs in RAAS activation and systemic blood pressure, the timing of which has been linked to feeding in dogs fed at a regular once daily time (Mochel, 2015). Observed circadian oscillations in renin activity, blood pressure and urinary electrolyte excretion are probably linked to the sodium retaining effects of AngII and ALD and the vasomotor effect of AngII. This chronobiologic effect is thought to involve the autonomic nervous system, dietary salt, and feeding-related hormones (such as ghrelin). The amount of sodium intake influences the tonic and phasic secretion of renin, with more sodium triggering a smaller degree of renin secretion. The timing of food (particularly sodium) intake appears to influence the timing of the renin secretion and circadian blood pressure peaks. ACE inhibition with benazepril was shown to alter RAAS dynamics by markedly reducing AngII and ALD release for approximately 5–10 hours. Therefore, the timing of ACE inhibitor administration with relation to food intake could have useful therapeutic implications (see p. 322).

The inhibition of ACE can reduce NH activation, promote vasodilation and diuresis, reduce ALD release, and reduce the

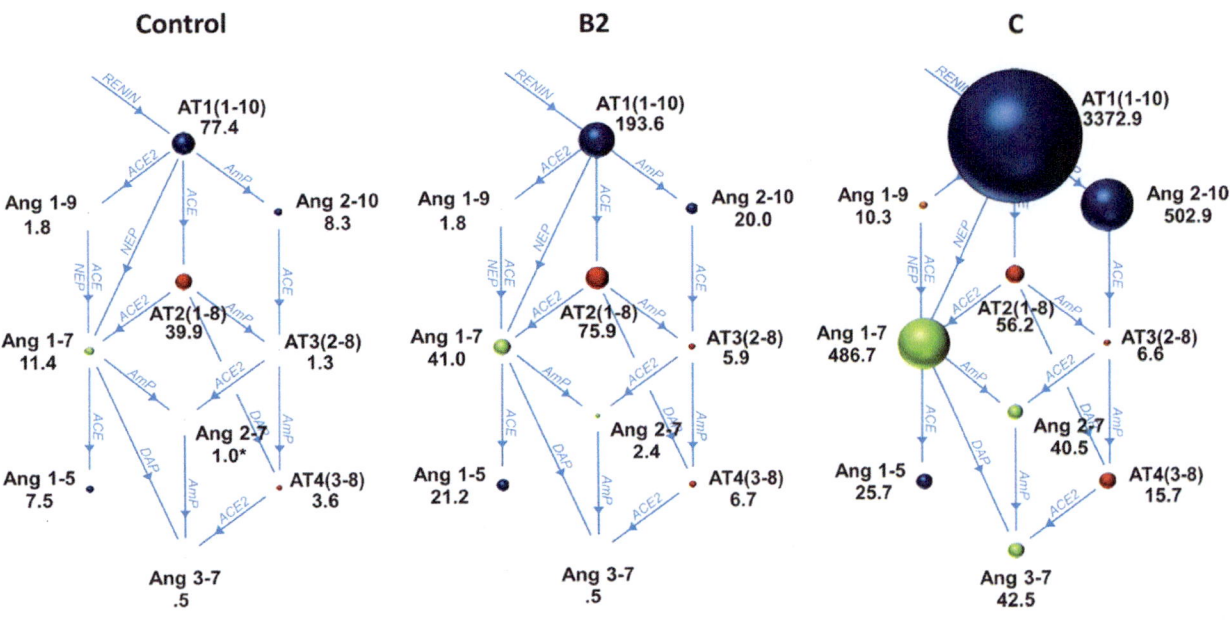

Figure 20.4 Renin–angiotensin system equilibrium analyses ("fingerprints"), created using liquid chromatography-mass spectrometry, from groups of healthy dogs (Control) and dogs with degenerative mitral valve disease classified as advanced preclinical (stage B2) or congestive heart failure (stage C). Stage C dogs had been treated with an ACE inhibitor, but Stage B2 dogs had not. Circle sizes are proportional to median equilibrium concentrations (pg/mL). See **Figure 20.3** legend for abbreviations. (Modified from Larouche-Lebel, et al. Plasma and tissue angiotensin-converting enzyme 2 activity and plasma equilibrium concentrations of angiotensin peptides in dogs with heart disease. J Vet Intern Med 2019;33:1571–1584.)

degradation of bradykinin (**Figure 21.2**, p. 321). However, ACE inhibitors do not block other enzymatic pathways that generate AngII. For example, ACE inhibition does not prevent volume overload (eccentric) myocardial hypertrophy in dogs, presumable because local tissue conversion to AngII depends largely on a chymase pathway. Furthermore, ACE inhibition does not totally suppress ALD release as heart failure progresses. Non-Ang-mediated pathways are presumed to increase further ALD production and lead to so-called ALD breakthrough. This phenomenon of incomplete RAAS suppression was found in almost one-third of dogs with DMVD being treated with an ACE inhibitor, whether CHF was present or not (Ames, 2017). An ACE gene polymorphism occurs in some dogs and it could reduce ACE activity somewhat (p. 321).

Drugs that block Ang1R directly present another potential strategy for opposing AngII effects (and increasing Ang1-7 and 1-9 generation), although ALD breakthrough still can occur despite use of an ARB. Presently there is much less clinical veterinary experience using ARBs in CHF therapy, although they are used with growing frequency to manage systemic hypertension, particularly in cats (p. 803). Other strategies aimed at counteracting the effects of RAAS activation have been tried, including the combinations of ACE inhibitor or ARB with a drug to inhibit the breakdown of natriuretic peptides (such as neprilysin; p. 309, below, and p. 333).

ALD secretion in CHF is stimulated by AngII, hyperkalemia, and chronically high plasma corticotrophin. Less important in increasing ALD release are circulating catecholamines, ETNs, and AVP (ADH). ALD binds to mineralocorticoid receptors to effect Na^+ and Cl^- reabsorption, as well as K^+ and H^+ secretion, in the renal collecting tubules; concurrent water reabsorption augments vascular volume. Increased ALD can promote hypokalemia and hypomagnesemia. Mineralocorticoid receptors in tissues other than the kidney also bind to ALD, including in the heart and vasculature. ALD interferes with baroreceptor function in heart failure; it also can potentiate the effects of catecholamines by blocking NE reuptake and degradation in peripheral nerve terminals. Like AngII, ALD produced locally in the CV system promotes inflammation and fibrosis. Chronic exposure contributes to pathologic cardiac and vascular (including coronary and renal) remodeling, fibrosis, and endothelial cell dysfunction. Reactive oxygen species generated by increased AngII and ALD expression contribute to cardiac and vascular remodeling in chronic heart failure. Reduced hepatic perfusion slows the clearance of ALD. In people with chronic heart failure, treatment with an ALD antagonist can increase survival time. This could be the case in companion animals also, although controversy remains.

Arginine Vasopressin (Antidiuretic Hormone) AVP, also known as ADH, is released from secretory granules within nerve terminals in the posterior pituitary gland. The AngII metabolite, AngIII(2-8) effects its release. The hormone's precursor (provasopressin) is synthesized by neurons in the hypothalamus, and then is converted into active AVP within transport vesicles which travel down the nerve axons to become the pituitary secretory granules. AVP structure is highly conserved among people, dogs, and cats.

This hormone directly causes vasoconstriction and also promotes free water reabsorption in the distal nephron. Vasopressin type-1A (V1A) receptors in the vasculature and heart mediate the vasoconstrictive and inotropic effects of AVP. Vasopressin type-2 (V2) receptors in the kidney mediate water reabsorption. Increased plasma osmolality and low blood volume are the normal stimuli for AVP release. Nonosmotic stimuli for AVP release occur with reduced effective circulating volume and low systemic arterial or renal perfusion pressure. The subsequent baroreceptor activation, sympathetic stimulation, and AngII production promote AVP's continued release in CHF. Excessive AVP (ADH) release, even as plasma osmolality falls and cardiac filling pressure rises, contributes to the dilutional hyponatremia that develops in some animals with severe or end-stage CHF. Hyponatremia is considered a poor prognostic sign. It also contributes to the progression of cardiac dysfunction. Increased circulating AVP has been demonstrated in dogs with DCM and DMVD. Drugs that block the effects of V2 receptors (such as tolvaptan) potentially can reverse dilutional hyponatremia.

Endothelin ETN-1 is one of several ETNs produced by the vascular endothelium. The normal function of these vasoconstrictor peptides is to maintain vascular tone, in opposition to endothelial-derived vasodilators such as NO and prostacyclin. ETN-1 is produced in a series of steps which lead to its conversion from an inactive precursor (proendothelin or "big" ETN) to the active ETN-1 via ETN-converting enzyme. ETN-1 is highly conserved across species.

Production of ETN is stimulated by hypoxia and vascular mechanical factors, such as stretch or low shear stress, and also by vasoactive substances, including AngII, AVP (ADH), NE, bradykinin, and cytokines such as tumor necrosis factor-alpha (TNF-alpha) and interleukin (IL)-1. ETN-1 acts on two receptors, ETN_A and ETN_B. The ETN_A receptor mediates smooth muscle vasoconstriction, increased myocardial contractility, ALD secretion, and renin suppression. In the normal situation, ETN-1 functions at the local vascular level, not as a circulating hormone. However, circulating ETN (and pro-ETN) concentrations increase in dogs, cats, and people with CHF, as well as in those with PH. Chronically increased ETN-1 contributes to adverse remodeling by promoting vascular smooth muscle and myocardial hypertrophy, increasing collagen synthesis, and stimulating further NH activation.

Cytokines and Inflammation Cytokines are endogenous peptides produced by various cells; they can act as autocrine, paracrine, and sometimes as endocrine mediators. Cytokines influence gene expression and protein synthesis. They are involved in modulating CV structure and function. Increased circulating concentrations occur in CHF and cytokine overexpression is thought to contribute to heart failure progression. In people, increased expression of TNF-alpha, IL-6, IL-1, IL-8, and transforming growth factor-beta are associated with disease severity and negative outcome. Other cytokines that might be involved include osteopontin and cardiotrophin-1. In dogs with DMVD, differences in the expression of various cytokines also occur compared to healthy dogs, especially with regard to IL-8 and transforming growth factor-beta$_1$. Chronic increases in sympathetic activity, AngII and ALD stimulate further cytokine production, although the initiating stimulus is unclear. TNF is a proinflammatory cytokine that contributes to cardiac remodeling, hypertrophy, and apoptosis. It also has negative inotropic effects. TNF is produced by macrophages, the heart, and other tissues in response to stress. While this initially can be an adaptive and protective response after ischemia and hemodynamic overload, the response becomes maladaptive over time. Exuberant production in the heart spills over and can cause secondary circulatory immune-stimulating effects. Proinflammatory cytokines stimulate inducible-NO synthase (iNOS) expression. However, this iNOS activation ultimately has negative inotropic and cytotoxic effects on the myocardium.

Increased concentration of C-reactive protein, an acute-phase marker of systemic inflammation, can occur with decompensated CHF. Elevated white blood cell (WBC) count and neutrophilia are manifestations of inflammation in some cases of advanced CHF. Even when the WBC count is within reference range, higher numbers of neutrophils, band neutrophils, and monocytes are reported in dogs with heart failure, compared to normal dogs. Mean serum C-reactive protein was positively correlated with total WBC and neutrophil counts in a group of dogs with decompensated CHF, although not in those with compensated heart failure and healthy dogs (Domanjko, 2018). In the overt CHF group, C-reactive protein concentration also correlated negatively with LV ejection fraction and positively with mitral (Doppler) E-wave velocity.

Several studies have sought to identify an association between markers of oxidative stress and CHF in dogs. However, despite any local effects, circulating antioxidant substances or their surrogates do not appear to be substantially altered among dogs with heart disease of various severity and healthy dogs.

Natriuretic Peptides and Other Endogenous Vasodilatory Substances Endogenous mechanisms which oppose the vasoconstrictor neurohormones also are invoked with cardiac dysfunction. These include the natriuretic peptides, NO, vasodilatory Ang metabolites (see section "Renin–Angiotensin–Aldosterone System" and **Figure 20.3**), adrenomedullin, and vasodilatory prostaglandins. Normally, a balance between vasodilatory and vasoconstrictor effects maintains circulatory homeostasis and renal solute excretion. However, the growing influence of vasoconstrictor mechanisms becomes predominant as heart failure progresses, despite increased activation of vasodilator mechanisms. The natriuretic peptides promote diuresis, natriuresis, and peripheral vasodilation. They antagonize the effects of the RAAS and also can inhibit fibrosis and smooth muscle hypertrophy, as well as alter (increase) vascular permeability. Overall, they tend to mitigate the progression of heart failure and reduce CV hypertrophy and fibrosis.

Natriuretic peptides play important physiologic roles in regulating blood volume and pressure. Natriuretic peptides can act as autocrine, paracrine or endocrine mediators. Atrial natriuretic peptide (ANP) and, to a minor degree, B-type (brain) natriuretic peptide (BNP) are produced by atrial myocytes. Mechanical stretch of the atrial wall stimulates their release. Production of BNP, and also ANP, in the cardiac ventricles markedly increases with myocardial dilation, increased transmural pressure, or ischemia. ANP and BNP synthesis also is stimulated by hypoxia, vasoconstrictor neurohormones (or their vasodilatory metabolites), and proinflammatory cytokines. Other natriuretic peptides have been identified as well. C-type NP (CNP) is secreted mainly from endothelial cells and fibroblasts in response to vascular injury. It has local vasodilatory and antiremodelling effects on the myocardium and vasculature. These natriuretic peptides are secreted in preprohormone form, then cleaved to a prohormone before being split into the active (C-terminal) product and an inactive N-terminal peptide (for example, NT-proANP and NT-proBNP). Circulating concentrations of ANP, BNP, and their N-terminal fragments increase in patients with heart failure (p. 291). Their elevation has correlated with pulmonary capillary wedge pressure and heart failure severity in dogs and cats.

Natriuretic peptide receptors (NPRs) are present in many tissues. These cell membrane receptors are coupled to guanylate cyclase; activation increases cyclic guanosine monophosphate (cGMP) production which mediates various pathways. ANP and BNP exert their effects via the NPR type-A. This receptor is found especially in the kidney, adrenal gland, lung, as well as other tissues. In the kidney, its activation reduces renal Na^+ transport in the inner medullary collecting duct, which promotes sodium and water excretion. NPR-A activation also mediates systemic and pulmonary arteriolar vasodilation, as well as inhibits both renin and ALD release. NPR type-B mediates the vasodilating effect of locally produced CNP. Natriuretic peptides are cleared via degradation by membrane-bound neutral endopeptidases (such as neprilysin) and other enzymes, or by binding to NPR type-C (clearance receptor). The N-terminal fragments of proANP and proBNP are cleared more slowly than the C-terminal fragments, perhaps because this depends on renal excretion.

There have been many attempts to leverage the beneficial effects of natriuretic peptides in CHF. Synthetic analogues of ANP and BNP have been tried in people to treat acute CHF, however without convincing benefit. Neutral endopeptidase inhibitors have been tried in chronic heart failure; alone, they have not shown benefit although natriuretic peptide concentrations might increase. This relates to the fact that neutral endopeptidase also degrades other vasodilators (such as bradykinin and adrenomedullin), as well as vasoconstrictors (such as AngII and ETN-1). When neutral endopeptidase is inhibited, the effects of the vasoconstrictor substances predominate and exacerbate RAAS activation. The strategy of combining an inhibitor of neutral endopeptidase with an ACE inhibitor seemed promising in animal studies; however, because both ACE and neutral endopeptidase break down bradykinin, their simultaneous inhibition magnified the effects of bradykinin and caused angioedema to occur at an unacceptable frequency in people. Subsequently, the combination of the neutral endopeptidase (neprilysin) inhibitor, sacubitril, and the ARB, valsartan, was explored. This combination of 'angiotensin receptor blocker and neprilysin inhibitor' (ARNI) enhances natriuretic peptide effects, blocks AngII effects at its main receptor, and leaves ACE available to metabolize bradykinin, which minimizes the risk of angioedema. In people, the sacubitril/valsartan combination has improved survival time and reduced hospitalizations for CHF, and has improved blood pressure control in hypertension. Experimentally, reduced cardiac hypertrophy and fibrosis also have been shown. ARNI therapy also appears to benefit people who have heart failure with preserved ejection fraction (that is, diastolic dysfunction). Application of ARNI therapy in veterinary patients with CHF is being explored.

NO (also known as endothelium-derived relaxing factor) is a functional antagonist of ETN and AngII. Endothelial-derived NO is produced in vascular endothelium from L-arginine, in response to endothelial-NOS (eNOS). NO mediates vasodilation by activating soluble guanylate cyclase to increase cGMP production. However, this process is impaired in CHF. At the same time, myocardial inducible-NOS (iNOS) expression is enhanced in heart failure. This myocardial NO release has negative effects on myocyte function through its consequences of reduced vasodilatory capacity, negative inotropic and chronotropic effects, and myocyte damage. However, Ang1-7, by stimulating MasR, also can activate the eNOS pathway as well as potentiate the effects of bradykinin.

Adrenomedullin is another peptide that is thought to play a role in counterbalancing the vasoconstrictive forces in heart failure. It is produced in the adrenal medulla, heart, lung, and other tissues. Adrenomedullin has natriuretic and vasodilatory effects; it also might have a positive inotropic effect. AngII stimulates adrenomedullin production. Elevated circulating concentrations have been observed in dogs with CHF caused by DMVD.

Intrarenal vasodilatory prostaglandins (prostacyclin) are produced to a much greater degree in the renal glomerular afferent (compared with the efferent) arterioles. By this means, they attenuate AngII's vasoconstrictive effects on afferent (but not efferent) arterioles. The use of prostaglandin synthesis inhibitors in severe heart failure potentially could cause afferent arteriolar resistance to increase. This could reduce glomerular filtration rate (GFR) and renal blood flow, as well as enhance Na^+ retention. However, the clinical importance of this in animals is not clear.

Other Factors The expression profiles of circulating microRNAs (miRNAs) become altered in heart failure. MiRNAs are post-transcriptional regulators of mRNA expression and protein production. In dogs with DMVD, distinct differences in expression profiles have been found between animals with CHF and healthy dogs. Cats with hypertrophic cardiomyopathy also show a distinct miRNA profile, somewhat similar to that in people with cardiac disease. MiRNA profiles might someday be useful as molecular biomarkers of CHF.

Serum homocysteine concentrations appear to be higher in dogs with DMVD, compared to normal dogs. These also were associated with stage of disease and correlated with cTnI, creatinine concentration, systolic blood pressure, and left atrial-to-aortic diameter ratio. Whether serum homocysteine concentration will be useful as an indicator of cardiac disease severity in dogs is not clear. However in cats, there appears to be no significant difference in homocysteine levels between those with cardiomyopathy and normal cats.

Vitamin D, as measured by serum 25(OH)D concentration, appears to be reduced in dogs with advanced heart disease or CHF compared to normal dogs. Inverse relationships between some measures of disease severity and 25(OH)D concentration have been noted. Similar findings are reported in people, suggesting a negative association between vitamin D status and disease severity. Vitamin D status in cats (as indicated by the sum of serum $25(OH)D_3$ and its prominent 3-epimer metabolite concentrations) was found to be lower in cats with cardiomyopathy compared to clinically normal cats, even after accounting for the effect of age. Low vitamin D status also has been associated with reduced survival time in people, dogs and cats with CV and other diseases. However, it is unclear whether low vitamin D status plays a role in heart failure progression or is merely an epiphenomenon.

Renal Responses

The balance (or imbalance) between vasoconstrictive-volume retentive stimuli and vasodilatory-natriuretic factors is reflected in the kidney. Sympathetic stimulation and AngII are important vasoconstrictors. AngII has greater effect on the efferent (compared to afferent) glomerular arterioles, which helps maintain GFR when cardiac output and renal blood flow are reduced. The higher oncotic and lower hydrostatic pressures that develop in the peritubular capillaries enhance fluid and Na^+ reabsorption. AngII also promotes renal cortical blood flow redistribution toward the juxtamedullary regions, where longer loops of Henle penetrate more deeply into the hypertonic medullary region. Thus, the effects of AngII increase salt and water retention in the proximal nephron and loop of Henle. AngII-induced ALD release stimulates further Na^+ and water retention at the distal convoluted tubule and collecting duct. Continued activation of these mechanisms promotes the accumulation of tissue edema and effusions. Reduction in GFR occurs as heart failure develops and worsens. Serum concentrations of cystatin-C and symmetric dimethylarginine (SDMA), two markers of declining GFR, were shown to increase progressively with advancing functional class of heart failure in dogs with DVMD. Elevated SMDA concentration in cats with CHF from cardiomyopathy also appears to be associated with shorter survival.

Afferent arteriolar vasodilation, mediated by intrarenal vasodilator prostaglandins, natriuretic peptides, and the effects of Ang1-7 and Ang1-9, can partially offset the effects of strong efferent vasoconstriction in heart failure. However, progressive reduction in renal blood flow can lead to renal insufficiency. There appears to be blunted renal responsiveness to natriuretic peptides over time in chronic CHF. Diuretic use can magnify azotemia and electrolyte loss by further reducing circulating volume and cardiac output. Diuretics, especially loop-diuretics, also exacerbate NH activation.

Connections between cardiac and kidney disease are widely recognized in human medicine, where disease involving one system provokes secondary abnormality in the other. This is known as cardiorenal syndrome; several subtypes are described. A major factor in cardiorenal syndrome in people is NH activation, especially the RAAS and AVP. Decreased cardiac output and renal perfusion activate baroreceptors and the RAAS, which stimulates AVP release (nonosmotic pathway). AVP activation of V2 receptors in the renal collecting ducts promotes fluid retention and worsening heart failure. V2 blockers (vaptans) antagonize the effects of AVP and can reduce volume overload and hyponatremia by promoting free water excretion.

The term cardiovascular–renal axis disorders (CvRDs) has been proposed to describe the situation of concurrent cardiac and renal disease in companion animals. Abnormal interactions between these systems could result from disease-, toxin-, or drug-induced structural or functional damage to the kidney or CV system. Although the extent and interrelationships involved have not been fully elucidated in animals, preliminary comparisons between the human cardiorenal syndrome subclassifications and CvRDs in veterinary patients and potential screening methods have been described (Orvalho, 2017). In patients with heart failure, renal injury could result from reduced perfusion, systemic venous congestion, extrinsic pressure from ascites, and the effects of NH activation. Renal perfusion can be further compromised by excessive dosing of diuretic or RAAS-blocking agents. Conversely, systemic hypertension secondary to underlying renal disease could exacerbate cardiac dysfunction. The prevalence of azotemia in dogs with cardiac disease has been estimated to range from 7 to over 24%. A higher prevalence of chronic renal disease has been observed in dogs with DMVD than in the general dog population. In one study of dogs with DMVD, the prevalence of chronic kidney disease with azotemia was ~25%; however, in the dogs with stage C and D CHF it was 32% (Martinelli, 2016). Correlation was found between the stage of heart disease/failure (**Table 20.2**) and International Renal Interest Society (IRIS) stage, although a majority of dogs in each cardiac group was nonazotemic in

Table 20.2 Assessment of Heart Disease and Failure Severity

ACVIM Heart Failure Staging System[a]
- A No apparent structural disease yet, but animal considered "at risk" for developing heart disease (for example, breed-associated risks include DCM for Doberman Pinschers and other large or giant breeds, and DMVD for Cavalier King Charles Spaniels and other small breeds, with age).
- B Structural cardiac abnormality is evident (such as a murmur or valve pathology typical for the underlying disease); however no clinical signs of heart failure have occurred.
    - B1 Asymptomatic disease, either without radiographic or echocardiographic cardiac chamber enlargement or with only mild remodeling, insufficient to justify therapy based on clinical trial evidence[b]
    - B2 Asymptomatic disease, with cardiac chamber enlargement (remodeling) sufficient to justify medical therapy to delay the onset of congestive heart failure (CHF)
- C Structural cardiac abnormality is evident and clinical heart failure signs have occurred, either in the past (resolved with therapy) or currently present. For animals with mild signs of heart failure decompensation, outpatient intensification of therapy could be appropriate. However, patients with severe congestive signs generally require hospital-based therapy.
- D Persistent or end-stage heart failure, with signs difficult to control or refractory to standard therapy (for example, requiring ≥ 6–8 mg/kg furosemide q12h). Similar to stage C, cases with relatively mild clinical signs might be managed at home. Those with more overt and severe signs should be hospitalized for more intensive therapy.

Modified New York Heart Association Functional Classification
- I Heart disease is present, but no evidence of heart failure or exercise intolerance; cardiomegaly is minimal to absent.
- II Heart disease is present; clinical signs of heart failure with moderate/strenuous exercise; radiographic cardiomegaly is present.
- III Signs of heart failure with normal activity or mild exercise (such as increased respiratory effort, cough, orthopnea); radiographic signs include cardiomegaly and mild to moderate pulmonary edema or pleural or abdominal effusion.
- IV Severe clinical signs of heart failure at rest or with minimal activity; marked radiographic signs of CHF and cardiomegaly.

International Small Animal Cardiac Health Council Functional Classification
- I Asymptomatic patient
    - Ia Signs of heart disease without cardiomegaly
    - Ib Signs of heart disease and evidence of compensation (cardiomegaly)
- II Mild to moderate heart failure; clinical signs of failure evident at rest or with mild exercise and adversely affect quality of life
- III Advanced heart failure; clinical signs of CHF immediately obvious
    - IIIa Home care is possible
    - IIIb Hospitalization recommended (cardiogenic shock, life-threatening edema, large pleural effusion, refractory ascites)

---

[a] Adapted from the American Heart Association/American College of Cardiology staging system by the Cardiology specialty of the American College of Veterinary Internal Medicine (ACVIM).
[b] With regard to dogs with DMVD, this means cardiac changes are not severe enough to meet current clinical trial criteria used to determine that treatment initiation is warranted (also see Chapter 29).
Abbreviations: DMVD, degenerative mitral valve disease; DCM, dilated cardiomyopathy; CHF, congestive heart failure.

---

this study. The severity of renal dysfunction, as well as cardiac disease, negatively affected survival time in this study; furosemide administration and advanced patient age also were associated with shorter survival.

Although current indicators of renal dysfunction, including SDMA, proteinuria, urine specific gravity, and serum creatinine are useful, mechanisms to identify renal injury at even earlier stages could be advantageous. The same is true for markers of cardiac disease. ACE inhibitors, ARB, and ALD antagonists can provide beneficial effects in both renal and cardiac disease. In patients with severe ascites, reducing systemic venous pressures with diuretics and inotropic support might improve renal function. Similarly, the increased intra-abdominal pressure of severe ascites can promote renal injury secondary to external compression; abdominocentesis can mitigate this by reducing intra-abdominal pressure.

Anemia is another abnormality also associated with chronic heart failure and renal dysfunction in people. A higher prevalence of anemia appears to occur in DMVD compared to healthy dogs. The prevalence of anemia in dogs with cardiac disease is estimated to range from 8% to over 23%. Increased prevalence of anemia has been associated with heart disease severity in some, but not all, reports. Anemia appears substantially more prevalent in DMVD dogs with azotemia, compared to nonazotemic dogs, and appears to be a negative prognostic indicator.

Exercise Capacity

Reduced exercise capacity and skeletal muscle atrophy develop with heart failure. Although cardiac output might be fairly normal at rest, the ability to increase cardiac output in response to exercise becomes impaired. Reduced diastolic filling, inadequate contractility reserve, valvular insufficiency, and compromised pulmonary function caused by edema or pleural effusion all contribute to decreased exercise tolerance.

Furthermore, abnormal peripheral vasodilatory responses are underappreciated; these impair skeletal muscle perfusion and induce exertional fatigue. Altered skeletal muscle metabolism secondary to chronic physical deconditioning also might contribute to fatigue. High sympathetic tone, AngII (both circulating and locally produced), and AVP can contribute to the reduction in skeletal muscle vasodilatory capacity that occurs in chronic heart failure. Increased vascular wall sodium content and interstitial fluid pressure promote vascular stiffening and compression. Impaired endothelium-dependent vasorelaxation, increased ETN production, and vascular wall remodeling induced by the effects of various NH vasoconstrictors also are implicated. Normal physiologic production of endothelial-dependent NO (mediated by eNOS) is downregulated in CHF. This contributes to endothelial dysfunction and reduced responsiveness in exercise. Treatment with an ACE inhibitor or ARB (and the combination sacubitril/valsartan), and possibly also spironolactone, could improve endothelial vasomotor function and exercise capacity. Pulmonary endothelial function is improved by ACE inhibitors in dogs with CHF.

Cardiac Cachexia Cardiac cachexia is the syndrome of progressive muscle wasting, with or without weight loss, associated with advanced heart disease and CHF. Evaluation of the cardiac patient's muscle condition score (not just body condition score) and body weight over time allow earlier identification. Those judged to have any degree of muscle loss can be considered to have cachexia. Muscle loss over the spine and gluteal region usually is noted first. Unintended weight loss of >5% over the prior 12 months also might signal cachexia. The pathogenesis of cardiac cachexia involves multiple factors, including the effects of proinflammatory cytokines, such as TNF-alpha, IL-1beta, and IL-6. These substances also suppress appetite and promote hypercatabolism. Increased energy requirements in the face of reduced food intake, as well as metabolic abnormalities, contribute to the development of cachexia. AngII is implicated in the process of skeletal muscle atrophy, also. Weakness and fatigue are amplified as lean body mass is lost in patients with cardiac cachexia; cardiac mass also is affected.

Cardiac cachexia typically is identified after CHF develops (**Figure 20.5**, and **Figure 2.1**, p. 35). It can affect all species. Obvious cachexia might be more common in animals with right-sided CHF signs (especially ascites), DCM, or chronic pericarditis. Frequently, cats with cardiac cachexia have chronic pleural effusions. Cardiac cachexia becomes most prominent in animals with long-standing, often refractory (Stage D) heart failure. Cardiac cachexia is associated with shortened survival time (Ineson, 2019; Santiago, 2020). Reduced immune function also has been documented in people with cardiac cachexia. Measures to optimize patient nutrition and food intake could slow the development of cardiac cachexia.

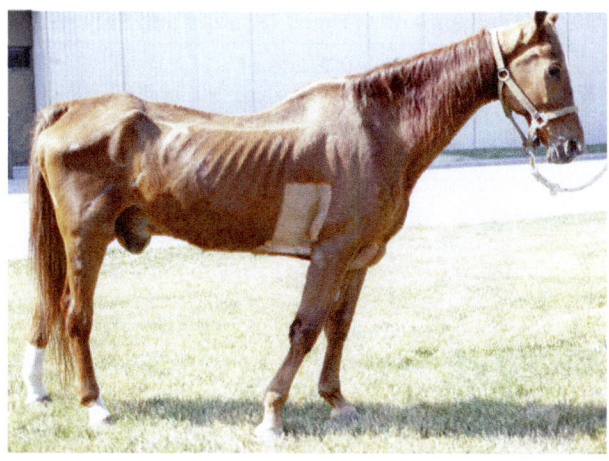

Figure 20.5 Severe cardiac cachexia in a 20-year-old American Saddlebred gelding with advanced myocardial failure. The horse had atrial fibrillation, severe tricuspid and moderate mitral regurgitation, and clinical signs of biventricular congestive heart failure. The owner reported that the horse was somewhat thin when purchased 2 months earlier, but that no other problems were evident then.

Clinical Manifestations of Congestive Heart Failure

Presenting Signs

The clinical signs of CHF result largely from chronic NH activation and renal compensation. Excessive volume retention and elevated ventricular filling pressures cause congestion ("backward" failure), manifested as tissue edema and body cavity effusions (**Table 20.1**). Most animals with clinical CHF develop resting tachycardia, and tachypnea at rest or with exertionin. Pulmonary venous congestion and edema occur as consequences of increased left atrial and LV filling pressures and are characteristic signs of left-sided CHF. Pulmonary edema is likely when mean filling pressure exceeds 20–25 mm Hg. However, the rate at which LV filling pressure rises can affect this. Experimentally, gradual increase to mean left atrial pressures of even 40 mm Hg might not be associated with overt pulmonary edema in dogs. Lymphatic capacity to remove interstitial fluid can increase tremendously when the rise in venous pressure is gradual. Likewise, signs of right-sided CHF, such as hepatic congestion and ascites, usually become evident when central venous pressure exceeds 15 mm Hg. Clinical signs typical for right-sided CHF also commonly occur with biventricular failure, as well as pure right heart disease. Pleural effusion is a common manifestation of biventricular failure, especially in cats and horses. Unlike in dogs and cats, subcutaneous edema along the ventral body wall and distal limbs is a frequent manifestation of CHF in horses.

The onset of CHF signs occurs gradually in many cases. Conversely, sudden onset of fulminant pulmonary edema is likely to follow rupture of major chordae tendineae. However, too often "acute" CHF is the culmination of progressive CHF signs that are recognized only after they have become severe. Additional information can be found in Chapters 9, 10, and 15–17, which focus on clinical problems associated with CHF, as well as other diseases. Low cardiac output ("forward" failure) can produce signs of poor exercise tolerance, weakness, prerenal azotemia, and syncope (**Table 20.1** and Chapters 7 and 8).

Cardiogenic Shock Cardiogenic shock can be defined as heart failure with a systolic blood pressure under 80 mm Hg, along with hypothermia, impaired peripheral perfusion, and elevated blood lactate. Most cases have concurrent pulmonary edema or pleural effusion. Profoundly impaired cardiac pump function can lead to cardiogenic shock. Severe DCM is the most common cause in veterinary patients. Other precipitating factors can include acute valvular disruption with massive regurgitation, sustained and severe brady- or tachyarrhythmias, overdose of a hypotensive or negative inotropic drug (especially with preexisting cardiac disease), and intracardiac flow obstruction (as with heartworm caval syndrome or an intracardiac tumor). Extracardiac causes of obstructed blood flow (such as cardiac tamponade, PH, or massive pulmonary embolism) can severely reduce cardiac output, too. Acute myocardial infarction is a rare cause of cardiogenic shock in animals, unlike in people, although it perhaps occurs more often in cats. Signs of cardiogenic shock relate to low cardiac output, arterial hypotension, and the compensatory mechanisms activated to increase vascular volume and pressure. Evidence of the animal's underlying disease (including a murmur, gallop sound, arrhythmia, or muffled sounds), as well as congestive signs, are likely.

Diagnosis

It is important to identify the underlying cardiac (or other) abnormality that led to the CHF signs, as well as any complicating factors, in the individual animal. This is especially critical in situations where standard heart failure therapy (diuretic, vasodilator, positive inotrope) is potentially harmful, such as cardiac tamponade (p. 713), or where other specific therapies are indicated (such as heartworm disease, severe PH, pulmonary thromboembolism, and some congenital malformations). The diagnostic process begins with a thorough history and CV examination (Chapter 2). Careful attention at this stage not only can reveal historical and physical signs suggestive of CHF, but also can help the clinician identify specific (objective) signs of cardiac disease, such as a murmur or arrhythmia. Without clear, objective signs of cardiac disease, a diagnosis of CHF is less certain.

The animal's sleeping or resting respiratory rate (RRR) provides important information. The authors recommend instructing owners of dogs (and cats) with preclinical, as well as more advanced, heart disease to monitor RRR at home and ideally during sleep (**Table 22.1**, p. 339). Dogs and cats without pulmonary edema (and without other inflammatory or infiltrative lung disease, which also can raise RRR) usually have a RRR less than 30 breaths/minute (and <25 breaths/minute during sleep). In heart disease patients, a RRR (ideally counted when sleeping) which becomes persistently more than 20% above that individual's normal baseline, and especially when over 40 breaths/minute, strongly suggests decompensated CHF. With regard to coughing in dogs particularly, the RRR is a historical parameter that can help differentiate CHF (or pulmonary parenchymal disease) from airway disease as the underlying cause (Chapter 9). Point-of-care lung ultrasound also helps the clinician assess the likelihood of underlying CHF (p. 80).

Following the physical examination and consideration of the patient's problems and suspected differential diagnoses, additional graphical tests (Chapters 3–5) help in further defining the underlying etiology of the clinical abnormalities (Chapters 7–19). Appropriate therapy can be selected once the diagnosis is established. When CHF is suspected but radiographic and other findings are inconclusive, a therapeutic trial of furosemide is reasonable. In dogs with substantial cardiomegaly from DMVD, the addition of pimobendan (assuming this has not already been prescribed) is another commonly used treatment. Respiratory signs stemming from pulmonary edema usually improve markedly or resolve shortly after instituting furosemide treatment (for example, 2 mg/kg q12 hr PO for a few days). In such cases, additional heart failure therapy should be started as well (Chapter 22). Furosemide as monotherapy is not recommended for chronic CHF management. In cases where minimal or no improvement occurs after furosemide therapy has begun, the cause of the clinical signs most likely is not CHF. Other chapters related to specific CV diseases provide additional information helpful for diagnosis and management.

Laboratory Tests Routine clinical laboratory tests are useful for identifying prerenal azotemia and other abnormalities associated with advanced cardiac disease, and to screen for concurrent non-cardiac disease. However, results often are non-contributory in animals with CHF. Tests for specific cardiac biomarkers, especially NT-proBNP and sometimes cTnI, can help the clinician differentiate underlying cardiac from non-cardiac disease and monitor cardiac disease progression. More information about these and other laboratory tests is in Chapter 19.

Assessment of Heart Disease and Heart Failure Severity

Heart Disease/Failure Staging System

Guidelines for clinical staging of heart failure are now in common use for veterinary patients (**Table 20.2**). This system, originally derived from that used by the American Heart Association and American College of Cardiology, sometimes is called the American College of Veterinary

Internal Medicine (ACVIM) staging system. It describes the progression of cardiac disease through four general stages over time. The importance of patient screening and early diagnosis is emphasized. The staging system provides a guide for coordinating appropriate (ideally, evidence-based) treatment to disease severity and clinical manifestations at each stage. Of note, this staging system also deemphasizes the term "congestive" in CHF, because edema and effusions are not consistently present at all times and stages. Nevertheless, attention to the patient's volume status is highly important. Progression through these stages essentially occurs in only one direction. Once an animal enters stage C, it cannot return to stage B (except perhaps in cases where surgical treatment is possible and successful).

Heart Failure Functional Classification Systems

The clinical severity of heart failure also has been described according to a modified New York Heart Association (NYHA) classification scheme and the International Small Animal Cardiac Health Council (ISACHC) criteria. These systems group patients into functional categories based on observations of clinical signs, rather than underlying cardiac disease progression or myocardial function. Such classification still could be helpful conceptually and for categorizing study patients; it also can complement the previously described staging system. In any case, identifying the underlying disease etiology and pathophysiology, as well as clinical CHF severity, is important for individualizing therapy.

Suggested Additional Reading and References

Also See Online Comprehensive Bibliography at: https://www.routledge.com/9781482246223.

Ames MK, Atkins CE, Eriksson A, et al. Aldosterone breakthrough in dogs with naturally occurring myxomatous mitral valve disease. J Vet Cardiol 2017;19:218–227

Ames MK, Atkins CE, Pitt B. The renin-angiotensin-aldosterone system and its suppression. J Vet Intern Med 2019;33: 363–382.

Badino P, Odore R, Re G. Are so many adrenergic receptor subtypes really present in domestic animal tissues? A pharmacological perspective. Vet J 2005;170:163–174.

Bonagura JD. Overview of equine cardiac disease. Vet Clin North Am Equine Pract 2019;35:1–22.

Choi BS, Moon HS, Seo SH, et al. Evaluation of serum cystatin-C and symmetric dimethylarginine concentrations in dogs with heart failure from chronic mitral valvular insufficiency. J Vet Med Sci 2017;79:41–46.

Cunningham SM, Rush JE, Freeman LM. Systemic inflammation and endothelial dysfunction in dogs with congestive heart failure. J Vet Intern Med 2012;26:547–557.

Domanjko Petric A, Lukman T, Verk B, et al. Systemic inflammation in dogs with advanced-stage heart failure. Acta Vet Scand 2018;60:20.

Du Bois P, Pablo Tortola C, Lodka D, et al. Angiotensin II induces skeletal muscle atrophy by activating TFEB-mediated MuRF1 expression. Circ Res 2015;117:424–436.

Eriksson AS, Haggstrom J, Pedersen HD, et al. Increased NT-proANP predicts risk of congestive heart failure in Cavalier King Charles spaniels with mitral regurgitation caused by myxomatous valve disease. J Vet Cardiol 2014;16:141–154.

Freeman LM. Cachexia and sarcopenia: emerging syndromes of importance in dogs and cats. J Vet Intern Med 2012;26:3–17.

Freeman LM, Sutherland-Smith J, Prantil LR, et al. Quantitative assessment of muscle in dogs using a vertebral epaxial muscle score. Can J Vet Res 2017;81:255–260.

Fu S, Ping P, Wang F, et al. Synthesis, secretion, function, metabolism and application of natriuretic peptides in heart failure. J Biol Eng 2018;12:2.

Gehlen H, Sundermann T, Rohn K, et al. Aldosterone plasma concentration in horses with heart valve insufficiencies. Res Vet Sci 2008;85:340–344.

Hamilton-Elliott J, Ambrose E, Christley R, et al. White blood cell differentials in dogs with congestive heart failure (CHF) in comparison to those in dogs without cardiac disease. J Small Anim Pract 2018;59:364–372.

Huh T, Larouche-Lebel É, Loughran KA, et al. Effect of angiotensin receptor blockers and angiotensin-converting enzyme 2 on plasma equilibrium angiotensin peptide concentrations in cats with heart disease. J Vet Intern Med 2020;n/a.

Ineson DL, Freeman LM, Rush JE. Clinical and laboratory findings and survival time associated with cardiac cachexia in dogs with congestive heart failure. J Vet Intern Med 2019;33: 1902–1908.

Jones ID, Fuentes VL, Boswood A, et al. Ultrasonographic measurement of flow-mediated vasodilation in dogs with chronic valvular disease. J Vet Cardiol 2012;14:203–210

Jung S, Bohan A. Genome-wide sequencing and quantification of circulating microRNAs for dogs with congestive heart failure secondary to myxomatous mitral valve degeneration. Am J Vet Res 2018;79:163–169.

Kanno N, Asano K, Teshima K, et al. Plasma adrenomedullin concentration in dogs with myxomatous mitral valvular disease. J Vet Med Sci 2012;74:739–743.

Kanno N, Hori Y, Hidaka Y, et al. Plasma atrial natriuretic peptide and N-terminal pro B-type natriuretic peptide concentrations in dogs with right-sided congestive heart failure. J Vet Med Sci 2016;78:535–542.

Keene BW, Atkins CE, Bonagura JD, et al. ACVIM consensus guidelines for the diagnosis and treatment of myxomatous mitral valve disease in dogs. J Vet Intern Med 2019;33(3): 1127–1140.

Kellihan HB, Stepien RL. Pulmonary hypertension in canine degenerative mitral valve disease. J Vet Cardiol 2012;14:149–164.

Kraus MS, Rassnick KM, Wakshlag JJ, et al. Relation of vitamin D status to congestive heart failure and cardiovascular events in dogs. J Vet Intern Med 2014;28:109–115.

Larouche-Lebel E, Loughran KA, Oyama MA, et al. Plasma and tissue angiotensin-converting enzyme 2 activity and plasma equilibrium concentrations of angiotensin peptides in dogs with heart disease. J Vet Intern Med 2019;33:1571–1584.

Lee CM, Jeong DM, Kang MH, et al. Correlation between serum homocysteine concentration and severity of mitral valve disease in dogs. Am J Vet Res 2017;78:440–446.

Linklater AKJ, Lichtenberger MK, Thamm DH, et al. Serum concentrations of cardiac troponin I and cardiac troponin T in dogs with class IV congestive heart failure due to mitral valve disease. J Vet Emerg Crit Care 2007;17:243–249.

Little CJ, Julu PO, Hansen S, et al. Non-invasive real-time measurements of cardiac vagal tone in dogs with cardiac disease. Vet Rec 2005;156:101–105.

Ljungvall I, Hoglund K, Tidholm A, et al. Cardiac troponin I is associated with severity of myxomatous mitral valve disease, age, and C-reactive protein in dogs. J Vet Intern Med 2010;24:153–159.

Macdonald PS. Combined angiotensin receptor/neprilysin inhibitors: a review of the new paradigm in the management of chronic heart failure. Clin Ther 2015;37:2199–2205.

Marcondes Santos M, Strunz CM, Larsson MH. Correlation between activation of the sympathetic nervous system estimated by plasma concentrations of norepinephrine and Doppler echocardiographic variables in dogs with acquired heart disease. Am J Vet Res 2006;67:1163–1168.

Martinelli E, Locatelli C, Bassis S, et al. Preliminary investigation of cardiovascular-renal disorders in dogs with chronic mitral valve disease. J Vet Intern Med 2016;30:1612–1618.

Mavropoulou A, Guazzetti S, Borghetti P, et al. Cytokine expression in peripheral blood mononuclear cells of dogs with mitral valve disease. Vet J 2016;211:45–51.

Mochel JP, Danhof M. Chronobiology and pharmacologic modulation of the renin-angiotensin-aldosterone system in dogs: what have we learned? Rev Physiol Biochem Pharmacol 2015;169:43–69.

Moesgaard SG, Klostergaard C, Zois NE, et al. Flow-mediated vasodilation measurements in Cavalier King Charles Spaniels with increasing severity of myxomatous mitral valve disease. J Vet Intern Med 2012;26:61–68.

Ohad DG, Rishniw M, Ljungvall I, et al. Sleeping and resting respiratory rates in dogs with subclinical heart disease. J Am Vet Med Assoc 2013;243:839–843.

Oliveira MS, Muzzi RA, Araujo RB, et al. Heart rate variability parameters of myxomatous mitral valve disease in dogs with and without heart failure obtained using 24-hour Holter electrocardiography. Vet Rec 2012;170:622.

Orvalho JS, Cowgill LD. Cardiorenal syndrome: diagnosis and management. Vet Clin North Am Small Anim Pract 2017;47:1083–1102.

Osuga T, Nakamura K, Morita T, et al. Vitamin D Status in different stages of disease severity in dogs with chronic valvular heart disease. J Vet Intern Med 2015;29:1518–1523.

Oyama MA. Neurohormonal activation in canine degenerative mitral valve disease: implications on pathophysiology and treatment. J Small Anim Pract 2009;50(Suppl 1):3–11.

Pierce KV, Rush JE, Freeman LM, et al. Association between survival time and changes in NT-proBNP in cats treated for congestive heart failure. J Vet Intern Med 2017;31:678–684.

Polizopoulou ZS, Koutinas CK, Ceron JJ, et al. Correlation of serum cardiac troponin I and acute phase protein concentrations with clinical staging in dogs with degenerative mitral valve disease. Vet Clin Pathol 2015;44:397–404.

Rasmussen CE, Falk T, Zois NE, et al. Heart rate, heart rate variability, and arrhythmias in dogs with myxomatous mitral valve disease. J Vet Intern Med 2012;26:76–84.

Reimann MJ, Ljungvall I, Hillstrom A, et al. Increased serum C-reactive protein concentrations in dogs with congestive heart failure due to myxomatous mitral valve disease. Vet J 2016;209:113–118.

Reimann MJ, Haggstrom J, Moller JE, et al. Markers of oxidative stress in dogs with myxomatous mitral valve disease are influenced by sex, neuter Status, and serum cholesterol concentration. J Vet Intern Med 2017;31:295–302.

Rossi F, Mascolo A, Mollace V. The pathophysiological role of natriuretic peptide-RAAS cross talk in heart failure. Int J Cardiol 2017;226:121–125.

Santiago SL, Freeman LM, Rush JE. Cardiac cachexia in cats with congestive heart failure: prevalence and clinical, laboratory, and survival findings. J Vet Intern Med 2020;34:35–44.

Santos RAS, Sampaio WO, Alzamora AC, et al. The ACE2/angiotensin-(1-7)/MAS axis of the renin-angiotensin system: focus on angiotensin-(1-7). Physiol Rev 2018;98:505–553.

Schober KE, Hart TM, Stern JA, et al. Effects of treatment on respiratory rate, serum natriuretic peptide concentration, and Doppler echocardiographic indices of left ventricular filling pressure in dogs with congestive heart failure secondary to degenerative mitral valve disease and dilated cardiomyopathy. J Am Vet Med Assoc 2011;239:468–479.

Smith KF, Quinn RL, Rahilly LJ. Biomarkers for differentiation of causes of respiratory distress in dogs and cats: part 1–Cardiac diseases and pulmonary hypertension. J Vet Emerg Crit Care 2015;25:311–329.

Spier AW, Meurs KM. Assessment of heart rate variability in Boxers with arrhythmogenic right ventricular cardiomyopathy. J Am Vet Med Assoc 2004;224:534–537.

Svete AN, Verk B, Seliskar A, et al. Plasma coenzyme Q10 concentration, antioxidant status, and serum N-terminal pro-brain natriuretic peptide concentration in dogs with various cardiovascular diseases and the effect of cardiac treatment on measured variables. Am J Vet Res 2017;78:447–457.

Verk B, Nemec Svete A, Salobir J, et al. Markers of oxidative stress in dogs with heart failure. J Vet Diagn Invest 2017;29:636–644.

Vinod P, Krishnappa V, Chauvin AM, et al. Cardiorenal syndrome: role of arginine vasopressin and vaptans in heart failure. Cardiol Res 2017;8:87–95.

Ware WA, Freeman LM, Rush JE, et al. Vitamin D status in cats with cardiomyopathy. J Vet Intern Med 2020;34(4):1389–1398.

Weber K, Rostert N, Bauersachs S, et al. Serum microRNA profiles in cats with hypertrophic cardiomyopathy. Mol Cell Biochem 2015;402:171–180.

Yandrapalli S, Aronow WS, Mondal P, et al. The evolution of natriuretic peptide augmentation in management of heart failure and the role of sacubitril/valsartan. Arch Med Sci: AMS 2017;13:1207–1216.

Yu IB, Huang HP. Prevalence and prognosis of anemia in dogs with degenerative mitral valve disease. BioMed Res Int 2016;2016:4727054.

Zois NE, Moesgaard SG, Kjelgaard-Hansen M, et al. Circulating cytokine concentrations in dogs with different degrees of myxomatous mitral valve disease. Vet J 2012;192:106–111.

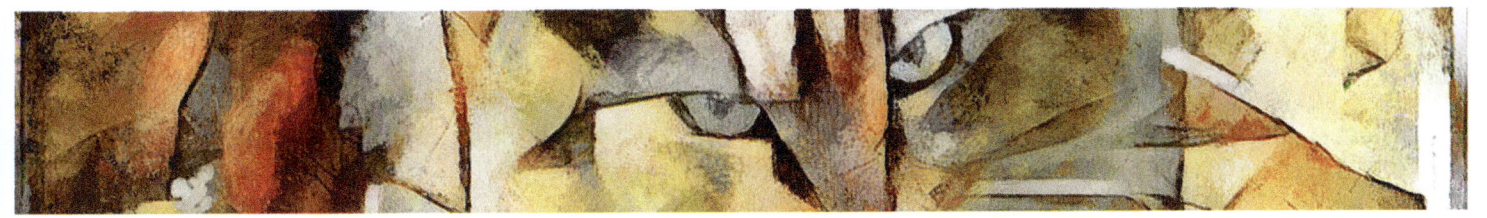

21
DRUGS FOR THE TREATMENT OF HEART FAILURE

Pharmacologic therapy for animals with heart failure involves a balanced combination of drugs. This chapter provides information about the most commonly used heart failure drugs, other agents which are useful in certain cases, and possible future treatment strategies. Specific guidelines for heart failure management and related information, including drug dosages, are described in Chapter 22 (see **Tables 22.2** and **22.3**, pp. 342 and 345).

Diuretics

Furosemide and Other Loop Diuretics

Furosemide (frusemide) is the diuretic used most often to control edema and effusions. It has been shown to reduce left atrial (LA) pressure in dogs with congestive heart failure (CHF) in a dose-dependent manner that is similar after IV and oral dosing (Suzuki, 2011). Although aggressive furosemide therapy is indicated for fulminant pulmonary edema, the lowest effective doses are administered at consistent time intervals for chronic CHF management. In cases where it is unclear if CHF underlies a recent onset of respiratory signs, a trial course of furosemide can be helpful. However, furosemide (or other diuretic) alone is not recommended as the sole treatment for chronic heart failure because it can exacerbate neurohormonal (NH) activation and impair renal function. Furosemide dosage, especially in chronic heart failure, depends on the patient's clinical status and should be guided by respiratory pattern, hydration, body weight, exercise tolerance, arterial blood pressure (BP), renal function, and serum electrolyte concentrations. In racehorses, IV furosemide has been used (where permitted), 1–2 hours prerace, to reduce exercise-induced pulmonary hemorrhage and epistaxis. Increased vascular capacitance, with reduced LA pressure, is thought to underlie its effectiveness for this purpose. Another potential use for furosemide includes treatment of hypercalcemia, because it increases renal Ca^{++} excretion.

Like other "loop" diuretics, furosemide inhibits active Cl^-, K^+, and Na^+ co-transport in the ascending limb of the loop of Henle. This promotes excretion of these electrolytes along with water (**Figure 21.1**); Ca^{++} and Mg^{++} also are lost in the urine. In addition, furosemide could promote salt loss by increasing total renal blood flow and preferentially enhancing renal cortical flow, provided counter-regulatory neurohormonal compensations do not supervene. Loop diuretics administered IV might increase systemic venous capacitance, possibly by stimulating renal prostaglandin release from the juxtaglomerular apparatus. Other loop diuretics include torsemide (see next section), bumetanide and ethacrynic acid. Loop diuretics produce greater peak diuresis compared to other classes of diuretics.

Furosemide is well-absorbed orally in dogs and moderately well-absorbed in cats. However, furosemide has poor oral bioavailability (~5%) in horses and PO dosing produces inadequate plasma concentrations to effect diuresis in that species. Transdermal absorption in cats is negligible (Sleeper, 2019). Furosemide is actively secreted into the urine in the proximal convoluted tubule, and rapidly reaches its site of action in Henle's loop. After IV administration, diuretic effects begin within 5 minutes, peak by 30–60 minutes and last about 2 hours. The plasma half-life is 1–2 hours in most species. Continuous rate infusion (CRI) can produce greater and more consistent diuresis compared to intermittent boluses within the first several hours after initiation, although diuresis over 24 hours might be comparable. In a group of dogs and cats with acute left-sided CHF, the median furosemide dose used in those receiving CRI furosemide was lower than that needed for animals treated by intermittent IV boluses (0.99 mg/kg/h and 1.19 mg/kg/h, respectively; Ohad, 2018).

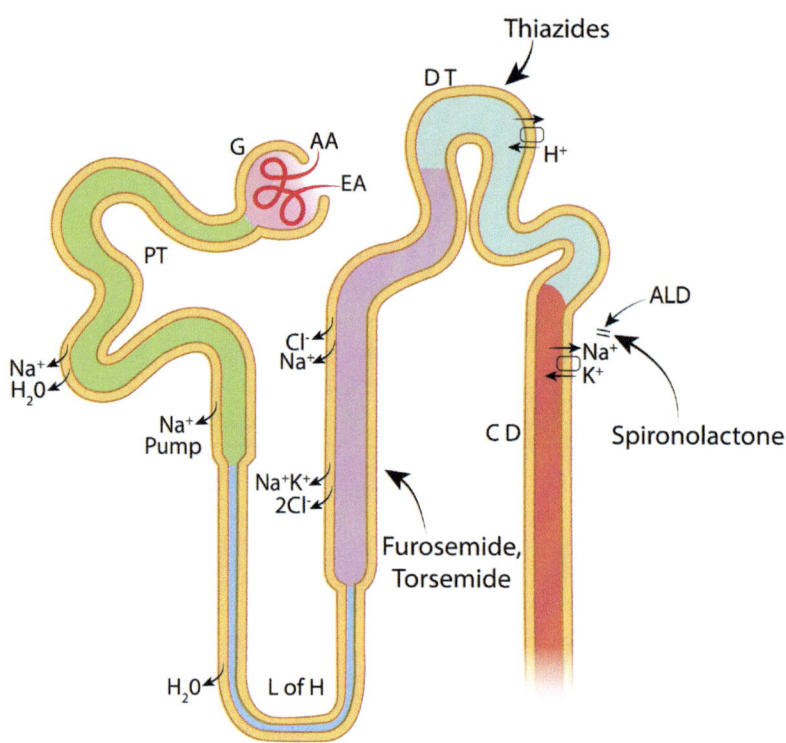

Figure 21.1 Simplified schematic of the nephron and major diuretic drug site of action. The "loop" diuretics promote loss of Na^+, Cl^-, K^+, (and water) in the thick ascending limb of the loop of Henle; they also promote Ca^{++} and Mg^{++} loss. Spironolactone's anti-aldosterone effect occurs at the level of the collecting ducts, where it promotes Na^+ loss and K^+ reabsorption. The thiazide diuretics act on the distal convoluted tubules to reduce Na^+ and Cl^- absorption; they also increase Ca^{++} absorption. AA, afferent arteriole; ALD, aldosterone; CD, collecting duct; DT, distal tubule; EA, efferent arteriole; G, glomerulus; L of H, loop of Henle; PT, proximal tubule.

Higher creatinine and total plasma protein levels were observed in the CRI group, suggesting potentially greater risk for dehydration and renal hypoperfusion. Clinically, lower CRI doses (0.66 mg/kg/h) often are used in dogs. In horses, the elimination half-live of furosemide delivered CRI was <0.5 hour, compared to between 1 and 2 hours after intermittent IV injection. In dogs, the effects of SC furosemide also peak at about 1 hour after injection and last about 4 hours. Oral dosing in dogs produces peak diuretic effect in 2 hours, with effects dissipating by about 6 hours. In a canine experimental model of mitral regurgitation, the time to maximal LA pressure reduction depended on dose and route of administration. Peak effect occurred earlier with IV dosing compared to PO (for example, maximal LA pressure decrease occurred 1 hour after 1 mg/kg IV compared to 4 hours after PO dosing); higher doses produced their greatest LA pressure declines later than smaller doses.

Caution is required in animals with underlying renal disease. Dosage reduction is necessary in animals that develop more than mild azotemia. Dehydration, azotemia, decreases in electrolyte concentrations, and alkalosis are the most common adverse effects. Reduction in serum chloride is the electrolyte abnormality observed most often in dogs and cats with acute and chronic loop diuretic therapy, although hypokalemia also is common with IV treatment and in patients not receiving renin-angiotensin-aldosterone system (RAAS) blocking drugs. Furosemide also can reduce serum Mg^{++} and Na^+ concentrations. In animals without anorexia or vomiting, the use of judicious doses is less likely to provoke major adverse effects. Animals with documented hypokalemia can be given a potassium supplement. However, serum potassium often is normal, and can even be mildly elevated with concurrent angiotensin converting enzyme (ACE) inhibitor and spironolactone therapy, or if renal disease is present.

Furosemide activates the RAAS. Although ACE inhibition can mitigate this, aldosterone (ALD) release and tissue conversion of angiotensin (Ang)I still can occur (see "Spironolactone"). Furosemide has minor potential for ototoxicity. Hypokalemia increases the risk for digoxin toxicity in patients receiving that drug. Rarely, furosemide might cause skin lesions, especially when repeatedly administered subcutaneously.

Diuretic resistance can occur with chronic therapy. This is predisposed by RAAS activation, insufficient oral absorption (especially in right-sided CHF), concurrent nonsteroidal anti-inflammatory drug administration, and by chronic kidney disease in some patients. A diuretic acting at a different segment of the nephron (such as spironolactone or a thiazide) sometimes is combined with furosemide for refractory CHF therapy. Multiple diuretic therapy ("sequential nephron blockade") can promote excessive volume contraction and

RAAS activation, as well as cause or exacerbate azotemia and electrolyte imbalances. Therefore, the indications for use should be clearly established and the lowest effective doses administered.

Torsemide Torsemide (torasemide) is an alternative agent that can be used in place of furosemide to provide enhanced diuresis in animals with refractory CHF. The drug is also veterinary-labeled for initial therapy of canine CHF in some countries. Torsemide acts similarly to furosemide to increase renal excretion of $2Cl^-$, Na^+, K^+, Ca^{++}, Mg^{++}, and water. However, it is about 10 times more potent than furosemide on a milligram basis and must be dosed accordingly. The advantages of torsemide reside mainly in its better bioavailability and prolonged duration of action when compared to furosemide. Torsemide can blunt the diuretic resistance that might occur with long-term and progressively increasing dosages of furosemide. Torsemide also exerts some ALD antagonist effects by reducing ALD's binding in distal tubule cells. In dogs, torsemide causes much greater Na^+ excretion compared to K^+ excretion (about 20:1); furosemide promotes Na:K excretion at about a 10:1 ratio. Because of its lesser excretion of K^+ compared to Na^+, replacing furosemide with torsemide at earlier stages of CHF progression might be useful in dogs. Some clinicians prescribe oral torsemide after initial parenteral furosemide diuresis. Once daily therapy can be effective in mild-moderate CHF. In cats, torsemide's Na:K excretion ratio is similar to that of furosemide; the drug can be effective in advanced CHF.

Torsemide is well-absorbed orally in dogs and cats. Its absorption reportedly is better and more consistent than that of furosemide. In humans, administration with food slows drug absorption and delays peak plasma concentration, although this doesn't influence total bioavailability and diuresis; this might be similar in animals. Peak plasma concentrations occur at about 1.5 hour post-dose in dogs. Diuresis begins within 1 hour, peaks at 2–4 hours post-dose, and lasts ~ 12 hours. Plasma half-life in dogs is ~8 hours. Renal tubular secretion of torsemide is slower and more prolonged than that of furosemide, which provides more sustained diuresis.

In healthy horses, a large (6 mg/kg) single oral dose produced peak plasma concentrations of ~10 mcg/mL (similar to those seen in dogs) within about 3 hours. Plasma concentrations among individual horses is quite variable over time; mean terminal half-life is about 9 hours (Agne, 2018). In contrast to oral furosemide, PO torsemide at 2 mg/kg q12h over 6 days can produce therapeutic serum concentrations and significant diuresis in horses. However, moderate prerenal azotemia as well as decreases in mean arterial BP and serum Na^+, K^+, and Cl^- are likely at this dose. A starting dose of 0.5–1 mg/kg PO q12h has been suggested for horses with CHF or other fluid overload states. Torsemide tablets can be crushed, mixed with an aliquot of water, and administered via nasogastric tube.

Adverse effects of torsemide are similar to those of furosemide. Because of its potency and frequent use at higher dosages in end-stage CHF, torsemide often induces azotemia and electrolyte disturbances. Accordingly, clinical laboratory tests should be reevaluated, generally within a week after initiating or increasing the dosage. In people, other adverse effects have included fatigue, weakness, hypotension, skin rash, atrial fibrillation (AF), gastrointestinal (GI) upset, and others.

Spironolactone

Spironolactone is increasingly administered in dogs and cats with chronic CHF, in combination with furosemide, pimobendan, and an ACE inhibitor. Besides a potential mild diuretic effect, as a mineralocorticoid receptor blocker, spironolactone is thought to confer a protective cardiovascular (CV) effect. The phenomenon of ALD escape (breakthrough) refers to ALD release that occurs despite ACE inhibition. This could involve reduced hepatic clearance, increased release stimulated by K^+ elevation or Na^+ depletion, effects of other NH modulators, and local tissue ALD production via myocardial chymase or other tissue enzymes. Spironolactone's anti-ALD effects are known to mitigate ALD-induced CV remodeling and fibrosis in people.

In dogs with experimental heart failure, spironolactone reduced ventricular fibrosis, arrhythmia propensity, and inflammatory cytokine gene overexpression. Whether chronic spironolactone therapy confers a survival benefit in dogs and cats with naturally occurring CHF, as it does in people, is not fully established. Spironolactone was associated with reduced morbidity-mortality risk in one study of dogs with degenerative (myxomatous) mitral valve disease (DMVD; Bernay, 2010). However, questions were raised about the definition of CHF and patient categorization methods used in that study. A small study using lower spironolactone doses failed to find a survival benefit (Schuller, 2011). In dogs with preclinical DMVD, spironolactone plus low-dose benazepril appeared to slow the rate of left heart remodeling; however, it did not delay the onset of CHF or improve survival in these dogs (Borgarelli, 2020). A preliminary study of spironolactone efficacy in feline CHF showed a trend for benefit (James, 2018); but larger, prospective studies are needed.

Spironolactone is a potassium-sparing agent that is a steroid analogue of ALD. As a competitive antagonist of ALD, spironolactone promotes Na^+ loss and K^+ retention in the distal renal tubule (**Figure 21.1**). It is most effective when circulating ALD concentration is high. It appears to lack diuretic effect in normal dogs at standard doses. In experimental canine studies it exerts a digitalis-like effect on arterial baroreceptors, increasing sensitivity to prevailing BP that might reduce neurohormonal activation. Spironolactone's onset of action is slow and peak effect occurs in 2–3 days. The drug is metabolized extensively in the liver. Canrenone is an active metabolite that has a long half-life.

Potassium-sparing diuretics are contraindicated in patients with preexisting hyperkalemia, and serum potassium should be monitored in patients receiving an ACE inhibitor or potassium supplement. Adverse effects generally relate to excess K⁺ retention and GI disturbances. Cutaneous excoriations have been reported in cats receiving higher dosages chronically. It is important to monitor for hyperkalemia and azotemia when using an ACE inhibitor and potassium-sparing diuretic together, because serious hyperkalemia can develop. However, in most cases, increases in K⁺ and blood urea nitrogen (BUN) are not clinically relevant. Metabolic acidosis is possible from excessive H⁺ retention and bicarbonate excretion. Spironolactone could decrease the clearance of digoxin, when used concurrently.

Eplerenone is another aldosterone antagonist with more selective action (and fewer endocrine side effects in people). In experimental heart failure, eplerenone significantly reduced ventricular remodeling and fibrosis. In dogs and cats, clinical experience is lacking and it is unclear whether this drug has advantages over spironolactone.

Thiazides

Hydrochlorothiazide (or chlorothiazide) sometimes is used as adjunctive diuretic therapy for refractory CHF, although its use has largely been supplanted by the availability of torsemide. When adding it to furosemide therapy, it is important to start with low doses, given once (daily or) every other day, in order to prevent rapid volume depletion and minimize electrolyte disturbances. If renal function and electrolyte levels remain stable, the drug can be continued if it is helping. Thiazides can reduce urine output in nephrogenic diabetes insipidus; they can be helpful in dogs with calcium oxalate bladder stones by reducing urinary Ca⁺⁺ excretion.

Thiazide diuretics block the sodium transporter and reduce Na⁺ and Cl⁻ absorption in the distal convoluted tubule, but they increase Ca⁺⁺ absorption. They cause mild to moderate diuresis and Na⁺, Cl⁻, K⁺, and Mg⁺⁺ excretion. When used with furosemide, thiazides prevent distal reabsorption of some Na⁺ that escaped the loop diuretic effect (sequential nephron blockade). Hydrochlorothiazide's diuretic effect begins within 2 hours, peaks at 4 hours, and lasts 12 hours. Chlorothiazide produces diuresis within 1 hour, with a peak effect in 4 hours and duration of 6–12 hours.

Thiazides reduce renal blood flow and should not be given to animals with azotemia. Adding a thiazide to other diuretics for end-stage CHF therapy can rapidly precipitate marked azotemia. Thiazides are relatively contraindicated with hyponatremia because they impair free-water clearance. Hypokalemia, other electrolyte disturbance, severe azotemia, and dehydration can occur, especially with excessive use or in patients with anorexia. Thiazides can cause hyperglycemia in diabetic or prediabetic animals by inhibiting conversion of proinsulin to insulin.

Angiotensin Converting Enzyme Inhibitors

ACE inhibitors are used in the treatment of chronic CHF of many dogs, cats and horses with valvular heart disease and cardiomyopathies. Several older studies demonstrating clinical efficacy of different ACE inhibitors in canine heart failure were published prior to the availability of the inodilator pimobendan; these drugs were administered at varying dosages. However, the incremental value of adding RAAS inhibition in dogs with DMVD and receiving a background therapy of pimobendan and furosemide has been challenged (Haggstrom, 2008; Wess, 2020). Unfortunately, clinical trials have not sufficiently addressed the efficacy of "quad-therapy" with pimobendan, a loop diuretic, and RAAS inhibition with spironolactone and an ACE inhibitor. This situation has confused the optimal treatment of canine CHF; a decision that in some countries revolves around the cost of multiple drug treatments. ACE inhibitors also are prescribed by some clinicians to delay the onset of CHF in dilated cardiomyopathy (DCM), as well as in dogs and horses with degenerative valve disease. Again, the value of ACE inhibition therapy (with or without spironolactone) for this purpose is controversial, as is optimal dosing for delaying or preventing CHF. Paralleling the canine situation is the lack of clear proof of benefit for this class of drugs in the treatment of cardiac diseases in cats and in horses.

By blocking conversion of the inactive precursor peptide AngI to active AngII through inhibition of ACE, these drugs oppose RAAS cascade effects (**Figure 21.2**). Thus, they ameliorate the negative vascular and renal effects of AngII, reduce ALD production, moderate other systemic NH responses, and potentially reduce abnormal CV remodeling. Plasma renin activity commonly increases because the negative feedback effect of AngII on its release is suppressed. ACE inhibitor use also can enhance alternative RAAS pathways (**Figures 20.3** and **20.4**, pp. 305 and 307). ACE inhibitors are less potent vasodilators than hydralazine and amlodipine, but have advantages because of their multiple effects to oppose NH activation. Some studies report sustained clinical improvement, and possibly lowered mortality rates, with ACE inhibitors in dogs with CHF from myocardial disease or volume overload caused by DMVD. Cats with diastolic dysfunction and horses with chronic valvular disease might benefit as well, although this is unclear. ACE inhibitors reduce ventricular arrhythmias and the rate of sudden death in people (and experimentally in animals) with myocardial disease and heart failure; one mechanism could be that AngII-induced enhancement of norepinephrine and epinephrine release is inhibited. The effects of drugs in this class are uncertain in horses, although ACE inhibitors have been used for management of CHF and in chronic valvular disease.

Although there are conflicting reports as to whether ACE inhibition can prevent ventricular remodeling and dilation in canine heart disease, ACE inhibitors might attenuate

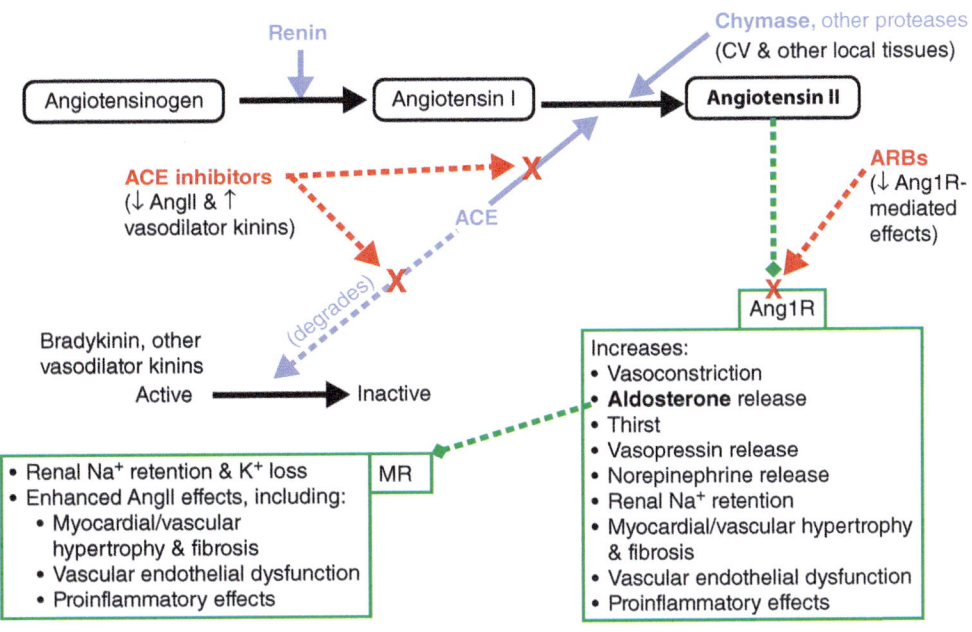

Figure 21.2 Simplified schematic of the renin-angiotensin-aldosterone system and related effects. Additional Ang peptides can be generated by other peptidases; some have other effects (Figure 20.3, p. 305). Figure 1.30 (p. 29) shows stimuli for renin release. ACE, angiotensin converting enzyme; ARBs, angiotensin (1) receptor blockers; Ang, angiotensin; Ang1R, angiotensin type 1 receptor; CV, cardiovascular; MR, mineralocorticoid receptor.

progressive left ventricular (LV) remodeling and secondary mitral regurgitation (MR) in DCM. ACE inhibitors could delay the onset of clinical heart failure in patients with myocardial dysfunction and this is strongly supported in animal models of cardiomyopathy. Reduced heart rate, cardiac filling pressure, peripheral vascular resistance, and improved cardiac output, have been variably reported. Secondary ALD inhibition can help reduce edema, as well as the direct, adverse CV effects. Some evidence indicates that ACE inhibitor use does not significantly delay the onset of CHF signs in dogs with preclinical DMVD, perhaps especially Cavalier King Charles Spaniels. However, for dogs with advanced preclinical DMVD and severe left heart enlargement, other evidence suggests an ACE inhibitor could provide benefit toward delaying CHF (Atkins, 2007); although this delay is relatively modest compared to pimobendan use in this setting (Boswood, 2016). Genetic variation could influence effects of the RAAS and response to ACE inhibitors. For example, ACE polymorphism was identified in a high percentage of Cavalier King Charles Spaniels (Meurs, 2018). Lower ACE activity was associated with the polymorphism compared to the wild-type gene sequence. There also is evidence suggesting ALD breakthrough could be more prevalent in dogs with the ACE polymorphism (Adin, 2020).

ACE inhibitors can lower BP, reduce proteinuria, and might slow progression of chronic renal disease in cats, and possibly in dogs. ACE inhibitors are considered agents of first choice for treating systemic arterial hypertension in dogs, although amlodipine is usually chosen first in cases with severely increased BP (p. 803). They can lower BP in some hypertensive cats, although amlodipine and the angiotensin receptor blocker (ARB) telmisartan are more effective for this purpose (p. 804). ARBs block AngII effects selectively at the angiotensin type 1 receptor (Ang1R) level. In theory, ARBs can allow relative increase of Ang2R effects, including vasodilation, while reducing risk of ALD breakthrough. Nevertheless, ALD production still can occur with ARB therapy. These agents previously have received little attention in the management of heart failure in companion animals and are used currently for treatment of systemic hypertension and chronic kidney disease. However, this situation might change given the successful use of combined ARB and neprilysin inhibitor therapy in human heart failure (p. 333, below).

Several ACE inhibitors are available. Most, except captopril and lisinopril, are prodrugs that are converted to their active form in the liver. Severe liver dysfunction interferes with this conversion. The ACE inhibitors used most often in animals are enalapril and benazepril. As a group, the ACE inhibitors have modest diuretic and vasodilatory effects; these occur as decreased AngII levels permit some arteriolar and venous dilation, reduce circulating ALD concentration, and reduce Na^+ and water retention. Vasodilation associated with ACE inhibitors also partially relates to the effects of vasodilator kinins such as bradykinin, which are degraded by ACE. In addition, increased generation of Ang1-7 and Ang1-9 (p. 306) could contribute. Local tissue ACE inhibition also could modulate vascular smooth muscle and myocardial remodeling, as well as promote local vasodilation. However, several other enzymes besides ACE can generate AngII locally, including myocardial chymase.

Adverse effects of ACE inhibitors include hypotension, GI upset, anorexia, azotemia, acute renal failure, and hyperkalemia (especially when used with a potassium-sparing diuretic or potassium supplement). AngII is important in mediating renal efferent arteriolar constriction, which maintains glomerular filtration when renal blood flow decreases. As long as cardiac output and renal perfusion improve with therapy, renal function usually is maintained. When administered without diuretics significant increases in serum BUN and creatinine are unlikely to occur in dogs. Reduced glomerular filtration is more likely to occur with excessive diuresis or vasodilation, volume depletion, chronic diuretic therapy, and severe myocardial dysfunction. Mild or moderate azotemia can be addressed by decreasing the diuretic dosage. If necessary, the ACE inhibitor dose also can be reduced, or the drug discontinued, especially when acute renal failure occurs. Occasionally, cautious fluid therapy is needed to restore kidney function (p. 348). Hypotension usually can be avoided with lower initial doses (for example, 50% of the projected dosage for 1 to 2 weeks). ACE inhibitors are not recommended in pregnant animals because of the potential for fetal injury. Other adverse effects associated with ACE inhibitors that are reported in people include rash, pruritus, impaired taste, proteinuria, cough, and neutropenia. Cough is a common ACE inhibitor side effect in people; it appears to be much less so in dogs, although this can be challenging to determine because cough frequently occurs in dogs with heart (as well as airway) disease. The mechanism of ACE inhibitor-induced cough is unclear; it could involve inhibition of endogenous bradykinin degradation and possibly, increased nitric oxide (NO) generation. NO can have an inflammatory effect on bronchial epithelial cells. Aspirin does not appear to reduce the beneficial effects of ACE inhibition in CHF; however, it is unclear if other nonsteroidal antiinflammatory drugs do.

Enalapril

Enalapril is one of the most commonly employed ACE inhibitors in animals. It has been used in multiple clinical studies in dogs, although very few in combination with the inodilator pimobendan. Enalapril is hydrolyzed in the liver to its most active form, enalaprilat. The drug is well-absorbed orally in dogs and bioavailability is not decreased by food. Peak ACE inhibiting activity occurs within 4–6 hours in dogs. Duration of action is 12–14 hours. Enalapril's effects are minimal by 24 hours at once daily dosing; consequently, dosing every 12 hours usually is recommended in dogs. Maximal activity in cats occurs within 2–4 hours after an oral dose, and some ACE inhibition (50% of control) persists for 2–3 days. Enalapril and its active metabolite are excreted in the urine. In horses, oral administration of enalapril produces no significant pharmacodynamic effect nor ACE activity suppression. However, IV enalaprilat does reduce ACE activity without changing hemodynamic response to exercise.

Enalapril does not cause significant adverse effects on renal function in dogs with advanced DMVD without CHF. However, renal failure and severe CHF prolong its elimination, so reduced dosage or benazepril are common, although unstudied, considerations in these patients. Injectable enalaprilat is available, although there is little veterinary experience with it.

Benazepril

Benazepril, like enalapril, is well-tolerated in CHF. It has improved exercise tolerance, clinical status, and survival in dogs with CHF, as reported in clinical studies that did not include pimobendan (BENCH study group, 1999); however, it was inferior to pimobendan in dogs with DVMD and CHF receiving a background therapy of furosemide and spironolactone (QUEST study, Häggström, 2008). Benazepril might slow renal function deterioration and partially mitigate hypertension in cats with renal disease. Only about 40% is absorbed when administered orally. Feeding does not affect absorption. Benazepril is metabolized to its active form (benazeprilat) in the liver. Peak ACE inhibition occurs within 2 hours of PO administration in dogs and cats. Complete ACE inhibition occurs in cats at doses of 0.25–0.5 mg/kg, with maintenance of >90% inhibition at 24 hours. Repeated dosing moderately increases drug plasma concentrations. Benazepril is eliminated equally in urine and bile in dogs, a theoretical but untested advantage for animals with CHF and renal disease. In cats, about 85% is excreted in the feces and only 15% in the urine. In healthy horses, oral doses (0.5–1 mg/kg) of benazepril produce more ACE inhibition than other ACE inhibitor drugs. Feeding does not appear to affect benazepril's pharmacokinetics in horses, nor does repeated dosing. A chewable benazepril formulation is available in some countries; combination products containing benazepril and pimobendan, and spironolactone and benazepril (Cardalis®, Ceva) also are available in many countries. The time of day when benazepril (or other ACE inhibitor) is administered potentially is important, at least in dogs fed once daily. This relates to circadian oscillations in RAAS activity and BP that have been demonstrated in dogs and presumably are present in other species (p. 306). Benazepril influences the dynamics of the RAAS by temporarily decreasing AngII and ALD for ~5–10 hours. For dogs fed in the morning, peak renin activity and BP were observed to occur in the evening and at night. Benazepril dosing at night provided optimal synchronization with this biological rhythm. Improved ACE inhibitor efficacy also was shown in mice and humans with night dosing. Although a dose range of 0.25 to 0.5 mg/kg, PO q24-12h daily, is listed in various sources, the optimal dosage range for CHF across species has not been determined.

Other ACE Inhibitors

Captopril was the first ACE inhibitor used clinically. This drug, in contrast to other ACE inhibitors, contains a sulfhydryl group, which might confer a beneficial free-radical scavenging effect although the clinical significance of this is unclear. Captopril appears less effective in reducing ACE activity than other ACE inhibitors in normal dogs. The drug is well-absorbed orally (75% bioavailable), but food decreases bioavailability by 30–40%. Hemodynamic effects appear within 1 hour, peak in 1–2 hours, and last <4 hours in dogs. Captopril is excreted in the urine. It requires q8h dosing, often caused anorexia, and rarely is used now.

Other ACE inhibitors that have been used in animals include ramipril, quinipril, imidapril, lisinapril, and fosinopril. Ramipril veterinary (Vasotop®, available outside the United States) is rapidly absorbed and converted to ramiprilat, although bioavailability is fairly low (similar to benazepril). Ramipril produces good ACE inhibition within 1–2 hours, which can last about 24 hours despite rapid clearance of free ramiprilat. Elimination is about 40% through the kidney and 60% by hepatic metabolism. Ramipril's pharmacokinetic properties are not significantly altered by moderate renal dysfunction. Both ramipril and quinapril can reduce ACE activity and BP in healthy horses, and appear to have some effect in horses with heart disease.

Imidapril also is comparable to enalapril and benazepril in efficacy. It appears to have a longer half-life, about 18–20 hours, in dogs. Imidapril's elimination is about 40% through the kidney and 60% by the liver. It is available in liquid form, although other ACE inhibitors can be compounded into suspension.

Lisinopril is a lysine analog of enalaprilat with direct ACE inhibiting effects. It is 25–50% bioavailable; absorption is not affected by feeding. Time to peak effect is 6–8 hours. Once daily lisinopril administration appears to be effective. Fosinopril is structurally different from other ACE inhibitors in that it contains a phosphinic acid radical (rather than sulfhydryl or carboxyl). It might be retained longer in myocytes. Fosinopril is converted to its active form (fosinoprilat) in the GI mucosa and liver. Elimination occurs equally by the kidney and liver. Its duration of action is >24 hours in people. Fosinopril might falsely lower serum digoxin measurements by radioimmunoassay tests.

Other Vasodilators used in Heart Failure

Drugs that produce varying degrees of systemic arterial vasodilation are mainstays of CHF therapy. Besides the ACE inhibitors (and potentially ARBs) and the inodilator pimobendan, described previously, drugs used less often include the Ca^{++} channel blocker amlodipine, hydralazine, and sodium nitroprusside. Arteriolar vasodilation reduces systemic vascular resistance, systemic arterial BP, and potentially LV afterload to increase forward cardiac output. Arterial (arteriolar) vasodilators might also diminish regurgitant fraction in animals with MR, thereby decreasing LA pressure, pulmonary congestion, and possibly LA size. Despite these potential benefits, these agents can cause clinically relevant hypotension and impaired tissue perfusion, especially in animals with low cardiac and heart rate reserves and in those already receiving ACE inhibitor and diuretic therapy. Therefore, low doses are used initially, with slow up-titration and regular monitoring of systemic BP. Other uses of arterial vasodilators are mainly for control of systemic hypertension (Chapter 38), including the ARBs (p. 332 and p. 807).

Venodilator drugs relax systemic veins. This increases systemic venous capacitance and allows for translocation of blood volume from the lungs, reducing cardiac filling pressures (preload) and pulmonary congestion. Some of these agents, such as topical nitroglycerin and oral isosorbide are mainly venodilators, although ACE inhibitors, sodium nitroprusside, and pimobendan have mixed arteriolar and venodilating action. The evidence for clinical benefit of venodilation in animals with CHF is largely theoretical, extrapolated from humans or experimental models, or based on clinical experience. This is particularly relevant to the various nitrates.

Hydralazine

Hydralazine is prescribed most often for afterload reduction in dogs with severe, acute CHF from DMVD (p. 560), especially after chordal ruptures. It reduces regurgitant volume and pulmonary venous pressure, and increases forward cardiac output. Hydralazine also can be used in the acute treatment of hypertension. Hydralazine or amlodipine (see next section) sometimes is added as adjunct therapy for additional afterload reduction in dogs with chronic refractory CHF; a low starting dose is used. If the initial dose is well-tolerated, the next dose can be increased to a maintenance level titrated to a systolic arterial BP of 90 mm Hg or above. In dogs with CHF that do not tolerate ACE inhibitors, hydralazine could be combined with a nitrate for chronic vasodilator therapy, although this is not commonly done today.

Hydralazine is classified as an arteriolar dilator, with little effect on veins. It promotes arteriolar smooth muscle relaxation by stimulating endothelial NO synthesis (**Figure 21.3**).

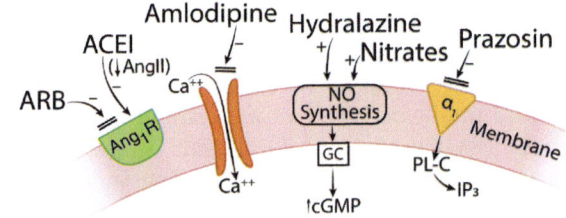

Figure 21.3 Vasodilator drug mechanisms. ACEIs reduce AngII formation. ARBs displace AngII from AT_1 receptors, blocking its effects. Amlodipine blocks membrane L-type Ca^{++} channels in vascular smooth muscle, leading to its relaxation. Hydralazine stimulates endothelial NO synthesis; consequently, increased cGMP formation mediates vascular smooth muscle relaxation. Nitrate drugs are metabolized to produce NO. Prazosin's alpha$_1$-adrenergic receptor blockade reduces IP_3 formation, leading to less Ca^{++} available for vascular smooth muscle contraction. ACEI, angiotensin converting enzyme inhibitor; ARB, angiotensin receptor blocker; AngII, angiotensin II; AT_1R, angiotensin type 1 receptor; cGMP, cyclic guanosine monophosphate; GC, guanylate cyclase; IP_3, inositol triphosphate; NO, nitric oxide; PL-C, phospholipase-C.

NO activates guanylate cyclase to increase cyclic guanosine monophosphate (cGMP) formation, which mediates relaxation of vascular smooth muscle. Hydralazine affects cerebral, coronary, splanchnic, and renal circulations more than skeletal muscle or skin vasculature; its effect on pulmonary arteries is negligible. Hydralazine is absorbed rapidly after oral administration; its onset of action is within 1 hour. Peak effect occurs within 3–5 hours and lasts up to 12 hours in dogs. Administration with food decreases bioavailability by >60%. First-pass hepatic metabolism is extensive; however, bioavailability in dogs increases over time as this mechanism becomes saturated. A small amount of hydralazine is excreted unchanged in the urine.

Clinical evaluation of the patient helps guide dosage titration of hydralazine. Increasing tachycardia, weakened pulses, lethargy, and poor peripheral perfusion can signal hypotension. Serial measurements of BP should be done, especially after dosage increase. Mean BPs under 70–80 mm Hg, or systolic pressures under 90–100 mm Hg are to be avoided. Jugular venous PO_2 can indicate directional changes in cardiac output; a venous PO_2 over 30 mm Hg is desirable. Hydralazine often causes reflex tachycardia and can precipitate marked hypotension; the dosage should be reduced if this occurs. Hydralazine can further increase NH activation and fluid retention in heart failure, which makes it less desirable than ACE inhibitors for long-term use. GI upset and anorexia also might occur. Hydralazine has not been well-evaluated clinically in cats or horses.

Amlodipine

Amlodipine sometimes is used as adjunctive therapy for acute or chronic CHF, especially in dogs with DMVD, where afterload reduction might reduce the severity of MR. Typically, it is added to furosemide, pimobendan, and RAAS inhibitor therapy. Amlodipine often is the drug of first choice for treating systemic arterial hypertension in cats, particularly when BP is severely elevated or there is target organ damage. It can be useful as an adjunct agent in hypertensive dogs, and might be effective as a single agent in some (see Chapter 38). Co-administration with an ACE inhibitor or telmisartan is common, especially in dogs and cats with systemic hypertension.

Amlodipine is a dihydropyridine L-type calcium channel-blocker (**Figure 21.3**). Its major effect is peripheral vasodilation, which also offsets any potential negative inotropic effect. However, it has no appreciable cardiac effects aside from reflex changes secondary to reduced BP. Amlodipine has good oral bioavailability and a long duration of action (at least 24 hours in dogs). Plasma concentration peaks in 3–8 hours; half-life is about 30 hours in dogs. Plasma concentrations increase with long-term therapy. Maximal effect develops over 4–7 days after therapy is begun in dogs. Because of the delay in achieving maximum effect, low initial doses and weekly BP monitoring during up-titration are recommended.

Amlodipine's effect on BP in cats lasts at least 24 hours. The drug generally has no significant effect on serum creatinine concentration or body weight in cats with chronic renal failure. The drug is metabolized in the liver although there is little first-pass elimination. Caution is warranted in animals with impaired liver function. Excretion is through the urine and feces.

Hypotension is possible with amlodipine, but it is less likely than with hydralazine because of the slower onset of action. Infrequently, inappetence, azotemia, lethargy, hypokalemia, reflex tachycardia, or weight loss could occur. Rarely, diffuse peripheral edema occurs and is a sign to immediately stop the drug. Gingival hyperplasia, typical of other calcium channel blockers, occurs sporadically in dogs and cats (**Figure 38.15**, p. 808). Amlodipine has not been evaluated in horses.

Prazosin

Prazosin is a selective alpha$_1$-adrenergic receptor-blocker that promotes arteriolar and venous dilation. It rarely is used for CHF because drug tolerance can develop over time and there are almost no clinical trial data. Additionally, the capsule sizes are inconvenient for small animals. However, prazosin sometimes is used in the management of systemic hypertension (Chapter 38).

Nitrates

Nitrates are metabolized in vascular smooth muscle to generate NO, which mediates vasodilation through activation of guanylate cyclase and formation of cGMP. Sodium nitroprusside is a potent dilator of both arteriolar and venous smooth muscle; it reduces afterload as well as preload on the heart. In contrast, other nitrates, including topical nitroglycerin ointment and orally stable isosorbide dinitrate, act as peripheral venodilators that potentially reduce cardiac filling pressures, without noticeable effect on the arterial vasculature. Nitrates effect blood redistribution in people, however there are few clinical veterinary studies on which to base any firm recommendations for clinical use. Isosorbide mononitrate does not appear to demonstrably shift blood volume to the splanchnic circulation, based on limited radionuclide data in dogs.

Sodium nitroprusside (for IV infusion) can be used in the treatment of fulminant CHF and also for some cases of acute hypertensive crisis. Sodium nitroprusside's effect on BP lasts less than 10 minutes, so the drug must be given by intravenous infusion. This agent should only be used when arterial BP and IV infusion rate can be constantly monitored. The initial dosage in CHF should be low (0.5-1.0 mcg/kg/minute) then titrated upward to maintain mean arterial pressure at about 70-80 mm Hg (at least >60 mm Hg) or systolic BP between 90 and 100 mm Hg. Higher dosages often are needed for treatment of systemic hypertension. Nitroprusside CRI usually is continued for only 12–24 hours. Nitroprusside should not be infused in the same line with other drugs, and it should be protected from light. Unfortunately, this drug has become quite expensive, further limiting its use. Nitroprusside is metabolized to a cyanide radical, and then further metabolized in the liver; elimination is via the urine, feces, and exhaled air. Profound hypotension is the major side effect of sodium nitroprusside. Cyanide toxicity can result from excessive or prolonged use (for example, >48 hours).

Nitroglycerin topical ointment (2%) has been used most often as an adjunct treatment for acute cardiogenic pulmonary edema. It is applied to the skin of the groin, axillary area, or ear pinna, although the efficacy of this treatment in CHF is unclear. An application paper or glove is used to measure the dose and avoid skin contact with the person applying the drug. Nitroglycerin ointment or oral isosorbide dinitrate also has been used infrequently in chronic CHF management, either added to standard therapy for refractory CHF or combined with hydralazine or amlodipine in animals that cannot tolerate ACE inhibitors.

There is extensive first-pass hepatic metabolism for these nitrates and oral efficacy is questionable. The transcutaneous route is used most often in animals, although nitroglycerin also is well-absorbed sublingually. Onset of action is within 1 hour, with variable duration of effect (from 2 to 12 hours). The half-life in dogs is unclear; it is under 5 minutes in people; however, metabolites have some activity. Dosage and absorption are variable. The self-adhesive, sustained release preparations might be useful, although they have not been systematically evaluated in small animals. Nitrate receptors can become saturated. Therefore, progressively higher IV doses of nitroprusside might be needed over time; additionally, response to topical nitroglycerin might improve with a nitrate-free interval of 6-12 hours (after wiping the ointment from the skin). Whether such intermittent treatment (with drug-free intervals) would prevent nitrate tolerance from developing in dogs and cats is unknown.

Hypotension also is possible with excessive or inappropriate use of topical or oral nitrates; however, this is not a common clinical problem compared to IV sodium nitroprusside, where BP must be carefully monitored. Chronic high dosages and frequent application or long-acting formulations are most likely to be associated with development of drug tolerance.

Positive Inotropic Agents

Pimobendan

Pimobendan is standard therapy for treatment of dogs with (stage C and D) heart failure caused by DCM or DMVD, in combination with diuretic, ACE inhibitor and other therapies appropriate for the individual case. Clinical trials in dogs with DCM or DMVD indicate improved clinical status and survival time with pimobendan. Compared to an ACE inhibitor, pimobendan has been associated with longer survival times; however, the value of co-administering these two drugs has not been sufficiently explored. Pimobendan also is used in cats with CHF from various cardiomyopathies, although there is some controversy regarding its use in hypertrophic cardiomyopathy. Other uses include treatment of heart failure associated with pulmonary hypertension, severe congenital disease, myocarditis, and infective endocarditis.

Pimobendan also is recommended for dogs with advanced preclinical (stage B2) DMVD, where it was shown to delay the onset of CHF by a median of over 15 months and to prolong survival (Boswood, 2016). Compared to placebo, there was no increase in adverse events. Furthermore, in dogs with stage B2 DMVD, reduction in heart size (as assessed by normalized LV diastolic dimension and LA/Ao) was seen after one month of pimobendan therapy and was associated with increased time to CHF (Boswood, 2018). Whether pimobendan produces significant beneficial effect for dogs in earlier preclinical (stage B1, with no or mild left heart enlargement) DMVD is not known; treatment currently is not advocated for these cases (Chapter 29).

Doberman Pinschers, and probably other dogs, with occult (pre-clinical) DCM can experience a delay in clinical CHF onset and prolonged survival with pimobendan (Chapter 32). The drug is often prescribed in dogs with occult DCM and ventricular arrhythmias treated with sotalol, because it might counter the negative inotropic effect of the antiarrhythmic drug. Pimobendan appears safe and helpful in cats with DCM or refractory CHF from other end-stage cardiomyopathies. These cats often have CHF characterized by a moderate to large pleural effusion. However, definitive evidence that it improves outcome in cats with hypertrophic cardiomyopathy and preserved LV systolic function – especially those with acute or chronic pulmonary edema – is lacking at present. Pimobendan theoretically could worsen severe dynamic LV outflow obstruction; caution is advised if used in cases so affected. Pimobendan was shown to improve some measures of LA function in studies of healthy cats (Baron Toaldo, 2020) and cats with HCM (Kochie, 2020). Pimobendan also might be helpful as adjunct therapy for severe pulmonary hypertension, mainly related to improvement of right heart function; the benefits of phosphodiesterase (PDE)-3 inhibition on pulmonary vasodilation are less certain (Morita, 2020).

Pimobendan is a (benzimidazole-pyridazinone derivative) non-sympathomimetic, non-glycoside inotropic drug with vasodilating properties (**Figure 21.4**). It is known as an "inodilator" because it increases contractility while also causing systemic and possibly pulmonary vasodilation. Pimobendan has an important calcium-sensitizing effect on the myocardial contractile proteins, which produces a dose-dependent increase in contractility; this particular mechanism does not involve greater myocardial O_2 consumption. Pimobendan also is a PDE-3 inhibitor. As such, it slows cyclic adenosine monophosphate (cAMP) breakdown and enhances adrenergic effects on Ca^{++} flux and myocardial contractility. Pimobendan's PDE-3 inhibition also causes endothelium-dependent systemic venous and arteriolar vasodilation. It can

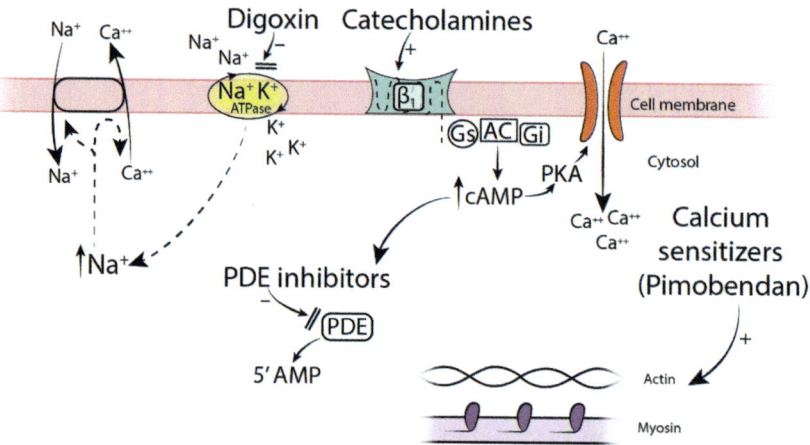

Figure 21.4 Schematic diagram showing mechanisms of action of commonly used positive inotropic drugs. Digoxin binds to ("poisons") the Na+K+ ATPase pump, which inhibits its activity and results in rising intracellular Na+ concentrations. This, in turn, causes the transmembrane Na+-Ca++ exchanger's usual direction (of moving Na+ in and Ca++ out) to slow and then reverse, which increases Ca++ entry (and Na+ extrusion); thus, more intracellular Ca++ becomes available for contraction. Catecholamines stimulate cardiac beta$_1$-adrenergic receptors, leading to Gs-mediated activation of AC and increased cAMP synthesis. cAMP stimulates PKA, which promotes increased Ca++ entry through membrane L-type Ca++ channels. Pimobendan sensitizes the contractile proteins to the prevailing Ca++ concentration within the cytosol; it also has PDE-inhibiting effects. PDE inhibitors act by blocking the enzyme PDE, which degrades cAMP, thereby increasing its concentration (and duration of action). AC, adenylyl cyclase; AMP, adenosine monophosphate; cAMP, cyclic adenosine monophosphate; Gi, inhibitory G-protein; Gs, stimulatory G-protein; Na+K+ ATPase, sodium-potassium-adenosine triphosphatase pump; PDE, phosphodiesterase; PKA, protein kinase A.

reduce LA pressure in animals with MR. In addition, the drug appears to have other beneficial effects by modulating NH and proinflammatory cytokine activation. Pimobendan has antiplatelet effects but only at much higher doses than used clinically, so it does not pose a risk for bleeding. Its direct effects on pulmonary arterial resistance in animals requires more study.

Pimobendan is available in different proprietary oral formulations (Vetmedin capsule and chewable tablets, Boehringer Ingelheim) for veterinary use, as well as unregulated compounded capsules and liquids. An intravenous preparation is available in some countries. Peak plasma concentrations occur within an hour of PO dosing in dogs. Tissue levels rise more slowly and persist longer than plasma levels. There is wide tissue distribution, with a delay from the time of peak plasma concentration to maximal effect on myocardial contractility. Increased dP/dt_{max} is observed for 8 or more hours after PO dosing. Bioavailability is about 60% in dogs, but this decreases in the presence of food. After IV injection (0.15 mg/kg) in healthy dogs, an increase in dP/dt_{max} occurred rapidly and was sustained for about an hour. SC injection of pimobendan does not appear to have significant hemodynamic effect. Pimobendan is highly protein-bound. Elimination is mainly via hepatic metabolism and biliary excretion; there is an active metabolite. The elimination half-life for pimobendan and its metabolite are ~0.5 and ~2 hours, respectively.

In normal horses, pimobendan (0.25 mg/kg) administered by nasogastric tube or IV was shown to increase heart rate by about 35% at about 2 hours post-dose (Afonso, 2016). Significant increase in ventricular contractility and decrease in ventricular filling pressure occurred by 1 hour after IV dose (as assessed from the right ventricle); similar but nonsignificant trends occurred after nasogastric administration. The lack of significance was attributed to inter-animal variability and small sample size. Bioavailability in horses is unknown. The heart rate increase was considered only a minor contributor to the enhanced cardiac performance after IV administration. This dose of pimobendan did not alter arterial BP in normal horses. Effects in horses with heart failure are unknown.

Pimobendan is generally well-tolerated in both dogs and cats. The occurrence of adverse effects appears similar to that of dogs treated with ACE inhibitors and might relate mainly to underlying heart failure, or the chewable vehicle in countries where that preparation is available. These include poor appetite, lethargy, diarrhea, dyspnea, azotemia, and weakness. Sporadic mild increase in serum alkaline phosphatase has occurred. Hyperactivity, hemorrhage, drooling, constipation, and diabetes mellitus have been reported as suspected adverse reactions. Ingestion of amounts far above the recommended dose could produce tachycardia and either hypotension or hypertension. Reported adverse effects in cats are uncommon, but have included agitation, anorexia, vomiting, and constipation.

Pimobendan does not appear to increase the frequency of ventricular arrhythmias and sudden death, as has occurred with other PDE inhibitors and inotropic drugs; however, studies of sufficient magnitude have not been completed to fully address that issue. Although more dogs with DMVD died suddenly in the pimobendan treatment limb of the EPIC trial (Boswood, 2016), that outcome was not definitive statistically and the dogs on pimobendan therapy also had a delayed onset of CHF and longer lifespan overall. Reports conflict about pimobendan's effect on heart rate. Concurrent calcium channel- or beta-blocker therapy might diminish the drug's positive inotropic effect, although to a lesser degree than with other PDE-3 inhibitors.

Digoxin

Digoxin now is used most often for the management of AF in dogs and in horses because of its vagomimetic effects. It rarely is used in cats. However, digoxin monotherapy is only moderately effective in slowing the ventricular response rate to AF (p. 411), especially in animals with CHF or during exertion. Furthermore, it does not cause conversion to sinus rhythm, although it can be an effective adjunct in managing horses with AF undergoing quinidine cardioversion (p. 413). Although pimobendan is the oral positive inotropic drug of first choice, digoxin could be used for animals with reduced myocardial contractility in which the expense or adverse effects of pimobendan are prohibitive. Digoxin also is used for CHF management in selected equine cases, and can be administered IV and in the feed. Digoxin can be added to diuretic, pimobendan, ACE inhibitor, and other therapy in the management of advanced heart failure, although this is mainly in cases with AF. Probably more importantly than its modest inotropic effect, digoxin favorably modulates baroreceptor function in CHF. By improving baroreceptor sensitivity, digoxin can blunt sympathetic and other excessive NH activation.

Digoxin increases the Ca^{++} available for contraction by inhibiting myocardial membrane Na/K-adenosine triphosphatase (ATPase) pump activity (**Figure 21.4**). The drug binds competitively to the extracellular K^+ site. Subsequent intracellular Na^+ accumulation promotes increased Ca^{++} entry via the transmembrane Na^+-Ca^{++} exchange mechanism. The drug's positive inotropic effect results from the increased Ca^{++} available to the contractile proteins. Digoxin does not increase cAMP. Digoxin has antiarrhythmic effects against some supraventricular tachyarrhythmias. These are mediated primarily by increased parasympathetic tone to the sinus and atrioventricular (AV) nodes and atria. The drug also has some direct effects which further prolong AV nodal conduction time and refractory period. These effects slow the sinus rate, reduce the ventricular response rate in AF, and could suppress atrial premature depolarizations.

Digoxin is well-absorbed orally, at ~60% for the tablet form and 75% for the elixir. The presence of food, kaolin–pectin compounds, antacids, and malabsorption syndromes decreases bioavailability. About 27% of the drug in serum is protein-bound. Digoxin is poorly lipid-soluble and skeletal muscle binding is high. Hepatic metabolism is minimal. Therapeutic serum concentrations occur in dogs within 2–4.5 days with every 12 hour dosing (half-life in dogs is ~23–39 hours). Steady state serum concentrations are achieved in ~7 days for dogs. Cats have more variable pharmacokinetics and the half-life ranges widely (~25 to over 78 hours).

The alcohol-based digoxin elixir is poorly palatable in cats and yields ~50% higher serum concentrations than the tablet form. Steady state concentrations are achieved in about 10 days with q48h dosing in cats with CHF. Digoxin is eliminated primarily by glomerular filtration and renal secretion in dogs; renal and hepatic elimination are thought to be equally important in cats. Serum digoxin concentration (and risk of toxicity, see next section) increases with renal dysfunction because of reduced total body clearance and volume of distribution. However, there appears to be no consistent correlation between degree of azotemia and serum digoxin concentration. Use of low doses and serum concentration monitoring are recommended for animals with renal disease.

In horses, oral digoxin bioavailability is only about 20%. Significant enterohepatic recycling might produce a second peak serum concentration. Serum concentrations of over 0.5 ng/mL could be achieved within 1–2 hours. Digoxin therapy often is begun with IV administration. Digoxin's half-life is variable and reportedly between 7 and 28 hours in horses. Steady state serum concentrations are achieved in 3–6 days. Quinidine therapy can increase serum digoxin concentrations (see "Digoxin Toxicity"), but practically, these two drugs are co-administered only briefly during cardioversion therapy of AF and during hospital monitoring.

Digoxin should be avoided in patients with serious preexisting ventricular tachyarrhythmias; if digoxin is deemed necessary, only lower doses should be used until the arrhythmia is controlled. The appearance of new tachyarrhythmias, especially with evidence of impaired conduction, can be a sign of digoxin toxicity, as can junctional tachycardia with AV dissociation. Digoxin is relatively contraindicated in the presence of sinus or AV nodal disease. It is not used in cats with hypertrophic cardiomyopathy because of its potential to worsen existing ventricular outflow obstruction and toxicity concerns. Digoxin is not indicated for treating pericardial disease. Although enhanced vagal tone might help suppress some ventricular arrhythmias, digoxin has potential arrhythmogenic effects that should be considered in animals with CHF.

Digoxin Toxicity Digoxin toxicity is more likely to occur with renal dysfunction, hypokalemia, and concurrent use of certain drugs. Renal function and serum electrolyte concentrations should be monitored during digoxin therapy. Hypokalemia promotes myocardial toxicity by leaving more membrane Na/K-ATPase binding sites available; conversely, hyperkalemia displaces digitalis from those binding sites. Hypercalcemia and hypernatremia potentiate both the inotropic and toxic effects of the drug. Hyperthyroidism and hypoxia could potentiate the toxic myocardial effects of the drug. Many drugs increase digoxin's serum concentration, although many of these are not used often now. Quinidine displaces the drug from skeletal muscle binding sites and reduces its renal clearance. Verapamil and amiodarone also can increase serum digoxin concentration; other drugs possibly do as well, including diltiazem, prazosin, spironolactone and triamterene. Drugs affecting hepatic microsomal enzymes also might have effects on digoxin metabolism. Neomycin and sulfasalazine decrease bioavailability.

Digoxin toxicity can cause GI signs, various cardiac arrhythmias, and sometimes central nervous system (CNS) signs. GI toxicity can develop before signs of myocardial toxicity and sometimes occurs with digoxin concentrations in the therapeutic range. GI signs include poor appetite or anorexia, depression, vomiting, borborygmus, diarrhea, and colic (horses). Direct effects of digoxin on chemoreceptors in the brainstem are responsible for some GI effects. CNS signs can include depression and disorientation. Because these also can be manifestations of hypotension or arrhythmias from underlying cardiac disease, digoxin serum concentration should be verified.

Myocardial toxicity can cause many cardiac rhythm disturbances, including ventricular tachyarrhythmias, supraventricular premature complexes and tachycardia, sinus arrest, Mobitz type I 2nd degree AV block, and junctional rhythms (**Figure 21.5**). Bigeminal rhythms are common. Myocardial toxicity can occur before any other signs are evident and can lead to collapse and death, especially in animals with myocardial failure. Therefore, the criteria of PR interval prolongation on electrocardiogram (ECG) or signs of GI toxicity should never be used to guide progressive dosing of digoxin. Digoxin can provoke spontaneous automaticity in myocardial cells by inducing late afterdepolarizations; cellular stretch, Ca^{++} overloading, and hypokalemia enhance this effect. Toxic concentrations further enhance automaticity by increasing cardiac sympathetic tone. The parasympathetic effects of slowed conduction and altered refractory period also facilitate reentrant arrhythmias.

Because of the risk for toxicity, dosage always should be conservative and measurement of serum digoxin concentration incorporated along with clinical and ECG monitoring. Therapy generally is begun using oral maintenance doses (except in horses where IV digoxin is recommended). Because digoxin has poor lipid solubility, doses should be based on the animal's estimated lean body weight; this is especially important in obese animals. Furthermore, the risk of toxicity is increased in animals with reduced muscle mass or cachexia, even at usual doses, because much of the drug is bound to skeletal muscle. There is only weak correlation between digoxin dose and serum concentration in dogs with heart failure. Conservative dosing and measurement of serum concentration help to prevent toxicity. In some dogs, toxicity seems to develop at relatively low dosages. For example, a total maximum daily dose of 0.25–0.375 mg/day is used initially for Doberman Pinschers, and a total of 0.5 mg or less for other large and giant breed dogs.

Digoxin usually is instituted at the oral maintenance dose in dogs; in situations where faster increase in serum concentration is deemed urgent and safer alternative agents are not available, some clinicians administer a loading (twice the PO maintenance) dose for the first 1 or 2 doses only. Alternatively, in such situations other clinicians give the first 1-2 (maintenance) doses IV. As a general rule, however, IV digoxin administration to dogs (and cats) is not recommended; other IV positive inotropic agents and oral pimobendan are safer and more effective than digoxin for rapid support of myocardial contractility, and alternate antiarrhythmic therapy usually is more effective for supraventricular tachycardias and AF (Chapter 25). Conversely, in horses, digoxin usually is administered IV. Animals with myocardial failure should not be given loading doses of digoxin because this could aggravate cellular Ca^{++} overloading and electrical instability.

Serum Digoxin Concentration Serum digoxin concentration measurement in dogs and horses is recommended at 1 week (or 10 days, in cats) after therapy is initiated or dosage is changed. Serum concentration also should be measured in patients that develop GI or other signs of potential toxicity, or reduced renal function, while on digoxin therapy. Although different approaches are used, the authors recommend that blood samples be drawn 8–12 hours after the previous dose (that is, at the time of "trough levels"). A serum concentration between 0.8 and 1.2 ng/mL is the target in companion animals, accepting that trough values between 0.5 and 1.5 ng/mL also can be effective and safe. This depends in part on co-therapies for CHF and AF. Although an upper-limit therapeutic serum concentration of 2 ng/mL (2.6 nmol/L) has been reported, this depends on when the sample is drawn. A greater risk for sudden death was found in people with serum digoxin concentrations toward the higher end of "therapeutic." If serum concentration is less than 0.8 ng/mL, the digoxin dose can be increased by 10–30% if heart rate control of AF is insufficient, and serum concentration measured the following week. If toxicity is suspected but serum concentration cannot be measured, the drug should be discontinued for 1–2 days and then reinstituted at half of the original dose. Subacute digoxin toxicity, manifested as hyporexia and progressive weight loss, is under-recognized in dogs with chronic AF and emphasizes the importance of serum monitoring.

Management of Digoxin Toxicity Treatment for digoxin toxicity depends on the manifestations. GI signs usually respond to drug withdrawal and correction of fluid or electrolyte disturbances. Abnormal AV conduction should resolve after drug withdrawal, although anticholinergic therapy might be needed. Digoxin-induced ventricular tachyarrhythmias often respond to lidocaine (p. 426). This agent reduces sympathetic tone and suppresses reentry and late afterdepolarizations, with little effect on sinus rate or AV node conduction. If lidocaine is ineffective, phenytoin (diphenylhydantoin) is the traditional drug of second choice in dogs for digoxin-induced ventricular tachyarrhythmias; it can be used in horses for the same purpose. Phenytoin has effects similar to lidocaine (p. 378). Also helpful is IV potassium supplementation, if serum K^+ concentration is <4 mEq/L (**Table 25.4**, p. 414).

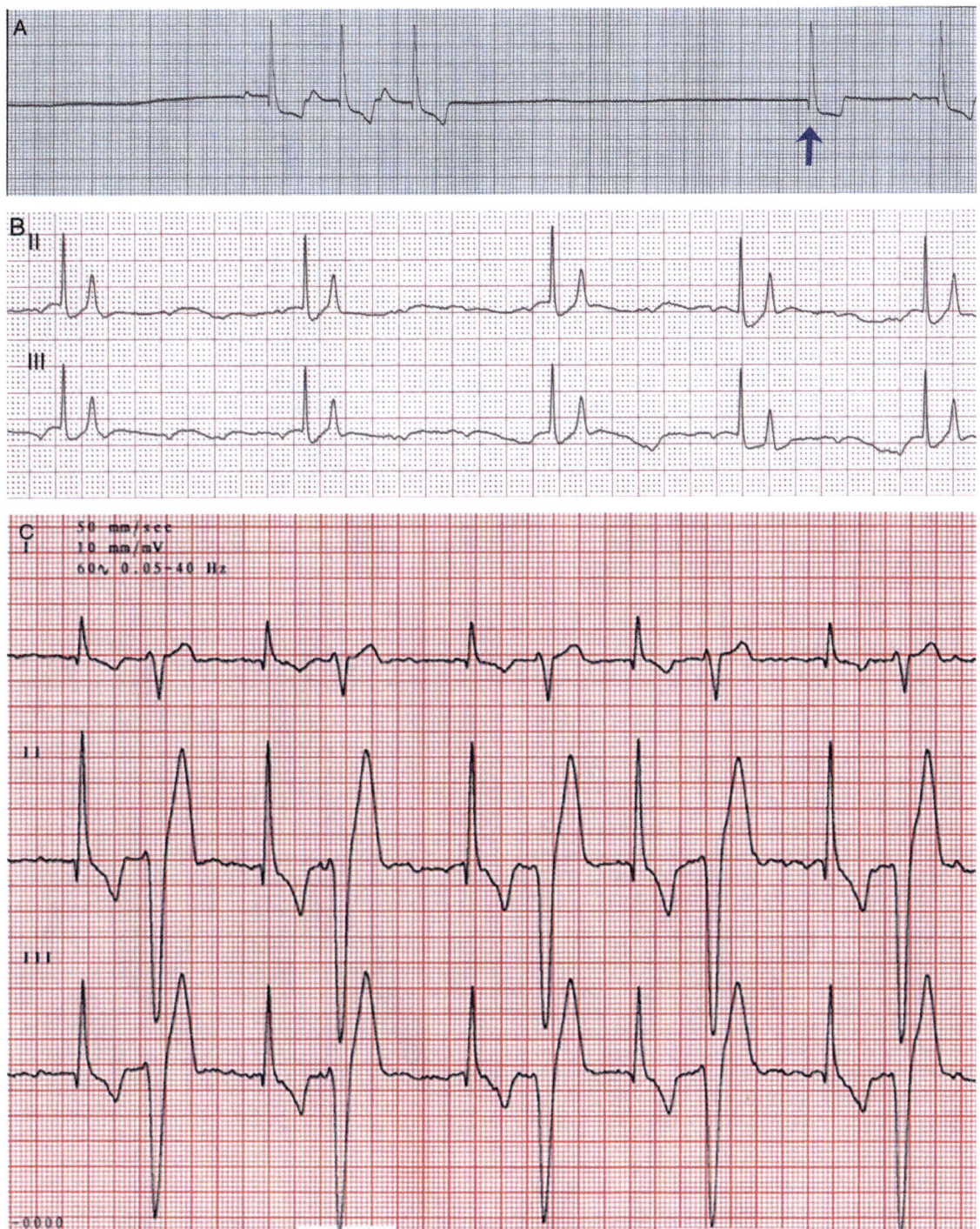

Figure 21.5 (A) Digoxin toxicity in an older Terrier-mix with degenerative mitral valve disease. This ECG shows periods of sinus arrest, sometimes interrupted by a junctional escape complex (arrow). Also note the 1st degree atrioventricular (AV) block, especially in the 2nd and 3rd complexes from the left (PR intervals ~0.18 second), as well as ST segment slurring and depression. This dog had other rhythms at different times, including intermittent atrial premature complexes, paroxysmal atrial tachycardia with high-grade 2nd degree AV block, and ventricular bigeminy. Serum digoxin concentration was 15 ng/mL. Lead II, 50 mm/s, 1 cm = 1 mV. (B) ECG from a 12-year-old, female Cocker Spaniel with lethargy and anorexia for a week; she had been treated with furosemide, digoxin, and enalapril for suspected left ventricular dilation. Increasing lethargy and respiratory effort, ascites, and the development of bradycardia prompted referral. The ECG shows a slightly irregular heart rate of ~40 beats/minute, abnormal P wave configuration with 2nd degree AV block, ST slurring and tented T waves. Echocardiography showed normal left heart size and function, moderate pulmonary hypertension, and a suspected thrombus in the right atrium. Serum digoxin concentration was in the toxic range; metabolic abnormalities included severe azotemia (blood urea nitrogen >100 mg/dl), hyperkalemia (K^+, 8.9 mEq/l), leukocytosis, and proteinuria. The ECG reflects effects of both digoxin and hyperkalemia (which presumably mitigated some digoxin effects). Leads II & III; 25 mm/s, 0.5 cm = 1 mV. (C) Ventricular bigeminy developed secondary to digoxin toxicity in an 11–year-old Weimaraner with atrial fibrillation. Leads I, II, & III; 50 mm/s, 1 cm = 1 mV.

Practically, IV magnesium supplementation is used more often to suppress malignant ventricular arrhythmias due to digitalis toxicity in dogs and horses (**Table 25.2**, p. 404). Cautious fluid therapy is indicated to correct dehydration and maximize renal function. Sometimes, a beta-blocker helps control ventricular tachyarrhythmias, but beta-blockers should not be used with AV conduction block or uncontrolled CHF. Quinidine is not used. The oral steroid-binding resin cholestyramine is useful only very soon after accidental digoxin overdose, because enterohepatic circulation of this drug is minimal. A preparation of digoxin-specific antigen–binding fragments (digoxin-immune Fab) derived from ovine anti-digoxin antibodies has been used rarely for severe digoxin overdose. The Fab binds with antigenic determinants on the digoxin molecule, preventing and reversing the pharmacologic and toxic effects of digoxin. The Fab–digoxin complex subsequently is excreted by the kidney. Each 38 mg vial will bind about 0.5 mg digoxin. For acute oral ingestion, the dose (1 vial for every milligram of digoxin consumed) is based on total digoxin intake. After prolonged overdose (steady state concentration), the following modified formula, taking the volume of distribution of digoxin in the dog into account, could be used: number of vials needed = body load of digoxin in mg/0.6. The body load of digoxin = (serum digoxin concentration in ng/mL/1,000) × 14 L/kg × body weight in kg.

Catecholamines

Dobutamine   Dobutamine, in conjunction with other therapy, is used for short term inotropic and BP support in dogs and cats with myocardial failure, as well as for anesthetic support of CV function in horses. It has lesser effect on heart rate and afterload than dopamine and is preferred over that drug. Dobutamine also is used for hypotension due to cardiogenic shock, unless the cause is vasodilation, which typically indicates another cause of hypotension such as sepsis. In those cases, dopamine, norepinephrine, or vasopressin tend to be used over dobutamine.

Dobutamine is a synthetic analog of dopamine. Catecholamines increase contractility and heart rate, especially at higher doses. Stimulation of cardiac beta$_1$-adrenergic receptors (coupled to G$_s$) activates adenylyl cyclase to increase cAMP synthesis, which stimulates a protein kinase A that in turn activates L-type Ca^{++} channels, leading to increased Ca^{++} influx and greater contractility (**Figure 21.4**). Dobutamine stimulates beta$_1$-receptors, but has only weak action on beta$_2$- and alpha-receptors; it does not stimulate dopaminergic receptors. The drug increases contractility, with minimal effects on heart rate and BP at lower infusion rates (3–7 mcg/kg/minute). Beta-receptor downregulation and uncoupling limit its effectiveness within a few days of administration such that higher dosages might be needed over time. Concurrent use of a beta-blocker also blunts the effect of dobutamine (and dopamine). Dobutamine's short half-life (<2 minutes) and extensive hepatic metabolism make it suitable only for IV administration, usually by CRI. The initial infusion rate should be low (about 2.5 mcg/kg/minute in dogs and cats, and lower in horses); this can be increased gradually over several hours to achieve greater inotropic effect, a targeted systolic arterial BP between 90 and 120 mm Hg, and signs of improved perfusion (such as increased body temperature). Heart rate, rhythm, and BP must be monitored closely.

At higher doses, dobutamine increases heart rate, myocardial oxygen demand and risk of ventricular arrhythmias. It could increase pulmonary and systemic vascular resistance. Although dobutamine is less arrhythmogenic than dopamine, at higher infusion rates (such as 10–20 mcg/kg/minute) it can precipitate supraventricular and ventricular arrhythmias. Development of sinus tachycardia or tachyarrhythmias should prompt a decrease in infusion rate. Adverse effects are more likely in cats; these also include nausea and seizures at relatively low doses.

Dopamine   Dopamine can be used for short-term support of myocardial contractility and BP, similar to dobutamine. Dopamine is an endogenous catecholamine (see "Dobutamine") that is a precursor to norepinephrine. Low-to-moderate doses enhance contractility and cardiac output. Dopamine stimulates beta- and also alpha-receptors at higher doses. At low doses (<2–5 mcg/kg/minute CRI) it also stimulates vasodilator dopaminergic D$_1$-receptors in the renal, mesenteric, coronary, and cerebral circulations. The drug's short half-life (<2 minutes) and extensive hepatic metabolism make it suitable only for IV administration, usually by CRI. By increasing renal blood flow, dopamine may enhance the renal clearance of other drugs. An initial IV infusion of 1 mcg/kg/minute can be titrated upward to desired clinical effect. The infusion rate should be decreased if sinus tachycardia or other tachyarrhythmias develop. At higher doses (such as 10–15 mcg/kg/minute), dopamine causes peripheral vasoconstriction and increases heart rate, O$_2$ consumption, and risk of ventricular arrhythmias. Dopamine mainly is used in anesthesia and critical care medicine, as opposed to CHF. It can be useful when there is a comorbidity such as sepsis or pancreatitis, where the action of a vasopressor is needed to maintain arterial BP.

Other Phosphodiesterase-3 Inhibitors

Amrinone was developed for short-term inotropic support in severe myocardial failure, but is no longer used today. *Milrinone*, a bipyrdine cardiac inotropic agent, is similar to but more potent than amrinone. Drugs in this class increase intracellular Ca^{++} by inhibiting PDE-3, an intracellular enzyme that degrades cAMP (**Figure 21.4**). This increases myocardial contractility and also causes vasodilation, because increased cAMP promotes vascular smooth muscle relaxation. Effects begin shortly after IV bolus injection. Constant infusion is required for sustained effect. The main indication for milrinone is as an inodilator for treatment of CHF, but there is little veterinary experience with the available IV preparation. Oral milrinone (0.5–1 mg/kg) was used in a clinical trial of dogs with myocardial failure and produced clinical, hemodynamic, and echocardiographic improvement. However, this formulation was withdrawn because of increased risk for sudden death in humans. Adverse effects include hypotension and tachycardia at high dosages, and potentially vomiting, diarrhea, hepatotoxicity, and thrombocytopenia (with prolonged use).

Other Drugs Used in Heart Failure

Sildenafil

Sildenafil citrate, and the related drug tadalafil, are selective PDE type-5 inhibitors that promote NO-mediated vasodilation in the pulmonary vasculature. These drugs prevent the breakdown of the intracellular vasodilator cGMP (p. 834). The main indication for PDE-5 inhibitors is for treatment of severe and symptomatic pulmonary arterial hypertension with associated signs of exertional collapse, syncope, or right-sided CHF. Sildenafil also is used as adjunct therapy in dogs with refractory (stage D) CHF, mainly in the setting of severe MR where a combination of postcapillary and precapillary pulmonary hypertension sometimes is observed. It occasionally has been used in cats and horses with severe pulmonary hypertension. This drug is discussed further in Chapter 39.

Beta-blockers in Chronic Heart Failure

Physicians and medical nurses who own an animal in heart failure often ask why a beta-blocker is not being prescribed for their pet. This question arises from the context that beta-blockers have the greatest positive impact of any medicine on cardiac-related survival in people. Specific beta-blockers prolong life and eventually improve heart function in humans (and some experimental animals) with heart failure caused by reduced ejection fraction (HFrEF), as well as some with heart failure associated with preserved ejection fraction but impaired diastolic function (HFpEF). While coronary artery disease, idiopathic DCM, and hypertension are major reasons for heart failure in people, there are other reasons for the discrepancy between species. For one, the actual definition of "heart failure" is different. In veterinary medicine, "heart failure" typically refers to the state of CHF, an advanced stage of cardiac dysfunction where sympathetic stimulation is needed to preserve CV function. In contrast, heart failure signs in people are typically less severe. Often there is minimal or no congestion, with clinical signs confined to exertional symptoms of tiring or breathlessness. Occult DCM in dogs is the veterinary disorder most similar to HFrEF in people, while preclinical HCM in cats and severe subaortic stenosis in dogs are probably the best veterinary examples of HFpEF. Although experimental studies in canine myocardial disease support the judicious use of beta-blockers in preclinical DCM, there currently are no clinical trial data to recommend the widespread use of beta-blockers for prevention or treatment of heart failure in dogs, cats or horses. Thus the usual, and accurate, response to these questions about beta-blockers for pets is: the value and indications for beta-blockers in veterinary patients with heart failure are unresolved, and these drugs can be dangerous in uncontrolled CHF.

Aside from treatment of arrhythmias (Chapter 25), there are limited situations where beta-blockers are used in the setting of heart failure. These include slowing of the heart rate (especially during AF) and reduction of myocardial O_2 consumption (especially in animals with severe ventricular concentric hypertrophy). As in people, there has been interest in the possibility that certain beta-blockers (such as carvedilol, metoprolol, and bisoprolol) might have cardioprotective effects in animals with preclinical heart disease or even overt heart failure, by reducing the adverse effects of chronic sympathetic activation. Yet, apart from arrhythmia control, their use in patients with myocardial failure seems counterintuitive. Especially in animals with marked systolic dysfunction and particularly in those with overt CHF, the negative inotropic effect of these agents is of concern. Nevertheless, in people with stable heart failure caused by systolic dysfunction (myocardial failure; HFrEF), long-term (>4 month) therapy with certain beta-blockers can improve cardiac function, reverse pathologic ventricular remodeling, and prolong survival. The 3rd generation beta-blocker carvedilol, and some 2nd generation agents (metoprolol, bisoprolol), have produced this survival benefit in people. The underlying molecular mechanisms are poorly understood. However, protection from the toxic effects of endogenous catecholamines could improve myocardial function with time, overcoming the negative inotropic effect of adrenergic blockade. In experimental heart failure models, metoprolol upregulates myocardial beta$_3$-adrenoreceptor expression, which can contribute to a beta$_1$-blocker-mediated cardioprotective effect. In MR-induced volume overload in dogs, metoprolol enhances myocardial beta$_3$-adrenoreceptor coupling with NO-stimulated cGMP signaling, although only in certain membrane microdomains. Unfortunately, veterinary clinical studies to date have shown no convincing benefit.

Although dogs and cats with advanced heart disease that are not yet in CHF might tolerate a beta-blocker fairly well, caution is warranted when using beta-blockers in animals with CHF, or even with preclinical myocardial dysfunction. Some patients experience clinical deterioration, including hypotension, bradycardia, and worsening failure. Considering the relatively short survival time for most dogs with overt CHF caused by DCM, perhaps this is one reason significant myocardial functional improvement has not been realized. Dogs and cats in heart failure are unlikely to tolerate moderate to high dosages of beta-blockers unless carefully up-titrated, and their use in uncontrolled CHF is discouraged. Regardless, small or uncontrolled studies of atenolol, metoprolol (long-acting), carvedilol, and bisoprolol have been published or presented. In an unpublished trial, bisoprolol given to dogs with stage B2 DMVD failed to delay CHF onset so the trial was stopped.

While beta-blocker initiation during the clinically occult stage of DCM in dogs and HCM in cats would appear rational as a myocardial protectant strategy, such benefit remains unproven. If carvedilol, metoprolol (long-acting), or atenolol is being considered for a dog with occult DCM, or stable compensated CHF (meaning no evidence of congestion for at least a week or more) caused by DCM, or chronic MR with myocardial dysfunction (that is, a DCM phenotype), low initial doses should be used. Frequent monitoring is important, especially during up-titration; if bradycardia, hypotension, or clinical CHF decompensation occurs, the dosage should be reduced or the drug discontinued. Whether individual patients might derive benefit from such therapy is unclear. Nevertheless, limited small studies to date have not demonstrated significant positive effects on outcome. Therefore, beta-blocker therapy cannot be advised as a blanket recommendation for heart failure treatment, especially in general small animal practice.

Carvedilol Carvedilol blocks $beta_1$-, $beta_2$-, and $alpha_1$-adrenergic receptors, has antioxidant effects, and decreases endothelin release. Carvedilol also has some Ca^{++} blocking properties and lacks intrinsic sympathomimetic activity. Carvedilol, and to a lesser extent metoprolol, was shown to reduce circulating proinflammatory cytokine levels in people with DCM. The attenuation or reversal of pathologic myocardial remodeling seen with carvedilol in human heart failure might be related partly to reduction in oxygen free radicals, which contribute to myocardial dysfunction and cell death. However the antioxidant effects of this drug might be far less in dogs, related to bioavailability and other factors. Carvedilol's combined beta-blockade reduces cardiac adrenergic activity without up-regulating beta-receptors. The $alpha_1$-blocking effect of carvedilol offsets its $beta_1$-blocking effect on contractility. In healthy dogs with normal myocardial function, low dose carvedilol causes minimal hemodynamic effect. Doses of 0.2–0.4 mg/kg in experimental MR lowered BP and heart rate within 3 hours without changing other hemodynamic parameters; values returned to baseline by 24 hours. IV carvedilol decreases systemic vascular resistance in dogs. Optimal plasma concentration is 100 ng/mL in people. IV infusion to a cumulative dose of 0.15–0.31 mg/kg can achieve that plasma level in dogs. Oral doses of 1.5 mg/kg in healthy dogs produce a wide range in peak plasma concentration, from well below to almost 2.5 times the human optimal level.

Anecdotal experience with carvedilol suggests an initial dose of 0.05–0.1 mg/kg q24h, with an eventual target of 0.2–0.3 mg/kg q12h might be tolerated. Higher dosages (0.6 mg/kg q12h) could be used in DMVD, but these dogs have largely preserved systolic function. The dosage is increased every 1–2 weeks, if possible, over a 2-month period, to a target dose, or as tolerated. Carvedilol is eliminated mainly through hepatic metabolism; the terminal half-life in dogs is <1–2 hours (shorter than in people) and the drug is highly protein-bound. A substantial nonselective beta-blocking effect lasts for 12 hours and some residual effect persists for up to 24 hours. An active metabolite is probably responsible. Although carvedilol is unproven as a cardioprotective drug in veterinary medicine, it sometimes is valuable when added to diltiazem to attain control of heart rate in canine CHF complicated by AF. The same conservative dosing guidelines as indicated above should be followed.

Metoprolol and Atenolol Metoprolol (long-acting) has been used in dogs with DMVD and DCM. The drug seems to be well-tolerated, but its long-term effect on myocardial function and survival is unknown. In an experimental dog model of ischemic DCM, three months of metoprolol treatment prevented progressive LV dilation, remodeling, and dysfunction. An initial metoprolol dose might be 0.1–0.2 mg/kg/day, with an eventual target of 1 mg/kg daily, if tolerated.

Atenolol, another 2nd generation beta-blocker, also produced beneficial effects on myocardial function in dogs with iatrogenic MR. Atenolol's heart rate reduction was thought to positively affect myocardial energetics. This drug often is used in cats with preclinical HCM and dynamic LVOT obstruction, although evidence of benefit on major endpoints such as CHF or survival is lacking (Schober, 2013). Similarly, in dogs with moderate to severe subaortic or pulmonary stenosis, the value of atenolol to mitigate effects on the affected ventricle has not been demonstrated in any controlled, prospective studies. Thus, the use of atenolol for feline HCM and for canine congenital heart diseases should be individualized, recognizing the lack of high-grade evidence showing benefit beyond the theoretical benefits associated with reductions in dynamic outflow obstruction, exercise heart rate, myocardial oxygen consumption, diastolic filling times, and ventricular ectopy.

Newer Therapies

Angiotensin Receptor Blockade and Natriuretic Peptide Potentiation Because there are alternative pathways besides ACE for AngII production, blockade of Ang1R presents another therapeutic possibility (**Figure 21.2**). These subtype-1 Ang receptors mediate AngII's CV effects. They are located mainly in vascular smooth muscle, kidney, heart, and adrenal gland tissue. ARBs, used in place of (or occasionally in combination with) an ACE inhibitor, have shown beneficial effects in people with CHF. Their clinical use in companion animals with CHF has not been well-studied. Valsartan is an ARB that has reduced preload and afterload in canine experimental HF. Telmisartan is another ARB that is used more as an antihypertensive agent, especially in cats (Chapter 38).

Exogenous natriuretic peptide administration has been tried successfully as adjunctive therapy in people with severe, acute CHF. This can reduce cardiac filling pressure and improve clinical signs of pulmonary edema. A synthetic canine B-type natriuretic peptide is being studied. It appears to be well-tolerated in healthy dogs and does increase plasma cGMP. However, its use and efficacy in dogs with CHF are not yet reported.

Blockade of other NH pathways activated in CHF presents possible new treatment strategies. These include the inhibition of neprilysin (a neutral endopeptidase that inactivates natriuretic peptides, angiotensins, and bradykinins (**Figure 21.6**), the combination of a neprilysin inhibitor with an ARB, and other approaches. In people with heart failure the use of an ARB and neprilysin inhibitor (a combination known as ARNI) has decreased the risk of death and hospitalization for CHF better than an ACE inhibitor (enalapril). Neprilysin degrades natriuretic peptides. The specific ARNI studied is the combination valsartan and sacubitril (Entresto, Novartis AG). In a preclinical study in healthy Beagle dogs with RAAS activation induced by low salt diet, this ARNI (sacubitril/valsartan, at 225 or 675 mg/day) reduced ALD levels significantly; valsartan alone also decreased ALD, but benazepril had minimal effect (Mochel, 2019). In addition, the higher ARNI dose produced a substantial increase in plasma cGMP concentration, reflecting the ability of neprilysin inhibition to magnify the effects of natriuretic peptide; benazepril and valsartan had no effect. At higher doses, there might be a rebound increase in ALD by 12 hours post-dose. In a small study of stage B2 DMVD dogs that were receiving pimobendan, 20 mg/kg of Entresto q12h PO for 30 days produced significantly lower rise in urinary ALD/creatinine ratio compared to dogs given placebo (12% vs 195%). Adverse effects were not seen (Newhard, 2018). Although clinical trial data are not yet available, anecdotal experience with Entresto in dogs (and cats) with refractory CHF appears positive. A dosage of 5-10 mg/kg q24(-12)h has been suggested; this dosage level reflects the combined total mg of sacubitril plus valsartan. ACE inhibitor therapy should be discontinued 2 days before instituting ARNI treatment. Whether sacubitril, in combination with an ARB, is more effective than the related neutral endopeptidase inhibitor ecadotril requires more study; the latter agent by itself failed in a canine study (unpublished) of advanced CHF.

Other Strategies Tolvaptan is a selective vasopressin V2-receptor antagonist. In people with CHF, and combined with conventional therapy, it can increase free water excretion and reverse hyponatremia without impairing renal function. In a small study in dogs with experimental CHF, it increased free water clearance and serum Na^+ concentration, and reduced pulmonary capillary wedge pressure without affecting systemic resistance, glomerular filtration rate, or plasma renin activity.

Ivabradine is a selective heart rate-lowering drug, as opposed to beta blockers, Ca^{++} channel blockers, and digoxin, which have other CV effects. Ivabradine slows the heart rate

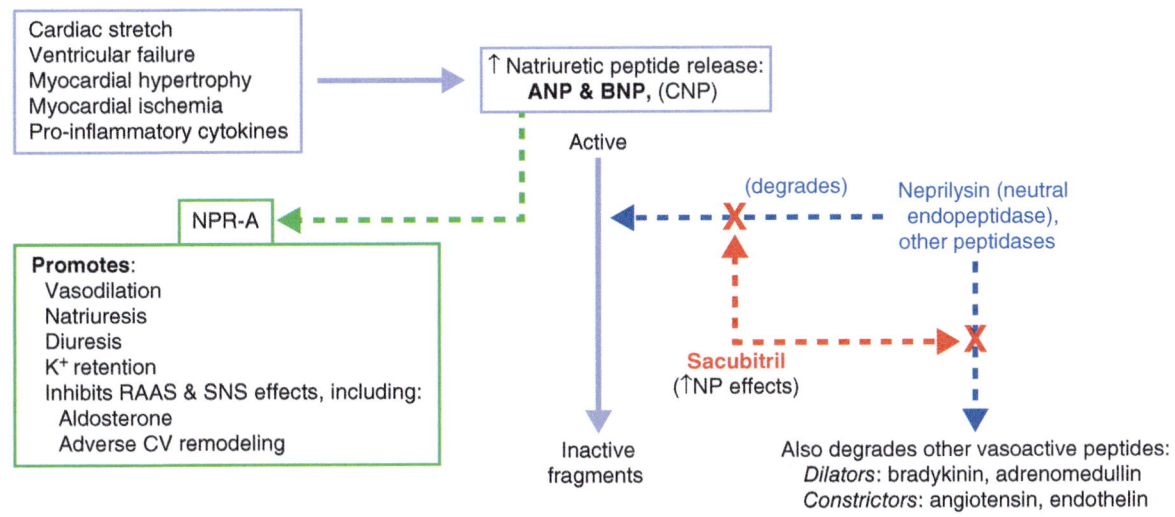

Figure 21.6 Simplified schematic of the natriuretic peptide system and related effects. The NPs are released as preprohormones, which are cleaved to prohormones and ultimately to inactive N-terminal fragments (such as NT-proBNP) and active C-terminal fragments, before degradation by neprilysin or other means. Sacubitril inhibits the action of neprilysin, thereby slowing NP degradation. Type-A NP receptors mediate the effects of ANP and BNP (via the 2nd messenger cyclic guanosine monophosphate). CNP is secreted mainly by endothelial cells and cardiac fibroblasts; it acts locally via type-B NP receptors to promote vasodilation and counteract cardiac remodeling. There also are type-C NP receptors (clearance receptors) that function to degrade NPs. ANP, atrial or A-type natriuretic peptide (mainly secreted by the atrial myocardium); BNP, brain or B-type natriuretic peptide (mainly secreted by the ventricular myocardium); CNP, C-type natriuretic peptide; CV, cardiovascular; NP, natriuretic peptide; NPR-A, type-A natriuretic peptide receptor; RAAS, renin-angiotensin-aldosterone system; SNS, sympathetic nervous system.

of patients in sinus rhythm by inhibiting the hyperpolarizing I_f (funny) current. This reduces the rate of spontaneous diastolic depolarization (automaticity) in sinus node cells, especially under the influence of sympathetic tone (p. 385). Elevated heart rate is an independent predictor of worse outcome in people with chronic heart failure. Ivabradine has improved clinical outcomes in people with chronic heart failure and elevated sinus heart rate. In those with severe myocardial failure, its effect to slow heart rate and increase ventricular filling time also appears to improve the hemodynamic response to dobutamine infusion. Heart rate reduction decreases myocardial oxygen requirements and allows for increased myocardial perfusion. This could be particularly important with hypertrophic myocardial disease, especially for cases where a beta-blocker might be detrimental. Ivabradine treatment in a canine experimental heart failure model reduced heart rate and was associated with improved cardiac function and reversal of several biochemical and molecular maladaptive changes. A dose-dependent reduction in heart rate occurred in a small number of dogs with preclinical, spontaneous DMVD given oral ivabradine. No adverse effects were seen. A dose of 1 mg/kg has been suggested for reducing heart rate in dogs with asymptomatic DMVD; twice that dose caused a significant decrease in BP (Pirintr, 2018). A number of feline studies have shown ivabradine to successfully reduce heart rate in cats in a similar manner to atenolol when dosed at 0.3 mg/kg PO q12h. However, this dose did not eliminate dynamic LVOT obstruction (Blass, 2014).

3-Hydroxy-3-methylglutaryl coenzyme A reductase inhibitors (statins) usually are prescribed for their cholesterol lowering effects in people. However, they also have antioxidant and anti-inflammatory effects, can improve endothelial function, and have other potentially beneficial cardiac effects apart from their influence on cholesterol. Lipophilic statins (atorvastatin, simvastatin) might improve survival in people with CHF. In a small study of healthy dogs and dogs with well-controlled CHF caused by DMVD, atorvastatin at 2 mg/kg q24hr was well-tolerated; it also decreased white blood cell count and systolic BP, as well as total serum cholesterol, in the CHF dogs (Cunningham, 2013). This short-term study could not address whether atorvastatin might improve CHF control and outcome in veterinary patients.

A small study using low-dose imatinib in dogs with pulmonary hypertension secondary to CHF found reduced cough, improved total clinical symptom score, and lowered LA/Ao ratio and Doppler-estimated pulmonary artery pressure with this drug. Imatinib is a tyrosine kinase inhibitor that inhibits the actions of platelet-derived growth factor. In experimental pulmonary hypertension studies, imatinib reduced pulmonary artery smooth muscle proliferation, reversed vascular remodeling, and promoted pulmonary vasodilation that were induced by platelet-derived growth factor. Its potential use in chronic heart failure requires further study. At higher doses, imatinib has antineoplastic effects against certain tumors.

Pentoxifylline is a methylxanthine drug with immunologic and hematologic properties, but with less potent chronotropic and inotropic effects than theophylline. It reportedly reduces inflammatory mediators, including tumor necrosis factor (TNF) and interleukin (IL)-1, and stimulates collagenase. It is not used often in CHF. Nevertheless, it has been associated with improved clinical signs and ventricular function in people with idiopathic DCM, when added to therapy with digoxin, ACE inhibitor, and carvedilol.

Cardiac resynchronization therapy, using artificial biventricular pacing, has improved systolic function, clinical status, and survival in people with abnormal intraventricular conduction and myocardial failure. The applicability of this therapy in dogs has not been well explored beyond experimental canine models. Stem cell transplantation is another emerging modality for human heart failure that could hold promise for veterinary patients. Gene therapy options to improve myocardial function might become available at some point in the future.

Suggested Additional Reading and References

Also See Online Comprehensive Bibliography at: https://www.routledge.com/9781482246223.

Adin D, Atkins C, Domenig O, et al. Renin-angiotensin aldosterone profile before and after angiotensin-converting enzyme-inhibitor administration in dogs with angiotensin-converting enzyme gene polymorphism. J Vet Intern Med 2020;34:600–606.

Agne GF, Jung SW, Wooldridge AA, et al. Pharmacokinetic and pharmacodynamic properties of orally administered torsemide in healthy horses. J Vet Intern Med 2018;32:1428–1435.

Afonso T, Giguere S, Rapoport G, et al. Cardiovascular effects of pimobendan in healthy mature horses. Equine Vet J 2016;48:352–356.

Afonso T, Giguere S, Rapoport G, et al. Pharmacodynamic evaluation of 4 angiotensin-converting enzyme inhibitors in healthy adult horses. J Vet Intern Med 2013;27:1185–1192.

Ames MK, Atkins CE, Pitt B. The renin-angiotensin-aldosterone system and its suppression. J Vet Intern Med 2019;33:363–382.

Arita S, Arita N, Hikasa Y. Therapeutic effect of low-dose imatinib on pulmonary arterial hypertension in dogs. Can Vet J 2013;54:255–261.

Atkins CE, Keene BW, Brown WA, et al. Results of the veterinary enalapril trial to prove reduction in onset of heart failure in dogs chronically treated with enalapril alone for compensated, naturally occurring mitral valve insufficiency. J Am Vet Med Assoc 2007;231:1061–1069.

Baron Toaldo M, Pollesel M, Diana A. Effect of pimobendan on left atrial function: an echocardiographic pilot study in 11 healthy cats. J Veter Cardiol 2020;28:37–47.

Beddies G, Fox PR, Papich MD, et al. Comparison of the pharmacokinetic properties of bisoprolol and carvedilol in healthy dogs. Am J Vet Res 2008;69:1659–1663.

BENCH Study Group. The effect of benazepril on survival times and clinical signs of dogs with congestive heart failure: Results of a multicenter, prospective, randomized, double-blinded, placebo-controlled, long-term clinical trial. J Vet Cardiol 1999;1:7–18.

Bernay F, Bland JM, Häggström J, et al. Efficacy of spironolactone on survival in dogs with naturally occurring mitral regurgitation caused by myxomatous mitral valve disease. J Vet Intern Med 2010;24:331–341.

Blass KA, Schober KE, Li X, et al. Acute effects of ivabradine on dynamic obstruction of the left ventricular outflow tract in cats with preclinical hypertrophic cardiomyopathy. J Vet Intern Med 2014;28:838–846.

Borgarelli M, Ferasin L, Lamb K, et al. Delay of appearance of symptoms of canine degenerative mitral valve disease treated with spironolactone and benazepril: the DELAY study. J Vet Cardiol 2020;27:34–53.

Boswood A, Gordon SG, Häggström J, et al. Longitudinal analysis of quality of life, clinical, radiographic, echocardiographic, and laboratory variables in dogs with preclinical myxomatous mitral valve disease receiving pimobendan or placebo: the EPIC study. J Vet Intern Med 2018;32:72–85.

Boswood A, Häggström J, Gordon SG, et al. Effect of pimobendan in dogs with preclinical myxomatous mitral valve disease and cardiomegaly: the EPIC study-a randomized clinical trial. J Vet Intern Med 2016;30:1765–1779.

Boyle KL, Leech E. A review of the pharmacology and clinical uses of pimobendan. J Vet Emerg Crit Care 2012;22:398–408.

Chetboul V, Pouchelon JL, Menard J, et al. Short-term efficacy and safety of torasemide and furosemide in 366 dogs with degenerative mitral valve disease: the TEST study. J Vet Intern Med 2017;31:1629–1642.

Cunningham SM, Rush JE, Freeman LM. Short-term effects of atorvastatin in normal dogs and dogs with congestive heart failure due to myxomatous mitral valve disease. J Vet Intern Med 2013;27:985–989.

Davis JL, Kruger K, LaFevers DH, et al. Effects of quinapril on angiotensin converting enzyme and plasma renin activity as well as pharmacokinetic parameters of quinapril and its active metabolite, quinaprilat, after intravenous and oral administration to mature horses. Equine Vet J 2014;46:729–733.

Gomez-Diez M, Munoz A, Caballero JM, et al. Pharmacokinetics and pharmacodynamics of enalapril and its active metabolite, enalaprilat, at four different doses in healthy horses. Res Vet Sci 2014;97:105–110.

Häggström J, Boswood A, O'Grady M, et al. Effect of pimobendan or benazepril hydrochloride on survival times in dogs with congestive heart failure caused by naturally occurring myxomatous mitral valve disease: the QUEST study. J Vet Intern Med 2008;22:1124–1135.

Harada K, Ukai Y, Kanakubo K, et al. Comparison of the diuretic effect of furosemide by different methods of administration in healthy dogs. J Vet Emerg Crit Care 2015;25:364–371.

Hezzell MJ, Boswood A, Lopez-Alvarez J, et al. Treatment of dogs with compensated myxomatous mitral valve disease with spironolactone-a pilot study. J Vet Cardiol 2017;19:325–338.

Hori Y, Taira H, Nakajima Y, et al. Inotropic effects of a single intravenous recommended dose of pimobendan in healthy dogs. J Vet Med Sci 2019;81:22–25.

James R, Guillot E, Garelli-Paar C, et al. The SEISICAT study: a pilot study assessing efficacy and safety of spironolactone in cats with congestive heart failure secondary to cardiomyopathy. J Vet Cardiol 2018;20:1–12.

Johansson AM, Gardner SY, Levine JF, et al. Pharmacokinetics and pharmacodynamics of furosemide after oral administration to horses. J Vet Intern Med 2004;18:739–743.

Johansson AM, Gardner SY, Levine JF, et al. Furosemide continuous rate infusion in the horse: evaluation of enhanced efficacy and reduced side effects. J Vet Intern Med 2003;17:887–895.

Kochie SL, Schober KE, Rhinehart J, et al. Effects of pimobendan on left atrial transport function in cats. J Vet Intern Med 2020.

Lake-Bakaar GA, Singh MK, Kass PH, et al. Effect of pimobendan on the incidence of arrhythmias in small breed dogs with myxomatous mitral valve degeneration. J Vet Cardiol 2015;17:120–128.

Lefebvre HP, Ollivier E, Atkins CE, et al. Safety of spironolactone in dogs with chronic heart failure because of degenerative valvular disease: a population-based, longitudinal study. J Vet Intern Med 2013;27:1083–1091.

Macdonald PS. Combined angiotensin receptor/neprilysin inhibitors: a review of the new paradigm in the management of chronic heart failure. Clin Ther 2015;37:2199–2205.

Marcondes-Santos M, Tarasoutchi F, Mansur AP, et al. Effects of carvedilol treatment in dogs with chronic mitral valvular disease. J Vet Intern Med 2007;21:996–1001.

McMurray JJ, Packer M, Desai AS, et al. Angiotensin-neprilysin inhibition versus enalapril in heart failure. N Engl J Med 2014;371:993–1004.

Meurs KM, Olsen LH, Reimann MJ, et al. Angiotensin-converting enzyme activity in Cavalier King Charles Spaniels with an ACE gene polymorphism and myxomatous mitral valve disease. Pharmacogenet Genomics 2018;28:37–40.

Mizuno M, Yamano S, Chimura S, et al. Efficacy of pimobendan on survival and reoccurrence of pulmonary edema in canine congestive heart failure. J Vet Med Sci 2017;79:29–34.

Mochel JP, Danhof M. Chronobiology and pharmacologic modulation of the renin-angiotensin-aldosterone system in dogs: what have we learned? Rev Physiol Biochem Pharmacol 2015;169:43–69.

Mochel JP, Peyrou M, Fink M, et al. Capturing the dynamics of systemic renin-angiotensin-aldosterone system (RAAS) peptides heightens the understanding of the effect of benazepril in dogs. J Vet Pharmacol Ther 2012.

Mochel JP, Teng CH, Peyrou M, et al. Sacubitril/valsartan (LCZ696) significantly reduces aldosterone and increases cGMP circulating levels in a canine model of RAAS activation. Eur J Pharm Sci 2019;128:103–111.

Morita T, Nakamura K, Osuga T, et al. Acute effects of intravenous pimobendan administration in dog models of chronic precapillary pulmonary hypertension. J Vet Cardiol 2020;32:16–27.

Newhard DK, Jung S, Winter RL, et al. A prospective, randomized, double-blind, placebo-controlled pilot study of sacubitril/valsartan (entresto) in dogs with cardiomegaly secondary to myxomatous mitral valve disease. J Vet Intern Med 2018;32:1555–1563.

Nishijima Y, Sridhar A, Viatchenko-Karpinski S, et al. Chronic cardiac resynchronization therapy and reverse ventricular remodeling in a model of nonischemic cardiomyopathy. Life Sci 2007;81:1152–1159.

O'Grady MR, Minors SL, O'Sullivan ML, et al. Effect of pimobendan on case fatality rate in Doberman Pinschers with congestive heart failure caused by dilated cardiomyopathy. J Vet Intern Med 2008;22:897–904.

Ohad DG, Segev Y, Kelmer E, et al. Constant rate infusion vs. intermittent bolus administration of IV furosemide in 100 pets with acute left-sided congestive heart failure: a retrospective study. Vet J 2018;238:70–75.

Onogawa T, Sakamoto Y, Nakamura S, et al. Effects of tolvaptan on systemic and renal hemodynamic function in dogs with congestive heart failure. Cardiovasc Drugs Ther 2011;25(Suppl 1):S67–76.

Oyama MA, Solter PF, Thorn CL, et al. Feasibility, safety, and tolerance of subcutaneous synthetic canine B-type natriuretic peptide (syncBNP) in healthy dogs and dogs with stage B1 mitral valve disease. J Vet Cardiol 2017;19:211–217.

Oyama MA, Sisson DD, Prosek R, et al. Carvedilol in dogs with dilated cardiomyopathy. J Vet Intern Med 2007;21:1272–1279.

Pirintr P, Limprasutr V, Saengklub N, et al. Acute effect of ivabradine on heart rate and myocardial oxygen consumption in dogs with asymptomatic mitral valve degeneration. Exp Anim 2018;67:441–449.

Qian M, Chen T, Zhou D, et al. Development of a new benazepril hydrochloride chewable tablet and evaluation of its bioequivalence for treatment of heart failure in dogs. J Vet Pharmacol Ther 2016;39:98–101.

Redpath A, Bowen M. Cardiac therapeutics in horses. Vet Clin North Am Equine Pract 2019;35:217–241.

Sabbah HN, Gupta RC, Kohli S, et al. Heart rate reduction with ivabradine improves left ventricular function and reverses multiple pathological maladaptations in dogs with chronic heart failure. ESC Heart Fail 2014;1:94–102.

Schober KE, Zientek J, Li X, et al. Effect of treatment with atenolol on 5-year survival in cats with preclinical (asymptomatic) hypertrophic cardiomyopathy. J Vet Cardiol 2013;15:93–104.

Schuller S, Van Israel N, Vanbelle S, et al. Lack of efficacy of low-dose spironolactone as adjunct treatment to conventional congestive heart failure treatment in dogs. J Vet Pharmacol Ther 2011;34:322–331.

Serrano-Rodriguez JM, Gomez-Diez M, Esgueva M, et al. Pharmacokinetics and pharmacodynamics of ramipril and ramiprilat after intravenous and oral doses of ramipril in healthy horses. Vet J 2016;208:38–43.

Sleeper MM. Status of therapeutic gene transfer to treat cardiovascular disease in dogs and cats. Vet Clin North Am Small Anim Pract 2017;47:1113–1121.

Sleeper MM, O'Donnell P, Fitzgerald C, et al. Pharmacokinetics of furosemide after intravenous, oral and transdermal administration to cats. J Feline Med Surg 2019;21:882–886.

Suzuki S, Ishikawa T, Hamabe L, et al. The effect of furosemide on left atrial pressure in dogs with mitral valve regurgitation. J Vet Intern Med 2011;25:244–250.

Trappanese DM, Liu Y, McCormick RC, et al. Chronic beta1-adrenergic blockade enhances myocardial beta3-adrenergic coupling with nitric oxide-cGMP signaling in a canine model of chronic volume overload: new insight into mechanisms of cardiac benefit with selective beta1-blocker therapy. Basic Res Cardiol 2015;110:456.

Uechi M, Matsuoka M, Kuwajima E, et al. The effects of the loop diuretics furosemide and torasemide on diuresis in dogs and cats. J Vet Med Sci 2003;65:1057–1061.

Wess G, Kresken JG, Wendt R, et al. Efficacy of adding ramipril (VAsotop) to the combination of furosemide (Lasix) and pimobendan (VEtmedin) in dogs with mitral valve degeneration: The VALVE trial. J Vet Intern Med 2020;34:2232–2241.

Yandrapalli S, Aronow WS, Mondal P, et al. The evolution of natriuretic peptide augmentation in management of heart failure and the role of sacubitril/valsartan. Arch Med Sci 2017;13:1207–1216.

Yata M, McLachlan AJ, Foster DJ, et al. Single-dose pharmacokinetics and cardiovascular effects of oral pimobendan in healthy cats. J Vet Cardiol 2016;18:310–325.

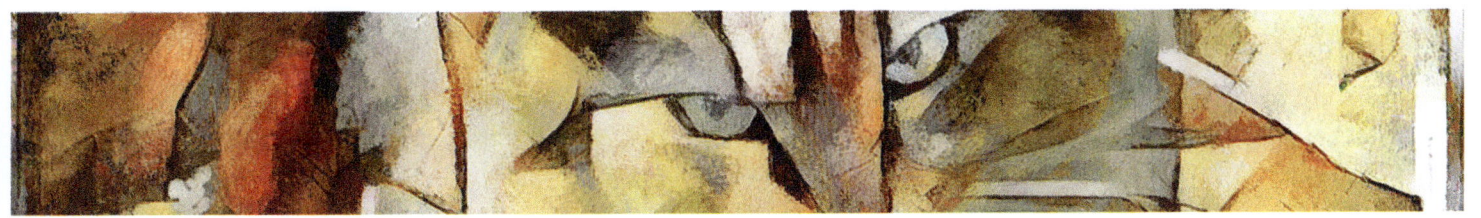

22
MANAGEMENT OF HEART FAILURE

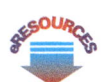

Heart failure entails abnormalities of cardiac systolic or diastolic function, or both. Especially in the earlier stages of disease, these can occur without evidence of abnormal fluid accumulation (congestion). Congestive heart failure (CHF) is characterized by high cardiac filling pressures, which lead to venous congestion and increased capillary fluid transudation (p. 25 and Chapter 20). The first step is to confirm the diagnosis of heart failure or CHF and determine the underlying cause. Several treatment principles are common to most etiologies of heart failure; however, it is important to consider the individual patient's underlying pathophysiologic abnormality(ies) when designing a treatment plan. **Figure 22.1** outlines a general approach to CHF management; chapters on specific diseases also should be consulted for more detail. The predominant or initiating pathophysiology (Chapter 20) in dogs and horses most often involves volume overload or primary myocardial failure, often complicated by arrhythmias such as atrial fibrillation (AF). Systolic pressure overload, as from systemic hypertension or other causes, is less common but can complicate preexisting heart disease. Reduced ventricular compliance stemming from hypertrophic or restrictive forms of cardiomyopathy (most common in cats) or concentric hypertrophy can involve additional treatment considerations. Finally, it is important to recognize when CHF signs have resulted from impaired filling caused by cardiac tamponade or constrictive pericardial disease, because the approach to therapy fundamentally differs from what is effective for most other causes of CHF.

Most current strategies for managing heart failure are oriented toward two major goals: (1) optimize hemodynamics by improving cardiac function and reducing venous pressure, and (2) modify the long-term consequences of neurohormonal (NH)–renal activations, including vasoconstriction, tissue injury, and excess fluid retention. Targeting the activation process itself, with the aim of minimizing progression of myocardial remodeling and dysfunction, also is a goal. The search for improvements in survival time, as well as functional status and quality of life, is a major impetus behind ongoing research. Inodilators, diuretics, modest dietary salt restriction, and some vasodilators help to control signs of congestion, while angiotensin converting enzyme (ACE) inhibitors, as well as aldosterone (ALD) and sympathetic antagonists, modulate NH responses. Treatment strategies center on controlling edema and effusions, improving cardiac output, reducing cardiac workload, supporting myocardial function, and managing arrhythmias or other complications that develop. The approach to these goals varies somewhat with different diseases, most notably those that mainly impair ventricular filling (Chapters 33 and 35). Besides arrhythmias, other complicating factors in animals with heart failure include azotemia, electrolyte abnormalities, and concurrent noncardiac abnormalities, particularly respiratory diseases, thyroid disorders, anemia and systemic infections. Some of these conditions are consequences of CHF or its therapy, some induce similar clinical signs, and others can precipitate CHF in previously compensated patients.

Considerations for Managing Preclinical Heart Disease

The use of specific cardiovascular (CV) drug therapy in animals with heart disease, but that have not yet experienced CHF, is sometimes controversial. Clearly, no therapy is indicated for animals merely at risk for heart disease (stage A; **Table 20.2**, p. 311), although periodic physical exam (and auscultation), blood pressure (BP) measurement, and other routine health maintenance regimens are recommended. Other tests, such as thoracic radiographs, echocardiography, or NT-proBNP measurement, might be indicated in some cases. For animals classified as stage B1 (Table 20.2), no therapy is recommended currently. For patients in stage B2, recommendations regarding cardiac therapy can vary depending on etiology. In some situations, there are differences of opinion among cardiologists.

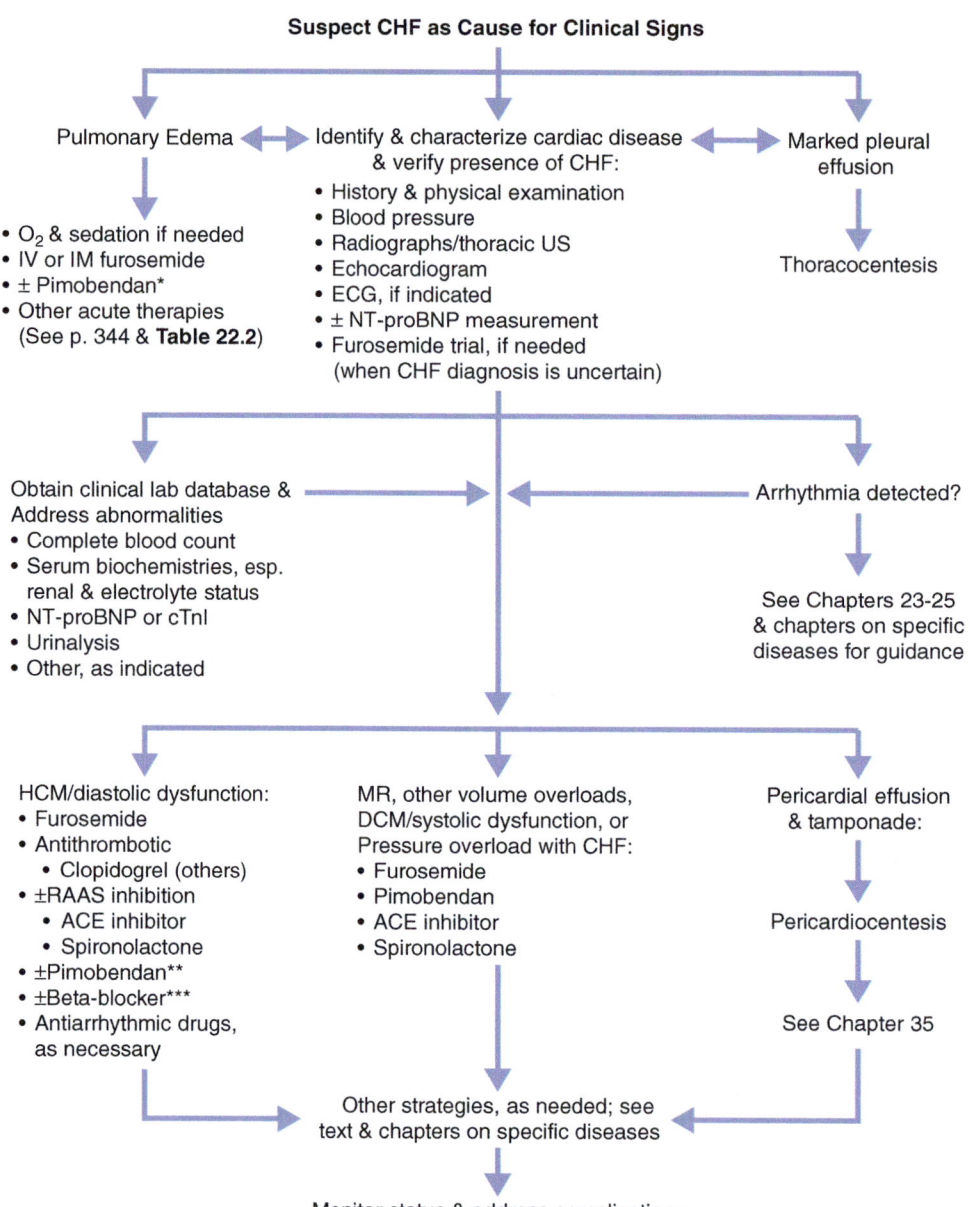

Figure 22.1 A general approach to CHF management. These are general guidelines and exceptions can occur. *Pimobendan indicated for heart failure with reduced ejection fraction (DCM phenotype), valvular heart diseases, pulmonary hypertension, and potentially for some patients with diastolic heart failure. **Pimobendan appears beneficial in some cats with HCM, especially those without murmurs and pleural effusions. ***Beta-blockers should not be given to animals with uncontrolled CHF; in selected cases, they might have value for controlling tachycardias or dynamic left ventricular outflow obstruction. ACE, angiotensin converting enzyme; CHF, congestive heart failure; cTnI, cardiac troponin I; DCM, dilated cardiomyopathy; ECG, electrocardiogram; esp., especially; HCM, hypertrophic cardiomyopathy; IV, intravenous; MR, mitral regurgitation; NT-proBNP, N-terminal probrain natriuretic peptide; RAAS, renin angiotensin aldosterone system; US, ultrasound.s

In any case, it is prudent to discuss with the owner of a stage B2 patient the early signs likely to be observed, should decompensated CHF develop. Especially when pulmonary edema is an expected CHF manifestation (based on the individual patient's disease), the authors recommend that owners begin to periodically monitor the animal's resting (preferably sleeping) respiratory rate (RRR) at home (**Table 22.1**, client guidelines). Pulmonary congestion and edema (as well as other pulmonary parenchymal diseases) increase lung stiffness; this leads to compensatory tachypnea, which minimizes the work of breathing. Accordingly, by RRR monitoring owners are alerted to increases in resting breathing rate, which often allows detection of CHF before it becomes critical. When this monitoring is begun during stage B2, owners can become comfortable with the procedure in a nonurgent setting, and it helps them determine the normal baseline RRR for that individual animal. This is particularly pertinent to dogs already receiving a drug aimed at delaying CHF onset,

Table 22.1 Client Guidelines for Resting Respiratory Rate (RRR) Monitoring

For Dogs and Cats at Increased Risk for Developing Congestive Heart Failure (Stage B2)
- Over the next week or two, please monitor your pet's resting (ideally sleeping) respiratory rate (RRR) at home whenever he/she is quietly sleeping, in order to determine his/her normal baseline RRR.
- Periodically monitor the RRR in the future to help detect early signs of congestive heart failure (fluid in the lungs; pulmonary edema), should it develop.
- See the specific instructions that follow regarding guidelines for monitoring.

For Dogs and Cats That Have Had a Prior Episode of Congestive Heart Failure with Pulmonary Edema, Now Resolved (Stage C or D)
- Please monitor your pet's resting (sleeping) respiratory rate (RRR) at home multiple times over the next several days to determine his/her normal (congestion-free) baseline rate, if not already known.
- Continue to monitor the RRR every 1–2 weeks, or more often, to help detect early signs of recurrent congestive heart failure (fluid in the lungs; pulmonary edema).

Instructions for Monitoring RRR
- While your pet is quietly sleeping (or almost sleeping) and without touching or disturbing him/her, count the number of breaths taken in 30 seconds. You can usually determine this by watching the chest move in and out (or by counting the "snores", if your dog makes noise while breathing during sleep).
- Multiply this number by 2 to obtain the number of breaths per minute.
- Keep track of this number, either by recording it in a calendar or logbook, or by using a smartphone respiratory rate monitoring app.
- Most dogs and cats with normal lungs have a RRR <30 breaths/min; very often it is <20/min.
- Once you have determined your pet's normal baseline RRR, continue to monitor the RRR periodically.

If RRR becomes Increased
- If your pet's RRR becomes persistently increased by >20% above his/her normal baseline, and especially if the RRR increases to 40 breaths/min or higher, contact your veterinarian right away.
- This could be an early indicator of congestive heart failure (pulmonary edema).

such as pimobendan or an ACE inhibitor, because pulmonary edema usually signals progression to stage C disease.

Pimobendan is recommended for dogs with advanced preclinical (stage B2) degenerative (myxomatous) mitral valve disease (DMVD) because it was shown to delay the onset of CHF signs and prolong survival (EPIC study, Boswood, 2016). The benefit of initiating renin-angiotensin-aldosterone system (RAAS) inhibitor therapy with an ACE inhibitor and/or spironolactone during preclinical (stage B) DMVD disease is unclear. Clinical trials have shown either no benefit (SVEP study, Kvart, 2002; and DELAY study, Borgarelli, 2020) or at best, modest prolongation to CHF (of about 4 months in the Vetproof trial, Atkins, 2007). The potential value of combining RAAS inhibition with a background therapy of pimobendan in DMVD has not been sufficiently addressed. This lack of data, and availability of cost-effective generic drugs, accounts for the different practices among cardiologists for dogs in this stage. Dogs with more advanced DMVD, and severe left atrial (LA) and left ventricular (LV) dilation, might gain some benefit toward delaying the onset of CHF or reducing the degree of cardiac remodeling (DELAY, Borgarelli, 2020). In the authors' view, a marked increase in radiographic or echocardiographic heart size that occurs over a relatively short (~6 month) period and radiographic evidence for pulmonary venous congestion (suggesting incipient CHF) are signals to start RAAS inhibitor therapy. Other reasons for prescribing an ACE inhibitor in dogs with stage B2 DMVD include systemic hypertension, chronic renal disease, and possibly, cough from main bronchus compression caused by marked LA enlargement. There are theoretical reasons why spironolactone might help delay CHF onset; however, it has not yet been shown to do so. The DELAY study, a prospective randomized, multicenter, single-blinded placebo-controlled study, of dogs with stage B2 DMVD, showed that the combination of spironolactone and benazepril did not significantly delay the onset of CHF (the primary study end-point). Nevertheless, multiple echocardiographic and radiographic indicators of disease progression were improved in the treatment group (Borgarelli, 2020). Similarly, although beta-blocker therapy might have theoretical benefit, it has not been shown to delay CHF onset in DMVD. In an unpublished multicenter prospective clinical study, bisoprolol failed to provide benefit.

In Doberman Pinschers with occult (stage B) dilated cardiomyopathy (DCM), pimobendan begun at the time of echocardiographic diagnosis delayed the onset of CHF (PROTECT study, Summerfield, 2012). Whether dogs of other breeds with preclinical DCM experience the same quantitative benefit from pimobendan at this stage of disease is unclear. However, the authors generally recommend starting pimobendan when echocardiography shows progressive deterioration in LV systolic function or there is an unambiguous decrease in estimates of ejection fraction (such as fractional shortening <15%

or 2D ejection fraction <40%) along with LV dilation. Clinical signs, such exercise intolerance, also might prompt at least a trial course of pimobendan, as would radiographic evidence for pulmonary venous congestion (or early edema). In addition, ACE inhibitor therapy usually is started in dogs with preclinical (occult) DCM once the diagnosis is confirmed, as well as in large-breed dogs with stage B2 DMVD and LV systolic dysfunction or marked cardiomegaly. Spironolactone can be added for more complete RAAS inhibition, although this has only been studied in experimental models. Some clinicians add a beta-blocker for "cardioprotection" (p. 331) in some cases; however, there is no convincing evidence it affects outcome.

In cats with preclinical cardiomyopathy, there currently is no evidence that any therapy delays the onset of CHF or ultimately affects survival. Nevertheless, it is prudent to offer antiplatelet therapy for cats with moderate or progressive LA enlargement in the hope of prevent arterial thromboembolism (ATE; p. 769). Some clinicians prescribe an ACE inhibitor, in an attempt to reduce continued myocardial remodeling, or a beta-blocker to reduce severe dynamic LV outflow obstruction or a tachyarrhythmia. However, evidence for clear long-term benefit currently is lacking.

For horses with known cardiac disease, important questions revolve around whether the animal is safe to ride or work. Reducing the intensity of the animal's physical activity generally is advised. In some cases, specific antiarrhythmic therapy might be indicated. Whether other medical therapy can delay CHF is unknown, and there is need for clinical trial evidence regarding use of an ACE inhibitor such as benazepril in equine stage B2 valvular disease.

Initial Signs of Congestive Heart Failure

The transition from stage B2 to stage C might not be clearly demarcated. Especially in dogs with DMVD, the development of pulmonary edema can be gradual and clinical signs might wax and wane for a time. The owner who routinely monitors RRR (as a strategy to help detect early pulmonary edema) is better positioned to notice a gradual but persistent increase in rate. Reduced exercise tolerance or the onset of coughing also might be noticed.

Cough is a common sign of CHF in dogs with DCM and horses with heart failure, but is much less common in cats. Cough due to concurrent bronchopulmonary diseases must always be considered, especially in small breed dogs with DMVD. Coughing also might relate to bronchial compression by a markedly enlarged left atrium. Thoracic radiographs are recommended to identify signs of pulmonary venous congestion or edema, as well as other bronchopulmonary or thoracic pathology. Both lateral views are useful for identifying left bronchial compression (left lateral view is best) and for measuring vertebral LA score in dogs (right lateral view is best; see p. 542). The latter is typically >2.8 vertebral bodies in dogs with CHF caused by DMVD. Lung ultrasound also can be helpful (by identifying B-lines; lung rockets) when radiographs cannot be obtained immediately (p. 80). In cases where radiographs (or lung ultrasound) are inconclusive for CHF or left bronchial compression, a trial of furosemide (such as 1–2 mg/kg/day) can be given for several days. When early CHF has caused the clinical signs, the patient usually responds to this therapy with improvements in RRR, coughing, and activity. If the patient responds positively and signs abate, furosemide therapy is continued, with the addition of pimobendan and an ACE inhibitor (± spironolactone). However, as pimobendan now is recommended for dogs with stage B2 DMVD (or unequivocal DCM) even before signs of CHF develop, many dogs will already be receiving pimobendan and potentially, RAAS inhibition. If results of a furosemide therapeutic trial are negative or equivocal, furosemide is discontinued and the patient monitored closely for increase in RRR or return of the cough. It should be noted that coughing from mainstem bronchus compression might respond to pimobendan or to furosemide, as both treatments reduce heart size.

When a dog with DMVD and cough or tachypnea does not clearly respond to furosemide (with or without pimobendan or ACE inhibitor cotherapy), further evaluation is indicated for airway disease (especially tracheal collapse; bronchomalacia/collapse; and idiopathic, allergic, or infectious bronchitis) and for pulmonary parenchymal disease (including neoplasia, heartworm disease, pneumonia, or chronic interstitial lung disease). Thoracic radiography and routine laboratory tests can exclude some of these potential diagnoses, but dynamic airway collapse, bronchitis, and interstitial pulmonary fibrosis often are missed without bronchoscopy or thoracic computed tomography (CT). Because these advanced tests are obtained infrequently, brief therapeutic trials to address airway inflammation can be considered and often are the most practical approach. Antimicrobials with anti-inflammatory effects and extended spectrum, especially doxycycline, can be given for 10 days (and continued for a total of 3 weeks if there is >50% improvement in cough). If antimicrobial therapy is unsuccessful, a short course of prednisone at anti-inflammatory dosages should be considered; a 5 to 7 day course usually is well-tolerated in dogs with DMVD and unlikely to cause fluid retention. A strongly favorable response suggests underlying airway disease. The frequency of coughing should be determined; occasional bouts need not be treated. However, severe coughing spells, cough associated with fainting, or debilitating cough can be suppressed with hydrocodone. As an additional note, dental disease is common in dogs with DVMD.

Acute Decompensated Congestive Heart Failure in Dogs and Cats

Acute CHF sufficient to demand emergent veterinary care usually is characterized by clinical signs of severe cardiogenic pulmonary edema, large pleural effusion, or both. In many cases, this situation represents the "tip of the iceberg," or a culmination of progressive heart failure signs that were mostly overlooked. At other times, fulminant pulmonary edema develops rapidly, secondary to an acute stressor such as ruptured chordae tendineae, the onset of AF, infective endocarditis, or an aortic thromboembolism. Patients that require acute hospital care are markedly "decompensated," in that compensatory mechanisms to maintain cardiac output and arterial BP, and prevent edema, have been overwhelmed. Although clinical features of acute CHF focus largely on pulmonary dysfunction, these signs can coexist with an abdominal effusion, subcutaneous edema (especially in horses), and various signs of low cardiac output, including cardiogenic shock. The latter is most common in cats. Acutely decompensated CHF can occur in stage C or D patients (**Table 20.2**, p. 311).

Acute CHF requires rapid detection and urgent therapy (**Table 22.2**). Treatment is aimed at rapidly clearing pulmonary edema, relieving compression atelectasis if present, improving oxygenation while reducing oxygen demand, and optimizing cardiac output. Medical therapy is required to manage pulmonary edema, while thoracocentesis is indicated for moderate- to large-volume pleural effusion in order to improve ventilation. Large-volume ascites, which impairs ventilation and compresses abdominal organs, also should be drained after any pulmonary issues are addressed. Enhancing cardiac output is a key feature of therapy and is critical in patients with cardiogenic shock. Animals with severe CHF are greatly stressed and fragile, which often is not noticed by the owner until the situation becomes critical. Unnecessary patient handling and repeated use of oral medications should be avoided whenever possible. Physical activity must be maximally restricted to reduce total oxygen consumption; cage confinement is preferred and sedation is nearly always in order. Environmental stresses, such as excess heat and humidity or extreme cold, must be avoided. When transported, small animals should be placed on a cart or carried with the head slightly above the abdomen and with minimal pressure placed on the chest and abdomen.

Oxygen Supplementation and Ventilation

Supplemental O_2 can be provided initially by face mask or improvised O_2 hood, and for longer-term, by using a nasal or nasopharyngeal catheter, oxygen cage, or endotracheal tube, if required. Whatever the method, care should be taken to avoid increasing patient distress. An oxygen cage with temperature and humidity controls is preferred for cats and small dogs; a setting of 65° F is recommended for normothermic animals. An O_2 flow rate of 6–10 L/minute usually is adequate. Concentrations of 50–100% O_2 might be needed initially; however, O_2 concentration should be reduced to 40% or less within 12 hours to avoid lung injury. Larger dogs and horses usually are managed with nasal oxygen; the tube should deliver humidified O_2 at a rate of 50–100 mL/kg/minute for dogs. High-flow oxygen delivery systems are now available and represent a potential alternative treatment to short-term ventilation in cases of respiratory failure. These units require significant sedation to assure patient tolerance.

Patients with severe pulmonary edema and impending respiratory failure might require intubation and can respond to short- or longer-term mechanical ventilation. Too often, patients with fulminant CHF "code" on admission due to respiratory failure, cardiac arrest, or both. Respiratory management in these cases demands an endotracheal tube, suctioning of frothy edema fluid in the airways, and at least short-term artificial ventilation with oxygen, during which time decisions about further treatments can be made. Often the heart rate increases substantially with intubation and oxygenation and consciousness resumes. In other cases, cardiac arrest from asystole or ventricular fibrillation leads to death unless a normal heart rhythm is established. In most general practices, the patient will either recover and be treated medically, stabilized and then transferred, or be euthanatized. Ventilator therapy is available in many advanced emergency centers, although few clients opt for this treatment. Mechanical ventilation allows time for medical therapy to take effect, helps to clear the lungs of edema fluid, and provides time for further LA dilation to occur (as in cases of acutely increased mitral regurgitation secondary to chordal rupture). Large airways are suctioned periodically, and positive end-expiratory pressure ventilation administered to clear small airways and expand alveoli. A reasonably good rate of survival to discharge has occurred at experienced centers following positive pressure ventilation in dogs and cats. Preexisting azotemia, oliguria, and the use of pentobarbital for anesthesia/sedation have been negative predictors of outcome. Continuous monitoring is essential for intubated animals. Positive airway pressure can adversely affect hemodynamics, by increasing RV afterload and reducing LV filling. Section "Suggested Additional Reading and References" contains sources for further information on assisted ventilation.

Diuretic Therapy

Circulating volume reduction and blood redistribution are strategies used to control cardiogenic pulmonary edema. Acute LA pressure elevation leads to alveolar flooding with low protein fluid. Alveolar epithelium also can serve as a site of higher protein fluid leak (Staub, 1976). Secondary capillary membrane injury caused by high venous pressures (West, 1995) leads to protein leakage and capillary rupture, manifested as pink or blood-tinged froth exiting the nares. Diuretic therapy is needed to quickly decrease pulmonary venous and capillary hydrostatic pressures. Reduction of venous pressures also helps reduce pleural and peritoneal effusion formation, both acutely and longer-term.

Although the optimal approach to in-hospital diuretic therapy requires better delineation and guidelines, IV furosemide offers rapid diuresis and is preferred in acute decompensation. The IV route also provides a mild venodilator effect.

Table 22.2 Management of Acute Decompensated Congestive Heart Failure in Dogs and Cats

Minimize Patient Activity and Stress!

- Provide cage or kennel rest and minimize movement
- Sedate
- Avoid excessive environmental heat & humidity (especially in oxygen cages)
- Carry or cart for transport (no activity allowed)
- Beware stressful procedures (such as radiography or arterial access)

Reduce Anxiety

- Butorphanol – Dogs: 0.15–0.3 mg/kg IM or IV, can repeat in 30–60 min if needed. Cats: 0.1–0.3 mg/kg IM (or IV). Use lower doses for initial IV administration. OR,
- Morphine – Dogs: 0.025–0.1 mg/kg IV boluses q2–3min to effect, or 0.1–0.5 mg/kg single IM or SC dose. Do not use in cats. OR,
- Acepromazine – Cats: 0.05–0.1 mg/kg SC; or 0.05–0.1 mg/kg IM with butorphanol. Dogs: 0.025–0.05 mg/kg IM, SC, or IV.

Enhance Oxygenation

- Check airway patency
- Provide supplemental O_2
- Postural support if needed (maintain sternal recumbency, extended neck with head elevation)
- If frothing is evident, suction airways if possible
  - Intubate and mechanically ventilate if needed
- Perform thoracocentesis if moderate to severe pleural effusion is present
- Perform abdominocentesis for tense ascites

Initiate Diuresis

- Furosemide - Dogs: 2 mg/kg IV, IM, or SC initial bolus, then repeat at 1–4 mg/kg q1–4h until RR decreases and diuresis begins; then reduce to 1–4 mg/kg q6–12h, depending on severity and response. If insufficient response to initial boluses or life-threatening edema, use 0.66–1 mg/kg/hour CRI over the next 6-12 hours until adequate diuresis ensues; then reduce the infusion rate by 50% or switch to lower dose boluses (see p. 344).
  - Cats: 1–2 mg/kg IV, IM, or SC initial bolus, then 1–2 mg/kg q1–4h until RR decreases, then q6–12h; OR, follow IV bolus with 0.33–0.66 mg/kg/h CRI until diuresis occurs and RR decreases, as per the dog.
- Provide access to water after diuresis is evident

Support Cardiac Pump Function (Inodilator)

- Pimobendan - Dogs: 0.2–0.3 mg/kg PO q8-12h, begin as soon as possible. Cats (extralabel): 0.2–0.3 mg/kg PO or 1.25 mg/cat q12h; usage for congestive heart failure therapy with systolic dysfunction, moderate to large pleural effusions, and right-sided failure; indications for use in HCM with pulmonary edema, especially with HOCM, require definition (see text).

Load Reduction (see indications and details in text)

- Inodilator (pimobendan, see above)
- Vasodilators: Nitrates
  - 2% Nitroglycerin ointment (for venodilation only) - Dogs: 1/4–1 inch (0.6–3.8 cm, or 3.75–15 mg) cutaneously, apply for 8 to 12 hours, wipe off, and reapply 8 to 12h later (can combine with hydralazine or amlodipine in dogs). Cats: ~1/8–1/4 inch (0.3–0.6 cm, ~1.9 to 3.75 mg) cutaneously, as per the dog. OR,
  - Sodium nitroprusside or IV nitroglycerin (if able to monitor ABP closely): 0.5–1 mcg/kg/min (initial) CRI in D_5W (for cats, dilute to 100–300 mcg/mL). Slowly titrate upward as needed: in Dogs up to 5(–15) mcg/kg/min for nitroprusside; 6 mcg/kg/min for nitroglycerin. In Cats up to 2 mcg/kg/min for nitroprusside. Monitor ABP; administer until systolic ABP ~90–100 mm Hg (or mean of >60 mm Hg). Protect from light, and do not give for more than 24 hours.
- Vasodilators: Arterial vasodilators[a] (do not co-administer with injectable nitrates)
  - Hydralazine - Dogs: initial 0.5–1.0 mg/kg PO, repeat in 2–3 hours (until systolic ABP is 90–110 mm Hg), then q12h (p. 344); OR, 0.05–0.1 mg/kg IV bolus, repeat q1–2h if needed. OR,
  - Amlodipine - Dogs: 0.05–0.1 mg/kg initially, to 0.3 mg/kg PO q12–24h with ABP monitoring. OR,
  - Enalapril – Dogs: 0.5 mg/kg PO q12–24h, (or other ACE inhibitor)
- ±Additional inotropic support (if myocardial systolic failure or persistent hypotension and cardiogenic shock):

Table 22.2 (Continued) Management of Acute Decompensated Congestive Heart Failure in Dogs and Cats

Additional Strategies (see indications and details in text)

- Dobutamine[b] - 1 mcg/kg/min initial CRI; titrate upward to effect q15–30min, as needed for 24–48 hours then wean off. Dogs: up to 20 mcg/kg/min. Cats: up to 10 mcg/kg/min. (Alternatively, can use dopamine[c] - Dogs: 1–10 mcg/kg/min CRI. Cats: 1–5 mcg/kg/min CRI. Start low, titrate to effect q15–30min, for 24–48 hours then wean off). (And/)OR,
- Milrinone (50 mcg/kg IV over 10 min initially; 0.375–0.75 mcg/kg/min CRI [human dose]).
- Digoxin (not generally used unless as adjunct for atrial fibrillation in dogs; see **Table 22.3** for dosing).
- Other hospital treatments – see text for details

For Diastolic Dysfunction (Cats with Hypertrophic Cardiomyopathy; see text for details)

- General recommendations, O_2 therapy, furosemide, and sedation (as above in this table)
- Thoracocentesis, if needed for moderate to large pleural effusion
- ±Nitroglycerin (cutaneously)
- ±Pimobendan (see above)
- ±Dobutamine (for cardiogenic shock; see above)
- Monitor and manage abnormalities and comorbidities, as possible (see below)
- (Delay ACE inhibitor until after appetite returns, see **Table 22.3**)

Monitor and Manage Clinical Abnormalities and Comorbidities, as Possible

- Observations:
  - Attitude & level of consciousness (sedation)
  - Respiratory rate, depth, pattern & effort (trends)
  - Urinary output (from diuretic therapy)
  - Heart rate and rhythm (from a monitor, see Chapter 25)
  - Water and food consumption
- Physical Diagnosis & Monitoring Procedures:
  - Temperature (rectal, axillary, otic, or toe-web and trends)
  - Arterial pulse rate and strength
  - Arterial blood pressure (noninvasive)
  - Cardiac & pulmonary auscultation
  - Hydration status (before and after diuresis)
  - Bladder size (palpation & ultrasound, before & after diuretics)
  - Body weight & changes with diuresis
  - Mucous membrane color & peripheral perfusion
  - O_2 saturation or arterial blood gas analysis
  - Point-of-care ultrasound (effusions, B-lines, vena caval size, cardiac chamber size & function)
- Clinical laboratory test monitoring:
  - PCV or complete blood count (exclude anemia and systemic inflammation)
  - Serum biochemistry tests, blood lactate, serum thyroxine, cardiac troponin, etc.
- ±Invasive pressure monitoring (infrequently performed):
  - Invasive ABP
  - Pulmonary arterial and pulmonary wedge pressures
- Diagnostic Imaging:
  - Serial thoracic radiography
  - Doppler echocardiography (cardiac chamber size & function, filling pressures)

[a] Used for afterload reduction in dogs with fulminant pulmonary edema that are not responding adequately to furosemide, especially those with mitral regurgitation (and when not administering sodium nitroprusside); ACE inhibitors are less potent and can promote renal failure during vigorous diuresis; generally reserved for chronic therapy
[b] Dilution of 250 mg dobutamine into 500 mL of D_5W or lactated Ringer's solution yields 500 mcg/mL; infusion at 0.6 mL/kg/hour provides 5 mcg dobutamine/kg/min (also see **Table 25.3**, p. 411 for CRI rate calculation).
[c] Dilution of 40 mg dopamine into 500 mL of D_5W or lactated Ringer's solution provides a solution of 80 mcg/mL; infusion at 0.75 mL/kg/hour provides 1 mcg dopamine/kg/min (also see **Table 25.3**, p. 411 for CRI rate calculation).

Abbreviations: ABP, arterial blood pressure; ACE, angiotensin converting enzyme; CRI, constant rate infusion; D_5W, 5% dextrose in water; HCM, hypertrophic cardiomyopathy; HOCM, hypertrophic obstructive cardiomyopathy; PCV, packed cell volume; RR, respiratory rate.

However, both SC and IM administration can be similarly effective if IV access cannot be established immediately. Some patients require aggressive initial doses or high cumulative doses administered at frequent intervals, or by constant rate infusion (CRI). Regardless of route, higher dosages of furosemide increase the risks for azotemia and acute kidney injury (p. 317). Additionally, once diuresis begins, time is needed before pulmonary edema is fully mobilized and pulmonary function returns toward normal; this can take hours or even days if there is secondary capillary injury. It is common practice to continue or even escalate high-dose furosemide in a patient that has not yet "responded" to the diuretic, in terms of respiratory function. However, whether this is reasonable in a patient that already has lost substantial body weight (through diuresis) can be questioned, and such therapy increases the risk for azotemia and electrolyte disturbances. Similarly, there is an increasing trend toward using furosemide CRI in decompensated CHF. This approach potentially can yield greater diuresis; however, there currently are no clinical patient trials comparing equivalent furosemide doses delivered by CRI to repeated bolus injections. Thus, the clinician should actively determine if diuresis is occurring, gauge the magnitude of fluid loss, and understand that a time lag commonly is observed between brisk diuresis and improvement in respiratory rate and effort. Beyond these determinations, comparing diuretic effectiveness (by dose or route of administration) is complicated by the complementary effects of sedation, oxygen delivery, other medical treatments, and time.

The veterinary formulation of furosemide (50 mg/mL) can be diluted to 10 mg/mL in 5% dextrose in water (D_5W), lactated Ringer's solution (LRS), or sterile water. Dilution to 5 mg/mL in D_5W or sterile water is an alternative. The patient's respiratory rate, effort, auscultation and thoracic imaging findings; urinary output; changes in bodyweight; and renal function and serum electrolyte concentrations are among the parameters that guide continued furosemide therapy. Once diuresis has begun and respiration improves, furosemide dosage should be reduced to prevent excessive volume contraction or electrolyte depletion.

Vasodilator Therapy

Vasodilator drugs can reduce pulmonary edema either by increasing systemic venous capacitance and lowering pulmonary venous pressure, or reducing systemic arterial resistance, or both. Although ACE inhibitors have greater advantage for long-term treatment, more immediate afterload reduction often is needed for patients with acute pulmonary edema, especially those with ruptured mitral chords or with concurrent systemic hypertension. The initial dose(s) of an arteriolar vasodilator should be low, with subsequent titration upward as needed, based on BP and clinical response. Besides BP monitoring, it is important to assess serum creatinine concentration within 24–48 hours after initiating arteriolar vasodilator therapy. Arteriolar vasodilation is not recommended for heart failure caused by diastolic dysfunction, especially with ventricular outflow obstruction.

Hydralazine or amlodipine, administered in combination with topical nitroglycerin (as a possible alternative to sodium nitroprusside) is used to treat life-threatening or refractory pulmonary edema caused by severe mitral regurgitation, systemic hypertension, or less often, DCM. These drugs can reduce the regurgitant fraction and lower LA pressure. Hydralazine also can be administered IV (at very low dose) for acute CHF. More often, an initial PO dose is repeated every 2–3 hours until systolic BP is 90–110 mm Hg or clinical improvement is obvious (**Tables 22.2** and **22.3**). The addition of 2% nitroglycerin ointment might provide a beneficial venodilating effect. Alternatives to hydralazine-nitroglycerin include amlodipine and an ACE inhibitor. However, these agents have slower onset of action and immediate effects are less pronounced (Chapter 21). Neither hydralazine nor amlodipine are recommended in the setting of LV outflow obstruction (including hypertrophic obstructive cardiomyopathy); they could exacerbate dynamic obstruction or precipitate hypotension and coronary ischemia, especially in cases with severe, fixed obstruction (such as congenital subaortic stenosis).

Sodium nitroprusside (p. 324) and IV nitroglycerin are potent arteriolar and venous dilators; BP must be monitored closely because these drugs can cause severe hypotension. There is more experience with nitroprusside, although administration of intravenous nitroglycerin in dogs has been reported (Achiel, 2000). These drugs are given by IV infusion, with the dose titrated to maintain mean arterial BP at about 80 mm Hg (at least >70 mm Hg) or systolic BP between 90 and 110 mm Hg. Nitroprusside CRI usually is continued for only 12–24 hours. Dosage adjustments might be needed because drug tolerance develops rapidly.

Topical nitroglycerin and orally administered nitrates act mainly on venous smooth muscle to increase venous capacitance and reduce cardiac filling pressure. The major indication for nitroglycerin is acute cardiogenic pulmonary edema. Nitrates are probably less effective in patients with severe ascites, and increased abdominal pressure on capacitance veins. Nitroglycerin ointment (2%) usually is rubbed onto the skin of the groin, axillary area, or ear pinna, although the efficacy of this in CHF is unclear. Persons applying the drug (or handling the animal) should take care to avoid skin contact with it (use application paper or glove). The ointment is preferred for smaller dogs and cats and delivers approximately 3.75 mg of nitroglycerine per ¼ inch of the 2% ointment. Transdermal nitrate patches (5 mg) applied for 12 hours/day have been used in larger dogs with anecdotal success. Such treatments are generally short-lived. A nitrate-free interval is recommended to overcome nitrate tolerance that is caused by depletion of sulfhydryl groups needed in the conversion of nitrates to nitric oxide. This involves removing the drug for 8 to 12 hours (wiping it from the skin) to allow saturated receptors to become re-sensitized to the nitrate.

Table 22.3 Drugs for Heart Failure Management

Drug	Dog	Cat	Horse
Diuretics			
Furosemide	*Acute CHF:* 2 mg/kg IV, IM or SC initial bolus, then 1–4 mg/kg q1–4h until RR decreases and diuresis begins, then reduce to 1–4 mg/kg q6–12h (depending on severity & response); OR, if inadequate response to initial boluses, 0.66–1 mg/kg/hour CRI for next 6 hours until RR decreases. *Maintenance:* 1–3+ mg/kg PO q8–24h (long term); use smallest effective dose. In refractory CHF, several intermittent 2 mg/kg SC doses/week, in place of PO doses, may be helpful (or use torsemide; see p. 319).	*Acute CHF:* 1–2 mg/kg IV, IM or SC initial bolus, then 1–2 mg/kg q1–4h until RR decreases, then q6–12h (depending on severity & response); OR follow IV bolus with 0.33–0.66 mg/kg/h CRI until RR decreases. *Maintenance:* 1–2 (to 3) mg/kg PO q8–12h; use smallest effective dose.	*Acute CHF:* 1–3 mg/kg IV or IM (or SC?) q6–8(–12)h to effect; OR 1–2 mg/kg IV loading, then 0.12 mg/kg/h CRI. *Maintenance:* 1–2 mg/kg IV or IM q6–24h. Not effective PO.
Torsemide	Dose at 1/8 to 1/12 of patient's total daily furosemide dose; administer in two divided doses	Dose at 1/10 to 1/12 of patient's total daily furosemide dose; administer in two divided doses (or 0.1–0.3 mg/kg PO q12h)	0.5 – 1 (up to 2?) mg/kg PO q12h (?)
Spironolactone	0.5–2 mg/kg PO q24h (or divided, q12h); target dose, 2 mg/kg/day	0.5–1 (to 2) mg/kg PO q24h (or divided, q12h)	2–4 mg/kg PO q24h
Hydrochlorothiazide	0.5–4 mg/kg PO q12–48h (start qod with low dose)	0.5–2 mg/kg PO q12–48h (start qod with low dose)	
Chlorothiazide	10–40 mg/kg PO q12–48h (start qod with low dose)	10–40 mg/kg PO q12–48h (start qod with low dose)	
ACE Inhibitors			
Enalapril	0.5 mg/kg PO q12–24h	0.25–0.5 mg/kg PO q(12–)24h	Little to no PO efficacy
Benazepril	0.25–0.5 mg/kg PO q(12–)24h	0.25–0.5 mg/kg PO q24(–12)h	0.5–1 mg/kg PO q24(–12)h
Captopril	0.5–2.0 mg/kg PO q8–12h	0.5–1.25 mg/kg PO q12–24h	
Lisinopril	0.25–0.5 mg/kg PO q(12–)24h	0.25–0.5 mg/kg PO q24h	
Fosinopril	0.25–0.5 mg/kg PO q24h		
Ramipril	0.125–0.25 mg/kg PO q24h		0.05–0.2 mg/kg PO q24h
Imidapril	0.25 mg/kg PO q24h		
Quinapril			0.125–0.5 mg/kg PO q24h
Other Vasodilators			
Hydralazine	*Acute CHF:* 0.5–1.0 mg/kg PO (initial), can repeat in 2–3h (see **Table 22.2**). OR, 0.05–0.1 mg/kg IV bolus, repeat q1–2h, if needed. Monitor BP. *Maintenance:* 0.5–2 (–3) mg/kg PO q12h (to 1 mg/kg initial)	2.5 (up to 10) mg/cat PO q12h	0.5–1.5 mg/kg PO q12h; OR, up to 0.5 mg/kg IV q(4–)12h
Amlodipine	0.05–0.1 mg/kg initially, to 0.3(–0.5) mg/kg PO q(12–)24h	0.3125–0.625 mg/cat PO q24(–12)h	
Nitroprusside	0.5–1 mcg/kg/min (initial) up to 5(–15) mcg/kg/min CRI (see **Table 22.2** & text)	0.5–1 mcg/kg/min (initial) up to 2 mcg/kg/min CRI (see **Table 22.2** & text)	
Nitroglycerin (for IV use)	*For acute CHF:* 0.5–1.0 mcg/kg/min initial CRI; titrate up in increments of 1–2 mcg/kg/min as needed, up to 10 mcg/kg/min		*For acute CHF:* 5 mcg/kg/min initial CRI; slowly titrate up (to 20 mcg/kg/min) as needed
Nitroglycerin 2% ointment (15 mg/inch)	0.25–1.5 inch (0.6–3.8 cm) cutaneously q4–6h for 24–48 hours	0.25–0.5 inch (0.6–1.3 cm) cutaneously q4–8h for 24–48 hours	

(Continued)

Table 22.3 (Continued)   Drugs for Heart Failure Management

Drug	Dog	Cat	Horse
Isosorbide dinitrate	0.5–2 mg/kg PO q(8–)12h		
Isosorbide mononitrate	0.25–2 mg/kg PO q12h		
Acepromazine	Not typically used as vasodilator	Not typically used as vasodilator	0.01–0.06 mg/kg IM q6–8h; or 0.1–1.0 mg/kg PO q8–12h. Dose to effect & monitor BP.
Positive Inotropic Agents			
Pimobendan	0.2–0.3 (up to 0.5) mg/kg PO q12h (to q8h); (0.15 mg/kg IV initial dose, if necessary & available)	As for dog, or 1.25 mg/cat PO q12h	(0.25 mg/kg IV q12h, if parenteral form available); PO bioavailability not established.
Digoxin	*Maintenance*: dogs <22 kg, 0.005–0.008 mg/kg PO q12h; dogs >22 kg, 0.22 mg/m^2 or 0.003–0.005 mg/kg PO q12h. Decrease by 10% for elixir. Maximum: 0.5 mg/day or 0.375 mg/day for Doberman Pinchers. *Loading* (see text for indications) PO: 1 or 2 doses at twice calculated maintenance; (IV [not recommended]: 0.01–0.02 mg/kg – give 1/4 of this total dose in slow boluses over 2–4 hours to effect)	*Maintenance*: 0.007 mg/kg (or 1/4 of 0.125 mg tab) PO q48h. Rarely used. *Loading* (see text for indications) PO: 1 or 2 doses at twice calculated maintenance; (IV [not recommended]: 0.005 mg/kg – give 1/2 of total, then 1–2 hours later give 1/4 dose bolus[es], if needed)	*Loading*: 0.0022 mg/kg IV q12 for two doses. *Maintenance*: 0.011 mg/kg PO q12h; (or 0.0022 mg/kg IV q24h). Commonly, 1 mg/horse given by slow IV push.
Dobutamine	1 mcg/kg/min initial CRI; titrate upward to effect q15–30min, as needed, up to 20 mcg/kg/min CRI. Wean down before discontinuing.	1 mcg/kg/min initial CRI; titrate upward to effect q15–30min, as needed, up to 10 mcg/kg/min CRI. Wean down before discontinuing.	1 mcg/kg/min initial CRI; titrate upward to effect q15–30min, as needed, up to 5 mcg/kg/min CRI. Wean down before discontinuing.
Dopamine	1–10 mcg/kg/min CRI; start low, titrate to effect q15–30min	1–5 mcg/kg/min CRI; start low, titrate to effect q15–30min	Not recommended
Milrinone	*Acute CHF*: 50 mcg/kg IV over 10 min initially; 0.375 to 0.75 mcg/kg/min CRI (human dose)	Same?	*Acute CHF*: 0.2 mcg/kg IV bolus, then 5–10 mcg/kg/min CRI;

Abbreviations: CHF, congestive heart failure; CRI, constant rate infusion; RR, respiratory rate.

Other Therapies for Acute Congestive Heart Failure

Mild sedation (**Table 22.2**) helps reduce patient anxiety. Butorphanol is preferred for dogs, cats, and horses in CHF. Morphine traditionally was administered to dogs with CHF, and its benefits can include slower, deeper breathing from respiratory center depression and blood redistribution away from the lungs via capacitance vessel dilation. However, morphine often induces vomiting and this can precipitate cardiac arrest. The drug is contraindicated in dogs with neurogenic edema because it can raise intracranial pressure. Morphine should not be used in cats.

Some dogs with severe pulmonary edema and bronchoconstriction might benefit from bronchodilator therapy although clinical response to albuterol inhalation has been disappointing overall and not systematically studied. Previously, the methylxanthine bronchodilator theophylline, or its amino salt, aminophylline, was used for canine CHF. Given slowly IV or by IM injection these drugs exert mild diuretic and positive inotropic actions, as well as a bronchodilating effect. Respiratory muscle contractility also is increased, potentially reducing fatigue. However, in light of currently available therapeutics, and lack of clinical trial data, bronchodilators are administered infrequently now unless there is clear evidence of bronchial narrowing such as wheezing, in which case, albuterol inhalation can be tried. Adverse effects include increased sympathomimetic activity and arrhythmias. If effective, the oral route can be used when respiration improves because gastrointestinal (GI) absorption is rapid.

Inotropic Support

Pimobendan is indicated for dogs with CHF caused by DMVD, infective endocarditis, DCM, pulmonary hypertension, and congenital heart disease. The drug has no direct effect on heart rate in AF. Pimobendan is likely to be effective in horses, but experience is lacking and drug cost too high for this species. The extra-label use of pimobendan in cats is best guided by point-of-care echocardiography. Most cardiologists agree that systolic dysfunction – whether global or segmental – constitutes an indication for its use in CHF. Treatment with pimobendan in cats with hypertrophic cardiomyopathy (HCM), especially in the setting of dynamic LV outflow obstruction, is more controversial and lacks high-grade evidence; there are proponents both for and against its use. Practical experience suggests that cats with CHF and in the following situations are reasonable candidates for treatment; these include: cats without a heart murmur, cats affected by moderate to large pleural effusions, and cats in cardiogenic shock (low temperature, BP and heart rate). Most cats falling into those clinical scenarios have end-stage HCM, DCM, restrictive cardiomyopathy, right ventricular (RV) cardiomyopathy, or transient myocardial thickening/myocarditis attended by some element of LV or RV systolic failure. Pimobendan also can augment LA transport function and cardiac output in these cats by improving atrial and RV contractility. Conversely, many cats with HCM suffering from acute pulmonary edema respond favorably to simple sedation, oxygen, furosemide, cage rest, and time. Regardless of species or cause, when pimobendan (PO or IV, where available) is indicated, the drug is started as soon as possible and continued orally as part of long-term heart failure management.

Additional positive inotropic therapy, mainly catecholamines, should be considered for dogs or cats with persistent hypotension or cardiogenic shock (p. 313) that is not caused by cardiac tamponade or constrictive pericarditis. Catecholamines can support arterial BP, increase cardiac output, and improve organ perfusion when myocardial failure or hypotension is severe (**Tables 22.2 and 22.3**, and p. 330). Most often, treatment for 24–48 hours with IV dobutamine (or dopamine, if dobutamine is unavailable) is initiated alongside pimobendan. This can stabilize the patient and assist the transition to oral therapy. Some dogs with DCM and cats with cardiogenic shock (from various types of cardiomyopathy) respond favorably to catecholamines. A low initial dose is used, then up-titrated to effect, with adjustments made every 15–30 minutes until CV status is more stable. Signs of excessive dosage include tachycardia and premature ectopic activity. When weaning off dobutamine (or dopamine), the dose is decreased by half every 2–4 hours and BP monitored to ensure that hypotension does not recur. Theoretically, another phosphodiesterase (PDE)-3 inhibitor drug (milrinone) also could be used for this purpose. This seems redundant with pimobendan, but might be considered in cases when there is overdosing of a beta-blocker.

Digoxin, along with pimobendan, is indicated for dogs with CHF and AF. Oral digoxin dosing is used most often. IV administration of digoxin is not recommended except in horses with CHF, or in dogs with a supraventricular tachyarrhythmia when other acute therapy is unavailable or ineffective (p. 408). Acidosis and hypoxemia associated with severe pulmonary edema, and hypokalemia secondary to IV furosemide administration, can increase myocardial sensitivity to digoxin-induced arrhythmias. If IV digoxin administration is deemed necessary, it must be given slowly (over at least 15 minutes), because rapid injection causes peripheral vasoconstriction. The calculated dose usually is divided, and boluses of one-fourth the calculated dose are given slowly over several hours. Contraindications to digoxin include complex ventricular tachyarrhythmias, bradyarrhythmias, and moderate or severe renal dysfunction (p. 327).

If new arrhythmias develop during IV inotropic therapy, the infusion rate should be reduced or the drug discontinued. In animals with AF, catecholamine infusion could increase the ventricular response rate by enhancing atrioventricular (AV) conduction, although the opposite also might be observed, perhaps related to improvement in BP. If dobutamine or dopamine is deemed necessary for such a case, diltiazem (**Table 25.2**, p. 403) is initiated to help reduce the heart rate. Digoxin, either PO (maintenance or loading dose) or given cautiously IV, are alternatives.

Heart Failure from Diastolic Dysfunction

When acute CHF is caused by HCM or similar pathophysiology, thoracocentesis (if needed), furosemide, and oxygen therapy are given as outlined previously. Topical nitroglycerin also can be used. Arteriolar vasodilators can be detrimental in animals with dynamic LV outflow obstruction, and are avoided. Pimobendan and other positive inotropic agents theoretically could worsen dynamic outflow obstruction, although adverse clinical effects appear to be uncommon with pimobendan (see discussion above for more details). ACE inhibitors at standard doses do not appear to worsen the LV outflow gradient, although this therapy usually is delayed until the patient is stabilized and eating again.

Although diltiazem and atenolol have theoretical advantages for improving diastolic heart failure by augmenting ventricular relaxation and ventricular filling time, respectively, as well as reducing demand ischemia to the left ventricle, neither drug is recommended in acute, uncontrolled CHF. This is true even in the setting of sinus tachycardia, which is managed by controlling underlying heart failure. In general, beta-blockers are not given to "wet" patients, and nonspecific beta-blockers could induce bronchoconstriction. Diltiazem is reserved for non-sinus supraventricular tachycardia or AF. Drugs that directly slow sinus rate, such as ivabradine (pp. 333 and 385) have not been sufficiently studied in cats or dogs with CHF.

In animals with an uncontrolled ventricular response rate to AF, therapy to reduce heart rate can help in managing acute CHF by increasing ventricular filling time and output. Judicious doses of IV or PO diltiazem, given in combination with (oral) digoxin, are used in dogs. Standard diltiazem is recommended for initial in-hospital (oral) dosing; a long-acting formulation can be substituted once the rate is under some control and the patient is eating. See pp. 411 and 413 for more details about management of AF.

Monitoring and Initial Follow-up

Repeated assessment is important to monitor the effectiveness of therapy and to recognize adverse effects, including hypotension, azotemia, or arrhythmias caused by the various drug treatments. Monitoring in dogs and cats can be crudely divided into the observations possible with the patient in an oxygen cage; those non- or minimally invasive procedures that require physical handling of the patient (outside of oxygen, unless there is a nasal cannula); and those procedures that are invasive or require transporting to another location. These procedures are outlined at the bottom of **Table 22.2**.

In addition to observations focused on attitude, responsiveness, and respiration, urinary output should be observed carefully, remembering that this is evidence of initial diuretic effectiveness. This determination might require palpation of the bladder or application of a cage-side ultrasound probe, as some patients simply refuse to void. Body weight also should be monitored closely; initial weight loss usually relates to diuretic therapy (with each ½ kg of weight loss approximating 500 mL of urinary output plus insensible water loss). This same relationship will hold when centesis removes large volumes of pleural or peritoneal fluid.

Cardiovascular and tissue perfusion variables are serially recorded. Heart rate and rhythm should be monitored, as should arterial BP, generally by indirect means because gaining arterial access is often difficult or impractical and can increase patient stress. A systolic BP of 100 to 110 mm Hg is a reasonable target, and systolic BP as low as 90 mm Hg might be optimal for some patients with acute CHF. Indirect measures of organ perfusion, such as capillary refill time, mucous membrane color, pulse oximetry, urine output, rectal and toe-web temperatures, and mentation can be useful. Blood lactate is an objective measure and decreases as tissue perfusion is improved. Pulse oximetry is helpful for monitoring oxygen saturation (SpO_2; Chapter 10). Supplemental O_2 should be given if SpO_2 is <90% or the patient is showing evidence of respiratory distress. Mechanical ventilation is indicated when there is evidence of respiratory fatigue in the setting of carbon dioxide retention (hypercarbia) and marked hypoxemia. Although stressful to obtain, arterial blood gas analysis more accurately assesses ventilation and oxygenation. Generally, severe hypoxemia corresponds to a SpO_2 <80% despite O_2 therapy, accepting that pulse oximetry readings can be inaccurate.

Point-of-care ultrasound imaging is employed at the time of admission to rapidly screen the heart for size, function and lesions, and to provide initial cardiac assessment, along with signalment and physical diagnosis. Peritoneal, pleural and pericardial effusions also are sensitive to ultrasound identification and can be semi-quantitated. Lung ultrasound can locate intrapulmonary B-lines (lung rockets). These often are diffuse and coalescing in severe pulmonary edema, and become more isolated with effective treatment. Nevertheless, B-lines are not specific for pulmonary edema and must be interpreted with other clinical findings. Radiography remains the standard for diagnosis of left-sided CHF in stabilized patients. In unstable patients, treatment for presumptive CHF should begin (with at least sedation, furosemide and oxygen) before radiographs are obtained. Resolution of radiographic evidence for pulmonary edema usually lags behind clinical improvement by a day or two, but it is common to see some radiographic improvement within 12 to 24 hours.

Serum biochemical testing every 12–24 hours is advised until the patient is eating and drinking well. Mild to moderate azotemia is common in the acute setting, and generally is ignored; although free access to water should be given when this occurs and the diuretic doses reduced, if feasible and in light of the effectiveness of diuresis. Hypokalemia, hypochloremia and metabolic alkalosis are common with aggressive diuresis, but usually improve once the patient is home. Maintaining the serum potassium concentration within the mid- to high-normal range is especially important for animals with atrial and ventricular arrhythmias (p. 349).

After diuresis has begun and respiratory signs start to abate, free-choice water is offered. Fluid administration, either SC or IV, generally is not advisable in patients with fulminant CHF. In most cases, gradual rehydration by free-choice water intake is preferred, even after aggressive diuretic therapy. However, cautious fluid therapy might be necessary for CHF patients with intrinsic kidney disease, acute kidney injury, marked hypokalemia, systemic hypotension, digoxin toxicity, persistent anorexia, or other serious systemic disease. Some animals require high cardiac filling pressures in order to maintain cardiac output, particularly those with myocardial failure or markedly reduced ventricular compliance (as from HCM or pericardial disease). Preload reduction produced by diuresis and vasodilation leads to inadequate cardiac output and hypotension in some CHF cases. CHF associated with myocardial infarction or pancreatitis is observed in some cats, which requires judicious IV fluid therapy; these patients also can develop cardiogenic shock without overt CHF. When fluid therapy is necessary, D_5W or a reduced sodium fluid (for example, 0.45% NaCl ±2.5% dextrose) with added KCl is administered at a conservative rate (such as 15–30 mL/kg/day IV). Alternatively, 0.45% NaCl or lactated Ringer's solution can be administered subcutaneously. When delivering a drug by CRI to an animal with decompensated CHF, the smallest fluid volume possible is used.

Central venous pressure (CVP) does not adequately reflect left heart filling pressures; therefore, it should not be used to guide fluid or diuretic therapy in cardiogenic pulmonary edema. Likewise, when right heart function is poor, CVP becomes a misleading indicator of circulating blood volume status. Although pulmonary capillary wedge pressure can reliably guide therapy in patients with pulmonary edema, indwelling pulmonary artery catheter placement and care require special equipment and training, meticulous attention to details, and close monitoring. It is a rare procedure even in academic centers. Doppler echocardiography can provide some noninvasive information about cardiac filling pressures, as can vena caval diameter and collapsibility, but these techniques require some training to use effectively.

Potassium supplementation at a maintenance rate is provided when needed by infusion of 0.05–0.1 mEq/kg/hour (or, more conservatively, 0.5–2.0 mEq/kg/day). For animals with hypokalemia, higher rates are used: 0.15–0.2 mEq/kg/hour for mild K^+ deficiency, 0.25–0.3 mEq/kg/hour for moderate deficiency, and 0.4–0.5 mEq/kg/hour for severe deficiency (or see **Table 25.4**, p. 414). Serum K^+ measurement after 4–6 hours is advised when supplementing for moderate to severe deficiency. Hyponatremia and worsened fluid retention can develop with low-sodium IV solutions in some patients, potentiated by free water retention and diuresis; a more balanced crystalloid solution might be needed.

Other supportive therapies for CHF and any underlying disease(s) depend on the individual patient situation. Careful monitoring and continued, but usually less intense, diuretic therapy are important to avoid recurrent pulmonary edema. Parenteral fluid administration, if necessary, is tapered then discontinued as the animal begins to resume oral food and water intake.

Chronic Heart Failure Management in Dogs

A summary of long-term canine heart failure management strategies is presented here. Readers also should consult chapters on specific diseases for additional information. Drug dosages are summarized in **Table 22.3**. While the treatment goals for acute CHF focus on oxygenation, rapid diuresis, drainage of large effusions, and improvement of cardiac function, chronic heart failure management additionally is focused on reducing maladaptive NH activity, myocardial remodeling, and progressive cardiac dysfunction. There is considerable debate about optimal therapy for chronic CHF caused by DMVD and DCM in dogs, but the authors believe there is sufficient overall evidence to recommend "quad therapy" consisting of: (1) *the inodilator pimobendan*, (2) *the loop diuretic furosemide (or torsemide)*, (3) *one of the studied ACE inhibitors (usually enalapril or benazepril)*, and (4) *spironolactone*.

Treatment selection in the "real world" must consider drug costs. In the United States, only pimobendan is without a readily available, approved generic equivalent and the yearly cost for that drug is considerable, especially in larger dogs. A proven generic formulation would be beneficial to many dog owners. Otherwise, generic ACE inhibitors, furosemide, and spironolactone are available and cost-effective. Where generic equivalents are largely available, there is little downside to "quad therapy," and that approach has been suggested in the ACVIM consensus report on DVMD (Keene, 2019). However cost considerations can scale treatment to "triple therapy" (dropping the spironolactone), or even dual therapy with furosemide and pimobendan, because those two drugs carry the strongest clinical trial evidence in dogs. But in those cases, RAAS inhibition is ignored (and likely activated), which is of particular concern in canine DCM and also relevant to advanced DMVD. Most veterinary clinical trials have been driven, at least in part, by pharmaceutical interests. These studies have not sufficiently addressed the value of "quad therapy" that includes aggressive RAAS inhibition (moderate to high-dose ACE inhibitor plus spironolactone) combined with the well-tested combination of furosemide and pimobendan. Adjunctive therapy in canine CHF should consider dietary management (with sufficient protein and sodium restriction), dietary ingredients in dogs with DCM, and possibly supplements. Dogs with severe, symptomatic pulmonary hypertension often benefit from the addition of sildenafil or tadalafil. Additional afterload reduction with amlodipine or hydralazine is useful in selected dogs with severe MR, or when CHF is complicated by systemic hypertension. Antiarrhythmic drugs including digoxin and diltiazem are added for AF, and other antiarrhythmic drugs considered on a case-by-case basis for other arrhythmias (Chapter 25).

Pimobendan improves clinical status and survival in dogs with DMVD and DCM receiving background therapy of furosemide and often spironolactone. Therapy with ACE inhibitors, certain beta-blockers, and the ALD antagonist spironolactone improve clinical status and survival in people with chronic heart failure and there are supporting data for RAAS inhibition in dogs at least, but not other species at this time (Chapter 21). Unfortunately, the commonly prescribed "quad therapy" combination of pimobendan, furosemide, ACE inhibitor and spironolactone has not been sufficiently evaluated. Most studies comparing pimobendan to ACE inhibition in dogs with DVMD have shown better outcomes with pimobendan, but have not addressed the incremental value of combining pimobendan with ACE inhibition (QUEST). However, one trial of dogs with CHF caused by DMVD showed no survival advantage of adding ramipril to furosemide and pimobendan, compared to treatment with the latter two agents alone (Wess, 2020). Whether these results are definitive is uncertain, considering study limitations (high diuretic doses) and unmeasured degree of RAAS inhibition used.

Drugs that simply reduce afterload (pure arteriolar vasodilators) have not been sufficiently studied and there is no evidence they will improve long-term survival. However, in patients with systemic hypertension or advanced CHF from DMVD, amlodipine or hydralazine should be considered. Therapy with an angiotensin receptor blocker (ARB) and neprilysin inhibitor combination (ARNI, p. 333) improves outcomes in people with heart failure; this requires further study in companion animals, as only preliminary reports are available at this time.

Long-term heart failure therapy must be tailored to the individual patient's needs by adjusting dosages or drugs used and by modifying lifestyle and diet. As the underlying heart disease progresses over time, therapy typically must be intensified. Cardiac arrhythmias that require specific antiarrhythmic therapy commonly develop (Chapter 25). Pleural effusion and large-volume ascites that accumulate despite medical therapy should be drained to facilitate respiration; medical therapy is intensified as possible to slow reaccumulation. If pericardial effusion compromises cardiac filling, it must be drained (p. 724).

Drug Therapy

Diuretic therapy remains fundamental to the management of chronic CHF because of its ability to prevent renal sodium retention and reduce recurrence of cardiogenic pulmonary edema and effusions (**Table 22.3** and Chapter 21). Furosemide continues to be the first-line diuretic in most situations because of its potent ability to promote both salt and water loss. Alternatively, torsemide can have potential advantages over furosemide in advanced or refractory cases, or even as a first-line agent in some (see section "Approach to Refractory CHF" and p. 319). The potassium-sparing agent spironolactone could enhance diuresis in animals with CHF and RAAS activation, but is mainly used for cardiac muscle protection. In healthy dogs, it exhibits little to no diuretic effect. Infrequently, a thiazide is combined with furosemide and spironolactone for more intense diuresis in patients with refractory heart failure (p. 354). However, diuretics (especially at high doses or in combination) can promote excessive volume contraction, azotemia, electrolyte depletion, and further activate the RAAS. Because diuretics can exacerbate preexisting dehydration, azotemia and electrolyte disturbances, the indication for their use in animals with such problems should be clearly established and the lowest effective doses used. Respiratory rate and pattern, hydration, body weight and condition, exercise tolerance, renal function, and serum electrolyte concentrations are used to monitor response to therapy. Monitoring the resting (sleeping) respiratory rate is particularly helpful in guiding this therapy (**Table 22.1**). Furosemide (or other diuretic) even with pimobendan will exacerbate NH activation and reduce renal function.

Although still controversial in DMVD, an ACE inhibitor is recommended for most causes of chronic CHF in dogs (**Table 22.3** and Chapter 21). Although ACE inhibitors have only modest diuretic and vasodilatory effects, their role in opposing the effects of NH activation in heart failure is thought to be important, certainly in dogs with DCM. A lower starting dose can be increased at the time of first recheck provided appetite, BP and renal function are adequate. An ARB, or ARNI combination, might be substituted for an ACE inhibitor, although clinical experience with this in dogs currently is too limited to unequivocally recommend this therapy.

The inodilator pimobendan improves clinical status and survival in dogs with CHF from DCM or DMVD when added to standard therapy (**Table 22.3** and Chapter 21). Pimobendan most often is used with an ACE inhibitor. However, if only one of these agents can be used in a particular dog for financial reasons, pimobendan is likely to have greater positive impact. Survival time and pulmonary edema recurrence rate were studied in dogs with CHF caused by DMVD using two dosage levels of pimobendan along with conventional diuretic and ACE inhibitor therapy, and compared to conventional therapy alone (Mizuno, 2017). Although the retrospective nature of the study precludes definitive conclusions, the median survival time was longest (~11 months) in dogs receiving standard to mildly increased doses of pimobendan (0.2–0.48 mg/kg q12h); dogs receiving low-dose pimobendan (0.05–0.19 mg/kg q12h) had lesser increase in median survival time (~9 months). However, survival time for dogs not receiving pimobendan was about 4½ months. A dose-dependent reduction in pulmonary edema recurrence rate also was observed.

Spironolactone is thought to be more useful for its anti-ALD effects in cardiac and other tissues than for its diuretic effect, although the latter probably is a helpful adjunct in patients with advanced heart failure. Because the phenomenon of ALD breakthrough appears to occur in almost a third of dogs with DMVD despite ACE inhibitor therapy, and probably occurs with other causes of heart failure as well, it is reasonable to add spironolactone to the chronic heart failure management regime when possible. Dogs with ACE gene polymorphism might be more likely to develop ALD breakthrough. Spironolactone could improve survival at doses of 2 mg/kg/day (Bernay, 2010), although not all animals tolerate this dose. Furthermore it is unlikely many dogs in that quoted study had severe CHF, based on the <8% cardiac mortality reported after nearly 15 months of therapy with spironolactone and considering some dogs diagnosed with heart failure were not even receiving any furosemide.

So-called "quad therapy" (furosemide, pimobendan, and ACE inhibitor, with spironolactone), is considered standard treatment by many cardiologists. As previously mentioned, this is not universally the case for management of DMVD, and issues of drug costs in some countries impede this multidrug approach. Other drugs can be useful for chronic heart failure management in certain cases, too. For example, in dogs with advanced DMVD when CHF is becoming difficult to control, the addition of amlodipine (or hydralazine) can improve forward cardiac output and reduce regurgitant fraction. This is especially relevant in dogs with elevated systemic BP. However, care must be taken to avoid hypotension. For dogs with CHF and AF, digoxin and diltiazem (or a beta-blocker) are added to baseline therapy (p. 411). CHF that is difficult to control with standard or initial drug therapies might respond to dosage intensification or other strategies described in section "Approach to Refractory CHF" (p. 354).

Some clinicians have prescribed a beta-blocker for patients with stable heart failure, in an effort to protect the myocardium from the adverse effects of continued catecholamine exposure. Although cardioprotective effects have been demonstrated in people with chronic heart failure and in experimental dog studies, clinical studies in dogs have shown no demonstrable survival benefit to date. Therefore, beta-blockers currently are not considered standard of care for chronic CHF in dogs. Nevertheless, an individual patient might have particular indication for use. If beta-blocker therapy is pursued, very low initial doses are used along with conventional CHF therapy as indicated; dosage up-titration must be done slowly (p. 331).

Dietary Considerations

A good quality diet with adequate calories and protein, and only moderate salt restriction is recommended for most patients with chronic heart failure. Good nutritional support can help prevent or delay cardiac cachexia (p. 312), which has been associated with worsened prognosis. Recording the patient's body weight, as well as body condition and muscle condition scores, at each visit will allow the clinician to monitor for deterioration and the need for more intensive attention to food intake and nutrition. An underlying cause for any decline or loss of appetite should be sought and addressed, as possible (see "Inappetence" section, below). Although energy requirements vary among animals, an intake of about 60 kcal/kg body weight should minimize chronic heart failure-associated weight loss in dogs. Protein restriction is not recommended unless indicated because of concurrent severe renal disease. For patients with hypokalemia (or even low-normal serum potassium), supplementing the diet with additional potassium-rich foods sometimes will raise serum potassium concentration acceptably; in other cases, a commercial potassium supplement is needed.

Mild to moderate dietary salt restriction usually is recommended to help control fluid accumulation and reduce necessary drug therapy. The NH changes in heart failure interfere with the kidney's ability to excrete sodium and water loads. However, markedly restricted salt intake can increase RAAS activation. It is unclear whether a moderately reduced-salt diet is necessary before overt CHF develops; nevertheless, avoiding high-salt table scraps or treats would seem prudent. High-salt foods include processed meats, canned fish, cheese, regular canned vegetables, breads, potato chips, pretzels, and other processed snack foods, as well as dog treats such as rawhide and biscuits.

Moderate salt restriction represents a sodium intake of about 30 mg/kg/day (about 0.06% sodium for canned food or 210–240 mg/100 g of dry food, or 50–80 mg sodium/100 kcal of dietary energy). Although diets for senior animals or those with renal disease usually provide this level of salt, their protein restriction is a drawback for many cases. Supplementing with additional protein (such as hard-boiled eggs or cooked chicken) is one strategy. A number of commercial prescription and other diets provide moderate salt reduction, along with adequate protein and omega-3 fatty acid supplementation. Some prescription cardiac diets have much greater sodium restriction (~13 mg sodium/kg/day, or about 90–100 mg sodium/100 g of dry food, or 0.025% sodium in a canned food). This might be helpful if the patient's CHF becomes increasingly refractory. Severe sodium restriction (such as 7 mg/kg/day) exacerbates NH activation and can contribute to hyponatremia, at least in dogs with DMVD not taking diuretics. Recipes for homemade low-salt diets are available; however, providing balanced vitamin and mineral content can be challenging. Consultation with a veterinary nutritionist can be helpful.

Dietary changes are best instituted gradually and after congestive signs have abated. For example, mix the new with the old diet in a 1:3 ratio for several days, then increase to 1:1 for several days, then 3:1, and finally the new diet alone). Supplementation of specific nutrients is important in some cases (see following paragraphs). In some regions, drinking water might contain relatively high sodium concentrations. Nonsoftened water or (where the public water supply contains more than 150 ppm of sodium) distilled water can be recommended to further decrease salt intake in patients with refractory CHF.

Grossly obese pets with heart disease might benefit from a weight-reduction diet, especially prior to CHF onset. Obesity increases metabolic demands on the heart and expands blood volume. Mechanical interference with respiration promotes hypoventilation, which could contribute to *cor pulmonale* and complicate preexisting heart disease. Conversely, animals in heart failure that are mildly overweight could have a survival advantage (similar to the obesity paradox described in people). Some evidence suggests dogs with heart failure that gain or maintain their weight live longer than those that lose weight.

Omega-3 Fatty Acids Dietary supplementation with fish oils, which are rich in omega-3 fatty acids (eicosapentaenoic acid, EPA, and docosahexaenoic acid, DHA) can reduce cytokine production, might improve endothelial function, and could have antiarrhythmic effects, among other benefits. Reduced cachexia and circulating interleukin-1 concentrations in dogs with DCM have been associated with EPA (27 mg/kg/day) and DHA (18 mg/kg/day) supplementation. Whether higher EPA and DHA doses would provide added benefit is not known; 30–40 mg/kg/day EPA and 20–25 mg/kg/day DHA have been suggested. Over-the-counter 1 gm fish oil capsules containing 180 mg EPA and 120 mg DHA could be used at about 1 capsule per 10 lbs body weight per day. Various veterinary formulations are available as well. The major limitation to this supplementation is the large number of medications already prescribed and the fact that some dogs simply refuse to ingest the capsules or oil. Concerns related to the potential for vitamin D toxicity with high-dose fish oil supplements remain unanswered. Cod liver oil and flax seed oil are not recommended as omega-3 fatty acid sources.

Other Dietary Supplements Taurine is important for normal myocardial function. Taurine is considered an essential nutrient for cats, although not for dogs, which can manufacture this amino acid. Nevertheless, inadequate protein intake or abnormal metabolic pathways might result in low taurine levels and potentially, myocardial dysfunction. The vast majority of dogs with CHF are not taurine-deficient; supplementation in these cases is unlikely to provide benefit. However, some dogs with DCM appear deficient in taurine and L-carnitine, most notably American Cocker Spaniels but also other breeds, including Golden Retrievers (p. 632). Although not all taurine-deficient Cocker Spaniels need both taurine and L-carnitine supplements, some appear to. Dogs fed protein-restricted, legume rich ("grain-free"), or vegetarian diets, as well as some exclusively lamb-rice, "novel protein," "off-brand," or "boutique" diets can become taurine deficient; furthermore, some develop DCM despite normal whole blood taurine concentrations. It is important to note that the large majority of dogs suspected to have diet-related DCM (p. 633) do not appear to be deficient in taurine, and not all "grain-free" diets lead to DCM. The optimal dose for taurine supplementation in deficient animals is unclear; 500–1000 mg every 8 hours for dogs under 25 kg and 1–2 g every 8–12 hours for dogs 25–40 kg have been suggested. Others recommend taurine supplementation at 500–1000 mg/day.

L-carnitine plays an essential role in transporting fatty acids into mitochondria for use in energy generation. Although L-carnitine deficiency was identified in a family of Boxers and a small number of Doberman Pinschers with DCM, its prevalence is thought to be low, and the number of affected dogs responsive to L-carnitine supplementation even lower. Some suggest a trial period of supplementation (at a higher dosage) might be worthwhile; however, this cannot be advanced as a blanket recommendation. Echocardiography should be repeated after at least 4 months of L-carnitine supplementation, to assess whether LV function has improved. If not, the supplement usually is discontinued, especially in view of its expense. The minimum effective dose of L-carnitine is not known; it may vary with the mechanism of deficiency, if deficiency is present. Several dose ranges have been suggested, including 50–100 mg/kg every 8–12 hours for systemic deficiency or 200 mg/kg every 8 hours for myopathic deficiency. Others use 1 g of oral L-carnitine every 8 hours for dogs under 25 kg and 2 g every 12 hours for dogs between 25 and 40 kg. About ½ teaspoonful of pure L-carnitine powder is the equivalent of 1 g. Both taurine and L-carnitine supplements can be mixed with food for easier administration. Dogs treated with L-carnitine might give off a peculiar odor.

Dogs being treated with a PDE-5 inhibitor, such as sildenafil, for severe pulmonary hypertension might benefit from extra L-arginine; however, this remains to be proven (p. 834). This amino acid is an important precursor in the endothelial production of nitric oxide, which is stimulated by PDE-5 inhibition. The optimal dose of L-arginine is unknown; suggested doses range from 100 mg/kg/day to between 250 and 500 mg q8h PO.

The role of other dietary supplements is unclear. Oxidative stress and free-radical damage probably play a role in the pathogenesis of myocardial dysfunction. Increased circulating cytokines in heart failure can promote oxidative stress; however, the role of supplemental antioxidant vitamins in animals with CHF is unclear. Coenzyme Q-10 is an antioxidant and cofactor involved in cellular energy production. Yet, convincing evidence that it provides any measurable benefit is completely lacking. Doses of 30(–90) mg PO q12h have been used in dogs with uncertain effect. Currently, the authors do not prescribe this supplement.

Inappetence Poor appetite is a common problem in patients with advanced heart failure, as is the development of cardiac cachexia. Caloric intake often is suboptimal even though energy needs are increased. Fatigue, increased respiratory effort, azotemia, adverse medication effects, and low diet palatability all can contribute to poor appetite. At the same time, poor splanchnic perfusion, bowel and pancreatic edema, and secondary intestinal lymphangiectasia in advanced CHF could reduce nutrient absorption and promote protein loss. Hypoalbuminemia and reduced immune function can develop. These factors, as well as concurrent renal or hepatic dysfunction, also can alter the pharmacokinetics of certain drugs.

Strategies that could help improve appetite include warming the food to enhance its flavor or adding small amounts of more palatable human foods (including nonsalted meats or gravy and low-sodium soup) or canned reduced-sodium dog or cat food. Sprinkling garlic powder or salt substitute (KCl) on the food might help, too. Handfeeding and providing small quantities of food several times a day sometimes will encourage an animal to eat more. An appetite stimulant drug also might help. Capromorelin (Entyce; Aratana Therapeutics) is a selective ghrelin receptor agonist that stimulates hunger shortly after its administration (3 mg/kg PO once daily), although long-term treatment has not been evaluated yet. This drug can cause severe polyuria/polydipsia and also can be unpalatable; placing the dose into an empty gelatin capsule can help. Mirtazapine is another drug that might provide some appetite stimulation.

Exercise

Strenuous exercise can provoke dyspnea and potentially serious cardiac arrhythmias in animals with CHF. Furthermore, during episodes of decompensation (especially with pulmonary edema), even mild exercise is to be avoided. In patients with chronic heart failure, skeletal muscle alterations occur that contribute to fatigue and dyspnea. Physical training can improve cardiopulmonary function and quality of life in patients with chronic, compensated heart failure. This is mediated partly by improved vascular endothelial function and enhanced flow-dependent vasodilation. However, it is difficult to know how much exercise is beneficial in an individual. Although some dogs might seem to self-regulate their activity to an appropriate degree, others clearly do not. Therefore, the authors recommend these guidelines for most patients, after pulmonary edema has fully resolved: Regular (not sporadic) mild to moderate activity is encouraged, as tolerated. This means that excessive respiratory effort or tiring does not develop during the activity. Strenuous bursts of activity should be avoided.

Long-Term Management of Diastolic Dysfunction

HCM and hypertensive cardiomyopathy are uncommon causes of CHF in dogs. The approach to therapy is similar to that used for cats with HCM (Chapter 33). Following management for acute CHF, if this is needed, furosemide is used at the lowest effective dose PO. An ACE inhibitor and spironolactone also are prescribed. The value of pimobendan is unknown and there are theoretical arguments for and against its use. A beta-blocker might be helpful in moderating heart rate and reducing dynamic LV outflow obstruction, if present, but only if CHF is well managed. In dogs with systemic hypertension or iatrogenic hyperthyroidism, treating the underlying disorder is critical to reduce LV thickening. Ventricular tachyarrhythmias usually are managed with sotalol, although other agents could be effective (p. 424). Exercise restriction and a diet moderately reduced in sodium are recommended as well.

Monitoring and Follow-up Evaluation

Client education and participation are crucial to successful long-term heart failure management. Early identification of complications is more likely when the owner has a good understanding of the underlying disease process, manifestations of CHF, and the purpose and potential adverse effects of each medication. Home monitoring of the pet's resting (ideally, sleeping) respiratory rate (RRR) is strongly recommended, especially when pulmonary edema is likely (**Table 22.1**). Most dogs and cats with normal lungs breathe at ≤30 breaths/minute when resting in the home environment; baseline RRR in some is under 20 breaths/minute. It is important for the owner to know the pet's normal, baseline RRR, and to monitor for changes periodically. Monitoring every few days, at minimum, is important for animals recovering from an episode of acute CHF; monitoring can be done less frequently in stable patients. A persistent increase in RRR (of >20% above that animal's normal baseline, and especially to >40 breaths/minute) usually is an early sign of decompensating left-heart failure. As pulmonary edema accumulates, increasing lung stiffness induces faster and shallower respirations. It is important to note that pulmonary infiltrative diseases and fibrosis will increase RRR, too. A persistent increase in resting heart rate also occurs with the heightened sympathetic tone of CHF; some owners are able to monitor for this, as well.

Periodic reevaluation is important (**Table 22.4**). The initial recheck visit after an episode of decompensated CHF usually is scheduled for within a week of hospital discharge (or diagnosis, if in-hospital therapy was not needed),

Table 22.4 Reevaluation of the Chronic Heart Failure Patient

Review Recent History
- Attitude and activity level
- Appetite and water intake
  - Verify patient's diet
- Respiratory (± heart) rate when resting/sleeping at home
- Any coughing? (Chapter 9):
  - How often and when does it occur?
  - Dry/honking or moist sound?
- Any episodes of respiratory distress? (Chapter 10)

Verify All Medications (prescription and nonprescription)
- Drug name(s)
  - Tablet size/liquid concentration
  - Dosage and frequency
- Any concerns about possible adverse drug effects?
- Any problems with medication administration?
- Have all doses been given as prescribed?
- Are any refills needed?

Physical Examination
- Thorough general examination
- Careful cardiovascular examination (Chapters 2, 11, and 13–17)
- Note heart rate and rhythm (Chapter 12)
- Note respiratory rate and effort
- Note changes since last examination:
  - Heart sounds/murmurs
  - Heart rhythm
  - Pulmonary sounds
  - Body weight/condition
  - Any abnormal fluid accumulation?

Laboratory and Other Testing
- Blood pressure
- Check renal function as well as serum Na^+ and K^+, at minimum
  - Periodically obtain a complete biochemistry panel, CBC, and urinalysis also, especially if other concerns
- ± Thoracic radiographs—obtain if suspect pulmonary edema (increased home RRR, pulmonary crackles, new or worsened cough) or other concerns based on history/physical examination (Chapters 2 and 3)
- ± ECG—obtain if an arrhythmia is suspected, an unexpectedly low or high heart rate is detected, or to document heart rate with atrial fibrillation (Chapter 5)
  - Ambulatory ECG monitoring, if indicated (to identify occult arrhythmias or assess antiarrhythmic therapy efficacy)
- ± Serum digoxin concentration (if this drug is being used)—indicated especially if therapy recently begun, dosage changed, or any signs suspicious for toxicity (p. 328)
- ±Echocardiography—if unexpected physical findings, or periodically to assess myocardial function and evidence for disease progression (Chapter 4)
- Heartworm testing and prophylaxis as indicated in endemic areas
- Other tests as indicated

Abbreviations: CBC, complete blood count; ECG, electrocardiogram; RRR, resting respiratory rate.

with the next follow-up in 3–4 weeks, or sooner if needed. Reevaluation every 3–4 months thereafter generally is recommended, unless problems develop. Some clinically stable animals might do well with rechecks every 4–6 months. However, complications (including arrhythmias and metabolic derangements) often accompany disease progression. Medication and dosage schedules should be reviewed with the owner at each visit. Problems with drug administration, including compliance in dosing as prescribed or adverse effects, should be ascertained. The animal's recent resting RRRs at home, current diet, appetite, and activity level, and any owner concerns should be discussed, as well. The overall focus for continued therapy is on quality of life for the patient, as well as the owner. The patient's comfort (including ability to sleep well and breathe easily), appetite, mobility, attitude, and family interactions are important considerations for owners.

A thorough physical examination, with emphasis on the CV system (Chapter 2), is important at each evaluation; this includes recording the patient's body weight and condition (including muscle condition). Depending on the patient's status, other tests might include a resting ECG or ambulatory monitoring (Chapter 5), thoracic radiographs (Chapter 3), complete blood count and serum biochemical tests, an echocardiogram (Chapter 4), serum digoxin concentration, or others. All these tests are not necessarily indicated in all cases nor at all visits. However, serum electrolyte (especially Na^+ and K^+) and creatinine (or urea nitrogen) concentrations should be monitored frequently. Mild azotemia commonly develops, with BUN usually increasing relatively more than serum creatinine. This might relate to intrarenal handling of urea nitrogen or to cardiac cachexia, with less breakdown of skeletal muscle creatinine. If the patient is stable, slight reduction in furosemide dosage (~25%) can be tried. Other medication adjustments (see next section) also might allow improved renal perfusion while still maintaining CHF control. Mild azotemia often is tolerable, as long as the patient is showing no adverse effects and appetite is maintained. Attentive at-home monitoring of the RRR, as well as other observations, helps guide determination of the lowest effective diuretic dosage. Moderate to severe azotemia requires reduction in diuretic dosage; it is a poor prognostic sign.

Electrolyte imbalances (especially hypo- or hyperkalemia, hypomagnesemia, and sometimes hyponatremia) can occur with the use of diuretics, ACE inhibitors, and salt restriction. Prolonged anorexia contributes to hypokalemia. However, potassium supplements should not be used without documented hypokalemia, especially when an ACE inhibitor and spironolactone are prescribed. Serum magnesium concentration does not accurately reflect total body stores, and supplementation might help animals that develop ventricular tachyarrhythmias while receiving furosemide and digoxin. Hyponatremia associated with severe CHF results from an inability to excrete free water (dilutional hyponatremia) rather than from a total body sodium deficit. It can be difficult to correct and is considered a poor prognostic sign. In some cases, it helps to reduce the furosemide or other diuretic dose, cautiously add or increase dose of an arteriolar vasodilator (to improve renal perfusion), or enhance inotropic support by increasing pimobendan dose or adding another inotrope. However, vigilant monitoring is needed to avoid worsened congestion, hypotension, and other potential adverse effects. The vasopressin receptor antagonist tolvaptan might be helpful in treating progressive hyponatremia; however, clinical experience in dogs is scant.

Many factors can exacerbate the signs of CHF, including physical exertion, infection, anemia, fluid administration, high-salt diet or dietary indiscretion, erratic medication administration, inappropriate medication dosage for the level of disease, cardiac arrhythmias, environmental stress, development or worsening of concurrent extracardiac disease (including systemic hypertension, hyperadrenocorticism, hypo- or hyperthyroidism, renal failure, neoplasia, pneumonia, pulmonary hypertension, anemia), and progression of the underlying heart disease. Repeated episodes of decompensated CHF occur relatively commonly in patients with chronic progressive heart failure.

Approach to Refractory CHF

Chronic heart failure management can be like a dance among intertwining players, including the ongoing disease progression and its various clinical manifestations, the patient's response to medications and dosages prescribed, and the numerous complications that can develop. Recurrent episodes of CHF usually respond initially to increased doses of furosemide. In addition, using an ACE inhibitor every 12 hours, rather than once daily, along with escalating doses of pimobendan are recommended in dogs with progressive CHF, provided renal function does not further deteriorate. Spironolactone, if not already being administered, should be added (spironolactone is not a substitute for loop-diuretic therapy). The usual target dose of spironolactone is 2 mg/kg/day, given in one or two divided doses; some patients might not tolerate this dose. When an arrhythmia is evident, appropriate antiarrhythmic therapy is used to maintain sinus rhythm as much as possible or, in the case of AF, to maintain adequate heart rate control (p. 411). If a beta-blocker is being administered for cardioprotection and CHF recurs, it should be discontinued.

The stage D heart failure classification generally implies that control of edema or effusions requires furosemide doses of over 8 mg/kg/day despite combination "quad" therapy, outlined earlier. Advanced CHF often is accompanied by reduced concentrations of serum electrolytes, especially Na^+, K^+, and Cl^-. High diuretic doses and the effects of chronic RAAS activation contribute. Low serum Na^+ and Cl^- concentrations could signal diuretic resistance. In dogs, serum Cl^- concentration appears to be more useful than Na^+ or K^+ in differentiating stage D, or refractory, CHF from stage

C. A serum Cl⁻ concentration <103.5 mmol/L predicted stage D CHF with 81% sensitivity and 75% specificity in one study (Adin, 2020).

Acute CHF recurrence that requires hospitalization is managed as outlined in **Table 22.2**. Several additional strategies for chronic CHF therapy are described here (and in **Table 22.5**). They usually are instituted one at a time (not necessarily in the order presented), then evaluated for effectiveness. As always, therapy must be tailored to the individual patient's needs. Furosemide dosage essentially is limited by renal function or by absorption and bioavailability. In patients with serum creatinine ≤2.5 mg/dL and BUN <80 mg/dL, especially those with acute pulmonary edema exacerbation, further increases in furosemide might be possible, at least temporarily. Serum creatinine should be rechecked in 1–2 days. Other strategies also can be tried for a more balanced approach. Substituting several intermittent 2 mg/kg SC furosemide doses/week, in place of oral doses, might be helpful. Practically, most cardiologists switch from furosemide to torsemide to improve diuretic delivery and bioavailability. This strategy should be considered in cases where progressively higher furosemide dosages are needed to control congestion, or ascites is developing. Increasingly, earlier institution is being pursued, before end-stage disease develops. Torsemide dosage is calculated as 1/8 to 1/12 of the patient's daily furosemide milligram dosage and given in two divided doses.

Another useful strategy is to increase the pimobendan frequency (to every 8 hours) or dosage (to 0.5 mg/kg/dose). Even higher dosages can be tolerated but their incremental value has not been studied. Additional afterload reduction using amlodipine (or hydralazine) can be helpful for dogs with DMVD, and sometimes (cautiously) those with DCM.

Table 22.5 Strategies for Managing Refractory Congestive Heart Failure in Dogs

The individual patient's clinical situation, including underlying cardiac pathophysiology and related complications (such as arrhythmia, pulmonary hypertension), as well as renal function, electrolyte status, current medications, and any concurrent disease condition(s) must be considered when deciding which treatment strategies to employ and when to institute them. The following are not necessarily listed in order of recommendation. See text (and Chapters 29 and 32) for additional information.

For All Cases

- Verify that basic CHF therapy is being provided (that is, furosemide, pimobendan, ACE inhibitor, and spironolactone at recommended doses, given twice daily), and that moderate dietary salt and exercise restrictions are followed.
- Verify that the dog is actually receiving the medications as prescribed.
- For dogs with moderate-marked pleural effusion or marked ascites, drain the fluid to improve ventilation and comfort. Dogs with ascites often have atrial fibrillation or pulmonary hypertension that will require management.

Treatment Intensification Options

- Increase the dose and/or frequency of furosemide (assuming that creatinine is ≤2.5 mg/dL and BUN <80 mg/dL), at least temporarily. Recheck renal function & electrolytes within a couple days.
- Add or increase spironolactone (to target dose of 2 mg/kg/day; consider starting lower), if not already being given. Recheck renal function and electrolytes in several days to a week.
- Increase pimobendan dose or administer original dose q8h, or both.
- If the furosemide dosage needed for edema control is approaching or exceeding 8 mg/kg/24 h, switch to torsemide (at an initial dose of 1/8 to 1/12 of the patient's prior total daily furosemide dosage, in two divided doses). Monitor renal function and electrolytes. If marked azotemia occurs, consider reducing ACE inhibitor dose and reducing torsemide by ~25%.
  - As an alternative to switching to torsemide, can substitute several furosemide (2 mg/kg) SC injections in place of oral doses intermittently throughout each week. Monitor renal function and electrolytes.
- Provide additional afterload reduction (especially for DMVD, but caution if DCM), starting with a low dose; amlodipine is usually preferred over hydralazine for chronic use.

Other Considerations and Strategies

- Provide antiarrhythmic therapy, if indicated (Chapter 25).
  - If atrial fibrillation is present, optimize heart rate (Chapter 25).
- Add sildenafil, if concurrent pulmonary hypertension, especially with signs of collapse or if there is ascites.
- If a beta-blocker, or other negative inotropic agent, is being used, reduce dosage or discontinue (preferably not abruptly).
- Consider adding digoxin (if not contraindicated), although this is not commonly done; monitor serum concentration, renal function, and serum potassium.
- For persistent congestive signs despite the above measures, can consider cautiously adding a third (thiazide) diuretic at low doses q24–48h; closely monitor renal function—severe derangement can develop within 1–2 days.
- Some respiratory signs might be caused by airway or other pulmonary conditions, rather than pulmonary edema. A cough suppressant, bronchodilator, antiinflammatory glucocorticoid, or other treatment could be helpful in such cases.

Abbreviations: ACE, angiotensin converting enzyme; CHF, congestive heart failure.

Low doses are used initially, gradually titrating upward if needed while monitoring BP. Amlodipine's effect on BP is not fully manifest for several days. An arteriolar vasodilator is not recommended in cases with dynamic or fixed ventricular outflow obstruction (such as subaortic stenosis). Possible adverse effects of arteriolar vasodilators include hypotension and impaired renal function, as well as reflex tachycardia (especially with hydralazine). In patients where ACE inhibitors and loop diuretics cannot be tolerated without high BUN and creatinine levels, it can be useful to reduce or even discontinue the ACE inhibitor and substitute amlodipine and spironolactone.

Dogs affected mainly by pulmonary arterial hypertension (including chronic heartworm disease or idiopathic pulmonary hypertension) usually present with exertional problems and ascites. For dogs with moderate to severe pulmonary hypertension, especially with body cavity effusions or signs of low cardiac output, the addition of sildenafil (1–3 mg/kg q8–12h PO) can help improve clinical status. When sildenafil is used, an L-arginine supplement might (or might not) be helpful (p. 834). In DMVD, a combined form of pulmonary hypertension (with both postcapillary and precapillary causes) is common. Once left heart failure has been optimally managed sildenafil can be carefully added to further reduce pulmonary hypertension. This is most helpful if there is exertional collapse, syncope or ascites. Sildenafil therapy is best guided by Doppler echocardiography.

More stringent dietary salt restriction might be useful; however, it is more important that the patient's appetite and food intake be maintained. The addition of a third diuretic (thiazide) could be considered; however, extremely conservative dosing and close attention to renal function and electrolyte concentrations are imperative because severe derangements can develop quickly (within 1–2 days). A low dose given only every other day or even less frequently (instead of q12–24h) is likely to be necessary to avoid serious azotemia and electrolyte abnormalities in patients with chronic refractory heart failure. Digoxin, if not previously used and not contraindicated, might be useful for additional inotropic support and its baroreceptor sensitizing effect, even in dogs with sinus rhythm. However, renal function, serum K^+ concentration, and appetite should be within acceptable levels, which rarely is the situation in Stage D CHF. Low doses and stringent monitoring are especially important to avoid digoxin toxicity in these compromised patients (p. 328). A decrease in appetite or onset of diarrhea or malaise can be an early sign of digoxin toxicity, as well as reduced renal function.

In some dogs, a persistent dry "airway" cough occurs without evidence of pulmonary edema. Massive LA enlargement and airway collapse exacerbate this. Chronic airway disease is a concurrent problem for many small dogs with DMVD. A cough suppressant (hydrocodone) can be helpful for these patients. However, it is important to continue monitoring RRR and otherwise observe for early signs of recurrent pulmonary edema. For dogs with persistent coughing caused by inflammatory, non-infectious airway disease, low doses of a glucocorticoid can help reduce cough severity and frequency. Because glucocorticoid therapy usually is avoided in animals with CHF, if deemed necessary, only the lowest effective doses should be used. Some cases benefit from a bronchodilator, although this could exacerbate sinus tachycardia or (other) arrhythmias.

Chronic Heart Failure Management in Cats

After the acute signs of heart failure have been controlled, the cat is transitioned to long-term therapy. Goals include preventing or at least slowing the accumulation of recurrent pulmonary edema and pleural effusion, reducing risk of arterial thromboembolism, and improving quality and length of life. The furosemide dosage used for acute CHF treatment is decreased as possible over the coming days to weeks to find the lowest effective dose for the individual patient. A common at-home starting dose for cats is 1–2 mg/kg q12–24h, with adjustment up or down as needed. As in dogs, the lowest diuretic dose at the longest time interval that will control congestive signs is the goal.

A drug to reduce risk of arterial thromboembolism is an important component of chronic heart failure therapy in cats. Clopidogrel is more effective than aspirin for this (p. 769) and therefore is recommended. Some clinicians add in small doses of aspirin and others, a factor Xa inhibitor such as rivaroxaban or apixaban. The bitter taste of clopidogrel complicates its administration (see following paragraph). An ACE inhibitor (usually benazepril) also is typically instituted using a conservative dose, after acute CHF signs have abated and the cat begins eating again. This agent is prescribed in an effort to reduce progressive maladaptive NH activity, myocardial remodeling and cardiac dysfunction. However, ACE inhibitors can depress appetite and promote azotemia. Many cats appear to do well for a variable time with these three medications (furosemide, clopidogrel, benazepril); sometimes, pimobendan and spironolactone also are added. However, the present lack of definitive evidence regarding optimal chronic heart failure therapy for cats is acknowledged. There are no sufficiently powered prospective studies of CHF therapy in cats and each of the available reports present limitations to interpretation. The addition of pimobendan to the treatment regime helps control CHF signs in some cats, especially those with reduced systolic function or end-stage cardiomyopathy. Pimobendan appears to have beneficial effects in many cats with HCM, as well. However, caution is warranted when dynamic LV outflow obstruction is present, because the combination of increased contractility with arteriolar dilation might exacerbate the obstruction. If pimobendan is used in a cat with LV outflow obstruction, heart rate and BP monitoring before and 2–3 hours after the initial dose is advised. Marked increase in heart rate or decrease in BP could indicate that pimobendan has exacerbated the obstruction. In general, cats in CHF without an obvious heart murmur are unlikely to have significant obstruction.

Administering medications to cats often is difficult for owners, especially if the drug is distasteful (examples include clopidogrel and spironolactone). Placing pills (or portions thereof) into pill-pockets, small (#4 or 5) gelatin capsules, or even little bits of cold butter can increase compliance in some cats. In others, compounding medications into strongly-flavored (such as chicken or tuna) suspensions is effective. However, in some cases, getting a cat to take just furosemide (and aspirin, if clopidogrel is totally refused) on a "close to prescribed" schedule must be considered success. Pimobendan is available in capsular form in most countries, but not the United States, and the tablet is large. Crumbling the chewable tablet into moist food (especially those containing "gravy") might facilitate administration.

Pleural effusion of more than mild amount should be drained to facilitate lung expansion. Medical therapy is intensified as possible to reduce fluid accumulation. Long-term heart failure therapy is tailored to the individual cat's (and owner's) needs by adjusting dosages or formulations, adding or substituting drugs (for example, adding spironolactone), and modifying lifestyle and diet. The owner's commitment and ability to medicate the cat are hugely important.

Management of Diastolic Dysfunction

In the past, a beta-blocker or calcium channel blocker routinely was advocated to address diastolic dysfunction caused by hypertrophic or restrictive cardiomyopathy in cats. Despite theoretical benefits, however, no overall survival benefit has been demonstrated so far with these agents (Chapter 33). Thus, beta-blocker and diltiazem are omitted from the long-term management of most cats with heart failure. Nevertheless, one of these drugs might present potential advantages for individual cats.

Calcium channel-blockers theoretically have beneficial effects in HCM by modestly reducing heart rate and contractility, thereby reducing myocardial O_2 demand (p. 384). The negative inotropic effect could be advantageous by reducing ventricular outflow obstruction, assuming this is not offset by vasodilation. Diltiazem could enhance myocardial relaxation also. Standard diltiazem requires dosing three times/day, which usually is impractical in cats; but sustained release preparations can produce either inadequate or excessive blood levels. Furthermore, adverse effects including inappetence, lethargy, and hepatotoxicity are fairly common. Diltiazem might be considered for heart rate control in a cat with AF, if atenolol or other beta-blocker cannot be used for some reason.

Beta-blockers are thought to have a greater ability to reduce heart rate and dynamic LV outflow obstruction compared with diltiazem. However, they also are not routinely used for most cats with chronic heart failure caused by diastolic dysfunction. A degree of concern exists that these agents might worsen outcome, although the evidence is not conclusive. Nevertheless, for cats with a tachyarrhythmia, a beta-blocker usually is the agent of first choice. A beta-blocker also might be used in a cat that has severe dynamic LV outflow obstruction, especially at higher heart rates, to reduce sympathomimetic influence on both heart rate and obstruction. By inhibiting catecholamine-induced myocyte damage, a beta-blocker might reduce myocardial fibrosis and stiffness. However, beta-blocker treatment does not appear to improve survival. Atenolol is the beta-blocker that has been used most commonly (p. 379). If prescribed, signs of recurrent CHF or bradycardia should prompt dosage reduction and possible discontinuation, although not abruptly.

Ivabradine, also has heart rate lowering effects (p. 385). Whether it will be useful for cats with CHF from diastolic dysfunction is presently unclear. IV ivabradine appears to mildly reduce both diastolic and systolic function.

Dietary and Other Recommendations

As for dogs, a good quality diet with adequate calories and protein are recommended for cats with chronic heart failure. Ideally, moderate sodium restriction would be enforced, but realistically most clinicians (and clients) simply want their cat to eat. Enticing a sick cat to accept a diet change, or even eat at all, often is difficult. If the techniques of gradual transitioning to a new diet, hand-feeding small amounts, or other strategies to improve appetite (as described for dogs, p. 352) are not effective, it is better to feed whatever diet the cat will eat. Capromorelin, mirtazapine (1.25–4 mg/cat PO q72h), or cyproheptadine (2 mg/cat PO) also might be effective adjuncts. The development of cardiac cachexia (p. 312) is of concern in cats, as well.

Most commercial and prescription cat foods are well-supplemented with taurine, which has dramatically reduced the prevalence of taurine-responsive DCM in cats. Nevertheless, blood taurine concentration should be measured in any cat diagnosed with DCM, because some cats are deficient, especially those eating "off-brands" or dog food. Cats with DCM and low (or unmeasured) taurine levels should be supplemented with 250–500 mg PO q12h. A high-taurine diet is also recommended, which could allow eventual discontinuation of the supplement (p. 682).

Monitoring and Follow-up Evaluation

Early identification of complications is more likely with an attentive owner who can recognize early signs of CHF and understands the purpose and potential adverse effects of each medication. Home monitoring of the cat's RRR is helpful for identifying early signs of recurrent pulmonary edema in cats, as it is in dogs (discussed previously, p. 338). However, pleural effusion often is associated with an increase in respiratory effort rather than rate. So observing for both respiratory effort and rate is especially important in cats. Recommendations for reevaluation are similar to those for dogs (p. 353). Azotemia is nearly impossible to avoid with twice daily dosing of medications and the emphasis is on preventing severe azotemia and related signs like anorexia.

Approach to Refractory CHF

As heart disease progresses, increasing doses of furosemide usually are needed. Drug administration can become more difficult, and the patient less cooperative, especially as medication frequency increases. For some cats, substituting a SC injection of furosemide for an oral dose every day or two is helpful. Torsemide has been used in cats with refractory CHF, in place of furosemide; it is dosed at 1/10 to 1/12 of the daily mg dosage of furosemide, divided into 2 daily doses. Based on the torsemide tablet size (5 mg), the drug might require compounding for accurate and safe feline dosing. Hypokalemia and azotemia are more likely at higher diuretic dosages. The addition (or dosage adjustment) of concurrent medications such as benazepril (or possibly an ARB instead), pimobendan, and spironolactone can help.

Hypokalemia might respond to the addition of spironolactone therapy or supplementing the diet with additional potassium rich foods, although some cats need a prescription potassium supplement. Preliminary study suggests a possible survival benefit with spironolactone in cats with chronic heart failure; however, evaluation in a larger population is needed. Digoxin almost never is used in cats now, and is not recommended.

Recurrent pleural effusion is common with advanced heart failure in cats. Repeated thoracocentesis could be required, which can become increasingly challenging over time. Pulmonary hypertension secondary to left heart failure is uncommon in cats; however, it has been documented in some cases. The need for intensified diuretic and other heart failure drug doses in cats with refractory CHF must be balanced against the renal function deterioration, electrolyte abnormalities, and inappetence that often develop. If azotemia or inappetence worsen, the doses of diuretic, ACE inhibitor, or other medications should be reduced or even discontinued for one to several days ("drug holidays"). Some cases might benefit from judicious doses of SC (or IV) fluid. Persistent cardiac arrhythmias should be addressed as appropriate (Chapter 25).

Management of Heart Failure in Horses

Acute Congestive Heart Failure

The most common reason for CHF in the horse is a combination of severe valvular disease and AF. Postcapillary pulmonary hypertension can occur with chronic left heart disease, leading to biventricular CHF with pleural effusion and subcutaneous edema. The other common presentation is that of acute pulmonary edema resulting from a mitral chordal rupture or infective endocarditis. The decision to pursue or continue CHF therapy is influenced by several considerations, which must be balanced against the costs and challenges of providing that treatment. Results of the clinical exam, echocardiography, electrocardiography, and other pertinent tests will inform that decision. As with small animals, it is important to define the underlying etiology and any complicating factors as clearly as possible. One consideration is the likelihood that enough functional improvement could occur with therapy to allow the patient to return to an adequate level of activity. For example, a horse with suspected myocarditis or myocardial dysfunction secondary to persistent tachyarrhythmia potentially might improve with treatment and time. Therapy might help maintain a broodmare's pregnancy to term or support a valuable stallion's ability to breed for a time. In some cases, an owner might seek to extend a horse's quality and length of life as a valued companion animal. However, even when arrhythmias and congestive signs can be controlled, caution must be used. Horses with heart failure are considered unsafe to ride, and should not be worked with any degree of intensity. Rupture of the pulmonary artery (from pulmonary hypertension) and probable arrhythmic causes of sudden death have occurred.

As for dogs and cats, therapeutic aims include improving oxygenation, resolving congestive signs, optimizing forward cardiac output, and controlling arrhythmias and other complicating factors. Furosemide is administered IV (1–2 mg/kg) and repeated as needed. Short-term intranasal O_2 delivery can be provided, if available. Flow rates of 5–10 L/minute are recommended. As for small animals, it is important to reduce stress and activity level. Minimizing environmental noise, commotion, heat and humidity (or excessive cold) could help. Mild sedation can reduce anxiety in animals with respiratory distress. Conservative doses of butorphanol or acepromazine usually are well-tolerated; however, agents that provoke vasoconstriction (such as the alpha$_2$ agonists xylazine and detomidine) can increase afterload and exacerbate mitral and aortic valve regurgitation. Horses with poor myocardial contractility or persistent hypotension can benefit from acute inotropic support with a dobutamine CRI, although this rarely is done. IV digoxin is recommended, whether the horse is in sinus rhythm or AF; generally, 1 mg will be given by slow IV push. IV pimobendan is available in some countries, but is likely to be cost-prohibitive.

Heart rate and rhythm should be assessed. If AF is present, the heart rate is likely to be high. This can exacerbate congestion and poor cardiac output. Digoxin also is indicated here to slow AV conduction and ventricular response rate. Attempted conversion using quinidine is not recommended (p. 413). Digoxin also helps support myocardial function; however, it must be used cautiously and monitored carefully because of the risk for proarrhythmia and other toxicity signs (p. 327). Severe preexisting ventricular tachyarrhythmia is a relative contraindication to using digoxin. Frequent ventricular premature beats or ventricular tachycardia can worsen CHF signs, as well as predispose to sudden death. Lidocaine can help manage these acutely. Magnesium sulfate or other strategies might be needed, also (p. 424). It is important to monitor serum electrolyte (especially K^+ and Mg^{++}) and renal function status, as well as BP.

Considerations for Ongoing Therapy

Furosemide can be continued IV, IM (or SC); 1 mg/kg q24–12h can be tried initially. However, furosemide dosage should be guided by clinical response and renal function. Oral furosemide administration is not effective in horses. Torsemide could be used PO (p. 319). The addition of an ACE inhibitor should be helpful for longer-term CHF therapy. Benazepril, ramipril, and quinapril are options for PO administration; however, enalapril is unlikely to be effective (p. 322). Digoxin can be continued; serum concentrations should be monitored. Oral pimobendan might be a consideration for its inodilator effects.

The prognosis for horses with progressive cardiac structural disease unfortunately is guarded to poor. Even if clinical signs resolve, the likelihood of returning to moderate or even mild work is questionable. Horses with heart failure are considered unsafe to ride or drive, but might survive as a companion animal or be used for reproduction.

Suggested Additional Reading and References

Also See Online Comprehensive Bibliography at: https://www.routledge.com/9781482246223.

Achiel R, Carver A, Sanders RA. Treatment of congestive heart failure with intravenous nitroglycerin in three dogs with degenerative valvular disease. J Am Anim Hosp Assoc. 2020;56:37-41

Adin D, Kurtz K, Atkins C, et al. Role of electrolyte concentrations and renin-angiotensin-aldosterone activation in the staging of canine heart disease. J Vet Intern Med 2020;34:53–64.

Ames MK, Atkins CE, Eriksson A, et al. Aldosterone breakthrough in dogs with naturally occurring myxomatous mitral valve disease. J Vet Cardiol 2017;19:218–227.

Atkins C, Bonagura J, Ettinger S, et al. Guidelines for the diagnosis and treatment of canine chronic valvular heart disease. J Vet Intern Med 2009;23:1142–1150.

Atkins CE, Keene BW, Brown WA, et al. Results of the veterinary enalapril trial to prove reduction in onset of heart failure in dogs chronically treated with enalapril alone for compensated, naturally occurring mitral valve insufficiency. J Am Vet Med Assoc. 2007;231:1061–1069.

Bernay F, Bland JM, Häggström J, et al. Efficacy of spironolactone on survival in dogs with naturally occurring mitral regurgitation caused by myxomatous mitral valve disease. J Vet Intern Med 2010;24:331–341.

Borgarelli M, Ferasin L, Lamb K, et al. Delay of appearance of symptoms of canine degenerative mitral valve disease treated with spironolactone and benazepril: the DELAY study. J Vet Cardiol 2020;27:34–53.

Boswood A, Häggström J, Gordon SG, et al. Effect of pimobendan in dogs with preclinical myxomatous mitral valve disease and cardiomegaly: the EPIC study-a randomized clinical trial. J Vet Intern Med 2016;30:1765–1779.

Davis JL, Gardner SY, Schwabenton B, et al. Congestive heart failure in horses: 14 cases (1984-2001). J Am Vet Med Assoc 2002;220:1512–1515.

Edwards TH, Erickson Coleman A, Brainard BM, et al. Outcome of positive-pressure ventilation in dogs and cats with congestive heart failure: 16 cases (1992–2012). J Vet Emerg Crit Care 2014;24:586–593.

Freeman LM. Beneficial effects of omega-3 fatty acids in cardiovascular disease. J Small Anim Pract 2010;51:462–470.

Freeman LM. Cachexia and sarcopenia: emerging syndromes of importance in dogs and cats. J Vet Intern Med 2012;26:3–17.

Gordon SG, Cote E. Pharmacotherapy of feline cardiomyopathy: chronic management of heart failure. J Vet Cardiol 2015;17(Suppl 1):S159–172.

Hezzell MJ, Boswood A, Lopez-Alvarez J, et al. Treatment of dogs with compensated myxomatous mitral valve disease with spironolactone-a pilot study. J Vet Cardiol 2017;19:325–338.

Hopper K, Powell LL. Basics of mechanical ventilation for dogs and cats. Vet Clin North Am Small Anim Pract 2013;43:955–969.

James R, Guillot E, Garelli-Paar C, et al. The SEISICAT study: a pilot study assessing efficacy and safety of spironolactone in cats with congestive heart failure secondary to cardiomyopathy. J Vet Cardiol 2018;20:1–12.

Johansson AM, Gardner SY, Levine JF, et al. Furosemide continuous rate infusion in the horse: evaluation of enhanced efficacy and reduced side effects. J Vet Intern Med 2003;17:887–895.

Kvart C, Häggström J, Pedersen HD, et al. Efficacy of enalapril for prevention of congestive heart failure in dogs with myxomatous valve disease and asymptomatic mitral regurgitation. J Vet Intern Med 2002;16:80–88.

Keene BW, Atkins CE, Bonagura JD, et al. ACVIM consensus guidelines for the diagnosis and treatment of myxomatous mitral valve disease in dogs. J Vet Intern Med 2019;33:1127–1140.

Leroux AA, Detilleux J, Sandersen CF, et al. Prevalence and risk factors for cardiac diseases in a hospital-based population of 3,434 horses (1994–2011). J Vet Intern Med 2013;27: 1563–1570.

Meurs KM, Olsen LH, Reimann MJ, et al. Angiotensin-converting enzyme activity in Cavalier King Charles Spaniels with an ACE gene polymorphism and myxomatous mitral valve disease. Pharmacogenet Genomics 2018;28:37–40.

Mizuno M, Yamano S, Chimura S, et al. Efficacy of pimobendan on survival and reoccurrence of pulmonary edema in canine congestive heart failure. J Vet Med Sci 2017;79(1):29–34.

Oyama MA, Peddle GD, Reynolds CA, Singletary GE. Use of the loop diuretic torsemide in three dogs with advanced heart failure. J Vet Cardiol 2011;13:287–292.

Peddle GD, Singletary GE, Reynolds CA, et al. Effect of torsemide and furosemide on clinical, laboratory, radiographic and quality of life variables in dogs with heart failure secondary to mitral valve disease. J Vet Cardiol 2012;14: 253–259.

Porciello F, Rishniw M, Ljungvall I, et al. Sleeping and resting respiratory rates in dogs and cats with medically-controlled left-sided congestive heart failure. Vet J 2016;207: 164–168.

Pouchelon JL, Jamet N, Gouni V, et al. Effect of benazepril on survival and cardiac events in dogs with asymptomatic mitral valve disease: a retrospective study of 141 cases. J Vet Intern Med. 2008;22:905–914.

Redpath A, Bowen M. Cardiac therapeutics in horses. Vet Clin North Am Equine Pract 2019;35:217–241.

Riesen SC, Schober KE, Smith DN, et al. Effects of ivabradine on heart rate and left ventricular function in healthy cats and cats with hypertrophic cardiomyopathy. Am J Vet Res 2012;73: 202–212.

Rishniw M, Ljungvall I, Porciello F, et al. Sleeping respiratory rates in apparently healthy adult dogs. Res Vet Sci 2012;93: 965–969.

Rishniw M, Pion PD. Is treatment of feline hypertrophic cardiomyopathy based in science or faith? A survey of cardiologists and a literature search. J Feline Med Surg 2011;13:487–497.

Rush JE, Freeman LM, Brown DJ, et al. Clinical, echocardiographic, and neurohormonal effects of a sodium-restricted diet in dogs with heart failure. J Vet Intern Med 2000;14:513–520.

Schwarzwald CC. Disorders of the cardiovascular system. In, Reed SM, Bayly WM, Sellon DC (editors), Equine Internal Medicine, 4th edition. Elsevier, St. Louis, MO; 2018, pp. 387–541.

Slupe JL, Freeman LM, Rush JE. Association of body weight and body condition with survival in dogs with heart failure. J Vet Intern Med 2008;22:561–565.

Staub NC, Gee M, Vreim C. Mechanism of alveolar flooding in acute pulmonary oedema. Ciba Found Symp 1976:255–272.

Summerfield NJ, Boswood A, O'Grady MR, et al. Efficacy of pimobendan in the prevention of congestive heart failure or sudden death in Doberman Pinschers with preclinical dilated cardiomyopathy (the PROTECT Study). J Vet Intern Med 2012;26(6):1337–1349.

Wess G, Kresken JG, Wendt R, et al. Efficacy of adding ramipril (VAsotop) to the combination of furosemide (Lasix) and pimobendan (VEtmedin) in dogs with mitral valve degeneration: The VALVE trial. J Vet Intern Med 2020;34:2232–2241.

West JB, Mathieu-Costello O. Vulnerability of pulmonary capillaries in heart disease. Circulation. 1995;9:622–631.

Wolf J, Gerlach N, Weber K, et al. Lowered N-terminal pro-B-type natriuretic peptide levels in response to treatment predict survival in dogs with symptomatic mitral valve disease. J Vet Cardiol 2012;14:399–408.

Section IV

Heart Rhythm Disturbances

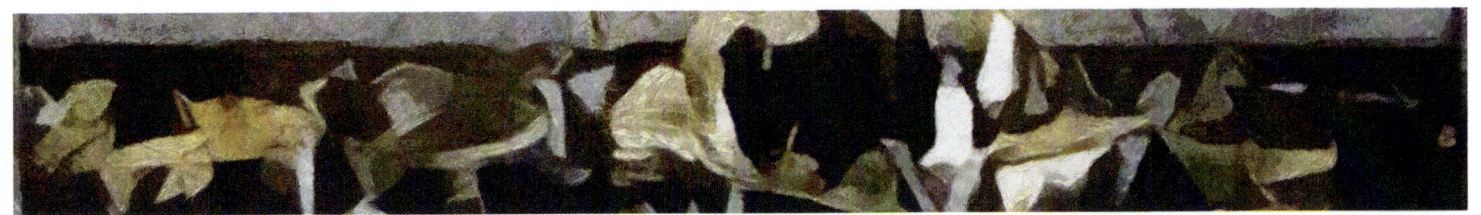

23

ARRHYTHMIAS
Pathophysiology and Clinical Associations

Multiple factors play a role in the development of abnormal cardiac rhythms. Alterations from the normal cardiac cell action potentials involving excitability, refractoriness, conduction, or automaticity predispose to arrhythmias. These changes are caused by cardiac structural or physiologic abnormalities, and can develop even without overt structural disease. Electrophysiologic changes create a so-called substrate for arrhythmogenesis. Changes in both structure (such as cell degeneration), and function (as with abnormal calcium transients), arise during cardiac remodeling from different diseases and heart failure (Chapter 20). Genetic and environmental factors, including drug therapies, also can be involved. Specific disorders associateded with arrhythmias include cardiomyocyte hypertrophy, cardiomyopathies with fat or fibrous tissue replacement of myocytes, abnormal ion channel structure or function, tissue inflammation, and congenital conduction anomalies, among other derangements. Differences in electrical properties across cardiac tissues are also relevant. For example, increasing heterogeneity of repolarization (refractoriness) or conduction velocities across different regions of ventricular myocardium (or from endocardium to epicardium), fosters conditions more favorable for arrhythmogenesis, including myocardial fibrillation.

Yet even with such underlying abnormalities, arrhythmias might not occur unless provoked by some triggering event. This could be an abrupt change in cardiac cycle length or instantaneous heart rate (HR) or a premature stimulus. Isolated or sustained arrhythmias can result when the underlying conditions are favorable. Additional modulating factors further influence whether an arrhythmia occurs or is sustained. These include changes in cardiac sympathetic or vagal tone, circulating catecholamine concentrations, systemic and local electrolyte disturbances, pH, and ischemia. For example, anger and aggressive behavior have been associated with increased susceptibility to arrhythmias and sudden arrhythmic death in dogs, as well as in people, particularly when coronary blood flow is compromised. Such modulating factors also influence the response to antiarrhythmic drugs. The sympathetic nervous system can potentiate arrhythmias caused by various mechanisms, including increased automaticity, triggered activity, and reentry. The specific mechanism underlying an arrhythmia is not always clear from the surface ECG. However, the ECG together with the overall cardiac workup, often does provide clues to the most likely underlying abnormality.

Electrophysiologic Mechanisms

The electrophysiologic mechanisms underlying cardiac arrhythmias generally involve abnormalities of impulse formation or impulse conduction, or a combination of these. Abnormalities in cellular excitability and refractoriness strongly influence cardiac conduction (**Figure 23.1**). The property of automaticity allows cardiac cells to generate action potentials spontaneously via diastolic (phase 4) depolarization, where a net inward current progressively brings the membrane to threshold potential. Multiple voltage- and time-dependent ion currents influence the level of automaticity, including the hyperpolarizing current I_f ("funny current," involving Na^+ and K^+), transient (I_{Ca-T}) and long-lasting (I_{Ca-L}) calcium currents, and the sodium-calcium exchange current (I_{NCX}). Sympathetic nervous activity strongly influences I_f and I_{Ca-L}. Abnormal impulse formation also occurs when cells depolarize spontaneously following a prior depolarization or trigger (see section "Triggered Activity").

Disorders of impulse conduction can involve conduction delay or block within the sinoatrial (SA) node or atrioventricular (AV) node, a major ventricular conduction pathway (bundle branch), or within small areas of myocardium. Accessory AV

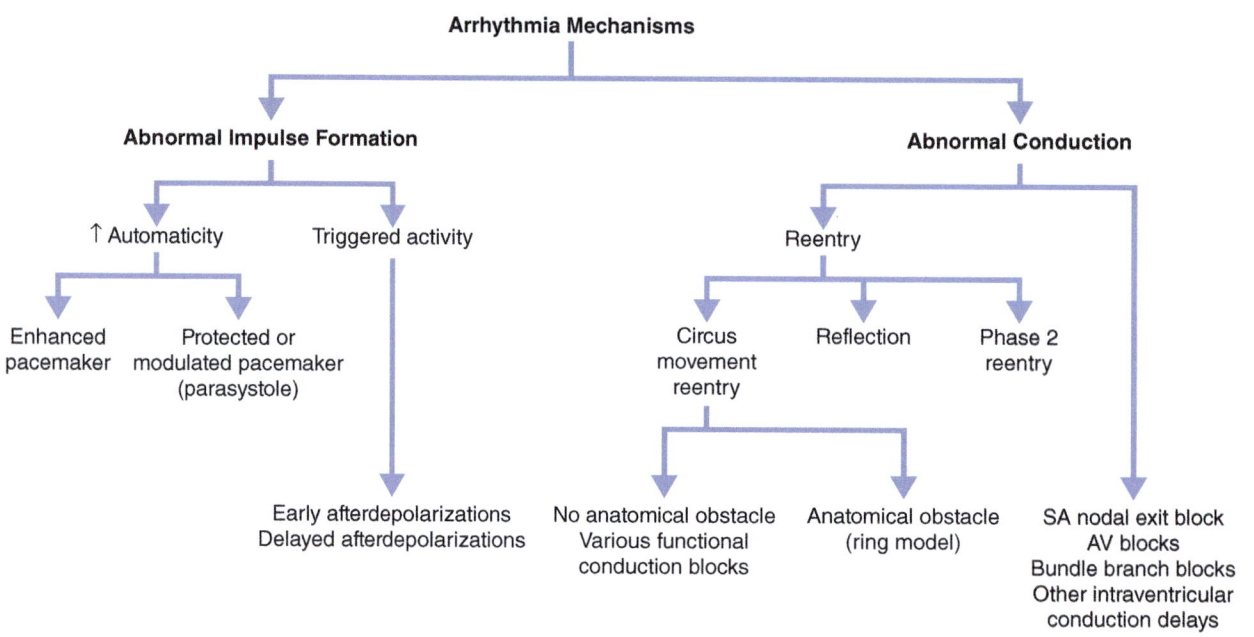

Figure 23.1 Abnormalities of electrical impulse formation or conduction, or both, can lead to cardiac arrhythmias. This diagram outlines major mechanisms of arrhythmogensis.

conduction pathways also can exist as congenital malformations. A bradyarrhythmia results when conduction fails in the SA or AV node, leading to asystole or more often, a slow escape rhythm to "rescue" the heart. Conversely, abnormal conduction is inherent to many atrial and ventricular tachyarrhythmias too. These include premature complexes, sustained tachycardias of multiple types, and myocardial flutter and fibrillation. These rhythms are induced by various forms of micro- and macro-reentry related to defined electrical reentry paths, circuit movements, or disordered reentry (fibrillation; see section "Reentry").

The sick sinus syndrome (SSS), preexcitation syndromes, and other arrhythmias can involve abnormalities of both impulse formation and conduction. The SSS, or bradycardia–tachycardia syndrome (p. 405), involves abnormal SA node activation (leading to sinus bradycardia and arrest), delays in AV node conduction (causing 1st and 2nd degree heart block), and variable disturbances in excitability (provoking junctional or atrial tachyarrhythmias and, sometimes, ventricular ectopy). Preexcitation involves an accessory conduction pathway that bypasses the AV node; faster conduction over the accessory pathway activates a portion of the ventricular myocardium early, before conduction can occur through the normal AV pathway. It also can allow a rapid reentrant tachycardia to be sustained over a macroreentry circuit involving the AV node and accessory pathway (p. 417).

Enhanced and Abnormal Automaticity

Abnormal impulse formation can include an inappropriate sinus node rate for the patient's physiologic needs, or discharge from ectopic (subsidiary or latent) pacemaker cells, which normally are overdrive suppressed. These are examples of enhanced normal automaticity. Increased automaticity is appropriate in the case of sinus tachycardia caused by heightened sympathetic tone or in a subsidiary pacemaker activated after sinus arrest or AV block. Conversely, decreased automaticity ultimately can cause bradycardia or asystole (arrest).

In contrast, abnormal automaticity involves spontaneous activation of atrial or ventricular cells that do not normally demonstrate pacemaker activity. The development of abnormal automaticity is thought to involve reduced (less negative) resting membrane potentials, possibly from impaired function or density of the I_{K1} channels. This can allow spontaneous and repetitive impulse generation, known as "depolarization-induced automaticity." Local tissue injury (as from ischemia or inflammation), hyperkalemia, and other factors can underlie this by partially depolarizing cell membranes. Increased sympathetic activity also increases abnormal (as well as normal) automaticity. Myocardial cells that develop abnormal or enhanced automaticity can generate depolarizations at a rate faster than cells with normal automaticity (as in the SA node). The resulting ectopic beats or sustained tachycardias can overdrive suppress or interfere with conduction of the normal sinus impulses. Accelerated idioventricular rhythms; atrial, junctional, and ventricular premature extrasystoles; and rapid atrial or ventricular tachycardias can arise from abnormal automaticity. Parasystole is a phenomenon of spontaneous automaticity where the abnormal focus can activate surrounding myocardium, but is protected from being overdrive suppressed itself by a faster rhythm (p. 149).

Triggered Activity

Triggered activity is another type of abnormal impulse formation. It entails abnormal depolarization or oscillation in transmembrane voltage either during or following a cardiac action potential. Collectively these are termed afterdepolarizations; if their amplitude is sufficient to reach threshold potential, a spontaneous action potential (a triggered response) is generated. These sometimes recur with each subsequent cycle and precipitate a tachyarrhythmia, which can terminate or progress to a polymorphic tachycardia or myocardial fibrillation. Two forms (subclasses) of triggered activity are described: early afterdepolarizations (EADs) and delayed afterdepolarizations (DADs; **Figure 23.2**). EADs interrupt the repolarization process during phases 2 and 3 of the cardiac action potential and occur when the net (+) transmembrane currents suddenly shift to an inward direction. Cardiac tissue injury, electrolyte disturbance, hypoxia, acidosis, ventricular hypertrophy, catecholamines, and heart failure can predispose to EADs. A slower HR and drugs that inhibit K^+ currents, or increase inward currents, increase the risk for EADs, as does a long-short cardiac cycle and T-wave alternans. Ventricular mid-myocardial cells (M cells) and Purkinje fibers are thought to be more susceptible to EADs than cells in epicardial or endocardial regions. However, a decrease in the repolarizing currents I_{Kr} and I_{Ks}, as occurs with conditions causing QT interval prolongation or with cardiomyopathy, can promote EADs in any area. EADs are thought to be the usual trigger for the polymorphic ventricular tachycardia known as *torsades de pointes* that is associated with long QT syndromes (**Figure 23.3**; also see **Figure 5.34**, p. 149), but also occurs in some cases of cardiomyopathy.

In contrast, DADs occur during phase 4 of the cardiac action potential, after repolarization, and when intracellular Ca^{++} levels are increased. These result in classic oscillatory afterpotentials that, if strong enough, can achieve threshold and induce a premature complex or ectopic tachycardia. Digoxin, catecholamines, and situations where "leaky" ryanodine receptors cause Ca^{++} overload increase the risk for DADs, especially at higher HRs. Clinical associations include ventricular hypertrophy, heart failure, and myocardial ischemia or infarction. These also are relevant to atrial arrhythmias. A form of triggered activity known as late phase 3 EADs, with characteristics of both EADs and DADs, also can occur and might underlie the onset of atrial fibrillation (AF). A shortened repolarization period combined with robust normal sarcoplasmic reticular Ca^{++} release could generate late phase 3 EADs, especially with simultaneous increases in sympathetic and vagal activation.

Reentry

Not all conduction blocks produce bradycardia. The phenomenon of reentry, which also involves abnormal conduction, can lead to premature beats and to rapid and sustained tachycardias. Reentry can occur within defined anatomic pathways (anatomic reentry) or because of functional electrophysiologic changes in adjacent tissues (functional reentry). The classic prerequisites for reentry are unidirectional

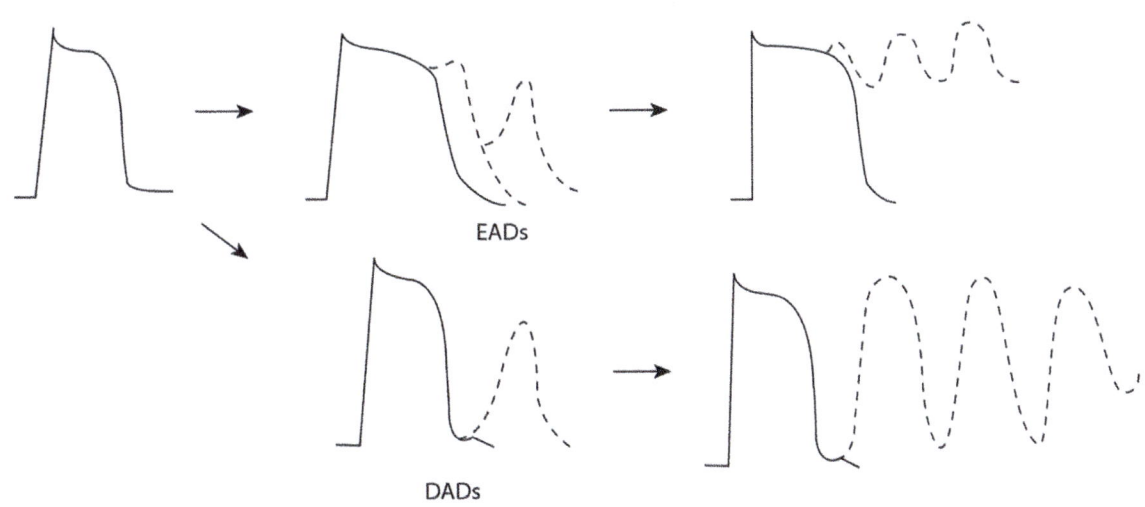

Figure 23.2 Oscillations in membrane potential sometimes occur following (triggered by) an action potential. If these are strong enough, they can trigger one or more additional action potentials. Triggered activity is a form of abnormal automaticity. Early afterdepolarizations (EADs; top) occur in late phase 2 or in phase 3, thereby interrupting the normal repolarization process. They are more likely to develop when repolarization is prolonged. Cell injury, altered electrolyte (especially hyperkalemia) or acid-base status, heart failure, cardiac hypertrophy, and antiarrhythmic or other drugs (especially those that inhibit K^+ currents) can predispose to EADs. EADs can induce arrhythmias that subsequently continue via a reentrant mechanism, such as *torsades de pointes* or ventricular fibrillation. Delayed afterdepolarizations (DADs; bottom) occur after the cell repolarizes, usually under conditions of increased intracellular Ca^{++}. This can develop with catecholamine or excessive digoxin exposure, and at increased heart rates. Myocardial hypertrophy and heart failure also can predispose to DADs (as well as reentrant arrhythmias). Like EADs, DADs can trigger ventricular tachycardia or fibrillation, which then is sustained by a reentrant mechanism. (Adapted from Coronel, 2013.)

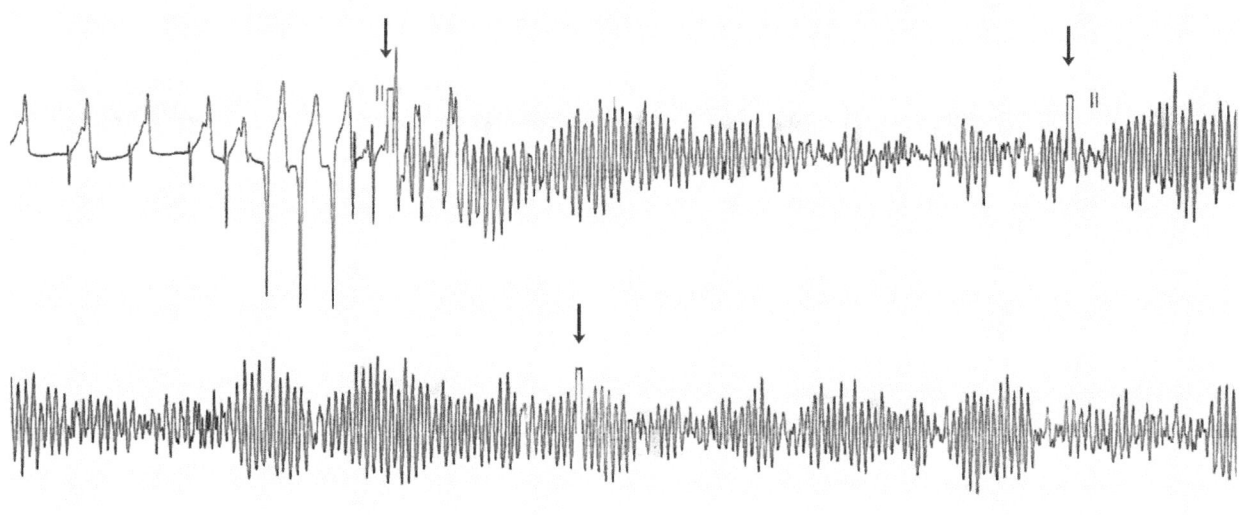

Figure 23.3 Continuous ECG recording shows the onset of *torsades de pointes* in a dog with congenital long QT syndrome. Lead II, compressed to 10 mm/s. Arrows indicate calibration marks automatically inscribed by the recording device; 1 cm = 1 mV.

current block, current propagation along another pathway, and sufficient (decremental) conduction delay to permit repolarization and subsequent reactivation of the previously blocked zone. It can involve small circuits (microreentry) or large circuits which often include the AV node or large parts of the atria (macroreentry). A characteristic of macroreentry is that the tachycardia can be "entrained" and either terminated or reset by a suitably timed external stimulus penetrating the circuit (Veenhuyzen, 2008). This interruption can occur spontaneously, from native activity, but more often is induced during an electrophysiology study. This concept also underlies the therapeutic benefit of electrocardioversion, which involves depolarizing part of a reentrant circuit to extinguish the arrhythmia. Reentry underlies many clinical arrhythmias, including atrial flutter (macro-reentry atrial tachycardia), AF, ventricular fibrillation (VF), many atrial and ventricular tachycardias, and AV reciprocating tachycardia.

There are several types of reentry. "Circus movement" reentry involves an activation wavefront that propagates around an anatomic or functional obstacle to reexcite the area of origin, as long as those cells have recovered from activation and can be excited again when next wavefront arrives (**Figure 23.4**). This is the classic mechanism for atrial flutter, also termed macro-reentrant atrial tachycardia. In contrast, with "reflection" and "phase 2 reentry," large differences of recovery from refractoriness exist between different sites. The site with delayed recovery excites neighboring cells that have already recovered, producing reentrant reexcitation. Reentry is not necessarily linear or planar but can involve three dimensional activation processes with anatomic or functional cores that are static or dynamic (**Figure 23.4**).

Circus movement involves an excitatory wave that progresses along a distinct pathway, returns to the point of origin, and then follows the same path again. Circus movement reentry requires two fundamental conditions in order for it to start and be maintained: (1) an area of unidirectional block (which allows the impulse to travel in only one direction along the circuit's pathway), and (2) a long enough circuit (and slow enough conduction around it) so that every site within the circuit is able to recover before the circulating wave of activation returns. Interruption (block) of the circuit at any point should terminate the circus movement and thus, the resulting arrhythmia. Whether reentry can be established depends on conduction velocity and refractoriness. The length of the circuit must be longer than or equal to the wavelength (that is, conduction velocity × refractory period). Slowing of conduction velocity (for example, by an antiarrhythmic drug) can facilitate reentry. Circus movement reentry typically requires a specific substrate, such as scar tissue, diseased myocardium, or accessory conducting fibers. It occurs in ischemic tissue (often affected by local hyperkalemia and acidosis), as well as in nonischemic myocardial disease. However, functional reentry also can occur without an anatomic obstacle. Premature impulses propagate only in the direction where the refractory period is shorter; this creates an arc of block or refractory core around which the impulse circulates to reexcite its site of origin. This is known as the "leading circle model." Spiral wave reentry is a similar and perhaps more likely concept, where reentrant activity forms three-dimensional scroll waves that can take on several configurations. Spiral wave activity can explain the ECG patterns of monomorphic and polymorphic ventricular tachycardia (VT), as well as VF. With monomorphic VT, the spiral wave is anchored and doesn't

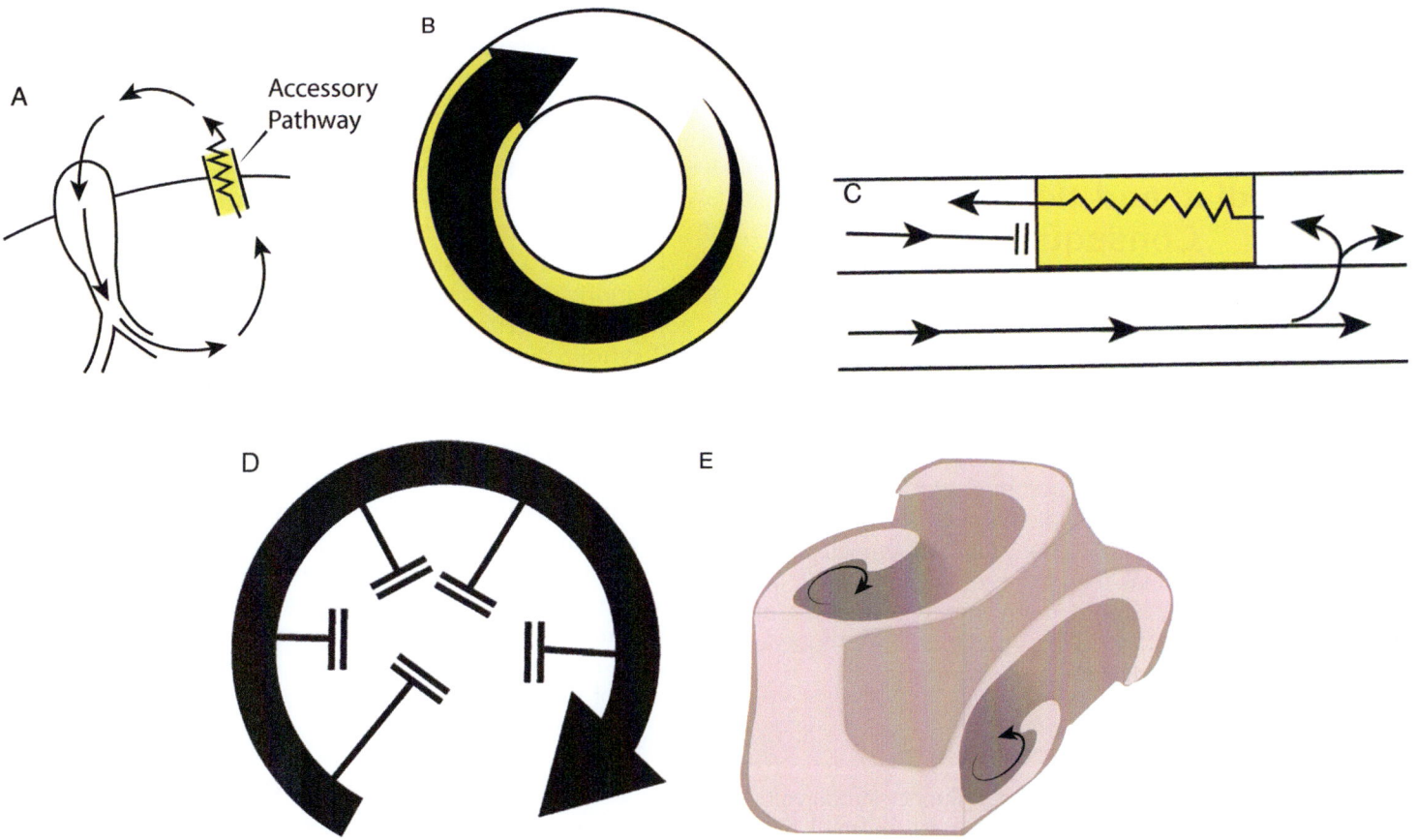

Figure 23.4 Schematic illustrations of circus movement reentry (A–D) and spiral (scroll) wave reentry (E). (A) Macro-reentrant circuit involving an accessory pathway in the Wolff-Parkinson-White syndrome (p. 153 and p. 417). Slower, retrograde conduction across the accessory pathway (on right) from ventricle to atrium, followed by antegrade conduction over the normal atrioventricular (AV) conduction system (on left), leads to sustained AV reciprocating tachycardia (orthodromic conduction direction illustrated here). (B) Another, so-called "ring model" of reentry, where the black arrow represents an activation wavefront circling around an (anatomical or functional) obstacle or core. The wavefront travels on to reexcite its site of origin. The yellow color indicates refractoriness of the previously depolarized myocardium; recovered tissue, ready to be depolarized again, is indicated in white. Conduction velocity and refractoriness are important for sustaining reentry. The circuit's path must be long enough to allow previously depolarized tissue to recover in time to be reexcited by the returning wavefront (see section "Reentry"). (C) Concept of circus movement in a linear bundle of tissue. The activation wavefront enters from the left in both upper and lower bundles; however, it is blocked (unidirectionally) in the upper bundle at the yellow-colored region. The successfully conducted wavefront (below) can cross over to activate the upper bundle distal to the area of unidirectional block. Slowed, retrograde conduction through this area can reexcite recovered tissue at upper left. (D) Concept of "leading circle" reentry around a core of functionally refractory tissue created by centripetal wavelets that collide with and block each other at the vortex of a circulating wavefront (block indicated by double bars). (E) Concept of "spiral waves" (rotors) that occur without an anatomical obstacle; this is represented here as three-dimensional "scroll waves." A scroll wave rotates around a central "filament" (or core, in two-dimensional description). The wave-break occurs as the wavefront meets the refractory tail of a previous activation, inducing scroll waves in circus movement around the wave-break site. The filament can take on different shapes. Scroll (spiral) waves can remain fairly stable (anchored) and create a monomorphic tachycardia; alternatively, they could drift in shape and path, causing polymorphic tachycardia, or break into multiple spirals and lead to fibrillation. (Adapted from Antzelevitch, 2013.)

drift within the ventricular myocardium; in polymorphic VT and VF, the spiral wave drifts within the myocardium. When a single spiral wave breaks up, multiple drifting spirals can occur which are continually extinguished and recreated. This could explain the degeneration of VT into VF.

Reentry can occur without circus movement by the mechanisms of "reflection" and "phase 2 reentry" when there are large differences in recovery from refractoriness between one site and another. The area with delayed recovery acts as a "virtual electrode" which excites already-recovered adjacent tissue, thus provoking reentrant arrhythmia. In reflection, slow anterograde conduction of the impulse in a fiber is followed by a retrograde wavefront that produces a "return extrasystole." Reflection is thought to result from "electrotonically mediated" impulse transmission moving to-and-fro across the same excitable segment, or across an inexcitable gap, which generates a closely coupled reflected reentry (Antzelevitch, 2013). This mechanism has been demonstrated in isolated atrial and ventricular myocardium and in Purkinje fibers. Phase 2 reentry also does not depend on circus movement; however, it can appear to be of focal origin. Phase 2 reentry requires marked spatial dispersion of repolarization. It occurs when the action potential dome propagates from a site (usually epicardial) where it is maintained to a site at which it is abolished, causing local epicardial reexcitation and a closely coupled extrasystole.

Cardiac and Hemodynamic Consequences

The hemodynamic effects of an arrhythmia depend on a number of factors. These include the ventricular activation rate, arrhythmia duration, temporal relation between atrial and ventricular contractions, sequence or coordination of ventricular activation, drug therapy, the animal's activity level, and effects of any underlying disease on cardiac function. Arrhythmias that compromise cardiac output (CO) and coronary perfusion promote hypotension, myocardial ischemia, impaired pump function, and sometimes, sudden death. These arrhythmias tend to be either very rapid (such as sustained ventricular or supraventricular tachycardias; **Figure 23.5**) or very slow (such as high-grade AV block with a slow or unstable ventricular escape rhythm).

Effects of Heart Rate

CO depends on HR and the factors that influence stroke volume (SV; p. 15). Within a physiologic range and in normal hearts, increases in HR are accompanied by increases in myocardial contractility and relaxation, and therefore, CO. However, excessively fast ventricular rates reduce CO once diastole becomes too short to support adequate ventricular filling. Conversely, when HR is excessively slow, CO might be inadequate to support the animal's activity level if SV cannot increase enough. Structural heart disease exacerbates these effects.

Inadequate CO can promote systemic hypotension and poor tissue perfusion. Hypotension also reduces coronary perfusion pressure (that is, mean aortic pressure minus right atrial pressure). Rapid tachycardias, in particular, promote myocardial ischemia because they reduce coronary perfusion pressure and markedly abbreviate diastole (when most coronary blood flow occurs). Thus, rapid VT could degenerate quickly into VF. Supraventricular tachycardia (SVT) could promote secondary ventricular arrhythmias related to poor myocardial perfusion, ischemia, and increased sympathetic stimulation.

Persistent tachycardia of either supraventricular or ventricular origin (with ventricular rates ≥180–200 beats/minute in dogs, or >100–120 beats/minute in horses) will cause myocardial systolic dysfunction within a few weeks. This is known as "tachycardia-induced cardiomyopathy" (TICM; p. 630). In addition, AF with an uncontrolled ventricular response rate and very frequent ventricular premature beats also can lead to myocardial failure. Therefore, the umbrella term of "arrhythmia-induced cardiomyopathy" sometimes is applied, rather than TICM. All these persistent tachyarrhythmias can produce myocardial structural and functional changes, chamber enlargement, and neurohormonal (NH) activation that mimic spontaneous cardiomyopathy. However, TICM usually is reversible if HR can be controlled within a few weeks of its onset.

Ineffective Atrial Contraction

The loss of effective atrial contraction (the atrial kick), which occurs with AF or atrial standstill, reduces maximum ventricular end-diastolic volume (preload). At slower heart rates, this is clinically inconsequential for most cases because the contribution of atrial contraction to total ventricular filling is relatively small. However as HR increases, the relative importance of atrial contraction also increases. The atrial kick can contribute up to 30% (or even more) of total ventricular end-diastolic volume at high HRs. Therefore, during exercise or with heart failure, the loss of atrial contraction can have a pronounced detrimental effect on CO.

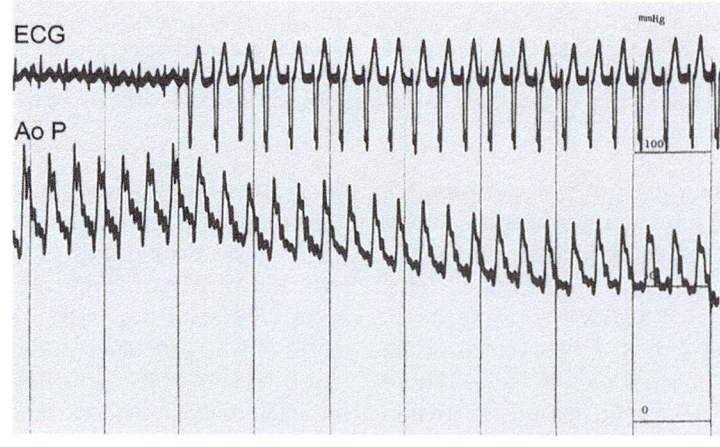

Figure 23.5 The electrocardiogram (ECG, top) shows the onset of sustained ventricular tachycardia, which leads to progressive decline in aortic blood pressure (AoP, bottom). Pressure scale, from 0 to 100 mm Hg, indicated on the right. (Image courtesy of Dr RL Hamlin.)

Loss of Atrioventricular Synchrony

AV synchrony is lost when the atria and ventricles beat at different rates. This can occur with various premature beats and abnormal tachycardias, during 3rd degree AV block (with a ventricular escape rhythm), and with accelerated ventricular-origin rhythms, including an artificially paced ventricular rhythm. With AV dyssynchrony, the temporal relationship between atrial and ventricular contractions varies. The atria might contract simultaneously with the ventricles, which essentially is an ineffective atrial contraction because no atrial blood can enter the ventricles when the AV valves are closed. Regurgitant pulse waves (cannon a waves; **Figure 15.5**, p. 264) might be visualized in the jugular veins or by Doppler echocardiographic recordings of the pulmonary veins. Conversely, an atrial contraction might, by chance, be perfectly timed to maximize ventricular filling prior to ventricular contraction. However, for most heartbeats, the AV timing will lie between these extremes and the atrial kick will range from suboptimal to absent. Consequently, CO can suffer.

Ventricular Dyssynchrony

In addition to AV dyssynchrony, both intra- and interventricular dyssynchrony can occur with arrhythmias. Interventricular dyssynchrony involves delayed or incoordinated activation and contraction of one ventricle compared to the other; it can be quantified by Doppler echocardiographic recordings of aortic versus pulmonary artery ejection times. Intraventricular dyssynchrony usually relates the activation sequence of the ventricular septum compared to the left ventricular free wall, as viewed by M-mode echocardiography or advanced tissue imaging methods including strain imaging. Ventricular tachyarrhythmias typically cause some degree of ventricular dyssynchrony; this can exacerbate the arrhythmia's negative impact on CO at any given HR. Left and right bundle branch blocks also cause dyssynchronous ventricular contractions, which could reduce CO depending on HR and myocardial function. Artificial cardiac pacing using a single ventricular lead similarly results in a degree of dyssynchronous ventricular activation and contraction. Especially in animals with underlying myocardial disease, ventricular dyssynchrony can contribute to deteriorating cardiac function, even without overt intraventricular conduction delay or ventricular tachyarrhythmias.

Clinical Causes and Associations of Arrhythmias

Arrhythmias are associated with many cardiac, as well as noncardiac, conditions (**Table 23.1**). Although the electrophysiologic mechanism of a particular arrhythmia might be uncertain, the clinical association is perhaps more important to understand since it influences prognosis and therapy. The multitude of associated conditions usually can be grouped into five general categories:

- Primary cardiac diseases (structural or electrical abnormalities, often genetically predisposed)
- Metabolic or endocrine disorders
- Autonomic nervous system-related arrhythmias
- Effects of drugs or toxins
- Noncardiac disorders that can induce arrhythmias by causing ischemia-reperfusion injury, cytokine release, altered autonomic traffic, or unknown mechanisms

The diagnostic workup for most arrhythmias includes a search for structural cardiac disease. Heart rhythm disturbances can be the initial manifestation of various cardiomyopathies, even before overt structural changes occur. The majority of cats with persistent arrhythmias, if not related to a metabolic or systemic disease, will have some form of cardiomyopathy. Congenital heart defects often are accompanied by arrhythmias, including subvalvular aortic stenosis in dogs. Animals with an anomalous AV nodal bypass tract (whether concealed or with overt preexcitation), including Labrador Retrievers with tricuspid valve dysplasia, are predisposed to macro-reentrant SVT. Heart size also is relevant; for example, even in otherwise normal hearts "lone" AF develops more easily in horses and large-breed dogs, related to their large atrial size and ability to maintain reentry. Myocardial stretch, hypertrophy, fibrosis, and ischemia can promote arrhythmias through various electrophysiologic mechanisms. Myocardial ischemia can alter the cellular environment of affected tissues, causing localized acidosis, hypoxia, and hyperkalemia; such changes are not necessarily manifested systemically. These metabolic derangements severely depress cell-to-cell conduction and can induce afterdepolarizations and triggered ectopy. In addition, clinicians should always consider iatrogenic causes of arrhythmias, including administration of L-thyroxine and drugs such as digoxin, sedatives, and sympathomimetic agents. Cardiotoxins and poisonous plants are important considerations, especially in horses. The large group of noncardiac disorders that cause arrhythmias includes sepsis, anemia, gastric dilatation, colic, and splenic disease (in dogs).

Understanding the arrhythmia's likely clinical association can guide the choice of specific treatments and duration of therapy, and might inform prognosis. Yet even healthy animals, especially of older age, are known to have occasional ventricular and supraventricular premature complexes. Clinically inapparent areas of myocardial fibrosis or inflammation might underlie these.

Autonomic imbalance, with either high sympathetic or vagal tone, can trigger atrial premature activity even in animals with apparently normal atrial structure. High vagal tone shortens the atrial action potential duration by opening acetylcholine dependent potassium channels. This can facilitate reentrant arrhythmias. Atrial premature activity could lead to sustained atrial tachycardia, flutter or AF, especially in animals with advanced underlying cardiac disease and atrial

Table 23.1 Factors Predisposing to Arrhythmias[a]

Cardiac
- Congestive heart failure, from any cause
- Cardiomyopathies, including
  - Arrhythmogenic right (or left) ventricular
  - Dilated
  - Hypertrophic
  - Restrictive and fibrotic forms
- Other myocardial disorders
  - Myocarditis (infectious or noninfectious)
  - Toxic injury (doxorubicin, ionophores, poisonous plants)
  - Myocardial ischemia and reperfusion injury
  - Myocardial fibrosis
  - Cardiac neoplasia, primary (hemangiosarcoma, others) and metastatic
  - Ventricular or atrial dilation or acute stretch
  - Myocardial trauma or cardiac contusion
  - Acquired or congenital ion channelopathies
- Mechanical stimulation (intracardiac catheter, pacing wire)
- Degenerative or infective valvular diseases
- Congenital heart diseases, especially
  - Ventricular outflow tract obstructions (aortic and pulmonary stenoses)
  - Mitral or tricuspid dysplasia
  - Accessory AV nodal bypass tracts (often concurrent with AV valve dysplasia)
- Pericarditis and pericardial effusions
- Pulmonary hypertension and cor pulmonale
  - Heartworm disease

Extracardiac
- High sympathetic tone or catecholamine effects (including drugs and pheochromocytoma)
- Central nervous system disease (causing increases in sympathetic or vagal stimulation)
- High vagal tone of other causes
- Drugs and toxins
  - Digoxin and digitalis-glycoside containing plants
  - Antiarrhythmic drugs
  - Catecholamines and sympathomimetic bronchodilators
  - Thyroid hormone supplementation
  - Sedatives, tranquilizers, and anesthetic agents
  - Poisonous plants including white snake root, oleander, taxus, avocado leaves, among others
  - Cardiotoxic drugs (including doxorubicin, ionophores)
  - Envenomations and insect toxins, including venomous snakebites, toad poisoning (*Buffo marinus*), cantharidin (blister beetles)
  - Cobalt
- Hypoxia
- Severe anemia
- Pulmonary disease (including cor pulmonale)
- Trauma (thoracic or abdominal)
- Fever
- Infections, sepsis or endotoxemia
- Systemic inflammatory disease
- Hypothermia
- Electrolyte imbalances, especially
  - Hypokalemia
  - Hyperkalemia
  - Hypomagnesemia
- Acidosis or alkalosis
- Electric shock
- Thoracic surgery
- Abdominal and gastrointestinal diseases, including
  - Gastric dilatation, with or without volvulus
  - Colic
  - Pancreatitis
  - Splenic mass or splenectomy, including
    - Hemangiosarcoma
  - Uremia and acute kidney injury
- Endocrine diseases, including
  - Hypoadrenocorticism
  - Hyper- or hypothyroidism
  - Diabetes mellitus
  - Pheochromocytoma

[a] Some factors fit into more than one category.
Abbreviation: AV, atrioventricular.

enlargement (remodeling). It might facilitate development of AF in horses and large-breed dogs without overt heart disease, too. Increased sympathetic (and reduced vagal) activity also can promote ventricular tachyarrhythmias.

Measures of heart rate variability (in time- or frequency-domain) can be derived from continuous ECG recordings to provide insight into the patient's underlying balance between sympathetic and vagal tone. Scatterplots of successive R-R intervals (Poincaré or Lorenz plots) obtained during sinus rhythm also reflect sympathovagal input. Certain visual patterns on such plots have been associated with various arrhythmias. For further detail, see sources in "Suggested Additional Reading and References" and the on-line Bibliography.

Accelerated idioventricular rhythms commonly appear after trauma, with primary gastrointestinal diseases, and after prolonged anesthesia, as well as in other circumstances. These generally are benign rhythms, with the ventricular-origin beat arising only during longer sinus intervals. In contrast, several clinical conditions are associated with frequent ventricular tachyarrhythmias and higher risk of sudden cardiac death. Most of these involve marked structural heart disease, although some do not. Sometimes a lethal arrhythmia (such as VF; **Figure 23.6**) is triggered by a single premature activation, without prior sustained arrhythmia and clinical manifestations. Often it is proceeded by a brief period of polymorphic ventricular tachycardia that soon degenerates

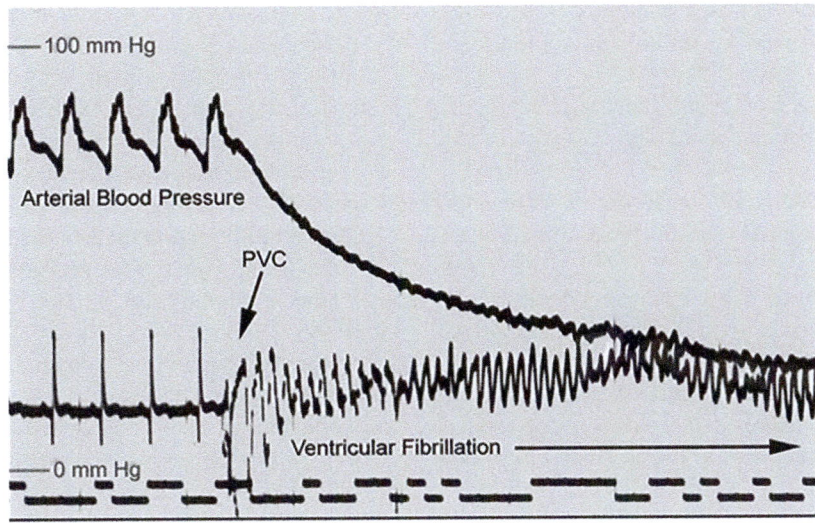

Figure 23.6 Electrocardiogram (bottom trace) from a dog that initially was in sinus rhythm. A single premature ventricular complex (PVC) provoked the onset of ventricular fibrillation. Arterial blood pressure (top trace) plummeted as soon as effective ventricular contractions ceased. (Image courtesy of Dr RL Hamlin.)

to fibrillation. Cardiomyopathies, especially in Doberman Pinschers and Boxers (Chapter 32), often convey a higher risk for sudden death, even in dogs with relatively normal myocardial function. Cardiac diseases associated with marked ventricular hypertrophy (and greater likelihood for ischemia) also are associated with sudden death. Severe subaortic stenosis (p. 480) and hypertrophic cardiomyopathy (p. 649 and p. 629) are examples.

Abnormalities of ion channels involved in cardiac depolarization or repolarization (channelopathies), or of cardiac sympathetic innervation or mitochondrial function, can underlie serious arrhythmias even in the absence of gross structural lesions. Familial ventricular arrhythmia syndromes in some lines of German Shepherd, Rhodesian Ridgeback, and Leonberger dogs are known to cause sudden arrhythmic death in affected young dogs (Moise, 1997; Meurs, 2016; Wiberg, 2020). Affected Rhodesian Ridgebacks typically are under 2–3 years of age and display an autosomal recessive inheritance pattern. An associated gene mutation was recently identified (Meurs, 2019). Acquired repolarization abnormalities associated with certain drugs (examples in **Table 5.7**, p. 158), electrolyte disturbances, and other conditions increase the risk of arrhythmias and even sudden death. Although rare, congenital QT interval prolongation with sudden death (long QT syndrome) was documented in a family of English Springer Spaniels (**Figure 5.56**, p. 159, and **Figure 23.3**); affected dogs had a mutated gene associated with the cardiac repolarizing current I_{Ks} (Ware, 2015).

In horses, lone AF is the arrhythmia most often requiring assessment and management. Ventricular arrhythmias seem less common than those of atrial origin, and are more likely to be associated with structural heart disease or serious systemic illness. Nevertheless, occasional ventricular premature complexes detected immediately postexercise, or that disappear during exercise, often are not of clinical concern. In contrast, those that persist or increase in frequency during exercise can not only reduce performance, but also could indicate greater risk for collapse. More complex ventricular tachyarrhythmias and rapid supraventricular tachyarrhythmias (including AF) pose a safety risk to horse and rider. Horses with these rhythm disturbances generally should not be ridden or worked (Chapters 30 and 34).

Suggested Additional Reading and References

Also See Online Comprehensive Bibliography at: https://www.routledge.com/9781482246223.

Abriel H, Zaklyazminskaya EV. Cardiac channelopathies: genetic and molecular mechanisms. Gene 2013;517:1–11.

Antzelevitch C, Burashnikov A. Mechanisms of cardiac arrhythmia. In, Gussak I, Antzelevitch C (editors), Electrical Diseases of the Heart. Springer-Verlag, London. 2013. pp. 93–128.

Blake RR, Shaw DJ, Culshaw GJ, et al. Poincaré plots as a measure of heart rate variability in healthy dogs. J Vet Cardiol 2018;20:20–32.

Bruler BC, Jojima FS, Dittrich G, et al. QT instability, an indicator of augmented arrhythmogenesis, increases with the progression of myxomatous mitral valve disease in dogs. J Vet Cardiol 2018;20:254–266.

Buhl R, Carstensen H, Hesselkilde EZ, et al. Effect of induced chronic atrial fibrillation on exercise performance in Standardbred trotters. J Vet Intern Med 2018;32:1410–1419.

Campbell FE, Atwell RB. Long QT syndrome in dogs with tick toxicity (Ixodes holocyclus). Aust Vet J 2002;80:611–616.

Coronel R, Wilders R, Verkerk AO, et al. Electrophysiological changes in heart failure and their implications for arrhythmogenesis. Biochim Biophys Acta 2013;1832:2432–2441.

Cruickshank J, Quaas RL, Li J, et al. Genetic analysis of ventricular arrhythmia in young German Shepherd dogs. J Vet Intern Med 2009;23:264–270.

DeProspero DJ, Adin DB. Visual representations of canine cardiac arrhythmias with Lorenz (Poincaré) plots. Am J Vet Res 2020;81:720–731.

Doytchinova A, Patel J, Zhou S, et al. Subcutaneous nerve activity and spontaneous ventricular arrhythmias in ambulatory dogs. Heart Rhythm 2015;12:612–620.

Dunnink A, Stams TRG, Bossu A, et al. Torsade de pointes arrhythmias arise at the site of maximal heterogeneity of repolarization in the chronic complete atrioventricular block dog. Europace 2017;19:858–865.

Flethoj M, Kanters JK, Haugaard MM, et al. Changes in heart rate, arrhythmia frequency, and cardiac biomarker values in horses during recovery after a long-distance endurance ride. J Am Vet Med Assoc 2016;248:1034–1042.

Gladuli A, Moise NS, Hemsley SA, et al. Poincaré plots and tachograms reveal beat patterning in sick sinus syndrome with supraventricular tachycardia and varying AV nodal block. J Vet Cardiol 2011;13:63–70.

Hamlin RL. Animal models of ventricular arrhythmias. Pharmacol Ther 2007;113:276–295.

Jesty SA, Jung SW, Cordeiro JM, et al. Cardiomyocyte calcium cycling in a naturally occurring German shepherd dog model of inherited ventricular arrhythmia and sudden cardiac death. J Vet Cardiol 2013;15:5–14.

Kalyanasundaram A, Li N, Hansen BJ, et al. Canine and human sinoatrial node: differences and similarities in the structure, function, molecular profiles, and arrhythmia. J Vet Cardiol 2019;22:2–19.

Kiryu K, Machida N, Kashida Y, et al. Pathologic and electrocardiographic findings in sudden cardiac death in racehorses. J Vet Med Sci 1999;61:921–928.

Kovach JA, Nearing BD, Verrier RL. Angerlike behavioral state potentiates myocardial ischemia-induced T-wave alternans in canines. J Am Coll Cardiol 2001;37:1719–1725.

Lyle CH, Blissitt KJ, Kennedy RN, et al. Risk factors for race-associated sudden death in Thoroughbred racehorses in the UK (2000–2007). Equine Vet J 2012;44:459–465.

Meurs KM, Friedenberg SG, Olby NJ, et al. A QIL1 variant associated with ventricular arrhythmias and sudden cardiac death in the juvenile Rhodesian Ridgeback dog. Genes 2019;10:168–178.

Meurs KM, Weidman JA, Rosenthal SL, et al. Ventricular arrhythmias in Rhodesian Ridgebacks with a family history of sudden death and results of a pedigree analysis for potential inheritance patterns. J Am Vet Med Assoc 2016;248:1135–1138.

Moise NS, Gilmour RF Jr., Riccio ML. An animal model of spontaneous arrhythmic death. J Cardiovasc Electrophysiol 1997;8:98–103.

Navas de Solis C. Exercising arrhythmias and sudden cardiac death in horses: review of the literature and comparative aspects. Equine Vet J 2016;48:406–413.

Obreztchikova MN, Sosunov EA, Anyukhovsky EP, et al. Heterogeneous ventricular repolarization provides a substrate for arrhythmias in a German shepherd model of spontaneous arrhythmic death. Circulation 2003;108:1389–1394.

Porteiro Vazquez DM, Perego M, Santos L, et al. Paroxysmal atrial fibrillation in seven dogs with presumed neurally-mediated syncope. J Vet Cardiol 2016;18:1–9.

Renier AC, Kass PH, Magdesian KG, et al. Oleander toxicosis in equids: 30 cases (1995–2010). J Am Vet Med Assoc 2013;242:540–549.

Shu C, Huang W, Zeng Z, et al. Connexin 43 is involved in the sympathetic atrial fibrillation in canine and canine atrial myocytes. Anatol J Cardiol 2017;18:3–9.

Veenhuyzen GD, Quinn FR. Principles of entrainment: diagnostic utility for supraventricular tachycardia. Indian Pacing Electrophysiol J 2008;8:51–65.

Ware WA, Reina-Doreste Y, Stern JA, et al. Sudden death associated with QT interval prolongation and KCNQ1 gene mutation in a family of English Springer Spaniels. J Vet Intern Med 2015;29:561–568.

Wiberg M, Niskanen JE, Hytonen M, et al. Ventricular arrhythmia and sudden cardiac death in young Leonbergers. J Vet Cardiol 2020;27:10–22.

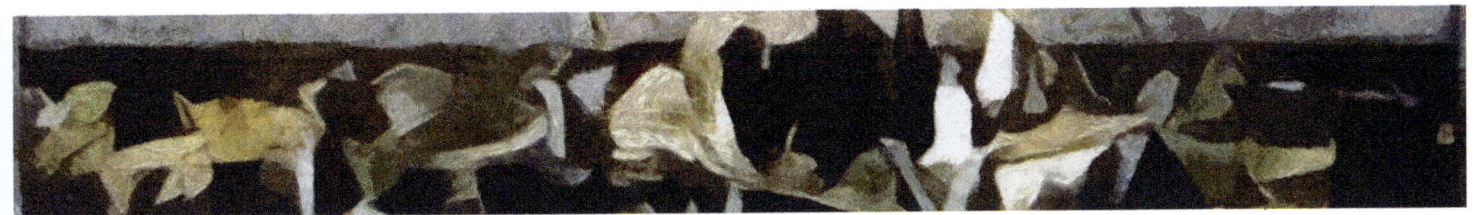

24
ANTIARRHYTHMIC THERAPIES

Antiarrhythmic drugs variously can suppress premature complexes and slow or terminate a tachycardia. These effects are achieved by terminating reentry, or preventing abnormal impulse formation or conduction (Chapter 23). Some antiarrhythmic drugs can stimulate pacemaker activity or enhance conduction in cardiac tissues. These actions can occur through modulation of tissue electrophysiologic properties or the autonomic nervous system. Unfortunately, antiarrhythmic drugs also can promote arrhythmias in certain patients, as well as cause noncardiac-related adverse effects.

Drug Classification Systems

The traditional (Vaughan Williams) antiarrhythmic drug classification scheme divides drugs into four classes based on their predominant electrophysiologic effect on cardiac action potentials (**Table 24.1**; **Figure 24.1**). This classification system is suboptimal, however, because it excludes some drugs with antiarrhythmic effects (such as digoxin and atropine), pigeonholes drugs with effects that bridge multiple classes, and groups some quite dissimilar drugs within the same class. Furthermore, its focus on electrophysiologic blocking mechanisms, rather than ion channel or receptor activation, has constrained its value as new information becomes available. Sometimes, a designation of Class V is used to group drugs with antiarrhythmic properties that work by mechanisms other than those described in the original four classes. A second classification scheme (the Sicilian Gambit) was proposed to categorize antiarrhythmic drugs by their actions on underlying arrhythmia mechanisms, with emphasis on how they affect ion currents, membrane pumps, and receptors. This approach has not markedly facilitated clinical arrhythmia management, especially in veterinary medicine where electrophysiologic studies rarely are done. Thus, the traditional classification system remains in common veterinary use, and will serve as the framework for this chapter. Nevertheless, another extensive categorization has been proposed which builds on the Vaughan Williams system, but also incorporates the electrophysiologic tenants of the Sicilian Gambit (**Table 24.2**; Lei, 2018). This newer classification system includes a Class 0 (for drugs that block the hyperpolarization-activated, HCN, channels, including the pacemaker or "funny" current, I_f).

Vaughan Williams class I agents have membrane-stabilizing effects that tend to slow conduction, as well as decrease automaticity and increase refractoriness (decrease excitability). The "traditional" ventricular antiarrhythmic drugs belong to this class. Class II consists of beta-adrenergic antagonists, which act by inhibiting catecholamine effects on the heart. Class III drugs are potassium channel blockers (nonspecific or targeted channels) that prolong the effective refractory period of cardiac action potentials without decreasing conduction velocity; these class III agents could be most effective in suppressing reentrant arrhythmias or in preventing (atrial and ventricular) fibrillation. Class IV contains calcium-entry blocking drugs. These are most useful for supraventricular tachyarrhythmias; ventricular arrhythmias usually are unresponsive to these drugs. More information about specific agents is found below. Suggested drug dosages are listed in **Table 25.2** (p. 402); methods for constant rate infusion (CRI) dosage are described in **Table 25.3** (p. 411).

Other drugs also can be useful against some arrhythmias. These include digoxin, anticholinergic agents, catecholamines, and some drugs not typically considered to have antiarrhythmic effects. These are included in the enhanced classification scheme shown in **Table 24.2**. Modification of certain modulating factors involved in arrhythmogenesis could prevent some arrhythmias. For example, factors involved in the cardiac remodeling associated with

Table 24.1 Traditional Classification of Antiarrhythmic Drugs

Class	Drug	Mechanism and ECG Effects
I		Decreases fast inward Na$^+$ current; membrane-stabilizing effects (slowed conduction, decreased excitability and automaticity)
Ia	quinidine, procainamide	Moderately slows conduction, increases action potential duration; can prolong QRS complex and QT interval
Ib	lidocaine, mexiletine, phenytoin	Little change in conductivity, decreases action potential duration; QRS complex and QT interval unchanged
Ic	flecainide, propafenone, encainide	Markedly slows conduction without change in action potential duration
II	propranolol, atenolol, metoprolol, esmolol, carvedilol, others	Beta-adrenergic blockade, reduces effects of sympathetic stimulation (no direct myocardial effects at clinical doses)
III	sotalol, amiodarone, ibutilide, dofetilide, dronedarone, others	Selectively prolongs action potential duration and refractory period; antiadrenergic effects; QT interval prolonged
IV	diltiazem, verapamil	Decreases slow inward Ca^{++} current (greatest effect on SA and AV nodes)
Other drugs with antiarrhythmic effects include:	digoxin	Antiarrhythmic action results mainly from indirect autonomic effects, especially increased vagal tone, as well as some direct effects
	atropine, other anticholinergic agents	Opposes vagal effects on SA and AV nodes
	some sympathomimetic agents	Increases sinus node activation and AV conduction
	ivabradine	Inhibits the I_f to reduce sinus node rate

various heart diseases (Chapter 20) can facilitate arrhythmia development, including catecholamines, free radicals, angiotensin II, cytokines, and nitric oxide. Suppression of these factors could reduce arrhythmia frequency or severity. Angiotensin converting enzyme (ACE) inhibitors, angiotensin receptor blocker (ARB) drugs, and omega–3 polyunsaturated fatty acids (in fish oil) can have "upstream" benefits on myocardial substrates; these have antiarrhythmic effects in people, and potentially in animals. For example, there is limited evidence for omega–3 fatty acids reducing ectopy in dogs with arrhythmogenic right ventricular cardiomyopathy (ARVC; also known as arrhythmogenic cardiomyopathy). Some evidence suggests that statin drugs also might play a role in arrhythmia suppression by virtue of their antioxidant and antiinflammatory properties; however, clinical veterinary experience with this is lacking. The increased survival in human heart failure patients receiving ACE inhibitors, spironolactone, and some beta-blockers is consistent with this concept.

Antiarrhythmic Drugs

While there are different approaches to classifying antiarrhythmic drugs, as noted previously, the following discussion uses the traditional four-class system of Vaughan Williams and includes additional comments about antiarrhythmic drugs that fall outside this system.

Class I Antiarrhythmic Drugs

These agents block membrane "fast" Na$^+$ channels and depress the action potential upstroke (phase 0). This slows conduction velocity, and could interrupt reentrant rhythms. Class I drugs are subclassified according to additional electrophysiologic characteristics that affect action potential duration and cell refractoriness and excitability. Agents in this class block cardiac Na$^+$ channels in what is termed a "use-dependent" manner. This behavior causes the drugs to bind increasingly to the Na$^+$ channels at faster stimulation rates; this property

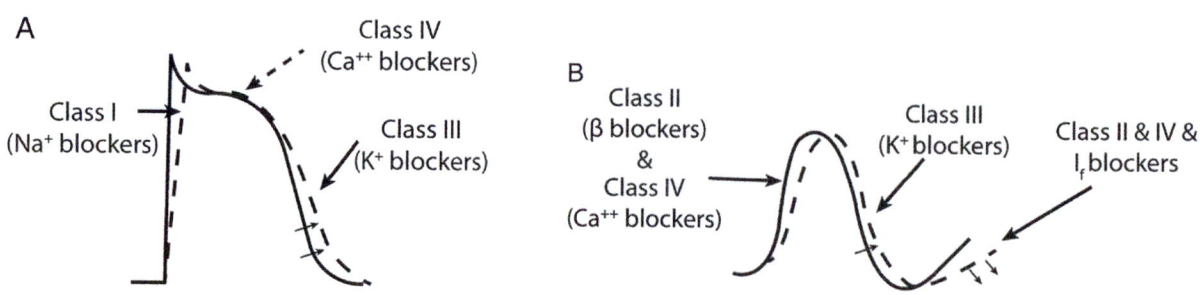

Figure 24.1 Schematic diagrams showing the major effects of antiarrhythmic drugs on (A) the fast response action potential and (B) the slow response (pacemaker) action potential.

Table 24.2 A Modernized Classification of Antiarrhythmic Drugs

Class	Description*	Example(s)
0	HCN channel blockers	Includes the I_f blocker, ivabradine
I	Voltage-gated, sodium channel blockers	Ia to Ic: similar to Vaughan Williams classification; Id – late current blocker (ranolazine)
II	Autonomic inhibitors and activators	Five subclasses that include beta-adrenergic blockers (atenolol, others) and activators (isoproterenol); muscarinic M_2 blockers (atropine, others) & activators (also includes digoxin); and adenosine A_1 receptor activators
III	Potassium channel blockers and openers	Three subclasses; IIIa – blockers of various K+ channels (including amiodarone, sotalol, ibutilide, and dofetilide). Also, metabolically dependent K+ channel openers or transmitter dependent K+ channel blockers (investigational drugs).
IV	Calcium handling modulators	Five subclasses of drugs that block (including diltiazem, flecainide & propafenone) or activate Ca^{++} movement
V	Mechanosensitive calcium blockers	Affect intracellular Ca^{++} signaling and afterdepolarizations (all drugs are investigational)
VI	Gap junction channel blockers	Drugs are investigational (carbenoxolone)
VII	Upstream target modulators	Reduce structural and electrophysiological remodeling; Includes ACE inhibitors, ARBs and omega-3 fatty acids

* This table provides only an overview of the scheme; see Lei M, Wu L, Terrar DA, et al. Modernized classification of cardiac antiarrhythmic drugs. Circulation 2018;138:1879–1896 for complete details.

Abbreviations: ACE, angiotensin converting enzyme; ARB, angiotensin receptor blocker; HCN, hyperpolarization-activated cyclic nucleotide-gated (channel); I_f, funny current.

is prominent in class Ib drugs. The kinetics of channel binding and dissociation vary for different class I drugs, which likely explains in part their efficacy against specific rhythm disturbances (**Table 24.1**). The electrophysiologic effects of class I drugs are extremely dependent on extracellular K+ concentration; hypokalemia can render these drugs ineffective, whereas moderate to severe (systemic or local) hyperkalemia and acidosis intensify their depressant effects on conduction. All these agents are contraindicated in animals with complete heart block and should be used only cautiously in animals with sinus bradycardia, sick sinus syndrome (SSS), and 1st or 2nd degree atrioventricular (AV) block.

Lidocaine Lidocaine hydrochloride (HCl; class Ib) generally is the agent of first choice for acute (intravenous, IV) therapy of ventricular tachyarrhythmias in dogs. It is used in cats and horses as well. Lidocaine usually is ineffective against supraventricular arrhythmias; however, it might induce conversion of recent onset, vagally mediated atrial fibrillation (AF) or supraventricular tachycardia (SVT) in some dogs, especially those with macro-reentrant SVT associated with an accessory pathway (Wright, 2019). Only lidocaine without epinephrine should be used for antiarrhythmic therapy. Lidocaine at standard doses has little effect on sinus rate, AV conduction velocity, and refractoriness. Lidocaine suppresses automaticity in normal Purkinje fibers and diseased myocardium, slows conduction, and reduces the dispersion of refractoriness, especially in ischemic tissues, thus reducing the likelihood of ventricular fibrillation (VF). Its effects are greater on diseased and hypoxic cardiac cells and at faster stimulation rates (use-dependence). Like other class I drugs, lidocaine's electrophysiologic effects are dependent on extracellular K+ concentrations; hypokalemia could make the drug ineffective, while moderate to severe hyperkalemia intensifies its depressant effect on cell-to-cell conduction. Lidocaine produces little or no depression of contractility when given slowly IV at therapeutic doses. Therapeutic plasma concentrations in people are 0.5–2 mcg/mL.

Lidocaine is metabolized rapidly in the liver; some metabolites are active and can contribute to toxicity. The drug is not effective orally (PO) because of almost complete first-pass hepatic elimination. Lidocaine is administered as slow IV boluses followed by CRI. Intramuscular (IM) administration could be considered if IV access is not possible, but IV is much preferred. Antiarrhythmic effects after an IV bolus occur within 2 minutes and abate within 10–20 minutes in dogs. CRI without a loading dose produces steady-state concentrations in 4–6 hours. The half-life is less than 1 hour in the dog, ~1.7 hours in cats, and ~3 hours in horses. In cats under isoflurane anesthesia, lidocaine's half-life is shorter (only ~1 hour) although higher initial serum concentrations are achieved; other pharmacokinetic properties also are affected by isoflurane anesthesia. Lidocaine has induced cardiodepressive effects and increased mean arterial blood pressure (BP) in isoflurane-anesthetized cats. In anesthetized horses, serum concentration rises rapidly after IV bolus and declines quickly after infusion is stopped, with a terminal half-life of ~1 hour +/−30 minutes. Protein binding of lidocaine is moderate. Hepatic disease and poor liver blood flow can slow lidocaine's extraction and metabolism, and predispose to toxicity, especially in cats and horses. Heart failure and drugs such as propranolol, cimetidine, chloramphenicol, halothane, and others can decrease liver blood flow and slow lidocaine clearance.

Excessively high doses of lidocaine can cause hypotension. Most often, however, lidocaine's toxic effects relate to the central nervous system (CNS). They include agitation, disorientation, mental depression, ataxia, muscle twitches, nystagmus, and generalized seizures. The latter might require diazepam (0.25–0.5 mg/kg IV) or a short-acting barbiturate. Nausea also can occur. Toxicity signs usually dissipate shortly after the drug is discontinued; a lower infusion rate can be reinstituted as needed. Arrhythmia worsening (proarrhythmia) occurs occasionally, as with any drug that has cardiac electrophysiologic effects. Cats are particularly sensitive to lidocaine's toxic effects; bradycardia and respiratory arrest can occur, along with seizures. There are anecdotal reports of respiratory depression and arrest after lidocaine administration to unconscious dogs and cats. Use of small IV boluses (0.5 mg/kg) at 5–10 minute intervals helps minimize severe toxicity in cats, as does controlled dosing via CRI. Lipid emulsion infusion has been used successfully to treat lidocaine toxicity in a cat. Similar to cats, horses also are relatively more sensitive to lidocaine's CNS toxic effects. Rapid administration or excessive doses (such as ≥1.5 mg/kg) can cause nervousness, excitement, sweating, tachycardia, and occasionally, seizure activity in horses.

Procainamide Procainamide HCl (Class Ia) is used infrequently today, despite long experience with the drug in veterinary medicine. Procainamide is similar to quinidine in its electrophysiologic effects; however, it causes less QT prolongation, less hypotension, and no interaction with digoxin. Procainamide has both direct and indirect (vagolytic) effects. It is indicated for ventricular (and sometimes supraventricular) tachyarrhythmias, but generally is less effective than quinidine for atrial tachyarrhythmias. However, IV administration sometimes terminates atrial flutter or fibrillation and can facilitate electrocardioversion in some horses and in dogs. Procainamide prolongs the effective refractory period and slows conduction in the accessory pathway of dogs with orthodromic AV reciprocating tachycardia. Procainamide should be used only cautiously in hypotensive animals.

Procainamide is well-absorbed orally in dogs although food may delay absorption; however, its half-life is only 2.5–4 hours (3–6 hours for sustained-release procainamide). Protein-binding is fairly low in dogs. In horses, procainamide's half-life is ~3.5–7 hours; PO bioavailability is low. The drug undergoes hepatic metabolism and renal excretion. The metabolite N-acetylprocainamide is not present to any significant degree in dogs and cats, although it is produced in horses. N-acetylprocainamide has class III-like effects and a longer half-life than procainamide. The drug induces lupus erythematosus in people (especially slow acetylators) and is rarely used now. Oral procainamide currently is not available in the United States, and IV formulations are quite expensive.

Rapid IV injection of procainamide can produce hypotension from cardiac depression and vasodilation, although to a lesser degree than quinidine. IM administration is effective and does not cause marked hemodynamic effects. Subcutaneous absorption of the drug has been documented in dogs. Procainamide CRI is useful for arrhythmias that respond to an IV bolus. In dogs without heart failure, a 2 mg/kg IV bolus administered slowly and repeated every five minutes can be given, up to a 15 to 20 mg/kg cumulative dosage. BP and ECG monitoring are recommended at higher dosages. Steady state concentration occurs in 12–22 hours. Therapeutic plasma range in dogs is 4–12 mcg/mL. Serum concentration could be measured 4–5 hours after an oral procainamide dose (or 8 hours after a sustained release preparation). In horses, graded IV doses appear well tolerated up to a cumulative dose of 10 mg/kg; however, arterial BP and the QRS and QT interval durations on ECG should be monitored. The drug has been used in a similar manner in cats. Procainamide often is administered with a beta-blocker or another class I agent (usually lidocaine) for treating refractory ventricular arrhythmias. Procainamide can increase the ventricular response rate to AF (because of its vagolytic effect) if used without digoxin or a beta- or calcium channel blocker.

Procainamide's toxic effects are similar to, but usually milder than, those of quinidine. Gastrointestinal (GI) upset and QRS or QT interval prolongation can occur. More serious toxic effects include hypotension, depressed AV conduction (sometimes causing 2nd or 3rd degree AV block), and worsening of arrhythmias, which can lead to polymorphic ventricular tachycardia (VT) and syncope or VF. IV fluids, phenylephrine or other catecholamines, or Ca^{++}-containing solutions can be used to treat hypotension. Adverse GI signs associated with oral procainamide (if available) might respond to dosage reduction. Long-term use has caused brown discoloration of the haircoat in Doberman Pinschers and Boxers.

Quinidine Quinidine (class Ia) is rarely used in small animals today, although it is still available for human use; chemical grade quinidine is (rarely) given for cardiac disease. A related drug, disopyramide, is available but causes significant myocardial depression, and mainly is used in humans to treat hypertrophic obstructive cardiomyopathy. Quinidine potentially is useful for treating ventricular and some supraventricular tachyarrhythmias if other drugs or strategies are unavailable or ineffective. Currently, quinidine's major veterinary indication is the conversion of lone AF to sinus rhythm in horses, and rarely, in large-breed dogs. It must be given cautiously, if at all, to animals with heart failure or abnormal serum K^+ concentration. Quinidine characteristically depresses automaticity and conduction velocity and prolongs the effective refractory period. Corresponding dose-dependent ECG changes (prolonged PR, QRS, and QT intervals) result from its direct electrophysiologic effects. However, the drug's vagolytic effects can offset its direct effects and increase the sinus rate or the ventricular response rate to AF. This latter complication is observed commonly in horses as atrial fibrillation organizes to a slower and more effective atrial flutter. As with other class I agents, hypokalemia reduces quinidine's antiarrhythmic effectiveness and might increase proarrhythmia.

The drug is well absorbed orally with little first-pass hepatic elimination. Peak effect usually occurs in 1–2 hours. It is highly protein-bound in dogs and cats; severe hypoalbuminemia can predispose to toxicity. Quinidine undergoes extensive hepatic metabolism. Its half-life is about 6 hours in dogs, 2 hours in cats, and 4–7 hours in horses. Anticonvulsants and other drugs that induce hepatic microsomal enzymes can speed quinidine's metabolism. Slow-release sulfate (83% active drug), gluconate (62% active drug), and polygalacturonate (80% active drug) salts of quinidine prolong the drug's absorption and elimination. The sulfate salt is absorbed more rapidly than the gluconate. Peak effect usually is achieved 1–2 hours after PO administration. In dogs, therapeutic blood concentrations (2.5–5 mcg/mL) are reached 12–24 hours after PO and IM administration. Chemical (analytical) grade quinidine sulfate often is purchased for use in horses and reconstituted in distilled water, because of the large amounts required. However, the drug is unavailable in some countries, which influences the preferred method for treating AF in this species.

Horses usually are treated by nasogastric tube every 2 hours for up to 5–6 doses to convert AF, although alternative dosing schemes (q6h) frequently are adopted if there is toxicosis. Treatment in experienced centers is associated with an 80 to 90% conversion success rate, depending on the duration of AF and the breed. Most horses tend to cardiovert after 2 to 4 doses, with each dose separated by 2 hours. However, that is not always the case and after five or six doses, or if severe adverse effects develop, the drug interval usually is increased to every 6 hours, if tolerated. IV digoxin might be needed to blunt the vagolytic effect on the AV node (see paragraphs that follow and p. 413). Between 10–50% drug absorption occurs within 2 hours in horses; a plasma concentration of 2–4 mcg/mL is thought to be therapeutic. Quinidine toxicity usually is associated with serum concentrations over 5 mcg/mL. Retrospective measurement of blood concentrations can be useful to determine if sufficient drug was administered to a horse, although the laboratories able to perform this test are highly limited. Experience indicates that with q2h dosing some horses will not convert, even after the usual upper limit of 6 doses; however, cardioversion occurs in some of these patients within 12 hours after the last dose.

Because of its propensity to cause vasodilation (via alpha-receptor blockade and possibly direct vasorelaxation) and myocardial depression, hypotension is a risk. Therefore, quinidine is not used IV in dogs and cats; it should be administered cautiously by that route in horses. The PO and IM routes usually do not cause adverse hemodynamic effects initially, but can do so with cumulative dosing and in animals with underlying cardiac disease. Quinidine toxicity extends from the drug's electrophysiologic, hemodynamic, and neural effects, as well as effects on GI function. ECG interval prolongations occur in a dose-related manner, although idiosyncratic reactions are possible with the first or second dose if the drug interacts with the HERG (human-ether-a-gogo related gene) potassium channel. Marked QT prolongation, right bundle branch block, or QRS widening to more than 25% of pretreatment duration suggest toxicity. AV conduction block and ventricular tachyarrhythmias also can result. Marked QT prolongation, whether dose-related or idiosyncratic, implies increased temporal dispersion of myocardial refractoriness, which predisposes to *torsades de pointes* (TdP), so-called quinidine-syncope, and to VF. Lethargy, weakness, and congestive heart failure (CHF) can result from quinidine's negative inotropic and vasodilatory effects (and subsequent hypotension). Cardiotoxicity and hypotension are partially reversed by sodium bicarbonate (0.5–1 mEq/kg IV), which temporarily reduces serum K^+ concentration and enhances quinidine's binding to albumin. Other adverse or toxic effects common with PO quinidine in dogs include the GI signs of nausea, vomiting, and diarrhea. Thrombocytopenia that is reversible after drug cessation is reported in people, as is hepatopathy. Severe hypoalbuminemia can predispose to toxicity. Protracted co-therapy of quinidine with digoxin increases the serum digoxin concentration by about two-fold by displacing digoxin from skeletal muscle-binding sites and decreasing its renal clearance. Cimetidine can predispose to toxicity by slowing the drug's elimination. Some Collie dogs or others deficient in P-glycoprotein might be especially sensitive to quinidine.

In horses, adverse effects of quinidine include many of the above, as well as apprehension, depression, anorexia, and nasal mucosal edema that can lead to upper airway obstruction (made worse by a nasogastric tube). Urticaria, paraphimosis, ataxia, hypotension, diarrhea, and colic also are seen. Diarrhea and anorexia can continue for up to three days with higher cumulative quinidine doses (such as >160 mg/kg). In rare cases, seizures, laminitis, or sudden death have occurred. Fortunately, many of these adverse effects are mild and tolerable and it is likely that treatment is abandoned too soon in many cases. Slowly walking the horse between doses can reduce some signs and if necessary, infusions of magnesium sulfate and the alpha-agonist phenylephrine can ameliorate severe ECG abnormalities or symptomatic hypotension. One common but manageable adverse effect is acceleration of the ventricular response rate with incremental quinidine doses. As noted previously, this stems from the combination of a vagolytic (anticholinergic) effect on the AV node concurrent with slowing of the atrial rate (often to flutter) that more effectively conducts to the ventricle. This can be mitigated in many horses by administering one or two IV doses of digoxin (usually 1 mg slowly IV for a 450 to 500 kg horse). Alternatively, quinidine can be stopped and the horse treated with digoxin for 2 (or 3) doses; then quinidine therapy is resumed the next day. Many horses will convert to sinus rhythm on this combination of therapy. The most severe quinidine adverse effect is polymorphic VT. When this develops, the horse is given magnesium sulfate and sodium bicarbonate (along with lidocaine) and quinidine is discontinued; these horses are best treated by electrocardioversion.

Mexiletine Mexiletine HCl (class Ib) is similar to lidocaine in its electrophysiologic, hemodynamic, toxic, and antiarrhythmic properties. It is used to treat ventricular tachyarrhythmias in dogs. It also is used in the chronic management of reentrant SVT associated with an accessory pathway. Mexiletine can suppress arrhythmias associated with repolarization abnormalities by decreasing late Na^+ influx during repolarization and thereby decreasing early afterdepolarizations (EADs). The combination of a beta-blocker or class III agent with mexiletine might be more effective and cause fewer adverse effects than mexiletine alone, because adverse effects can occur at doses producing subtherapeutic mexiletine serum concentrations. When used together, mexiletine counteracts the action potential prolongation caused by sotalol. When administered with mexiletine, sotalol appears to mildly increase mexiletine plasma concentration.

Mexiletine is well-absorbed orally (<10% first-pass elimination), although antacids, cimetidine, and narcotic analgesics reportedly slow its absorption in people. The drug is highly protein-bound. Mexiletine undergoes hepatic metabolism, influenced by liver blood flow, and renal excretion, which is slower if the urine is alkaline. Some metabolites appear to have activity similar to the parent compound, at least in people, which could contribute to toxicity. Hepatic microsomal enzyme inducers could accelerate its clearance. The half-life in dogs is about 4.5–7 hours. Therapeutic serum concentrations are thought to be 0.5–2.0 mcg/mL (as in people). The effects of this drug in cats are not known. Toxic effects are similar to those of lidocaine. In dogs, adverse effects have included vomiting, anorexia, tremor, ataxia, disorientation, sinus bradycardia, and thrombocytopenia. Reversible rear-limb weakness has been observed in a small number of dogs. Administration with food can reduce GI side-effects.

Phenytoin Phenytoin sodium is an anticonvulsant drug that has electrophysiologic effects similar to those of lidocaine. It also has some Ca^{++} channel inhibitory and CNS effects that could contribute to its effectiveness against digoxin-induced arrhythmias. Phenytoin can be used in dogs and horses to treat digoxin-induced ventricular tachyarrhythmias that are unresponsive to lidocaine. The drug is not used in cats because even low doses can produce toxicity. Phenytoin also has been used successfully in horses with VT refractory to lidocaine and procainamide. Other contraindications to its use are the same as those for lidocaine. Rapid IV injection is avoided because the propylene glycol vehicle can depress myocardial contractility and cause vasodilation, hypotension, respiratory arrest, and arrhythmia exacerbation. Slow IV infusion and PO administration do not cause relevant hemodynamic disturbance; however, phenytoin's oral bioavailability is poor. The drug is ~80% bound to albumin in dogs. The half-life is only about 3–7 hours in the dog, about 8 hours in horses, and 42–108 hours in cats. Therapeutic plasma range is ~9–16 mcg/mL. Hepatic metabolism occurs; phenytoin induces hepatic P450 enzymes and increases its own metabolism. Coadministration of cimetidine, chloramphenicol, and other drugs that inhibit microsomal enzyme activity increases phenytoin's serum concentration. Manifestations of phenytoin toxicity include bradycardia, AV block, VT, and cardiac arrest, as well as GI (anorexia, vomiting) and CNS signs (depression, nystagmus, disorientation, and ataxia). High plasma concentrations can cause adverse effects such as excitement and recumbency.

Class Ic Agents In general, class Ic agents markedly slow cardiac conduction velocity but have minimal effect on sinus rate or refractoriness. However, high doses depress automaticity in the sinus node and specialized conducting tissues. Drugs in this class are considered mainly for the management of difficult atrial arrhythmias, including suppression and cardioversion of AF. However, veterinary clinical trials are lacking and these drugs should not be used in the setting of heart failure or systolic dysfunction. Proarrhythmia is a serious potential adverse effect of the class Ic agents, which have been associated with increased mortality in people; this has occurred in both canine and equine cases too. Therefore these agents must be used with caution and only for serious arrhythmias refractory to other therapy.

Flecainide can prolong sinus cycle length, AV nodal conduction time, and refractoriness. Flecainide (and *encainide*) have a blocking effect on the delayed rectifier potassium current (I_K) similar to class III agents, although this effect to prolong repolarization is mitigated by their Na^+ channel blocking action, so little change in action potential duration occurs. However, at high plasma concentrations flecainide can prolong the QT interval. Its ability to increase the ventricular effective refractory period and reduce conduction velocity produce greater risk for proarrhythmia and sudden death in patients with prior myocardial damage or infarction. It also has been shown to increase the defibrillation threshold. In horses, flecainide has variable effectiveness for converting spontaneously occurring AF to sinus rhythm. Acute AF might be more responsive. Flecainide (2 mg/kg) slowed AF rate and terminated acute, experimentally induced AF in horses, although it did not change atrial effective refractory period or AF vulnerability (Haugaard, 2015). Both IV and PO flecainide have successfully converted AF in horses; however, quinidine and electrocardioversion are more tested options for this. Flecainide can prolong ventricular repolarization time, which could increase risk for ventricular arrhythmia. Although AF conversion with PO flecainide might be successful, TdP is a risk. Sudden death also can occur in horses when it is used for other arrhythmias, such as atrial tachycardia (Dembek, 2014). In view of flecainide's potential to induce dangerous arrhythmias, quinidine should be tried first. Flecainide should be used only as a last resort and with great caution. The drug's half-life after IV injection is about 6 hours in horses. Besides the risk for polymorphic VT and sudden death, adverse effects of flecainide in horses include agitation, and prolonged QRS and QT durations. Vasodilation and myocardial depression can cause severe hypotension after IV injection, especially in animals with underlying cardiac disease. In dogs, bradycardia, intraventricular conduction disturbance, and consistent, although transient, hypotension, as well as nausea, vomiting, and anorexia, have occurred.

Propafenone increases AV nodal functional refractory period, slows intraatrial conduction, and reduces ventricular excitability and triggered activity; it has less effect on the QT interval. Propafenone also has weak beta- and calcium channel blocking activity, and a vagolytic effect. It can be effective against incessant atrial tachycardia; in people it also is used for other atrial and ventricular tachyarrhythmias. However, propafenone's ability to convert AF in horses is poor. In a dog model, propafenone was shown to increase defibrillation energy requirements. This drug is highly protein-bound, undergoes extensive hepatic metabolism, and has active metabolites which appear to have greater antiarrhythmic effects than the parent compound. In dogs, the half-life after an IV dose is about 1 hour. Within 24 hours of propafenone dosing in dogs, ~65% is excreted in the bile and ~20% in the urine. In the horse, propafenone has a high clearance rate with elimination half-life of 1–2 hours; IV injection produces very low plasma concentrations. Propafenone increases the serum concentration of concurrent digoxin, metoprolol, and warfarin. Cimetidine slightly increases propafenone concentrations. Adverse effects in people include lightheadedness, nausea, vomiting, and proarrhythmia. In cases of propafenone toxicity, injection of an alkalinizing solution (such as Na^+ bicarbonate) can increase propafenone metabolism. Overall, there is scant experience and no clinical trial data to support its routine use in veterinary medicine.

Ranolazine is a drug with multiple ionic effects that is approved in people for treating chronic angina. It mainly blocks persistent or late inward Na^+ current, which can reduce intracardiac Ca^{++} concentrations and myocardial O_2 requirements. Ranolazine also inhibits the rapid component of the delayed repolarizing current (I_{Kr}; a class III effect), which prolongs action potential and QT interval durations. At high doses, it can mildly affect the I_{L-Ca}. Ranolazine could reduce occurrence of AF, and other supraventricular or ventricular arrhythmias. There is little veterinary experience with this drug.

Class II Antiarrhythmic Drugs

Class II consists of the beta-adrenergic blocking agents. The antiarrhythmic effect of beta-blockers relates to $beta_1$-receptor blockade rather than direct electrophysiologic effects. $Beta_1$-receptors, located primarily in the myocardium, mediate increases in contractility, heart rate (HR), AV conduction velocity, and automaticity in specialized fibers. $Beta_2$-receptors in extracardiac regions mediate bronchodilation and vasodilation, as well as renin and insulin release. There also are some $beta_2$-receptors in the heart, varying with species (few in the dog). The L-type calcium channels and funny current (I_f) channels are regulated by $beta_1$-receptors, and the suppression of these ion currents probably is what underlies the antiarrhythmic action of the beta-blockers. Consequently, these drugs slow HR and increase AV conduction time and refractoriness. They also reduce myocardial oxygen demand, potentially improving so-called demand ischemia. They are unlikely to directly affect repolarization. By decreasing the force of myocardial contraction, beta-blockers can reduce dynamic left ventricular outflow obstruction, as in hypertrophic obstructive cardiomyopathy (HOCM). However, depression of myocardial contractility is a major concern in patients with heart failure. Also, in patients with heart failure and $beta_1$-receptor downregulation, an increase in relative responsiveness to $beta_2$ stimulation affects diastolic Ca^{++} fluxes, which could magnify the risk for ventricular tachyarrhythmias and VF.

"Nonselective" beta-blockers inhibit catecholamine binding to both $beta_1$- and $beta_2$-receptors. Other beta-blockers are more selective and antagonize primarily one or the other receptor subtype. First generation beta-blockers (such as propranolol) have nonselective beta-blocking effects. Second generation agents (including atenolol, metoprolol, and esmolol) are relatively $beta_1$ selective; these are the agents used most often in treating heart disease. Third generation beta-blockers (such as carvedilol) affect both $beta_1$ and $beta_2$-receptors but also exert other effects, such as blocking $alpha_1$-receptors. A few beta-blockers have some degree of intrinsic sympathomimetic activity. Although the pharmacokinetics for most beta-blockers are well known, plasma concentrations do not always correlate with pharmacodynamic (beta-blocking) effects. Lipid and water solubility of various beta-blockers are relevant to hepatic and renal elimination, respectively. Thus, reduced hepatic blood flow in heart failure, anesthesia, or shock especially affects the elimination of lipophilic agents, while renal failure impacts that of hydrophilic beta-blockers.

Beta-receptor blockers sometimes are used in animals with congenital or acquired ventricular outflow tract obstruction (Chapters 27 and 33), systemic hypertension (Chapter 38), and supraventricular and ventricular tachyarrhythmias, especially those provoked by increased sympathetic tone. They also are used for other diseases or toxicities associated with excessive sympathetic stimulation, including hyperthyroidism. A beta-blocker could be administered to slow the ventricular response rate to AF, usually in combination with digoxin (or added with caution to digoxin and diltiazem). In cats, beta-blockers are considered the first line antiarrhythmic agent for both supraventricular and ventricular tachyarrhythmias. In dogs, the combination of a beta-blocker with a class I agent can produce better ventricular tachyarrhythmia suppression than either agent alone. Beta-blockers magnify the depression of AV conduction produced by digoxin, class I antiarrhythmic drugs, and calcium channel-blockers such as diltiazem. These combinations can provide better rate control but carry the risk of more severe AV block or depression of contractility (with diltiazem). Long-term therapy with certain beta-blockers can improve cardiac function and prolong survival in people (and experimental animals) with stable heart failure; however, clinical studies in animals with heart failure so far have not demonstrated measurable advantage, although some individuals might benefit (p. 331).

Beta-blocker effects depend on the level of sympathetic activation, so individual patient response can be quite variable. Initial doses should be low, with gradual uptitration as needed according to the animal's response. These drugs must be used cautiously in patients with severe myocardial disease, because increased sympathetic drive might be required to support cardiac output. In such patients, beta-blocker administration could markedly depress cardiac contractility, conduction, or HR. In these cases, prior institution of inotropic support is advised.

Beta-blockers generally are contraindicated in animals with sinus bradycardia, SSS, high-grade AV block, and untreated or severe CHF. The simultaneous use of a beta-blocker and calcium channel-blocker usually is avoided because marked decreases in HR and myocardial contractility could result. However, dogs with well-controlled CHF often can tolerate small, incremental doses if needed to better control rate response in AF. Theoretically, because of beta-receptor upregulation (increased number or affinity of receptors) during long-term beta-blockade, abrupt discontinuation of therapy could result in serious cardiac arrhythmias; this is certainly an issue in people with coronary artery disease. For that reason, gradual dosage reduction is recommended before stopping beta-blocker therapy in most cases. However, if a patient develops acute CHF, as sometimes occurs in cats previously prescribed atenolol for HOCM, the drug is discontinued immediately. Nonselective beta-blockers could promote bronchoconstriction by their $beta_2$ antagonism and increase peripheral vascular resistance, because of unopposed alpha-adrenergic effects. Lipophilic beta-blockers, such as propranolol, might cause depressed attitude and disorientation because of CNS effects. Conversely, drug clearance of water-soluble agents like atenolol could be reduced in patients with renal failure. Other adverse effects of beta-blockers can include lethargy, fatigue, anorexia, vomiting, diarrhea, hypotension, onset or recurrence of CHF, sinus bradycardia, and AV block. In diabetic animals, beta-blockers can mask early signs of acute hypoglycemia (such as tachycardia and BP changes) and reduce insulin release in response to hyperglycemia. Some animals cannot tolerate even small doses of a beta-blocker. The effects of excessive beta-blockade can be mitigated by catecholamine (dobutamine or dopamine) infusion, atropine, and if necessary, milrinone or glucagon, which increase cyclic adenosine monophosphate (cAMP) and intracellular Ca^{++}, independent of beta-receptor stimulation.

Propranolol Propranolol HCl is the prototypical nonselective beta-blocker, although it is used infrequently now. Propranolol should be avoided in patients with pulmonary edema because of the potential for bronchoconstriction from $beta_2$-receptor antagonism, as well as myocardial depression. Propranolol's $beta_2$-receptor blocking effects also make it relatively contraindicated in patients with asthma or chronic small airway disease. Propranolol has a relatively low oral bioavailability because of extensive first-pass hepatic metabolism, although long-term use and higher doses can saturate hepatic enzymes and increase bioavailability. Propranolol decreases hepatic blood flow, prolonging its own elimination and that of other drugs that depend on liver blood flow for their metabolism (such as lidocaine). Feeding delays PO absorption and enhances drug clearance by increasing hepatic blood flow. In horses, PO administration rarely produces therapeutic plasma concentrations because of propranolol's low bioavailability. The half-life of propranolol is only about 1.5 hours in dogs, 0.5–4.2 hours in cats, and 1.2–1.7 hours (IV use) in horses. However, active metabolites exist that can extend the drug's antiarrhythmic effects. Peak plasma concentration is higher in hyperthyroid compared to euthyroid cats. IV propranolol is used mainly for refractory VT, in conjunction with a class I drug, and for acute management of atrial or junctional tachycardia. However, esmolol is a better choice for evaluating the effects of beta-blockade in many circumstances.

Atenolol Atenolol is a selective $beta_1$-blocker. It is the beta-blocker used most commonly in dogs and cats. The half-life of atenolol is slightly over 3 hours in dogs and about 3.5 hours in cats. Oral bioavailability in both species is 90%. Atenolol is excreted in the urine; renal impairment delays clearance. Its beta-blocking effects are evident for over 12 hours, but are gone by 24 hours in normal cats. Similarly, atenolol's effect at 24 hours after dosing is minimal in dogs. Twice daily dosing is recommended for both species. This hydrophilic drug does not readily cross the blood–brain barrier, so adverse CNS effects are unlikely. Increased drug accumulation can potentially occur in renal failure, though. Weakness from reduced CO or worsening of heart failure can occur, as with other beta-blockers. This drug has not been evaluated sufficiently in horses.

Metoprolol Metoprolol tartrate is another longer acting $beta_1$-selective agent. The long-acting formulation is one of the few beta-blockers shown to prolong survival in people with heart failure. It has been suggested as a cardioprotectant in dogs with dilated cardiomyopathy (DCM) and chronic valvular disease. Clinical efficacy remains unproven, although experimental heart failure studies in dogs with myocardial dysfunction suggest possible improvement in pump function over time (p. 331). Metoprolol is well absorbed orally, but bioavailability is reduced by a large first-pass effect. There is minimal protein-binding. The drug is metabolized in the liver and excreted in the urine. Half-life is 1.6 hours in dogs, and 1.3 hours in cats. Both standard and long-acting formulations are available.

Esmolol Esmolol HCl is an ultra-short acting agent with beta$_1$-receptor selectivity and a half-life of less than 10 minutes. Esmolol is metabolized rapidly by blood esterases. Its major metabolite has only weak beta-blocking effects. Steady state occurs in 5 minutes with, or 30 minutes without, an IV loading dose. Effects dissipate within 10–20 minutes of CRI cessation. Although somewhat expensive, this drug can be helpful for acute treatment of tachyarrhythmias and severe dynamic left ventricular outflow obstruction (as in HOCM). It also is useful to "test" the effectiveness of a beta-blocker against an arrhythmia prior to beginning oral therapy.

Other Beta-blocking Drugs Other beta-blocking drugs are available. Their basic effects are similar, although their relative selectivity for beta$_1$-receptors and their pharmacologic characteristics vary. Certain beta-blockers, particularly carvedilol and metoprolol, have improved cardiac function and survival in people with heart failure (p. 331). Nonselective (1st generation) agents and some later-generation agents do not appear to confer these survival benefits. Agents with intrinsic sympathomimetic activity appear to have deleterious effects. Timolol mainly is used to treat glaucoma; however, ophthalmic administration does produce some systemic effects. In healthy cats, 1 drop of 0.5% timolol ophthalmic solution produced a drop in mean HR of 25 beats/minute, with sporadic transient 1st degree AV block (Gunther-Harrington, 2016).

Class III Antiarrhythmic Drugs

These agents prolong action potential duration and effective refractory period without decreasing conduction velocity. They act mainly by inhibiting the repolarizing potassium channel I_K (delayed rectifier), and potentially other potassium channels as well. The effects of some drugs in this class (such as amiodarone) are greater at higher HRs; this is the characteristic of "use-dependence" (also observed with lidocaine). Other agents exhibit reverse use-dependence (such as sotalol), with greater effects at slower HRs. Class III drugs can be effective for refractory ventricular arrhythmias, especially those caused by reentry. They can have antifibrillatory effects on atrial and ventricular tissues. Currently available agents share some characteristics of other antiarrhythmic drug classes in addition to their class III effects.

Sotalol Sotalol HCl is a nonselective beta-blocker with class III effects at higher doses. It is effective against ventricular and some supraventricular tachyarrhythmias. It may be more effective in preventing AF than terminating it because its effect to prolong refractory period is more pronounced at slower HRs. However, its beta-blocking effect helps control ventricular rate in animals with AF. Sotalol often is used in dogs with ventricular tachyarrhythmias, especially when supraventricular tachyarrhythmias are concurrent. It can be effective in cats with severe ventricular tachyarrhythmias, as well. In horses, sotalol sometimes is used after AF conversion in an attempt to suppress atrial premature activity and maintain sinus rhythm; the drug generally is tapered then discontinued before training is resumed. Sotalol also might be helpful against recurrent VT in horses.

Sotalol's beta-blocking effects (from the l-isomer) occur at lower doses, are about 30% of the potency of propranolol, and are important to sotalol's antiarrhythmic effectiveness. d-Sotalol alone has no beta-blocking effect. Instead, it prolongs repolarization; however, nonuniformity of this is thought to underlie the increased risk for proarrhythmia and death seen with this isomer. The racemic mixture is used clinically. Sotalol prolongs the refractory period by selectively blocking the rapid component (I_{Kr}) or HERG channel of the delayed rectifier current responsible for repolarization. Sotalol can increase triggered activity (EADs); it can cause TdP at high doses or, in the presence of hypokalemia, at slow HRs. Fortunately, this appears to be less common in animals than in people, yet it still demands consideration and supports the need for Holter ECG monitoring to detect proarrhythmia once a dose is established. Dogs appear to require much higher doses than people to manifest solalol's class III effects. Doses that are used clinically in dogs might produce mainly beta-blocking effects. Experimentally, in hypokalemic dogs, coadministration of mexiletine reduced sotalol's proarrhythmic potential. Sotalol often is used to treat VT in Boxers with ARVC, but it is not advised as therapy for Boxers or other breeds with bradycardia-associated (vasovagal, neural, neurocardiogenic) syncope. The latter syndrome is an underappreciated reason for transient loss of consciousness in dogs (Perego, 2020), and in the authors' experience, beta-blockers and sotalol often worsen the clinical signs. Sotalol also was shown to induce VT in young German Shepherd Dogs affected with inherited ventricular tachyarrhythmias; it should be avoided as a sole agent in these animals (Gelzer, 2010). It can be combined with mexiletine, however.

The bioavailability of sotalol is high with negligible first-pass effect, although absorption is reduced with food. The half-life is ~5 hours in dogs, with peak concentration at ~3 hours post dose. It is eliminated unchanged by the kidneys; renal dysfunction prolongs elimination. Sotalol's beta-blocking effects last longer than its plasma half-life. The drug usually has minimal hemodynamic effects, although it can cause hypotension. Slowed sinus rate and 1st degree AV block can occur. In horses, sotalol has modest PO bioavailability (48%), with maximal absorption at about 1 hour. The elimination half-life is about 15 hours. Dose-dependent increase in plasma concentrations occur, but do not appear to cause progressive increases in effective refractory period or QT interval prolongation.

In horses with AF, sotalol decreases ventricular response rate (that is, HR) and increases QT interval duration. When administered (at 2 mg/kg q12h) for several days prior to electrical cardioversion, fewer shocks and lower energy were required for conversion, although not all animals converted to sinus rhythm. Unfortunately, prevention of AF recurrence in horses receiving sotalol after electrocardioversion has been unimpressive. Sotalol can cause transient sweating in horses, especially at higher PO doses.

Some dogs with DCM experience worsened myocardial function on sotalol, and this can (rarely) precipitate CHF. However, sotalol has less negative inotropic effect than propranolol; myocardial depression often is countered by the concurrent use of pimobendan. Sotalol's ability to prolong action potential duration could theoretically confer a mild positive inotropic effect related to increased intracellular Ca^{++}, but this might not be realized at doses used in dogs. Other adverse effects of sotalol can include hypotension, depression, nausea, vomiting, diarrhea, and bradycardia. The PR interval on ECG often prolongs slightly during sotalol therapy, especially at dosages in the 2-3 mg/kg PO q12h range, but higher grades of AV block are uncommon. There are a few anecdotal reports of aggression that resolved after sotalol was discontinued. Overall, sotalol appears to be the most frequently used oral antiarrhythmic drug, and it carries a relatively low adverse-effect profile in dogs. It is used increasingly in cats (compounded) and in horses for suppression of ventricular ectopy.

Amiodarone Amiodarone HCl is a unique Class III agent with nonspecific potassium channel (I_k) blocking properties. While it prolongs the action potential duration and effective refractory period in both atrial and ventricular tissues, it also shares properties with all three other antiarrhythmic drug classes. Amiodarone is an iodinated benzofuran compound that has effects on Na^+, K^+, and Ca^{++} channels. It also has noncompetitive alpha$_1$- and beta-blocking properties. Its beta-blocking and class Ib-like effects occur soon after administration. However, maximal class III effects, with action potential and QT interval prolongation and reduced Purkinje fiber automaticity, are achieved after weeks of oral administration. In contrast to other class III drugs, which tend to induce EADs, amiodarone can abolish these afterdepolarizations. Its Ca^{++} channel-blocking effects might contribute to the reduced triggered activity. Amiodarone's action potential prolongation is more uniform across ventricular tissues than that of other agents and the rate of TdP occurrence associated with amiodarone is lower than with other drugs; however it is still a risk. Amiodarone also might reduce the dispersion of repolarization that accompanies myocardial failure. The effective refractory period is prolonged to a greater extent in the atria than ventricles. Yet an experimental study in dogs showed that the early repolarization period was not prolonged, which might explain its reduced proarrhythmic potential even though it prolongs the QT interval.

Therapeutic doses slow the sinus rate, decrease AV conduction velocity, and minimally depress myocardial contractility and BP. Indications for amiodarone include refractory tachyarrhythmias of both atrial and ventricular origin, especially reentrant arrhythmias using an accessory pathway. Amiodarone has shown variable effectiveness in converting AF to sinus rhythm in dogs and horses, preventing postoperative AF in dogs (with tricuspid dysplasia), and preventing recurrent AF in horses after successful cardioversion.

Amiodarone's pharmacokinetic characteristics are complex and species dependent. There is delayed onset of action and prolonged time to steady state (>10 weeks). The drug concentrates in myocardial and other tissues (especially fat), and an active metabolite (desethylamiodarone) accumulates. The drug is metabolized in the liver. The half-life in dogs after a single PO dose is ~7.5 hours, but increases to 3.2 days with long-term use, suggesting steady state will require at least 3 weeks of regular oral dosing before it develops. As a result, loading doses often are used for the first two weeks of therapy. In the horse, after a single IV dose, rapid distribution to well-perfused tissue is followed by slow accumulation in fat with almost 100 days required for drug elimination. Most is eliminated as desethylamiodarone in the urine. After single IV dose (5 mg/kg) median terminal half-life of ~51 hours for amiodarone and ~75 hours for desethylamiodarone are reported. Peak plasma concentrations occurred in less than 3 hours; however, they were low (<0.1 mcg/mL). After a single PO dose in horses, absorption is slow and highly variable, although peak plasma concentration 7 hours post dose reportedly is higher than after IV administration. Median half-life after PO administration is ~24 hours for amiodarone and ~59 hours for its metabolite. The drug is highly protein bound. Therapeutic serum concentrations (human) for both amiodarone and desethylamiodarone are thought to be 0.5–2.0 mcg/mL. Amiodarone can be compounded into an oral suspension for easier dosing in small animals.

Even after initial IV use, oral loading doses (typically, twice the projected maintenance dosage) generally are given once per day for 7–14 days (or the maintenance dose is administered twice daily for that duration). Experimentally, PO loading doses (25 mg/kg q12h) of amiodarone in normal dogs lowered HR and prolonged PR and QT intervals; however, maintenance doses (of 30 mg/kg/day) caused no significant ECG or echocardiographic changes in normal dogs. Steady state was reached only after 11 weeks of treatment, highlighting the variable pharmacokinetics observed even within species. Adverse effects are likely to increase at these dosages, or in patients with structural heart disease; lower loading and maintenance doses are strongly recommended (8 to 10 mg/kg PO daily as a maintenance dose). If those fail, some dogs will experience better rhythm control with higher doses but the risk of hepatotoxicity and other adverse effects probably increases. Experimentally, IV amiodarone administered to normal dogs did not decrease myocardial contractility (dP/dt_{max}) until cumulative doses of 12.5 and 15 mg/kg were reached (given in 2.5 mg/kg increments q15min). However, the potential for more profound cardiac depression and hypotension with IV amiodarone is of concern in animals with myocardial disease.

Slow IV bolus administration can suppress ventricular arrhythmias in dogs. However, the older ("standard") IV formulation often precipitates hypotension and anaphylactic-like reactions, related to solvents (polysorbate 80 and benzyl alcohol) used to keep the drug in solution. Acute therapy for hypersensitivity reactions has included stopping IV amiodarone and using diphenhydramine (1 mg/kg IV), a corticosteroid (such as prednisolone 1-2 mg/kg IV), IV fluids and other supportive care as needed. Although antihistamine pretreatment, conservative dosing, and slow injection over 10-20 minutes have been helpful in some cases, the use of this IV amiodarone formulation is NOT currently recommended. Instead, a newer preservative-free formulation (Nexterone; Baxter Healthcare) without polysorbate 80 and benzyl alcohol is available and should be used when IV amiodarone administration is indicated. A retrospective study in dogs given the premixed formulation of Nexterone identified no adverse effects; in most cases, a 2 mg/kg IV bolus was administered over 10 min, followed by CRI of 0.8 mg/kg/h for 6 hours, and then decreased to 0.4 mg/kg/h for 18 hours (median 9 h, range 0-29 h; Levy, 2016). In horses, IV administration using a loading dose infused over an hour, followed by maintenance infusion for 1-2 days has been used for converting AF or preventing recurrent AF after cardioversion. The authors have used both Nexterone and standard, diluted amiodarone in this species. Amiodarone use is not sufficiently described in cats.

Many potential side-effects occur with long-term amiodarone use, including depressed appetite, GI upset, pneumonitis, pulmonary fibrosis, hepatopathy, thyroid dysfunction, positive Coomb's test, thrombocytopenia, and neutropenia. Some of these resolve with drug discontinuation or dosage reduction. Hepatotoxicity appears common and somewhat dose related in Doberman Pinschers. Collie dogs, or others with P-glycoprotein deficiency, might be especially sensitive to amiodarone. Adverse effects in horses after IV infusion have included hind limb weakness, leg shifting, diarrhea, and bilrubinemia. Other adverse effects noted with long-term use in people include corneal microdeposits, photosensitivity, bluish skin discoloration, and peripheral neuropathy. Amiodarone can increase serum concentrations of digoxin, diltiazem, and, possibly, procainamide and quinidine.

Other Class III Agents

Dronedarone is a noniodinated benzofuran, similar to amiodarone, but designed to overcome some of the side effects of that iodinated drug. It is used in people with AF and atrial flutter, to help maintain sinus rhythm, and for ventricular arrhythmias. High doses have a cardiodepressant effect. The drug also can slow AV and intraventricular conduction, consistent with Ca^{++} and Na^+ blocking effects as well as its class III activity. Dronedarone has greater effect on the atrial myocardium with regard to effective refractory period prolongation, consistent with its greater action against atrial arrhythmas. It causes dose-related prolongation of repolarization, with increasing risk for TdP. In an experimental model of AF in dogs, dronedarone (20 mg/kg q12h PO for 7 days) significantly lengthened the atrial action potential duration and effective refractory period; the duration of induced AF was shortened (Saengklub, 2017). Dronedarone is highly protein-bound; its bioavailability after oral administration in dogs is fairly low (14-22%) despite a good absorption rate. The drug undergoes extensive metabolism and is excreted mainly in the feces. There are conflicting experimental reports about whether chronic oral dosing (at 20-25 mg/kg q12h) prolongs the corrected QT interval in dogs. Oral dronedarone administration in dogs (20 mg/kg q12h) over several days slows AV conduction; it might reduce BP and HR. The drug appears to have negligible effect on myocardial function in conscious normal dogs. However, IV administration (2.5 mg/kg) to anesthetized normal dogs did depress contractility, cardiac output, and relaxation, in addition to prolonging AV conduction time and increasing systemic vascular resistance. Therefore, caution is warranted in animals with preexisting cardiac disease. The most common side effects reported in humans are diarrhea, nausea and abdominal pain, so short-term usage is the rule.

Ibutilide fumarate is a blocker of the rapid repolarizing potassium channel Kv 11.1 (HERG). It is used for converting recent onset AF in people; however, there is little veterinary experience with it. Experimental studies in dogs have shown that ibutilide causes SA and AV nodal suppression, increases atrial and ventricular refractoriness and repolarization dispersion, prolongs the QT interval, and induces EADs, especially in people with reduced left ventricular ejection fraction. It appears to have only a 50% success rate for converting acutely induced AF; doses effective in terminating AF also increase myocardial refractoriness and QT duration. Ibutilide has caused TdP in dogs with experimental AV block and cardiomyopathy. Besides its class III effects, ibutilide also activates a slow inward Na^+ current. The drug is cleared mainly through the kidney.

Dofetilide is related to ibutilide and selectively blocks the rapid component of the repolarizing K^+ current, especially in atrial tissue. It prolongs atrial action potential duration. Dofetilide is used in people for acute conversion of AF and to suppress recurrent AF and other atrial tachyarrhythmias. However, its efficacy might depend on the duration and underlying mechanism of AF; it could be more effective in preventing rather than terminating AF. Dofetilide also tends to induce EADs and TdP, especially in animals with cardiac remodeling and greater repolarization dispersion. Abnormal calcium handling within myocardial cells increases beat-to-beat variability in ventricular repolarization, which increases risk for TdP. Dofetilide was shown to increase short-term beat-to-beat variability in QT duration in animals with intact autonomic function and endogenous HR oscillations; this was associated with increased risk for ventricular arrhythmias, including TdP. It appears to prolong the QT interval to a greater degree in dogs than in people at comparable doses. In an equine model of acute AF, dofetilide, in combination with ranolazine, was more effective than either drug alone; no change in atrial effective refractory period was noted with either drug or the combination (Carstensen, 2018). Dofetilide is well-absorbed orally in dogs, but has some first pass hepatic metabolism. The drug is about 50% protein-bound. The half-life is about 4.5 hours. Dofetilide undergoes hepatic metabolism mediated by cytochrome p450; there are weakly active metabolites. Clearance is by both hepatic and renal (unchanged) routes. In dogs, QT prolongation, ventricular premature complexes and right bundle branch block can occur at doses of 0.3 mg/kg. Dofetilide does not appear to exacerbate left ventricular dysfunction.

Vernakalant blocks yet another potassium channel (KV1.5), an ultrarapid repolarizing current. It also exerts mostly atrial-specific activity and was developed for rapid conversion of AF in humans.

Class IV Antiarrhythmic Drugs

Class IV contains calcium channel blocking agents. This diverse group of drugs reduces cellular Ca^{++} influx by blocking transmembrane L-type Ca^{++} channels. Calcium channel-blockers as a group can cause coronary and systemic vasodilation, as well as diminish myocardial contractility and potentially, enhance relaxation; however, various agents differ in these effects. Some calcium channel-blockers (the nondihydropyridines: diltiazem and verapamil) have antiarrhythmic effects, especially on tissues that depend on the slow inward Ca^{++} current, particularly the sinus and AV nodes. They slow the sinus rate, increase AV nodal refractory period, and can interrupt some arrhythmias caused by abnormal automaticity, triggered mechanisms, and reentry. These agents are most effective against supraventricular tachyarrhythmias, although they might suppress some ventricular arrhythmias dependent on abnormal Ca^{++} fluxes (as in the wide-QRS fascicular tachycardia of humans). Initial doses should be low, with hemodynamic monitoring when given IV, then increased as needed to effect or to maximal recommended dosage. Side effects of these agents can include reduced contractility, vasodilation, hypotension, depression, anorexia, lethargy, bradycardia, and AV block. Calcium channel-blockers usually are not prescribed concurrently with a beta-blocker, although they could be used together with cautious up-titration of the beta-blocker. An overdose or exaggerated response to a calcium channel-blocker is treated with supportive care; atropine (**Table 25.2**, p. 402) for bradycardia or AV block; dopamine or dobutamine (**Table 22.2**, p. 343) and furosemide (**Table 22.3**, p. 345) for heart failure; and dopamine or IV calcium salts for hypotension.

Dihydropyridine calcium channel-blockers have little to no direct cardiac effect and are not helpful against arrhythmias. These agents act as vasodilators. Amlodipine besylate is used most commonly; it often is recommended as the first line antihypertensive agent in cats, and is used in some hypertensive dogs too (p. 803). Amlodipine also is useful in dogs with chronic refractory heart failure (p. 349).

Diltiazem Diltiazem HCl is a benzothiazepine calcium channel-blocker. It causes dose-dependent slowing of sinus node activity, increases AV nodal refractory period, and can block some arrhythmias caused by abnormal automaticity, triggered mechanisms, and reentry. Some effects on the sinus node are blunted if there is reflex sympathetic stimulation from a fall in BP. Diltiazem's channel-blocking effect in the AV node is greater at faster rates (use-dependence). Diltiazem also causes potent coronary and mild peripheral vasodilation, perhaps varying across species. It is preferred over verapamil because it has less negative inotropic effect; diltiazem also does not interfere with digoxin elimination. Diltiazem is indicated for supraventricular tachyarrhythmias. It can be used as a CRI after IV bolus injections, if necessary; however, it more often is continued as an oral formulation. Arterial BP should be monitored during IV administration and conservative doses used, especially in animals with reduced myocardial function. Diltiazem commonly is used in combination with digoxin to further slow the ventricular response rate to AF in dogs. Diltiazem is the agent used in those cats with hypertrophic cardiomyopathy that are thought to benefit from calcium channel blockade (p. 672). Contraindications to diltiazem include sinus bradycardia, AV block, SSS, digoxin toxicity, severe myocardial failure, and systemic hypotension.

Diltiazem's bioavailability is only about 43% in dogs because of extensive first-pass metabolism. Effects peak within 2 hours after PO dosing and last at least 6 hours in dogs. Conventional diltiazem's bioavailability is greater in cats than in dogs. The half-life in dogs is just over 2 hours, but is extended with long-term PO use because of its enterohepatic circulation. The half-life in cats is about 2–3 hours; plasma concentrations peak within 30–90 minutes and effects last for 8 hours although much pharmacokinetic variability exists among individual cats. The therapeutic range is 50–300 ng/mL. Oral diltiazem at 5 mg/kg in normal dogs with experimentally induced acute AF can produce therapeutic blood levels (32–100 ng/mL) within 3 hours after dosing and without significant hemodynamic detriment; however, animals with heart disease might not tolerate such high doses. Diltiazem is metabolized in the liver; active metabolites exist. Drugs that inhibit hepatic enzyme systems (such as cimetidine) reduce diltiazem's metabolism. Diltiazem ER is a sustained-release preparation; the 240 mg capsules contain four tablets of 60 mg each. Doses of 30–60 mg q24h produced serum concentrations >200 ng/mL for 24 hours in cats, although some cats on the lower dose reached <50 ng/mL by 24 hours (Wall, 2005). The 60 mg dose (~9–15 mg/kg) caused lethargy, GI signs and weight loss in about a third of cats on chronic therapy. Another sustained-release preparation (Cardizem CD capsules) at 10 mg/kg daily in cats produces plasma concentrations that peak in 6 hours and remain in the therapeutic range for 24 hours. Sustained-release diltiazem might have less efficacy in preventing sinus tachycardia compared with atenolol. The bioavailability of PO diliazem in the horse is unclear.

Diltiazem administered IV at 0.4–0.9 mg/kg to dogs with experimentally induced AF, produced plasma concentrations between 68 and 117 ng/mL and HRs closest to the animals' baseline sinus rhythm (Miyamoto, 2000). However, dogs with heart disease or failure are unlikely to tolerate such high doses. Accordingly, the authors suggest much lower IV doses (typically 0.05 to 0.1 mg/kg IV every 5 to 10 minutes with BP monitoring, up to 0.4 to 0.5 mg/kg cumulative dose). In horses, intermittent SA and AV nodal depression and mild impairment of systolic and diastolic function, as well as decreased systemic vascular resistance, were reported with IV diltiazem. Cumulative doses to 2 mg/kg resulted in plasma concentrations between 390 and 910 ng/mL; some horses developed significant hypotension and nodal suppression at these doses (Schwarzwald, 2005). Effective IV diltiazem doses in horses appear to range from 0.125 to 1.125 mg/kg.

Severe adverse effects are uncommon at therapeutic doses, although anorexia, nausea, bradycardia, and, rarely, other GI, cardiac, or neurologic effects can occur and are probably under-recognized (and attributed to other drugs or complications of CHF). Adverse effects could be more common in cats, including anorexia with weight loss, vomiting, lethargy, and evidence of hepatopathy. Anecdotally, some cats become aggressive or show other personality change when treated with diltiazem. Concurrent use of diltiazem and a beta-blocker can cause sudden fall in sinus rate or serious AV block. Toxic effects include reduced myocardial contractility, hypotension, lethargy, bradycardia and AV block. Therapy needed for diltiazem toxicity might include atropine, calcium gluconate, dopamine, glucagon, and temporary pacing. Use of high-dose insulin and IV lipid emulsion therapy also have been used successfully.

Verapamil Verapamil HCl is a phenylalkylamine, with potent cardiac effects, that generally is avoided in companion animals. It causes dose-related slowing of the sinus rate and AV conduction. By prolonging nodal tissue refractoriness it can abolish reentrant SVT and slow the ventricular response rate to AF. Verapamil's half-life in dogs is ~2.5 hours. It is poorly absorbed and undergoes first-pass hepatic metabolism, resulting in low PO bioavailability. The pharmacokinetics in cats are similar to dogs, although more variable. Verapamil has important negative inotropic and some vasodilatory effects that can precipitate hypotension, heart failure, and even death in animals with underlying myocardial disease. Arterial BP should be monitored if this drug is used. Verapamil should not be administered to animals with heart failure and rarely is used clinically in other animals. Verapamil is contraindicated with myocardial failure, CHF, sinus bradycardia, AV block, SSS, and digoxin toxicity. The concurrent use of verapamil and a beta-blocker can cause a sudden decrease in sinus rate or complete AV block. Toxic effects of verapamil include sinus bradycardia, AV block, hypotension, reduced myocardial contractility, and cardiogenic shock. The negative inotropic effects of verapamil might be reversed with IV calcium salts, sympathomimetic drugs, or milrinone (**Table 22.2**, p. 343). Atropine might mitigate bradycardia or AV block precipitated by verapamil. Verapamil reduces the renal clearance of digoxin.

Other Drugs with Antiarrhythmic Effects

Digoxin Although digoxin typically is considered a positive inotropic drug, it is useful for slowing the ventricular response rate in AF, atrial flutter, and potentially, focal atrial tachycardias. Digoxin also can suppress some supraventricular premature depolarizations. These effects are mediated by an increase in parasympathetic tone, which mainly affects the SA and AV nodes and atrial tissue, as well as direct effects that prolong AV nodal conduction and refractory period. See p. 327 for more information on this drug.

Ivabradine Ivabradine is a selective inhibitor of the "funny current" (I_f), that flows through the HCN channel and plays a major role in diastolic depolarization of sinus node cells. This current is especially active when the diastolic potential is hyperpolarized by sympathetic tone and beta-receptor activation. By reducing the rate of diastolic depolarization, the drug decreases HR. Ivabradine's main use in people is for treating inappropriate sinus tachycardia and reducing ischemia by decreasing myocardial oxygen demand and prolonging coronary perfusion time. The drug reportedly does not significantly affect conductivity, repolarization, or refractoriness of the AV node, atrial or ventricular myocardium, or His-Purkinje system. However, effects on the AV node require better delineation, and because I_f also is present in ventricular Purkinje cells, ivabradine might potentially have other antiarrhythmic effects. The reduction in sinus rate is dose-dependent; however, extreme bradycardia caused by ibravadine appears to be rare, which probably relates to redundant pacemaker currents in the sinus node. Overall, ivabradine exerts minimal negative effects on inotropy and BP. Nevertheless, reduced systolic and diastolic function were observed in a small study of anesthetized cats with hypertrophic cardiomyopathy (Riesen, 2012). While ivabradine's effects would appear limited to slowing the HR during sinus rhythm, there are sporadic human reports of its successful use in treating automatic atrial or junctional tachycardias. Furthermore, in a small study of induced AF in older dogs, ivabradine prolonged the effective refractory period in certain left atrial regions, reduced susceptibility to AF induction, and shortened AF duration (Li, 2015).

Ivabradine and its major active metabolite appear to reach peak plasma concentrations in ~1 hour after oral dosing in dogs and cats, with peak negative chronotropic effect in ~3 hours. Plasma half-life of ivabradine is ~2 hours in dogs and ~3.5 hours in cats. Ivabradine is metabolized by hepatic cytochrome P450 enzyme pathways. Dosing (0.1-0.3 mg/kg PO) at 12 hour intervals appears appropriate in healthy cats. The drug should be avoided in patients with SSS. Ivabradine seems to be well-tolerated in people and experimental animals; some people have experienced minor, transient visual disturbances. Ivabradine now is commercially available in the United States, although so far there is little clinical veterinary experience with this agent (also see p. 333).

Other Agents *Magnesium sulfate* (or chloride) can demonstrate antiarrhythmic effects, even when serum Mg^{++} concentrations are normal. The membrane stabilizing actions and antiarrhythmic effects of this ion are incompletely understood, but likely relate to actions on repolarizing K^+ currents and reduction of potassium conductance, including inward rectifying currents that can cause EADs. Regardless of mechanism, magnesium sulfate therapy for ventricular (or atrial) ectopy is especially relevant in these clinical settings: patients with hypomagnesemia or hypokalemia; ventricular tachycardia related to quinidine or digitalis toxicoses; and in VT or TdP associated with QT interval prolongation. In many veterinary intensive care units, a magnesium infusion is started if initial boluses of lidocaine do not sufficiently suppress ventricular ectopy, whether from cardiac disease or systemic illness. Although this "second-line" treatment approach might be logical and usually is well-tolerated, the overall response rate to empirical magnesium therapy is largely unstudied, at least in companion animals. Dosing generally follows guidelines established in veterinary critical care settings and can include emergency bolus injections (such as 0.15 to 0.3 mEq/kg bodyweight of elemental magnesium for dogs; 1 gm/minute to 25 grams of $MgSO_4$ for horses) followed by a CRI infusion of approximately 0.5 – 1.0 mEq/kg bodyweight over 24h (Humphrey, 2015).

Fish oil supplements are considered "upstream modulators" of ventricular arrhythmias, acting on the myocardial substrate (**Table 24.2**). Preliminary data suggest omega-3 fatty acids can reduce ventricular arrhythmias in Boxers with ARVC. More data are needed.

Adenosine is an endogenous purine nucleoside that briefly opens specific K^+ channels and indirectly impedes the L-type Ca^{++} current, with greatest effect on SA and AV nodes. By transiently depressing AV node activity, in people it can terminate reentrant SVTs and is useful in the differential diagnosis of wide-QRS tachycardias (helping to distinguish VT from SVT with ventricular aberrancy). Adenosine must be administered rapidly IV into a central vein; it is degraded within seconds by enzyme systems in the vascular endothelium and blood cells. However, body weight-adjusted doses more than twice comparable human doses have been ineffective in dogs. Therefore, the use of adenosine as an antiarrhythmic agent cannot be recommended.

Anticholinergic Drugs

Atropine Sulfate and Glycopyrrolate These agents increase sinus rate and AV conduction when vagal tone exerts excessive influence on nodal function. Parenteral atropine or glycopyrrolate is used when necessary for sinus bradycardia or AV block induced by anesthesia, CNS lesions, and certain other diseases or toxicities. Atropine is a competitive muscarinic (M_2) receptor antagonist that is used to test for underlying vagal influence in animals with AV block, sinus bradycardia, or sinus arrest (also see section "Atropine Response Test"). A dose of 0.04 mg/kg can largely abolish parasympathetic tone in normal dogs. Atropine's effect peaks within 5 minutes after IV administration, but is more delayed when injected by other routes. It is metabolized in the liver and excreted in the urine. Glycopyrrolate has a longer duration of action than atropine, without centrally mediated effects.

The response to atropine relates to prevailing vagal tone and the health of the cardiac impulse-forming and conduction system. Normally, atropine increases HR and improves AV conduction, although there can be a time lag between the onset of these effects, during which the increasing atrial rate can overwhelm AV conduction and briefly cause 1st- or 2nd degree AV block, especially after IV administration. Conceptually, sinus bradycardia and AV blocks that are vagally mediated should resolve with atropine; whereas the drug should exert little effect on bradyarrhythmias caused by intrinsic disease of the sinus node or AV conduction system. However, this is an oversimplification, because vagal influence can further depress SA and AV nodal responsiveness in the presence of preexisting conduction system disease.

Experience indicates that atropine administration rarely affects complete (3rd degree) AV block, aside from increasing the P wave (sinus) rate or infrequently, releasing a faster escape rhythm. Atropine's effects in 2nd degree AV block range from minimal to substantial, depending on the overall contribution of vagal input. With intrinsic AV conduction system disease, atropine will increase sinoatrial discharge and atrial rate, but the severity of AV block often increases as more atrial impulses fail to reach the ventricle. Conversely, complete resolution of AV block suggests the cause is vagally-mediated. Yet, even with improved AV conduction, 1st degree AV block can persist, which suggests some role for intrinsic conduction disease. This finding often occurs in dogs genetically predisposed to AV conduction disease, but prior to the onset of complete AV block.

In sinus node dysfunction or with SSS, the response to atropine also is variable. Development of normal sinus rhythm does not definitively indicate that the sinus node is structurally normal, but does suggest vagal influence to the sinus bradycardia or pauses. However, a failure of the SA node to respond with an increased HR, or the emergence of an ectopic supraventricular pacemaker (often with negative P' waves), supports a diagnosis of intrinsic SA node disease. Vagolytic drugs, including atropine and oral anticholinergics, can aggravate paroxysmal atrial and junctional tachyarrhythmias (especially in canine SSS), leading to overdrive suppression of the SA node and subsequent periods of sinus arrest. Atropine crosses the blood-brain barrier and could cause CNS effects such as excitement or sedation. Other adverse effects, also observed with the chronic use of oral anticholinergics, might include vomiting, dry mouth, decreased GI motility, constipation, keratoconjunctivitis sicca, mydriasis-induced photophobia, increased intraocular pressure, and drying of respiratory secretions. In horses, anticholinergic drug administration can precipitate ileus and colic.

Atropine Response Test An atropine response test is used to determine the degree of vagal influence on sinus and AV nodal functions. It is valuable for both a preanesthetic evaluation in dogs or cats with sinus bradycardia or 2nd degree AV block and as a diagnostic tool to detect intrinsic SA nodal or AV conduction disease. This test reveals the impact of vagal input on those bradyarrhythmias. The IV, IM, and SC routes of atropine administration are used by different cardiologists; each approach has merit and currently, there is no accepted standard. Parenteral atropine – especially if administered IV – can transiently exacerbate vagally mediated AV block when the atrial rate increases faster than cells in the AV node can respond to the drug. Additionally, in dogs with SSS, paroxysmal sinus or ectopic atrial tachycardias can occur, alternating with protracted periods of sinus arrest. For these reasons, many cardiologists prefer IM (or SC) atropine administration, with a follow up ECG recorded 20-30 minutes later. Some bradyarrhythmias that respond to parenteral atropine (or glycopyrrolate) do respond at least partially to oral anticholinergic agents, like hyoscyamine, but this is variable.

Following a baseline ECG recording, atropine is administered (0.04 mg/kg). A second recording is obtained 5–10 minutes after IV injection or 20-30 minutes after IM or SC injection. If the HR has not increased by at least 50%, another ECG is recorded 10 to 15 minutes after the prior ECG, as improvement in AV conduction can lag after initial administration of the drug in some cases. The sinus node rate for most dogs will increase to >150/minute, although based on a study of six larger breed dogs receiving 0.04 mg/kg IV, a rate of 135/minute or higher might be another benchmark of response. Conversely, many dogs develop sinus tachycardia with atrial rates >200/minute. In cases of sinus node dysfunction, an increase in HR might occur from release of a subsidiary supraventricular pacemaker from vagal influence; therefore, P wave morphology should be scrutinized. All of this suggests that the response to atropine in dogs is variable, and depends on the initial HR and prevailing parasympathetic tone, the route of atropine administration, the type of bradyarrhythmia, and probably the species and breed, as well. Thus, results of the atropine response test demand clinical interpretation, as opposed to a dogmatic analysis.

Other Anticholinergic Agents *Propantheline bromide* and *hyoscyamine sulfate* are used commonly for long-term anticholinergic therapy in dogs; other oral anticholinergic agents also are available. Oral absorption of propantheline is variable; individual dosage is adjusted to effect and must be tailored to minimize adverse effects. Food could decrease the drug's absorption. Potential adverse effects are as described for atropine. *Scopalamine* (butylscopalamine, scopolamine butylbromide, hyoscine) has been used in horses for spasmodic colic; it reduces GI motility but only briefly (~30 minutes or less). It might provide short-term HR support in vagally mediated bradycardia; however, effective infusion rates are not established.

Sympathomimetic Drugs

Isoproterenol Isoproterenol HCl is a beta-receptor agonist (or receptor activator of Class IIb, in **Table 24.2**) that has been used for the acute treatment of symptomatic AV block and bradycardia refractory to atropine. However, its use is not recommended because artificial pacing is safer and more effective, and other catecholamines can better support hemodynamics. It also has been used to shorten the refractory period in TdP, but it could exacerbate this rhythm disturbance (therefore, magnesium salts are preferred). PO administration is not effective because marked first-pass hepatic metabolism prevents achievement of effective blood levels. Because of its strong affinity for beta$_2$-receptors, isoproterenol can cause vasodilation and hypotension, in contrast to other catecholamines such as dopamine or norepinephrine that potentially can increase both HR and vascular resistance to support BP. Isoproterenol is not used in patients with heart failure or cardiac arrest. Isoproterenol can be strongly arrhythmogenic, like other catecholamines.

Bronchodilator Drugs The oral bronchodilator terbutaline sulfate is a beta$_2$-receptor agonist. It can have a mild stimulatory effect on HR, depending in part on the density of beta$_2$-receptors within the SA node. As an antiarrhythmic, terbutaline is potentially valuable as a 2nd or 3rd-line therapy for patients with symptomatic hyperkalemia, because beta stimulation reduces serum K$^+$, probably by stimulation of skeletal muscle sodium-potassium ATPase.

The methylxanthine bronchodilators, aminophylline and theophylline, can increase HR in some dogs with SSS, especially when used at higher dosages. This action presumably occurs by inhibiting degradation of the 2nd messenger of the beta-receptor (cAMP). Anxious behavior, panting, polydipsia and polyuria are common adverse effects.

Epinephrine Epinephrine is not considered an antiarrhythmic agent, but it can treat asystole or sinus bradycardia in the setting of cardiac arrest. It is a potent catecholamine that causes cardiac stimulation and vasoconstriction through activation of alpha- and beta-adrenergic receptors. Epinephrine is used in the context of cardiopulmonary resuscitation (CPR; p. 428), mainly to help support BP although it also can stimulate the sinus node and latent escape pacemakers, and enhance AV nodal conduction. Similar to terbutaline, its beta agonism can lower serum potassium concentration, which might make it useful in resuscitation of patients with urinary obstruction, Addison's disease, and other causes of severe hyperkalemia. Conversely, epinephrine can be strongly proarrhythmic and induce VF. Low-dose epinephrine is administered at 0.01 mg/kg IV (or intraosseous, IO) using the 1:1000 (1 mg/mL) dilution; this can be repeated a couple of times at 4-minute intervals, as needed. Endotracheal administration (via a long catheter) is an alternative route, dosed at 0.02 mg/kg. Epinephrine sometimes is given at a high dose (0.1 mg/kg IV or IO; or 0.2 mg/kg endotracheally) during protracted CPR; however, survival generally has not been good.

Other Drugs

Phenylephrine Phenylephrine HCl is an alpha-adrenergic agonist that increases BP by causing peripheral vasoconstriction. In terms of arrhythmia management, a baroreflex-mediated increase in vagal tone slows AV conduction and might terminate SVT. In horses with severe quinidine toxicity and hypotension, infusion of this drug can support arterial BP and reduce other signs of vasodilation. Phenylephrine's pressor effect begins rapidly after IV injection and persists for up to 20 minutes. The drug is contraindicated in patients with hypertension or VT. Extravasation can cause ischemic necrosis of surrounding tissue.

Edrophonium Edrophonium chloride is a short-acting anti-cholinesterase with nicotinic and muscarinic effects. The drug is used primarily for diagnosing myasthenia gravis, although its effect of slowing AV conduction might potentially help diagnose and terminate some cases of acute SVT. Edrophonium's effect begins within 1 minute and lasts up to 10 minutes after IV injection. Yet because of adverse cholinergic effects, this drug is rarely if ever considered for use in cardiac patients. These effects include GI (vomiting, diarrhea, salivation), respiratory (bronchospasm, respiratory paralysis, edema), cardiovascular (bradycardia, hypotension, cardiac arrest), and muscular (twitching, weakness) signs. They are treated with atropine and supportive care.

Vagal Maneuver

A vagal maneuver is a physical procedure, generally involving the application of external pressure, and designed to stimulate a reflex vagal surge to the heart. The afferent limb involves either baroreceptor reflexes or the trigeminal nerve. The main indication is for an unexplained SVT or for therapy of a known macro-reentrant SVT that uses the AV node. This procedure usually is tried initially, during preparations for IV catheter placement and other therapy. There is no standardization of the maneuver nor any prospective clinical studies regarding its effectiveness during SVT in animals. A successful vagal maneuver can help the clinician differentiate among tachycardias caused by an ectopic automatic focus, a reentrant circuit involving the AV node, or excessively rapid sinus node activation. Conceptually, increasing vagal tone should transiently slow the rate of sinus tachycardia and allow normal P waves to be seen, although an ectopic atrial tachycardia might slow also. A reentrant tachycardia involving the AV node could be abruptly terminated by a vagal maneuver, provided the increasing AV nodal refractoriness blocks further conduction within the circuit. Finally, if a regular SVT is caused by an automatic ectopic atrial focus (focal atrial tachycardia) or atrial flutter, the vagal maneuver might transiently slow or intermittently block AV conduction sufficiently to expose the abnormal atrial P' or flutter (F) waves.

A vagal maneuver can be performed by massaging the carotid sinus region (with gentle continuous pressure over the carotid sinuses, just caudodorsal to the larynx), or by applying firm (but gentle) bilateral ocular pressure, over closed eyelids, for 15–20 seconds. Other strategies for increasing vagal tone can include progressive and firm digital pressure applied to the face or the nasal planum (especially in cats), or potentially applying iced water or an icepack to the face to stimulate the diving reflex (as in deep sea mammals). Carotid sinus massage is not advised in patients that might have carotid atherosclerosis or other abnormality that could predispose to thromboembolic stroke; however, these rarely are relevant in companion animals. The ocular pressure technique is contraindicated in animals with eye disease. There can be a considerable lag between the application of pressure and the vagal response; for example, it can take 20 seconds or more after removal of pressure to see a response in the cat.

Although a vagal maneuver might be ineffective initially in many cases, it can be repeated after antiarrhythmic drug administration, an opioid, or if the rhythm disturbance persists. In addition, an IV drug that increases vagal tone, or decreases sympathetic tone, can potentiate the vagal maneuver. Such agents include propranolol, esmolol, edrophonium chloride, and phenylephrine; morphine sulfate (0.2 mg/kg IM) also has been suggested. IV fluids are administered concurrently to maintain BP and enhance endogenous vagal tone; however, patients with known or suspected heart failure should receive only a small volume slowly, if at all. Further cardiac diagnostic tests are indicated once conversion is achieved or the ventricular rate falls below 190–200 beats/minute (in dogs).

Pacing Therapy

Cardiac pacing is an advanced, referral procedure and only the basics of cardiac pacing are considered in this volume. Most of the information in this section pertains to dogs, but some comments specific to cats and horses also are included. Interested readers are referred to more detailed veterinary references (Santilli, 2019; Estrada, 2019; DeForge, 2019; Orton, 2019; and other articles in the recent veterinary journal issue focused on this subject, see Pariaut, 2019).

Temporary and permanent artificial cardiac pacing therapies are indicated for bradyarrhythmias, especially high-grade 2nd and 3rd degree AV blocks, SSS with frequent episodes of syncope, and persistent atrial standstill. These disorders are infrequently responsive to medical management. Some canine patients with neural (that is, vasovagal, reflex-mediated, or neurocardiogenic) syncope benefit from specialized pacing modes, although this indication needs more study. Pacing cannot completely mitigate hypotension caused by vasodilation in reflex-mediated syncope. Currently, cardiac resynchronization pacemaker therapy for DCM is considered experimental.

Pacing systems consist of a current source, the pulse generator (pacemaker), and lead(s) that connect the pacemaker to the heart. Most pacing leads are designed for human adult or pediatric use but can be adapted to animals. Pacemakers used for veterinary patients include devices manufactured specifically for animals and human pacemakers that are donated (often with expired shelf-life) or that have been previously used, explanted, and resterilized. Often forgotten is the requirement for compatible external programming devices (computers) to optimize pacing therapy. Some factors that limit the use of pacing therapy include the expense involved with the procedure, concurrent disease, the availability of an appropriate pulse generator with compatible pacing leads, and available operators with appropriate training.

Temporary pacing can involve transvenous leads, transcutaneous thoracic electrodes, or esophageal pacing leads (to pace the atria). Each of these must be attached to an external pacing system. Transcutaneous and transesophageal pacing are painful and must be performed under general anesthesia; as such, they are reserved for intraoperative use during permanent pacemaker implantation, or for backup pacing in patients with a high risk of bradyarrhythmia during general anesthesia for other procedures. The main indications for temporary transvenous pacing are: 1) to manage the hemodynamically unstable patient, especially one with intermittent VT that results in overdrive suppression of ventricular escape rhythms; 2) to assess the effects of a normal HR on pre-existing CHF or severe azotemia, prior to embarking on a permanent pacing system; and 3) to provide HR and BP support during general anesthesia for permanent pacemaker implantation. The temporary lead can be inserted under mild sedation and local anesthesia through the left jugular vein (reserving the right jugular for the permanent lead) or into a femoral or saphenous vein. It is removed once the permanent lead is in place. Transthoracic external pacing (or transesophageal atrial pacing in animals with normal AV conduction) provides an alternative means of supporting HR during permanent pacemaker implantation. In patients with SSS and an intact AV conduction system, transesophageal pacing could be considered but this is less reliable than temporary transcutaneous or transvenous pacing.

A thorough patient workup is indicated before permanent pacemaker implantation. Some underlying conditions (including severe myocardial dysfunction or endocarditis) are associated with a poor prognosis, even after pacing. Animals with CHF complicated by a bradyarrhythmia often do improve with pacing, if the cause relates to periods of prolonged bradycardia; however, prognosis is less favorable if CHF is mainly due to severe structural heart disease, such as from degenerative (myxomatous) mitral valve disease, DCM or persistent atrial standstill. Even moderate to severe degrees of azotemia will improve with pacing, if it is mainly "pre-renal"; but this might not be known until after the procedure or temporary pacing. There are numerous medical and practical considerations involved with identifying optimal patients for pacing, and offering an accurate prognosis for outcome. The specialist consultant should discuss these issues with the client and referring veterinarian. Operators should be intimately familiar with the extensive issues related to technical specifications, procedural steps, system programming, and follow-up (Pariaut, 2019 and others in this journal issue).

Pacemaker therapy is well established in veterinary patients for the aforementioned symptomatic bradycardias. Permanent implantation can be achieved via the jugular transvenous route with a right ventricular (RV) or right atrial (RA) endocardial lead implant (or both) depending on the heart rhythm and operator preferences. The procedure is performed under anesthesia and fluoroscopic guidance, and the pulse generator is implanted under subcutaneous muscle in or around the neck. Single-chamber, RV permanent transvenous pacing is used most commonly today, with the pacing lead tip typically located at the RV apex (see p. 175 and Estrada, 2019, for procedural details; also see **Figures 6.11** & **6.12**, pp. 175 & 176; and **Figures 24.2** & **24.3**). Many single-chamber pacemakers are programmed to a rate-response mode, such that patient movement can trigger a faster HR within programmable ranges. Isolated RA pacing has been done for SSS with intact AV conduction, but can be challenging because of the small size of many veterinary patients. Dual-chamber (RA and RV) pacing can maintain AV synchrony and HR responsiveness to stress in complete AV block, provided SA nodal function is normal. This is especially reasonable for larger breed, active dogs without structure heart disease and at low risk of AF. Epicardial pacing systems are advantageous in some cases (Orton, 2019) and both single- and dual-chamber epicardial pacing system have been described in dogs. This approach is particularly logical for cats, small dogs, in severe right heart disease, or when thoracic or abdominal surgery also are needed. Placement of an epicardial electrode during abdominal surgery often can be done using a transdiaphragmatic approach, with the pulse generator secured within the abdominal cavity or thoracic wall. Permanent endocardial and epicardial pacing is performed

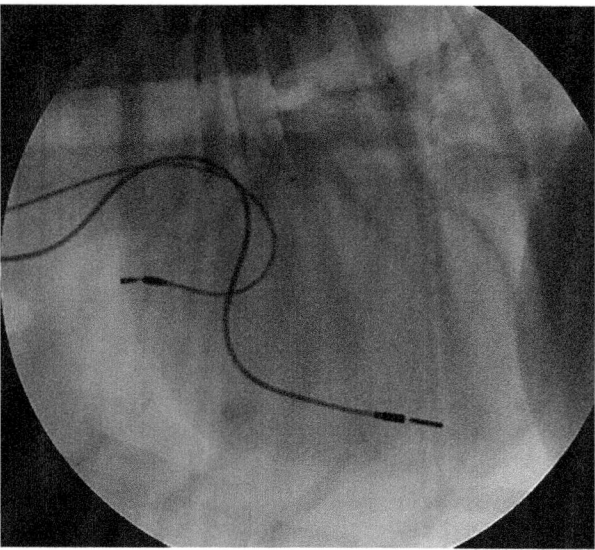

Figure 24.2 Fluoroscopic image showing a dual chamber pacing system in a young dog with 3rd degree AV block. Properly coordinating the timing of ventricular stimulation (pacing lead at lower right) after atrial stimulation (atrial lead at upper left) simulates a normal "AV conduction" interval. This creates a more physiologic synchronization of atrial and ventricular contraction and can improve cardiac output.

rarely in ponies, miniature donkeys, and adult horses, but the procedure is feasible (van Loon, 2001). Overall, major complication rates and survival times appear similar for both transvenous (endocardial) and epicardial pacing, although large dogs might be more likely to experience major complications with epicardial pacing.

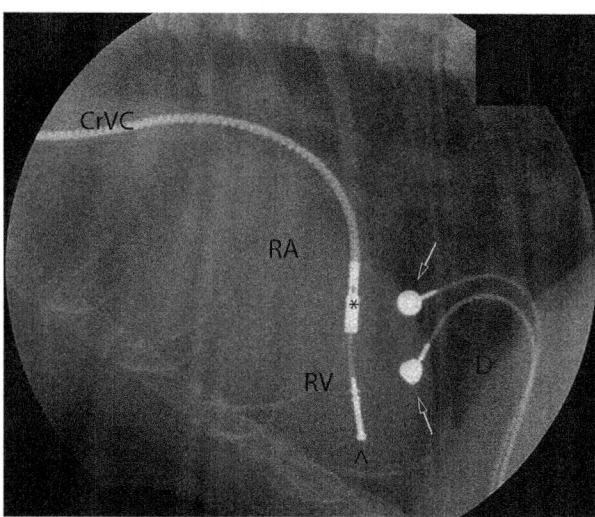

Figure 24.3 Epicardial and permanent transvenous pacing leads in a middle-aged cat with complete AV block. The initial bipolar epicardial leads (arrows) failed because fibrous tissue developed (causing exit block). The system was replaced with a permanent endocardial bipolar lead and cervical pulse generator (not shown). The proximal (*) and distal (^) electrodes of the endocardial lead are outlined, along with the approximate regions of the right atrium (RA) and right ventricle (RV). CrVC, cranial vena cava; D, diaphragm.

For cats that require artificial pacing, the epicardial approach might be better. Chylothorax (presumably from venous obstruction or right-sided CHF) has occurred subsequent to transvenous pacing in cats, although this does not always happen. Before pacing a cat, several issues should be reviewed, including: 1) whether any clinical signs are present (such as syncope, or events that might be interpreted as partial seizures); 2) if there is any underlying disease (such as a cardiomyopathy); 3) whether a stable escape rhythm is present or not; and 4) the likelihood that most cats with 3rd degree AV block have prolonged survival even without artificial pacing. If pacing is pursued in cats, low profile pacemakers and leads should be selected as often as possible. See p. 175 and section "Suggested Additional Reading and References" for more details about pacemaker implantation.

A pacemaker's functional mode is identified by a three (or more) letter code. The first letter refers to the chamber that is paced and the second to the chamber where endogenous electrical activity is sensed. The third letter describes the response to sensed activity (**Table 24.3**). The VVI mode was traditionally used in animals, although the DDD and VDD modes are preferred in people and have been used in dogs. Current pacemakers have multiple programmable features, including rate responsiveness to patient activity; the VVIR mode is probably used most often now in canine pacing. Proper adjustment of the various programmable parameters (both before and after implantation) is important to optimize pacing stability and battery life.

Although single chamber (RV endocardial) pacing is used most often in dogs, and clearly offers satisfactory symptomatic and longevity results in the majority of cases, there are potential negative consequences. Single chamber RV pacing also is associated with dyssynchronous right and left ventricular activation, similar to left bundle branch block, and (with complete AV block) atrial-ventricular dyssynchrony. These can reduce cardiac output and could contribute to progressive ventricular dysfunction. The concern is heightened in large-breed dogs, more prone to DCM, and when pacing is continuous, as with complete AV block. Dual chamber (atrial and ventricular) pacing can be an option for reducing AV dyssynchrony but involves longer procedural times, more cost, and can be more challenging to implant or program. There are some single lead systems that allow both atrial sensing and sequential ventricular (VDD) pacing; however, these leads are long, with inappropriate electrode spacing for most dogs. AV sequential pacing is more physiologic, but challenging to program in sinus node dysfunction. Furthermore, it does not reduce interventricular dyssynchrony or mitigate the effects of chronic RV pacing on ventricular function. Those two issues can only be addressed by developing alternative pacing sites, but where the lead also might be less stable (such as RV outflow tract pacing), or by invoking appropriate sleep and hysteresis modes during programming, to reduce pacing during rest and sleep. Biventricular pacing ("cardiac re-synchronization therapy") can improve left ventricular

Table 24.3 Revised Pacemaker Nomenclature

NBG[a] Code

I	II	III	IV	V
Chamber paced	Chamber sensed	Response to sensing	Programmability, rate modulation	Multipace Site
0 = none	0 = none	0 = none	0 = none	0 = none
A = atrium	A = atrium	T = triggered		A = atrium
V = ventricle	V = ventricle	I = inhibited		V = ventricle
D = dual (A ± V)	D = dual (A + V)	D = dual (T and I)	R = rate modulation	D = dual (A + V)
S = Single (A or V)[b]	S = Single (A or V)[b]			

[a] The North American Society of Pacing and Electrophysiology and the British Pacing and Electrophysiology Group (see Bernstein, 2002).
[b] Manufacturer's designation only.

performance and is a beneficial strategy in people with cardiomyopathy and preexistent left bundle branch block. This involves positioning one lead in the right ventricle and inserting a second lead into a coronary vein to pace the left ventricle. The potential role for biventricular pacing in animals with myocardial failure remains to be explored.

Complications associated with pacing therapy can be common, but often are related to operator and hospital experience. Major complications have occurred in 12 to 33% of cases. Operator experience as well as the relative health and size of the patient substantially influence outcomes. For example, in a high-volume research setting, the rate of major complications, including infection and lead dislodgement, was under 5.5% (Swanson, 2018). In a study of 105 dogs at an experienced university center, the major and minor complication rates were 13% and 11% respectively, with most major complications related to lead dislodgement or sensing issues. Lead dislodgement, with loss of sensing or pacing, appears to be particularly common in large breed dogs and with passive fixation leads. Major complications also can include infection, associated either with the lead wire or pulse generator; RV perforation; VT; profound bradycardia; vena caval thrombosis and stricture; chylothorax; generator failure (or battery depletion); cardiac arrest; and others. Some of these are undoubtedly related to anesthetic management or failure to provide backup (transvenous or transcutaneous) pacing. Minor complications include seroma formation at the generator site (which can become more problematic), muscle twitch, minor ventricular or atrial arrhythmias, and mild hemorrhage, among others. Mean survival time after pacemaker implantation in dogs reportedly is between 2 and 3 years, although many cases live much longer. The underlying disease process is influential, as are comorbidities since the majority of these patients are older.

The potential role of pacing therapy with an implantable cardioverter defibrillator device to interrupt tachyarrhythmias or provide defibrillation shocks currently is undefined, and this is not recommended. Aside from challenges involving device availability, human algorithms, advanced programming requirements, and other technical issues, there is a propensity for T-wave (as well as R-wave) oversensing. This causes inaccurate rhythm assessment by the device and can trigger inappropriate (and painful) defibrillation shocks to the patient.

Cardioversion and Defibrillation

Electrical conversion of a supraventricular or ventricular tachyarrhythmia to sinus rhythm can occur via external or internal current delivery. Arrhythmias dependent on impulse reentry are most susceptible to termination. These include AF, atrial flutter, reentrant AV nodal tachycardia, AV reciprocating tachycardia using an accessory pathway, and many VTs. The effectiveness of the electric shock depends on simultaneous depolarization of the entire myocardium, possibly with refractory period prolongation; this interrupts reentrant circuits and allows sinus rhythm to be reestablished. The timing of the shock used for electrical cardioversion must be synchronized to one of the patient's endogenous QRS complexes (R waves), otherwise there is high risk of inducing a lethal arrhythmia. In contrast, the electric shock used to attempt defibrillation in patients with VF is unsynchronized. The energy delivered during electrical cardioversion generally is less than that required for defibrillation. Both monophasic and biphasic (positive followed by negative) energy waveforms have been used for cardioversion and defibrillation. Biphasic cardioverter/defibrillators use lower energy shocks that can be more effective and safer than devices producing monophasic shocks.

Cardioversion

External cardioversion in dogs is accomplished by a direct current (DC) shock applied via cardioverter/defibrillator paddles (or adhesive cardioversion pads) positioned on the thorax overlying the heart and synchronized to the patient's R wave (to avoid inducing VF). Appropriate equipment and operator training are necessary for successful cardioversion. Except in emergency situations, general anesthesia is used prior to

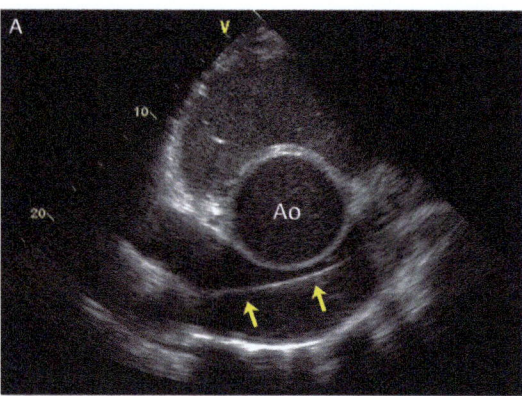 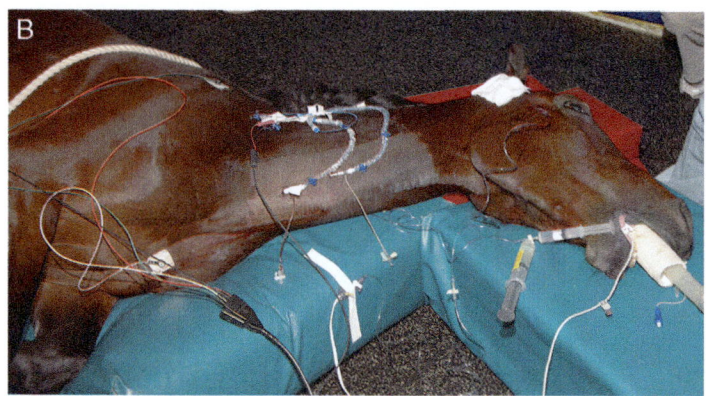

Figure 24.4 (A) Echocardiographic image showing an electrode catheter (arrows) positioned in the left pulmonary artery in preparation for transvenous electrical cardioversion of atrial fibrillation in a horse. Ao, aorta. (B) After both electrode catheters have been inserted (through the jugular vein) and secured in position, general anesthesia is induced. Catheter position should be verified before applying direct current shock(s), synchronized to the patient's QRS complexes.

shock delivery. Cardioversion of AF might be more successful with antiarrhythmic drug pretreatment and after serum potassium and magnesium concentrations are optimized. In dogs, amiodarone loading or sotalol therapy for a week or two has been recommended, but there are no prospective studies regarding this. Even after successful cardioversion, arrhythmias can recur. Sinus rhythm is less likely to be maintained in animals with structural heart disease, such as cardiomyopathy, and in those with long-standing AF. Cardioversion should be used only cautiously in animals with known sinus node dysfunction unless a pacemaker or endocardial cardioversion leads are in place, because sinus rhythm might not adequately resume postconversion. The presence of an intraatrial thrombus is one contraindication for electrical cardioversion in animals with AF, because reestablishment of sinus rhythm and atrial contraction could lead to systemic arterial embolization. Electrical cardioversion should not be done in patients with digoxin-induced tachyarrhythmias. Shock-associated hemolysis does not appear to be a clinical concern, at least in dogs undergoing biphasic cardioversion.

The initial cardioversion shock "dose" used for dogs depends on the rhythm, the size of the animal, operator preference, and to some degree, the available equipment. Uniform prospective studies are lacking. Personal experience indicates that low energy levels (~1 J/kg) often are sufficient for converting sustained VT; if that is ineffective, higher doses can be used. A higher energy dose often is needed to cardiovert AF, and an initial 2 J/kg shock is suggested; this is increased by ~50% until cardioversion or the highest energy output is obtained (see p. 412 for additional details).

In horses, transvenous electrical cardioversion can successfully convert AF (**Figure 25.8**, p. 416). The procedure requires specialized catheters and advanced training. The two electrode catheters are placed percutaneously into the jugular vein using local anesthetic, with the horse sedated and standing. One catheter is positioned with its tip in the left pulmonary artery; the tip of the other catheter is positioned in the right atrium. Catheter placement can be guided by the pressures and intracardiac electrogram recorded at the catheter tip and by echocardiography (**Figure 24.4**). The catheters are secured at their insertion site, then general anesthesia is induced. Catheter positioning is verified radiographically before or ideally after the horse is positioned in lateral recumbency, and before proceeding with cardioversion. Shocks are synchronized with the patient's QRS complexes (R waves), as in transthoracic cardioversion. The initial energy used can vary, but an initial dose of 0.2-0.3 J/kg is suggested. Complications related to either anesthesia or the applied current can occur. Transient AV block has occurred rarely. See "Suggested Additional Reading and References" for sources of further details about electrical cardioversion.

Intracardiac Electrical Mapping and Catheter Ablation

Various tachyarrhythmias that depend on a focal anatomical area for their continuation potentially can be treated by catheter ablation. These arrhythmias include automatic or reentrant atrial and AV junctional tachycardias, atrial flutter (and fibrillation), and AV reentrant tachycardia involving an accessory pathway. Most often, catheter ablation procedures utilize radiofrequency energy to create small point or linear lesions or scars that interrupt the circuit (Chapter 23) and prevent arrhythmia continuation. Radiofrequency current produces heat, which causes coagulation necrosis and disrupts the electrophysiologic function of the affected tissue. In some cases, cryoablation catheters are used to destroy focal areas of tissue by freezing. Prior to ablation, intracardiac electrical mapping is used to identify the anatomical origin of the arrhythmia, guide the ablation procedure, and assess its effectiveness. General anesthesia is required and procedure time can be lengthy, depending on the methodology of mapping. Intracardiac electrophysiologic study and ablation require specialized equipment and subspecialized training. These procedures are available at some referral centers. Catheter ablation might not be possible in patients too small to accommodate the mapping or ablation catheters. However, for cases suited to this treatment, it can provide freedom from the need for long-term antiarrhythmic drug therapy and complications associated with tachycardia-induced cardiomyopathy.

Defibrillation

Defibrillation can be an important component of advanced life support therapy for cardiopulmonary arrest. It is indicated only for certain cardiac rhythms that are likely to respond to defibrillation (so-called "shockable" rhythms). Such rhythms include VF and pulseless VT. The goal of defibrillation is to stop chaotic, ineffective ventricular activation by depolarizing the myocardium all at once so that, upon repolarization, normal coordinated electrical activation and contraction can resume. Defibrillation can be done with either biphasic or monophasic current. Biphasic defibrillation can more effectively convert VF and uses lower current. Recommended initial energy level for biphasic external defibrillation is 2–4 J/kg (and for internal defibrillation, 0.2–0.4 J/kg). For monophasic defibrillation, an initial recommended setting is 4–6 J/kg for external (and 0.5–1 J/kg for internal) defibrillation.

When a shockable cardiac rhythm has been identified, CPR should be continued while the defibrillator is being charged and other preparations made prior to shock delivery. The manufacturer's instructions should be followed closely. Care must be taken to avoid inadvertent shocks to personnel and equipment. After defibrillator discharge, CPR immediately is resumed for 2 minutes before the ECG and pulses are reassessed. If rhythm conversion did not occur, defibrillation should be repeated using an energy level 50% higher than the previous dose, followed by CPR for another 2 minutes before cardiac status is reassessed. This sequence can be repeated to a maximum dose of 10 J/kg, as long as a shockable rhythm exists. If multiple defibrillation shocks have not produced an effective rhythm, IV amiodarone or lidocaine might be helpful. In situations where no defibrillator is available, a precordial thump could be tried to attempt mechanical defibrillation; this involves an abrupt, strong blow to the chest wall over the heart. Unfortunately, it usually is unsuccessful.

Some cardiac rhythms that occur during cardiac arrest are unlikely to respond to defibrillation. These so-called "non-shockable" rhythms, include ventricular asystole and "pulseless electrical activity." The latter entails ventricular-origin waveforms (generally at rates <200/minute) which produce no evidence of myocardial contraction. Electrical-mechanical dissociation is an older name for this. Defibrillation is not recommended for ventricular asystole and pulseless electrical activity. Instead, CPR with epinephrine and other supportive measures are advocated. See "Suggested Additional Reading and References" for more detailed information about CPR guidelines.

Suggested Additional Reading and References

Also See Online Comprehensive Bibliography at: https://www.routledge.com/9781482246223.

Bernstein AD, Daubert JC, Fletcher RD, et al. The revised NASPE/BPEG generic code for antibradycardia, adaptive-rate, and multisite pacing. North American Society of Pacing and Electrophysiology/British Pacing and Electrophysiology Group. Pacing Clin Electrophysiol 2002;25:260–264.

Boller M, Fletcher DJ. RECOVER evidence and knowledge gap analysis on veterinary CPR. Part 1: evidence analysis and consensus process: collaborative path toward small animal CPR guidelines. J Vet Emerg Crit Care 2012;22:S4–S12.

Broux B, De Clercq D, Decloedt A, et al. Pharmacokinetics and electrophysiological effects of sotalol hydrochloride in horses. Equine Vet J 2018;50:377–383.

Carstensen H, Kjaer L, Haugaard MM, et al. Antiarrhythmic effects of combining dofetilide and ranolazine in a model of acutely induced atrial fibrillation in horses. J Cardiovasc Pharmacol 2018;71:26–35.

Cushing DJ, Cooper WD, Gralinski MR, et al. Comparison of the cardiac electrophysiology and general toxicology of two formulations of intravenous amiodarone in dogs. Cardiovasc Toxicol 2009;9:126–133.

De Clercq D, van Loon G, Tavernier R, et al. Use of propafenone for conversion of chronic atrial fibrillation in horses. Am J Vet Res 2009;70:223–227.

De Clercq D, Baert K, Croubels S, et al. Evaluation of the pharmacokinetics and bioavailability of intravenously and orally administered amiodarone in horses. Am J Vet Res 2006;67:448–454.

Decloedt A, Broux B, De Clercq D, et al. Effect of sotalol on heart rate, QT interval, and atrial fibrillation cycle length in horses with atrial fibrillation. J Vet Intern Med 2018;32:815–821.

DeForge WF. Cardiac pacemakers: a basic review of the history and current technology. J Vet Cardiol 2019;22:40–50.

Dembek KA, Hurcombe SD, Schober KE, et al. Sudden death of a horse with supraventricular tachycardia following oral administration of flecainide acetate. J Vet Emerg Crit Care 2014;24:759–763.

Estrada AH, Maisenbacher HW 3rd, Jones AE, et al. Transvenous pacing implantation: techniques, tips, and lessons learned along the way. J Vet Cardiol 2019;22:51–64.

Fletcher J, Boller M. Cardiopulmonary arrest and CPR. In, Ettinger SJ, Feldman EC, Côté E (editors). Textbook of Veterinary Internal Medicine. 8th edition. Elsevier, St. Louis, MO. 2017. pp. 581–586.

Fletcher DJ, Boller M, Brainard BM, et al. RECOVER evidence and knowledge gap analysis on veterinary CPR. Part 7: clinical guidelines. J Vet Emerg Crit Care 2012;22:S102–S131.

Gelzer AR, Kraus MS, Rishniw M, et al. Combination therapy with mexiletine and sotalol suppresses inherited ventricular arrhythmias in German Shepherd dogs better than mexiletine or sotalol monotherapy: a randomized cross-over study. J Vet Cardiol 2010;12:93–106.

Genovese DW, Estrada AH, Maisenbacher HW, et al. Procedure times, complication rates, and survival times associated with single-chamber versus dual-chamber pacemaker implantation in dogs with clinical signs of bradyarrhythmia: 54 cases (2004–2009). J Am Vet Med Assoc 2013;242:230–236.

Gunther-Harrington CT, Ontiveros ES, Hodge TE, et al. Effects of 0.5% timolol maleate ophthalmic solution on heart rate and selected echocardiographic indices in apparently healthy cats. J Vet Intern Med 2016;30:733–740.

Haugaard MM, Pehrson S, Carstensen H, et al. Antiarrhythmic and electrophysiologic effects of flecainide on acutely induced atrial fibrillation in healthy horses. J Vet Intern Med 2015;29:339–347.

Hesselkilde EZ, Carstensen H, Haugaard MM, et al. Effect of flecainide on atrial fibrillatory rate in a large animal model with induced atrial fibrillation. BMC cardiovascular disorders 2017;17:289.

Hildebrandt N, Stertmann WA, Wehner M, et al. Dual chamber pacemaker implantation in dogs with atrioventricular block. J Vet Intern Med 2009;23:31–38.

Humphrey S, Kirby R, Rudloff E. Magnesium physiology and clinical therapy in veterinary critical care. J Vet Emerg Crit Care (San Antonio) 2015;25:210–225.

Jackson BL, Adin DB, Lehmkuhl LB. Effect of atenolol on heart rate, arrhythmias, blood pressure, and dynamic left ventricular outflow tract obstruction in cats with subclinical hypertrophic cardiomyopathy. J Vet Cardiol 2015;17(Suppl 1):S296–305.

Johnson MS, Martin MW, Henley W. Results of pacemaker implantation in 104 dogs. J Small Anim Pract 2007;48:4–11.

Jung SW, Newhard DK, Harrelson K. Transvenous electrical cardioversion of atrial fibrillation in two dogs. J Vet Cardiol 2017;19:175–181.

Kraus MS, Thomason JD, Fallaw TL, et al. Toxicity in Doberman Pinchers with ventricular arrhythmias treated with amiodarone (1996–2005). J Vet Intern Med 2009;23:1–6.

LeBlanc NL, Agarwal D, Menzen E, et al. Prevalence of major complications and procedural mortality in 336 dogs undergoing interventional cardiology procedures in a single academic center. J Vet Cardiol 2019;23:45–57.

Lei M, Wu L, Terrar DA, et al. Modernized classification of cardiac antiarrhythmic drugs. Circulation 2018;138:1879–1896.

Levy NA, Koenigshof AM, Sanders RA. Retrospective evaluation of intravenous premixed amiodarone use and adverse effects in dogs (17 cases: 2011–2014). J Vet Cardiol 2016;18:10–14.

Li YD, Ji YT, Zhou XH, et al. Effects of ivabradine on cardiac electrophysiology in dogs with age-related atrial fibrillation. Med Sci Monit 2015;21:1414–1420.

Lichtenberger J, Scollan KF, Bulmer BJ, et al. Long-term outcome of physiologic VDD pacing versus non-physiologic VVI pacing in dogs with high-grade atrioventricular block. J Vet Cardiol 2015;17:42–53.

Matsukura S, Nakamura Y, Cao X, et al. Anti-atrial fibrillatory versus proarrhythmic potentials of amiodarone: a new protocol for safety evaluation in vivo. Cardiovasc Toxicol 2017;17:157–162.

McGurrin MK, Physick-Sheard PW, Kenney DG. How to perform transvenous electrical cardioversion in horses with atrial fibrillation. J Vet Cardiol 2005;7:109–119.

McGurrin MK, Physick-Sheard PW, Kenney DG, et al. Transvenous electrical cardioversion of equine atrial fibrillation: technical considerations. J Vet Intern Med 2005;19:695–702.

McGurrin MK, Physick-Sheard PW, Kenney DG. Transvenous electrical cardioversion of equine atrial fibrillation: patient factors and clinical results in 72 treatment episodes. J Vet Intern Med 2008;22:609–615.

Miyamoto M, Nishijima Y, Nakayama T, et al. Cardiovascular effects of intravenous diltiazem in dogs with iatrogenic atrial fibrillation. J Vet Intern Med 2000;14:445–451.

Moise NS, Pariaut R, Gelzer AR, et al. Cardioversion with lidocaine of vagally associated atrial fibrillation in two dogs. J Vet Cardiol 2005;7:143–148.

Noszczyk-Nowak A, Michalek M, Janiszewski A, et al. Analysis of haematological and biochemical blood parameters after electrical cardioversion of atrial fibrillation in dogs. J Vet Res 2018;62:109–112.

Orton EC. Epicardial pacemaker implantation in small animals. J Vet Cardiol 2019;22:65–71.

Oyama MA, Sisson DD, Lehmkuhl LB. Practices and outcome of artificial cardiac pacing in 154 dogs. J Vet Intern Med 2001;15:229–239.

Pariaut R. Special issue: cardiac pacing. J Vet Cardiol 2019;22:1.

Pariaut R, Moise NS, Koetje BD, et al. Lidocaine converts acute vagally associated atrial fibrillation to sinus rhythm in German Shepherd dogs with inherited arrhythmias. J Vet Intern Med 2008;22:1274–1282.

Pedro B, Lopez-Alvarez J, Fonfara S, et al. Retrospective evaluation of the use of amiodarone in dogs with arrhythmias (from 2003 to 2010). J Small Anim Pract 2012;53:19–26.

Perego M, Porteiro Vazquez DM, Ramera L, et al. Heart rhythm characterisation during unexplained transient loss of consciousness in dogs. Vet J 2020;263:105523

Preiss EE, Kenney DG, McGurrin MK, et al. Influence of electrode position on cardioversion energy requirements during transvenous electrical cardioversion in horses. Am J Vet Res 2011;72:1193–1203.

Ramadeen A, Laurent G, dos Santos CC, et al. N-3 polyunsaturated fatty acids alter expression of fibrotic and hypertrophic genes in a dog model of atrial cardiomyopathy. Heart Rhythm 2010;7:520–528.

Redpath A, Bowen M. Cardiac therapeutics in horses. Vet Clin North Am Equine Pract 2019;35:217–241.

Riesen SC, Schober KE, Smith DN, et al. Effects of ivabradine on heart rate and left ventricular function in healthy cats and cats with hypertrophic cardiomyopathy. Am J Vet Res 2012;73:202–212.

Risberg AI, McGuirk SM. Successful conversion of equine atrial fibrillation using oral flecainide. J Vet Intern Med 2006;20:207–209.

Rishniw M, Kittleson MD, Jaffe RS, et al. Characterization of parasympatholytic chronotropic responses following intravenous administration of atropine to clinically normal dogs. Am J Vet Res 1999;60:1000–1003.

Robinson SJ, Feary DJ. Sudden death following oral administration of flecainide to horses with naturally occurring atrial fibrillation. Aust Equine Vet 2008;27:49–51.

Rodrigo R, Vinay J, Castillo R, et al. Use of vitamins C and E as a prophylactic therapy to prevent postoperative atrial fibrillation. Int J Cardiol 2010;138:221–228.

Rozanski EA, Rush JE, Buckley GJ, et al. RECOVER evidence and knowledge gap analysis on veterinary CPR. Part 4: advanced life support. J Vet Emerg Crit Care 2012;22(Suppl 1):S44–64.

Saengklub N, Limprasutr V, Sawangkoon S, et al. Acute effects of intravenous dronedarone on electrocardiograms, hemodynamics and cardiac functions in anesthetized dogs. J Vet Med Sci 2016;78:177–186.

Saengklub N, Limprasutr V, Sawangkoon S, et al. Dronedarone attenuates the duration of atrial fibrillation in a dog model of sustained atrial fibrillation. Exp Anim 2017;66:251–258.

Santilli RA, Giacomazzi F, Porteiro Vazquez DM, et al. Indications for permanent pacing in dogs and cats. J Vet Cardiol 2019;22:20–39.

Saunders AB, Miller MW, Gordon SG, et al. Oral amiodarone therapy in dogs with atrial fibrillation. J Vet Intern Med 2006;20:921–926.

Savelieva I, Kourliouros A, Camm J. Primary and secondary prevention of atrial fibrillation with statins and polyunsaturated fatty acids: review of evidence and clinical relevance. Naunyn Schmiedebergs Arch Pharmacol 2010;381:1–13.

Schwarzwald CC, Bonagura JD, Luis-Fuentes V. Effects of diltiazem on hemodynamic variables and ventricular function in healthy horses. J Vet Intern Med 2005;19:703–711.

Schwarzwald CC, Hamlin RL, Bonagura JD, et al. Atrial, SA nodal, and AV nodal electrophysiology in standing horses: normal findings and electrophysiologic effects of quinidine and diltiazem. J Vet Intern Med 2007;21:166–175.

Smith CE, Freeman LM, Rush JE, et al. Omega-3 fatty acids in Boxer dogs with arrhythmogenic right ventricular cardiomyopathy. J Vet Intern Med 2007;21:265–273.

Sun JL, Han R, Guo JH, et al. Effect of ibutilide on the canine cardiac conduction system. Cell Biochem Biophys 2012;64:161–168.

Swanson LE, Huibregtse BA, Scansen BA. A retrospective review of 146 active and passive fixation bradycardia lead implantations in 74 dogs undergoing pacemaker implantation in a research setting of short term duration. BMC Vet Res 2018;14:112.

Syring RS, Costello MF, Poppenga RH. Temporary transvenous cardiac pacing in a dog with diltiazem intoxication. J Vet Emerg Crit Care 2008;18:75–80.

Takahashi Y, Ishikawa Y, Ohmura H. Treatment of recent-onset atrial fibrillation with quinidine and flecainide in Thoroughbred racehorses: 107 cases (1987-2014). J Am Vet Med Assoc 2018;252:1409-1414.

Thomasy SM, Pypendop BH, Ilkiw JE, et al. Pharmacokinetics of lidocaine and its active metabolite, monoethylglycinexylidide, after intravenous administration of lidocaine to awake and isoflurane-anesthetized cats. Am J Vet Res 2005;66:1162–1166.

van Loon G, Blissitt KJ, Keen JA, et al. Use of intravenous flecainide in horses with naturally-occurring atrial fibrillation. Equine Vet J 2004;36:609–614.

van Loon G, Fonteyne W, Rottiers H, et al. Dual-chamber pacemaker implantation via the cephalic vein in healthy equids. J Vet Intern Med 2001;15:564–571.

Visser LC, Kaplan JL, Nishimura S, et al. Acute echocardiographic effects of sotalol on ventricular systolic function in dogs with ventricular arrhythmias. J Vet Intern Med 2018.

Visser LC, Keene BW, Mathews KG, et al. Outcomes and complications associated with epicardial pacemakers in 28 dogs and 5 cats. Vet Surg 2013;42:544–550.

Wall M, Calvert CA, Sanderson SL, et al. Evaluation of extended-release diltiazem once daily for cats with hypertrophic cardiomyopathy. J Am Anim Hosp Assoc 2005;41:98–103.

Wess G, Thomas WP, Berger DM, et al. Applications, complications, and outcomes of transvenous pacemaker implantation in 105 dogs (1997–2002). J Vet Intern Med 2006;20:877–884.

Wiedemann N, Hildebrandt N, Wurtinger G, et al. Follow-up of troponin I concentration in dogs with atrioventricular block and dual-chamber pacing in a case-matched study. J Vet Cardiol 2017;19:247–255.

Wijnberg ID, Ververs FF. Phenytoin sodium as a treatment for ventricular dysrhythmia in horses. J Vet Intern Med 2004;18:350–353.

Wright KN, Connor CE, Irvin HM, et al. Atrioventricular accessory pathways in 89 dogs: clinical features and outcome after radiofrequency catheter ablation. J Vet Intern Med 2018;32:1517–1529.

Wright KN, Knilans TK, Irvin HM. When, why, and how to perform cardiac radiofrequency catheter ablation. J Vet Cardiol 2006;8:95–107.

Wright KN, Nguyenba T, Irvin HM. Lidocaine for chemical cardioversion of orthodromic atrioventricular reciprocating tachycardia in dogs. J Vet Intern Med 2019;33:1585–1592.

Zhou SX, Fang C, Zheng SX, et al. Effect of amiodarone on dispersion of ventricular repolarization in a canine congestive heart failure model. Clin Exp Pharmacol Physiol 2012;39:241–246.

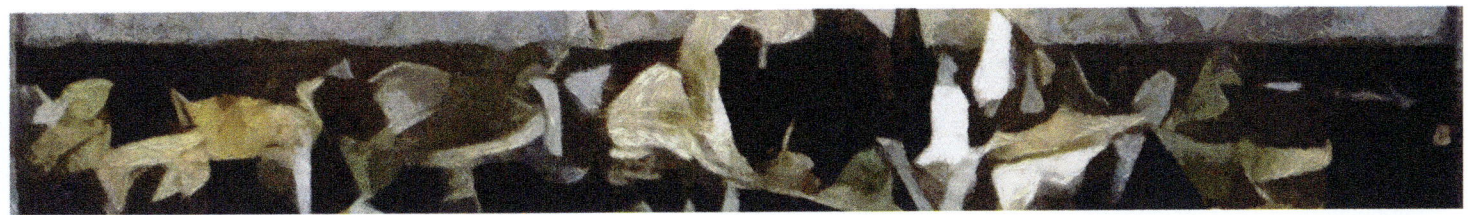

25
MANAGEMENT OF CARDIAC ARRHYTHMIAS

Cardiac arrhythmias present a number of challenges for the clinician. Some arrhythmias clearly produce serious and potentially fatal hemodynamic compromise, while others cause no clinical problems. Some might portend increased risk for sudden arrhythmic death. A complex interplay of factors influence the heart's rhythm (Chapter 23). Some factors are modifiable, which could reduce arrhythmia occurrence or severity even without antiarrhythmic drugs. In all cases, any identified predisposing conditions should be managed, as possible. Besides identifying the presence and type of arrhythmia in a patient, the clinician must decide whether antiarrhythmic drug therapy is warranted, and if so, which drug is likely to be most effective, and whether the therapeutic benefits outweigh potential risks and cost. Before prescribing an antiarrhythmic drug, the clinician should understand the properties and potential adverse effects of that agent (Chapter 24).

Whether antiarrhythmic drug therapy should be used for arrhythmias that cause no clinical signs is not always clear. Individual circumstances often influence that decision. When ventricular structure and function are normal in animals with asymptomatic ventricular ectopy, there generally is less advocacy for antiarrhythmic drug use. However, this conservative approach might not be advisable for animals with a condition known to be associated with sudden death. Nevertheless, there is agreement that arrhythmias causing acute clinical signs, or hypotension in an anesthetized or critically ill patient, should be treated. Likewise, therapy is indicated for persistent tachycardias because of their negative long-term effect on myocardial function. Antiarrhythmic therapy is unlikely to suppress all abnormal beats; however, reduced frequency and repetitive rate of a tachycardia and restoration of normal hemodynamic status can be signs of treatment success. Some antiarrhythmic therapies could reduce the risk for sudden death. Yet it is important to recognize that even apparently complete arrhythmia suppression does not necessarily provide total protection against a lethal arrhythmia and sudden cardiac death.

Initial Management Considerations

Patient Assessment

All aspects of the patient's clinical situation should be considered (**Table 25.1**). Signalment, medical history, findings from a complete physical examination, and other available clinical data provide important information (also see Chapter 12). Signalment can be particularly important because some breeds have an increased prevalence of diseases associated with sudden arrhythmic death, including Boxers (arrhythmogenic right ventricular cardiomyopathy, ARVC) and Doberman Pinschers (dilated cardiomyopathy, DCM). When cardiac output becomes inadequate for the animal's level of activity, weakness, lethargy, syncope, or pre-syncope are likely to occur (Chapter 8). An arrhythmia's immediate effects on cardiac function are manifest by the presence or absence of these clinical signs, as well as the patient's peripheral perfusion, mentation, pulse quality, and arterial blood pressure (BP). The onset or exacerbation of congestive heart failure (CHF) can be another consequence of arrhythmias. Of greatest concern are arrhythmias that cause marked hemodynamic compromise, as well as those that occur in situations known to be associated with sudden death. Conversely, especially in animals with normal heart size and function, some arrhythmias can be fairly benign. These could include pronounced sinus pauses, isolated premature beats, accelerated idioventricular rhythm, brief episodes of paroxysmal tachycardia at a moderate heart rate (HR), and intermittent low-grade atrioventricular (AV) block (Chapters 5 and 12). The abolition of arrhythmias during exercise often is a favorable sign; whereas, their provocation with exertion is concerning, and in a horse, potentially dangerous to people.

Table 25.1 Approach to the Patient with an Arrhythmia

Identify and Define the Arrhythmia

- See Tables 5.3, p. 140, and 12.2, p. 238, and Figure 12.7, p. 243
- An extended recording period might be necessary (ambulatory ECG or prolonged in-hospital monitoring)

Evaluate the Patient

- History, physical exam findings, laboratory tests (especially electrolytes), cardiac & respiratory function, acid/base status, other tests as indicated
- Correct what can be corrected

Decide Whether to Use Antiarrhythmic Drug or Other Therapy

- Consider case context & clinical signs (see text)
- Consider benefits versus risks of therapeutic options
- Define individual patient goals for antiarrhythmic drug therapy, if used

Initiate therapy as needed and determine effectiveness

- Assess arrhythmia control
  - Continuous ECG monitoring for acute cases
  - Consider repeated Holter studies, or other ECG monitoring for chronic cases
- Assess the patient
  - Blood pressure, cardiac function, peripheral perfusion, resolution of clinical signs
- Adjust drug dose(s) or try alternate agent(s) as necessary (see text)
- Restrict exercise and provide ancillary support, as appropriate

Monitor and Follow-up

- Continue monitoring heart rhythm & rate
- Manage underlying disease or other abnormalities, as possible
- Monitor for adverse drug effects & other complications
- Periodically reassess need for continued therapy

In all cases, a search for underlying conditions potentially associated with the arrhythmia (**Table 23.1**, p. 370) and an accurate electrocardiographic (ECG) rhythm diagnosis, along with monitoring of the patient's rhythm and clinical status, are warranted. Echocardiography can provide important information in animals with suspected structural or genetically-predisposed cardiac diseases, and thoracic radiographs permit evaluation for cardiomegaly, signs of CHF, pulmonary hypertension, and noncardiac disorders (such as metastatic neoplasia) that might incite rhythm disturbances. When myocarditis or other acute cardiac insult is suspected, measuring cardiac troponin (cTnI) concentration is helpful; although, severe arrhythmias that promote myocardial ischemia can secondarily elevate cTnI concentrations. When a noncardiac disorder is suspected or clear evidence of primary heart disease is lacking, an ECG, complete blood count (CBC), routine serum chemistry profile with electrolytes (especially K^+ and Mg^{++}), cTnI, and at least a screening echocardiogram are advised. Thoracic radiography and abdominal ultrasonography, especially with careful splenic evaluation, also might be useful.

Rhythm Diagnosis

Accurate ECG interpretation is important for defining the origin, timing, and severity of arrhythmias and for guiding treatment decisions. However, this can be challenging and findings on one resting ECG recording could potentially be misleading. Cardiac arrhythmias can vary tremendously in frequency and severity over time. Critical arrhythmias easily can be missed on a routine ECG. Holter or other ambulatory ECG monitoring (with an event or implantable loop recorder) allows the clinician to better assess arrhythmia frequency and severity, as well as treatment efficacy. This is especially important in patients with weakness or syncopal episodes.

Single-lead ECG recordings often are adequate for rhythm analysis, as long as P waves are clearly seen. These could be acquired from lead II, a thoracic (or base-apex) lead, or with a smartphone app (**Figures 12.8** and **12.9**, p. 244). There usually is good correlation between rhythm diagnosis from smartphone app and standard 6 lead ECG recordings, however multiple-lead (3–9 lead) recordings are useful in many cases. For example, multiple leads recorded sequentially or simultaneously, as well as special lead systems, can be helpful when P waves are difficult to identify; this often occurs in cats and during narrow-QRS tachycardias in dogs. The morphology of P waves in multiple leads also is instructive with a "supraventricular tachycardia" (SVT). Sometimes just moving the forelimb electrodes to the thorax (left arm to left apex, right arm to the craniodorsal right cardiac base, and selecting lead I) and increasing the sensitivity of the recording to 20 mm/mV can help the clinician identify P waves. Additionally, recording more than one lead simultaneously can help in differentiating artifacts from rhythm disturbances, when this is unclear. Esophageal leads or intracardiac electrograms might record difficult-to-see P waves better in some cases, but these are rarely used.

Arrhythmia identification begins with a left-to-right visual scan of the entire ECG recording (**Table 5.3**, p. 140). Normal P-QRS-T waveforms are identified, HR determined, and an orientation to the overall rhythm obtained. Because some ECG artifacts can resemble rhythm disturbances (p. 161), close evaluation is warranted to avoid misinterpretation. For example, multiple "blips" or small baseline deflections might be mistaken for ectopic P (P′) waves, but if they occur regularly and are superimposed on true P waves, their artifactual nature will be recognized.

Ectopic (abnormal) complexes are identified and classified, as possible, by origin (supraventricular or ventricular), site (right or left ventricle), and timing (premature or escape). Variations in P wave size and morphology might indicate an ectopic atrial focus, but could simply be a normal wandering pacemaker (p. 143). QRS-T complexes that are wider or markedly different from sinus QRS complexes are more likely to be ventricular in origin, but could represent supraventricular impulses conducted aberrantly within the ventricle. For example, exercise ECGs in horses often show premature complexes of different morphology; however, determining the atrial or ventricular origin of the impulses can be challenging. Clues to the electrophysiologic mechanism underlying ectopic complexes, such as an automatic focus or reentry, also might be evident, although this often is speculative. More information on the general approach to ECG interpretation and descriptions of common rhythm disturbances are in Chapter 5. **Table 12.2** (p. 238) provides guidelines for differential diagnoses based on the rhythm's rate and regularity.

Rapid and regular narrow-QRS tachycardias generally involve atrial or AV junctional tissues. When a fast rhythm involves at least one of these tissues, the generic "SVT" term often is used. However SVT represents a nonspecific diagnosis, which might be caused by sinus tachycardia, a focal atrial tachycardia (FAT), macro-reentrant atrial tachycardia (that is, atrial flutter) with regular AV conduction, an AV reciprocating (or other possibly reentrant AV nodal) tachycardia, or a junctional (nodal) tachycardia. Moreover, a ventricular tachycardia (VT) originating high in the interventricular septum also can produce relatively narrow QRS complexes. Differentiation can be challenging, especially because P waves might not be seen well (or at all), if buried in preceding QRS or ST-T waveforms. A vagal maneuver (p. 388) or drug that acts on the AV node might help define or even interrupt the arrhythmia. It is important to differentiate sinus tachycardia from other tachyarrhythmias, either by interrupting the circuit and breaking the SVT or by blocking P′ or flutter (F) waves in the AV node. Sinus tachycardia should improve when the underlying cause for high sympathetic tone is addressed. Ectopic rhythms with a rapid ventricular rate (for example, >200 to 250 beats/minute in dogs and >100 to 120 beats/minute in horses) usually require immediate intravenous (IV) antiarrhythmic drug therapy.

Wide-QRS tachycardias can present a diagnostic challenge, too. If the rhythm is fairly regular, a ventricular origin is most likely. However, a SVT with aberrant ventricular conduction (such as a major bundle branch block; p. 153) also must be considered, especially if there is no response to initial ventricular antiarrhythmic drug therapy. Irregular, wide-QRS tachycardias without visible P waves usually are atrial fibrillation (AF) with concurrent ventricular aberrancy (**Figure 25.1**), or rarely, antegrade conduction down an accessory pathway with complete ventricular preexcitation. Moreover, VT can be somewhat irregular (especially multiform VT), and unrelated sinus P waves might not be clearly visualized if the ventricular rate is rapid. ECG features consistent with VT, and that are helpful for differentiating it from a supraventricular tachyarrhythmia with aberrancy, include the presence of fusion or capture complexes (p. 148), evidence for AV dissociation, and multiple wide-QRS configurations. A vagal maneuver might help identify whether AV dissociation is present, although the maneuver infrequently works. Termination of the tachyarrhythmia by a vagal maneuver suggests a reentrant SVT, although rarely, termination of VT secondary to triggered activity might occur. Subtle physical exam findings that suggest AV dissociation (and a ventricular-origin tachycardia) can include intermittently strong jugular pulsations from "cannon a waves" (p. 262), variable intensity first (S_1) heart sounds resulting from beat-to-beat differences in how open the AV valve leaflets are when ventricular contraction begins, and split second (S_2) heart sounds caused by dyssynchronous ventricular contraction. Echocardiography might be valuable if the ventricular activation sequence can be identified; however, this requires advanced tissue Doppler and strain methodologies.

Decision to Treat

Standards for choosing and continuing antiarrhythmic therapy are not clearly defined for many situations. Questions remain regarding which patients should receive antiarrhythmic drug therapy and which strategies would be most effective in suppressing arrhythmias, as well as preventing sudden death. Nevertheless, isolated supraventricular or ventricular premature beats generally are hemodynamically unimportant, and thus do not require specific drug therapy unless frequent (perhaps ~10–20% of total beats on a 24h Holter

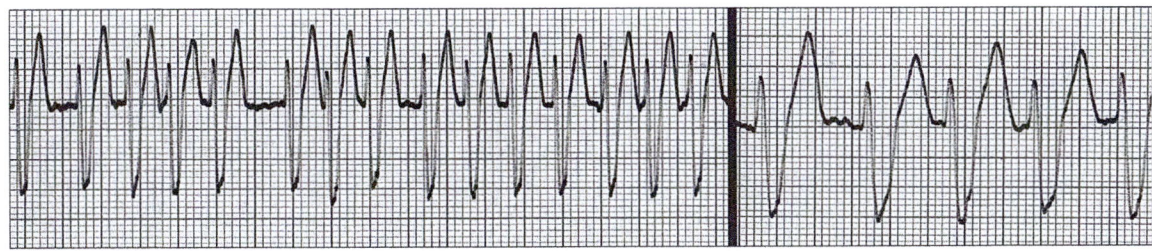

Figure 25.1 ECG from a female German Shepherd Dog with dilated cardiomyopathy. The wide-QRS tachycardia could be mistaken for ventricular tachycardia; however, its irregularity and the absence of P waves are more typical for atrial fibrillation, which is the ECG diagnosis here. Aberrant ventricular conduction (right bundle branch block) caused the wide, negative QRS configuration. Lead aVF, 25 mm/s (left), and 50 mm/s (right).

ECG). Antiarrhythmic therapy is indicated when rhythm disturbances cause clinical signs or hemodynamic instability, or when the risk of a lethal arrhythmia is thought to be high. For example, patients under general anesthesia or critically ill are more likely to be treated, especially if arterial BP is affected. Control of persistent tachycardia also can prevent tachycardia-induced cardiomyopathy (TICM; p. 630). In an asymptomatic animal without apparent cardiac structural changes, yet still thought to have a disease associated with increased risk of sudden death, antiarrhythmic therapy for an occasional complex ventricular arrhythmia might appear compelling. However, whether (or which) antiarrhythmic therapy will prolong survival is unclear. Some antiarrhythmic drugs also have antifibrillatory activity, but others do not. Furthermore, sudden cardiac death can result from asystole or pulseless electrical activity (PEA; previously known as electrical–mechanical dissociation), rather than ventricular fibrillation (VF). Antiarrhythmic drugs might suppress potentially life-saving ventricular escape rhythms.

In the presence of heart failure or cardiac structural disease, ventricular tachyarrhythmias are thought to increase the risk of sudden death. However, some antiarrhythmic agents also have the potential to increase mortality by inducing more arrhythmias (proarrhythmic effect). In people with severe left ventricular (LV) dysfunction, the only antiarrhythmic agents shown to reduce death caused by arrhythmias are beta-blockers and amiodarone. Some drugs used to treat heart failure in people are more effective in reducing sudden death than antiarrhythmic drugs *per se*; besides beta-blockers, these (so-called "upstream modulators") include angiotensin converting enzyme (ACE) inhibitors, angiotensin receptor-blockers (ARBs), aldosterone receptor-blockers, omega-3 polyunsaturated fatty acids, and statins. ACE inhibitors and ARBs also might protect from the angiotensin II-induced atrial structural and electrical remodeling associated with AF in patients with heart disease. Artificial pacing clearly is an effective interventional therapy for animals with symptomatic bradyarrhythmias (p. 388 and p. 175). Electrical cardioversion and intracardiac electrical mapping with catheter ablation are other strategies that can abolish some tachyarrhythmias in animals (p. 391). Unfortunately, aside from treatment of accessory pathways, there is little experience thus far with ablation for AF, atrial flutter, or ventricular tachycardias in veterinary patients. Some people with heart failure benefit from cardiac resynchronization therapy (biventricular pacing) to improve ventricular coordination or cardioverter/defibrillator implantation; whether these therapies will become important in veterinary medicine remains to be seen.

The decision to use antiarrhythmic drug therapy must take into account the animal's clinical status (see previous paragraphs), underlying disease(s), serum electrolyte concentrations, current medications, and the potential benefits and risks of specific drugs (Chapter 24). Treatment goals for the individual patient also should be defined. An obvious immediate goal is to restore hemodynamic stability. Complete conversion to sinus rhythm and correction of underlying disease might, or might not, be achievable goals. Successful therapy against a tachyarrhythmia usually means sufficient reduction in frequency (perhaps by ≥70–80%), complexity, or repetitive rate of ectopic beats to restore normal hemodynamic status and eliminate clinical signs. However, even apparently complete conversion to sinus rhythm does not assure protection from sudden death. Antiarrhythmic agents with greater antifibrillatory activity (such as class III drugs) are thought to provide increased protection; however, such agents also can have proarrhythmic effects (Chapters 23 and 24) and do not prevent other lethal arrhythmias such as asystole. An understanding of what antiarrhythmic therapy can and cannot do, especially over the long term, is important for the patient's owner, as well as the clinician.

Potential adverse effects of an antiarrhythmic drug must be considered against the desired benefits. Besides their expense, antiarrhythmic drugs can have multiple adverse effects beyond proarrhythmia. Furthermore, proarrhythmic effects can be more pronounced in the presence of hypokalemia or hypomagnesemia, myocardial dysfunction, CHF, and other causes of increased sympathetic tone (Chapter 24). Careful monitoring of the patient and the ECG is warranted to determine drug effectiveness. Dosage adjustments or alternate antiarrhythmic agents might be needed. Monitoring for adverse drug effects and other complications continues in importance during chronic therapy. Antiarrhythmic therapy that is initially effective sometimes loses efficacy over time. Repeated Holter monitoring can help assess arrhythmia control.

General Supportive Measures

Exercise restriction and stress avoidance can reduce sympathetic activation (which often exacerbates arrhythmias) and cardiac workload. Ideally, the impact of exertion on an arrhythmia should be evaluated by Holter ECG, or in horses, a suitable exercise test. Treatment for concurrent cardiac or extracardiac disease could further reduce arrhythmias; therefore, abnormalities that can be corrected should be. **Table 23.1** (p. 370) lists conditions commonly associated with various arrhythmias. Hypokalemia, moderate to severe hyperkalemia, and hypomagnesemia predispose to ventricular arrhythmias by affecting cell electrophysiologic properties. Electrolyte abnormalities can reduce the effectiveness or enhance the proarrhythmic side effects of many antiarrhythmic drugs. Hypomagnesemia is more likely in animals with decreased serum albumin, K^+, total CO_2, and urea nitrogen, as well as those with cardiovascular disease. Patients with a total body deficit of Mg^{++} could have a normal serum concentration. Regional myocardial increases in K^+ can occur during myocardial ischemia. Some therapies, including the "upstream therapies" noted previously and other treatment for CHF or preclinical cardiac diseases, might provide ancillary antiarrhythmic effects.

Sinus Rhythm Disturbances

Normal pacemaker activity resides within the cells of the sinoatrial node, in the right atrium. Normal sinus discharge rates vary across species (p. 237). Numerous extracardiac factors affect sinus node function and rate, including the autonomic nervous system, hormones, body temperature, oxygen tension, pH, age, stretch, structural heart disease, and drugs.

Sinus Tachycardia

High sympathetic tone or drug-induced vagal blockade causes sinus tachycardia by increasing the rate of phase 4 diastolic depolarization in sinoatrial cells. Sinus tachycardia is physiologic when associated with exercise, and relates to workload and degree of conditioning. Maximal sinus HR can approach 250 beats/minute in elite equine athletes, and 300 to 310 beats/minute in dogs treated with the beta-agonist isoproterenol. However, such HRs rarely are encountered during sinus tachycardia in veterinary settings. Arbitrarily, sinus rates exceeding 50 (horses), 180 (dogs), and 240 (cats) beats/minute during a resting ECG are consistent with sinus tachycardia. Extreme sinus tachycardia, even >300 beats/minute, could be observed with thyrotoxicosis or ingestion of exogenous stimulants (particularly in cats). A HR >250 beats/minute in a dog, or >280 beats/minute in a cat, should raise suspicion for another SVT such as FAT, as should the presence of a perfectly regular HR or the presence of any blocked P waves. Sinus tachycardia usually demonstrates some variation, including an acceleration (warm-up) and deceleration in rate, as opposed to an abrupt onset or termination. In horses and in dogs, sinus tachycardia can be somewhat irregular probably related to activation of baroreceptors.

After confirming a diagnosis of sinus tachycardia, management is focused on identifying and treating the underlying conditions responsible for heightened sympathetic tone. These might include anxiety, pain (including insufficient analgesia during procedures), fever, anemia, thyrotoxicosis, infection, hypovolemia, hypotension, shock, heart failure, the ingestion of stimulants or toxins (such as chocolate and caffeine), or drugs (including catecholamines, anticholinergics, theophylline, and related agents). Many causes, such as colic or pancreatitis, could involve more than one operative mechanism. Whether inappropriate sinus tachycardia occurs in animals, as reported in humans, is unknown. If the underlying stimulus for sinus tachycardia can be identified and alleviated, sympathetic tone and the sinus rate should decrease.

Often, a bolus of IV fluid (10-15 ml/kg of balanced electrolyte solution) is administered to patients in urgent and critical care settings because hypovolemia frequently causes sinus tachycardia. Such therapy can help reverse hypotension and increase vagal tone; however, fluid therapy usually is inappropriate in the face of edema (as in CHF) or systemic arterial hypertension. In some patients, an analgesic (such as butorphanol) might be administered to assess the influences of pain or anxiety. Otherwise, sinus tachycardia rarely is treated with drugs.

Some situations where sinus tachycardia might be treated with a beta-blocker are severe thyrotoxicosis in cats (prior to benefit of antithyroid therapy) or when thyrotoxicosis cannot be suitably managed because of client constraints. Beta-blockers can be useful to mitigate sinus tachycardia in some toxicoses (check with Poison Control or other reference textbooks) and in pheochromocytoma (in combination with an alpha-blocker, p. 806). When evaluating the influence of a beta-blocker in hospital settings, the potential for a sudden drop in BP should be anticipated. Esmolol, as a short-acting drug, can be useful as a trial therapy in these situations. Elevated resting HR in people with chronic heart failure is associated with worse outcome; the selective I_f (funny current)-blocker ivabradine can reduce HR and has improved clinical outcomes in specific scenarios. Whether similar benefit might be obtained in animals with chronic heart failure is presently unknown.

Sinus Bradycardia

Increased vagal tone slows sinus discharge rate. This occurs normally in resting or sleeping animals and should resolve with stimulation or exertion. Vagal tone also controls HR through baroreceptor reflexes, and slows or suppresses the sinus node during neural (reflex-mediated) syncope. Persistent sinus bradycardia can relate to excessive vagal tone, administration of certain drugs (including digoxin toxicity, xylazine, thorazine tranquilizers, some anesthetic agents, medetomidine, calcium entry blockers, beta-blockers, and parasympathomimetic drugs), hyperkalemia, hypoglycemia, hypothyroidism, hypothermia, and pathology within the heart (**Table 12.2**, p. 238, and Chapter 5). Notably, cats in cardiogenic shock often demonstrate sinus bradycardia, as opposed to the anticipated sinus tachycardia. Increased vagal tone can occur with airway obstruction or other respiratory diseases, brain injury or intracranial mass lesion, elevated cerebrospinal fluid pressure, ocular or periocular injury or manipulation (the oculocardiac reflex), compression of the carotid sinus region(s), and sometimes with gastrointestinal (GI) disease. Hypotension accompanies sinus bradycardia in some cases.

Many cases of sinus bradycardia require no therapy as long as BP and perfusion are maintained. The rhythm is more dangerous in patients under general anesthesia or in those with critical illnesses. When bradycardia is induced by anesthesic or other drugs, that agent should be discontinued or its dosage reduced. Atropine commonly is given if there is a concern about increased vagal tone; however, this therapy is not always effective (as often noted in cats with shock). Additional measures might be indicated, too, such as passive warming; IV fluid support; calcium salts or dobutamine for calcium channel-blocker overdose; or dobutamine, dopamine or atropine for beta-blocker toxicity. Underlying disease should be addressed, as possible. Dogs that manifest clinical signs of bradycardia usually have a HR lower than 40 to 50 beats/minute with pronounced underlying disease. Because sinus bradycardia and sinus bradyarrhythmia (slow sinus arrhythmia) are uncommon in cats, a search for underlying cardiac, pulmonary, or systemic disease (including hyperkalemia), or causes of shock is warranted.

When associated with clinical signs, such as weakness, exercise intolerance, syncope, or worsening cardiac disease, sinus bradycardia is treated initially with anticholinergic or adrenergic drug therapy (**Table 25.2**, **Figure 25.2**, and p. 386). An atropine response test (p. 387) can reveal the extent to which excessive vagal tone underlies the bradycardia and thus, whether an oral anticholinergic agent might be useful. If medical therapy does not improve symptomatic bradycardia, temporary or permanent artificial pacing might be indicated (p. 388 and p. 175).

Table 25.2 Dosages of Antiarrhythmic Drugs

Drug	Dosage
Class I	
Lidocaine	*Dog*: 2 mg/kg initial boluses slowly IV (over 2 min), up to 8 mg/kg (over ≥10 min, stop if vomiting or tremors); or rapid IV infusion at 0.8 mg/kg/min; if effective, 25–80 mcg/kg/min CRI; can use IT for CPR. *Cat*: 0.2–0.5 mg/kg initial bolus slowly IV; can repeat boluses of 0.15–0.25 mg/kg, up to total of 2(–4) mg/kg unless adverse effects; if effective, 10–40 mcg/kg/min CRI. *Horse*: 0.25–0.5 mg/kg slowly IV; repeat in 5–10 min, to effect, up to total dose of 1.5(–2) mg/kg; if effective, can use 30–50 mcg/kg/min (0.03–0.05 mg/kg/min) CRI.
Procainamide	*Dog*: 2 mg/kg IV over 2 min; repeat if needed, up to cumulative dose of 20 mg/kg; 10–50 mcg/kg/min CRI; 6–20 (up to 30) mg/kg IM q4–6h; (PO, if available, 10–20 mg/kg q8–12h [sustained-release]). *Cat*: 1–2 mg/kg IV over 2 min, repeat if needed, up to cumulative dose of 10 mg/kg; 10–20 mcg/kg/min CRI; 7.5–20 mg/kg IM (or PO) q(6–)8h. *Horse*: 1 mg/kg/min IV, up to maximum total dose of 20 mg/kg.
Quinidine	*Dog*: 6–20 mg/kg IM q6h (loading dose, 14–20 mg/kg); 6–16 mg/kg PO q6h; or 8–20 mg/kg PO q8h for sustained action preparations. *Cat*: 6–16 mg/kg IM or PO q8h. *Horse*: 22 mg (sulfate)/kg, in 3–4 L water, PO by NG tube q2h for up to 4(–6) doses, see p. 413.
Mexiletine	*Dog*: 4–6 (–8) mg/kg PO q8h.
Phenytoin	*Dog*: 10 mg/kg slowly IV; 20–50 mg/kg PO q8h. *Cat*: do not use. *Horse*: 7.5 (or 5–10) mg/kg IV; can follow with 1–5 mg/kg IM (or PO maintenance dose) q12h. 20 mg/kg PO q12h (loading) for 3–4 doses, then 10–15 mg/kg PO q12h (maintenance dose).
Propafenone	*Dog*: 4–5 (up to 8) mg/kg PO q8h (start low). *Horse*: 0.5–2 mg/kg IV (in D5W) slowly IV over 5–15 min, followed by 0.07 mg/kg/min CRI for up to 2 h; 2 mg/kg PO q8h.
Flecainide	*Dog*: 1–2 (up to 3?) mg/kg PO q(8–)12h, start low (not advised with CHF or impaired ventricular function). *Horse*: 0.2 mg/kg/min IV, up to total dose of 1–2 mg/kg (per day); 3–4(–6) mg/kg PO by NG tube q(4??–)24h for up to 4 days. Can cause sudden death, use only with caution & in dogs, consider combining with a beta-blocker.
Class II	
Atenolol	*Dog*: 0.2–1 mg/kg PO q12 (–24)h; start low in cases with impaired ventricular function. *Cat*: same; or 6.25 (–12.5) mg/cat PO q12 (–24)h. *Horse*: 0.5–1.5 mg/kg PO q12h
Propranolol	*Dog*: 0.02 mg/kg initial bolus slowly IV (up to maximum 0.1 mg/kg); initial PO dose, 0.1–0.2 mg/kg PO q8h, up to 1 mg/kg q8h. *Cat*: same IV instructions; 2.5 up to 10 mg/cat PO q8–12h. *Horse*: 0.03–0.16 mg/kg IV; PO dosing unlikely to be effective in horses, although 0.38–0.78 mg/kg PO q8h has been used.
Metoprolol	*Dog*: initial dose, 0.1–0.2 mg/kg PO q24(–12)h, up to 1(–2) mg/kg q8(–12)h. *Cat*: 2 up to 15 mg/cat PO q 8(–12)h, start low. *Horse*: 0.1–0.3 mg/kg PO q12h (up to 1 mg/kg); caution in heart failure.

Table 25.2 (Continued)   Dosages of Antiarrhythmic Drugs

Drug	Dosage
Esmolol	*Dog*: 50–100 mcg/kg (0.05–0.1 mg/kg) IV, can repeat up to total of 500 mcg/kg (0.5 mg/kg) over 5 min (loading dose); if needed, follow with infusion of 25–50 (up to 200) mcg/kg/min (0.025–0.05 [up to 0.2] mg/kg/min). Use low doses if myocardial failure. *Cat*: same. *Horse*: 200–500 mcg/kg (0.2–0.5 mg/kg) IV over 2–5 min (loading dose), followed by infusion of 25–100 mcg/kg/min (0.025–0.1 mg/kg/min), titrate to effect.
Class III	
Sotalol	*Dog*: 1–2.5 (–5?) mg/kg PO q12h. *Cat*: 10(–20) mg/cat PO q12h (or 2[–4] mg/kg PO q12h). *Horse*: 1 mg/kg PO q12h for 1st day, then 2–3 mg/kg PO q12h.
Amiodarone	*Dog*: PO loading doses of 10(–15) mg/kg PO q12h for 4(–7) days, then give same dose q24h for 7 days; then decrease to maintenance doses of 5–7.5 mg/kg PO q24h; for IV administration, use Nexterone (1.5 mg/mL) at 3–5 mg/kg slowly IV over 15 min, then can use 0.05 mg/kg/min CRI, if needed. Do not use standard older injectable formulation—see text (p. 383); monitor BP. *Horse*: 5(–6.5) mg/kg infused IV over 1h, then 0.83(–1.1) mg/kg/h for 23 h (prior to DC cardioversion for AF); or for converting AF, continue at 1.9 mg/kg/h for 30h or to effect. PO doses of 10 mg/kg q24h have been used, with unclear efficacy.
Class IV	
Diltiazem	*Dog*: Acute IV for rapid rate control of AF: 0.05–0.15 mg/kg IV over 2–5 min, can repeat if needed. Acute IV for SVT: 0.1–0.2 mg/kg over 2–5 min IV, can repeat to cumulative IV dose of 0.3–0.4(–0.7??) mg/kg; monitor BP. CRI: 0.002–0.006 mg/kg/min (or 0.12–0.36 mg/kg/h). PO loading dose: 0.5 mg/kg PO followed by 0.25 mg/kg PO q1h to a total of 1.5(–2.0) mg/kg or conversion. Oral maintenance: initial dose 0.5–1 mg/kg (up to 2–3 mg/kg) PO q8h. Extended release (diltiazem ER): 1–4 (up to 6) mg/kg PO q 12h. *Cat*: Acute IV for uncontrolled AF or rapid SVT: 0.05–0.1 mg/kg slowly IV, can repeat up to 0.25 mg/kg total. Or regular diltiazem, 1.5–2.5 mg/kg (or 7.5–10 mg/cat) PO q8h; Extended release preparations: diltiazem ER, 30 mg/cat/day (½ of a 60 mg controlled-release tablet within the 240 mg gelatin capsule), can increase to 60 mg/day in some cats if necessary; Cardizem-CD, 10 mg/kg/day. *Horse*: 0.125 mg/kg slowly IV over 2 min, can repeat q10min to effect, up to 1.25 mg/kg total dose.
Verapamil (not recommended)	*Dog*: initial dose, 0.02–0.05 mg/kg slowly IV, can repeat q5min up to total of 0.15(–0.2) mg/kg; 0.5–2 mg/kg PO q8h (see text; diltiazem preferred). *Cat*: initial dose, 0.025 mg/kg slowly IV, can repeat q5min up to total of 0.15(–0.2) mg/kg; 0.5–1 mg/kg PO q8h (see text; diltiazem preferred). *Horse*: 0.025–0.05 mg/kg IV q30min, up to 0.2 mg/kg total dose (see text; diltiazem preferred).
Anticholinergic	
Atropine	*Dog*: 0.02–0.04 mg/kg IV, IM, SC; can give IT for CPR; 0.04 mg/kg PO q6–8h. *Cat*: same. *Horse*: 0.01–0.02 mg/kg IV, IM, SC.
Glycopyrrolate	*Dog*: 0.005–0.01 mg/kg IV or IM; 0.01–0.02 mg/kg SC. *Cat*: same. *Horse*: 0.005–0.01 mg/kg IV.
Hyoscyamine	*Dog*: 0.003–0.006 mg/kg PO q8h; or (large dogs) extended release tablets, 0.01mg/kg PO q12h. *Cat*: 0.003–0.005 mg/kg PO q8h.
Propantheline	*Dog*: 0.25–0.5 mg/kg (or 3.73–7.5 mg/dog) PO q8–12h. (Some clinicians have used up to 3 mg/kg PO q8h).
Scopolamine	*Horse*: 0.1–0.2 mg/kg IV.
Sympathomimetic	
Dobutamine	*Dog*: 1–5 mcg/kg/min (up to 20 mcg/kg/min) CRI, start low. *Cat*: 1–5 mcg/kg/min (up to 10 mcg/kg/min) CRI, start low. *Horse*: 1–5 mcg/kg/min CRI (start low), titrate up to effect unless adverse signs.
Isoproterenol	*Dog*: 0.04–0.08 mcg/kg/min CRI. *Cat*: same.

(Continued)

Table 25.2 *(Continued)* Dosages of Antiarrhythmic Drugs

Drug	Dosage
Theophylline, extended release	*Dog*: 10 mg/kg PO q12h. *Cat*: 10–15 mg/kg PO q24h (in evening).
Terbutaline	*Dog*: 0.14 mg/kg, or (1.25–)2.5 up to 5 mg/dog, PO q8–12h. *Cat*: 0.1–0.2 mg/kg, or 0.625–1.25 mg/cat, PO q12h; 0.01 mg/kg SC, can repeat once in 5–10 min, if needed. *Horse*: not recommended.
Other Agents	
Digoxin	*Dog*: 0.003–0.005 (–0.011) mg/kg PO q12h (or see **Table 22.3**, p. 346 and text, p. 327). *Cat*: see **Table 22.3**. *Horse*: 0.0022 mg/kg IV q12h for 2 doses (IV loading), then 0.0022 mg/kg IV q24h (IV maintenance); 0.011 mg/kg PO q12h (PO maintenance).
Magnesium sulfate (MgSO$_4$)	*Dog*: 25–40 mg/kg (diluted in D5W) slow IV bolus, followed by same dose infused over a 12–24h period. *Cat*: same? *Horse*: 2–6 mg/kg/min IV q2min to effect, or maximum total dose of 55(–100) mg/kg.
Edrophonium	*Dog*: 0.05 to 0.1 mg/kg IV (have atropine and endotracheal tube available).
Phenylephrine	*Dog*: 0.004 to 0.01 mg/kg IV. *Cat*: same? *Horse*: 0.1–0.2 mcg/kg/min CRI, start low and titrate to effect or maximum total dose of 0.01 mg/kg.

Abbreviations: AF, atrial fibrillation; BP, blood pressure; CPR, cardiopulmonary resuscitation; CRI, constant rate infusion; D$_5$W, 5% dextrose in water; IT, intratracheal; NG, nasogastric; SVT, supraventricular tachycardia.

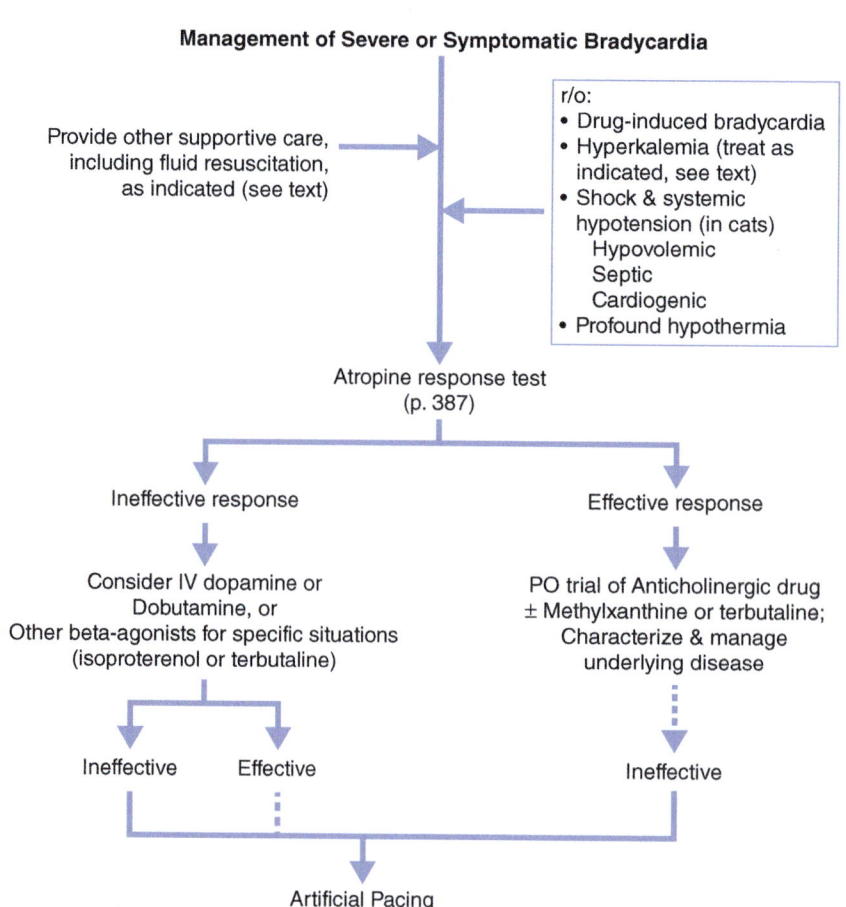

Figure 25.2 Approach to managing the patient with a severe bradyarrhythmia. These are general guidelines and exceptions can occur. For further information, see text section relevant to the individual patient's ECG diagnosis and **Table 25.2** for drug doses. IV, intravenous; PO, oral; r/o, rule out.

Sinus Node Dysfunction

The term sinus node dysfunction implies disease of the sinoatrial node, but this does not necessarily involve overt clinical signs. This disorder is mainly confined to the dog, and is revealed by a prolonged sinus node recovery time following rapid atrial pacing. Practically, sinus node dysfunction usually is manifest as periods of sinus pause or arrest (or sinoatrial block) or inappropriately slow sinus rhythm (or sinus arrhythmia) for the clinical context. Some animals with sinus node dysfunction are variably responsive to anticholinergic drug therapy, suggesting a component of abnormally enhanced vagal tone. Whether animals with a normal atropine response truly have sinus node dysfunction is controversial. Less so is the definition of sick sinus syndrome (SSS), which is a syndrome of clinical signs related to sinus node dysfunction. With either diagnosis, periods of sinus arrest are typical although robust escape activity often prevents clinical signs. Additional abnormalities of heart rhythm and cardiac conduction can occur, as well.

Sick Sinus Syndrome The SSS is described mainly in dogs. It is most common in older female Miniature Schnauzers in the United States; although West Highland White Terriers and Cocker Spaniels also have increased prevalence. Geographic variation exists in breeds most affected by SSS, with highest prevalence reported in West Highland White Terriers in the United Kingdom. SSS also occurs in male dogs, as well as in dogs of other small breeds including Dachshunds, Pugs, Miniature Poodles, and other purebred and mixed-breed dogs. SSS is extremely rare in cats and horses.

Sudden episodes of weakness or syncope are the typical clinical manifestations; these usually follow periods of sinus bradycardia or asystole caused by sinus arrest with insufficient escape activity. The syncopal episodes sometimes are accompanied by convulsive activity (Stokes–Adams seizures), which can mimic neurologic- or metabolic-induced seizure activity. Intermittent premature complexes or runs of SVT are common, and these might be followed by long pauses before sinus node activity resumes, consistent with prolonged sinus node recovery time (**Figure 25.3**; also **Figures 5.40**, p. 151 and **12.6**, p. 241). Variable AV conduction block (especially 1st and 2nd degree blocks) and prolonged pauses before an escape complex appears occur in some cases, suggesting more widespread conduction system dysfunction. Intermittent periods of accelerated atrial or junctional rhythms and variable junctional or ventricular escape rhythms can occur. Some affected dogs also have paroxysmal supraventricular tachyarrhythmias, prompting the alternate name "bradycardia–tachycardia syndrome" (**Figure 12.6**). Paroxysms of rapid SVT can underlie some episodes of weakness or collapse in these cases. While the ECG abnormalities are dramatic in dogs with advanced SSS, resting ECG findings might be equivocal or even normal in some with early disease. Concurrent degenerative AV valve disease is common in these older, small breed dogs. CHF, if present, usually relates to the AV valve insufficiency, although the arrhythmias might be a complicating factor.

An atropine response test (p. 387) is indicated for dogs with persistent sinus bradycardia or periods of sinus arrest. This also is clinically relevant prior to any anesthetic procedure. Medical therapy with an anticholinergic agent, methylxanthine bronchodilator, or terbutaline sometimes can ameliorate or reduce clinical signs of SSS, especially in earlier stages. Response to oral anticholinergic agents usually is correlated with positive response to IV atropine challenge, although there are exceptions. In a relatively large retrospective report, medical therapy provided long-term relief of clinical signs in over half of dogs so treated (Ward, 2016). Dogs with a higher average HR at presentation responded better to medical treatment. However, controlled prospective studies that include detailed ambulatory monitoring are needed to

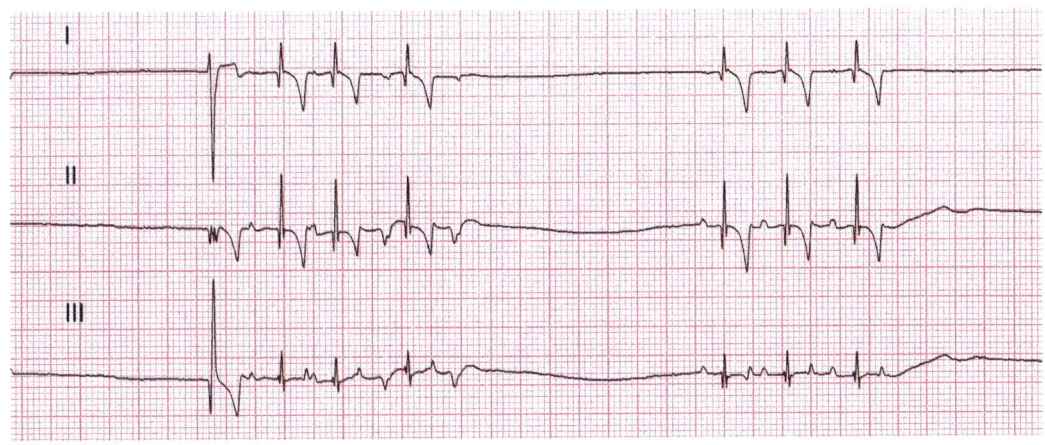

Figure 25.3 ECG from a 9-year-old, male Miniature Schnauzer with a history of syncope caused by sick sinus syndrome. This strip shows an initial period of sinus arrest which is interrupted by a ventricular escape complex. A sinus P wave then appears, which is conducted with 1st degree AV block, followed by another. However, the next two atrial depolarizations have negative, ectopic P′ waves; the first is conducted but the next is not (2nd degree AV block). After another period of sinus arrest, three more sinus complexes appear before sinus arrest recurs. Leads I, II, & III; 25 mm/s; 1 cm = 1 mV.

confirm which patients are most likely to benefit from medical therapy. Syncope can be sporadic in early disease and medication eventually can become ineffective. Furthermore, drugs used to accelerate the sinus rate also can exacerbate tachyarrhythmias, so caution is advised.

When clinical signs are frequent or severe and uncontrolled by medical therapy, SSS is best managed by permanent artificial pacing. Dogs with tachycardia-bradycardia forms of SSS can receive more aggressive medical therapy for SVTs, if needed, after successful pacemaker implantation. Without pacing, drugs that suppress supraventricular tachyarrhythmias can magnify the bradycardia in this syndrome. Digoxin and beta-blockers are relatively contraindicated for this reason; in addition, digoxin toxicity can mimic the ECG changes seen with SSS. Nevertheless, as long as sinus node function is not further depressed, some dogs with SSS might tolerate conservative doses of diltiazem or digoxin for paroxysmal SVT even without permanent pacing.

The prognosis for SSS, especially with cardiac pacing, is good. SSS in itself is an uncommon direct cause of death in dogs. More likely causes of death or euthanasia relate to CHF from degenerative (myxomatous) mitral valve disease, various noncardiac diseases (including renal failure or cancer), and infrequently, complications associated with pacing. However, euthanasia requested because of recurrent weakness and syncope caused by SSS (in dogs treated only medically) is probably underestimated.

Atrial Rhythm Disturbances

Atrial (supraventricular) tachyarrhythmias include atrial premature complexes (APCs or PACs); FATs, stemming from various electrophysiologic mechanisms; various forms of macro-reentrant atrial tachycardia (atrial flutter); AV reentrant (reciprocating) tachycardias (AVRT) involving the AV node and an accessory pathway; and AF (p. 409). AV nodal reentrant tachycardia has been induced experimentally in dogs, but not reported clinically as far as we know. Junctional tachycardia is uncommon (aside from digoxin toxicity) and might be confused with an atypical FAT coming from the left- or the caudoventral right atrium. Several factors could predispose to supraventricular tachyarrhythmias; these should be minimized as far as possible (**Table 23.1**, p. 370). FAT and reentrant atrial or AV tachycardias can be quite rapid, with atrial rates often exceeding 300 impulses/minute in dogs and cats, and with ventricular response rates similarly high if there is 1:1 AV conduction. Although some cases might be relatively asymptomatic on presentation, rapid SVT commonly causes weakness or syncope. Tachypnea or respiratory distress can be another sign, especially in cats and horses. Affected animals often have structural heart disease or will develop a cardiomyopathy in the future. One report in dogs also found a male preponderance and a median age of 9 years (Finster, 2008). In horses, atrial arrhythmias often occur in the absence of overt structural disease, although microscopic atrial lesions and functional electrophysiologic disturbances are likely present in many cases. In standardbred horses, AF has slight heritable and male predispositions (Kraus, 2018).

Atrial arrhythmias, including isolated APCs, reportedly are the most common rhythm abnormalities affecting horses. Their prevalence in apparently normal horses is unclear, but could range from <3% to ~28% at rest. During and immediately after exercise, the frequency of atrial arrhythmias often increases. Especially in horses with poor or reduced performance, it is important to determine if transient episodes of atrial (or ventricular) tachyarrhythmias occur during exercise. APCs that are confined to the post-exercise period and cause no clinical signs are likely to be benign and related to changes in autonomic balance immediately after exercise.

Atrial tachycardias as a group can arise from an abnormal automatic focus or a micro- or macro-reentrant mechanism within the atrial tissues, pulmonary veins, AV node, or a congenital accessory conduction pathway (see sections "Atrioventricular Reentrant (Reciprocating) Tachycardia" and "AV Junctional Rhythms," p. 417 on). These rhythms often produce a regular ventricular rhythm, in contrast to AF (see p. 409). However, non-regular (intermittent) AV conduction of FAT or atrial F waves will result in an irregular ventricular response rate. Rather than simply grouping these as "SVTs," the precise rhythm abnormality should be sought if possible, because the underlying mechanism can influence response to treatment. Although these tachyarrhythmias typically have a normal QRS configuration (narrow and upright in lead II and negative in lead aVR), if a major bundle branch block (p. 153) or other intraventricular conduction disturbance is present, the resulting wide and abnormal QRS configuration can mimic VT.

Intracardiac electrophysiologic testing usually is needed to clearly identify the specific arrhythmia mechanism and its anatomical origin. However, a report describing surface ECG characteristics of FAT compared with orthodromic AVRT (p. 417) in dogs identified several features that could help differentiate these arrhythmias (Santilli, 2008). Dogs with FAT generally had faster HRs and less QRS alternans during the onset of the tachycardia, compared to those with orthodromic AVRT. However, QRS alternans does occur with paroxysmal atrial tachycardias and the ventricular response rates can overlap, such that these distinctions are not absolute. Among other details, P′ wave polarity usually was positive in the caudal (II, aVF) and chest leads of dogs with FAT, supporting an origin near the cristae terminalis. In contrast, dogs with orthodromic AVRT had negative P′ waves in leads II and aVF and positive P′ waves in lead aVR. Unfortunately, P waves can be difficult to identify clearly with rapid tachycardias.

Rapid atrial tachycardias, whether originating from one or more automatic foci or a form of intraatrial reentry, often are associated with underlying heart disease. They can cause serious hemodynamic compromise, especially in cases with preexisting cardiac disease, and they are difficult to suppress with antiarrhythmic therapy. There are three general approaches for managing atrial rhythm disturbances, namely: (1) suppression of atrial ectopy or paroxysmal tachycardias; (2) conversion of a sustained atrial tachyarrhythmia to sinus rhythm; and (3) control of the ventricular response rate by blocking AV nodal conduction. Antiarrhythmic drugs in all four drug classes variously are used to achieve each of these purposes (Chapter 24). Electrocardioversion is used in dogs and horses to convert AF and less often, atrial flutter or FAT. Spatial mapping of atrial arrhythmias followed by catheter ablation of the substrate is a potentially curative therapy for some atrial arrhythmias, but currently underdeveloped in veterinary practice. Some infrequent arrhythmias could be ignored if there are no associated clinical signs, although the likely cause should be investigated. However, paroxysmal atrial tachycardias or even frequent APCs can degenerate into AF. Furthermore, a sustained or frequently recurring tachycardia of any origin can lead to profound myocardial dysfunction within a period of weeks (TICM, p. 630).

Atrial Premature Complexes

Occasional APCs do not require antiarrhythmic therapy. 24-hour Holter or telemetry monitoring can be used to assess arrhythmia frequency and screen for runs of sustained or exercise induced arrhythmias. This is especially important in animals with clinical signs that could be caused by arrhythmias. However, APCs that are numerous at rest (for example, >10% of total beats) or associated with atrial disease and enlargement are of greater clinical importance because they could trigger an atrial tachycardia or AF. In horses especially, factors that can facilitate the onset of atrial tachyarrhythmias include larger atrial size, the common occurrence of focal atrial fibrosis, and the ability of high vagal tone to shorten atrial action potential duration and refractoriness. Structural heart disease further exacerbates this risk. Atrial arrhythmias also can be paroxysmal and underlie poor performance during exercise.

The optimal therapy for suppressing APCs is unknown. For frequent APCs in dogs, diltiazem, digoxin, sotalol, or a pure beta-blocker are initial options for treatment (**Table 25.2** and **Table 22.3**, p. 346). The potential for drug-induced depression of myocardial function should be considered when selecting treatments for patients with heart failure or systolic dysfunction. Digoxin often is considered for dogs and horses with heart failure. If the arrhythmia is not sufficiently controlled with digoxin, in addition to an ACE inhibitor and other CHF therapy, another drug can be added or substituted. For cats with hypertrophic cardiomyopathy (HCM) or hyperthyroidism, a beta-blocker (such as atenolol) or class III drug with beta-blocking properties (compounded sotalol) is recommended, although diltiazem could be a reasonable alternative. In horses with frequent APCs that trigger AF, or that occur after AF conversion, oral sotalol could be tried; quinidine and procainamide are only suitable for acute therapy.

Atrial Tachycardia

FAT can arise from either atrium or the pulmonary veins. It often is confused with sinus tachycardia when the origin is near the cristae terminalis and the resulting P' waves are positive in the caudal limb and left lateral chest leads. FAT also can be confused with atrial flutter, especially typical "reversed" (clockwise circuit) and atypical (not engaging the cavo-tricuspid isthmus) forms of flutter. The presence of a rapid atrial rate (approaching or exceeding 300 impulses/minute in the dog or cat) argues for a diagnosis of FAT, macro-reentrant atrial tachycardia (atrial flutter), or AVRT. FAT or flutter is especially likely when physiological antegrade AV nodal block is present, either during sustained tachycardia or near the termination of a tachycardia paroxysm. These arrhythmias also occur in horses, although at much lower rates; FAT often is observed during quinidine conversion of AF to sinus rhythm. These tachycardias can be paroxysmal or sustained in nature. Rarely, there is multifocal atrial tachycardia (not addressed here). The optimal treatment for atrial tachycardias is uncertain. Therapy frequently is a clinical exercise in trial and error.

Paroxysmal (Nonsustained) Atrial Tachycardia Diltiazem usually is tried first in dogs (and sometimes cats). Even if the tachycardia is not adequately suppressed, AV nodal depression and ventricular rate control might be achieved. Diltiazem can be combined with digoxin (in dogs) or cautiously, with a beta-blocker in an effort to further suppress the ectopy or control ventricular rate. Alternatively, sotalol or amiodarone can be tried. These class III agents have the potential both to suppress FATs, and to slow AV conduction for HR control. Recurrent atrial tachycardia that is refractory to these drugs might respond to procainamide, quinidine, or a class Ic agent, such as propafenone or flecainide (see Chapter 24 for drug details). A FAT that occurs in a horse during quinidine sulfate treatment for AF can be treated with digoxin if the ventricular response rate exceeds 90 to 120 beats/minute, depending on the clinical signs. If this is not effective, IV diltiazem could be tried; however, BP should be monitored closely. Evaluation for underlying cardiac or metabolic abnormalities and general supportive care are indicated, as for all arrhythmias.

Sustained Atrial Tachycardia Sustained, rapid atrial tachycardia requires urgent therapy. A **vagal maneuver** (p. 388) usually is tried first in small animals to increase vagal tone to the AV node (**Figure 25.4**). If successful, it can offer both diagnostic and therapeutic benefits. An IV catheter should be placed as soon as possible. Unless the animal is in heart failure, IV fluid administration is begun to help support BP and increase endogenous vagal tone. Although a FAT and atrial flutter often are not suppressed, increasing vagal tone to the sinoatrial node can transiently slow sinus tachycardia, while vagal-induced blocking of AV conduction can reveal ectopic P' or F waves and transiently slow the ventricular rate. Flutter rate might also change slightly (including increasing) during a vagal maneuver. An AVRT that uses the AV node might be

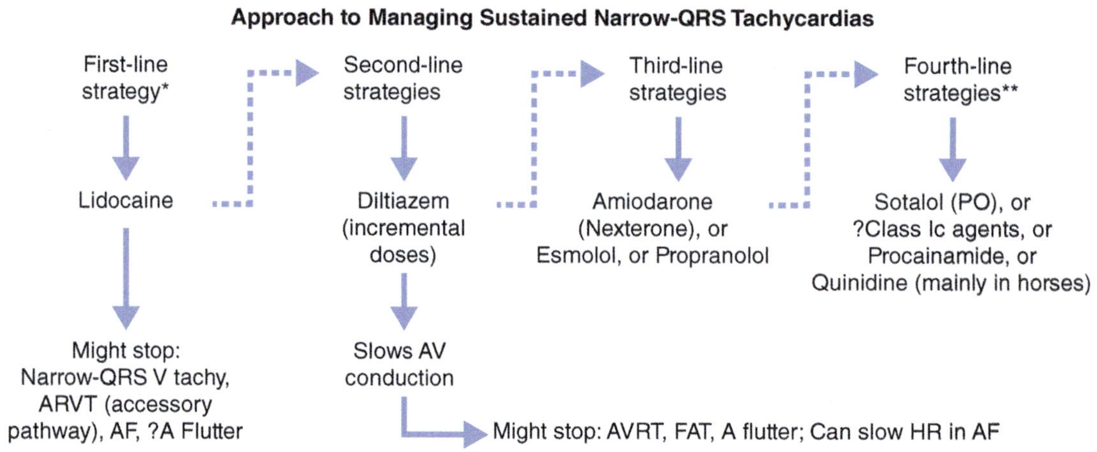

Approach to Managing Sustained Narrow-QRS Tachycardias

First-line strategy* → Lidocaine → Might stop: Narrow-QRS V tachy, ARVT (accessory pathway), AF, ?A Flutter

Second-line strategies → Diltiazem (incremental doses) → Slows AV conduction → Might stop: AVRT, FAT, A flutter; Can slow HR in AF

Third-line strategies → Amiodarone (Nexterone), or Esmolol, or Propranolol

Fourth-line strategies* → Sotalol (PO), or ?Class Ic agents, or Procainamide, or Quinidine (mainly in horses)

Figure 25.4 General guidelines for managing sustained narrow-QRS tachycardias. Narrow-QRS tachycardias most commonly are supraventricular, indicating that at least one component of the arrhythmia involves atrial muscle or atrioventricular (AV) tissues. Regular narrow-QRS tachycardias include: focal atrial tachycardia (FAT), atrial (A) flutter with regular A:V conduction; junctional tachycardia, AV reentrant (reciprocating) tachycardia (AVRT, usually orthodromic, employing an accessory pathway), and AV nodal reentrant tachycardia. Nexterone is preservative free amiodarone. *If initial strategy is not effective, try a next-level therapy. **Avoid beta-blockers if depressed LV function or heart failure is present; Class Ic agents are potentially dangerous and should be avoided in patients with depressed LV function or heart failure; quinidine is most relevant to the horse. See text for further information, especially regarding treatment of AF, and **Table 25.2** for drug doses. AF, atrial fibrillation; HR, heart rate; PO, oral; V tachy, ventricular tachycardia.

broken as antegrade AV conduction is required for maintenance of the circuit. Treatment for sustained atrial tachycardia in horses is largely the same as for AF (see section "Atrial Fibrillation Management in Horses," below). Digoxin can be administered IV to slow AV nodal conduction in horses with heart failure or hemodynamic instability.

If the vagal maneuver is unsuccessful, diltiazem (IV or PO loading) usually is administered next (**Figure 25.5**). Slow bolus injection of a beta-blocker (such as esmolol or propranolol) is an alternative therapy; its negative inotropic effect also is of concern in animals dependent on high underlying sympathetic tone. Lidocaine (IV) is rarely effective in FAT, compared to interrupting orthodromic AVRT (p. 417), where the accessory pathway can be blocked. If diltiazem, beta-blocker, or lidocaine therapy does not suppress a sustained FAT, IV procainamide might be helpful (if available). A refractory AV node-independent FAT or macro-reentrant tachycardia (flutter) might respond to sotalol or IV amiodarone. The combination of a calcium channel- and beta-blocker could be (cautiously) considered in animals with a refractory FAT and reasonably normal myocardial function and BP; however, the dose of the second agent should be low to avoid hypotension. IV digoxin generally is less effective than a calcium channel-blocker and its potential adverse effects render it much less desirable. Digoxin's onset of action is slower and, while it increases vagal tone, IV administration can increase central sympathetic output. Some class Ic agents, as well as synchronized direct current (DC) cardioversion, also have been used successfully for acute therapy. Short-term conversion of SVT to sinus rhythm using IV amiodarone was reported in a horse; arrhythmia recurrence subsequently was treated successfully with transvenous electrical cardioversion. Other drugs that theoretically might be useful for the acute treatment of refractory atrial (supraventricular) tachycardias include the alpha$_1$-agonist phenylephrine, which reflexly increases vagal tone, or the anticholinesterase edrophonium chloride; however, these are not recommended.

Long-term therapy used for FAT in dogs and cats depends on whether any prior treatment(s) effectively suppressed the ectopic rhythm. If so, an oral form of that drug is continued. If suppression is incomplete, another drug potentially could be added for ventricular rate control. When rate control is the main goal, long-acting diltiazem, a beta-blocker, digoxin, or often, some combination of these drugs, could be effective. In some cases, amiodarone or sotalol, (or a class Ic drug such as propafenone), is effective in achieving both rhythm and, when needed,

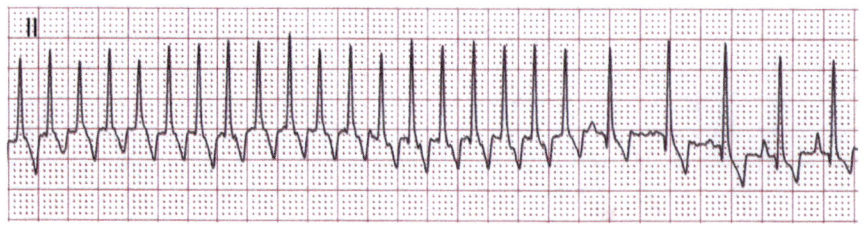

Figure 25.5 A rapid supraventricular tachycardia (~300 beats/min) in an older dog converted to sinus rhythm (at right side of image) after IV diltiazem administration. Lead II, 25 mm/s, 1 cm = 1 mV.

rate control (**Table 25.2**). FATs can be unrelenting (**Figure 25.6**) and very often the therapeutic target becomes ventricular rate control (see "Atrial Fibrillation" section). While sotalol and amiodarone can help with this, the high sotalol doses often needed and amiodarone's adverse effects profile present disadvantages to their use solely for rate control. Alternatively, a patient with persistent FAT could be a candidate for catheter ablation, although details of this treatment currently are scant in veterinary practice. Another possible strategy for HR control could be AV node ablation, followed by permanent pacemaker implantation; this would be another rare form of veterinary treatment.

Atrial Flutter and Fibrillation

Atrial Flutter Atrial flutter is a form of macro-reentry atrial tachycardia. It is especially common in cases of severe right atrial dilation and stretch. This can occur with some forms of right ventricular cardiomyopathy (especially in English Bulldogs), cor pulmonale, and congenital right heart disease. Typical atrial flutter involves a counterclockwise circuit around the right atrium (the cavo-tricuspid isthmus). It produces sawtooth flutter (F) waves, without a clear isoelectric shelf, at rates >300 impulses/minute (and sometimes >450/minute) in unsedated dogs. The flutter rate in horses usually is 170–275 impulses/minute. The condition is rare in cats. It is unusual for all atrial waves to be conducted into the ventricles, although a regular AV conduction sequence, such as a 2:1 (F:QRS) pattern is common and can result in a regular ventricular rate. Variable AV conduction also can occur; this can change rapidly as a result of vagal input and decremental and concealed conduction within the AV node. Flutter likely can develop reorganization and circuit movement of impulses, arising from pulmonary vein rotors or spiral waves (p. 366). This seems plausible for explaining the alternating atrial "flutter-fibrillation" that sometimes is observed in horses. In dogs with right atrial dilation, it is likely that a FAT or even APC's might trigger on the onset of flutter.

Drugs that slow conduction and prolong effective refractory period are likely to interrupt the underlying reentrant circuit. Experimentally in dogs, class Ic sodium channel blockers such as ibutilide, flecainide, and encainide have converted atrial flutter to sinus rhythm. More traditional agents including quinidine and procainamide (where available) and amiodarone can work in some cases, especially for flutter of acute onset. If drug therapy does not convert the arrhythmia, ventricular rate control becomes the goal and drug(s) that slow AV conduction are used, as for AF (discussed in the following paragraphs) or refractory FAT. Atrial flutter often degenerates to AF, which actually can make rate control easier.

Electrical cardioversion might be effective in cases without structural heart disease. Intracardiac overdrive pacing is another strategy that has been used to convert atrial flutter in the horse. In the future, electrical mapping followed by radiofrequency catheter ablation might be used to create atrial or pulmonary venous scars and so abolish atrial flutter.

Atrial Fibrillation AF is probably the most common sustained arrhythmia in horses and dogs. It can develop with structural heart disease (especially with atrial dilation), or in the absence of clinically detectable cardiac disease (lone AF). In humans, AF often is classified as: *paroxysmal*, if it is short-lived and spontaneously converts to sinus rhythm; *persistent*, when the AF will not spontaneously convert but it still is of short duration; and *permanent*, when it persists for more than seven days (this exact time interval might not be applicable to animals). Because a certain "critical mass" of atrial tissue is needed to sustain this arrhythmia, the incidence is higher in animals of larger body size or atrial size. AF is comparably rare in cats and usually requires severe atrial dilation to be sustained in this species. AF rarely occurs in foals or in puppies under a year old. It is seen infrequently in ponies and in weanling horses. An inherited predisposition to AF might occur in some lines of Standardbred horses (Kraus, 2018). Larger body weight and AV valve insufficiency (especially with atrial enlargement) convey increased risk. Draft and warmblood horses appear to develop AF more often than horses of smaller breeds. Likewise in dogs, AF prevalence is greater in those of large and (especially) giant breeds, as well as in dogs with atrial enlargement caused by cardiac disease.

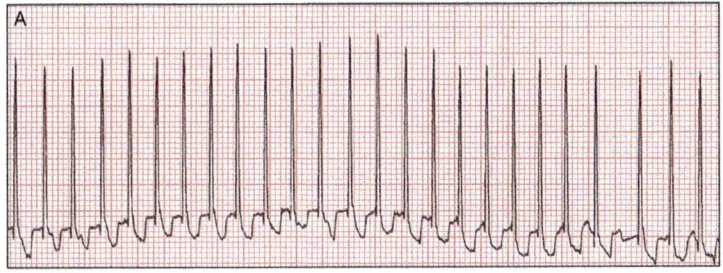
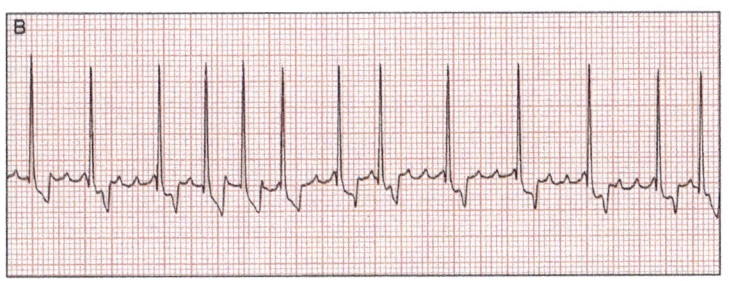

Figure 25.6 (A) Sustained atrial tachycardia (or atypical atrial flutter) in a 9-month-old female Jack Russell Terrier with cardiomegaly and myocardial failure. The ventricular rate is ~280/minute, with 2:1 AV conduction of P′ waves (except briefly at right of strip). (B) The focal atrial tachycardia persisted (atrial rate ~460/minute) despite therapy with digoxin, diltiazem, sotalol and enalapril, although variable AV block produced a reasonable heart rate (~140/minute). Congestive signs had resolved and she had resumed her normal energetic activity. Amiodarone later was used instead of sotalol; however, this only intermittently suppressed the tachycardia. Nevertheless, heart rate control allowed the dog to live well for 13 more years. Lead II, 25 mm/s, 1 cm = 1 mV.

A basic understanding of the electrophysiology underlying AF could be useful for its treatment (DeCloedt, 2020). Unlike the macro-reentrant atrial circuits associated with flutter, AF involves a multiple wavelet (or unstructured) form of atrial reentry. Theories of AF generally include at least four key components: 1) Predisposing factors – such as ion channel abnormalities or altered autonomic tone; 2) triggers – a rapidly firing focus in a pulmonary vein or atrium; 3) susceptible substrate for fibrillation – sufficient atrial mass, or stretched or fibrotic atrial myocardium; and 4) various perpetuating factors – that can modify the trigger or the substrate and thereby, maintain AF.

A number of factors beyond atrial size can predispose to and perpetuate AF. Focal areas of atrial inflammation or fibrosis could promote AF development and continuation in horses and large dogs without atrial enlargement. Channelopathies are largely unexplored in animals, as are pulmonary vein rotors arising from myocardial sleeves; these probably are triggers for AF, especially in animals with "lone" AF or "flutter-fib." Furthermore, parasympathetic stimulation opens acetylcholine-responsive K^+ channels, predisposing to AF by shortening atrial action potential and refractory period durations. Animals with increased vagal tone or vago-sympathetic imbalance might have increased dispersion of refractoriness, as can those with atrial stretch. Furosemide-induced potassium loss, as well as overt hypokalemia, can induce APC's or FAT. These rhythms might precipitate the onset of AF in race horses or animals with CHF. Metabolic alkalosis (as from bicarbonate administration) and epinephrine lower serum K^+, and thyrotoxicosis (natural or iatrogenic) is a known predisposing factor for APCs and AF in humans and animals. When AF is sustained, progressive atrial myocardial remodeling occurs over time and involves structural, electrical, and functional changes that perpetuate AF. Consequently, chronic AF is associated with reduced likelihood of conversion to sinus rhythm and, if conversion is achieved, greater chance for AF recurrence.

Some horses, most dogs, and virtually all cats with AF have significant underlying cardiac disease, with marked enlargement of one or both atria. Chronic mitral valve regurgitation, usually related to degenerative valve disease, is the most common cause for left atrial enlargement in dogs and horses. DCM and untreated congenital heart disease are other diagnostic considerations. Most cats with AF have some form of advanced or end-stage cardiomyopathy. The ventricular response rate is instructive; AF with resting tachycardia indicates increased basal sympathetic tone, often relating to significant underlying cardiac disease or overt CHF. Because successful cardioversion and maintenance of sinus rhythm are difficult to achieve in the face of atrial enlargement or CHF, the usual therapeutic goals for these patients are to: 1) slow AV nodal conduction (with drug therapy), and 2) manage underlying disease (to reduce sympathetic tone). The ventricular response rate to AF depends on AV nodal conduction velocity and recovery rate, which are influenced greatly by prevailing sympathetic tone. A slower HR allows more time for ventricular filling and lessens the relative importance of (the now absent) atrial contraction to ventricular filling.

Most horses with AF have a negative workup for other cardiac problems. The echocardiogram in these cases is normal or shows only borderline atrial dilation and equivocally reduced LV ejection fraction. These subtle echocardiographic changes become normal with successful cardioversion, although atrial mechanical function can take weeks to normalize (as evaluated by advanced tissue imaging methods). Lone AF in dogs occurs sporadically in apparently normal large and giant breeds; it seems especially common in Irish Wolfhounds. The arrhythmia often is an incidental finding. Male dogs are affected more often than females. There could be a familial predisposition in some cases. Additionally, giant breed dogs undergoing general anesthesia seem at higher risk for acutely developing AF. This might relate to vagomimetic opioids administered during the procedure, atrial ectopy, or occult myocardial disease. Dogs with lone AF are better candidates for cardioversion to sinus rhythm. When underlying cardiac structure and function are normal, resting HR should be normal as well, although ambulatory ECG (Holter) monitoring sometimes reveals inappropriately fast exercise HRs. Affected dogs can develop DCM over time, so continued monitoring of these cases is important (p. 611).

Paroxysmal, or short-lived, AF in horses has been associated with high intensity exercise. It seems comparably rare in dogs, although it does occur sometimes in the aforementioned anesthesia scenario. As defined previously, paroxysmal AF indicates that spontaneous conversion to sinus rhythm will occur, often within 24 to 48 hours of AF onset. Frequently, drug therapy is given credit for the conversion, but the potential for spontaneous return to normal rhythm is one reason why cardioversion therapy sometimes is delayed for a day after the observed onset of AF.

Although cardiac output and BP often are normal at rest, AF is likely to reduce exercise performance, especially with moderate to strenuous work. In equine athletes, exercise-induced pulmonary hemorrhage, respiratory distress, ataxia, collapse, CHF, and skeletal myopathy are potential comorbidities or consequences of AF. Horses with AF have higher HRs during exercise than those in sinus rhythm. Some horses with lone AF develop a rapid HR even with modest exercise. Experimentally induced AF in Standardbred trotters not only decreased exercise performance, AF increased mean maximum HR during treadmill exercise to over 300 beats/minute (and, in some horses, instantaneous maximum HR to over 450 beats/minute); in contrast, the mean maximum HR in control horses was about 220 beats/minute (Buhl, 2018). Furthermore, abnormally wide QRS complexes, couplets and paroxysmal tachycardia with R-on-T timing also occurred in the AF group of this study. Weakness, collapse, and even sudden death has been associated with AF in horses. Rapid ventricular response rates with exercise also can induce aberrant ventricular conduction or ventricular premature complexes (VPCs), which could precipitate more serious arrhythmias, especially if quinidine is being administered. Permanent AF therefore presents a safety issue in some horses. This can be difficult to predict, and some clinicians believe horses with permanent AF should be retired from athletic work if conversion is unsuccessful, or not attempted. However, many horses with chronic AF seem to perform light to moderate work without issue. There are no suitable prospective studies addressing this point. At minimum, recommendations include an exercise ECG to assess the effects of exercise on AF ventricular response rate and clinical signs, and to limit use of the horse to an informed adult rider. Serial follow-up and monitoring also are indicated in horses that continue to work. Several HR variability calculations based on HR monitor recordings can help distinguish recurrent AF from sinus rhythm, especially during exercise (Broux, 2017).

Holter monitoring of dogs with AF undergoing rate control therapy has shown that ECGs recorded in the hospital are not highly predictive of HRs recorded at home. Patients with AF have higher HRs related to stress and excitement during hospital visits. However, dogs with AF and an in-hospital HR over 155 beats/minute are unlikely to have adequate rate control at home, and therapy should be provided or intensified. In-hospital HRs <150 beats/minute in dogs (or <180 beats/minute in cats) are thought to be desirable, because the presumption is that the HR will be much lower at home. The ideal *target HR* depends on the species and probably the underlying disease. For 20–25 kg dogs, an in-clinic HR of about 130–145 beats/minute might be an appropriate target. The animal's HR at home will be less than this; home HRs of 70–120 beats/minute in dogs and 80–140 beats/minute in cats are probably acceptable, with higher rates suitable when there is CHF. Holter monitoring to estimate a true 24-hour mean HR, not simply a 1-minute average, might yield prognostic information, as well as guide the intensity of therapy aimed at HR control. A retrospective study in dogs with AF reported a ten-fold longer survival time (mean of 1037 days) when mean 24-hour HR was under 125 beats/minute, compared to when mean HR was over 125 beats/minute (mean of 105 days; Pedro, 2018). The authors concur with that general message, but highlight that other treatments cannot be standardized in retrospective studies, and that better rate control might simply indicate less severe CHF, as opposed to of intensive HR control. As an alternative to Holter monitoring, periodic at-home HR checks also can be obtained using a smartphone ECG app, ideally recorded at rest and immediately after exercise. Whether obtained in-clinic, by Holter monitoring, or at home with a smartphone app, using an ECG recording to document the ventricular rate is important. HR estimation by auscultation or palpation can be quite inaccurate, depending on the skill of examiner, as well as the degree of tachycardia. Femoral pulses **never** should be used to assess HR in animals with AF because of frequent pulse deficits.

Animals with ventricular preexcitation (p. 153) that develop AF are at increased risk for VF, especially if the antegrade refractory period in the accessory pathway is brief. AV nodal blocking drugs (calcium channel blockers, digoxin, and possibly beta-blockers) are not advised in this special situation because these could paradoxically increase the ventricular response rate if impulses travel more rapidly or preferentially down the accessory pathway. This could trigger VF. Electrocardioversion is recommended; otherwise, amiodarone or mexiletine can be used to slow conduction in the accessory pathway. Sotalol (or procainamide, if available) are other options.

Atrial Fibrillation Management in Dogs Rapid HR reduction during AF sometimes is indicated, such as when resting HR exceeds 200–240 beats/minute with CHF or during general anesthesia. In these situations, the IV route provides rapid onset and precise dosage control. Low dose(s) of IV diltiazem (starting with 0.05 mg/kg; **Table 25.2**), administered with caution, usually are tolerated and effective. Although diltiazem has lesser negative inotropic effect than verapamil or an IV beta-blocker, conservative doses and slow IV injection should be used, especially in patients suspected to have poor myocardial contractility. By slowing the HR, diltiazem can improve ventricular filling and performance and reduce myocardial O_2 requirement. The risks are that some animals could experience hypotension or worsening heart failure. IV digoxin generally is avoided in dogs with decompensated CHF, although some cardiologists occasionally use it for initial HR control in AF. Although cautious use of IV esmolol is an alternative for rapid HR reduction, this should be limited to lone AF, because beta-blockers generally are contraindicated in untreated CHF. Furthermore, in patients with AF that need dobutamine or another catecholamine to support myocardial function (**Tables 25.2** and **25.3**), a beta-blocker should be avoided. The alternative, and often more practical choice, to IV therapy for HR control is PO loading dose(s) of standard diltiazem, or PO

Table 25.3 Formulas for Constant Rate Infusion

Method 1 (Allows for fine-tuning fluid as well as drug administration rate)

- Determine desired drug infusion rate: mcg/kg/min × kg body weight = mcg/min (A)
- Determine desired fluid infusion rate: ml/hour ÷ 60 = ml/min (B)
- (A) ÷ (B) = mcg/min ÷ ml/min = mcg drug/ml of fluid
- Convert from mcg to mg of drug needed (1 mcg = 0.001 mg)
- mg drug/ml fluid × ml of fluid in bag (or bottle or burette) = mg of drug to add to fluid bag

Method 2 (For total dose over a 6-hour period, must also calculate fluid volume and administration rate)

- Total dose in mg to infuse over a 6-hour period = body weight (kg) × dose (mcg/kg/min) × 0.36.

Method 3

- Drug dose (mcg/kg/min) × body weight (kg) = mg drug to add to 250 ml fluid to administer at drip rate of 15 ml/hour.

Method 4 (For lidocaine—faster but less helpful if fluid rate is important or fine drug dosage adjustments are needed)

- For CRI of 44 mcg/kg/min of lidocaine, add 25 ml of 2% lidocaine to 250 ml of D5W
  - Infuse at 0.25 ml/25 lb of body weight/min.

digoxin. Diltiazem can be given every 1 or 2 hours until the desired HR slowing is achieved. A maintenance or loading oral dose of digoxin also can be used (**Table 22.3**, p. 346).

Long-term oral therapy for AF in dogs with CHF typically includes the combination of diltiazem plus digoxin, as long as the latter is not contraindicated. Combined treatment is more effective for long-term HR control than either drug alone. Digoxin alone does not sufficiently control the HR, because increases in sympathetic tone from CHF, exercise, or excitement can override the vagal effect of digoxin on AV conduction. Most cardiologists prescribe a long-acting preparation of diltiazem and titrate the dosage upward as needed to adequately slow the HR. Simultaneous use of diltiazem and the usual dose of a beta-blocker is not recommended in heart failure because reduced contractility and AV nodal depression could lead to hypotension. However small doses of carvedilol (uptitrated every two weeks) usually are tolerated and the combination of these three drugs will better manage HR in some dogs. This therapy demands that CHF be under excellent control, that serum digoxin is measured and falls within the nontoxic (therapeutic) range, and that the diltiazem dosage has been optimized. Other therapy for CHF should be continued or instituted, as indicated.

Alternate drugs that have been used instead of diltiazem or a (standard) beta-blocker for HR control in dogs with AF, include amiodarone and sotalol. These would be reasonable considerations in dogs with AF and concurrent ventricular ectopy. Occasionally, conversion to sinus rhythm might occur in response to amiodarone, or even diltiazem therapy. Fish oil and ACE inhibitors have been shown to reduce the risk of AF in experimental canine models; improved intraatrial conduction and downregulation of genes associated with adverse atrial remodeling might be mechanisms.

Of course, not all dogs develop AF in the setting of CHF or advanced cardiac disease. Paroxysmal AF in medium to large dogs without structural heart disease could occur in association with anesthesia, hypothyroidism, iatrogenic hyperthyroidism, rapid removal of large-volume pericardial effusion, GI disease, or atrial distension induced by volume infusion. Changes in autonomic balance can provoke the onset of AF. Acute AF without signs of heart disease or failure might convert to sinus rhythm spontaneously, or in response to electrical cardioversion or drug therapy (see following paragraphs). Conversion is more likely with AF of recent onset and normal atrial size.

Regarding lone AF, it is not known if dogs with permanent AF but consistently slow HR response have comparable survival times to those converted to sinus rhythm. For dogs that do not convert spontaneously to sinus rhythm, electrical cardioversion should be considered; if unsuccessful (or not available), diltiazem or a beta-blocker can help control HR, especially during exercise, if a Holter ECG shows an excessive HR over the course of the day or with activity. Alternatively, if the ventricular rate is consistently low at rest, these dogs could be monitored periodically without therapy. Many of these dogs have preclinical DCM and rapid HRs could accelerate deterioration of myocardial function, however a possible advantage of a beta-blocker for rate control in lone AF is the potential for additional cardiac muscle protection, as well as the availability of generic formulations.

Pharmacologic cardioversion of recent onset AF to sinus rhythm in dogs has been achieved with a number of drugs, including amiodarone (IV or PO), diltiazem (IV or PO for ~3 days), sotalol, propafenone and other Class Ic agents. Also, acute-onset AF associated with high vagal tone could convert with IV lidocaine. If effective, the drug is either discontinued or, if available in oral formulation, continued for an indefinite period of time after sinus rhythm is achieved, as for electrical cardioversion. Previously, the class Ia drugs procainamide and quinidine also were used for attempted cardioversion in large dogs without signs of heart disease, but quinidine especially could provoke serious adverse effects (p. 376). In people with recent-onset AF, ibutilide has been effective; however, this agent is known to increase dispersion of ventricular repolarization and has provoked TdP in dogs with experimental cardiomyopathy. Experimentally in dogs, a ranolazine IV bolus followed by infusion converted a majority of dogs to sinus rhythm, but clinical experience presently is lacking. Other drugs used successfully to convert AF in people include flecainide and dofetilide. Magnesium supplementation is useful in some people with AF and rapid ventricular rate.

Electrical cardioversion (see p. 391) of AF is a therapeutic option for some dogs, especially those with lone AF or select cases without advanced heart disease. Several methods have been used successfully. The DC shock is synchronized with endogenous electrical activity (R wave) to avoid stimulation during the cardiac vulnerable period and precipitation of VF. Biphasic transthoracic current delivery combined with amiodarone (or other drug) therapy, appears highly effective in dogs. Prior to the cardioversion procedure, careful echocardiographic examination for intracardiac thrombi is advised. Thromboembolism post-AF conversion is a common complication in people and while rare, has occurred in some dogs. Cardioversion using transesophageal and right atrial electrodes also has been tried. Multiple complicating factors related to the animal or the equipment can prevent successful DC cardioversion. Furthermore, reversion to AF at some point after successful conversion is common, and might occur within seconds to months after a successful procedure. This is especially likely in dogs with long standing AF or underlying heart disease. If repeated attempts at electrical cardioversion fail, pharmacologic HR control becomes the therapeutic goal. Catheter ablation procedures have been variably successful in controlling experimental AF in dogs. The Suggested Additional Reading list contains more in-depth references for the interested reader.

Atrial Fibrillation Management in Cats A beta-blocker or diltiazem can provide HR control in cats with AF. For cats with systolic dysfunction or uncontrolled CHF, diltiazem usually is chosen, along with pimobendan for inotropic support and diuretic and RAAS inhibition to control congestive signs. Digoxin is rarely, if ever, used in cats now due to high risk of toxicosis. Compounded atenolol could be cautiously added to diltiazem and the dosage uptitrated to gain better HR control, if needed.

Atrial Fibrillation Management in Horses Most horses with AF have lone AF and conversion to sinus rhythm is the usual treatment goal. It is particularly important to attempt AF conversion if average HR exceeds 220 beats/minute during exercise or if ventricular arrhythmias occur. The exception to this recommendation is the horse with significant structural heart disease, especially if CHF is present. Horses with AF and a resting HR greater than ~60 beats/minute are more likely to have significant underlying cardiac disease and could be in CHF, although other causes for high sympathetic tone also should be investigated. It is important to identify the duration of AF, if possible. Thorough physical and auscultatory examinations, along with echocardiography, are recommended. The previously mentioned possible risk or potentiating factors for AF should be considered. Treatment for horses with AF and CHF is aimed at slowing the HR and controlling signs of congestion, rather than attempting cardioversion to sinus rhythm. Furosemide, digoxin, and possibly an ACE inhibitor (such as benazepril) are used in this situation. Quinidine therapy is not recommended because risks are higher for therapeutic failure and development of adverse effects, including hypotension, QRS prolongation, and tachyarrhythmia. Long-term prognosis for horses in CHF is poor.

Lone AF, in contrast, carries a high likelihood of cardioversion to sinus rhythm. Two approaches are used, namely electrocardioversion (p. 392) and pharmacologic conversion using quinidine sulfate (p. 377). It is important that cardioversion by either means be done in a controlled setting with continuous ECG monitoring. Horses with lone AF or with mild atrial enlargement are candidates for either treatment approach. Quinidine is recommended in cases where general anesthesia is not advisable or when electrical cardioversion is unavailable. When the onset of AF is recent, typically within the prior 24 to 48 hours, cardioversion often is delayed for a day or two, in case sinus rhythm resumes spontaneously (paroxysmal AF). After successful cardioversion, serum electrolyte measurement and continued ECG monitoring over the following 2–3 days are advised, even with spontaneous conversion. Successful conversion of lone AF with quinidine occurs about 80 to 90% of cases if the AF is of recent onset (generally within a few months). However, AF probably will recur in about one of four horses. The breed may also influence the likelihood of recurrence. With either pharmacologic or electrical cardioversion, over 40% of horses with structural cardiac disease, faster HRs, or AF of long-standing duration are likely to fail conversion or to develop AF recurrence.

A number of successful *quinidine protocols* have been used over the years (**Figure 25.7A**) and the recommended one involves administering quinidine sulfate by nasogastric tube at 22 mg/kg every 2 hours, starting in the early morning and continuing for 2 to 4 (potentially up to 6) doses thereafter. Most horses convert after 2 or 3 doses, and if signs of mild toxicity develop, most experienced clinicians monitor and manage these until 5 or 6 total doses have been given. However, should severe or unmanageable toxicity signs occur, quinidine must be stopped. Despite limited availability, measurement of plasma quinidine concentration can be instructive if conversion fails or toxicity occurs. This determination can indicate if sufficient drug was administered and absorbed. The therapeutic concentration range is 2–5 mcg/mL (6.2–15.4 micromol/L); toxicity is likely at higher plasma concentrations. Some horses convert hours after the last dose, as the blood concentration falls. If the maximal number of doses is administered without success, digoxin is given and then repeated the next morning. At that time, the quinidine dosing interval is extended to every 6 hours until conversion or signs of toxicity appear (p. 377). This extended dosing interval helps reduce quinidine toxicity. The total cumulative quinidine dose should not exceed 180 mg/kg. Because quinidine can predispose to digoxin toxicity, serum digoxin concentration should be measured if this drug is administered for longer than 24 hours (p. 328). It is important to ensure good hydration and electrolyte balance, particularly of K^+ and Mg^{++}, especially if the treatment period extends beyond 12 hours. IV fluid support might be needed if the horse is not drinking well. Horses that seem uncomfortable can be slowly walked between doses.

The clinician should anticipate quinidine's vagolytic and other adverse effects. This includes procuring and calculating treatment doses that might be needed to manage complications (including injectable digoxin, $MgSO_4$, $NaHCO_3$, lidocaine, phenylephrine and IV crystalloid fluids). Close monitoring of the ECG and the patient helps prevent serious toxicity. A pretreatment ECG should be recorded and the QRS duration measured; QRS prolongation to >25% of baseline is a sign of quinidine toxicity (from sodium channel blocking). The QT interval also should be evaluated, although prolongation of repolarization is observed less often. Besides the ECG changes, depressed attitude, inappetence, reduced drinking, mild colic, diarrhea, nasal edema, and hypotension are among the adverse effects that can develop during quinidine therapy. These signs should resolve after discontinuing the drug. Rarely, seizure activity, hypotension, CHF, laminitis, urticaria, or sudden death have occurred.

Cumulative doses of quinidine can increase HR significantly prior to AF conversion, due to simultaneous slowing of the atrial rate along with accelerated AV conduction that allows more fibrillation waves to reach the ventricles. High-strung horses might be more likely to experience excessively increased HR during quinidine therapy. Some increase in HR is anticipated after 2 or 3 doses; however, once the HR exceeds 80 to 90/minute either quinidine therapy should stop or IV digoxin be administered slowly (0.0022 mg/kg or about 1 mg for a 450 kg horse) to depress AV conduction and ventricular response rate. If the response to digoxin is good, quinidine treatment can be continued.

Table 25.4 Strategies for Refractory Ventricular Tachycardia in the Dog

Reevaluate the ECG

- Could the rhythm have been incorrectly diagnosed initially? (For example, SVT with aberrant intraventricular conduction can mimic VT)

Assess serum K^+ (and Mg^{++}) concentration

- Hypokalemia reduces class I antiarrhythmic drug efficacy and can predispose to some arrhythmias. Strive for a serum K^+ concentration in the high normal range.
    - If serum K^+ concentration is <3 mEq/L, can infuse KCl at 0.5 mEq/kg/h
    - If serum K^+ is between 3 and 3.5 mEq/L, can infuse KCl at 0.25 mEq/kg/h
- If serum Mg^{++} concentration is <1.0 mg/dL, can administer $MgSO_4$ (or $MgCl_2$), diluted in D_5W, at 0.75–1.0 mEq/kg/day, by CRI

Maximize the dose of lidocaine

Start $MgSO_4$ infusion, if not already done

- $MgSO_4$ could help suppress ventricular tachyarrhythmias associated with digoxin toxicity or suspected *torsades de pointes* (**Table 25.2**)

Try an alternative antiarrhythmic strategy

- Sotalol (PO) – either with lidocaine or alone, or
- Amiodarone (IV or PO loading), or
- A beta-blocker with a class I drug (such as esmolol, propranolol, or atenolol with lidocaine, procainamide or quinidine), or
- A class Ia drug with a class Ib drug (such as procainamide with lidocaine or mexiletine)

Consider that the antiarrhythmic drug(s) might be having a proarrhythmic effect

- Proarrhythmia can occur with any drug, directly or by changing heart rate
- Polymorphic ventricular tachycardia (including *torsades de pointes*) can occur with quinidine, procainamide, and other drug toxicities

Consider (if available) or refer for electrocardioversion[a]

If the arrhythmia is well-tolerated

- Continue supportive care and correct other abnormalities as possible
- Monitor (± continue the most effective antiarrhythmic drug)

---

[a] DC cardioversion (see p. 391) could be attempted for refractory VT, if the equipment is available. ECG synchronization and anesthesia or sedation are required. High-energy, nonsynchronized shock (defibrillation) can be used for rapid polymorphic VT or flutter degenerating into VF.
Abbreviations: CRI, constant rate infusion; D_5W, 5% dextrose in water; ECG, electrocardiogram; SVT, supraventricular tachycardia; VT, ventricular tachycardia.

Some horses have developed severe tachycardia during quinidine treatment, with HRs approaching 300 beats/minute. It can be difficult to know in some cases if the rhythm is simply accelerated conduction of AF or atrial flutter along with VPCs, or if a ventricular tachyarrhythmia has assumed control of the ventricles. Multiform VT and TdP represent the most extreme rhythm disturbances and sudden death is possible (**Figure 25.7B**). In these cases, quinidine is discontinued, digoxin is held in reserve, and IV fluid is administered to support blood pressure and increase vagal tone. IV $MgSO_4$ should be given to suppress quinidine-induced ventricular tachyarrhythmias. Administration of sodium bicarbonate (1 mEq/kg IV) helps counteract quinidine's Na^+ channel blocking effect by increasing extracellular Na^+ concentration and pH, which increases the drug's protein binding; extracellular ionized Ca^{++} is reduced, as well. Lidocaine often is co-administered to observe the effect. Severe hypotension might require a pressor agent such as IV phenylephrine. It should be noted that despite the potential for severe quinidine toxicosis, the success rate for conversion of lone AF at experienced centers has been 80 to 90%. It is likely higher in horses with acute AF that is managed promptly and where quinidine therapy is not stopped for only minor complications.

Alternative drug therapy can be considered if AF does not respond to quinidine, or recurs quickly. An IV amiodarone infusion could be tried, although infusion of long duration might be needed. Amiodarone has been less effective for AF conversion in horses than quinidine or electrical cardioversion. For horses that develop AF during general anesthesia or fail electrical cardioversion at the highest energy levels, procainamide (1 mg/kg IV, up to maximum of 20 mg/kg) could be tried (with shocks repeated). Flecainide has variable effectiveness in chronic AF and can cause life-threatening arrthythmias and sudden death, so it generally is not recommended except as a last resort. However, recent-onset AF might convert in response to IV flecainide, followed by oral doses as needed (Takahashi, 2018). Nevertheless, even with acute-onset AF, flecainide's efficacy is much less than that of quinidine. Propafenone (2 mg/kg) has not been effective for AF conversion. Dofetilide or ranolazine might be future considerations but currently there is insufficient experience with these agents in horses.

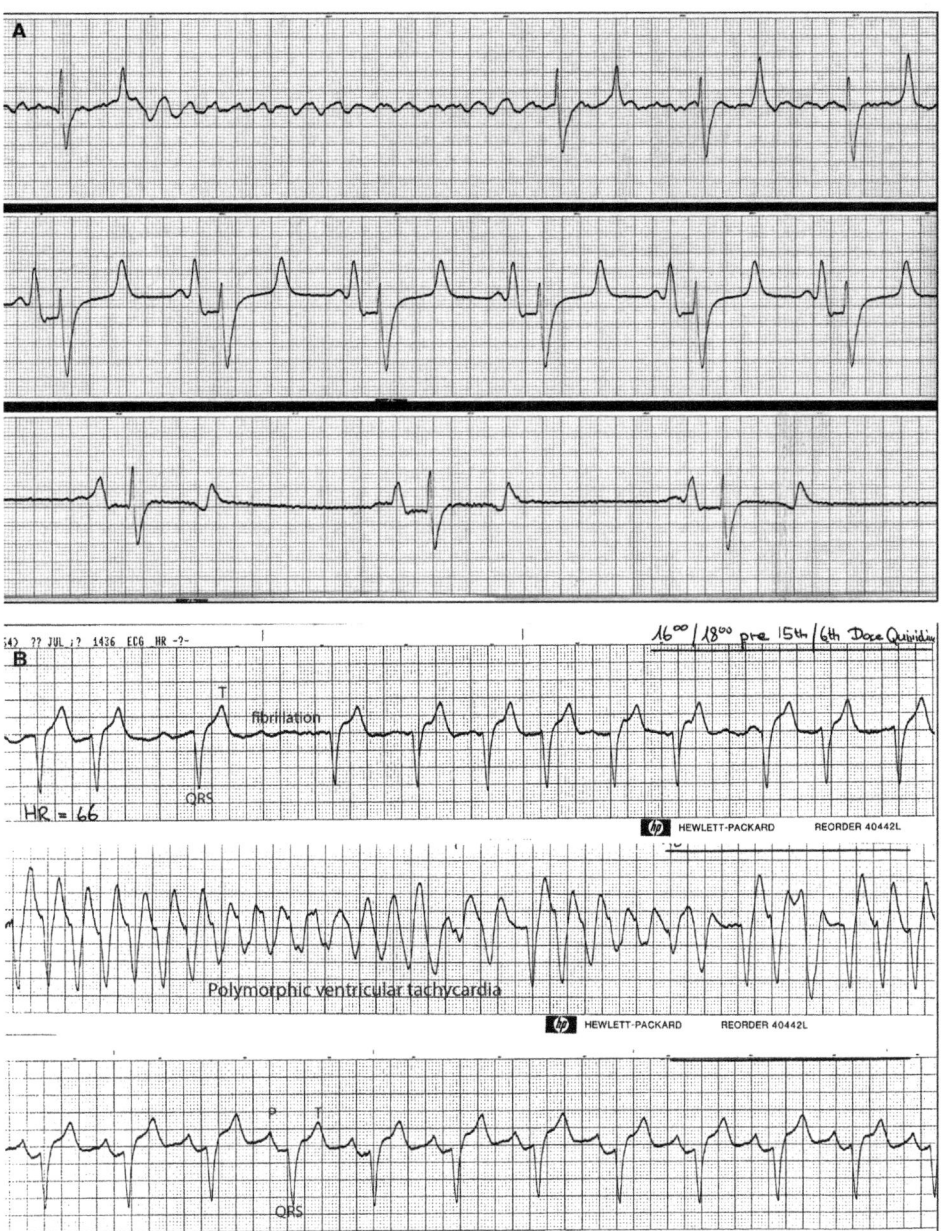

Figure 25.7 (A) Atrial fibrillation (AF, top strip) in a clinically normal horse being treated with quinidine via nasogastric tube; the long cycle following the first QRS complex shows drug-induced coarsening of baseline fibrillation waves prior to conversion to sinus tachycardia (middle strip). The sinus rate subsequently returned to normal (bottom strip). Base-apex lead, 50 mm/s. (B) AF (top strip) in a mule being treated with quinidine sulfate; the AF persisted despite multiple doses. Note the increased ventricular rate response, likely from quinidine's vagolytic effects on the AV node. *Torsades de pointes* (middle strip), a form of polymorphic ventricular tachycardia, then developed. Note the wide-QRS complexes of varying morphology and direction. After successful treatment that included sodium bicarbonate, magnesium sulfate, and lidocaine, the *torsades* abated and conversion to sinus rhythm occurred (bottom strip), presumably as quinidine blood levels were falling. Base apex lead, 25 mm/sec.

Electrical cardioversion (p. 392) is a good primary option and is highly effective in converting AF to sinus rhythm in horses with lone AF, a well-controlled ventricular rate, and minimal atrial enlargement (**Figure 25.8**). It also can be considered when quinidine is contraindicated, fails to convert the rhythm, or causes adverse reactions. AF recurrence might be more frequent than with quinidine conversion, but this could relate to the predominant patient population treated this way. Pretreatment with amiodarone or sotalol prior to electrical cardioversion could enhance conversion rate and reduce AF recurrence, at least in the short term. Adjunctive antiarrhythmic therapy requires further study. As noted previously, the addition of IV procainamide sometimes leads to successful electrocardioversion after previous attempts have failed.

After successful cardioversion by any method, ECG monitoring (preferably continuously) over the following 24 hours is recommended to identify any atrial arrhythmias. Serum K^+ and Mg^{++} concentrations should be verified; if low, supplementation

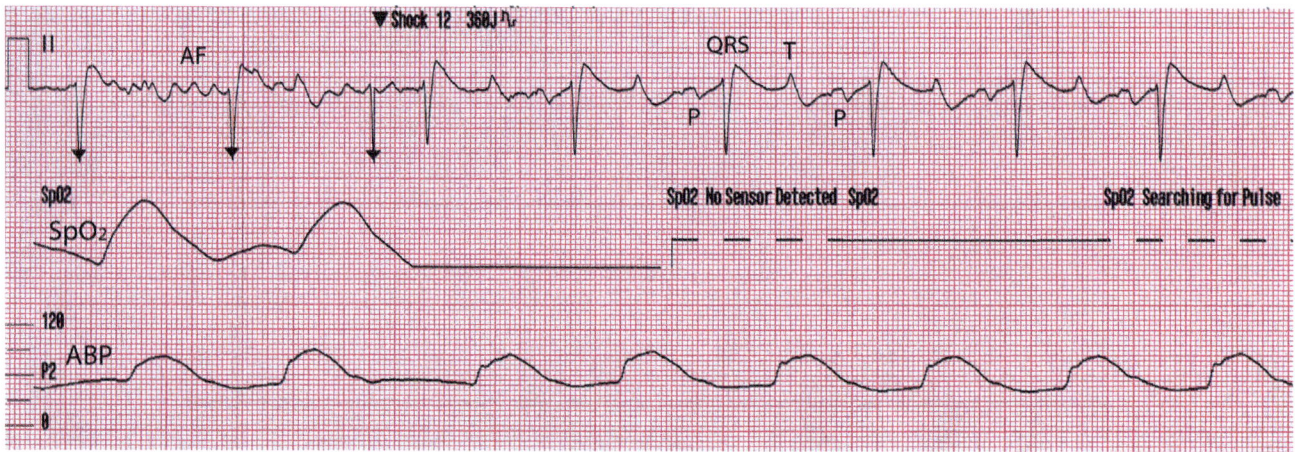

Figure 25.8 Transvenous electrocardioversion of atrial fibrillation (AF) in a horse. A relatively high energy level (360J) was eventually needed for cardioversion to sinus rhythm (P-QRS-T). Although the system was set for a synchronized biphasic shock during the QRS complexes (see the markers on the first two QRS complexes), the cardioverter-defibrillator actually discharged just prior to the third QRS complex. This was sufficient to terminate AF and initiate sinus rhythm; however, had this shock occurred on the T wave, it might have precipitated ventricular fibrillation. The pulse oximetry (SpO$_2$) sensor became dislodged from the horse during the shock. ABP, systemic arterial blood pressure (facial artery catheter).

might help reduce risk of AF recurrence. Follow-up echocardiography is used to evaluate atrial size, ventricular function, and valve competence. LV contractility usually normalizes within several days, unless underlying cardiac disease is present. Return of left atrial contractile function could take several weeks and might not fully normalize; poor atrial function could indicate a higher risk for recurrent AF. Sotalol (1 mg/kg initially, then 2–3 mg/kg PO q12h) sometimes is begun or continued after cardioversion in hope of suppressing atrial ectopy, which could trigger recurrent AF. The efficacy of this is unclear at present and it is often unsuccessful. Prior to resuming work or training, the sotalol dose is reduced and then discontinued. Horses with normal cardiac size and function, and in which AF was short-lived, can return to training in a relatively short time; many racing horses have returned to the track within 2 weeks of conversion. In contrast, at least 4 to 6 weeks of rest after cardioversion are advocated for horses that had AF of long duration, or that demonstrate persistent atrial arrhythmias, sinus tachycardia, or poor left atrial function. Episodes of AF could become increasingly frequent, and resistant to conversion, with progressive atrial disease. Holter and exercise ECG are recommended when feasible for long-term follow-up.

Atrial Standstill

Loss of atrial electrical activation occurs as a consequence of severe hyperkalemia or from extensive replacement fibrosis of atrial myocardium. It is important to exclude hyperkalemia as a cause for a flat baseline with absent P waves, as this is treatable and reversible. Hyperkalemia usually induces bradycardia, however in cats, the HR might be normal or even rapid and the rhythm could be confused with VT. A similar ECG pattern to hyperkalemia, with absent P waves, that is unresponsive to atropine occasionally is observed in cats with cardiogenic shock. However, atrial activity returns if the shock is managed successfully. Whether this rhythm represents a transient form of atrial standstill or sinus arrest with escape activity is uncertain.

Persistent atrial standstill, also called silent atrium, is characterized by loss of effective atrial electrical and mechanical activities and an absence of P waves. A junctional or ventricular escape rhythm controls the heart in these cases (**Figure 25.9**). The baseline can be flat, show

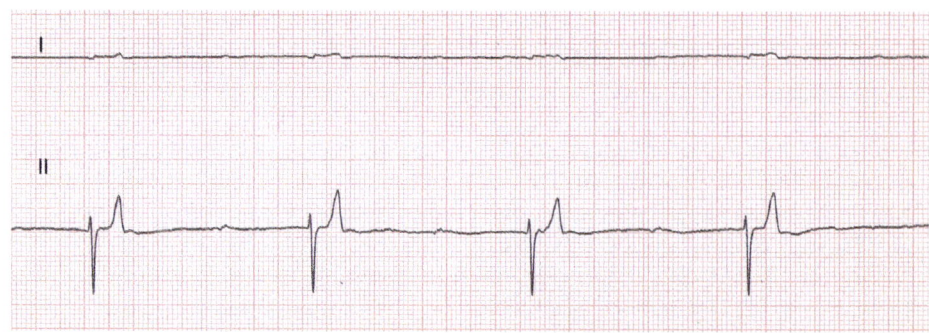

Figure 25.9 Atrial standstill in a 13-year-old female Dachshund. There is a ventricular escape rhythm (~30 beats/min). Low-amplitude baseline deflections might represent residual activity in an isolated area of atrial muscle, or artifact. Artificial pacing was recommended.

tiny undulations reminiscent of AF, or have small regular atrial deflections that represent ineffective depolarizations in isolated remnants of atrial muscle. This bradyarrhythmia is rare in dogs and extremely rare in cats. Most cases reported originally occurred in English Springer Spaniels; some of these dogs were thought to have a muscular dystrophy (fascioscapulohumeral type). However, idiopathic atrial myopathy (with progressive myocyte loss, inflammatory cell infiltrate, and fibrosis) or other diseases of the atrial myocardium also could result in atrial standstill. Besides English Springer Spaniels, Labrador Retrievers might be overrepresented; a variety of other breeds have been affected, as well. Persistent atrial standstill most often affects young adults. There might be a slight female predisposition. Organic disease of the atrial myocardium can progress to involve the ventricular myocardium and sometimes leads to CHF. Therefore, persistent atrial standstill could foreshadow a progressive cardiac disorder. Partial atrial standstill (where one atrium retains some electromechanical function) is possible, although rare. Clinical signs of syncope, lethargy, or CHF are typical.

Medical treatment for persistent atrial standstill usually is unrewarding, aside from managing CHF should that be present. However, an anticholinergic drug or infusion of dopamine or another catecholamine could temporarily accelerate the escape rhythm (**Figure 25.2**). Terbutaline (PO) might also have some beneficial effect; but if this provokes ventricular tachyarrhythmias, the drug should be discontinued or its dosage reduced. Ventricular antiarrhythmic drugs are contraindicated (prior to pacemaker implantation) because they could suppress the escape rhythm. Permanent pacemaker implantation is the treatment of choice. If the right ventricle is healthy, aside from some dilation, transvenous pacing usually is appropriate. However, when right ventricular function is impaired, a left ventricular epicardial lead might be preferable. Patient survival after pacing appears to be much better than previously thought; median survival time in a group of 20 dogs after pacing was about 28 months, although there was a wide range in outcomes (Cervenec, 2017). Some cases have lived many years longer. CHF at the time of atrial standstill diagnosis does not appear to shorten survival time, although progressive ventricular dysfunction could negatively affect outcome.

Atrioventricular Reentrant (Reciprocating) Tachycardia

AVRT involves a reentrant circuit comprised of the AV node, ventricular myocardium, an accessory conduction pathway (bypass tract), and atrial myocardium. These tachycardias can be very rapid, leading to clinical signs. Dogs with tricuspid valve malformations are probably at higher risk, especially Labrador Retrievers. Cases where conduction down the accessory pathway also occurs during sinus rhythm are considered to have "preexcitation syndrome," and the eponym Wolff–Parkinson–White (WPW) syndrome is commonly applied. In this syndrome, the accessory conduction pathway lies outside the AV node. This is the most common form of preexcitation (p. 153). Often there is no overt ventricular preexcitation during sinus rhythm and the accessory pathway is considered "concealed," conducting only during the AVRT. The vast majority of these accessory pathways in dogs are located on the right side of the heart (Santilli, 2007). Some animals have more than one accessory pathway. In people, a similar type of reentrant tachycardia can develop within the AV node and is called AV nodal reentrant tachycardia. This only has been induced experimentally in dogs so far; its occurrence in cats and horses is unknown.

Orthodromic AVRT is the most common pattern. It develops when a ventricular impulse is conducted backward (retrograde) through the accessory pathway into the atrium, then the impulse travels down the AV node in the normal (orthodromic) direction to reenter the ventricles (**Figure 23.4A**, p. 367). The resulting SVT can be initiated by either an atrial or a ventricular premature complex, provided the impulse enters and conducts through only one of the AV pathways. Because the refractory periods of AV nodal cells and accessory pathways cells usually are different, premature beats are a likely trigger of AVRT. Changes in autonomic traffic might represent another trigger. The authors have observed AVRT where a sudden prolongation in PR interval preceded the tachycardia; whether this is a form of AV nodal reentrant tachycardia is uncertain and would require electrophysiologic verification.

Once initiated, the AVRT macroreentry circuit can perpetuate itself, causing a rapid and regular SVT with attendant acute clinical signs (**Figure 25.10**). HRs approaching 400 beats/minute can occur, depending on the refractory periods of the pathways. Persistent AVRT leads to TICM (p. 630). The QRS complexes with orthodromic AVRT usually are of normal (narrow) configuration, unless an intraventricular conduction disturbance (such as a major bundle branch block) causes aberrancy. However, in occasional cases, the direction of the macroreentrant circuit is reversed, so that ventricular-to-atrial conduction occurs retrograde through the AV node and atrial-to-ventricular conduction occurs across the accessory pathway. This is known as *antidromic AVRT*. The QRS complexes associated with antidromic AVRT are wider than normal because of complete ventricular preexcitation. Antidromic AVRT could easily be confused with VT.

Because this is a macro-reentrant circuit, blocking conduction in any of the four limbs can at least temporarily break the tachyarrhythmia. An electrical shock (electrocardioversion) can accomplish this in the atrial and ventricular muscle, but drug therapy is chosen first and acts more selectively on the AV node, the accessory pathway or both tissues. Importantly, these tissues have dissimilar electrophysiologic properties, so they often respond differently to an antiarrhythmic drug. The AV node is richly innervated with autonomic nerves, but innervation is inconsistent in the accessory pathway. Orthodromic AVRT might respond to a vagal maneuver if AV conduction slows enough to break the reentry cycle

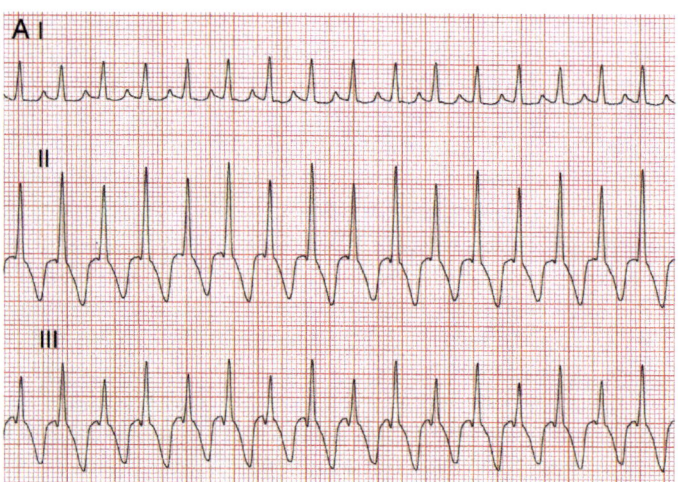
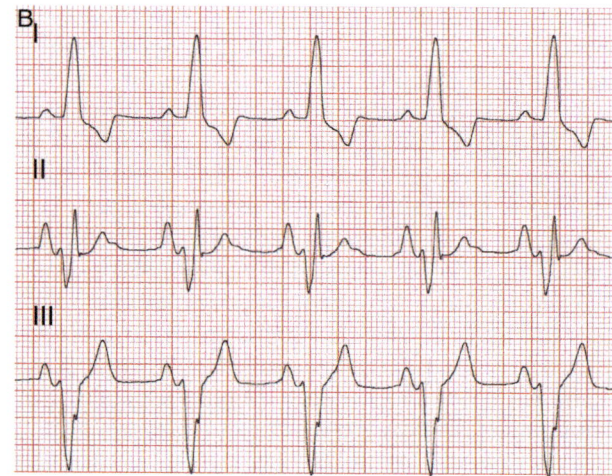

Figure 25.10 A 7-year-old mixed breed dog was presented for intermittent tachycardia and weakness. (A) ECG recorded during an episode shows a rapid and regular, narrow-complex tachycardia at ~340 beats/min (with electrical alternans). The tachycardia ceased after several IV doses of diltiazem. (B) The ECG complexes during sinus rhythm show ventricular preexcitation, indicating that the dog has Wolff–Parkinson–White syndrome with orthodromic AV reciprocating tachycardia (A). The short PR intervals are better-appreciated in leads II & III (PR ~ 0.06 sec); ventricular pre-excitation widens the initial part of the QRS complex and deviates the electrical axis. Leads I, II & III, 50 mm/s, 1 cm = 1 mV.

there. Drugs that slow conduction or prolong the refractory period of the AV node, bypass tract, or potentially both tissues, also interrupt the tachycardia. When a vagal maneuver fails to interrupt the tachycardia, IV diltiazem (acting on the AV node) or esmolol (potentially acting on both tissues) can be tried, although these are not used initially in the setting of preexisting AF (see p. 411) and only cautiously in CHF. Vagal maneuvers can be repeated after these drugs are given. For some cardiologists the preferred initial treatment involves delaying conduction in the accessory pathway with procainamide (if available) or lidocaine; lidocaine was highly effective in a retrospective case study (Wright, 2018). Amiodarone also might be effective. When the patient is in sinus rhythm, ventricular function should be evaluated echocardiographically to screen for TICM; if present, medical therapy as appropriate for dogs with occult (or overt) DCM is indicated.

The definitive treatment for ARVT involves intracardiac electrical mapping and radiofrequency catheter ablation of the accessory pathway(s). Consultation with a specialist who has expertise in such procedures and the detailed nuances of these arrhythmias is recommended. Ablation can successfully abolish refractory AVRT in dogs, essentially correcting a congenital heart defect (Santilli, 2006; Wright, 2018; **Figure 25.11**). Although the availability of this procedure is limited to a small number of referral centers, it is an excellent therapeutic option to avoid or reverse TICM, prevent signs related to SVT, and minimize the expense and potential adverse effects of chronic antiarrhythmic drug therapy. Catheter ablation therapy might not be possible in smaller dogs and cats because of intracardiac mapping catheter size.

When accessory pathway ablation is not an option, long-term oral antiarrhythmic therapy will likely be needed in patients with preexcitation syndrome. However, the optimal chronic therapy for AVRT is undetermined. Class Ic and III drugs are used most often in people. Although procainamide (and quinidine) lengthen the accessory pathway's refractory period and high-dose PO procainamide, with or without a beta-blocker or diltiazem, has successfully prevented recurrent AVRT in some cases, oral procainamide is unavailable and quinidine generally is avoided in small animals. These arrhythmias can vary in terms of mechanism, triggers, and response to drug therapy. Strategies that might be effective include a beta-blocker, sotalol, amiodarone, mexiletine (with or without a beta-blocker), possibly propafenone, or quinidine combined with a beta-blocker (**Table 25.2**). Although digoxin slows AV conduction, it can decrease the refractory period of the accessory pathway; therefore, it is avoided with

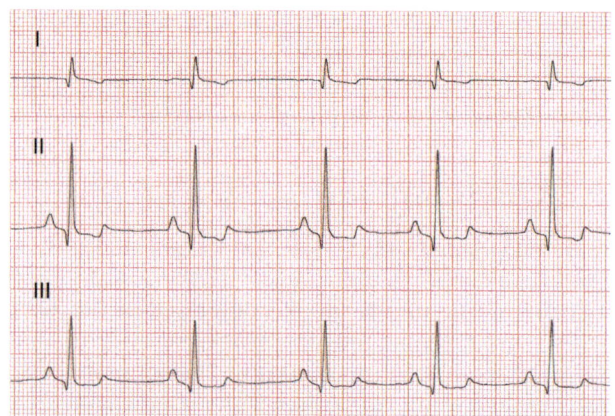

Figure 25.11 The dog of **Figure 25.10** was referred for intracardiac electrical mapping and accessory pathway ablation. The ECG complexes normalized after the successful procedure; no further episodes of orthodromic AV reciprocating tachycardia occurred. Leads I, II & III, 50 mm/s, 1 cm = 1 mV.

preexcitation syndromes. In addition, if the patient is thought to be at increased risk for developing AF, diltiazem, digoxin, and possibly beta-blockers should not be used.

AV Junctional Rhythms

Ectopic complexes and rhythms can arise in different levels of the AV junctional region. These include normal escape (subsidiary pacemaker) activity, observed during AV blocks, as well as abnormal premature complexes and tachycardias. Junctional QRS complex morphology generally is consistent with the normal sinus QRS configuration for each animal. AV conduction disturbances of varying degree and mechanism also are common. These often relate to conduction blocks with resultant escape activity (see "Atrioventricular Blocks" section); however, functional interference with atrial impulse conduction ("AV dissociation") due to abnormal AV junctional impulse formation also is important. An older label for these fast ectopic rhythms is "nodal" tachycardia, although the compact AV node is not thought to exhibit automaticity. Functional (longitudinal) dissociation of the AV node into two pathways, which can permit a reciprocating tachycardia, was demonstrated experimentally in dogs, although not yet conclusively proven to occur in veterinary practice. Automatic cells in the AV junction normally are overdrive-suppressed by faster sinus node activity. However, in cases of sinus node dysfunction or proximal AV block, automatic cells can generate junctional escape complexes to activate the heart. This is a normal rescue mechanism to support cardiac function and should not be suppressed by antiarrhythmic drug therapy. The rate of a junctional escape rhythm generally is faster than that of ventricular escape activity, often around 60 beats/minute in the dog and likely much faster in the cat.

Abnormal premature junctional activity also can occur and cause junctional premature complexes, an ectopic junctional tachycardia, or an accelerated junctional ("idionodal") rhythm. Labrador Retrievers appear predisposed to many of these junctional rhythms (Perego, 2012), as well as to structural AV blocks. Digoxin toxicity is another well-known cause of such rhythms. The mechanism underlying a particular junctional arrhythmia could involve abnormal automaticity or a reentrant circuit involving the AV node, although the surface ECG cannot differentiate these. It also can be challenging to distinguish junctional rhythms from "high" ventricular rhythms (originating in the dorsal septum); comparing the initial vector of the ectopic QRS complexes with that of normally conducted sinus complexes using multiple leads might be helpful.

Enhanced junctional rhythms and junctional ("nodal") tachycardias often discharge at a similar or slightly higher rate than the normal sinus node, for example, ~100–160 beats/minute in dogs or ~60–80 beats/minute in horses. These rhythms are typically, but not invariably, regular. Most result in a functional form of AV dissociation (with independent atrial and ventricular activations), sometimes with the junctional impulse causing retrograde capture of the atria. Atrial and ventricular rates can be similar and appear related for variable intervals, probably from BP (baroreceptor) or mechanical influences of ventricular pumping on the sinus node. This is termed "*isorhythmic AV dissociation*"; the two pacemakers either depolarize during the refractory period or more likely, collide near the AV node. This AV relationship can occur as a transient hookup ("accrochage") or more persistent relationship ("synchrony," usually of the so-called type I, with slight migrations of the P wave back and forth over the QRS complex).

Antiarrhythmic therapy is not indicated for occasional junctional premature beats or necessary for relatively slow junctional rhythms, although if these are persistent the loss of AV synchrony and potential for pulmonary venous backflow should be considered. Therapeutic strategies for paroxysmal or sustained junctional tachycardia and frequent junctional premature complexes generally are similar to those described for atrial (supraventricular) tachycardias. When there clearly is AV dissociation associated with a higher ventricular rate, but uncertainty regarding a ventricular origin, lidocaine, procainamide, or sotalol could be tried. For example, in horses, junctional and high ventricular tachycardias could be confused and initial treatment with a ventricular antiarrhythmic agent is recommended. If the HR with a junctional rhythm is slow, conduction system function should be confirmed, for example with atropine or exercise.

Atrioventricular Blocks

AV conduction disturbances vary in cause and severity (**Figures 25.12–25.14**; also see p. 151, and **Figures 5.42–5.46**, and **5.66**). They can be functional, as discussed for junctional tachycardias, or secondary to vagal tone, drugs, or structural disease. For example, high vagal tone, including the normal baroreceptor reflex in horses (and perhaps in some dogs) can slow and block AV conduction. AV blocks can occur with use (or toxicity) of drugs such as alpha$_2$-agonists, opioids, digoxin, and antiarrhythmic agents, as well as from organic diseases of the AV node and surrounding conduction tissues. Multifocal conduction disease that affects both proximal left and right bundle branches can also produce all degrees of AV block. Some diseases that have been associated with abnormal AV conduction include aortic valve endocarditis, HCM, hyperthyroidism (perhaps as an age-related comorbidity), infiltrative myocardial disease (including tumors), and myocarditis. Evidence of any AV conduction disturbance should prompt further diagnostic evaluation, including with echocardiography. Idiopathic AV blocks occur most often in middle-aged to older dogs and cats; sometimes they are revealed during general anesthesia for a surgical or dental procedure. AV blocks also can be transient and the predominant rhythm can change, even abruptly, from 3rd to 2nd to 1st degree block (Santilli, 2016). Myocarditis might underlie some cases of transient AV block, especially in younger animals.

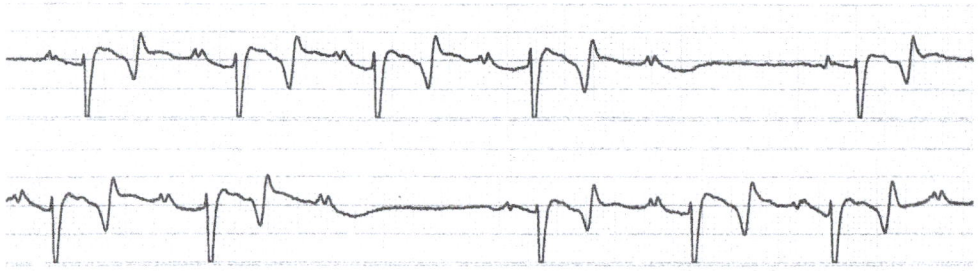

Figure 25.12 Variable 1st degree and Mobitz type I (Wenckebach) 2nd degree atrioventricular (AV) block in a 2-year-old Belgian gelding. This is a common rhythm seen in normal horses. It reflects relatively high vagal tone at rest, is related to baroreceptor activation, and requires no treatment. The AV block disappeared once the horse became active. Base-apex lead, 25 mm/s.

The occurrence of AV blocks seems, at least subjectively, to be higher in certain canine breeds, including the German Shepherd, Labrador Retriever, Cocker Spaniel, Afghan, Chow-Chow, Dalmatian, English Bulldog, Pug, and Dachshund, and with likely regional predilection. Congenital 3rd degree heart block also is reported in dogs. Symptomatic AV block is less common in cats; yet CHF can occur if the escape rhythm is too slow. Although the literature suggests that most feline cases are associated with cardiomyopathy, AV block often is observed in old cats without detectable organic heart disease. It likely is missed in many because escape rhythm rates are faster in this species. In horses, 1st degree

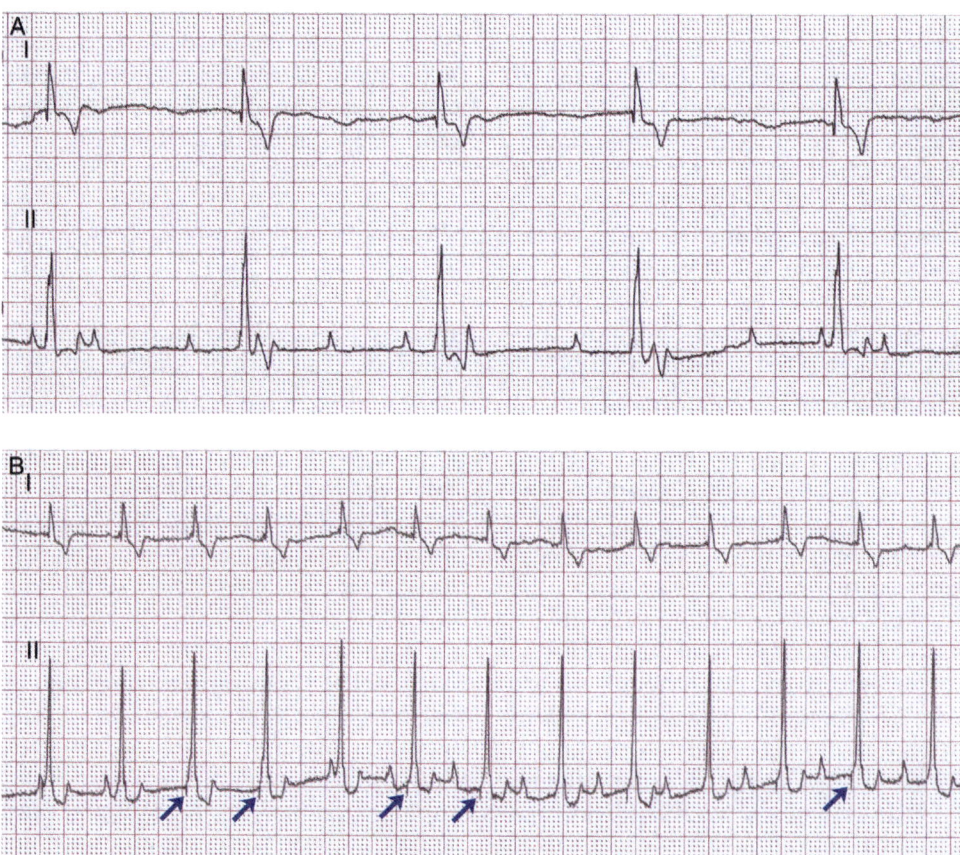

Figure 25.13 (A) Complete (3rd degree) AV block with a ventricular escape rhythm (~40 beats/min) discovered in a 13-year-old, female German Shepherd referred for removal of a large intra-abdominal mass. Note the positive ventricular escape complex configuration; ventricular-origin complexes can be of any shape, size and polarity. (B) A permanent transvenous pacing system was implanted. This ECG shows ventricular-paced QRS complexes at a rate of 100 beat/min. A small pacing artifact is visible at the onset of most complexes (arrows); bipolar pacemakers create a much smaller pacing artifact than unipolar systems and it is not always clearly visible on the surface ECG. Nonconducted sinus P waves are present in the background on both ECGs. A few weeks later, a (~15 cm) omental mass was removed during exploratory laparotomy. The dog recovered uneventfully; the mass was a benign lipoma. Leads I & II, 25 mm/s; 1 cm = 1 mV.

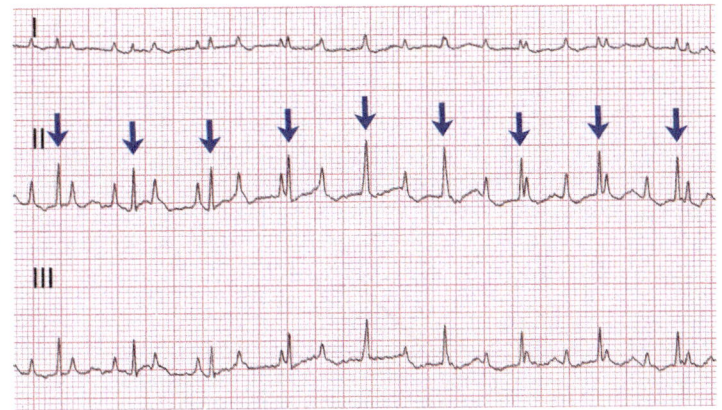

Figure 25.14 AV dissociation caused by 3rd degree AV block in a 6-year-old cat. The ventricular escape rhythm (arrows) was stable and, at 110 beats/min, caused no signs of lethargy or collapse. No treatment is needed at this time. The 5th and 6th QRS complexes from the left are taller than the others because they occur simultaneously with the prominent P waves. Leads I, II, & III; 25 mm/s; 1 cm = 1 mV.

and intermittent 2nd degree (often Mobitz I or Wenckebach) AV block are normal variations associated with high vagal tone (**Figure 25.12**; also **Figure 14.4**, p. 257). The AV block should disappear with an increase in excitement or activity, as vagal tone decreases. Persistent AV block during exercise is considered abnormal. Overall, organic causes of AV block in horses are rare compared to the dog and the cat.

Whether clinical signs result from AV block relates to the overall ventricular rate, stability of the escape rhythm, comorbidities, and underlying cardiac function. 1st degree AV block and 2nd degree AV block with occasional nonconducted P waves cause no clinical signs and need no treatment. However, a search for the underlying cause (such as high vagal tone or medication affecting AV conduction) and appropriate disease management are indicated. Dogs with high-grade 2nd degree (multiple blocked P waves in sequence) and 3rd degree (complete) AV blocks are more likely to display lethargy, exercise intolerance, weakness, syncope, and other signs of low cardiac output. These high-grade AV blocks also are associated with increased risk for sudden death. Low output signs in dogs become severe with HRs consistently below 40 beats/minute. CHF develops secondary to chronic bradycardia in some cases, especially if other cardiac disease such as advanced degenerative valvular disease is present. Although some dogs seem fairly asymptomatic, they still are likely to be at increased risk for sudden death, and most clients will remark on improved exercise capacity and general quality of life after permanent pacing.

The clinical workup usually will involve the following: routine laboratory tests (CBC, biochemical profile, serum thyroxine, and urinalysis with urine protein to creatinine ratio, if there is proteinuria); thoracic radiographs (to screen for CHF and exclude a comorbidity such as metastatic neoplasia); echocardiography; and often, abdominal ultrasonography to screen for comorbidity or assess kidney size in azotemic patients. Increased cTnI concentration can occur with high-grade AV block; this might persist shortly after pacemaker implantation but usually diminishes over time. Markedly elevated cTnI concentrations should prompt consideration of myocarditis or other infiltrative disease such as neoplasia. Findings that might modify the therapeutic approach include substantial proteinuria that could predispose to atrial or pacing lead thrombosis or intra-abdominal neoplasia requiring surgical intervention, where pacing by abdominal and epicardial routes could be most practical.

Cats with persistent 3rd degree AV block usually have a ventricular escape rhythm between 90 and 120 beats/minute and so most are relatively asymptomatic (**Figure 25.14**). Cats that have syncope associated with AV block are likely to have intermittent high-grade 2nd or 3rd degree AV block, or recent-onset AV block where a stable escape rhythm is not yet established (**Figure 5.66**, p. 163). In these cats, ventricular subsidiary pacemakers are overdrive suppressed during periods of relatively normal AV conduction; when AV block suddenly occurs (or recurs), a delay in escape rhythm activation often ensues. The resulting period of ventricular asystole could be long enough to cause weakness or syncope. Pacing can help these cats. However, because normal sinus rhythm might be present between episodes (although often with 1st degree block), a mistaken diagnosis of "seizure disorder" often is made. For cats with 3rd degree AV block and a stable escape rhythm, the patient's ventricular rate and comorbidities determine the outcome. A heart rate <90 beats/minute is likely to produce signs of inactivity and perhaps, CHF. Similarly, hyperthyroidism, moderate anemia, systemic hypertension, and possibly chronic kidney disease (especially with fluid therapy) predispose to CHF in cats with otherwise stable AV block. Manifestations of these include hypervolemia, jugular distension, and pleural effusion. Management of underlying systemic disease, along with judicious medical therapy for CHF (low-dosage furosemide, pimobendan, RAAS inhibition), and control of systemic hypertension if present, usually provides control of clinical signs without the need for pacing.

High-grade AV blocks are rare in horses, and they occasionally improve or resolve spontaneously. When AV block is diagnosed in conjunction with a high resting atrial rate, the clinician should consider a FAT with physiologic AV block. When multiple P waves are blocked at rest, vagal influence is still a potential cause, and that can be evaluated with care during modest exercise with ECG recording. If mild exercise does not eliminate the block, atropine administration helps exclude a vagal component (with consideration of adverse effects in this species). In the horse with transient AV block, the importance of suitable follow-up is emphasized. The horse should only be ridden by an adult who is aware of the potential for sudden recurrence of AV block, which can lead to collapse or sudden death. Horses with clinical signs caused by AV block, or in which the AV block persists after atropine or exercise challenge, should be rested and reevaluated. These animals are considered unsafe to use. Their prognosis is likely to be poor, although successful long-term pacing in a few adult horses (one of the authors' cases surviving for >10 years) and a number of miniature donkeys has been reported.

Patients with an AV block usually receive an atropine challenge. However, IV and PO anticholinergic drugs are widely ineffective in high-grade 2nd degree and complete (3rd degree) AV block. Artificial pacing usually is needed in these cases (p. 388, p. 175; **Figures 25.2** and **25.13**). An emergency infusion of dopamine, dobutamine, or isoproterenol (**Tables 25.2** and **25.3**) might increase the ventricular escape rate in these animals; however, such therapy also can provoke ventricular tachyarrhythmias. Although isoproterenol is probably most effective for improving AV conduction or escape activity, it also causes vasodilation and generally is avoided. Moderate and even severe azotemia can occur in dogs with complete AV block and slow escape activity (20-30/minute); the azotemia might normalize with pacing. Although temporary transvenous pacing for 2-3 days, to observe its effect in dogs with CHF or marked azotemia might seem logical, the attendant costs often rival those of permanent pacing. One situation where prompt temporary transvenous pacing is recommended involves the patient with AV block and a paroxysmal ventricular tachycardia that overdrive suppresses the escape rhythm, causing periods of asystole and syncope. Interestingly, after permanent pacing the ventricular tachycardia often abates in such cases. Animals with both 2nd degree AV block and conduction of their sinus impulses with bundle branch block have such high probability of multifocal conduction system disease that elective pacing might be considered before complete AV block develops.

Chronic medical therapy for high-grade AV block generally is unsuccessful, aside from managing comorbidities or CHF. Underlying structural disease (such as cardiomyopathy, endocarditis, myocarditis, fibrosis, trauma) is present in most cases, although this might not be detectable antemortem. Occasional cases have functional AV block (as with digoxin toxicity, alpha$_2$-agonist anesthetics, hyperkalemia). Rarely, an animal with myocarditis might show improved AV conduction in response to antiinflammatory glucocorticoid treatment; however, reports of "successful" treatment are uncontrolled and the labile nature of AV block in some patients must be appreciated.

Ultimately, the vast majority of patients with symptomatic or persistent high grade 2nd and 3rd degree AV block benefit from artificial pacing; outcomes generally are good, with acceptable complication rates (p. 391). Cats (in contrast to dogs) with complete AV block might survive for years without artificial pacing, even with underlying cardiac disease or heart failure at presentation. Many cats with consistent 3rd degree AV block and a stable ventricular escape rhythm exhibit no obvious clinical signs (**Figure 25.14**). Pacing therapy can be pursued for recurrently symptomatic cats, especially those with sudden periods of complete AV block and asystole.

Ventricular Rhythm Disturbances

Ventricular tachyarrhythmias (p. 147 on), other than sporadic VPCs, often indicate underlying cardiac or systemic disease (**Table 23.1**, p. 370). Guidelines for instituting ventricular antiarrhythmic therapy often are based on so-called "modified Lown criteria," related to the frequency, rate, and prematurity of ectopy, along with variability of QRS configurations. Rapid paroxysmal or sustained VT (for example, at rates >150–200 beats/minute in dogs, or >100–120 beats/minute in horses) are more likely to cause hemodynamic instability, myocardial ischemia, and potentially progress to a lethal arrhythmia (**Figure 25.15**). Other characteristics of "complex" or "malignant" ventricular arrhythmias, which are thought to imply electrical instability and greater risk of degeneration into a lethal rhythm, include multiform (polymorphic) QRS configuration (**Figures 5.32** and **5.35**, p. 149) and close coupling of VPCs to the preceding complexes (R-on-T phenomenon). As noted in Chapter 23, other variables such as QT interval, heart rate, varying long-short cardiac cycles, and autonomic traffic, as well as drug effects and underlying anatomic substrate, also can impact arrhythmogenesis and risk for syncope or sudden cardiac death.

Ventricular tachyarrhythmias that cause signs of hypotension or inadequate cardiac output should be treated. Considerations regarding the animal's underlying disease also are important. Animals thought to have a disease associated with sudden cardiac death (such as DCM) often are treated earlier and more aggressively. For all patients with serious arrhythmias, it is important to identify and address underlying cardiac or systemic abnormalities and to minimize sympathetic activation (as from pain, anxiety, fever, hypovolemia). Exercise restriction is wise. General goals for managing a ventricular tachyarrhythmia are to: (1) optimize cardiac output by controlling HR and rhythm as possible, (2) provide supportive care as needed, and (3) avoid adverse effects of antiarrhythmic therapy. Paroxysmal or sustained VT can degenerate into increasingly unstable rhythms. However, as previously noted, successful reduction in the number of VPCs or paroxysms of VT with antiarrhythmic drugs does not necessarily prevent sudden cardiac death.

Ventricular Premature Complexes

Occasional VPCs in an otherwise asymptomatic animal are unlikely to cause hemodynamic disturbance and generally are not treated. 24-hour Holter ECG studies suggest that most younger dogs and cats have only low numbers of true VPCs (not simply "ectopics") and some have none during the recording period. Most veterinarians have seen healthy animals with normal laboratory tests and structurally normal hearts (by echocardiography) that have occasional VPCs, especially older animals. The authors do not claim to know the answers to: "how many VPC's are normal?" or "at

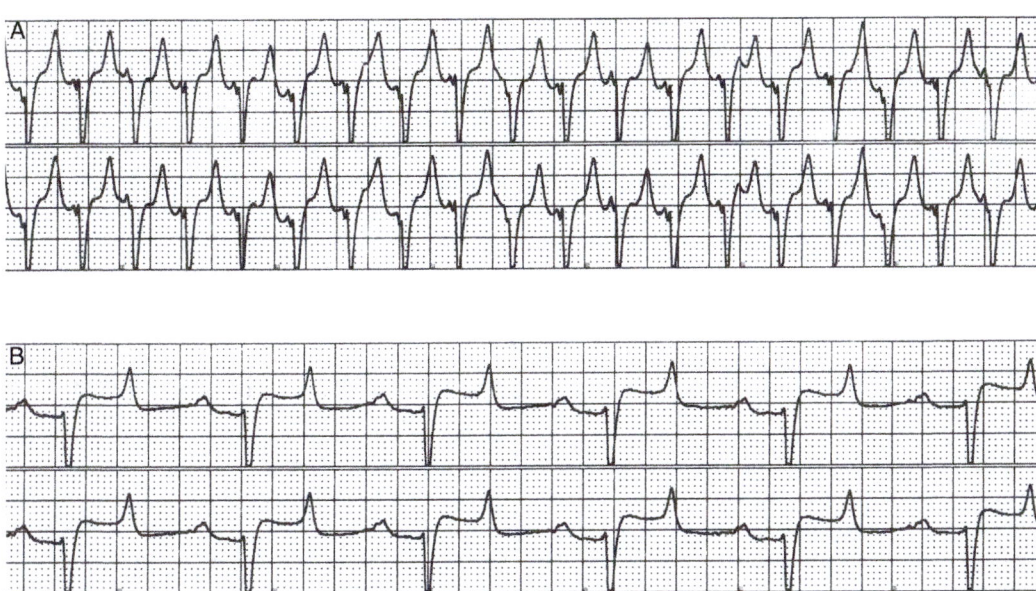

Figure 25.15 (A) ECG from a 10-year-old Quarterhorse gelding presented for lethargy and inappetance. The rhythm is ventricular tachycardia (VT) at a heart rate of ~160 beats/min. Two boluses of lidocaine (0.25 mg/kg each) converted the VT to normal sinus rhythm (~40 beats/min) with occasional monomorphic ventricular premature complexes. (B) ECG recorded later the same day shows sinus rhythm. Echocardiographic findings were unremarkable, except for mild aortic regurgitation. Recurrent VT occurred periodically over the following three years. An underlying cause could not be identified. Base-apex lead (recorded simultaneously on two channels), 25 mm/s.

what VPC frequency should treatment be started?" It might be remembered that 1440 isolated VPCs (clearly abnormal) averages to only 1 VPC/minute over 24 hours. The relative percentage is probably more relevant than isolated numbers. For example (at least in people), if 10% to 20% of total heartbeats are VPCs, there is greater likelihood that ventricular dysfunction (TICM) could develop. Other clinical findings can modify the approach. Even moderately frequent VPCs might not require antiarrhythmic drug treatment if underlying heart size and function are normal.

VPCs also occur in some apparently normal horses; these include what are considered normal immediate post-exercise VPCs. But VPCs that occur during exercise are of greater concern, especially if frequent or in a horse with poor performance. Although a horse with occasional VPCs might be cautiously acceptable as a mount for an informed adult following suitable work-up and exercise ECG, its use by a child or as a lesson horse is not advised.

Especially when there is underlying cardiac disease, VPCs with a short coupling interval (R-on-T timing) following the preceding QRS (whether normal or ectopic) are thought to portend increased risk for electrical instability and VF. Repetitive VPCs and VT, especially at a rapid rate, can lead to hypotension and electrical instability. Antiarrhythmic drug therapy as outlined later in this section generally is instituted in animals with frequent VPCs (example >10-20% of total beats), and especially those with short coupling intervals, closely timed couplets, repetitive VPCs, or an underlying disease associated with sudden death.

A search for underlying cardiac structural disease and systemic disorders is indicated in animals with more that occasional monomorphic VPCs. Therapy for the patient's cardiac and non-cardiac abnormalities should be provided, as appropriate. Animals with frequent VPCs also should be rested for several weeks to months, and periodically reevaluated. It might be possible to wean down then discontinue antiarrhythmic therapy if the underlying cause has resolved.

Accelerated Idioventricular Rhythm

Accelerated idioventricular rhythm (**Figure 5.36**, p. 149, and **Figure 32.25**, p. 643) and ventricular parasystole (p. 149) tend to be well-tolerated, benign rhythms. Similar to an accelerated junctional rhythm, accelerated idioventricular rhythms occur at rates slightly above the patient's normal sinus rate. They become overdrive suppressed when the sinus rate increases above that of the abnormal rhythm. Fusion complexes are common. Specific antiarrhythmic therapy usually is unnecessary, unless the ventricular rate increases markedly or the animal shows hemodynamic compromise, as might occur under general anesthesia. In such cases, lidocaine generally is used first. If this rhythm develops during anesthesia, reduction in anesthetic dosage (and that of any catecholamine being infused) might resolve it. When an underlying abnormality or disease is identified, therapy is directed at that condition. This includes electrolyte (especially K^+ and Mg^{++}) or acid-base imbalances and fluid losses. An accelerated idioventricular rhythm that occurs subsequent to thoracic trauma, such as being hit by a car (p. 641), typically resolves spontaneously with time. Horses that are apparently healthy otherwise and in which the accelerated idioventricular rhythm becomes suppressed as the sinus rate increases during exercise, probably can be used or ridden cautiously by an adult. However, because of uncertainty over possible underlying myocardial disease and risk of collapse during exercise, such horses should not be used as a lesson horse or ridden by children.

Ventricular Tachycardia

Nonsustained (Paroxysmal) Ventricular Tachycardia
Rapid and frequent paroxysms (bursts) of VT are treated more aggressively than isolated VPC's or accelerated idioventricular rhythms; strategies used are as described for sustained VT (see "Therapy of Ventricular Arrhythmias"). The approach to managing brief and intermittent paroxysms of VT, whether identified in the hospital or by ambulatory ECG, depends on the clinical situation. Heart failure patients that develop frequent or repetitive VPCs, might need additional antiarrhythmic drug therapy. Similarly, patients receiving digoxin for supraventricular tachyarrhythmias, might need other antiarrhythmic therapy in addition to digoxin withdrawal. Digoxin is not used to treat ventricular tachyarrhythmias specifically; it can predispose to ventricular, as well as other, arrhythmias (p. 328).

Sustained Ventricular Tachycardia VT is considered "sustained" if it lasts for >15–30 seconds. The QRS morphology in lead II usually suggests the origination site of the tachycardia (positive, suggesting a right ventricular origin; negative, left ventricular), although these are not absolute guidelines. VT can be monomorphic or polymorphic, including TdP. The rate and morphology of the tachycardia, as well as patient comorbidities, determine the hemodynamic consequences and urgency of treatment. Sustained VT, as for frequent or rapid paroxysmal VT, is treated aggressively because it can cause severe hypotension, with resulting clinical signs, or further destabilization of an anesthetized or critical care patient. It is important to pay close attention to the cardiac rhythm, ideally by continuous ECG monitoring in the hospital. The patient's BP, serum electrolytes, oxygenation, pain level, circulating blood volume, and acid/base status should be assessed and corrected as appropriate. Likewise, underlying systemic and cardiac disease should be identified and managed, as possible. The following section describes antiarrhythmic strategies.

Therapy for Ventricular Arrhythmias

When the ventricular rhythm disturbance is caused by primary cardiac disease there is reasonable expectation for lifelong therapy, or at minimum, monitoring. If the ventricular ectopy is secondary to other systemic disease, treatment might only be needed in the short-term. As for other arrhythmias, a thorough patient work-up is indicated to identify underlying abnormalities and complicating factors. The arrhythmia's hemodynamic consequences can be assessed by clinical signs, physical examination, BP and estimates of tissue perfusion, such as blood lactate. The frequency, rate, timing and complexity of the ventricular rhythm helps clarify the urgency of treatment, and whether an in-hospital or outpatient approach should be used.

In-hospital Therapy for Ventricular Arrhythmias For dogs, cats, and horses with sustained VT, IV lidocaine usually is the first-choice antiarrhythmic agent. Dosages vary across species (**Table 25.2**). Lidocaine can suppress arrhythmias from multiple underlying mechanisms and it has minimal adverse hemodynamic effects. Lidocaine's effect following IV boluses lasts about 10–15 minutes, so a CRI is warranted if the drug is effective. Small supplemental IV boluses can be administered with the CRI to maintain therapeutic concentrations until steady state is achieved. If necessary, IV infusion can be continued for several days. Ancillary KCl supplementation (if serum K^+ is <4 mmol/L; <4 mEq/L) in small animals with or without $MgSO_4$ may increase antiarrhythmic efficacy.

If lidocaine has not adequately suppressed the VT after maximal recommended doses, several other strategies can be tried (**Figures 25.16** to **25.18** and **Table 25.4**; also see Chapter 24). Generally, each antiarrhythmic drug is added or substituted in turn and its efficacy assessed; if deemed inadequate, the dose is increased (within accepted limits) or another antiarrhythmic drug chosen. Magnesium salts (sulfate or chloride) often are administered as a second line treatment for hospital therapy of VT due to their nonspecific effects on membrane stability and on afterdepolarizations, including TdP. Oral sotalol can be added to a concurrent lidocaine CRI; if the arrhythmia responds, the lidocaine dose can be tapered over some hours then discontinued. This approach is relevant to dogs, cats and horses. These therapies sometimes slow the rate of the VT before conversion occurs, especially with sustained VT. For refractory VT, IV loading doses of amiodarone are recommended for dogs (using Nexterone®) and for horses (using preservative-free or standard formulation). The original (standard) formulation of IV amiodarone is not recommended for dogs because it can induce marked hypotension and hypersensitivity reactions, mainly related to the solvents it contains (p. 383). More experience is needed regarding amiodarone use in cats. If lidocaine, magnesium, sotalol, and amiodarone fail, there are other, although less desirable, options. Any of these treatments could be successful, but unfortunately is a clinical trial and error exercise for each patient (see **Figures 25.16** to **25.18** and paragraphs that follow).

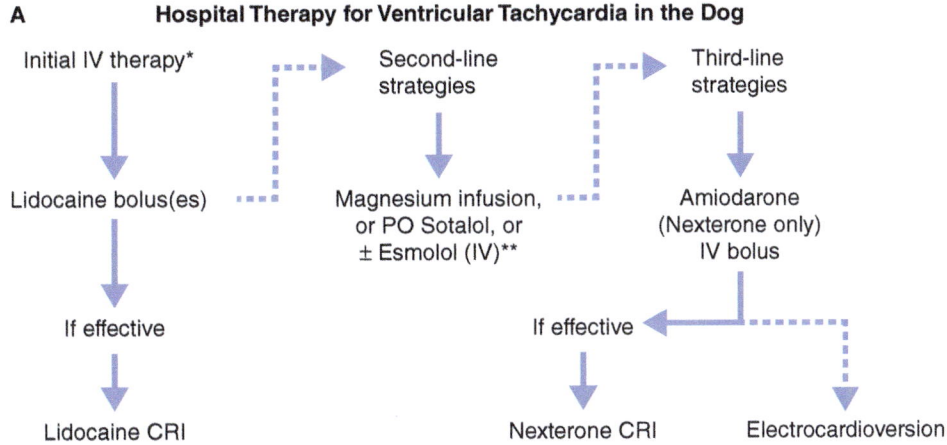

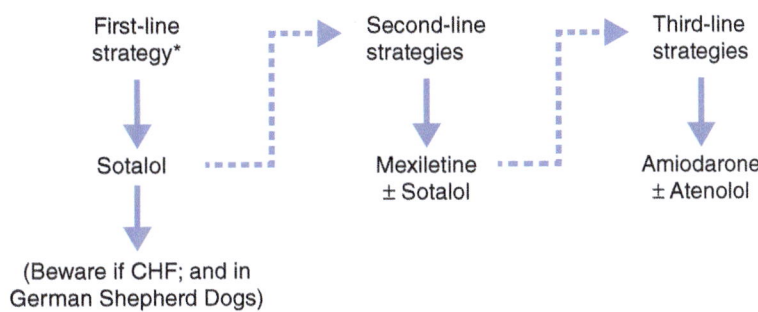

Figure 25.16 (A) Approach to in-hospital management for ventricular tachycardia in the dog. (B) Strategies for longer-term oral therapy in dogs with persistent ventricular tachyarrhythmias. These are general guidelines and exceptions can occur. See text for further information and **Table 25.2** for drug doses. *If initial strategy is not effective, try a next-level therapy. **Amiodarone (preservative free), also is a reasonable second-line IV drug for dogs; beta-blockers should not be given IV in the setting of uncontrolled CHF. CRI, constant rate infusion; IV, intravenous; PO, oral.

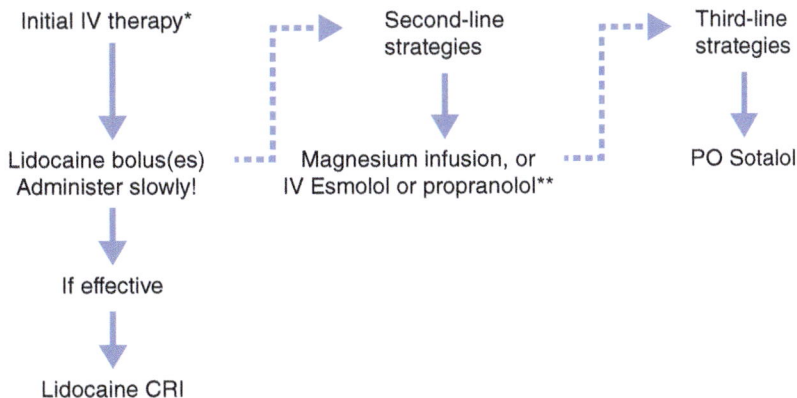

Figure 25.17 Approach to in-hospital management for ventricular tachycardia in the cat. These are general guidelines and exceptions can occur. See text for further information and **Table 25.2** for drug doses. *If initial strategy is not effective, try a next-level therapy. **Beta-blockers should not be given IV in the setting of uncontrolled CHF. CRI, constant rate infusion; IV, intravenous; PO, oral.

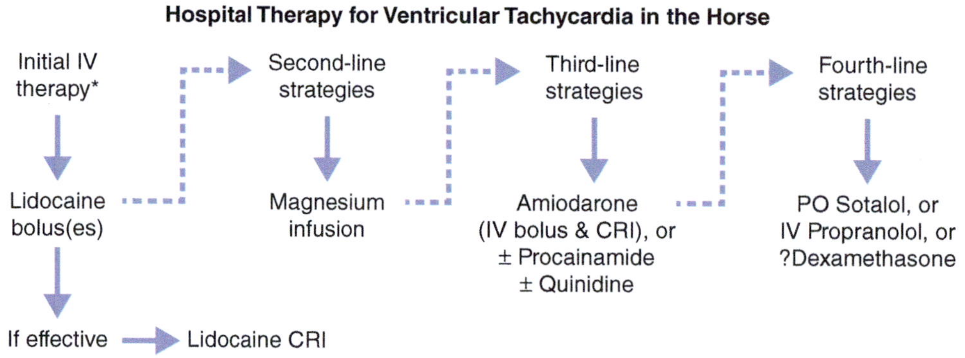

Hospital Therapy for Ventricular Tachycardia in the Horse

```
Initial IV          Second-line          Third-line            Fourth-line
therapy*    ---->   strategies   ---->   strategies    ---->   strategies
   |                    |                    |                     |
   v                    v                    v                     v
Lidocaine   ----->  Magnesium    ----->  Amiodarone    ----->  PO Sotalol, or
bolus(es)           infusion             (IV bolus & CRI), or  IV Propranolol, or
   |                                     ± Procainamide        ?Dexamethasone
   v                                     ± Quinidine
If effective  ---->  Lidocaine CRI
```

Figure 25.18 Approach to in-hospital management for ventricular tachycardia in the horse. These are general guidelines; exceptions can occur. See text for further information and **Table 25.2** for drug doses. *If initial strategy is not effective, try a next-level therapy. CRI, constant rate infusion; IV, intravenous; PO, oral.

Ventricular tachyarrhythmias related to digoxin toxicity often respond to IV lidocaine. In dogs or horses (only), if these arrhythmias are refractory to lidocaine, phenytoin can be tried slowly IV (to avoid hypotension). Phenytoin has been used PO to treat or prevent digoxin-induced ventricular arrhythmias. If the serum potassium concentration is <4 mmol/l (<4 mEq/l), IV potassium supplementation also is indicated for digitalis toxicity. Magnesium supplementation can help suppress these arrhythmias as well. MgSO$_4$ has been used in dogs at 25–40 mg/kg slow IV bolus, followed by infusion of the same dose over 12–24 hours.

A patient with refractory VT must be carefully assessed; a cardiologist should be consulted when feasible. Sometimes prior antiarrhythmic therapy will sufficiently slow a monomorphic VT or suppress a recurrent paroxysmal VT to the point where no additional therapy is given, aside from supportive treatment and "watchful waiting." When treatment still is needed, procainamide (IV and followed by a CRI, if effective) can be effective useful three species; however, the drug is not widely available and could be cost prohibitive. The IV use of a beta-blocker can be considered, especially esmolol for cats and dogs or propranolol for horses. Quinidine (PO) is a consideration for horses. Electrocardioversion can be effective for refractory VT in the dog (**Figure 25.19** and p. 392), and perhaps overdrive pacing with a transvenous catheter should be tried in selected cases of nonresponsive VT in horses. Precordial thumps (a sharp, firm, focal blow to the thorax) could be considered as a last resort in patients that are unconscious (coding) or receiving sufficient analgesia. A precordial thump might interrupt VT or a reentrant circuit causing antidromic ARVT; but these also can induce VF.

Chronic Therapy for Ventricular Arrhythmias Once in-hospital IV or oral antiarrhythmic therapy is effective, a decision must be made regarding longer-term treatment. Likewise, such decisions are needed during outpatient reevaluations for patients with recurrent VPC's or VT. It is helpful to consider 4 major goals (whether attainable or not). These are to: (1) prevent sudden cardiac death; (2) prevent or reduce hypotension and its clinical signs; (3) prevent TICM; and (4) preserve cardiac function in patients with structural heart disease. Some guidance for decisions about ongoing therapy are contained in prior sections, as well as chapters on specific cardiac diseases. In addition, the possible increases in survival time and quality of life must be balanced against the cost, inconvenience, and potential adverse effects of antiarrhythmic drugs. Unfortunately, there are no prospective and sufficiently controlled studies that document prolonged survival with antiarrhythmic drugs. But clinical experience indicates that ventricular ectopy often can be suppressed and that clinical signs, such as syncope, can be reduced in some patients.

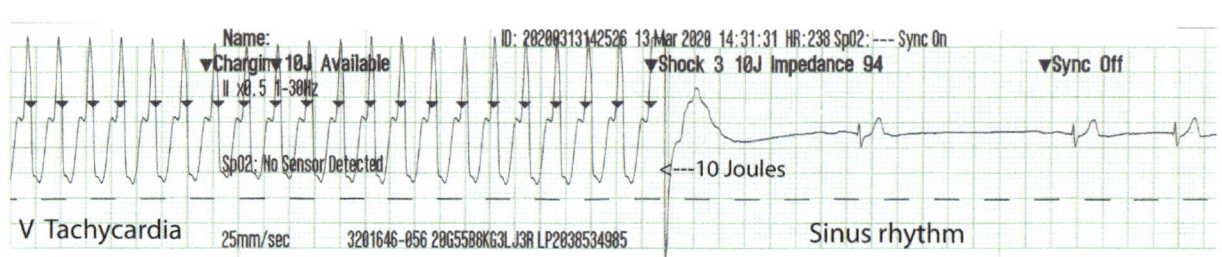

Figure 25.19 Successful electrocardioversion in a Boxer dog with sustained monomorphic ventricular tachycardia (VT) that was nonresponsive to lidocaine, magnesium chloride, esmolol, sotalol, and Nexterone®. The dog maintained sinus rhythm, which suggests that this was a reentrant VT. The dog was discharged on a combination of oral amiodarone and atenolol.

When the decision is made to pursue short- or long-term outpatient antiarrhythmic therapy, one or sometimes two oral drugs will be needed (**Table 25.2**; also see Chapter 24). *Sotalol* frequently is chosen for initial PO monotherapy, unless it was previously tested and ineffective in the hospital. *Sotalol* can be administered to dogs, cats, and horses. Another common antiarrhythmic choice for dogs is the class Ib agent *mexiletine*, either given *alone or with sotalol* (or another beta-blocker). Response to lidocaine in the hospital theoretically should translate to potential benefit with mexiletine. For animals with poor myocardial contractility, caution is advised when instituting sotalol (or another beta-blocker) because of the drug's negative inotropic effect. Occasionally, *atenolol* is used as monotherapy, mainly to suppress isolated VPCs in dogs and cats thought related to increased sympathetic tone. If these treatments are not adequately effective for cats or for horses, there are few good alternative options and a specialist should be consulted. Oral *amiodarone* is a reasonable 2nd or 3rd choice option for dogs; but it usually is not the agent of first choice for long term therapy because of its potential for adverse effects over time. Amiodarone also requires a long time to reach steady state, such that initial (PO or IV) loading doses often are needed. The class III agents appear to have greater antifibrillatory effects than the class I drugs. It is emphasized that sotalol and amiodarone are quite different drugs, even if lumped together as class III antiarrhythmics, and they are not interchangeable.

A beta-blocker can help prevent ventricular, as well as supraventricular, tachyarrhythmias that are provoked by sympathetic stimulation or catecholamines. Beta-blockers have protected people (and experimental dogs) with myocardial ischemia or infarction against VF. However, standard beta-blockers (such as atenolol) alone have not been adequately effective in suppressing ventricular tachyarrhythmias in Doberman Pinschers with DCM. A beta-blocker can be used in combination with a class I agent such as mexiletine; however, in animals with myocardial failure the negative effect on ventricular contractility can be clinically important.

Upstream treatments for arrhythmias are therapies that act directly on the substrate (myocardium) and less so on the responsible electrophysiologic mechanisms. For animals with structural heart disease or CHF, an ACE inhibitor, mineralocorticoid receptor blocker (spironolactone), and fish oil (omega-3 fatty acids) supplementation might also reduce arrhythmia severity. Fish oil supplement appears to reduce the frequency of ventricular tachyarrhythmias in Boxers with ARVC. Perhaps this might be helpful in other animals with VT, as well. Glucocorticoid therapy (dexamethasone) often is given to horses with ventricular arrhythmias in hope of treating myocarditis or systemic inflammation. There are anecdotal reports of response to this therapy, but scientific evidence currently is lacking and this is not recommended as a routine treatment.

Three canine breeds - Boxers and English Bulldogs with ARVC (p. 624; also **Figures 32.17** and **32.18**) and Doberman Pinchers with DCM constitute a substantial number of cases that veterinarians manage for ventricular ectopy. Other breeds, including younger German Shepherds and Rhodesian Ridgebacks also develop inherited forms of ectopy. There is considerable empirical experience for treating some of these breeds. In Boxers and English Bulldogs with ARVC, sotalol alone or mexiletine combined with sotalol or atenolol can significantly decrease the number of VPCs, as well as arrhythmia complexity. Doberman Pinschers with DCM and VT often respond to sotalol. However, myocardial function in some dogs with DCM has worsened with sotalol. Mexiletine or amiodarone could be effective alternative antiarrhythmic agents, although amiodarone's prolonged half-life and its array of potential adverse effects are concerns (p. 383). On the positive side, amiodarone might have less proarrhythmic effect and confer greater antifibrillatory protection compared to other agents. For German Shepherd Dogs with familial ventricular tachyarrhythmias, sotalol is not recommended as the sole antiarrhythmic agent. Sotalol monotherapy can worsen arrhythmia frequency and severity in these dogs (Gelzer, 2010), perhaps because the afterdepolarizations responsible appear to be worse with slower heart rates. Instead, for affected German Shepherds, mexiletine combined with sotalol is recommended. There is insufficient information yet about optimal treatment of Rhodesian Ridgebacks, but the standard drugs followed by Holter monitor follow-up to assess benefit and proarrhythmia are logical choices.

Beyond sotalol, mexiletine, amiodarone, and atenolol, other oral antiarrhythmic options are relatively poor, due in part to lack of drug availability or lack of efficacy and safety data. Quinidine and procainamide rarely are used today in dogs. Nevertheless, the combination of mexiletine with quinidine might be effective against arrhythmias refractory to each agent alone. Group Ic drugs, such as flecainide and propafenone have been prescribed inconsistently and are potentially dangerous in the setting of structural heart disease. Although catheter ablation or implantable cardioverter defibrillators have been used to treat some dogs with VT, these are not widely available; furthermore, defibrillator algorithms are inadequate for animals and cause too many inappropriate shocks.

Animals on long-term antiarrhythmic therapy should be reevaluated frequently. Besides assessing treatment efficacy, it is important to screen for adverse drug effects and disease progression. Although not always possible to obtain, pre- and posttreatment 24- to 48-hour ambulatory ECG recordings provide the best objective indicator of antiarrhythmic drug efficacy, as well as reduction in clinical signs, if any. Based mainly on human studies, an effective antiarrhythmic drug should produce at least a 70–80% reduction in arrhythmia frequency. Ideally, the complexity of the arrhythmia also will decrease. Total suppression of ectopy is unrealistic in many, if not most, cases. Intermittent ECG recordings cannot truly differentiate between drug effect, or lack thereof, and the marked spontaneous variability that can occur in arrhythmia frequency. Nevertheless, in-hospital ECG recordings often are used in an attempt to monitor arrhythmias and drug effects. Less ideally, clients could be instructed to obtain multiple ECG recordings using a smartphone app; this might yield a rough estimate of arrhythmic event frequency (either single or paroxysms) and like outpatient ECGs, could reveal if the drug is not having sufficient effect. Subsequently, the decision to continue or discontinue successful oral antiarrhythmic therapy is based on the individual's clinical situation. Considerations should include underlying cardiac status, any concurrent systemic abnormalities, current antiarrhythmic drug (or combination) efficacy, drug dosage(s), and any adverse effects that have developed.

Horses without marked structural cardiac disease might be able to return to work if episodes of VT resolve after a period of antiarrhythmic (and any other indicated) therapy and a couple months of rest. Horses that continue in sinus rhythm after the antiarrhythmic drug is discontinued, should be further assessed with 24-hour Holter monitoring, exercise ECG testing, and echocardiography before the decision is made whether to return them to work. Another exercise ECG is advised after full workload has been reached. Annual 24-hour Holter monitoring and exercise ECGs also have been recommended in these horses. It is not clear whether horses with complex ventricular arrhythmias or clinical signs from VT can safely return to work in the future. Recurrent VT is probably more likely to occur in animals with structural heart disease, evidence for myocardial fibrosis, or moderate to severe aortic regurgitation. Therefore, strenuous work is not recommended for these horses; also, they should not be used by children or as lesson horses.

Torsades de Pointes TdP is a form of polymorphic VT associated with underlying QT prolongation (p. 149), either acquired or, rarely, from an inherited channelopathy. TdP typically is preceded by a period of slow HR with prolonged QT intervals (for example, >0.25 seconds in dogs); its onset is triggered by a VPC during the ventricular repolarization period (long-short cycle sequence). TdP is characterized by a rapid VT of continuously changing amplitude and polarity (as if its axis is "rotating around a point"; **Figure 23.3**, p. 366). It usually occurs as a brief paroxysm; however, it can degenerate into VF. Anything that causes QT interval prolongation (with increased dispersion of refractoriness) can predispose to TdP, including hypokalemia, hypocalcemia, antiarrhythmic drug toxicity (especially some class Ia, Ic and III agents), other drugs, myocardial disease, and other acquired or congenital long QT syndromes. When TdP is suspected, all drugs that can prolong the QT interval should be discontinued and electrolyte imbalances corrected. Slow IV injection of $MgSO_4$ (**Table 25.2**) might suppress the arrhythmia. Isoproterenol or ventricular pacing can also be effective for TdP when baseline HR is slow; however, isoproterenol infusion can provoke VF if the rhythm is not really TdP, so this usually is not advised. Polymorphic VT that is not associated with underlying QT prolongation might respond to amiodarone.

Ventricular Flutter and Fibrillation

VF (p. 150 and **Figure 5.38**) usually is preceded by VT, TdP, or ventricular flutter (**Figure 5.39**, p. 150). Severe myocardial disease, including myocardial anoxia or ischemia, trauma, severe electrolyte imbalance, or shock often exists in these patients. Effective ventricular contractions cease during VF and circulatory collapse quickly ensues. Immediate cardiopulmonary resuscitation (CPR, **Table 25.5**), followed by high-energy, unsynchronized electrical defibrillation (p. 393) are indicated. Other treatments (such as a precordial thump, KCl and $CaCl_2$, or class III agents) rarely are effective without defibrillation.

Lethal Arrhythmias and Cardiopulmonary Arrest

Several arrhythmias produce no effective ventricular contractions and so are incompatible with life. These include VF (above), pulseless VT (a rapid VT at >200 complexes/minute lacking effective ventricular ejection), other PEA, and ventricular asystole. Immediate CPR is indicated when cardiopulmonary arrest is detected.

The approach to an unresponsive patient should begin with a rapid assessment for airway patency and spontaneous breathing ("A" & "B"). Verification of apnea and (ideally) tracheal intubation should be completed within 10 seconds of discovering an unresponsive patient. Taking time to check for circulation ("C") currently is not recommended, especially if it delays CPR beyond the initial 10 seconds for AB assessment. If there is any doubt about the presence of cardiopulmonary arrest, CPR should be started immediately rather than doing further assessment. The two main components of CPR are basic life support (BLS; chest compressions, positive pressure ventilation) and advanced life support (ALS; drug and fluid therapy, defibrillation). These entail 5 main steps, which should be accomplished in the order presented (**Table 25.5**). Ideally, the 5-step cycle is completed within the first 2 minutes of CPR. Repeated 2-minute BLS cycles are interspersed with brief periods to check for return of spontaneous circulation, evaluate the patient's ECG rhythm, and administer drug or defibrillation therapy, as appropriate. An in-depth discussion of these issues is outside the scope of this text. More detailed guidelines for CPR are described in the papers from the Reassessment Campaign on Veterinary Resuscitation (RECOVER) and other recent references (see "Cardiopulmonary Resuscitation" subheading of section "Suggested Additional Reading and References").

Table 25.5 Cardiopulmonary Resuscitation Outline

Initial Assessment (5–10 sec)

- Airway (A): Examine oral cavity, clear obstructions, verify airway patency, use laryngoscope if possible
- Breathing (B): Check for spontaneous breathing (chest excursions, lung sounds, hold glass slide up to nares, etc.)

Basic Life Support (2-Min Cycles)

- 1. Chest compressions[a]:
  - Position most animals on firm surface in lateral recumbency, so that rescuer's hands can be positioned directly below his/her shoulders:
    - Narrow-chested dogs (chest width < depth): compress directly over the heart with both hands (one over the other, fingers interlaced, elbows locked)
    - Round-chested dogs (chest width ≈ depth): compress over widest portion of chest with both hands (one over the other, fingers interlaced, elbows locked)
    - Cats and small dogs or puppies: compress directly over the heart using one hand wrapped around sternum (thumb on one side of the chest, fingers on the other; support patient's back with other hand)
    - Position barrel-chested dogs (chest width > depth) in dorsal recumbency: compress over sternum with both hands (one over the other, fingers interlaced, elbows locked)
  - Compress chest: by one-third to one-half its width at a rate of 100-120 compressions/min for all dogs & cats
    - Allow chest to fully recoil between each compression
    - Continue uninterrupted for a full 2 min
  - Recommend changing to another rescuer for each 2-min cycle to reduce fatigue
- 2. Ventilation:
  - Place, verify, inflate cuff, and secure endotracheal tube as soon as possible (ideally, do not interrupt chest compressions)
  - Give one breath every 6 seconds (10 breaths/min), with an inspiratory duration of 1 second, simultaneously with chest compressions
  - If endotracheal tube not available, can try mouth-to-snout or mask-to snout ventilation; after every 30 chest compressions, pause briefly to apply two quick breaths (30:2 ratio)

Advanced Life Support

- 3. Initiate monitoring:
  - Attach ECG, assess rhythm for brief (3–5 sec) period between each 2-min BLS cycle (see Chapter 5).
  - If available, attach end-tidal CO_2 monitor (>15 mm Hg suggests adequate chest compressions; sudden rapid rise can accompany return of spontaneous circulation)
- 4. Obtain vascular access:
  - Place IV catheter and verify patency as soon as possible; use venous cut-down technique if necessary (cephalic or jugular). Alternatively, place interosseous catheter.
- 5. Administer reversal agents, if patient has been given an:
  - Opioid: give naloxone (0.04 mg/kg IV or IO)
  - Benzodiazepine: give flumazenil (0.01 mg/kg IV or IO)
  - $Alpha_2$ agonist: give atipamezole (0.1 mg/kg IV or IO) or yohimbine (0.1 mg/kg IV or IO)

Continue the 2-min BLS cycles interspersed with

- Cardiac rhythm assessment, and
- Drug (or defibrillation shock) administration, as appropriate, based on ECG rhythm and other findings.

ECG Rhythm Assessment

- If relatively consistent QRS complexes (of any configuration) are seen:
  - Check for signs of cardiac contraction (apical beat, arterial pulse) & estimate QRS complex rate/min:
    - If no evidence for circulation with <200 complexes/min: PEA is likely → non-shockable rhythm; try vasopressor (below), ± anticholinergic agent (see **Table 25.2**).
    - Vasopressor therapy options include:
      - Vasopressin at 0.8 U/kg IV, IO, or via endotracheal tube q4min, or
      - Epinephrine (1:1000; 1 mg/ml dilution) at 0.01 mg/kg IV, IO, or via endotracheal tube (at 0.02 mg/kg); can repeat q4min for a couple times (see p. 387). Reported doses for horses include 0.01–0.05 mg/kg IV (or 0.1–0.5 mg/kg via endotracheal tube), or
      - Norepinephrine at 0.05–1 mcg/kg/min CRI to effect, or
      - Phenylephrine (see **Table 25.2**)
    - If no evidence for circulation with >200 complexes/min: pulseless VT likely → shockable rhythm; prepare for defibrillation (see p. 393)
- If no consistent QRS complexes are seen:
  - Ventricular fibrillation evident → shockable rhythm; prepare for defibrillation (p. 393)
  - Essentially flat baseline → asystole; non-shockable rhythm; try vasopressor, ± anticholinergic therapy (see earlier).

Note: See Fletcher, et al. (2012; RECOVER, part 7: Clinical guidelines) and section "Suggested Additional Reading and References" for more details.

[a] External chest compression usually is ineffective with pericardial effusion/tamponade, pleural space disease, rib fractures, other thoracic wall defects, or in very large (or round-chested) animals, including giant breed dogs and adult horses.

Abbreviations: BLS, basic life support; ECG, electrocardiogram; IO, interosseous; PEA, pulseless electrical activity; VT, ventricular tachycardia.

Suggested Additional Reading and References

Also See Online Comprehensive Bibliography at: https://www.routledge.com/9781482246223.

Bellei MH, Kerr C, McGurrin MK, et al. Management and complications of anesthesia for transvenous electrical cardioversion of atrial fibrillation in horses: 62 cases (2002–2006). J Am Vet Med Assoc 2007;231:1225–1230.

Bright JM, Martin JM, Mama K. A retrospective evaluation of transthoracic biphasic electrical cardioversion for atrial fibrillation in dogs. J Vet Cardiol 2005;7:85–96.

Bright JM, Zumbrunnen J. Chronicity of atrial fibrillation affects duration of sinus rhythm after transthoracic cardioversion of dogs with naturally occurring atrial fibrillation. J Vet Intern Med 2008;22:114–119.

Broux B, De Clercq D, Decloedt A, et al. Heart rate variability parameters in horses distinguish atrial fibrillation from sinus rhythm before and after successful electrical cardioversion. Equine Vet J 2017;49:723–728.

Buhl R, Carstensen H, Hesselkilde EZ, et al. Effect of induced chronic atrial fibrillation on exercise performance in Standardbred trotters. J Vet Intern Med 2018;32:1410–1419.

Carstensen H, Hesselkilde EZ, Haugaard MM, et al. Effects of dofetilide and ranolazine on atrial fibrillatory rate in a horse model of acutely induced atrial fibrillation. J Cardiovasc Electrophysiol 2019;30:596–606.

Cervenec RM, Stauthammer CD, Fine DM, et al. Survival time with pacemaker implantation for dogs diagnosed with persistent atrial standstill. J Vet Cardiol 2017;19:240–246.

Cote E. Feline arrhythmias: an update. Vet Clin North Am Small Anim Pract 2010;40:643–650.

De Clercq D, Decloedt A, Sys SU, et al. Atrial fibrillation cycle length and atrial size in horses with and without recurrence of atrial fibrillation after electrical cardioversion. J Vet Intern Med 2014;28:624–629.

De Clercq D, van Loon G, Baert K, et al. Treatment with amiodarone of refractory ventricular tachycardia in a horse. J Vet Intern Med 2007;21:878–880.

De Clercq D, van Loon G, Baert K, et al. Effects of an adapted intravenous amiodarone treatment protocol in horses with atrial fibrillation. Equine Vet J 2007;39:344–349.

De Clercq D, van Loon G, Schauvliege S, et al. Transvenous electrical cardioversion of atrial fibrillation in six horses using custom made cardioversion catheters. Vet J 2008;177:198–204.

De Clercq D, van Loon G, Tavernier R, et al. Use of propafenone for conversion of chronic atrial fibrillation in horses. Am J Vet Res 2009;70:223–227

Decloedt A, Schwarzwald CC, De Clercq D, et al. Risk factors for recurrence of atrial fibrillation in horses after cardioversion to sinus rhythm. J Vet Intern Med 2015;29:946–953.

Decloedt A, Van Steenkiste G, Vera L, et al. Atrial fibrillation in horses part 1: Pathophysiology. Vet J 2020;263:105521.

Decloedt A, Verheyen T, Van Der Vekens N, et al. Long-term follow-up of atrial function after cardioversion of atrial fibrillation in horses. Vet J 2013;197:583–588.

Dicken M, Gordon SJ, Mayhew IG. The use of phenytoin in two horses following conversion from atrial fibrillation. N Z Vet J 2012;60:210–212.

Durando MM. Cardiovascular causes of poor performance and exercise intolerance and assessment of safety in the equine athlete. Vet Clin North Am Equine Pract 2019;35:175–190.

Estrada AH, Pariaut R, Moise NS. Avoiding medical error during electrical cardioversion of atrial fibrillation: prevention of unsynchronized shock delivery. J Vet Cardiol 2009;11:137–139.

Finster ST, DeFrancesco TC, Atkins CE, et al. Supraventricular tachycardia in dogs: 65 cases (1990–2007). J Vet Emerg Crit Care 2008;18:503–510.

Flethoj M, Kanters JK, Haugaard MM, et al. Changes in heart rate, arrhythmia frequency, and cardiac biomarker values in horses during recovery after a long-distance endurance ride. J Am Vet Med Assoc 2016;248:1034–1042.

Frye MA, Selders CG, Mama KR, et al. Use of biphasic electrical cardioversion for treatment of idiopathic atrial fibrillation in two horses. J Am Vet Med Assoc 2002;220:1039–1045, 1007.

Gelzer AR, Kraus MS, Rishniw M. Evaluation of in-hospital electrocardiography versus 24-hour holter for rate control in dogs with atrial fibrillation. J Small Anim Pract 2015;56:456–462.

Gelzer AR, Kraus MS, Rishniw M, et al. Combination therapy with mexiletine and sotalol suppresses inherited ventricular arrhythmias in German shepherd dogs better than mexiletine or sotalol monotherapy: a randomized cross-over study. J Vet Cardiol 2010;12:93–106.

Gelzer AR, Kraus MS, Rishniw M, et al. Combination therapy with digoxin and diltiazem controls ventricular rate in chronic atrial fibrillation in dogs better than digoxin or diltiazem monotherapy: a randomized crossover study in 18 dogs. J Vet Intern Med 2009;23:499–508.

Greet V, Sargent J, Brannick M, et al. Supraventricular tachycardia in 23 cats; comparison with 21 cats with atrial fibrillation (2004-2014). J Vet Cardiol 2020;30:7–16.

Guglielmini C, Chetboul V, Pietra M, et al. Influence of left atrial enlargement and body weight on the development of atrial fibrillation: retrospective study on 205 dogs. Vet J 2000;160:235–241.

Guglielmini C, Goncalves Sousa M, Baron Toaldo M, et al. Prevalence and risk factors for atrial fibrillation in dogs with myxomatous mitral valve disease. J Vet Intern Med 2020;34:2223–2231.

Hanka J, van den Hoven R, Schwarz B. Paroxysmal atrial fibrillation and clinically reversible cor pulmonale in a horse with complicated recurrent airway obstruction. Tierarztliche Praxis Ausgabe G, Grosstiere/Nutztiere 2015;43:109–114.

Haugaard MM, Pehrson S, Carstensen H, et al. Antiarrhythmic and electrophysiologic effects of flecainide on acutely induced atrial fibrillation in healthy horses. J Vet Intern Med 2015;29:339–347.

Jesty SA, Kraus MS, Gelzer AR, et al. Effect of transvenous electrical cardioversion on plasma cardiac troponin I concentrations in horses with atrial fibrillation. J Vet Intern Med 2009;23:1103–1107.

Johnson MS, Martin M, Smith P. Cardioversion of supraventricular tachycardia using lidocaine in five dogs. J Vet Intern Med 2006;20:272–276.

Johnson MS, Martin MW, Henley W. Results of pacemaker implantation in 104 dogs. J Small Anim Pract 2007;48:4–11.

Kellum HB, Stepien RL. Third-degree atrioventricular block in 21 cats (1997–2004). J Vet Intern Med 2006;20:97–103.

Kraus MS, Gelzer AR, Rishniw M. Detection of heart rate and rhythm with a smartphone-based electrocardiograph versus a reference standard electrocardiograph in dogs and cats. J Am Vet Med Assoc 2016;249:189–194.

Kraus M, Physick-Sheard P, Brito LF, et al. Marginal ancestral contributions to atrial fibrillation in the Standardbred racehorse: comparison of cases and controls. PLoS One 2018;13:e0197137.

Leroux AA, Detilleux J, Sandersen CF, et al. Prevalence and risk factors for cardiac diseases in a hospital-based population of 3,434 horses (1994–2011). J Vet Intern Med 2013;27:1563–1570.

Marly-Voquer C, Schwarzwald CC, Bettschart-Wolfensberger R. The use of dexmedetomidine continuous rate infusion for horses undergoing transvenous electrical cardioversion–A case series. Can Vet J 2016;57:70–75.

McAulay G, Borgeat K, Sargent J, et al. Phenotypic description of cardiac findings in a population of dogue de Bordeaux with an emphasis on atrial fibrillation. Vet J 2018;234:111–118.

McGurrin MK, Physick-Sheard PW, Kenney DG. Transvenous electrical cardioversion of equine atrial fibrillation: patient factors and clinical results in 72 treatment episodes. J Vet Intern Med 2008;22:609–615.

McGurrin MKJ. The diagnosis and management of atrial fibrillation in the horse. Vet Med 2015;6:83–90.

Meurs KM, Weidman JA, Rosenthal SL, et al. Ventricular arrhythmias in Rhodesian Ridgebacks with a family history of sudden death and results of a pedigree analysis for potential inheritance patterns. J Am Vet Med Assoc 2016;248:1135–1138.

Navas de Solis C, Reef VB, Slack J, et al. Evaluation of coagulation and fibrinolysis in horses with atrial fibrillation. J Am Vet Med Assoc 2016;248:201–206.

Noszczyk-Nowak A, Michalek M, Kaluza E, et al. Prevalence of arrhythmias in dogs examined between 2008 and 2014. J Vet Res 2017;61:103–110.

Pariaut R. Atrial fibrillation: current therapies. Vet Clin North Am Small Anim Pract 2017;47:977–988.

Pedro B, Dukes-McEwan J, Oyama MA, et al. Retrospective evaluation of the effect of heart rate on survival in dogs with atrial fibrillation. J Vet Intern Med 2018;32:86–92.

Penning VA, Connolly DJ, Gajanayake I, et al. Seizure-like episodes in 3 cats with intermittent high-grade atrioventricular dysfunction. J Vet Intern Med 2009;23:200–205.

Perego M, Ramera L, Santilli RA. Isorhythmic atrioventricular dissociation in Labrador Retrievers. J Vet Intern Med 2012;26:320–325.

Physick-Sheard PW. Seek and ye shall find: cardiac arrhythmias in the horse. Equine Vet J 2013;45:270–272.

Physick-Sheard P, Kraus M, Basrur P, et al. Breed predisposition and heritability of atrial fibrillation in the Standardbred horse: a retrospective case-control study. J Vet Cardiol 2014;16:173–184.

Preiss EE, Kenney DG, McGurrin MK, et al. Influence of electrode position on cardioversion energy requirements during transvenous electrical cardioversion in horses. Am J Vet Res 2011;72:1193–1203.

Reef VB, Bonagura J, Buhl R, et al. Recommendations for management of equine athletes with cardiovascular abnormalities. J Vet Intern Med 2014;28:749–761.

Risberg AI, McGuirk SM. Successful conversion of equine atrial fibrillation using oral flecainide. J Vet Intern Med 2006;20:207–209.

Robinson SJ, Feary DJ. Sudden death following oral administration of flecainide to horses with naturally occuring atrial fibrillation. Aust Equine Vet 2008;27:49–51.

Ryan N, Marr CM, McGladdery AJ. Survey of cardiac arrhythmias during submaximal and maximal exercise in Thoroughbred racehorses. Equine Vet J 2005;37:265–268.

Santilli RA, Giacomazzi F, Porteiro Vazquez DM, et al. Indications for permanent pacing in dogs and cats. J Vet Cardiol 2019;22:20–39.

Santilli RA, Perego M, Crosara S, et al. Utility of 12-lead electrocardiogram for differentiating paroxysmal supraventricular tachycardias in dogs. J Vet Intern Med 2008;22:915–923.

Santilli RA, Porteiro Vazquez DM, Vezzosi T, et al. Long-term Intrinsic Rhythm Evaluation in Dogs with Atrioventricular Block. J Vet Intern Med 2016;30:58–62.

Santilli RA, Spadacini G, Moretti P, et al. Radiofrequency catheter ablation of concealed accessory pathways in two dogs with symptomatic atrioventricular reciprocating tachycardia. J Vet Cardiol 2006;8:157–165.

Santilli RA, Spadacini G, Moretti P, et al. Anatomic distribution and electrophysiologic properties of accessory atrioventricular pathways in dogs. J Am Vet Med Assoc 2007;231:393–398.

Saunders AB, Miller MW, Gordon SG, et al. Oral amiodarone therapy in dogs with atrial fibrillation. J Vet Intern Med 2006;20:921–926.

Schauvliege S, van Loon G, De Clercq D, et al. Cardiovascular responses to transvenous electrical cardioversion of atrial fibrillation in anaesthetized horses. Vet Anaesth Analg 2009;36:341–351.

Schwarzwald CC. Disorders of the cardiovascular system. In, Reed SM, Bayly WM, Sellon DC (editors). Equine Internal Medicine. 4th edition. Elsevier, St. Louis, MO. 2018. pp. 387–541.

Schmitt KE, Lefbom BK. Long-term management of atrial myopathy in two dogs with single chamber permanent transvenous pacemakers. J Vet Cardiol 2016;18:187–193.

Slack J, Boston RC, Soma LR, et al. Occurrence of cardiac arrhythmias in Standardbred racehorses. Equine Vet J 2015;47:398–404.

Takahashi Y, Ishikawa Y, Ohmura H. Treatment of recent-onset atrial fibrillation with quinidine and flecainide in Thoroughbred racehorses: 107 cases (1987–2014). J Am Vet Med Assoc 2018;252:1409–1414.

Trachsel DS, Bitschnau C, Waldern N, et al. Observer agreement for detection of cardiac arrhythmias on telemetric ECG recordings obtained at rest, during and after exercise in 10 Warmblood horses. Equine Vet J 2010;42(Suppl 38):208–215.

Usechak PJ, Bright JM, Day TK. Thrombotic complications associated with atrial fibrillation in three dogs. J Vet Cardiol 2012;14:453–458.

van Loon G. Cardiac arrhythmias in horses. Vet Clin North Am Equine Pract 2019;35:85–102.

van Loon G, De Clercq D, Tavernier R, et al. Transient complete atrioventricular block following transvenous electrical cardioversion of atrial fibrillation in a horse. Vet J 2005;170:124–127.

Verheyen T, Decloedt A, van der Vekens N, et al. Ventricular response during lungeing exercise in horses with lone atrial fibrillation. Equine Vet J 2013;45:309–314.

Vezzosi T, Buralli C, Marchesotti F, et al. Diagnostic accuracy of a smartphone electrocardiograph in dogs: comparison with standard 6-lead electrocardiography. Vet J 2016;216:33–37.

Vollmar AC, Fox PR. Long-term outcome of Irish Wolfhound dogs with preclinical cardiomyopathy, atrial fibrillation, or both treated with Pimobendan, benazepril hydrochloride, or methyldigoxin monotherapy. J Vet Intern Med 2016;30:553–559.

Ward JL, DeFrancesco TC, Tou SP, et al. Outcome and survival in canine sick sinus syndrome and sinus node dysfunction: 93 cases (2002–2014). J Vet Cardiol 2016;18:199–212.

Wiedemann N, Hildebrandt N, Wurtinger G, et al. Follow-up of troponin I concentration in dogs with atrioventricular block and dual-chamber pacing in a case-matched study. J Vet Cardiol 2017;19:247–255.

Wright KN, Connor CE, Irvin HM, et al. Atrioventricular accessory pathways in 89 dogs: clinical features and outcome after radiofrequency catheter ablation. J Vet Intern Med 2018;32:1517–1529.

Cardiopulmonary Resuscitation

Boller M, Fletcher DJ. RECOVER evidence and knowledge gap analysis on veterinary CPR. Part 1: evidence analysis and consensus process: collaborative path toward small animal CPR guidelines. J Vet Emerg Crit Care 2012;22:S4–S12.

Boller M, Fletcher DJ, Brainard BM, et al. Utstein-style guidelines on uniform reporting of in-hospital cardiopulmonary resuscitation in dogs and cats. A RECOVER statement. J Vet Emerg Crit Care 2016;26:11–34.

Brainard BM, Boller M, Fletcher DJ, et al. RECOVER evidence and knowledge gap analysis on veterinary CPR. Part 5: monitoring. J Vet Emerg Crit Care 2012;22(Suppl 1):S65–84.

Fletcher DJ, Boller M, Brainard BM, et al. RECOVER evidence and knowledge gap analysis on veterinary CPR. Part 7: clinical guidelines. J Vet Emerg Crit Care 2012;22(Suppl 1): S102–131.

Holmes AC, Clark L. Changes in adherence to cardiopulmonary resuscitation guidelines in a single referral center from January 2009 to June 2013 and assessment of factors contributing to the observed changes. J Vet Emerg Crit Care 2015;25: 801–804.

Hopper K, Epstein SE, Fletcher DJ, et al. RECOVER evidence and knowledge gap analysis on veterinary CPR. Part 3: basic life support. J Vet Emerg Crit Care 2012;22(Suppl 1):S26–43.

Kneba EJ, Humm KR. The use of mental metronomes during simulated cardiopulmonary resuscitation training. J Vet Emerg Crit Care 2020;30:92–96.

Maton BL, Smarick SD. Updates in the American Heart Association guidelines for cardiopulmonary resuscitation and potential applications to veterinary patients. J Vet Emerg Crit Care 2012;22:148–159.

McIntyre RL, Hopper K, Epstein SE. Assessment of cardiopulmonary resuscitation in 121 dogs and 30 cats at a university teaching hospital (2009–2012). J Vet Emerg Crit Care 2014;24: 693–704.

McMichael M, Herring J, Fletcher DJ, et al. RECOVER evidence and knowledge gap analysis on veterinary CPR. Part 2: preparedness and prevention. J Vet Emerg Crit Care 2012;22(Suppl 1):S13–25.

Muir WW, Hubbell JAE. Cardiopulmonary resuscitation. In, Muir WW, Hubbell JAE (editors). Equine Anesthesia—Monitoring and Emergency Therapy. Saunders Elsevier, St. Louis, MO. 2009, pp 418–429.

Rozanski EA, Rush JE, Buckley GJ, et al. RECOVER evidence and knowledge gap analysis on veterinary CPR. Part 4: advanced life support. J Vet Emerg Crit Care 2012;22(Suppl 1): S44–64.

Smarick SD, Haskins SC, Boller M, et al. RECOVER evidence and knowledge gap analysis on veterinary CPR. Part 6: postcardiac arrest care. J Vet Emerg Crit Care 2012;22(Suppl 1):S85–101.

Section V

Cardiovascular Diseases

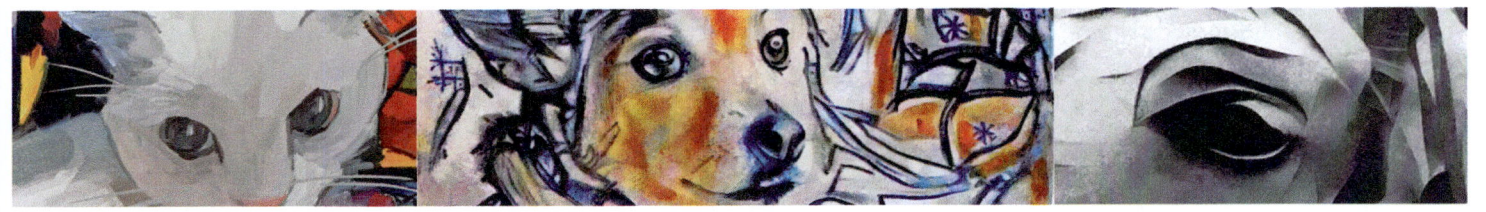

26
CONGENITAL CARDIAC SHUNTS

Congenital Cardiovascular Disease in General

Congenital cardiovascular (CV) malformations comprise a wide spectrum of inherited and developmental abnormalities. The most common malformations affect cardiac valves (or valve regions) or directly connect the left and right sides of the circulation. Multiple anomalies occur in some patients. This chapter describes the most common defects that cause shunting between the systemic and pulmonary circulations. Cardiac malformations that cause valvular insufficiency, stenosis, and ventricular outflow obstructions are discussed in Chapter 27. Other CV defects occur sporadically and have variable effects on the heart, circulation, or other organ systems (see Chapter 28).

To describe congenital heart disease as "shunts" or "valvular malformations" is practical, although somewhat inelegant. Pediatric cardiologists and surgeons often classify cardiac malformations based on the segmental analysis method, described by Van Praagh et al. and subsequently modified (Van Praagh, 1970). This analysis describes the visceroatrial situs (the laterality of the abdominal organs and atria); the direction of the primitive cardiac loop; and the relationship of the aorta and pulmonary artery (PA). These are designated by three letters, S = situs solitus (normal), D = right (dexter), L = left; normal is (S, D, S). Additionally, the arrangements can be concordant or discordant in terms of the atrio-ventricular and ventricular to arterial relationships. The morphology also can be abnormal, with various cardiac segments malaligned or malformed. This classification has been described in the veterinary literature for both cats and horses (Scansen, 2015a; Schwarzwald, 2008). Although this is a standard for defining congenital heart defects, it is uncommonly used in veterinary medicine for a variety of reasons. Considering our focus is the veterinary student and practicing veterinarian, we will not discuss defects in terms of the segmental analysis, and refer the interested reader to the references list for more detail.

In general, purebred animals have a higher rate of congenital malformations than mixed-breed animals. Certain species and breed predispositions, as well as geographical variation in prevalence, have been observed with many congenital defects (**Table 26.1** and **Table 27.1**, p. 478). Most malformations are thought to have a genetic basis, although causative mutations are defined in relatively few cases. The overall prevalence of congenital cardiac disease in the general canine population might be at least 0.5–0.85%. In dogs specifically evaluated for cardiac disease, malformations of the heart and great vessels represent an estimated 16–24% of cases. However, in a large population of mixed-breed dogs screened at a shelter, the lower prevalence of 0.13% was reported (Schrope, 2015). Among various surveys of prevalence, patent ductus arteriosus (PDA), subaortic stenosis (SAS), and pulmonic stenosis (PS) are consistently the most common cardiac defects in dogs; their relative ranking depends on the survey reported and likely the criteria used to diagnose SAS. Scansen (2014) summarized results from multiple canine and feline surveys of congenital heart disease. Among 4,694 dogs, PDA (25.7%), SAS (23.5%) and PS (22.1%) comprised nearly three fourths of all cases. Other congenital cardiac shunts had much lower incidence, at 8.8% for ventricular septal defect (VSD), 2.3% for tetralogy of Fallot (T of F) and 1.9% for isolated atrial septal defect (ASD). It is likely that ASDs are underrepresented, as some surveys were reported prior to the widespread use of echocardiography with Doppler. Patent foramen ovale (PFO) is not considered a true ASD. Malformations (dysplasia) of the AV valves (8.9%, see Chapter 27), persistent right aortic arch and other vascular

Table 26.1 Breed Predispositions for Common Congenital Shunts

Defect	Breed
Patent ductus arteriosus	Australian Shepherd, Belgian Shepherd, Bichon Frise, Cavalier King Charles Spaniel, Chihuahua, Cocker Spaniel, Collie, Doberman Pinscher, English Springer Spaniel, German Shepherd Dog, Keeshond, Kerry Blue Terrier, Labrador Retriever, Maltese, Newfoundland, Pomeranian, Poodle (Toy and Miniature), Shetland Sheepdog, Welsh Corgi, Yorkshire Terrier. Females > males
Ventricular septal defect	English Bulldog, English Springer Spaniel, French Bulldog, German Shepherd Dog, Keeshond, Pinscher, West Highland White Terrier. Cats and horses also
Atrial septal defect	Boxer, Doberman Pinscher, Samoyed, Standard Poodle
Tetralogy of Fallot	English Bulldog, Keeshond

Note: Breeds not listed in order of malformation prevalence.

ring anomalies (3.3%; see Chapter 28), and other defects also have lower incidence. There is a male predisposition toward SAS and mitral valve dysplasia, and a strong female predisposition toward PDA in most canine breeds. Undoubtedly, some of the most severe and complicated malformations observed in children are underreported in these canine surveys; affected puppies are likely to die before ever seeing a veterinarian.

In cats, the overall prevalence of congenital cardiac disease is less clear; it could be between 0.2–1%, although an estimated prevalence of only 0.14% was reported in mixed-breed cats examined at a shelter (Schrope, 2015; Payne, 2015). An estimated 6–8% of cats specifically evaluated for cardiac disease have a congenital defect (Tidholm, 2015). About 10% of affected cats have more than one cardiac malformation. Combined data from multiple reports suggest that of a total of 435 cats, VSD (18.4%) is most common, followed by PDA (11.3%), tricuspid valve dysplasia (10.8%), mitral valve dysplasia (10.1%), atrioventricular septal defect (AVSD, 9.7%), aortic stenosis (7.1%), T of F 6.9%, isolated ASD (6%), vascular ring anomalies (5.3%), pulmonary stenosis (3.9%), and other defects (~10% combined). The least common congenital CV defects in cats include endocardial fibroelastosis (reported mainly in Burmese and Siamese cats), double-chamber right ventricle, and various malformations of the great vessels. Some defects, such as supravalvular AS and endocardial fibroelastosis, are probably overrepresented in particular surveys and these are rarely seen today. Pulmonic and aortic stenosis, VSD, and endocardial fibroelastosis appear to be more prevalent in male cats.

Likewise, the prevalence of congenital cardiac disease in horses is unclear but estimated to be relatively low at 0.1–0.5% (Hall, 2010). About 3–4% of horses evaluated specifically for cardiac disease have a congenital malformation (Marr, 2010). Defects involving shunts and the presence of multiple defects appear common. VSD is the cardiac malformation identified most often in horses; ASD, PDA, and T of F, as well as other complex defects, also occur. Valvular malformations in horses include AV (especially tricuspid) valve dysplasia or atresia, and rarely, pulmonary valve atresia or stenosis. The prevalence of congenital heart defects appears higher in Arabian horses; other breeds that might be overrepresented include Standardbreds, Welsh Mountain Ponies, and Morgan horses.

Many animals are asymptomatic at initial diagnosis, even when the underlying defect is severe. Clinical signs generally involve reduced exercise tolerance, signs of left- or right-sided congestive heart failure (CHF; **Table 20.1**, p. 300), stunted growth, intermittent weakness or syncope, or cyanosis. Once clinical signs of congenital heart disease are manifest, the situation often is severe enough to warrant urgent therapy. Most congenital heart diseases are identified in young animals, although some defects are discovered only later, when the animal is older. An unknown number of animals die from CV malformations before or shortly after birth.

Most congenital cardiac defects cause an audible murmur (**Figures 11.3** and **11.4**, pp. 229 and 234), although some do not. Murmur intensity (loudness) sometimes relates to the defect's severity (such as with SAS and PS), but in other situations a softer murmur might indicate more a severe problem, because other factors can modify murmur intensity. Serious anomalies that typically are associated with no (or only a very soft) murmur include: shunts where systemic and pulmonary pressures are closely equilibrated; "reversed" shunts with marked erythrocytosis (polycythemia) and hyperviscosity; some cases of tricuspid valve dysplasia, with torrential regurgitation and minimal systolic pressure gradient; pure stenosis of an AV valve (p. 480); vascular ring anomalies; cor triatriatum dexter (p. 511); and some others. Soft "innocent" murmurs also are relatively common in young animals (p. 228). Other physical findings, along with radiographic and electrocardiographic (ECG) abnormalities, can be useful when evaluating an animal with suspected congenital disease. However, echocardiography with Doppler provides greater diagnostic accuracy in the hands of a skilled sonographer. Additional diagnostic tests, such as cardiac catheterization, selective angiography, blood gas analysis, computed tomography (CT) with contrast, and magnetic resonance imaging (MRI) also might be useful in selected cases. Notably, vascular anomalies beyond the heart usually are best evaluated by CT (or standard) angiography or MRI.

Pathophysiology

Left-to-Right Shunting

Abnormal systemic-to-pulmonary shunts most commonly involve a PDA, VSD, or ASD. The volume and direction of blood flow through the shunt is a function of the pressure gradient across the communication and the defect's size. In general, small caliber defects maintain the normal pressure differential between the left and right sides. Conversely, extremely large (unrestrictive) defects can result in equilibration of pressures across the defect. The pulmonary vasculature normally is a low-pressure and low-resistance system. The pulmonary system can accommodate a substantial increase in flow volume while maintaining relatively low resistance (and pressure), as it normally does during exercise. Therefore, the shunt direction in the majority of animals with these defects is "left-to-right" (L-to-R), that is, from systemic to pulmonary sides of the circulations, and PA pressures usually are maintained near normal values despite the increased flow. As long as pulmonary vascular resistance remains relatively low, and there are no other obstructive lesions on the right side, these shunts cause pulmonary overcirculation. This imposes a volume overload on the left heart (with PDA and VSD; **Figure 26.1**) or right heart (with ASD). L-to-R shunts cause total blood volume and cardiac output to increase in response to the partial diversion of blood away from the systemic circulation.

If pulmonary vascular resistance increases, however, so will PA pressures, as PA pressure depends on the product of flow and resistance. Pulmonary hypertension (PH) not only increases pressure in the PA, it also leads to increases in right ventricular (RV) systolic and diastolic pressures, along with right atrial (RA) pressures. This reduces the magnitude of L-to-R shunting and usually decreases the radiographic size of pulmonary vessels, especially towards the lung periphery. PH also can develop from the combined effects of increased pulmonary blood flow and left heart failure. In these cases, the left heart is essentially unable to pump the extra volume it receives from the shunt; consequently, left ventricular (LV) diastolic and left atrial pressures increase. This is one outcome of PDA, VSD and potentially, an ASD (when part of an AVSD with mitral regurgitation, MR). In these settings, pulmonary vascular markings appear engorged on radiographs and often, congestive heart failure (CHF) is present. PH in such cases usually will respond to medical management for CHF and shunt closure, when possible. Combinations of increased pulmonary resistance, L-to-R shunting (flow), and left heart failure occur, which presents a challenge when assessing the relative contribution of each component. Concurrent valvular lesions on the right side of the heart also can diminish L-to-R shunting. For example, PS increases pressures in the right ventricle and right atrium; this reduces and can even reverse shunting across a VSD, ASD or PFO. Tricuspid valve malformations, whether associated with stenosis or severe

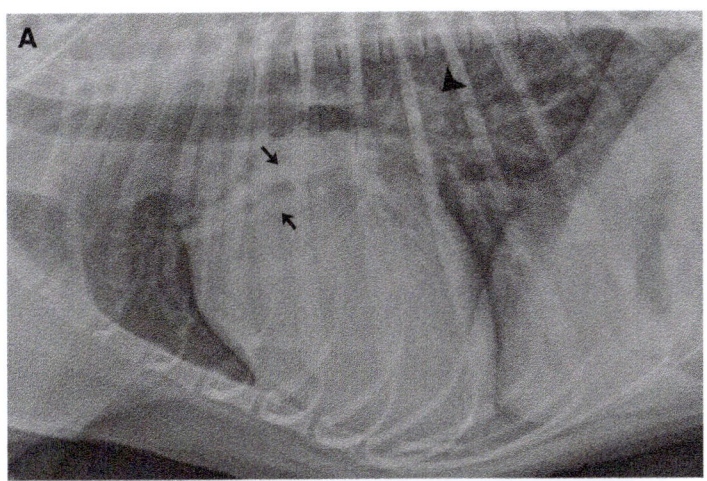

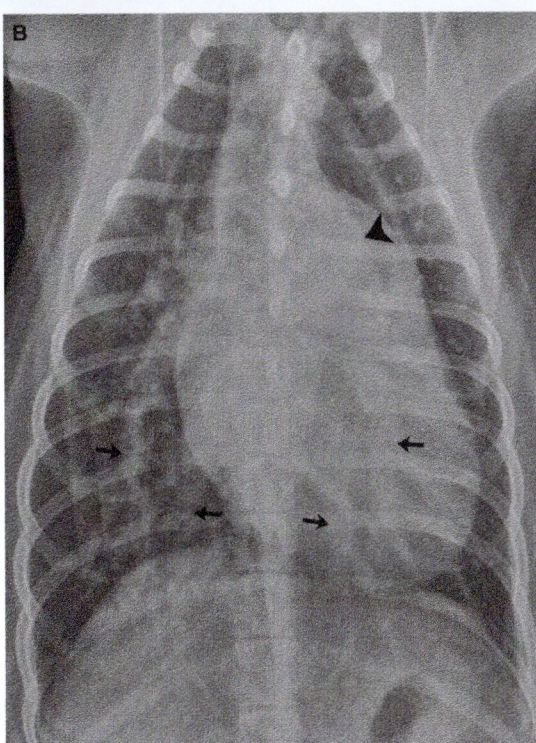

Figure 26.1 Lateral (A) and dorsoventral (B) thoracic radiographs from a 7-month-old female English Springer Spaniel with patent ductus arteriosus show left-sided cardiomegaly and pulmonary overcirculation. The small arrows indicate lobar pulmonary vessels; the dorsal (A) and lateral (B) vessels are arteries. Marked left atrial enlargement is evident on lateral view (arrowhead). On DV view, a prominent bulge ("ductus bump," arrowhead) is visible in the cranial descending aorta.

regurgitation, can increase RA pressure sufficiently to reduce (or reverse) shunting at the atrial level.

Right-to-Left Shunting

R-to-L shunting generally occurs either from PH caused by increased vascular resistance or from an obstructive lesion in the right side of the heart. In each situation, right-sided

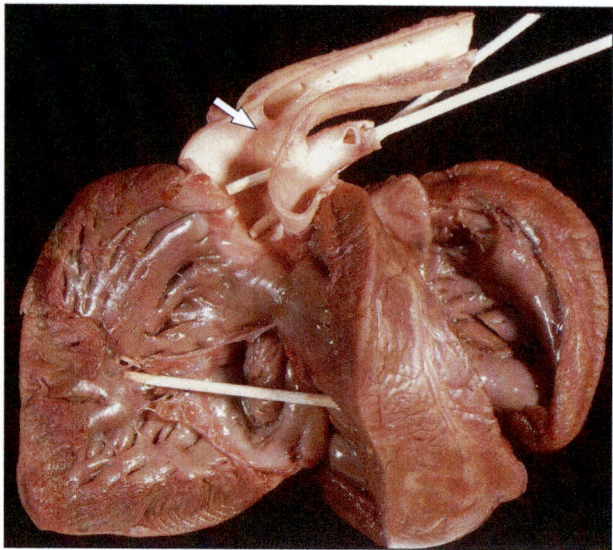

Figure 26.2 Specimen from a young, female Cocker Spaniel with "reversed" patent ductus arteriosus (PDA). The hypertrophied right ventricle is open from inflow to outflow regions; the cut extends into the dilated pulmonary trunk, through the large PDA (arrow), and into the descending aorta. Wooden probes are inserted at the pulmonary artery bifurcation.

pressure exceeds that on the left during at least part of the cardiac cycle. PH develops in a small proportion of animals with a shunt, including PDA, VSD, ASD, AVSD, aorticopulmonary window, and other less common defects. The associated defect generally is quite large in cases that develop reversed shunting (**Figures 26.2** and **26.3**). A large shunt probably interferes with the normal postnatal decline in pulmonary vascular resistance, and could promote the irreversible histologic changes in pulmonary vascular walls that lead to increased resistance. These changes include intimal thickening, medial hypertrophy, and characteristic plexiform lesions (**Figure 39.4**, p. 818).

Whenever pulmonary pressure exceeds that of the systemic circulation, the shunt reverses direction and deoxygenated blood flows into the aorta. Depending on the relative pressure differences, this could occur only during a portion of the cardiac cycle (either in diastole or in systole), which creates a so-called bidirectional shunt. Bidirectional shunting (or an increase in the volume of R-to-L shunting) can occur during exercise, as well as other times when systemic resistance (and pressure) fall relative to the pulmonary system. It appears that the vascular changes associated with PH develop at an early age, although rare exceptions might occur. There does seem to be some species difference in the rate of pulmonary vascular injury and remodeling, and the associated PH, with these being accelerated in dogs and more gradual, and potentially reversible, in cats.

The term Eisenmenger's (patho)physiology refers to this PH with shunt reversal. Defects that cause R-to-L shunting sometimes are described as cyanotic or complex congenital defects. Pathophysiologic and clinical sequelae of reversed shunts resemble those produced by T of F, although the impediment to pulmonary flow with T of F occurs at the pulmonary valve, rather than the pulmonary arteriolar level. Systolic pressure overload (whether caused by PH, PS, or double-chambered right ventricle) produces RV concentric hypertrophy, as well as some degree of RV dilation. In contrast to T of F, PH leads to dilation of the pulmonary annulus, pulmonary trunk, and large lobar pulmonary arteries. Secondary pulmonary and tricuspid valve regurgitation, from annular dilation, often adds an extra volume load on the right heart. The RV hypertrophy contributes to increasing ventricular wall stiffness and diastolic pressures. In cases with tricuspid valve malformation, R-to-L shunting at the atrial level occurs when an ASD is concurrent or the foramen ovale maintains patency. Similarly, the intra-atrial obstruction and RA pressure elevation of cor triatriatum dexter (Chapter 28) can cause R-to-L flow across a PFO.

Reversed shunts cause hypoxemia by allowing deoxygenated blood to reach the systemic circulation. Physical exertion exacerbates R-to-L shunting and cyanosis because peripheral vascular resistance decreases as skeletal muscle blood flow increases. Chronic renal hypoxia stimulates erythropoietin release and secondary erythrocytosis, as a mechanism to increase blood oxygen-carrying capacity. Visible cyanosis, which occurs with 50 g/L (5 g/dL) or more of desaturated hemoglobin (Chapter 13), becomes more likely as the hematocrit rises. Additionally, blood viscosity and resistance to flow also rise along with hematocrit. Severe erythrocytosis (with packed cell volume, PCV, well over 65%; **Figure 19.1**, p. 288) can lead to microvascular sludging, poor tissue oxygenation, and intravascular

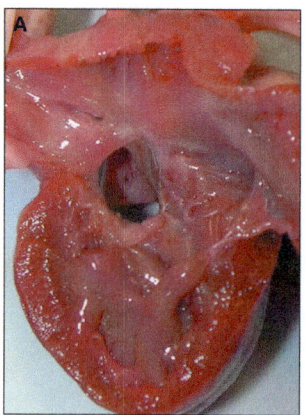
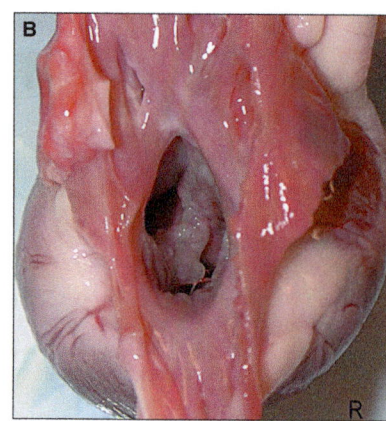

Figure 26.3 (A) View from the right showing right ventricular (RV) hypertrophy and large atrioventricular (AV) septal defect, with malformed tricuspid valve, in a 5-month-old kitten. The enlarged right atrium (RA) and auricle are at the top. Pulmonary hypertension caused right-to-left shunting. (B) Top-down view from RA through the common AV annulus showing top of the interventricular septum, with malformed septal tricuspid and mitral (bridging) leaflets. The left ventricle is to the upper left of the septal ridge, the RV opening is below.

thrombosis. The clinical effects of hyperviscosity include weakness, cerebrovascular events (hemorrhage, stroke), seizures, cardiac arrhythmias, syncope, reduced kidney function, metabolic acidosis, clotting abnormalities, and iron deficiency. Because hyperviscosity also reduces blood flow turbulence (p. 23), shunt-associated murmurs become softer. Affected animals often have no audible murmur at the time of diagnosis, especially if obstructive lesions reduce blood flow substantially.

Collateral blood flow to the lungs can arise from bronchial arteries of the systemic circulation. These small tortuous vessels can increase the radiographic opacity of the central lung fields. Rarely, PH can lead to vascular rupture and hemoptysis. R-to-L shunts also might allow venous emboli to cross into the arterial system, causing a stroke or other paradoxical arterial embolization. Despite the RV pressure overload, signs of right-sided CHF are uncommon with reversed shunts because the shunt acts as a "pop-off" valve for the right heart. Nevertheless, right-sided CHF does develop in sporadic cases, especially when tricuspid insufficiency or secondary myocardial failure exists.

Patent Ductus Arteriosus (Left-to-Right Shunting)

PDA is one of the most common congenital CV defects in dogs, although not in cats and horses. The L-to-R shunting PDA is by far the most common presentation. The ductus arteriosus is a fetal vessel, originating from the left 6th embryonic arch which extends between the proximal descending aorta and the origin of the left PA at the pulmonary trunk. Before birth, the ductus conveys blood from the PA into the aorta, thus bypassing the non-inflated fetal lungs. After birth, as breathing begins, pulmonary vascular resistance falls with lung inflation. The reduced pulmonary arterial pressure causes ductal flow to change direction, now bringing oxygenated blood from the aorta into the ductus; this inhibits local vasodilatory prostaglandin release. Smooth muscle in the wall of the normal ductus then constricts to close the ductus arteriosus. Functional closure of the ductus occurs within hours after birth; structural changes over several days to a week or so cause permanent closure. In puppies, closure should be complete by 7–10 days of age. In horses, physiologic or functional closure reportedly occurs between 48 and 72 hours of age, with complete anatomic closure by 4 days of age.

PDA occurs when the ductus fails to constrict (**Figures 26.4 and 26.5**). As described in dogs (Buchanan, 2003), ductal wall structural abnormalities involve variably reduced mural smooth muscle and increased elastic tissue, similar to the aortic wall. This structure renders the ductus unable to constrict normally after birth; neither will it respond to prostaglandin inhibitors like indomethacin or aspirin.

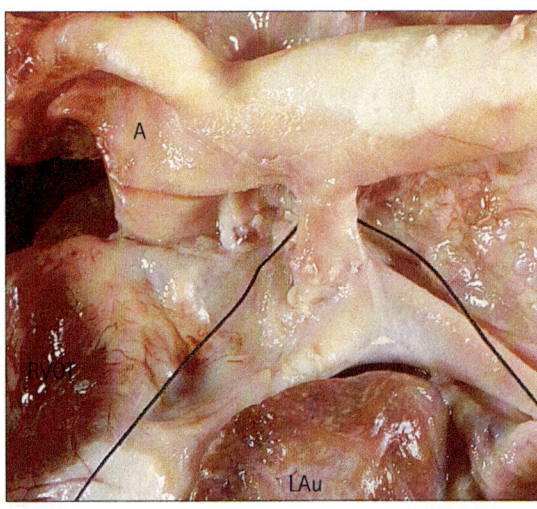

Figure 26.4 A suture has been passed around the patent ductus arteriosus in this autopsy specimen from a dog. The ductus connects the proximal descending aorta with the pulmonary artery. A, aorta; LAu, left auricle; RVOT, right ventricular outflow tract. Cranial is to the left.

Such abnormalities in ductal wall morphology occur in dogs with inherited (as well as apparently sporadic) PDA, suggesting common genetic defect(s). A spectrum of patent ductus size and morphology can occur. The mildest is an incomplete, clinically inapparent form ("*forme fruste*") of PDA, where ductal closure occurs only at the pulmonary side. This creates a ductus diverticulum from the aorta, but no shunt (or murmur). A ductus diverticulum is visible only with angiography or on postmortem examination (**Figure 26.6**).

Fully patent ductal morphology in dogs has been classified into four general types based on angiocardiographic

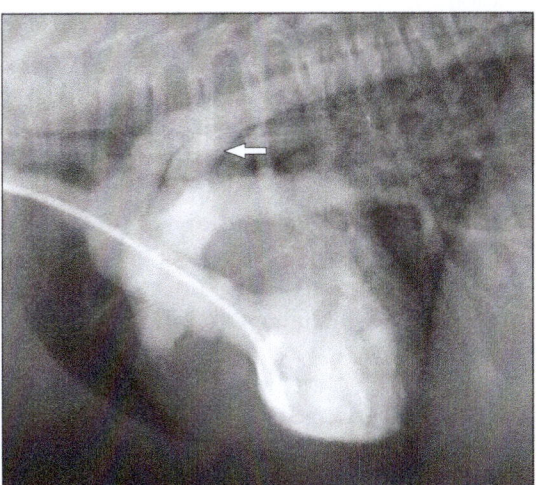

Figure 26.5 Left ventricular angiocardiogram in a dog. Radiopaque dye is present in the left ventricle, aorta, a large left-to-right shunting patent ductus arteriosus (arrow), and pulmonary artery. The engorged pulmonary vasculature also is highlighted.

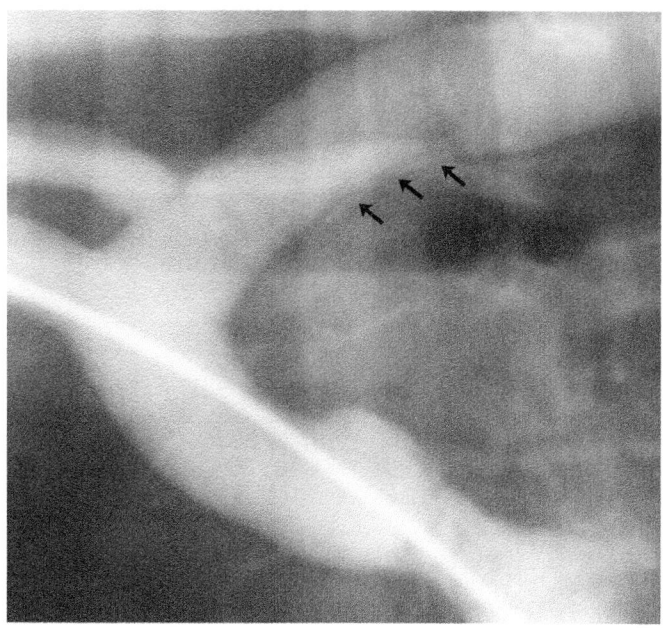

Figure 26.6 Left ventricular angiocardiogram from a dog with mild subaortic stenosis also shows the presence of a ductus diverticulum (arrows). Because the ductus has closed on the pulmonary artery side, there is no flow through this incomplete form of ductus arteriosus.

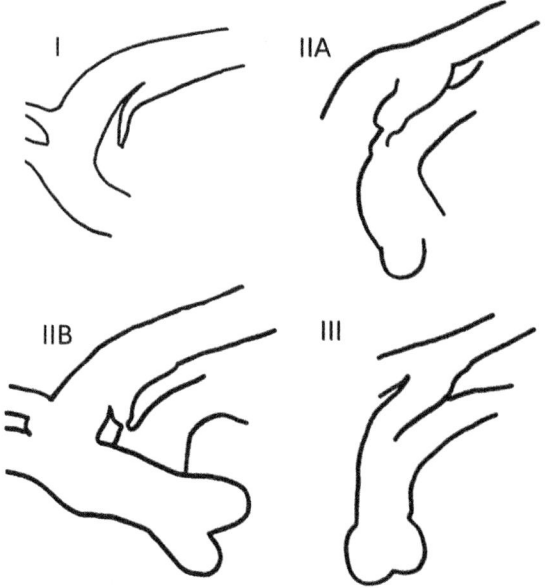

Figure 26.7 Morphologic classification of patent ductus arteriosus. Type I (upper left) shows gradual ductal tapering from aorta to pulmonary artery (PA). Type IIA (upper right) shows nearly parallel ductal walls extending from the aortic side with abrupt narrowing near the PA. Type IIB ductus (lower left) has a conical ductal shape with abrupt narrowing near the PA insertion. Type III (lower right) has a wide tubular shape with little to no tapering. (Modified from Miller MW, Gordon SG, Saunders AB, et al. Angiographic classification of patent ductus arteriosus morphology in the dog. J Vet Cardiol 2006;8:109–114.)

appearance (Miller, 2006). This classification depends on the degree of ductal tapering, as well as the presence (or absence) and location of abrupt ductal narrowing (**Figure 26.7**). Type I PDA displays gradual ductal tapering from the aorta toward the point of pulmonary insertion; this appears to be the least common morphology in dogs. Type IIA ductus has nearly parallel ductal walls extending from the aortic side with abrupt narrowing (of >50%) near the pulmonary insertion site. Type IIA morphology is the most common form in dogs, occurring in over half of PDA cases. Type IIB morphology, found in about one-third of affected dogs, displays a conical ductal shape with abrupt narrowing (of >50%) near the PA insertion. Type III PDA morphology has a tubular appearance, with little to no decrease in diameter. The type III ductus generally is wider at its pulmonary insertion point compared to other ductal morphologies. The type III PDA might be more common in German Shepherd dogs, although not all reports concur. Other, more unusual PDA morphologies also have been reported, including a rare intramural form with an extended conical tunnel within the aortic wall, which connects the aortic opening of the shunt to the more proximal PA opening. Two additional classification categories recently were proposed to describe PDA morphology that did not fit into the previously described types I–III. These include type IV, where the ductus contains several narrowed areas, and type V, which encompasses other unusual morphologies (Doocy, 2018).

When the ductus is fully patent, blood shunts continuously (throughout the cardiac cycle) from descending aorta into the PA (**Figure 26.5**), because aortic pressures normally are higher during both systole and diastole. As with other systemic-to-pulmonary communications, the shunt flow volume depends on the pressure gradient between the two circulations and ductal diameter. Typically, the volume of blood "run-off" from aorta into the PA is sufficient to cause a rapid decrease in aortic diastolic pressure. This widens the aortic (arterial) pulse pressure, creating the hyperkinetic arterial pulse quality characteristic of PDA (p. 255).

The L-to-R shunt imposes a volume overload on the pulmonary circulation, left atrium, and left ventricle (**Figure 26.1**). While compensatory mechanisms (increased heart rate, volume retention, increased LV preload) maintain systemic blood flow, the hemodynamic burden on the ventricle can be great because it must pump the increased volume into the relatively high-pressure aorta. LV and mitral annulus dilation in turn cause MR and further volume overload. Excess fluid retention, ventricular distensibility and myocardial contractility reduction associated with extreme volume overload, and arrhythmias contribute to the development of left-sided CHF. Clients often overlook the clinical signs until the situation is critical.

High-velocity L-to-R flow can injure the pulmonary endothelium and cause jet lesions (**Figure 26.8**). In rare cases, dissection of the pulmonary arterial or ductal wall can occur, either naturally or during ductal closure procedures, even in

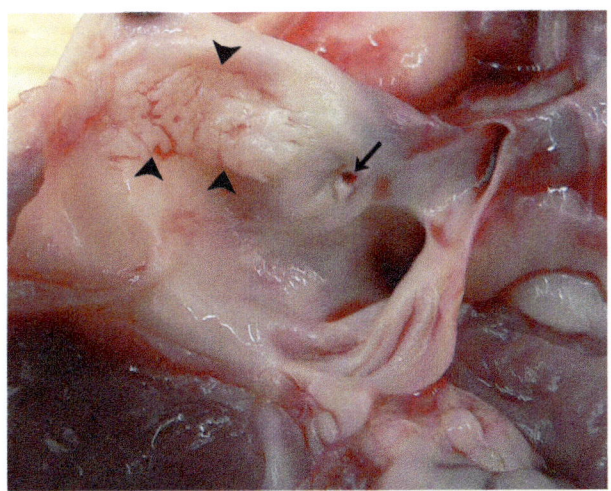

Figure 26.8 Open main pulmonary artery showing a large jet lesion (arrowheads) in a dog with patent ductus arteriosus. The small arrow points to the ductal opening.

the absence of PH. Ductal flow into the false lumen formed between intimal and medial layers causes the intima to balloon into the true pulmonary arterial lumen, which could obstruct forward flow. Rarely, the obstruction could become severe enough to cause RV pressure overload and possibly lead to right-sided CHF signs. PDA is considered a predisposing factor for infective endocarditis in people; the infection usually involves the ductus or PA. Although rare in animals, aortic endocarditis has been reported in a dog with PDA.

In some cases, excessive pulmonary blood flow with transmission of aortic pressure induces pulmonary vascular changes that lead to increased pulmonary resistance and pressure. If, at any time, the PA pressure rises close to aortic pressure, little shunting occurs; however, if PA pressure exceeds aortic pressure, the shunt will reverse (p. 449). Depending on the relative pressures across the ductus throughout the cardiac cycle, bidirectional shunting also can occur.

Other malformations occasionally cause hemodynamic and clinical abnormalities similar to PDA, including an aorticopulmonary window (between ascending aorta and PA) and major aortopulmonary collateral arteries connecting the aorta or its branches to the pulmonary circulation. These have occurred in dogs, and can mimic a L-to-R shunting PDA. These aberrant shunts might possibly persist from an embryologic systemic-to-pulmonary vascular plexus that normally regresses during pulmonary arterial system development. They can cause a relatively soft continuous murmur at the left heart base (similar to PDA) or they could be silent, leading only to functional MR from LV dilation. Echocardiography in such cases might show some continuous retrograde pulmonary arterial flow as well as turbulence in more peripheral pulmonary arteries, without evidence of a discrete PDA. Acquired aorticopulmonary anastomoses that develop subsequent to R-to-L shunts or pulmonary disease are possible, also. These are seen best with standard angiography or CT angiography.

Clinical Features

The prevalence of PDA is higher in certain breeds of dog, with the majority of cases involving small breeds (**Table 26.1**). A polygenic inheritance pattern is probably responsible. The prevalence is approximately three times greater in female than in male dogs. Most PDAs in dogs are isolated defects, however an estimated 10% of cases have concurrent congenital malformations, usually either PS or SAS. The great majority of affected animals are presented at a young age, usually when less than 6 months to a year old. Occasionally, a previously undiagnosed PDA is discovered in an older animal; typically, the shunt is small in these cases. About one-third of dogs that are diagnosed with PDA as adults (≥5 years of age) have concurrent degenerative mitral valve disease; arrhythmias also are common (Boutet, 2017). A few cases have some degree of PH or another defect. While L-to-R shunting occurs in most of these, in cases of severe PH the shunt is usually bidirectional. A substantial number of dogs have incipient or overt left-sided CHF; these are treated with furosemide and pimobendan. Prompt ductal closure is indicated in such cases; subsequently, most can be weaned off medical therapy. Dogs with moderate PH, not severe enough to cause persistent (complete) R-to-L shunting, also can do well after ductal closure.

PDA is much less common in cats compared to dogs, although it likely is underdiagnosed. Isolated PDA is rare in the horse. The average age at diagnosis for cats is ~6 months, although as with dogs, some are diagnosed as middle-aged to older adults. There appears to be no sex predilection in this species. About half of cats with PDA have concurrent CV defect(s). The majority of affected cats are asymptomatic at diagnosis. Between 37% and >45% have some degree of PH, although less than half of these appear to have R-to L-shunting (Wustefeld-Janssens, 2016; Bascunan, 2017). Clinical signs, including CHF, are common in cats with PH.

Although many dogs with PDA are apparently asymptomatic at first diagnosis, critical evaluation reveals reduced exercise ability, tachypnea, or cough in a substantial number of cases. If the ductus is not closed, signs of left-sided CHF are highly likely to develop over time, generally within a year of diagnosis. Progressive LV dysfunction, generalized cardiomegaly, and atrial fibrillation (AF) or other arrhythmias can occur with time; this can mimic the presentation of dilated cardiomyopathy (DCM). Nevertheless, some animals with a small shunt flow have lived well for >10 years without intervention. It is likely that many puppies with a large and unrestrictive PDA die of CHF before seeing a veterinarian, unless they develop pulmonary vascular disease.

Physical findings with L-to-R shunting PDA generally include hyperkinetic (bounding) arterial pulses (**Figure 26.9**), pink mucous membranes, and normal jugular vein appearance. The left apical impulse can be displaced caudally

442 Cardiovascular Diseases

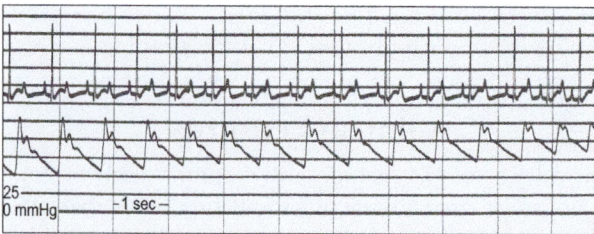

Figure 26.9 Simultaneous ECG (top) and femoral arterial pressure recording (bottom). Patent ductus arteriosus causes a widened pulse pressure (seen at the left side of this recording). During surgical ligation of the ductus, the pulse pressure narrows as blood run-off into the pulmonary artery is curtailed (ligation complete at the right side). (Original recording courtesy of Dr D Riedesel; from Ware WA & Ward JW. Congenital cardiac disease. In, Nelson RW & Couto GC (editors). Small Animal Internal Medicine. 6th edition. Elsevier, St. Louis, MO. 2019. p. 102.)

because of left heart enlargement. A continuous murmur, heard best at the dorsal left base over the PA (**Figure 11.3**, p. 229), is characteristic of L-to-R PDA. A continuous precordial thrill accompanies loud murmurs. However, in a relatively large survey of cats with PDA, a continuous murmur was heard only in slightly more than half of cases; a systolic murmur was identified in the rest (Bascunan, 2017). This probably relates to the faster heart rate as well as the substantial number of cats with PH. Sometimes, a PDA murmur trails off toward end-diastole and is described (incorrectly) as a "long" systolic murmur.

Diagnostic Tests

Typical radiographic findings include cardiac elongation (left heart dilation), left atrial (LA) and auricular enlargement, and pulmonary overcirculation (**Table 26.2**; **Figure 26.1**; and **Figure 3.17B**, p. 60). Characteristically, there is a bulge in the cranial descending aorta ("ductus bump"). The main pulmonary trunk can be enlarged as well. Occasionally, a triad of three bulges representing pulmonary trunk, aorta, and left auricle (located in that order from the 1 o'clock to 3 o'clock position) is evident on DV radiograph. Some animals have more generalized cardiomegaly, although LV enlargement is largely responsible (**Figures 26.10** and **26.11**). Especially in

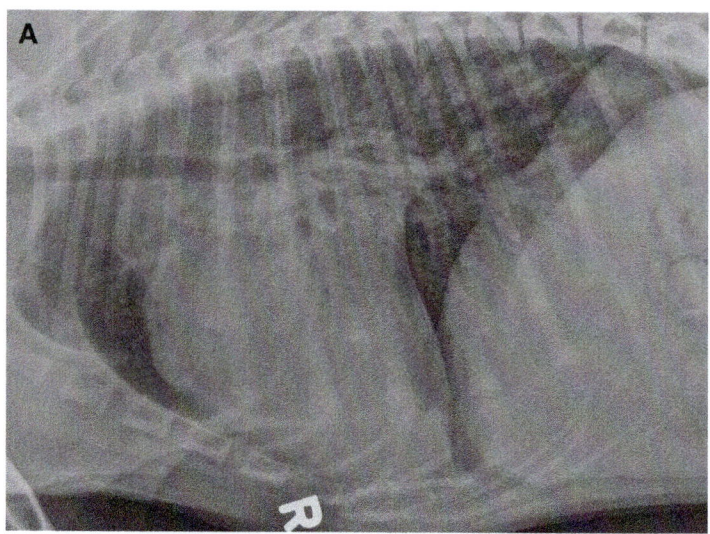

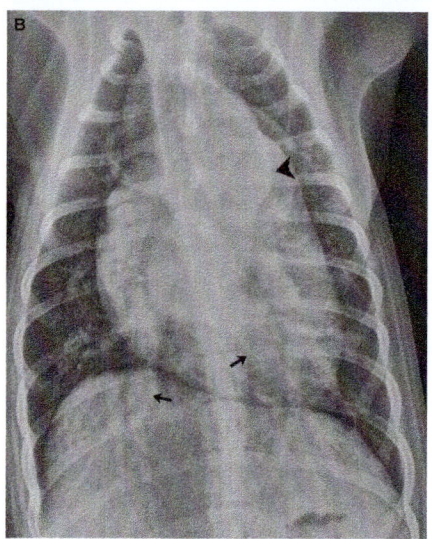

Figure 26.10 Right lateral (A) and DV (B) radiographs from a 6-month-old female Irish Setter with patent ductus arteriosus show marked left heart enlargement, a prominent ductus bump in the aorta (B; arrowhead), main pulmonary artery dilation and pulmonary overcirculation. Although the dog was asymptomatic, venous congestion (indicated by the wider caudal pulmonary veins compared to their accompanying arteries; arrows, B) suggested impending congestive heart failure. Furosemide was administered and the ductus was closed successfully.

Table 26.2 Characteristic Radiographic Findings in Dogs and Cats with Congenital Shunts

Defect	Heart	Pulmonary Vessels	Other
Patent ductus arteriosus	LAE, LVE; left auricular bulge; ± increased cardiac width	Overcirculated; lobar vein often > lobar artery	Bulge(s) in descending aorta + pulmonary trunk; ± pulmonary edema
Ventricular septal defect	LAE, LVE; ± RVE	Overcirculated	Pulmonary edema; ± pulmonary trunk bulge (large shunt)
Atrial septal defect	RAE, RVE	± Overcirculated	Pulmonary trunk bulge
Tetralogy of Fallot	RVE, RAE	Undercirculated; ± prominent bronchial collateral vessels	Normal to small pulmonary trunk; ± cranial aortic bulge on lateral view

Abbreviations: LAE, left atrial enlargement; LVE, left ventricular enlargement; RAE, right atrial enlargement; RVE, right ventricular enlargement.

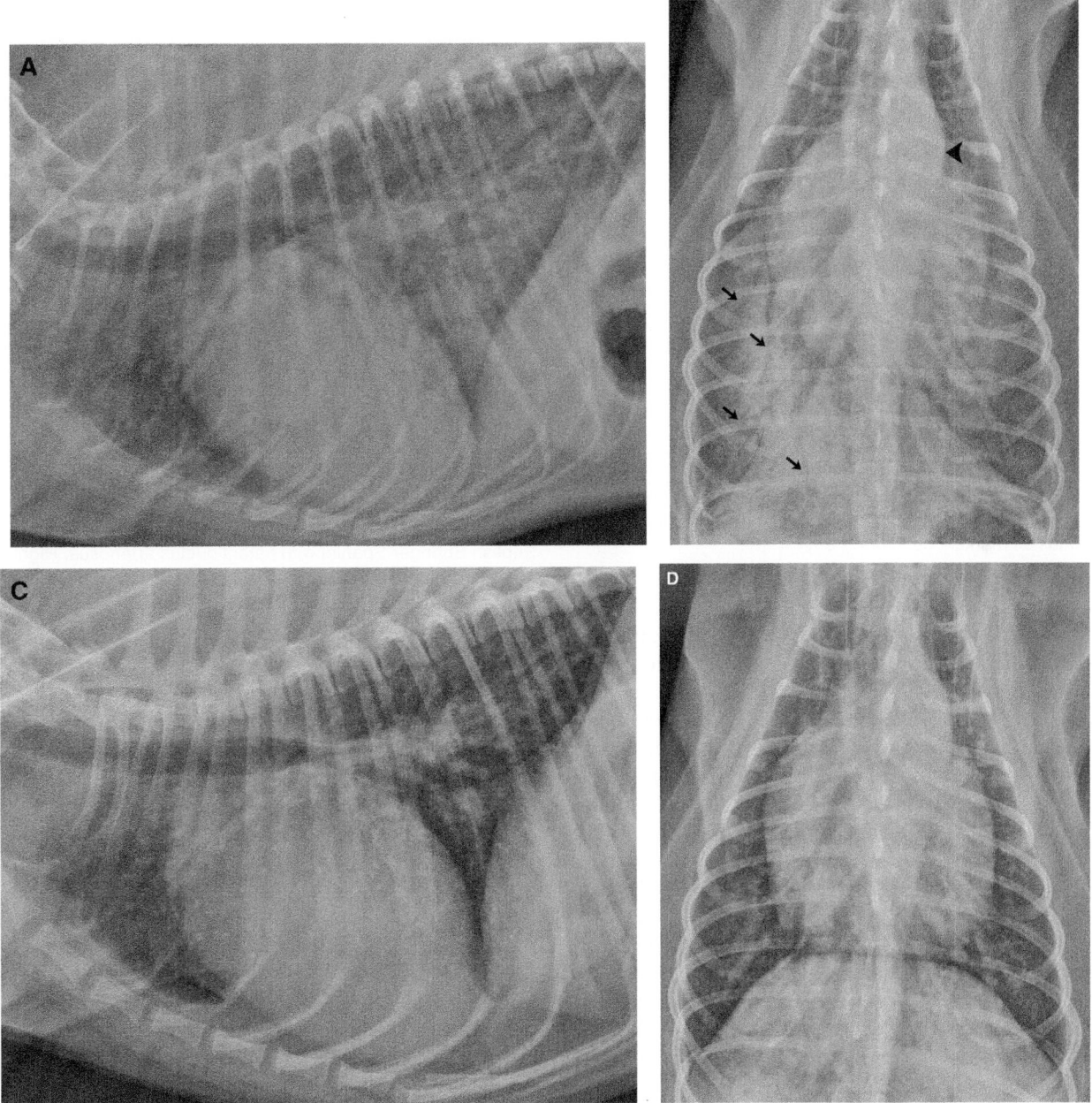

Figure 26.11 (A–D) A 3½-year-old female Sheltie was presented for rapidly worsening dyspnea. The owners reported no prior problems and were unaware of the dog's murmur. A loud continuous murmur and pulmonary crackles were heard. Lateral (A) and DV (B) radiographs show moderate generalized cardiomegaly (VHS >13v), engorged lobar pulmonary arteries and veins, and a pulmonary alveolar pattern consistent with severe left-sided congestive heart failure (CHF). Air bronchograms (arrows, B) are prominent in right middle and caudal lung lobes. The ductus bump (arrowhead, B) is less prominent in this dog. Two weeks after beginning CHF therapy (C, D), pulmonary edema is almost resolved and overall heart size is smaller (VHS ~12v). Generally, only a few days of CHF therapy are recommended before ductal closure because some dogs don't respond to medical treatment. This dog has a more rounded cardiac shape than shown in **Figures 26.1** and **26.10**.

those with poor LV myocardial function, the radiographic (as well as echocardiographic) appearance can be similar to that of DCM. Evidence of overcirculation and pulmonary edema accompanies left-sided heart failure; frequently the lobar pulmonary vein is larger than the accompanying artery. Cardiac CT angiography or MRI can help better define the anatomy in complex cases.

Characteristic ECG findings include wide P waves, tall R waves and often, deep Q waves in leads II, aVF, and left precordial leads (**Figure 26.12**). ST-T segment changes secondary to LV enlargement can occur. A minority of patients have arrhythmias such as AF or ventricular premature complexes (VPCs). However, the ECG can be normal in some cases.

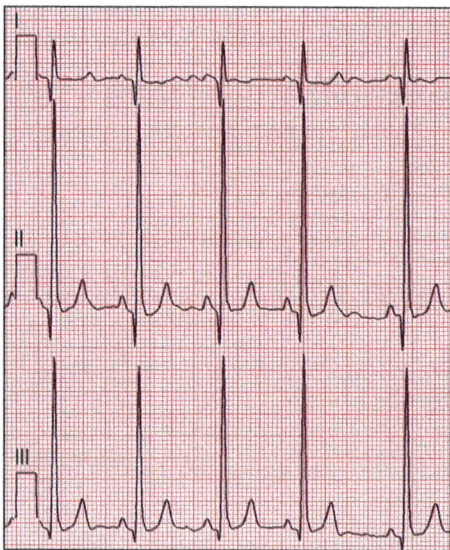

Figure 26.12 Tall QRS complexes (R wave, 4.8 mV) with deep Q waves are common in patent ductus arteriosus, as seen here in a small mixed-breed dog. Leads as marked, 50 mm/s, 1 cm = 1 mV.

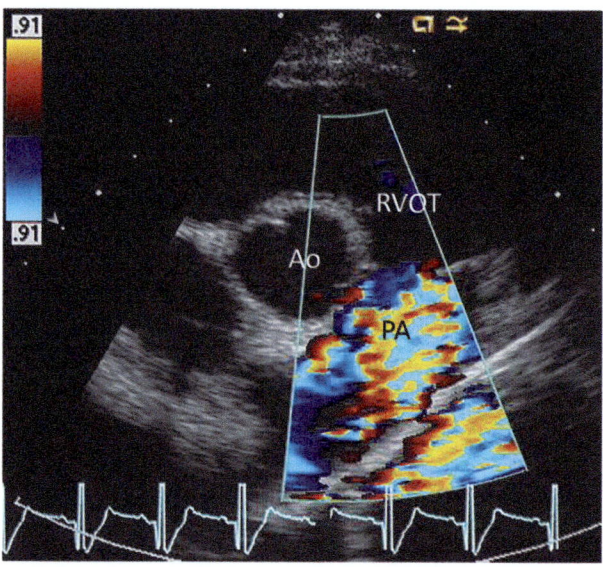

Figure 26.13 Color-flow Doppler image during diastole shows a turbulent flow jet into the dilated pulmonary trunk, in a 7-month-old female English Springer Spaniel with patent ductus arteriosus. Right parasternal short-axis view. Ao, aorta; PA, pulmonary artery; RVOT, right ventricular outflow tract. Mirror image artifact is lateral to the PA.

The plasma concentration of the N-terminal B-type (brain) natriuretic peptide prohormone (NT-proBNP) could be elevated. This has been correlated with heart size, murmur grade, and heart failure class. Ductal closure leads to significant decline in plasma NT-proBNP concentrations.

Echocardiography documents dilation of the left heart, aorta, and pulmonary trunk. LV systolic function indices usually are normal, but LV function can decline over time, especially in larger dogs. LV systolic function should be assessed with 2D volume estimates and calculation of ejection fractions, not just the M-mode fractional shortening, which can substantially underestimate global LV systolic function. The ductus itself often can be visualized between the PA and descending aorta, especially in right and left cranial parasternal views. Transthoracic echocardiography (TTE) tends to overestimate the minimal ductal diameter, compared to angiography and transesophageal echocardiography (TEE). A significant, although weakly correlated, relationship was found between angiographic and 2D TEE measures of minimal ductal diameter and ductal ampulla diameter. Nevertheless, one study found that 2D TEE measurements generally do not correlate well with various other imaging modalities used, indicating that measurements by different methods are not interchangeable (Doocy, 2018). Based on 3D TEE imaging, the ductal pulmonary ostium and ampulla had an oval shape in about three-fourths of these study dogs. Doppler echocardiographic studies document continuous turbulent flow into the PA and are used to estimate the aortic-to-PA pressure gradient (**Figures 26.13–26.16**). A large L-to-R shunt can increase LV outflow tract velocity substantially, with maximal velocities approaching 3 m/s in some cases. This makes it challenging to recognize mild SAS in these dogs.

Cardiac catheterization, done prior to transcatheter ductal occlusion, demonstrates the wide aortic pulse pressure. Although not usually measured in these cases, oximetry will reveal higher oxygen content in the PA than in the right ventricle (an oxygen "step-up"). Angiocardiography documents L-to-R shunting through the ductus and the relevant ductal anatomy (**Figure 26.5**).

Management

Closure of the L-to-R PDA is needed for the vast majority of dogs to prevent CHF and a shortened lifespan. Ideally, this is accomplished as soon as the diagnosis is confirmed and when the patient is younger, with less adverse cardiac remodeling. Several surgical and transcatheter occlusion techniques have been described. After ductal occlusion, a drop in heart rate can occur abruptly (with surgical closure) or within several minutes (with device closure) because of a reflex baroreceptor response, as the previously shunted blood now expands aortic volume. Diastolic and mean blood pressures also are higher after shunt occlusion. Because the original shunt volume now is confined in the aorta, LV function can appear worse immediately following ductal closure, as LV afterload is increased. Cardiac function generally improves with time and as LV diastolic volume decreases. A soft residual systolic murmur might be heard, originating from concurrent MR; this usually resolves as LV size normalizes, provided the valve is structurally normal. Unless CHF was present before ductal closure, therapy for this usually is not necessary.

The presence of CHF could increase risk for death or an unsuccessful procedure, so ductal occlusion is recommended as early as possible. Patients with CHF or arrhythmias should be treated for those prior to PDA closure. However, experience indicates that medical therapy for severe pulmonary

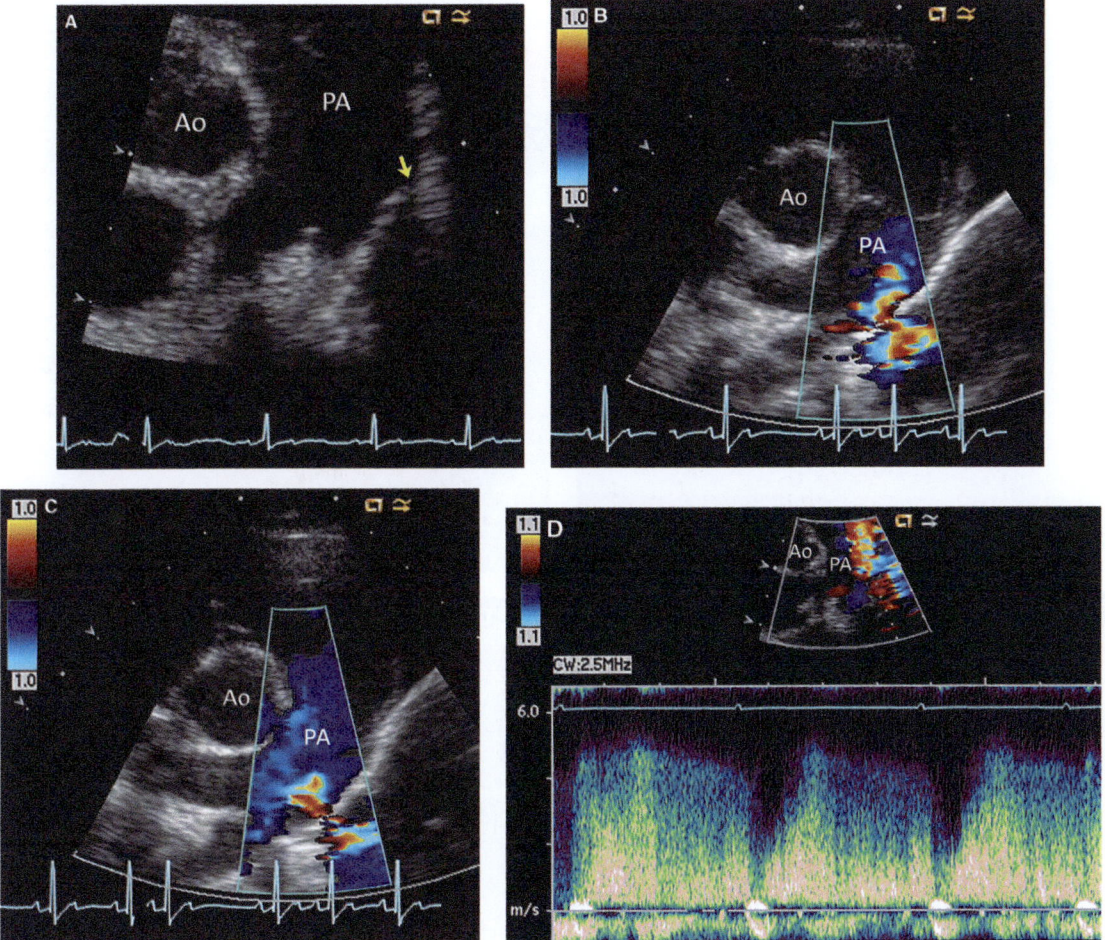

Figure 26.14 (A) A small ductal opening into the PA (arrow) is visible on this echocardiographic image from a 5-month-old female American Water Spaniel with patent ductus arteriosus (PDA). Continuous flow (B, diastole; C, systole) into the PA is evident (with mirror image artifact laterally), in a slightly modified view from (A). (D) Continuous-wave Doppler image reveals a peak ductal flow velocity of about 5 m/s into the PA, indicating that PA pressures are normal. Ao, aortic root; PA, pulmonary artery. (Images from left cranial short-axis view).

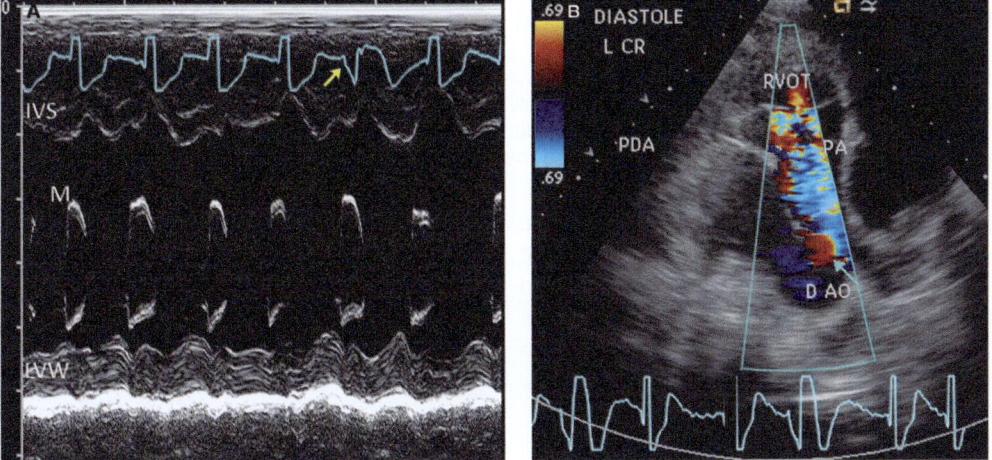

Figure 26.15 Patent ductus arteriosus, over time, leads to poor myocardial function, cardiac arrhythmias and congestive heart failure; this can mimic dilated cardiomyopathy, as in this 4-year-old female Labrador Retriever. (A) M-mode echocardiogram at the mitral valve level reveals left ventricular dilation, reduced motion of IVS and LVW, and wide mitral E-point-septal separation. The electrocardiogram (at top) shows atrial fibrillation with a rapid ventricular response rate and one ventricular premature complex (arrow). (B) Color-flow Doppler image in diastole documents continuous ductal flow into the PA (arrow); left cranial long-axis view. D AO, descending aorta; IVS, interventricular septum, LVW, left ventricular wall; M, anterior mitral leaflet; PA, pulmonary artery; RVOT, right ventricular outflow tract.

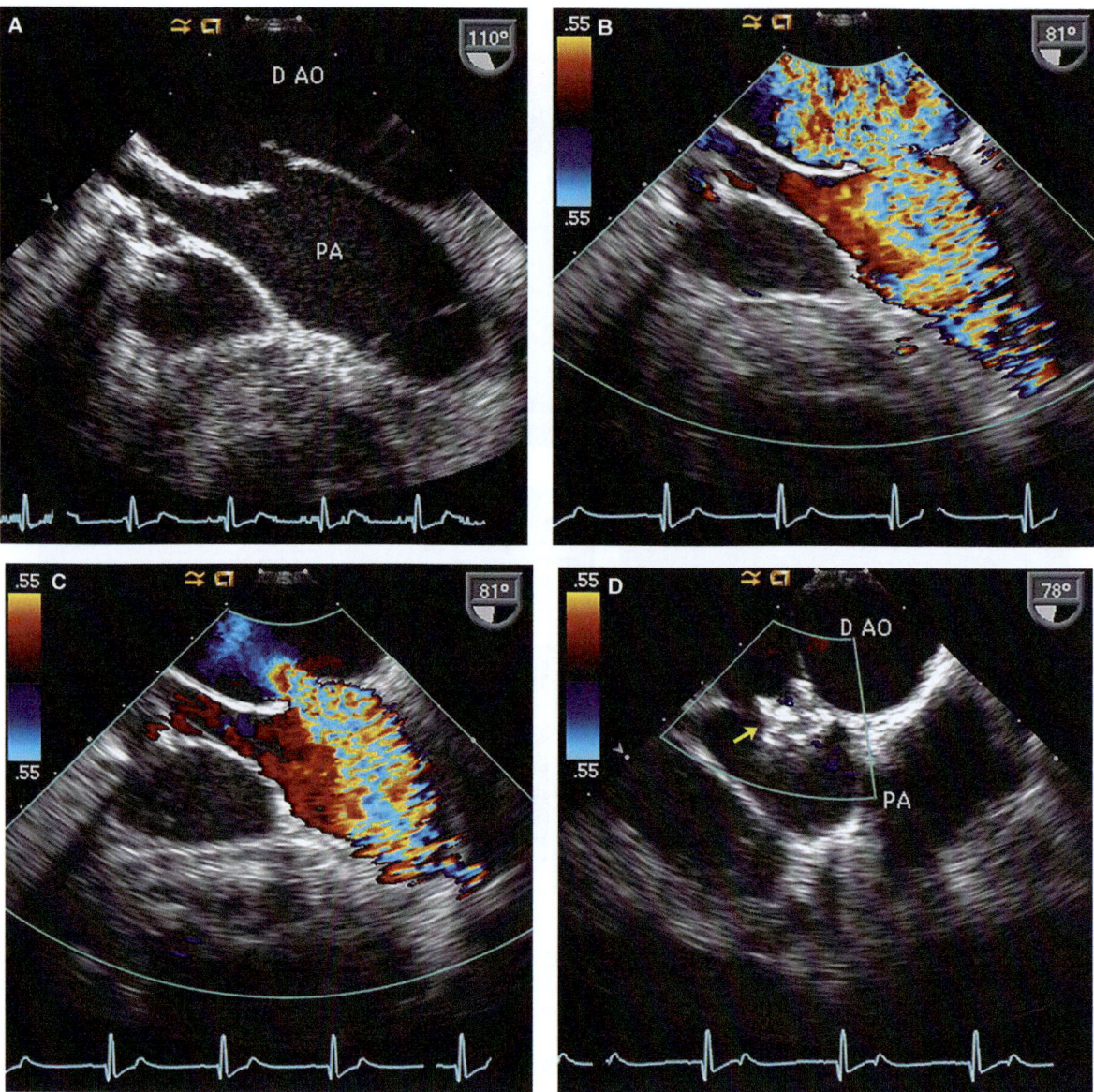

Figure 26.16 (A) A patent ductal opening into the PA usually can be visualized more clearly with 2D transesophageal echocardiography (TEE), compared to transthoracic echocardiography. Left-to-right ductal flow is evident using color Doppler in systole (B) and diastole (C) in an adult female English Springer Spaniel; same view as in (A). (D) Placement of an Amplatz Canine Duct Occluder (ACDO) successfully stopped ductal flow in this dog; slightly different TEE probe angulation shows the ACDO device (arrow). D AO, descending aorta; PA, pulmonary artery.

edema is, at best, stabilizing and that ductal closure should be pursued promptly, if not emergently. Heart failure therapy still might be needed for weeks or even months after successful closure in some animals with complicated disease, particularly those with a DCM phenotype or AF. If AF is present then cardioversion can be considered at the time of ductal closure (p. 391). CHF at initial presentation was identified as a negative prognostic sign in some, but not in all studies. Marked LA enlargement is associated with an increased risk of perioperative death (Saunders, 2014). Animals with PH, but that still have some L-to-R shunting, might realize improvement or resolution of the PH after ductal closure. However, for cases with severe PH and continuous or bidirectional R-to-L shunting unresponsive to sildenafil or tadalafil, ductal closure is contraindicated.

Transcatheter Ductal Occlusion Transcatheter PDA occlusion is performed at many centers with high rates of success. The Amplatz canine duct occluder (ACDO; **Figures 26.16D** and **26.17**; and **Figure 6.15**, p. 180) has advantages over coils or other occlusion devices, although it is not suitable for all cases. The ACDO is a self-expanding nitinol mesh device designed for the typical canine ductal morphology. The ACDO is inserted through an arterial delivery catheter that has been positioned in the ductus. When deployed, the ACDO takes the shape of a flattened disk on

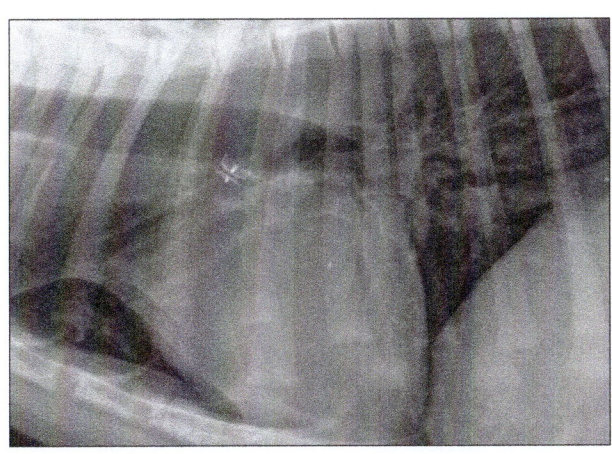

Figure 26.17 The patent ductus arteriosus of this 6-month-old German Shepherd Dog was closed using a catheter-delivered Amplatz Canine Duct Occluder.

one end and a cupped disk on the other, separated by a short narrow waist. The flat disk is deployed within the PA and brought snug against the ductal opening to the PA, so that the waist of the device straddles the ductal opening. Then the cupped disk is deployed within the ductal ampulla.

Other ductal occlusion methods that have been used successfully include wire coils (single or multiple) that incorporate thrombogenic Dacron tufts, and other vascular occluding devices including plugs placed within the ductus. The ACDO is easier to place, is associated with fewer complications, and has a higher rate of initial occlusion success compared to other transcatheter techniques. However, because of size limitations, occlusion using a coil, small vascular plug, or surgery might be necessary in small puppies, toy breed dogs, and cats. Vascular access for transcatheter ductal occlusion usually is via the femoral artery, although a brachial artery approach also is described. A transvenous approach can be used for retrograde device (coil, small vascular plug, or ACDO) delivery into the ductus; this often is the preferred access in patients with small femoral artery size. See Chapter 6 for additional details.

Accurate determination of ductal morphology and minimal internal ductal diameter are critical for appropriate device selection and sizing during transcatheter closure, in order to effectively achieve ductal occlusion and minimize risk of device embolization. There is no good correlation between patient size or weight and ductal diameter, so measurements are important in each case. Although TTE can provide an estimate of minimum ductal diameter and ductal morphology during planning for the transcatheter approach (and the occlusion device sizes likely to be needed), TTE tends to overestimate minimal ductal diameter. Therefore, other measurements also are needed during the occlusion procedure. Fluoroscopy and angiography generally are used for final device sizing, although TEE often provides even better visualization of ductal anatomy, with the advantage of reducing radiation and radiopaque contrast exposure. Often,

both techniques are employed; as noted, TEE is considered more accurate for measuring minimal ductal diameter than TTE. The 2D mode should be used for measurement because color-flow Doppler imaging results in overestimation (on both TTE and TEE). TEE alone has been used successfully to guide ACDO placement and assess occlusion. However, probe size might not be appropriate or imaging clarity adequate for all cases, so fluoroscopy with angiography might still be required. Infrequently, TTE is used to guide ACDO placement, although visualization often is less optimal. Intracardiac and 3D echocardiography modes present other possible options for guiding ductal closure, although equipment availability is a limitation.

Transcatheter occlusion might not be possible or suitable for some patients. Usually this includes very small dogs and cats, although some operators are successful with device closure in dogs even smaller than 2.5 kg. Patients with a large type III ductus, and those with pulmonary arterial or ductal wall dissection, should have the ductus surgically ligated. Ductal closure in cats usually is by surgical ligation, although coil embolization also can be successful. A low-profile ACDO device (Stauthammer, 2015) currently is unavailable, but a type 4 Amplatz vascular plug can be delivered via a standard (0.038" lumen) catheter. Although ACDO placement has been successful in some dogs with type III ductus, effective placement might be elusive, especially when the ductus is large. Coil occlusion is not advised for type III ductus and surgical ligation usually is recommended.

Complications have occurred in about 1–3% of ACDO patients, in contrast to the 25–33% complication rate reported in patients undergoing coil procedures. Major complications associated with transcatheter procedures include hemorrhage at the femoral artery puncture site, hemorrhage from aortic puncture by a catheter stylet, systemic arterial coil embolization with visceral ischemic injury, and death. Major hemorrhage and systemic coil embolization are associated with high risk of mortality. Minor complications associated with coil techniques have included coil embolization into the PA (with occurrence rates of 0–46%), minor hemorrhage, coil protrusion into the aorta, hemolysis with hemoglobinuria and thrombocytopenia, and seroma or infection at the femoral arterial puncture site. Usually no clinical adverse effects result from coil embolization into a PA, although coil retrieval can be pursued when straightforward. Ductal recanalization can occur, especially with coil occlusion. Device infection with its associated thrombosis, hematogenous pneumonia, and septicemia, seem rare but have been reported. Treatment involves medical therapy for the infection, with surgical coil removal and ductal resection. Reported complications associated with ductal occlusion in cats include hemorrhage, left-sided laryngeal paralysis, voice change, fever, chylothorax, and death (Hutton, 2015).

Surgical Ductal Ligation Surgical ligation was the standard for ductal closure until the ACDO device became available, and it is an excellent treatment in the hands of a surgeon sufficiently trained and experienced with the operation. Ligation is recommended most often now for cats, for dogs too small for interventional devices, for dogs with type III ductal anatomy, and when an experienced interventional cardiologist is unavailable. Previously, surgical success rates at specialty centers consistently exceeded 92%. However, today surgical success rates and complications depend very much on the experience of the operator. One obvious downside to the proliferation of (less invasive) catheter-based interventions has been the decline in number of surgeons who are highly proficient and experienced with this operation. The reported rate of major complications has been greater for surgical (10–12%) compared to transcatheter (0–4%) procedures in some more recent reports (Singh, 2012; Ranganathan, 2018). Success and complication rates are very surgeon-specific and major complication rates have been as low as 1% and as high as 40% or greater over various referral centers (unpublished observations).

Older and larger dogs have increased risk of death with surgical ligation according to some, but not all, studies. Similarly, some studies report no relation between PDA-associated MR prior to surgery and the probability of survival, while others indicate an association between concurrent MR and increased mortality. The rate of minor complications is comparable between open surgical and transcatheter approaches in some reports.

There are several surgical techniques for PDA occlusion. The most common are the standard ductal dissection technique and the Jackson-Henderson technique, approached via left lateral thoracotomy. The standard ductal dissection technique, compared to the Jackson-Henderson technique, has been associated with fewer intraoperative complications and a lower rate of residual ductal flow. Use of vascular clips rather than suture ligatures can be successful; however, incomplete ductal closure or clip slippage and persistent ductal flow can occur, especially with a large ductus. Other techniques described include intrapericardial PDA dissection and ligation, and a thoracoscopic approach using titanium ligation clips.

Beyond failure to sufficiently occlude the ductus, major surgical complications include severe intraoperative hemorrhage (in 0–12% of cases), lung lobe damage requiring lobectomy, cardiac arrest, respiratory insufficiency requiring ventilator therapy, mesenteric torsion, chylothorax, infection, pneumothorax, arrhythmias, and heart failure. Surgical mortality most often relates to massive hemorrhage. Minor complications associated with surgery can include left forelimb lameness, suture reaction, postoperative hypoxia, incisional seroma, minor hemorrhage, transient mild hemoptysis, and recurrent laryngeal nerve damage leading to laryngeal paralysis. Residual ductal flow following the procedure contributes to persistent volume overload and could predispose to ductal recanalization or endocarditis.

Changes and Prognosis Following Ductal Closure

Residual shunting, silent to auscultation, is commonly noted by color Doppler in the immediate postoperative period. This is true with both device and surgical closure procedures, although the amount of residual flow with an ACDO is much less than for older coil-based occlusion techniques. From a practical standpoint, the absence of a postoperative continuous murmur indicates effective ductal closure and a successful procedure, regardless of residual flow visualized by color Doppler. Residual flow immediately post-procedure occurs in about one-quarter to one-half of coil occlusion cases, especially with moderate to larger ductal diameter or when only a single coil is deployed. However, final cumulative closure rates are much higher. Use of more than one coil for a larger ductus reduces the rate of residual shunt, but increases risk of coil embolization. When a continuous murmur persists, the procedure should not be considered fully successful; however, if the shunt is sufficiently attenuated then significant hemodynamic improvement can occur. Dogs with faint to soft residual murmurs of PDA often develop complete ductal closure over time, although this is less likely if the post-procedure murmur is moderate to loud.

Ductal recanalization can occur after surgical ligation as well as after transcatheter occlusion. In dogs, the frequency of PDA recanalization after surgical treatment is estimated to be between 1 and 19%. It is likely that some cases of "recanalization" in the literature were simply lack of sufficient closure at the time of surgery. When a continuous murmur persists and Doppler studies show significant shunting then coils can be used to achieve complete occlusion. A small residual flow does not appear to affect survival.

After successful occlusion, significant regression of cardiac enlargement (remodeling) generally occurs over time. Radiographic heart size decreases post-closure, although it might not completely normalize. The dilation in the ascending and cranial descending aorta (ductus bump) usually persists. QRS complex voltage tends to decrease after closure, as left heart enlargement regresses. The pre-closure increase in aortic outflow velocity should resolve post-closure. Aortic and pulmonic valve insufficiencies, if present, tend to persist, probably because of valve annulus dilation.

Residual ductal flow that is audible, or a concurrent acquired heart disease, reduces the regression of remodeling changes, as does impaired systolic function prior to ductal closure. LV systolic dysfunction improves after closure in about half of cases, although poor baseline fractional shortening is unlikely to normalize. It is emphasized, however, that fractional shortening is only one method for estimating LV systolic function, and reduced values should be substantiated by other 2D methods for assessing LV ejection fraction and systolic function. Dogs with severe MR, AF, large residual shunt, or marked aortic regurgitation (AR) post-occlusion are more likely to have persistent left heart dilation and reduced LV function, as are dogs that are older at time of ductal closure. Although LV function might not normalize after occlusion, many of these dogs have no clinical signs. Any long-term medical treatment should be determined on a case by case basis. Acquired (degenerative, myxomatous) mitral valve disease commonly develops in older dogs with PDA, even in some of larger breeds; this can interfere with reverse remodeling.

Long-term prognosis generally is good to excellent after successful ductal closure, with a normal life span expected, especially in young dogs without other complications. Factors associated with decreased survival time after successful closure include concurrent congenital heart malformation(s), clinical signs of CHF, and severe MR that persists after ductal closure (usually related to concurrent left heart enlargement and acquired heart disease). Long-term prognosis is particularly poor for dogs with all of these conditions. One large case review (Saunders, 2014) reported that, in dogs without other congenital malformations, ductal closure produced a median lifespan 10 years longer than if the ductus had not been closed (12 vs. 2 year median survival time). In dogs with concurrent congenital disease, PDA closure increased survival time by a mean of 6 years. PDA closure in cats generally yields a good long-term outcome. Mean survival time after ductal closure in cats with PDA alone appears to be about 2.5 years. Survival time is shorter in those with multiple defects (Wustefeld-Janssens, 2016). The procedure complication rate appears to be <15%, but can include death (Bascunan, 2017).

Conversely, for most dogs where the ductus is not closed, CHF is the eventual outcome and usually develops within a year of diagnosis. Cats not treated also might be more likely to die eventually of cardiac disease. Precapillary PH can occur in either species. Shunt reversal in dogs is unlikely to occur after four to six months of age. In cats, progressive increase in pulmonary vascular resistance can occur, and can respond to sildenafil and eventual ductus closure.

Reversed Patent Ductus Arteriosus (Right-to-Left Shunting)

Animals with "reversed" PDA (rPDA) represent a small fraction of all PDA cases. Female Cocker Spaniels may be at increased risk. Animals with rPDA generally have a large ductal diameter. Increased pulmonary vascular resistance, associated with reactive vasoconstriction and pulmonary arteriopathy lesions, induces precapillary PH. Whenever PA pressure exceeds aortic pressure, shunt flow reverses direction. With severe PH, flow reversal can be continuous throughout the cardiac cycle. However, bidirectional shunting is observed most often during color Doppler imaging, with flow direction determined by whichever pressure is higher at any instant. Exercise usually reduces systemic vascular resistance, facilitating R-to-L shunting. Conversely, O_2 therapy and sildenafil usually can reduce pulmonary vascular resistance and increase L-to-R shunting. Pulmonary arterial reactivity, compared to fixed anatomic arterial wall changes, determines the responsiveness of these vessels to therapeutic interventions.

The sequelae of rPDA generally are similar to those seen with other causes of reversed shunting (p. 437) and include RV hypertrophy with dilation, and main PA dilation. However, an important difference with rPDA relates to the ductus' anatomical location distal to the aortic arch (**Figure 26.5**). With rPDA, the cranial body receives normally oxygenated blood via the brachycephalic trunk and left subclavian artery, which arise from the aortic arch (upstream from the ductus). Deoxygenated blood from the pulmonary trunk flows through the ductus into the cranial descending aorta (**Figure 26.18**). Therefore, signs

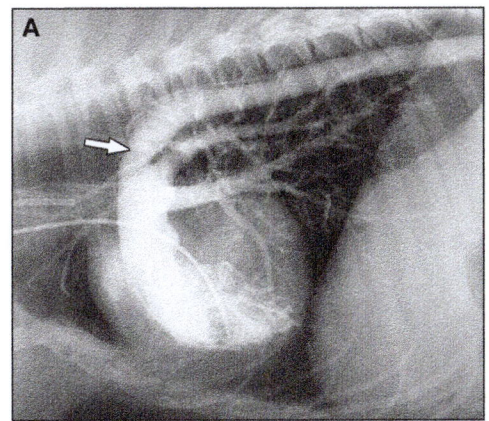 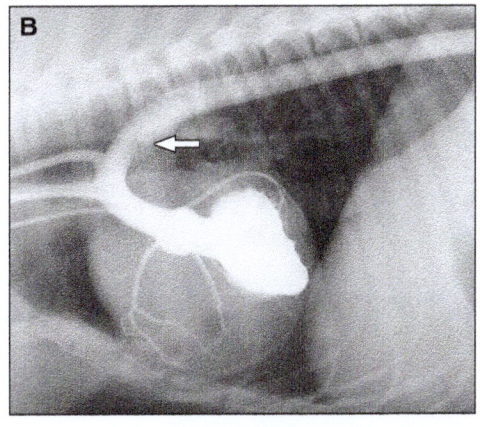

Figure 26.18 Right (A) and left (B) ventricular angiocardiograms from an 8-month-old female Cocker Spaniel with reversed patent ductus arteriosus. (A) Opacified blood flows from the hypertrophied right ventricle (RV) to the dilated pulmonary trunk and into the descending aorta via the large ductus (arrow). (B) The relatively small left ventricle appears perched atop the large RV. Note that the brachycephalic and left subclavian arteries exit the aorta upstream from the area of the ductus (arrow). Dilution of dye within the descending aorta results from mixing with unopacified blood entering from across the ductus. (From Ware WA & Ward JW. Congenital cardiac disease. In, Nelson RW & Couto GC (editors). Small Animal Internal Medicine. 6th edition. Elsevier, St. Louis, MO. 2019. p. 115.)

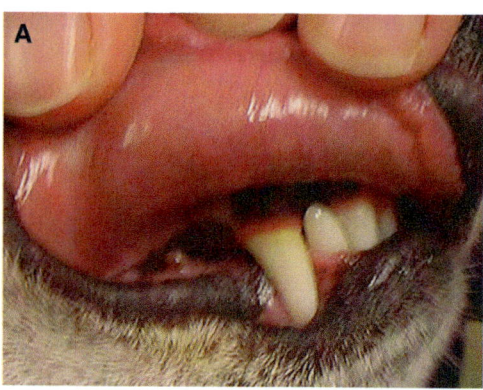 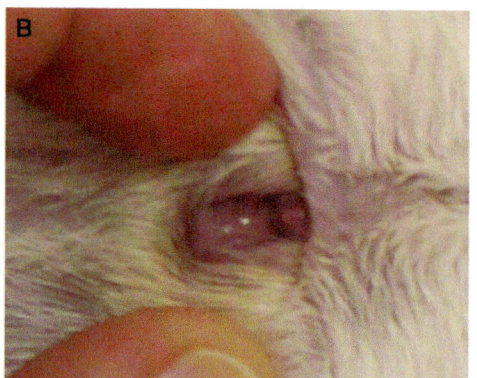

Figure 26.19 The oral mucous membranes (A) are pink, however, caudal (vaginal) membranes (B) are cyanotic in a female Rat Terrier with reversed patent ductus arteriosus. This is known as differential cyanosis.

of hypoxemia, such as weakness and cyanosis, are manifest in the caudal body. *Differential cyanosis* refers to the finding of cyanotic caudal membranes (vulvar, preputial) while cranial (oral) membranes remain pink; it is a hallmark of rPDA (**Figure 26.19**).

Clinical Features

The history and clinical presentation in patients with rPDA are similar to those associated with T of F and other reversed shunts. Exercise intolerance, shortness of breath, collapse (especially with exercise or excitement), syncope and seizures are common complaints. However, an important diagnostic clue with rPDA is progressive weakness or collapse particularly in the hindlimbs, usually associated with activity (**Figure 26.20**). This can be confused with clinical signs of myasthenia gravis. In severe rPDA cases seizures, cough, hemoptysis, and sudden death also can occur.

Cyanosis (typically differential cyanosis) might be evident at rest or only with exercise or excitement. If the hematocrit is only mildly elevated, or mucous membranes are pigmented, cyanosis can be difficult to identify. Other subtle physical examination findings include a pronounced right precordial impulse and jugular pulsations (giant a waves).

Femoral pulses are normal. There is no continuous murmur with rPDA. A soft systolic murmur might be heard at the left heart base, although often no murmur is audible because of increased blood viscosity or minimal pressure gradient across the shunt. The S_2 sound can be split or loud and "snapping," as is common with PH (**Figure 26.21**). A gallop sound is heard occasionally. Overt right-sided CHF is rare, although sporadic cases of rPDA-associated CHF, with systemic venous congestion and ascites, have occurred in dogs, and especially in cats with rPDA (Greet, 2021).

Diagnostic Tests

A complete blood count (CBC) usually shows an increased PCV in animals with predominantly R-to-L shunting. In cases where the diagnosis is in question, comparison of blood gas results from caudal (for example, metatarsal) and cranial (such as auricular) arteries can confirm the presence of differential hypoxemia. Supplemental O_2 administration does not substantially improve hypoxemia in cases of R-to-L shunt.

Thoracic radiographs usually show right heart enlargement, a prominent pulmonary trunk, and a bulge in the descending aorta (ductus bump; **Figure 26.22**). The lobar

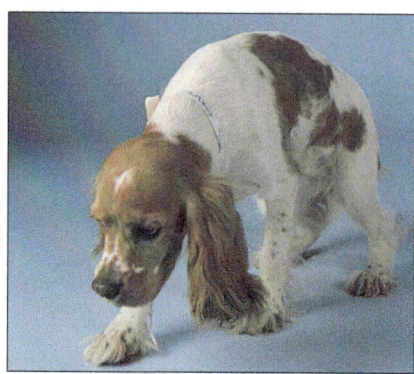

Figure 26.20 Hindlimb weakness was the presenting complaint in the dog of **Figure 26.18**.

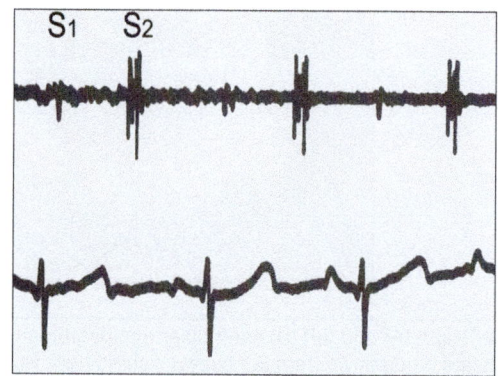

Figure 26.21 Phonocardiogram (top) depicts the relatively loud, snapping, and split S_2 sound recorded from the dog of **Figure 26.18**. No murmur was audible. Lead II electrocardiogram (at bottom); the dog's right axis deviation caused the abnormal QRS configuration.

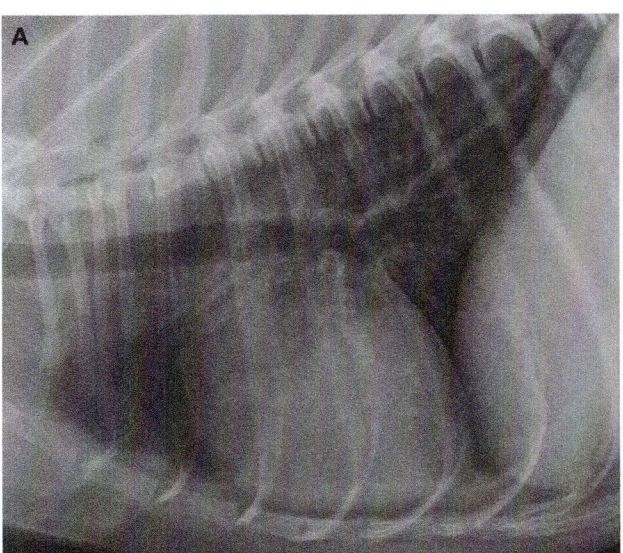
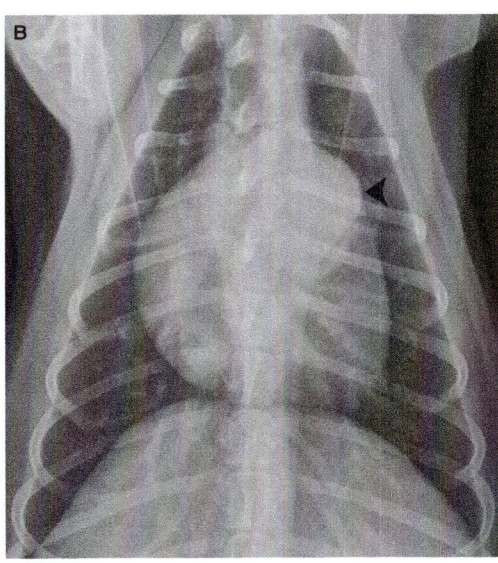

Figure 26.22 Lateral (A) and dorsoventral (B) thoracic radiographs from a 6-year-old female mixed-breed dog with reversed patent ductus arteriosus. Note the right ventricular enlargement (both views) and large ductus bump (B, arrowhead).

pulmonary arteries might appear tortuous and proximally widened; sometimes the caudal vena cava is dilated (**Figure 26.23**). The left heart usually is not enlarged with rPDA. The ECG typically indicates RV and, sometimes, RA enlargement, with a right axis deviation (**Figure 26.24**).

Echocardiography demonstrates the RV hypertrophy and enlargement, with septal flattening and a widened pulmonary trunk. In some cases, the large ductus creates the appearance of a trifurcation of the main PA (**Figure 26.25**). In other cases, it can be difficult to clearly distinguish the ductus because of surrounding lung. Color Doppler shows a normal flow pattern toward the left and right PA branches, rather than a continuous retrograde jet into the main PA. However, if pulmonary and systemic pressures are nearly equivalent, bidirectional shunting is evident at different times during the cardiac cycle. High-velocity pulmonary regurgitation often is seen, secondary to pulmonary annular dilation and high PA pressures. Generally, rPDA is documented by imaging the abdominal aorta during a venous echocontrast injection (saline bubble

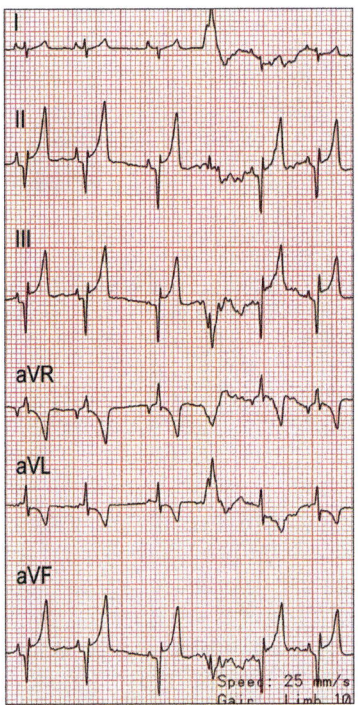

Figure 26.23 Lateral radiograph from an 8-year-old female Boston Terrier newly diagnosed with reversed patent ductus arteriosus. Note the prominent caudal lobar pulmonary arteries and distended caudal vena cava. This dog's presentation was atypical because she had overt signs of right-sided congestive heart failure (ascites).

Figure 26.24 ECG from a young Cocker Spaniel with reversed PDA shows sinus rhythm with one ventricular premature complex (4th QRS from left), cranial axis deviation, RV hypertrophy (S wave in lead I), and secondary ST & T wave changes in caudal leads.

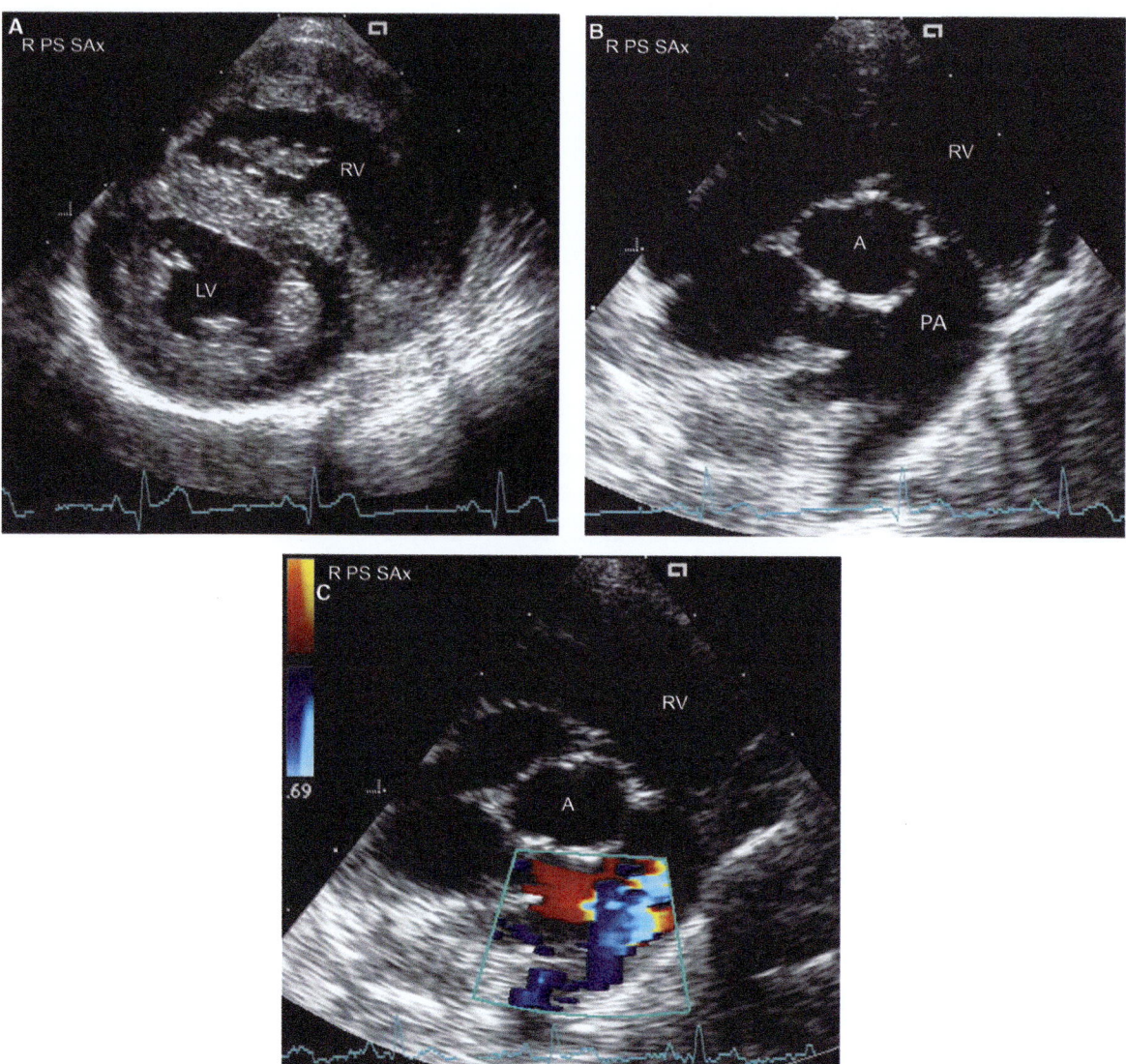

Figure 26.25 (A) Right parasternal short-axis view (R PS SAx) at the ventricular level from a male Sheltie puppy with reversed patent ductus arteriosus. The right ventricular wall is thicker than the left and the septum is mildly flattened. (B) At the heart base, the PA appears to separate into three branches in this dog (from top to bottom: right and left lobar arteries and the large ductus). (C) Same orientation as in (B); color-flow Doppler shows that flow through the ductus (coded blue) is moving away from transducer and out of the main PA (toward the descending aorta). A, aorta; LV, left ventricle; PA, pulmonary artery; RV, right ventricle.

study; **Figure 26.26**). One also might be able to see bubbles flowing from the main PA through a large ductus into the cranial descending aorta, especially using the left cranial views. Measurement of a tricuspid (or pulmonary) regurgitation jet peak velocity allows estimation of RV systolic and (in the absence of PS or other RV outflow obstruction) PA pressures (p. 828).

Although the diagnosis generally is evident from echo-Doppler study and other clinical tests, cardiac catheterization and angiography can confirm the diagnosis, and the severity of PH and systemic hypoxemia (**Figure 26.18**). Cardiac catheterization is especially valuable in cases where the shunt still is largely L-to-R and the responses to pulmonary vasodilators or transient occlusion of the ductus with a balloon catheter might be evaluated. Nuclear scintigraphy (with 99mTc-macroaggregated albumin) occasionally has been used as a diagnostic tool, as well. A sharp cut-off in radioactivity occurs at the level of forelimbs and neck with rPDA, because the shunt flows from PA into the descending aorta.

Management

Ductal closure generally is contraindicated in animals with severe PH and shunt reversal. In such cases, ductal closure is likely to promote development of fatal hypotension from acute RV failure, rather than clinical improvement. Similar to a pressure "pop-off" valve, the rPDA allows increasing shunt volume to flow from the pulmonary to systemic circulation, especially during exercise or other times when pulmonary

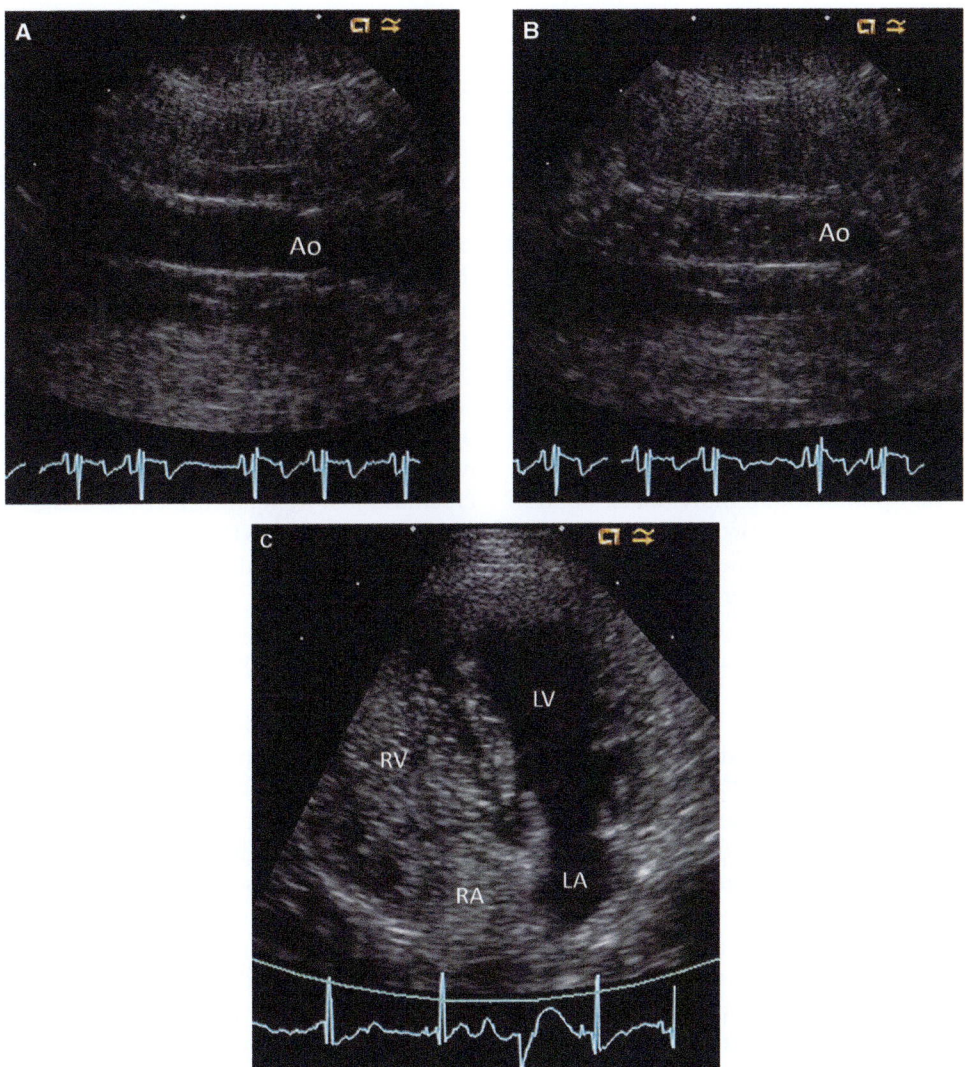

Figure 26.26 Echocontrast studies from the dog of **Figure 26.22**. (A) The abdominal aorta is shown just before an injection of agitated sterile saline into a cephalic vein. (B) Shortly after the injection, echo-"bubbles" appear in the aorta, verifying a right-to-left shunt (the microbubbles cannot pass through the lung). (C) Left apical four-chamber cardiac image recorded immediately after another injection of agitated saline. There is opacification of the RA and RV, as expected; however, no bubbles appear in the left heart indicating that the shunt is extracardiac. Ao, (abdominal) aorta; LA, left atrium; LV, left ventricle; RA, right atrium; RV, right ventricle.

resistance increases even further (compared to systemic resistance). Exceptions to this general contraindication can occur in animals with lesser degrees of PH, where predominantly L-to-R shunting occurs, or when PH responds well to treatment with a phosphodiesterase-5 (PDE-5) inhibitor such as sildenafil. In some of these cases, blocking the excess flow (L-to-R shunting) through the pulmonary circulation has allowed pulmonary vascular resistance and pressure to decline. Cats with severe PH and CHF (including right-sided CHF) have been successfully treated with surgical ligation if predominately L-to-R shunting is present at catheterization.

Medical therapy for rPDA involves exercise restriction, PDE-5 inhibitor therapy aimed at reducing pulmonary vascular resistance, and management of secondary erythrocytosis to minimize signs of hyperviscosity. Hydration is important to prevent hemoconcentration, so sufficient fresh water should be provided. This is especially crucial for dogs that are crated or otherwise might have restricted access. Lightly salting the food can encourage fluid intake. Parenteral fluid therapy is indicated for patients that develop gastrointestinal signs sufficient to prevent drinking. Additionally, fluid therapy often is administered when phlebotomy is performed. Exercise restriction also is important because exercise-induced decreases in systemic vascular resistance facilitate greater R-to-L shunting.

PDE-5 inhibitors reduce pulmonary resistance via nitric-oxide-dependent vasodilation, and thereby can reduce PH and severity of R-to-L shunting. In some patients, clinical signs improve quite dramatically. Sildenafil citrate is the PDE-5 inhibitor used most commonly. Doses of 1–3 mg/kg q8 or 12 hours generally are well-tolerated and improve clinical status in some cases (see p. 834 for more information). Other (non-PDE-5 inhibitor) vasodilator drugs produce greater systemic effects than those on the pulmonary vasculature; therefore, they are of little benefit and can even be detrimental. Low-dose antiplatelet therapy (with clopidogrel or aspirin) also might be helpful in animals with PH and reversed shunt, but this is not well studied.

Periodic phlebotomy, and infrequently, hydroxyurea therapy are used to prevent the hematocrit from rising excessively (in most cases, this means >65%). Alternatively, periodic hirudotherapy (use of medicinal leeches) has been described to manage erythrocytosis; the authors do not have personal experience with this method. Ideally, the patient's PCV is maintained at a level where signs of hyperviscosity (including rear limb weakness, shortness of breath, lethargy) are minimal. A PCV of about 62% sometimes is recommended, however this might not be optimal for all individuals. Caution is needed to avoid a PCV that is too low for the particular patient (usually less than ~55%). One method for phlebotomy is to remove 5–10 mL blood per kg body weight and administer an equal volume of isotonic fluid. Another technique involves removing 10% of the circulating blood volume initially without fluid replacement. Circulating blood volume (mL) is calculated as 8.5% × body weight (kg) × 1000 g/kg × 1 mL/g. After 3–6 hours of cage rest, an additional volume of blood is removed if the patient's initial PCV was >60%. This additional volume would be 5–10% of the circulating blood volume if initial PCV was between 60 and 70%, or an additional 10–18% if initial PCV was >70% (Côté, 2001).

Hydroxyurea (40–50 mg/kg by mouth q48h or three times/week) has been used as an alternative or adjunct to periodic phlebotomy in some dogs with refractory secondary erythrocytosis. Consultation with an oncologist is advised before using this drug. The CBC and platelet count should be monitored weekly or biweekly to start. Dosage adjustments are made as needed over time to maintain the desired PCV. Adverse effects of hydroxyurea can include anorexia, vomiting, bone marrow hypoplasia, alopecia, and pruritus. The dose can be divided q12h on treatment days, or administered twice weekly, or at <40 mg/kg depending on the patient's response.

Long-term prognosis generally is poor for animals with rPDA. Nevertheless, some patients have been managed successfully well into middle age and beyond. Complications from chronic hypoxemia and hyperviscosity are common, as is sudden death.

Ventricular Septal Defect (Left-to-Right Shunting)

Interventricular septal formation during fetal development proceeds from the apical region and extends dorsally. Simplistically, the growing septal tissues fuse with the septal portion of the atrioventricular cushions and conus arteriosus development of which continues as the truncus arteriosus and from which the great arteries are derived. The normal interventricular septum consists mostly of a large muscular wall that separates the two ventricles. Frequently, the ventricular septum is referred to as having inlet and outlet parts; however, much of the RV inflow septum is in anatomic continuity with the LV outflow septum, so this designation is at best relevant only to the right side. Within the right ventricle, the muscular ridge known as the supraventricular crest (*crista supraventricularis*) delineates inlet and outlet segments of the right ventricle. A trabecular band – most prominent in horses – extends from near the apical RV septum and joins the supraventricular crest and the muscular infundibulum that projects toward the pulmonary valve. The septum beyond the supraventricular crest is a freestanding muscular sleeve that is unrelated to the LV outflow tract when development is normal. At the dorsal RV inlet septum, caudal to the supraventricular crest and just beneath the cranial edge of the septal tricuspid leaflet is the comparably tiny membranous (fibrous) portion of the interventricular septum. This fibrous septum extends to the left side just below the right and noncoronary cusps of the aortic valve. Thus, the membranous septum relates the subaortic LV outflow tract to the atrioventricular septum on the right side. Each of the aforementioned structures are relevant to understanding the pathology, as well as the echocardiographic and clinical features of VSDs. Traditionally, VSDs are classified by location as perimembranous, juxta- or subarterial, inlet, or muscular. Modern classifications classify VSDs not just on "geography," but also by the structures adjacent to the defect's borders and the defect's relationship to the conduction system, as emphasized by Anderson and colleagues (1984). In reality, there is considerable variation among VSDs and some defects demonstrate characteristics of more than one type.

Most VSDs in dogs, cats and horses are perimembranous (infracristal), situated ventral to the right and noncoronary cusps of the aortic valve on the left (**Figure 26.27**) and located beneath the cranial edge of the septal tricuspid leaflet (at the junction of the septal and parietal leaflets) on the right. Typically, the aortic valve leaflets and septal tricuspid leaflet are in continuity across the defect, although persistent muscular tissue sometimes is found below the aortic valve in what are termed central perimembranous VSDs. Depending on the location of the perimembranous VSD, the septal tricuspid and anterior mitral leaflets might be in continuity across the defect. Large septal defects can be perimembranous, but also extend substantially toward the RV inlet or outlet; the latter is usual with T of F. There can be a variable degree of malalignment between the supraventricular crest and RV outlet septum, relative to the trabecular band and aortic root. In such cases, aortic valve leaflets might be visible through the VSD, and prolapse of the right or noncoronary aortic cusp can occur. Although a prolapsed aortic cusp can partially occlude the VSD, this also fosters aortic regurgitation. This situation seems especially prevalent in horses, where some degree of aortic-to-septal malalignment is common. It also occurs in dogs, for example, in English Springer Spaniels

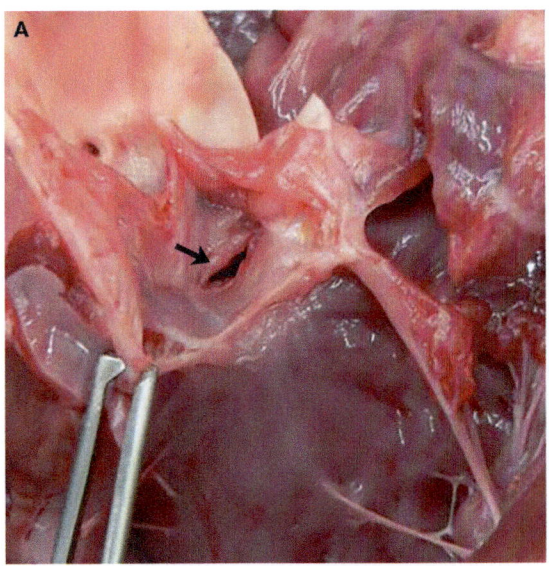
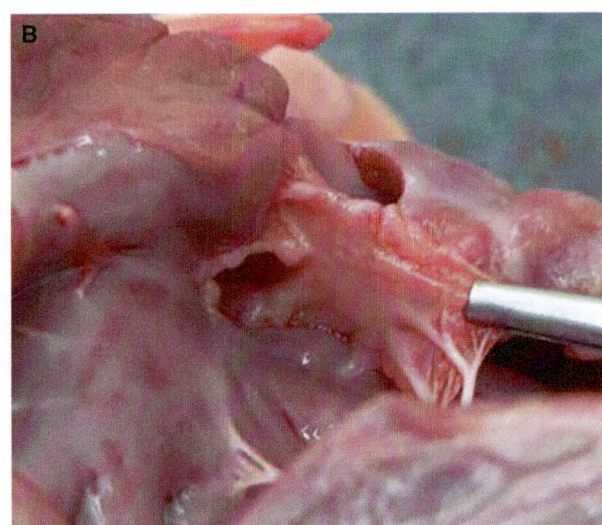

Figure 26.27 (A) A typical location for ventricular septal defect (VSD, arrow) is just ventral to the noncoronary and right coronary cusps of the aortic valve in the membranous septum. (B) On the right, the VSD opens under the cranial edge of the septal tricuspid valve leaflet. Specimen is from a 4-month-old male Golden Retriever that also had severe subaortic stenosis; the prominent fibrous ring is visible ventral to the VSD in (A).

with a large malalignment VSD. When a membranous VSD is beneath the edge of the septal tricuspid leaflet, scarring of the leaflet, fibrous tissue proliferation, or both might partially or completely occlude it. In the latter case, a ventricular septal aneurysm is formed (Thomas, 2005). A large unrestrictive, perimembranous VSD that extends into the supraventricular crest is a typical component of the T of F/pulmonary atresia complex.

Other VSD locations are less common in dogs, cats and horses. Abnormal fusion or absence of the pulmonary infundibular sleeve produces a supracristal, juxtarterial VSD. This places the aortic and pulmonary valves in fibrous continuity. When the VSD is located directly under the pulmonary valve, it often is termed an "uncommitted" defect (as well as a subarterial and subpulmonic VSD, just to make the nomenclature more confusing!). This appears to be the second most common type of VSD in dogs, and a defect observed in horses, as well. These lesions are likely to reduce support for the aortic valve leaflets and allow Venturi hydraulics to suck the right coronary cusp into the defect. A marked prolapse of the right coronary cusp, or an aortic root aneurysm protruding into the subarterial VSD, can result; consequently, severe aortic regurgitation with its accompanying diastolic murmur develops in some animals. Another form of VSD involves malformation of the embryonic AV septum and endocardial cushions. This causes an inlet VSD, located ventral to the septal tricuspid or bridging AV valve leaflet (see "Atrioventricular Septal Defect"). Rarely, a VSD can involve the muscular inlet or trabecular portions of the interventricular septum, in the inlet, mid- or apical, or outlet ventricular regions. Such defects are bordered by muscle. Even rarer is the Gerbode defect, a LV-to-RA shunt (or LV-to-RV and then -to-RA shunt, via tricuspid regurgitation). The Gerbode defect can occur as a congenital lesion, or be secondary to infective endocarditis or thoracic trauma. All these have occurred in dogs.

A VSD often is associated with other complex congenital heart lesions, that are largely beyond the scope of this textbook. A VSD is found in double-outlet right ventricle, where both great vessels originate from the right ventricle. The location of the VSD is variable and might be related to one, or uncommitted to either, of the great arteries which can be normally related, transposed, or exhibit malpositioning relative to each other. Persistent truncus arteriosus is a malformation where partitioning of the fetal common trunk does not occur and the pulmonary circulation stems directly from the truncal vessel (also see Chapter 28). It has occurred more frequently in horses and cats. Most often, the type I (single PA) form is seen, although a mature dog was reported with type III (with two PA branches). The common truncal valve can be abnormal (including quadricuspid) and there is no pulmonary valve. The common arterial trunk supplies blood to coronary, pulmonary and systemic circulations. As with T of F, some affected animals have marked hypoxemia with erythrocytosis; although, if pulmonary circulation is sufficient the patient could be relatively asymptomatic or exhibit signs of a L-to-R shunt.

As pulmonary resistance declines after birth, a VSD imposes a volume overload on the lungs and left heart. The more common "high" septal defects (perimembranous or juxta-arterial) allow the shunt volume to flow across the defect from the left ventricle into the PA, such that most of the systolic work is performed by the left ventricle. Unlike with an ASD, the right ventricle is not volume overloaded and RV enlargement is variable and frequently absent. In contrast, the left atrium and left ventricle collect the shunt volume and perform additional volume work. The shunt volume depends on the defect's size and the relative pressures on either side. Most flow occurs in systole because the pressure gradient across the VSD is highest then. With a restrictive (small) VSD, there is a large systolic pressure gradient (with normal LV and RV pressures), high-velocity shunting (~4.5 to 5 m/s), and a comparably small shunt volume. Small defects usually are clinically unimportant, although some left heart enlargement can be anticipated. Moderate to large defects cause substantial left heart enlargement and predispose to left-sided or biventricular CHF. When a VSD becomes unrestrictive, pressures across the defect equilibrate and both ventricles function essentially as a common chamber, leading to the development of RV hypertrophy and enlargement. Pulmonary vascular injury that results in severe precapillary PH and shunt reversal (Eisenmenger's VSD) is more likely to occur with such nonrestrictive defects (p. 460). Shunt flow volume (as well as direction) associated with a large defect depends mainly on the relative vascular resistances (and therefore pressures) in the pulmonary and systemic circulations. Shunt reversal also is more likely with concurrent PS (see section "Tetralogy of Fallot"), or in the setting of an intra-RV obstruction called double-chambered right ventricle. The latter defect often is associated with a VSD, and might stem from a RV myocardial tissue response to the high-velocity jet crossing the VSD.

As noted, AR occurs in some animals with a VSD, especially those with a large perimembranous malalignment defect or a juxta-arterial (subpulmonic) defect. The AR results from inadequate anatomic support for the aortic root, with prolapse of the right or noncoronary cusp of the aortic valve into the defect. AR places an additional volume load on the left ventricle and is perhaps the most common reason for CHF in dogs with otherwise restrictive VSDs.

The conduction system of the heart might be affected by a VSD, depending on its location relative to the apex of the triangle of Koch. Although AV block is rare, other conduction defects might be seen. In the uncommon situation of operative closure of a VSD, the surgeon must be cognizant that inexact suture placement can cause iatrogenic AV block, necessitating external cardiac pacing. Congenital VSD, like PDA, is considered a risk factor for endocarditis in people. Vegetative lesions tend to occur on the right (downstream) side of the shunt where turbulence is greater. Endocarditis associated with congenital VSD has been observed only rarely in dogs.

Clinical Features

VSD appears to be more prevalent in some canine breeds (**Table 26.1**); it could have an increased association with PS and with double-chambered right ventricle. VSD is the most common congenital defect reported in cats and in horses. Arabian horses have a higher prevalence of VSD, as well as congenital heart defects in general. Standardbreds also might be overrepresented. VSD can occur as an isolated defect or it can accompany other malformations. Concurrent defects, especially T of F, were found in half of the foals examined in one case series (Hall, 2010).

Most dogs and cats do not see a veterinarian until 6 to 8 weeks of age and it is likely that many with an unrestrictive VSD die from CHF before that visit. The vast majority of dogs and cats with VSD, that are seen by cardiologists, have a small restrictive defect which rarely causes clinical signs and can be an incidental finding. But even small septal defects are likely to produce some left-sided cardiomegaly. In children, isolated VSDs with approximately 1.5-to-1, pulmonary-to-systemic, flow ratios usually are well-tolerated. Thus, mild to moderate cardiomegaly should not raise an immediate call for medication or PA banding. Larger L-to-R shunts are likely to cause reduced exercise tolerance and potentially can lead to left-sided CHF, although this is rare in dogs without concurrent defect(s) or audible AR. Horses and cats seem more likely to survive with larger septal defects, and might develop CHF or more gradually progressive PH in the future.

Physical examination findings with L-to-R VSD include pink membranes, normal jugular vein appearance, normal to caudally displaced left precordial impulse (from cardiomegaly), and possibly, a precordial thrill where the murmur is loudest. Characteristic auscultatory findings include a holosystolic murmur, usually loudest at the cranial right sternal border (corresponding to the direction of shunt flow for perimembranous VSD). However, the murmur's point of maximal intensity (PMI) can vary, depending on the anatomical location of the VSD. For example, the murmur PMI of juxta-arterial VSD is at the cranial left base, while that of a muscular VSD or a partially closed defect with a fibrous baffle might be focused near the right apical area. A large L-to-R shunt volume also causes relative or functional PS, accompanied by a systolic ejection murmur at the left base and possibly a split S_2. When AR accompanies the VSD, a corresponding diastolic decrescendo murmur might be heard at the left base; however, if the AR jet is angled toward the right ventricle, the diastolic murmur might be louder over the right hemithorax. Marked AR also causes hyperkinetic arterial pulses.

Diagnostic Tests

Radiographic findings depend on VSD size and shunt volume (**Table 26.2**). Large L-to-R shunts cause left heart enlargement and pulmonary overcirculation; however, RV enlargement also occurs if the defect is very large, pulmonary vascular resistance increases causing PH, or there is any degree of RV outflow obstruction. A large shunt volume can dilate the main pulmonary trunk (**Figure 26.28**), as can PH, although Eisenmenger's pathophysiology is associated with reduced peripheral pulmonary vascular markings.

The ECG could be normal or it might suggest LA or LV enlargement. Sometimes, "fractionated" or splintered QRS complexes are seen, suggesting intraventricular conduction disturbance. An RV enlargement pattern usually indicates a very large defect, PH, concurrent RV outflow tract obstruction,

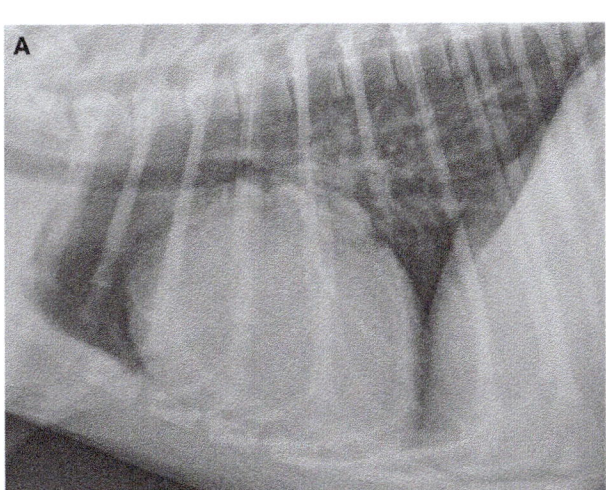
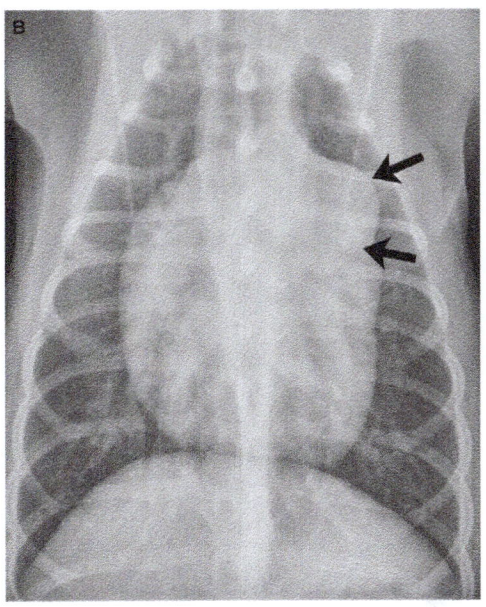

Figure 26.28 Lateral (A) and DV (B) thoracic radiographs from a 5-month-old small, mixed breed dog with a ventricular septal defect. There is mild cardiomegaly (VHS 10.7v), with some left atrial enlargement, and prominent lobar pulmonary vessels. The large main pulmonary artery bulge (B, arrows) is attributed to increased pulmonary flow (and relative pulmonic stenosis). The pulmonary valve appeared normal on echocardiogram.

or an AVSD, although it also could result from a partial or complete right bundle branch block (RBBB) caused by the defect.

Echocardiography reveals left heart dilation, with or without RV enlargement (expected in animals with a large shunt). Perimembranous defects are best visualized in two orthogonal views. The first is just below the aortic valve and adjacent to the septal tricuspid leaflet in the right parasternal long-axis plane optimized for the LV outflow tract. The second is the right parasternal, short-axis view at the level of the aorta or aortic root. These two imaging planes often depict any AR jet that might be present, and provide good alignment for measuring the peak shunt velocity in most cases (**Figures 26.29–26.32**). Because echo "drop-out" is common at the thin membranous septum (especially with 3D imaging) more than one scanning plane always should be used to evaluate a suspected VSD. Doppler studies should

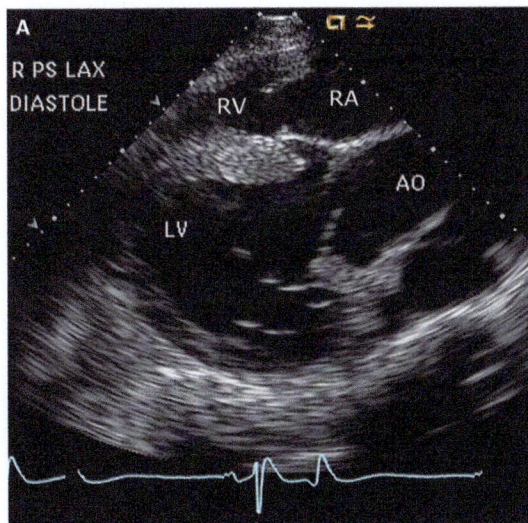
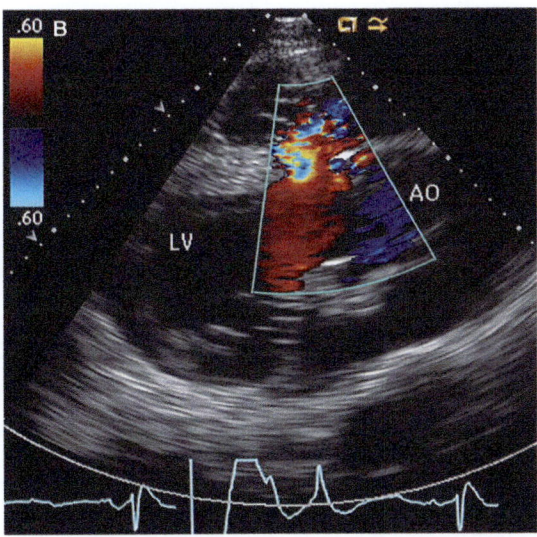

Figure 26.29 A small perimembranous ventricular septal defect (VSD) was an incidental finding in this 7-month-old American Saddlebred colt presented for signs of colic. (A) Off-angle right parasternal long-axis view optimized to show the VSD (just ventral to the aortic root and left of the septal tricuspid valve leaflet); the LV appears foreshortened. Left heart size and function were normal. (B) Color-flow Doppler image in systole showing flow accelerating toward the VSD (with color aliasing), then becoming turbulent into the right ventricle. AO, aorta; LV, left ventricle; RA, right atrium; RV, right ventricle. VSD often is an incidental finding in mature horses.

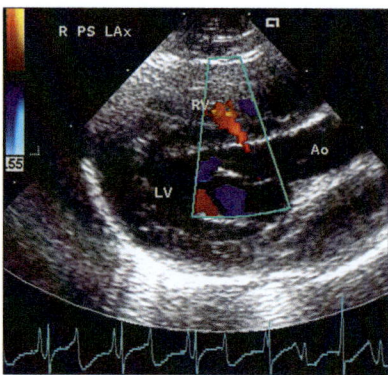

Figure 26.30 Small left-to-right flow through a ventricular septal defect in a 6-month-old female cat. Right parasternal long-axis view. Ao, aorta; LV, left ventricle; RV, right ventricle.

verify the shunt flow. Although the VSD anatomy often is complex, a useful clinical ratio is the defect's maximal diameter to that of the aortic root. Defects that are <40% of short-axis aortic diameter (that includes one valve sinus) usually are well-tolerated; however, the supporting findings of high-velocity L-to-R shunting and only mild-moderate left heart enlargement also should be present. Occasionally, a membranous septal aneurysm (intact or perforated) is identified along the VSD edge; it appears as a hyperechoic thin membrane bulging into the right ventricle.

The right parasternal short-axis view at the heart base is best for differentiating a perimembranous from a juxta-arterial VSD, based on the origin of the flow disturbance on color Doppler. In contrast, the true inlet VSD, part of an AVSD, is imaged best in the left apical 4-chamber view or in a right parasternal long-axis image optimized for the two ventricular inlets. Apical, short- and long-axis views focused more ventrally are best for identifying a muscular VSD (**Figure 26.33**). Other scanning planes might be needed for optimal visualization of shunt size and flow velocity (and direction). Color Doppler interrogation of the basilar septum using the aforementioned views might also reveal small perimembranous or muscular VSDs that are not evident by 2D scanning alone. Assuming good alignment with flow (Chapter 4), when RV systolic pressure is normal, peak VSD flow velocity generally exceeds 4.5 m/s, which correlates to an estimated pressure gradient of 80 mm Hg across the septum. With large shunt flows, pulmonary outflow velocity often is mildly increased, reflecting relative PS.

Echocardiography has supplanted invasive diagnosis, although cardiac catheterization and angiocardiography can be used to measure intracardiac pressures and identify a VSD. An oximetry run reveals the typical step-up in oxygen content within the RV outflow tract. Angiography delineates the abnormal blood flow (**Figure 26.34**).

Management

Small defects sometimes close spontaneously within the first 2 years of life, either from myocardial hypertrophy around the VSD or from a seal formed by the septal tricuspid leaflet, fibrous tissue, or a prolapsed aortic valve leaflet. Animals with a small to moderate-sized defect often have a relatively normal life span. Large L-to-R shunts, with or without concurrent AR, can progress to left-sided CHF. In other cases with a large VSD, PH with shunt reversal develops, usually at an early age (see next section). Animals that develop left-sided CHF are managed medically (Chapter 22). Systemic arterial hypertension will exacerbate L-to-R shunting, so patients should be periodically screened and treated appropriately if hypertensive.

Definitive therapy for VSD has required cardiopulmonary bypass or hypothermia and intracardiac surgery. However, VSD occlusion using a catheter-delivered device is possible in some cases and an interventional cardiologist can

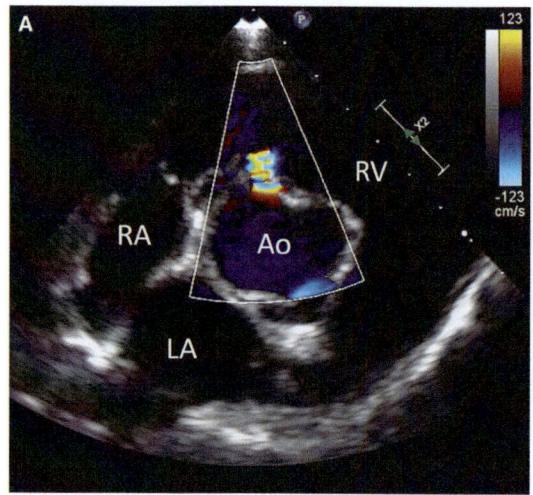
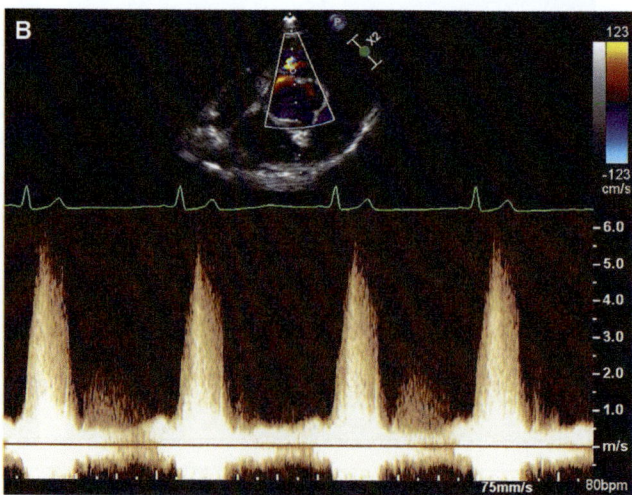

Figure 26.31 (A) Color-flow Doppler image from a 5-year-old female Labrador Retriever shows early systolic flow through a perimembranous ventricular septal defect (VSD); the turbulent jet enters the RV just under the septal tricuspid leaflet. (B) The high-velocity (>5 m/s) continuous-wave Doppler flow across the defect, and the normal left atrial size (A) indicate that the VSD is small and restrictive. Right parasternal short-axis view. Ao, aorta; LA, left atrium; RA, right atrium; RV, right ventricle.

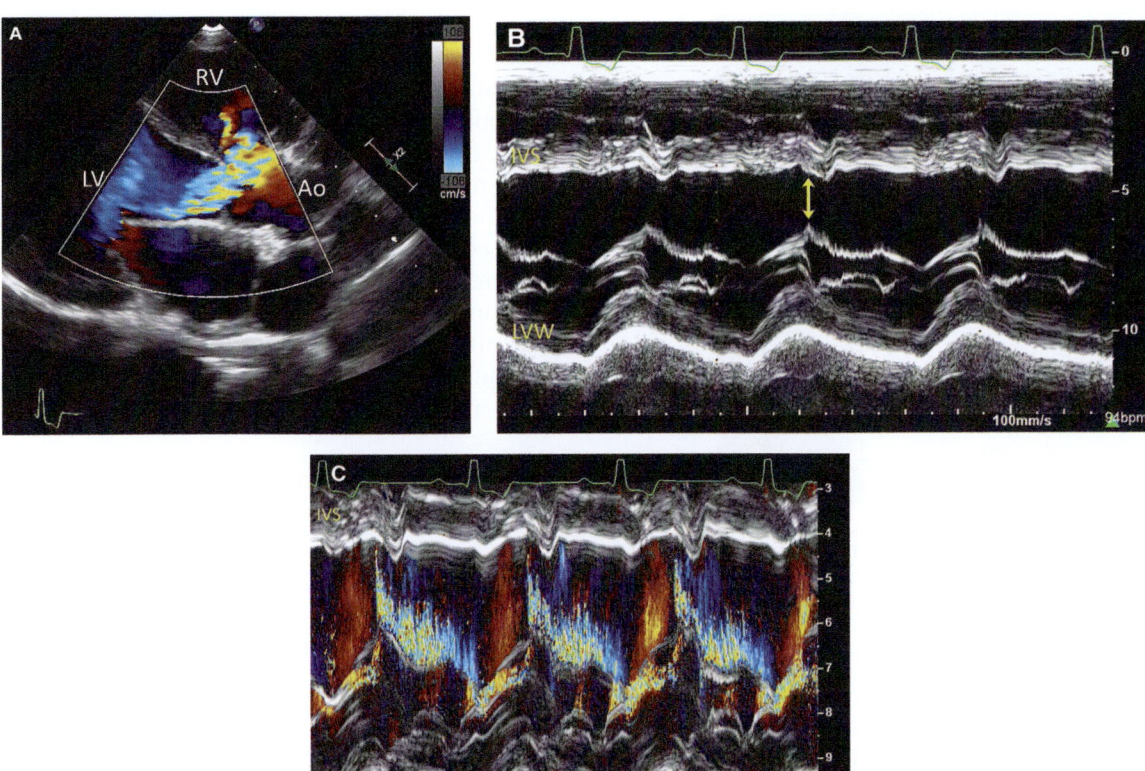

Figure 26.32 (A) Severe aortic regurgitation (AR) is evident on this diastolic color Doppler image from a 1-year-old female German Shepherd with a ventricular septal defect and prolapsing aortic leaflet. The regurgitant jet angles along the anterior mitral leaflet, preventing it from opening fully. Moderately severe valvular aortic stenosis (AS), moderate left heart enlargement, and declining systolic function also were present. Right parasternal long-axis view. (B) M-mode image at the mitral valve level shows the wide E-point-septal separation (arrow) and diastolic mitral leaflet flutter caused by the AR jet. (C) Color M-mode image from the same position shows the turbulent AR flow against the anterior mitral leaflet throughout diastole. The dog also had mitral regurgitation, as indicted by the turbulent flow signal between the two mitral leaflets during systole. ECG trace at top for timing. Ao, aorta; IVS, interventricular septum; LV, left ventricle; LVW, left ventricular wall; RV, right ventricle.

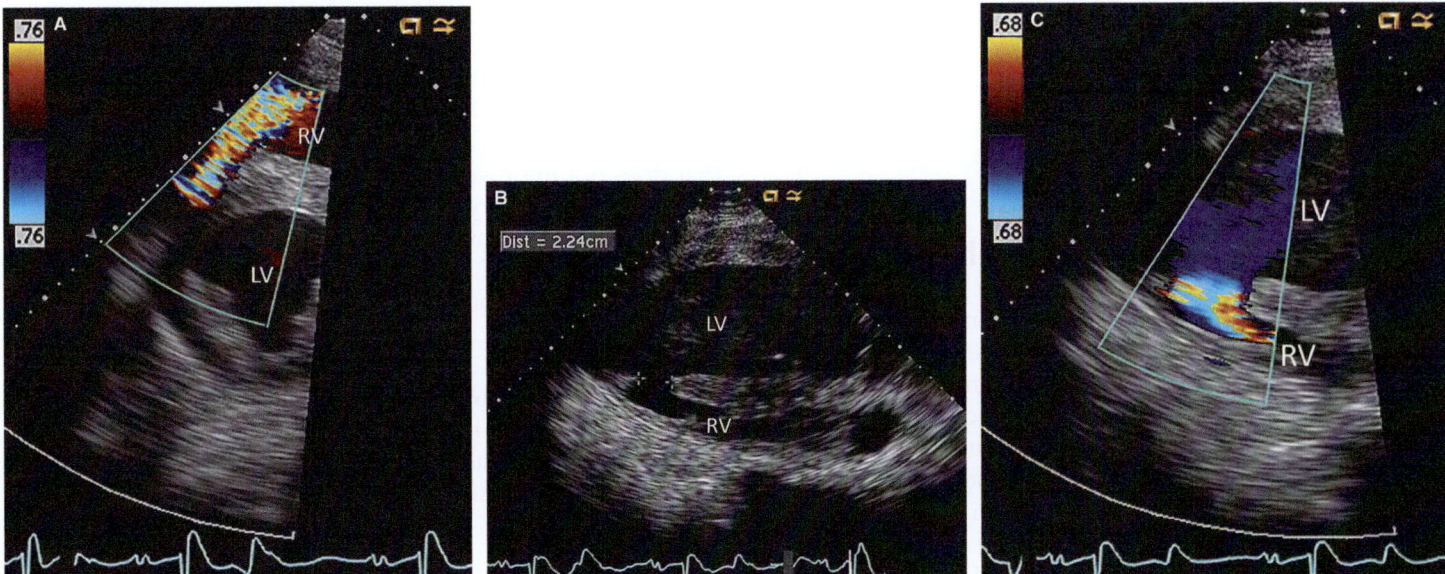

Figure 26.33 A large muscular ventricular septal defect (VSD) was identified in a 1-year-old Paint gelding presented for evaluation of a murmur. The 5/6 systolic murmur was loudest over the caudal right precordium, rather than the more typical cranial right sternal border. (A) Color-flow Doppler image near the cardiac apex shows a left-to-right turbulent flow jet in systole; right parasternal short axis view. (B) Long axis image from the left chest wall shows the location and diameter (2.24 cm) of the VSD. (C) Color-flow image depicts flow from LV to RV through the defect. The increased flow also caused main pulmonary artery enlargement (not shown). LV, left ventricle; RV, right ventricle.

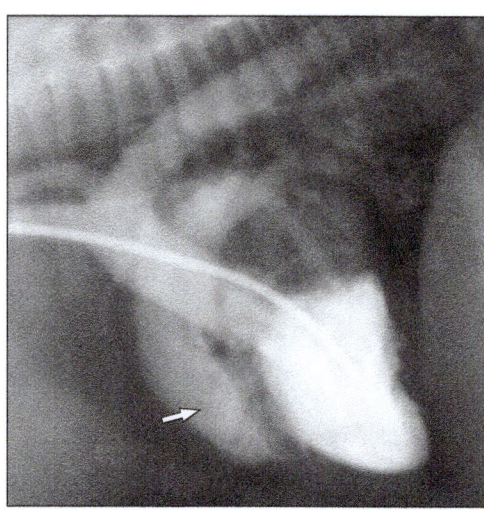

Figure 26.34 Left ventricular angiocardiogram shows dye in the right ventricular outflow tract (arrow) and pulmonary arteries, as well as in the left ventricle and aorta, in a 4-month-old Chow Chow with a ventricular septal defect.

be consulted if that is a consideration. Several techniques are described, including hybrid surgical and catheter-based approaches for occlusion device delivery (p. 184). The defect must include sufficient tissue rims and the thickness of the myocardium must be considered in muscular VSDs. Complications related to thoracotomy or transvascular access are possible, in addition to the potential for LV outflow tract obstruction and systemic embolization. A large L-to-R shunt sometimes is palliated by placing a constrictive band around the pulmonary trunk to create mild supravalvular PS. This increase in outflow resistance raises RV systolic pressure in response, reduces the systolic LV to RV pressure gradient, and consequently reduces shunt volume. However, an excessively tight band can cause shunt reversal (functionally analogous to a T of F). This procedure usually is reserved for unrestrictive defects or cases where CHF has developed.

Reversed Ventricular Septal Defect (Right-to-Left Shunting)

Animals that develop severe PH with shunt reversal generally have a large defect. Similar to rPDA cases, an initially large shunt flow is thought to damage the pulmonary vasculature and prevent normal postnatal decline in pulmonary resistance, producing vascular lesions that can progressively increase pulmonary vascular resistance and pressure (p. 437). The direction of shunt flow depends on the relative pressures in the right and left ventricles during different phases of the cardiac cycle. Shunt flow might be bidirectional or R-to-L throughout the cycle. A large defect coupled with severe PH can produce a large R-to-L shunt volume; however, when ventricular pressures are closely matched, there is little shunt flow. The PH and shunt reversal associated with a VSD is sometimes called "Eisenmenger's complex" after the original description, although the more general term "Eisenmenger's (patho)physiology" often is applied to reversal of any shunt from pulmonary vascular injury and PH.

In contrast to rPDA, intracardiac R-to-L shunts (rVSD, rASD) promote hypoxemia throughout the systemic circulation, including the coronary vasculature. Coronary hypoxemia, coupled with RV concentric hypertrophy, promotes myocardial ischemia, which exacerbates RV stiffness and arrhythmia risk. As with other R-to-L shunts, systemic hypoxemia stimulates erythropoiesis and increase in hematocrit. In addition, R-to-L shunts increase the risk for systemic embolization of venous thrombi.

Clinical Features

Poor exercise stamina, increased respiratory rate and effort, cyanosis (especially with exercise), and collapse or seizures are common signs, as with other R-to-L shunts. Cyanosis, when evident, is equally intense throughout the body, in contrast to the differential cyanosis of rPDA. Jugular distension or pulsations, reflecting increased RV filling pressure with or without TR, and a prominent right precordial impulse often are evident. There might be a soft systolic murmur or no murmur, depending on the amount of shunt flow and also the degree of hyperviscosity. The S_2 sound can be split or loud and "snapping," as is common with PH.

Diagnostic Tests

Thoracic radiographs usually show right heart enlargement, with a prominent main pulmonary trunk and lobar pulmonary arteries that might appear tortuous but with attenuated peripheral arterial filling. The caudal vena cava can be dilated. ECG findings usually include criteria for RV and sometimes RA enlargement, with a right axis deviation. QRS complexes can appear splintered or show other conduction disturbances. As with other R-to-L shunts, rVSD causes arterial hypoxemia that does not improve substantially with supplemental O_2, as well as secondary erythrocytosis.

Echocardiography demonstrates the RV hypertrophy, RV dilation and septal flattening, as well as a widened RV outflow tract and pulmonary trunk. The VSD itself usually is easily visualized with 2D imaging (**Figure 26.35**). Doppler or echocontrast (bubble) study confirms the intracardiac R-to-L shunt (**Figure 26.36**). If a tricuspid (or pulmonary) regurgitation jet is present, measurement of its peak velocity allows estimation of RV systolic and, in the absence of PS, PA pressures (p. 828). Peak shunt velocity estimates the systolic RV to LV pressure gradient.

Management

Surgical closure or palliative PA banding generally is contraindicated when severe PH and shunt reversal exists. Therapy involves exercise restriction, use of a PDE-5 inhibitor

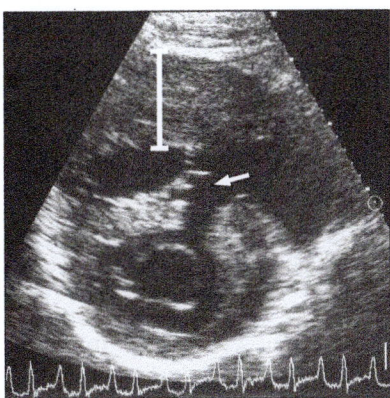

Figure 26.35 Right parasternal short-axis view at the mitral valve level from a cat with a reversed ventricular septal defect. The large septal defect (arrow) and severe right ventricular wall hypertrophy (bar) are evident. The open mitral valve is evident within the left ventricle.

(in attempt to reduce pulmonary vascular resistance and pressure), and management of secondary erythrocytosis to minimize signs of hyperviscosity (p. 454). Long-term prognosis is poor. Complications generally relate to chronic hypoxemia and hyperviscosity. Sudden death is common.

Atrial Septal Defects

During fetal development, the interatrial septum forms from the growth and fusion of two septa. The *septum primum* grows downward from the sinus venosus on the dorsal atrial wall toward the ventricles. During this process, oxygenated venous blood returning from the umbilicus through the caudal vena cava preferentially enters the left atrium across the *ostium primum*, which is the (interatrial) communication ventral to septum primum. This flow provides the oxygen supply to the fetus. Eventually, this first opening will close as septum primum fuses with the endocardial cushions. However before this occurs, perforations develop in the mid-dorsal part of the septum primum which then coalesce to form a second interatrial communication, the *ostium secundum*. Subsequently, a second atrial septum (*septum secundum*) develops from the dorsal atrial wall and grows downward to the right of septum primum, also eventually joining the endocardial cushions at the AV junction. The septum secundum develops in a way that abuts and overlaps the ostium secundum, creating an ovoid depression known as the *fossa ovalis*. However, this does not seal the ostium secundum shut in the fetus and the overlap allows the septum primum to function as a "flap valve." The higher RA (compared to LA) pressure in the fetus pushes this "flap" open, creating a path for flow across what now is termed the *foramen ovale*. This maintains the fetal R-to-L interatrial shunting and preferential return of more-oxygenated blood from the caudal vena cava to the left heart. After birth, when pulmonary resistance drops and LA pressure rises above that in the right atrium, the flap-like opening is pressed closed, blocking flow across it and functionally closing the foramen ovale. Anatomical closure usually follows, but not always (see section "Patent Foramen Ovale").

Developmental failure in one or more atrial septal components, or abnormal development or fusions to the endocardial cushions, can cause an ASD. Ostium primum ASDs are located in the ventral interatrial septum; they occur when the septum primum does not fuse normally with the AV cushions. Ostium primum defects often are large. They can occur in isolation or as a component of the partial or complete AVSD (see section "Atrioventricular Septal Defect").

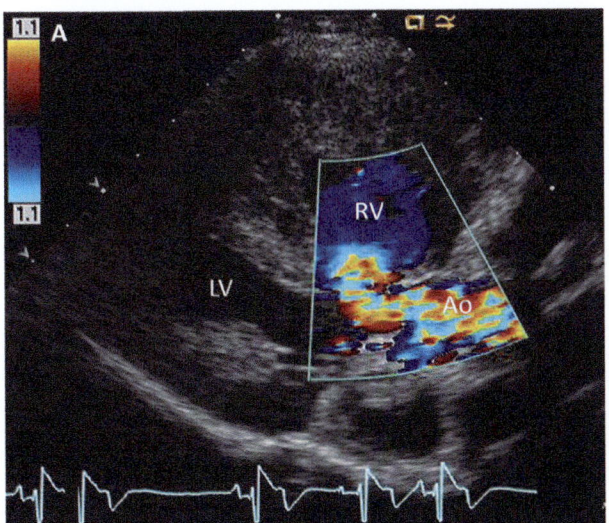 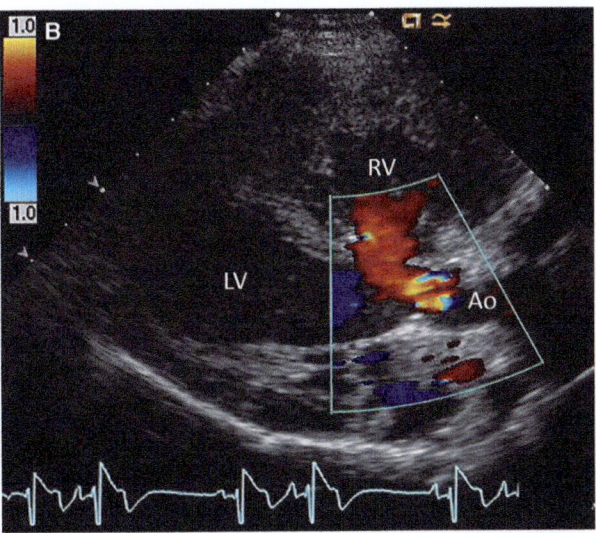

Figure 26.36 Right parasternal long axis images from a 10-month-old female Brussels Griffon with reversed ventricular septal defect (VSD), as well as subaortic stenosis (SAS). (A) Right-to-left flow through the perimembranous VSD occurs in systole. (B) In diastole, however, there is low-velocity left-to-right flow (coded red) through the septal defect; this is aided by mild aortic regurgitation associated with the SAS. Severe right ventricular hypertrophy also is evident. Ao, aorta; LV, left ventricle; RV, right ventricle.

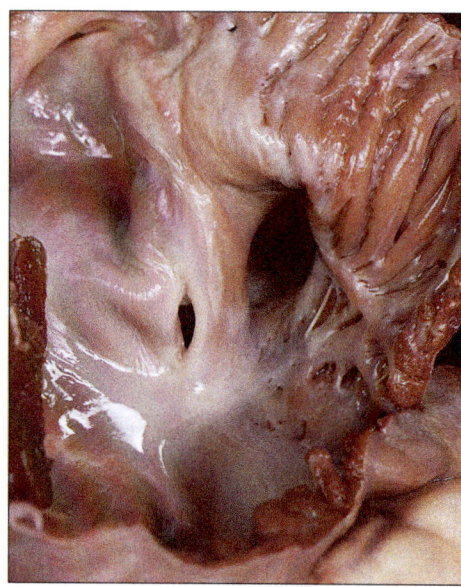

Figure 26.37 Small secundum-type atrial septal defect, seen from the right, in a young dog with multiple cardiac malformations. The right auricle is to the upper right and right ventricle is at bottom of the photo.

Ostium secundum ASDs are located in the mid-interatrial septum (**Figure 26.37**); these occur from deficits in the tissues that normally close the foramen ovale. A PFO is located in the same area as a secundum ASD, but is not considered a true ASD (see "Patent Foramen Ovale"). An uncommon, but perhaps overlooked, type of ASD are the sinus venosus defects. In animals, these usually are located dorsally (and cranial to the fossa ovalis) near the origin of the right pulmonary veins. These veins often drain directly across the defect, allowing L-to-R shunting. A fourth type of ASD is the "unroofed" coronary sinus that communicates blood earmarked for the right atrium directly into the left atrium; this is rare. Although not technically a form of ASD, anomalous pulmonary venous connections can create a similar pathophysiology; pulmonary venous malformations that direct some pulmonary venous drainage into the vena cava or right atrium are observed sporadically in companion animals.

The pathophysiology associated with an isolated secundum defect depends on the size of the opening and the pressure gradient across it. With small (restrictive) defects, the interatrial pressure gradient usually is normal and L-to-R shunting occurs. RA and RV volume overloading and pulmonary overcirculation occur to a degree dependent on shunt volume. If the ASD is small, there is minimal hemodynamic consequence. Large defects can cause clinically important L-to-R shunting with RA, RV, and pulmonary volume overloading and dilation. Although excess pulmonary flow returns to the left atrium, most is shunted directly into the right atrium, so LA enlargement typically is minimal, unless there is concurrent MR (for example, from mitral valve dysplasia or an AVSD).

Pressures in both atria are relatively low; therefore, no murmur arises from the interatrial shunt itself because turbulence is minimal. However, an abnormally large RV stroke volume can cause a murmur of relative PS. Splitting of the second heart sound (S_2) might be heard because the ASD shunt flow promotes delayed pulmonary valve closure and early aortic valve closure. ASDs characteristically cause "fixed splitting" of the S_2, which means splitting occurs during both inspiration and expiration, and that the timing between pulmonary and aortic components does not vary significantly over the respiratory cycle. Conditions that increase RA pressure reduce the L-to-R shunting and potentially can promote shunt reversal (see "Reversed Atrial Septal Defect" and "Patent Foramen Ovale," below). ASDs often are associated with other cardiac anomalies. They are thought to be more common in cats than in dogs, although the Boxer appears to be predisposed. An acquired ASD, secondary to tearing of the atrial septum (most likely in area of the fossa ovalis) could occur as an uncommon complication in dogs with advanced degenerative (myxomatous) mitral valve disease; right-sided CHF has been a rare sequela of this situation.

Clinical Features of Left-to-Right Shunting Atrial Septal Defect

The secundum ASD is more common in dogs; primum defects are recognized more often in cats. There are sporadic reports of both defects in horses. Certain breeds of dog appear predisposed to ASD particularly Boxers and Standard Poodles (**Table 26.1**). A genetic basis is suspected, although not clarified. In people, autosomal dominant inheritance is most common, but some mutations are autosomal recessive.

The clinical history often is nonspecific. Physical findings are generally unremarkable with a small isolated ASD. Clinical signs associated with large ASDs can include exercise intolerance, syncope, cough, dyspnea, and signs of right-sided CHF. A large L-to-R shunt is likely to cause a murmur of relative PS and fixed splitting of the S_2 (see pathophysiology discussion, above). Rarely, a soft diastolic murmur of relative tricuspid stenosis might be audible.

Diagnostic Tests in Left-to-Right Shunting Atrial Septal Defect

Right heart enlargement, with or without pulmonary trunk dilation, is radiographically evident with large shunts (**Table 26.2**). The pulmonary circulation could appear increased unless high pulmonary resistance has developed. The left heart is not enlarged unless another defect such as mitral dysplasia or an AVSD is present.

The ECG can be normal or it might show RV and RA enlargement patterns. Animals with an ostium primum defect (often as part of an AVSD) could have an RV enlargement or RBBB pattern and possibly left cranial axis deviation in the frontal plane, likely from interruption of the conduction pathways. AF can develop, especially with marked atrial enlargement. Sometimes other arrhythmias occur.

RA and RV dilation, with or without paradoxical interventricular septal motion, can be seen with 2D and M-mode echocardiography. Large ASDs are visualized more easily. However, the thinner fossa ovalis region of the interatrial septum sometimes is confused with a septal defect, because echo dropout also occurs here. Doppler echocardiography might reveal smaller shunts that are not evident on 2D examination, as well as demonstrate flow patterns with larger defects (**Figures 26.38** and **26.39**). Normal caudal vena caval inflow tracks along the atrial septum and can be confused with flow across an ASD. Larger shunt flows cause an increase in pulmonary outflow velocity (relative PS). A sinus venosus defect easily can be missed, unless multiple long- and short-axis images of the dorsal atrial septum are obtained and pulmonary venous drainage is carefully interrogated by color Doppler. Cardiac catheterization with oximetry shows an oxygen step-up at the level of the right atrium and RV inlet. The

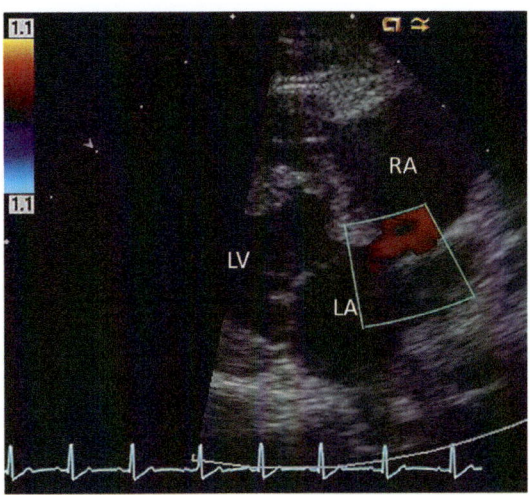

Figure 26.38 Right parasternal long-axis view with color-flow Doppler imaging reveals low-velocity left-to-right flow through a small secundum atrial septal defect in a 3-month-old male English Bulldog. The right atrium is mildly enlarged. LA, left atrium; LV, left ventricle; RA, right atrium.

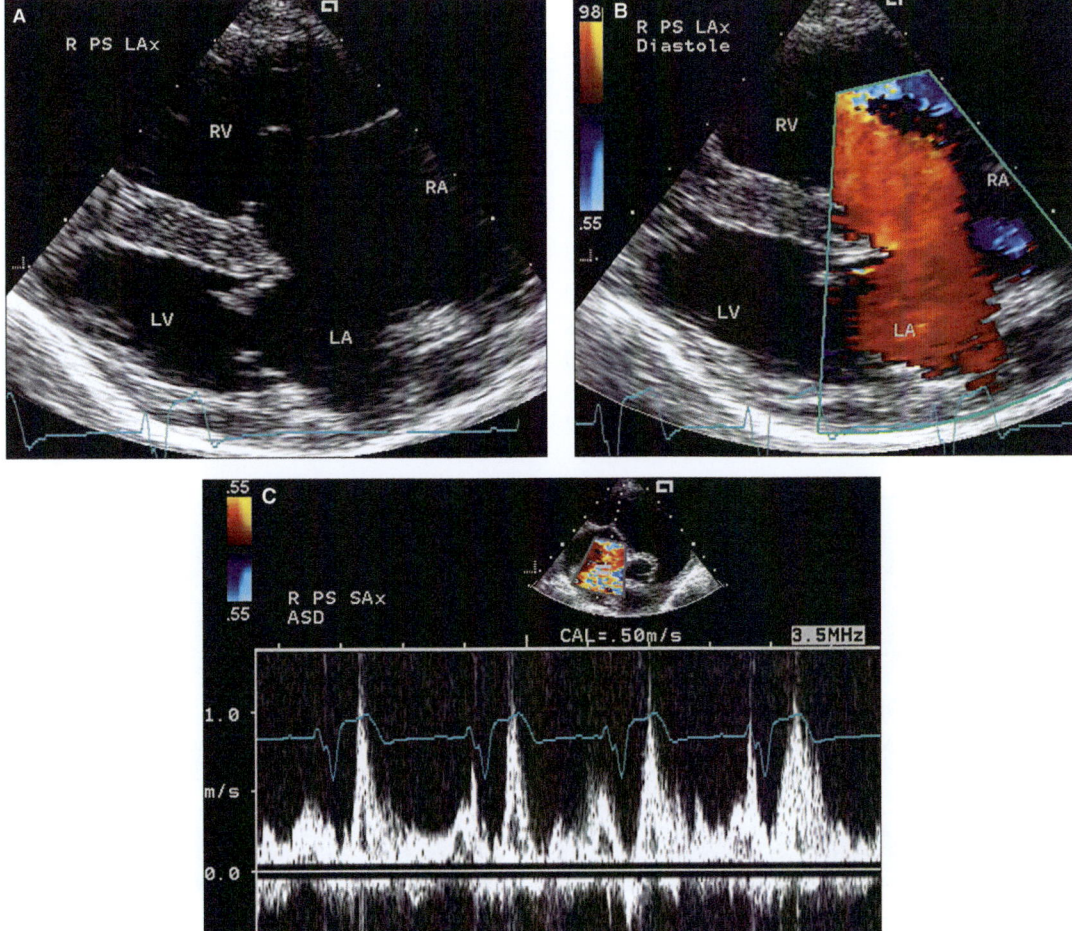

Figure 26.39 (A) A large atrial septal defect (ASD) with RA and RV dilation is evident on right parasternal long-axis view in an 8-year-old female mixed-breed dog. The dog also had mitral and tricuspid regurgitation. (B) Color-flow imaging shows a wide band of low-velocity flow from LA to RA through the ASD in this diastolic frame. (C) Pulsed-wave Doppler with the sample volume placed at the interatrial septum (in short-axis view) shows variable left-to-right flow across the ASD throughout the cardiac cycle. LA, left atrium; LV, left ventricle; RA, right atrium; RV, right ventricle.

shunt becomes evident after radiopaque contrast injection into the PA, or when the catheter passes across the ASD from right to left atrium.

Reversed Atrial Septal Defect (Right-to-Left Shunting)

R-to-L shunting across an ASD (or PFO) can occur with concurrent PS, marked TR, tricuspid valve stenosis, or PH. A large ASD essentially creates a common atrial chamber. Large L-to-R shunt volumes are more likely to induce PH. In humans, pulmonary vascular injury and PH develop more gradually (over decades) with an ASD, compared to a VSD; this might also be the case in animals. As with other R-to-L shunts, there is increased risk for systemic embolization of venous thrombi with a reversed ASD (rASD) or PFO. When PH underlies the R-to-L shunt, sequelae are similar to those with rVSD and rPDA. If pulmonary and systemic pressures are nearly equivalent, bidirectional shunting can occur at different times during the cardiac cycle. If the shunting stems from a right-sided obstructive lesion, other therapeutic options might be available. For information about PS, TR, and tricuspid stenosis, see Chapter 27.

Clinical Features and Diagnostic tests for Right-to-Left Shunting ASD

Reduced exercise tolerance, hypoxemia, shortness of breath, collapse, and cyanosis can occur, as with other reversed shunts. Intracardiac shunts cause equally intense cyanosis throughout the body. However if the hematocrit is normal or only minimally elevated, or mucous membranes are pigmented, cyanosis might be difficult to identify. There can be jugular distension or pulsation. The right precordial impulse often is pronounced. Arterial pulses generally are normal. The rASD itself is unlikely to cause a murmur; however, concurrent PS, AV valve insufficiency, or other defect could do so. The S_2 sound could be split, or loud and "snapping," with PH.

Thoracic radiographs usually show an enlarged right heart and often a prominent pulmonary trunk. With PH, the proximal lobar pulmonary arteries can appear dilated and tortuous. The left atrium might be mildly enlarged. Sometimes the caudal vena cava is quite dilated. The ECG usually indicates RV and sometimes RA enlargement, with a right axis deviation.

When PH underlies the R-to-L shunt, echocardiography demonstrates RV hypertrophy and dilation with septal flattening throughout the cardiac cycle, as well as a widened RV outflow tract and pulmonary trunk. Unlike L-to-R shunting ASD, paradoxical septal motion usually is absent. Especially in cases with PH, the ASD is seen easily with 2D imaging (**Figure 26.40**), unless it is a sinus venosus type defect (**Figure 26.41**). When PS is the cause of RV pressure overload, echocardiographic findings are similar but the RV outflow tract and pulmonary annulus often are narrowed, with increased pulmonary outflow velocity (p. 495). When primary TR underlies the increased RA pressure, RA and RV dilation occur, without concentric hypertrophy. If the primary pathophysiology is tricuspid stenosis, RA but not RV dilation is expected (Chapter 27). Doppler or echocontrast (bubble) study can confirm the intracardiac R-to-L shunt. Bidirectional shunting might be evident at different times during the cardiac cycle, depending on relative intra-atrial pressures. Measurement of the peak velocity of a tricuspid (or pulmonic) regurgitation jet allows estimation of RV systolic and, in the absence of PS, PA pressures (p. 828). The peak shunt velocity allows estimation of the maximal RA to LA pressure gradient.

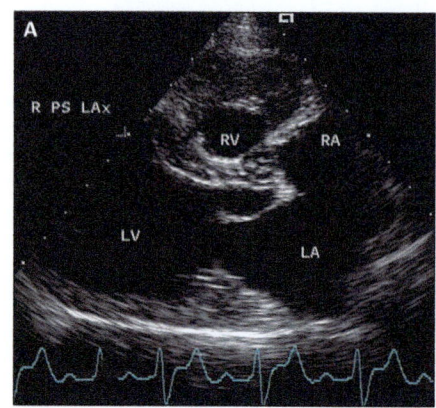 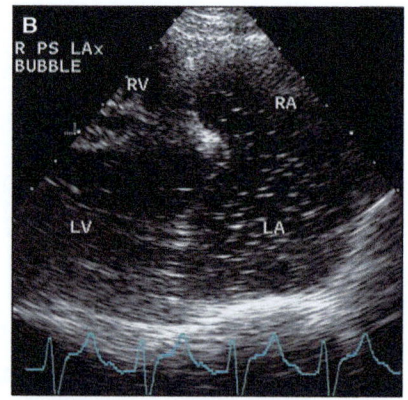

Figure 26.40 (A) A large atrial septal defect (ASD) is visible in this 18-month-old Akita with a history of exercise intolerance and cyanosis. Severe pulmonary hypertension had caused the shunt to reverse and marked RV hypertrophy to develop. (B) A bubble (echocontrast) study using an IV bolus of agitated saline shows that bright "bubbles" have moved from RA to LA across the ASD; some bubbles also are present in the LV. Right parasternal long-axis four-chamber view. LA, left atrium; LV, left ventricle, RA, right atrium; RV, right ventricle.

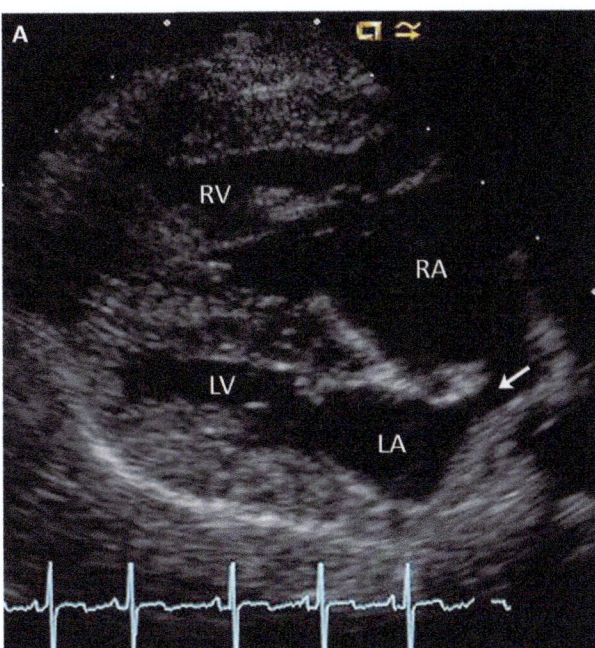 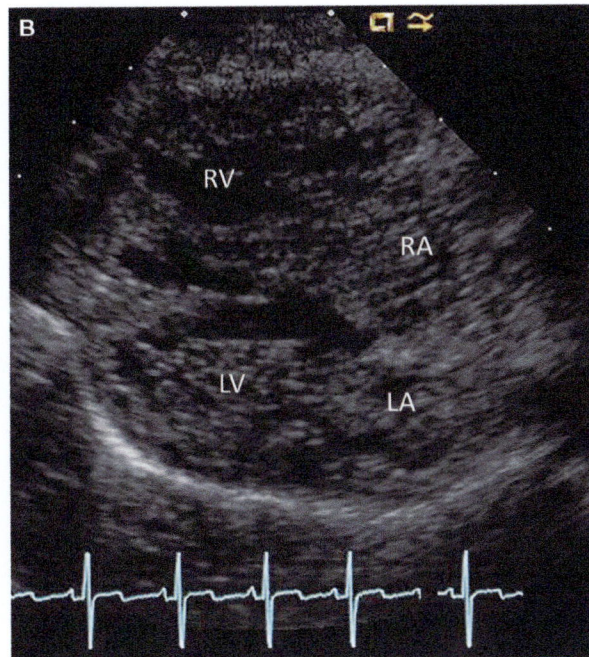

Figure 26.41 A 2-year-old female Bichon Frise had shortness of breath and cyanosis after short periods of play; a murmur of tricuspid regurgitation and loud S₂ were heard on cardiac auscultation. (A) Right parasternal long-axis four-chamber view shows a sinus venosus-type atrial septal defect (ASD, arrow) about 4 mm in diameter, with right atrial and ventricular dilation and right ventricular hypertrophy. The large papillary muscle in the RV and mildly thickened tricuspid valve could relate to tricuspid dysplasia, or be consequences of the dog's severe pulmonary hypertension (estimated pulmonary artery systolic pressure >140 mm Hg) and secondary ventricular hypertrophy. (B) Echo-bubble study documents the intracardiac right-to-left shunt (reversed ASD), with almost instantaneous opacification of all four cardiac chambers. LA, left atrium; LV, left ventricle, RA, right atrium; RV, right ventricle.

Management of Atrial Septal Defect

Medical management is indicated if CHF develops. Large L-to-R shunts could be treated surgically with cardiopulmonary bypass and a patch graft. Transcatheter closure of septum secundum defects, or a hybrid surgical-transcatheter approach, also has been successful in dogs, assuming there are sufficient tissue rims to hold the device and venous return is not obstructed. Complications are similar to those for other shunt occlusion procedures. Although complete ASD closure might not occur initially, residual shunt flow could decrease or cease over time. Prognosis for animals with an ASD is variable and depends on shunt size, whether other defects are present, and pulmonary vascular resistance. A large defect is more likely to cause CHF or PH.

Surgical closure or palliative PA banding is contraindicated when PH underlies shunt reversal. For cases with PS, tricuspid stenosis, or cor triatriatum dexter, balloon valvuloplasty could effectively reduce rASD shunting. Surgical approaches for the palliation of PS or for tricuspid valve repair could be appropriate in some cases. Medical therapy for rASD involves exercise restriction and management of secondary erythrocytosis to minimize signs of hyperviscosity (p. 454). For cases with PH, PDE-5 inhibitor therapy aimed at reducing pulmonary vascular resistance (and pressure) is used. Therapy for right-sided CHF signs occasionally might be needed.

Patent Foramen Ovale

Persistent patency of the foramen ovale can allow R-to-L shunting when RA pressures rise, as operative in the fetus. Conversely and uncommonly, if marked LA stretch prevents the foramen ovale from closing, L-to-R shunting could ensue. A PFO differs from a true ASD inasmuch as the tissue components of the normal fossa ovalis are present, but either high RA or LA pressure prevents sealing of the fetal communication. A PFO usually is clinically silent, because LA pressure normally slightly exceeds RA pressure.

Anatomical closure of the foramen ovale normally follows the functional closure that occurs immediately after birth. In neonatal dogs and cats, a small tunnel extending from the RA entry of the caudal vena cava is evident (MacDonald, 1995). In foals, fusion and anatomic closure occurs within 2–9 weeks of age, and during that interval, a mobile LA membrane that appears at postmortem as a tubular, fenestrated "finger cot" (MacDonald, 1988) is quite visible by 2D echocardiography. In the neonate, a PFO can permit R-to-L shunting in cases of lung immaturity or severe pneumonia with persistent PH. This is observed most often in foals, since newborn puppies and kittens do not receive comparable veterinary care. However, in some animals anatomic closure of the foramen ovale never occurs, especially in the setting of previously mentioned right-sided lesions. The uncommon malformation of cor triatriatum dexter (Chapter 28) also can be associated with a R-to-L shunting PFO, as the high-pressure caudal RA chamber often communicates in this way with the left atrium. Additionally, marked LA dilation secondary to PDA, or a cardiomyopathy in cats, rarely can lead to stretching of a foramen ovale and maintenance of its patency; this can create a L-to-R shunt visible by color Doppler. Finally, as noted previously, dogs with chronic severe MR could develop a tear in the atrial septum resulting in a functional L-to-R shunt.

The overall incidence of PFO in healthy companion animals previously was thought to be low; however, probe-patent foramen ovale might be more common in mature dogs and cats than previously suspected. The data differ depending on the study sample, method and intensity of PFO evaluation, and concurrent diseases. For example, in one study only 0.2% of nearly 1000 canine congenital heart disease cases were reported to have a PFO (Oliveira 2011). Yet, using contrast echocardiography, 39% of dogs with PS were discovered to have a functional PFO with R-to-L shunting (Fujii, 2012; also see Chapter 4). Most cases of PFO are not evident antemortem, however, because the normally higher LA pressure keeps the septal membrane flap pressed closed over the foramen. If RA pressure rises to exceed LA pressure (as can occur with PH, PS, or marked TR), interatrial R-to-L shunting results. Management principles are as described for ASD above.

Atrioventricular Septal Defect

The normal AV septum is the portion of tissue that joins the ventral atrial septum and dorsal ventricular septum. There is a normal longitudinal offset, with the mitral valve inserting more dorsally compared to the tricuspid valve attachment at the septum. The left side of the AV septum functions as part of the ventricular septum; whereas, the right side is located between the atrial septum and right AV valve. This geography places the AV septum at the junction of the atria, ventricles, and AV valves. Although the embryogenesis is contested, the structures near the AV septum are formed largely from fetal endocardial cushion(s) that normally partition the embryonic AV canal. Previously, this malformation has been called an endocardial cushion defect, common AV canal, or AV canal defect.

AVSDs are uncommon congenital malformations caused by abnormal fetal development in this region. These defects involve a spectrum of simple to complex malformations that can variously include: the dorsal (inlet) ventricular septum, ventral (primum) atrial septum, the AV valves, and the ventricular outlets. There are different classification systems, but the majority of AVSDs seen in animals are partial or transitional defects. Features of a complete AVSD include: a large primum ASD, an inlet VSD, and a common (usually five-leafleted) AV valve with two common or "bridging" mitral-tricuspid valve leaflets located between the two septal defects. This common AV valve bridges the defect; there is fusion of the septal mitral and tricuspid leaflets and variable or no anchoring of the cranial (anterior) leaflet to the interventricular septum. One or both AV valves can be cleft or otherwise malformed. An incomplete AVSD has variable combinations of VSD, ASD, and AV valve malformations. The most commonly observed form in the cat is a partial AVSD consisting of a primum ASD and bridging septal leaflet. These malformations have been reported rarely in the horse. Rarely, a leftward-shift in the ventral interatrial septal border attaches in such a way that it obstructs LA emptying, opens the RA to both ventricles, and functionally creates what is called a "double-outlet right atrium" (Durham, 2014). This causes a variable degree of inflow obstruction dorsal to the left AV valve (supravalvular mitral stenosis), which can lead to pulmonary edema. It should be distinguished from supravalvular mitral ring and cor triatriatum sinister. Additionally, the LV outflow tract can be elongated, as it no longer is wedged between the two AV valves. If there is a secundum ASD, it can fuse with the primum defect to create a common atrium.

Enlargement of the right ventricle (and its atrium) is common, especially with a large ASD, as shunting is usually L-to-R at the atrial level. LV dilation also occurs, especially when there is a partial AVSD with VSD. LA dilation is less common, but can occur when AV valve insufficiency causes regurgitation into that chamber. There is interatrial communication in many cases of AVSD, even when interatrial septal length is relatively normal; this implies that ventricular septal deficiency also causes atrial communication. Some cases of AVSD have delayed RV or left anterior fascicular conduction. This possibly results from malpositioning of the AV conduction system, because the AV node and His bundle are anatomically close to the inflow septum.

AVSDs have been classified into so-called Rastelli types according to AV valve structural characteristics. Type A is most common; the chordae tendineae of the septal (anterior, superior) leaflet of the common AV valve attach to the crest of the interventricular septum. In Rastelli type B, the left anterior (superior) leaflet chordae attach to anomalous papillary muscles that originate from the inlet VSD, within the RV. Type C involves the left anterior (superior) leaflet bridging the inlet VSD to the RV.

Clinical Features

AVSDs occur most often in cats and comprise an estimated 5–10% of feline congenital heart disease cases. AVSDs also occur occasionally in dogs and horses. There is no apparent sex predilection. Most cases are diagnosed within the first year of life. In one case series of cats with AVSD, about three-quarters of the cases had a partial AVSD, while the remaining one-quarter had complete AVSD. Of cats with partial AVSD, about half had an ASD and half had a VSD.

AVSD often leads to left-sided or biventricular CHF, although some cases develop severe PH with R-to-L shunting. A history of dyspnea or tachypnea is common. Occasionally, syncope, signs of right-sided CHF, or cyanosis occur. Some animals are asymptomatic at initial diagnosis. A systolic murmur is common; it can be loudest either low on the left or near the right sternal border region. Occasionally, a diastolic murmur is present.

Diagnostic Tests

Radiographs show cardiomegaly. There might be pulmonary infiltrates consistent with edema, or caudal vena caval dilation and dilated or tortuous pulmonary vessels (**Figure 26.42**). On ECG, most cases have sinus rhythm, although supraventricular tachycardia also is reported. Many cases have widened P waves (P mitrale), with or without tall P waves (P pulmonale). Intraventricular conduction disturbances are common,

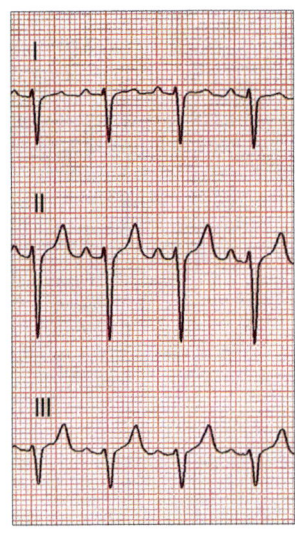

Figure 26.43 Electrocardiogram from the kitten of **Figure 26.42** shows sinus rhythm with a right axis deviation. Large QRS complexes and wide P waves also are present. Leads as marked; 50 mm/s, 1 cm = 1 mV.

especially partial or complete RBBB; occasionally, a left anterior fascicular block pattern is present (**Figure 26.43**).

Echocardiography demonstrates the intracardiac anatomic defects and secondary chamber enlargement, which can be marked. RV hypertrophy and a widened pulmonary trunk accompany PH. Doppler studies show AV valve regurgitation and abnormal shunting (**Figure 26.44**). An echo-contrast (bubble) study also can confirm the presence of intracardiac R-to-L shunting.

Management

Primary repair using open-heart surgery techniques is reported in dogs. Without repair, long-term prognosis is poor although occasional animals could live well into adulthood. Prognosis is worse for complete AVSD compared to partial AVSD. Many affected animals develop signs of CHF, although some die suddenly and some develop signs related to R-to-L shunting caused by PH.

Tetralogy of Fallot

The Tetralogy of Fallot is one of a group of genetically and embryologically related cardiac malformations that in older veterinary literature are referred to as conotruncal defects. A spectrum of defects was described in Keeshonden (Patterson, 1974). So-called grade 1 conotruncal defects include subclinical malformations of the RV conal septum, including ventricular septal aneurysm and absence of the papillary muscle of the conus. Grade 2 conotruncal defects include an infundibular VSD or PS, combined with grade 1 defects. Grade 3 conotruncal defects consist of the complete T of F. In the original theory, malformations of the fetal conus and truncus arteriosus combined to produce abnormal alignment of

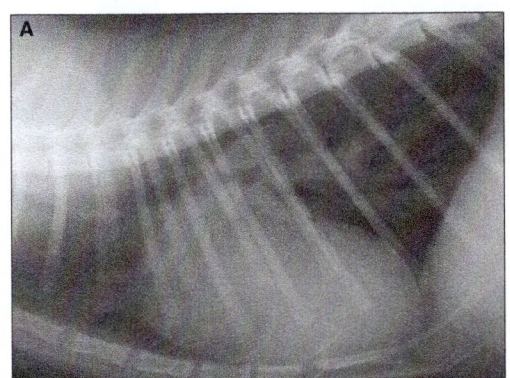
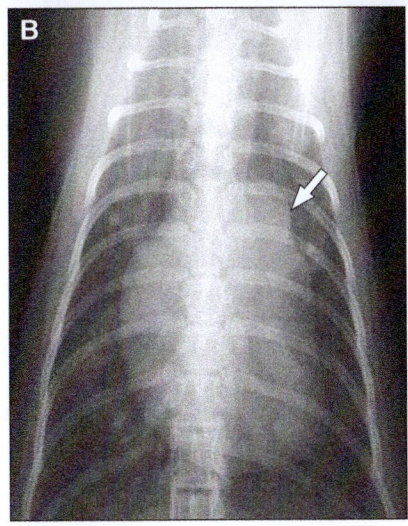

Figure 26.42 Lateral (A) and DV (B) radiographs from a kitten with a reversed-shunting AV septal defect indicate massive cardiomegaly with right heart predominance. Dilated and tortuous pulmonary vessels are evident on both views, with a bulge in the area of the main pulmonary artery (arrow, B).

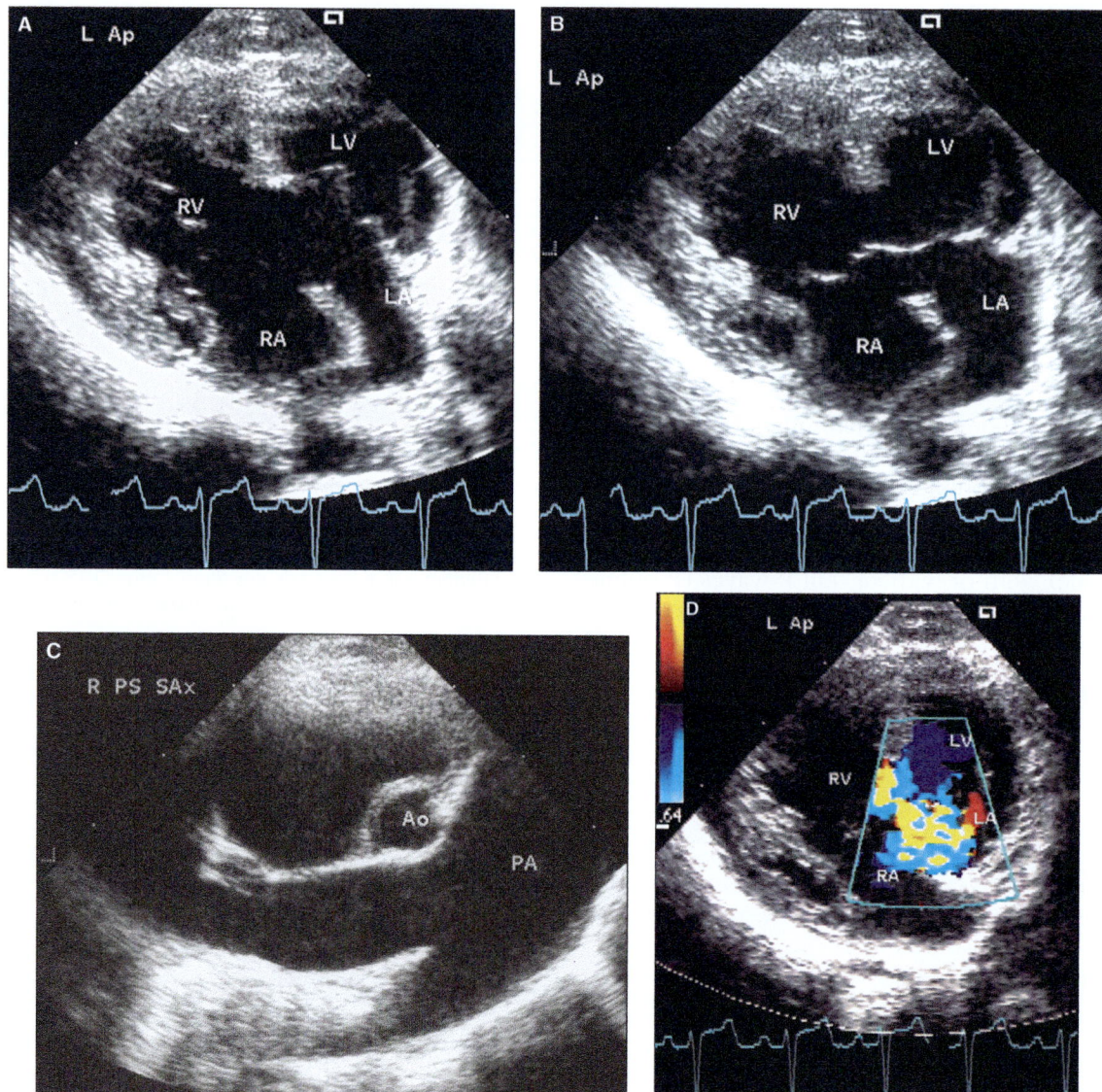

Figure 26.44 (A, B) Left apical 4-chamber views from a kitten with a reversed AV septal defect show a large primum (low) atrial septal defect (ASD) merged with a high ventricular septal defect (VSD). Malformed AV valves are visible, open in diastole (A) and closed in systole (B); note that the septal leaflets insert at the same level, also the right ventricular hypertrophy. (C) Right parasternal short-axis view at the heart base reveals massive pulmonary artery dilation (secondary to pulmonary hypertension) in this case. (D) Color flow Doppler demonstrates right-to-left shunting (systole, left apical view as in A and B). Ao, aorta; LA, left atrium; LV, left ventricle; PA, pulmonary artery; RA, right atrium; RV, right ventricle.

the developing ventricular septum with the ventricular outlet region. Meanwhile, asymmetrical partitioning of the truncus arteriosus produced a large dextropositioned aorta and small PA. Patterson's sentinel publication highlighted the T of F in the veterinary literature, but other theories and nomenclature have superseded. A persistent truncus arteriosus also was reported in this colony; however, the defect is unrelated to T of F and probably stems from an abnormality in truncal partitioning, from anlagen derived in part from the neural crest.

The modern theory of abnormal cardiac development in T of F indicates that each of the important components can be explained by one major malformation: the cranioventral displacement of the RV outflow septum during development.

The anomalies that comprise the T of F are: an unrestricted VSD, RV outflow obstruction (typically subvalvular) with PS, cranial and rightward shifting (malalignment) of the aortic root, and secondary RV hypertrophy. Extreme malpositioning and muscular ingrowth of the subpulmonary septum can result in a pulmonary atresia, characterized by complete obstruction to pulmonary outflow with vestigial pulmonary valve and PA. In this case, there is one functional great artery (the aorta) coming from both ventricles; in older literature, this condition is referred to as "pseudotruncus arteriosus."

The VSD associated with T of F often is quite large and unrestrictive, related to abnormal shifting of the infundibular septum and absence of normal tissue near the trabecular

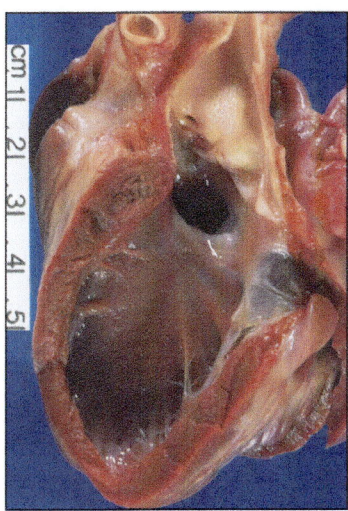

Figure 26.45 The large ventricular septal defect, with overriding aorta above, is seen from the left in this postmortem specimen from an English Springer Spaniel puppy with tetralogy of Fallot.

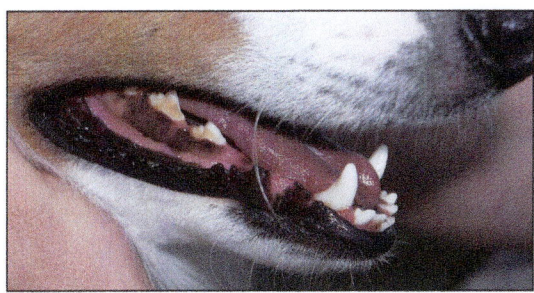

Figure 26.46 Mildly cyanotic tongue in a 2-year-old male Collie with tetralogy of Fallot. (Image courtesy of Dr JO Noxon.)

bands and supraventricular crest (**Figure 26.45**). The cranial and rightward shift (dextroposition) of the aortic root causes it to override the VSD. The two ventricular pressures equalize in systole. RV concentric hypertrophy develops secondary to the systolic pressure overload imposed by PS and systemic arterial pressure. The amount of RV-to-aortic shunting depends on the degree of outflow resistance caused by the PS (which is usually fixed or static) compared with the level of systemic arterial resistance (which can vary). The R-to-L shunt volume increases with exercise and other causes of reduced systemic arterial resistance. The RV outflow obstructive lesion(s) classically involves the subvalvular infundibulum although the pulmonary valve also can be hypoplastic and stenotic. Infundibular hypertrophy can cause additional, dynamic outflow obstruction and is a potential target for beta-blocker therapy. In T of F, the PA often is hypoplastic and can be atretic, as fits the moniker "tet-pulmonary atresia." The left heart chambers tend to be small because inflow from the pulmonary circulation is poor. Aortic arch anomalies also occur in some animals. An ASD might coexist, creating a so-called pentalogy of Fallot. Pulmonary vascular resistance generally is normal with T of F, because the PS protects the pulmonary arterial system; however, PH can develop from systemic collateral circulation. Other features associated with T of F are similar to those of other reversed shunts, including the possibility of venous to systemic thromboembolism.

Pulmonary atresia has been reported in cats, horses and dogs. In this condition, pulmonary perfusion must occur either through a PDA, the bronchial arteries, or other systemic-to-pulmonary shunts, including multiple aorticopulmonary collateral vessels. The latter occur in some animals even without pulmonary atresia. Pulmonary collateral vessels can be of varying size, which can cause different levels of perfusion and perfusion pressure across different areas of the lungs. Pulmonary vascular injury and regional (lobar) pulmonary hypertension might occur in these cases.

Clinical Features

Historically, T of F was recognized most widely in the Keeshond breed in earlier literature. However, this defect occurs in terriers and other dog breeds (**Table 26.1**), as well as in cats and horses. The inheritance pattern for T of F, studied in the Keeshond, previously was thought to be autosomal recessive, with alleles at modifying loci affecting severity. However, inheritance appears to be more complex and involves predisposing genes on three different chromosomes.

Most animals with T of F have exhibited clinical signs by the time of diagnosis. Common findings in the patient history include syncope, exertional weakness, tachypnea, cyanosis, seizures, and stunted growth. Signs of right-sided CHF usually do not develop, but could occur in sporadic cases, especially when marked TR or a restrictive VSD also exists. Chylous pleural effusion secondary to CHF sometimes occurs in affected cats.

Physical findings vary with the relative severity of the disease components. Cyanosis might be present at rest in some animals (**Figures 26.46** and **26.47**, also see **Figure 13.5**, p. 249). Others have pink mucous membranes at rest, although

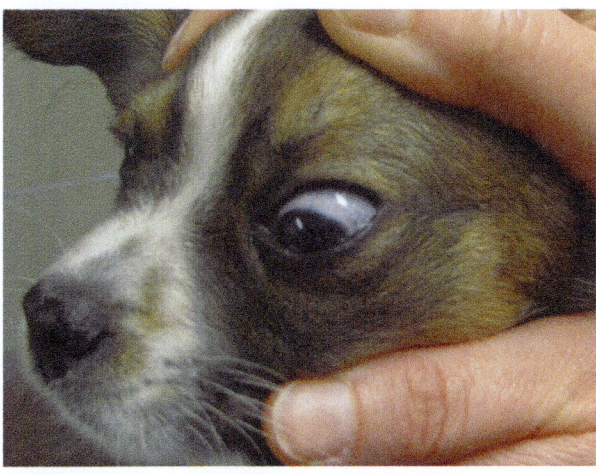

Figure 26.47 Cyanosis is apparent in the sclera of this 2-month-old, mixed-breed dog with tetralogy of Fallot.

cyanosis usually becomes evident with exercise. The right precordial impulse can be equal to or stronger than that on the left. A precordial thrill might be palpable at the right sternal border or left basilar area, depending on murmur intensity in those areas. Jugular pulsations could be present. Auscultation most often reveals a systolic ejection murmur at the left base compatible with PS. In addition or instead, a holosystolic murmur loudest at the right sternal border, compatible with a VSD, might be heard if the defect is restrictive. However, in cases with pulmonary atresia, the left basilar murmur is absent. Some animals have no discernible murmur because of pulmonary atresia, hyperviscosity associated with erythrocytosis (p. 23), and/or systolic pressure equalization between right and left ventricles.

Diagnostic Tests

Arterial hypoxemia and an elevated hematocrit are the usual laboratory abnormalities. Radiographically, the heart might be of normal size or small, with RV prominence. The left auricle and atrium are small, which can create a straight cardiac border between 1 and 3 o'clock on the VD projection ("boot-shaped" heart). However, cardiomegaly with RV enlargement is present in some cases (**Table 26.2**). The main PA typically is small, although sometimes a bulge is evident. Pulmonary vascular markings are reduced; but compensatory enhancement of the bronchial circulation can increase overall pulmonary opacity. On lateral views, the malpositioned aorta appears to bulge cranially and the hypertrophied RV displaces the left heart dorsally, mimicking left heart enlargement, especially on the left lateral view (**Figure 26.48**). Caudal caval distension can be prominent (**Figure 26.49**). An RV enlargement pattern is typical on ECG, although left axis deviation occasionally is noted in affected cats.

Echocardiography shows the typically large perimembranous, outlet VSD, meaning there is anatomic continuity between the rim of the defect and the septal tricuspid leaflet. The large aortic root is shifted cranially and rightward to straddle the ventricular septum. There is a variable degree of PS (typically severe), and RV hypertrophy (**Figure 26.50**). Most cases of true T of F have subvalvular or infundibular stenosis, and it can be challenging to distinguish a case with a large perimembranous VSD and valvular PS from T of F unless the aortic anatomy is carefully evaluated. Hypertrophy of the RV outflow area can be severe and contribute to outflow obstruction. The left heart usually appears small, except in so-called "pink tet" where the PS is less severe and pulmonary flow more normal. The PA can be difficult to image when hypoplastic, and is not evident at all when atretic. Mitral valve systolic anterior motion (SAM) occasionally occurs in association with high RV systolic pressure, RV hypertrophy and altered LV geometry in dogs with T of F (as well as those with PS or PH). There might be minimal hemodynamic effect from mitral SAM in such cases; however, if this dynamic LV outflow obstruction markedly increases LV systolic pressure, it could contribute to myocardial ischemia, especially during times of high heart rate.

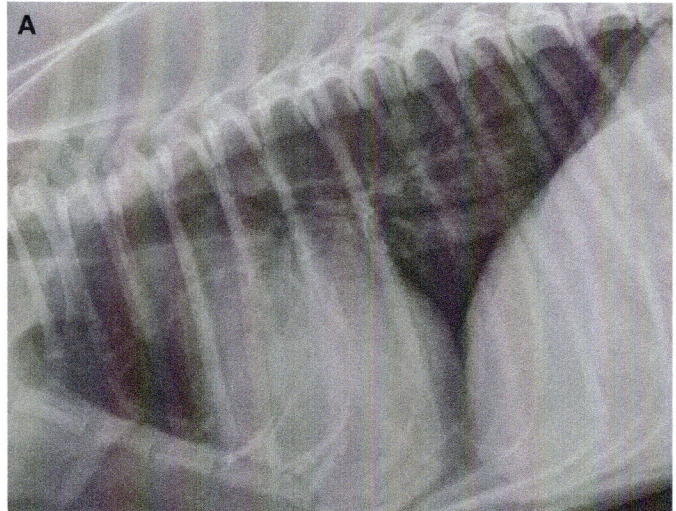
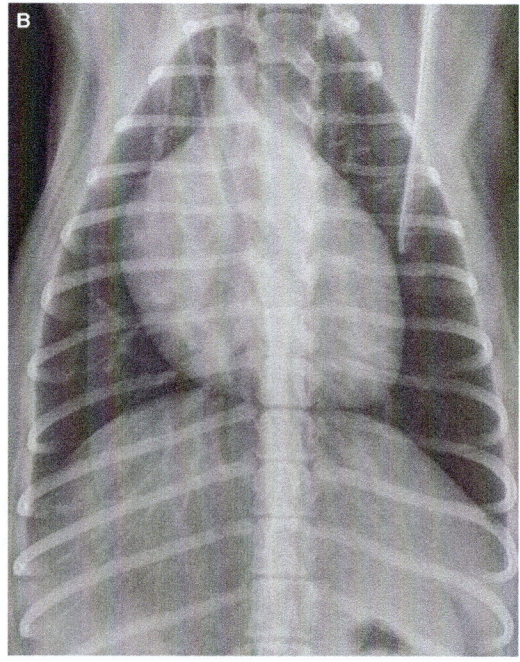

Figure 26.48 Lateral (A) and DV (B) radiographs from a 2-year-old male Yorkshire Terrier with tetralogy of Fallot, as well as left ventricular outflow obstruction. There is mild cardiomegaly with right ventricular prominence, attenuated pulmonary vasculature, and widening in the area of the ascending aorta (A).

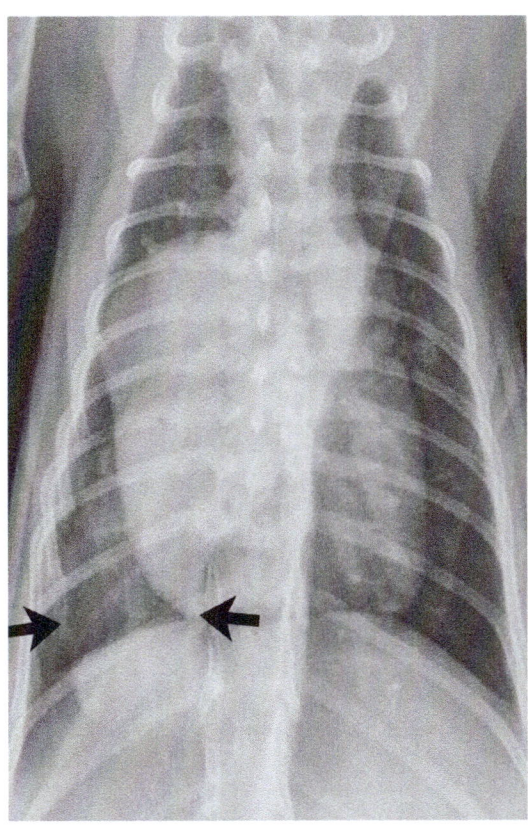

Figure 26.49 Dorsoventral radiograph shows massive right ventricular enlargement in a 4-month-old kitten with tetralogy of Fallot. The caudal vena cava is extremely distended (between arrows); this is more easily appreciated on the kitten's lateral view (see **Figure 3.18**, p. 61).

Doppler studies reveal the RV-to-aortic shunt that can be bidirectional or predominately R-to-L (or possibly L-to-R) along with the increased outflow velocity of PS (unless there is pulmonary atresia). An echocontrast study or angiocardiogram also can document the R-to-L shunt. Although cardiac catheterization can demonstrate RV and LV pressure equalization, decreased aortic O_2 saturation, and other angiographic features, it is rarely done (**Figures 26.51** and **26.52**). If surgical palliation or correction are contemplated, CT angiography is recommended to measure the size of the pulmonary arteries and identify aorticopulmonary collateral vessels.

Management

Definitive repair for T of F requires open-heart surgery. Various palliative procedures increase pulmonary blood flow by surgically creating a L-to-R shunt, although this risks overloading the left heart and causing pulmonary edema. Techniques used have included anastomosing the left subclavian artery to the PA (Blalock–Taussig procedure) either directly or via artificial shunt, creating a window between the ascending aorta and PA (Potts procedure), or creating an aortic to right PA shunt (Waterston–Cooley procedure). In cases of valvular stenosis, pulmonary balloon valvuloplasty potentially can serve as a palliative procedure by decreasing resistance to flow across the pulmonary valve, thereby reducing R-to-L shunting. If a PDA is also present it will serve to increase pulmonary blood flow and the vessel might be stented to better perfuse the lung.

Maintaining hydration is essential; free access to water and lightly salting the food might encourage more fluid intake. Periodic phlebotomy helps manage severe erythrocytosis and clinical signs associated with hyperviscosity (including

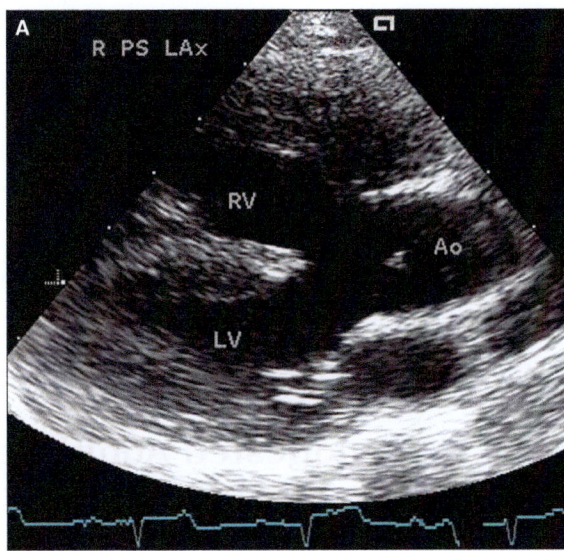 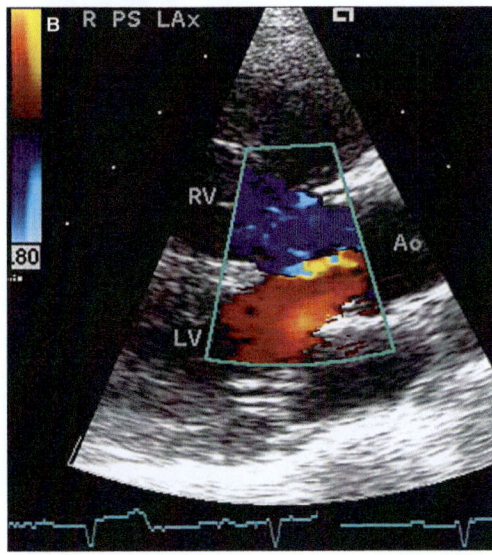

Figure 26.50 (A) Right parasternal long-axis image from the dog of **Figure 26.45**, with tetralogy of Fallot, shows the large ventricular septal defect with wide overriding aortic root. (B) Color flow Doppler demonstrates flow from both ventricles entering the aorta. Ao, aorta; LV, left ventricle; RV, right ventricle.

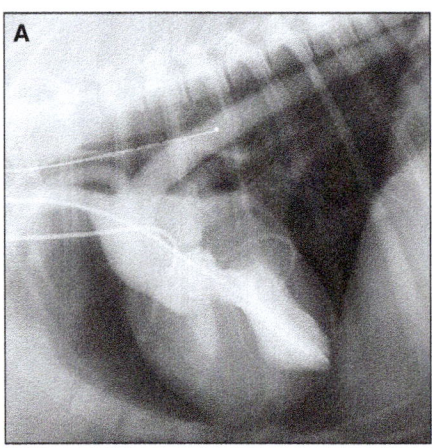 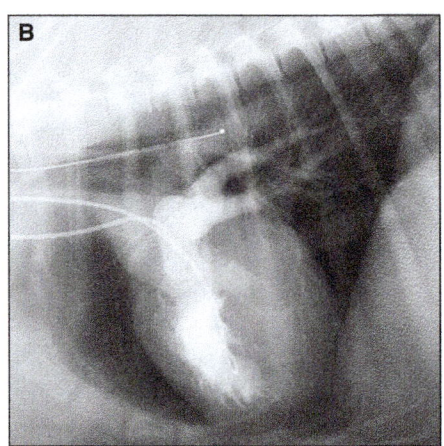

Figure 26.51 Angiocardiograms from the dog of **Figure 26.46**. (A) Left ventricular (LV) injection shows a large aortic root overriding the hypertrophied interventricular septum. Bidirectional shunting is evident from the dye seen in the right ventricular (RV) outflow region and pulmonary arteries. The hypertrophied right ventricle has lifted the LV apex dorsally. (B) RV injection through the same catheter as in (A), which was passed from the carotid artery to the ascending aorta then into the right ventricle; dye in the aorta and left ventricle documents right-to-left shunting. Poststenotic dilation of the main pulmonary artery is evident. (Images courtesy of Drs JO Noxon and S McNeel.)

weakness, shortness of breath, seizures). A volume of blood is withdrawn, and sometimes replaced with isotonic fluid, to maintain the hematocrit at a level where clinical signs are minimal (see p. 454). Excessive reduction in hematocrit can exacerbate signs of hypoxia. Alternatively, hydroxyurea might be used to control erythrocytosis in some cases (p. 454).

A beta-adrenergic blocker also might help some animals with T of F that have a component of dynamic RV outflow tract obstruction. In theory, propranolol is the best beta-blocker for this purpose because of its potent negative inotropy, strong beta-receptor inverse agonism, and the potential for some peripheral vasoconstriction by blocking beta-2 receptors. In most countries, atenolol is more practical based on available dosing sizes and twice-daily administration. Reduction of sympathetic tone, RV contractility, RV (dynamic muscular) outflow obstruction, and myocardial oxygen consumption, along with increased peripheral vascular resistance, are purported benefits of nonspecific beta-blocker therapy in children (and presumably, animals) with T of F. Exercise restriction is important to help minimize R-to-L shunting. Drugs with systemic vasodilator effects should be avoided.

The prognosis for T of F can depend on the degree of PS and erythrocytosis. Progressive hypoxemia, erythrocytosis and hyperviscosity, arrhythmias, and sudden death at an early age are common. Mean survival time was slightly under 2 years in a case series of dogs and cats; however, for patients with soft or no murmurs, mean survival was just over 3 months (Chetboul, 2016). This is consistent with the concept that marked secondary erythrocytosis and hyperviscosity, severe PS or pulmonary atresia, or a combination of these findings worsens the prognosis. Nevertheless, mildly affected animals or those that have undergone a successful palliative surgical shunting procedure have lived well into middle age. CHF is uncommon with T of F.

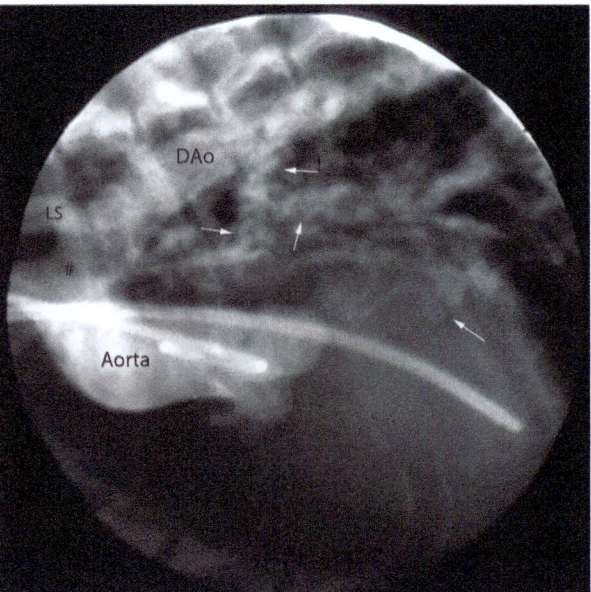

Figure 26.52 Aortic root angiographic contrast injection in a cat with pulmonary atresia and prominent systemic collateral vessels (arrows). These are multiple dilated and tortuous vessels that develop in response to reduced pulmonary blood flow. # aortic arch; LS left subclavian artery; DAo descending aorta.

Suggested Additional Reading and References

Also See Online Comprehensive Bibliography at: https://www.routledge.com/9781482246223.

Achen SE, Miller MW, Gordon SG, et al. Transarterial ductal occlusion with the Amplatzer vascular plug in 31 dogs. J Vet Intern Med 2008;22:1348–1352.

Anderson RH, Becker AE, Freedom RM, et al. Sequential segmental analysis of congenital heart disease. Pediatr Cardiol. 1984;5:281–287.

Aramaki Y, Chimura S, Hori Y, et al. Therapeutic changes of plasma N-terminal pro-brain natriuretic peptide concentrations in 9 dogs with patent ductus arteriosus. J Vet Med Sci 2011;73: 83–88.

Bascunan A, Thieman Mankin KM, Saunders AB, et al. Patent ductus arteriosus in cats (*Felis catus*): 50 cases (2000–2015). J Vet Cardiol 2017;19:35–43.

Baumgartner C, Glaus TM. Congenital cardiac diseases in dogs: a retrospective analysis. Schweiz Arch Tierheilkd 2003;145: 527–533, 535–526.

Blossom JE, Bright JM, Griffiths LG. Transvenous occlusion of patent ductus arteriosus in 56 consecutive dogs. J Vet Cardiol 2010;12:75–84.

Bomassi E, Libermann S, Bille C, et al. Patent ductus arteriosus in a family of Chihuahuas. J Small Anim Pract 2011;52:213–219.

Bonagura JD. Overview of equine cardiac disease. Vet Clin North Am Equine Pract 2019;35:1–22.

Boutet BG, Saunders AB, Gordon SG. Clinical characteristics of adult dogs more than 5 years of age at presentation for patent ductus arteriosus. J Vet Intern Med 2017;31:685–690.

Buchanan JW. Prevalence of cardiovascular disorders. In, Fox PR, Sisson D, Moise NS (editors). Textbook of Canine and Feline Cardiology. 2nd edition. WB Saunders, Philadelphia, PA. 1999. pp. 457–470.

Buchanan JW, Patterson DF. Etiology of patent ductus arteriosus in dogs. J Vet Intern Med 2003;17:167–171.

Buergelt CD. Equine cardiovascular pathology: an overview. Anim Health Res Rev 2003;4:109–129.

Bureau S, Monnet E, Orton EC. Evaluation of survival rate and prognostic indicators for surgical treatment of left-to-right patent ductus arteriosus in dogs: 52 cases (1995–2003). J Am Vet Med Assoc 2005;227:1794–1799.

Chetboul V, Charles V, Nicolle A, et al. Retrospective study of 156 atrial septal defects in dogs and cats (2001–2005). J Vet Med A Physiol Pathol Clin Med 2006;53:179–184.

Chetboul V, Pitsch I, Tissier R, et al. Epidemiological, clinical, and echocardiographic features and survival times of dogs and cats with tetralogy of Fallot: 31 cases (2003–2014). J Am Vet Med Assoc 2016;249:909–917.

Chetboul V, Roche-Catholy M, Pun-Garcia A, et al. The variety of phenotypes behind 'double outlet right ventricle': clinical and imaging presentations in four dogs and a cat. J Vet Cardiol 2020;31:51–60.

Côté E, Ettinger SJ. Long-term clinical management of right-to-left ('reversed') patent ductus arteriosus in 3 dogs. J Vet Intern Med 2001;15:39–42.

Das S, Yool DA, French AT, et al. An unusual morphology of patent ductus arteriosus in a dog. J Small Anim Pract 2012;53:353–356.

De Lange L, Vera L, Decloedt A, et al. Prevalence and characteristics of ventricular septal defects in a non-racehorse equine population (2008-2019). J Vet Intern Med 2021. doi: 10.1111/jvim.16106. (Epub ahead of print. PMID: 33742468.)

De Monte V, Staffieri F, Caivano D, et al. Heart rate and blood pressure variations after transvascular patent ductus arteriosus occlusion in dogs. Res Vet Sci 2017;113:73–78.

Doocy KR, Nelson DA, Saunders AB. Real-time 3D transesophageal echocardiography-guided closure of a complicated patent ductus arteriosus in a dog. J Vet Cardiol 2017;19: 287–292.

Doocy KR, Saunders AB, Gordon SG, et al. Comparative, multidimensional imaging of patent ductus arteriosus and a proposed update to the morphology classification system for dogs. J Vet Intern Med 2018;32:648–657.

Durham J, Maisenbacher H. Double-outlet right atrium in a 9 year-old cat. J Vet Cardiol. 2014;16:127–131.

Falcini R, Gaspari M, Polveroni G. Transthoracic echocardiographic guidance of patent ductus arteriosus occlusion with an Amplatz(R) canine duct occluder. Res Vet Sci 2011;90: 359–362.

Fujii Y, Aoki T, Takano H, et al. Arteriovenous shunts resembling patent ductus arteriosus in dogs: 3 cases. J Vet Cardiol 2009;11:147–151.

Fujii Y, Nishimoto Y, Sunahara H, Takano H, Aoki T. Prevalence of patent foramen ovale with right-to-left shunting in dogs with pulmonic stenosis. J Vet Intern Med 2012;26:183–185.

Goodrich KR, Kyles AE, Kass PH, et al. Retrospective comparison of surgical ligation and transarterial catheter occlusion for treatment of patent ductus arteriosus in two hundred and four dogs (1993–2003). Vet Surg 2007;36:43–49.

Gordon SG, Saunders AB, Achen SE, et al. Transarterial ductal occlusion using the Amplatz canine duct occluder in 40 dogs. J Vet Cardiol 2010;12:85–92.

Greet V, Bode EF, Dukes-McEwan J, et al. Clinical features and outcome of dogs and cats with bidirectional and continuous right-to-left shunting patent ductus arteriosus. J Vet Intern Med 2021;35:780–788.

Hall TL, Magdesian KG, Kittleson MD. Congenital cardiac defects in neonatal foals: 18 cases (1992–2007). J Vet Intern Med 2010;24:206–212.

Hariu CD, Saunders AB, Gordon SG, et al. Utility of N-terminal pro-brain natriuretic peptide for assessing hemodynamic significance of patent ductus arteriosus in dogs undergoing ductal repair. J Vet Cardiol 2013;15(3):197–204.

Henrich E, Hildebrandt N, Schneider C, et al. Transvenous coil embolization of patent ductus arteriosus in small (</=3.0 kg) dogs. J Vet Intern Med 2011;25:65–70.

Hildebrandt N, Schneider C, Schweigl T, et al. Long-term follow-up after transvenous single coil embolization of patent ductus arteriosus in dogs. J Vet Intern Med 2010;24:1400–1406.

Hutton JE, Steffey MA, Runge JJ, et al. Surgical and nonsurgical management of patent ductus arteriosus in cats: 28 cases (1991–2012). J Am Vet Med Assoc 2015;247:278–285.

Lee SA, Lee SG, Moon HS, et al. Isolation, characterization and genetic analysis of canine GATA4 gene in a family of Doberman Pinschers with an atrial septal defect. J Genet 2007;86:241–247.

Macdonald AA, Fowden AL, Silver M, et al. The foramen ovale of the foetal and neonatal foal. Equine Vet J 1988;20:255–260.

Macdonald AA, Johnstone M. Comparative anatomy of the cardiac foramen ovale in cats (Felidae), dogs (Canidae), bears (Ursidae) and hyaenas (Hyaenidae). J Anat 1995;186:235–243.

Markovic LE, Scansen BA. Effect of calibration methods on the accuracy of angiographic measurements during transcatheter procedures in dogs. J Vet Intern Med 2018;32(3):956–961.

Marr CM. Cardiac murmurs: congenital heart disease. In, Marr CM (editor). Cardiology of the Horse. 2nd edition. Saunders Elsevier, Edinburgh. 2010. pp. 193–205.

Miller MW, Gordon SG, Saunders AB, et al. Angiographic classification of patent ductus arteriosus morphology in the dog. J Vet Cardiol 2006;8:109–114.

Nguyenba TP, Tobias AH. Minimally invasive per-catheter patent ductus arteriosus occlusion in dogs using a prototype duct occluder. J Vet Intern Med 2008;22:129–134.

Oliveira P, Domenech O, Silva J, et al. Retrospective review of congenital heart disease in 976 dogs. J Vet Intern Med 2011;25:477–483.

Oyama MA, Sisson DD. Evaluation of canine congenital heart disease using an echocardiographic algorithm. J Am Anim Hosp Assoc 2001;37:519–535.

Patterson DF, Pyle RL, Van Mierop L, et al. Hereditary defects of the conotruncal septum in Keeshond dogs: pathologic and genetic studies. Amer J Cardio 1974;34:187e205.

Payne JR, Brodbelt DC, Luis Fuentes V. Cardiomyopathy prevalence in 780 apparently healthy cats in rehoming centres (the CatScan study). J Vet Cardiol 2015;17(Suppl 1):S244–257.

Peddle GD, Buchanan JW. Acquired atrial septal defects secondary to rupture of the atrial septum in dogs with degenerative mitral valve disease. J Vet Cardiol 2010;12:129–134.

Porciello F, Caivano D, Giorgi ME, et al. Transesophageal echocardiography as the sole guidance for occlusion of patent ductus arteriosus using a canine ductal occluder in dogs. J Vet Intern Med 2014;28:1504–1512.

Ranganathan B, LeBlanc NL, Scollan KF, et al. Comparison of major complication and survival rates between surgical ligation and use of a canine ductal occluder device for treatment of dogs with left-to-right shunting patent ductus arteriosus. J Am Vet Med Assoc 2018;253:1046–1052.

Reef VB. Evaluation of ventricular septal defects in horses using two-dimensional and Doppler echocardiography. Equine Vet J Suppl 1995:86–95.

Sanders RA, Olivier NB. Alternative methods for the measurement of the minimal ductal diameter of a patent ductus arteriosus in a dog. J Vet Cardiol 2016;18:372–376.

Saunders AB, Achen SE, Gordon SG, et al. Utility of transesophageal echocardiography for transcatheter occlusion of patent ductus arteriosus in dogs: influence on the decision-making process. J Vet Intern Med 2010;24:1407–1413.

Saunders AB, Gordon SG, Boggess MM, et al. Long-term outcome in dogs with patent ductus arteriosus: 520 cases (1994-2009). J Vet Intern Med 2014;28:401–410.

Saunders AB, Miller MW, Gordon SG, et al. Pulmonary embolization of vascular occlusion coils in dogs with patent ductus arteriosus. J Vet Intern Med 2004;18:663–666.

Saunders AB, Miller MW, Gordon SG, et al. Echocardiographic and angiographic comparison of ductal dimensions in dogs with patent ductus arteriosus. J Vet Intern Med 2007;21:68–75.

Scansen BA. Cardiac interventions in small animals: areas of uncertainty. Vet Clin North Am Small Anim Pract 2018;48:797–817.

Scansen BA. Equine congenital heart disease. Vet Clin North Am Equine Pract 2019;35:103–117.

Scansen BA, Cober RE, Bonagura JD. Congenital heart disease. In Bonagura JD & Twedt DC (editors), Kirk's Current Veterinary Therapy XV. Elsevier Saunders, St. Louis. 2014; pp756–761.

Scansen BA, Schneider M, Bonagura JD. Sequential segmental classification of feline congenital heart disease. J Vet Cardiol. 2015a; Suppl 1:S10–52.

Scansen BA, Simpson EM, Lopez-Alvarez J, et al. Pulmonary artery dissection in eight dogs with patent ductus arteriosus. J Vet Cardiol 2015b.

Schneider M, Hildebrandt N, Schweigl T, et al. Transthoracic echocardiographic measurement of patent ductus arteriosus in dogs. J Vet Intern Med 2007;21:251–257.

Schneider M, Schneider I, Hildebrandt N, et al. Percutaneous angiography of patent ductus arteriosus in dogs: techniques, results and implications for intravascular occlusion. J Vet Cardiol 2003; 5:21–27.

Schrope DP. Atrioventricular septal defects: natural history, echocardiographic, electrocardiographic, and radiographic findings in 26 cats. J Vet Cardiol 2013;15:233–242.

Schrope DP. Prevalence of congenital heart disease in 76,301 mixed-breed dogs and 57,025 mixed-breed cats. J Vet Cardiol 2015;17:192–202.

Schwarzwald CC. Sequential segmental analysis – a systematic approach to the diagnosis of congenital cardiac defects. Equine Vet Educ 2008;20:305–309.

Seibert RL, Maisenbacher HW 3rd, Prosek R, et al. Successful closure of left-to-right patent ductus arteriosus in three dogs with concurrent pulmonary hypertension. J Vet Cardiol 2010;12:67–73.

Singh MK, Kittleson MD, Kass PH, et al. Occlusion devices and approaches in canine patent ductus arteriosus: comparison of outcomes. J Vet Intern Med 2012;26:85–92.

Stanley BJ, Luis-Fuentes V, Darke PG. Comparison of the incidence of residual shunting between two surgical techniques used for ligation of patent ductus arteriosus in the dog. Vet Surg 2003;32:231–237.

Stauthammer CD, Olson J, Leeder D, et al. Patent ductus arteriosus occlusion in small dogs utilizing a low profile Amplatz(R) canine duct occluder prototype. J Vet Cardiol 2015;17:203–209.

Thomas WP. Echocardiographic diagnosis of congenital membranous ventricular septal aneurysm in the dog and cat. J Am Anim Hosp Assoc 2005;41:215–220.

Tidholm A. Retrospective study of congenital heart defects in 151 dogs. J Small Anim Pract 1997;38:94–98.

Tidholm A, Ljungvall I, Michal J, et al. Congenital heart defects in cats: a retrospective study of 162 cats (1996-2013). J Vet Cardiol 2015;17(Suppl 1):S215–219.

Van Israel N, Dukes-McEwan J, French AT. Long-term follow-up of dogs with patent ductus arteriosus. J Small Anim Pract 2003;44:480–490.

Van Praagh R. Nomenclature and Classification: Morphologic and segmental approach to diagnosis. In: Moller JH, Hoffman JIE (editors), Pediatric Cardiovascular Medicine. New York, Churchill Livingstone; 1970:275–288.

Werner P, Raducha MG, Prociuk U, et al. The keeshond defect in cardiac conotruncal development is oligogenic. Hum Genet 2005;116:368–377.

Wesselowski S, Saunders AB, Gordon SG. Relationship between device size and body weight in dogs with patent ductus arteriosus undergoing amplatz canine duct occluder deployment. J Vet Intern Med 2017;31:1388–1391.

Wesselowski S, Saunders AB, Gordon SG. Anatomy, baseline characteristics, and procedural outcome of patent ductus arteriosus in German shepherd dogs. J Vet Intern Med 2019;33:471–477.

Wustefeld-Janssens BG, Burrow R, Motskula P, et al. Clinical findings and treatment outcomes for cats diagnosed with patent ductus arteriosus in the UK: a retrospective study of 19 cases (2004-2012). Vet Rec 2016;179:17.

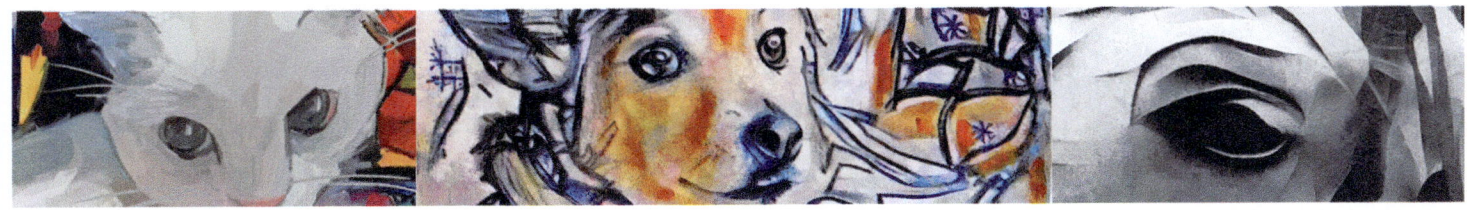

27
CONGENITAL VALVULAR MALFORMATIONS

Malformations of cardiac valves and their adjacent or support structures are common, especially in dogs. Defects that involve the semilunar valve regions mainly cause ventricular outflow obstruction, although mild, and usually inaudible, valvular regurgitation commonly coexists. Outflow obstructive lesions can occur at the semilunar valve itself, just below the valve (subvalvular), or in the proximal great vessel (supravalvular). In the left heart, stenosis below the aortic valve (subaortic) is most common in dogs. In contrast, malformations at the pulmonary valve leaflet and annulus level occur most often in companion animals; this can include tethering of the leaflets to the pulmonary artery at the upper reaches of the valve. Subvalvular (infundibular) narrowing from muscular hypertrophy is a frequent accompaniment. Sporadically, isolated stenotic lesions occur above the pulmonary valve or in a major branch pulmonary artery rather than the pulmonary valve region. Defects of the atrioventricular (AV) valves and related structures usually cause valve regurgitation. AV valve stenosis (or supravalvular ring), causing ventricular inflow obstruction, occurs only in a small minority of cases. Some animals have a combination of two or more congenital cardiac malformations, which might include valvular lesion(s), shunt(s), or other defects. These could occur sporadically or represent a breed or familial predilection (**Table 27.1**). Tetralogy of Fallot (T of F) in Keeshond dogs is a well-known example (p. 467). In some regions, Boxer dogs seem predisposed to concurrent aortic stenosis (AS) and pulmonic stenosis (PS), with a male predominance.

Various clinical case surveys of congenital heart disease (CHD) report subaortic stenosis (SAS), or even valvular PS, to be the most common congenital heart malformation in dogs, rather than patent ductus arteriosus (PDA, Chapter 26). However, predisposition to these different malformations varies among breeds and geographic regions. In a compilation of multiple canine studies, the percentage of 4,694 dogs with CHD, indicated PDA at 25.7%, SAS at 23.5% and PS at 22.1% of cases, followed by ventricular septal defect (VSD) at 8.8% (Scansen, 2014). The overall prevalence of valvular malformations appears lower in cats and horses, compared to dogs. In the previously noted survey, tricuspid valve dysplasia (TVD) and mitral valve dysplasia (MVD) represented 10.8% and 10.1% of 435 feline cases, respectively. Additionally, AV valve malformation is a component of both partial and complete AV septal defects (p. 466). Tricuspid and pulmonary valve malformations are observed sporadically in horses, whereas left-sided valvular malformations are rare. Therefore, this chapter is focused on dogs and cats, unless otherwise noted. Nevertheless, the principles of pathophysiology relevant to dogs and cats do apply to the horse (also see Chapter 30).

As with congenital shunts (Chapter 26), many animals show no clinical signs before the discovery of a heart murmur alerts the clinician to a potential problem. Especially with defects causing ventricular outflow obstruction, murmur intensity generally correlates with severity. When clinical signs are evident, the prognosis usually is guarded to poor unless intervention or other therapy can be provided expeditiously. Such signs most commonly include reduced exercise tolerance and evidence for left- or right-sided congestive heart failure (CHF), depending on the lesion. Stunted growth, intermittent weakness or syncope, sudden death, and occasionally, cyanosis also occur in some cases.

Severe defects are relatively straightforward to identify. However, screening of potential breeding animals can be challenging, especially with regard to AS variants and AV valve dysplasia. The facts that some animals have a soft murmur without structural disease and that certain mild defects (or genetic predisposition to them) might not cause an audible murmur are confounding factors. This is augmented by the lack of autopsy-proven correlations to Doppler echocardiography, such that this examination sometimes can yield equivocal findings. It is especially challenging to separate murmurs of trivial to mild AS from innocent murmurs, which also are relatively common in young animals. Innocent murmurs (p. 228) typically are soft, systolic ejection murmurs heard best

Cardiovascular Disease in Companion Animals 477

Table 27.1 Breed Predispositions for Congenital Valvular Malformations

Defect	Breed
Subaortic stenosis	Bouvier des Flandres, Boxer, Dogue de Bordeaux, English Bulldog, German Shepherd Dog, German Shorthaired Pointer, Golden Retriever, Great Dane, Newfoundland, Rottweiler, Samoyed; males > females, at least in some breeds
Aortic stenosis (valvular)	Boxer, Bull Terrier; ? males > females
Pulmonic stenosis	Airedale Terrier, American Staffordshire (Pitbull) Terrier, Bassett Hound, Beagle, Boxer, Boykin Spaniel, Chihuahua, Chow Chow, Cocker Spaniel, English Bulldog (males > females), Fox Terrier(?), French Bulldog, Labrador Retriever, Mastiff, Newfoundland, Samoyed, Schnauzer (Miniature, Standard), Pinscher (?), Scottish Terrier, West Highland White Terrier; also, other terrier and spaniel breeds; males > females, at least in some breeds
Mitral dysplasia	Boxer, Bull Terrier, Dalmation, German Shepherd Dog, Golden Retriever, Great Dane, Mastiff, Newfoundland, Rottweiler(?); cats (especially Sphynx, others); males > females
Tricuspid dysplasia	Border Collie, Boxer, Dogue de Bordeaux, English Bulldog, German Shepherd Dog, Golden Retriever, Great Dane, Labrador Retriever, Old English Sheepdog, Weimaraner; other large breeds; Chartreux cats; males > females

Note: Breeds not listed in order of malformation prevalence.

at the left heart base (over the aortic valve area); their intensity can vary with heart rate or body position. They can sound similar to those pathologic murmurs, but often are of shorter duration, although this could be difficult to discern without phonocardiography. Innocent puppy murmurs often diminish with time and "classically" disappear by about 4 months of age. However, this is an oversimplification. Soft ejection murmurs are common in mature large-breed dogs. Some of these breeds are prone to (sub)aortic stenosis (including; Boxers, Bull terriers, and others), but others are not (such as Greyhounds). Simply stated, cardiologists have developed largely arbitrary diagnostic guidelines to separate soft pathologic from physiologic murmurs and much work needs to be done. Murmurs associated with significant valvular malformations usually persist and many become louder as the animal grows. This is typical of SAS but also can be seen with PS and AV valve malformations. Careful evaluation at full maturity is especially important in animals intended for breeding, because those with a congenital cardiac malformation should not be bred.

Pathophysiology

Ventricular Outflow Obstruction

Ventricular outflow obstruction, whether caused by a fixed stenotic lesion or muscular (dynamic) obstruction during systole, imposes a systolic pressure overload on the affected ventricle. Concentric hypertrophy is the ventricle's response to chronic systolic pressure overload (p. 16; **Figure 27.1**). However, some dilation of the affected ventricle can occur if there is ventricular failure, concurrent valvular regurgitation, or a shunt that increases venous return. Downstream from the stenosis, measured pressure is normal unless altered by abnormally increased vascular resistance. The high pressure generated within the ventricle serves as a source of potential energy, which is converted to kinetic energy as red cells accelerate and are rapidly ejected across the stenosis. Downstream, turbulent flow and pressure fluctuations within the wake of this high velocity jet produce a systolic murmur and disturbed blood flow, as recorded by Doppler echocardiography (echo). The turbulence and dissipation of energy from the high-velocity flow jet distends the proximal great vessel (post-stenotic dilation; p. 23). However, aortopathy and pulmonary arteriopathy also can occur independently from a severe stenosis in some breeds, and in part, might be genetically programmed. The magnitude of the systolic pressure difference (pressure gradient, PG) across the stenotic area is related to the severity of obstruction, as well as ventricular contractile strength and stroke volume. A common error made when assessing the severity of stenosis by Doppler echo is

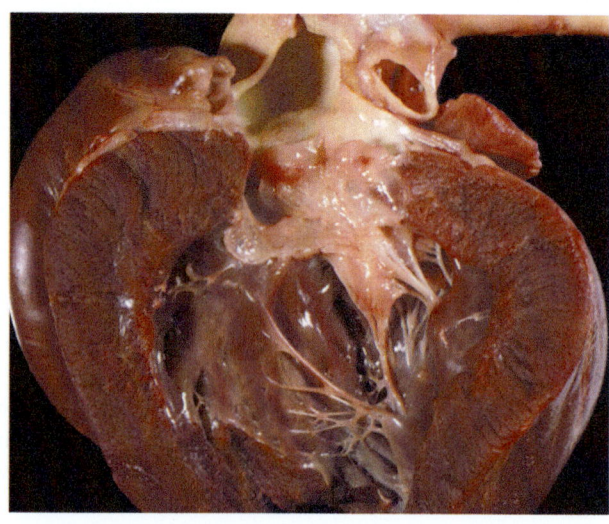

Figure 27.1 Myocardial concentric hypertrophy is a major consequence of ventricular outflow obstruction. Marked left ventricular (LV) hypertrophy is evident in this specimen from a dog with severe subaortic stenosis. A wide fibrous ring encircles the LV outflow tract, including the ventricular side of the anterior mitral leaflet, in this case.

emphasizing the PG while neglecting the importance of flow. Secondary (or primary) AV valve regurgitation imposes an additional volume load on the affected ventricle, as semilunar valve regurgitation sometimes can as well.

Concentric hypertrophy impairs myocardial relaxation, reduces ventricular compliance, and impairs diastolic filling (because of increased ventricular stiffness). This increases reliance on atrial contraction in late diastole; the development of atrial fibrillation (AF) can precipitate CHF. Even when sinus rhythm is maintained, progressive diastolic and systolic dysfunction from chronic pressure overload will increase filling pressures and predispose to congestive signs. Concentric hypertrophy and increased systolic pressure also impair coronary blood flow. High intraventricular pressure can even cause coronary arterial flow reversal during systole. Subendocardial to mid-myocardial regions are at greatest risk for inadequate perfusion and myocardial ischemia, which leads to the development of replacement fibrosis over time. These factors further increase myocardial stiffness and can trigger arrhythmias, as well as contribute to impaired systolic function, CHF and low output signs.

Furthermore, sudden increases in intraventricular systolic pressure related to outflow obstruction and sympathetic stimulation can activate ventricular mechanoreceptors (baroreceptors), inappropriately triggering reflex bradycardia and vasodilation. The combination of outflow obstruction, paroxysmal tachyarrhythmias, or inappropriate bradycardia secondary to ventricular baroreceptor stimulation can cause exercise intolerance, syncope, and sudden death even in the absence of CHF. These low-output signs are most often associated with severe outflow tract obstruction.

Plasma N-terminal probrain natriuretic peptide (NT-proBNP) concentration might be elevated in animals with a malformation that causes ventricular outflow obstruction; however, this test alone is not adequately sensitive to consistently differentiate innocent from pathologic murmurs. In a recent study involving Cairn Terriers, although mean NT-proBNP was significantly higher in puppies with congenital disease, some animals with severe PS showed no increase in NT-proBNP (Marinus, 2017).

Semilunar Valve Regurgitation

Doppler echo usually reveals trivial to mild semilunar valve regurgitation associated with outflow tract obstructions. More significant aortic and pulmonary valve regurgitation occurs when the valve itself is malformed; this is of greater concern on the left side because of the higher aortic pressures. Mild aortic valve regurgitation (AR) commonly accompanies SAS, VSD, PDA, and T of F, largely related to aortic root dilation in these conditions, or prolapse of an aortic valve into the VSD (Chapter 26). Likewise, mild to moderate pulmonary valve regurgitation (PR) is common in congenital PS. Mild AR and PR usually are inaudible. Trivial PR is common in most normal animals, also.

Isolated congenital AR and PR occur rarely. These can be associated with abnormal valve leaflet formation (sporadically, this could include a quadricuspid or bicuspid aortic valve; **Figure 27.2**) or annular dilation. Moderate to severe AR imposes a volume overload on the left ventricle, increases stroke volume, and eventually can lead to left-sided CHF. A large stroke volume can cause an ejection murmur (of relative valve stenosis) even in the absence of structural stenosis. In combination with the diastolic murmur of AR, this produces a "to-and-fro" murmur (p. 231). Marked AR also produces hyperkinetic or bounding arterial pulses, as the rapid diastolic backflow from aorta to ventricle causes arterial diastolic pressure to fall quickly, widening the pulse pressure (p. 255). In the case of PR, because pulmonary artery pressures normally are low, the hemodynamic consequences are better tolerated; usually there is minimal to no murmur. Yet with severe PR, right ventricular (RV) eccentric hypertrophy does develop and a diastolic murmur might become audible. This often is noted after balloon valvuloplasty for valvular PS. Humans with chronic PR can develop RV dysfunction and heart failure, but this seems less common in dogs. Pulmonary hypertension in combination with moderate to severe PR can produce a to-and-fro murmur and potentially, could lead to right-sided CHF; although, in the context of a right-to-left (R-to-L) shunt, CHF is unlikely.

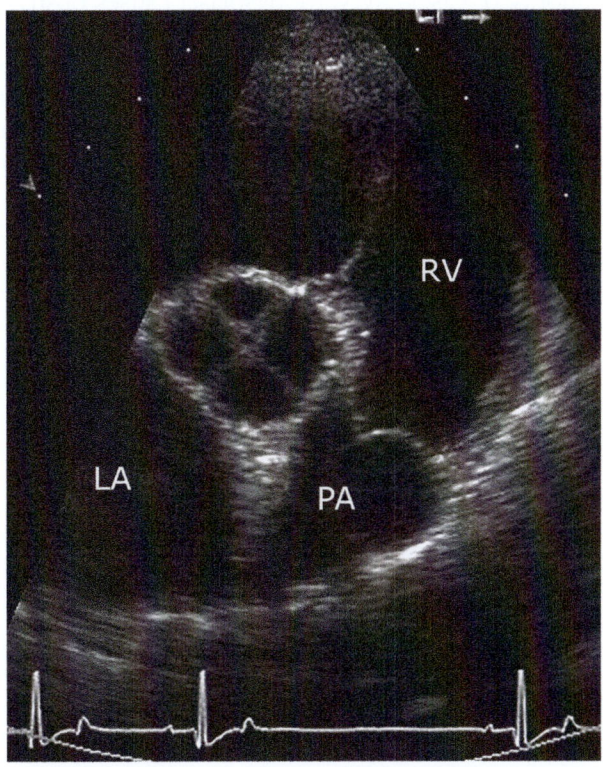

Figure 27.2 Quadricuspid aortic valve malformation in a young Boxer dog. Mild-moderate aortic regurgitation also was present in this case. Right parasternal short-axis view. LA, left atrium; PA, pulmonary artery; RV, right ventricle.

Atrioventricular Valve Regurgitation

Congenital malformation (dysplasia) of AV valves and their support structures usually cause valvular regurgitation (insufficiency), although some cause stenosis (see next section). Together these account for about 25% of feline CHD, if valvular malformations associated with AV septal defects also are included. AV dysplasia is less common in dogs (about 10% of CHD) and sporadically is observed in foals and young horses. Subtle mitral valve malformations probably are underdiagnosed in all three species. AV valve regurgitation imposes a volume overload on the affected side of the heart, leading to atrial and ventricular dilation (eccentric hypertrophy). The pathophysiology and clinical sequelae are similar to those of chronic degenerative (myxomatous) valve disease (Chapter 29).

Mitral valve malformations can cause valve leaflet systolic anterior motion (SAM) and dynamic left ventricular (LV) outflow obstruction in both dogs and cats; this can lead to concentric LV hypertrophy, as well as secondary mitral regurgitation (MR). Beta-blocker therapy often resolves this situation, unlike the LV hypertrophy caused by hypertrophic cardiomyopathy or fixed SAS. After the animal matures, gradual withdrawal of beta-blocker therapy usually is possible. Residual thickening of the mitral leaflets typically is evident.

Atrioventricular Valve Stenosis

In a minority of cases, AV valve dysplasia causes obstruction to ventricular inflow. Some degree of AV valve insufficiency usually is present, as well. AV valve stenosis produces a small but significant diastolic pressure gradient and turbulent flow across the narrowed area (**Figure 27.3**). The increased atrial pressure upstream from the stenosis leads to secondary atrial dilation and hypertrophy, and often, CHF. The valve leaflets themselves usually are thickened, malformed and fused or tethered to shortened chordae tendineae. Hypoplasia of the valve annulus is possible, especially in *cor triatriatum dexter* (Chapter 28), where downstream stenosis of both tricuspid and pulmonary valves also can occur. Rarely, supravalvular mitral stenosis occurs, involving a fibrous or fibromuscular membrane just upstream from the AV valve or, in some cases of AV septal defect, a leftward shift of the ventral interatrial septal edge (p. 466). Supravalvular mitral stenosis is different from the defect known as *cor triatriatum sinister* (p. 512) or double outlet right atrium, although the hemodynamic consequences are similar.

Aortic Stenosis

Subvalvular narrowing caused by a fibrous or fibromuscular ring is the usual cause of AS in dogs (**Figures 27.1** and **27.4**) and it occurs in some cats. SAS is exceedingly rare in horses. Valvular stenosis or supravalvular AS also occurs uncommonly. Valvular AS can be caused by a fused, bicuspid aortic valve. Bull terriers and Boxers seem more prone to valvular AS, although they often have SAS. Valvular AS is characterized by variably thickened and usually fused leaflets; the valve annulus sometimes is narrowed.

The severity of SAS varies widely, ranging from subtle subclinical fibrous tissue ridges to a complete fibrous ring that causes severe obstruction within the LV outflow tract (LVOT). While the obstructive lesion appears as a thin protruding ridge ventral to the aortic valve in many cases, others have an elongated, tunnel-like obstruction. These lesions cause so-called "fixed" or anatomic obstruction. The ascending aorta often is dilated. It frequently forms a more acute (aorto-septal) angle with the dorsal ventricular septum

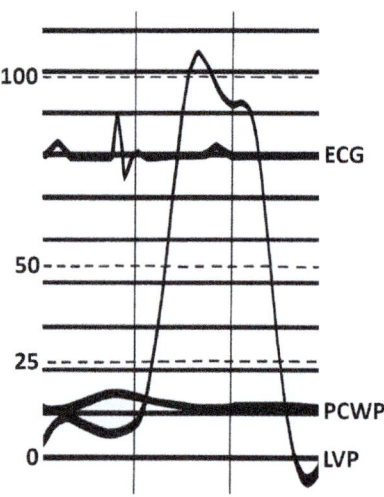

Figure 27.3 Simultaneous pulmonary capillary wedge pressure (PCWP) and left ventricular pressure (LVP) recordings represent the diastolic pressure gradient between left ventricle and left atrium in a 6-year-old female Irish Setter-mix with mitral valve stenosis. The transmitral gradient is greatest in early diastole. Pressure scale on left (mm Hg). ECG, electrocardiogram.

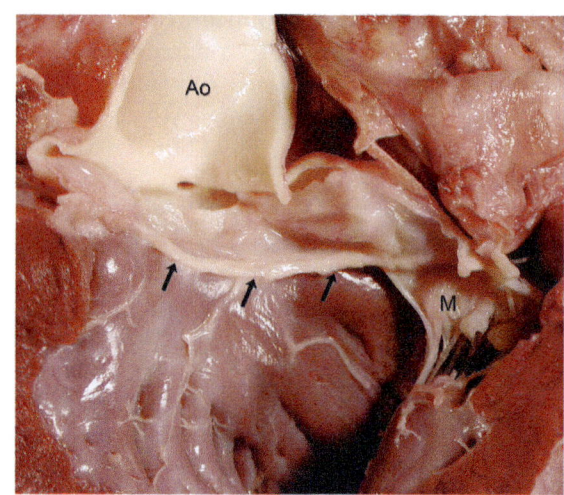

Figure 27.4 A band of fibrous tissue (arrows) extends around the left ventricular outflow tract and involves the anterior mitral leaflet (M) in this postmortem specimen from a dog with subaortic stenosis. Ao, aorta.

(as viewed from the right). This angle might be relevant to the development of the subaortic ridge, as has been suggested in Golden Retriever dogs (and in children), in that the shear forces which develop during blood ejection are thought to stimulate subvalvular tissue growth. This also supports the concept of an independent aortopathy in some cases. LVOT narrowing from dynamic obstruction between the ventricular septum and anterior mitral leaflet (with SAM), with or without a discrete subvalvular ridge, also has been noted, especially in Golden Retrievers but in other canine breeds and cats also. Malformation (dysplasia) of the mitral valve apparatus can coexist and contribute to fixed or dynamic obstruction. Dynamic LVOT obstruction also can occur in other CHD, likely from reduced LV volume.

Three grades of SAS severity, based on postmortem examination, originally were described in Newfoundland dogs (Pyle, 1976). Grade 1 (mild, subclinical) SAS consists of small, pale, and slightly raised nodules on the septal endocardium below the aortic valve. Dogs with grade 1 SAS might have no murmur; there is no significant systolic PG. Grade 2 (moderate) SAS involves a narrow ridge of pale, thickened endocardium that partially extends around the LVOT; affected dogs have a soft murmur and small systolic PG. Grade 3 (severe) SAS is characterized by a fibrous ridge or band that encircles the LVOT below the aortic valve; this fibrous ring can involve the cranioventral (anterior) mitral leaflet and the base of the aorta. Similar lesions occur in many other breeds with SAS; in some dogs, the anterior mitral leaflet is enveloped in the fibrous band (tunnel). Aortic valve thickening also can occur.

The obstructive lesion of SAS develops during the first few months of life. There often is no audible murmur at an early age. In some affected dogs, no murmur is detected until 1 or even 2 years of age; the obstruction might possibly continue to worsen beyond that age. Exercise or excitement generally increases the murmur's intensity. These factors, and the common occurrence of physiologic murmurs in some dog breeds that have a high prevalence of SAS, make definitive diagnosis of mild cases and genetic counseling to breeders challenging. Some SAS cases have concurrent defect(s) such as mitral dysplasia, PDA, or aortic arch abnormalities.

The severity of stenosis determines the degree of LV systolic pressure overload and influences the resulting concentric hypertrophy. The higher-velocity turbulent flow across the stenosis produces a systolic ejection murmur and promotes post-stenotic dilation of the ascending aorta, brachiocephalic artery, and aortic arch. SAS with fixed stenosis leads to a delayed, late-rising arterial pulse that feels weak (hypokinetic) on palpation (p. 255).

Coronary perfusion is compromised in dogs with severe SAS (also see p. 21). High LV systolic wall tension compresses and can reverse the direction of flow in small coronary arteries. In addition, intramural coronary arteries commonly are narrowed, perhaps as an adaptive response, but which further compromises coronary perfusion. Myocardial capillary density can become inadequate in the face of progressive concentric hypertrophy as well. These factors contribute to myocardial ischemia, cell death, and development of replacement fibrosis, especially in subendocardial and mid-myocardial regions.

Any AR or MR, caused by concurrent malformation or secondary ventricular changes, adds a component of LV volume overload on top of the systolic pressure load. Left-sided CHF in patients with SAS can be consequent to a combination of increased LV stiffness (diastolic dysfunction, from the effects of myocardial hypertrophy and ischemia), myocardial systolic failure (the cardiomyopathy of overload), MR, AR, and tachyarrhythmias, including ventricular ectopy and AF. Syncope and sudden death are common with severe (S) AS. In most cases, the proximate cause is probably a ventricular tachyarrhythmia provoked by ischemia or increased sympathetic tone. However, a bradyarrhythmia triggered by ventricular mechanoreceptor activation (from excessive intraventricular systolic pressure) also can occur. SAS predisposes to aortic valve endocarditis because of jet lesion injury to the LV side of the valve leaflets or concurrent AR (**Figures 31.7**, **31.10**, and **31.13**, pp. 599, 601, and 602, respectively.).

Clinical Features

SAS is more common in larger canine breeds (**Table 27.1**). At least in Boxers, SAS has a male predominance. It is thought to be inherited as an autosomal dominant trait (Boxers and Newfoundlands) with incomplete penetrance and variable phenotypic expression; however, another inheritance pattern is possible. An autosomal recessive pattern was suggested in Dogue de Bourdeax and a survey of Golden Retrievers suggested possible autosomal recessive or polygenic inheritance. A genetic mutation in the phosphatidylinositol-binding clathrin assembly protein (PICALM) gene has been identified that is strongly associated with SAS development in Newfoundland dogs, and in the few non-Newfoundland dogs with SAS tested (Stern, 2014). PICALM is involved in embryonic cardiac morphogenesis, particularly in LV outflow region development. Pedigree evaluation in this Newfoundland study supported an autosomal dominant pattern of inheritance, but also suggested that dogs with equivocal SAS could produce affected dogs when bred to normal animals. Clinical experience indicates that parents without obvious murmurs can produce a litter with multiple affected puppies.

Many affected animals are asymptomatic on initial presentation. Others show signs of reduced stamina, episodic weakness or collapse, stunted growth, and sometimes, left-sided CHF. Low output signs in dogs with severe SAS can result from an inability to increase cardiac output adequately with activity, tachyarrhythmias, or abrupt reflex bradycardia with hypotension. Severe SAS can cause sudden death without premonitory signs. Historical complaints of fatigue, exertional weakness, syncope, or sudden death occur in about one-third of dogs with SAS. Dyspnea is the most commonly reported sign in cats with SAS. Concurrent MR, AR, other cardiac malformations, and aortic valve endocarditis increase the risk for left-sided CHF.

Physical findings depend on the severity of the obstructive lesion. Moderate to severe stenosis often produces the characteristic weak and late-rising femoral pulses, a precordial thrill low on the left heart base, and a harsh systolic ejection murmur. There might be an especially strong and caudally displaced precordial impulse on the left, caused by LV hypertrophy. Normal jugular vein appearance is expected. Signs of pulmonary edema or arrhythmias might be present. The systolic ejection murmur originates at or just below the aortic valve area on the left hemithorax (**Figure 11.3**, p. 229). This murmur radiates equally, or more loudly, to the right heart base because the ascending aorta angles rightward into the aortic arch. With moderate to severe stenosis, a precordial thrill often is palpable at the right base in addition to that in the aortic valve area, because of turbulence in the ascending aorta. The murmur also can be heard fairly well over the carotid arteries. In severe cases, it might be softly audible on top of the patient's head as it radiates to the calvarium. In mild cases, a soft, poorly radiating ejection murmur at the left and, sometimes, the right heart base might be the only detectable abnormality. Murmur grade and time to peak intensity generally correlate with the severity of outflow obstruction. Projection of the murmur from the subaortic area to the apex can cause confusion with MR. Concurrent AR could produce a soft diastolic murmur at the left base (creating a "to-and-fro" murmur), especially when there is severe aortic root dilation or infective endocarditis. However, the mild AR associated with most cases of SAS is inaudible and only recognized on echo study.

The diagnosis of mild SAS can be challenging. Because the obstructive lesion of SAS develops as the animal grows to full adult size, there may be no or only a soft murmur at a young age. This is especially common in giant breeds like the Newfoundland. In addition, mild SAS murmurs are easily confused with innocent or nonpathological functional murmurs, which can sound similar and are quite common in many breeds predisposed to SAS. In a study involving Boxers, the absence of a murmur, or only a soft one, detected between 2 and 3 months of age correlated fairly well with aortic velocities under 2.4 m/s; velocities were similar at 1 year of age, although the correlation was not perfect (Jenni, 2009). Judgement regarding potential breeding animals should be reserved until the dog is fully mature.

Diagnostic Tests

Routine clinical laboratory tests typically are non-contributory. Increases in cardiac troponin (cTn) I concentration are modestly correlated with LV hypertrophy in dogs with SAS, although values can range widely. Increased NT-proBNP concentration also occurs with LV hypertrophy from experimental LV outflow obstruction. How these tests would be used clinically in SAS is uncertain.

Radiographic abnormalities (**Table 27.2**) often are subtle, especially in milder cases. The LV can appear normal or enlarged. A prominent cranial waist in the cardiac silhouette (lateral projection) and cranial mediastinal widening are manifestations of post-stenotic dilation in the ascending aorta (**Figures 27.5** and **27.6**). Some cases show left atrial (LA) enlargement, especially with concurrent MR. Thoracic radiographs can be normal with mild SAS.

The electrocardiogram (ECG) often is normal as well, although some cases show evidence of LV concentric hypertrophy (left axis deviation; **Figure 27.7**) or enlargement (tall complexes). ST segment depression resulting from myocardial ischemia or other changes secondary to hypertrophy might be present in the caudal leads (II and aVF) and left precordial leads (**Figure 5.54**, p. 157). A post-exercise ECG could reveal further ischemic ST segment changes, although Holter or event monitoring is more likely to show these. Ventricular tachyarrhythmias also are common, especially with exertion (**Figure 27.8**).

Echocardiography confirms the extent of LV hypertrophy and subaortic narrowing. Most patients with moderate to severe disease have a discrete subaortic tissue ridge or tunnel evident on 2D imaging; however, this can be subtle,

Table 27.2 Characteristic Radiographic Findings with Common Congenital Valvular Malformations

Defect	Heart	Pulmonary Vessels	Other
Subaortic stenosis	± LAE, LVE	Normal	Wide cranial cardiac waist (dilated ascending aorta)
Pulmonic stenosis	RAE, RVE; reverse D	Normal to undercirculated	Pulmonary trunk bulge; ± asymmetric pulmonary artery branch diameters; ± caudal vena caval dilation & R-CHF signs
Mitral dysplasia	LAE, LVE	± Venous hypertension	± Pulmonary edema
Tricuspid dysplasia	RAE, RVE; ± globoid shape	Normal	Caudal vena caval dilation; ± R-CHF signs

Findings within a specific diagnosis are quite variable; in some cases, findings also could relate to other valvular lesions, concurrent shunts, or congestive heart failure. R-CHF signs include: pleural effusion, hepatomegaly, ascites.
Abbreviations: LAE, left atrial enlargement; LVE, left ventricular enlargement; RAE, right atrial enlargement; R-CHF, right-sided congestive heart failure; RVE, right ventricular enlargement.

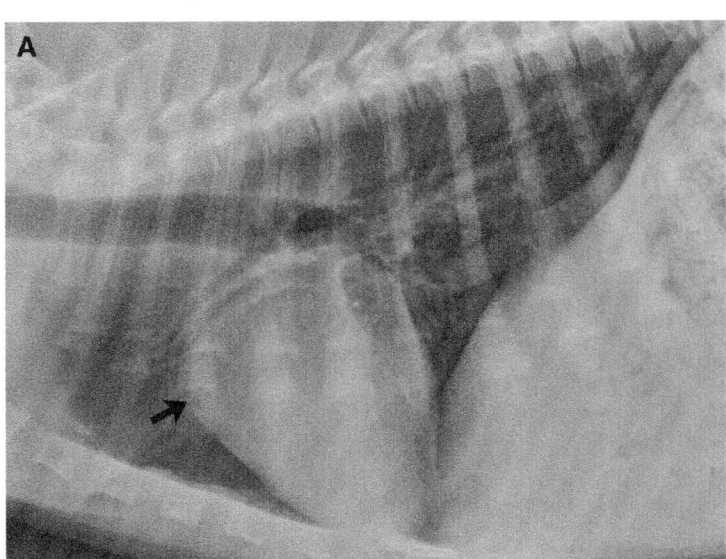
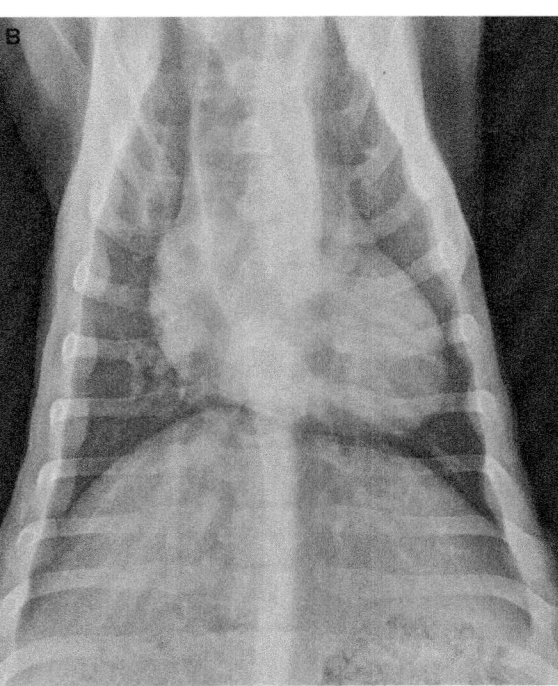

Figure 27.5 Lateral (A) and dorsoventral (B) radiographs from a 2-month-old female German Shepherd with severe subaortic stenosis (Doppler gradient ~145 mm Hg). Although the overall cardiac size is normal on lateral projection (VHS ~10.5v), the wide cranial waist (arrow) is consistent with post-stenotic dilation of the ascending aorta. The DV view shows some cardiac widening, with the apex elongated leftward.

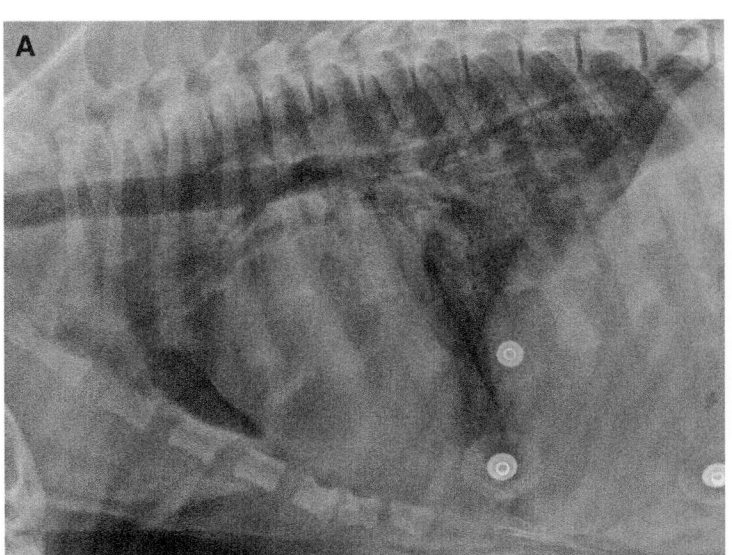
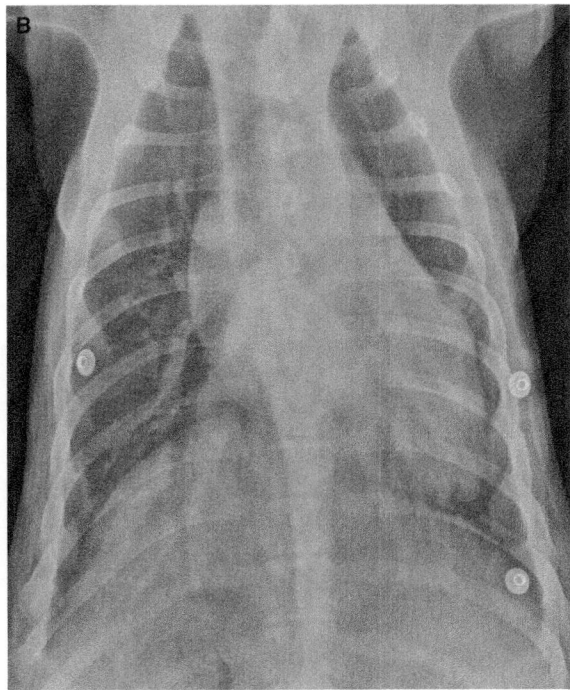

Figure 27.6 Lateral (A) and dorsoventral (B) radiographs from a 3-month-old male Newfoundland with severe subaortic stenosis (Doppler gradient ~118 mm Hg). On presentation, the puppy was in congestive heart failure, with rapid paroxysmal ventricular tachycardia. These images were obtained the following day; there is mild residual pulmonary edema, and pulmonary venous distension (B). The cardiac silhouette shows marked left ventricular and atrial enlargement (VHS ~13v), with a wide cranial cardiac waist. Three ECG electrodes are on the chest wall.

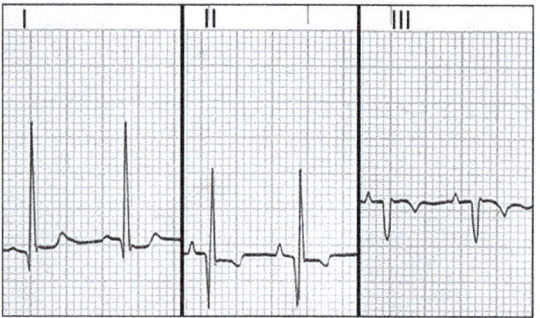

Figure 27.7 Electrocardiogram from a 1-year-old female Mastiff with subaortic stenosis shows sinus rhythm with a left axis deviation. Leads as marked; 25 mm/s, 1 cm = 1 mV.

ambiguous, or inapparent in mild cases (**Figures 27.9** and **27.10**). Grade 1 lesions usually are not identifiable on echo (or cardiac catheterization). M-mode and 2D findings might be normal or equivocal in affected animals with milder grade 2 lesions. In ambiguous cases, some examiners focus on a linear hyperechoic echo on the dorsal ventricular septum; however, many healthy dogs without a murmur demonstrate this hyperechoic tissue signal. It is possible that transesophageal echo might better identify dogs with subtle subaortic or aortic valvular lesions, although currently this is rarely pursued. The challenge of visualizing a subaortic obstruction has increased reliance on Doppler imaging for the diagnosis; however as noted later, the mildly elevated LV outflow velocities of borderline cases overlap with those of normal animals.

2D imaging can reveal LV subendocardial and papillary muscle hyperechogenicity (presumably from fibrosis) in animals with severe obstruction (**Figures 27.11** and **27.9**). Partial mid-systolic closure of the aortic valve can be evident on fast frame 2D or by M-mode imaging with severe SAS when there also is dynamic LV outflow obstruction caused by mitral valve SAM (**Figures 27.12** and **27.13**). Post-stenotic dilation of the ascending aorta (**Figure 27.14** and **27.10**), variable aortic valve thickening, and LA enlargement are other potential findings. Even LA wall thickening (representing hypertrophy), secondary to increased LV stiffness and elevated atrial pressure, might be evident in cases with severe (S)AS.

Other approaches to identifying and quantifying SAS using 2D imaging have been undertaken, although these are not widely used. Calculations of LV outflow effective orifice area could be used (p. 122). However, the likelihood that this approach can clearly differentiate mild SAS from unaffected dogs with equivocally elevated LV outflow velocity is questionable. Nevertheless, in a study of Golden Retriever puppies,

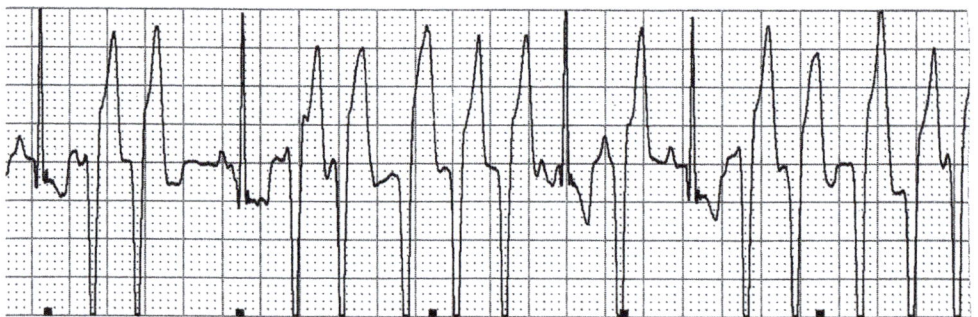

Figure 27.8 Electrocardiogram recorded shortly after emergency admission on the puppy of **Figure 27.6**. Frequent ventricular premature complexes and paroxysmal ventricular tachycardia, with only intermittent sinus complexes, are present in this tracing. Lead II, 25 mm/s, 1 cm = 1 mV.

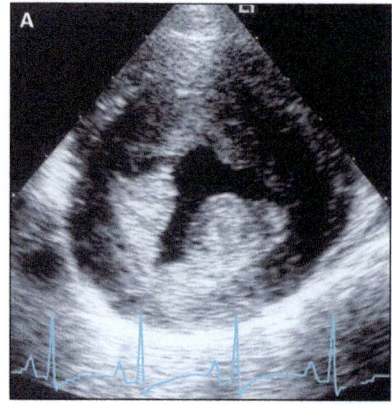 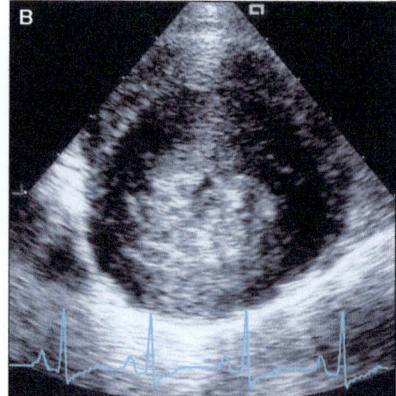

Figure 27.9 Right parasternal short-axis echocardiographic images at end-diastole (A) and in systole (B) from a 4-month-old female Golden Retriever with severe subaortic stenosis. There is marked left ventricular (LV) hypertrophy, with increased echogenicity of LV papillary muscles and subendocardial to mid-LV wall. In systole, the LV lumen is almost obliterated.

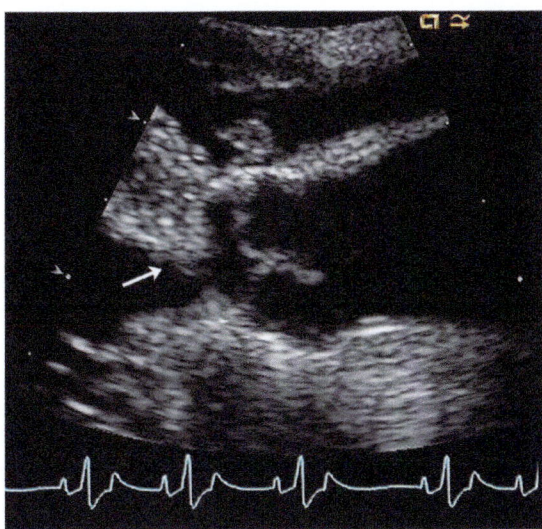

Figure 27.10 A prominent subaortic ridge (arrow) is evident in this 4-year-old male Boxer with subaortic stenosis. On presentation, the dog had rapid ventricular tachycardia, which responded to lidocaine. Left ventricular (LV) outflow systolic pressure gradient was ~74 mm Hg; however, LV systolic function also was mildly reduced. Right parasternal long-axis view in diastole.

the LV outflow effective orifice area indexed to body surface area was shown to predict development of SAS at adulthood, based on the diagnostic criterion of an aortic ejection velocity of 2.3 m/s or greater (Javard, 2014). The indexed effective orifice area in these dogs did not change during growth; puppies with values less than 1.46 cm²/m² had SAS as adults. This study also evaluated peak LV outflow velocities; puppies with values higher than 2.3 m/s were 100% specific, although only moderately sensitive for a diagnosis of SAS in adulthood, emphasizing the postnatal development of this lesion which has also been shown in the original Newfoundland colony studies.

Additional investigations have evaluated the angle formed by the interventricular septum and ascending aorta, as this might contribute to the development and the progression of

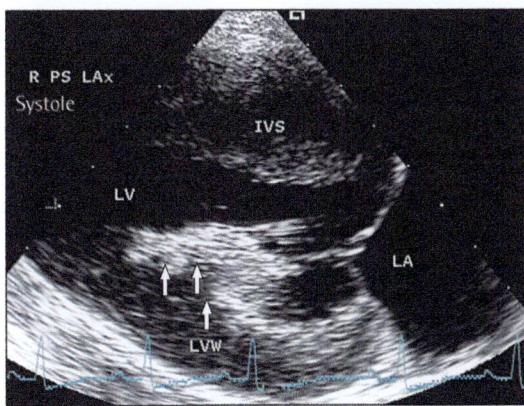

Figure 27.11 Marked hyperechogenicity (arrows) in this hypertrophied papillary muscle and the surrounding myocardium suggests chronic ischemia with fibrosis. IVS, interventricular septum; LA, left atrium; LV, left ventricle; LVW, left ventricular wall.

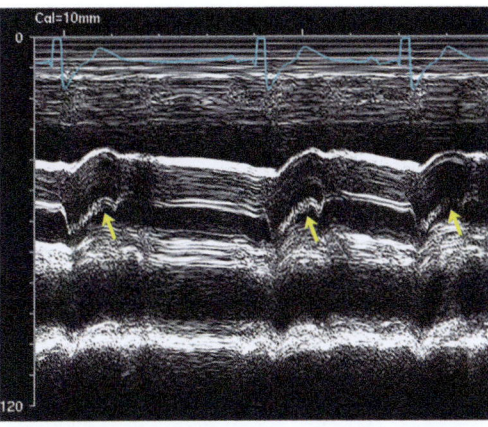

Figure 27.12 M-mode echocardiogram at the aortic root level, from an 11-month-old female Newfoundland with severe subaortic stenosis (pressure gradient >280 mm Hg). The high-velocity, turbulent flow crossing the aortic valve during systole caused coarse fluttering of the leaflets. Mid-systolic partial valve closure (arrows) also is evident and results from dynamic obstruction in the left ventricular outflow tract. ECG trace is at top of image.

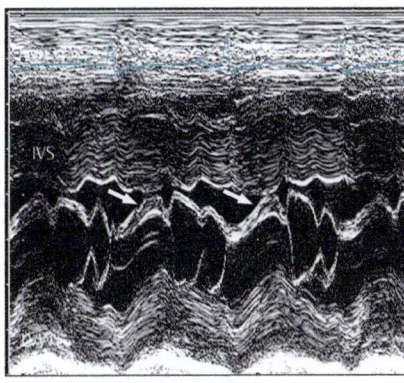

Figure 27.13 M-mode echocardiogram from a 4-month-old female German Shepherd with severe subaortic stenosis (pressure gradient >215 mm Hg). Mitral valve systolic anterior motion (SAM, arrows) indicates a component of dynamic, as well as the fixed, left ventricular outflow obstruction in this case. Note the hypertrophied left ventricular free wall (LVW) and interventricular septum (IVS); cm marks along left edge.

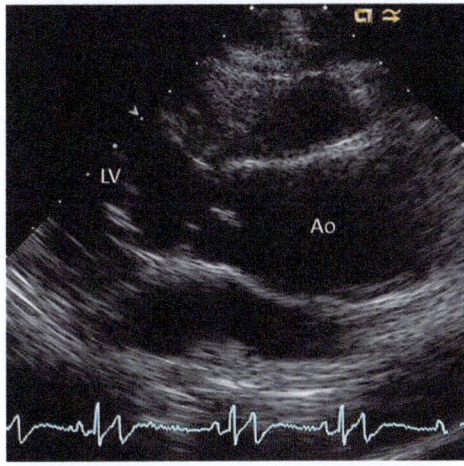

Figure 27.14 Prominent ascending aortic dilation is visible in this diastolic left cranial long-axis image of the aortic root and ascending aorta from a 4-year-old male Newfoundland with moderately severe subaortic stenosis.

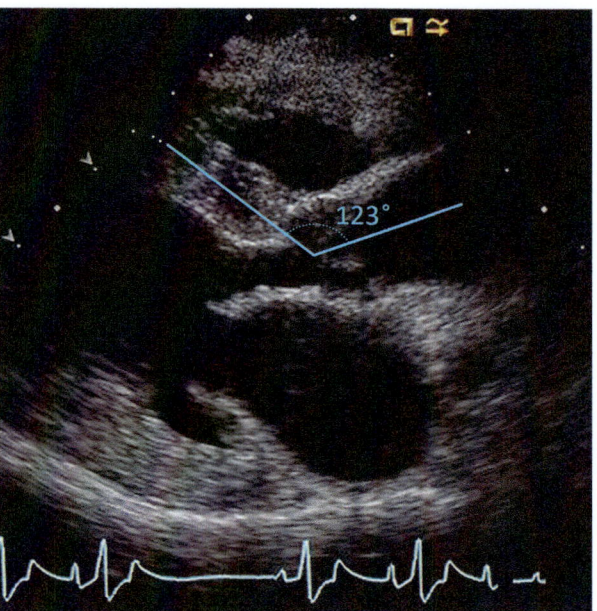

Figure 27.15 The aorto-septal angle is narrow (~123°) in the Boxer of Figure 27.10.

SAS. This aorto-septal angle (AoSA) can be estimated using the right parasternal long-axis view. The AoSA was shown to be smaller in Boxer, Dogue de Bordeaux, and Golden Retriever breeds with SAS compared to normal dogs (**Figure 27.15**). The aortic angulation is steeper in dogs with more severe SAS. In the Boxer study, although some overlap in AoSA measurements between normal and affected dogs occurred, an AoSA <140° was found only in Boxers with SAS (Quintavalla, 2010). However, the predictive value of this measurement could not be established. The best "cut-off" value for AoSA to separate normal from SAS might be different among breeds or species. A study in Golden Retrievers found most dogs with SAS had an AoSA <145° and AoSAs were smaller as SAS severity increased; there was no significant change in AoSA with growth of the dog (Belanger, 2014). These are interesting data, but interobserver repeatability has not been reported and the cut-offs used to diagnose SAS were based on an LVOT velocity without an anatomical standard. Nevertheless these findings are intriguing both in terms of pathogenesis and potential for recognizing younger dogs who might not serve as good breeding stock.

Color and spectral Doppler echo permit detection of systolic flow acceleration that originates below the aortic valve and turbulence that extends into the aorta, as well as the high systolic outflow velocity that characterizes outflow tract stenoses (**Figures 27.16** and **27.17**). Doppler studies might also reveal AR and MR. Mild AR is almost always present in SAS, perhaps from slight thickening of the leaflets facing higher velocity flow, or related to aortic root dilation or aortopathy. It usually is holodiastolic in unambiguous cases of SAS. Spectral Doppler can show LV diastolic function abnormalities, which also are common in animals with SAS. Stenosis severity typically is estimated using continuous-wave (CW) Doppler. Currently, an estimated peak instantaneous gradient of 80 mm Hg or higher is considered severe (S)AS. Unfortunately, older studies have mixed gradients obtained by cardiac catheterization with those by Doppler imaging, but these are not interchangeable, as discussed later. Many consider a peak instantaneous Doppler gradient between 50 and 80 mm Hg as "moderate" stenosis. These are somewhat arbitrary but do generally relate to prognosis, especially in larger breeds of dogs.

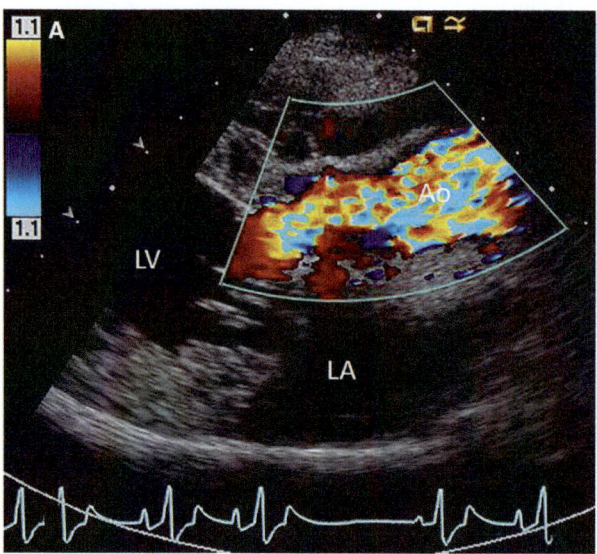
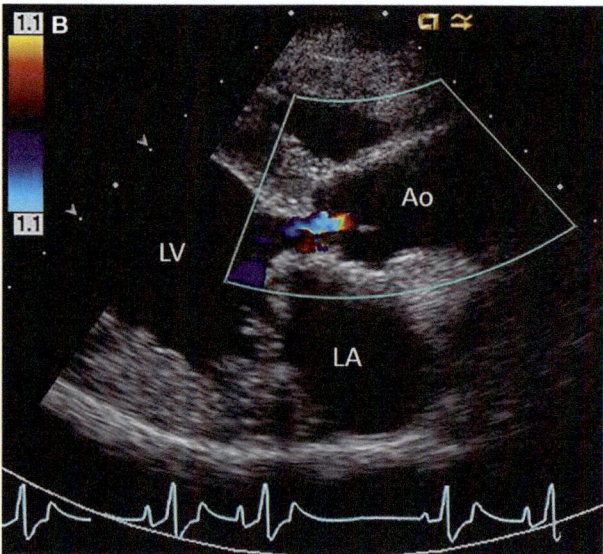

Figure 27.16 (A) Systolic turbulence originates in the narrowed left ventricular outflow tract of a dog with severe subaortic stenosis (SAS). (B) Diastolic frame from the same case shows mild aortic regurgitation, which is common with SAS. Right parasternal long-axis, color-flow Doppler images. Ao, aorta; LA, left atrium; LV, left ventricle.

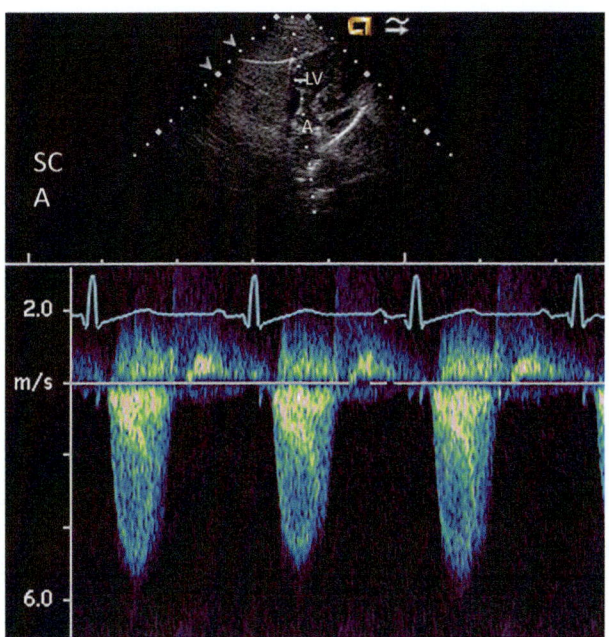

Figure 27.17 Continuous-wave (CW) Doppler flow profiles (bottom) indicate maximal left ventricular outflow velocity of ~5.5 m/s (instantaneous pressure gradient of ~120 mm Hg) in a 2-month-old male Rottweiler puppy with subaortic stenosis. Given the young age of this puppy, outflow obstruction severity would be expected to worsen as he grows. An aortic insufficiency signal is present above the CW baseline during diastole. Subcostal position; 2D image (top) shows good alignment of Doppler cursor with outflow tract and ascending aorta. A, aorta; LV, left ventricle.

Interrogation of the LVOT from more than one position is important to achieve the best possible alignment with blood flow. It is critical not to overpower or apply excessive gain to the velocity spectrum as these artificially inflate the velocity and gradient (p. 124). Multiple spectra should be averaged in dogs with pronounced sinus arrhythmia because velocities preceded by a long R-R interval are higher. The subcostal (subxiphoid) position usually yields the highest velocity signals, although in some animals the left apical position is better (p. 113). Assuming optimal echo beam alignment, most unsedated dogs without a heart murmur demonstrate aortic velocities of ≤1.9 m/s by CW Doppler and <1.7 by pulsed-wave (PW) Doppler. Velocities consistently exceeding 2.4 m/s in a calm dog are considered diagnostic of (S)AS by most cardiologists; however, others use lower cut-off values. Peak velocities between 1.9 and 2.4 m/s are often labeled as equivocal, suggesting mild (S)AS might be present if other supportive evidence can be found. This issue mainly is of concern when selecting animals for breeding. Yet velocities in this equivocal range (1.9–2.4 m/s) also could stem from breed-related differences in LVOT anatomy or response to sympathetic stimulation. Certainly, a higher aortic ejection velocity indicates a greater *liability* for aortic stenosis; however, there are no confirmatory autopsy studies, and a single velocity cut-off within the equivocal range cannot conclusively establish the diagnosis in the absence of a clear anatomic lesion. For example, mild increases in peak LV outflow velocity associated with increased stress are evident in both normal and SAS-affected Boxers. This is attributed to an increase in stroke volume during stress.

Stroke volume markedly affects the velocity and derived PG, and increased flow also augments the murmur. This can be readily tested by jogging the dog and immediately repeating auscultation. Simply administering a catecholamine such as dobutamine to a normal dog (without a murmur) can increase the aortic velocity to at least 2.4 m/s. Similarly, sympathetic activation (including the stress of an unsedated echo exam) and other causes of increased stroke volume (fever, anemia, PDA, bradycardia) will increase outflow velocity. Conversely, volume depletion, myocardial failure, cardiodepressant drugs, and heavy sedation or anesthesia will reduce the PG. This influence of flow is relevant both to assessment of severity in moderate to severe SAS, as well as to appreciating the challenges of diagnosing borderline to mild SAS.

Substantial controversy revolves around the Doppler echo findings indicating mild SAS in the absence of a clear anatomic lesion. These include: a mild increase in LV outflow velocity (with suggested cut-off values for AS ranging from 2.0 to 2.5 m/s); identifying RBC velocity acceleration proximal to the aorta; finding LVOT turbulence; and detecting aortic valve insufficiency of an unspecified degree or duration. Each of these listed criteria for SAS are reasonable, but also fail to mitigate the following arguments. It is true that most dogs with left-sided ejection murmurs and otherwise normal echo studies have increased LVOT velocities (typically between 1.7 and 2.4 m/s). Unfortunately, most Doppler echo studies of "normal" dogs have excluded animals with cardiac murmurs, and therefore, those that might have a nonpathological, functional murmur. Secondly, it is normal to identify a systolic velocity step-up in the LVOT using PW Doppler in dogs without any murmur at all. Color flow Doppler can detect "turbulence" but this variance encoding is not specific for disease and highly dependent on transducer and instrument settings. Moreover, looking for spectral broadening on PW Doppler is challenging when it is minimal, in most dogs with ejection velocities <2.4 m/s, or is created artificially by poor angulation or improper power and gain settings. Lastly, trivial and silent AR can be seen in many healthy dogs by color Doppler imaging; this becomes more likely with higher LVOT velocities, age, and sedation. All of these issues create confusion and frustration when attempting to differentiate mild SAS from normal dogs with a functional murmur, and begs the question of "what is normal breed variation?" In one study, almost three-quarters of Dogue de Bordeaux had a left basilar systolic murmur, but less than 20% had a peak aortic velocity exceeding 2.5 m/s (Hollmer, 2008). The authors have experienced similar findings when screening other breeds, including Boxer dogs and Bouvier de Flanders dogs at shows or so called "cardiac health" clinics. Some breeds such as Boxers, Bull Terriers, Golden Retrievers, and Dogue

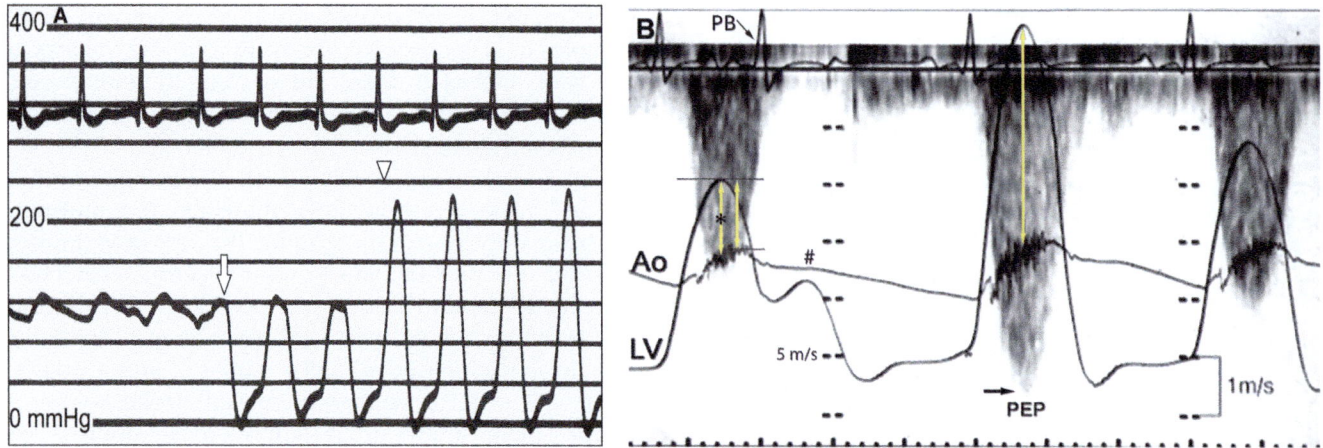

Figure 27.18 (A) Electrocardiogram (top) and pressure (bottom) recordings obtained during cardiac catheterization in a 2-year-old female German Shorthaired Pointer with severe subaortic stenosis (SAS). The catheter tip is in the ascending aorta at the left side of the trace (pressure range indicated in mm Hg). As the catheter is pushed just past the aortic (Ao) valve, left ventricular (LV) diastolic and normal systolic (arrow) pressures are recorded; the LV systolic pressure is normal for these 2 cycles because the catheter tip is above (downstream from) the stenosis. Continued catheter advancement deeper into the ventricle, past the subvalvular obstruction, reveals that the peak LV systolic pressure is well over 200 mm Hg (arrowhead). (B) Simultaneous CW Doppler echocardiogram and LV and Ao pressures recorded in a dog with SAS. The cardiac cycle on the left shows the instantaneous gradient (*) recorded by maximal CW Doppler velocity ($4V^2$); the gradient indicated by the yellow arrow just to its right is the "peak to peak" gradient. After a premature beat (PB), a pulse deficit (#) occurs, followed by a post-extrasystolic potentiated beat (PEP). This stronger contraction produces a higher gradient between LV and Ao pressures (and higher ejection velocity, horizontal arrow below), estimated as >100 mm Hg. The cardiac cycle on the right shows reduced pressure gradient and maximal Ao flow velocity. Ao pressure recording made with a filtered micromanometer catheter to record Ao turbulence (an intracardiac murmur), which superimposes high frequency oscillations on the systolic limb of the Ao pressure curve. Study recorded with Dr LB Lehmkuhl.

de Bordeaux have generally smaller LV outflow tract dimensions or ascending aortas. Hydraulic principles indicate that a small aorta will predispose to increased ejection velocity and therefore, a systolic murmur at the aortic valve and left base. These details might seem pedantic when considering a mature dog with a soft, early-peaking aortic ejection murmur and maximal aortic velocity <2.5 m/s, that is unlikely to experience any cardiac health issues from these findings. However, our ability to accurately screen and classify potential breeding dogs for SAS certainly is challenged, even with detailed echo studies.

Cardiac catheterization and angiocardiography can be used to measure PG in the LVOT and outline the obstructive lesion prior to an interventional procedure (**Figures 27.18–27.20**). Angiography also highlights the post-stenotic aortic dilation, coronary anatomy, and any AR, MR or left-to-right shunts. The Doppler-estimated maximal instantaneous PG in an unanesthetized animal usually is 40–50% higher than the PG recorded during cardiac catheterization under general anesthesia. The negative inotropic effects of sedatives and anesthesic agents contributes to this marked difference by reducing stroke volume. In addition, the peak-to-peak PGs used in direct measurements are somewhat lower than the instantaneous PGs derived during Doppler studies (**Figure 27.18B**; p. 122). Mean PGs, measured simultaneously in dogs with SAS, have been compared and are largely equivalent; therefore, the differences relates mainly to LV stroke volume.

Management

Affected animals should not be bred. For cases with mild to moderate SAS, avoiding prolonged strenuous activity and using antibiotic prophylaxis prior to procedures with the potential to cause bacteremia (such as dentistry) generally are recommended, although the efficacy of these recommendations is unclear. For animals with moderate to severe SAS, marked exercise restriction is recommended, in addition to antibiotic prophylaxis prior to "dirty" procedures or

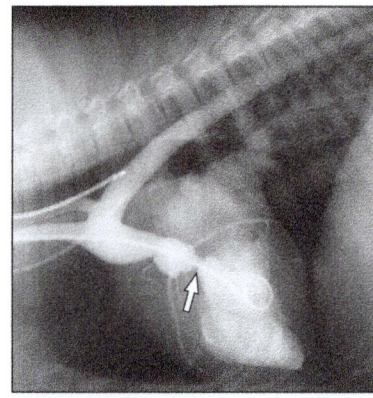

Figure 27.19 Left ventricular (LV) angiocardiogram from a 5-month-old male German Shepherd pup shows a fairly discrete subaortic narrowing (arrow). LV hypertrophy, left atrial enlargement, and modest post-stenotic dilation of the ascending aortic also are visible.

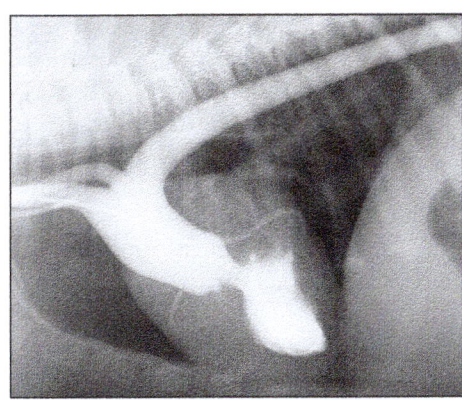

Figure 27.20 Left ventricular (LV) angiocardiogram from a 4-month-old male Rottweiler pup shows a tunnel-like subaortic stenosis, with marked post-stenotic aortic dilation that extends into the brachycephalic trunk. LV hypertrophy and a prominent left circumflex coronary artery are evident.

any wounds. A beta-blocker (such as atenolol, 0.5 to 1 mg/kg PO q12h) often is prescribed in severe SAS cases. Beta-adrenergic blockers have been advocated in hope of reducing myocardial oxygen demand (and ischemia) and minimizing the frequency and severity of arrhythmias. This also could be beneficial if the patient has a component of dynamic LVOT obstruction, although that is uncommon. Animals with severe stenosis, marked ST segment depression, frequent ventricular ectopy, or a history of syncope theoretically might be more likely to benefit from this therapy. Yet, a retrospective investigation of 50 dogs with SAS showed no difference in survival time between those treated with atenolol and those not (Eason, 2014). Clearly, prospective studies are needed regarding this matter. Nevertheless, therapy for frequent or complex ventricular tachyarrhythmias using sotalol is appropriate. Likewise, AF or other arrhythmias should be treated as indicated (Chapter 25). It is unclear whether angiotensin converting enzyme (ACE) inhibitor therapy is helpful. Theoretically, it could be harmful if blood and coronary perfusion pressures are reduced. Medication for CHF is prescribed, if that develops.

Various techniques have been employed to reduce LVOT obstruction in dogs with severe SAS, including cardiopulmonary bypass and open-heart surgery to access the lesion directly. Although surgical resection of the stenotic region can significantly reduce the LV systolic PG and possibly improve exercise ability, it has not effectively reduced the risk of sudden death or improved long-term survival. Other surgical procedures aimed at bypassing or dilating the obstruction have been of limited benefit and associated with multiple complications.

Transcatheter balloon dilation (alone) of the stenotic area has reduced the measured gradient in some dogs, but partial restenosis often develops over time. Some improvement in clinical signs might be noted, although no survival benefit was documented with this procedure when compared to treatment with atenolol (Meurs, 2005). A newer cutting-balloon technique could help achieve greater dilation and reduce the likelihood of restenosis; however, other concerns and potential complications remain. This technique uses a balloon catheter with thin cutting blades (artherotomes) that are fixed longitudinally along the surface of the balloon; these score the surrounding tissue when the balloon is inflated. When followed by use of a standard high-pressure balloon catheter, these thin cuts should allow greater dilation of the stenotic tissue (**Figure 6.17**, p. 183). When properly done, the combined cutting-balloon and high-pressure balloon technique has reduced the PG and clinical signs in some dogs (Kleman, 2012; Sykes, 2020). However, there are significant technical limitations related in part to the size of available cutting-balloons and the lack of prospective studies. At present, it is unclear whether overall long-term survival is significantly increased, and many cardiologists consider it a salvage procedure only. The patient's AoSA could influence the degree to which the PG can be reduced and how well the reduction is maintained over time following combined cutting- and high-pressure balloon dilation (Shen, 2017). Complications of transcatheter balloon dilation include ventricular tachycardia and fibrillation, aortic endocarditis, LV perforation, aortic regurgitation, aortic annulus rupture, and arterial rupture or avulsion.

Prognosis Animals with AS are at increased risk for sudden death as well as left-sided CHF, especially when the LV outflow gradient is more severe. The overall prevalence of sudden death in dogs with SAS appears to be just over 20%. Sudden death usually occurs during or shortly after a period of exercise or excitement and likely relates to ventricular tachycardia – fibrillation, or sudden onset of bradycardia and asystole. Exercise intolerance and syncope might or might not occur prior to sudden death. As noted previously, there also is increased risk for aortic valve endocarditis in animals with SAS. Infective endocarditis and CHF might be more likely to develop later. Atrial and ventricular arrhythmias and worsened MR are complicating factors.

Dogs with mild stenosis (PG < 50 mm Hg) are more likely to live longer and without clinical signs. Some can have a normal lifespan, although sudden death and endocarditis also can occur. The prognosis with severe stenosis (variously defined as maximal Doppler instantaneous gradient of >80 to 100 mm Hg, or a mean gradient of 55 to 60 or greater) is guarded. In a retrospective study, >50% of severely affected dogs died suddenly before 3 years of age and many before 2 years. A higher PG at diagnosis was associated with increased risk of death in another study (Eason, 2014). These reports vary in terms of disease severity and methods used to assess PGs, making comparisons difficult. One report of dogs with SAS on medical therapy (usually beta-blocker) showed an average lifespan of ~4.5 years. Factors that negatively affect prognosis include severe stenosis (high PG), MR, AR, aortic endocarditis, CHF, and AF. Breed or body size also might be relevant.

Pulmonic Stenosis

PS usually is an isolated defect, although it can accompany other cardiac malformations, as well as contribute to the T of F (see Chapter 26). Although PS is common in dogs, it is relatively uncommon in cats, and rare in horses. Valvular stenosis is the most common form of PS. Valve dysplasia (or "atypical PS," in humans) occurs more frequently than simple fusion of pulmonic valve leaflets. Patterson's original work in Beagle dogs described three main components: valve thickening, asymmetrical and partially fused leaflets, and variable hypoplasia of the valve annulus (Patterson, 1981; **Figure 27.21**). This description still is relevant, but should be further expanded by describing the following: any fixed (fibrous) or dynamic (muscular) subvalvular obstructions; any tethering or adherence of the leaflets to the pulmonary artery; the degree of pulmonary leaflet thickening and mobility; the anatomy of the supravalvular pulmonary trunk and branches; the size and function of the right ventricle and right atrium; the structure and function of the tricuspid valve; any abnormalities of systemic venous return; proximal aortic and coronary artery anatomy; secondary effects of RV hypertrophy on the left ventricle, such as dynamic LVOT obstruction; and the presence of any ventricular or atrial defects with R-to-L shunting. Canine PS has been classified as type A, characterized by leaflet fusion with a central opening and dome-like valve appearance during systole, and type B, characterized by dysplastic, thick and hypomobile leaflets with annulus hypoplasia. Although this categorization is useful and might influence the selection of any interventional catheterization, these two types do not fully describe the spectrum of lesions observed in this disease nor the related issues that should be considered in affected patients. Additionally, type A is not the same as "typical" PS of children where the leaflets are minimally thickened, mobile and dome in systole. Unlike children, some dogs with type A PS exhibit extremely dysplastic and thick valve leaflets. Primary supravalvular and subvalvular stenotic lesions are much less common in animals. Isolated branch stenosis or absence is considered rare. Bicuspid pulmonary valve with stenosis has been reported in horses.

The systolic pressure overload caused by RV outflow obstruction stimulates concentric hypertrophy proximal to the obstruction. Myocardial ischemia and its sequelae (including arrhythmias, CHF, and sudden death) are likely with severe hypertrophy. RV outflow tract (infundibular) hypertrophy can contribute a component of dynamic RV outflow obstruction, especially with excitement and exercise. Post-stenotic dilation of the main pulmonary trunk occurs to a variable degree that is not always consistent with the type of stenosis. Secondary right atrial (RA) and RV dilation are common. Tricuspid regurgitation (TR), secondary to annulus dilation or concurrent tricuspid dysplasia, also predisposes to atrial arrhythmias (including AF) and congestive failure. Patients with a patent foramen ovale (PFO) or atrial septal defect (ASD) can develop R-to-L shunting if RA pressure rises above LA pressure.

A single anomalous coronary artery, thought to contribute to the outflow obstruction, occurs in association with PS in some breeds (English Bulldogs, Boxers, and possibly others). As described in Bulldogs, this aberrant coronary artery usually is of the R2A type (Buchanan, 2001). The abnormal left coronary vessel that arises from the single ostium travels in a "pre-pulmonic" path, passing over the RV outflow tract just proximal to the pulmonary valve region, in the area of (and often contributing to) a subvalvular obstruction (**Figures 27.22 and 27.23**). The practical significance is that

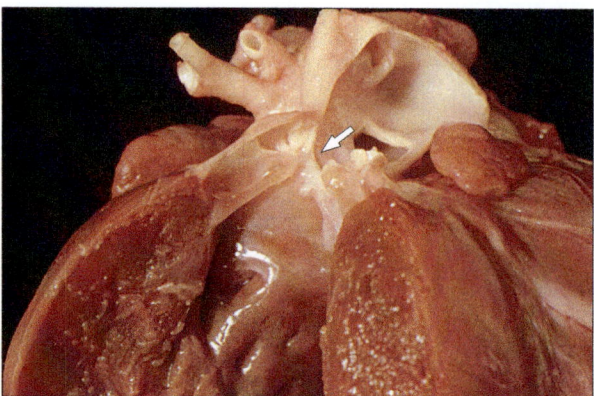

Figure 27.21 Postmortem specimen opened through the right ventricular (RV) outflow tract into the pulmonary artery, from a 4-month-old male Miniature Schnauzer with a severely dysplastic pulmonary valve. The thick, malformed valve lacks clearly demarcated leaflets and has only a tiny orifice (arrow). Note the marked RV hypertrophy.

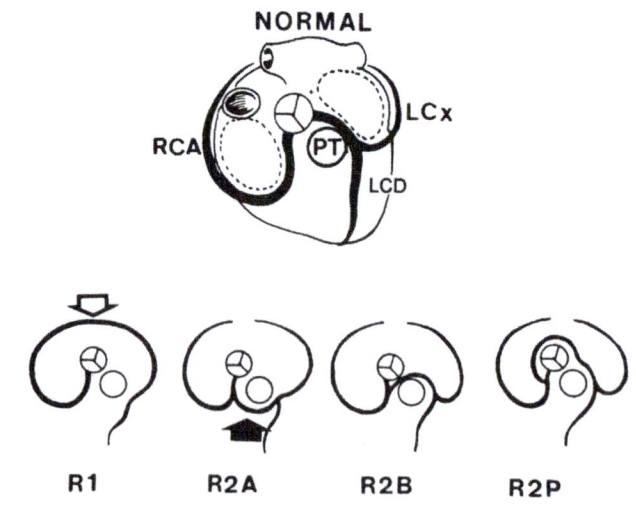

Figure 27.22 Illustration on top shows the normal anatomical arrangement of the major coronary arteries. Several variations of abnormal single right coronary artery distribution (bottom row) are described in people. The R2A variant (arrow) is known to occur most often in dogs, particularly English Bulldogs. This variant involves a circumpulmonary left coronary branch, which can constrict the pulmonary valve area and contribute to right ventricular outflow obstruction. (From Buchanan JW. Pulmonic stenosis caused by single coronary artery in dogs: Four cases (1965–1984). J Am Vet Med Assoc 1990;196:115–120.)

this coronary anomaly limits the potential effectiveness of balloon valvuloplasty, and excessive pressure on the vessel can result in coronary ischemia and death during the procedure. Other coronary anomalies also have been described with PS. R2A type abnormalities have been found in Bulldogs unaffected by other CHD (Scansen, 2017). Coronary anatomy should be verified prior to any planned palliative procedure (see "Management" section).

Infundibular obstruction of the right ventricle most often stems from RV hypertrophy secondary to valvular PS. However, primary infundibular stenosis can occur in both dogs and cats; the obstructive lesion can be in the form of a fibrous diaphragm or fibromuscular or muscular narrowing. Primary infundibular stenosis might have an increased prevalence in Golden Retrievers and Siberian Huskies. Prognosis is guarded for animals with severe infundibular stenosis. Balloon valvuloplasty might be helpful in some cases. Another uncommon but well recognized variant of RV obstruction is a fibromuscular partition within the body of the ventricle, separating inflow and outflow tracts to create a "double-chambered" right ventricle (DCRV; **Figure 27.24**). The DCRV causes clinical and pathophysiologic signs similar to those of congenital valvular PS. In some cases, there is a related or spontaneously closed VSD. There is considerable discussion about the precise lesions and RV locations separating these two defects, especially in cats, and some would classify several published

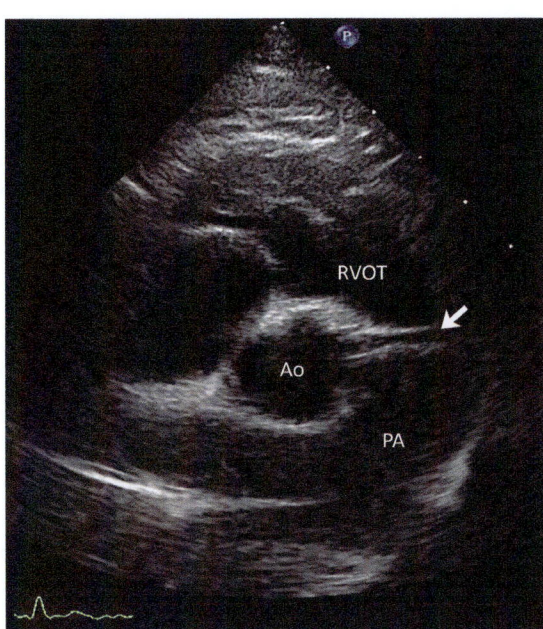

Figure 27.23 Abnormal coronary artery (arrow), consistent with the R2A coronary anomaly, crosses over the pulmonary valve region in this 6-month-old female English Bulldog with severe pulmonic stenosis (Doppler gradient 114 mm Hg). Right parasternal short axis echocardiographic view. (Image courtesy of Dr JL Ward.)

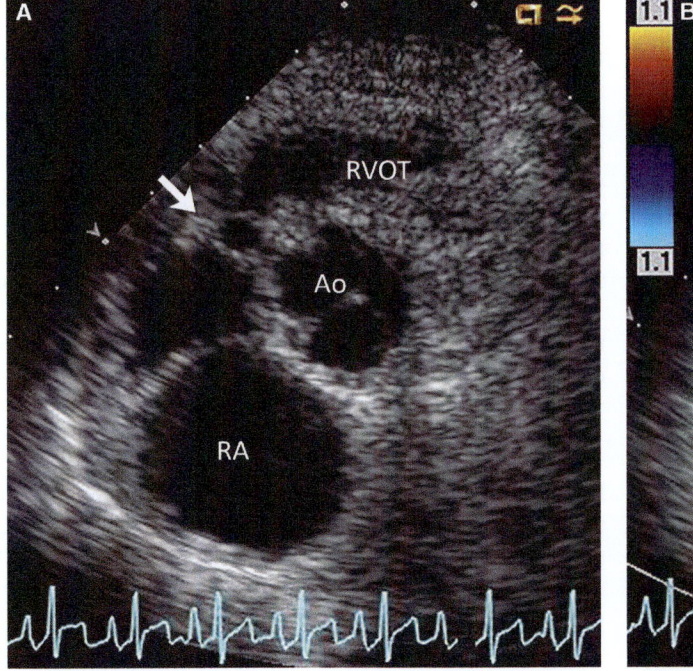
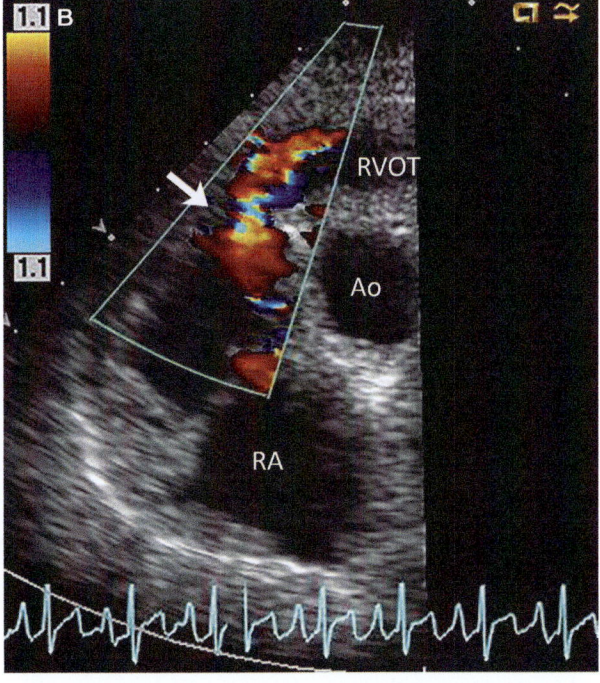

Figure 27.24 2D echocardiographic image from a 3-year-old female English Bulldog with double-chambered right ventricle. The dog began having syncope with exercise and excitement over the prior 5 months. A loud left basilar systolic murmur was heard. (A) Focal mid-chamber right ventricular (RV) fibromuscular stenosis (arrow) is present. The proximal RV wall (upstream from the stenosis) is hypertrophied and the RA is dilated. Wall thickness in the RVOT and pulmonary valve structure were normal (not seen in this image because of transducer angulation). Peak pulmonary outflow velocity was normal. (B) Color-flow Doppler image in systole shows turbulent flow past the stenotic area (peak velocity 5.35 m/s; pressure gradient ~114 mm Hg). Modified left cranial short-axis view, angled to optimize inflow and mid-RV region. Ao, aorta; RA, right atrium; RVOT, RV outflow tract region.

cases of infundibular stenosis as DCRV. Regardless, the prognosis is guarded for animals with severe obstruction due to infundibular stenosis or DCRV. Both CHF and sudden death have occurred. Catheter-based procedures might be helpful in selected cases, but this is uncertain, and an interventional cardiologist should be consulted. Open heart surgical repair would be the treatment of choice.

Shunting can occur in conjunction with PS. When RA pressure is elevated, a patent foramen ovale (PFO) or atrial septal defect (ASD) will cause R-to-L shunting at the atrial level. R-to-L shunting via a PFO appears to be more common in animals with severe PS as well as TR; it is minimal to absent with mild PS. A VSD might permit R-to-L shunting, if RV pressure exceeds that on the left side at any time during the cardiac cycle. Most VSDs seen in cases of RV outflow obstruction are perimembranous (below the aortic valve and adjacent to the septal tricuspid leaflet) or infracristal; however, defects in other locations, including the muscular septum, have been observed. A large membranous defect in association with subvalvular PS and hypoplasia of the pulmonary valve are typical of T of F (see Chapter 26). Pulmonary atresia (also known as pseudotruncus arteriosus) occurs uncommonly. It usually is associated with a hypoplastic right ventricle and tricuspid valve. Pulmonary atresia causes R-to-L shunting through a VSD (or PFO); pulmonary flow would occur through bronchial arterial collaterals (**Figure 26.52**, p. 472) or a PDA. Clinical findings in such cases are similar to those with T of F. Pulmonary atresia with a VSD is a form of T of F. This malformation is recognized most often in Arabian horses and in cats; pulmonary atresia with an intact interventricular septum occurs in rare cases.

Mitral SAM, with dynamic LVOT obstruction and eccentric MR jet(s), occasionally occurs in association with high RV systolic pressure and altered LV cavity size in dogs with PS. It also might be seen in T of F. Mitral SAM in these situations could relate to changes in LV geometry or function secondary to reduced pulmonary venous return, or to increased sympathetic tone caused by poor stroke volume. Whether any resulting LV systolic pressure increase contributes to clinically relevant hemodynamic impairment or myocardial ischemia is unclear.

Clinical Features

PS is more common in small breeds of dog, although larger breeds, such as Boxers and Labrador Retrievers, also are affected (**Table 27.1**). It occasionally occurs in cats and rarely in horses. Many cases are asymptomatic at the time of diagnosis. However, severe stenosis often is associated with the development of secondary TR, right-sided CHF, arrhythmias, exertional syncope, and sometimes sudden death. Hypoxemia, cyanosis, and secondary erythrocytosis can occur in cases with R-to-L shunting. Yet even in animals with severe stenosis, these signs might not develop for several years. Sudden death associated with severe PS seems much less common than with SAS.

Physical findings characteristic of moderate to severe stenosis include a prominent right precordial impulse, normal

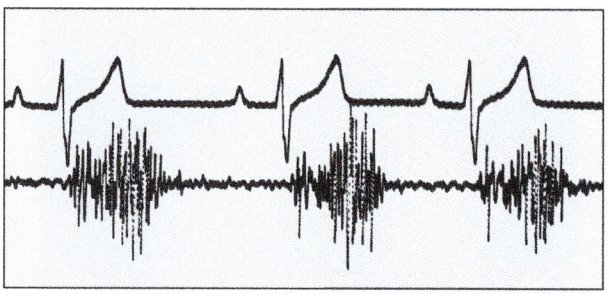

Figure 27.25 Phonocardiogram (bottom) depicts the systolic ejection (crescendo-decrescendo) murmur of a dog with pulmonic stenosis. Simultaneous lead II ECG (top) shows QRS complexes that reflect a right axis deviation, caused by RV hypertrophy.

(or slightly diminished) femoral pulses, pink mucous membranes, and in some cases, prominent jugular pulses (either large "cv waves" caused by TR or more commonly, prominent "a waves" caused by increased RV stiffness; see **Figures 15.3** and **15.4**, p. 263). Concurrent CHF also produces jugular vein distension, as well as ascites and sometimes, pleural effusion or chylothorax. A precordial thrill at the dorsal left base is likely with severe PS because of increased murmur intensity and proximity of the pulmonary trunk to the thoracic wall; however, this might not always be evident, especially in barrel-chested or obese individuals. The systolic ejection murmur is heard best from the left cranial thorax over the pulmonary valve and extending into the pulmonary trunk high at the left base, where it might be loudest (**Figure 27.25**). PS murmur grade and time to peak murmur intensity generally correlate with stenosis severity. The intensity of the murmur (and stenosis severity) tends to be consistent from early in life to maturity. The murmur sometimes radiates cranioventrally and to the right, but usually is not heard over the carotid arteries. An early systolic click is audible in occasional cases; this probably results from abrupt checking of a fused valve as it opens. A right apical holosystolic murmur of secondary (or dysplasia-induced) TR, or an arrhythmia, might be heard in some cases. Animals with a concurrent PFO, or atrial or ventricular septal defect, could have reduced O_2 saturation and even visible cyanosis, especially with exercise, because of R-to-L shunting.

Diagnostic Tests

Routine laboratory tests generally are non-contributory or non-specific. NT-proBNP is likely to be elevated in severe symptomatic PS, but not in mild PS. Increased plasma NT-proBNP concentrations have been correlated with Doppler pressure gradient in dogs with PS (Kobayashi, 2014). About a third of dogs with severe PS had an increase in cTnI, as well as C-reactive protein, in one study (Saunders, 2009). When R-to-L shunting is identified by echo, the packed cell volume should be determined and followed.

Typical radiographic features are outlined in **Table 27.2**. **Figures 27.26–27.28** illustrate some of the variability in radiographic appearance. The heart might not appear very

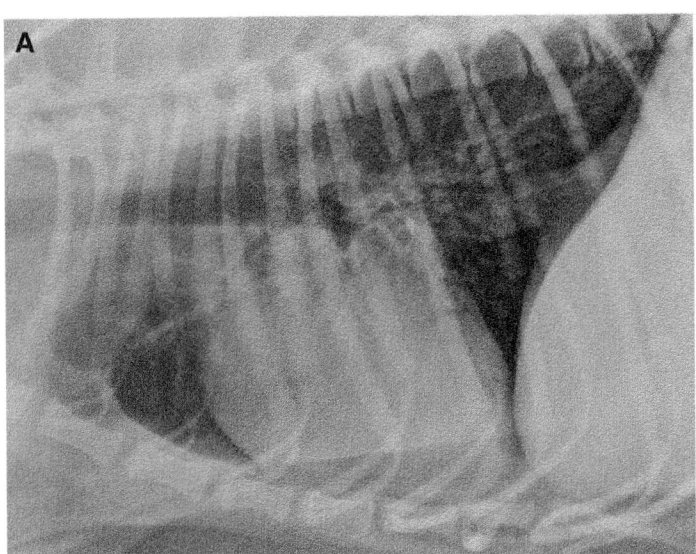
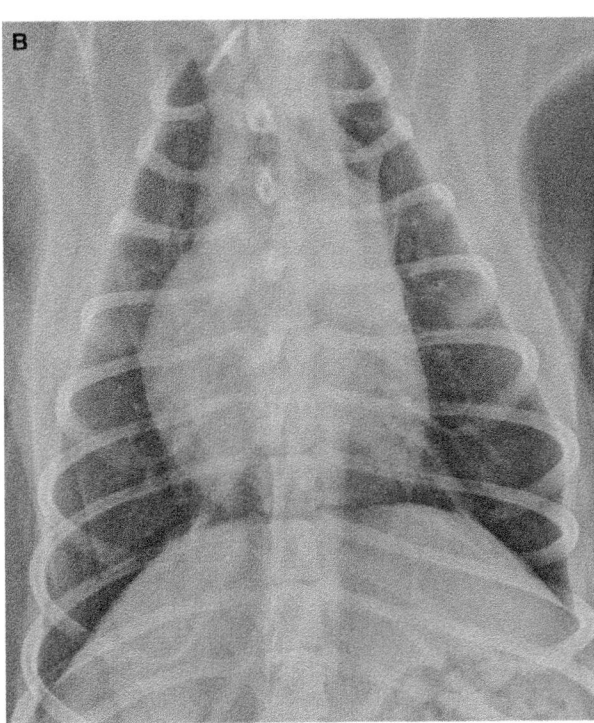

Figure 27.26 (A) Lateral radiograph from a 1-year-old male Cavelier King Charles Spaniel appears normal in terms of overall size (VHS 9.9v) despite the dog's severe pulmonic stenosis (Doppler gradient ~86 mm Hg). (B) Dorsoventral view suggests right ventricular enlargement; however, the main pulmonary artery segment is not prominent in this case.

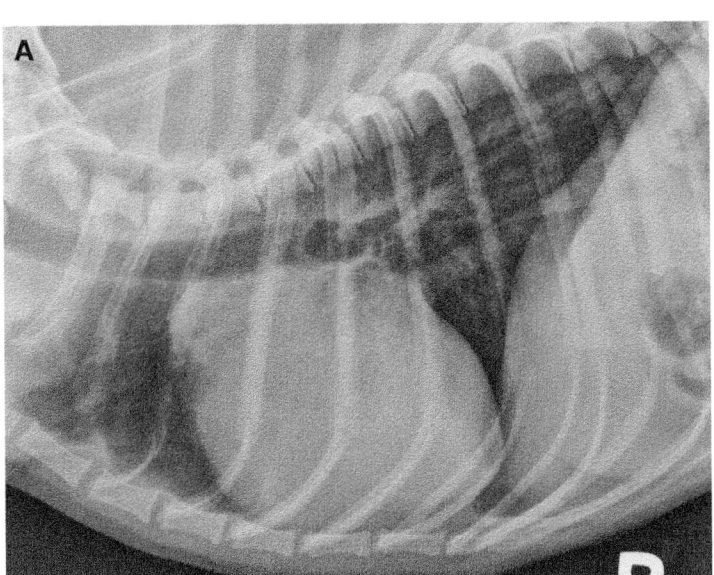
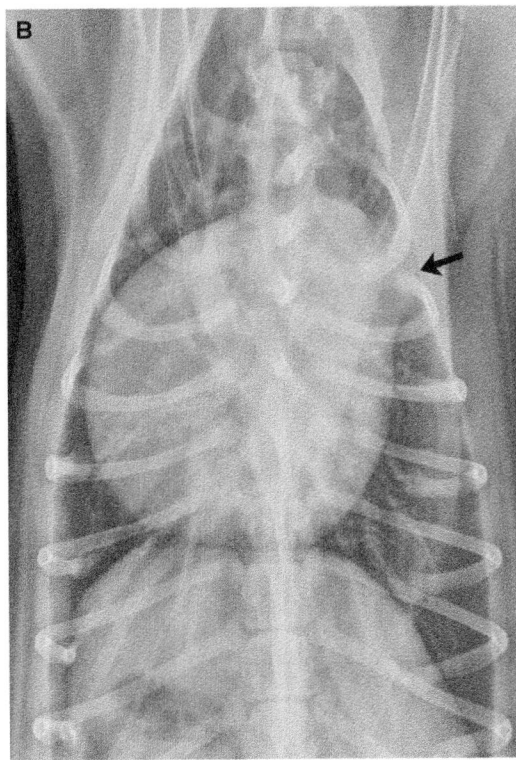

Figure 27.27 Lateral (A) and dorsoventral (B) radiographs from an asymptomatic, 4-year-old male Dachshund with a thick, dysplastic pulmonary valve and severe stenosis. Balloon valvuloplasty, when the dog was 8 months old, achieved only modest reduction in the pressure gradient (from 105 to ~79 mm Hg). Marked right heart enlargement is present, with apex elevation off the sternum (A) and a large pulmonary artery bulge (B, arrow).

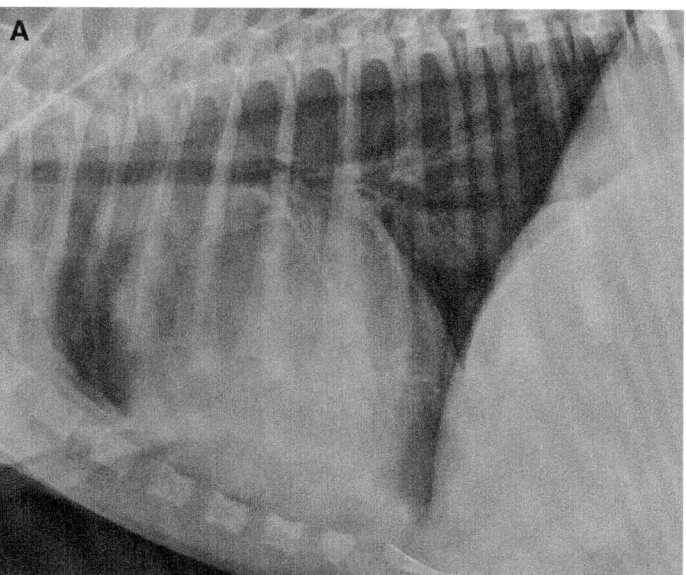
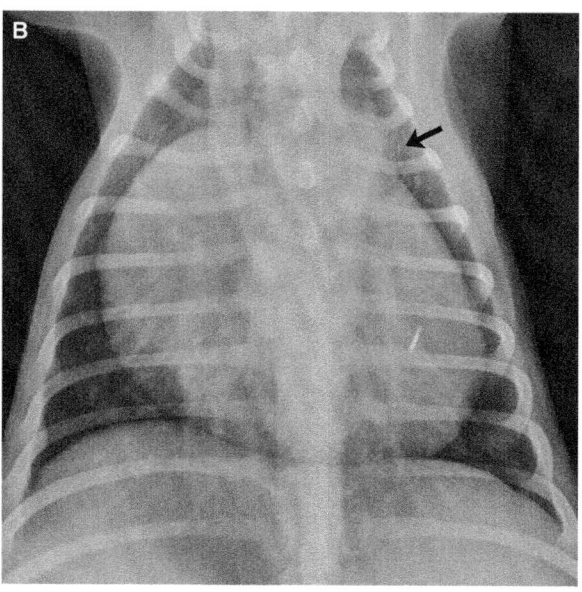

Figure 27.28 Lateral (A) and dorsoventral (B) radiographs from a 3-month-old male mixed breed dog with severe pulmonic stenosis (Doppler gradient ~120 mm Hg). Severe right-sided cardiomegaly is accompanied by a small main pulmonary artery bulge (B, arrow), attenuated pulmonary vasculature, mild caudal vena caval distension, and moderate ascites (not seen on these cropped images) from right-sided congestive heart failure.

enlarged unless there is concurrent TR or impending CHF. However, marked concentric RV hypertrophy usually changes the cardiac shape and shifts the apex dorsally and leftward. The cardiac silhouette can assume a "reverse D" shape on DV or VD view. A pulmonary trunk bulge (post-stenotic dilation) is seen best at the 1 o'clock position on a DV or VD view, although its size does not correlate with pressure gradient severity. Turbulence can preferentially extend into the left or right pulmonary artery branch, causing that segment to appear dilated. Caudal vena caval dilation can be evident, especially with overt right-sided CHF.

The ECG features of moderate to severe PS typically include a right axis deviation, because of the RV hypertrophy and enlargement (**Figure 27.29**). Sometimes an RA enlargement pattern (*p pulmonale*), tachyarrhythmias, or ST segment elevation also are present (**Figure 5.53**, p. 157). Some animals with mild to moderate, or even severe, PS have a normal mean electrical axis, although RV enlargement could be indicated by an S wave in Lead I, prominent S wave in the lower left precordial leads, or an rSr' appearance to lead V_1 (**Figure 27.30**).

Echocardiographic findings are compatible with the lesions previously described in this section. Moderate to severe

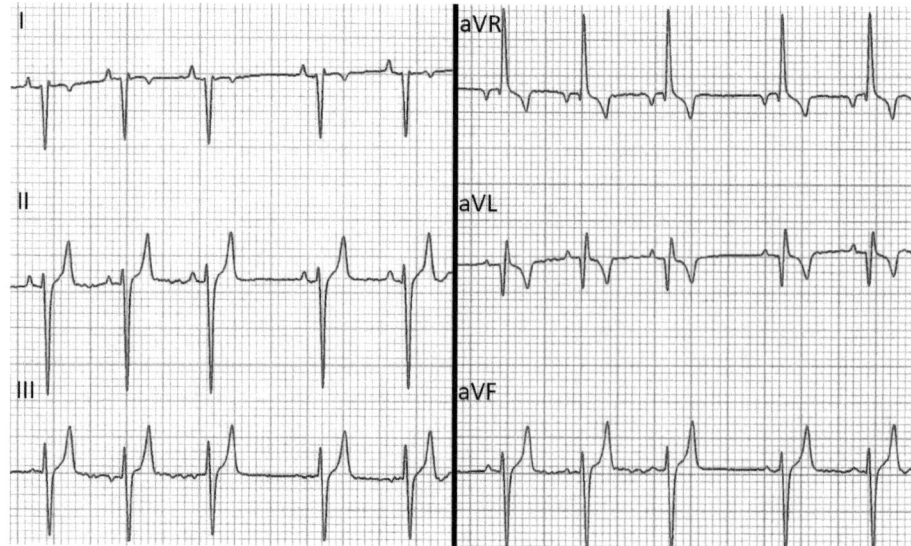

Figure 27.29 Electrocardiogram from the dog of **Figure 27.27** shows sinus arrhythmia at a heart rate ~120 beats/min. There is a pronounced right axis deviation, with large QRS complexes (note ½ standard calibration). Leads as marked; 25 mm/s, 0.5 cm = 1 mV.

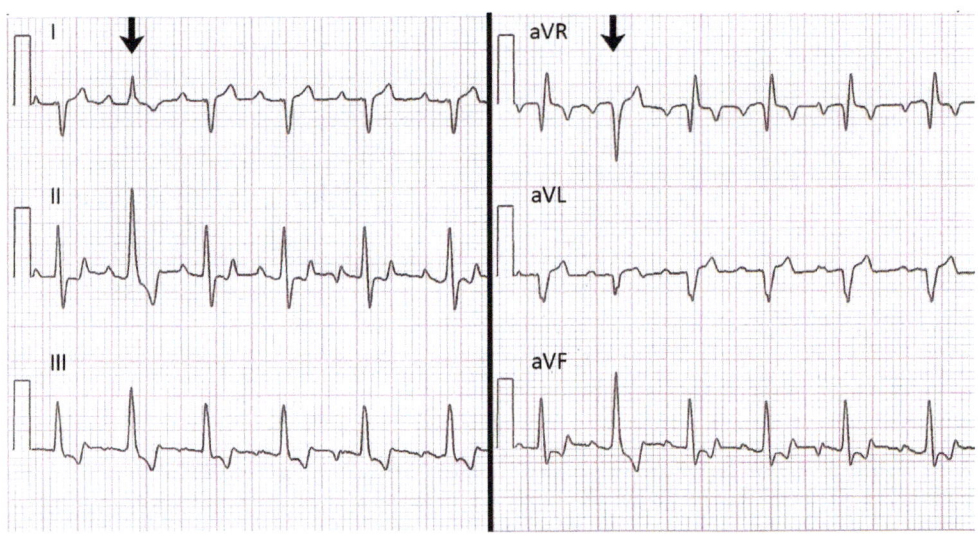

Figure 27.30 This ECG from an 8-year-old male English Bulldog with severe pulmonic stenosis (Doppler gradient ~129 mm Hg) shows clear evidence for right ventricular enlargement (note especially the S wave in lead I); however, the mean electrical axis is between 90° and 120°, or only borderline rightward (see p. 155). A ventricular premature complex (arrows) is present, with a background of sinus rhythm at ~150 beats/min. Leads as marked, recorded simultaneously; 25 mm/s, 1 cm = 1 mV.

stenosis is heralded by RV wall, papillary muscle and septal hypertrophy, as well as RV chamber enlargement. The interventricular septum often appears flattened, causing the left ventricle to look "D-shaped" on short-axis views, as higher RV pressure pushes it toward the left (**Figures 27.31** and **27.32**). A reduction in RV systolic function might be evident based on decreased tricuspid annular plane systolic excursion (TAPSE; p. 94). RA enlargement is common and explained by RV diastolic or systolic dysfunction, TR, or increased systemic venous pressures. These RV and RA findings generally are more pronounced with more severe outflow obstruction. Increased venous pressures can cause the caudal vena cava to appear distended, with reduced respiratory variation in diameter.

In type A PS, the pulmonary annulus is normal in diameter with leaflets that dome into the PA during systole (**Figure 27.33**). In type B PS, the annulus is hypoplastic. However, as noted above this binary classification oversimplifies the spectrum of disease. Dysplastic valve leaflets are thickened, often asymmetrical, fused, or otherwise malformed; they also can show systolic doming (**Figure 27.34**). The RV outflow area can be narrowed and difficult to visualize clearly. Other lesions include fixed subvalvular obstruction, apparent tethering of the dorsal leaflet edges to the PA wall, and echoes suggesting fibrous tissue or rudimentary valvular tissue extending inward from the medial or lateral edges of the valve region. Multiple levels of obstruction can be observed, as often occurs in French Bulldogs. In patients

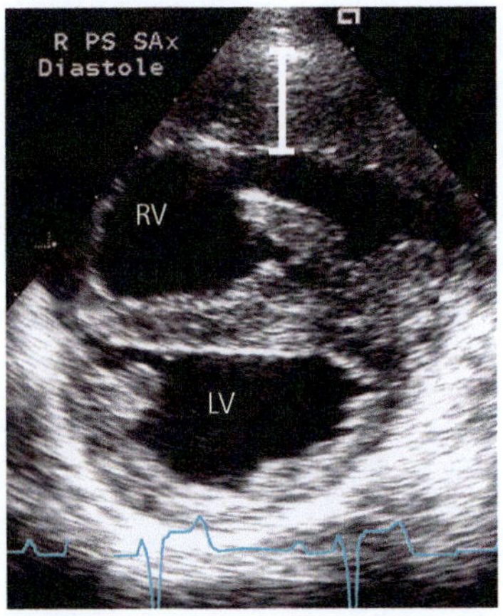

Figure 27.31 Right ventricular pressure overload caused by pulmonic stenosis led to severe hypertrophy of the free wall (bar), dilation of the RV, and septal flattening toward the LV (here in diastole) in a 2-year-old male mixed breed dog (Doppler gradient 126 mm Hg); right parasternal short-axis view. LV, left ventricle; RV, right ventricle.

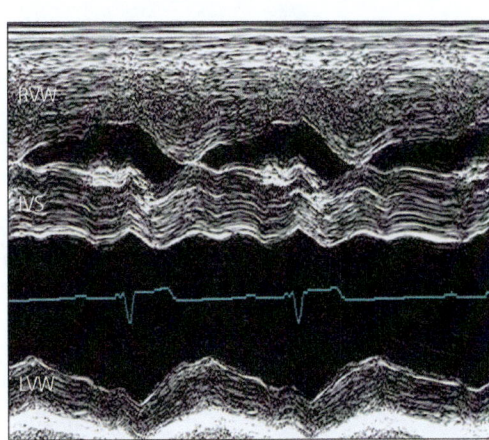

Figure 27.32 M-mode image from a 3-year-old female Brittany Spaniel with severe pulmonic stenosis shows right ventricular hypertrophy and flattened septal motion. IVS, interventricular septum; LVW, left ventricular wall; RVW, right ventricular wall.

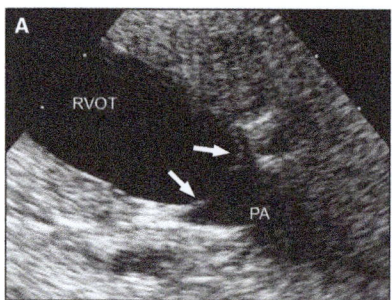 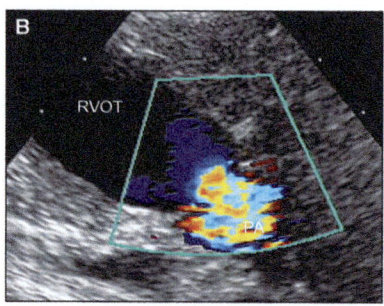

Figure 27.33 (A) Systolic doming of the pulmonary valve (arrows) in the dog of **Figure 27.31**. The valve is relatively thin, although the leaflets appear fused. (B) Color-flow Doppler image in systole shows blood flow acceleration proximal to the valve orifice and turbulence, distal. Left cranial short-axis view. PA, pulmonary artery; RVOT, right ventricular outflow tract.

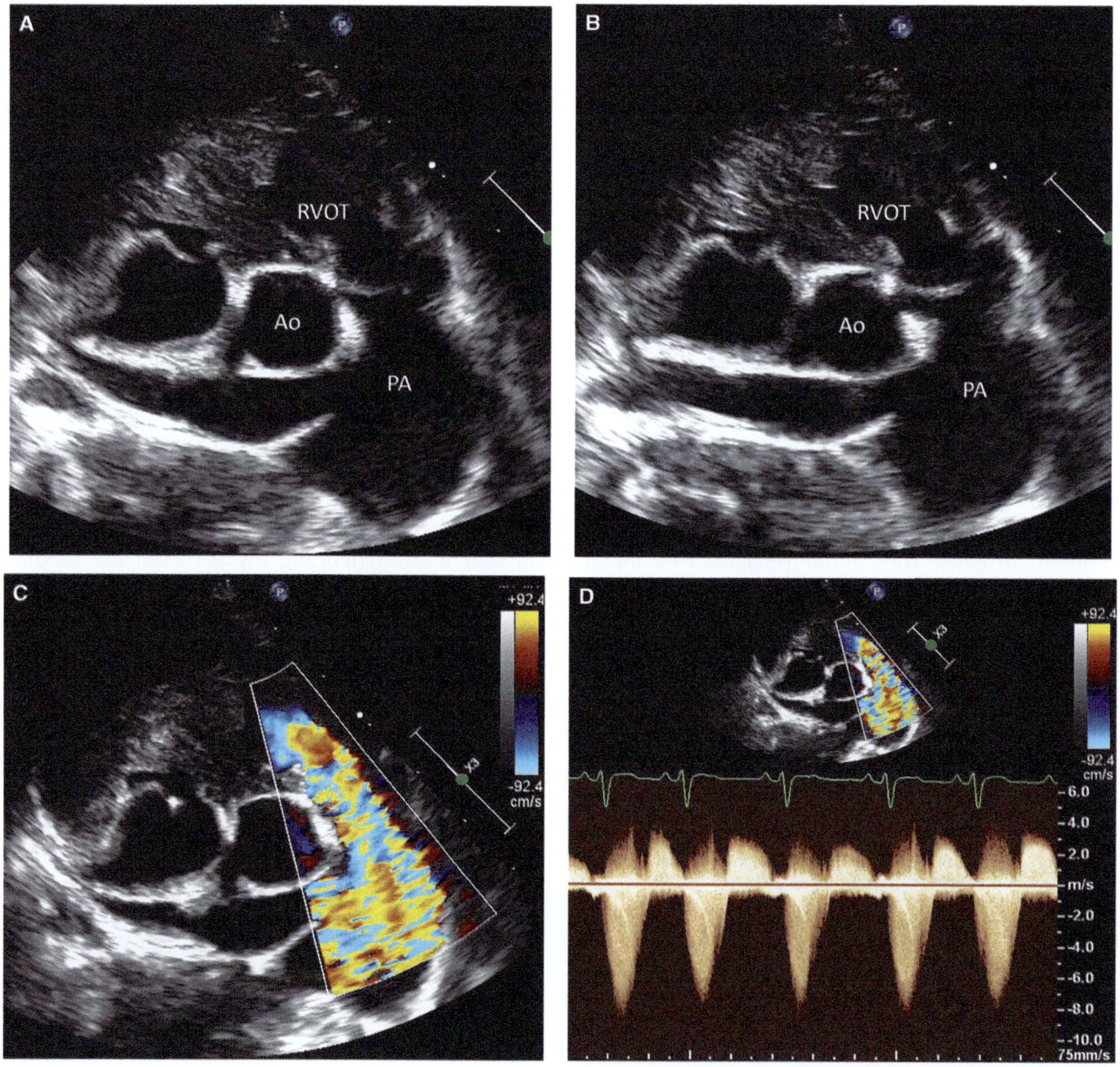

Figure 27.34 Pulmonic stenosis with severely dysplastic valve in a 6-month-old male Jack Russell Terrier. The thick, poorly mobile valve leaflets are shown in diastole (A) and systole (B). There is a large post-stenotic dilation of the pulmonary artery (PA). Color-flow in systole (C) shows turbulent flow from narrowed valve orifice into the dilated main PA. Continuous-wave Doppler (D) shows peak systolic velocity >7 m/s at modal velocity (pressure gradient >200 mm Hg). A faint, dynamic obstruction profile is superimposed (best seen in second cardiac cycle). Pulmonary insufficiency is evident in diastole.

with an aberrant coronary artery, the pulmonary annular region's appearance on (transthoracic) echo often raises suspicion for a coronary malformation (**Figure 27.23**). However, findings can be inconclusive and require coronary angiography or transesophageal echo for confirmation (see "Management" section). Post-stenotic dilation of the main pulmonary trunk usually is evident and can extend into one or both branch PAs. In some animals with PS (or other causes of high RV systolic pressure), mitral valve SAM might be observed. This is more likely when the LV size is small (with pseudohypertrophy from poor filling) or from severe interventricular septal hypertrophy. Varying amounts of pleural effusion, pericardial effusion, and ascites accompany marked right heart dilation in most cases of CHF. Paradoxical septal motion (**Table 4.2**, p. 91) might be noted in such cases as well, from extensive RV volume overload. In dogs with a PFO, an echo "bubble" study, with saline contrast injected into a peripheral vein, can further delineate caval entry into the right heart as well as R-to-L shunting.

Doppler evaluation, along with anatomic and functional findings, provides an estimate of lesion severity (**Figure 27.34**). Color-flow Doppler can help localize the initial site of stenosis (valvular, sub- or supravalvular, or dynamic), although multiple levels of obstruction often are evident from spectral Doppler recordings. Prominent pulmonary valvular insufficiency is common, and can be severe, especially after balloon valvuloplasty. Every possible view of the RV outflow region and pulmonary trunk should be interrogated to determine anatomy and peak outflow velocity (with CW Doppler), because the orientation of the maximum velocity jet is not necessarily the same as that for normal pulmonary flow. Color-flow Doppler aids in aligning the CW Doppler cursor used for measurement, is better for identifying concurrent PR or TR, and when properly processed (by lowering velocity scales and filters), this modality can efficiently identify most R-to-L shunts. Similar to SAS, the PS is considered mild if the maximal instantaneous Doppler-derived PG is under 50 mm Hg, moderate when the Doppler gradient is between 50 and 79 mm Hg, and severe if it exceeds 80 mm Hg. These cutoffs have not been rigorously tested in terms of prognosis, especially in smaller breeds that often seem to tolerate higher pressure gradients.

As with AS, the derived pressured gradients depend on ventricular stroke volume, a point that is too often overlooked when assessing lesion severity or the response to an interventional procedure. Calculating the pulmonary valve effective orifice area and the pulmonary to aortic VTI ratio are less dependent on flow and can be used to estimate PS severity. The valve area must be indexed to body size. These methods are especially recommended for patients undergoing balloon valvuloplasty (p. 122), as well as when systolic ventricular function is impaired. They also are relevant when cardiac output is increased by sympathetic tone or by a successful valve procedure. For example, even in the absence of a dynamic infundibular obstruction, atenolol therapy can decrease PG in dogs with PS simply by reducing stroke volume. This does not make PS "better" and does not alter indexed pulmonary valve orifice area or other relatively flow-independent indices (Nishimura, 2018). The pulmonary to aortic (PA/Ao) VTI ratio also is recommended, and obtained by recording CW Doppler across each outlet valve and comparing to areas under the spectral envelopes (at similar instantaneous heart rates). The VTI relates directly to the mean pressure gradient across each valve, which in turn, depends on stroke volume (flow) and valvular cross-sectional area. For example, a PA/Ao VTI that decreases from 7.7 to 3.1 suggests a technically successful procedure, even if the maximal PS gradient only decreases by 40%. These points are relevant also to sedation, which both withdraws sympathetic tone and can depress myocardial function. In the aforementioned study, butorphanol did not alter PG or the more flow-independent indices.

The systolic PG across the stenotic valve (or other obstruction), the right heart filling pressures, and other anatomic features can be determined by cardiac catheterization and angiocardiography, too (**Figures 27.35–27.37**). These procedures usually are confined to patients undergoing catheter balloon valvuloplasty. As with AS, catheter-estimated systolic PGs in anesthetized animals often are 40% to 50% lower than those recorded by Doppler echo in the awake patient. It can be challenging to assess the effectiveness of a balloon procedure by catheter-derived pressures because the abrupt reduction in RV afterload can, in turn, cause worsening dynamic obstruction.

Management

For cases with mild to moderate PS, periodic reevaluation and echo with no specific therapy usually are recommended. Avoiding prolonged, strenuous exercise is prudent. It is

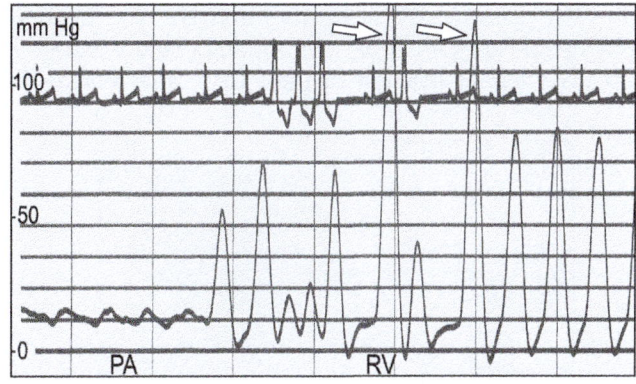

Figure 27.35 Electrocardiogram (top) and pressure (bottom) recording obtained during cardiac catheterization in a dog with pulmonic stenosis. At left, the catheter tip was within the PA; normal PA pressure was recorded. As the catheter was pulled back into the RV, a brief paroxysm of ventricular tachycardia and an isolated ventricular premature beat occurred before the rhythm stabilized and baseline RV systolic pressure became evident (right side of trace). Note the poor systolic pressure generation in response to the ectopic ventricular complexes. The sinus complexes that follow them stimulate greater systolic pressure generation than otherwise would have occurred (postextrasystolic potentiation; arrows). PA, pulmonary artery; RV, right ventricle. Pressure scale on left.

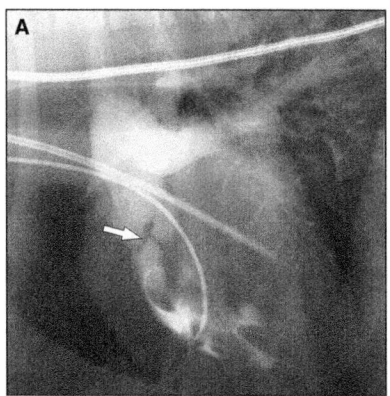 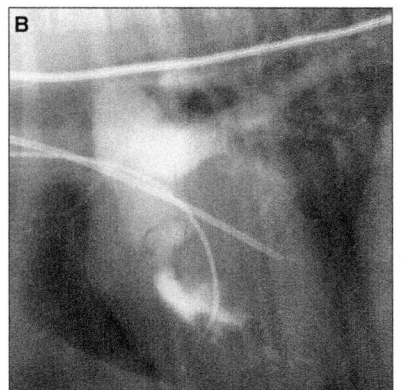

Figure 27.36 Right ventricular (RV) angiocardiographic images in diastole (A) and systole (B) from a 1-year-old male Vizsla with pulmonic stenosis. The thickened pulmonary valve leaflets appear as a filling defect (arrow, A). Doming of the thickened and fused leaflets (B) occurs during systole. Post-stenotic dilation of the pulmonary trunk and proximal lobar pulmonary arteries and RV hypertrophy are evident.

important to monitor for progression of RV hypertrophy, which can worsen dynamic outflow obstruction, and for the onset or progression of TR, arrhythmias or other problems. For animals with moderate to severe stenosis, exercise should be restricted. A beta-blocker (atenolol) might be helpful, especially if infundibular hypertrophy and dynamic outflow obstruction are identified or in cases where exertional ectopy occurs. Signs of CHF are managed medically (Chapter 22). Animals with PS should not be bred, even if the malformation is mild.

Palliation for severe PS by balloon valvuloplasty is recommended in most cases. This procedure has been shown to reduce clinical signs and improve survival in dogs with severe PS. Balloon dilation also is recommended for some cases with moderately severe PS, especially those with marked TR or clinical signs, such as exercise intolerance or exertional collapse. Valvuloplasty can improve quality of life and reduce risk for CHF in such cases (p. 177). Patients with CHF have been successfully treated after medical stabilization of failure. Some (but not all) dogs gain resolution of their CHF, and reduction or elimination of CHF drug therapy might be possible. The procedure can be beneficial even if there is severe TR or AF, however, these complications reduce the likelihood of long-term benefit.

The goal of palliative valvuloplasty is to reduce the PG into the mild range or at least by 50% of the original PG. Perhaps a more realistic goal would be a doubling of effective cross-sectional area or halving of the PA/Ao VTI ratio, although these measures are reported less often. Balloon valvuloplasty is most successful in patients with normal pulmonary annulus size and thin, fused leaflets (**Figure 27.38**). Animals with thick, dysplastic leaflets and a hypoplastic annulus are less likely to have optimal results; sometimes little to no reduction in PG is achieved. The use of high-pressure (burst pressure between 12 and 18 atmospheres) balloon catheters for pulmonary valvuloplasty was reported to be highly effective in reducing PG in dogs. Valve morphology and degree of RV hypertrophy did not appear to affect success rate using this equipment; however, pulmonary valve annulus diameter was negatively correlated with the degree of post-procedural PG reduction (Belanger, 2018). Whether cutting balloon dilation, followed by high-pressure pulmonary balloon valvuloplasty, could improve results for dogs with a dysplastic pulmonary valve is under investigation. Poor balloon valvuloplasty results are more likely with severe infundibular obstruction or DCRV malformations, and it is uncertain if these procedures should even be recommended. Infundibular hypertrophy and dynamic RV outflow obstruction can complicate palliative procedures and cause post-procedural obstruction, although the "suicide ventricle" is probably overemphasized and this can regress over time. For some complicated obstructions, intracardiac stenting extending into the pulmonary artery has been employed; however, this requires more study and careful case selection. Operators should anticipate more PR following a successful procedure. This might in fact be one reason why RV size increases and dynamic obstruction decreases in the long-term. This regurgitation is audible as a diastolic murmur in many dogs. Whether this affects long-term prognosis, as it does in humans, is uncertain.

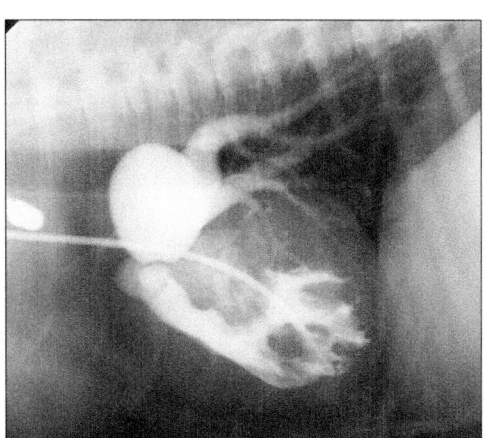

Figure 27.37 A thick, dysplastic pulmonary valve, with asymmetrical valve sinuses, large post-stenotic pulmonary trunk dilation, and right ventricular hypertrophy are evident. Angiocardiogram from a 3-year-old female West Highland White Terrier with severe pulmonic stenosis.

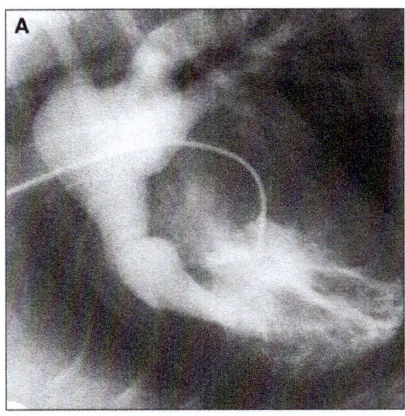 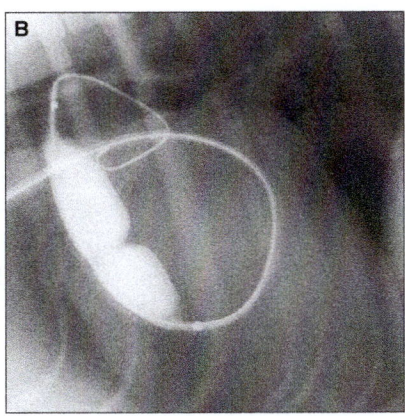 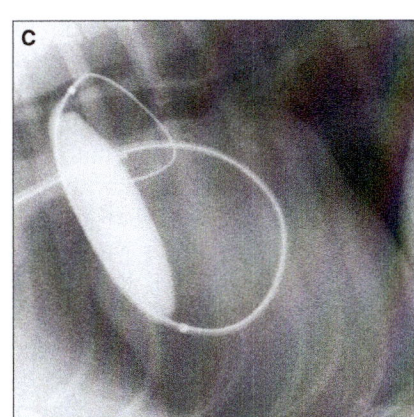

Figure 27.38 (A) Baseline right ventricular angiocardiogram from a 1.5-year-old Brittany Spaniel with severe pulmonic stenosis (Doppler gradient ~210 mm Hg) prior to balloon valvuloplasty. (B) The stenotic valve creates a "waist" in the partially filled balloon of the dilation catheter. (C) Full inflation of the balloon dilates the stenotic valve. A couple subsequent inflations during the procedure verified that the waist did not recur. Doppler gradient the following day was 75 mm Hg.

It is important to verify normal coronary anatomy prior to balloon valvuloplasty, particularly in English Bulldogs and Boxers where prevalence of anomalous coronary anatomy is increased (**Figures 27.22** and **27.23**). While echo studies (transthoracic and particularly, transesophageal) can identify the presence and origin of a coronary malformation, and depict the initial path of a coronary vessel, echo cannot show the arterial arborization as effectively as traditional or computed tomographic (CT) angiography. In many larger referral centers, CT angiography is used to screen for coronary anomalies in suspicious cases before embarking on cardiac catheterization. The presence of a single anomalous coronary artery generally is a contraindication to palliative surgical procedures, and probably a non-indication to perform balloon valvuloplasty. These procedures have caused death secondary to transection, compression or avulsion of the left coronary branch. Nevertheless, conservative balloon valvuloplasty has been tried, and while patients can survive the procedure, only mild reduction in PG has been demonstrated thus far.

Balloon valvuloplasty is performed under general anesthesia with fluoroscopic and angiographic guidance (see Chapter 6). It has been performed in cats and in foals. In some cases, transthoracic or transesophageal echo is used to guide the procedure. Usually a balloon:annulus ratio of 1.2 to 1.5 is selected; for some large dogs, a double balloon technique can be appropriate, and experience suggests that a 1.5 ratio (or even higher) is sometimes more effective for reducing the obstruction; however, this depends greatly on anatomy and the type of balloon selected. In dogs with severe PS, an additional decrease in PG might occur within the few months following balloon valvuloplasty. However, in a minority of cases, restenosis occurs and can be successfully treated in most cases (Winter, 2021). Various methods have been considered to reduce the potential for restenosis, including external beam radiation therapy, but far more study

is needed (Nagata, 2020). Complications of balloon valvuloplasty can include hemorrhage, hypotension, cardiac puncture, arrhythmias, pulmonary artery dissection, hypoxemia, and death. The overall rate of major complications associated with pulmonary balloon valvuloplasty in 117 cases from one institution was 11% (LeBlanc, 2019). CHF increases the risk of complications.

Various surgical and hybrid procedures also have been used for palliation of moderate to severe PS in dogs. These have included closed and open patch-graft techniques to expand the pulmonary valve and subvalvular area, depending on the type of obstructive lesion in the individual patient. Significant reduction in PG is possible, although results can be variable and the procedures carry significant risks. Cardiopulmonary bypass is required for open pulmonary valve commissurotomy. Use of a RV-to-pulmonary artery valved conduit to bypass severe PS also has been described. Balloon valvuloplasty usually is attempted before surgical procedures in patients with valvular PS because it is generally less risky. In the future, another possible treatment option might be transcatheter pulmonary valve implantation.

Balloon dilation of supravalvular PS or peripheral pulmonary artery stenosis has been tried but generally appears less successful than for valvular stenosis. Intravascular stents have been employed to treat supravalvular pulmonic stenosis in some dogs. These also might be applicable for peripheral or main pulmonary artery stenosis.

Prognosis The prognosis for patients with PS usually depends on stenosis severity. Those with mild PS typically have a normal life span, as do many with moderately severe PS. Because mild PS generally has a good long-term prognosis, valvuloplasty is not advocated in this group. Dogs with moderate PS often show no clinical signs and have fairly low cardiac mortality. It is not clear whether balloon valvuloplasty improves survival in these asymptomatic dogs or in the dogs that do have clinical signs associated with moderate PS. There is a tendency to be more aggressive in recommending valvuloplasty for larger breed dogs with moderate PS.

Animals with severe stenosis often die within 3 years of diagnosis. Balloon valvuloplasty usually can prolong survival and improve clinical signs in dogs with severe PS. When balloon valvuloplasty is not done (or is unsuccessful), greater severity of PS is associated with worse survival. Presence of TR also is linked with greater risk of cardiac death (Francis, 2011). In addition, the presence of clinical signs, AF or other tachyarrhythmias, and CHF, especially at a young age, worsen the outcome. Prognosis is considered guarded to poor in these animals. Type B PS morphology also has been associated with poorer prognosis; this probably relates to stenosis severity. Marked reduction in PG during balloon dilation is more difficult to achieve when dealing with a hypoplastic, dysplastic valve or multiple levels of obstruction.

Mitral Dysplasia

The AV valves originate embryologically from the endocardial cushions and ventricular walls through a process of endomyocardial tissue infolding and diverticulation. AV valve malformation (dysplasia) often involves multiple abnormalities of the valve leaflets, as well as of their supporting structures. These can include: shortened, thickened, cleft, and fused or rolled leaflets; fusion of leaflets or related structures to the ventricular or septal wall; short or long, fused or thickened chordae; leaflets connecting directly to a papillary muscle with little to no chordal interface; and malformed, malpositioned, or fused papillary muscles. MVD (and also TVD) can occur as components of partial or complete AV septal defect, or as isolated abnormalities. Alternatively, affected animals also could have a secundum ASD or other defect, such as pulmonary valve dysplasia. MVD accompanies SAS in some dogs, particularly Bull Terriers. Occasionally, dynamic LVOT obstruction occurs in dogs with a mild mitral malformation, in the absence of the fixed LVOT obstruction characteristic of SAS. Such dynamic obstruction can resolve as the animal grows to adult size.

Valvular regurgitation is the usual functional abnormality. Its extent ranges from mild to severe. The pathophysiology and sequelae are similar to those in animals with acquired MR (Chapter 29). LV function declines over time in patients with mitral dysplasia, as it does with acquired MR. In contrast, stenosis of the mitral valve orifice is relatively uncommon. When present, it usually coexists with regurgitation. Mitral stenosis (MS) causes LV inflow obstruction because the effective mitral orifice area is restricted during ventricular filling. The resulting increase in LA pressure, although fairly mild, leads to LA dilation which can become massive. Abbreviated diastole, as occurs with exercise or tachyarrhythmias, increases the diastolic pressure gradient across the valve and can lead to abrupt onset of pulmonary congestion or even edema. AF, pulmonary hypertension, and left-sided CHF are common outcomes of MVD.

Other causes of mitral inflow obstruction occur sporadically. Supravalvular MS (supravalvular ring) is uncommon; it can occur as an isolated defect or in association with an AV septal defect, where it can be confused with double-outlet right atrium. Supravalvular MS involves an obstructive fibrous or fibromuscular shelf above the mitral valve, yet ventral to the atrial appendage and foramen or fossa ovale (in contrast to *cor triatriatum sinister*; p. 512). The pathophysiology is the same as for valvular MS. Supravalvular MS and double-outlet right atrium have been reported in cats; the Siamese breed could be overrepresented. Severe LA enlargement with signs of CHF or pulmonary hypertension, as well as aortic thromboembolism, are common in MS.

Clinical Features

MVD occurs most commonly in larger breeds of dog, and also in cats (**Table 27.1**). English Springer Spaniels also might be predisposed. MVD is thought to have a heritable basis. It is a common congenital defect in Sphynx cats. Concurrent cardiac malformations are common, including TVD and septal defects.

Except for the young age of the affected animal, the clinical signs associated with MVD with predominately MR are similar to those in older dogs with degenerative (myxomatous) mitral valve disease (p. 538). Severely affected animals also might have stunted growth. Severity of signs depends on the degree of MR, as well as whether MS coexists. Exercise intolerance, cough, respiratory distress caused by left-sided CHF, and atrial arrhythmias, especially AF, commonly develop. The onset of AF or supraventricular tachycardia is likely to provoke decompensated CHF. Collapse or syncope occurs in some cases. The systolic murmur of MR is heard best at the left apex, although it can radiate craniodorsally or to the right.

Severe MS typically causes signs of low cardiac output and pulmonary edema; secondary pulmonary hypertension could promote the development of right-sided congestive signs, as well (especially in cats). With MS, a soft diastolic murmur or opening snap of the mitral valve might be audible, rarely. The diagnosis of mild MS depends on echocardiographic screening.

Diagnostic Tests

The radiographic, ECG, and catheterization findings associated with MVD are similar to those found in dogs with degenerative mitral valve disease (p. 541). Although chamber enlargements will be similar, 2D echo will demonstrate the valve malformation, as opposed to typical changes of degenerative valve disease. Radiographic signs of pulmonary congestion and edema commonly are present. LA enlargement can be massive, especially with concurrent MS (**Figure 27.39**, also see **Figure 3.12**, p. 56). Some cats with

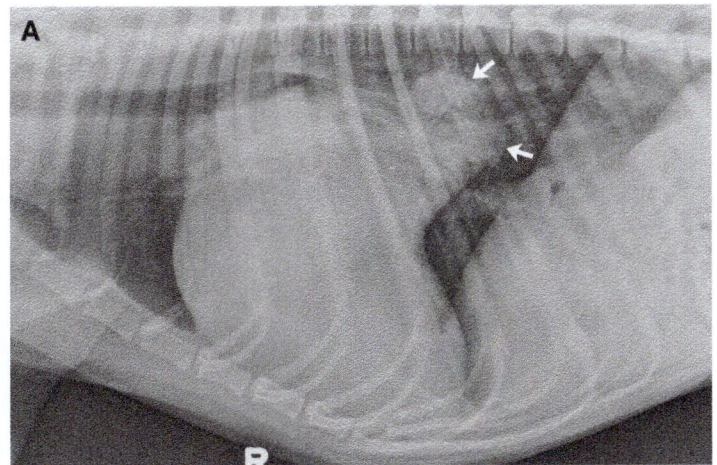

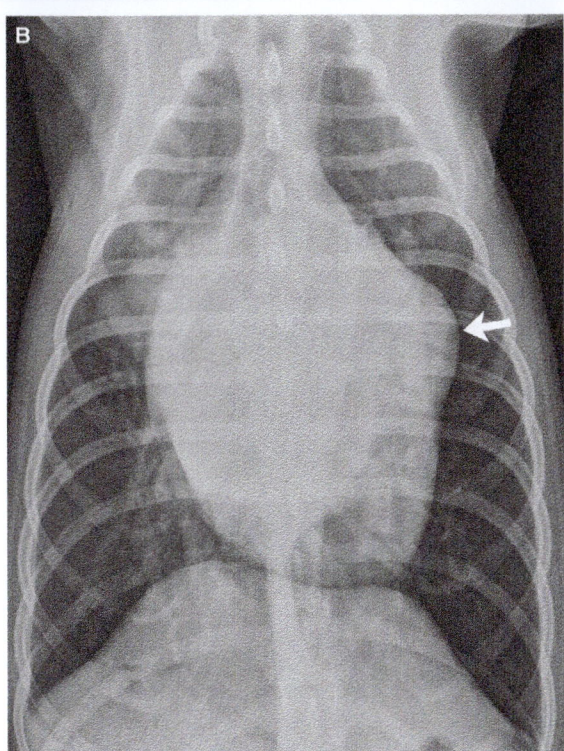

Figure 27.39 Lateral (A) and DV (B) radiographs from a 2-year-old female Labrador Retriever with mitral dysplasia. Valve regurgitation and stenosis both were present. There is severe left heart enlargement (VHS ~13.5v), with massive dorsocaudal left atrial protrusion (A, arrows) and a large left auricular bulge (B, arrow). The dog had been in atrial fibrillation for over a year and was being treated for congestive heart failure. These radiographs show no evidence of pulmonary edema.

MS have dilated pulmonary arteries as well as veins, right heart enlargement, and pleural effusion; even ascites occurs sometimes, secondary to severe pulmonary hypertension. ECG abnormalities are variable but can include atrial and ventricular tachyarrhythmias, as well as criteria for atrial and ventricular enlargement.

Echo can depict the left heart chamber dilation and mitral apparatus malformations, such as abnormal attachments,

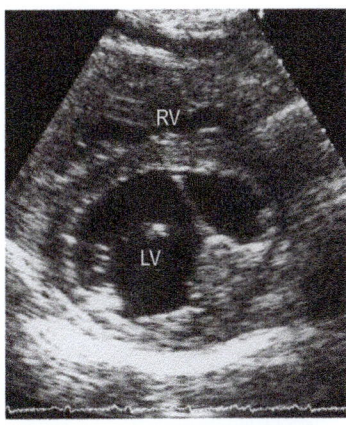

Figure 27.40 Right parasternal short-axis echocardiogram shows asymmetrical papillary muscles and abnormal chordae (or false tendon) in a cat with mitral dysplasia. LV, left ventricle; RV right ventricle.

shape, motion, and function (**Figures 27.40–27.47**). There can be multiple MR jets. MS is characterized by abnormal mitral valve motion. 2D imaging shows restricted leaflet separation and diastolic doming of leaflet tips toward the LV. M-mode studies show parallel (concordant) mitral leaflet motion and decreased E-to-F slope. Doppler studies indicate increased mitral inflow velocities, with increased diastolic transmitral PG and prolonged mitral inflow time (pressure half-time, p. 125). Both E waves and A waves are increased, and if atrial function is well-preserved the A wave velocity can exceed 2 m/s. Cardiac catheterization also will document the diastolic PG between LA pressure (or its proxy, pulmonary

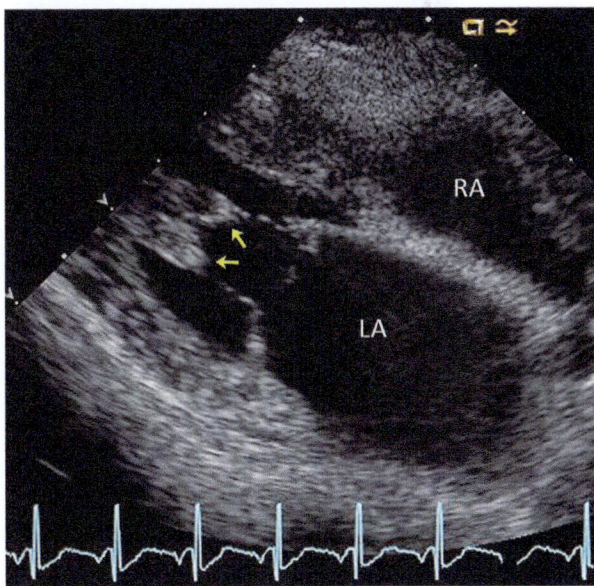

Figure 27.41 A malformed, double-headed papillary muscle (arrows) found in a 7-year-old Standard Poodle. The dog also had mild mitral regurgitation and leaflet thickening; however, it was unclear whether mitral dysplasia or degenerative mitral valve disease caused the latter two findings. Right parasternal long-axis view. LA, left atrium RA, right atrium.

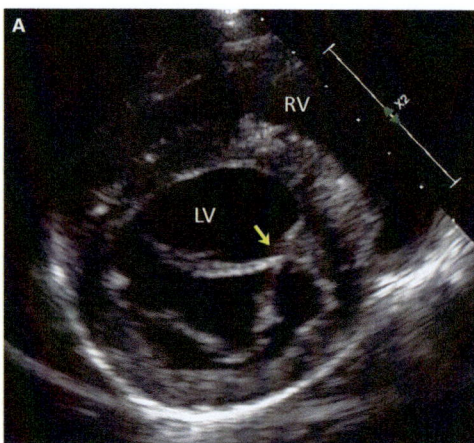
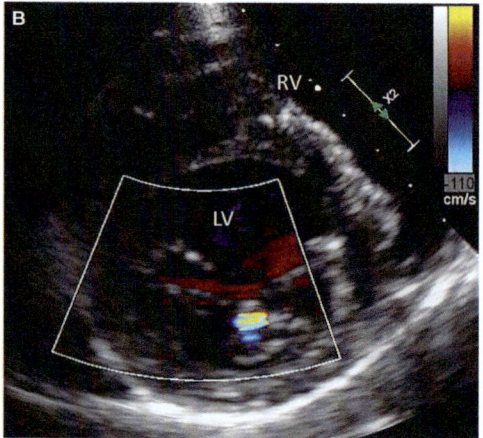

Figure 27.42 Mild mitral dysplasia in a 2-year-old female Labrador Retriever. (A) Papillary muscle-chordal malformation at the cranial aspect of the anterior leaflet caused this region to appear tethered (arrow). (B) Nevertheless, the associated mitral regurgitation is only minimal, as shown by the tiny systolic flow disturbance with color flow Doppler imaging. Right parasternal short axis view. LV, left ventricle; RV right ventricle.

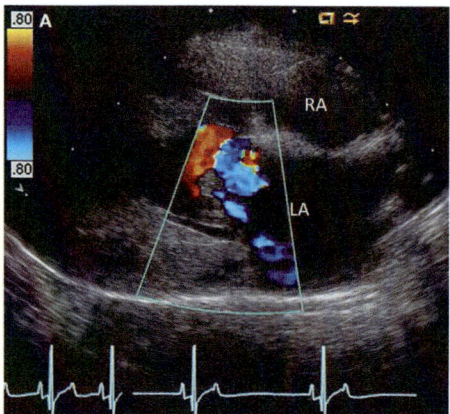
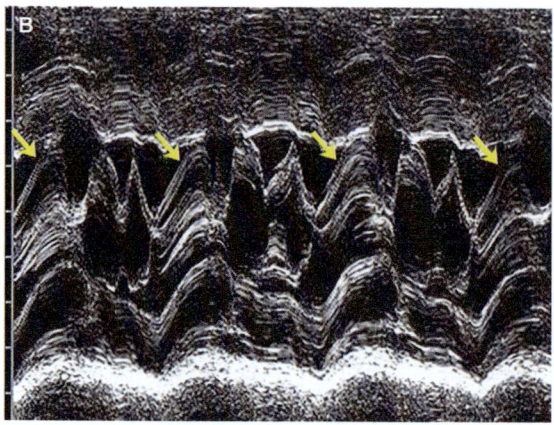

Figure 27.43 Mild mitral dysplasia in a 5-month-old female Sheltie. (A) The anterior leaflet is thick and knobby (outlined by color Doppler signal). Minimal mitral regurgitation (MR) occurred at rest, although, mild excitement would provoke dynamic left ventricular (LV) outflow obstruction with its characteristic caudally directed mitral regurgitant jet. There also was mild LV hypertrophy. Right parasternal long-axis view. LA, left atrium; RA, right atrium. (B) M-mode image at the mitral valve level shows systolic anterior motion (SAM, arrows). Atenolol treatment abolished the SAM. Atenolol was discontinued when the dog was a young adult; follow-up echocardiogram a year later showed no evidence for dynamic LV outflow obstruction and only minimal MR.

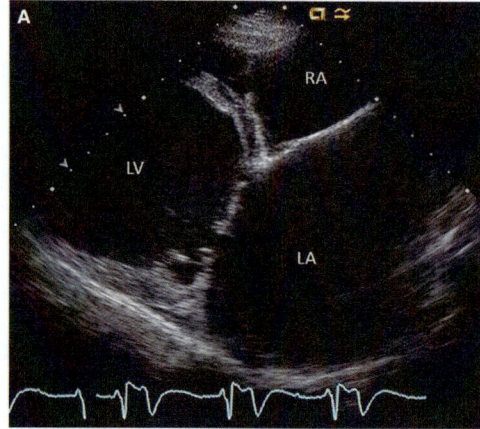
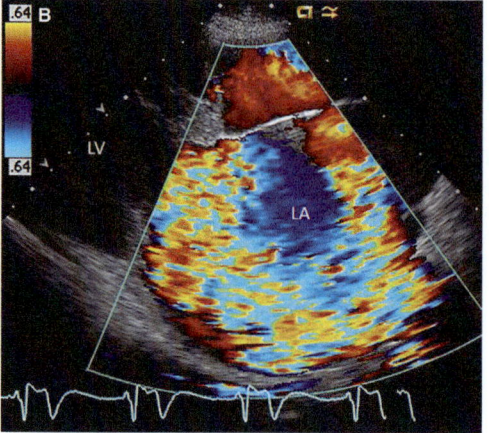

Figure 27.44 (A) Mitral dysplasia caused severe mitral regurgitation, with massive left heart dilation, early congestive heart failure, and moderate pulmonary hypertension in a 4-year-old Golden Doodle. This systolic frame shows a wide gap between the closed mitral leaflets. (B) Color Doppler depicts a wide band of MR-induced turbulence swirling into and around the LA. The dog also had tricuspid valve dysplasia. Right parasternal long axis view. LA, left atrium; LV, left ventricle; RA, right atrium. **Figure 3.12** (p. 56) shows this dog's radiographs.

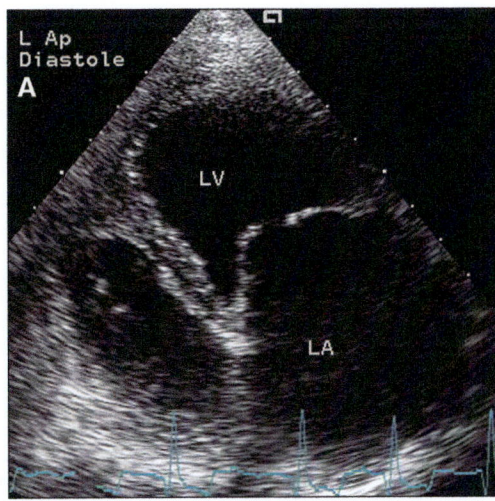
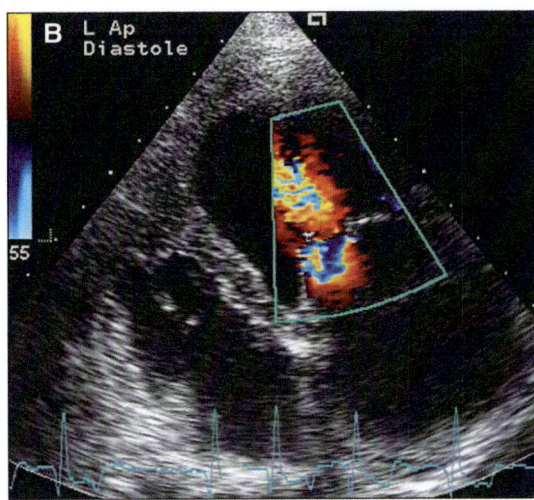

Figure 27.45 (A) Diastolic left apical image shows restricted mitral leaflet opening in a 7-year-old female Labrador Retriever with pulmonary edema. Mitral dysplasia caused valve stenosis and regurgitation. LA and LV are markedly dilated. ECG (at bottom) shows atrial fibrillation. (B) Color Doppler frame in diastole depicts flow acceleration toward the stenotic valve, then turbulence into the LV. LA, left atrium; LV, left ventricle.

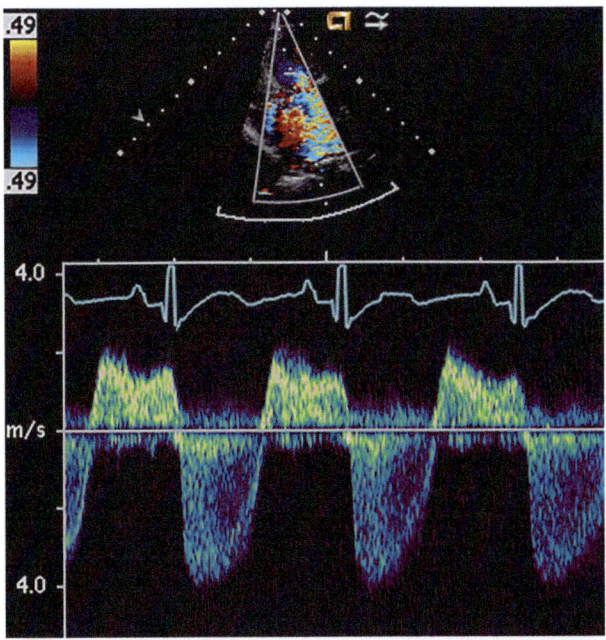

Figure 27.46 Continuous-wave Doppler through the mitral orifice shows elevated inflow velocity (with slowed E wave deceleration) throughout diastole, the diastolic transmitral pressure gradient. The time required for peak gradient to fall by one half (pressure half-time) can be used to estimate mitral stenosis severity; but mitral regurgitation (MR), which increases the maximum diastolic gradient, and ventricular compliance can limit the calculation's accuracy. MR peak velocity in this dog is ~4 m/s; it occurs in early systole, suggesting elevated LA pressure.

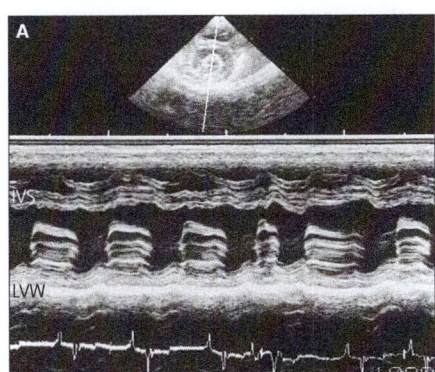
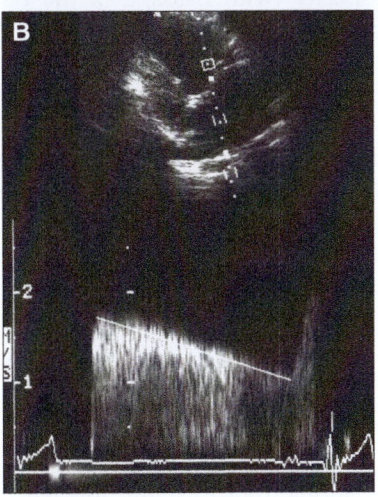

Figure 27.47 (A) M-mode image at the mitral valve level from a 6-year-old female Irish Setter with mitral stenosis shows the characteristic parallel motion of both mitral leaflets. The leaflets are thickened. The ECG (bottom) shows sinus rhythm with one atrial premature complex. IVS, interventricular septum; LVW, left ventricular wall. (B) Pulsed-wave Doppler image of mitral inflow during one cycle from this dog illustrates slow decline in diastolic transvalvular velocity (prolonged pressure half-time) and enhanced atrial contraction velocity. Left apical position.

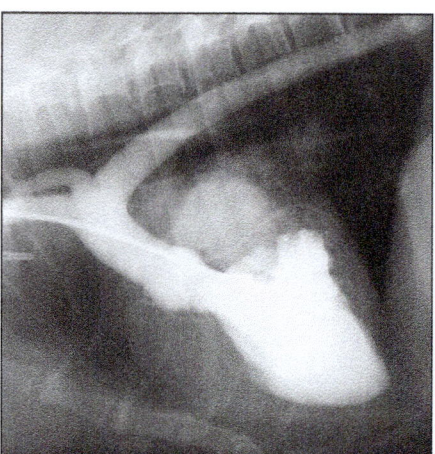

Figure 27.48 Left ventricular angiocardiogram in diastole, from dog of **Figure 27.47**. Note the thickened, stenotic mitral valve with restricted opening ("V"-shaped filling defect in left ventricle). Concurrent mitral regurgitation allowed dye into the atrium. (From Lehmkuhl, 1994.)

capillary wedge pressure) and LV diastolic pressure, although this is rarely done now. Angiocardiography can illustrate some structural consequences (**Figure 27.48**).

Management

Medical therapy involves exercise restriction and management of arrhythmias and CHF, as indicated (Chapters 25 and 22). Surgical mitral valve reconstruction or replacement using cardiopulmonary bypass might be an option. Surgical strategies for MS could include cardiopulmonary bypass and open mitral commissurotomy, a hybrid balloon-thoracotomy surgical procedure without bypass, or a transvascular mitral balloon valvuloplasty (with passage of the balloon catheter transseptally from right to left atrium).

Prognosis If the mitral malformation causes only mild to moderate MR, the patient can do well for years. However, the prognosis is poor with severe MR or with significant MS, unless successful surgical correction or palliation occurs. Sixty percent of dogs with moderate to severe MS died or were euthanized before 2½ years of age in one study (Lehmkuhl, 1994). However, some cats with mitral valve malformations, including stenosis, have survived to 8 years of age or more.

Tricuspid Dysplasia

An estimated 25–30% of cases with TVD have concurrent cardiac malformations; these usually involve MVD or septal defects, although some have concurrent PS. This figure depends in part on the criteria used to define tricuspid valve malformation by echo. Malformations of the tricuspid valve and its support apparatus are similar to those of MVD (see preceding discussion), and **Figures 27.49** and **27.50**). In some cases, the tricuspid valve appears to be displaced ventrally into the ventricle (an Ebstein-like anomaly). However, this point is debated

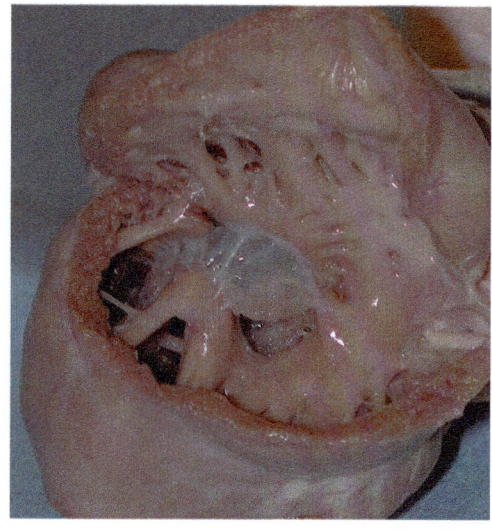

Figure 27.49 Open right ventricle (free wall on top) from a young Labrador Retriever puppy with severe tricuspid dysplasia. This view from the ventricular side shows the lateral leaflet fused directly to a broad, multi-segmented papillary muscle complex.

because frequently the septal leaflet fails to delaminate from the ventricular septum; while this displaces the leaflet coaptation point from the annular plane, this is not necessarily accompanied by downward displacement of the right atrium. The prevalence of accessory conduction pathways and overt ventricular pre-excitation (Wolff–Parkinson–White syndrome; p. 153) is probably increased in such animals. TVD can cause severe TR, but many milder cases are diagnosed only by echo and are silent to auscultation. This situation creates a potential for over-diagnosis of TVD considering the common finding of (silent) tricuspid regurgitation by Doppler imaging across species. The pathophysiologic features of moderate to severe

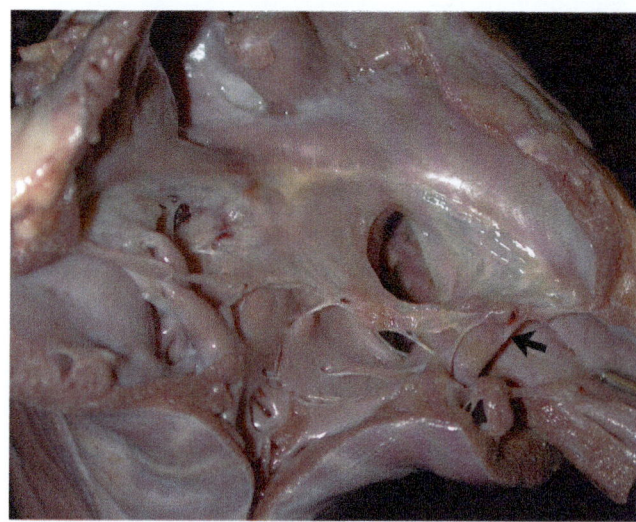

Figure 27.50 View from the open right atrium of another Labrador Retriever puppy with tricuspid dysplasia. Note the large cleft in the lateral leaflet and the wide papillary muscle (arrow) underneath that is fused directly to the caudal aspect of the leaflet.

TVD relate to right heart volume overload, with RA and RV dilation likely starting in utero and progressing with growth. Increasing RV end-diastolic pressure eventually results in right-sided CHF, which often is precipitated by the onset of atrial flutter or AF. A small percent of cases present mainly for signs of R-to-L shunting across an ASD or PFO.

TVD with stenosis, and especially tricuspid valve atresia, occur only rarely and might be more common in cats and foals. These severe obstructive lesions are similar to MS but also have significant potential for causing R-to-L shunting at the interatrial septal level (via a PFO or ASD). This can lead to severe cyanosis and metabolic acidosis, along with RA and coronary sinus enlargement. Animals with tricuspid atresia that do not concurrently have a VSD (which, by L-to-R flow, would allow pulmonary perfusion), must obtain pulmonary flow through a PDA or systemic collaterals (bronchial arteries). In dogs, tricuspid stenosis can occur in conjunction with a hypoplastic right heart syndrome which includes cor triatriatum dexter, tricuspid stenosis, small right ventricle, and pulmonary stenosis.

Clinical Features

TVD is relatively uncommon compared to other CHDs; it is more likely to occur in larger dog breeds, especially the Labrador Retriever. Border Collies also might be overrepresented, especially in the United Kingdom. TVD might occur more often in males, although this is not reported consistently. Cats also are affected; the Chartreux breed is noted to have higher risk in Europe. An autosomal dominant mode of inheritance with reduced penetrance, or perhaps more likely, an autosomal recessive pattern have been proposed in dogs. There are reports in Arabian and Arabian-crossbred horses of tricuspid stenosis or atresia, as well as multiple other defects. Tricuspid malformations have occurred in other breeds too, including Standardbred horses.

The historical signs and clinical findings vary. Signs might not occur until the dog is older or has developed an atrial arrhythmia. In mildly to moderately severe cases, the animal might be asymptomatic or only mildly exercise intolerant. However, fatigue, ascites, dyspnea from pleural effusion, anorexia, and cardiac cachexia frequently develop in severe cases. Syncope or collapse can occur, especially in cases with tricuspid stenosis or severe TR. In patients with severe tricuspid stenosis and a PFO, cyanosis is likely.

Physical features can include a systolic murmur of TR and jugular vein pulsations; but the murmur of tricuspid stenosis is virtually never heard. Murmur intensity in TVD might not correlate with the severity of TR. Although a soft murmur might be missed, an audible murmur is not always present, especially in puppies. Even with severe TR, the murmur grade can underestimate severity because with wide-open TR, the systolic PG across the tricuspid valve is relatively low. Jugular vein distension, muffled heart and lung sounds, and ballottable abdominal fluid develop in animals with CHF. Over time, pleural effusion associated with CHF can become chylous. Supraventricular tachyarrhythmias are common; these can include re-entrant AV tachycardias over an accessory pathway, as well as the more common atrial flutter or AF.

Diagnostic Tests

Right heart enlargement is visible radiographically (**Figure 27.51** and **Figure 3.15**, p. 57). Sometimes, the cardiac silhouette is quite large and round, similar to that seen with pericardial effusion or DCM. At other times, the left apex is displaced so caudally and to the left that LV enlargement is

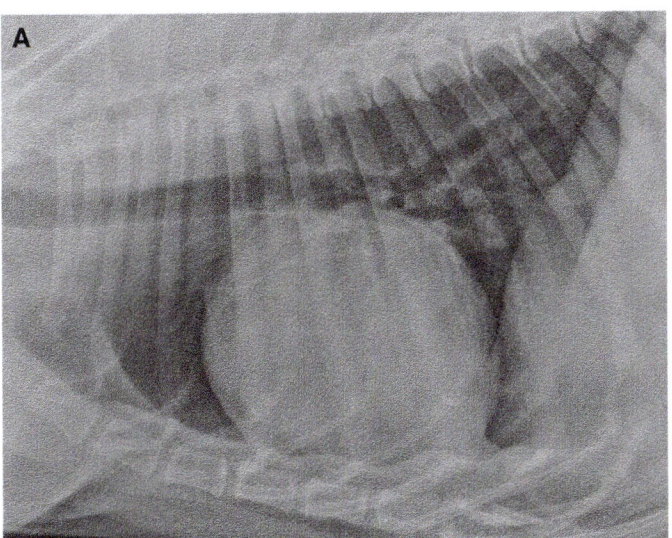
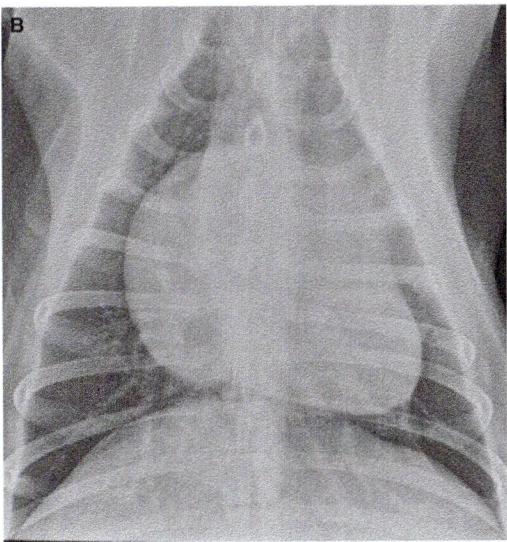

Figure 27.51 (A) Lateral radiograph from a 7-year-old male Labrador Retriever with tricuspid dysplasia and severe tricuspid regurgitation. The enlarged heart looks quite round in this view, which could suggest dilated cardiomyopathy or pericardial effusion; (contrast with Figure 3.15A, p. 57). (B) However, the DV view shows a large bulge in the right ventricular area, with a well-defined but displaced left ventricular apex. Echocardiography revealed normal left heart size and function, with severe right atrial and ventricular dilation and malformed tricuspid apparatus.

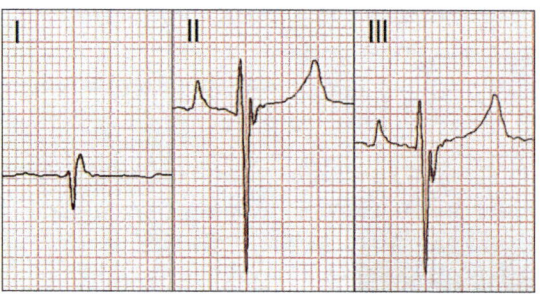

Figure 27.52 The QRS complexes appear splintered, especially in leads II and III, in a male Labrador Retriever with tricuspid dysplasia. Leads as marked; 50 mm/s, 1 cm = 1 mV.

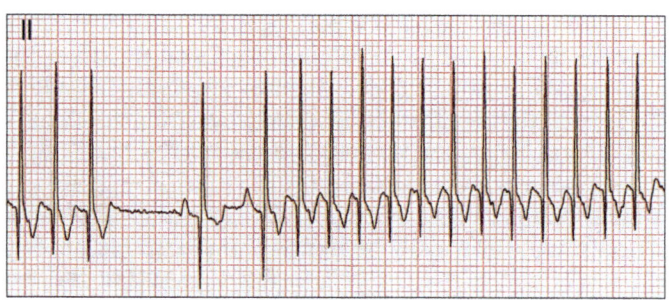

Figure 27.53 Paroxysmal atrioventricular reciprocating tachycardia in a 3-month-old female Labrador Retriever with tricuspid dysplasia and congestive heart failure. Lead II, 25 mm/s, 1 cm = 1 mV.

erroneously diagnosed. Caudal vena caval distension, pleural or peritoneal effusion, and hepatomegaly often are evident. The ECG usually shows RV and occasionally RA enlargement criteria, especially S-waves in leads I and the lower left precordial leads. The QRS complexes might appear splintered (**Figure 27.52**). Focal atrial tachycardia, flutter or AF often develops. Evidence for ventricular pre-excitation rarely is present; rapid AV reciprocating tachycardia (p. 417) can occur in animals with an accessory pathway (**Figure 27.53**).

Echo depicts the often massive right heart dilation (**Figures 27.54–27.57**). Malformations of the valve apparatus usually are visible in multiple views. The left apical four-chamber view appears to be especially useful; typically in dogs, it shows a normal tricuspid annulus (slightly ventral to the mitral annular plane), adherence of the septal leaflet to the ventricular septum, and a wide TR jet seen by color Doppler that originates from an apical location in the ventricle. The papillary muscles often appear abnormal or multiheaded. Less often, short chords or overt stenosis are seen. Echocardiographic features of tricuspid stenosis are similar to those of MS. Tricuspid stenosis with only minimal regurgitation causes marked atrial, but not ventricular, enlargement.

Intracardiac electrocardiography is necessary to confirm the presence of Ebstein's anomaly, which is suggested by ventral displacement of the tricuspid valve annulus; this involves recording atrial pressures at the same location (dorsal to the tricuspid valve annulus) as documenting a ventricular electrogram.

Management

Medical management involves exercise restriction and treatment of CHF and arrhythmias, as needed (Chapters 22 and 25). Periodic thoraco- or abdominocentesis also might be required. For persistent chylous pleural effusion in dogs, thoracic duct ligation, with or without passive pleuroperitoneal shunting, has been tried along with pleural ports, with varying success.

Surgical bioprosthetic tricuspid valve replacement using cardiopulmonary bypass has been tried in dogs at specialized centers. Potential complications associated with valve replacement surgery include tachyarrhythmias, complete AV

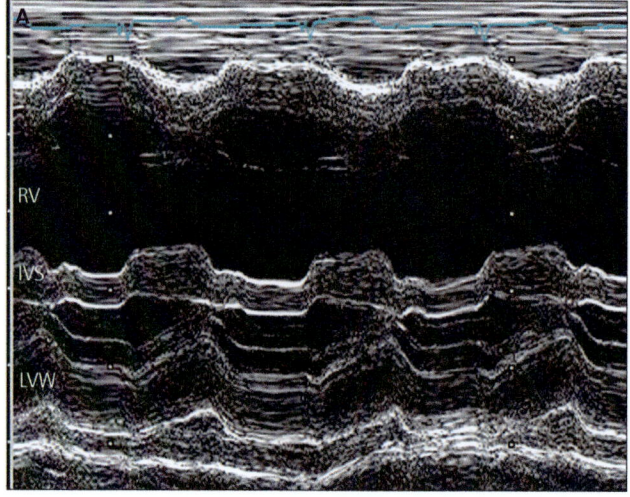
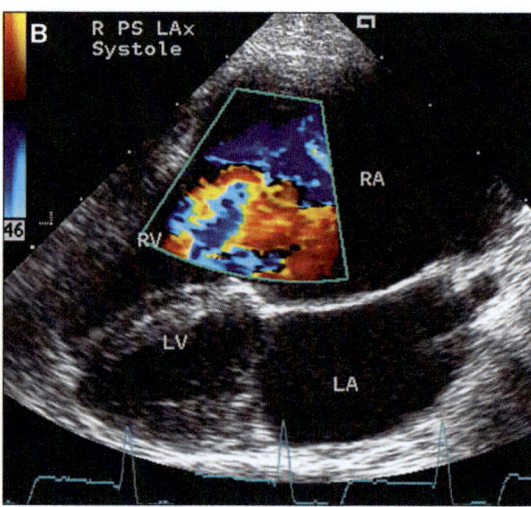

Figure 27.54 (A) Severe right ventricular dilation with paradoxical septal motion is evident in this M-mode echocardiogram from a male cat with tricuspid dysplasia and congestive heart failure. (B) Color-flow Doppler image in systole shows this cat's marked tricuspid regurgitation and huge RA. Right parasternal long-axis view. IVS, interventricular septum; LA, left atrium; LV, left ventricle; LVW, left ventricular wall; RA, right atrium; RV, right ventricle.

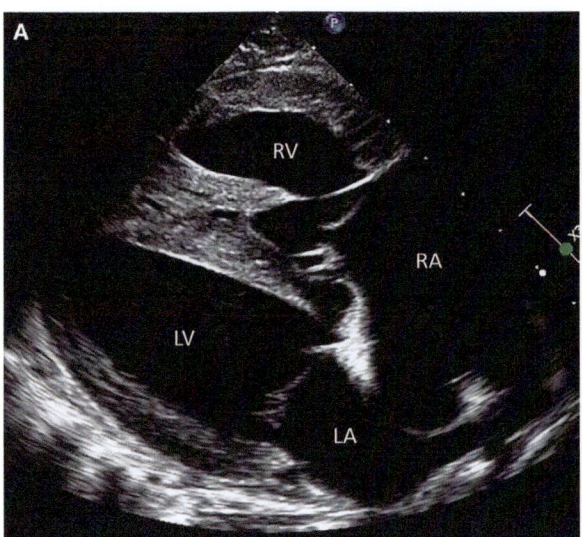
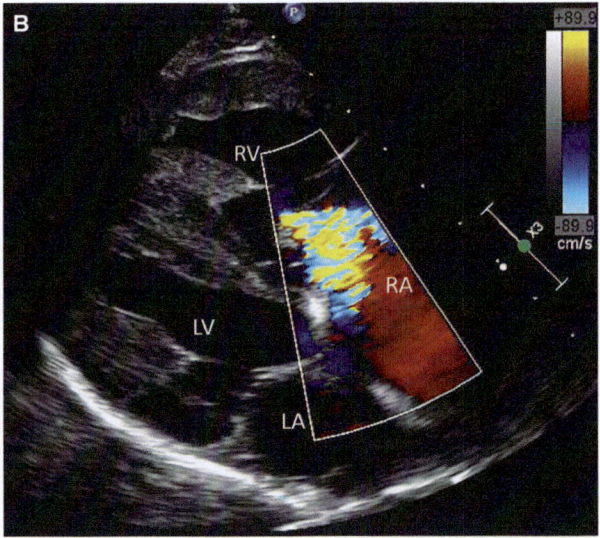

Figure 27.55 (A) Right parasternal long axis, four-chamber view from a 1-year-old dog with tricuspid dysplasia reveals a large, malformed and perforated papillary muscle complex, along with severe dilation of the RA. This systolic frame shows that the tricuspid leaflets do not fully coapt. Concurrent, severe pulmonic stenosis caused the right ventricular free wall hypertrophy. (B) Color-flow Doppler image in systole shows the regurgitant jet originating from the gap between the closed tricuspid leaflets. LA, left atrium; LV, left ventricle; RA, right atrium; RV, right ventricle.

block, thrombosis, inflammatory pannus, endocarditis, and death. However, in dogs that survive to discharge, intermediate outcome, at least, can be good.

Tricuspid stenosis in dogs potentially can be managed successfully with balloon valvuloplasty. Clinical improvement is likely, although signs could recur over time in some cases. One potential complication is worsening of pre-existing TR; this can accelerate the development of right-sided CHF. Surgical palliation of tricuspid stenosis also has been tried in dogs.

Prognosis The prognosis is guarded for animals with a functionally severe defect and marked cardiomegaly. Right-sided CHF commonly develops in these cases. However, survival times can be quite variable. Many animals with mild to moderately severe tricuspid dysplasia live for 8 years or more, and surprisingly, even some with severe TR can do so. AF and right-sided CHF are negative prognostic indicators. Syncope appears to indicate increased risk for cardiac death.

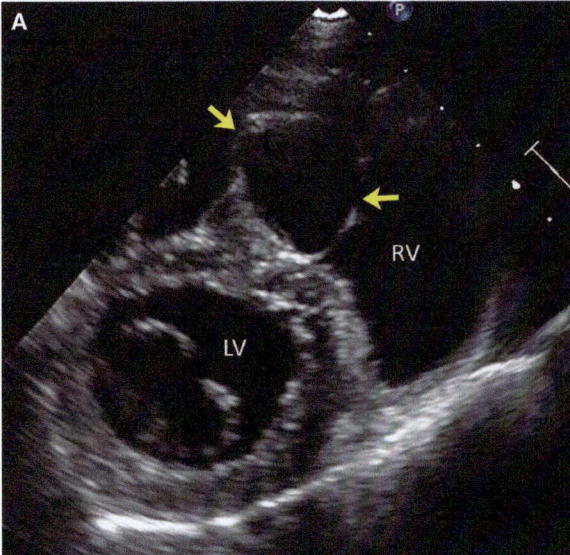
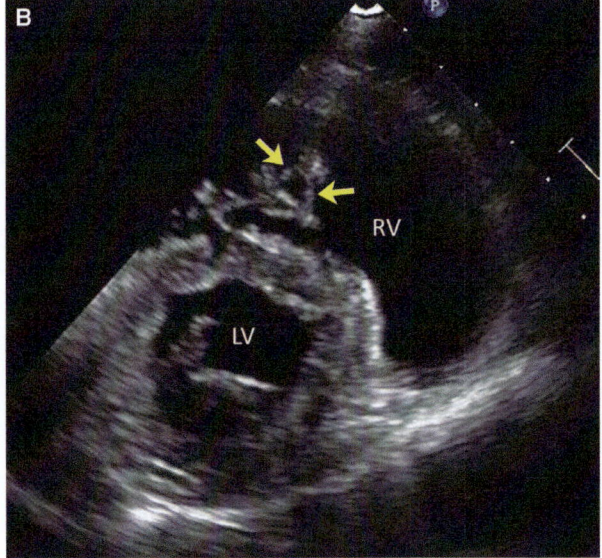

Figure 27.56 (A) Diastolic 2D echocardiographic frame shows the open tricuspid valve leaflets (arrows) in a 6 year old male Boxer with tricuspid dysplasia. (B) In systole, a prominent gap (arrows) is evident between the thickened leaflets. Right parasternal short axis view. LV, left ventricle; RV, right ventricle.

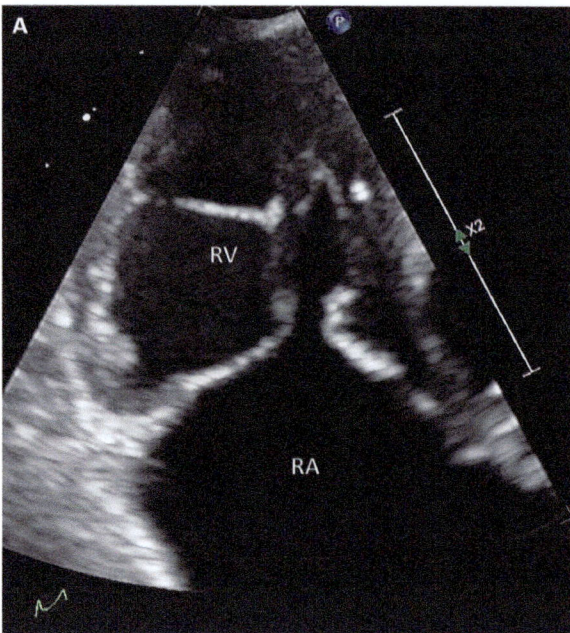 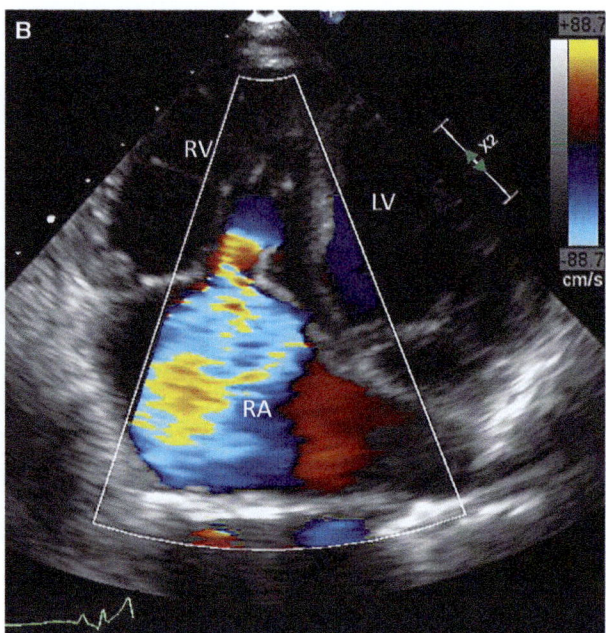

Figure 27.57 (A) Left apical view in systole shows abnormal papillary muscle structure, thickened valve leaflets that do not fully close, and dilation of the RA in a 1½ year old male Labrador Retriever with tricuspid dysplasia. (B) Color Doppler depicts severe tricuspid regurgitation originating from the apically displaced coaptation points of the valve. This is a common finding with this malformation. The dilated caudal vena cava enters the RA at the lower right aspect of the image. LV, left ventricle; RA, right atrium; RV, right ventricle.

Suggested Additional Reading and References

Also See Online Comprehensive Bibliography at: https://www.routledge.com/9781482246223.

Aoki T, Sunahara H, Sugimoto K, et al. Peripheral pulmonary artery stenosis in three cats. J Vet Med Sci 2015;77:487–491.

Arai S, Griffiths LG, Mama K, et al. Bioprosthesis valve replacement in dogs with congenital tricuspid valve dysplasia: technique and outcome. J Vet Cardiol 2011;13:91–99.

Arndt JW, Oyama MA. Balloon valvuloplasty of congenital mitral stenosis. J Vet Cardiol 2013;15:147–151.

Bayly WM, Reed SM, Leathers CW, et al. Multiple congenital heart anomalies in five Arabian foals. J Am Vet Med Assoc 1982;181:684–689.

Belanger MC, Cote E, Beauchamp G. Association between aortoseptal angle in Golden Retriever puppies and subaortic stenosis in adulthood. J Vet Intern Med 2014;28:1498–1503.

Belanger C, Gunther-Harrington CT, Nishimura S, et al. High-pressure balloon valvuloplasty for severe pulmonary valve stenosis: a prospective observational pilot study in 25 dogs. J Vet Cardiol 2018;20:115–122.

Borenstein N, Chetboul V, Passavin P, et al. Successful transcatheter pulmonary valve implantation in a dog: first clinical report. J Vet Cardiol 2019;26:10–18.

Bristow P, Sargent J, Luis Fuentes V, et al. Outcome of bioprosthetic valve replacement in dogs with tricuspid valve dysplasia. J Small Anim Pract 2017;58:205–210.

Bristow P, Sargent J, Luis Fuentes V, et al. Surgical treatment of pulmonic stenosis in dogs under cardiopulmonary bypass: outcome in nine dogs. J Small Anim Pract 2018;59:38–44.

Buchanan JW. Pathogenesis of single right coronary artery and pulmonic stenosis in English Bulldogs. J Vet Intern Med 2001;15:101–104.

Bussadori C, Amberger C, Le Bobinnec G, et al. Guidelines for the echocardiographic studies of suspected subaortic and pulmonic stenosis. J Vet Cardiol 2000;2:15–22.

Bussadori C, DeMadron E, Santilli RA, et al. Balloon valvuloplasty in 30 dogs with pulmonic stenosis: effect of valve morphology and annular size on initial and 1-year outcome. J Vet Intern Med 2001;15:553–558.

Caivano D, Birettoni F, Fruganti A, et al. Transthoracic echocardiographically-guided interventional cardiac procedures in the dog. J Vet Cardiol 2012;14:431–444.

Caivano D, Dickson D, Martin M, et al. Murmur intensity in adult dogs with pulmonic and subaortic stenosis reflects disease severity. J Small Anim Pract 2018;59:161–166.

Campbell FE, Thomas WP. Congenital supravalvular mitral stenosis in 14 cats. J Vet Cardiol 2012;14:281–292.

Chetboul V, Petit A, Gouni V, et al. Prospective echocardiographic and tissue Doppler screening of a large Sphynx cat population: reference ranges, heart disease prevalence and genetic aspects. J Vet Cardiol 2012;14:497–509.

Chetboul V, Poissonnier C, Bomassi E, et al. Epidemiological, clinical, and echocardiographic features, and outcome of dogs with Ebstein's anomaly: 32 cases (2002-2016). J Vet Cardiol 2020;29:11–21.

Eason BD, Fine DM, Leeder D, et al. Influence of beta blockers on survival in dogs with severe subaortic stenosis. J Vet Intern Med 2014;28:857–862.

Estrada A, Moise NS, Erb HN, et al. Prospective evaluation of the balloon-to-annulus ratio for valvuloplasty in the treatment of pulmonic stenosis in the dog. J Vet Intern Med 2006;20:862–872.

Famula TR, Siemens LM, Davidson AP, et al. Evaluation of the genetic basis of tricuspid valve dysplasia in Labrador Retrievers. Am J Vet Res 2002;63:816–820.

Fonfara S, Martinez Pereira Y, Swift S, et al. Balloon valvuloplasty for treatment of pulmonic stenosis in English Bulldogs with an aberrant coronary artery. J Vet Intern Med 2010;24:354–359.

Francis AJ, Johnson MJ, Culshaw GC, et al. Outcome in 55 dogs with pulmonic stenosis that did not undergo balloon valvuloplasty or surgery. J Small Anim Pract 2011;52:282–288.

Fujii Y, Nishimoto Y, Sunahara H, et al. Prevalence of patent foramen ovale with right-to-left shunting in dogs with pulmonic stenosis. J Vet Intern Med 2012;26:183–185.

Fujiwara M, Harada K, Mizuno T, et al. Surgical treatment of severe pulmonic stenosis under cardiopulmonary bypass in small dogs. J Small Anim Pract 2012;53:89–94.

Griffiths LG, Bright JM, Chan KC. Transcatheter intravascular stent placement to relieve supravalvular pulmonic stenosis. J Vet Cardiol 2006;8:145–155.

Grint KA, Kellihan HB. Pulmonary artery dissection following balloon valvuloplasty in a dog with pulmonic stenosis. J Vet Cardiol 2017;19:182–189.

Gunther-Harrington CT, Phillips KL, Visser LC, et al. Non-electrocardiographic-gated computed tomographic angiography can be used to diagnose coronary artery anomalies in Bulldogs with pulmonary valve stenosis. Vet Radiol Ultrasound 2019;60:38–46.

Hollmer M, Willesen JL, Jensen AT, et al. Aortic stenosis in the Dogue de Bordeaux. J Small Anim Pract 2008;49:432–437.

Javard R, Belanger MC, Cote E, et al. Comparison of peak flow velocity through the left ventricular outflow tract and effective orifice area indexed to body surface area in Golden Retriever puppies to predict development of subaortic stenosis in adult dogs. J Am Vet Med Assoc 2014;245:1367–1374.

Jenni S, Gardelle O, Zini E, et al. Use of auscultation and Doppler echocardiography in Boxer puppies to predict development of subaortic or pulmonary stenosis. J Vet Intern Med 2009;23:81–86.

Johnson MS, Martin M. Results of balloon valvuloplasty in 40 dogs with pulmonic stenosis. J Small Anim Pract 2004;45:148–153.

Kander M, Paslawska U, Staszczyk M, et al. Retrospective analysis of co-occurrence of congenital aortic stenosis and pulmonary artery stenosis in dogs. Pol J Vet Sci 2015;18:841–845.

Kleman ME, Estrada AH, Maisenbacher HW 3rd, et al. How to perform combined cutting balloon and high pressure balloon valvuloplasty for dogs with subaortic stenosis. J Vet Cardiol 2012;14:351–361.

Kobayashi K, Hori Y, Chimura S. Plasma N-terminal pro B-type natriuretic peptide concentrations in dogs with pulmonic stenosis. J Vet Med Sci 2014;76:827–831.

Koplitz SL, Meurs KM, Bonagura JD. Echocardiographic assessment of the left ventricular outflow tract in the Boxer. J Vet Intern Med 2006;20:904–911.

Laborda-Vidal P, Pedro B, Baker M, et al. Use of ECG-gated computed tomography, echocardiography and selective angiography in five dogs with pulmonic stenosis and one dog with pulmonic stenosis and aberrant coronary arteries. J Vet Cardiol 2016;18:418–426.

Lake-Bakaar GA, Griffiths LG, Kittleson MD. Balloon valvuloplasty of tricuspid stenosis: a retrospective study of 5 Labrador Retriever dogs. J Vet Intern Med 2017;31:311–315.

LeBlanc NL, Agarwal D, Menzen E, et al. Prevalence of major complications and procedural mortality in 336 dogs undergoing interventional cardiology procedures in a single academic center. J Vet Cardiol 2019;23:45–57.

Lehmkuhl LB, Ware WA, Bonagura JD. Mitral stenosis in 15 dogs. J Vet Intern Med 1994;8:2–17.

Locatelli C, Spalla I, Domenech O, et al. Pulmonic stenosis in dogs: survival and risk factors in a retrospective cohort of patients. J Small Anim Pract 2013;54:445–452.

Marinus SM, van Engelen H, Szatmari V. N-terminal pro-B-type natriuretic peptide and phonocardiography in differentiating innocent cardiac murmurs from congenital cardiac anomalies in asymptomatic puppies. J Vet Intern Med 2017;31:661–667.

Martin JM, Orton EC, Boon JA, et al. Surgical correction of double-chambered right ventricle in dogs. J Am Vet Med Assoc 2002;220:770–774, 768.

Meurs KM, Lehmkuhl LB, Bonagura JD. Survival times in dogs with severe subvalvular aortic stenosis treated with balloon valvuloplasty or atenolol. J Am Vet Med Assoc 2005;227:420–424.

Minors SL, O'Grady MR, Williams RM, et al. Clinical and echocardiographic features of primary infundibular stenosis with intact ventricular septum in dogs. J Vet Intern Med 2006;20:1344–1350.

Nagata K, Coleman AE. Outcomes after combined percutaneous balloon valvuloplasty and external beam radiation therapy for the treatment of congenital pulmonic stenosis in four dogs. J Vet Cardiol 2020;28:1–10.

Navalon I, Pradelli D, Bussadori CM. Transesophageal echocardiography to diagnose anomalous right coronary artery type R2A in dogs. J Vet Cardiol 2015;17:262–270.

Navarro-Cubas X, Palermo V, French A, et al. Tricuspid valve dysplasia: a retrospective study of clinical features and outcome in dogs in the UK. Open Vet J 2017;7:349–359.

Nishimura S, Visser LC, Belanger C, et al. Echocardiographic evaluation of velocity ratio, velocity time integral ratio, and pulmonary valve area in dogs with pulmonary valve stenosis. J Vet Intern Med 2018.

Ohad DG, Avrahami A, Waner T, et al. The occurrence and suspected mode of inheritance of congenital subaortic stenosis and tricuspid valve dysplasia in Dogue de Bordeaux dogs. Vet J 2013.

Oliveira P, Domenech O, Silva J, et al. Retrospective review of congenital heart disease in 976 dogs. J Vet Intern Med 2011;25:477–483.

Oyama MA, Sisson DD. Cardiac troponin-I concentration in dogs with cardiac disease. J Vet Intern Med 2004;18:831–839.

Paige CF, Abbott JA, Pyle RL. Systolic anterior motion of the mitral valve associated with right ventricular systolic hypertension in 9 dogs. J Vet Cardiol 2007;9:9–14.

Patterson DF, Haskins ME, Schnarr WR. Hereditary dysplasia of the pulmonary valve in beagle dogs. Pathologic and genetic studies. Am J Cardiol 1981;47:631–641.

Pyle RL, Patterson DF, Chacko S. The genetics and pathology of discrete subaortic stenosis in the Newfoundland dog. Am Heart J 1976;92:324–334.

Quintavalla C, Guazzetti S, Mavropoulou A, et al. Aorto-septal angle in Boxer dogs with subaortic stenosis: an echocardiographic study. Vet J 2010;185:332–337.

Ramos RV, Monteiro-Steagall BP, Steagall PV. Management and complications of anaesthesia during balloon valvuloplasty for pulmonic stenosis in dogs: 39 cases (2000 to 2012). J Small Anim Pract 2014;55:207–212.

Reist-Marti SB, Dolf G, Leeb T, et al. Genetic evidence of subaortic stenosis in the Newfoundland dog. Vet Rec 2012;170:597.

Reller MD, McDonald RW, Gerlis LM, Thornburg KL. Cardiac embryology: basic review and clinical correlations. J Am Soc Echocardiogr 1991;4:519e532.

Ristic JM, Marin CJ, Baines EA, et al. Congenital pulmonic stenosis a retrospective study of 24 cases seen between 1990–1999. J Vet Cardiol 2001;3:13–19.

Saunders AB, Smith BE, Fosgate GT, et al. Cardiac troponin I and C-reactive protein concentrations in dogs with severe pulmonic stenosis before and after balloon valvuloplasty. J Vet Cardiol 2009;11:9–16.

Scansen B. Coronary artery Anomalies in animals. Vet Sci 2017;4:20.

Scansen BA. Equine congenital heart disease. Vet Clin North Am Equine Pract 2019;35:103–117.

Scansen BA, Cober RE, Bonagura JD. Congenital heart disease. In Bonagura JD & Twedt DC (editors), Kirk's Current Veterinary Therapy XV. Elsevier Saunders, St. Louis. 2014; pp756–761.

Schober KE, Fuentes VL. Doppler echocardiographic assessment of left ventricular diastolic function in 74 Boxer dogs with aortic stenosis. J Vet Cardiol 2002;4:7–16.

Schrope DP. Primary pulmonic infundibular stenosis in 12 cats: natural history and the effects of balloon valvuloplasty. J Vet Cardiol 2008;10:33–43.

Serres F, Chetboul V, Sampedrano CC, et al. Quadricuspid aortic valve and associated abnormalities in the dog: report of six cases. J Vet Cardiol 2008;10:25–31.

Shen L, Estrada AH, Cote E, et al. Aortoseptal angle and pressure gradient reduction following balloon valvuloplasty in dogs with severe subaortic stenosis. J Vet Cardiol 2017;19:144–152.

Staudte KL, Gibson NR, Read RA, et al. Evaluation of closed pericardial patch grafting for management of severe pulmonic stenosis. Aust Vet J 2004;82:33–37.

Stern JA, Meurs KM, Nelson OL, et al. Familial subvalvular aortic stenosis in Golden Retrievers: inheritance and echocardiographic findings. J Small Anim Pract 2012;53:213–216.

Stern JA, White SN, Lehmkuhl LB, et al. A single codon insertion in PICALM is associated with development of familial subvalvular aortic stenosis in Newfoundland dogs. Hum Genet 2014;133:1139–1148.

Sutherland BJ, Pierce KV, Heffner GG, et al. Surgical repair for canine tricuspid valve dysplasia: Technique and case report. J Vet Cardiol 2020;33:34–42.

Sykes KT, Gordon SG, Saunders AB, et al. Palliative combined cutting and high-pressure balloon valvuloplasty in six dogs with severe, symptomatic subaortic stenosis. J Vet Cardiol 2020;31:36–50.

Tidholm A. Retrospective study of congenital heart defects in 151 dogs. J Small Anim Pract 1997;38:94–98.

Tobias AH, Stauthammer CD. Minimally invasive per-catheter occlusion and dilation procedures for congenital cardiovascular abnormalities in dogs. Vet Clin North Am Small Anim Pract 2010;40:581–603.

Visser LC, Nishimura S, Oldach MS, et al. Echocardiographic assessment of right heart size and function in dogs with pulmonary valve stenosis. J Vet Cardiol 2019;26:19–28.

Winter RL, Rhinehart JD, Estrada AH, et al. Repeat balloon valvuloplasty for dogs with recurrent or persistent pulmonary stenosis. J Vet Cardiol 2021;34:29–36.

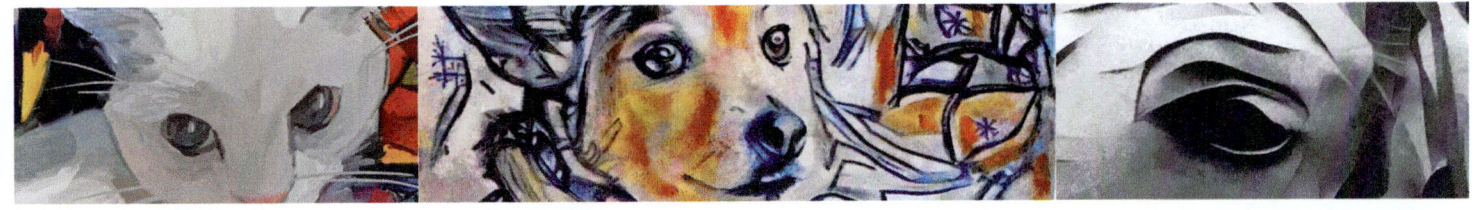

28
OTHER CARDIOVASCULAR MALFORMATIONS

Primary Contributor, Brian A. Scansen

A myriad of variably complex congenital cardiovascular malformations can occur in animals. The most common malformation involving the great vessels is patent ductus arteriosus (PDA; Chapter 26). Other direct communications between aorta and pulmonary artery, such as aortopulmonary window, occur only sporadically and have a similar pathophysiology as PDA. This chapter focuses on additional, less common congenital cardiac and vascular malformations. Some of these have dramatic clinical consequences.

Cor Triatriatum

The term *cor triatriatum* refers to anomalous atrial partitioning during fetal development. This leads to a persistent fetal structure which functionally divides either the right (dexter) or left (sinister) atrium into two chambers. Although uncommon, *cor triatriatum dexter* (CTD) has been reported most frequently in dogs, and the condition is seen with some regularity by veterinary cardiologists. Both conditions are rare in cats, with published cases dominated by *cor triatriatum sinister*, although this defect can be confused with other feline malformations. Both conditions are exceedingly rare in foals.

Cor Triatriatum Dexter

The intra-atrial membrane of CTD results from failure of the embryonic right sinus venosus valve to regress. Typically, caudal vena cava and coronary sinus empty into the caudal right atrial (RA) chamber, while cranial cava and tricuspid orifices are within the cranial RA chamber. Obstruction to venous flow through the abnormal membrane increases hydrostatic pressure within the caudal RA chamber, caudal cava, and abdominal structures. Although in absolute terms, the intra-RA pressure gradient is small, the resulting chronic pressure elevation within the caudal vena cava produces caudal venous congestion and often massive ascites. In patients with a patent foramen ovale (PFO), right-to-left flow occurs through the foramen. Concurrent tricuspid and pulmonary valve dysplasias occur in some cases. When the intra-atrial communication is highly restrictive, downstream development of right heart structures can be impaired, with subsequent hypoplasia of tricuspid valve, right ventricle, and pulmonary valve.

Clinical Features There are multiple reports of CTD in dogs in the veterinary literature (Nadolny, 2019). Large- or medium-sized breeds seem affected most often. The most prominent clinical sign is persistent ascites that develops at an early age (**Figure 28.1**). Exercise intolerance, lethargy, distended cutaneous abdominal veins, and sometimes diarrhea are reported also (**Figure 28.2**). Neither a cardiac murmur nor jugular venous distension are features of this anomaly, unless concurrent valve malformation exists. Cyanosis can be severe with a PFO.

Diagnostic Tests Thoracic radiographs show a distended caudal vena cava without generalized cardiomegaly. Massive ascites can displace the diaphragm cranially (**Figure 28.3**). The ECG generally is normal. Echocardiography reveals the abnormal intra-RA membrane, with dilation of caudal RA chamber, caudal vena cava, and hepatic veins. Doppler studies show the flow disturbance within the right atrium and allow estimation of the pressure gradient across the abnormal membrane (**Figure 28.4**). Right-to-left shunting across a PFO frequently is evident. Computed tomography (CT)- and standard angiocardiography often are performed prior to or during an interventional procedure. These will outline the intra-RA obstruction and secondary dilation caudally

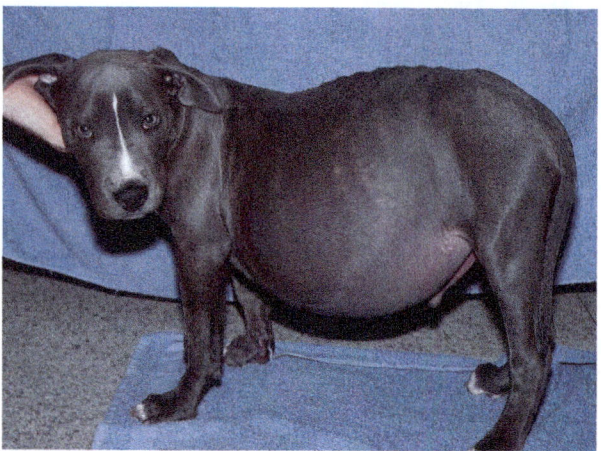

Figure 28.1 Massive ascites in a 5-month-old male Pit Bull Terrier with cor triatriatum dexter.

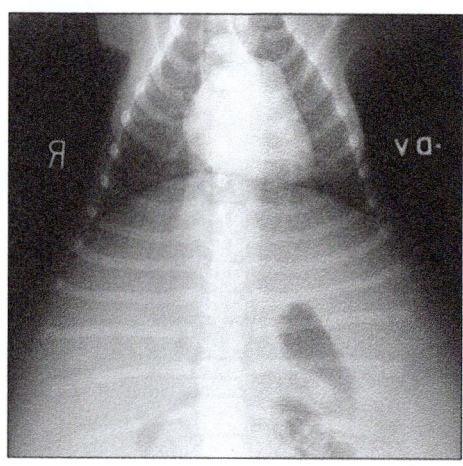

Figure 28.3 Dorsoventral radiograph from the dog of **Figure 28.2** shows a normal-sized cardiac silhouette, but caudal vena caval distension and massive ascites.

(**Figures 28.5** and **28.6**). Saline contrast echocardiography, performed from a saphenous vein, illuminates the various atrial chambers and any right-to-left shunt across a PFO. However, if caudal venous pressures are excessive, saline contrast might not transit to the atrium but instead appear in the cranial right atrial chamber; this confusing finding is caused by collateral circulation, with the contrast draining through the azygous vein.

Management Successful therapy requires enlarging the membrane orifice to relieve the flow obstruction. Percutaneous balloon dilation of the membrane orifice can accomplish this, if the balloon is large enough (or several balloon catheters are used simultaneously) to eliminate the obstruction (**Figures 28.7** and **28.8**). A cutting balloon technique also has been used, followed by a larger high-pressure balloon. Transvenous stent implantation across the membrane is reserved for resistant lesions. Surgical excision of the abnormal membrane is another therapeutic option.

Cor Triatriatum Sinister

This malformation involves an (oblique) fibromuscular partition within the left atrium. The pulmonary veins empty into the dorsal compartment and a variably sized opening in the membrane allows flow into the ventral compartment adjacent to the mitral valve. The left auricle communicates with the ventral compartment, while the fossa ovalis usually is within the dorsal compartment. This malformation has occurred concurrently with a persistent left cranial vena cava (PLCVC) or atrioventricular (AV) septal defect in cats.

The embryological origin of cor triatriatum sinister might relate to failure of the common pulmonary vein to regress normally; however, this has not been fully clarified and other mechanisms are possible. Cor triatriatum sinister is considered a different congenital malformation than supravalvular mitral stenosis; the location of the left auricle in relation to the obstructive membrane allows differentiation. Nevertheless, the resulting pathophysiology is essentially the same for both of these left ventricular (LV) inflow obstructive lesions. Restricted flow across the abnormal membrane raises pressure within the dorsal compartment and pulmonary veins, which promotes pulmonary venous congestion and pulmonary edema. The size of the opening in the partitioning membrane is the major determinant of the pressure gradient between dorsal and ventral left atrial (LA) compartments. Pulmonary hypertension also is likely.

Clinical Features Cor triatriatum sinister has been reported sporadically within the veterinary literature, mostly in cats. Clinical signs develop at a relatively young age and stem from pulmonary congestion and edema, although low output signs also could occur. Historical complaints include tachypnea, dyspnea, and reduced activity. Pulmonary crackles, with or without a cardiac murmur, are auscultatory findings. The magnitude of the pressure gradient across the intra-LA membrane influences the severity of clinical signs and at what age they develop.

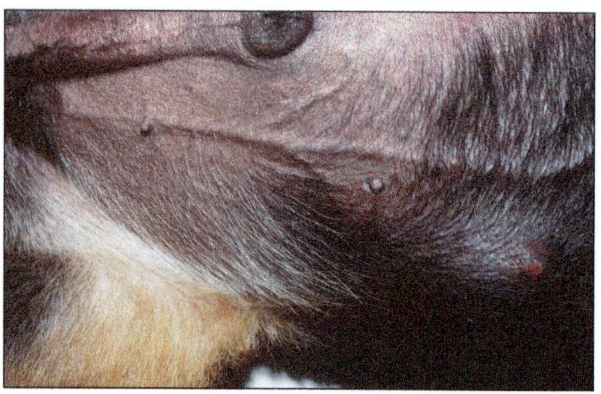

Figure 28.2 Distended abdominal veins signal high venous pressure in the caudal body of this 5-month-old male Rottweiler with cor triatriatum dexter. The jugular and other veins that drain into the cranial vena cava appeared normal.

Other Cardiovascular Malformations 513

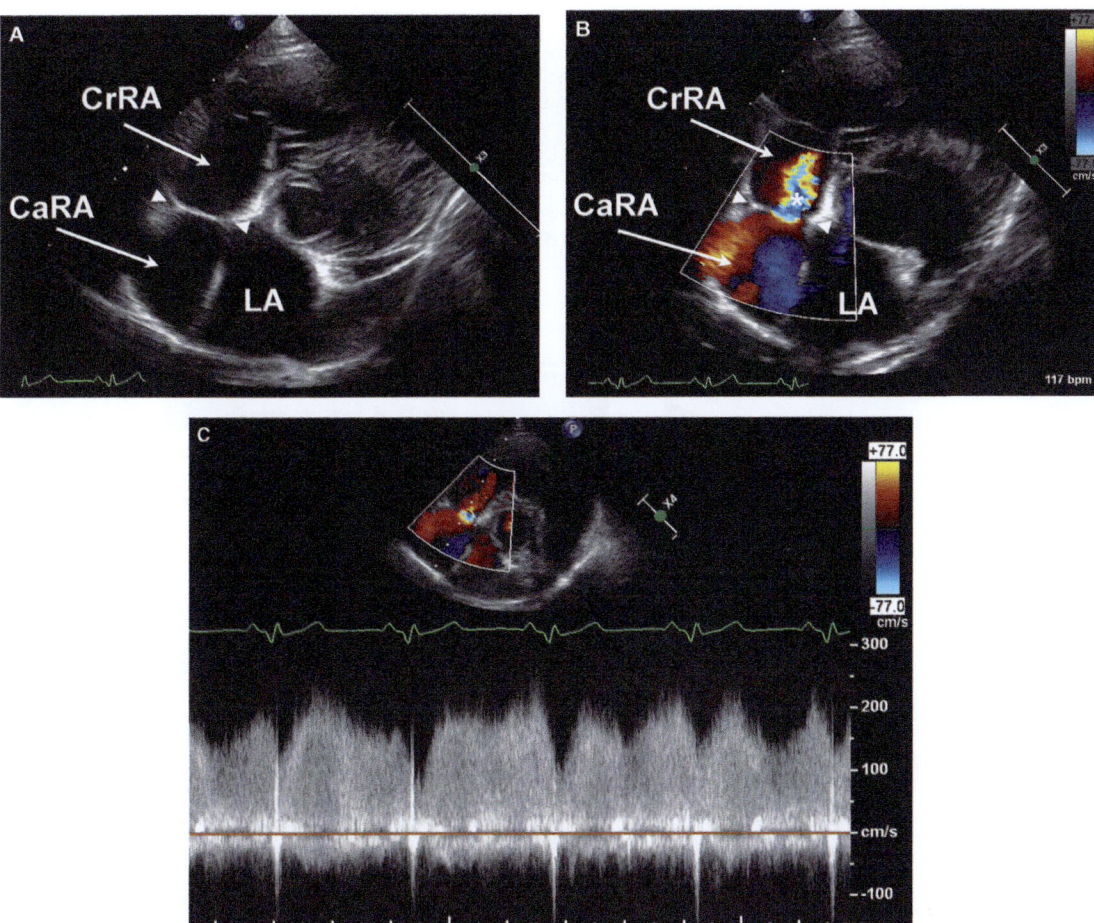

Figure 28.4 Two-dimensional short-axis echo images at the heart base without (A) and with (B) color-flow Doppler imaging from a dog with cor triatriatum dexter. The abnormal membrane (between the *white arrowheads*) divides the right atrium into cranial (CrRA) and caudal (CaRA) chambers. (B) Blood flow in the CaRA accelerates toward the membrane's opening, then becomes turbulent (*) as it enters the CrRA. (C) Spectral Doppler interrogation shows a peak velocity of ~2 m/s across the obstructing membrane. LA, left atrium.

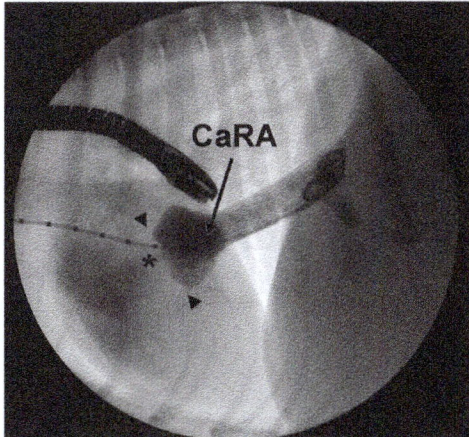

Figure 28.5 Angiographic image from a dog with cor triatriatum dexter demonstrates the dilated caudal right atrial chamber and caudal vena cava. The obstructing membrane lies between the arrowheads; the asterisk denotes the cranial right atrial chamber. A transesophageal echocardiography probe is dorsal to the heart. CaRA, caudal right atrium.

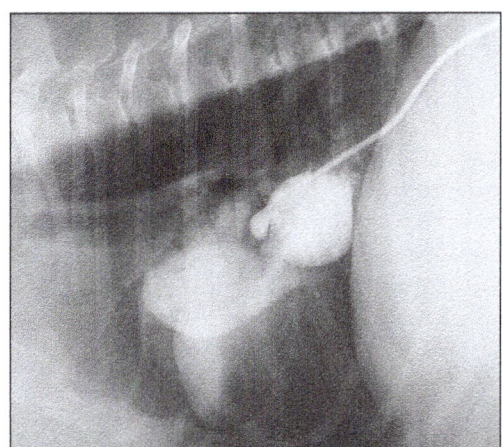

Figure 28.6 Caudal vena caval angiocardiogram, from the puppy of **Figure 28.1**, shows an irregular filling defect created by the abnormal intra-atrial membrane. Upstream from the obstruction, the increased filling pressure has distended the caudal right atrial chamber and proximal caudal vena cava.

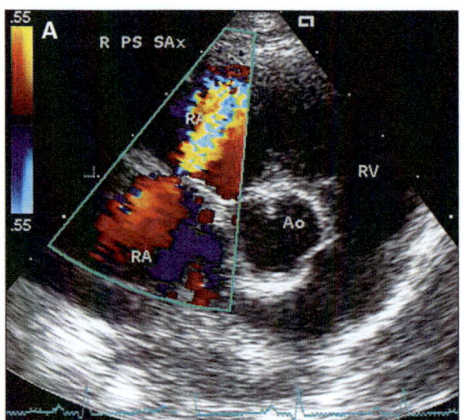
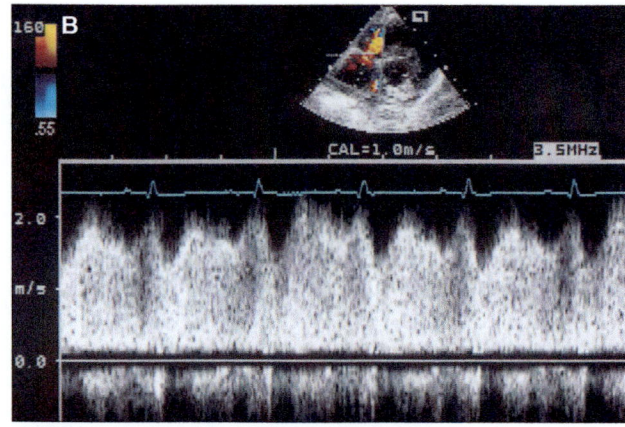

Figure 28.7 (A) Right parasternal short-axis color-flow image from the puppy of Figure 28.1 prior to balloon dilation procedure. Low-velocity flow in the caudal RA chamber moves toward (coded *red*) the abnormal membrane, then becomes turbulent in the cranial chamber. (B) Pulsed-wave Doppler image, sampled at the cranial side of the membrane, shows increased flow velocity throughout the cardiac cycle, with estimated mean gradient ~11 mm Hg. Note velocity scale on left. Ao, aorta; RA, right atrium; RV, right ventricle.

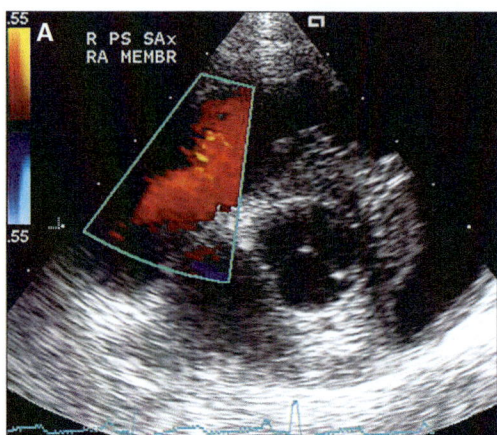
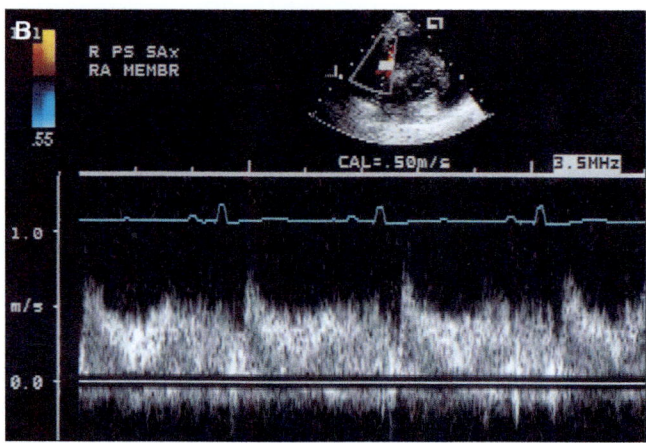

Figure 28.8 (A) Same patient and view as in Figure 28.7 after triple-balloon dilation of the abnormal right atrial membrane. Low-velocity laminar flow is present throughout the right atrium now. (B) Post-dilation, pulsed-wave Doppler shows much reduced intra-right atrial velocity (note different scale on left compared to in Figure 28.7B; estimated mean gradient ~1 mm Hg). The puppy's clinical signs resolved and did not recur.

Diagnostic Tests Radiographs show cardiomegaly, especially involving the LA region. Pulmonary venous distension and infiltrates of pulmonary edema are likely to be present. Echocardiography provides the diagnosis by revealing the membranous partition with dilation of the dorsal LA compartment, communication of the ventral compartment with the LA appendage, and a turbulent flow jet across the opening in the LA membrane and into the ventral compartment. As noted, this defect can be confused with a supravalvular mitral ring, which shares many similar pathophysiologic characteristics but might not be amenable to similar catheter based procedures. Another defect that can confuse the diagnosis of cor triatriatum sinister is an AV septal defect with double-outlet right atrium (Durham, 2014; also p. 466). This malformation is caused by extreme left-dorsal displacement of the atrial septum, which obstructs pulmonary venous return; left atrial blood communicates with the right atrium through an ostium primum atrial septal defect that opens into both ventricles. A bridging septal AV valve leaflet also might be present.

Management Medical therapy for left-sided congestive heart failure (CHF) signs might provide temporary palliation, but it cannot address the causative structural abnormality. A hybrid surgical approach with (cutting and standard) balloon dilation of the LA membrane has been used successfully to enlarge the membrane opening and relieve the pressure gradient in a cat (Stern, 2013). However, the small body size of cats precludes a transvascular balloon catheter approach. Unless the intra-LA pressure gradient is reduced sufficiently for pulmonary edema to resolve, long-term prognosis is poor.

Endocardial Fibroelastosis

This is a rare congenital abnormality characterized by diffuse fibrosis and elastic thickening of the endocardium. Little is known about the pathogenesis; it is potentially genetic in people and is observed with a number of congenital heart defects. A unifying theory is that of aberrant endothelial to mesenchymal transition that results in a dense endomyocardial layer of collagen and elastin. The left side of the heart is affected most often, with both hypertrophy and dilation described. Most reports involve cats, especially Burmese and Siamese. However, endocardial fibroelastosis also occurs sporadically in other species, including the dog and horse. Clinical signs relate to left-sided or biventricular heart failure, which typically develops early in life. A gallop sound and murmur of mitral regurgitation might be audible. Criteria for LV and LA enlargement are seen on radiographs, ECG, and echocardiogram. Evidence for reduced LV myocardial function and increased stiffness is expected. Definitive antemortem diagnosis is difficult. Postmortem descriptions have differed somewhat from observations in human infants. It is suspected that some reported feline cases might actually have been due to dilated cardiomyopathy caused by taurine deficiency, with secondary subendocardial fibrosis from chamber dilation.

Vascular Developmental Considerations

Aortic Arch Embryology and Anatomy

The great vessels and their principal branches begin developing during initial cardiac loop formation. They arise from a set of paired arches that derive from the aortic sac. These paired embryologic vessels surround the esophagus and trachea and connect with paired dorsal aortae; eventually, only one dorsal aorta will persist. During development, not all the aortic arches are present simultaneously; rather, they develop and atrophy during various developmental stages. There are six primary arch vessels, with intersegmental arteries sometimes considered as 7th arch vessels. The first two pairs of arches typically atrophy and disappear. Although they are not important for cardiovascular development, their remnants contribute to arteries in the head. The 3rd arches form the common carotid arteries and proximal internal carotid artery segments. The portion of the dorsal aorta between the 3rd and 4th arches is called the carotid duct; it also atrophies and disappears. The right 4th arch forms the proximal aspect of the right subclavian artery. The left 4th arch becomes the definitive aortic arch. The 5th arches normally do not persist in mammals (although they do in reptiles); rarely, anomalous vessels in animals might relate to their persistence. The proximal segment of the left 6th arch forms the pulmonary trunk and left pulmonary artery while the distal segment forms the muscular *ductus arteriosus*. The proximal segment of the right 6th arch develops into the proximal right pulmonary artery; the distal segment typically atrophies. The intersegmental (7th) arteries arise from the dorsal aorta caudal to the 6th arch; they supply blood to the forelimbs, cranial to the first rib. These paired intersegmental arteries navigate along the dorsal aorta via the tension that is created between the cranially developing forelimbs and 1st rib and the caudal expansion of the growing heart. After the right (7th) intersegmental grows to the right 4th aortic arch, these two arterial segments develop into the right subclavian artery and the right 4th arch separates from the aorta. The left (7th) intersegmental ends at the craniodorsal aspect of the left 4th aortic arch, where it develops into the left subclavian artery. In the normal mammal, all of the mature aortic arch structures lie to the left of the esophagus and trachea.

There are species differences in final aortic arch anatomy. Horses (and ruminants) have only one vessel (the brachiocephalic trunk) that branches cranially from the ascending aorta. Dogs and cats (as well as pigs, rabbits, and mice) have two cranial vessels: the brachiocephalic trunk and left subclavian artery. In contrast, people (and European hamsters and rats) have three cranial branches: the brachiocephalic trunk (often called the innominate artery), and the right common carotid and left subclavian arteries.

Venous Embryology and Anatomy

Development of the venous system is more complex than that of the arterial system. There are three fetal venous systems which contribute to the animal's final venous anatomy: the vitelline, umbilical, and cardinal vein systems. The vitelline veins return blood from the yolk sac. They develop into portions of the hepatic sinusoids, as well as the hepatic section of the caudal vena cava. The umbilical veins carry blood from the placenta. Portions of the umbilical veins contribute to intrahepatic segments of the portal vein and to the falciform ligament. The cardinal vein system has multiple components: the cranial (or anterior) cardinal, caudal (or posterior) cardinal, subcardinal, and supracardinal paired venous segments. These collect venous return from the fetus itself. Segments of these three venous systems variably regress, fuse or persist to form the venae cavae, azygous vein, and portal venous system.

The anterior or cranial cardinal veins deserve specific mention. Normally, the paired anterior cardinal veins fuse to form the right-sided cranial vena cava. The portion of left anterior cardinal vein caudal to this fused segment atrophies, except for a section that persists to form the oblique vein of the left atrium, which drains into the coronary sinus. The atrophied portion becomes the ligament of Marshall, which is an anatomic structure crossing the dorsal border of the left atrium. These structures can be used as anatomical reference points with regard to coronary venous anomalies. Sometimes the caudal aspect of the left anterior cardinal vein does not atrophy normally, but rather remains as a persistent left cranial vena cava (see section by that name, p. 524, which enters into the coronary sinus.

As with the arterial system, there are species differences in final venous anatomy that are relevant during angiographic interpretation and surgical procedures. Normally, dogs and cats have only a right azygous vein; however, an anomalous left azygous vein occasionally persists and drains into the coronary sinus. The hemiazygous vein is a normal structure that originates around the level of the left renal vein or left phrenicoabdominal vein. It collects blood from the left intercostal veins, courses cranially to the left of the vertebral column, and crosses midline to terminate in the azygous vein in the caudal thorax; it is not the same as a left azygous vein.

Vascular Ring Anomalies

Several arterial malformations arising from the embryonic aortic arches occur in animals. Some of these can entrap the esophagus (and occasionally the trachea also) within a vascular ring over the heart base. As a historical note, the original human medical term for a vascular ring anomaly was *dysphagia lusoria* (from the Greek *dysphagia lusus natural*, meaning difficulty eating and freak of nature).

The common pathophysiology of vascular ring malformations relates to esophageal constriction at the level of the heart base. With restricted passage of solid food, the esophagus dilates cranial to the ring. Regurgitation is common and some food can be retained in the cranial esophagus for a prolonged time. Affected animals are at increased risk for aspiration pneumonia. Occasionally, esophageal dilation caudal to the stricture occurs as well, indicating that altered esophageal motility might also be a factor. Additional vascular anomalies, such as a persistent left cranial vena cava or PDA, sometimes coexist with a vascular ring anomaly. The most common clinical presentation is a young animal with dysphagia. Vascular ring anomalies appear to be more common in dogs; they are rare in cats and horses.

Persistent Right Aortic Arch

The persistent right aortic arch (PRAA) is the most common vascular ring anomaly in companion animals. It encloses the esophagus dorsally and to the right with the aortic arch, to the left with the *ligamentum arteriosum* (or PDA), and ventrally with the base of the heart (**Figure 28.9**). It results from persistence of the right 4th aortic arch with absence of the left 4th aortic arch. The intersegmental arteries track forward along the aorta as usual; however, the left (instead of the right) arch separates from the dorsal aorta. Consequently, the right 4th aortic arch matures and a left-sided ductus arteriosus and pulmonary artery entrap the esophagus and trachea within a vascular ring (**Figure 28.10**). PRAA occurs most often in dogs; however, cats, horses, and other species sometimes are affected by this malformation (**Figure 28.11**). PRAA appears to be familial, with an increased incidence in German Shepherd Dogs, Irish Setters, and possibly Great Danes.

Other Vascular Ring Anomalies

Double Aortic Arch Another vascular ring anomaly, recognized sporadically in dogs and cats, is the double aortic arch. Here, both the left and right 4th arches remain attached to the dorsal aorta during development, entrapping the esophagus and trachea; the ligamentum also contributes to the constriction of these structures (**Figure 28.12**). One of the arches can be atretic or less well-developed than the contralateral arch. Tracheal stenosis, malformed tracheal rings, and associated respiratory signs might accompany a double aortic arch anomaly.

Right Ductus Arteriosus The normal ductus arises from the distal left 6th arch. However, regression of the left 6th arch with persistence of the right 6th arch produces the right

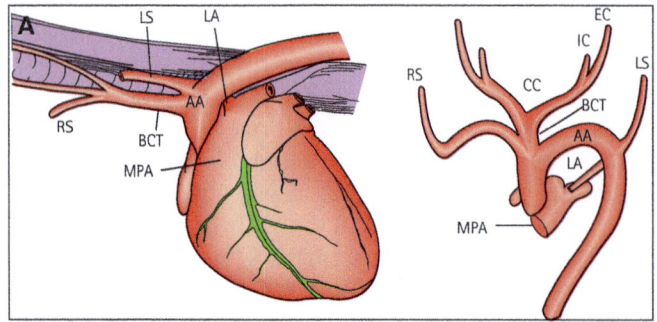 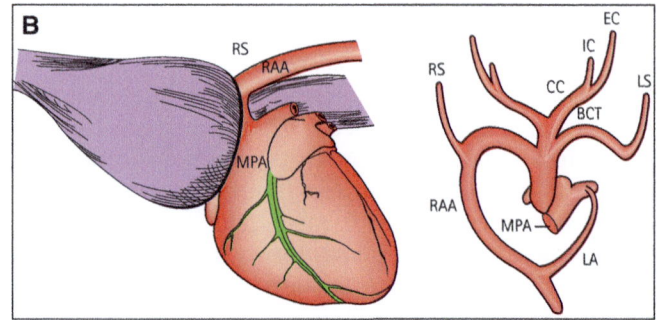

Figure 28.9 **(A)** Diagram of normal vessel formation from embryonic aortic arches. **(B)** Diagram of the persistent right aortic arch. AA, aortic arch; BCT, brachycephalic trunk; CC, common carotid; EC, external carotid; IC, internal carotid; LA, ligamentum arteriosum; LS, left subclavian; MPA, main pulmonary artery; RAA, right aortic arch; RS, right subclavian. (Modified after Ellison GW. Vascular ring anomalies in the dog and cat. Compend Cont Educ Pract Vet. 1980;11:693–705.)

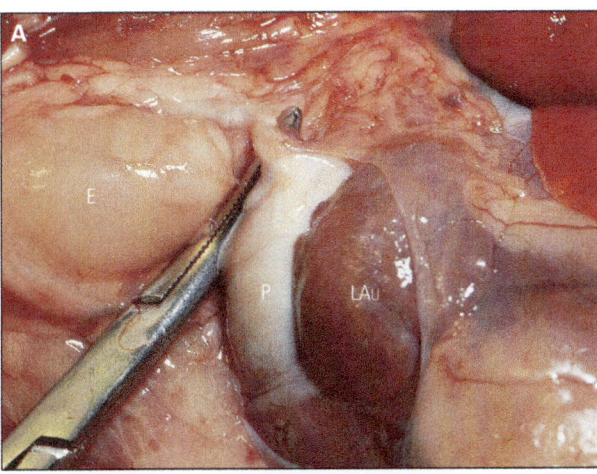
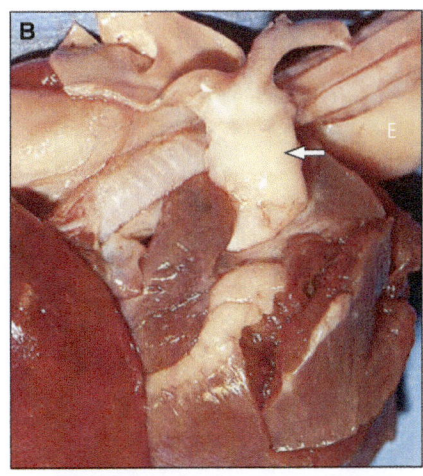

Figure 28.10 (A) Postmortem *in situ* view from the left in a 7-week-old female Chow Chow-mix with a persistent right aortic arch, as well as patent ductus arteriosus (PDA) and ventricular septal defect. Hemostat tip is under the PDA; the dilated cranial esophagus (E) is to the left. The main pulmonary artery (P) and left auricle (LAu) are in the center of the image. (B) View from the right shows the right aortic arch (*arrow*) crossing over the trachea and esophagus; the dilated cranial esophagus is to the upper right in the photo.

ductus arteriosus (or ligamentum arteriosum). The combination of a normal left 4th aortic arch and a right ductus (or ligamentum) is another cause of esophageal and tracheal entrapment. This anomaly has occurred sporadically in dogs, cats, and other species.

Aberrant (Retroesophageal) Subclavian Arteries Abnormal subclavian artery anatomy can cause partial tracheoesophageal compression. A retroesophageal left subclavian artery occurs concurrently in about one-third of dogs with PRAA (Buchanan, 2004). It develops when the left (7th) intersegmental artery, as it is being pulled forward along the dorsal aorta, fails to reach the left 4th arch before the latter separates from the dorsal aorta. Consequently, the left subclavian artery develops in an abnormally caudal position and must cross over the esophagus dorsally to reach the left forelimb (**Figure 28.13**). This causes dorsal esophageal compression, in addition to the constriction caused by the PRAA and left-sided ductus (or ligamentum). Surgical division of the

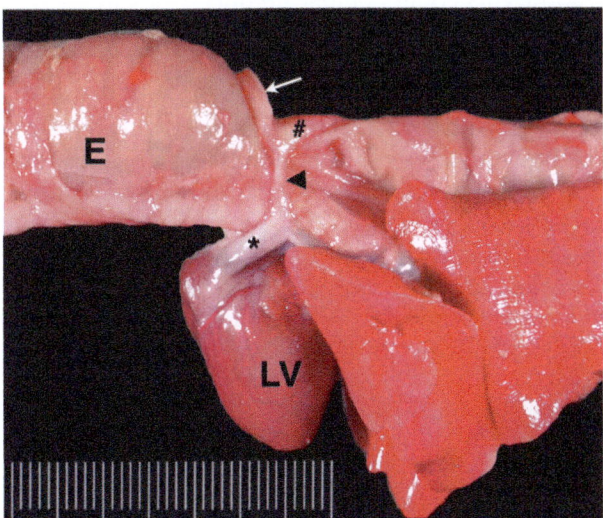

Figure 28.11 Left lateral, postmortem image from a cat with persistent right aortic arch. Cranial is to the left in the image. The esophagus (E) is severely dilated cranial to the constricting band formed by the right-sided aorta (#), ligamentum arteriosum (*black arrowhead*), and pulmonary artery (*). A retroesophageal left subclavian artery (*white arrow*) also is present. LV, left ventricle.

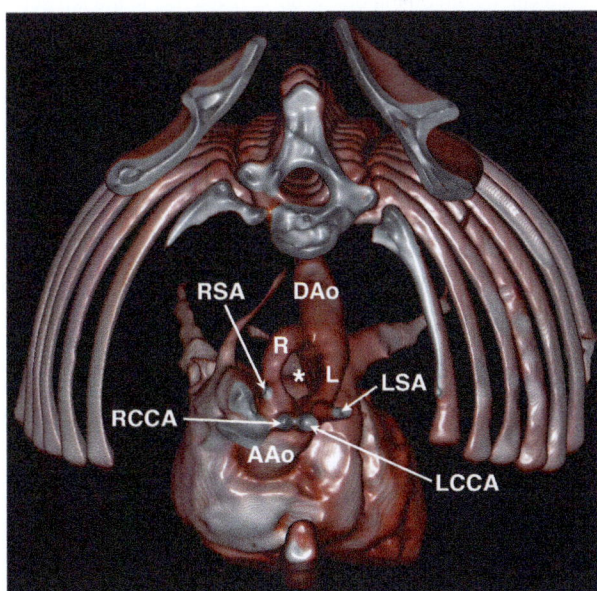

Figure 28.12 Three-dimensional, volume-rendered reformat from a computed tomography angiography scan of a dog with double aortic arch. The great vessels are seen from a direct cranial perspective, looking caudally. The ascending aorta (AAo) and descending aorta (DAo) are connected by both a left (L) and right (R) aortic arch. These give rise to the left common carotid artery (LCCA), left subclavian artery (LSA), right common carotid artery (RCCA), and right subclavian artery (RSA). The asterisk (*) marks the vascular ring through which the esophagus and trachea pass.

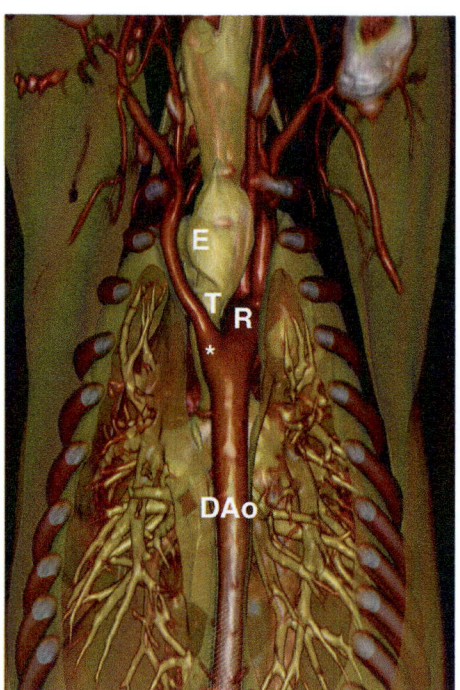

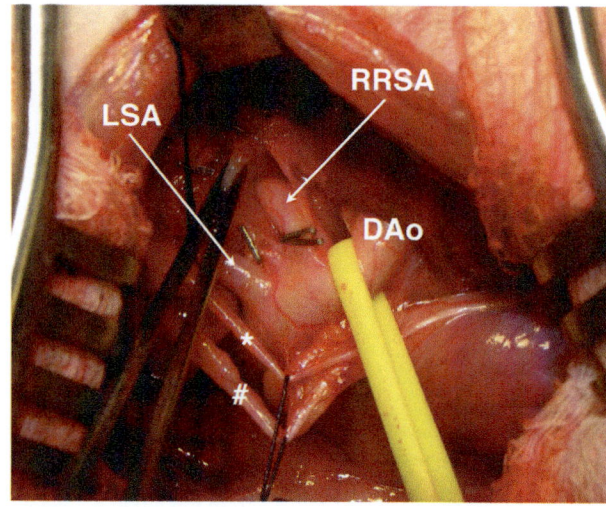

Figure 28.13 Three-dimensional, volume-rendered reformat from a computed tomography angiography scan in a dog with persistent right aortic arch and retroesophageal left subclavian artery. From dorsal perspective: the right side of the body is to the right in the image. Air-filled structures are colored *yellow*; vascular and bony structures are *red*. The aortic arch (R) ascends to the right of the trachea (T) and a dilated, air-filled esophagus (E) before continuing as the descending aorta (DAo). A prominent diverticulum on the dorsal aorta gives rise to the left subclavian artery (*), which passes dorsal to the esophagus and trachea.

Figure 28.14 Intraoperative photograph from a cat with a dilated cranial esophagus. Left thoracotomy revealed a left aortic arch. Upon further dissection, and with retraction of the phrenic nerve (#), vagus nerve (*), and descending aorta (DAo), the dorsal course of the retroesophagal right subclavian artery (RRSA) is visible. The left subclavian artery (LSA) is in normal position.

retroesophageal left subclavian artery might be required to relieve signs related to esophageal compression.

A retroesophageal right subclavian artery in the presence of a normal left 4th arch might also cause dorsal esophageal compression. This abnormality occurs when the right (7th) intersegmental artery, as it is pulled forward along the dorsal aorta, fails to reach the right 4th arch before the latter separates from the dorsal aorta. This vascular ring anomaly can present an unexpected finding at surgery when a normal left aortic arch and left ligamentum arteriosum are discovered. However, further dissection reveals the right subclavian artery arising from the dorsal aorta and crossing over the esophagus. This anomaly has been reported in dogs and has been seen by the author (BAS) in a cat with signs of esophageal compression (**Figure 28.14**).

Additional anomalies of subclavian anatomy can occur, including an isolated left subclavian artery (attached to the aortic arch via an atretic, non-patent segment) that causes esophageal compression; in this situation, flow through the subclavian artery is supplied by retrograde flow from the left vertebral artery via the circle of Willis. Alternatively, the left subclavian artery could arise from a PDA rather than from the dorsal aorta; this could complicate ductal closure.

Clinical Features

Most animals with a vascular ring anomaly are presented at a young age, usually within 6 months of weaning. The history typically includes frequent regurgitation beginning after the introduction of solid food, because the vascular ring prevents the food from passing normally through the esophagus (**Figure 28.15**). Stunted growth is common. Some animals appear clinically normal although thin; however,

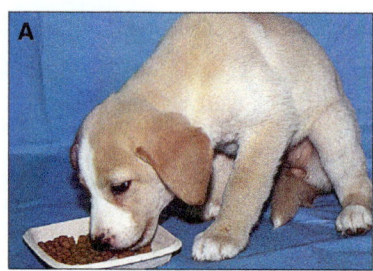
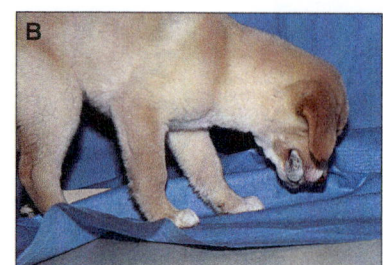
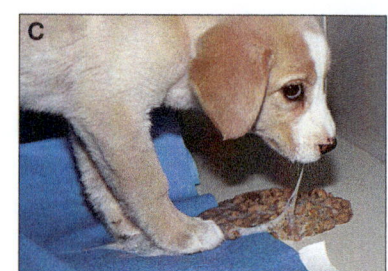

Figure 28.15 In this puppy with a persistent right aortic arch, eating solid food (A) is soon followed by regurgitation (B, C).

progressive debilitation generally develops. A breed predilection is suspected in German Shepherd, Great Dane, and Irish Setter dogs.

There is no cardiac murmur unless another cardiac defect, such as a PDA, is concurrent. Respiratory signs such as cough, wheezing, and cyanosis usually signal secondary aspiration pneumonia, although a double aortic arch might cause stridor and other respiratory signs secondary to tracheal stenosis. Aspiration pneumonia often causes fever, as well as respiratory signs. A dilated cervical esophagus (containing food or gas) sometimes is palpable at the thoracic inlet.

Diagnostic Tests

Thoracic radiographs can indicate the presence of a vascular ring defect. Air or food often is evident in the dilated cranial esophagus and there might be evidence of aspiration pneumonia. Leftward deviation of the trachea near the cranial heart border (DV or VD view) is a consistent radiographic sign of PRAA (**Figure 28.16**), but not of megaesophagus (Buchanan, 2004). Focal tracheal narrowing and ventral displacement cranial to the heart (lateral view), as well as cranial mediastinal widening, also are common. A barium swallow depicts the esophageal stricture over the heart base along with cranial esophageal dilation, with or without caudal esophageal dilation (**Figure 28.17**). Esophagoscopy could help rule out intraluminal esophageal constriction and can support a vascular cause of compression; a pulsatile vessel might be evident adjacent to the level of constriction. However, esophagoscopy does not provide confirmatory evidence as to the precise anatomy of the vascular ring nor of concurrent arterial or venous anomalies.

Angiography, either selective, nonselective, or with contrast-guided cross-sectional imaging (CT, or magnetic resonance imaging, MRI) will confirm the diagnosis and delineate the venous and arterial anatomy. A nonselective angiogram (injection of contrast into a peripheral vein) is the simplest of these methodologies. The left cephalic vein is the best site for contrast injection because this will reveal a persistent left

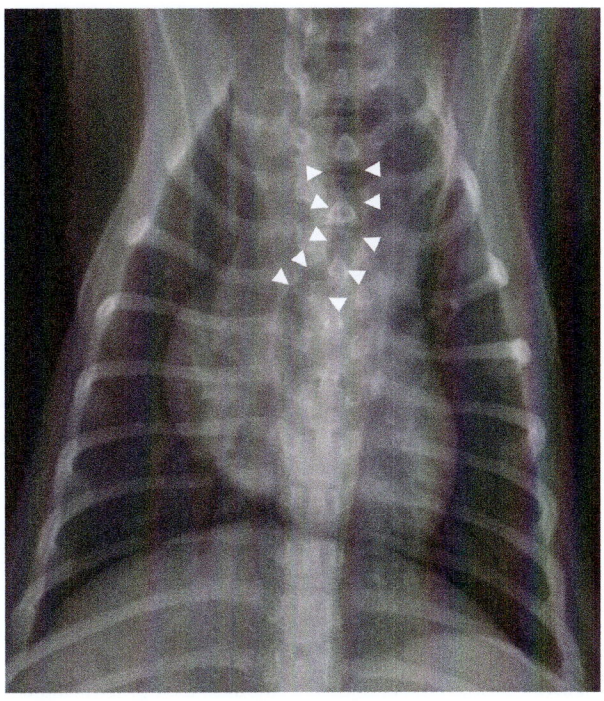

Figure 28.16 Ventrodorsal thoracic radiograph from a 12-week-old Australian Shepherd with persistent right aortic arch. The leftward deviation of the trachea at the heart base (*arrowheads*) is considered pathognomonic for a right-sided aortic arch.

cranial vena cava, if present. Use of digital subtraction angiography and suspended respirations will optimize the diagnostic yield. Fluoroscopic cine images are captured from the time of injection until the dye has circulated to the left heart and the aortic arch is apparent. The position of the ascending aorta as it crosses the tracheal bifurcation defines the arch. If the aorta ascends to the left of the trachea, the animal has a left 4th arch; if it ascends to the right, a diagnosis of PRAA can be made (**Figure 28.18**). Care should be taken to evaluate the cranial branches in addition to the arch laterality to screen for retroesophageal subclavian arteries or other malformations. Advanced imaging techniques have been described

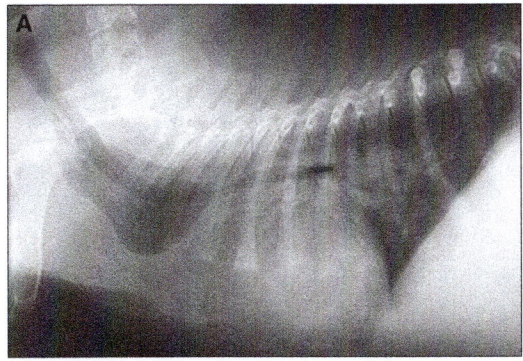 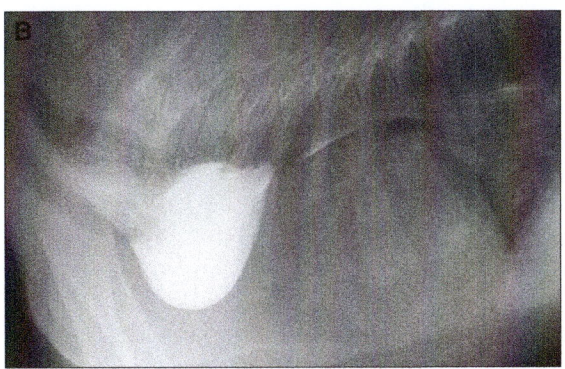

Figure 28.17 (A) An air-filled esophageal dilation, cranial to the heart base, is present in this lateral radiograph from a Chow Chow-mix puppy. Concurrent patent ductus arteriosus and ventricular septal defect caused cardiomegaly in this case. (B) A barium swallow illustrates the extent of esophageal dilation.

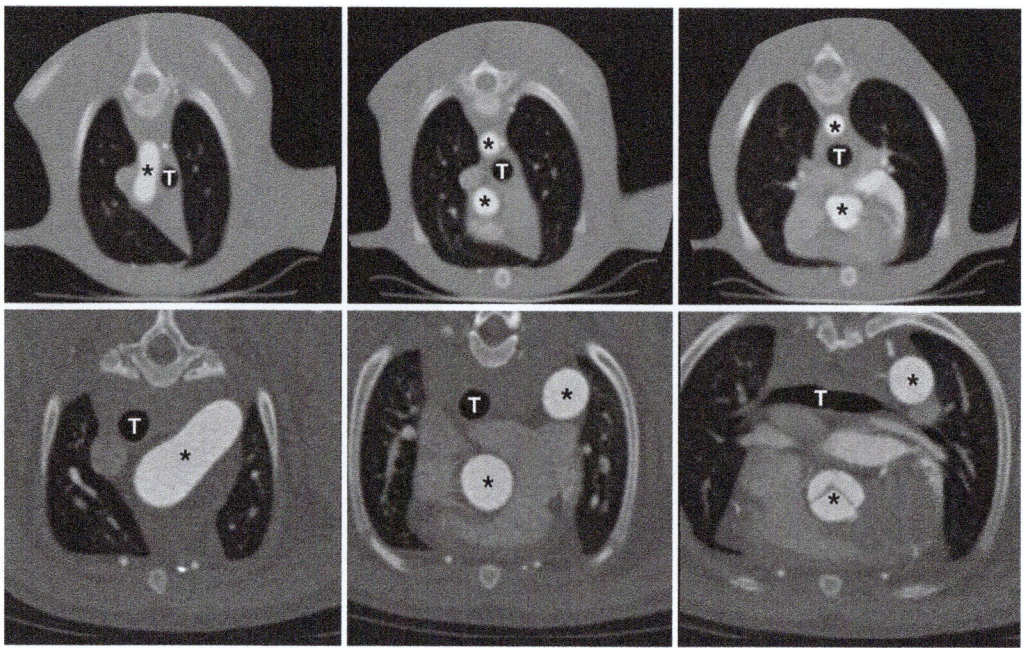

Figure 28.18 Transverse images of computed tomography angiography studies from two different dogs (*top*, *bottom*). Sections through the thorax from the aortic arch (leftmost images) and back caudally to the aortic valve are shown. *Top* series: the transverse aortic arch lies to the right of the trachea, indicating persistence of the right 4th aortic arch in this case. *Bottom* series: the transverse aortic arch is left of the trachea in this dog, indicating persistence of the normal left 4th aortic arch. Asterisks (*) mark the aorta (ascending, transverse arch, and descending); T, trachea.

in animals, and are commonly employed in people to define aortic arch laterality and associated anomalies. CT angiography can highlight the vascular anatomy and provide the surgeon with a three-dimensional, volume-rendered image of the anomaly (Henjes, 2011); it can even allow for rapid printing of patient-specific anatomy.

Management

The treatment of choice for vascular ring anomalies is surgical division of the offending vascular structure. In most cases, the constriction is relieved after the ductus (or ligamentum arteriosum) is divided, via a left fourth intercostal thoracotomy. If the animal has a double aortic arch, the surgical approach is to divide one of the aortic arches, whichever is least functional. Thoracoscopic dissection of the ligamentum is another approach described in dogs with PRAA (Townsend, 2016).

In rare cases, the surgeon finds a normal left arch upon opening the thorax. If a vascular anomaly is the cause of the clinical signs, it could be because of aberrant subclavian anatomy (as in **Figure 28.14**) or an atypical right ductus (or ligamentum). The existence of such cases further argues for appropriate presurgical imaging, because a right thoracotomy might be required. With respect to aberrant subclavian anatomy, the vascular ring often is not complete, although dorsal compression of the esophagus still can occur; palliation of this is done by ligation and division of the offending artery. After subclavian ligation, blood flow to the ipsilateral limb occurs via retrograde flow through the vertebral artery. Although "subclavian steal syndrome" (with headache, visual deficits, and other signs) can occur in people after such procedures, this has not been recognized in animals. A right ligamentum arteriosum is a remnant of the right 6th aortic arch. It can coexist with any of the other arch abnormalities and cause independent vascular ring compression of the esophagus. Ventrally, the right ligamentum attaches to the right pulmonary artery. Dorsally, it could attach directly to the aorta, to a retroesophageal right subclavian artery, or to an atretic or functional right 4th arch. These all can be dissected from the dorsal aspect, then separately ligated and divided, as appropriate.

Medical management consists of giving frequent, small, semisolid or liquid meals in an upright position for an indefinite time. Most dogs become clinically normal after successful surgery; however, some experience persistent regurgitation, indicating a permanent esophageal motility disorder.

Other Aortic Arch Anomalies

Truncus Arteriosus Communis

Truncus arteriosus, or common arterial trunk, is a congenital abnormality in which only one great vessel arises from the heart. It develops when no septation occurs within the embryologic truncus arteriosus; consequently, there is no division

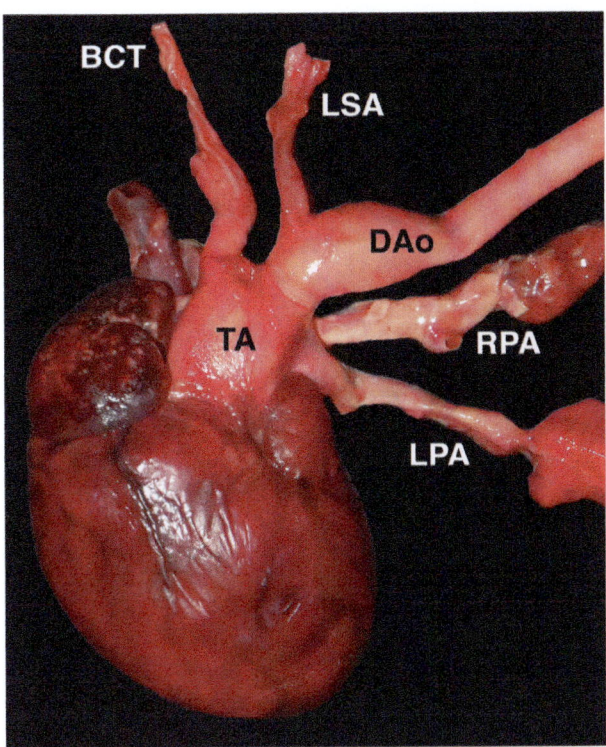

Figure 28.19 Photograph of the heart from a cat with truncus arteriosus communis. A single great vessel, the truncus arteriosus (TA), exits the heart and gives rise to the cranial branch vessels including the brachiocephalic trunk (BCT) and left subclavian artery (LSA), the descending aorta (DAo), and the left (LPA) and right (RPA) branch pulmonary arteries.

perfusion to the descending aorta. LV hypertrophy develops secondary to the systolic pressure overload. Severe collateral development can occur. Sporadic cases of coarctation have been described in dogs, cats, and a few other domestic species, usually in conjunction with other congenital defects (**Figure 28.21**). Therapy in humans involves either stenting the narrowed segment or surgical reconstruction of the arch; this has not been reported in animals.

Tubular Hypoplasia of the Aorta

Tubular hypoplasia refers to a segmental narrowing of the aortic arch to less than half of its normal diameter, rather than a discrete tissue ridge causing obstruction, as with coarctation. Tubular hypoplasia can occur anywhere along the aortic arch. One of the authors (BAS) has observed this in a horse (as well as a cow and alpaca). This malformation usually occurs in conjunction with other congenital defects, rather than as a solitary lesion.

Interruption of the Aorta

Interruption of the aortic arch is analogous to the most extreme form of coarctation. The descending aorta is anatomically separate from the arch in this malformation. Blood flow to the descending aorta and caudal half of the body occurs via ductal flow and the development of collateral vessels. There are only sporadic canine and equine reports of this congenital defect.

between ascending aorta and pulmonary artery. The truncus exits the heart through a common ventriculoarterial junction, then gives rise directly to the systemic, pulmonary, and coronary circulations (**Figures 28.19** and **28.20**). The left and right pulmonary arteries exit the common trunk at variable locations (classified traditionally according to the scheme of Collette and Edwards, 1949). Truncus now is considered to occur in two principal forms: aortic dominant or pulmonary dominant (Russell, 2011). There can be various malformations of the truncal valve. Truncus arteriosus has been identified in dogs, cats, and horses, among other species.

Coarctation of the Aorta

This congenital defect causes a focal narrowing of the aorta. It is rare in animals, although common in children. The coarctation is a ridge of tissue at the aortic isthmus (the junction of the arch and descending aorta), adjacent to where the ductus or ligamentum attaches. Often it is immediately distal to the left subclavian artery, although variable pre-ductal or post-ductal locations along the aorta are possible. Causes of coarctation are unclear; it might occur secondary to ectopic ductal tissue or abnormal pre-ductal flow. When severe, the coarctation causes hypertension in the cranial limbs but poor

Other Causes of Aortic Dilation

"Annuloaortic ectasia," "aortic aneurysm," and "aortic dissection" are terms that describe conditions of aortic dilation distinct from the post-stenotic dilation that occurs with sub-aortic stenosis. Mild ascending aortic dilation occurs commonly in older cats, for reasons that are not well defined, but could relate to systemic hypertension. Severe aortic aneurysm has occurred rarely in dogs, often as an incidental finding (**Figure 28.22**). Typically, large breeds of dog are affected. A family of Leonberger dogs with the condition was identified and potential comparison to human Marfan syndrome was suggested (Chetboul, 2003). In Marfan syndrome, abnormalities in the fibrillin-1 gene result in cystic medial necrosis of the aorta with subsequent aneurysmal dilation; (a similar aortic aneurysmal condition, with fibrillin-1 gene mutation, also was identified in cattle). Aortic dissection and rupture leading to sudden death is the most common cause of mortality in people with Marfan syndrome. Aortic dissection or rupture is rare in small animal patients with aortic aneurysm. There are sporadic case reports of aortic dissection in cats with hypertension (**Figure 37.13**, p. 785). Sporadic reports of aortic dissection in dogs have been associated with aortic aneurysm or suspected elastin dysplasia, or secondary to tumor infiltration.

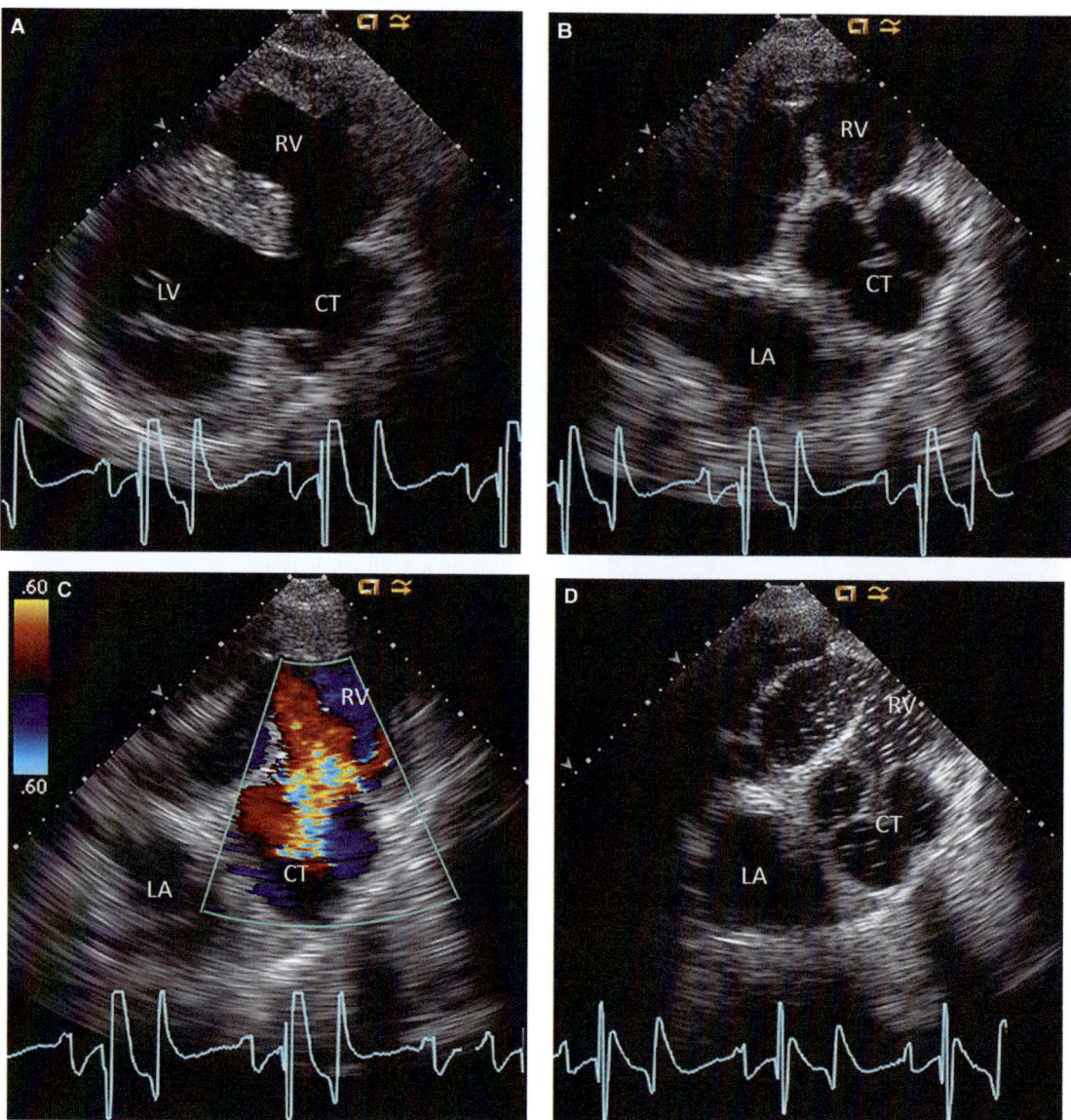

Figure 28.20 Right parasternal short-axis echo images from a 7-month-old Arabian foal with common arterial trunk. (A) Both the LV and RV open into one large great vessel (CT). No normal right ventricular outflow region is evident, instead the RV appears to end bluntly near the CT. (B) At the heart base, only one great vessel is visible. (C) Color-flow Doppler image in systole shows the RV emptying into the CT. (D) An echo-bubble study shows RV-to-CT flow with no bubbles in the LA. CT, common trunk; LA, left atrium; LV, left ventricle; RV, right ventricle.

Idiopathic aortic dilation without LV outflow tract obstruction is encountered sporadically in middle-aged to older canine breeds prone to subvalvular aortic stenosis. This usually involves the ascending aorta, arch and proximal descending aorta. It can appear as a heart base mass radiographically. This likely represents a form of inherited aortopathy, a disorder observed in children. It has been observed in the Rottweiler, Newfoundland, and Golden Retriever breeds in particular. Affected dogs are normotensive and might have a soft ejection murmur yet normal LV outflow velocity. Some aortic regurgitation is visible on color Doppler imaging, probably from annular dilation. It appears to be a benign condition.

Aortocardiac and Aortopulmonary Fistulae

An intracardiac fistula, or anomalous connection between cardiac chambers or great vessel, is identified occasionally. Most often this occurs in horses, between the aortic root and right atrium or ventricle. This aortocardiac fistula can develop subsequent to rupture of an aortic sinus of Valsalva (p. 784). The cause is uncertain, although both congenital and acquired etiologies are suspected. Presenting signs can relate to a new continuous heart murmur or the onset of CHF.

Arteriovenous Malformations

Direct connection between the high-pressure systemic arterial system and the low-pressure venous system can cause significant morbidity. Arteriovenous (A-V) malformations consist of disorganized tangles of vessels with A-V shunts that lack an intervening capillary bed (**Figure 28.23**). Such A-V malformations have an identifiable nidus with feeding vessels. In contrast, A-V fistulae consist of direct A-V communications without an intervening nidus. These connections often are congenital, although acquired fistulae do occur. Abnormal A-V communications appear most frequently in the liver of dogs, although they can develop in any organ system. Variable and somewhat confusing terminology has been used in the literature, including A-V fistula(e), A-V malformation(s), telangiectasia, and Osler–Weber–Rendu syndrome. However, the terms hemangioma or angioma are inappropriate for this condition because the suffix "oma" implies neoplastic origin; malformations are developmental or acquired vascular disruptions. Vascular tumors have cells with increasing mitotic activity. In contrast, malformations (which also can grow) contain mature, nonproliferating cells and grow by distension, bleeding, thrombosis, or enlargement of smaller vessels.

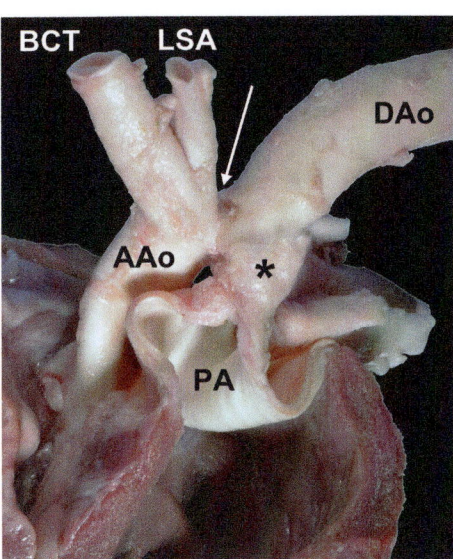

Figure 28.21 Coarctation of the aorta in an alpaca cria (from cranial left orientation). The right ventricular outflow tract and pulmonary trunk (PA) are open. A ductus arteriosus (*) connects the PA to the descending aorta (DAo). A focal constriction (arrow) between the ascending aorta (AAo) and DAo, just downstream from the left subclavian artery (LSA), is the site of coarctation. BCT, brachycephalic trunk.

Arteriovenous and Venovenous Malformations

Anomalous connections between the left and right sides of the systemic circulation occur and can result in clinical disease. Similarly, communications between two normally separate venous systems (such as portal and systemic veins) also can develop sporadically in animals.

Portosystemic Vascular Anomalies

Portosystemic shunts (venovenous connections) occur commonly in dogs and are thought to be more prevalent in the Yorkshire Terrier, Pug, Miniature and Standard Schnauzer, Maltese, Pekingese, Shih Tzu, and Lhasa Apso breeds. Portosystemic shunts occasionally are identified in cats, horses, and other species. These shunts can lead to hepatic encephalopathy, as well as other signs. They can involve a single intrahepatic portocaval shunt vessel, a single extrahepatic

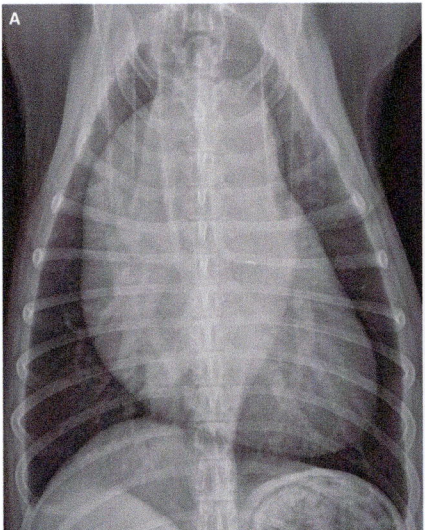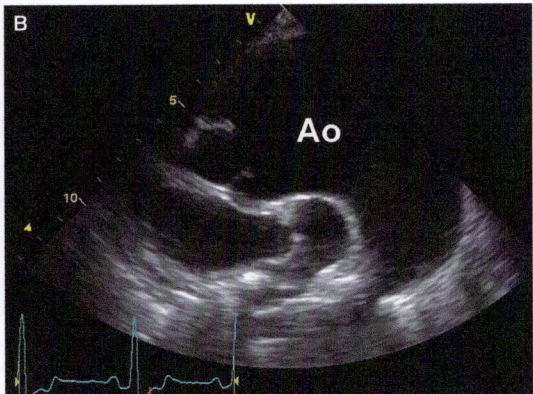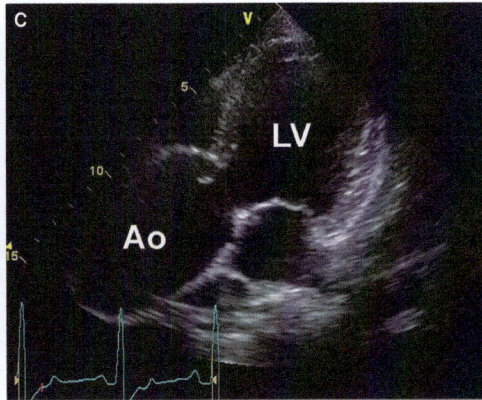

Figure 28.22 Ventrodorsal thoracic radiograph (A), right parasternal long-axis echocardiographic image (B), and left apical three-chamber echo image (C) from a dog with severe aneurysmal dilation of the ascending aorta. Ao, ascending aorta; LV, left ventricle.

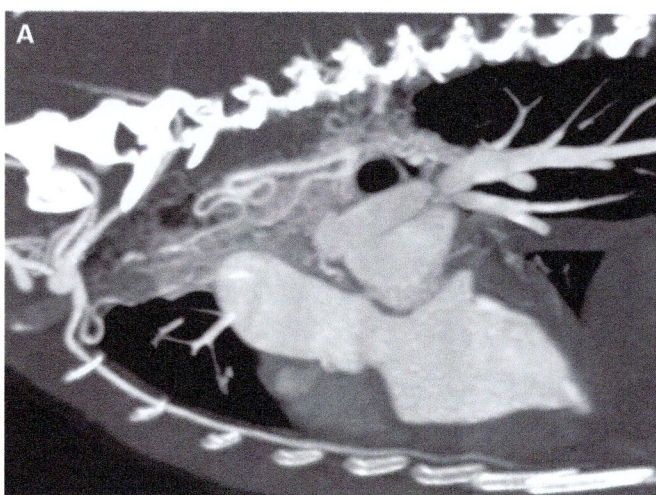
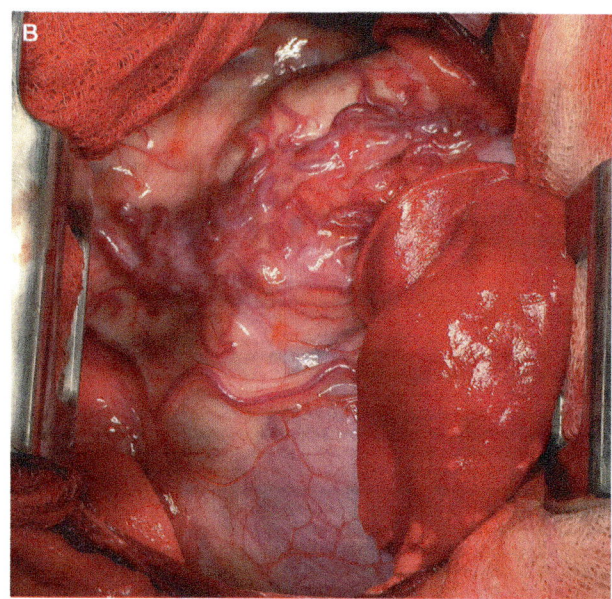

Figure 28.23 Maximum intensity projection, sagittal reformat, from a computed tomography angiography scan (A) and intraoperative photograph (B) from a dog with a thoracic arteriovenous (A-V) malformation, which surrounds the heart base and great vessels. The complex of anomalous vessels arose from systemic arteries and drains into the pulmonary circulation, causing left-to-right shunting and left-sided volume overload.

portocaval or portoazygous shunt, portal vein atresia with multiple secondary portal-caval anastamoses, or portal vein hypoplasia (formerly known as microvascular dysplasia).

Venous Malformations

Congenital anomalies of the venous system often are incidental findings and rarely cause clinical signs. Yet they can be important in certain situations. For example, venous anomalies can create confusion for surgeons unfamiliar with their existence. They also could complicate catheter placement for transcatheter procedures or diagnostic angiography. In some cases, they might impact adjacent structures and cause disease. Transpositional venous anomalies are common in animals with transpositional arterial anomalies, such as PRAA.

Persistent Left Cranial Vena Cava Dogs, cats, and horses normally have only a right cranial vena cava. The PLCVC is a fetal venous remnant. Because of its embryologic origin, it courses lateral to the left AV groove and empties into the coronary sinus at the caudal aspect of the RA (**Figures 28.24** and **28.25**). When the left anterior cardinal vein fails to regress, a PLCVC results. The left cranial vena cava could occur singularly; however more often, both left and right cranial cavae are present (**Figure 28.26**). The size of a PLCVC usually is inversely proportional to the size of a co-existent right cranial cava. Both complete and incomplete forms of PLCVC have been described in the dog (Buchanan, 1963).

The PLCVC generally poses no clinical problem for the animal, although it might be possible for a partially atretic PLCVC to cause megaesophagus. Of most clinical relevance, a PLCVC can complicate surgical exposure of other structures at the left heart base during left thoracotomy (**Figure 28.27**). The PLCVC crosses over and could obscure the ligamentum arteriosum (or patent ductus), especially when the PLCVC is large. Therefore, this anomalous vessel must be isolated and gently retracted ventrally to expose the ligamentum (ductus). Because the PLCVC appropriately returns blood to the RA, it should not be ligated.

The presence of a PLCVC also presents challenges during right heart catheterization, when approached via the left jugular vein, because of how this anomalous vessel courses caudally around the left side of the heart before reaching the coronary sinus. Most venous interventions performed from the cranial half of the body are approached through the

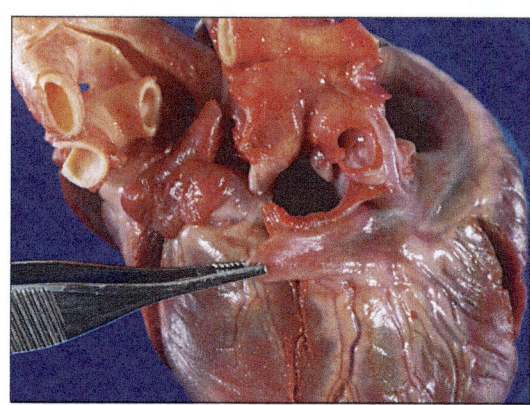

Figure 28.24 Left dorsal aspect of the heart from an English Springer Spaniel with multiple congenital defects. Forceps grasp the transected edge of a persistent left cranial vena cava. This vessel courses along the atrioventricular junction caudal to the left atrium (cut open, above) and enters the caudal right atrium at the coronary sinus.

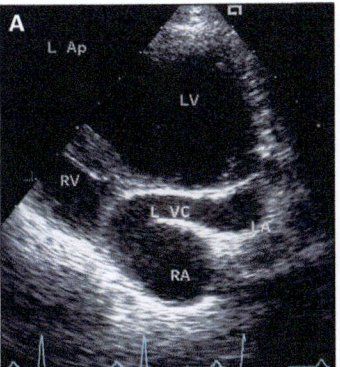 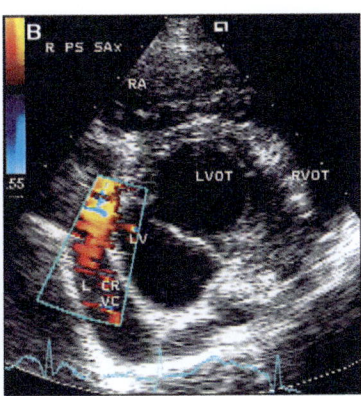 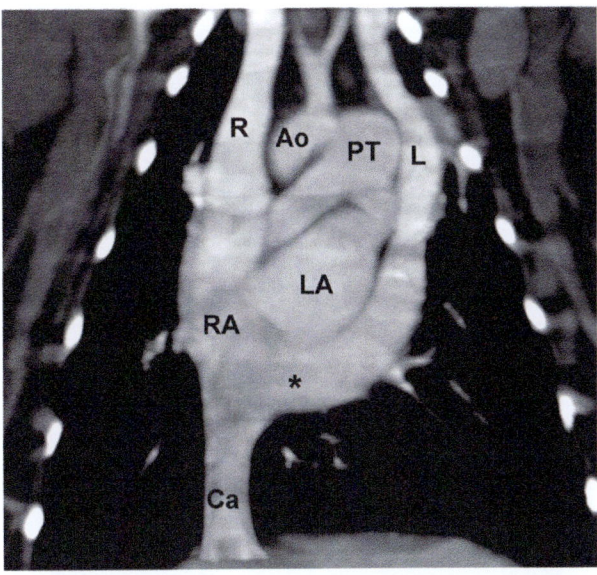

Figure 28.25 (A) Modified left apical four-chamber view (angled caudally) in a 9-month-old male Rottweiler shows a persistent left cranial vena cava (L VC) as it enters the RA, just caudal to the LA. (B) Modified right short-axis view with color-flow Doppler from the same dog. Flow within the persistent left cranial vena cava (L CR VC) moves around the caudal atrioventricular junction toward the RA. LA, left atrium; LV, left ventricle; L VC and L CR VC, persistent left cranial vena cava; LVOT, left ventricular outflow tract; RA, right atrium; RV, right ventricle; RVOT, right ventricular outflow tract.

right jugular vein; therefore, a PLCVC might not be identified unless noticed during echocardiography or other imaging. Nonetheless, pacemaker implantation and heartworm extraction have been done through a PLCVC, although these are technically more challenging than via the standard route.

Left Azygous Vein Although normally present in some species, a left azygous vein typically is absent in dogs and cats. When present, it is a remnant of the left supracardinal

Figure 28.26 Maximum intensity projection, dorsal reformat, from a computed tomography angiography scan of a dog with a persistent left cranial vena cava. Both the normal right (R) and persistent left (L) cranial venae cavae enter into the right atrium (RA); the left enters caudal to the left atrium (LA) at the coronary sinus (*). The caudal vena cava (Ca), pulmonary trunk (PT), and a portion of the aortic arch (Ao) also are visible.

system which enters the coronary sinus. However, it does not usually obscure the ligamentum (ductus) if there is no PLCVC. A left azygous vein occurs sporadically in dogs (**Figure 28.27**); occasionally, it is the sole source of caudal venous return if there is concurrent interruption of the caudal vena cava.

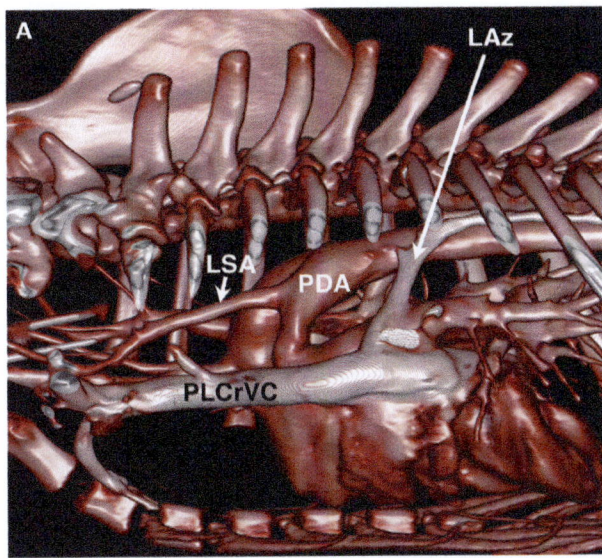 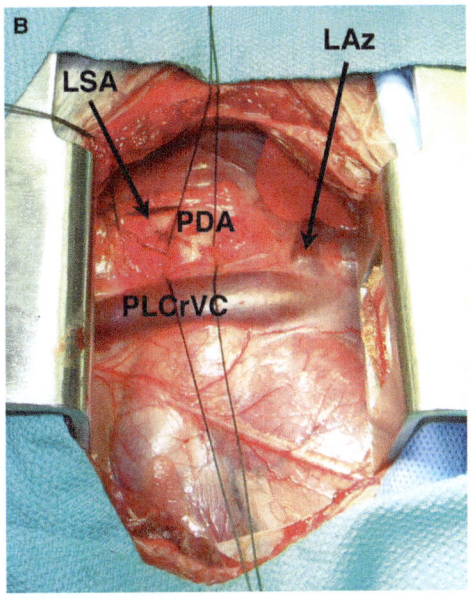

Figure 28.27 Three-dimensional, volume-rendered reformat from a computed tomography (CT) angiography scan (A) and intraoperative photograph (B) from the same dog with a vascular ring anomaly. The volume-rendered CT image shows the anatomy at the time of surgery, including a persistent right aortic arch, left-sided patent ductus arteriosus (PDA) from which arises the left subclavian artery (LSA), and the venous malformations of a persistent left cranial vena cava (PLCrVC) and left azygous vein (LAz).

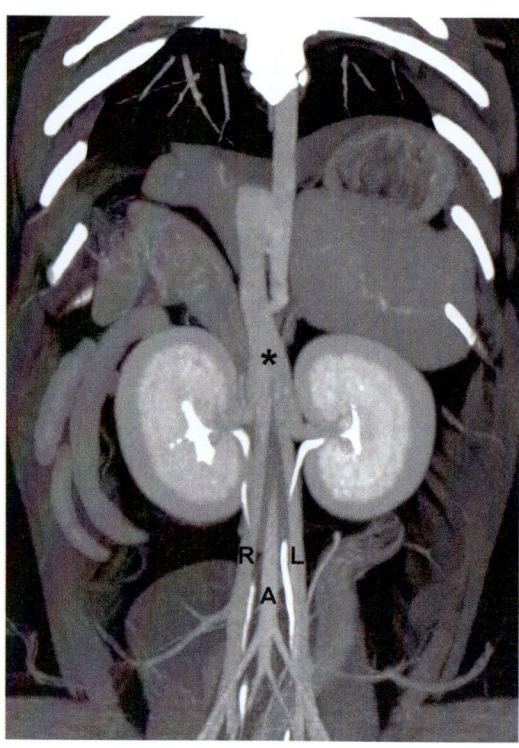

Figure 28.28 Maximum intensity projection, dorsal reformat from a computed tomography angiography scan of a dog with duplication of the caudal vena cava. The right (R) and left (L) caudal vena cavae can be seen as separate vascular structures on either side of the descending aorta (A) until they join together at the confluence of the renal veins (*).

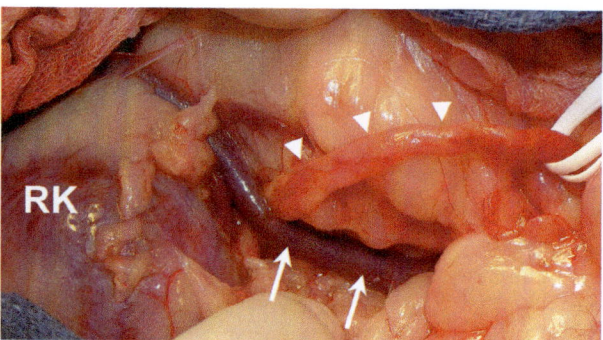

Figure 28.29 Intraoperative photograph from a cat with ureteral obstruction and a retrocaval right ureter. The caudal vena cava (*arrows*) developed ventral to the right ureter (*arrowheads*), causing the ureter to course dorsal to the cava and resulting in a ureteral constriction. RK, right kidney.

Anomalies of the Caudal Vena Cava Numerous abnormalities of the caudal vena cava have been observed. The caudal vena cava can display duplication, leftward transposition, or interruption with azygous continuation; these malformations also might be associated with portosystemic shunting. Most do not cause clinical signs unless portocaval shunting is concurrent. Caudal caval anomalies might become evident during surgical exploration or diagnostic imaging studies (**Figure 28.28**).

Venous Aneurysms Vascular aneurysms, in general, are rare in veterinary patients and venous aneurysms appear especially rare. However, such anomalies do occur (often for unknown reason) and could produce unexplained vascular shadows or apparent masses on standard imaging studies. A large aneurysm of the cranial vena cava was reported in a dog. Large aneurysms associated with caudal vena caval interruption also have been seen (BAS). Venous varicosis, a condition of tortuous and dilated veins, is rare in dogs and cats. When present, venous varices can accompany A-V fistulae or be a consequence of chronic venous obstruction. Four pathways for collateral venous flow in the setting of caudal vena caval obstruction in dogs have been described (Specchi, 2014). Orbital varix, or aneurysmal dilation of a normal vein around or behind the eye, is another venous dilation that can occur as a congenital anomaly; interventional occlusion is possible.

Retrocaval Ureter Also known as circumcaval ureter, this rare anomaly occurs when the subcardinal (rather than the supracardinal) vein persists at the level of the kidney and forms the renal segment of the caudal vena cava. In such cases, the caudal vena cava forms ventral to the ureter (**Figure 28.29**). This alters the ureteral course and causes gradual ureteral obstruction and hydronephrosis. There are sporadic reports of this condition in dogs and cats. The ureteral obstruction can be treated by surgical transection and anastamosis of the ureter after it has been repositioned ventral to the cava. Alternatively, long-term ureteral stenting or subcutaneous ureteral bypass could be done, particularly in cats, where ureteral reconstruction is associated with greater morbidity.

Suggested Additional Reading and References

Also See Online Comprehensive Bibliography at: https://www.routledge.com/9781482246223.

Adam FH, German AJ, McConnell JF, et al. Clinical and clinicopathologic abnormalities in young dogs with acquired and congenital portosystemic shunts: 93 cases (2003–2008). J Am Vet Med Assoc 2012;241:760–765.

Barncord K, Stauthammer C, Moen SL, et al. Stent placement for palliation of cor triatriatum dexter in a dog with suspected patent foramen ovale. J Vet Cardiol 2016;18:79–87.

Belanger R, Shmon CL, Gilbert PJ, et al. Prevalence of circumcaval ureters and double caudal vena cava in cats. Am J Vet Res 2014;75:91–95.

Bertolini G, Diana A, Cipone M, et al. Multidetector row computed tomography and ultrasound characteristics of caudal vena cava duplication in dogs. Vet Radiol Ultrasound 2014;55:521–530.

Birettoni F, Caivano D, Bufalari A, et al. Transthoracic ultrasound guided balloon dilation of cor triatriatum dexter in 2 Rottweiler puppies. J Vet Cardiol 2016;18:385–390.

Bristow P, Lipscomb V, Kummeling A, et al. Health-related quality of life following surgical attenuation of congenital portosystemic shunts versus healthy controls. J Small Anim Pract 2018.

Bruehschwein A, Foltin I, Flatz K, et al. Contrast-enhanced magnetic resonance angiography for diagnosis of portosystemic shunts in 10 dogs. Vet Radiol Ultrasound 2010;51:116–121.

Brunson BW, Case JB, Ellison GW, et al. Evaluation of surgical outcome, complications, and mortality in dogs undergoing preoperative computed tomography angiography for diagnosis of an extrahepatic portosystemic shunt: 124 cases (2005–2014). Can Vet J 2016;57:59–64.

Buchanan JW. Persistent left cranial vena cava in dogs: angiocardiography, significance, and coexisting anomalies. J Amer Vet Radiol Soc 1963;4:1–8.

Buchanan JW. Tracheal signs and associated vascular anomalies in dogs with persistent right aortic arch. J Vet Intern Med 2004;18:510–514.

Campbell FE, Thomas WP. Congenital supravalvular mitral stenosis in 14 cats. J Vet Cardiol 2012;14:281–292.

Case JB, Marvel SJ, Stiles MC, et al. Outcomes of cellophane banding or percutaneous transvenous coil embolization of canine intrahepatic portosystemic shunts. Vet Surg 2018;47:O59–O66.

Chetboul V, Tessier D, Borenstein N, et al. Familial aortic aneurysm in Leonberg dogs. J Am Vet Med Assoc 2003;223:1159–1162, 1129.

Choi SY, Song YM, Lee YW, et al. Imaging characteristics of persistent left cranial vena cava incidentally diagnosed with computed tomography in dogs. J Vet Med Sci 2016;78:1601–1606.

Chuzel T, Bublot I, Couturier L, et al. Persistent truncus arteriosus in a cat. J Vet Cardiol 2007;9:43–46.

Cinti F, Della Santa D, Borgonovo S, et al. Aberrant right subclavian artery causing megaoesophagus in three cats. J Small Anim Pract 2018;60:571–574

Collett RW, Edwards JE. Persistent truncus arteriosus: a classification according to anatomic types. Surg Clinics North Amer 1949;29:1245–1270.

Cuddy LC, Maisenbacher HW, Vigani A, et al. Computed tomography angiography of coarctation of the aorta in a dog. J Vet Cardiol 2013;15:277–281.

Culp WTN, Griffin MA, Case JB, et al. Use of percutaneous transvenous coil embolization in the treatment of intrahepatic portosystemic shunts in four cats. J Am Vet Med Assoc 2020;257:70–79.

Cushing TL. Endocardial fibroelastosis in a quarterhorse mare. J Comp Pathol 2013;149:318–321.

Durham J, Maisenbacher H. Double-outlet right atrium in a 9 year-old cat. J Vet Cardiol 2014;16:127–131.

Ferrigno CR, Ribeiro AA, Rahal SC, et al. Double aortic arch in a dog (*Canis familiaris*): a case report. Anat Histol Embryol 2001;30:379–381.

Fukushima K, Kanemoto H, Ohno K, et al. Computed tomographic morphology and clinical features of extrahepatic portosystemic shunts in 172 dogs in Japan. Vet J 2014;199:376–381.

Fujii Y, Aoki T, Takano H, et al. Arteriovenous shunts resembling patent ductus arteriosus in dogs: 3 cases. J Vet Cardiol 2009;11:147–151.

Henjes CR, Nolte I, Wefstaedt P. Multidetector-row computed tomography of thoracic aortic anomalies in dogs and cats: patent ductus arteriosus and vascular rings. BMC Vet Res 2011;7:57.

Holt D, Heldmann E, Michel K, et al. Esophageal obstruction caused by a left aortic arch and an anomalous right patent ductus arteriosus in two German Shepherd littermates. Vet Surg 2000;29:264–270.

Johnson MS, Martin M, De Giovanni JV, et al. Management of cor triatriatum dexter by balloon dilatation in three dogs. J Small Anim Pract 2004;45:16–20.

Jung S, Orvalho J, Griffiths LG. Aortopulmonary window characterized with two- and three-dimensional echocardiogram in a dog. J Vet Cardiol 2012;14:371–375.

Keene BW, Tou S. Cor triatriatum. In, Weisse C and Berent A (editors), Veterinary Image-Guided Interventions. Wiley-Blackwell. Ames, IA. 2015. pp. 604–609.

Krebs IA, Lindsley S, Shaver S, et al. Short- and long-term outcome of dogs following surgical correction of a persistent right aortic arch. J Am Anim Hosp Assoc 2014;50:181–186.

Leblanc N, Defrancesco TC, Adams AK, et al. Cutting balloon catheterization for interventional treatment of cor triatriatum dexter: 2 cases. J Vet Cardiol 2012;14:525–530.

Mankin KM. Current concepts in congenital portosystemic shunts. Vet Clin North Am Small Anim Pract 2015;45:477–487.

Morgan KRS, Bray JP. Current diagnostic tests, surgical treatments, and prognostic indicators for vascular ring anomalies in dogs. J Am Vet Med Assoc 2019;254:728–733.

Markovic LE, Scansen BA, Potter BM. Role of computed tomography angiography in the differentiation of feline truncus arteriosus communis from pulmonary atresia with ventricular septal defect. J Vet Cardiol 2017;19:514–522.

Marr CM, Reef VB, Brazil TJ, et al. Aorto-cardiac fistulas in seven horses. Vet Radiol Ultrasound 1998;39:22–31.

Nadolny KE, Kellihan HB, Scansen BA, et al. Cor triatriatum dexter in 17 dogs. J Vet Cardiol 2019;23:129–141.

Nakao S, Tanaka R, Hamabe L, et al. Cor triatriatum sinister with incomplete atrioventricular septal defect in a cat. J Feline Med Surg 2011;13:463–466.

Nelson NC, Nelson LL Imaging and clinical outcomes in 20 dogs treated with thin film banding for extrahepatic portosystemic shunts. Vet Surg 2016;45:736–745.

Nicolson G, Daley M, Makara M, et al. Partial anomalous pulmonary venous connection with suspected pulmonary hypertension in a cat. J Vet Cardiol 2015;17(Suppl 1):S354–359.

Noden DM, De Lahunta A. The Embryology of Domestic Animals: Developmental Mechanisms and Malformations. Williams & Wilkins, Baltimore, MD. 1985.p. 367.

Nucci DJ, Hurst KC, Monnet E. Retrospective comparison of short-term outcomes following thoracoscopy versus thoracotomy for surgical correction of persistent right aortic arch in dogs. J Am Vet Med Assoc 2018;253:444–451.

Oliveira P, Domenech O, Silva J, et al. Retrospective review of congenital heart disease in 976 dogs. J Vet Intern Med 2011;25:477–483.

Palerme JS, Brown JC, Marks SL, et al. Splenosystemic shunts in cats: a retrospective of 33 cases (2004–2011). J Vet Intern Med 2013;27:1347–1353.

Parry AT, White RN. Comparison of computed tomographic angiography and intraoperative mesenteric portovenography for extrahepatic portosystemic shunts. J Small Anim Pract 2017;58:49–55.

Plesman R, Johnson M, Rurak S, et al. Thoracoscopic correction of a congenital persistent right aortic arch in a young cat. Can Vet J 2011;52:1123–1128.

Russell HM, Jacobs ML, Anderson RH, et al. A simplified categorization for common arterial trunk. J Thorac Cardiovasc Surg 2011;141:645–653.

Saunders AB, Winter RL, Griffin JF, et al. Surgical management of an aberrant left subclavian artery originating from a left patent ductus arteriosus in a dog with a right aortic arch and abnormal branching. J Vet Cardiol 2013;15:153–159.

Scansen BA. Equine congenital heart disease. Vet Clin North Am Equine Pract 2019;35:103–117.

Scansen BA, Schneider M, Bonagura JD. Sequential segmental classification of feline congenital heart disease. J Vet Cardiol 2015;17(Suppl 1):S10–52.

Scansen BA, Townsend KL, McLoughlin MA. Variants of anomalous left subclavian artery anatomy in dogs with persistent right aortic arch: isolation, hypoplasia, ductal origin, and lateral origin from the ascending aorta. Vet Surg 2014;43:E199.

Scollan K, Salinardi B, Bulmer BJ, et al. Anomalous left-to-right shunting communication between the ascending aorta and right pulmonary artery in a dog. J Vet Cardiol 2011;13:147–152.

Sebastian-Marcos P, Fonfara S, Borgeat K, et al. Anatomical anomalies and variations of main thoracic vessels in dogs: a computed tomography study. J Vet Cardiol 2019;21:57–66.

Serrano G, Charalambous M, Devriendt N, et al. Treatment of congenital extrahepatic portosystemic shunts in dogs: a systematic review and meta-analysis. J Vet Intern Med 2019;33:1865–1879.

Serres F, Chetboul V, Sampedrano CC, et al. Ante-mortem diagnosis of persistent truncus arteriosus in an 8-year-old asymptomatic dog. J Vet Cardiol 2009;11:59–65.

Sherman A, Kim S, Craft W, et al. Micro-arteriovenous malformation causing spontaneous metacarpal pad hemorrhage in a dog. Can Vet J 2018;59:659–662.

Sleeper MM, Durando MM, Miller M, et al. Aortic root disease in four horses. J Am Vet Med Assoc 2001;219:491–496, 459.

Specchi S, d'Anjou MA, Carmel EN, et al. Computed tomographic characteristics of collateral venous pathways in dogs with caudal vena cava obstruction. Vet Radiol Ultrasound 2014;55:531–538.

Specchi S, Rossi F, Weisse C, et al. Canine and feline abdominal arterioportal communications can be classified based on branching patterns in computed tomographic angiography. Vet Radiol Ultrasound 2018.

Stern JA, Tou SP, Barker PC, et al. Hybrid cutting balloon dilatation for treatment of cor triatriatum sinister in a cat. J Vet Cardiol 2013;15:205–210.

Strickland R, Tivers MS, Adamantos SE, et al. Incidence and risk factors for neurological signs after attenuation of single congenital portosystemic shunts in 253 dogs. Vet Surg 2018;47:745–755.

Taulescu M, Palmieri C, Leach J, et al. Multiple congenital cardiovascular defects including type IV persistent truncus arteriosus in a Shetland pony – short communication. Acta Vet Hung 2016;64:360–364.

Tivers MS, Lipscomb VJ, Brockman DJ. Treatment of intrahepatic congenital portosystemic shunts in dogs: a systematic review. J Small Anim Pract 2017;58:485–494.

Tobias KM, Rohrbach BW. Association of breed with the diagnosis of congenital portosystemic shunts in dogs: 2,400 cases (1980–2002). J Am Vet Med Assoc 2003;223:1636–1639.

Townsend S, Oblak ML, Singh A, et al. Thoracoscopy with concurrent esophagoscopy for persistent right aortic arch in 9 dogs. Vet Surg 2016;45:O111–O118.

Traverson M, Lussier B, Huneault L, et al. Comparative outcomes between ameroid ring constrictor and cellophane banding for treatment of single congenital extrahepatic portosystemic shunts in 49 dogs (1998–2012). Vet Surg 2018;47:179–187.

Tremolada G, Longeri M, Polli M, et al. Persistent right aortic arch and associated axial skeletal malformations in cats. J Feline Med Surg 2013;15:68–73.

Valiente P, Trehy M, White R, et al. Complications and outcome of cats with congenital extrahepatic portosystemic shunts treated with thin film: thirty-four cases (2008–2017). J Vet Intern Med 2020;34:117–124.

Vedrine B, Durieux F. Aberrant left subclavian artery in a Beagle puppy with a persistent right aortic arch. Use of cone beam computed tomography to diagnose a vascular ring anomaly. Top Companion Anim Med 2017;32:76–79.

Weisse C. Hepatic arteriovenous malformations (AVMs) and fistulas. In, Weisse C and Berent A (editors), Veterinary Image-Guided Interventions. Wiley-Blackwell. Ames, IA. 2015.

Weisse C, Berent AC, Todd K, et al. Endovascular evaluation and treatment of intrahepatic portosystemic shunts in dogs: 100 cases (2001–2011). J Am Vet Med Assoc 2014;244:78–94.

White RN, Burton CA, Hale JS. Vascular ring anomaly with coarctation of the aorta in a cat. J Small Anim Pract 2003;44:330–334.

Yoon H, Kim J, Kwon GB, et al. Imaging diagnosis-computed tomographic angiography characteristics of multiple vascular anomalies in a senior dog with late-onset regurgitation. Vet Radiol Ultrasound 2018;59:E44–E49.

Zwingenberger AL, Spriet M, Hunt GB. Imaging diagnosis-portal vein aplasia and interruption of the caudal vena cava in three dogs. Vet Radiol Ultrasound 2011;52:444–447.

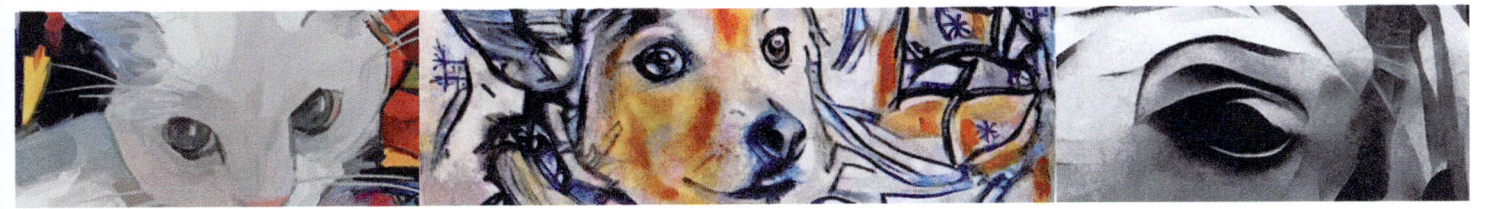

29

DEGENERATIVE VALVULAR DISEASE OF THE DOG

Chronic degenerative (myxomatous) atrioventricular (AV) valve disease is the most common heart disease and cause of congestive heart failure (CHF) in dogs. Older descriptors for this condition include endocardiosis, mucoid valvular degeneration, and chronic valvular fibrosis. Overall, this condition is estimated to account for more than 70% of canine cardiac disease. Most middle-aged to older dogs have at least some evidence of degenerative valve changes, although it is most common in dogs weighing <20 kg. Reported prevalence varies depending on type of practice (general versus specialty), whether studies were based on necropsy or clinical examination, and the age and breed distribution of dogs surveyed. It is clear that the prevalence of degenerative valvular disease in dogs increases with age. In smaller breeds, essentially all middle-aged to older individuals are affected to some degree.

The mitral valve, especially the anterior leaflet, usually is the most affected. About 50–60% of cases have only mitral valve involvement. Therefore, the disease typically is referred to as degenerative (or myxomatous or chronic) mitral valve disease (DMVD; or MMVD or CMVD). Nevertheless, both AV valves are involved in about one-third of cases. Isolated degenerative disease of the tricuspid valve is uncommon. Aortic or pulmonic valve thickening also occurs in some older animals; however, valve insufficiency, if present, usually is only mild (a minor color Doppler finding), and rarely audible.

DMVD is characterized by a prolonged preclinical phase, where valve lesions might only be apparent on postmortem exam. Early lesions appear grossly as small nodules on the free margins of the valve. Progressive accumulation of glycosaminoglycans (GAGs; previously known as acid-staining mucopolysaccharides) and other substances within the leaflets, along with collagen and elastin degeneration, cause nodular thickening, deformity, and weakening of the valve and its chordae tendineae. Eventually, valve insufficiency (regurgitation) develops. Progressive worsening of the regurgitation and secondary volume overloading of the adjoining atrium and ventricle follow.

The typical initial clinical manifestation of DMVD is the onset of a mitral regurgitation (MR) murmur (p. 229) when the animal is middle-aged or older. Auscultatory evidence of DMVD in the form of systolic clicks sometimes is heard in relatively young dogs of breeds at high risk, such as the Cavalier King Charles Spaniel and Dachshund. The severity of valve regurgitation and subsequent atrial and ventricular enlargement usually increases over a period of years. While many affected dogs remain asymptomatic, others eventually develop CHF and other complications. Cardiac enlargement accelerates fastest during the 6–12 months before CHF onset. In these dogs, CHF often is the cause of death, although sudden death, or a non-cardiac cause of death, occurs in some. Multiple complications can arise in dogs with advanced DMVD. However, appropriate therapy can extend survival, potentially even for several years after CHF develops. Despite the large number of dogs affected by DMVD, infective endocarditis is rare in this population. There is no convincing evidence that DMVD increases the risk for valve infection, although the effects of chronic inflammation elsewhere in the body might trigger some mediators of valve thickening.

The Normal Mitral Valve

Normal mitral (or tricuspid) function depends not only on valve leaflet structure and integrity, but also on other components of the valve apparatus. These include the chordae tendineae, papillary muscles, and valve annulus, where the leaflets attach at the AV junction. Myocardial function also can influence valve function. The three-dimensional contour of the normal mitral annulus is "saddle-shaped" rather than flat. The raised areas are oriented cranially (where anterior mitral and aortic leaflets meet in fibrous continuity) and caudally; the depressed areas are medial and lateral. This annular curvature is thought to decrease peak stress on the leaflets. The AV leaflets normally are thin and translucent, especially at the free margins. The mitral valve has two main leaflets (anterior/septal and posterior/parietal or mural). The valve's atrial surface is smooth. The ventricular surface is irregular because of the multiple chordal attachment points. Branched chordae connect the leaflets to the papillary muscles and sometimes directly to the ventricular wall. Commissural (or first-order, primary, or marginal) chordae attach to the leaflet free margins; mitral leaflet (or second-order chordae) attach to the ventricular aspect of the leaflets. Each leaflet receives chordae that originate from both anterior and posterior papillary muscles.

Histologically, normal valve leaflet structure encompasses four layers: atrialis, spongiosa, fibrosa, and ventricularis (**Figure 29.1**). The leaflets are covered on both sides by a layer of valve endothelial cells (VECs), with its basement membrane of various proteins, including laminins, type IV collagens, and a heparin sulfate proteoglycan. The atrialis faces the atrium; blood flows over this surface into the ventricle. The atrialis is a thin layer composed of elastin and collagen; it supports valve movement and helps mitigate the shear forces of blood flow across the valve. Also present in the atrialis, and the spongiosa and fibrosa layers as well, are fibroblastic mesenchymal cells known as valve interstitial cells (VICs). Both VICs and VECs are important in the formation and maintenance of normal valve extracellular matrix (ECM) and the pathogenesis of DMVD. The ECM is a dynamic network comprising collagens, elastin, fibronectin, laminin, proteoglycans, and glucosamines. Proteoglycans are important to the formation and organization of the spongiosa and fibrosa. VICs and VECs also produce matrix metalloproteinases (MMPs) as well as tissue inhibitors of MMPs (TIMPs). A balance between MMPs and TIMPs is important for normal ECM and valve function. VICs are fairly quiescent in normal valves, having only homeostatic functions. The valve spongiosa layer also is rich in proteoglycans and GAGs, with loose collagen, elastic fibers, and VICs. Functionally, this helps resist the compressive forces on the valve during systole and contributes to valve flexibility. The fibrosa layer, toward the ventricular side of the valve, is the thickest layer. It contains densely organized collagen fibers and is continuous with the chordae tendineae, as well as the fibrous cardiac skeleton. This layer provides tensile strength while the valve is closed, and allows flexure during opening. The ventricularis is a thin layer containing elastic and collagen fibers and covered by endothelium that is continuous with that covering the chordae. The chordae tendineae have a core of densely packed collagen fibers aligned longitudinally in the direction of the mechanical load, with some elastic fibers and fibroblasts. There are chordae of various thicknesses. The fibrosa and ventricularis, along with the chordae, provide important tensile strength against the powerful pressure generated during ventricular contraction and protect against valve leaflet prolapse into the atrium. A few cardiomyocytes, as well as small nerves and vessels, extend part way into the mitral leaflets from the atrial wall. For additional details of normal mitral valve structure and changes that occur with DMVD, see the Suggested Additional Reading and References list (including the excellent reviews by Fox, 2012; Markby, 2017; and Oyama, 2020).

Pathophysiology

The pathogenesis of myxomatous valvular degeneration involves multiple factors. Of major importance are: (1) the activation of VICs into a myofibroblast phenotype; (2) abnormal functioning, transformation, and some loss of VECs; and (3) dysregulation of valve ECM. Activated VICs produce catabolic enzymes that contribute to disturbed proteoglycan and collagen synthesis, which then leads to abnormal valvular remodeling. As the disease progresses, the spongiosa layer becomes thicker, while the fibrosa is diminished and collagen and elastin fibers disrupted (Oyama, 2020).

Although the structural and cellular changes in DMVD are understood fairly well, the underlying molecular mechanisms and biochemical changes involved are less clear. Various studies have identified differential expression of multiple genes in DMVD. Many genes are upregulated, while others are downregulated. Several gene families and signaling pathways appear to be involved in VIC transformation, as well as in VEC transformation, MMP production, and dysregulation of ECM protein synthesis. Some of the downregulated genes relate to formation of force-resistant collagen bundles or to certain MMPs involved in collagen maturation and elastic fiber formation. Decreased gene expression for important basement membrane components also occurs, which likely enhances the potential for VEC migration and transformation. Changes in the expression of

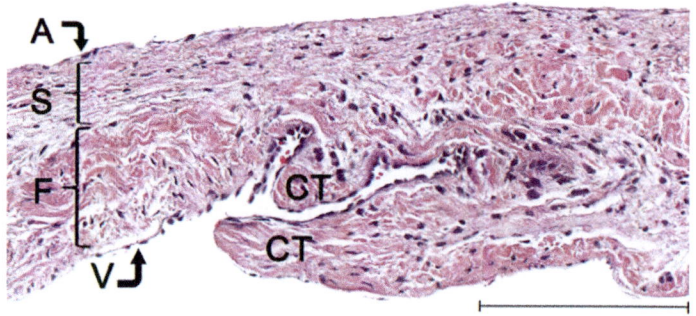

Figure 29.1 Photomicrograph showing the proximal third of the normal posterior mitral leaflet from a 3-year-old German Shepherd dog. The thin atrialis layer (A) lies on the inflow (atrial) side of the valve; it has a layer of endothelial cells overlying elastin fibers. The spongiosa (S) contains glycosaminoglycans, proteoglycans, and fine collagen fibers; this layer is present from valve annulus to free edge. The fibrosa (F) consists of dense, circumferentially oriented collagen fibers which extend into the valve annulus proximally; distally, these collagen fibers continue to form the central core of the chordae tendineae. The ventricularis (V), on the ventricular side of the valve, is a thin layer of elastic and collagen fibers covered by endothelium. Bar = 200 μm. (From Fox, 2012.)

genes related to various other biological functions occur in DMVD too. For example, reduced gene expression related to sarcoplasmic reticular calcium reuptake has been shown in dogs with DMVD and appears correlated with heart failure severity, as well as indicators of left heart size. Some expression changes involve genes associated with epithelial proliferation, ossification, oxidative stress, interleukins (ILs), interferons, tumor necrosis factor (TNF), and cardiovascular development, among other functions. There appears to be increased expression of genes related to inflammation, leading to increased expression of toll-like receptors and ILs which function in the control of inflammatory processes, as well as other biological pathways. However, inflammatory processes do not appear to be central to DMVD development. Although small increases in macrophage and mast cell numbers appear toward the base of the valve, they are not in areas more directly affected by degenerative changes. Nevertheless, it is unclear if mast cells play a role in pathogenesis.

Dysregulation of micro-ribonucleic acids (miRNAs) also could play an important role in DMVD pathogenesis. MiRNAs are a class of small, non-coding RNAs which are involved in controlling gene expression and helping maintain intracellular homeostasis. Changes in miRNA expression profiles can occur related to aging, DMVD, and CHF caused by DMVD. Altered expression of several miRNAs in DMVD influences genes associated with the ECM, and cell migration and differentiation. MiRNAs can negatively regulate gene expression by promoting degradation of messenger RNA transcripts or inhibiting protein translation. Differences between total plasma miRNA profiles and miRNA contained in circulating exosomes were found in dogs with DMVD. Exosomal miRNA expression levels might be more specific than total plasma levels; increases in certain exosomal miRNA were noted in dogs that had developed CHF. Circulating (plasma) miRNA expression profiles also can show differences between healthy dogs and those with DMVD, with several miRNAs upregulated and others downregulated in dogs with CHF. However, the specific miRNAs upregulated were different from those identified in exosomal miRNA profiling. Although miRNA expression patterns might have future potential as molecular biomarkers in dogs with CHF caused by DMVD, much additional study is needed.

Similarly, proteomic studies in dogs with DMVD have shown changes in affected animals. For example, several serum proteins appear to be differentially expressed in healthy Cavalier King Charles Spaniels (CKCS) compared to those with DMVD of varying severity. Whether assays for altered protein patterns will provide a useful means of detecting or monitoring progression of DMVD remains to be discovered.

Valvular Changes

Chronic mechanical stress on the valve leaflets from repeated impact is thought to play a role in initiating the process of myxomatous degeneration and contributing to its progression. The normal saddle-shape of the mitral valve probably helps mitigate mechanical stresses on the valve throughout the cardiac cycle. The morphology of the mitral valve, even in healthy CKCS, was shown to have a flatter three-dimensional (3D) shape compared to other breeds of dog (Menciotti, 2018). It is possible that this morphologic difference might confer reduced ability to withstand mechanical valve stress and thus contribute to early valve degeneration. The mitral valve annulus in various pure- and mixed-breed dogs with DMVD appears more circular, flatter, and less "saddle-shaped" than in healthy dogs.

Alterations in VIC and VEC phenotype and function are fundamental to the degenerative process. These disrupt normal ECM homeostatic mechanisms and lead to characteristic changes in the organization, quantity, and distribution of ECM components. Activated VICs appear to be the major mediators of myxomatous degeneration. The activation of these cells involves a process of transformation from their normal fibroblastic phenotype into a myofibroblastic, alpha-smooth muscle actin (alpha-SMA)-positive staining form. This transformation can be measured by the increased expression of alpha-SMA on immunohistochemistry and reverse transcriptase polymerase chain reaction (RT-PCR) testing. Activated VICs comprise a dynamic cell population, influenced by mechanical forces and external stimulation. VIC activation initially occurs in the atrialis layer; as the disease progresses, VICs in deeper layers also become activated.

The interaction between normal VEC and VIC cell types is important to valve ECM homeostasis. Endothelial cell signaling has modulating effects on ECM production. Endothelial damage and dysfunction are thought to play a role in DMVD pathogenesis. The basement membrane is important for maintaining integrity of the endothelium and damage to it probably contributes to the endothelial damage and cell loss seen. Early in the disease, increased as well as altered expression of basement membrane components develops. Areas of basement membrane splitting, VEC detachment, denuding, and apoptosis occur. Mechanisms related to VEC damage are thought to be involved in the abnormal ECM remodeling leading to myxomatous degeneration. For example, denuded VECs promote release of vasoactive substances such as endothelin (ETN) which can stimulate fibroblast proliferation and increased collagen production. Activation of pathways involved in endothelial function, including ETN-1 signaling and increased nitric oxide synthase (NOS) expression, appear to be involved in DMVD pathogenesis. Greater numbers of ETN-1 receptors have been found on affected valves. Platelet abnormalities also have been identified but are of unclear significance.

An endothelial to mesenchymal transition also occurs in DMVD, where VECs that migrate into the valve stroma develop increased expression of the myofibroblast marker alpha-SMA, and also of the endothelial marker, platelet endothelial cell adhesion molecule 1. The phenotypic changes that occur in these VECs are affected by changes within the valve stroma. Proliferation of activated, myofibroblastic VICs is evident near the valve surface, especially in areas of endothelial damage. However, in areas of advanced myxomatous change there are fewer activated VICs.

The increase in alpha-SMA-positive cells promotes ECM remodeling within the valve. Both VICs and VECs can produce components of the ECM and catabolic enzymes including MMPs and TIMPs. Altered activity of the various catabolic ECM enzymes such as MMPs, collagenases, and elastases occurs during the process of valve degeneration. Important in the normal ECM remodeling process, both MMPs and TIMPs increase in quantity as the valve degenerates. Altered gene expression for certain MMPs and TIMPs has been found in diseased valves compared to normal ones, a fact consistent with the concept that these enzymes are involved in ECM metabolic changes. Alterations in distribution and degree of MMP and TIMP expression contribute to the accumulation of ECM components and subsequent changes in valve structure and function. Several mediators are known to increase activity of MMPs, including angiotensin (Ang) II, ETN-1, norepinephrine and other catecholamines, TNF-alpha, IL-1beta, and possibly oxidative and mechanical stresses. Altered collagen expression occurs and is associated with progressive thickening of the valve spongiosa layer as deposition of GAGs, proteoglycans, and other components increases. The normal layered arrangement of collagen within the fibrosa becomes deranged and attenuated (**Figure 29.2**).

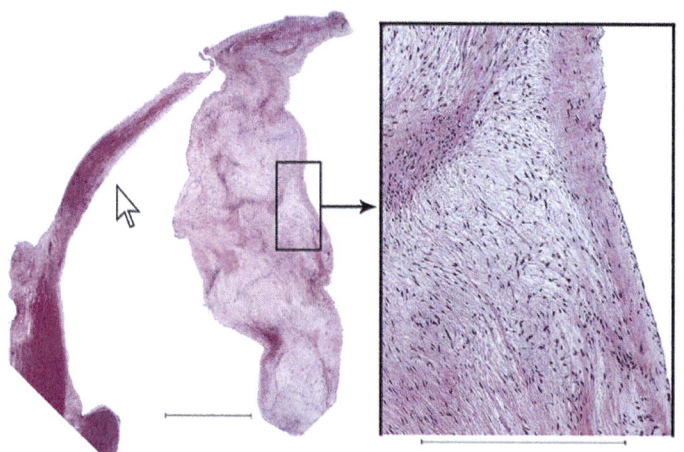

Figure 29.2 Photomicrograph of the distal posterior mitral leaflet from a 12-year-old male Maltese with advanced mitral valve disease (Whitney stage IV). The most prominent structural features are: increased thickness of the spongiosa (caused by glycosamine and proteoglycan deposition) and degeneration of the fibrosa. The leaflet's normal layered arrangement is totally disrupted. Collagen bundles in the fibrosa have disintegrated; their scattered remnants form swirls throughout the thickened valve leaflet stroma. These changes contribute to increased valve opacity and focal nodular thickening along leaflet edges that are visible grossly. Higher magnification (box on right) shows a granular-appearing spongiosa, associated with marked increase in glycosaminoglycan deposition. Stellate and spindle-shaped cells, along with scant mononuclear infiltration, lie within the increased myxomatous content. On the left side of the image is a large, second-order chord (arrow) associated with this leaflet. Hematoxylin and eosin stain. Bar on left = 1 mm; bar under magnified box = 500 μm. (From Fox, 2012.)

Collagen turnover is reduced and GAG infiltration disrupts collagen bundles. It is collagen fiber orientation that essentially determines the distribution and degree of mechanical strain in the valve leaflet throughout systole and diastole. This strain in turn influences various cellular functions, including remodeling, proliferation, cell migration, and apoptosis. The altered collagen fibril organization results in mechanically weaker and less flexible valves. Myxomatous degeneration of the chordae reduces their tensile strength and can predispose to rupture.

Transforming growth factor -beta (TGF-beta) and serotonin (5-HT) signaling appear to be involved in DMVD pathogenesis. Localized production of TGF-beta occurs in affected canine valves, and expression of TGF-beta subtypes and their receptors is increased. The larger TGF-beta family includes subfamily components, such as TGF-beta1-3 and bone morphogenic proteins, some of which play a role in valve cusp development. These presumably are also involved in DMVD pathogenesis, because they can regulate some ECM and endothelial-to-mesenchymal changes. For example, bone morphogenic protein 6 appears to be consistently upregulated in DMVD. This and related proteins function via various pathways, ultimately leading to effects that modify cellular actin organization, and cell migration, differentiation, and survival. Immunohistochemistry and RT-PCR studies have shown variably increased expression of TGF-beta1-3 and TGF-beta2 receptors in DMVD; however, the exact role of TGF-beta in disease pathogenesis remains unclear.

Serotonin gene expression is increased in DMVD, as is expression of tryptophan hydroxylase 1 (a rate-limiting enzyme for the serotonergic pathway). Affected valves also demonstrate increased 5-HT2B receptor gene expression, suggesting an important role for serotonin in DMVD pathogenesis. Serotonergic signaling can induce VIC proliferation and ECM production, although it apparently does not cause increase in alpha-SMA expression in these cells. It also affects TGF-beta signaling. 5-HT is produced locally in canine mitral valves and can be derived from platelet activation. Higher 5-HT concentrations have been found in dogs with mild DMVD, compared to normal dogs, although concentrations are reduced in severe DMVD. Breed differences in 5-HT concentrations are known to occur. Healthy CKCS were shown to have higher levels of 5-HT than other breeds. Higher 5-HT concentrations occur in healthy Newfoundlands and Belgian Shepherds, as well.

AngII might have a role in the pathogenesis of valvular changes in DMVD, although this remains to be clarified. Changes in protein or gene expression related to angiotensins have not been identified. Nevertheless, there could be interaction between AngII and 5-HT; experimental models (in mouse and pig) have shown that combined stimulation with 5-HT and AngII induces valve remodeling and increased alpha-SMA expression (Markby, 2017). Changes in circulating cytokine concentrations also occur, including increases in IL-8 associated with DMVD disease severity. Increase in inflammatory cytokines in human CHF has been associated with worsening disease progression and prognosis.

Mitral valve prolapse is common and might be important in the pathogenesis of the disease, at least in some breeds. Mitral valve prolapse occurs when redundant valve tissue between the chordal attachments bulges toward the atrium during systole. A high prevalence of mitral prolapse occurs in clinically normal dogs of some predisposed breeds. The degree of prolapse has been associated with disease severity. In some cases prolapse might be related to chordal laxity or secondary or tertiary chordal ruptures.

Valve Lesion Severity A histologic grading system for DMVD is described in **Table 29.1**. Myxomatous changes are most severe in the free edge to distal third of the valve leaflets. The leaflets thicken and lengthen as DMVD progresses. Reduced cell density develops in areas affected by myxomatous degeneration compared to normal areas. Connective tissue derangement and decreased density worsen with increasing disease severity. As the valve structure changes, leaflet apposition in systole becomes abnormal, leading to regurgitation and altered hemodynamic forces that provoke further tissue damage. In dogs with DMVD, there is a reduced number of nerve fibers associated with the myocardial cells at the base of the valve leaflets; however, it is unclear whether disease or aging is the cause.

Mitral valve lesions also are classified according to the severity of their macroscopic appearance (Whitney classification; **Table 29.2**). This is based on the degree of leaflet nodularity, thickening, and deformity (**Figure 29.3**). Early gross changes consist of small thickened areas along valve edges (**Figure 29.4**). These can progress to large areas of nodular, yet smooth-surfaced thickening along the leaflets, especially in areas of contact. In advanced disease, portions of chordae near the leaflets become thickened and elongated. Mild (Whitney type 1) lesions can develop in young dogs, even at 1–2 years of age. Type 1 and 2 lesions often are seen

Table 29.2 Whitney Classification of Gross Valve Lesions

Type 1
- A few small, discrete nodules present at valve contact points

Type 2
- Larger nodules that tend to coalesce at leaflet edges
- Areas of diffuse leaflet opacity might be present

Type 3
- Larger nodules, coalescing into irregular, plaque-like, smooth-surfaced deformities
- Lesions also extend into chordae

Type 4
- Gross valve distortion with "ballooning" of leaflets
- Proximally thickened chordae which could be ruptured

Note: From Whitney, 1974.

Table 29.1 Histologic Grading System for Degenerative Mitral Valve Disease

Mild Disease
- Activated valve stromal cells (VICs) evident
- Proliferation of endothelial and fibroelastic elements within the atrialis layer
- Irregular splitting of collagen and laminin in endothelial basement layer of the atrialis, with protrusion into the atrialis
- Breakdown of normal collagen layers in the atrialis and spongiosa
- Nodular proteoglycan deposition into the fibrosa

Moderate Disease
- Moderate increase in GAG and proteoglycan deposition in the spongiosa layer
- Mild disruption of collagen bundles in the fibrosa
- Decreased connective tissue density
- Distal valve leaflets are most affected by these changes; proximal (annular) half of leaflet still normal

Severe Disease
- Marked increase in GAG and proteoglycan deposits leading to displacement of the fibrosa
- Collagen bundle disruption in distal half of leaflets
- Fibroblastic proliferation in atrialis and fibrosa layers

Abbreviations: GAG, glycosaminoglycan; VICs, valve interstitial cells.

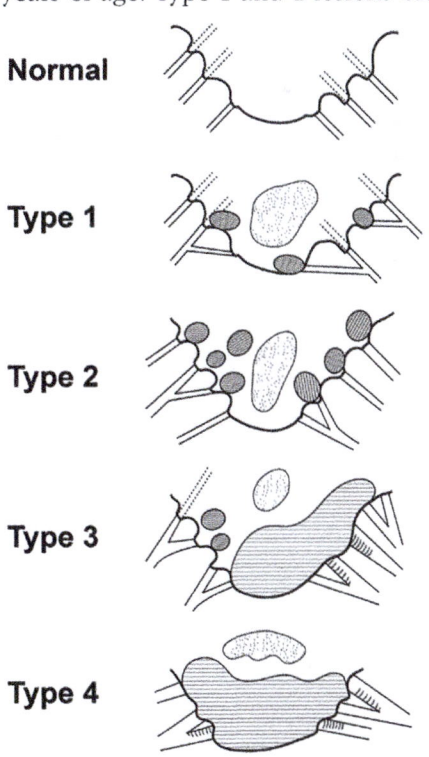

Figure 29.3 The four-grade Whitney classification scheme for chronic mitral valve lesions. The hatched areas represent locations of nodular or diffuse valve thickening and billowing. The dotted areas indicate regions of opacity caused by myxomatous degeneration. (From Borgarelli & Buchanan, 2012.)

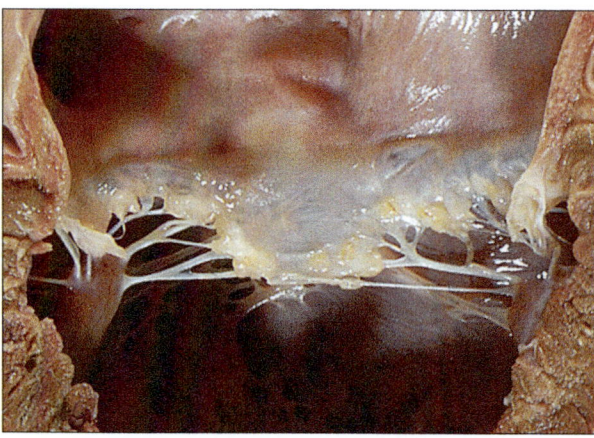

Figure 29.4 Specimen from a Cocker Spaniel with early signs of degenerative mitral valve disease shows nodular thickening along the free margins of the mitral valve.

in dogs under 5 years of age and usually are not clinically significant. Advanced (type 3 or 4) lesions occur in an estimated 75–97% of dogs aged 9 years and older (**Figure 29.5**, also **Figure 32.24C**, p. 642).

Myocardial and Chamber Remodeling

Disruption of normal valvular structure and function leads to valvular leakage and its progressive consequences. This usually worsens slowly, over months to years. Left atrial (LA) pressure increases occur mostly at end-systole, from regurgitant v (or c-v) waves. Atrial compliance allows mean LA pressure to remain relatively normal, unless MR suddenly worsens (as with chordal rupture). However, over time progressive rise in ventricular diastolic and mean LA pressures can lead to overt CHF (Chapter 20).

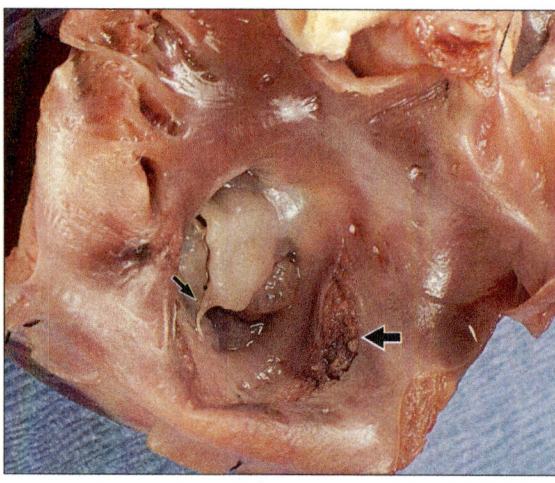

Figure 29.5 View from the enlarged left atrium shows marked mitral valve thickening, especially of the anterior (cranioventral) leaflet, with a ruptured chorda tendinea (small arrow). A partial-thickness left atrial tear also is visible (larger arrow). Specimen from a male Chihuahua with advanced degenerative mitral valve disease that died from fulminant pulmonary edema. (Image courtesy of Dr M Miller.)

As DMVD advances, worsening valve regurgitation leads to greater atrial and ventricular wall stress in diastole, which stimulates eccentric myocardial hypertrophy. Dilation also increases preload, which activates the Frank-Starling mechanism (p. 15) to maintain forward flow. Isovolumic contraction no longer exists now, because regurgitation starts as soon as LV pressure begins to rise. By the time of aortic valve opening, the LV volume is smaller, chamber walls have thickened, and peak wall stress is comparably lower than for volume overloads like PDA or AR, where ejection begins only after aortic valve opening. Valve regurgitation is well-tolerated for 4 to 6 years in most cases, as long as the regurgitant volume increases only gradually. However, the increased myocardial diastolic stretch induces myocyte lengthening as well as degradation of the collagen weave and ECM between myocytes. This promotes slippage of adjacent myocytes and contributes to progressive chamber enlargement. Genes important for normal myocardial collagen and ECM formation and maintenance become downregulated in DMVD, while those involved with ECM remodeling and collagen loss are upregulated. Increased chymase production in the myocardium and the effects of MMPs play an important role in intercellular collagen loss. Chymase is released from mast cells in response to myocardial stretch, especially in the earlier stages of DMVD. Chymase has significant antifibrotic actions because it activates MMPs and kallikrein and degrades fibronectin, although it also has some profibrotic effects. Furthermore, chymase appears to have adverse effects on cardiomyocyte myofibrillar structure and function.

Because chymase also catalyzes the conversion of AngI to AngII, increased chymase production within the myocardium promotes increased local AngII production. This likely contributes to continued left ventricular (LV) remodeling and dilation. Angiotensin converting enzyme (ACE) inhibitors do not effectively reduce myocardial AngII concentration or decrease LV remodeling in DMVD, presumably because the renin–Ang system has a limited role in LV remodeling during low-pressure volume overload states. The loss of myocardial interstitial collagen and downregulation of genes associated with collagen and ECM production also could explain why ACE inhibitors and other agents with antifibrotic activity have not effectively prevented LV dilation in some studies, although the recent DELAY study showed a tendency for less adverse remodeling with combined renin–angiotensin–aldosterone system (RAAS) inhibition (benazepril plus spironolactone; Borgarelli, 2020). Nevertheless, ACE inhibitors might reduce endothelial AngII formation, when catalyzed by ACE, and these drugs are helpful during CHF management, based on some clinical trials (Chapters 21 and 22). In late-stage DMVD, after dilation develops, chymase activity appears to be minimal.

In summary, MR causes a low-pressure volume overload resulting in LV and LA dilation (eccentric hypertrophy) with loss of interstitial collagen. LV dilation and geometric change also could impair the normal ventricular systolic twisting and untwisting that contribute to effective pumping and filling. As the LV becomes more enlarged and spherical, the mitral annulus dilates, and the function of the mitral apparatus decreases; this leads to even greater MR. Thus, the advanced LV dilation and remodeling of severe DMVD exacerbates MR, further increases LV wall stress (when compensatory hypertrophy is inadequate), and can promote decompensation to CHF. Although individual myocyte contractile function might be depressed, global LV function (and fractional shortening) usually appears vigorous, at least in smaller dogs, as MR increases LV preload and decreases peak wall stress, one measure of afterload.

Local cardiac sympathetic activity increases with advancing DMVD. Myocardial AngII promotes catecholamine release into the interstitium. Circulating catecholamine concentrations also can increase. Adrenergic activation is thought to have a role in the LV remodeling process, although beta-blocker treatment does not appear to attenuate LV dilation and collagen loss in natural cases of MR, despite some potential benefits in acute, experimental disease in dogs.

LV systolic function appears well-maintained overall, as measured by conventional ejection phase indices, although differences often are observed between smaller (<20 kg) and larger-sized dogs. However, precise ventricular systolic and diastolic function assessment in primary MR is nearly impossible with current echocardiographic techniques. Thus, LV fractional shortening, fractional area change, and ejection fraction all show increased values. This usually is explained by reduced LV wall stress (afterload), increased preload, and sympathetic nervous system support, the latter activated in heart failure. Estimates of isovolumic LV function (dP/dt_{max}) can be derived from the MR jet's velocity slope (Chapter 4), but because regurgitation begins early in systole (and true isovolumic contraction is lacking) their validity can be challenged. Clinical studies of spontaneous MR have demonstrated that fractional shortening and ejection fraction actually increase along with the regurgitant volume. Even dogs with severe signs of CHF and low aortic output typically show hyperdynamic LV systolic function when a comprehensive assessment is performed. Although this point is controversial, the authors believe that reliance on the end-systolic LV minor diameter and its calculated derivatives (normalized end-systolic dimension and end-systolic volume index) for systolic function assessment is unreliable; these overestimate LV volumes once the ventricle is dilated. Even tissue indices of LV function, such as myocardial strain and early diastolic recoil (e'), are hyperdynamic in DMVD, demonstrating the important influence of increased preload on ventricular function tests. Similarly, right ventricular (RV) systolic function is hyperdynamic, probably related to septal tethering to the left ventricle. Nevertheless, experimental studies do indicate that chronic volume overloading eventually reduces myocyte contractility, although conclusive demonstration of this might be impossible except in larger canine breeds where a dilated cardiomyopathy (DCM) phenotype can develop in the presence of severe MR. Mechanisms underlying depressed contractility might involve oxygen free radicals, as well as the effects of chronic neurohormonal activation. While long-term beta-blockade has improved myocyte contractility experimentally, it does not appear to delay CHF onset in clinical cases of DMVD. Over time, declining contractility can exacerbate ventricular dilation and valve regurgitation and, therefore, can worsen congestive failure.

Diastolic function, as measured by echocardiography, also appears enhanced in DMVD. The LA v wave associated with MR raises end-systolic pressure in the atrium, which then enhances early diastolic filling of the LV. The increasing mitral inflow (E wave) velocity in progressive MR (recorded by pulsed-wave Doppler) reflects this. Maximum inflow velocities <1 m/s generally suggest only mild or mild-moderate MR. Dogs at higher risk of pulmonary edema typically have inflow velocities >1.3 m/s. Estimation of LV filling pressure from the ratio of E/e' also is challenging, because e' is enhanced by increased preload too. Thus, extremely high E/e' ratios (typically >12 or 13) are required before one can reliably predict increased LV filling pressures by echocardiography.

Cardiac remodeling generally is quite advanced before signs of CHF develop. Compensatory increases in blood volume and heart size, along with preserved global ventricular function, allow most dogs to remain asymptomatic for a prolonged period. However, as the MR and neurohormonal activation (p. 303) worsen, regurgitant v wave amplitude and mean LA pressure increase, which in turn raises pulmonary venous and capillary hydrostatic pressures. Reduced cardiac output leads to volume expansion that further increases venous pressures. Post-capillary pulmonary hypertension (PH) increases RV afterload. In addition, slowed blood flow transit can be measured through the lungs. When pulmonary lymphatic capacity is exceeded, overt pulmonary edema develops. The onset of clinical CHF signs can be gradual or, especially with rupture of a major chorda tendinea, sudden and severe. A component of diurnal rhythm also influences the fluctuations in LA pressure, which rises slightly during the day and decreases at night, as shown in experimental canine MR. Additionally, abrupt increases in LA pressure can occur during excitement or with exertion. Therefore, restricting activity and excitement could help reduce LA pressure spikes in dogs with advanced DMVD. Pulmonary edema predominates in most cases with CHF; however, combinations of tricuspid regurgitation (TR), PH (see "Other Pathophysiologic Changes," below) and atrial fibrillation (AF) can promote the congestive signs of ascites or infrequently, pleural effusion.

Natriuretic peptides help counter the effects of systemic RAAS activation in preclinical disease (Chapter 20). Higher natriuretic peptide concentrations are associated with more severe MR; circulating concentrations are especially high with CHF. Yet, extremely high values also have been observed in dogs with compensated disease and marked cardiomegaly. Other biomarkers such as cardiac troponins (cTns) and adrenomedullin also increase in advanced disease. The rise in cTnI concentration with progressive heart failure has been attributed to ongoing myocardial injury and cardiac remodeling. Adrenomedullin is a peptide with vasodilating and natriuretic effects, similar to the natriuretic peptides; its plasma concentration correlates with those of atrial natriuretic peptide, as well as LA-to-aortic root diameter ratio (LA/Ao), and LV diameter in DMVD. The sodium-calcium exchanger (NCX-1) could function as a cardiac biomarker too, although this has not been widely explored. Compared to normal dogs, NCX-1 expression increases in those with moderate to severe DMVD; this marker is not correlated with renal function.

Chronic AV valve disease has been associated with intramural coronary arteriosclerosis, narrowing, and focal myocardial fibrosis. While these changes are present to some degree in older dogs generally, they reportedly are more prevalent in those with DMVD, compared to age matched controls (Falk, 2010). Perivascular fibrosis of small intramural vessels and mild to moderate interstitial fibrosis occur despite an overall decrease in myocardial collagen content and ECM turnover in DMVD. Greater degrees of myocardial fibrosis and intramural arteriolar luminal narrowing have been associated with higher cTnI concentrations. Focal areas of myocardial fibrosis and necrosis appear to be more prominent in LV papillary muscles and sub-endocardial regions, locations at higher risk for demand ischemia. Arteriolar changes in these areas involve proliferation of vascular fibroblasts and smooth muscle, with hyalinization of the vessel walls. To the degree that these vascular lesions cause arteriolar stenosis or occlusion, they can promote local myocardial ischemic injury and replacement fibrosis. Papillary muscle fibrosis could further reduce mitral valve function in DMVD. Such changes might accelerate the development of LV failure and reduce survival time in dogs with DMVD. Intramural arterial narrowing also was associated with more frequent ventricular ectopy and increased likelihood of sudden death.

Progressive LA enlargement, along with LV dilation, is a hallmark of DMVD. The LA enlargement observed by echocardiography and radiography relates to both an increase in chamber volume and changes in its shape. Pulmonary venous dilation also becomes obvious with progressive LA dilation and remodeling. This might relate in part to eccentric jets of MR that preferentially engage specific pulmonary veins. Some dogs develop massive LA dilation even before signs of CHF appear. Although some cases never show clinical signs of heart failure, moderate to severe LA enlargement indicates an increased risk for CHF and poorer prognosis (**Figure 29.6**). The LA has reservoir, conduit, and contractile functions that influence LV filling and pump function. With advancing DMVD, progressive increases in LA pressure and volume and deterioration in atrial contractile function occur. These are reflected in part by increasing transmitral E wave velocity and decreasing A wave velocity. CHF in dogs with DMVD is associated with reduced LA contractile function, as well as late diastolic strain, based on echocardiographic assessments (p. 103).

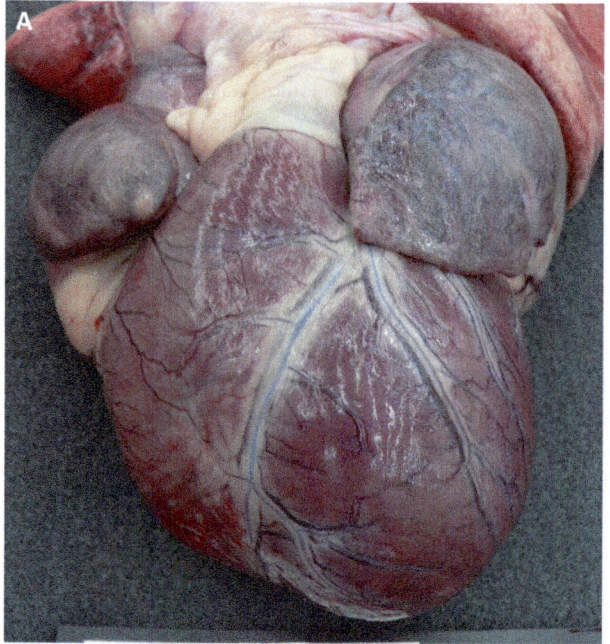
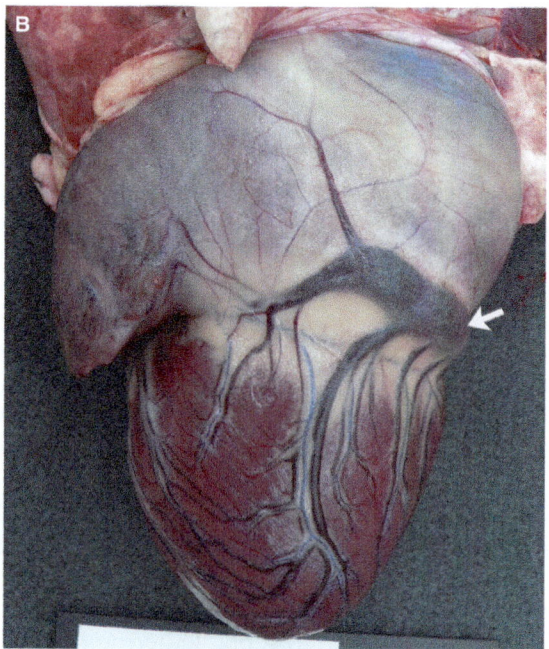

Figure 29.6 (A) Cranial view of the heart from a 12-year-old male German Shorthair Pointer with long-standing degenerative mitral valve disease, atrial fibrillation and biventricular congestive heart failure. There is massive left atrial enlargement (left auricle at top right of image), as well as dilation of all chambers. Left ventricular function was well-preserved on initial presentation ~3 years prior to death, but had progressively deteriorated. (B) Caudal view shows severe biatrial enlargement (left atrium at top left of image). The great coronary vein and coronary sinus (arrow) are markedly distended, consistent with chronically increased right heart filling pressure.

Atrial tachyarrhythmias, including AF, are more likely to develop with atrial enlargement. While the overall prevalence of AF in dogs with DMVD is low, based mainly on the small size of affected dogs, significant risk factors for AF have been identified by multivariable regression analyses. These include: increased LA size and LA to aortic root diameter (LA/Ao) ratio, advanced disease (ACVIM stage C & D; see Table 20.2, p. 311), increased body weight (size), increased early mitral filling velocity, and reduced LV fractional shortening (Guglielmini, 2020). An increase in fibrosis around the pulmonary veins, along with decreased connexion expression, could underlie increased susceptibility to AF, as seen in a dog model of MR. Tachyarrhythmias of either atrial or ventricular origin can reduce forward cardiac output and exacerbate congestive signs.

High-velocity MR jets can injure the LA endothelium, causing focal thickening and fibrotic "jet lesions." Severe endocardial trauma also can lead to partial- or full-thickness tearing of the LA wall (**Figure 29.5**). Histologic findings in these areas include endomyocardial degeneration, fibrosis, and necrosis, with hemorrhage and some inflammation. Multiple variable-thickness tears can develop in affected dogs. Of dogs with LA tear lesions, slightly more than half are estimated to have non-perforating lesions; about one-third have some degree of intrapericardial bleeding caused by a full-thickness tear (p. 562). Stretching or tearing near the fossa ovalis can lead to acquired atrial septal defect (ASD).

Other Pathophysiologic Changes

Pulmonary arterial pressures increase in many dogs with DMVD. An estimated 40% of cases are affected to some degree. PH is more common in dogs with advanced (stage C and D) disease. Chronically increased pulmonary venous and pulmonary capillary wedge pressures cause so-called post-capillary PH (Chapter 39). This typically is of mild to moderate severity. However, reactive pulmonary arterial vasoconstriction or remodeling secondary to hypoxia or concurrent lung disease (pre-capillary PH) can lead to marked increase in pulmonary vascular resistance and severe PH. Neurohormonal changes associated with heart failure, including increased ETN-1 release, along with reductions in endothelial nitric oxide (NO) production and NO-dependent vasodilation, are thought to contribute to pulmonary vascular remodeling and PH in some patients with chronic MR. Especially when RV function is compromised, the increase in RV afterload imposed by PH can lead to both right-sided congestive and low cardiac output signs, including exertional collapse and syncope. Clinical (Doppler) underestimation of PH severity is likely in such cases (p. 561). A substantial number of dogs with chronic MR and CHF develop auscultation findings that are compatible with interstitial pulmonary fibrosis. These dogs have diffuse lung crackles but no obvious edema radiographically. Whether this is related to elevated LA pressures and pulmonary congestion or a comorbidity is uncertain. Regardless, widespread pulmonary fibrosis can confuse the clinical examination, and it increases lung stiffness, which contributes to exercise intolerance and resting tachypnea.

Histologically, post-capillary PH can promote hypertrophy of the tunica media, along with intimal fibrosis, in muscular pulmonary arteries. Pulmonary veins show similar mural changes, along with dilation. Pulmonary capillary dilation, mural thickening, and basement membrane rupture might be evident with red blood cell (RBC) leakage into alveolar spaces, especially if LA pressure suddenly increases. Fibrosis seems a common comorbidity, of undetermined mechanisms. Marked pulmonary lymphatic dilation also is typical.

There is evidence that systemic vascular endothelial function and vasodilatory responses become impaired with advanced DMVD and CHF, as demonstrated by Doppler assessment of brachial artery flow. Increased levels of ETN, AngII, and vasopressin are likely contributors. An increase in systemic inflammation, as indicated by increased circulating C-reactive protein concentrations, and possibly in oxidative stress might also play roles in reducing normal vascular responsiveness in advanced cardiac disease and CHF. Systemic inflammation is thought to inhibit normal vasodilatory endothelial NO production, while increasing maladaptive inducible NOS activity.

Alterations in the concentrations of other circulating substances also occur in DMVD. For example, increases in the adipokine, leptin, were found in dogs with advanced (stage C) DMVD compared to normal dogs. Although results for circulating adiponectin are conflicting, there appears to be a shift in myocardial adiponectin isoform types in dogs with advanced DMVD. Galectin-3 is a marker of fibrosis. Increases in myocardial galectin-3 expression, percentage of fibrosis in the LV myocardium, and plasma galectin-3 concentration were identified in dogs with DMVD compared to normal.

Clinical Features

Clinical signs of DMVD occur most commonly in middle-aged and older small to mid-sized breeds. Disease prevalence and severity increase with age. Clinical estimates of prevalence have varied widely. An audible MR murmur occurs in 30 to over 90% of small-breed dogs aged 10 years or older. However, necropsy surveys suggest that almost all older small breed dogs have some myxomatous degenerative valve changes. Over 60% of Dachshunds without an audible murmur had some MR by color Doppler imaging in one study (Garncarz, 2017). The number of dogs affected increased with age and more males than females had MR. Yet many dogs were less than 5 years old. Mild mitral valve thickening and prolapse also were common in that study. In clinically normal Whippets, almost 30% had a soft to moderate MR murmur and almost 40% had some MR on echocardiogram; as expected, prevalence increased with age (Stepien, 2017). Younger onset is common in some breeds, especially CKCS and also in some Whippets and Bull Terriers (although the latter breed also is prone to congenital mitral malformations). CKCS historically have developed CHF more often and at a younger age than other breeds. Between 40 and 60% of CKCS aged 4 years or older have a MR murmur, and essentially all individuals over 10 years of age are affected.

A review of auscultation and pedigree records from a large number of 4–5 year old CKCS found that presence and severity of MR murmur (as an indicator of DMVD severity) was highly heritable. The specific genetic cause is unknown. DMVD could involve a complex autosomal polygenic trait with variable penetrance. Genome-wide association studies in CKCS have not found a single major gene effect. Regions on chromosomes 13 and 14 were associated with the disease, although there are conflicting data about whether several gene loci are involved. In Whippets, a significant association of DMVD was found on chromosome 15, with suspected association also on chromosome 2. These results further support a genetic basis for DMVD severity in this breed. So far, no potential pathological variants in canine genes orthologous to those associated with human myxomatous mitral valve disease have been found in dogs with DMVD. Selective breeding of dogs without a murmur could reduce the prevalence of DMVD in CKCS. Unfortunately, the efficacy of voluntary breeding guidelines to reduce disease prevalence, or at least increase the age of onset, in CKCS is questionable because of inconsistent breeder compliance. Nevertheless, in breeds with high risk for DMVD, yearly screening of animals intended for breeding is encouraged. Dogs that develop MR during the normal age range for breeding should not be bred again.

Other breeds with increased DMVD prevalence include Cocker Spaniels, Dachshunds, Beagles, Toy and Miniature Poodles, Miniature Schnauzers, Chihuahuas, Pomeranians, various terrier breeds (especially Yorkshire, Jack Russell, Boston, Fox, Norwich), Pekingese, Shih Tzus, Miniature Pinschers, and Border Collies. Some large-breed dogs also develop DMVD, although the degree of valve thickening and prolapse tends to be less pronounced than in small-breed dogs. German Shepherds might be overrepresented. Larger-breed dogs also are prone to DCM (which could coexist), or they might be more susceptible to myocardial dysfunction secondary to chronic volume overload. Without longitudinal studies of larger dogs affected initially with mild MR, this relationship cannot be determined with certainty.

The overall prevalence of MR murmurs and DMVD might be similar in males and females. However, some studies have shown an earlier onset, faster progression, greater severity, and a higher prevalence of CHF in males compared to females. An estimated 30% of all dogs with DMVD will eventually develop CHF. However, for CKCS, cardiac disease as the cause of death probably occurs in over 40%. Table 20.2 (p. 311) outlines the staging system commonly used for describing clinical disease severity.

Physical Findings

Many dogs with DMVD display no clinical signs, even when the disease is fairly advanced. In those that do, early clinical signs of (impending or overt) CHF usually include reduced exercise tolerance and tachypnea or cough with exertion. However, a persistent increase in baseline (resting) respiratory rate (RRR) often signals the onset of pulmonary interstitial edema before other signs of overt CHF, and radiographic changes, develop. Therefore, owner monitoring of RRR while the animal is sleeping can provide a useful early warning system (Table 22.1, p. 339). Coughing might occur at night and in the early morning, as well as with activity. Yet CHF, as indicated by radiographic evidence for pulmonary edema, is not always associated with coughing. An abnormal radiographic airway pattern (suggesting chronic airway disease) and enlarged LA size, but not pulmonary edema, were significantly associated with coughing in one study (Ferasin, 2013). In dogs with CHF, intermittent episodes of symptomatic pulmonary edema interspersed with periods of compensated heart failure can occur over months. However, a persistent cough without progressive increase in respiratory rate and effort usually is associated with airway disease, rather than CHF. Severe pulmonary edema causes obvious respiratory distress, often with a soft, moist cough. This is especially true in larger dog breeds, where coughing can be quite prominent along with radiographic pulmonary edema. Signs of severe pulmonary edema can develop gradually or acutely.

Transient weakness or acute collapse (syncope) can occur secondary to arrhythmias, coughing, marked PH, or a full-thickness atrial tear. The right-sided congestive signs of abdominal distension (ascites, hepatomegaly, tachypnea from diaphragmatic pressure) and infrequently, respiratory distress from pleural effusion are associated with severe TR, PH, or both. Development of AF makes right-sided CHF even more likely. Gastrointestinal (GI) signs might accompany splanchnic congestion. Only rarely does noticeable peripheral tissue edema develop in dogs with DMVD, and these cases invariably have ascites or moderate to severe hypoalbuminemia.

Cardiovascular examination findings in preclinical cases often are normal, with the exception of the MR murmur (see below). Heart rate and rhythm generally are normal in earlier stages of disease. Statistically, the heart rate increases with worsening stage of MR, yet this often occurs within the normal range. Heart rates over 130 beats/minute have been associated with greater risk for CHF. Sinus tachycardia is more typical as CHF develops. A follow-up review of EPIC study data indicated that the most pronounced changes (from baseline values), which occurred just prior to first CHF event, were increases in heart rate, in-clinic respiratory rate, and at-home RRR, although increase in radiographic vertebral heart size (VHS) was the earliest variable to begin changing (Boswood, 2020). Decreases in body temperature and weight also were observed prior to CHF onset.

Arrhythmias are more likely to occur with advanced disease. Mucous membrane color and peripheral perfusion usually remain normal even with CHF, unless severe pulmonary edema impairs tissue oxygenation. Normal arterial pulse strength is expected, although pulse deficits (p. 256) accompany some tachyarrhythmias. The jugular veins generally appear normal with MR alone. However, marked TR and especially PH often cause jugular pulsations that are accentuated after exercise, with excitement, or during abdominojugular (hepatojugular) reflux testing (p. 37). Concurrent jugular vein distension reflects increased right heart filling pressure.

MR produces a harsh (mixed frequency), holosystolic *murmur* loudest at or immediately dorsal to the left apex, over the mitral area. The murmur can radiate in any direction (p. 229). However, MR murmur characteristics can vary depending on the stage of disease and hemodynamic factors. Some MR murmurs sound like a musical tone or "whoop." With mild MR, a soft decrescendo murmur might be audible only in early to mid-systole (proto- or protomesosystolic). Exercise and excitement increase the intensity of soft MR murmurs, probably by increasing blood pressure (BP). As noted previously, some dogs with echo evidence of MR have no audible murmur. Estimates from individual breed studies suggest that 20–45% of dogs with mild MR identified by color Doppler echocardiography might not have a murmur. In such cases, an audible murmur might become evident with excitement and faster heart rate. Soft, grade 1 and 2/6 (localized) murmurs are associated with less severe disease in asymptomatic dogs. Moderate to loud murmurs radiate more widely over the thorax, and generally are associated with more advanced DMVD and increased risk for CHF. However, loud murmurs (grades 5 and 6/6) with a precordial thrill also are common in dogs without obvious clinical signs. Furthermore, with massive MR and severe heart failure, the systolic pressure difference between left ventricle and left atrium decreases and the murmur can become softer or even difficult to hear, especially in patients with respiratory distress. Audio signal analysis techniques for evaluating MR severity in dogs have been reported, but are not used clinically.

A mid- to late *systolic click* is heard in some dogs with DMVD and presumably is associated with mitral (or tricuspid) valve prolapse. A mitral or tricuspid (if louder on the right) click can be the first audible sign of degenerative valvular disease, usually before a murmur develops (**Figure 29.7**). The click might be fixed or vary in timing during systole, and multiple clicks might be heard. Many of these dogs will show valvular regurgitation if examined by color Doppler, although this information is of little incremental clinical value. A systolic click also might be heard concurrently with the MR murmur in some dogs. It is important to differentiate a systolic click from a gallop sound. Gallop sounds occur during diastole and in dogs, usually signal heart failure. Clicks are higher pitched and systolic in timing (p. 231). In some dogs

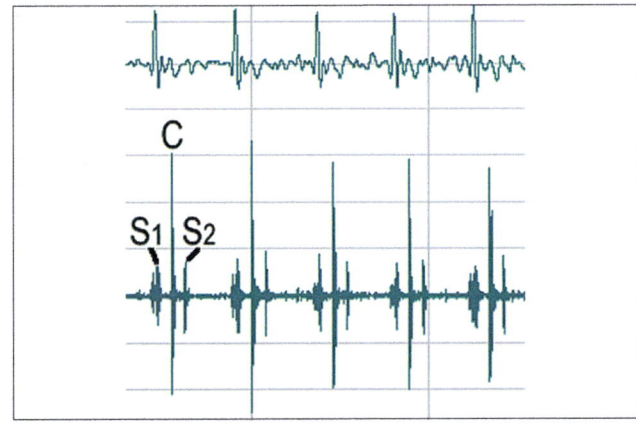

Figure 29.7 Phonocardiogram (bottom) depicts a loud mid-systolic click (C), but no murmur in a 6-year-old female Cavalier King Charles Spaniel with early degenerative mitral valve disease. The ECG (top) shows sinus rhythm, with much baseline artifact.

with advanced DMVD and myocardial dysfunction, an S_3 gallop sound might be evident at the left apex as a soft "thud" immediately following the murmur. However, this can be difficult to appreciate because the loud systolic murmur tends to "distract" the ear, and the S_3 can be confused with the second heart sound, which usually is obscured at the apex. A TR murmur is similar to that of MR, but is loudest at the tricuspid valve area (right apex). The presence of jugular vein pulsations, a precordial thrill over the right apex, and a different quality to the murmur heard over the tricuspid region can help the clinician differentiate TR from a MR murmur that radiates to the right chest wall.

Loud breath sounds and soft inspiratory crackles, especially in the ventral lung fields, develop with pulmonary edema. Fulminant pulmonary edema is likely to cause widespread inspiratory, as well as early expiratory, crackles and expiratory wheezes. However, concurrent primary pulmonary disease (especially interstitial fibrosis) can produce loud, coarse crackles or other abnormal lung sounds in some dogs with MR, so the presence of these sounds does not necessarily indicate CHF. Sinus tachycardia is common (although not always present) with CHF because of heightened sympathetic tone. Conversely, a pronounced sinus arrhythmia with normal heart rate often accompanies chronic pulmonary disease. Pleural effusion usually attenuates pulmonary sounds along the ventral thorax, but this is relatively uncommon in DMVD.

A "clinical severity score" was proposed to predict the likelihood of subsequent cardiac death from DMVD based on the number of certain historical and physical exam findings that were identified as independent risk factors on multivariate analysis. These include: history of cough, exercise intolerance, decreased appetite, breathlessness, syncope, murmur louder than 3/6, heart rate exceeding 135 beats/minute, and presence of regular sinus rhythm (rather than sinus arrhythmia). Progressively higher scores (greater number of factors present) appear to be moderately accurate in predicting future death from CHF (López-Alvarez, 2015). Maintaining normal sinus arrhythmia was a negative predictor for CHF in this study. Other prognostic indicators are discussed later (p. 565).

Several other diseases sometimes are confused with advanced DMVD and CHF, especially in dogs with a prominent heart murmur but otherwise compensated disease. These include tracheal collapse, chronic bronchitis, bronchomalacia with bronchial collapse, bronchiectasis, pulmonary fibrosis, pulmonary neoplasia, pneumonia, pharyngitis, heartworm disease, DCM in larger breeds, and infective endocarditis. The cough caused by major airway collapse often is described as a "honking" cough.

Complicating Factors

Various outcomes and complications provoke acute and chronic clinical signs in dogs with previously compensated DMVD. The most common problems are exercise intolerance, subtle weight loss, and the respiratory signs of tachypnea, distress, and cough caused by pulmonary edema or airway compression. Rupture of diseased chordae tendineae can acutely increase regurgitant volume and sometimes precipitates fulminant pulmonary edema, with or without low cardiac output signs (p. 562). As previously noted, ascites usually occurs with some combination of PH, severe TR, or AF and is frequently associated with cardiac cachexia. Chronic respiratory disease is another common complicating factor. Although LA enlargement extensive enough to impinge on a mainstem bronchus can stimulate persistent coughing in the absence of CHF, bronchial narrowing and collapse often are associated with concurrent inflammatory airway disease (p. 563).

Exertional collapse and syncope occur in many dogs, as well. These acute signs of low cardiac output could indicate progressive valvular regurgitation, severe PH, or a tachyarrhythmia that reduces cardiac output. Besides potentially precipitating pulmonary edema or collapse, tachyarrhythmias also increase myocardial oxygen demand. Frequent atrial premature beats, focal atrial tachycardias, and AF are the most common arrhythmias in dogs with DMVD, but ventricular tachyarrhythmias also occur in some dogs. Sudden bradycardia, especially with excitement, might represent an exaggerated neurocardiogenic (vasovagal) response and can cause weakness or syncope in some dogs. PH is a common consequence or independent comorbidity in dogs with advanced DMVD (p. 537, p. 561, and Chapter 39). A full-thickness LA tear typically causes intrapericardial bleeding; depending on the presence and severity of acute cardiac tamponade, it can cause transient weakness or profound hypotension, collapse and death (p. 562). **Table 29.3** lists some additional causes of CHF decompensation and low output signs.

Table 29.3 Some Complicating Factors in Degenerative Mitral Valve Disease.

For Acutely Worsened Pulmonary Edema and Congestion, Consider:

- Arrhythmias
  - Frequent atrial premature complexes
  - Paroxysmal atrial/supraventricular tachycardia
  - Atrial fibrillation
  - Ventricular tachyarrhythmias
  - Severe bradyarrhythmia (reflex-mediated or another cause)
  - Consider possibility of drug-induced exacerbation
- Ruptured chordae tendineae
- Iatrogenic volume overload
  - Excessive volume of IV fluid or blood transfusion
  - High-sodium fluids
- Excessive salt intake (food or liquid source)
- Erratic or improper medication administration
- Insufficient medication dosage for stage of disease
- Increased cardiac workload
  - Physical exertion
  - Anemia
  - Infections/sepsis
  - Hypertension
  - Disease of other organ systems (including pulmonary, renal, liver, endocrine)
  - Hyperthyroidism (usually iatrogenic in dogs)
  - Hot, humid or excessively cold environment
  - Other environmental stresses
- Moderate to severe pulmonary hypertension
- Myocardial (contractility) failure

For Signs of Weakness or Collapse, Consider:

- Arrhythmias (see above)
- Severe mitral or tricuspid regurgitation; worsening heart failure
- Pulmonary hypertension
- Ruptured chordae tendineae
- Cough-syncope
- Left atrial tear
  - Intrapericardial bleeding with cardiac tamponade
- Increased cardiac workload (see above)
- Medications (especially diuretics and vasodilators)

Diagnostic Tests

Clinical Laboratory Tests

Clinical laboratory data can be normal, or might reflect changes consistent with CHF, the effects of medications, or concurrent extracardiac disease. Given the older age of most dogs with DMVD, renal dysfunction and other systemic diseases are common. Dogs with severe CHF can have elevated serum pancreatic lipase immunoreactivity, presumably related to poor tissue perfusion. Elevated serum C-reactive protein concentrations have been observed in advanced DMVD with

CHF. Serum homocysteine concentration was positively correlated with DMVD severity, as well as with cTnI and creatinine concentrations, systolic BP, and LA/Ao ratio. Some of these parameters also are risk factors for CHF.

Circulating natriuretic peptide concentrations tend to reflect increasing disease severity; however, this is a generality and initiation of therapy never should be based only on natriuretic peptide results. High N-terminal probrain natriuretic peptide (NT-proBNP) concentration is associated with more severe disease and increased risk for CHF, with concentrations ≥1500 pmol/L being an independent risk factor for first onset CHF (PREDICT study, Reynolds, 2012). Dogs with N-terminal proatrial natriuretic peptide (NT-proANP) concentrations >1000 pmol/L had a median time to CHF onset of 11 months, compared to about 4½ years for dogs with concentrations ≤1000 pmol/L (Eriksson, 2014). Circulating natriuretic peptide concentrations typically are high in dogs with overt CHF, especially those with more severe failure. Decreasing NT-proBNP concentration following CHF therapy might have prognostic value in dogs with DMVD; values <965 pmol/L post-therapy have been associated with longer survival time (Wolf, 2012). In people with CHF, treatment protocols aimed at reducing NT-proBNP improve clinical outcome. In dogs with DMVD and stable CHF, diuretic and pimobendan dose escalation can decrease NT-proBNP concentrations within a few weeks (Hezzell, 2018). It should be noted, however, that elevated plasma NT-proBNP concentrations sometimes are found in healthy dogs and that breed differences must be considered (Sjöstrand, 2014). Impaired renal function is known to increase natriuretic peptide levels and intact females tend to have higher NT-proBNP compared to intact males. Controlled exercise testing has shown that NT-proBNP concentration increases, compared to pre-exercise baseline, in healthy dogs as well as in those with preclinical DMVD, although increases are more pronounced in the latter (Wall, 2018). Nevertheless, progressive MR leads to increased myocardial stretch and higher levels of natriuretic peptides; it is quite common in specialty practice to see dogs with values >2000 pmol/L yet not be in overt CHF. Thus, natriuretic peptide tests are useful for staging and for assessing risk for CHF, but are themselves insufficient for establishing a diagnosis of CHF or compelling therapy.

Cardiac troponins are biomarkers for myocardial cell injury or necrosis. Currently, these assays are not routinely performed in dogs with DMVD. A number of studies have evaluated cTnI concentrations in dogs with chronic MR, mostly using standard assays. Mild cTnI elevation occurs with exercise in some dogs with DMVD. Usually though, increased cTnI concentrations are confined to dogs with moderate to severe DMVD, especially when clinical signs are progressive. Persistently elevated cTnI has been associated with worsening clinical status, increased cardiac size, and MR severity. Yet, one study of dogs with CHF reported that decreasing cTnI concentration over time was associated with higher risk for cardiac death (Chan, 2019). Increased cTnI could be a marker for myocardial fibrosis in chronic heart disease; cTnI also is increased in advanced DMVD with PH, especially in patients showing clinical decompensation. However, cTnI elevations can occur with renal disease, age, and also with increasing C-reactive protein.

Plasma lactate concentration can rise in dogs with CHF, consistent with some level of tissue hypoperfusion. In people with heart failure, iron deficiency and anemia are associated with poorer outcomes. Concurrent renal disease is a common comorbidity, often made worse by diuretic therapy and RAAS inhibition. The relationship among these factors in dogs with DMVD is less defined. However, in dogs with DMVD low serum iron concentration is most likely to occur in those with advanced disease and acute CHF (Savarese, 2018).

Radiography

Thoracic radiography is recommended when a moderately loud (3/6) MR murmur is first discovered, in order to establish a baseline for the individual patient and assess hemodynamic significance. This is especially important given the normal variation in cardiac shape and size among breeds (Chapter 3). Radiographs in dogs with early (stage B1) DMVD typically are within normal limits. Progressive LA and then LV enlargement develop as MR severity increases. This gradually elevates the trachea and left mainstem bronchus dorsally (**Figures 29.8–29.11**; also **Figure 3.13**, p. 56). The vertebral heart size (VHS; p. 47) and vertebral LA size (VLAS) increase with the growing volume overload. However, especially in early disease, VHS does not always correlate well with echocardiographic evidence for cardiac enlargement. In coughing dogs with DMVD, a VHS ≤11.4v suggests a non-cardiac cause; dogs with cardiac or mixed-origin cough tend to have higher VHS. One retrospective study of stage B dogs found a VHS >11.7 to be specific for predicting echocardiographic left heart enlargement sufficient to meet stage B2 status, while a VHS ≤10.8 excluded dogs with such enlargement; however, the VHS for over 40% of the study dogs was in between these values (Poad, 2020). Cardiac size, as indicated by VHS as well as echocardiographic LA and LV dimensions, increases most rapidly within the 6–12 months (and especially the last few months) preceding CHF onset. Practically, a VHS "velocity" (rate of change/month) of ~0.1 vertebral body unit/month often predicts high risk for pulmonary edema.

Left mainstem bronchus elevation and ventrodorsal narrowing commonly occur in dogs with severe LA dilation. Fluoroscopy can show dynamic mainstem bronchus collapse associated with coughing, or even quiet breathing, in such cases (**Figure 9.4**, p. 205). On dorsoventral (DV) view, LA enlargement tends to increase the angle formed by the bifurcation of the main bronchi (sometimes called the "bow-legged cowboy sign"). However, this angle is not a highly

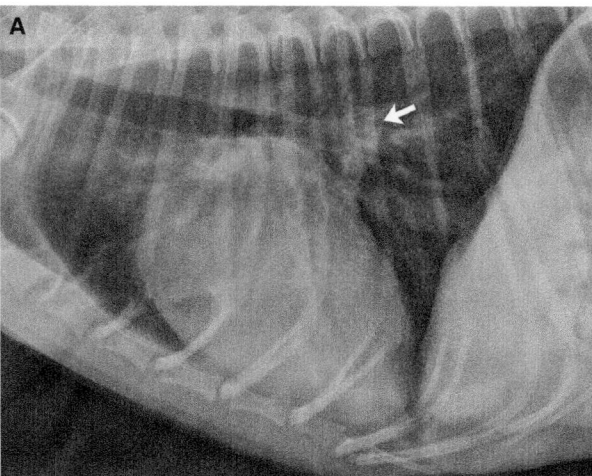
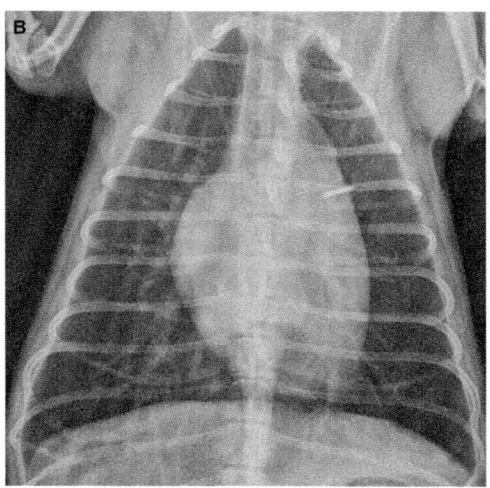

Figure 29.8 Lateral (A) and dorsoventral (B) thoracic radiographs from a 9-year-old male Maltese with stage B2 degenerative mitral valve disease show mild cardiomegaly (VHS 10.9v), with mild to moderate left atrial enlargement (A, arrow). There is no evidence for cardiac decompensation. A microchip is visible over the left cranial aspect of the heart (B).

sensitive indicator of LA enlargement because of its variability and the degree of overlap between dogs with normal and enlarged left atria.

LA size can be estimated using a vertebral heart scoring system (Malcolm, 2018). On right or left lateral view, VLAS is determined by extending a line from the center of the most ventral aspect of the carina to the most caudal aspect of the LA, where it joins the dorsal border of the caudal vena cava (**Figure 29.12**). From the cranial edge of the 4th thoracic vertebra, a line of the same length is extended parallel to the spine (as for the VHS method); the VLAS often is expressed in vertebral body units (v) to the nearest 0.1 vertebra, although some advocate using fractions of 0.25 vertebra. The VLAS showed moderately good correlation with echocardiographic LA/Ao ratios in that study, with a VLAS ≥2.3 to 2.5 suggesting LA enlargement. Two other studies in small-breed dogs with preclinical DMVD (Stepien, 2020; Mikawa, 2020) evaluated the utility of VLAS for differentiating stage B1 from stage B2 disease, as defined by echocardiographic criteria of (short-axis) LA/Ao ≥1.6 and normalized LV internal diameter in diastole (LVIDdN) ≥1.7 (Boswood, 2016). In both studies, VLAS correlated well with the echocardiographic LA/Ao ratio and also with LVIDdN. Based on receiver operator characteristic analysis, both studies identified an "optimal" VLAS cut-off of

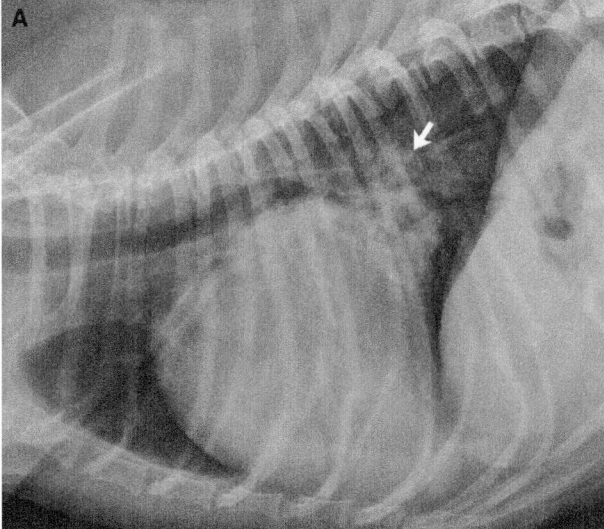
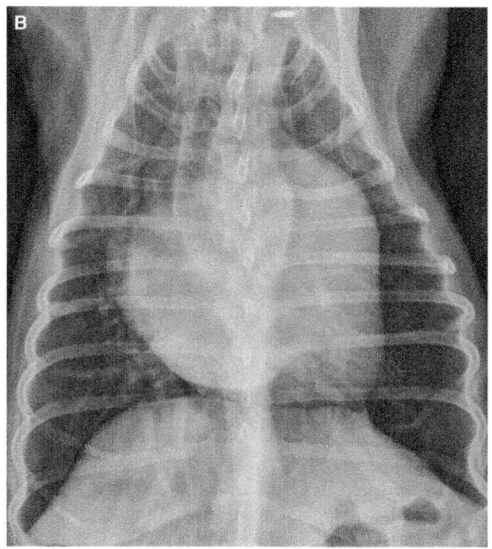

Figure 29.9 Lateral (A) and dorsoventral (B) thoracic radiographs from a 7-year-old male Shih Tzu with stage C degenerative mitral valve disease. Pulmonary edema has resolved, although mild pulmonary venous congestion persists (A, see cranial lobar vessels). Moderate generalized cardiomegaly with dorsal tracheal displacement, narrowed mainstem bronchi, and a large left atrial bulge (A, arrow) are present. There is fluid in the caudal esophagus.

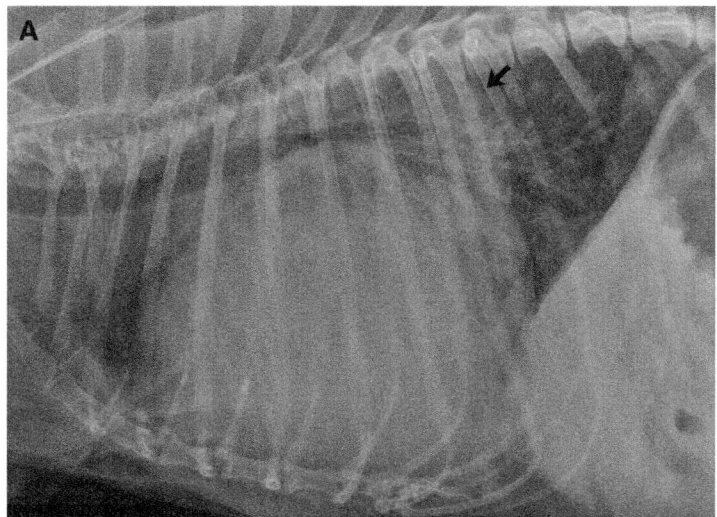

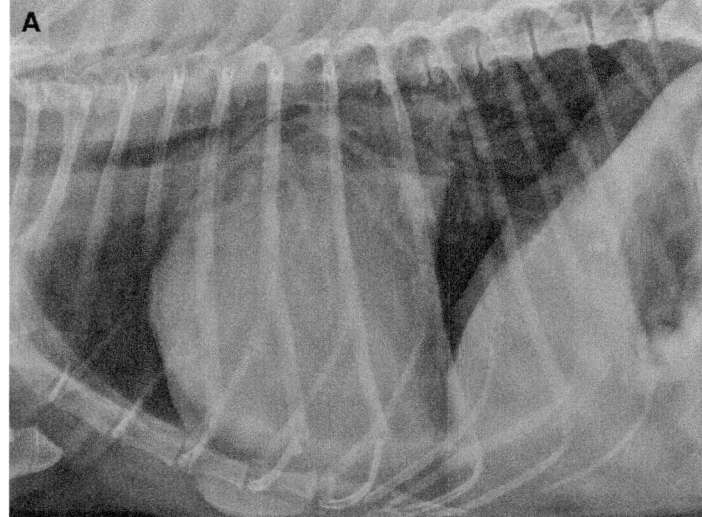

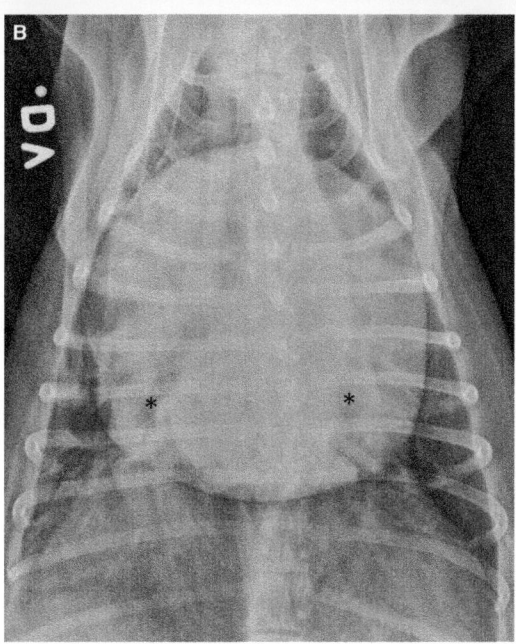

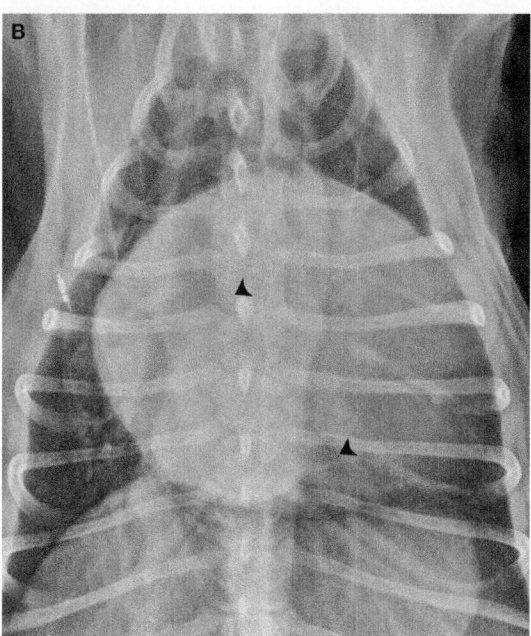

Figure 29.10 Radiographs show massive enlargement of the cardiac silhouette (VHS ~15.5v) in a 12-year-old male Cocker Spaniel with advanced degenerative mitral valve disease, atrial fibrillation, pulmonary hypertension, and moderate tricuspid regurgitation. (A) Lateral projection shows the huge left atrium (LA, arrow) abutting the spine and compressing the carina and mainstem bronchi. (B) On DV view, the mainstem bronchi (*) are widely separated as they curve around the LA. The left bronchus is harder to see because of greater compression by the LA. Pulmonary lobar arteries and veins are enlarged, consistent with both venous congestion and pulmonary hypertension. There is no evidence for pulmonary edema. The dog had (only) a minimal volume of pericardial effusion.

Figure 29.11 Right lateral (A) and DV (B) radiographs from an 11-year-old male mixed-breed dog presented for increased cough frequency. There is severe left atrial and ventricular enlargement, with marked dorsal airway compression (A), but no evidence for pulmonary edema. Although the positioning is slightly rotated (B), the compressed left mainstem bronchus seems to disappear from just distal to the carina to the caudal left atrial border (between arrowheads). See **Figure 3.13** (p. 56) for left lateral view from this case.

≥2.5v for distinguishing stage B2 from B1 dogs; however, a VLAS ≥3.0 or 3.1v had much better specificity (96 or 100%, respectively) for identifying small-breed dogs with LA/Ao ≥1.6 and LVIDdN ≥1.7. In addition, the combination radiographic variable of VHS + VLAS showed maximum specificity at ≥14.75v (positive predictive value, 93%) for identifying true stage B2 disease in small-breed dogs (Stepien, 2020).

Mild to moderate MR alone generally does not cause right heart enlargement. Because LV enlargement usually is more dominant, and the enlarging left heart can compress and displace the right heart, an increase in sternal contact on lateral view is not a reliable sign of right heart enlargement in DMVD. Nevertheless, variable right-sided cardiomegaly occurs with chronic TR, as well as PH.

Pulmonary venous congestion is a common early sign of left-sided CHF, so the diameter of lobar pulmonary veins

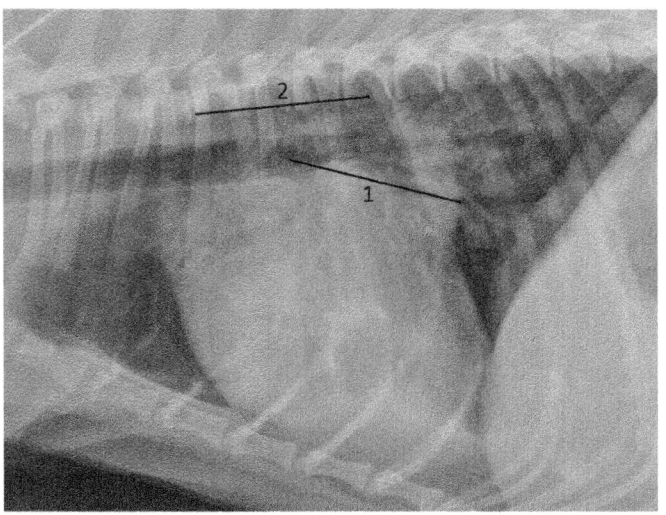

Figure 29.12 Method of vertebral left atrial size (VLAS) measurement, using a right lateral projection from an 11-year-old female Cavalier King Charles Spaniel-Maltese mix. A line (1) is drawn from the center of the most ventral aspect of the carina to the caudal aspect of the left atrium, where it joins the dorsal border of the caudal vena cava. A line of the same length (2) is extended caudally from the cranial edge of the 4th thoracic vertebra; this represents the VLAS (expressed in vertebral-body units to the nearest 0.1 vertebra, v). The VLAS in this dog is 3.6v.

should be compared with that of their accompanying artery (**Figure 3.17D**, p. 60). However, venous size must be interpreted with some caution. For example, on left lateral view the cranial pulmonary vein often is slightly larger than its accompanying pulmonary artery; if this is not also evident on the right lateral projection, it might be normal variation. Additionally, regurgitant jets sometimes directly enter pulmonary veins; this can distend the affected veins, as seen by echocardiography. Nevertheless, if multiple pulmonary veins are wider than their satellite arteries, a presumptive diagnosis of pulmonary congestion can be made. In dogs with moderately severe DMVD, the right caudal pulmonary vein often is larger than in normal dogs. A ratio of right caudal pulmonary vein diameter to 9th rib diameter (where they cross) that is >1.22 was suggested to indicate venous congestion, because in about two-thirds of normal dogs the vein slightly exceeds 9th rib diameter (Oui, 2014).

Pulmonary vascular definition diminishes as lung edema begins to accumulate. Progressive interstitial and then alveolar fluid infiltrates accumulate as edema worsens. Although the radiographic distribution of cardiogenic pulmonary edema in dogs classically is described as perihilar, dorsocaudal, and bilaterally symmetric, many dogs have an asymmetrical pattern (**Figure 29.13**; also **Figures 3.19–3.21**, pp. 62 & 63). Asymmetry might relate to differences in pulmonary lymphatic drainage or in the angulation of the MR jet, although some clinicians dispute the latter. In one report, an asymmetric pulmonary edema pattern was associated with eccentric MR jet angulation, while symmetric edema opacities were present in dogs with a centrally oriented MR

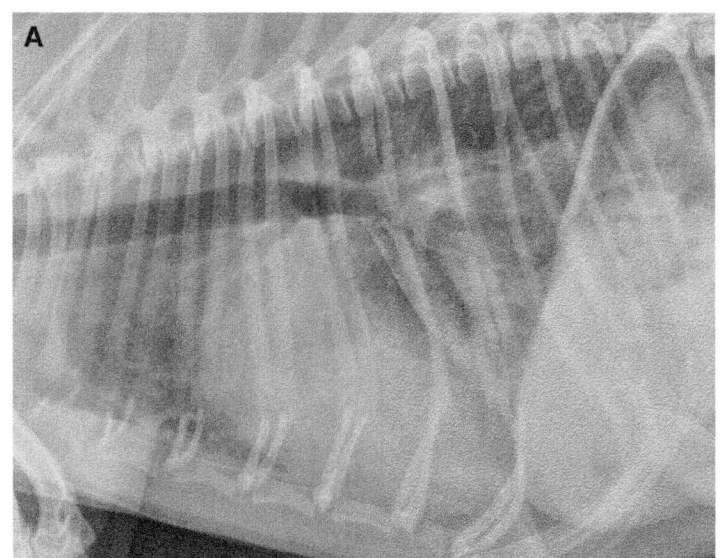
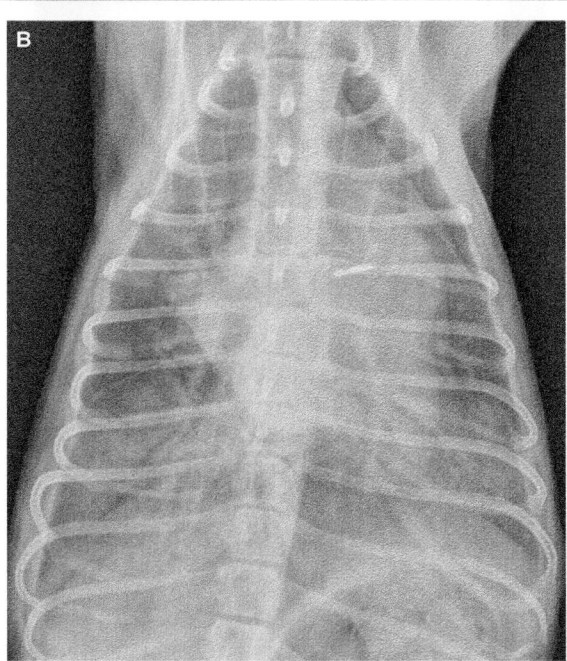

Figure 29.13 Lateral (A) and dorsoventral (B) radiographs from the dog of **Figure 29.8**, three months later, after the onset of respiratory distress caused by congestive heart failure. The increase in pulmonary opacity is widespread, although most intense in the caudodorsal lung fields. Several air bronchograms are evident, especially in the right caudal lobe (B). A pleural fissure line is visible between the right middle and caudal lung lobes. The caudal vena cava is border-effaced.

jet (Diana, 2009). However, other factors might be relevant considering that venous drainage from caudal left and right (and accessory) lung lobes enter the canine left atrium as a confluence, yet asymmetric patterns most often are observed in the right caudal lobe. The presence and severity of pulmonary edema do not necessarily correlate with the degree of cardiomegaly. Acute, severe MR (for example, precipitated by chordae tendineae rupture) can produce widespread cardiogenic edema with minimal LA enlargement. High hydrostatic capillary pressures can cause pulmonary capillary membrane rupture; alveolar infiltrates with a granular appearance suggest red blood cells within alveolar spaces. Conversely, MR that worsens slowly can lead to massive LA enlargement without evidence for congestive failure. Small pleural effusions, evident as prominent fissure lines, also are common in acute, severe left-sided CHF. Initial signs of right-sided CHF include caudal vena caval distension, prominent pleural fissure lines, and hepatomegaly; subsequently, ascites develops and occasionally, a more prominent pleural effusion.

Electrocardiography

An increase in mean heart rate, or overt sinus tachycardia, is present in many dogs with symptomatic DMVD, although anxiety associated with the clinic visit might underlie this in some without CHF. Arrhythmias also are common with advanced disease and they could precipitate clinical signs (**Table 29.3**). Supraventricular tachyarrhythmias, such as frequent premature complexes, paroxysmal or sustained supraventricular tachycardia, and AF are more likely with LA enlargement and CHF (**Figures 29.14** and **29.15**). Dogs with AF have increased likelihood of developing ascites and pleural effusion, especially when moderate to severe TR exists (Ward, 2018). Ventricular tachyarrhythmias are common in dogs with advanced DMVD, compared to those with preclinical disease. Some QT interval prolongation often accompanies ventricular dilation in dogs with DMVD, although the

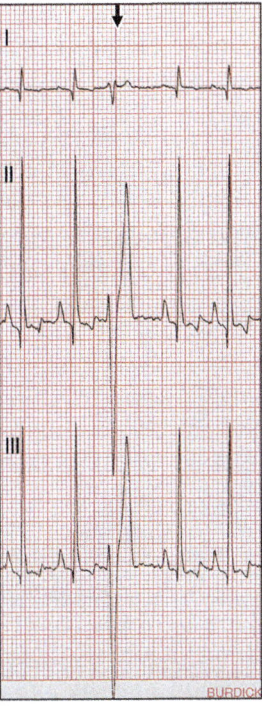

Figure 29.16 ECG from a 14-year-old mixed-breed dog with degenerative mitral valve disease shows sinus rhythm with a ventricular premature complex (arrow). Wide P waves (~0.07 sec) suggest left atrial enlargement. Tall R waves (~3.7 mV) and wide QRS complexes (~0.07 sec) suggest left ventricular enlargement. Leads I, II, & III; 25 mm/s, 1 cm = 1 mV.

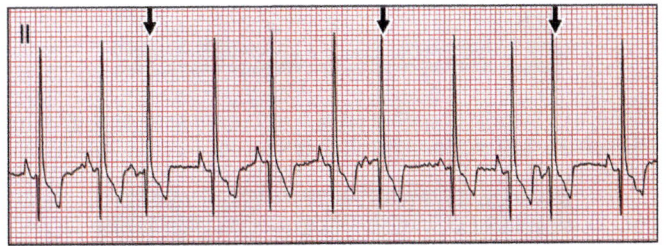

Figure 29.14 Sinus rhythm, with atrial premature complexes (arrows), and wide P waves (~0.06 sec) in a 9-year-old female Miniature Schnauzer with degenerative mitral valve disease, mild pulmonary edema, cough and syncope. Lead II, 25 mm/s, 1 cm = 1 mV.

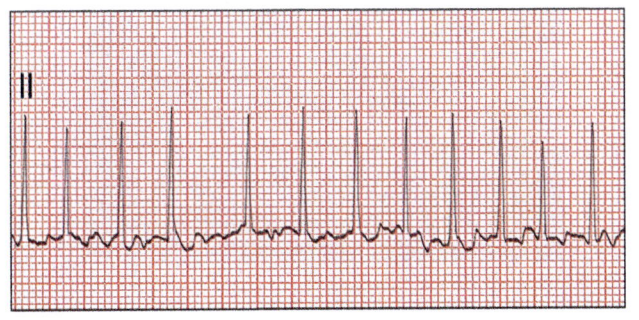

Figure 29.15 Atrial fibrillation in a geriatric dog with long-standing degenerative mitral valve disease. Lead II, 25 mm/s, 1 cm = 1 mV.

effects of increasing heart rate could mask this. Calculating a heart rate corrected QT (QTc) could help reveal this, especially on serial ECGs in individual patients. In addition to QT prolongation, variability or instability in the repolarization process (QT instability) increases with disease severity and CHF (Brüler, 2018). This can magnify the risk for ventricular arrhythmias and sudden death.

The ECG is much less sensitive than echocardiography for detecting cardiac chamber enlargement. Although criteria for LA or biatrial enlargement and LV dilation (p. 156 and **Figures 29.14** and **29.16**) are classic ECG changes, they often are absent. Occasionally, an S wave in Lead I or other finding characteristic of RV enlargement is present in dogs with severe TR.

Echocardiography

Echocardiography can reveal valve structural changes, chamber enlargement and remodeling, severity of valvular regurgitation, alterations in ventricular function, and estimates of intracardiac pressures. An experienced echocardiographer not only can verify the cause of the patient's murmur and quantitate chamber dimensions, but also can provide information about complicating factors such as the presence of PH, RV dysfunction, deteriorating myocardial contractility, and abnormal diastolic function and filling pressures.

Increased preload and reduced afterload in primary MR can obfuscate the assessment of myocardial contractility and ventricular systolic and diastolic functions.

Left Heart Evaluation In early DMVD, the echo exam is likely to show only mild mitral leaflet thickening, with or without a small MR jet, and normal chamber sizes. As the disease progresses, affected valve cusps become thicker and might appear knobby (**Figures 29.17-29.18**). Smooth thickening is characteristic of DMVD, in contrast to the rough and irregular vegetative valve lesions typical of infective endocarditis (p. 599). In some cases however, it can be impossible to differentiate between degenerative and infective thickening with echocardiography. Mild mitral prolapse occurs with early DMVD in some dogs. Mitral prolapse is more common in males and older dogs; it usually involves the anterior or both leaflets, rather than posterior alone. Due to the saddle shape of the mitral valve, prolapse is best assessed from the right parasternal long-axis position, although severe prolapse will be obvious in apical views, as well (**Figures 29.19-29.20**). Prolapse severity tends to increase with worsening MR and heart failure status, and in some cases, might stem from small chordal ruptures. Sometimes, a ruptured chord or flail leaflet tip is evident during systole (**Figure 29.21**). When a leaflet tip points or bends towards the dorsal atrial wall in systole, a chordal rupture is highly likely. Similarly, eversion of the anterior mitral leaflet towards the aortic valve in diastole is a proven sign of chordal rupture. With high quality, fast frame-rate 2D imaging, small cords often are observed flipping above the valve leaflet into the left atrium. Mitral leaflet prolapse also might be caused by (probably secondary or tertiary) chordal rupture, although this has not been established.

Echocardiography documents the degree of atrial and ventricular dilation secondary to the chronic volume overload

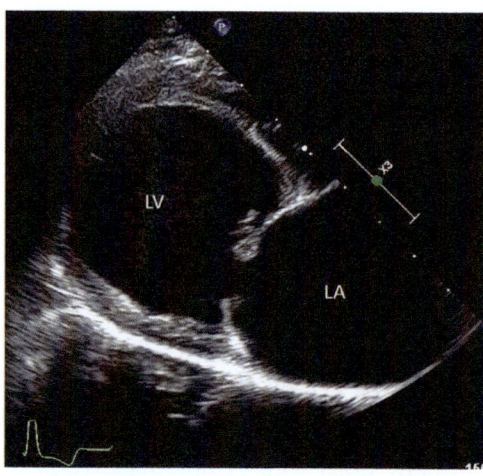

Figure 29.18 The mitral leaflets are markedly thickened and knobby in this 9-year-old female Cavalier King Charles Spaniel with compensated stage D mitral valve disease, pulmonary hypertension, and severe left heart dilation. Right parasternal long-axis, diastole. LA, left atrium; LV, left ventricle.

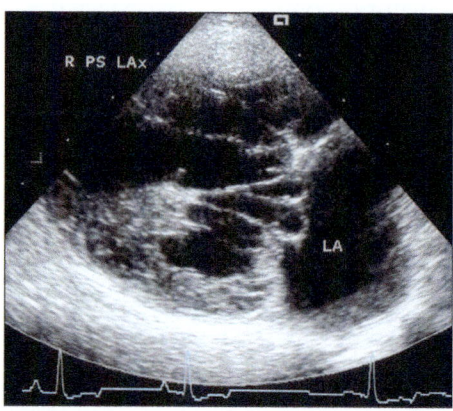

Figure 29.19 Systolic frame showing two areas of mitral prolapse in a terrier. Right parasternal long-axis. LA, left atrium.

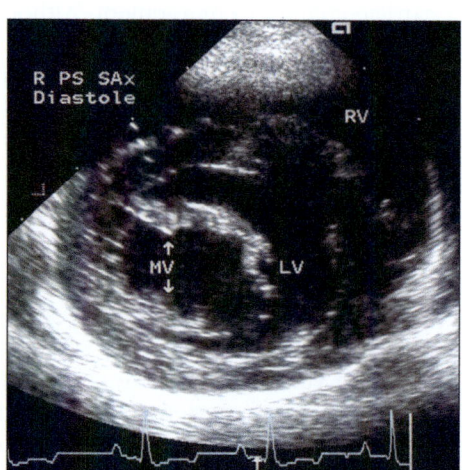

Figure 29.17 2D image in diastole, from a 16-year-old female terrier-mix, shows thickening of both mitral leaflets. Right parasternal short-axis. LV, left ventricle; MV, mitral valve; RV, right ventricle.

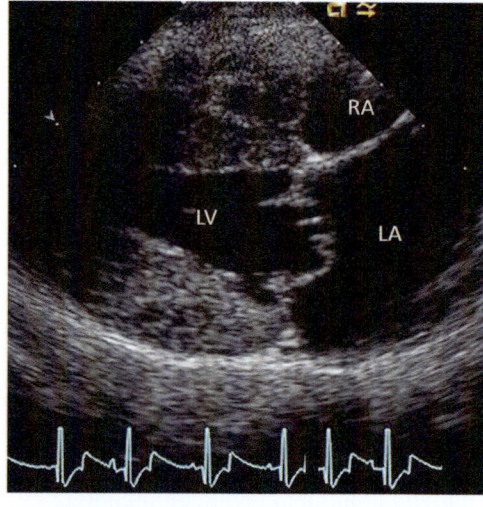

Figure 29.20 Prominent systolic mitral valve prolapse in an older Cavalier King Charles Spaniel with degenerative mitral valve disease, moderately enlarged LA, and early congestive heart failure. Right parasternal long-axis view. LA, left atrium; LV, left ventricle; RA, right atrium.

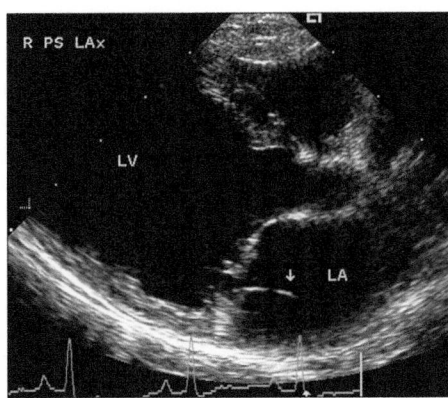

Figure 29.21 Flail mitral chord (arrow) in an older male Maltese with pulmonary congestion. The LV is severely dilated. Right parasternal long-axis, early systole. LA, left atrium; LV, left ventricle.

of AV valve regurgitation. LA size and LA/Ao ratio increase with advancing DMVD severity and have been negatively correlated with clinical outcome (**Figures 29.22–29.25**). LA volume measurement might be more accurate than dimensions, especially as the LA remodels, because linear dimensions and LA/Ao ratio can overestimate atrial size in this situation. However, accurate LA volume determination is difficult and wide variations in LA volume index have been reported in normal dogs of different breeds. Several methods can be used to estimate LA size and function (p. 103). Reduced LA function accompanies advancing DMVD and increasing LA size. Based on echocardiographic area-length calculations of LA volumes, an active LA emptying fraction <24% appears to suggest the presence of CHF in dogs with DMVD. However, a maximum LA volume <2.25 mL/kg was highly sensitive and specific for excluding CHF (Hollmer, 2017). LA longitudinal strain during atrial contraction is reduced in DMVD dogs with CHF, compared to those with preclinical disease.

Much attention is directed to the left atrium in DMVD, yet LV diastolic volume also must increase as the ventricle collects both the normal venous return and the regurgitant volume. Based on the confidence intervals of the hazards in the EPIC clinical trial, normalized diastolic LV diameter actually was a better predictor of pimobendan benefit in dogs with

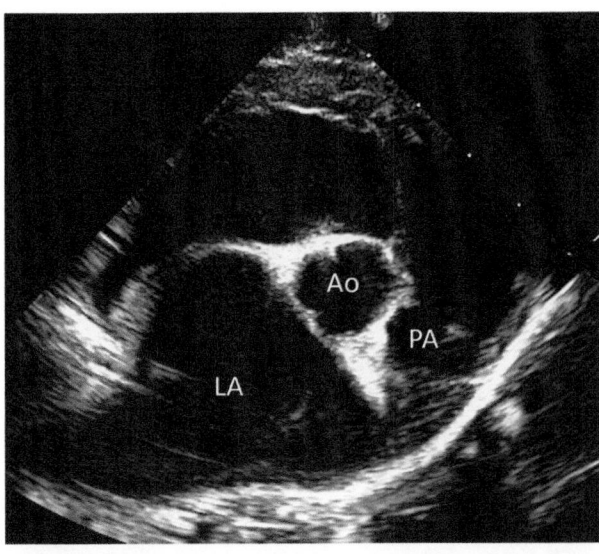

Figure 29.23 Severe left atrial enlargement (LA/Ao ~2.1) in a 10-year-old female Havanese with compensated stage C mitral valve disease. Right parasternal short-axis. Ao, aorta; LA, left atrium; PA, (proximal) pulmonary artery.

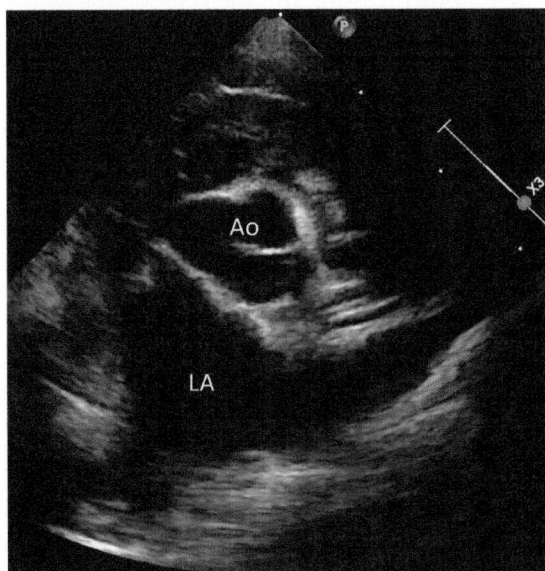

Figure 29.22 Minimal left atrial enlargement is present in this 15-year-old female Miniature Poodle with stage B1 mitral valve disease (LA/Ao ~1.5). Right parasternal short-axis view. Ao, aorta; LA, left atrium.

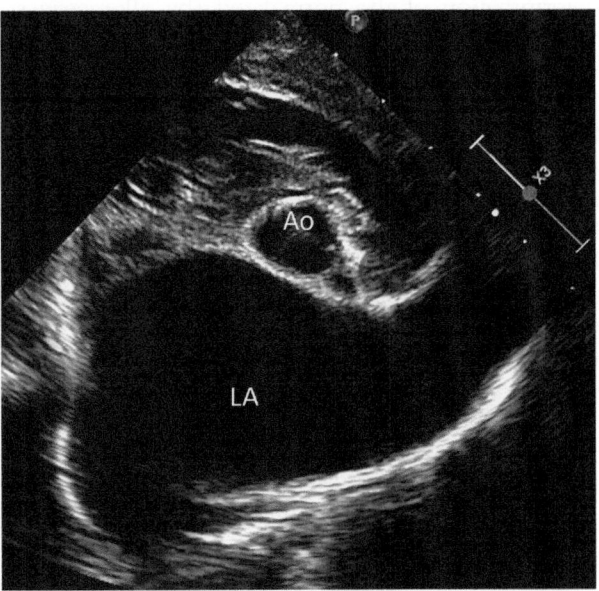

Figure 29.24 Massive left atrial enlargement (LA/Ao ~4) in a 9-year-old male mixed-breed dog with stage C degenerative mitral valve disease, mild congestive signs, and moderate pulmonary hypertension. Right parasternal short-axis view. Ao, aorta; LA, left atrium.

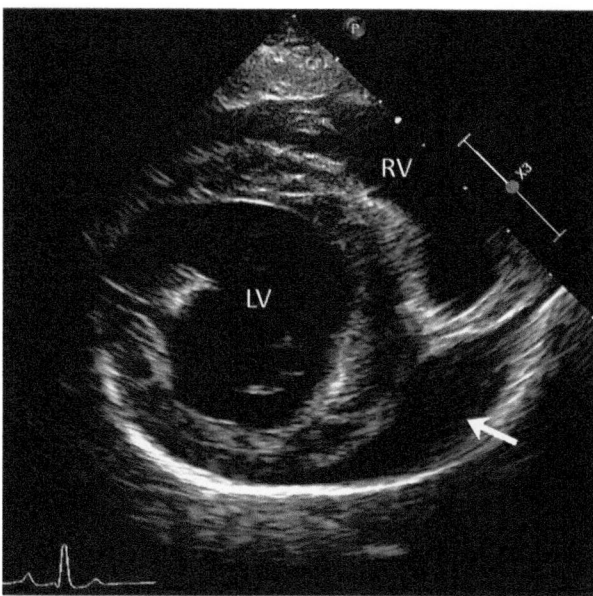

Figure 29.25 In dogs with severe left atrial enlargement, the distended left auricle (LAu) expands ventrally and cranially. During short-axis 2D imaging at the ventricular level, an enlarged LAu (arrow) might be misinterpreted as pericardial effusion. This image is from the dog of **Figure 29.11**, with stage B2 mitral valve disease. Right parasternal short-axis view. LV, left ventricle; RV, right ventricle.

stage B2 disease, compared to the LA/Ao (Boswood, 2016). In the PREDICT clinical trial, a ratio of diastolic LV internal dimension to aortic root diameter (LVIDd)/Ao) ≥3 was identified as an independent risk factor for first onset CHF (Reynolds, 2012). Increased LVIDd also has been associated with a negative outcome.

Determination of the normalized (by allometric scaling to body weight) LVIDd (LVIDdN or LVEDDN) is useful for identifying cardiomegaly, comparing serial examinations, and deciding if therapy should be initiated in the preclinical state. The LVIDdN used in the EPIC trial was based on a multibreed study with a large number of sighthounds; it used an allometric scaling exponent of 0.294, as LVEDdN = LVIDd (cm)/weight (kg)$^{0.294}$ (p. 95). A recent study of >6,000 dogs not classified as sighthounds suggested a scaling exponent of 0.32 might be more generalizable (Esser, 2020). Using those data, LVIDdN >1.65 indicates that "LV dilation" is present. The EPIC trial (using the 0.294 exponent) defined this entry criterion as LVIDdN ≥1.7; for a 10 kg dog, that would mean an LVIDd of 3.35 cm or greater. However, if the 0.32 exponent is used, a LVIDd of 3.55 cm would be needed to achieve an LVEDdN = 1.7. This 2 mm difference in minor dimension seems trivial, but for many dogs with stable DMVD, this dimension does not change by more than 1–2 mm in a year. The differences become proportionately greater with larger body sizes (for example, a 3 mm difference for a 15 kg dog). Anyone performing echocardiography should be intimately familiar with these details.

This degree of cardiomegaly might or might not concur with a patient's short-axis LA/Ao, and both chambers should be enlarged based on clinical trial criteria before any therapy is initiated (see "Management" section). Especially in dogs with preclinical disease, other indices can be more sensitive indicators of MR severity, compared to the short-axis LA/Ao ratio and LVIDdN, which are one-dimensional measures. Such indices include the calculated mitral regurgitant fraction, effective regurgitant orifice area (EROA), and ratio of MR flow to aortic flow. In one study, the one-dimensional measures were insensitive to MR severity at regurgitant fractions <50% (Larouche-Lebel, 2019). Furthermore, not until the EROA (normalized to body surface area) was ≥0.347 and MR/aortic flow ratio was ≥0.79 did a strong association between MR severity and LA/Ao ≥1.6 or normalized LVIDd ≥1.7 appear.

As the left ventricle enlarges secondary to progressively worsening MR, it becomes more spherical in shape. This occurs mainly near the mid-chamber and chordal levels, where the LVIDd and LVIDs (minor) dimensions are measured. This remodeling can foster overestimation of LV size, especially when the radius obtained from that measurement is cubed. Ventricular wall thickness typically is normal, although in advanced disease it might be somewhat reduced. However, the LVIDd/LV wall ratio often is significantly increased, especially in larger-breed dogs, which probably increases wall stress (afterload) based on LaPlace's relationship. The rate at which cardiac dimensions increase can be a useful indicator of impending CHF.

Comparisons of the right pulmonary vein and artery diameters, made from the right parasternal long-axis four-chamber view, can help clarify whether CHF is present in cases where this is unclear. Normally, the ratio of pulmonary vein to pulmonary artery diameters is about 1. An increased pulmonary vein diameter, where it joins the left atrium, is commonly observed; this can be explained by both the increase in venous pressure and the remodeling of the dorsal atrial septum and LA wall that often occurs with severe MR. A ratio >1.7 strongly predicted CHF in one study of dogs with varying stages of DMVD (Merveille, 2015). This pulmonary vein/artery ratio is especially useful in ruling out the risk for CHF, but it is emphasized that pulmonary vein size at that location depends on a number of factors.

The motion of LV wall and septum usually appears vigorous when MR is moderate to severe. The large LV diastolic volume and increasing filling pressures displace the ventricular septum toward the right ventricle in diastole; thus, the septum contracts from a more rightward location than normal. A septal systolic amplitude (the downward movement in mm) that exceeds LV freewall systolic amplitude is the opposite of normal, and an underappreciated feature of moderate to severe LV volume overload. In most cases, overall LV pump function is well-preserved. Little to no mitral E-point-septal separation and high shortening and ejection fractions are typical, even in the presence of CHF (**Figures 29.26–29.28**). Most small dogs die or are euthanatized before any obvious LV systolic dysfunction is measured (also see previous discussion). Although the diastolic LV dimension increases, the

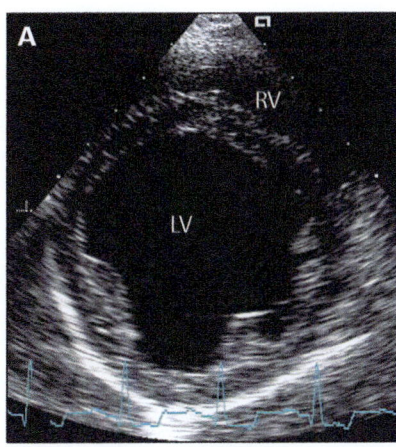 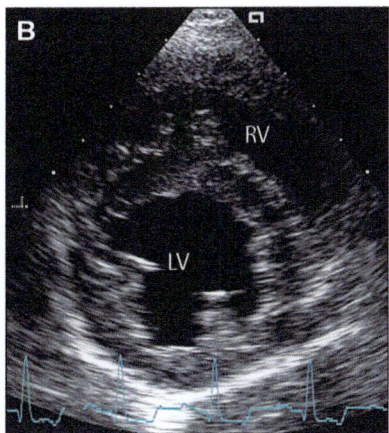

Figure 29.26 (A) End-diastolic 2D short-axis frame from an old dog with advanced degenerative mitral valve disease shows a dilated LV with normal wall thickness. (B) Systolic frame. Well-preserved systolic function, increased preload, and reduced afterload (from mitral regurgitation) yield vigorous ventricular wall motion and normal systolic chamber dimension. Right parasternal short-axis view. LV, left ventricle; RV, right ventricle.

concept of LV end-systolic volume index (ESVI) proposes that if myocardial contractility is normal the end-systolic volume (normalized to body size) should remain normal. As such, an increased ESVI obtained by a method of discs (see p. 104; or by 3D imaging) implies impaired myocardial contractility. However, use of an LV end-systolic linear dimension (as from M-mode examination) to derive the ESVI is unreliable once the LV dilates. Declining systolic function might be identified on serial echo exams, but progressive alterations in ventricular loading conditions can interfere with this detection.

Strain (deformation) imaging using 2D speckle tracking in dogs with DMVD has depicted increases in peak systolic and early diastolic radial and global circumferential strain. This reflects the hyperdynamic motion shown by increased LV fractional shortening, and implies well-preserved LV systolic function; although altered loading conditions, effects of compensatory mechanisms, or both could contribute. Reports conflict about the effects of DVMD on LV longitudinal strain and strain rate; increases might occur with moderate to severe disease, but in advanced heart failure with severe LA and LV enlargement there appears to be decline to levels similar to mildly affected dogs. Clinical benefit from detecting reduced strain in dogs with overt CHF is doubtful, unless prognostic value can be shown. Decreases observed during CHF tend to remain within reference limits or higher. Without serial exams, any decline will not be evident.

Color-flow Doppler imaging is the most sensitive way of demonstrating the presence of mitral or tricuspid regurgitation. Assessment should include at least three planes: parasternal long-axis, apical four chamber, and apical two chamber. Jets can appear quite different in these projections. The two chamber view is underutilized and often most effective for revealing the size of the regurgitant jet. Small jets of MR often are evident even in dogs without an obvious heart murmur, although such information is relevant only to breeders or people screening for the earliest onset of DMVD. It is more challenging to assess silent TR found by color Doppler imaging without 2D confirmation of tricuspid valve disease, because mild TR can be a physiologic event. Color Doppler shows the origin, direction, and extent of disturbed flow

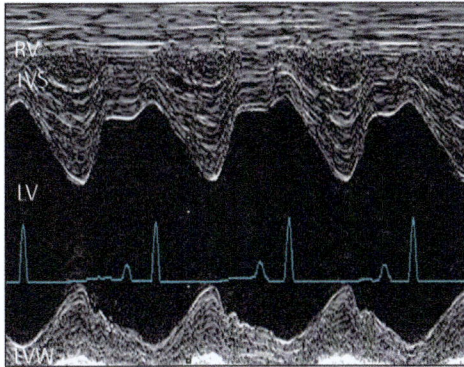

Figure 29.27 M-mode echo shows vigorous LVW and IVS motion, with high fractional shortening (57%), in an older mixed-breed dog with chronic mitral valve disease and normal systolic function. IVS, interventricular septum; LV, left ventricle; LVW, left ventricular wall; RV, right ventricle.

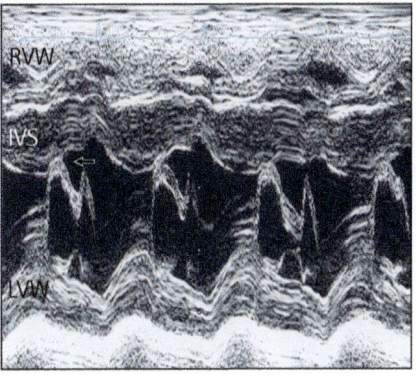

Figure 29.28 M-mode in an old Poodle shows thick septal (anterior) mitral leaflet echoes with virtually no E-point-septal separation (arrow), consistent with well-preserved LV systolic function. IVS, interventricular septum; LVW, left ventricular wall; RVW, right ventricular wall.

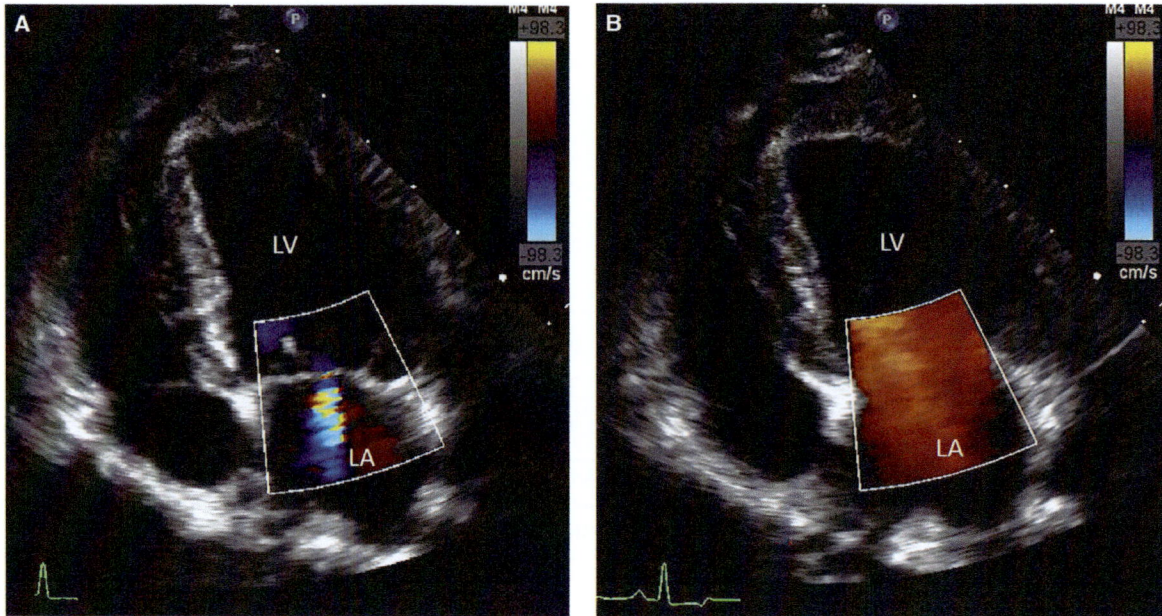

Figure 29.29 (A) Systolic color-flow Doppler image from a 3-year-old mixed-breed dog with stage B1 mitral valve disease and mild mitral regurgitation. The regurgitant jet causes only a small flow disturbance within the LA; the origin of the jet at the regurgitant orifice (vena contracta) is narrow. (B) Diastolic frame shows uniform low-velocity flow into the LV. Left apical view. LA, left atrium; LV, left ventricle.

entering the atrium (**Figures 29.29–29.31**). The flow disturbance always should be timed using spectral Doppler or color M-mode to prevent a false positive diagnosis of MR or TR, caused by presystolic regurgitation or valve closure signals, which can appear as a blue "flash" during 2D color imaging.

Additionally, color-flow Doppler allows semiquantitative assessment of MR severity based on analysis of the proximal isovelocity surface area (PISA), the width of the regurgitant jet at the valve annulus (vena contracta), and the atrial area affected by the disturbed flow pattern. However, without widespread availability of cardiac surgery for dogs, assessing the severity of MR from color Doppler (as opposed to the easily measured chamber remodeling) is of uncertain clinical value aside from acute chordal rupture, where remodeling

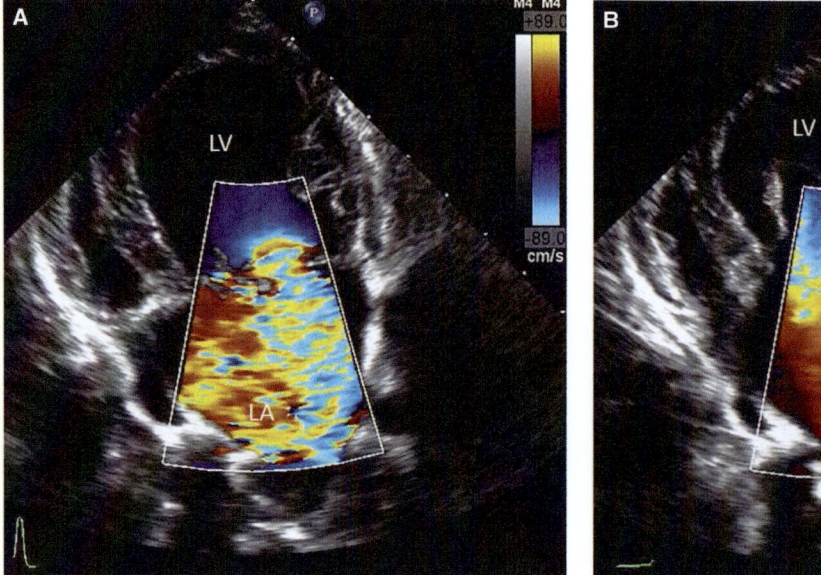
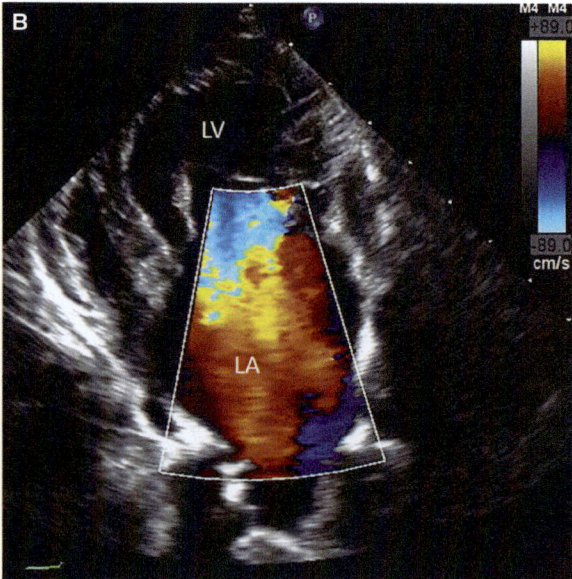

Figure 29.30 (A) Systolic color-flow Doppler image from a 9-year-old male mixed-breed dog with advanced degenerative mitral valve disease. The left heart is greatly dilated. Severe mitral regurgitation creates flow disturbance throughout the LA. The vena contracta is wide and there appears to be more than one regurgitant jet. The thickened valve leaflets are visible, surrounded by the color signal. (B) Diastolic frame shows early mitral inflow of increased velocity, with color aliasing. Left apical view. LA, left atrium; LV, left ventricle.

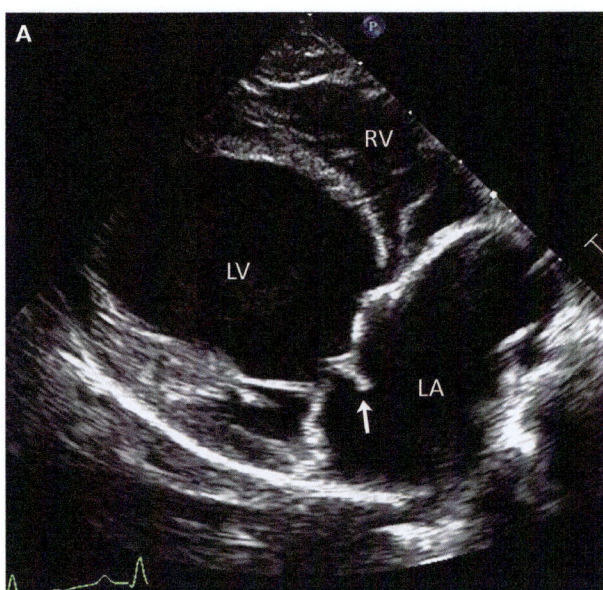 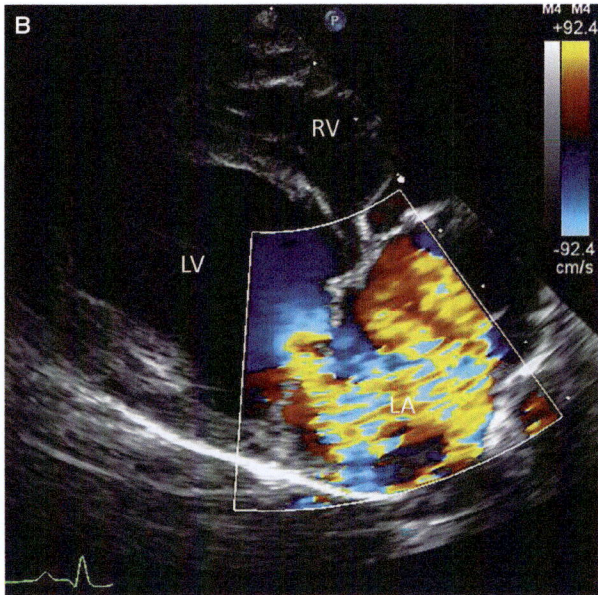

Figure 29.31 (A) Flail, thickened mitral leaflet tip (arrow) in a 10-year-old female Havanese with stage C degenerative mitral valve disease. (B) Color-flow image shows severe mitral regurgitation originating from the same area. The large jet of disturbed flow angles caudally then swirls around dorsocranially within the huge LA. Right parasternal long-axis view, systole. LA, left atrium; LV, left ventricle; RV, right ventricle.

might be minimal. Currently, therapy for preclinical DMVD is based on chamber remodeling, not color Doppler grading, although it is logical to use all available information when assessing severity. There are significant limitations to each of the color-Doppler approaches, especially the (atrial) receiving-chamber analysis (See Chapter 4). An eccentric jet that involves only a small area within the left atrium frequently is associated with moderate to severe LA dilation. Therefore, grading the severity of MR solely through receiving chamber analysis is discouraged. MR severity can vary with cardiac cycle length and systemic arterial BP. Additionally, ventricular ectopic contractions can magnify the degree of MR, which could relate to a change in cycle length or dyssynchronous papillary muscle function.

The PISA method has been described as a more accurate estimate of MR severity than the LA area of disturbed flow (see p. 121 and **Figure 4.36**). Flow acceleration occurs as blood moves toward the regurgitant orifice; at a specific distance (radius, "r") from the regurgitant orifice, a hemispheric surface at constant flow appears as the signal aliases. By measuring the "r" of this hemisphere (from valve orifice to aliased signal), the area of the hemisphere can be calculated ($2\pi r^2$). This area × the aliasing velocity = volume of regurgitant flow/second = instantaneous flow rate (cm^3/second). The effective regurgitant orifice area (EROA, in cm^2) = instantaneous flow rate/peak MR velocity, as measured by spectral Doppler. In addition, the regurgitant volume can be estimated as EROA × the velocity time integral (VTI) of the MR jet. But there are many assumptions and potential sources of inaccuracy with these calculations, especially if there are multiple MR jets, an angled jet flattened PISA hemisphere, MR velocity underestimation by an off-angle Doppler beam, and variable "r" during systole.

The EROA also could be calculated from the narrowest part of the proximal MR jet (the vena contracta) using 2D color-flow imaging. This is a relatively simple measurement, and has been correlated to concurrent remodeling. However, this vena contracta measurement assumes that the EROA is circular, which is unlikely. Evaluation using real-time 3D echo indicates that calculations using vena contracta diameter underestimate the EROA, especially as it enlarges (Tidholm, 2017). It is possible to assess MR severity using cardiac magnetic resonance imaging (MRI); however, this is largely impractical compared to echo indices and requires general anesthesia.

Continuous wave (CW) Doppler interrogation of MR peak velocity (**Figure 29.32**) verifies the timing of the flow

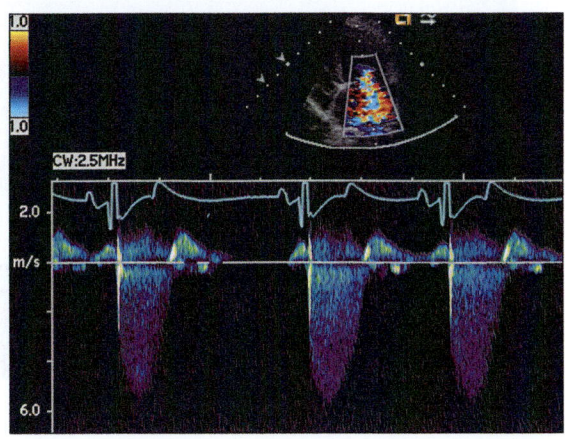

Figure 29.32 CW Doppler shows high-velocity mitral regurgitation (>5 m/s) in a geriatric dog with chronic mitral valve disease. Left apical view.

disturbance. It should be recorded from at least three planes to assure optimal alignment to regurgitant flow. The CW Doppler examination provides semiquantitative information about the severity of MR, in terms of a weak versus dense velocity spectrum and a rounded versus an early-peaking regurgitant profile (**Figure 4.37**, p. 124). CW Doppler also is used in the calculation of regurgitant orifice area by the PISA method. Theoretically, the maximal MR velocity can provide an approximation of systolic arterial BP (using the Bernoulli relationship); however, this method does not give consistent enough results to be used in lieu of BP measurement. Nevertheless, a maximum MR velocity of <4.5 m/s suggests either systemic hypotension, a high LA pressure, or both problems, and is compatible with severe regurgitation (or another cause of hypotension). A maximal MR velocity >6.5 m/s is an indication to reassess BP for systemic hypertension. The MR jet acceleration rate also could be used to estimate LV systolic function (dP/dt_{max}). Likewise, a crude index of ventricular relaxation ($-dP/dt_{max}$) might be approximated by the rate of MR velocity decline, as an estimate of diastolic function. However, the value of these estimates is uncertain because an eccentric jet angle, mid-to-late MR from mitral prolapse, and severe MR (with no isovolumic contraction period and increased filling pressures) all can affect these measurements.

Pulsed wave (PW) Doppler imaging of mitral inflow velocity, tissue Doppler imaging (TDI) of lateral or septal annulus velocity, and the ratio of early mitral inflow to annular velocities have been done with the aim of characterizing LV diastolic function and LV filling pressure (see p. 127 and **Table 4.13**). Discrimination of disease-induced, mild diastolic dysfunction is difficult because most older dogs have a delayed relaxation pattern of mitral inflow (E/A <1). This finding is clinically useful because when E<A, filling pressures are normal and the risk of CHF is low. Pseudonormal and restrictive inflow patterns occur in many dogs with advanced DMVD, especially those with CHF (**Figures 29.33–29.35**). A mitral E velocity >1 m/s is common with advanced DMVD and peak velocities >1.3 or 1.4 m/s indicate a higher risk for CHF. Some dogs with CHF and a restrictive inflow pattern do show improvement to a pseudonormal pattern after CHF therapy, but this is uncommon because the LA v wave raises end-systolic LA pressure, which is quickly transferred back to the LV during early filling in the form of kinetic (velocity) energy. Thus, the mitral inflow pattern by itself is not a sensitive correlate for identifying pulmonary edema, although it can provide insight about relative risk for CHF. The usefulness of the early mitral inflow to annular tissue velocity ratio, E/Ea (also expressed as E/e′ or E/Em), for predicting high LA filling pressure and CHF in DMVD also is limited, compared to DCM. Age-related ventricular relaxation impairment, effects of volume overload (increased preload with preserved systolic function) on early diastolic myocardial tissue velocities, and MR-induced LA pressure elevation perturb the early diastolic recoil (see p. 127). Although some have suggested that an incredibly high E/Ea (of >18–19) can detect CHF with high specificity in dogs with DMVD, this index has fairly low sensitivity (56%; Kim, 2015; Suzuki, 2011a), and is nearly double that used for predicting CHF in DCM. The authors believe values >13 or 14 are more realistic but this needs more study. Some have shown that E/Ea is not a useful indicator of CHF in volume overload disease. Nonetheless, this ratio and LA pressure both decrease after furosemide therapy. In contrast

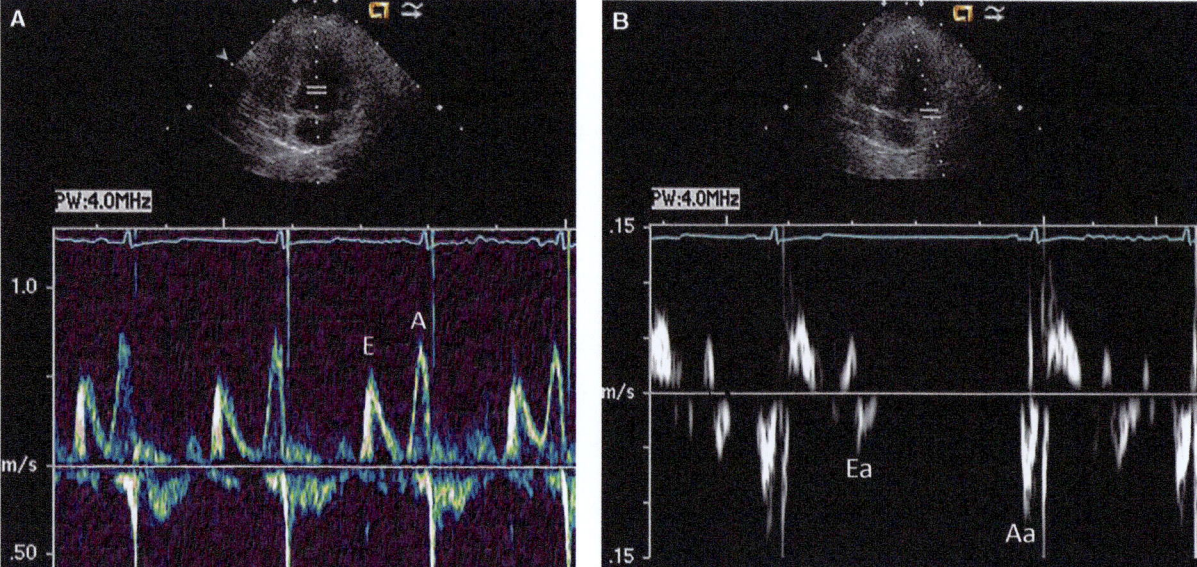

Figure 29.33 Pulsed-wave Doppler image of mitral inflow velocities (A) and Doppler tissue imaging at the lateral mitral annulus (B) show a delayed relaxation pattern of left ventricular filling in a 9-year-old male Toy Poodle with stage B1 mitral valve disease. This pattern of mild diastolic dysfunction is common in healthy older dogs also. The lower velocity E wave indicates left ventricular filling pressure is relatively normal. A, late diastolic mitral inflow velocity (from atrial contraction); Aa, late diastolic annular motion; E, early diastolic mitral inflow velocity; Ea, early diastolic annular motion.

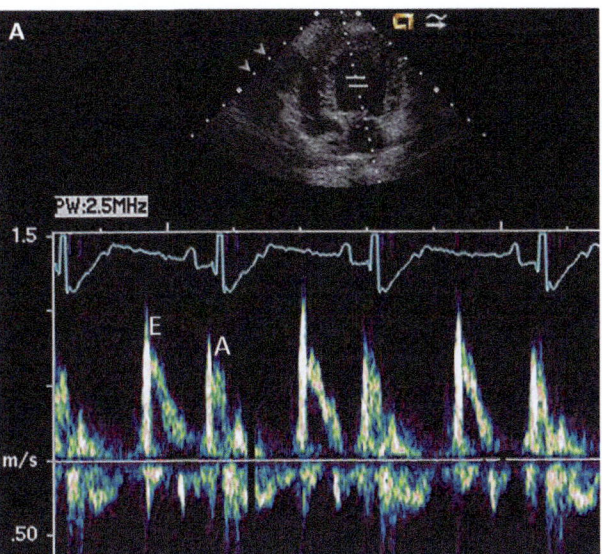
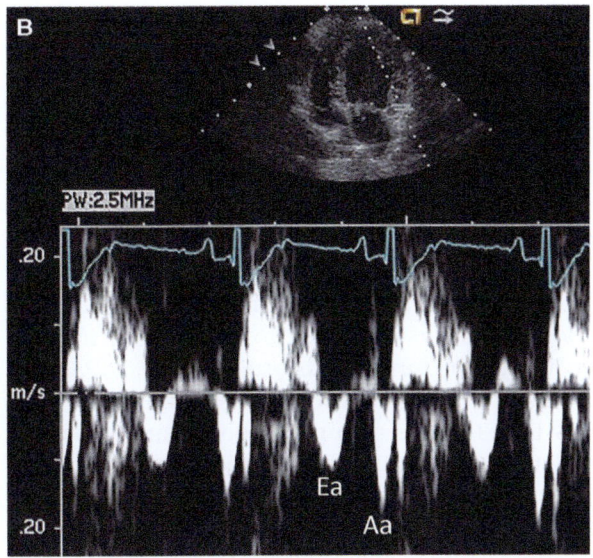

Figure 29.34 Pulsed-wave Doppler image of mitral inflow velocities (A) and Doppler tissue imaging at the lateral mitral annulus (B) indicate a pseudonormal pattern of left ventricular filling in a 10-year-old mixed-breed dog with advanced stage B2 mitral valve disease. This pattern would signal moderate diastolic dysfunction with increasing filling pressures in a dog with dilated cardiomyopathy, but the same interpretation cannot be applied here. With primary MR, the E wave no longer reflects the mean LA pressure (which predicts CHF) and instead is dominated by the end-systolic LA pressure caused by the regurgitant v wave. This is the most common pattern seen in dogs with MR. A, late diastolic mitral inflow velocity (from atrial contraction); Aa, late diastolic annular motion; E, early diastolic mitral inflow velocity; Ea, early diastolic annular motion.

to E/Ea, the ratio of early mitral inflow velocity to isovolumic relaxation time (E/IVRT) was shown to be more sensitive and specific for identifying elevated LA (LV filling) pressure in dogs with MR, as well as in those with DCM, experimental pacing-induced CHF, and volume loading. This index combines peak mitral E velocity (determined mainly by LV filling pressure and relaxation) and IVRT (dependent largely on LV relaxation rate but also shortened by high filling pressures). In normal dogs subjected to volume loading, a peak E/IVRT >2.2 was sensitive and specific for predicting mean LA pressures ≥15 mm Hg. Subsequently, an E/IVRT >2.5 was proposed as a cut-off value for predicting CHF in dogs with

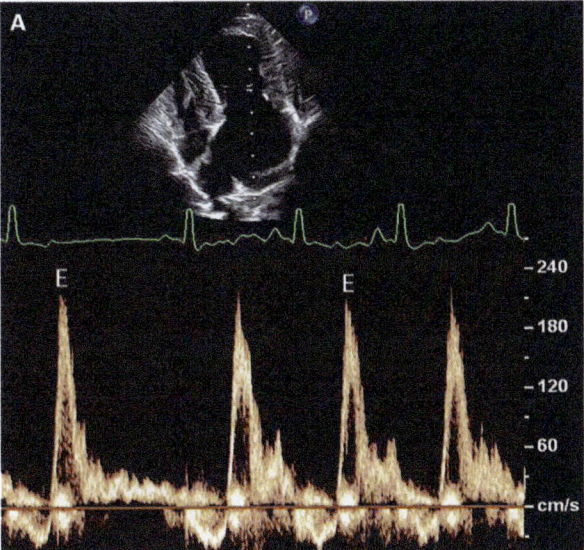
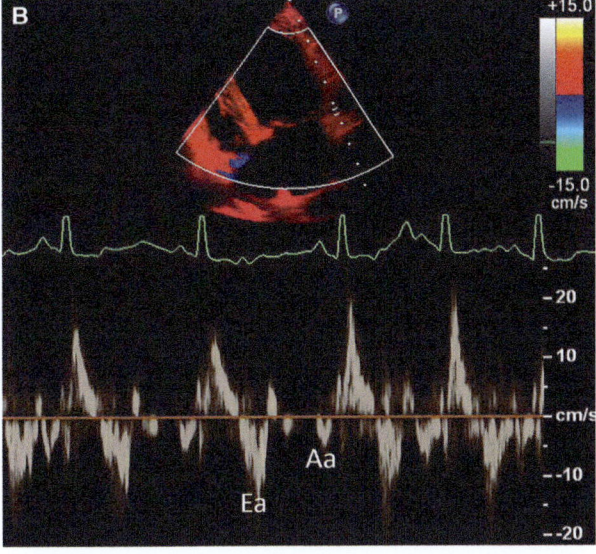

Figure 29.35 A restrictive pattern of LV filling is evident in this older mixed-breed dog with decompensated stage C mitral valve disease and pulmonary hypertension. This pattern typically indicates advanced diastolic dysfunction - a noncompliant left ventricle with high filling pressures, especially if deceleration time also is short and E>>>A. (A) The increased pulsed wave Doppler E velocity suggests elevated LA pressure. The elevated LV end-diastolic pressure minimizes the A velocity (obscured by artifact here). (B) Doppler tissue image at the lateral mitral annulus reflects a similar velocity pattern. Aa, late diastolic annular motion; E, early diastolic mitral inflow velocity; Ea, early diastolic annular motion. Left apical two-chamber view. LA, left atrial; LV, left ventricular.

DMVD (Schober, 2010). This ratio requires more clinical study in spontaneous cases of MR before it can be widely adopted.

Right Heart Evaluation RV and RA dilation develop with advancing TR and PH. RV chamber dilation is more prominent than RV wall hypertrophy in dogs with PH secondary to DMVD. Marked RV pressure or volume overload sometimes causes septal flattening or paradoxical septal motion Table 4.2, p. 91. The tricuspid annular plane systolic excursion (TAPSE; p. 94), an index of RV function influenced by body size, does not in itself appear to be reduced in dogs with DMVD. RV systolic function (as estimated by TAPSE, RV strain and strain rate) appears to be increased in late preclinical (stage B2) DMVD, similar to the hyperdynamic changes seen in the LV (Chapel, 2018). Similarly, the relatively weight-independent ratio of TAPSE to aortic root diameter (TAPSE/Ao) correlates positively to LA/Ao. Deterioration in RV function is likely after CHF develops, and especially with PH.

Spectral Doppler measurement of TR peak velocity is the easiest way to estimate the likely presence and severity of PH (pp. 126, 828, and **Figure 39.15**, p. 831). Using the TR jet's maximal velocity (Vmax), the Bernoulli relationship (4 × peak velocity^2) estimates the systolic pressure gradient (PG) between the RA and RV. The systolic RV pressure then is estimated as the (RA-to-RV) PG plus RA pressure; RA pressure usually is estimated as 5–10 mm Hg, or the measured central venous pressure is used. Because RV systolic pressure approximates pulmonary artery systolic pressure when there is no RV outflow obstruction, this can reveal the presence and severity of PH. It is important to identify the true maximum velocity by interrogating the TR jet from every available echo view. When a measurable TR jet is not present, other echo parameters can suggest PH, including pulmonary annulus dilation, pulmonary regurgitation jet velocity, right pulmonary artery distensibility index (RPADI), decreased pulmonary flow acceleration time to deceleration time (AT/DT), increased diastolic RV internal dimension (RVIDd) corrected for body weight, and increased LA/Ao (see Chapters 4 and 39). In addition, the TAPSE/Ao ratio correlates negatively to TR Vmax. With normal RV function, this ratio is >0.65; but it decreases with PH. An adjusted TAPSE/Ao ratio, which accounts for effects of bodyweight and severity of MR, provided greater sensitivity for identifying PH in dogs with moderate to severe DMVD (Caivano, 2018a). Reduced RV function associated with PH also might be detected by calculating the fractional shortening of the RV outflow tract. In dogs with normal RV systolic function, values >44% are expected. In dogs with DMVD and PH, this index of RV function was inversely related to PH severity, as assessed by TR Vmax (Caivano, 2018b).

Mild transudative pericardial effusion develops in some patients with right-sided CHF signs. In dogs where a full-thickness LA tear has occurred, pericardial fluid (blood) with or without signs of cardiac tamponade (p. 721) is likely to be evident.

Systemic Vascular Function Doppler ultrasound also can identify systemic vascular function abnormalities in dogs with DMVD. Doppler assessment of femoral artery flow resistance indices has demonstrated increased blood flow impedance. This is consistent with the increase in endogenous vasoconstrictors and vascular stiffening that accompany neurohormonal activation. Progressive DMVD and increasing LVIDd also have been associated with decreased flow-mediated vasodilation, which implies endothelial dysfunction.

Management

Management goals for dogs with preclinical DMVD are to delay the onset of CHF, as possible, and to detect and address early signs of decompensation before fulminant pulmonary edema develops. For dogs that already have developed CHF (stage C), goals are to control signs of congestion, enhance forward blood flow and reduce regurgitant volume, moderate excessive neurohormonal activation, provide good quality of life, and extend survival time. **Table 29.4** outlines general management strategies for DMVD based on disease progression; additional details are in Chapters 21 and 22.

Preclinical (Stage B) Degenerative Mitral Valve Disease

DMVD often is diagnosed before signs of CHF develop. This usually is based on hearing a murmur of MR in a dog without evidence for (congestive) heart failure. It is important to assess the severity of MR and cardiac remodeling to help estimate the current risk for CHF (see previous section). This will inform discussions with the client regarding the disease, its likely progression, and recommendations related to drug therapy, monitoring, and reevaluation visits. Although echocardiography is the preferred tool for identifying dogs that have developed stage B2 disease, when it is unavailable, radiographic criteria (including VLAS and VHS + VLAS) can be used (see p. 541, above). Measurement of NT-proBNP also can be helpful. Nevertheless, especially as the disease advances, echocardiography can become increasingly important for assessing cardiac chamber size, valvular structure and function, and other parameters.

Stage B1 Dogs in this stage have either no detectable cardiomegaly or enlargement that is mild and not proven to benefit from any therapy. This definition is modified from the original ACVIM consensus panel that considered stage B1 dogs as having only normal heart size. BP measurement, with thoracic radiographs and plasma NT-proBNP or echocardiography, generally are done yearly to monitor dogs with stage B1 disease (**Table 20.2**, p. 311). For large-breed dogs with suspected DMVD, reevaluation at 6-month intervals often is advised because their risk for more rapid myocardial

Table 29.4 General Management Guidelines for Dogs with Degenerative Mitral Valve Disease

No (or Mild) Cardiac Remodeling, No Clinical Signs of Disease, and No Proven Therapy—Stage B1

- Yearly examinations
  - Thoracic radiographs plus NT-proBNP or echocardiography (or all three)
    - Consider reevaluation at 6-month intervals for large-breed dogs
  - Blood pressure measurement
  - Routine preventative healthcare:
    - Vaccinations, as appropriate
    - Heartworm testing and prophylaxis, as appropriate for geographical region and travel history
    - Routine clinical laboratory tests (hemogram, serum chemistries, urinalysis, if indicatetd)
    - Dental prophylaxis, as needed
- Manage concurrent medical problems
- Owner education about DMVD, clinical signs of disease, early signs of CHF, and how to monitor RRR[a]
- Dietary considerations
  - Avoid high salt foods
  - Consider mild to moderate salt restriction
- Provide adequate protein and caloric intake
  - Maintain (or work toward) normal body weight/condition

Cardiac Remodeling Sufficient to Initiate Therapy but Without Clinical Signs of CHF—Stage B2

- Cardiac and routine preventative health care evaluations as for stage B1
  - Increase cardiac recheck frequency to every 6 months (or more often, depending on disease progression)
- Begin pimobendan therapy at 0.2 to 0.3 mg/kg PO q12h
- Consider RAAS inhibition? (see text for details)
- Manage concurrent medical problems
- Owner education as for stage B1
  - Owner should determine the dog's normal RRR, and regularly monitor RRR for changes
- Dietary considerations as for stage B1

Mild or Moderate Signs of CHF have Developed, Either Currently or Previously—Stage C Disease[b]

- Guidelines as for stages B1 & B2, above, plus:
- Furosemide, dosed as needed
- Continue pimobendan therapy
- RAAS inhibition (see text for details)
  - ACE inhibitor
  - Spironolactone
- No exercise until after CHF signs abate, then gradually introduce regular mild (to moderate) activity, as tolerated
- Moderate dietary salt (sodium) restriction
- Frequent home monitoring of RRR, as well as attitude, activity, appetite, cough, and other signs
- Increase reevaluation visit frequency (see p. 353)
- Antiarrhythmic therapy, if indicated

Acute, Severe Signs of CHF (Pulmonary Edema) are Present—Stage C or D Disease[c]

- Hospitalize and provide supplemental oxygen
- Sedation (butorphanol)
- Minimize handling
- Furosemide to induce a brisk diuresis; parenterally (IV, IM, CRI, as indicated)
- Pimobendan (consider q8h dosing until stable) – PO or IV (where available)
- Vasodilator therapy based on clinical assessment and initial response to therapy:
  - IV sodium nitroprusside, or topical or IV nitroglycerin
  - Hydralazine (PO or IV) or amlodipine ± topical nitroglycerin
- Antiarrhythmic therapy, if indicated
- Thoracocentesis, if large-volume pleural effusion
- Abdominocentesis, if tense ascites
- ± Bronchodilator (such as theophylline or albuterol; rarely used)
- ± Additional inotropic support if hypotensive (IV dobutamine or dopamine)
- Close monitoring of vital signs, diuresis, respiratory rate & effort, heart rate & rhythm, & renal function

(Continued)

Table 29.4 (Continued)   General Management Guidelines for Dogs with Degenerative Mitral Valve Disease

Chronic, Refractory CHF Not Requiring Hospitalization—Stage D Disease[b],[d]
- Verify that stage C recommendations are followed, with optimized doses and medication compliance
- Increase furosemide dose or frequency (guided by renal function) or use torsemide instead of furosemide; might be able to decrease dose slightly after signs abate
- Increase pimobendan frequency (to q8h) and dosage
- Add an arteriolar vasodilator (amlodipine or hydralazine; monitor blood pressure)
- Add (or maximize dose of) spironolactone
- Further restrict dietary salt intake and activity level
- Thoraco- (or abdomino-) centesis, as needed
- Manage arrhythmias, if present
- Add sildenafil (1–3 mg/kg PO q8-12h) if moderate to severe PH persists despite aggressive treatment of left heart failure; most often used when right-sided CHF or low cardiac output signs are present
- Consider adding digoxin, if not currently prescribed (monitor serum concentration, as well as renal function & electrolytes) – not commonly used except in cases of atrial fibrillation
- Consider adding a thiazide diuretic (only with great caution & close monitoring of creatinine & electrolytes)
- Cough suppressant, if persistent airway cough without pulmonary edema

[a] See Table 22.1 (p. 339). Monitoring RRR in Stage B1 is optional, as the likelihood of developing CHF will be very low at this stage in most dogs.
[b] See Tables 22.3 (p. 345) and 22.4 (p. 353), and Chapter 22 text for further details and doses. Most of these dogs will be treated as outpatients, or briefly hospitalized and released the same day.
[c] See Table 22.2 (p. 342) and Chapter 22 text for further details and doses. These patients have either life-threatening or unstable CHF that requires hospitalization for stabilization.
[d] Also see p. 354.

Abbreviations: ACE, angiotensin converting enzyme; CHF, congestive heart failure; DMVD, degenerative mitral valve disease; PH, pulmonary hypertension; RRR, resting (sleeping) respiratory rate.

contractility deterioration development of a DCM phenotype is greater. Routine preventative healthcare should be continued, including heartworm prevention, appropriate vaccinations, dental prophylaxis, and so on. Identification of and management for concurrent medical problems is important, as is owner education regarding DMVD and early signs of CHF.

Clients should be taught how to monitor their pet's RRR, to establish that animal's normal baseline rate; periodic RRR monitoring can help screen for early signs of decompensation (Table 22.1, p. 339). However, aggressive RRR monitoring is more appropriate for dogs in stage B2, as progression to CHF from stage B1 typically involves years.

No specific cardiac therapy is recommended for dogs in stage B1 at this time. If BP is elevated, the underlying cause should be investigated and an ACE inhibitor (or other therapy) prescribed to normalize BP and reduce cardiac afterload. Normal activity level and diet can be maintained at this stage, although avoidance of high-salt foods and treats is prudent. Other recommendations during this preclinical phase might include weight reduction for obese dogs; however, being mildly overweight is not considered problematic and might be of benefit.

Stage B2   Dogs with stage B2 DMVD have left heart enlargement and remodeling without clinical signs of CHF. Monitoring and routine healthcare recommendations for these dogs are similar to those for stage B1, except for more intense home RRR monitoring and sometimes, increased reevaluation frequency. Usually though, the most important trigger for added therapy is the client's detection of clinical CHF signs. In this regard, the RRR is a sensitive indicator of CHF in dogs with DMVD. A persistent increase in RRR of 20% or more above the individual's normal baseline could signal decompensating CHF. This is especially so if the RRR exceeds 40 breaths/minute. It is known that sleeping rates are lower than awake resting rates. Dogs with subclinical left heart disease typically have sleeping respiratory rates under 25/minute. Ideally, the client should maintain consistency by monitoring RRR either when the pet is resting quietly or sleeping; the authors recommend the latter.

Pimobendan is recommended for these dogs with preclinical cardiac remodeling (ACVIM Consensus, Keene, 2019). Compared with placebo, pimobendan at standard (international) label dosages of 0.2 to 0.3 mg/kg PO q12h was shown to delay the onset of CHF (by a median of 15 months), as well as prolong survival without clearly increasing adverse events (EPIC study, Boswood, 2016). The cardiac enlargement criteria used for inclusion in this landmark study were: radiographic VHS >10.5v, and echocardiographic (short-axis, diastolic) LA/Ao ≥1.6 and normalized LVIDd ≥1.7. Subsequent data analysis from these study dogs showed that reductions in LV size and LA/Ao were seen after a month of pimobendan therapy. Furthermore, decreased cardiac size was associated with increased time to CHF or cardiac-related death (Boswood, 2018). However, it is important to note that because radiographic VHS in some breeds normally ranges higher than 10.5v, echo criteria are considered more reliable for assessing LA and LV enlargement. Without an echocardiogram, a VHS of at least 11.7v plus VLAS >3.0v, ideally with demonstration of progressive VHS increase of ~0.1 v/month (over a period of 6 to 12 months), is suggested as an indication for initiating pimobendan therapy.

It is unclear whether additional medical therapy, besides pimobendan, is warranted for stage B2 DMVD. There are conflicting opinions among veterinary cardiologists with regard to blocking the RAAS at this stage with an ACE inhibitor and spironolactone. No significant delay in CHF onset was shown for CKCS given a relatively low dose of enalapril (Kvart, 2002). Although the same could be true for most other dogs, enalapril has reduced LVIDd and MR severity, as well as BP and sympathetic tone in dogs with preclinical DMVD. For dogs with advanced DMVD and more severe left heart enlargement, an ACE inhibitor could provide some benefit in delaying CHF (Atkins, 2007; Pouchelon, 2008). An ACE gene polymorphism is known to occur in some dogs and is associated with decreased ACE activity. It has high prevalence in the CKCS breed, with over 50% of studied dogs homozygous for the polymorphism (Meurs, 2018). The variant gene is associated with lower ACE activity, even in the presence of advanced DMVD, which could affect ACE inhibitor efficacy. In any case, for DMVD dogs with systemic hypertension, ACE inhibition is recommended as first line therapy to control BP; otherwise, there is no clear consensus.

Whether adding spironolactone to an ACE inhibitor can improve outcome in preclinical DMVD also is unclear. A prospective randomized, multicenter, single-blinded placebo-controlled (DELAY) study, of dogs with stage B2 DMVD, showed that the combination of spironolactone and benazepril did not significantly delay the onset of CHF (the primary study end-point). However, several echo- and radiographic indicators of disease progression were better in the treatment group (Borgarelli, 2020). Previous evidence in similar cases suggested that spironolactone might delay left heart enlargement; however, differences between treated and control groups were not significant. The decision to block the RAAS with an ACE inhibitor, ± spironolactone, depends in part on one's perspective about these studies and perhaps as importantly, on the cost of the different medications. In countries where RAAS inhibitors are generic, the potential benefit might "tip the scale" toward adding these to pimobendan. In contrast, a high cost for all three drugs would favor prioritization of pimobendan use, based on its much stronger evidence.

Another area of at least minor controversy relates to the recommended reevaluation frequency for dogs with stage B2 disease that are already receiving pimobendan (± RAAS inhibition) therapy. Considering that the average dog will not develop CHF for 15 months or longer, it is unlikely that a scheduled examination can be timed to "catch" incipient CHF. More importantly, there presently are no studies showing that augmentation of treatment during stage B2 is useful, even in the setting of progressive cardiomegaly (in an asymptomatic dog). Thus, one can reasonably argue that the next *cardiac* examination could be delayed until the client recognizes clinical signs of heart failure. However, others believe that regular cardiac reevaluations are important and might heighten a client's awareness for CHF, if substantial disease progression is revealed by thoracic radiography, echocardiography, or rising NT-proBNP concentrations. Practically, these examinations add considerably to the medical costs of care. Furthermore, Doppler echocardiography performed by a specialist is needed to provide detailed information about cardiac enlargement, function, regurgitation, filling pressures and other complicating factors. Realistically, only a small percentage of dogs with DMVD ever see a cardiologist. Without supporting data, a blanket recommendation for reassessment during stage B2 cannot be advanced. Perhaps a reasonable compromise is (at least) yearly screening for cardiovascular disease, including BP measurement, a basic echocardiogram or thoracic radiographs to observe for progression in heart size, and other diagnostic tests appropriate for routine health maintenance and other medical problems. Clients should be advised about the importance of home monitoring, as discussed previously, and encouraged to return their dog promptly should any clinical signs of possible heart failure be observed, whether exercise intolerance, collapsing, increase in coughing or RRR, or other signs.

In addition to more attentive home monitoring, regular (mild to moderate) exercise should be maintained, as tolerated. Strenuous exercise that provokes shortness of breath or excessive fatigue is to be avoided. Gradual transition to a diet mildly to moderately reduced in salt, but also well balanced and with adequate protein content, is recommended.

Investigation of other therapies for potential usefulness in preclinical DMVD is ongoing. It is emphasized that mechanistic and pathophysiologic benefits, while intriguing, are not substitutes for the major therapeutic endpoints that include delaying the onset of CHF, improving quality of life in heart failure, and increasing longevity. Without clinical trial data, starting any of the following treatments in preclinical disease cannot be recommended. Currently, beta-blocker therapy is not recommended as a strategy to delay CHF onset in dogs with DMVD. No clinical benefit toward this goal has been shown (including in a large multicenter clinical trial), despite evidence from experimental dog models of chronic MR indicating improved myocardial function with $beta_1$-blocker treatment. Sildenafil might possibly have benefit in preclinical DMVD, however more convincing evidence is needed. Preliminary data suggest it could mitigate some echo and NT-proBNP changes associated with disease progression. Sildenafil also improved heart rate variability (assessed by both time- and frequency-domain parameters) in a group of preclinical DMVD dogs, which suggests that the drug could improve sympathetic-vagal balance in these patients. Ivabradine, in a small single dose study of dogs with preclinical DMVD, reduced heart rate and a measure of myocardial oxygen consumption in a dose-dependent manner; at 1 mg/kg PO, it did not adversely affect BP. Another drug with possible potential in preclinical DMVD is the combination neprilysin inhibitor (sacubitril) and Ang receptor blocker (ARB, valsartan) marketed for human CHF (Entresto; Novartis AG; see p. 333). In a small clinical study, dogs with stage B2 DMVD treated with this combination for a month showed a markedly attenuated increase in urinary aldosterone to creatinine ratio compared to dogs given placebo. This suggests effective RAAS inhibition. However, the combined product was not tested against simple ACE inhibition or ARB therapy. Thus, additional studies of each of these agents in preclinical DMVD are needed.

Onset of Congestive Heart Failure (Stage C)

The clinical manifestations of heart failure in any individual do not necessarily develop in an orderly sequence. Congestive signs can appear gradually in some dogs, often preceded by exercise intolerance and subtle tachypnea. In others, fulminant pulmonary edema or episodes of syncope occur. Therapy must be guided by clinical status and the nature of any complicating factors. Medical therapy is the mainstay for dogs that have developed stage C heart failure. Surgical valve repair or replacement is a potential option for a tiny percentage of cases, and is increasingly available at specialized referral centers. Nevertheless, the practical treatment of CHF in almost all cases is medical. Clinical compensation for months to even years is sometimes possible with appropriate therapy, although frequent reevaluation and medication adjustments become necessary as the disease progresses. Intermittent episodes of decompensation (congestive signs) are common over time; often these can be managed successfully.

From the authors' perspective, and despite a number of study limitations, there are sufficient data to support the use of four medications in the chronic treatment of canine CHF: a loop diuretic, pimobendan, an ACE inhibitor, and spironolactone. There are challenges in interpreting clinical trial data based on: the criteria used for diagnosis, the severity of cases, relatively low enrollment numbers, issues related to prolonged enrollment and oversight of major endpoints, and the reality that many pharmaceutical-sponsored studies seem designed to pit one drug versus another. Unfortunately, no clinical trial has sufficiently tested the combination of all four medications, at least to our satisfaction. This situation is reflected clearly in the varying views of different cardiologists about the relative merits of these treatments, individually and in combination. Furosemide and pimobendan undoubtedly exert the strongest hemodynamic benefits in both acute and chronic CHF. These two drugs are most likely to control clinical signs of disease. However, this combination also activates the RAAS, and here the use of ACE inhibitors and spironolactone (and potentially ARBs) becomes more relevant for long-term therapy. With this opinion stated, we discuss the various treatment combinations.

Furosemide, pimobendan, and RAAS inhibition with an ACE inhibitor have long been considered as standard, "triple therapy" for dogs that have developed CHF (Chapter 22). This has been recommended by the ACVIM consensus panel, although not unanimously by its participants. Increasingly, spironolactone is included for "quad therapy." Torsemide can be substituted for furosemide, especially in dogs requiring higher diuretic doses or those with ascites. Pimobendan is well-tolerated and appears to confer greater benefit when compared to an ACE inhibitor for long-term heart failure management. Some studies have demonstrated the benefits of RAAS inhibition compared to diuretic therapy alone. Unfortunately, the combination of pimobendan with full RAAS inhibition, using higher doses of an ACE inhibitor and spironolactone, has not been sufficiently evaluated. In the authors' opinion, the European label doses for ACE inhibitors probably are too low; there is evidence that a greater effect is observed with higher doses. Both pimobendan and ACE inhibitors have been shown to reduce LA pressure in models of MR, but pimobendan improves cardiac function better than benazepril, at least over the short term. Pimobendan also prolongs the time before an increase in CHF therapy intensification is needed (Häggström, 2013). Pimobendan, in addition to other standard heart failure therapy, increases survival time in stage C DMVD. Standard (label) doses appear more effective in reducing recurrent pulmonary edema than lower doses and experience indicates that increasing the frequency and daily dose can be beneficial in progressive (stage D) CHF. Pimobendan can decrease average heart rate without (apparently) increasing frequency of tachyarrhythmias in DMVD dogs. ACE inhibition and pimobendan generally are used together for heart failure caused by DMVD, although whether their benefits are additive is unclear because no studies have sufficiently addressed this point. One study in dogs with first-onset CHF found that ramipril combined with pimobendan and furosemide provided no improvement in survival time, compared to pimobendan and furosemide alone (Wess, 2020); however, confirmatory studies using different (and higher doses) of enalapril or benazepril are needed to verify this finding. A fixed-dose combination formulation containing pimobendan and benazepril (Fortekor Plus®; Elanco) was non-inferior in efficacy and induced less vomiting than in control groups given the drugs separately. In a yet-to-be published clinical trial (FDA filings are available), a fixed dose of benazepril and spironolactone (Cardalis®; Ceva) plus furosemide was superior to furosemide. Unfortunately, pimobendan was not evaluated in this study.

Spironolactone often is added to furosemide, pimobendan and ACE inhibitor therapy for chronic CHF management. Spironolactone might reduce the risk of cardiac death or euthanasia because of CHF in dogs with DMVD. In general, spironolactone does not appear to significantly increase risk for adverse events, including hyperkalemia, azotemia, or death from cardiac or renal disease. However, individual dogs have developed serum electrolyte disturbances, azotemia, or both while taking this drug, so measuring these clinical variables at 1–2 weeks after initiating spironolactone therapy, and periodically thereafter, is recommended. Because ACE inhibition does not always adequately suppress the RAAS, aldosterone breakthrough can occur. Based on urine aldosterone:creatinine ratios, this appears to develop in almost a third of DMVD dogs, with or without CHF, being treated with an ACE inhibitor (Ames, 2017). Although the mechanism of aldosterone breakthrough is not clear, use of a mineralocorticoid receptor blocker such as spironolactone is likely to be especially helpful in these cases.

Digoxin is used only rarely in dogs with DMVD. Its main indication is for heart rate control in dogs with AF, usually in combination with diltiazem (p. 411). Digoxin also might suppress some other supraventricular tachyarrhythmias. Digoxin sometimes is added to the treatment regimen in stage D patients to help support myocardial function and improve baroreceptor function, as long as there are no contraindications to its use. Unfortunately, azotemia is common in late stages of CHF and precludes the use of this drug. Digoxin can be used with pimobendan. If digoxin is administered, conservative doses always should be used and serum concentrations measured to avoid toxicity (p. 328).

Newer treatment possibilities for dogs with advanced DMVD are continually being explored (also see "Strategies for End-Stage or Refractory Heart Failure," below). For example, sildenafil clearly is indicated for dogs with signs of moderate to severe PH that do not respond to standard therapy for CHF. Whether sildenafil might improve outcomes in other stage C patients is unknown. The same question remains for newer drugs such as ivabradine, sacubitril-valsartan, and others.

Exercise should not be allowed until after signs of congestive failure abate. However, in chronic compensated disease, regular mild to moderate activity is thought to be beneficial. Strenuous exercise is best avoided. At-home monitoring is important because decompensation often occurs unexpectedly. A persistent increase in the RRR or heart rate can signal early decompensation. Chronic pulmonary congestion does stiffen the lungs, though, and some increase in sleeping respiratory rate should be expected at this stage. As long as the sleeping respiratory rate is <30 breaths/minute, usually the dog is stable. If decompensated CHF develops, therapy is intensified or adjusted as needed while searching for any complicating factors that can be addressed. **Table 29.4** and Chapter 22 contain strategies for modifying or intensifying CHF therapy.

Dogs with a persistent dry cough stemming from primary airway disease or mainstem bronchus compression, and without pulmonary edema, might require antitussive therapy (such as hydrocodone bitartrate, 0.25 mg/kg PO q8–12h; or butorphanol, 0.5 mg/kg PO q6–12h). When noninfective, inflammatory bronchial disease underlies chronic coughing, a conservative course of anti-inflammatory glucocorticoid therapy can provide relief. The lowest effective doses should be used, especially if repeated course(s) or ongoing therapy is needed.

Mild to Moderate Signs of CHF Early signs of decompensation usually include a persistent increase in RRR at home. Shortness of breath, increased respiratory effort or excessive panting with previously tolerated levels of exercise, or decreased interest in exercise and food also are likely to occur. A new or worsened cough might be noted as well. A careful history and physical exam, thoracic radiographs, echocardiography, and lung ultrasound can help the clinician differentiate CHF from other causes of respiratory signs. The NT-proBNP test might be helpful if a baseline measurement previously was obtained; however, many dogs with compensated valvular disease and cardiomegaly also have significantly elevated natriuretic peptide concentrations. Conversely, a low NT-proBNP value would strongly argue against CHF. BP measurement and other lab tests also are important for identifying complications.

The aggressiveness of CHF therapy is guided by the individual patient's clinical signs and response to treatment. Parenteral and then oral furosemide is instituted when clinical signs and radiographic evidence of pulmonary edema appear. Higher and more frequent doses are indicated for more severe edema. When CHF signs are controlled, furosemide dosage and frequency gradually are reduced to find the lowest effective levels for long-term therapy in that patient. Although in some cases, furosemide alone might be prescribed initially as a therapeutic trial (see following paragraphs), furosemide continuation as monotherapy is not recommended for chronic heart failure treatment.

Mild clinical signs, with pulmonary venous congestion or minimal radiographic evidence for pulmonary edema, often respond well to PO furosemide (at about 1–2 mg/kg q12h), an ACE inhibitor given q24h, and pimobendan at standard doses (**Table 22.3**, p. 345). A diet moderately reduced in salt is recommended. If the client can restrict activity at home, the patient generally will be more comfortable there. No exercise should be allowed until the next reevaluation visit, usually in 5–7 days unless problems arise sooner. At that time, if all CHF signs have resolved, mild (to moderate) activity can be gradually reintroduced, medications continued and the potential addition of RAAS inhibition addressed. The frequency of subsequent reevaluations depends on the patient's clinical status. Recheck exams should assess clinical signs, RRR, and any issues with medication compliance at home, as well as BP, renal function, and serum electrolytes. Depending on the severity of clinical findings and disease progression, other tests such as repeat thoracic radiographs, ECG, NT-proBNP, or an echocardiogram could be appropriate. However, for most dogs in general small animal practice, a BP, "renal & electrolyte panel," and possibly follow-up thoracic radiographs will be all that is required for practical management, especially if the patient is doing well.

Some dogs show clinical signs that suggest early CHF, but have no clear radiographic (or other) evidence for pulmonary edema, making the diagnosis in doubt. In some of these cases, pulmonary venous distension might be evident, suggesting imminent CHF. It is relevant that pulmonary congestion (even without overt radiographic edema) also can increase RRR. Alternatively, there might be interstitial lung edema that would only be evident by computed tomography. If it is unclear whether respiratory signs stem from heart failure or a noncardiac cause, an initial therapeutic furosemide trial (1–2 mg/kg PO q8–12h for 3–5 days) is useful. In most cases, these dogs already should be receiving pimobendan, as they would previously have passed through stage B2 to reach this point; but if not, pimobendan is started along with the furosemide. Plasma NT-proBNP measurement also could help clarify if CHF has developed, assuming the patient's baseline value is known and results are returned soon enough. Cardiogenic pulmonary edema usually responds rapidly to furosemide. If CHF was the cause the owner should see resolution of the increased respiratory rate and effort, as well as (cardiogenic) cough, within a day or so. In these cases, standard triple or quad therapy then can be instituted, along with recommendations for moderate dietary salt and exercise restriction. Depending on the individual patient, it might be possible to reduce the dose of furosemide somewhat, using RRR monitoring as a guide. On the other hand, coughing or other respiratory signs that persist despite the furosemide trial usually means a diagnosis of CHF is unlikely, even if the dog has advanced DMVD. Chronic airway disease such as bronchitis, tracheal collapse, or left bronchial compression would be most likely if the radiographs exclude pulmonary neoplasia or pneumonia. Although this therapeutic trial can be helpful, confusion is still possible in some cases because a cough from airway irritation could resolve spontaneously, or the furosemide might have a mild anti-inflammatory or antitussive effect.

Severe Signs of CHF Acute, decompensated CHF with fulminant pulmonary edema and shortness of breath at rest is a true emergency. Aggressive therapy, with gentle handling, is crucial in these fragile patients. Cage rest, sedation, supplemental oxygen, pimobendan, and high-dose parenteral furosemide (such as 2 mg/kg q1–4h initially until there is substantial diuresis) are usual treatments. Optionally, vasodilator therapy can be initiated, especially for "white-out" lungs or other signs of severe pulmonary edema (**Table 29.4**, **Table 22.2**, p. 342, and Chapter 22, p. 340). Pimobendan is begun (or continued) as soon as possible; the dosing frequency can be increased to q8h during hospitalization. When more aggressive load reduction is indicated, both arteriolar and venous dilation can be achieved with IV nitroprusside or IV nitroglycerin, provided BP can be closely monitored to avoid hypotension (and maintaining systolic BP at 85 to 90 mm Hg or higher). Nitroprusside has become expensive in many countries. Alternatively, PO (or low dose IV) hydralazine can be used for acute afterload reduction because of its direct and rapid arteriolar vasodilating effect. A smaller dosage is used in animals already receiving an ACE inhibitor (**Table 22.3**, p. 345). Amlodipine is another potential afterload reducer, but has slower onset of action. Although amlodipine can significantly decrease LA pressure and mitral regurgitant jet severity compared to an ACE inhibitor, up to four days are required for its full effect. Topical nitroglycerin ointment can be used alone or in combination with an arteriolar dilator, in an attempt to reduce pulmonary venous pressure through systemic venodilation and translocation of pulmonary blood volume.

For the control of supraventricular tachyarrhythmias (particularly AF), diltiazem alone or combined with digoxin is the usual initial treatment choice (**Table 25.2**, p. 402). Chapter 25 contains details of this therapy. For dogs with DMVD that require BP support or have poor myocardial function, other more potent inotropic agents (such as dobutamine) can be given IV, if prior treatment was ineffective or if the patient is in cardiogenic shock (**Table 22.3**, p. 345). Heart rate and rhythm should be monitored.

Mild sedation is provided to reduce patient anxiety (**Table 22.2**, p. 342). It is important to minimize patient handling. Radiographs and other diagnostic procedures should be postponed as much as possible until the patient's respiratory condition is more stable. In dogs with moderate- to large-volume pleural effusion, thoracocentesis is indicated as soon as possible to improve pulmonary function. Ascites that is severe enough to impede respiration also should be drained. Although used uncommonly now, a bronchodilator (such as theophylline or aminophylline) might be considered to address possible bronchospasm induced by severe pulmonary edema; it might also support respiratory muscle function. Close monitoring for the patient's response to therapy (urinary output in particular) and any adverse effects (including hypotension, azotemia, electrolyte abnormalities, arrhythmias, drug toxicity, and so on) is important for optimizing care. See Chapter 22 (p. 348) for additional information. Mild to moderate azotemia is common after aggressive diuretic therapy. In most patients, slow oral "self-rehydration" is effective and mild azotemia is well tolerated. Parenteral fluid therapy is avoided whenever possible, because it can exacerbate congestive signs, (p. 348).

Transition to Home Care After the patient has been stabilized, medications are adjusted over a period of several days to weeks in order to optimize the home treatment regimen for that animal. In general, most treatments will be given twice daily once the patient is stable. The usual medications at the time of hospital discharge are pimobendan, furosemide, and an ACE inhibitor. Spironolactone often is added at the first recheck visit, but could be prescribed at the time of hospital release, especially if the combination product is being used. Furosemide is titrated to the lowest dose and longest dosing interval that control signs of congestion. RRR monitoring over time helps guide this treatment. An ACE inhibitor generally is used for chronic therapy. If another vasodilator was administered initially, the ACE inhibitor can be dosed once daily (or at a half dosage) to start, as the patient is weaned off the other (arteriolar) vasodilator. The ACE inhibitor dosing can be increased to q12h over the next several days to a week. Client education about the purpose and potential adverse effects of prescribed medications, RRR monitoring, diet, activity restrictions, follow-up schedule, and other recommendations is important.

Monitoring Heart Failure Therapy Continued monitoring is essential, especially for renal function, serum electrolyte concentrations, BP, recurrent congestive signs, and other complications. Intermittent arrhythmias can cause CHF decompensation, or episodes of transient weakness or syncope. Cough-induced syncope, atrial rupture, or other causes of poor cardiac output also can occur. Despite the likely periodic recurrence of CHF signs, with effective management many dogs with DMVD enjoy a good quality of life for several months to years after signs of CHF first appear. Dogs with recently diagnosed or decompensated heart failure should be reevaluated more frequently (usually within a week's time) until their condition is stable (**Table 22.4**, p. 353). Dogs with chronic heart failure that appears well controlled can be checked less often, although usually at least three to four times per year. Whenever a diuretic dosage is increased, it is prudent to reevaluate renal function within 1 to 2 weeks.

Strategies for End-Stage or Refractory (Stage D) Heart Failure Recurrent, acute CHF should be treated in-hospital as described previously (**Table 22.2**, p. 342). Pleural and abdominal effusions are drained as needed to maintain patient comfort. Other strategies for intensifying home therapy are described in Chapter 22 (p. 354). Current recommendations for sildenafil are noted below (p. 562; also see Chapter 39). Various other drugs might prove helpful in the future for dogs with DMVD and CHF. These could include the combination of sacubitril-valsartan (p. 333), statin drugs, ibravadine, carperitide, or others. Further research will help determine their role.

Mitral Valve Repair and Other Interventions

The potential options for surgical repair of the mitral valve in dogs with DMVD are expanding, yet realistically for the average dog owner, remain prohibitively expensive. Various mitral annuloplasty and artificial chordal reconstruction techniques using cardiopulmonary bypass have been explored, often with excellent results (Uechi, 2012). Procedures using porcine bioprosthetic valves also have been tried. Some techniques have been unrewarding, such as a partial external mitral annuloplasty procedure not requiring cardiopulmonary bypass, but with high perioperative mortality and minimal improvement in MR severity in survivors. Nevertheless, surgical treatments for DMVD are becoming more successful despite the many technical challenges. Long-term clinical improvement in cardiac size and function is possible following successful mitral valve repair, which would allow discontinuation of CHF therapy in some dogs. In cases that previously were in stage C heart failure, reclassification into stage B could be reasonable. Currently, only a small number of surgical centers around the world have the necessary expertise, facilities, and staffing to accomplish canine mitral valve repair with acceptably low complication rates, but this number is expected to grow.

The potential for catheter- or hybrid-based procedures is an active area of investigation, with a number of centers attempting to develop a catheter-delivered device that can clip or somehow attenuate the mitral orifice. None currently are available, and issues of thrombosis on the device must be overcome. An interesting approach that has been used experimentally and in some clinical canine cases is the creation of an interatrial septal opening (an acquired ASD) to decompress the left atrium. While this might seem counterintuitive, and would only increase pulmonary blood flow, there does seem to be clinical benefit based on preliminary data (Allen, 2021). Even more novel devices, that might alter pulmonary lymphatic drainage in CHF, are under investigation.

Complications and Comorbid Conditions

Pulmonary Hypertension PH of varying degree is estimated to occur in 14–53% of dogs with DMVD. Its presence and severity increase with advancing DMVD severity; PH is identified more often in dogs with stage C compared to stage B2 disease. PH associated with DMVD usually is of mild to moderate severity, and most of this can be attributed to increasing LA and pulmonary venous pressures stemming from left heart failure. About half of the cases have mild PH, and another quarter to a third are graded as moderately severe. Yet, an estimated 10–20% of dogs with DMVD have severe PH. An estimated pulmonary systolic pressure >55 mm Hg has been linked with a poorer outcome. When associated with DMVD, PH usually develops secondary to chronic pulmonary venous hypertension (so-called post-capillary PH). However, pre-capillary increase in pulmonary vascular resistance can result from hypoxia-induced pulmonary arteriolar vasoconstriction caused by pulmonary edema or concurrent pulmonary disease, especially interstitial pulmonary fibrosis. Furthermore, reactive pulmonary vascular remodeling and narrowing could contribute to chronically increased pulmonary artery pressures, especially in dogs with more severe disease (p. 819). The development of moderate to severe PH increases right heart strain and promotes RV dilation (and hypertrophy); it contributes to tricuspid annulus dilation and worsening TR.

Patients with mild to moderate PH might be asymptomatic, or they could show exercise intolerance or other clinical signs consistent with DMVD. With severe PH, clinical signs often include cough, respiratory difficulty, exertional collapse, syncope, and ascites; some cases manifest cyanosis. The precise mechanism for cough, respiratory difficulty, and cyanosis has not been clearly defined and it might simply relate to underlying cardiac or respiratory disease. The increase in RV afterload (and preload from TR) can change the predominantly left-sided heart failure patient to one with signs of mainly right-sided CHF (ascites, and sometimes pleural effusion and mild pericardial effusion), as well as low cardiac output (lethargy, weakness, syncope, prerenal azotemia). Concurrent arrhythmias, especially AF, exacerbate these signs. When PH is severe, the patient's systolic murmur often is as loud or louder over the tricuspid (rather than the mitral) region. In addition, a tympanic or even split S_2 might be audible over the pulmonary valve area, although this is challenging to hear through the murmur. Pulmonary crackles are a frequent finding and can relate either to pulmonary edema or chronic interstitial lung or small airway disease in these dogs. Diagnosis of PH generally is by echocardiography, but radiographic findings can be suggestive (see p. 554 and Chapters 4 and 39).

Management of dogs with DMVD and PH first centers on standard CHF therapy, to reduce pulmonary venous pressure by controlling pulmonary edema and optimizing forward cardiac output. Another possible benefit of pimobendan, besides support of myocardial function and systemic vasodilation, is the potential to induce pulmonary vasodilation through its phosphodiesterase-3 (PDE-3) inhibiting effect, although this effect was not significant in experimental canine models of pulmonary hypertension. Sometimes the pimobendan dose or administration frequency, or both, is increased in the hope of achieving this effect, or more likely, improving RV function and forward flow, which has been well demonstrated in similar models.

Additional therapy with a PDE-5 inhibitor (such as sildenafil or tadalafil) generally is reserved for dogs with severe PH that have persistent right-sided congestive signs or collapse/syncope. It presently is unclear whether the addition of a PDE-5 inhibitor to CHF therapy in cases with less severe PH would improve clinical status or survival, but clinical signs often improve. Sildenafil (1 to 3 mg/kg PO q 8-12h) usually is started at a lower dose, and then titrated upward over several days to a week based on clinical response. Concurrent administration of an L-arginine supplement might enhance sildenafil's efficacy because this amino acid is a substrate for NO production; however, this is not certain (p. 834). Ideally, the Doppler TR Vmax and other echo observations, such as improved left heart filling, are used to assess therapeutic effectiveness. Nevertheless, reduction in TR Vmax or RV size is not always documented despite clinical improvement in activity tolerance and quality of life. Even though sildenafil primarily affects the pulmonary vasculature, systemic BP should be monitored, especially in patients receiving another vasodilator along with an ACE inhibitor. When evidence for left heart failure is minimal, and especially when left heart size has become more normal, consideration might be given to stopping an ACE inhibitor but continuing spironolactone.

Another concern in dogs with severe PH and advanced DMVD, is that the initiation of sildenafil therapy (especially at higher doses) could exacerbate pulmonary venous hypertension and induce pulmonary edema. The likely mechanism relates to rapid reduction in pulmonary vascular resistance with marked secondary increase in pulmonary blood flow. Such triggering of clinical pulmonary edema seems to be uncommon, especially when sildenafil therapy is begun only after initial treatment for left-sided CHF and in dogs with symptomatic PH that persists after initial left heart failure treatment. Nevertheless, close monitoring for increasing RRR, cough, and other respiratory signs is warranted.

Arrhythmias Atrial ectopy and supraventricular tachyarrhythmias are a common complication as DMVD advances. Paroxysmal or sustained tachyarrhythmias can precipitate weakness, syncope and congestive signs in a previously stable patient. An arrhythmia might be evident on physical exam and further identified on resting ECG. However, ambulatory ECG monitoring might be needed for definitive diagnosis; it also can help guide antiarrhythmic therapy. Home monitoring of heart rate and rhythm using a smartphone ECG app can be quite useful, especially for patients with AF. In some cases, an intermittent bradyarrhythmia or ventricular tachycardia underlies episodic weakness and syncope. See Chapter 25 for arrhythmia management.

Ruptured Chordae Tendineae Chordal rupture is estimated to occur in 15–20% of cases, although small chordal ruptures might be more common; definitive echocardiographic criteria for this complication have not been established through sufficient autopsy studies. Echocardiographic findings of chordal rupture were noted earlier in this chapter. (p. 546) Chordal ruptures usually involve the anterior leaflet (**Figures 29.5, 29.21,** and **29.31**). Affected animals tend to be older male, small-breed dogs; chordal rupture also occurs in females occasionally. Rupture of a commissural (primary or marginal) chord usually leads to severe and acute pulmonary edema, and prognosis frequently is poor in such cases. However, rupture of minor chordae might not precipitate overt CHF. This sometimes is an incidental finding on echocardiogram or at necropsy. Factors that influence clinical outcome include the size and location of the ruptured chord, regurgitant orifice size, LA compliance, LV function, and heart rate. Some dogs survive for over a year with minor chordal rupture.

Left Atrial Tears There appears to be a higher prevalence of LA tears in older male Miniature Poodles, Cocker Spaniels, CKCS, Dachshunds, and Shetland Sheepdogs. Mixed-breed dogs also can be affected. The increased risk for males does not appear to hold in CKCS. Full-thickness tearing of the LA wall is a major, although uncommon, complication of DMVD. Acute intrapericardial bleeding typically causes rapid onset of cardiac tamponade (p. 713) and can be fatal. The predominant clinical manifestation is acute weakness or collapse;

other common signs include cough, dyspnea, and respiratory or cardiac arrest. Additionally, any cardiac murmur might be softer than previously noted. Although signs of cardiac tamponade are common, these might be absent in cases with only minor intrapericardial bleeding.

Most of these cases have advanced DMVD, with severe LA enlargement, atrial jet lesions, and often, ruptured commissural chordae tendineae. Nevertheless, some dogs with only moderate LA enlargement experience an LA tear. Thoracic radiographs can show an acutely increased VHS. Pericardial effusion is apparent on echocardiography in almost all cases, except when the tear occurs in the atrial septum. Clots could be evident in the pericardial fluid, which also can be of a mixed echoic appearance (**Figure 29.36**). Echocardiography also might show an intraluminal thrombus attached to the LA wall, associated with a partial or full-thickness tear (**Figure 29.37**). Rarely, a tear develops in the interatrial septum rather than the LA wall, causing an acquired ASD. Left-to-right shunting usually occurs in such cases; however, if there is severe TR or PH, right-to-left shunting through the acquired ASD could cause hypoxemia and acute respiratory distress.

If tamponade is present, a judicious attempt at pericardiocentesis can help relieve this, although the decrease

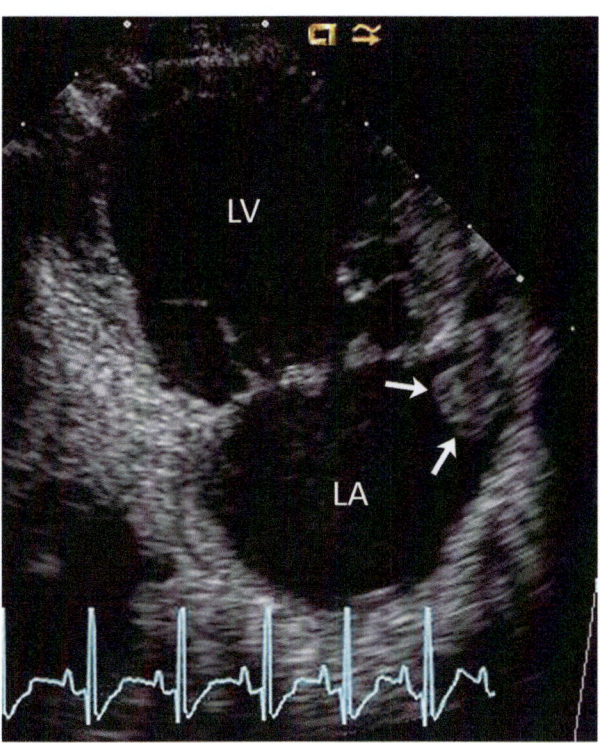

Figure 29.37 Echocardiography revealed a ~1.6 × 1 cm soft-tissue mass (arrows) adhered to the wall of the left atrium/auricle in a 13-year-old female Miniature Schnauzer with advanced stage C degenerative mitral valve disease and history of multiple collapse episodes. This mass is most likely a mural thrombus, formed secondary to a partial left atrial tear. No pericardial effusion was evident in this case.

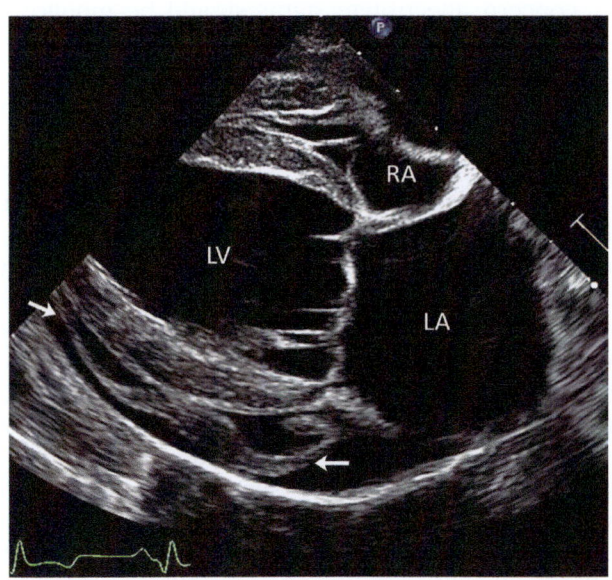

Figure 29.36 A full-thickness left atrial tear occurred in this 9-year-old male Sheltie with advanced degenerative mitral valve disease. A long thrombus (arrows) extends within the pericardial fluid (hemorrhage) from ventral LA toward the ventricular apex. Although the volume of pericardial fluid is only modest, the collapsed right atrial wall indicates cardiac tamponade is present. Because this dog's clinical status appeared relatively stable, conservative therapy was pursued, without pericardiocentesis. The dog was discharged from hospital a couple days later. Occasional episodes of syncope with excitement occurred over the following 3 weeks; the dog was subsequently lost to follow-up. Many cases of acute left atrial rupture rapidly lead to death. Right parasternal long-axis view, systole. LA, left atrium; LV, left ventricle; RA, right atrium. (Image courtesy of Drs S Murphy & J Ward.)

in intrapericardial pressure could trigger further bleeding, especially if a clot seal is disturbed. Removal of just a small volume of pericardial blood (10-20 ml) often will stabilize BP. Prognosis generally is guarded following an atrial tear. Yet, while some dogs die despite aggressive supportive care, a surprising number can survive to hospital discharge. Conservative treatment involves cage rest, BP support, and continued CHF therapy, as indicated. Some pericardial fluid is aspirated if hypotension or other signs of cardiac tamponade are present. With time, the rupture might seal and pericardial blood be reabsorbed. For dogs with echo evidence of an intraluminal thrombus in the LA, there is presumably increased risk for arterial thromboembolism. Dogs that survive an episode of LA rupture are prone to another.

Chronic Respiratory Disease Chronic bronchitis and collapsing trachea are common in older small-breed dogs. Chronic airway disease (bronchitis) with bronchomalacia can predispose to major bronchial collapse, similar to tracheal collapse. These conditions often coexist with LA enlargement, which itself can lead to left mainstem bronchus compression between the atrium and aorta (**Figure 9.2**, p. 204). Signs associated with primary airway disease sometimes are difficult to differentiate from those of bronchial compression or

CHF, although major airway compression or collapse usually causes a dry, "honking" cough. Results of at-home RRR monitoring, change in exercise tolerance and activity level, and thoracic radiographs are helpful in discerning the etiology. For dogs that develop a new or worsening cough (especially a dry, honking cough), yet still maintain a normal RRR at home, empiric therapy (such as with a bronchodilator, antibiotic trial, or lastly, anti-inflammatory doses of glucocorticoid) could be tried, if further diagnostic testing is not pursued. The latter might include radiographs with airway fluoroscopy, tracheal wash or bronchoscopy with bronchoalveolar lavage, and culture of airway secretions. For persistent dry cough in the absence of pulmonary edema, a cough suppressant (hydrocodone or another antitussive) can be helpful; this might be needed only intermittently, when the dog is having a "bad day" of coughing. It is important that the owner continue to monitor RRR and be alert to possible episodes of recurrent pulmonary edema.

Chronic interstitial pulmonary fibrosis also seems to be a common comorbidity in dogs with DMVD. The clinical signs of pulmonary fibrosis include tachypnea, exertional fatigue, hypoxemia, and often, a soft cough. Although these clearly are similar to signs of CHF, pulmonary fibrosis is suspected when there are diffuse or ventrally located inspiratory crackles in a dog with radiographically clear lungs. The pathogenesis of fibrosis in these cases is uncertain; PH often is present, as well. It is conceivable that recurrent pulmonary congestion might predispose to this condition but that is speculative. There is no specific treatment as pulmonary fibrosis represents an end-stage of lung injury, a form of scarring. Regardless of these limitations, appreciating this condition is important so that intensified CHF therapy is not given inadvertently or inappropriately.

Abnormal Blood Pressure Systemic arterial hypertension is another comorbidity that often is associated with renal or endocrine disease in dogs with DMVD (see Chapter 38). Because systemic hypertension can exacerbate MR and cardiac workload, BP measurement at each visit is advised. If elevated, and if the ACE inhibitor dose already is maximized, an arteriolar vasodilator (such as amlodipine) could be added to the dog's therapy. Alternatively, the ARB, telmisartan, could be effective in place of an ACE inhibitor (p. 803). Care should be taken to verify that the high BP readings are not just related to excitement.

Conversely, hypotension can occur with overdose of an arteriolar vasodilator, dehydration, persistent arrhythmias, or poor contractility. Although uncommon, LA rupture with cardiac tamponade causes acute and profound hypotension (see section "Left Atrial Tears").

Renal Dysfunction and Other Systemic Problems Impaired renal function is common in this older population and links between renal and cardiac dysfunction could relate to several mechanisms. The term "cardiovascular-renal axis disorders" has been proposed for the situation of concurrent cardiac and renal disease in companion animals (p. 310); in people this is known as cardiorenal syndrome. One proven cause of cardiorenal syndrome in dogs is severe right-sided CHF, because the elevated vena caval and intra-abdominal pressures will impair renal function. There is a concept that RAAS activation in CHF causes or exacerbates renal dysfunction, but more information is needed regarding this. In many cases, azotemia is simply a consequence of diuretic therapy and strictly speaking, this is not a syndrome but an adverse effect of drug therapy. It is important to verify that the patient does not have a treatable underlying disease that might be contributing to renal dysfunction, such as an ascending urinary tract infection.

It can be difficult to balance renal and cardiac function in dogs that need diuretic therapy for CHF and yet are azotemic. Treatment goals include using the lowest effective doses of furosemide, along with optimizing forward cardiac output and renal perfusion with pimobendan. As long as the patient is feeling and eating well, and the current intensity of therapy is needed to control edema, mild azotemia is acceptable. Both serum creatinine and blood urea nitrogen (BUN) should be followed; the latter is often a better marker of renal function since many of these dogs have reduced muscle mass. In general, a BUN <50 mg/dL is of low concern. Electrolyte status should be monitored as well. Hypochloremia is anticipated with loop diuretic use. Hypokalemia is less common in patients receiving RAAS inhibition. When an azotemic patient is being treated with digoxin, serum digoxin concentrations should be checked more often, to avoid toxicity. Digoxin dosage reduction or drug discontinuation might be needed. The dose or frequency of the loop diuretic and any ACE inhibitor can be decreased if necessary, as inhibition of Ang II in some dogs is associated with substantial azotemia, although this is probably overstated. Increasing pimobendan to q8h dosing might help by improving renal perfusion. BP should be monitored and elevated BP controlled, as possible. An arteriolar vasodilator (such as amlodipine) added to standard CHF therapy can help improve forward cardiac output and renal perfusion, as long as hypotension can be avoided. In cases of moderate to severe azotemia, it may be reasonable to discontinue the ACE inhibitor and administer amlodipine, as well as reduce the diuretic dosage. Although spironolactone is a diuretic it has minimal diuretic effects, at least in healthy dogs; it might be continued for some downstream RAAS inhibition. Whenever diuretic dosages are decreased, close monitoring (of RRR and other signs) is required.

Thyrotoxicosis and anemia both increase the demand for cardiac output and might lead to cardiac decompensation. Hyperthyroidism in dogs usually is iatrogenic and related to over-supplementation with thyroid hormone, or inappropriate treatment of dogs where a diagnosis of hypothyroidism has not been conclusively established by appropriate testing (for example, sick euthyroid dogs). Hypothyroidism can depress myocardial function, so a reasonable target for dogs with CHF and established hypothyroidism is to aim for a low to mid-therapeutic range on follow-up thyroid testing.

Similar to hyperthyroidism, anemia causes peripheral vasodilation and increases the demand for cardiac output. Although mild anemia is unlikely to be problematic, if the hematocrit is below 25% consideration should be given to more aggressive diagnostic testing and treatment. Anemia has been associated with increased serum creatinine and chronic kidney disease, as well as CHF severity and worse prognosis. Any dog receiving a nonsteroidal anti-inflammatory drug (NSAID) or aspirin should be evaluated for possible GI bleeding.

Osteoarthritis is common in this group of canine patients and management often is needed to maintain quality of life and mobility. In general, corticosteroids are not used chronically for joint pain; instead, NSAIDs usually are effective in controlling clinical signs. However, NSAIDs also are relatively contraindicated in patients receiving diuretics or those in heart failure. This is especially true of cyclooxygenase inhibitors. Additionally, some NSAIDs can reduce the effectiveness of diuretics by decreasing delivery to the proximal tubule. Clients should be advised of the potential interactions and complications of combining cardiac therapy and NSAIDs. Nevertheless, to maintain quality of life it is often necessary to prescribe an NSAID to these older dogs. Some of the newer formulations, such as grapiprant (Galliprant®, Elanco), a prostaglandin E_2, EP4 prostenoid receptor antagonist might be safer in the setting of heart failure or renal disease, although the drug is not without adverse GI effects even in otherwise healthy dogs. Pain control with gabapentin also is appropriate and more heart-friendly; however, its effectiveness usually decreases over time.

Cardiac cachexia occurs to varying degrees in dogs with chronic CHF caused by DMVD. This is especially likely in dogs with ascites, but even those with chronic left heart failure tend to lose body weight and muscle mass over time. For this reason, body weight should be carefully measured at each examination, food intake assessed, and a body condition score and muscle mass estimation recorded at follow-up examinations. A diet with sufficient quality protein is important for these patients. Reduced appetite and anorexia commonly occur with chronic heart failure and exacerbate the development of cachexia. In some patients, appetite stimulants such as capromorelin (Entyce®, Elanco) might be needed (p. 352). Clinicians frequently associate specific drugs with anorexia. Realistically, probably any medication could directly or indirectly reduce appetite. Most notorious is digoxin. Inhibitors of RAAS also might cause anorexia, although too often these drugs are discontinued and never reinitiated to better assess their effect on appetite. Even the proprietary form of pimobendan (Vetmedin® chewable tabs, Boehringer-Ingelheim Vetmedica) occasionally is associated with GI upset, which might relate to the chewable vehicle. Diltiazem, used to control AF, is probably under recognized for its potential to depress appetite.

Prognosis

The prognosis for dogs with DMVD can be quite variable. Many dogs remain asymptomatic for years and some never develop CHF. More than 70% of dogs with preclinical disease lived over 6 years in one study (Borgarelli, 2012). Others suggest that median survival for dogs with stage B2 disease is a little over 2 years. Risk factors for first-onset CHF relate mainly to increased heart size, and are associated with high circulating NT-proBNP concentrations. One study identified NT-proBNP concentrations ≥1500 pmol/L and end diastolic LV dimension indexed to aortic root diameter (LVIDd/Ao) ≥ 3 as independent risk factors for first-onset CHF in stage B dogs with DMVD, with congestive failure likely to occur within the subsequent 3–6 months (PREDICT; Reynolds, 2012). Besides echo-derived measures, a VHS >12v also emerged as an independent risk factor. Although the LA/Ao ratio was significantly associated with CHF in a retrospective cohort, the specificity of the predictive regression equation derived from this variable, with NT-proBNP concentration, was suboptimal when applied prospectively. However, it did correctly predict future CHF in over 69% of dogs tested. Other researchers also have noted the correlation of natriuretic peptide levels with measures of LA and LV size in DMVD, and have identified NT-proBNP elevation as a risk factor for CHF onset within a year. Additionally, the rate of increase in VHS and echo measures of left heart size is greatest in the 6–12 months preceding clinical CHF onset.

Survival times in dogs with moderate CHF and good medical management have ranged from ~1–3 years, although the therapy used, complications that develop, or even breed could influence this. For example, young CKCS (especially males) with moderate to severe MR and increasing (normalized) systolic LVID have higher risk for cardiac death when they are older. Despite periodic episodes of decompensated CHF or other complications, quality of life can be good most of the time for dogs with DMVD that respond well to CHF therapy. Nevertheless, some dogs die or are euthanized during the first onset of CHF. For dogs with advanced CHF, a median survival time between 6 and 9 months is more likely. Estimates of cardiac death associated with DMVD have ranged from around 40% to almost 70% of cases. However, evolving management strategies for CHF are becoming more effective in controlling clinical signs and increasing survival time. Medical care provided through collaboration between the patient's primary care veterinarian and a board-certified veterinary cardiologist was shown to increase survival time in small-breed dogs with DMVD, compared with primary care management only.

Prognostic indicators of reduced survival after CHF onset include high circulating NT-proBNP concentration, as well as indices of left heart (especially LA) enlargement. Decrease in circulating NT-proBNP concentration following CHF therapy is thought to be a positive sign. Dogs that had reduction in NT-proBNP to <965 pmol/L after initial CHF therapy were more likely to survive over the next year, compared to dogs with higher post-treatment NT-proBNP concentration

(Wolf, 2012). LA enlargement is a highly significant echocardiographic predictor of reduced survival. Various indices of LA size and function remain significant predictive indicators upon multivariate analysis. In one study, peak mitral inflow (E) velocity >1.3 m/s was an even stronger predictor, conveying an over fourfold increased risk of death (Baron Toaldo, 2018). Some echocardiographic variables advance over time in dogs that die from DMVD, but remain more stable in those that do not (Hezzell, 2012a). Besides progressive LA enlargement, these have included indices of declining myocardial contractility (such as body weight-normalized LV end systolic dimension and MR Vmax) and worsening diastolic function (increased mitral E velocity and E/A ratio).

In situations where echocardiographic evaluation is not available, other factors might help the clinician estimate prognosis. In a study involving almost 900 dogs with presumptive diagnosis of DMVD in primary care settings, findings associated with increased risk for cardiac-related death were high circulating NT-proBNP and cTnI concentrations, increased heart rate, a loud murmur, exercise intolerance, and treatment with a potent diuretic (Mattin, 2019). High circulating concentrations (and rate of increase) of serum cTnI are associated with death from DMVD, especially in combination with increased NT-proBNP, LV enlargement, and advancing age (Hezzell, 2012b). Increased cTnI likely reflects greater myocardial fibrosis. The development of AF in larger dogs with DMVD also has been associated with higher risk for cardiac-related death. But in these dogs with AF, good heart rate control (<160 beats/minute) was linked with increased median survival time; in contrast, survival time was markedly shorter for dogs with AF and uncontrolled heart rate (Jung, 2016). The situation in smaller dogs that develop AF is likely to be similar. PH, as indicated by TR Vmax > 55 mm Hg, has been identified as a negative prognostic indicator by some, although not all, investigators (Borgarelli, 2015). Cardiac cachexia also is a negative prognostic indicator (p. 312). Nevertheless, certain findings associated with disease progression or death in some reports or on univariate analysis have not necessarily been independent prognostic indicators. Depending on the study, these have included older age, male gender, loud murmur, more severe valve lesions and degree of valve leaflet prolapse, MR severity, ruptured chordae, LV enlargement, and reduced LV systolic function.

Suggested Additional Reading and References

Also See Online Comprehensive Bibliography at: https://www.routledge.com/9781482246223.

Allen JW, Phipps KL, Llamas AA, et al. Left atrial decompression as a palliative minimally invasive treatment for congestive heart failure caused by myxomatous mitral valve disease in dogs: 17 cases (2018-2019). J Am Vet Med Assoc 2021;258:638–647.

Ames MK, Atkins CE, Eriksson A, et al. Aldosterone breakthrough in dogs with naturally occurring myxomatous mitral valve disease. J Vet Cardiol 2017;19:218–227.

Atkins CE, Keene BW, Brown WA, et al. Results of the veterinary enalapril trial to prove reduction in onset of heart failure in dogs chronically treated with enalapril alone for compensated, naturally occurring mitral valve insufficiency. J Am Vet Med Assoc 2007;231:1061–1069.

Atkins C, Bonagura J, Ettinger S, et al. Guidelines for the diagnosis and treatment of canine chronic valvular heart disease. J Vet Intern Med 2009;23:1142–1150. (ACVIM Consensus Statement).

Aupperle H, Disatian S. Pathology, protein expression and signaling in myxomatous mitral valve degeneration: comparison of dogs and humans. J Vet Cardiol 2012;14:59–71.

Baron Toaldo M, Romito G, Guglielmini C, et al. Prognostic value of echocardiographic indices of left atrial morphology and function in dogs with myxomatous mitral valve disease. J Vet Intern Med 2018;32:914–921.

Bernay F, Bland JM, Häggström J, et al. Efficacy of spironolactone on survival in dogs with naturally occurring mitral regurgitation caused by myxomatous mitral valve disease. J Vet Intern Med 2010;24:331–341.

Besche B, Blondel T, Guillot E, et al. Efficacy of oral torasemide in dogs with degenerative mitral valve disease and new onset congestive heart failure: The CARPODIEM study. J Vet Intern Med 2020;34:1746-1758.

Birkegard AC, Reimann MJ, Martinussen T, et al. Breeding restrictions decrease the prevalence of myxomatous mitral valve disease in Cavalier King Charles Spaniels over an 8- to 10-year period. J Vet Intern Med 2016;30:63–68.

Bonagura JD, Schober KE. Can ventricular function be assessed by echocardiography in chronic canine mitral valve disease? J Small Anim Pract 2009;50(Suppl 1):12–24.

Borgarelli M, Abbott J, Braz-Ruivo L, et al. Prevalence and prognostic importance of pulmonary hypertension in dogs with myxomatous mitral valve disease. J Vet Intern Med 2015;29:569–574.

Borgarelli M, Buchanan JW. Historical review, epidemiology and natural history of degenerative mitral valve disease. J Vet Cardiol 2012;14:93–101.

Borgarelli M, Crosara S, Lamb K, et al. Survival characteristics and prognostic variables of dogs with preclinical chronic degenerative mitral valve disease attributable to myxomatous degeneration. J Vet Intern Med 2012;26:69–75.

Borgarelli M, Lanz O, Pavlisko N, et al. Mitral valve repair in dogs using an ePTFE chordal implantation device: a pilot study. J Vet Cardiol 2017;19:256–267.

Borgarelli M, Ferasin L, Lamb K, et al. Delay of appearance of symptoms of canine degenerative mitral valve disease treated with spironolactone and benazepril: the DELAY study. J Vet Cardiol 2020;27:34–53.

Boswood A, Häggström J, Gordon SG, et al. Effect of pimobendan in dogs with preclinical myxomatous mitral valve disease and cardiomegaly: the EPIC study—a randomized clinical trial. J Vet Intern Med 2016;30:1765–1779.

Boswood A, Gordon SG, Häggström J, et al. Longitudinal analysis of quality of life, clinical, radiographic, echocardiographic, and laboratory variables in dogs with preclinical myxomatous mitral valve disease receiving pimobendan or placebo: the EPIC study. J Vet Intern Med 2018;32:72–85.

Boswood A, Gordon SG, Häggström J, et al. Temporal changes in clinical and radiographic variables in dogs with preclinical myxomatous mitral valve disease: the EPIC study. J Vet Intern Med 2020;34:1108–1118.

Brüler BC, Jojima FS, Dittrich G, et al. QT instability, an indicator of augmented arrhythmogenesis, increases with the progression of myxomatous mitral valve disease in dogs. J Vet Cardiol 2018;20:254–266.

Caivano D, Dickson D, Pariaut R, et al. Tricuspid annular plane systolic excursion-to-aortic ratio provides a bodyweight-independent measure of right ventricular systolic function in dogs. J Vet Cardiol 2018a;20:79–91.

Caivano D, Rishniw M, Birettoni F, et al. Right ventricular outflow tract fractional shortening: an echocardiographic index of right ventricular systolic function in dogs with pulmonary hypertension. J Vet Cardiol 2018b;20:354–363.

Carlsson C, Häggström J, Eriksson A, et al. Size and shape of right heart chambers in mitral valve regurgitation in small-breed dogs. J Vet Intern Med 2009;23:1007–1013.

Chan IP, Wu SY, Chang CC, et al. Serial measurements of cardiac troponin I in heart failure secondary to canine mitral valve disease. Vet Rec 2019;185:343.

Chapel EH, Scansen BA, Schober KE, et al. Echocardiographic estimates of right ventricular systolic function in dogs with myxomatous mitral valve disease. J Vet Intern Med 2018;32:64–71.

Chetboul V, Serres F, Tissier R, et al. Association of plasma N-terminal pro-B-type natriuretic peptide concentration with mitral regurgitation severity and outcome in dogs with asymptomatic degenerative mitral valve disease. J Vet Intern Med 2009;23:984–994.

Chompoosan C, Buranakarl C, Chaiyabutr N, et al. Decreased sympathetic tone after short-term treatment with enalapril in dogs with mild chronic mitral valve disease. Res Vet Sci 2014;96:347–354.

Crosara S, Borgarelli M, Perego M, et al. Holter monitoring in 36 dogs with myxomatous mitral valve disease. Aust Vet J 2010;88:386–392.

Cunningham SM, Rush JE, Freeman LM. Systemic inflammation and endothelial dysfunction in dogs with congestive heart failure. J Vet Intern Med 2012;26:547–557.

Cunningham SM, Rush JE, Freeman LM. Short-term effects of atorvastatin in normal dogs and dogs with congestive heart failure due to myxomatous mitral valve disease. J Vet Intern Med 2013;27:985–989.

Diana A, Guglielmini C, Pivetta M, et al. Radiographic features of cardiogenic pulmonary edema in dogs with mitral regurgitation: 61 cases (1998–2007). J Am Vet Med Assoc 2009;235:1058–1063.

Dickson D, Caivano D, Matos JN, et al. Two-dimensional echocardiographic estimates of left atrial function in healthy dogs and dogs with myxomatous mitral valve disease. J Vet Cardiol 2017;19:469–479.

Dillon AR, Dell'Italia LJ, Tillson M, et al. Left ventricular remodeling in preclinical experimental mitral regurgitation of dogs. J Vet Cardiol 2012;14:73–92.

Ebisawa T, Ohta Y, Funayama M, et al. Plasma atrial natriuretic peptide is an early diagnosis and disease severity marker of myxomatous mitral valve disease in dogs. Res Vet Sci 2013;94:717–721.

Eriksson A, Hansson K, Häggström J, et al. Pulmonary blood volume in mitral regurgitation in cavalier King Charles spaniels. J Vet Intern Med 2010;24:1393–1399.

Eriksson AS, Häggström J, Pedersen HD, et al. Increased NT-proANP predicts risk of congestive heart failure in Cavalier King Charles Spaniels with mitral regurgitation caused by myxomatous valve disease. J Vet Cardiol 2014;16:141–154.

Esser LC, Borkovec M, Bauer A, et al. Left ventricular M-mode prediction intervals in 7651 dogs: Population-wide and selected breed-specific values. J Vet Intern Med 2020;34:2242–2252.

Falk T, Jonsson L, Olsen LH, et al. Associations between cardiac pathology and clinical, echocardiographic and electrocardiographic findings in dogs with chronic congestive heart failure. Vet J 2010;185:68–74.

Falk T, Ljungvall I, Zois NE, et al. Cardiac troponin-I concentration, myocardial arteriosclerosis, and fibrosis in dogs with congestive heart failure because of myxomatous mitral valve disease. J Vet Intern Med 2013;27:500–506.

Ferasin L, Crews L, Biller DS, et al. Risk factors for coughing in dogs with naturally acquired myxomatous mitral valve disease. J Vet Intern Med 2013;27:286–292.

Fox PR. Pathology of myxomatous mitral valve disease in the dog. J Vet Cardiol 2012;14:103–126.

French AT, Ogden R, Eland C, et al. Genome-wide analysis of mitral valve disease in Cavalier King Charles Spaniels. Vet J 2012;193:283–286.

Garncarz M, Parzeniecka-Jaworska M, Hulanicka M, et al. Mitral regurgitation in Dachshund dogs without heart murmurs. J Vet Res 2017;61:363–366.

Guglielmini C, Diana A, Pietra M, et al. Use of the vertebral heart score in coughing dogs with chronic degenerative mitral valve disease. J Vet Med Sci 2009;71:9–13.

Guglielmini C, Civitella C, Diana A, et al. Serum cardiac troponin I concentration in dogs with precapillary and postcapillary pulmonary hypertension. J Vet Intern Med 2010;24:145–152.

Guglielmini C, Goncalves Sousa M, Baron Toaldo M, et al. Prevalence and risk factors for atrial fibrillation in dogs with myxomatous mitral valve disease. J Vet Intern Med 2020;34:2223–2231.

Häggström J, Boswood A, O'Grady M, et al. Longitudinal analysis of quality of life, clinical, radiographic, echocardiographic, and laboratory variables in dogs with myxomatous mitral valve disease receiving pimobendan or benazepril: the QUEST study. J Vet Intern Med 2013;27:1441–1451.

Han D, Choi R, Hyun C. Canine pancreatic-specific lipase concentrations in dogs with heart failure and chronic mitral valvular insufficiency. J Vet Intern Med 2015;29:180–183.

Han RI, Black A, Culshaw G, et al. Structural and cellular changes in canine myxomatous mitral valve disease: an image analysis study. J Heart Valve Dis 2010;19:60–70.

Hezzell MJ, Boswood A, Moonarmart W, et al. Selected echocardiographic variables change more rapidly in dogs that die from myxomatous mitral valve disease. J Vet Cardiol 2012a;14:269–279.

Hezzell MJ, Boswood A, Chang YM, et al. The combined prognostic potential of serum high-sensitivity cardiac troponin I and N-terminal pro-B-type natriuretic peptide concentrations in dogs with degenerative mitral valve disease. J Vet Intern Med 2012b;26:302–311.

Hezzell MJ, Boswood A, Lopez-Alvarez J, et al. Treatment of dogs with compensated myxomatous mitral valve disease with spironolactone—a pilot study. J Vet Cardiol 2017;19:325–338.

Hezzell MJ, Block CL, Laughlin DS, et al. Effect of prespecified therapy escalation on plasma NT-proBNP concentrations in dogs with stable congestive heart failure due to myxomatous mitral valve disease. J Vet Intern Med 2018;32:1509–1516.

Hoglund K, Häggström J, Hanas S, et al. Interbreed variation in serum serotonin (5-hydroxytryptamine) concentration in healthy dogs. J Vet Cardiol 2018;20:244–253.

Hollmer M, Willesen JL, Tolver A, et al. Left atrial volume and function in dogs with naturally occurring myxomatous mitral valve disease. J Vet Cardiol 2017;19:24–34.

Hori Y, Iguchi M, Hirakawa A, et al. Evaluation of atrial natriuretic peptide and cardiac troponin I concentrations for assessment of disease severity in dogs with naturally occurring mitral valve disease. J Am Vet Med Assoc 2020;256:340–348.

Hori Y, Yamashita Y, Sakakibara K, et al. Usefulness of pericardial lung ultrasonography for the diagnosis of cardiogenic pulmonary edema in dogs. Am J Vet Res 2020;81:227–232.

Ineson DL, Freeman LM, Rush JE. Clinical and laboratory findings and survival time associated with cardiac cachexia in dogs with congestive heart failure. J Vet Intern Med 2019;33:1902–1908.

Ishikawa T, Tanaka R, Suzuki S, et al. Daily rhythms of left atrial pressure in beagle dogs with mitral valve regurgitation. J Vet Intern Med 2009;23:824–831.

Ishikawa T, Tanaka R, Suzuki S, et al. The effect of angiotensin-converting enzyme inhibitors of left atrial pressure in dogs with mitral valve regurgitation. J Vet Intern Med 2010;24:342–347.

Jung S, Bohan A. Genome-wide sequencing and quantification of circulating microRNAs for dogs with congestive heart failure secondary to myxomatous mitral valve degeneration. Am J Vet Res 2018;79:163–169.

Jung SW, Sun W, Griffiths LG, et al. Atrial fibrillation as a prognostic indicator in medium to large-sized dogs with myxomatous mitral valvular degeneration and congestive heart failure. J Vet Intern Med 2016;30:51–57.

Kanno N, Asano K, Teshima K, et al. Plasma adrenomedullin concentration in dogs with myxomatous mitral valvular disease. J Vet Med Sci 2012;74:739–743.

Keene BK, Atkins CE, Bonagura JD, et al. Updated ACVIM consensus guidelines for the diagnosis and therapy of chronic valvular heart disease in dogs. J Vet Intern Med 2019;33(3):1127–1140.

Kellihan HB, Stepien RL. Pulmonary hypertension in canine degenerative mitral valve disease. J Vet Cardiol 2012;14:149–164.

Kijtawornrat A, Komolvanich S, Saengklub N, et al. Long-term effect of sildenafil on echocardiographic parameters in dogs with asymptomatic myxomatous mitral valve degeneration. J Vet Med Sci 2017;79:788–794.

Kim JH, Park HM. Usefulness of conventional and tissue Doppler echocardiography to predict congestive heart failure in dogs with myxomatous mitral valve disease. J Vet Intern Med 2015;29:132–140.

Kim HS, Kang JH, Jeung EB, et al. Serum concentrations of leptin and adiponectin in dogs with myxomatous mitral valve disease. J Vet Intern Med 2016;30:1589–1600.

Kim HT, Han SM, Song WJ, et al. Retrospective study of degenerative mitral valve disease in small-breed dogs: survival and prognostic variables. J Vet Sci 2017;18:369–376.

Kim YH, Choi GJ, Park C. Rate of left ventricular pressure change by Doppler echocardiography in dogs with chronic mitral valve disease at different stages of congestive heart failure. Vet Radiol Ultrasound 2018;59:758–766.

King JN, Hirakawa A, Sonobe J, et al. Evaluation of a fixed-dose combination of benazepril and pimobendan in dogs with congestive heart failure: a randomized non-inferiority clinical trial. J Vet Sci 2018;19:117–128.

Kvart C, Häggström J, Pedersen HD, et al. Efficacy of enalapril for prevention of congestive heart failure in dogs with myxomatous valve disease and asymptomatic mitral regurgitation. J Vet Intern Med 2002;16:80–88.

Lake-Bakaar GA, Singh MK, Kass PH, et al. Effect of pimobendan on the incidence of arrhythmias in small breed dogs with myxomatous mitral valve degeneration. J Vet Cardiol 2015;17:120–128.

Lake-Bakaar GA, Mok MY, Kittleson MD. Fossa ovalis tear causing right to left shunting in a Cavalier King Charles Spaniel. J Vet Cardiol 2012;14:541–545.

Larouche-Lebel É, Loughran KA, Oyama MA. Echocardiographic indices and severity of mitral regurgitation in dogs with preclinical degenerative mitral valve disease. J Vet Intern Med 2019;33:489–498.

Lee CM, Jeong DM, Kang MH, et al. Correlation between serum homocysteine concentration and severity of mitral valve disease in dogs. Am J Vet Res 2017;78:440–446.

Lee JS, Pak SI, Hyun C. Calcium reuptake related genes as a cardiac biomarker in dogs with chronic mitral valvular insufficiency. J Vet Intern Med 2009;23:832–839.

Lefbom BK, Peckens NK. Impact of collaborative care on survival time for dogs with congestive heart failure and revenue for attending primary care veterinarians. J Am Vet Med Assoc 2016;249:72–76.

Lefebvre HP, Ollivier E, Atkins CE, et al. Safety of spironolactone in dogs with chronic heart failure because of degenerative valvular disease: a population-based, longitudinal study. J Vet Intern Med 2013;27:1083–1091.

Ljungvall I, Ahlstrom C, Hoglund K, et al. Use of signal analysis of heart sounds and murmurs to assess severity of mitral valve regurgitation attributable to myxomatous mitral valve disease in dogs. Am J Vet Res 2009;70:604–613.

Ljungvall I, Hoglund K, Tidholm A, et al. Cardiac troponin I is associated with severity of myxomatous mitral valve disease, age, and C-reactive protein in dogs. J Vet Intern Med 2010;24:153–159.

Locatelli C, Piras C, Riscazzi G, et al. Serum proteomic profiles in CKCS with mitral valve disease. BMC Vet Res 2017;13:43.

López-Alvarez J, Elliott J, Pfeiffer D, et al. Clinical severity score system in dogs with degenerative mitral valve disease. J Vet Intern Med 2015;29:575–581.

Lord P, Hansson K, Kvart C, et al. Rate of change of heart size before congestive heart failure in dogs with mitral regurgitation. J Small Anim Pract 2010;51:210–218.

Lord PF, Hansson K, Carnabuci C, et al. Radiographic heart size and its rate of increase as tests for onset of congestive heart failure in Cavalier King Charles Spaniels with mitral valve regurgitation. J Vet Intern Med 2011;25:1312–1319.

Lu CC, Liu MM, Culshaw G, et al. Gene network and canonical pathway analysis in canine myxomatous mitral valve disease: a microarray study. Vet J 2015;204:23–31.

Madsen MB, Olsen LH, Häggström J, et al. Identification of 2 loci associated with development of myxomatous mitral valve disease in Cavalier King Charles Spaniels. J Hered 2011;102(Suppl 1):S62–67.

Malcolm EL, Visser LC, Phillips KL, et al. Diagnostic value of vertebral left atrial size as determined from thoracic radiographs for assessment of left atrial size in dogs with myxomatous mitral valve disease. J Am Vet Med Assoc 2018;253:1038–1045.

Markby G, Summers K, MacRae V, et al. Comparative transcriptomic profiling and gene expression for myxomatous mitral valve disease in the dog and human. Veterinary Sciences 2017;4:34.

Mattin MJ, Boswood A, Church DB, et al. Prognostic factors in dogs with presumed degenerative mitral valve disease attending primary-care veterinary practices in the United Kingdom. J Vet Intern Med 2019;33:432–444.

Mavropoulou A, Guazzetti S, Borghetti P, et al. Cytokine expression in peripheral blood mononuclear cells of dogs with mitral valve disease. Vet J 2016;211:45–51.

Menciotti G, Borgarelli M, Aherne M, et al. Mitral valve morphology assessed by three-dimensional transthoracic echocardiography in healthy dogs and dogs with myxomatous mitral valve disease. J Vet Cardiol 2017;19:113–123.

Menciotti G, Borgarelli M, Aherne M, et al. Comparison of the mitral valve morphologies of Cavalier King Charles Spaniels and dogs of other breeds using 3D transthoracic echocardiography. J Vet Intern Med 2018;32:1564–1569.

Merveille AC, Bolen G, Krafft E, et al. pulmonary vein-to-pulmonary artery ratio is an echocardiographic index of congestive heart failure in dogs with degenerative mitral valve disease. J Vet Intern Med 2015;29:1502–1509.

Meurs KM, Friedenberg SG, Williams B, et al. Evaluation of genes associated with human myxomatous mitral valve disease in dogs with familial myxomatous mitral valve degeneration. Vet J 2018;232:16–19.

Meurs KM, Olsen LH, Reimann MJ, et al. Angiotensin-converting enzyme activity in Cavalier King Charles Spaniels with an ACE gene polymorphism and myxomatous mitral valve disease. Pharmacogenet Genomics 2018;28:37–40.

Mikawa S, Nagakawa M, Ogi H, et al. Use of vertebral left atrial size for staging of dogs with myxomatous valve disease. J Vet Cardiol 2020;30:92–99.

Misbach C, Chetboul V, Concordet D, et al. Basal plasma concentrations of N-terminal pro-B-type natriuretic peptide in clinically healthy adult small size dogs: effect of body weight, age, gender and breed, and reference intervals. Res Vet Sci 2013;95(3):879–885.

Mizuno M, Yamano S, Chimura S, et al. Efficacy of pimobendan on survival and reoccurrence of pulmonary edema in canine congestive heart failure. J Vet Med Sci 2017;79:29–34.

Moesgaard SG, Klostergaard C, Zois NE, et al. Flow-mediated vasodilation measurements in Cavalier King Charles Spaniels with increasing severity of myxomatous mitral valve disease. J Vet Intern Med 2012;26:61–68.

Moonarmart W, Boswood A, Luis Fuentes V, et al. N-terminal pro B-type natriuretic peptide and left ventricular diameter independently predict mortality in dogs with mitral valve disease. J Small Anim Pract 2010;51:84–96.

Nakamura K, Kawamoto S, Osuga T, et al. Left atrial strain at different stages of myxomatous mitral valve disease in dogs. J Vet Intern Med 2017;31:316–325.

Nam SJ, Han SH, Kim HW, et al. The cardiac biomarker sodium-calcium exchanger (NCX-1) can differentiate between heart failure and renal failure: a comparative study of NCX-1 expression in dogs with chronic mitral valvular insufficiency and azotemia. J Vet Intern Med 2010;24:1383–1387.

Nelson OL, Wood RM, Häggström J, et al. Myocardial adiponectin isoform shift in dogs with congestive heart failure–a comparison to hibernating Brown bears (*Ursus arctos horribilis*). Vet Sci 2017;4.

Newhard DK, Jung S, Winter RL, et al. A prospective, randomized, double-blind, placebo-controlled pilot study of sacubitril/valsartan (entresto) in dogs with cardiomegaly secondary to myxomatous mitral valve disease. J Vet Intern Med 2018;32:1555–1563.

O'Leary CA, Wilkie I. Cardiac valvular and vascular disease in Bull terriers. Vet Pathol 2009;46:1149–1155.

Orton EC, Lacerda CM, MacLea HB. Signaling pathways in mitral valve degeneration. J Vet Cardiol 2012;14:7–17.

Oui H, Oh J, Keh S, et al. Measurements of the pulmonary vasculature on thoracic radiographs in healthy dogs compared to dogs with mitral regurgitation. Vet Radiol Ultrasound 2015;56(3):251–256.

Oyama MA, Chittur SV. Genomic expression patterns of mitral valve tissues from dogs with degenerative mitral valve disease. Am J Vet Res 2006;67:1307–1318.

Oyama MA, Elliott C, Loughran KA, et al. Comparative pathology of human and canine myxomatous mitral valve degeneration: 5HT and TGF-beta mechanisms. Cardiovasc Pathol 2020;46:107196.

Paiva RM, Garcia-Guasch L, Manubens J, et al. Proximal isovelocity surface area variability during systole in dogs with mitral valve prolapse. J Vet Cardiol 2011;13(4):267–270.

Pat B, Chen Y, Killingsworth C, et al. Chymase inhibition prevents fibronectin and myofibrillar loss and improves cardiomyocyte function and LV torsion angle in dogs with isolated mitral regurgitation. Circulation 2010;122:1488–1495.

Pedersen HD, Häggström J, Falk T, Mow T, Olsen LH, Iversen L, Jensen AL. Auscultation in mild mitral regurgitation in dogs: observer variation, effects of physical maneuvers, and agreement with color Doppler echocardiography and phonocardiography. J Vet Intern Med 1999;13(1):56e64.

Pirintr P, Limprasutr V, Saengklub N, et al. Acute effect of ivabradine on heart rate and myocardial oxygen consumption in dogs with asymptomatic mitral valve degeneration. Exp Anim 2018;67(4):441–449.

Pirintr P, Saengklub N, Limprasutr V, et al. Sildenafil improves heart rate variability in dogs with asymptomatic myxomatous mitral valve degeneration. J Vet Med Sci 2017;79:1480–1488.

Poad MH, Manzi TJ, Oyama MA, et al. Utility of radiographic measurements to predict echocardiographic left heart enlargement in dogs with preclinical myxomatous mitral valve disease. J Vet Intern Med 2020;34:1728–1733.

Polizopoulou ZS, Koutinas CK, Dasopoulou A, et al. Serial analysis of serum cardiac troponin I changes and correlation with clinical findings in 46 dogs with mitral valve disease. Vet Clin Pathol 2014;43:218–225.

Poser H, Berlanda M, Monacolli M, et al. Tricuspid annular plane systolic excursion in dogs with myxomatous mitral valve disease with and without pulmonary hypertension. J Vet Cardiol 2017;19:228–239.

Pouchelon JL, Jamet N, Gouni V, et al. Effect of benazepril on survival and cardiac events in dogs with asymptomatic mitral valve disease: a retrospective study of 141 cases. J Vet Intern Med 2008;22:905–914.

Reimann MJ, Häggström J, Mortensen A, et al. Biopterin status in dogs with myxomatous mitral valve disease is associated with disease severity and cardiovascular risk factors. J Vet Intern Med 2014;28:1520–1526.

Reimann MJ, Ljungvall I, Hillstrom A, et al. Increased serum C-reactive protein concentrations in dogs with congestive heart failure due to myxomatous mitral valve disease. Vet J 2015;209:113–118.

Reimann MJ, Moller JE, Häggström J, et al. R-R interval variations influence the degree of mitral regurgitation in dogs with myxomatous mitral valve disease. Vet J 2014;199:348–354.

Reineke EL, Burkett DE, Drobatz KJ. Left atrial rupture in dogs: 14 cases (1990–2005). J Vet Emerg Crit Care 2008;18:158–164.

Reynolds CA, Brown DC, Rush JE, et al. Prediction of first onset of congestive heart failure in dogs with degenerative mitral valve disease: the PREDICT cohort study. J Vet Cardiol 2012;14:193–202.

Sakarin S, Rungsipipat A, Surachetpong SD. Galectin-3 in cardiac muscle and circulation of dogs with degenerative mitral valve disease. J Vet Cardiol 2016;18:34–46.

Sargent J, Connolly DJ, Watts V, et al. Assessment of mitral regurgitation in dogs: comparison of results of echocardiography with magnetic resonance imaging. J Small Anim Pract 2015;56:641–650.

Sargent J, Muzzi R, Mukherjee R, et al. Echocardiographic predictors of survival in dogs with myxomatous mitral valve disease. J Vet Cardiol 2015;17:1–12.

Savarese A, Probo M, Locatelli C, et al. Iron status in dogs with myxomatous mitral valve disease. Pol J Vet Sci 2018;21:507–515.

Schober KE, Bonagura JD, Scansen BA, et al. Estimation of left ventricular filling pressure by use of Doppler echocardiography in healthy anesthetized dogs subjected to acute volume loading. Am J Vet Res 2008;69:1034–1049.

Schober KE, Hart TM, Stern JA, et al. Detection of congestive heart failure in dogs by Doppler echocardiography. J Vet Intern Med 2010;24:1358–1368.

Schober KE, Hart TM, Stern JA, et al. Effects of treatment on respiratory rate, serum natriuretic peptide concentration, and Doppler echocardiographic indices of left ventricular filling pressure in dogs with congestive heart failure secondary to degenerative mitral valve disease and dilated cardiomyopathy. J Am Vet Med Assoc 2011;239:468–479.

Serres F, Chetboul V, Tissier R, et al. Chordae tendineae rupture in dogs with degenerative mitral valve disease: prevalence, survival, and prognostic factors (114 cases, 2001–2006). J Vet Intern Med 2007;21:258–264.

Serres F, Pouchelon JL, Poujol L, et al. Plasma N-terminal pro-B-type natriuretic peptide concentration helps to predict survival in dogs with symptomatic degenerative mitral valve disease regardless of and in combination with the initial clinical status at admission. J Vet Cardiol 2009;11:103–121.

Sjöstrand K, Wess G, Ljungvall I, et al. Breed differences in natriuretic peptides in healthy dogs. J Vet Intern Med 2014;28:451–457.

Smith DN, Bonagura JD, Culwell NM, et al. Left ventricular function quantified by myocardial strain imaging in small-breed dogs with chronic mitral regurgitation. J Vet Cardiol 2012;14:231–242.

Soares FB, Pereira-Neto GB, Rabelo RC. Assessment of plasma lactate and core-peripheral temperature gradient in association with stages of naturally occurring myxomatous mitral valve disease in dogs. J Vet Emerg Crit Care 2018;28:532–540.

Stepien RL, Kellihan HB, Luis Fuentes V. Prevalence and diagnostic characteristics of non-clinical mitral regurgitation murmurs in North American Whippets. J Vet Cardiol 2017;19:317–324.

Stepien RL, Rak MB, Blume LM. Use of radiographic measurements to diagnose stage B2 preclinical myxomatous mitral valve disease in dogs. J Am Vet Med Assoc 2020;256:1129–1136.

Stern JA, Hsue W, Song KH, et al. Severity of mitral valve degeneration is associated with chromosome 15 loci in Whippet dogs. PLoS One 2015;10:e0141234.

Sun Q, Tang M, Pu J, et al. Pulmonary venous structural remodeling in a canine model of chronic atrial dilation due to mitral regurgitation. Can J Cardiol 2008;24:305–308.

Suzuki S, Ishikawa T, Hamabe L, et al. The effect of furosemide on left atrial pressure in dogs with mitral valve regurgitation. J Vet Intern Med 2011a;25:244–250.

Suzuki S, Fukushima R, Ishikawa T, et al. The effect of pimobendan on left atrial pressure in dogs with mitral valve regurgitation. J Vet Intern Med 2011b;25:1328–1333.

Suzuki S, Fukushima R, Ishikawa T, et al. Comparative effects of amlodipine and benazepril on left atrial pressure in dogs with experimentally-induced mitral valve regurgitation. BMC Vet Res 2012;8:166.

Suzuki R, Matsumoto H, Teshima T, et al. Left ventricular geometrical differences in dogs with various stages of myxomatous mitral valve disease. J Small Anim Pract 2013;54:234–239.

Swift S, Baldin A, Cripps P Degenerative valvular disease in the Cavalier King Charles Spaniel: results of the UK Breed Scheme 1991-2010. J Vet Intern Med 2017;31:9–14.

Takemura N, Toda N, Miyagawa Y, et al. Evaluation of plasma N-terminal pro-brain natriuretic peptide (NT-proBNP) concentrations in dogs with mitral valve insufficiency. J Vet Med Sci 2009;71:925–929.

Tarnow I, Olsen LH, Kvart C, et al. Predictive value of natriuretic peptides in dogs with mitral valve disease. Vet J 2009;180:195–201.

Tidholm A, Bodegard-Westling A, Hoglund K, et al. Real-time 3-dimensional echocardiographic assessment of effective regurgitant orifice area in dogs with myxomatous mitral valve disease. J Vet Intern Med 2017;31:303–310.

Tidholm A, Hoglund K, Häggström J, et al. Diagnostic value of selected echocardiographic variables to identify pulmonary hypertension in dogs with myxomatous mitral valve disease. J Vet Intern Med 2015;29:1510–1517.

Trafny DJ, Freeman LM, Bulmer BJ, et al. Auscultatory, echocardiographic, biochemical, nutritional, and environmental characteristics of mitral valve disease in Norfolk terriers. J Vet Cardiol 2012;14:261–267.

Uechi M. Mitral valve repair in dogs. J Vet Cardiol 2012;14:185–192.

Uechi M, Mizukoshi T, Mizuno T, et al. Mitral valve repair under cardiopulmonary bypass in small-breed dogs: 48 cases (2006–2009). J Am Vet Med Assoc 2012;240:1194–1201.

Vezzosi T, Mannucci T, Pistoresi A, et al. Assessment of lung ultrasound B-lines in dogs with different stages of chronic valvular heart disease. J Vet Intern Med 2017;31:700–704.

Wall L, Mohr A, Ripoli FL, et al. Clinical use of submaximal treadmill exercise testing and assessments of cardiac biomarkers NT-proBNP and cTnI in dogs with presymptomatic mitral regurgitation. PLoS One 2018;13:e0199023.

Ward J, Ware W, Viall A Association between atrial fibrillation and right-sided manifestations of congestive heart failure in dogs with degenerative mitral valve disease or dilated cardiomyopathy. J Vet Cardiol 2019;21:18–27.

Wess G, Kresken JG, Wendt R, et al. Efficacy of adding ramipril (VAsotop) to the combination of furosemide (Lasix) and pimobendan (VEtmedin) in dogs with mitral valve degeneration: The VALVE trial. J Vet Intern Med 2020;34:2232–2241.

Wesselowski S, Borgarelli M, Bello NM, et al. Discrepancies in identification of left atrial enlargement using left atrial volume versus left atrial-to-aortic root ratio in dogs. J Vet Intern Med 2014;28:1527–1533.

Whitney JC. Observations on the effect of age on the severity of heart valve lesions in the dog. J Small Anim Pract 1974;15:511–522.

Wolf J, Gerlach N, Weber K, et al. Lowered N-terminal pro-B-type natriuretic peptide levels in response to treatment predict survival in dogs with symptomatic mitral valve disease. J Vet Cardiol 2012;14:399–408.

Wolf J, Gerlach N, Weber K, et al. The diagnostic relevance of NT-proBNP and proANP 31-67 measurements in staging of myxomatous mitral valve disease in dogs. Vet Clin Pathol 2013;42:196–206.

Yamamoto Y, Suzuki S, Hamabe L, et al. Effects of a sustained-release form of isosorbide dinitrate on left atrial pressure in dogs with experimentally induced mitral valve regurgitation. J Vet Intern Med 2013;27:1421–1426.

Yang VK, Loughran KA, Meola DM, et al. Circulating exosome microRNA associated with heart failure secondary to myxomatous mitral valve disease in a naturally occurring canine model. J Extracell Vesicles 2017;6:1350088.

Yokoyama S, Kanemoto I, Mihara K, et al. Treatment of severe mitral regurgitation caused by lesions in both leaflets using multiple mitral valve plasty techniques in a small dog. Open Vet J 2017;7:328–331.

Yu IB, Huang HP. Prevalence and prognosis of anemia in dogs with degenerative mitral valve disease. Biomed Res Int 2016;2016:4727054.

Zois NE, Tidholm A, Nagga KM, et al. Radial and longitudinal strain and strain rate assessed by speckle-tracking echocardiography in dogs with myxomatous mitral valve disease. J Vet Intern Med 2012;26:1309–1319.

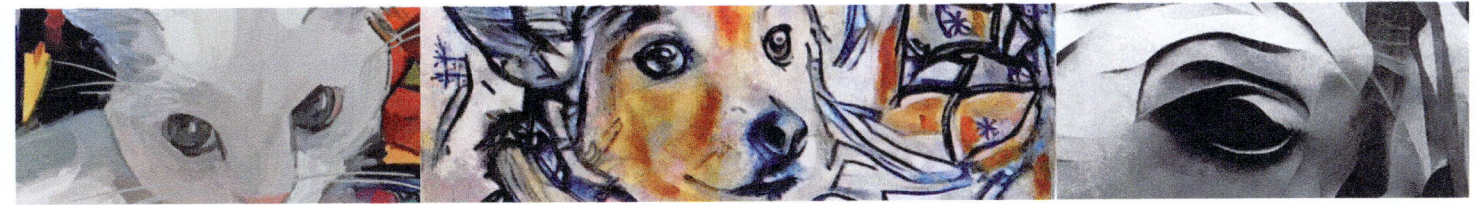

30
VALVULAR HEART DISEASE OF THE HORSE

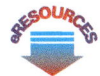

Heart murmurs are heard often during cardiac auscultation of horses. These frequently arise from diseases of the cardiac valves. As in other animal species, the atrioventricular (AV) valves are a complex functional apparatus of leaflet, chordal, fibrous, and muscular structures that close the valves in systole and control their opening during diastole. The aortic and pulmonary valves are composed of a valve ring with three semilunar leaflets that open during systole and close in diastole. The normal morphology of the four cardiac valves and their support structures is described further in Chapter 1 (p. 7). Cardiac murmurs caused by mitral regurgitation (MR), aortic regurgitation (AR), and tricuspid regurgitation (TR) are common in horses. Conversely, murmurs of valvular stenosis are quite rare. It is important to distinguish pathological (organic) from physiological (functional) systolic and diastolic heart murmurs.

Many organic murmurs in the horse seem to be associated with minimal, if any, impact on work performance. However, an objective assessment requires comprehensive integration of the work history, physical examination findings, heart rhythm, and echocardiographic (echo) imaging. Another special consideration relevant to horses relates to safety. The clinical issues, therefore, include determination of: the most likely source of the murmur, the underlying morphology of the lesion, any impact on performance, and the relative risk of any valvular disease to horse and rider (or driver).

Causes of Equine Valvular Disease

Table 30.1 summarizes potential causes of valvular heart disease (VHD) in the horse. Important lesions arise largely from acquired diseases and lead to valvular insufficiency. The most common etiology is degenerative valve disease, which mainly affects the mitral and aortic valve leaflets (**Figure 30.1**). Other causes of MR and TR, include malformations (likely under-recognized), infective endocarditis, chordal ruptures, and for TR, pulmonary hypertension (PH). AR can be secondary to a number of valvular and aortic root diseases (**Figures 30.1–30.3**), but most often it stems from degenerative valvular changes in older horses. Uncommon etiologies of AR include infective endocarditis, (congenital) malalignment ventricular septal defect (VSD), and rupture of a sinus of Valsalva with aortic-to-cardiac fistula (p. 784).

Valvar stenosis is rare in horses. When it occurs, it typically involves either pulmonary or tricuspid valve malformations or complete atresia of the inflow or outflow tract. Acquired valvular stenosis can develop with large vegetations or scarring from infective endocarditis (see Chapter 31) or ill-defined noninfective valvulitis (**Figure 30.4**). Progressive training-associated valvular regurgitation is common in high-performance horses, with TR and MR representing the most common of the auscultatory manifestations. The etiology and clinical significance of training-associated VHD in performance horses remains undetermined. Perhaps high-intensity training accelerates degenerative processes or causes adaptive changes in the valve or subvalvular support structures. These could include physiological hypertrophy or transient pulmonary or systemic hypertension, which might alter valvular structure or function.

Additional causes of cardiac murmurs in horses, including cardiomyopathies, are summarized in **Tables 30.1** and **30.2**. Ventricular chamber enlargement or papillary muscle lesions such as scars can cause so-called functional AV valve insufficiency. This terminology should not be confused with (normal) functional or physiological murmurs. Lastly, heart rhythm disturbances such as premature beats can induce transient AV valve regurgitation. Long diastolic periods accompanying sinoatrial or 1st- and 2nd-degree AV blocks foster diastolic AV valve regurgitation that is considered physiological; this is often silent.

Table 30.1 Causes of Equine Valvular Heart Disease

Mitral Valve Disease

- Mitral regurgitation (MR)
  - Malformations
    - Dysplasia of the valvular apparatus
    - Atrioventricular septal defects (including bridging leaflets)
    - Developmental hamartoma of the valve
  - Valvular degeneration and myxomatous change
  - Mitral valve prolapse
  - Ruptured chordae tendineae
  - Infective endocarditis
  - Training-related[a]
  - Functional[b] MR caused by congenital heart disease, cardiomyopathy, left heart dilation, or injury to papillary muscle(s)
  - Noninfective valvulitis[c]
  - Idiopathic
- Mitral stenosis
  - Rare congenital or developmental disorder
  - Secondary to infective endocarditis or valvulitis

Tricuspid Valve Disease

- Tricuspid regurgitation (TR)
  - Malformations
    - Dysplasia of the valvular apparatus
  - Atrioventricular septal defects
  - Training-related[a]
  - Infective endocarditis
  - Functional[b] TR caused by pulmonary hypertension, congenital heart disease, cardiomyopathy, or other causes of right heart dilation
  - Constrictive pericarditis
- Tricuspid stenosis
  - Rare congenital disorder, including tricuspid atresia in the extreme form
  - Secondary to infective endocarditis

Aortic Valve Disease

- Aortic regurgitation
  - Malformations
    - Congenital valve disease or fenestrations
    - Leaflet prolapse into a ventricular septal defect
  - Valvular degeneration, including aortic valve prolapse and leaflet tears
  - Infective endocarditis
  - Rupture of the aorta into the right atrium, ventricular septum, or right ventricle[d]
  - Systemic hypertension
- Aortic stenosis
  - Rare congenital malformation
  - Secondary to infective endocarditis or valvulitis

Pulmonary Valve Disease

- Pulmonary regurgitation
  - Pulmonary hypertension
  - Infective endocarditis
  - Other causes of pulmonary artery dilation[d]
- Pulmonic or RV outflow tract stenosis
  - Rare congenital disorder
  - Tetralogy of Fallot, including pulmonary atresia
  - Secondary to infective endocarditis
  - Supravalvular obstruction from a pulmonary neoplasm
  - Subvalvular obstruction from dissection or tumor of the ventricular wall

[a] The mechanisms for training-associated valvular regurgitation are unresolved.
[b] The descriptor "functional" in this setting does not indicate physiological, but a functional consequence of disease affecting the valve support apparatus.
[c] Poorly characterized thickening of valves with evidence for inflammation, but without histologic features of infective endocarditis or evidence of an active valve infection.
[d] Cardiac murmurs also occur with rupture of the aorta into the pulmonary artery (aortopulmonary fistula); however, such murmurs are not due to primary valve disease. Pulmonary regurgitation might develop from pulmonary hypertension or dilation of the pulmonary valve annulus.

Pathophysiology of Valvular Regurgitation

Valvular regurgitation is driven by the pressure gradient from source to sink and modified by the size and morphology of the regurgitant orifice. Hemodynamic features characterized from hydraulic experiments and visualized by color Doppler echo imaging include: 1) flow acceleration toward the regurgitant orifice (proximal flow convergence); 2) a narrow vena contracta spanning the regurgitant orifice; and 3) transmission of a high-velocity jet into the receiving chamber with associated flow disturbance or "turbulence" (**Figures 30.5** and **30.6**). These abnormalities can be appreciated only with Doppler echocardiography (see p. 121); however, the dynamics are fundamental to understanding auscultatory and echo features of all forms of valvular heart disease. Chronic valve regurgitation also can cause the effective regurgitant orifice to widen over time due to scarring from jet effects.

Hemodynamically significant valve regurgitation triggers cardiac remodeling (**Figures 30.6** and **30.7**). Similar to the situation in dogs with mitral valve disease (see Chapter 29), MR induces left ventricular (LV) eccentric hypertrophy and left atrial (LA) dilation, along with histological remodeling of these chambers. Increasing LA pressure at end systole (the "v wave") enhances LV filling and preload, but moderate to severe MR also can induce post- and possibly reactive pre-capillary PH. Increasing ventricular preload (Frank–Starling effect, p. 15) and myocardial hypertrophy increase total LV stroke volume, allowing the compensated ventricle to pump both the normal venous return and the regurgitant volume overload.

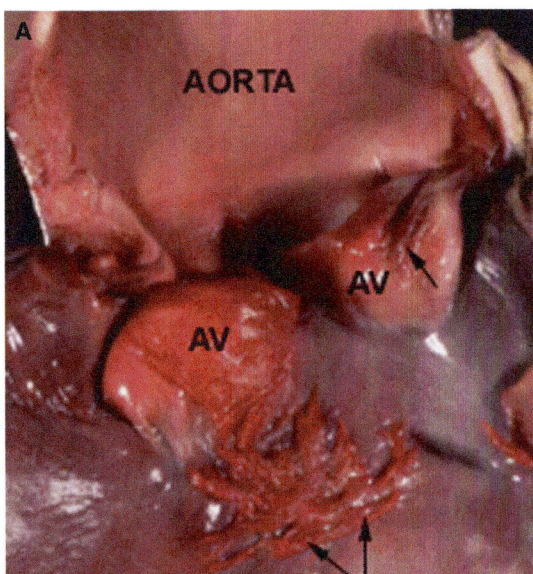

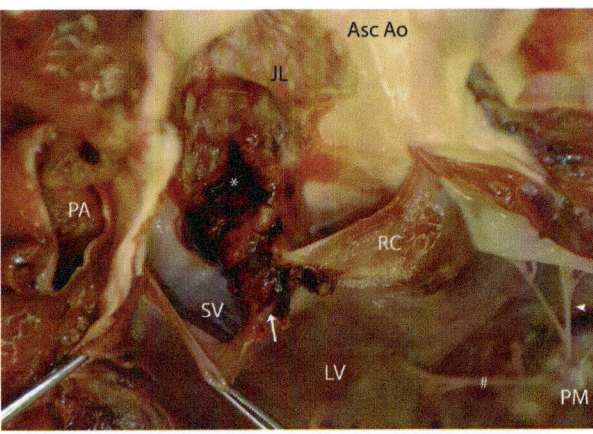

Figure 30.2 Infective endocarditis with aortic root abscess. Aortic valve leaflets are evident. A hemorrhagic vegetation (arrow) extends from a leaflet edge near the commissure of the right (RC) and noncoronary cusps into the root of the aorta (*). Jet lesions (JL) are evident at the root of the ascending aorta (Asc Ao). The tip of a papillary muscle (PM), with chordae tendineae (arrowhead) and false tendon (#) extending from it, is at lower right. LV, left ventricle; PA, transected pulmonary artery; SV, sinus of Valsalva.

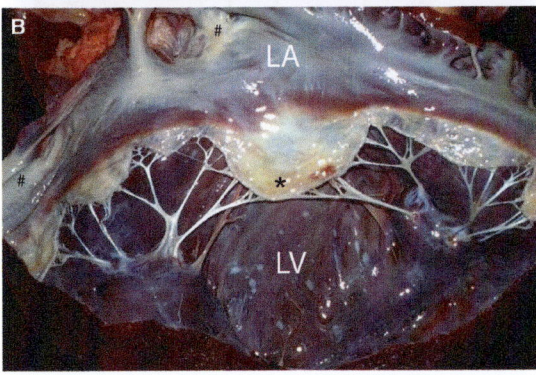

Figure 30.1 (A) Postmortem image of aortic valve degeneration, associated with valve prolapse and aortic regurgitation, in an older horse. Section shows the left ventricular outflow tract, two aortic valve (AV) leaflets, and aortic root. Linear thickenings (upper arrow), as well as general valvular thickening, are present. A prominent jet lesion caused by aortic regurgitation is evident (lower arrows). (B) Opened left ventricle (LV) from another horse showing discoloration and thickening (myxomatous change) on the anterior (*) mitral valve leaflet. The edges of the posterior leaflets also are affected. Jet lesions (#) are present in the left atrium (LA).

AR also exerts a volume load on the left ventricle, which leads to either eccentric or a mixed form of hypertrophy with increased LV mass. Compensatory changes such as hypertrophy, increased preload, and tachycardia can maintain cardiac output. The left ventricle pumps the normal venous return plus the regurgitant volume with each beat. The ascending aorta can dilate, most likely because of the large forward stroke volume. With progressive AR, increasing diastolic backflow into the ventricle widens the arterial pulse pressure and leads to hyperdynamic pulses in the facial and other peripheral arteries. The LV end diastolic pressure increases while aortic diastolic pressure declines. The left atrium also enlarges in horses with chronic AR, because of concurrent mitral valve disease, secondary (functional) MR related to chamber dilation, or from LV diastolic or systolic failure.

The workload on the left ventricle is theoretically greater with AR than with MR, assuming equal regurgitant volumes.

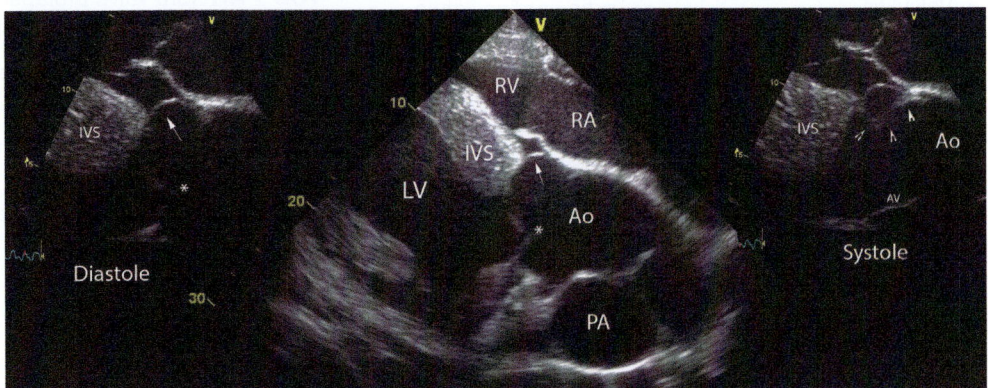

Figure 30.3 Two-dimensional echocardiographic images of aortic valve prolapse into a perimembranous ventricular septal defect (VSD). The central panel and upper left inset show the diastolic prolapse of a leaflet into the VSD (arrow). Aortic valve coaptation in diastole is indicated (*). The right upper inset shows an opened left aortic valve cusp (AV) and opening of the prolapsed leaflet (arrowheads). Ao, aorta; IVS, interventricular septum; LV, left ventricle; PA, pulmonary artery; RA, right atrium; RV, right ventricle.

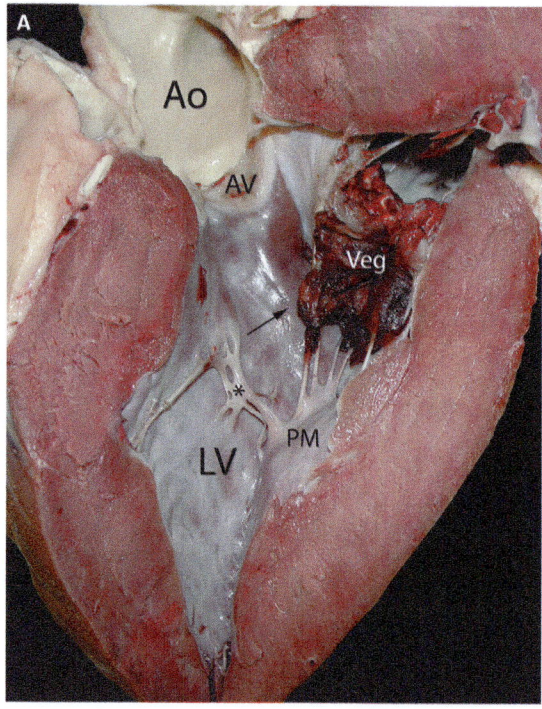
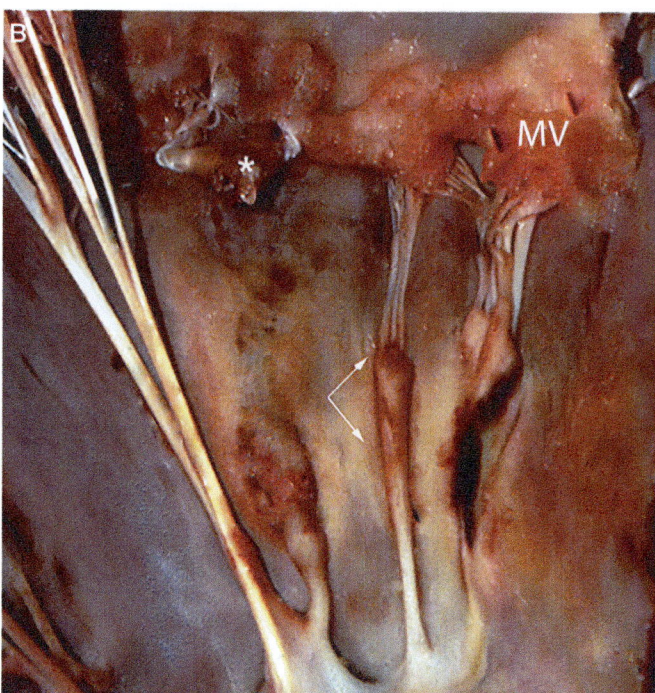

Figure 30.4 (A) Opened left ventricle (LV) demonstrating a large vegetation (Veg) on the mitral valve (arrow) in a horse with infective endocarditis. The lesion appears as a hemorrhagic thrombus on both leaflets and surfaces of the mitral valve. A papillary muscle (PM), false tendon (*), aortic valve cusp (AV), and ascending aorta (Ao) also are visible. (B) Poorly defined valvulitis with severe destruction of the mitral valve (MV) and many of the chordae tendineae in another horse. Notice the transition in thickness (arrows) and morphologic changes to the various mitral valve chords, as well as chordal avulsion (*) and adhesions to the myocardium. Portions of the myocardium are markedly discolored.

Table 30.2 An Overview of Cardiac Murmurs in the Horse

Systolic Murmur PMI: Right Side	Systolic Murmur PMI: Left Side	Diastolic Murmur	Continuous Murmur or Systolic + Diastolic Murmurs
PMI ventral → Perimembranous Ventricular septal defect (**VSD**[a]) PMI tricuspid or dorsal → **TR** • Congenital • Training-related[a] • Degenerative • Endocarditis • Pulmonary hypertension • Cardiomyopathy	Holosystolic or crescendo; apical or mitral area → **MR** • Congenital • Degenerative[a] • Endocarditis • Valvulitis • Ruptured chords • Cardiomyopathy Ejection; PMI over aortic or pulmonic area (craniodorsal base), Grade 1–3/6 → • **Functional/Physiologic**[a] Grade 4/6 or louder → • Subarterial **VSD** or **PS**	Holodiastolic, left-sided → **AR** • Degenerative[a] • Endocarditis • VSD • Aortic-cardiac fistula Protodiastolic, left/right-sided → • **Functional** filling murmur[a] Presystolic, left or right-sided → • **Functional** filling murmur after atrial contraction	Continuous over the heart or pulmonary artery → • **Aortic-cardiac fistula** • **Aortic-PA fistula** Systolic + diastolic → • **VSD + AR** from valve prolapse Systolic + diastolic with PMI over the aortic valve → • Infective endocarditis **Aortic ejection + AR** murmurs Systolic over left apex + diastolic over the aortic valve → • Degenerative[a] or infective mitral + aortic valvular disease **MR + AR** Continuous at left craniodorsal base in a foal or with complex CHD → • **PDA**, or other • **Aorticopulmonary shunt** Multiphasic "murmurs" → • **Pericardial friction rubs**

[a] Most common reasons; see **Table 30.1** for a more complete listing of potential causes of equine heart murmurs.

Abbreviations: AR, aortic regurgitation; CHD, congenital heart disease; MR, mitral regurgitation; PA, pulmonary artery; PDA, patent ductus arteriosus; PMI, point of maximal (murmur) intensity; PS pulmonary stenosis; TR, tricuspid regurgitation; VSD, ventricular septal defect.

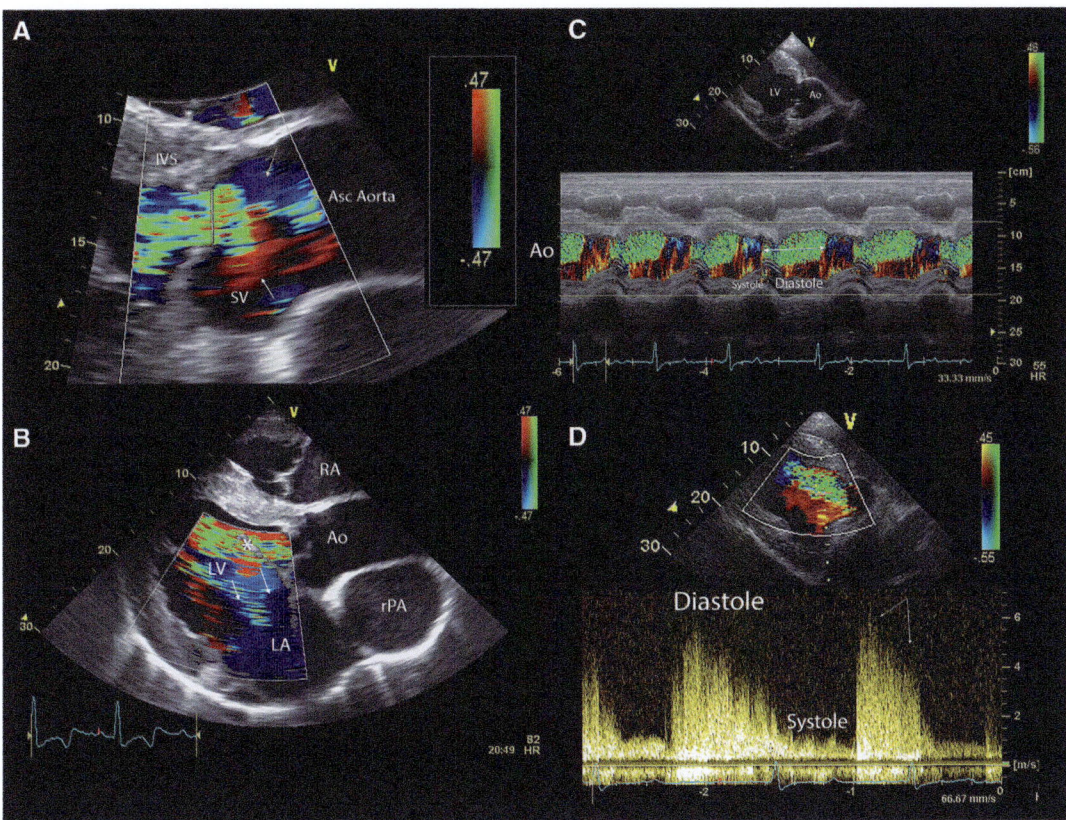

Figure 30.5 Color Doppler images showing the hemodynamics of valvular regurgitation. This horse had congestive heart failure from severe aortic regurgitation (AR), as well as mitral regurgitation (not shown). The cause was noninfective valvulitis (see **Figure 30.14**). (A) Proximal flow convergence of blood into the regurgitant orifice is color-coded (arrows) as blue (moving away from probe) and red (toward the probe). This flow accelerates and becomes turbulent (encoded green) to form the vena contracta (not well visualized to the right of the line) and receiving chamber turbulence within the regurgitant valve orifice. Asc, ascending; IVS, interventricular septum; SV, sinus of Valsalva. (B) The receiving chamber (left ventricle, LV) shows a wide jet area of turbulence (green); the increased ventricular pressure directs blood toward the open mitral orifice (arrows) and left atrium (LA). The right pulmonary artery (rPA) is dilated because of post-capillary pulmonary hypertension. *, open mitral leaflet; Ao, aorta; RA, right atrium. (C) Color M-mode shows the holodiastolic timing of the AR (double-headed arrow). Color M-mode combines the depth and time resolution of M-mode with color-flow mapping along the line of interrogation (shown in the small 2D reference image, above). (D) Continuous-wave Doppler echocardiography records the high-velocity diastolic flow. Peak AR velocity is ~6 m/sec, corresponding to a normal or slightly high aortic pressure in early diastole; however, the pressure half-time (arrows) is short, indicating severe AR with rapidly increasing left ventricular diastolic pressure. See Chapter 4 (p. 124) for more details.

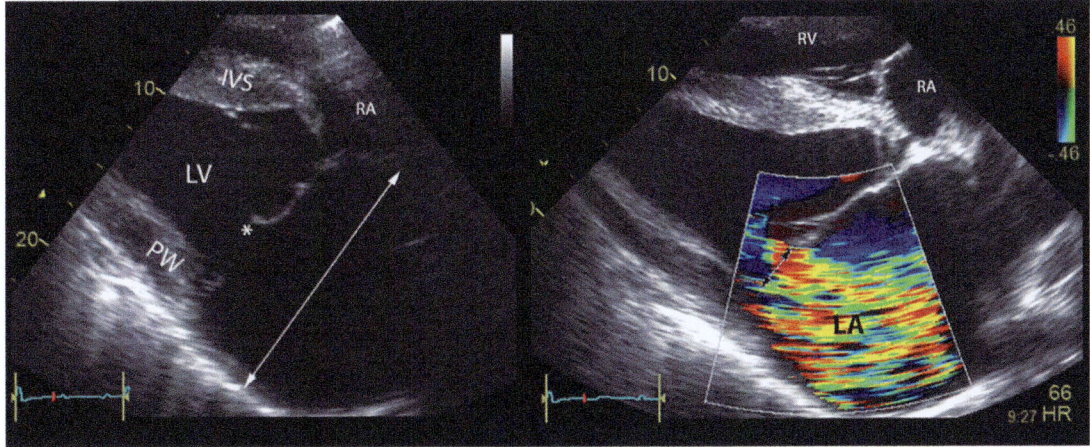

Figure 30.6 Left heart enlargement in a weanling colt with mitral valve hemartomas. The left atrium (LA) is severely dilated; the white arrow shows mid-chamber diameter (left panel). Color Doppler (right panel) displays turbulence-encoding, extending from left ventricle (LV) into the LA across a wide regurgitant orifice (black arrow). IVS, interventricular septum; PW, posterior wall; RA, right atrium; RV, right ventricle.

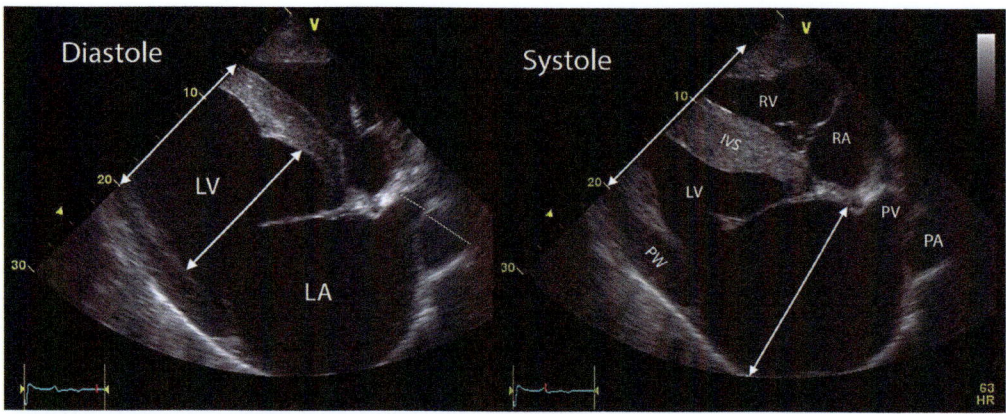

Figure 30.7 Left-sided cardiomegaly and hyperdynamic systolic function of left ventricle (LV) associated with volume overload from chronic mitral regurgitation in an adult horse. Diastolic frame (left) shows the LV is mildly dilated (~13.5 cm, arrows). In systole (right) the LV markedly shortens and the interventricular septum (IVS) and posterior wall (PW) thicken. The left atrium (LA) is moderately dilated (~16 cm, arrows). The right pulmonary artery (PA) is more dilated than the adjacent right vein (PV); this horse also had pulmonary hypertension. RA, right atrium; RV, right ventricle.

In both situations, the ventricle pumps an extra volume with each cardiac cycle. However, with MR, part of the LV stroke volume regurgitates into the lower pressure left atrium before the aortic valve opens. Although the mitral orifice does pose a resistance to flow, the partial LV chamber emptying prior to aortic ejection allows the ventricle to decrease in volume and increase in wall thickness, thus reducing peak LV wall stress (one estimate of ventricular afterload). During ventricular compensation, these adaptations are manifested on echo exam as hyperdynamic LV motion (**Figure 30.7**). In contrast, with AR, the regurgitant volume must be ejected back into the higher-pressure arterial system. Consequently, moderate to severe chronic AR is likely to induce greater LV mass development, myocardial tissue change, and risk for heart failure. Fortunately, most horses with AR exhibit only mild regurgitation, based on the degree of ventricular remodeling and a low incidence of congestive heart failure (CHF) associated with this condition.

With TR, the changes described above for MR are mirrored in the right atrium and ventricle. When TR is associated with vigorous training, regurgitant jet size and murmur intensity can increase over time. When TR is caused by chronic PH, a greater degree of right ventricular (RV) wall thickening (concentric or mixed hypertrophy) is likely.

The role of neural and hormonal activation (including sympathetic neural, renin–angiotensin–aldosterone, and arginine vasopressin systems) in the pathogenesis of ventricular remodeling in horses with VHD is largely unexplored. Limited studies of renin–angiotensin–aldosterone system (RAAS) hormones and natriuretic peptides have been reported. Standard assays of cardiac troponins generally show normal concentrations or "trickle" elevations. Thus, the overall value of measuring biomarkers or inhibiting vasoconstrictor/sodium-retaining/growth-promoting systems with drugs is presently unknown. Changes in ventricular cellular composition, especially interstitial fibrosis, potentially could increase the risk of ventricular arrhythmias in horses with significant MR or AR. Ventricular ectopy and sudden cardiac death have been reported in some horses with chronic AR (Reef, 2014).

Clinical Features

The most relevant clinical sign of equine valvular disease is the presence of a *cardiac murmur* (**Figure 30.8**) that typically is loudest over the affected valve area. The principles applied to auscultation in dogs (see Chapter 11) also are appropriate when examining horses. These include identifying the *timing* of the murmur in the cardiac cycle, locating the *point of maximal murmur intensity* (PMI), grading the *loudness* or *intensity* of the murmur, and further defining the murmur by its *configuration* ("shape"), thoracic *radiation*, and sound *quality*. In general, the heart sounds and murmurs of horses tend to be softer than comparable sounds in dogs, although some murmurs are very loud.

Cardiac Murmurs

The loudness of cardiac murmurs is influenced by the physical characteristics of the thorax, the breed, and the individual animal. Intensity also relates to the relative pressure difference between the source and receiving chamber. A faint or soft murmur is more likely to indicate mild disease, especially in an asymptomatic horse. However, murmur intensity sometimes correlates poorly with severity. For example, a murmur of TR associated with PH often is louder simply because RV systolic pressure is elevated. The murmur of MR in a horse with left-sided failure typically is holosystolic, but can have a decrescendo configuration and be relatively soft because of reduced pressure differences between the left ventricle and atrium, as well as the progressive systolic increase in LA pressure (v wave). Conversely, a small VSD can cause a very loud murmur because the normal interventricular pressure

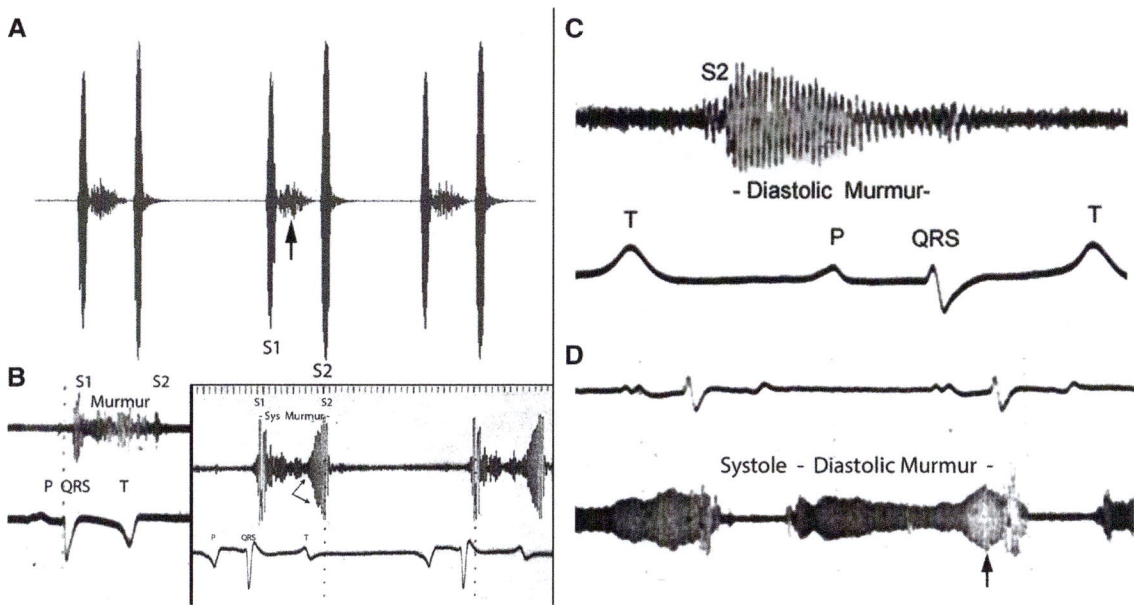

Figure 30.8 Phonocardiograms (PCGs) of equine cardiac murmurs. (A) Brief systolic ejection (functional) murmur (arrow). (B) Holosystolic murmur in a foal with a ventricular septal defect (left) and systolic murmur of mitral regurgitation (right), with a mid- to late systolic peak (arrows) typical of prolapse. (C) Holodiastolic, vibratory diastolic murmur of aortic regurgitation (AR). (D) Holodiastolic murmur of AR with presystolic accentuation (arrow). S_1, first heart sound; S_2, second heart sound. Electrocardiograms also shown in panels B, C, and D.

difference of ~100 mm Hg is maintained. Musical murmurs of AR, with their harmonic vibrations of tissue structures, often project across the thorax even when the regurgitant volume is relatively small.

Systolic Murmurs A soft- to moderate-intensity, left-sided ejection murmur that is loudest over the aortic valve, pulmonary valve, or great vessels is most likely functional (physiological), caused by the rapid ejection of blood. The first and second heart sounds (S_1 and S_2) are clearly detectable with most ejection murmurs. These murmurs assume a crescendo-decrescendo quality, typically peaking in early- to mid-systole. In contrast, a mid- to late-systolic murmur that is loudest over the mitral area is typical of MR and usually related to valve prolapse. Severe MR and TR (and the typical VSD) can generate loud, holosystolic murmurs that obscure S_1 and S_2.

Diastolic Murmurs A brief early- or late-diastolic murmur usually is a normal finding, especially in trained athletes. The protodiastolic functional murmur is associated with rapid ventricular filling; this murmur can have a low-pitched, whistling, vibratory, or creaking ("rusty gate") quality. When a presystolic functional murmur associated with atrial contraction is present, it is very brief and easily confused with a pericardial rub. Conversely, a holodiastolic murmur loudest over the aortic valve area is likely to indicate AR, especially when the murmur's character is musical, buzzing, or cooing (**Figure 30.8**). Continuous or combined systolic and diastolic murmurs are most often related to a VSD with secondary aortic valve prolapse, or caused by rupture or fistulation of the aorta into the heart or pulmonary artery. Some key features of cardiac murmur auscultation in horses are summarized in **Table 30.2**.

Other Clinical Findings

Historical aspects important for VHD assessment include evidence for any decline in performance or clinical signs of CHF, such as ill-defined anxiety or colic-like behavior, resting tachypnea, protracted recovery from exercise, or ventral edema (see Chapter 20). With infective endocarditis, the horse typically demonstrates signs of systemic inflammation that can include constitutional illness, fever, polyarthritis, or metastatic infection or infarction (see Chapter 31). With right-sided endocarditis, there might be evidence of prior or ongoing jugular thrombophlebitis and of concurrent hematogenous (metastatic) pneumonia.

Physical examination of the *arterial and jugular pulses* can be instructive. As noted above, hemodynamically significant AR causes hyperdynamic arterial pulses. With experience, this abnormality can be palpated or it can be measured objectively with a tail cuff and oscillometric blood pressure device. With moderate to severe TR, the jugular venous pulse can be abnormal, with "giant c-v waves" progressing more than one-third of the distance up the neck during late systole (p. 262). An elevated resting pulse rate unexplained by pain, fever, or anxiety might signal the presence of cardiac decompensation or heart failure with associated sympathetic activation.

The presence of cardiac rhythm disturbances, especially atrial fibrillation (AF) or ventricular premature complexes (VPCs), in the setting of valvular disease has been associated with cardiac remodeling, which predisposes to these electrical disturbances. The onset of AF, in the setting of previously compensated valvular insufficiency, can precipitate CHF. This is the most common scenario when CHF is identified in this species.

Although a small minority of horses with VHD experience CHF, the associated clinical signs can develop rapidly. For example, pulmonary edema could occur with acute rupture of major chordae tendineae or when endocarditis causes left-sided cardiac disease. In horses with compensated VHD, the stresses of pregnancy, anemia, infection, or heavy work might precipitate CHF. In addition to persistent resting sinus tachycardia (>60/minute in a mature horse), clinical signs can include tachypnea that progresses to respiratory distress, cough, pulmonary crackles, and antemortem nasal frothing (**Figure 31.6**, p. 597). Acute left heart failure often is confused with pleuropneumonia in horses (**Figures 30.9** and **30.10**). Some horses with CHF develop signs of colic. Even with left-sided VHD, signs of biventricular CHF commonly occur, especially secondary to AF or PH (p. 819). Right-sided failure causes signs of jugular vein distension and pulsation, subcutaneous edema in ventral regions and lower limbs, pleural effusion, and ascites.

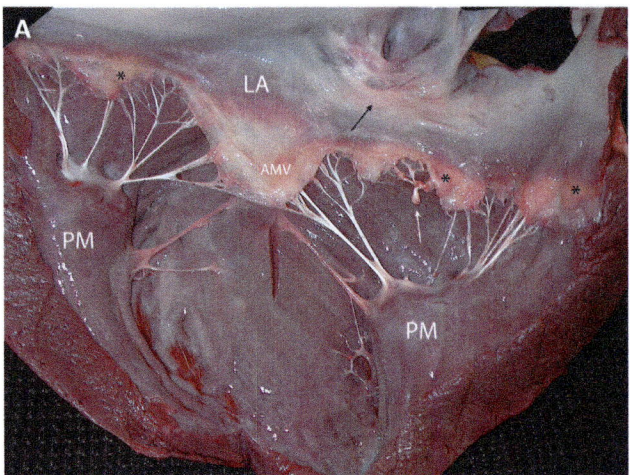

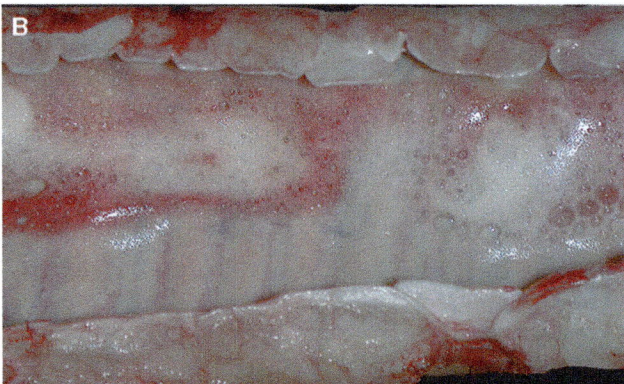

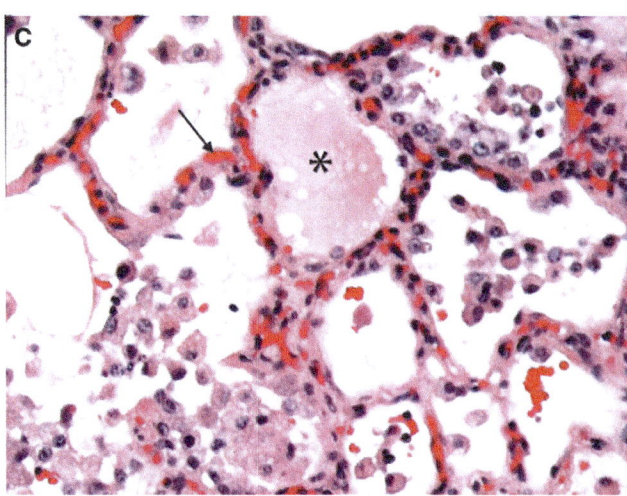

Figure 30.9 (A) Ruptured chorda tendineae (white arrow) in the posterior mitral valve leaflet of a horse with severe mitral regurgitation and congestive heart failure (CHF). Jet lesions (black arrow) are evident in the wall of the left atrium (LA). The valve itself has degenerative thickenings (*) in the anterior mitral leaflet (AMV) and the multiple cusps of the posterior leaflet (which is cut). PM, papillary muscle. (B) Intra-tracheal froth from pulmonary edema in the same horse. (C) Photomicrograph of the lung from another horse with CHF caused by mitral valve disease. There is congestion of red blood cells (arrow) and proteinaceous hyaline-staining edema fluid in some air spaces (*).

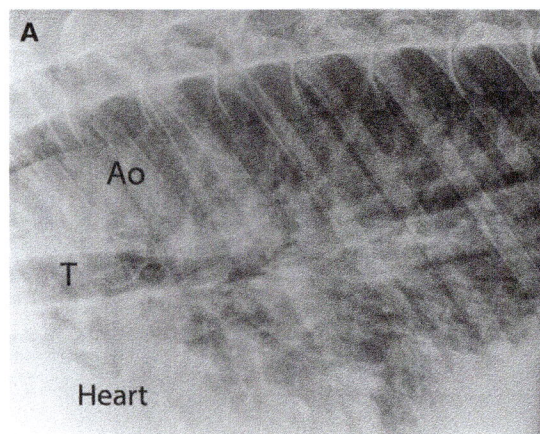

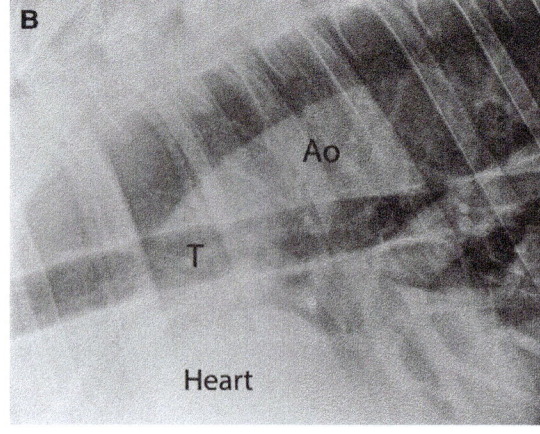

Figure 30.10 Congestive heart failure in an adult horse with severe mitral valve disease. (A) Thoracic radiograph at initial presentation shows a prominent vascular pattern with pulmonary interstitial opacities. (B) Follow-up examination after medical therapy (image centered cranial to prior radiograph). Vascular markings and perihilar infiltrates of edema are reduced. Ao, descending aorta; T, trachea.

Clinical Outcomes and Overall Risk Assessment

Table 30.3 summarizes various consequences of equine valvular disease. Gauging the risks of VHD to a rider or driver can be challenging, considering that many horses with auscultatory and Doppler echo evidence of valvular insufficiency still perform at high levels. However, after evaluations for orthopedic, respiratory, neurologic, infectious, and hematologic diseases have proved negative, the focus of suspicion in an underperforming horse logically shifts to the heart. This is especially so when a moderate to loud murmur characteristic of MR, AR, or TR is heard, or when a non-vagal arrhythmia is evident. For horses with AF in which cardioversion has been successful, maintenance of sinus rhythm can be more challenging when MR or TR causes persistent atrial dilation. The presence of VPCs is always worrisome in terms of risk assessment, especially in older horses with significant AR.

Veterinarians who examine horses with abnormal cardiac findings are encouraged to review the joint American and European Colleges of Veterinary Internal Medicine (ACVIM/ECVIM) consensus statement guidelines (Reef, 2014) for evaluating sports horses with cardiac disease. These guidelines recommend a comprehensive approach for assessing the severity of VHD including work history, inspection, physical diagnosis, and select imaging and laboratory tests appropriate for the clinical setting. The potential for nonsustained or paroxysmal rhythm disturbances, including atrial tachycardia, atrial flutter and AF, is one emphasis of the guidelines. Risk for collapse or sudden death from ventricular ectopy in horses with VHD, especially older horses with chronic AR, is another point of emphasis. The recommended approach to evaluation usually incorporates some form of extended and, ideally, exercise electrocardiography (ECG) as a component of risk and safety assessment (**Figures 30.11** and **30.12**). The guidelines stress the critical roles of echo, clinical, and ECG assessments. Echo findings with valvular diseases are summarized in the next section and in Chapter 4.

Diagnostic Tests

Echocardiography in Valvular Heart Disease

The two-dimensional (2D) and M-mode (grayscale) modalities are used most often in general practice, and these are fundamental for recognition of valve anatomy, thickness, motion, and cardiac remodeling in horses with VHD. Color or spectral Doppler echocardiography is needed to confirm abnormal flow patterns and might require referral. The colorized M-mode exam is an excellent way to determine the precise timing, duration, and depth of a "turbulent" color flow signal (**Figures 30.5** and **30.13**). Doppler echo imaging is highly sensitive, such that clinically irrelevant jets of valvular regurgitation often are identified. Accordingly, clinicians must auscultate skillfully and learn to integrate grayscale imaging, clinical findings, and their knowledge of cardiac diseases and diagnostic imaging. The potential for functional (physiologic, athletic) murmurs must always be considered in horses.

Valvular thickening is a nonspecific finding, but it can occur with both congenital and acquired valvular diseases (**Figures 30.14-30.17**). Degenerative disease creates variable amounts of thickening, ranging from borderline to severe. Infective endocarditis is similarly variable. Valvular lesions should be visualized in multiple imaging planes from both right- and left-sided thoracic windows. Occasionally, a valve appears overtly thickened with octave imaging but less so when the imaging mode is changed from harmonics to fundamental frequency.

A typical feature of acute or subacute endocarditis (affecting any of the valves) is an oscillating thrombus. Focal lesions of vegetative endocarditis generally appear on the valve surface facing normal blood flow (**Figure 30.15**); in other words on the atrial surfaces of the mitral and tricuspid valves and on the ventricular surfaces of the aortic and pulmonary valves. Large vegetations penetrate the entire valve stroma extending to either side. Vegetations also can envelop mitral or tricuspid valve chords, leading to rupture and a flail leaflet. Although endocarditis most

Table 30.3 Potential Outcomes of Equine Valvular Heart Disease

Outcome	Comments
Apparent tolerance of the lesion	• Majority of cases in mature horses • No overt influence on exercise performance or safety
Reduced exercise capacity	• Often creates a diagnostic dilemma related to the cause(s) of poor performance
Colic-like signs	• Usually related to heart failure or a tachyarrhythmia when cardiac in origin
Heart rhythm disturbances	• Atrial ectopy: APCs, atrial flutter, AF • Can precipitate CHF • Ventricular ectopy: VPCs, ventricular tachycardia (more common with aortic regurgitation?) • Low potential for sudden (arrhythmic) cardiac death
Left-sided CHF	• Peracute left-sided CHF is often confused with pneumonia
Right-sided CHF	• Ventral edema with jugular venous distension • Often develops secondary to left heart disease with superimposed AF or pulmonary hypertension
Post-capillary pulmonary hypertension from left heart disease	• Predisposes to right-sided CHF • Rarely, the pulmonary artery will rupture

Abbreviations: AF, atrial fibrillation; APCs, atrial premature complexes; CHF, congestive heart failure; VPCs, ventricular premature complexes. Other details are discussed within different section of text in this chapter.

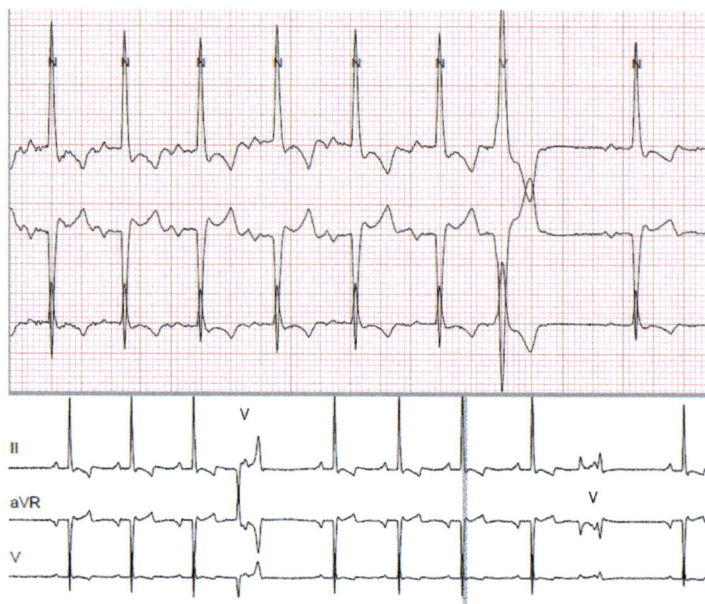

Figure 30.11 Ambulatory (Holter) electrocardiogram from a horse with aortic regurgitation showing the development of multiform ventricular premature complexes (V). Normal sinus complexes (N) are indicated in the upper disclosure strip. The three leads were recorded simultaneously.

often causes valve regurgitation, secondary granulomatous reaction and scarring caused by endocarditis (or sterile "valvulitis") can sometimes create an acquired valvular stenosis.

Table 30.4 summarizes some of the key variables for echo assessment of equine VHD. For most general equine practitioners, the key elements will be structure, motion, and quantitation of cardiac size and function using 2D imaging. More detail requires Doppler techniques. An overview of those methods applicable to the horse is summarized here and described in fuller detail in Chapter 4.

Mitral Regurgitation Structural and motion abnormalities often are evident in primary mitral valve disease. The equine mitral valve has a complicated structure. There is a large anterior (cranioventral or septal) leaflet that forms the caudal-dorsal border of the LV outflow tract and extends farther into the chamber when viewed by 2D echocardiography. The posterior (caudodorsal or mural) leaflet demonstrates a greater circumference around the mitral ring. There are usually three distinctive cusps to this leaflet (left, posterior and right) not unlike the P1-P2-P3 designation used for the human

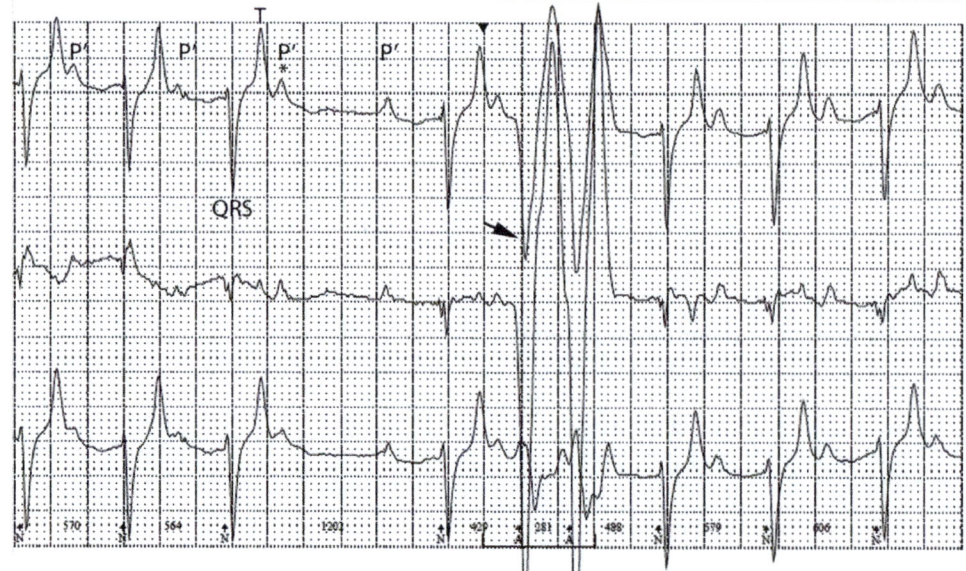

Figure 30.12 Electrocardiogram from a 15-year-old gelding with valvular disease showing an ectopic (focal) atrial tachycardia, with 1st- and occasional 2nd-degree (*) atrioventricular block and a ventricular couplet (arrow). P′, ectopic atrial depolarizations; QRS, (normal) ventricular waveforms.

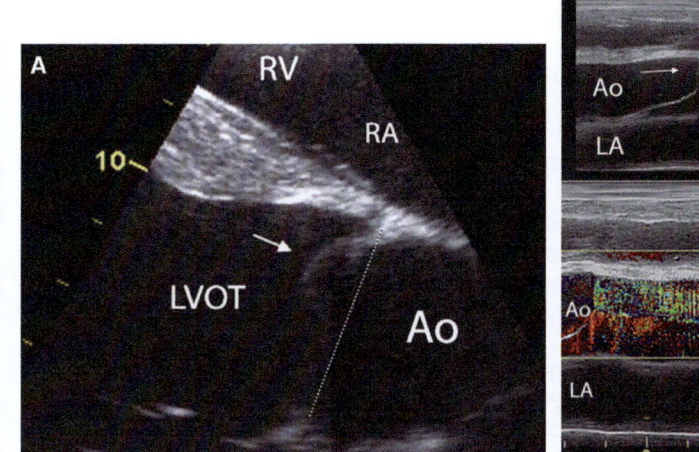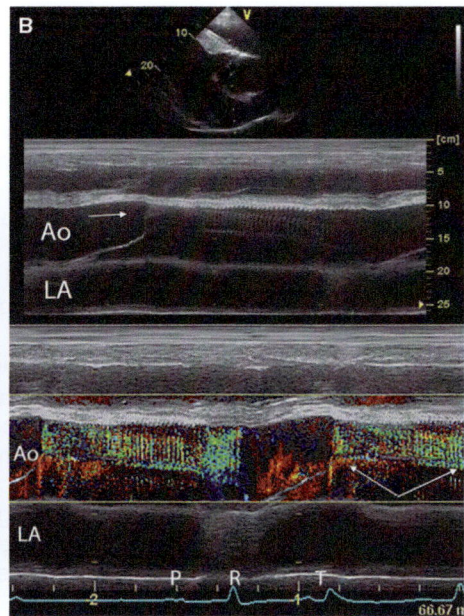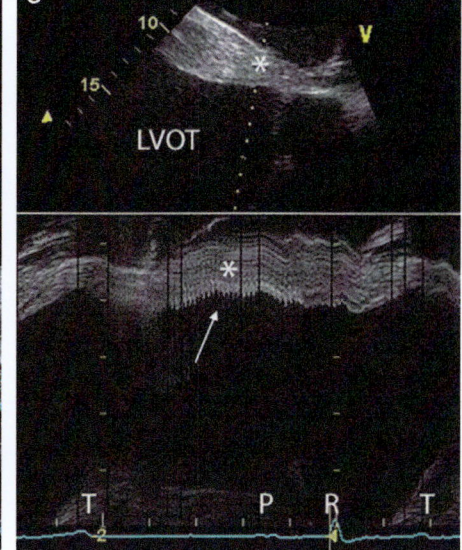

Figure 30.13 Echocardiographic images from a horse with degenerative aortic valve disease, with valve prolapse and regurgitation. (A) 2D image shows prolapse of the near-field (right) aortic valve leaflet (arrow) into the left ventricular outflow tract (LVOT), relative to the approximate annular plane (dotted line). (B) M-mode image at the aortic root (top) shows diastolic fluttering of the aortic valve (arrow) and proximal aortic wall. Color M-mode image (bottom) shows that turbulence related to the regurgitation is holodiastolic (arrows). (C) M-mode image (bottom) shows diastolic fluttering (arrow) of the basilar interventricular septum (*), at the level shown in the 2D image above. Electrocardiogram waveforms (P, R, T) indicated in (B) and (C). Ao, aorta; LA, left atrium; RA, right atrium; RV, right ventricle.

mitral valve. This valve is especially prone to over-interpretation as "thickened" or "prolapsing." Conversely, it is likely that we miss subtle mitral valve malformations, inflammatory thickenings, and leaflet prolapse caused by minor chordal ruptures. Such lesions might explain the finding of MR in some relatively young animals that seemingly would be too young for valvular degeneration. The clinician should look for diffuse or focal thickenings of the leaflet edges (cusps), focal vegetative lesions, and focal areas of prolapse beyond the annular plane when there is auscultatory or Doppler evidence of MR.

Abnormalities of valve motion might be identified by high frame-rate 2D imaging or by directing an M-mode cursor across the valve structure. Both right and left-sided imaging planes should be used, especially to evaluate the various components of the posterior leaflet. Specific findings might include valve prolapse beyond the annular plane, restricted valve motion, a flail or torn leaflet with vibration or chaotic

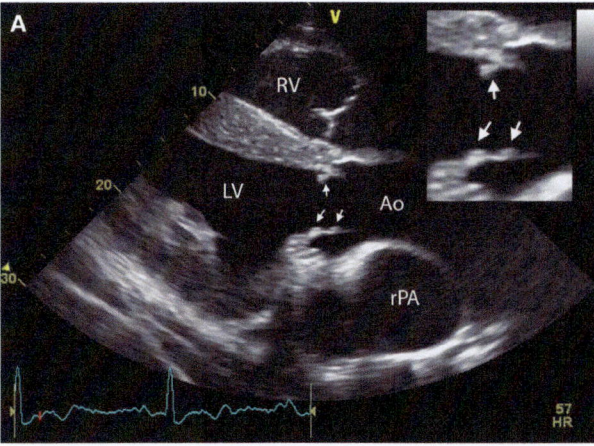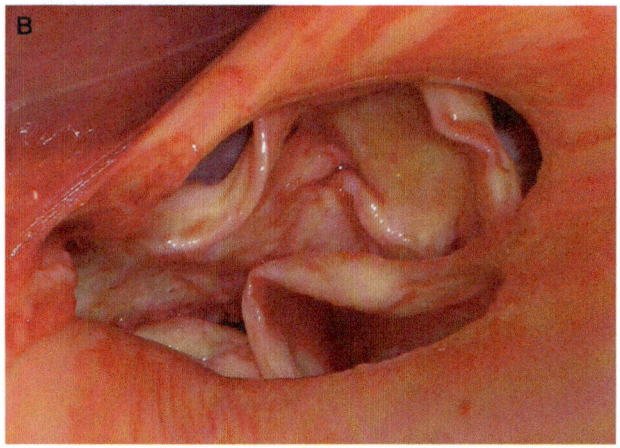

Figure 30.14 (A) 2D echocardiographic imaging shows severe aortic valvular thickening (arrows; main image and enlarged inset) that led to both aortic regurgitation and mild stenosis, in a 13-year-old Paint horse mare. The right pulmonary artery (rPA) is dilated because of pulmonary hypertension. Ao, aorta; LV, left ventricle; RV, right ventricle. (B) Postmortem image of this horse's aortic valve from the supravalvular (aortic) perspective. There was nonbacterial valvular inflammation, as well as myxomatous changes of both the aortic and mitral valves.

Table 30.4 Echocardiographic Assessment of Equine Valvular Heart Disease[a]

Echo Finding	Echo Modality	Comments

Nature of the valve lesion	2D imaging
	3D imaging
		• Often subtle or equivocal in degenerative disease
		• Prolapse of mitral valve might be seen (usually posterior leaflet)
		• Assess signs of lesion severity including:
		  • Gross malformation[b]
		  • Leaflet thickening (mild/moderate/severe)
		  • Leaflet tenting (mitral valve)
		  • Evidence of valvular or chordal vegetation
		  • Ruptured mitral or tricuspid chord
		  • Flail leaflet
		  • Gross failure of leaflet coaptation

Abnormal valve motion	2D imaging
	M-mode imaging
		• Diastolic fluttering (aortic regurgitation)
		  • Aortic or mitral valve valve (eccentric jet)
		  • Aortic root or ventricular septum
		• Leaflet prolapse
		  • Mitral or aortic (evaluate in long-axis planes)
		• Chaotic valvular motion (flail leaflet)
		• Reduced opening excursion or premature closure

Cardiac remodeling	2D imaging M-mode imaging 3D imaging	• Ventricular enlargement • Atrial enlargement • Altered LV or LA chamber shape (sphericity) • Altered LA chamber shape (dilated pulmonary veins & atrial septal distraction) • Serial examinations are important for assessment
Great vessel dilation	2D imaging 3D imaging	• Pulmonary artery in pulmonary hypertension • Aorta in aortic regurgitation

Left ventricular systolic function	2D imaging
	M-mode imaging
	3D imaging
	Tissue Doppler
	Advanced methods (strain)
		• Normal vs. hyper- or hypodynamic
		• Abnormal ventricular septal motion
		  • Exuberant – LV volume overload
		  • Paradoxical – RV volume overload
		• Follow progression of systolic function over time

Left ventricular diastolic function and filling pressures	M-mode imaging
	PW Doppler
	Tissue Doppler
	Advanced methods (strain)
		• Diastolic function is uncommonly assessed in horses
		• Normal transmitral inflow velocity suggests normal LA & pulmonary venous pressures
		• Increased transmitral flow (E) from moderate to severe MR or increased venous pressures
		• Mitral valve abnormalities (M-mode):
		  • Premature mitral closure: severe AR
		  • Delayed closure: elevated diastolic pressures (CHF)

Valvular function[a]	2D imaging Doppler imaging Color flow PW spectral CW spectral Color M-mode	• Correlate to auscultation! • Correlate to 2D imaging of valve & supporting tissues • Identify the flow disturbance(s) with color Doppler • Time the duration of the event using Doppler imaging or color Doppler M-mode • Evaluate for proximal flow convergence • Estimate the vena contracta size • Evaluate jet direction, area, and distance into the receiving chamber • Inspect the contour of the spectral flow profile • Measure the maximal and mean velocities • Estimate pressure gradients • Assess pressure half-time (AR) • Assess decrease in aortic dimension from early to late diastole (AR)
Pulmonary artery pressures	2D imaging CW Doppler	• Evaluate pulmonary trunk and branches for dilation • Measure velocity of any TR or PR jets • Compare right pulmonary artery to vein

[a] See text, section "Echocardiography in Valvular Heart Disease" and Chapter 4 for more details regarding these methods.
[b] Quadricuspid or supernumerary aortic valve leaflets can be misdiagnosed when the 2D imaging plane crosses into the sinus of Valsalva superficial to the valve commissure. This artifact was reported as aortic valve malformations in several case reports, probably in error.

Abbreviations: AR, aortic regurgitation; CHF, congestive heart failure; CW, continuous wave; LA, left atrial; LV, left ventricular; MR, mitral regurgitation; PR, pulmonary regurgitation; PW, pulsed wave; RV, right ventricular; TR, tricuspid regurgitation.

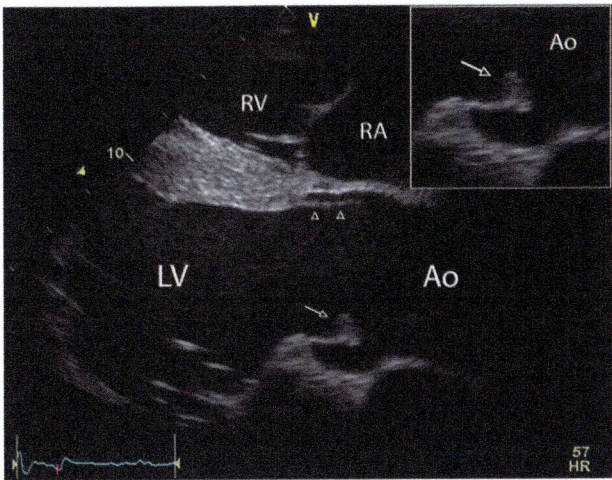

Figure 30.15 Focal vegetation on the aortic valve (arrow; main image and enlarged inset), seen with 2D imaging. The inset shows more clearly that the vegetation is located along the leaflet's ventricular surface, which is typical for focal aortic vegetations. Compare the affected leaflet to the open near-field leaflet (triangles). Ao, aorta; LV, left ventricle; RA, right atrium; RV, right ventricle.

motion, and high-frequency valvular vibrations associated with a regurgitant jet. In some horses with severe MR and ventricular dilation, the leaflet coaptation seems to occur more apically, which likely is related to apical displacement of the papillary muscles. This finding also occurs with the dilated cardiomyopathy phenotype; although in most cases of primary valve disease, LV systolic function is preserved.

The flow dynamics of a regurgitant jet have been noted previously (also see **Figure 30.5**); analysis of this information is discussed more fully in Chapter 4. Color Doppler assessment involves receiving chamber analysis (jet length or area relative to atrial chamber area), measurement of the vena contracta (jet width), and analysis of the proximal isovelocity surface area (PISA), an advanced technique. The first method is used most often in practice (**Figure 30.6**). However, there are substantial technical limitations involved with processing of jet area in the horse, and high potential to over- or underestimate severity when only this method is used.

Continuous-wave (CW) Doppler studies of MR (**Figure 30.16**) can identify both MR and potentially, elevated LA pressure. The red blood cell (RBC) velocity at the envelope

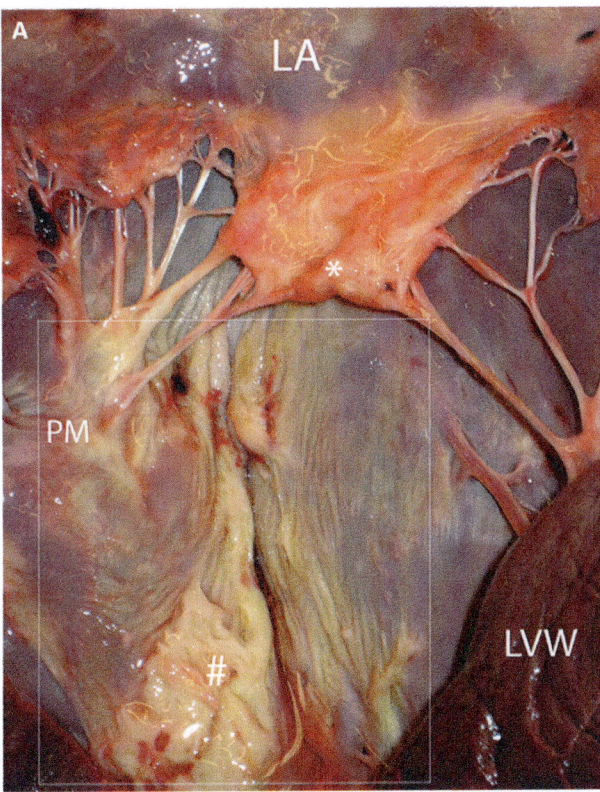
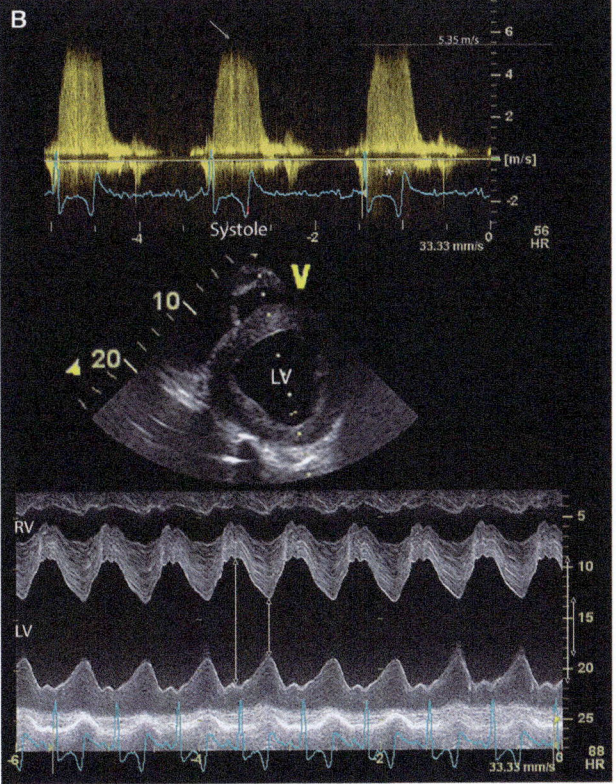

Figure 30.16 (A) Severe myxomatous mitral valve thickening (*) that led to mitral regurgitation (MR) in the horse of **Figure 30.14**. There also are extensive white, raised fibrotic jet lesions in the left ventricle (box and #) caused by concurrent aortic regurgitation. LA, left atrium; LVW, left ventricular wall; PM, papillary muscle. (B) Upper panel: continuous-wave Doppler recording from another horse with a high-velocity MR jet, recorded from the right thorax with flow moving toward the transducer (arrow). Horses often have multiple jets of MR and these can be highly eccentric. Another jet (moving away from the transducer) is faintly captured in the opposite direction (*), although this can also be observed as an artifact. The center, 2D image shows an M-mode cursor crossing the left ventricle (LV) of a horse with severe MR, recorded from the right thorax. The M-mode recording at bottom depicts the hyperdynamic nature of left ventricular contraction with severe MR. Diameter measurements of the minor axis of the LV are shown in diastole (left arrow) and systole (right arrow). RV, right ventricle. See Chapter 4 (p. 104 and **Figures 4.27 & 4.28**) for additional methods of assessing LV size and function.

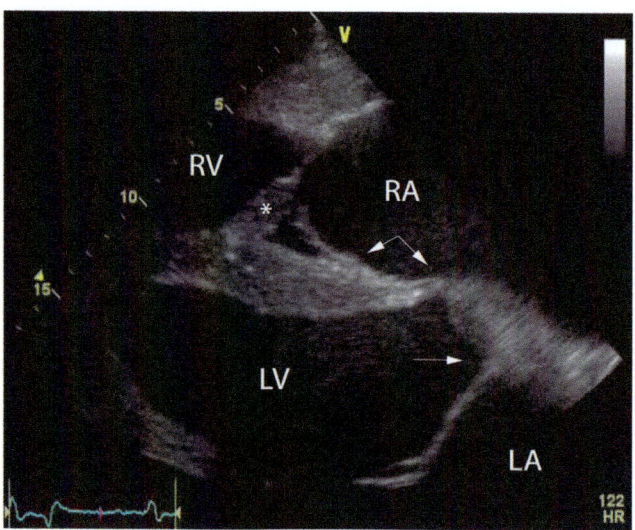

Figure 30.17 2D (long-axis) image from the right thorax shows tricuspid valve dysplasia in a 2-year-old Tennessee walking horse. Note the: tethering of the septal tricuspid leaflet to the ventricular septum (double arrow), relatively short chordal-to-papillary muscle (*) attachments, dilated right atrium (RA), and ventrally displaced septal tricuspid leaflet attachment, compared to the anterior mitral leaflet hinge point (single arrow). LA, left atrium; LV, left ventricle; RV, right ventricle.

of the jet relates to instantaneous pressure difference or gradient. The CW velocity spectrum of MR in most normotensive horses has a rounded peak and maximum of about 5–6 m/s, assuming tight cursor alignment to regurgitant flow. With severe LV systolic dysfunction, systemic hypotension, or high LA pressure, both peak velocity and rate of velocity change are reduced. The envelope of the CW Doppler changes to a more abrupt peak with a rapid velocity deceleration, indicating a marked increase in LA pressure (and reduction in LV to LA pressure gradient). High-velocity early diastolic filling (E) waves suggest hemodynamically significant MR or elevated LA pressure, especially when the deceleration time is short. In contrast, a low- to normal-velocity E wave suggests low ventricular filling pressure. Obtaining good cursor alignment with inflow is critical to avoid underestimating velocities and this is challenging in some horses.

The finding of moderate to severe PH in the setting of chronic MR (or AR) is a poor prognostic sign (**Figures 30.7** and **30.14**). Most cases will have an audible murmur of TR and a high-velocity TR jet on Doppler imaging (see "Tricuspid Regurgitation," below). In these cases, performance and safety are reduced. There also is a small, but finite potential for pulmonary artery rupture.

Aortic Regurgitation Aortic valve abnormalities evident on 2D imaging in horses with AR might include general thickening, linear thickenings (bands), hyperechoic beads on the leaflet surface, or vegetative lesions. The latter can be diffuse or focal in distribution. Motion abnormalities often are observed in AR. These include valve prolapse beyond the annular plane in degenerative VHD (**Figure 30.14**), a torn leaflet with vibration or chaotic motion, and high-frequency vibrations as structures are impinged by the regurgitant jet. The most common findings are leaflet prolapse (of the near field leaflet that can appear as a double line in diastole) and less often, an apparent tearing of the far field leaflet. However, imprecise imaging planes can mimic prolapse or quadricuspid valve leaflets. The typical musical or buzzing murmur of AR is associated with diastolic fluttering of the aortic valve, aortic root, anterior mitral leaflet, or ventricular septum; these are best observed with M-mode imaging because of its high sampling rate (**Figure 30.13**). Diastolic fluttering holds diagnostic but no obvious prognostic value. Lastly, 2D or M-mode aortic root measurements show both increased systolic diameter and greater relative change from early to late diastole when the regurgitant volume is large. A dilated pulmonary artery is suggestive of PH.

Doppler studies of AR demonstrate the diastolic reversal of flow into the LV outflow tract. Trivial, silent AR is common in horses of all ages, and often is augmented at end-diastole and with training. Mild to moderate AR that is audible is a frequent finding in older horses. It can be documented by color and spectral Doppler imaging. Similar to MR, the Doppler assessment of AR includes color Doppler imaging of jet area, vena contracta width, or PISA, which will appear close to the valve in mild AR or far from it with severe regurgitation. Jets of AR are often highly eccentric, such that jet area might be difficult to characterize. CW Doppler studies of AR (**Figure 30.5**) show a high-velocity diastolic regurgitant jet. As discussed in Chapter 4, the maximal velocity of AR and the slope of velocity change during diastole (quantified by the pressure half-time) can be used to assess severity. A steep slope (short pressure half-time) implies more rapid equilibration of the aortic and LV diastolic pressures. The utility of CW Doppler for assessing severity assumes cursor alignment closely parallel to the AR jet; however, this is challenging to achieve in horses because of a lack of apical imaging planes and translational motion of the heart as the ventricles fill.

Assessment of Left Heart Chambers It would be surprising to identify a normal LA or LV chamber size in a horse with moderate to severe MR or AR. Increased LV diastolic size is compatible with ventricular dilation and volume overload. It also is an indication for more regular evaluations, careful monitoring of exercise capacity, and an exercise ECG. One challenge relates to the assessment of a well-conditioned horse, because the "athletic equine heart" also involves morphologic changes that include increased ventricular luminal size and mass, as well as increased incidence of valvular regurgitation (Young, 1999). Another obstacle is the "first examination" after discovery of MR or TR, where there is no baseline study for comparison. As summarized by Schwarzwald (2019), there are limited reference ranges established for equine echo measurements across different breeds (see Chapter 4). Whenever a "reference standard" is used, the examiner must be careful to consider the physiological state, heart rate, age, weight, breed, influence of sedation, and the training history of that horse before deciding if there is chamber "remodeling" or not. Ultimately, when the initial examination suggests normal or equivocally enlarged ventricular and atrial size, the *progression of enlargement* becomes more important, along with other clinical and imaging findings that delineate disease severity and ventricular function. Some M-mode motion abnormalities relate to heart failure. Premature mitral valve closure (before the middle of the QRS complex) might indicate an AR jet is impinging on the anterior leaflet, or a short cardiac cycle has occurred related to an arrhythmia. However, this finding can mean that LV end diastolic pressure exceeds LA pressure - an ominous sign. Similarly, increased mitral E-point to septal separation, in the setting of MR and a dilated and hypodynamic LV, is a poor prognostic finding indicating reduced transmitral flow. Again, this must be distinguished from insufficient mitral opening caused by an eccentric AR jet, which can be readily seen once the color Doppler is activated. Delayed closure of the mitral leaflet in a horse with sinus rhythm suggests an elevated LV diastolic pressure; this "B-shoulder" is a sign of elevated end diastolic LA (and LV) pressure.

Beyond the nature of the valvular lesion itself, perhaps most pivotal in the horse with degenerative VHD is quantitation of LV and LA chamber sizes by 2D and M-mode studies. As discussed previously, ventricular dilation (eccentric hypertrophy) is the major finding indicating hemodynamically important MR and AR. LA size is another marker of MR severity. However, LA diameter represents both volume and remodeling of shape in this lower-pressure chamber, including dilation of pulmonary venous entries. In severe left-sided CHF, a more rounded, turgid LA appearance might be seen. In cases of AR, the major load is on the left ventricle, although the atrium might enlarge to a variable degree from LV dysfunction, fluid retention, or concurrent MR.

LV volume can be estimated in a number of ways. Subjectively, 2D echo imaging might demonstrate rounding of the normally pointed equine apex. Objectively, a minor dimension can be measured by M-mode, 2D, or with emerging 3D imaging modalities (**Figures 30.6**, **30.7**, and **30.16**). Linear dimensions from interventricular septum to posterior LV wall and long-axis areas traced at end diastole and end systole are used most often to estimate LV size, volumes, and systolic function. The inability to readily image from the LV apex is a limitation. A modified, slightly tilted long-axis image from the right thorax, optimized for the left ventricle should be used to trace LV areas and estimate volumes by method of discs. Doppler methods can assess severity of regurgitation, assuming available equipment and operator training.

Following chronic MR and AR progression in horses involves serial determinations of LV diameters, LV and LA areas, and LV volumes. Consistency in acquiring and measuring these is critical and can be problematic with multiple observers. The measurement line – be it a 2D caliper or M-line – should be at the insertion level of the chordae tendineae to the papillary muscles, intersect the walls at roughly right angles, and bisect the cross-sectional LV area into equal parts. The subaortic septal concavity poses point of error; this is readily observed from a long-axis image optimized for the LV inlet (see **Figure 30.7**). The authors recommend obtaining long- and short-axis images and digitally storing the method of measurement for future reference and comparison. Comparing the LV diastolic dimension by M-mode (short-axis) to the LV internal diameter measurement from a right parasternal long-axis image provides an internal check on angulation. These measurements should be within 5–10% of each other.

Other factors should be considered when measuring heart size. One is the effect of sedation with alpha-2 agonist drugs, which increase arterial blood pressure and slow heart rate, or with acepromazine, which can reduce blood pressure. These effects can alter LV size and systolic function in some horses. Accordingly, images should be obtained prior to any necessary sedation for assessment of chamber size and function. Other factors include the effects of hydration status and heart rate, especially in exercise studies. Lastly, some degree of LV and RV enlargement occurs secondary to training in high-performance animals.

Regarding the left atrium, both subjective inspection for changes in shape and chamber measurements are useful. However, the LA dimension obtained from the standard M-mode right parasternal short-axis view at the heart base is an unreliable measure of LA size, because the cursor crosses the junction of the atrial body and appendage. The authors prefer to measure the left atrium from the 2D parasternal long-axis view, optimized for the LV inflow tract, with the aorta excluded from the plane (see Chapter 4); measurements are made at maximal LA volume (end systole) roughly parallel to the mitral annulus. An alternative approach is the short-axis diameter or area at the level of the aorta. More advanced evaluations of atrial size and function, such as atrial strain, are largely investigational. Ultimately, LA size depends on mitral valve function, pulmonary venous pressure and return, and ventricular function. Moderate to severe MR, diastolic or systolic ventricular failure, volume retention, and heart rate all can influence LA size. The development of lone AF also mildly increases LA (and right atrial, RA) diameter and area in some horses. The ratios of aortic root diameter (as an internal index) to LA and LV diameters are potentially useful indices for MR. The aorta must be measured consistently; currently there are no accepted standards.

Indices of systolic heart function include the ejection fraction (from long-axis 2D or from 3D images), fractional shortening (from M-mode), and fractional area change (from short-axis 2D images). However, in chronic valvular disease these calculations are misleading, because increased LV preload improves echo measures of LV systolic function and in MR, reduced wall stress also might occur (see "Pathophysiology of Valvular Regurgitation") even in the presence of impaired contractility. There are no load-independent measures of systolic function available and even advanced methods, such as tissue Doppler imaging and speckle strain deformation (Chapter 4), are affected by LV loading conditions, becoming hyperdynamic when preload is high. Hyperdynamic systolic ventricular function can occur even in the setting of left-sided CHF, especially with acute MR, such as from infective endocarditis or rupture of primary chordae tendineae. With chronic volume overload, LV function indices tend to progress from normal to hyperdynamic and then back to normal, although some horses demonstrate progressive signs of myocardial failure (as a "cardiomyopathy of volume overload"). Exuberant ventricular septal motion, relative to the LV free wall, commonly is evidence of LV volume overload. This relates to alterations in LV geometry with rightward deviation of the septum during diastole, which promotes greater leftward movement during systole. It is a common feature of moderate to severe MR and AR and, in the authors' view, a negative prognostic sign.

Assessment of LV diastolic function and ventricular filling pressure also is complicated by altered loading conditions. These measures often are hyperdynamic until severe regurgitation has developed, especially in primary MR. Moderate to severe MR produces an abrupt increase in LA pressure related to the simultaneous arrival of the regurgitant stroke volume and pulmonary venous return. This transiently increases LA pressure and contributes somewhat disproportionately to early LV filling, which influences the transmitral flow and "artificially" increases the initial velocity of the filling (mitral E) wave and tissue Doppler e′ (also called E′ or Ea) wave. LA function sometimes is estimated using the same imaging methods applied to the left ventricle. Atrial function might be especially important in horses with AF, with respect to risk of AF recurrence or mechanical recovery following cardioversion from more sustained AF (Decloedt, 2013).

Tricuspid Regurgitation TR is a common Doppler imaging finding. In most cases, it is physiologic or training-related and is ignored. The typical TR jet, seen from the right parasternal long- and short-axis planes optimized for the LV outflow tract, is a thin eccentric jet directed toward the aorta. It is unlikely to be of clinical consequence and often silent to auscultation. Even larger, more central or laterally directed jets uncommonly progress to overt clinical disease or atrial arrhythmia, although the influence of exercise-induced changes in pulmonary artery pressures on TR needs further study. Some horses do exhibit a particularly loud murmur with a wide jet, larger vena contracta, and more distant PISA. If evidence of poor performance exists in these cases, more suspicion is directed toward the tricuspid valve. Sporadic cases develop atrial flutter or AF with an obviously enlarged RA chamber. TR also can be a functional consequence of PH, which frequently is a sequela of moderate to severe MR or severe interstitial lung disease.

RV and RA size and function assessments are challenging because of the complex anatomy of these chambers and difficulties in finding good acoustic windows. Measurements of internal diastolic and systolic dimensions, fractional linear or area changes, tricuspid annular plane systolic excursion (TAPSE), and segmental tissue velocities, time intervals, and myocardial strain have been investigated in horses, but there is no accepted standard for assessing the right ventricle. Again, serial examinations performed in a consistent manner are likely to be most valuable.

When TR peak velocity exceeds ~3.2 m/s at rest (in the absence of RV outflow obstruction), PH is likely. Normally, pulmonary regurgitation in horses is considered physiologic; however, in cases of PH the pulmonary regurgitation jet velocity also is increased (to >2.5 m/s). Other methods for identifying PH (Chapter 39) include pulmonary trunk (and major branch) dilation, abbreviated pulmonary acceleration time to ejection time (AT/ET), and the ratio of right pulmonary artery to vein diameters (increased with PH; **Figure 30.7**).

Other Diagnostic Tests

Routine clinical laboratory tests usually are non-contributory to diagnosis or assessment in equine VHD. However, infective endocarditis (Chapter 31) is an exception because it incites signs of systemic inflammation and potentially, secondary organ dysfunction. Cardiac troponins are mildly elevated in many horses with severe VHD, or once CHF has supervened. A marked elevation in these biomarkers should prompt consideration of myocarditis or cardiac muscle toxicosis (see Chapter 34). Presently, the measurement of natriuretic peptides for staging of VHD or for the diagnosis of CHF is not routine.

If there is any doubt regarding the horse's underlying cardiac rhythm, a resting (base-apex) ECG should be recorded. In some cases, 24-hour ambulatory (Holter) ECG monitoring can reveal intermittent rhythm disturbances (Navas de Solis, 2020). Exercise ECG testing is important for assessing whether an arrhythmia might be impairing performance in the equine athlete, or could pose increased risk to a rider. Accepting that exercise ECGs can be challenging to obtain and might involve referral, this test is especially important in horses with chronic VHD and AF that cannot be cardioverted to sinus rhythm, yet continue to be ridden. Rhythm analysis during exercise also is recommended in older horses with moderate to severe VHD, especially for those with AR.

Thoracic radiographs usually are unavailable for horses, and when obtained, are not always helpful in the diagnostic evaluation of VHD. Although radiographs can indicate cardiomegaly, pulmonary congestion, pulmonary edema (**Figure 30.10**), pleural effusion, or other lung pathology such as pneumonia, both echocardiography and thoracic ultrasonography are more practical diagnostic tests, and usually provide more information.

Management

Most horses with degenerative VHD are asymptomatic and require no treatment. As noted, the major challenge in these animals is deciding if the valve disease has affected performance or constitutes a risk for falling, injury, or death to the horse or rider. It is imperative to re-examine horses at predetermined intervals to evaluate for progressive changes in performance, chamber remodeling, or echo findings that suggest impending heart failure or PH development. The risk of AF or ventricular ectopy is the other prime consideration. Some horses are amazingly stable for years, despite having a moderately loud murmur and some degree of cardiac enlargement. However, any new changes in work capacity or clinical signs, such as unexplained stumbling or falling, should prompt immediate reevaluation.

When advanced MR or TR has caused demonstrable cardiac remodeling (cardiomegaly or altered geometric shape), some clinicians prescribe an angiotensin converting enzyme (ACE) inhibitor, hoping to delay adverse chamber remodeling. Benazepril is used most often in horses because of its more favorable kinetics. (Notably, enalapril has poor oral absorption in horses). Despite the theoretical benefits of ACE inhibition and aldosterone receptor antagonists on cardiac remodeling and reduction of arrhythmia, no efficacy data have been published in horses. Currently, such treatment is not considered standard of care, although it is employed by some clinicians.

Cardiac arrhythmias can complicate chronic VHD. AF usually can be cardioverted to sinus rhythm with quinidine or by transvenous electrocardioversion (pp. 392 and 415). However, there is substantial potential for reversion back to AF, especially with LA enlargement or persistent LA myocardial dysfunction. The most common precipitator of CHF in horses is the superimposition of AF on moderate to severe chronic valvular disease. As in other species, this rhythm can lead to sudden decompensation. When CHF occurs, management is medical (p. 358). Horses that have developed CHF should never be used, except perhaps for reproduction. Ventricular arrhythmias have been observed in some horses with chronic AR, and this is a potential risk to horse and rider. Accordingly, when such horses are used, an exercise ECG is strongly recommended and any signs of stumbling or sudden weakness should prompt an immediate cardiac examination.

Prognosis

There are some obvious concerns in terms of prognosis. For example, clinical signs of CHF or onset of AF in a horse with an enlarged heart would create great concerns regarding the use and longevity of the animal. Similarly, certain 2D or M-mode findings portend a negative outcome. Examples include: a flail leaflet or large vegetative lesion; moderate to severe ventricular and atrial remodeling; pulmonary artery dilation; low ventricular ejection fraction; a B-shoulder on mitral valve M-mode echocardiogram; and premature closure of the mitral valve (prior to the QRS complex) in a horse with AR. Assuming the recordings are technically correct, some Doppler echo features indicate moderate to severe valvular disease, as noted previously. For example, a short AR pressure half-time or a low velocity, early peaking CW Doppler envelope of MR would indicate severe valvular insufficiency. However, these are relatively dramatic findings and a minority of horses exhibit such advanced disease.

More challenging to assess are the horses with valvular heart disease that have no, or only borderline, cardiac enlargement based on standard echo exams and that are either performing as intended or show mildly decreased performance of unclear cause. The rider profile also is a consideration. Special concerns relate to the horse that performs strenuous work, is ridden by children, or is used as a lesson horse for inexperienced riders.

Suggested Additional Reading and References

Also See Online Comprehensive Bibliography at: https://www.routledge.com/9781482246223.

Berthoud D, Schwarzwald CC. Echocardiographic assessment of left ventricular size and systolic function in Warmblood horses using linear measurements, area-based indices, and volume estimates: A retrospective database analysis. J Vet Intern Med 2021; 35:504–520.

Bishop SP, Cole CR, Smetzer DL. Functional and morphologic pathology of equine aortic insufficiency. Path Vet 1966; 3:137–158.

Blissitt KJ, Bonagura JD. Colour flow Doppler echocardiography in horses with cardiac murmurs. Equine Vet J Suppl 1995;19:82–85.

Blissitt Long KJ, Bonagura JD, Darke PG. Standardised imaging technique for guided M-mode and Doppler echocardiography in the horse. Equine Vet J 1992;24(3):226–235.

Bonagura JD. Overview of equine cardiac disease. Vet Clin North Am Equine Pract 2019;35:1–22.

Buhl R, Ersbøll AK, Eriksen L, Koch J. Use of color Doppler echocardiography to assess the development of valvular regurgitation in standardbred trotters. J Am Vet Med Assoc 2005;227(10):1630–1635.

Buhl R, Ersbøll AK, Eriksen L, Koch J. Sources and magnitude of variation of echocardiographic measurements in normal Standardbred horses. Vet Radiol Ultrasound 2004;45(6):505–512.

Decloedt A. Pericardial disease, myocardial disease, and great vessel abnormalities in horses. Vet Clin North Am Equine Pract 2019;35(1):139–157. doi:10.1016/j.cveq.2018.12.005.

Decloedt A, Verheyen T, Van Der Vekens N, et al. Long-term follow-up of atrial function after cardioversion of atrial fibrillation in horses. Vet J 2013;197(3):583–588.

Decloedt A, De Clercq D, Ven Sofie S, et al. Echocardiographic measurements of right heart size and function in healthy horses. Equine Vet J 2017;49(1):58–64.

Durando MM. Cardiovascular causes of poor performance and exercise intolerance and assessment of safety in the equine athlete. Vet Clin North Am Equine Pract 2019;35:175–190.

Hallowell GD, Bowen M. Reliability and identification of aortic valve prolapse in the horse. BMC Vet Res 2013;9:9.

Helwegen MM, Young LE, Rogers K, et al. Measurements of right ventricular internal dimensions and their relationships to severity of tricuspid valve regurgitation in national hunt thoroughbreds. Equine Vet J Suppl 2006;36:171–177.

Huesler IM, Mitchell KJ, Schwarzwald CC. Echocardiographic assessment of left atrial size and function in warmblood horses: reference intervals, allometric scaling, and agreement of different echocardiographic variables. J Vet Intern Med 2016;30(4):1241–1252.

Imhasly A, Tschudi PR, Lombard CW, et al. Clinical and echocardiographic features of mild mitral valve regurgitation in 108 horses. Vet J 2010;183(2):166–171.

Keen JA. Examination of horses with cardiac disease. Vet Clin North Am Equine Pract 2019;35(1):23–42. doi:10.1016/j.cveq.2018.12.006.

Koenig TR, Mitchell KJ, Schwarzwald CC. Echocardiographic assessment of left ventricular function in healthy horses and in horses with heart disease using pulsed-wave tissue Doppler imaging. J Vet Intern Med 2017;31(2):556–567.

Marr CM. Equine acquired valvular disease. Vet Clin North Am Equine Pract 2019;35:119–137.

Marr CM, Reef VB. Physiological valvular regurgitation in clinically normal young racehorses: prevalence and two-dimensional colour flow Doppler echocardiographic characteristics. Equine Vet J Suppl 1995;19:56–62.

Navas de Solis C. Ventricular arrhythmias in horses: Diagnosis, prognosis and treatment. Vet J 2020;261:105476.

O'Gara P, Sugeng L, Lang R, et al. The role of imaging in chronic degenerative mitral regurgitation. JACC: Cardiovasc Imag 2008;1(2):221–237.

Patteson MW, Gibbs C, Wotton PR, et al. Echocardiographic measurements of cardiac dimensions and indices of cardiac function in normal adult thoroughbred horses. Equine Vet J Suppl 1995;19:18–27.

Reef VB. Assessment of the cardiovascular system in horses during prepurchase and insurance examinations. Vet Clin North Am Equine Pract 2019;35(1):191–204. doi:10.1016/j.cveq.2018.11.002.

Reef VB, Bain FT, Spencer PA. Severe mitral regurgitation in horses: clinical, echocardiographic and pathological findings. Equine Vet J 1998;30(1):18–27.

Reef VB, Bonagura J, Buhl R, et al. Recommendations for management of equine athletes with cardiovascular abnormalities. J Vet Intern Med 2014;28(3):749–61. (Joint ACVIM/ECVIM Consensus Statement).

Sleeper MM, Durando MM, Holbrook TC, et al. Comparison of echocardiographic measurements in elite and nonelite Arabian endurance horses. Am J Vet Res 2014;75(10):893–898.

Schwarzwald CC. Equine echocardiography. Vet Clin North Am Equine Pract 2019;35(1):43–64.

Stevens KB1, Marr CM, Horn JN, et al. Effect of left-sided valvular regurgitation on mortality and causes of death among a population of middle-aged and older horses. Vet Rec 2009;164(1):6–10.

van Loon G. Cardiac arrhythmias in horses. Vet Clin North Am Equine Pract 2019;35(1):85–102.

Ven S, Decloedt A, Van Der Vekens N, et al. Assessing aortic regurgitation severity from 2D, M-mode and pulsed wave Doppler echocardiographic measurements in horses. Vet J 2016;210:34–38.

Vörös K. Quantitative two-dimensional echocardiography in the horse: a review. Acta Vet Hung 1997;45(2):127–136.

Young LE. Cardiac responses to training in 2-year-old thoroughbreds: an echocardiographic study. Equine Vet J Suppl 1999;30:195–198.

Zucca E, Ferrucci F, Croci C, et al. Echocardiographic measurements of cardiac dimensions in normal Standardbred racehorses. J Vet Cardiol 2008;10(1):45–51.

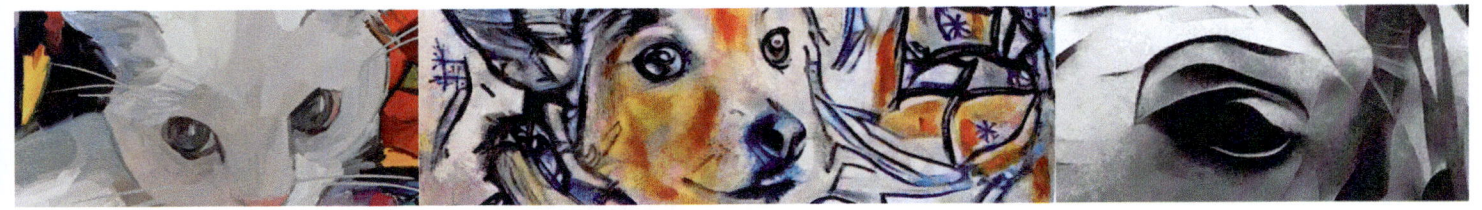

31
INFECTIVE ENDOCARDITIS

Infection of the cardiac valves and other endocardial tissue is relatively uncommon. However, when it does occur, the cardiac and systemic consequences usually are severe. Infective endocarditis is diagnosed more often in dogs than in cats. It is quite uncommon in horses also, although its relative prevalence compared to dogs or other species is not known. Endocarditis can be difficult to diagnose, especially before severe valve damage has occurred. Congestive heart failure (CHF) is a common sequela. Other consequences include thromboembolism (TE), multiorgan infection and abcessation, immune-mediated polyarthritis and glomerulonephritis, various arrhythmias, and sometimes, sudden death. Because of the widely disparate manifestations, endocarditis sometimes is called the "great imitator."

Invasion and infection of the endocardial surface occurs from bacteria or other microbes present in blood flowing past it. Successful therapy depends on rapid, aggressive, and long-term antimicrobial treatment with agent(s) effective against the invading organism, combined with appropriate management of concurrent disease sequelae. Even with efficacious antimicrobial treatment, severe valve damage or myocardial involvement can lead to CHF or sudden death.

Endocarditis usually involves the aortic, mitral, or both valves in dogs, cats, and horses. This could relate to an increased risk for endothelial damage from the higher left heart pressures. Infective endocarditis of the tricuspid valve is rare in small animals and uncommon in horses; pulmonary valve involvement is even more rare. Jugular thrombophlebitis, or another septic focus, could be the source of tricuspid (as well as other) valve endocarditis. The use of unsterile needles for IV injection has been associated with tricuspid valve endocarditis in humans (drug abusers) and in some other species.

Recurrent bacteremia can result from infections of the skin, mouth, urinary tract, prostate gland, lungs, gut, or other organs, and also from prolonged IV catheter placement. Dentistry procedures are known to cause transient bacteremia in a high percentage of cases, although endocarditis rarely is reported as a consequence. Other procedures (including endoscopy, urethral catheterization, anal surgery, and other so-called "dirty" procedures) are presumed to cause transient bacteremia in some cases.

Predisposing Factors

Endothelial damage, with secondary platelet and fibrin aggregation, probably serves as a nidus for circulating bacterial colonization in most cases of endocarditis. Highly virulent organisms or a heavy bacterial load increase the risk of cardiac infection. Normal valves might be invaded by virulent bacteria; however, previously damaged valves are more vulnerable, especially with persistent bacteremia. Mechanical valve trauma could result from turbulent blood flow (jet lesions) or endocardial injury from a catheter extending into the heart. Subaortic stenosis (SAS) is associated with an increased risk for aortic valve endocarditis. Damage to endothelium on the ventricular side of the aortic valve, caused by the high-velocity systolic jet is thought to be an important predisposing factor in SAS; the association with even mild aortic regurgitation (AR) likely increases the risk. Other congenital malformations considered to increase endocarditis risk in people include patent ductus arteriosus (PDA) and ventricular septal defect (VSD). Only sporadic cases of endocarditis are reported in animals with these defects. Aortic endocarditis has occurred in a dog with membranous ventricular septal aneurysm perforated by a small VSD. Endocarditis also can develop subsequent to implantation of an occlusion device to treat PDA or a septal defect, a valve replacement or reconstructive bioprosthetic device, or a pacemaker lead. Device-associated infection is possible following surgery despite perioperative antibiotic use. However, postprocedural endocarditis is highly unlikely when aseptic surgical technique and new sterile catheters and implanted devices are used, even without prophylactic antibiotics. Nevertheless, a future episode of bacteremia, associated with other systemic infection, could lead to secondary infection around an implanted device. Rare cases of endocarditis caused by foreign body (such as a grass awn or porcupine quill) migration into the heart are documented. Fungal, as well as bacterial, organisms can be involved in such cases.

Other predisposing factors could involve infection in another organ, including prostatitis, urinary tract infection, pneumonia, septic arthritis, diskospondylitis, dermatitis, or an abcess. Diseases that impair immune responses, such as diabetes mellitus and hyperadrenocorticism, or cause hypercoagulability or endothelial disruption probably increase the endocarditis risk. The possible effect of immunosuppressive therapy in predisposing to infective endocarditis is unclear. Findings related to a possible link between periodontal disease or dental procedures and endocarditis in dogs have been mixed. One retrospective study of dogs with endocarditis found that none had undergone an oral procedure within 3 months prior to diagnosis, and no difference was found in prevalence of oral infection between these dogs and a group of controls without endocarditis (Peddle, 2009). However, the endocarditis dogs were more likely to have had nonoral surgery requiring general anesthesia within 3 months of the endocarditis diagnosis, as well as a new heart murmur or change in intensity of an existing murmur. Preexisting heart disease was not found to be a risk factor. Another retrospective review of dogs with periodontal disease did suggest association between severity of oral disease and risk of cardiovascular conditions, including endocarditis, and cardiomyopathy (Glickman, 2009). However, in this study, the methods used to arrive at these cardiac diagnoses were not indicated, a surprisingly high number of cases were identified as having hypertrophic cardiomyopathy (although none were identified with SAS), and the prevalence of degenerative (myxomatous) mitral valve disease (DMVD) in the population was not identified. Nevertheless, in a small necropsy study of dogs with periodontal disease that grossly appeared to have endocarditis on postmortem exam, about 20% of cases had identical enterococci in both oral and cardiac samples (Semedo-Lemsaddek, 2016).

There is no convincing evidence that DMVD is a predisposing factor for endocarditis in dogs. Considering the high prevalence of both DMVD and progressive periodontal disease in small to medium-sized dogs, the sometimes "sudden" recognition of a previously undiagnosed mitral regurgitation (MR) murmur in dogs with DMVD, the echocardiographic findings of mitral valve thickening with or without chordal rupture in DMVD, and the uncommon occurrence of verified endocarditis in these breeds, a clear association between DMVD and infective endocarditis seems unlikely.

Pathophysiology

Multiple factors play a role in the development of infective endocarditis. These include endothelial damage, disturbed blood flow, hemostatic and immune responses, bacteremia, and bacterial virulence. Mechanical or inflammatory injury to endothelial surfaces facilitates microbial adhesion and invasion. Endothelial disruption stimulates platelet activation and a local coagulation response, with resulting aggregate of fibrin, platelets, red blood cells (RBCs) and leukocytes. Circulating bacteria adhere to and colonize this initially sterile thrombus, leading to the growth of vegetative lesions. Fibronectin, produced by endothelial cells, platelets and fibroblasts after endothelial injury, is thought to enhance bacterial adherence; many pathogenic bacteria possess surface receptors for this glycoprotein. Bacterial clumping, promoted by agglutinating antibodies, could facilitate attachment to the valves also. Vegetations consist mainly of aggregated platelets, fibrin, blood elements, inflammatory cells, necrotic valve tissue and bacteria, although bacteria might not be identified following antibiotic therapy (**Figures 31.1–31.4**).

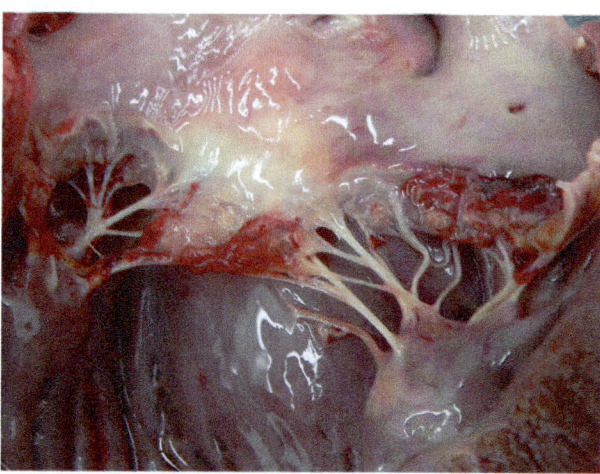

Figure 31.1 Infective endocarditis of the mitral valve, in a 10-year-old female Labrador Retriever. Clinical abnormalities included an inflammatory leukogram, azotemia, icterus, pancreatitis, pulmonary edema, multiple electrolyte abnormalities, and disseminated intravascular coagulation. Roughened hemorrhagic areas are visible on the mitral leaflets. Neutrophilic infiltrate, hemorrhage and fibrin disrupted the valve leaflet structure. Multiple infarcts and colonies of cocci were found in the kidneys.

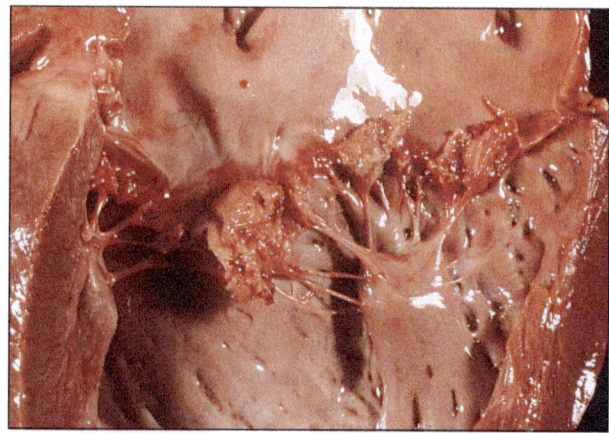

Figure 31.2 Vegetative lesions have destroyed most of the normal mitral valve structure in this dog with infective endocarditis. (Image courtesy of Dr R Myers.)

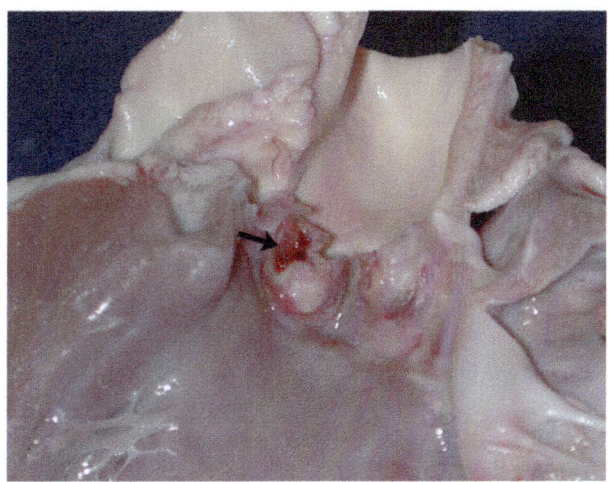

Figure 31.3 Aortic valve endocarditis in a 2-year-old female German Shepherd with congestive heart failure, renal failure and other metabolic abnormalities. Several tan nodules distort the valve leaflets and there is a 2 mm hole in one cusp (arrow). A heavy pure culture of *E. coli* was isolated from the kidney.

Colonizing bacteria can secrete enzymes that damage valve tissue and promote vegetative lesion proliferation. Organisms such as *Staphylococcus* species (spp.) and *Streptococcus* spp. have more adhesive ability, can increase tissue factor production and platelet aggregation, and are resistant to the bactericidal effect of platelet-derived proteins. Additional fibrin deposited over bacterial colonies protects them from normal host defenses and many antibiotics. Some organisms, including *S. aureus* and *Bartonella* spp., are internalized by endothelial cells, conferring more protection from the immune system. *Bartonella* organisms also escape the immune system by entering RBCs.

Endothelial damage and mechanical valve trauma can cause nonbacterial thrombotic endocarditis too. This is a sterile accumulation of platelets and fibrin on the valve surface. Nonseptic (so-called "bland") emboli can arise from such vegetations and cause infarction elsewhere. Bacteremia could cause a secondary infective endocarditis at these sites. This might be most relevant to right-sided endocarditis.

Cardiac Consequences

Endocarditis lesions (vegetations) typically develop along valve leaflet margins on the lower-pressure side of an affected valve, or at a location downstream from disturbed blood flow. Common sites include the ventricular surface of aortic valve leaflets with SAS, the atrial surface of the mitral valve, and the right ventricular side of a VSD. In severe cases, much of the valve stroma and endocardium are affected on both sides of the valve (**Figure 30.4A**, p. 576). However, "secondary" cardiac infections can occur, as when aortic endocarditis causes AR followed by seeding of the infection to the mitral valve's ventricular surface (**Figure 31.4**). Vegetations associated with a PDA would most likely affect ductal or proximal pulmonary artery endothelium or tissue around a ductal occlusion device.

Although vegetations usually involve the valve leaflets, in some cases lesions can extend into and damage adjacent cardiac tissues, such as chordae tendineae, sinuses of Valsalva, mural endocardium, and myocardium. Valve leaflet deformity, perforation, tearing, or chordal rupture causes valve insufficiency (**Figures 31.3–31.5**). Flail leaflet motion leads to severe valve regurgitation, with its secondary consequences. Some vegetations also are large enough to obstruct flow across an affected valve area, causing clinically relevant

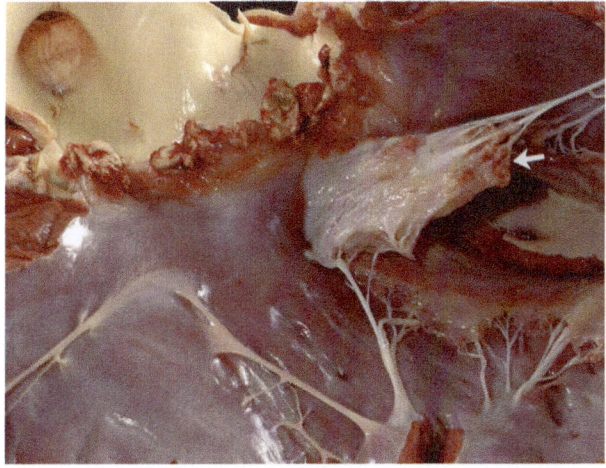

Figure 31.4 Infective endocarditis destroyed the aortic valve cusps in this horse with congestive heart failure. Small vegetations are present on the anterior mitral leaflet (arrow) also.

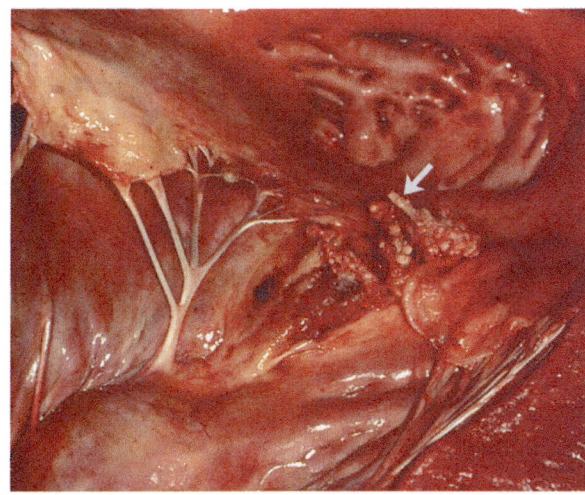

Figure 31.5 Rupture of a major chorda tendinea (arrow), secondary to infective endocarditis of the mitral valve in a 10-year-old Quarter Horse mare. Vegetations on the posterior leaflet are rough and irregular. The resulting severe mitral regurgitation led to acute left-sided congestive heart failure with fulminant pulmonary edema. Gram stain of a vegetation sample showed chains of cocci. Alpha-hemolytic colonies and mixed coliforms grew on culture; however, definitive identification was not available.

stenosis. This can occur with healed endocarditis and valve scarring, too. Newer vegetations, especially, are more friable, so embolization of other organs is common. With time, the lesions become fibrous and might calcify.

Mitral or aortic valve destruction commonly produces increasingly worse valve regurgitation and secondary volume overload. Signs of CHF can develop acutely or gradually, depending on the extent and progression of valve damage, as well as whether both mitral and aortic valves or other predisposing factors are involved. Left ventricular (LV) filling pressure and left atrial (LA) pressure can rise relatively quickly, causing rapid onset of pulmonary edema. Aortic endocarditis is especially likely to cause acute CHF with fulminant pulmonary edema. Left heart enlargement (secondary remodeling) might be minimal at the time of CHF onset if valve damage has progressed rapidly. In the minority of cases where aortic vegetative lesions also cause stenosis, cardiac workload and likelihood of CHF are further increased.

Extension of infection into the myocardium, myocardial infarction and abscessation caused by coronary embolization, and systemic inflammatory responses can provoke arrhythmias and compromise cardiac function. Aortic valve endocarditis in particular can extend into the surrounding atrioventricular (AV) nodal tissues, with potential for partial or complete AV block. Brady- or tachyarrhythmias can cause weakness, syncope, exacerbation of CHF signs, and sudden death. In rare cases, bacterial invasion and destruction of adjacent cardiac tissue might lead to an intracardiac perforation, such as a LV outflow tract to right atrial communication (Gerbode defect, p. 455) or LV outflow-to-LA communication along the mitral annulus.

Systemic Consequences

Both cell-mediated and humoral immune responses are activated in response to invading microorganisms. Circulating immune complex deposition and complement activation damage various tissues, especially glomerular and synovial basement membranes and dermis. Sterile (immune-mediated) polyarthritis, glomerulonephritis, vasculitis, and other immune-mediated organ damage are common.

Fragments of vegetative lesions often break loose and cause infarction or metastatic infection and abcessation in multiple organs, which contribute to the diverse clinical signs of endocarditis. Septic emboli and local abscess formation also can lead to recurrent bacteremia and fever. Septic arthritis, diskospondylitis, urinary tract infections, as well as renal and splenic infarctions are common. Skeletal muscle, brain, lymphoid and other tissues are affected, too. Meningitis appears to be a common consequence of endocarditis (Sykes, 2006). Postmortem studies suggest TE occurs in most cases, although clinical evidence of TE is found in slightly less than half. Mitral valve endocarditis is thought to be associated with TE more often. Larger and more mobile vegetations, as assessed echocardiographically, are associated with a higher rate of embolic events in people and this is presumably the same in animals. Emboli can be septic or bland (noninfective). In dogs, renal and splenic infarcts are identified most often. Myocardial, brain, and peripheral vascular obstructions occur frequently, although clinical vascular encephalopathy seems to be relatively uncommon in dogs. **Table 31.1** lists some consequences of infective endocarditis.

Causative Organisms

The organisms identified as causing endocarditis in dogs have most often been *Staphylococcus* spp., *Streptococcus* spp., or *Escherichia coli*. Other organisms isolated from infected valves in dogs have included *Corynebacterium* (*Arcanobacterium*) spp., *Pasteurella* spp., *Pseudomonas aeruginosa*, *Erysipelothrix rhusiopathiae* (also identified as *E. tonsillaris*), *Enterococcus* spp., *Serratia marcescens*, *Rhodococcus equi*, and others. Rare fungal infections also have been identified in dogs, usually in association with a foreign body. Various *Bartonella* spp., especially *B. vinsonii* subsp. *berkhoffii* and *B. henselae*, have been identified in dogs as well as cats with endocarditis. Compared to dogs, there are few reports of endocarditis in cats. Besides *Bartonella* spp., organisms reported in cats include *Streptococcus* spp., *Staphylococcus* spp., *E. coli, Pseudomonas, Pasturella* spp., and others. Organisms found in horses with endocarditis are most commonly *Streptococcus* spp., and *Actinobacillus* spp. However, many others have included *Pasteurella* spp., *E. coli, Staphylococcus* spp., *Rhodococcus equi, Pseudomonas* spp., and *S. marcescens*.

Streptococcal endocarditis might be more likely to affect the mitral valve, as well as be associated with polyarthritis. Viridans group Streptococci are particularly adept at binding to certain proteins on circulating platelets and thereby are carried to areas of damaged endocardium. *Bartonella* is an important cause of culture-negative endocarditis in some geographic areas. Dogs infected with *Bartonella* can harbor more than one species; they also might be coinfected with *Ehrlichia, Babesia,* and *Rickettsia* spp. Yet in dogs with endocarditis from other more common bacteria, coinfection with *Bartonella* appears to be rare. *Bartonella* spp. are facultative intracellular bacteria, with a preference for vascular endothelium and possibly RBCs and other cells (monocytes, macrophages); this helps them avoid destruction by the immune system. Relapsing bacteremia can occur, especially during stress or immunosuppression. Valvular endocarditis is just one consequence of *Bartonella* infection; others include polyarthritis and granulomatous or lymphocytic inflammation in lymph nodes, liver, spleen and many other tissues, as well as vasoproliferative tumors. Chronic *Bartonella* infection also has been associated with reduced immune function, including decreased monocyte phagocytic ability, reduced (CD8+) lymphocyte number and adhesion molecule expression, and inhibited B-cell antigen presentation.

Table 31.1 Potential Sequelae of Infective Endocarditis

Cardiac

- Valve insufficiency or stenosis
  - Murmur
  - Congestive heart failure
- Coronary embolization (aortic valve[a])
  - Myocardial infarction
  - Myocardial abscess
  - Myocarditis
  - Decreased contractility (segmental or global)
  - Arrhythmias
- Myocarditis (direct invasion by microorganisms)
  - Arrhythmias
  - Atrioventricular conduction abnormalities (aortic valve[a])
  - Decreased contractility
- Pericarditis (direct invasion by microorganisms)
  - Pericardial effusion
  - Cardiac tamponade (?)

Renal

- Infarction
  - Reduced renal function
- Abscess formation and pyelonephritis
  - Reduced renal function
  - Urinary tract infection
  - Renal pain
- Glomerulonephritis (immune-mediated)
  - Proteinuria
  - Reduced renal function
  - Systemic hypertension

Musculoskeletal

- Septic arthritis
  - Joint swelling and pain
  - Lameness
- Immune-mediated polyarthritis
  - Shifting-limb lameness
  - Joint swelling and pain
- Septic osteomyelitis
  - Bone pain
  - Lameness
- Myositis
  - Muscle pain
  - Hypertrophic pulmonary osteopathy

Nervous System

- Abscesses
  - Associated neurologic signs
- Encephalitis and meningitis
  - Associated neurologic signs

Vascular System

- Vasculitis
  - Thrombosis
  - Petechiae and small hemorrhages (including in eye, skin)
- Thromboembolic obstruction
  - Ischemia of tissues served, with associated signs

Pulmonary

- Pulmonary emboli (tricuspid or pulmonic valves, rare[a,b])
  - Pneumonia (tricuspid or pulmonic valves, rare[a,b])

General Systemic

- Sepsis
- Fever
- Anorexia
- Malaise and depression
- Shaking ("shivering")
- Vague pain
- Inflammatory leukogram
- Increased fibrinogen and inflammatory markers (horses)
- Mild anemia
- Increased serum globulin and decreased albumin
- ± positive antinuclear antibody test
- ± positive blood cultures

[a] Diseased valve most commonly associated with abnormality.
[b] Endocarditis of the tricuspid or pulmonic valve is rare in dogs and cats, and uncommon in horses.

About 20% of canine endocarditis cases could be caused by *Bartonella* alone, depending on the geographic region (Breitschwerdt, 2003). In dogs, *B. vinsonii* subsp. *berkhoffi* is known to cause endocarditis, as well as myocarditis, polyarthritis, meningoencephalitis, and granulomatous inflammation in lymph nodes and other tissues. *B. vinsonii* subsp. *berkhoffi* also can infect cats and has been associated with feline endomyocarditis-LV endocardial fibrosis. Other Bartonella species, especially *B. henselae*, also are associated with endocarditis and myocarditis in dogs, cats, and potentially other species. Cats, wild canids, rodents, and other species can serve as reservoir hosts for different *Bartonella* spp. There are several arthropod vectors, including ticks and fleas; in addition, the infection could be transmissible by scratches and bites from infected animals, which present important zoonotic potential. Repeated exposure to blood or body fluids of reservoir hosts, or even the feces of arthropod vectors, might present infection risk. Conversely, humans are considered the main reservoir host for *B. quintana*; yet this organism has been identified in dogs, cats and other species and has been associated with endocarditis in dogs. While subclinical *Bartonella* infections are common in cats, sporadic cases of endocarditis, myocarditis, and inflammation in other tissues occur this species, too. As in dogs, cats can harbor more than one *Bartonella* spp. simultaneously.

Endocarditis-causing *Bartonella* spp. preferentially appear to affect the aortic valve, although the mitral valve occasionally is involved. *Bartonella* infection appears less likely to cause fever. It often is associated with worse survival. Histologically, *Bartonella* endocarditis lesions look different from other bacterial vegetations and include a combination of fibrosis, mineralization, endothelial proliferation, neovascularization, and variable inflammation. *Bartonella* organisms might be found within endothelial cells and extracellularly. Serologic and polymerase chain reaction (PCR) techniques, in combination with clinical findings, are needed for definitive diagnosis of *Bartonella* endocarditis. Blood cultures usually are negative, even with long incubation using specialized culture media. However, in a small study of military dogs with culture-negative (endo/myo)carditis, PCR testing of postmortem valve or tissue samples identified *Bartonella* DNA in over 70% of the cases with endocarditis (Davis, 2020).

Clinical Features

The prevalence of infective endocarditis in dogs is low; it has been variably estimated at 0.05–0.08% (to over 6%, a figure that must reflect some sampling bias). Most cases are middle-aged, medium- or large-breed dogs. Male dogs appear to be affected at a rate twice that of females. The prevalence of endocarditis increases with age. More than three fourths of cases in one large survey were over five years of age (Sykes, 2006). Most reports suggest larger (>15 kg) dogs are at greater risk. German Shepherd Dogs and possibly Boxers, Golden Retrievers, and Labrador Retrievers might be overrepresented. The aortic valve is involved in about half of canine cases and the mitral valve in slightly more (Sykes, 2006). Both valves are affected in some cases. As noted, SAS is a risk factor for aortic valve endocarditis.

Cats rarely are diagnosed with infective endocarditis; prevalence has been estimated at 0.006–0.018%. Although cats of any age can be affected, a median age of 9 years was reported (Palerme, 2016). There does not appear to be a sex or breed predilection for endocarditis in cats. Aortic valve infection occurs in more than half of cases, sometimes in conjunction with mitral infection. Mitral valve endocarditis can occur alone, too. Horses also are uncommonly diagnosed with endocarditis and risk factors are not well understood. Young and male horses might be at greater risk, although some reports suggest no age or sex predisposition. The mitral valve is thought to be affected most often, followed by the aortic, or both valves simultaneously. Sporadic cases of endocarditis involving the right heart also occur in horses, as well as other species.

Although some affected animals have evidence of past or concurrent infection, a clear history of predisposing factors usually is absent. Immunocompromised animals might be at greater risk for endocarditis. The clinical signs of infective endocarditis are quite variable and can relate to the underlying infection, immune-mediated effects, arterial TE, and progressive valvular or myocardial dysfunction. These signs often are of recent onset. In one canine survey, clinical signs were present for a median duration of 10 days prior to hospitalization (Sykes, 2006). In a feline case series, the median duration of clinical signs prior to presentation was only 2.5 days (Palerme, 2016).

Physical Findings

Infective endocarditis can mimic immune-mediated disease. Nonspecific signs of endocarditis include lethargy, weight loss, inappetence, recurrent fever, respiratory signs, tachycardia, and weakness. Lameness is a common presenting complaint and was reported in over 50% of canine cases in one survey (Sykes, 2006). Likewise, lameness or paresis occurred in over 38% of cats (Palerme, 2016). Lameness can involve one or more limbs and be consistent or vary over time ("shifting leg lameness"). Lameness and joint swelling could relate to immune-mediated polyarthritis, septic arthritis, TE, or a combination. Palpable joint effusion might be present. Arthrocentesis can yield a suppurative fluid, which should be cultured, although immune-mediated arthritis is more common than septic joint disease. The majority of animals with bacterial endocarditis are febrile or have waxing and waning temperature spikes. Nevertheless, some are normothermic. Endocarditis caused by *Bartonella* spp. might not be associated with fever. Evidence for multiorgan dysfunction and suspected TE is common with endocarditis. Seizures or other neurologic signs occur less often, but could affect about a quarter of canine cases. So-called vascular encephalopathy, with acute neurologic deficits, occurs only sporadically in dogs with endocarditis.

In all species, cardiac signs from left-sided CHF or arrhythmias can predominate; fulminant pulmonary edema occurs in some cases (**Figure 31.6**). About 25–40% of dogs develop CHF. In contrast, over two-thirds of cats with endocarditis exhibit signs of CHF (from pulmonary edema, pleural effusion, or both) by the time of diagnosis. Alternatively, cardiac signs in animals with endocarditis might be overshadowed by systemic signs of infarction, infection, or immune-mediated damage. Some animals show signs of sepsis. Vomiting, and epistaxis occasionally are reported. Hypertrophic osteopathy is a rare clinical association of bacterial endocarditis in dogs. Manifestations of *Bartonella* endocarditis are similar to those caused by other bacteria and also can include immune-mediated hemolytic anemia, neutrophilic or granulomatous meningoencephalitis, neutrophilic polyarthritis, cutaneous vasculitis, or uveitis.

The combination of fever, lameness, and a cardiac murmur (especially if new, altered in quality, or diastolic in timing) should strongly raise suspicion of infective endocarditis. A cardiac murmur is evident in most endocarditis cases, including 59–96% of affected dogs. However, if the endocarditis lesion(s) have caused only minimal or no valve regurgitation, or stenosis, no murmur might be heard. Endocarditis can develop in animals with a known murmur from other cardiac disease. Yet it is important to remember that a "new" murmur might indicate noninfective acquired disease (such

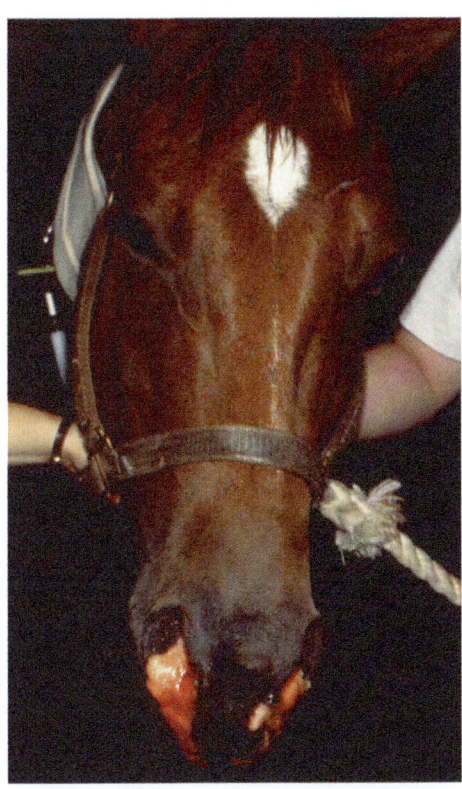

Figure 31.6 Fulminant pulmonary edema drips from the nares of the mare in **Figure 31.5**. This horse initially had a sudden onset of paroxysmal coughing, which progressed over 24 hours to severe respiratory distress. At presentation, sinus tachycardia, a grade 5/6 systolic murmur over the mitral region, and loud pulmonary crackles were heard on auscultation. Despite therapy for heart failure, the mare died the following day.

as degenerative valve disease or cardiomyopathy), previously undiagnosed congenital disease, or physiologic alterations (as with fever or anemia). While a change in murmur quality or intensity over a short time frame might indicate active valve damage, physiologic causes of murmur variation are common. Nevertheless, the onset of a diastolic murmur at the left heart base is highly suspicious for aortic valve endocarditis and clinically important valve regurgitation, especially if fever or other signs are present. Animals with SAS and aortic endocarditis typically have a combination of systolic ejection and diastolic decrescendo murmurs, known as a "to-and-fro" murmur (p. 231), although the diastolic component might be quite soft. Aortic vegetations that partially obstruct the valve orifice, as well as cause regurgitation, can cause the same type of murmur. Even without an obstructive LV outflow lesion, a soft systolic murmur might be heard because of the increased stroke volume associated with moderate to severe AR.

Severe AR produces hyperkinetic ("bounding") arterial pulses (p. 255). Cardiac arrhythmias are common, especially ventricular (or supraventricular) tachyarrhythmias. AV conduction disturbances, including complete AV block, can occur and are most often associated with aortic valve endocarditis. Signs of pulmonary edema sometimes develop acutely and without marked cardiomegaly, especially in animals with aortic valve involvement. CHF in an unexpected clinical setting, or in an animal with a murmur of recent onset, should raise suspicion for infective endocarditis, especially if other suggestive signs are present.

Diagnostic Tests

Definitive antemortem diagnosis of endocarditis can be difficult, especially because of its diverse clinical signs, rapid progression, and often elusive confirmatory testing. A presumptive diagnosis of infective endocarditis usually is based on two or more positive blood cultures, in addition to echocardiographic evidence of either vegetative lesions or valve destruction (see the following paragraphs). It can be difficult to identify bacteria. If there is echocardiographic evidence of vegetations or valve destruction, especially of the aortic valve, combined with other criteria (**Table 31.2**), endocarditis is likely even when blood cultures are negative or only intermittently positive.

Clinical laboratory findings in all species usually reflect the presence of inflammation. Neutrophilia with a left shift is typical of acute endocarditis; mature neutrophilia with or without monocytosis develops with time. Variable thrombocytopenia (mild to marked) occurs in over half of affected dogs, as does mild nonregenerative anemia. In dogs diagnosed with bartonellosis, thrombocytopenia, eosinophilia, and monocytosis have been reported. Evidence for disseminated intravascular coagulation (DIC) might be present in association with endocarditis. Common biochemical findings in dogs include hypoalbuminemia, elevated liver enzymes, azotemia, acidosis, and hyperglobulinemia. In cats, elevated blood urea nitrogen and hypoalbuminemia are likely. In horses, hyperglobulinemia, hypoalbuminemia, hyperfibrinogenemia, and leukocytosis, with or without anemia, are common. Urinalysis often shows hematuria, proteinuria and pyuria. A urine culture should be done to search for microorganisms (although a positive culture might not yield the microorganism responsible for endocarditis). Urine protein/creatinine ratio is useful in cases with proteinuria; a high ratio can signal increased risk of TE from hypercoagulability related to urinary loss of plasma antithrombin. Rheumatoid factor and antinuclear antibody tests might be positive in dogs with subacute or chronic bacterial endocarditis.

Blood Cultures

Blood cultures should be collected, although they could be negative in an estimated 40–70% of cases. Prior antibiotic use increases the likelihood of negative culture results. Yet negative culture results do not rule out infective endocarditis, especially with chronic endocarditis, recent antibiotic

Table 31.2 Criteria for Diagnosis of Infective Endocarditis[a]

Definite Endocarditis by Pathologic Criteria
- Pathologic (postmortem) lesions of active endocarditis with evidence of microorganisms in vegetation (or embolus) or intracardiac abscess

Definite Endocarditis by Clinical Criteria
- 2 major criteria (see "Major Criteria"), or
- 1 major and 2–3 minor criteria, or
- 5 minor criteria

Possible Endocarditis
- Findings consistent with infective endocarditis that fall short of "definite" but not "rejected" (see "Rejected Diagnosis of Endocarditis")

Major Criteria
- Positive blood cultures
  - At least 2 separate blood cultures positive for a microorganism typical for infective endocarditis
  - Persistently positive blood cultures (≥3) for organism consistent with endocarditis (including common skin contaminants). Samples either drawn >12 hours apart or ≥3 cultures drawn at least 1 hour apart.
- Positive echocardiographic findings
  - Vegetative lesion (especially an oscillating mass) on heart valve or support structure or in path of regurgitant jet
  - Destructive valve lesion
  - Evidence for cardiac abscess
  - New valvular regurgitation, especially more than mild aortic regurgitation (increase or change in preexisting murmur is not sufficient evidence)

Minor Criteria
- Subaortic stenosis, or other predisposing heart condition (p. 591)
- Fever
- Thromboembolic disease (arterial emboli, septic infarcts, intracranial hemorrhage)
- Immune-mediated disease (polyarthritis, glomerulonephritis, vasculitis, positive antinuclear antibody or rheumatoid factor tests)
- Positive blood culture not meeting Major Criteria
- Echocardiogram consistent with infective endocarditis but not meeting Major Criteria
- High seroreactivity (titer ≥1:1024) or positive PCR test for *Bartonella* spp.[b]
- Medium or large-size dog (>15 kg)[b]
- New and worsening heart murmur
- Chronic indwelling catheter
- Immunocompromised status
- Repeated nonsterile IV drug administration (rare)

Rejected Diagnosis of Endocarditis
- Firm alternative diagnosis for clinical manifestations
- Resolution of infective endocarditis signs within ≤4 days of antibiotic therapy
- No pathologic evidence of infective endocarditis at surgery or necropsy

[a] Adapted from modified Duke criteria for diagnosis of infective endocarditis in people (Li, 2000).
[b] Proposed criterion for use in dogs.

therapy, intermittent bacteremia, or infection by fastidious or slow growing organisms. Ideally, 3–4 blood samples of at least 10 mL are collected aseptically over a 24-hour period for bacterial culture, with more than an hour elapsing between collections. Smaller sample volumes might be required in small dogs and cats. Sampling during a fever spike or, if antibiotic therapy has already been given, at the expected time of trough drug concentration might increase diagnostic yield. For critical patients, an abbreviated sampling period of 3–4 hours might be selected before beginning empiric antibiotic therapy. Different venipuncture sites should be used for each sample. Blood collection from an indwelling IV catheter is not recommended. Both aerobic and anaerobic cultures have been recommended, although the value of routine anaerobic culture is questionable. Use of lysis centrifugation tubes might enhance the diagnostic yield from blood cultures. Prolonged incubation (3–4 weeks) is recommended because some bacteria grow slowly.

Bartonella spp. are an important cause of culture-negative endocarditis in some regions. These organisms are especially difficult to identify on blood cultures. Use of specialized culture conditions and an enriched insect cell culture medium (Bartonella alpha Proteobacteria growth medium; BAPGM) or heart infusion agar could increase the likelihood of growing these organisms. Blood can be aseptically collected in plastic ethylene diamine tetraacetic acid (EDTA) tubes then frozen at −70°C until plated.

Molecular and Serologic Testing

Molecular testing using PCR amplification of specific *Bartonella* gene segments is an important diagnostic tool. Yet PCR amplification directly from blood or other body fluid samples often does not identify *Bartonella* deoxyribonucleic acid (DNA) because of low circulating bacterial levels or intermittent bacteremia, and bacterial sequestration within endothelial cells and vegetative lesions. Positive results are more likely in immunosuppressed patients. A combined technique using preenrichment culture of aseptically collected blood (or body fluid or surgical tissue samples) in BAPGM followed by a high-sensitivity PCR assay can increase diagnostic yield and is commercially available[a]. Aseptic handling of samples is important to avoid contamination.

Serologic (including immunofluorescent antibody, IFA; or enzyme-linked immunosorbent assay, ELISA), as well as PCR, testing also can help identify bartonellosis, depending on the clinical scenario. *Bartonella* infection can cause variable seroreactivity. Some cases develop high titers to *Bartonella* spp. but others (~half of dogs) might not be seroreactive. The particular *Bartonella* species involved might influence seroreactivity. Seroreactivity (for example, a titer ≥1:64) to *B. vinsonii* subsp. *berkhoffii* in a dog with clinical

[a] Galaxy Diagnostics Inc. (Research Triangle Park, NC, USA; http://www.galaxydx.com).

signs of disease is evidence for exposure and likely an active *Bartonella* infection (Breitschwerdt, 2010). However, follow-up culture or PCR documentation of infection has been recommended. Dogs with a positive *Bartonella* antibody titer also could be positive for other tick-borne diseases such as *Anaplsma phagocytophilum*, *Ehrlichia canis*, or *Rickettsia rickettsia*, so screening for other tick-borne disease is advised.

Because of the high rate of subclinical infection in cats (a common reservoir host), interpreting seroreactivity or a positive PCR or culture result in this species is more difficult. Positive tests can occur in healthy cats as well as those sick from bartonellosis. However, in sick cats, these tests along with response to treatment can help support a diagnosis of bartonellosis.

Use of PCR techniques to identify nucleic acid of other bacteria in vegetations or blood can be a helpful adjunct to blood cultures. One study found that using both standard blood cultures and a PCR technique aimed at the bacterial 16s gene yielded a positive diagnosis in over 60% of cases, even though the same organism was identified by both tests individually in only about 10% of cases (Meurs, 2011). Nevertheless, even when bacteria are identified by PCR, this does not yield information on minimal inhibitory concentration for various antimicrobial drugs.

Postmortem histologic identification of organisms causing endocarditis usually is done with hematoxylin and eosin, Gram, and modified Steiner's stains. A fluorescence in-situ hybridization technique has been described that could provide additional diagnostic sensitivity, especially for *Streptococcus* and *Staphylococcus* spp. In acute endocarditis or other infections caused by *Bartonella,* silver stains might detect the organism. PCR testing of postmortem samples from infected valves might confirm *Bartonella* infection; however, potential for cross-contamination in the pathology laboratory is a concern.

Radiography and Electrocardiography

Radiographic findings might be unremarkable when valve damage is minimal. When acute, severe valve regurgitation has caused CHF, evidence for pulmonary venous congestion and edema could be present with minimal to no cardiac chamber enlargement. Other cases show evidence of cardiomegaly, with or without pulmonary edema, or other organ involvement (for example, diskospondylitis). Hypertrophic pulmonary osteopathy involving the long bones, along with pulmonary infiltrates, has occurred rarely in dogs with endocarditis.

The ECG could be normal or document tachyarrhythmias, a conduction disturbance, or evidence of myocardial ischemia. Premature ventricular complexes are common. These can indicate myocardial injury from infarction or myocarditis, or altered electrical activity related to systemic inflammation.

Echocardiography

Echocardiography is especially supportive of an endocarditis diagnosis when an oscillating thrombus and abnormal valve motion are identified. Aortic and mitral valves are most often affected. Lesion visualization depends on size and location, as well as image resolution quality. False negative and false-positive "lesions" can appear, so cautious interpretation of images is important. Transesophageal echocardiography (TEE) could provide greater sensitivity for visualizing valve lesions than transthoracic imaging; however, it also requires general anesthesia.

Early lesions consist of valve thickening, often with enhanced echogenicity. Vegetations appear as irregular, dense masses that can be rough, shaggy, or have long flailing tendrils (**Figures 31.7–31.9**). These essentially are infected thrombi. Chronic lesions appear hyperechoic and occasionally calcified (**Figure 31.10**). Multiple valves can be involved. Although chronic degenerative AV valve disease can look similar in some cases, especially those with markedly thickened and knobby mitral leaflets, degenerative valve disease causes relatively smooth thickening. Degenerative valve disease also is more likely to occur in small-breed dogs, whereas infective endocarditis usually occurs in medium- to large-breed dogs. As valve destruction progresses, ruptured chordae, flail leaflet tips, or other abnormal valve motion can be seen (**Figures 31.8** and **31.9**). AR can cause visible diastolic fluttering of the aortic valve, or the anterior (septal) mitral valve leaflet, if the regurgitant jet impinges on this leaflet (**Figure 31.11**). Marked AR also can impair diastolic opening of this mitral leaflet, mimicking mitral stenosis. Moderate to severe AR seen with color Doppler in any case should strongly raise suspicion for aortic valve endocarditis in a dog or cat, and a horse under 10 years of age. AR also leads

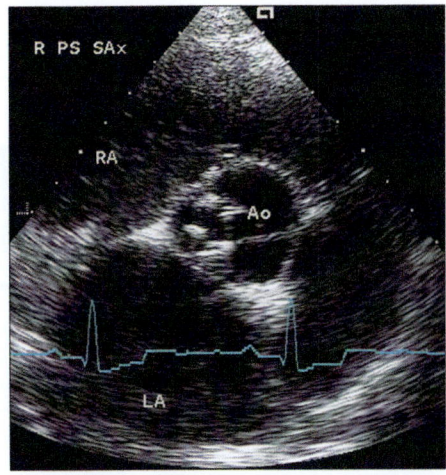

Figure 31.7 Several small, bright nodules on aortic valve cusps of a 2-year-old female Rottweiler with severe subaortic stenosis are suspected vegetations. The dog had poor exercise tolerance, but no other clinical signs at the time of exam. Sudden death occurred 3 weeks later; postmortem exam was not available. Right parasternal short-axis image. Ao, aortic root; LA, left atrium; RA, right atrium.

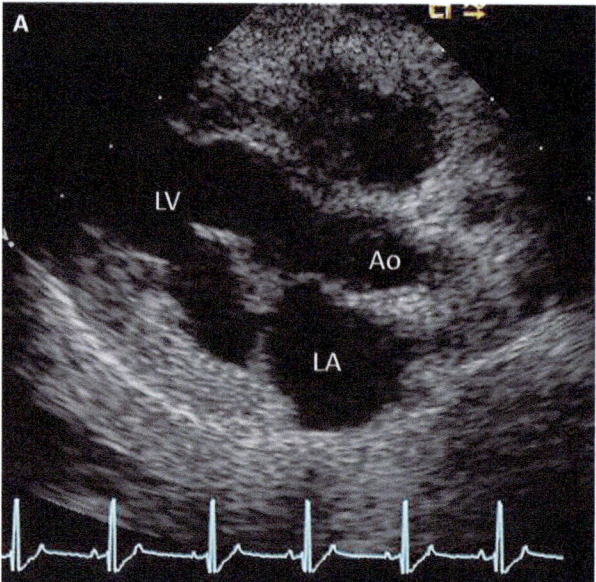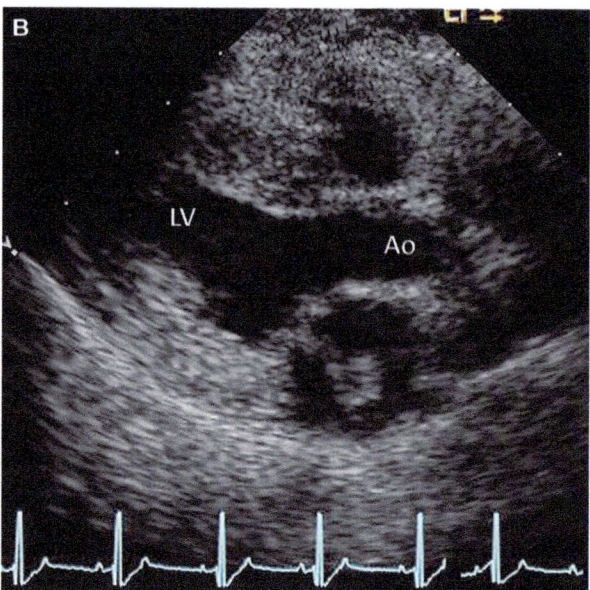

Figure 31.8 An 11-year-old Minature Schnauzer, presented for syncope, nonregenerative anemia, and weight loss, had a grade 6/6 mitral regurgitation murmur. Rather than the expected echo findings typical for chronic myxomatous mitral valve disease, a large pedunculated vegetative lesion is attached to the mitral valve. The vegetation extends far into the LV during diastole (A), then flips into the LA in systole (B). The minimal LA and LV enlargement suggests, a fairly acute process. Right parasternal long-axis view. Ao, aorta; LA, left atrium; LV, left ventricle.

to increased systolic stroke volume, which can increase LV outflow velocity. Concurrent SAS or obstructive aortic vegetations can further increase LV outflow velocity, sometimes dramatically (**Figures 31.12** and **31.13**).

Other cardiac sequelae include chamber enlargement from volume overload, myocardial dysfunction, and arrhythmias. The degree of LV dilation depends on the severity and chronicity of aortic or mitral valve insufficiency. Spontaneous echocontrast ("smoke") sometimes appears within the left heart chambers and could indicate increased risk for TE. This might be associated with hyperfibrinogenemia. Rarely, tissue destruction can cause an acquired cardiac septal defect (p. 594). In cases where endocarditis is strongly suspected, yet echo findings are negative or equivocal, another echocardiographic evaluation in several days to a week or so might show developing vegetative lesions.

Management

Aggressive, prolonged therapy with bactericidal antibiotics capable of penetrating fibrin is indicated, because bacteria can be sequestered within thrombotic layers and protected from leukocytes (zone of localized agranulocytosis). Appropriate supportive care for systemic illness or cardiac related complications also is needed. Drug choice ideally is guided by

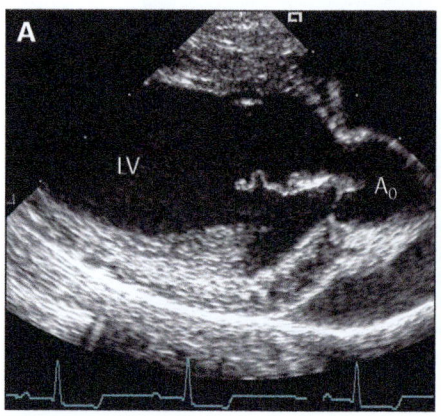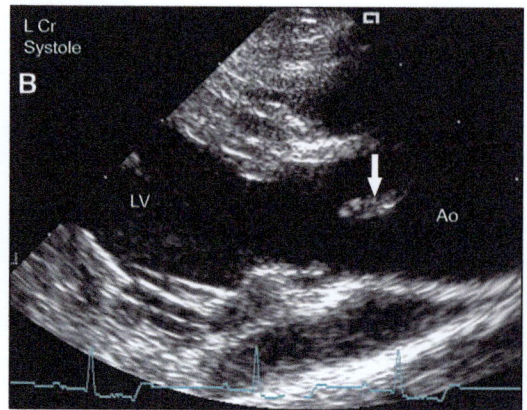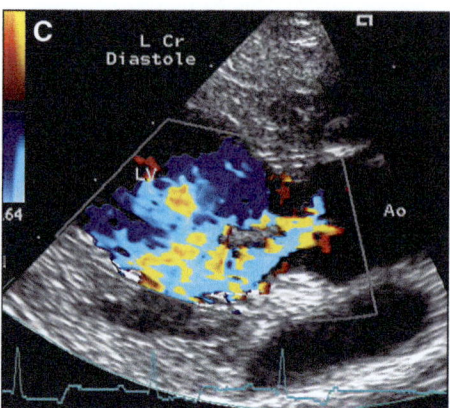

Figure 31.9 (A) A long, extremely mobile vegetative lesion is on the aortic valve of a 6-year-old Pomeranian with fever, syncope, and hypertension. Right parasternal long-axis, diastole. (B) The vegetation (arrow) flips into the aorta in systole. (C) Color Doppler shows severe aortic regurgitation (AR) during diastole. The vegetation is visible within the AR flow signal. B & C, left cranial long-axis. Ao, aorta; LV, left ventricle.

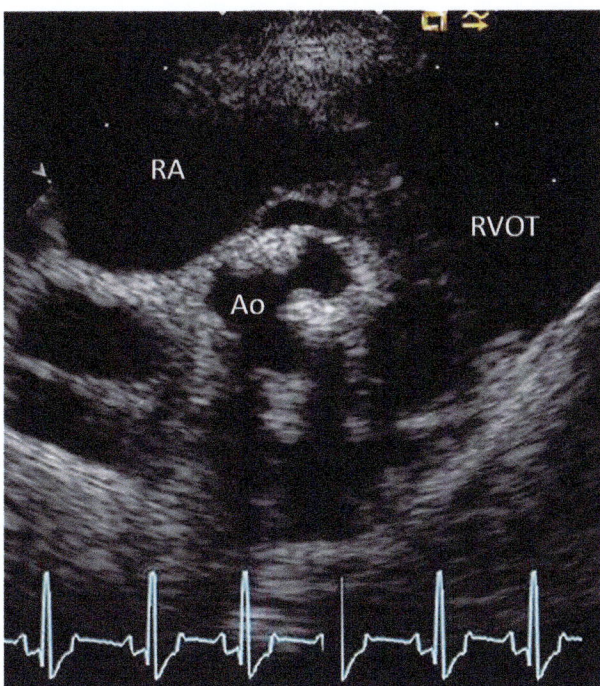

Figure 31.10 Echocardiography reveals vegetations, which are especially bright and appear calcified, on the aortic valve leaflets in a 7-year-old female Tibetan Terrier. Acoustic shadows extend deep to the two visible vegetative lesions. The aortic valve orifice is markedly compromised (also see **Figure 31.13**). Right parasternal short-axis view. Ao, aortic root; RA, right atrium; RVOT, right ventricular outflow tract.

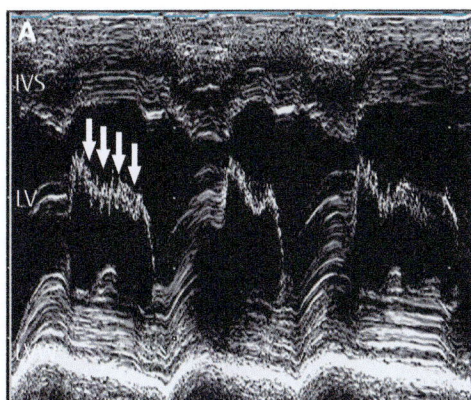

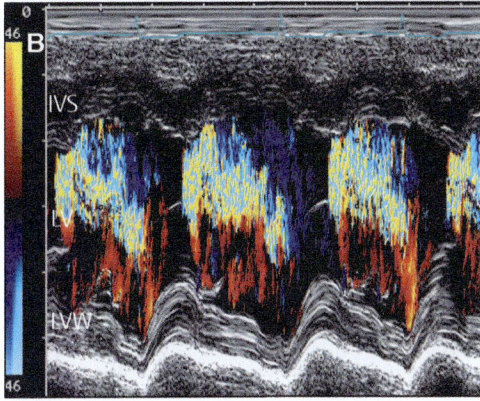

Figure 31.11 (A) Aortic regurgitation (AR) caused diastolic flutter (arrows) of anterior mitral leaflet in the dog of **Figure 31.9**. (B) Color M-mode shows the AR turbulence striking the mitral leaflet throughout diastole. IVS, interventricular septum; LV, left ventricle; LVW, left ventricular wall.

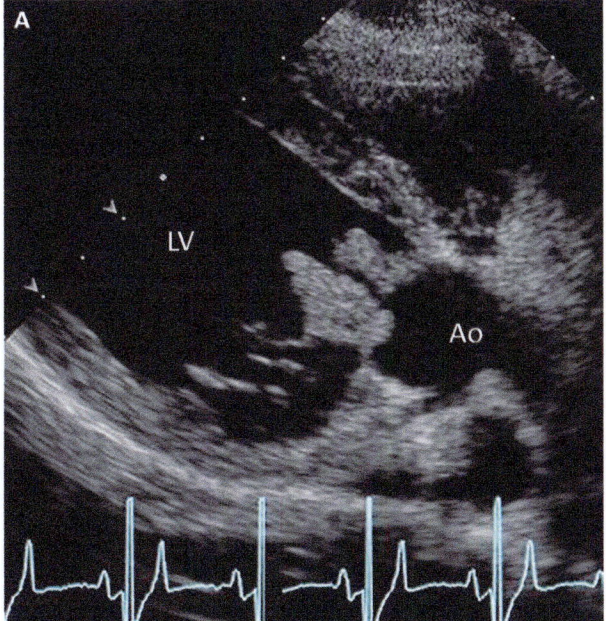

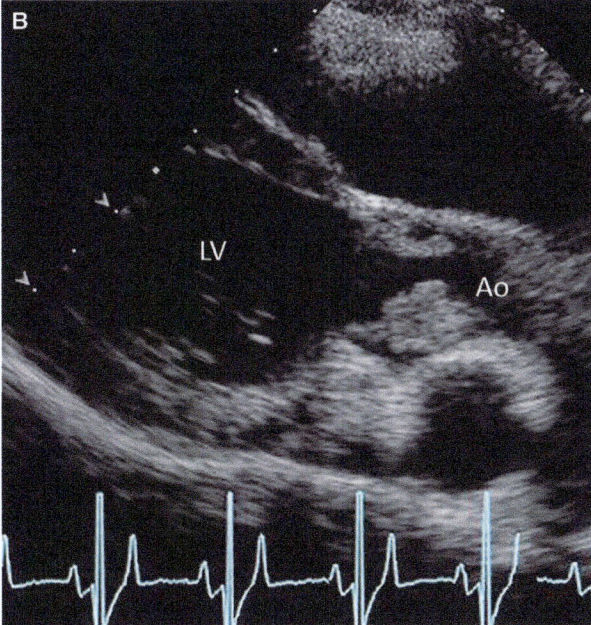

Figure 31.12 Large vegetations on the aortic leaflets not only caused severe aortic regurgitation during diastole (A), but also aortic stenosis (B, systole; pressure gradient ~70 mm Hg) in this male Flat Coated Retriever with infective endocarditis. The mild left ventricular dilation and mildly reduced systolic function (end systolic volume index 46 mL/m^2) evident on this echo exam progressed over time; however, the dog ultimately died from complications of cancer that was diagnosed 9 months later. Right parasternal long-axis view. Ao, aorta; LV, left ventricle.

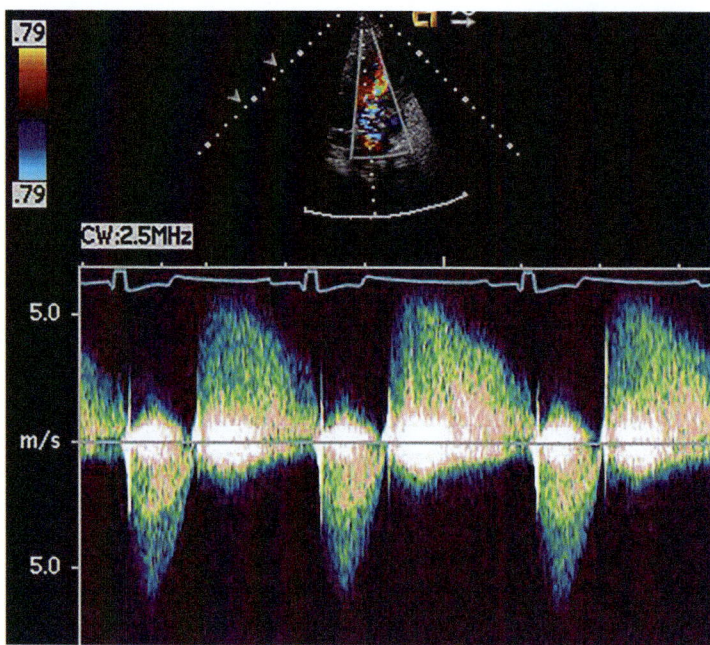

Figure 31.13 A to-and-fro murmur, with loud systolic component, was heard in the dog of **Figure 31.10**. Continuous wave (CW) Doppler (subcostal position) reveals severely increased aortic outflow velocity (>6 m/s), consistent with concurrent aortic stenosis. Severe aortic regurgitation (AR) also is evident. Note the steep slope and rapid velocity deceleration profile (short pressure half-time). Diabetes mellitus was diagnosed 2 years ago; the dog now was ketoacidotic.

Table 31.3 Suggested Empirical Antimicrobial Therapy for Endocarditis[a]

Initial Empirical Therapy

- Dog, Cat:
  - Either: ampicillin (22–40 mg/kg IV q6–8h); cefazolin (22–33 mg/kg IV q8h); ceftriaxone (20 mg/kg IV q12h); or ticarcillin/clavulanate (50 mg/kg IV q6h)
  - With: enrofloxacin (5–10 mg/kg IV q12h)
  - (A less favored alternative to enrofloxacin, and only if renal function is normal, is: amikacin, 7–10 mg/kg IV q12h [or 20 mg/kg q24h]; provide fluid support & discontinue after 5–10 days)
- Horse:
  - Penicillin 50,000 iu/kg q8h IV (or 22,000 iu/kg q6h IV)
  - With: gentamicin, 6.6 mg/kg IV q24h

Oral Continuation Therapy

- Dog, Cat:
  - Either: amoxicillin/clavulanate (20–25 mg/kg PO q8h); or cephalexin (25–30 mg/kg PO q8h)
  - With: enrofloxacin (2.5–5 mg/kg PO q12h)

[a] Modify therapy as necessary based on positive blood culture and susceptibility test results. If poor response to therapy consult with an expert on infectious diseases. See text for further information.

culture and sensitivity test results. However, to avoid treatment delay broad-spectrum combination therapy usually is started immediately after blood and urine culture samples (and blood for potential *Bartonella* testing) are obtained. Therapy can be altered if necessary when culture results are available. Animals with negative culture results should be continued on the broad-spectrum regimen. Testing for *Bartonella* spp. (serology, specialized culture & PCR) is advisable in dogs and cats with culture-negative endocarditis, with appropriate shift in antimicrobial strategy made for animals with positive test results (see the next paragraphs). Initial, empiric broad-spectrum combination therapy for infective endocarditis usually includes a beta-lactam antibiotic, such as a cephalosporin or synthetic penicillin derivative (amoxicillin or amoxicillin/clavulanate), with a fluoroquinolone or an aminoglycoside (in horses; **Table 31.3**). The former provides coverage for a Gram positive spectrum and the latter, Gram negative. Clindamycin or metronidazole provides added anaerobic coverage. For horses, initial empiric therapy with penicillin and an aminoglycoside has been recommended; penicillin given by constant rate infusion (CRI) could be more effective than intermittent boluses. Bacterial resistance to some antibiotics including enrofloxacin, penicillin, ampicillin, and potentially others is increasing in some areas. When blood cultures are negative in a patient recently treated with a fluoroquinolone (or other antibiotic), choosing a different antimicrobial drug is probably wise.

Antibiotics are best administered IV for the first week (or longer) to obtain higher and more predictable blood concentrations, although this often is impractical in small animals. Oral therapy can be used thereafter in dogs and cats, assuming clinical and laboratory abnormalities are improved. Oral bioavailability of some agents is quite good, including >75% for amoxicillin, >90% for amoxicillin/clavulanate, and >90% for fluoroquinolones. However, for multiple-drug resistant bacteria requiring therapy with imipenem, SC administration following an initial 1–2-week course of IV administration has been recommended.

Antimicrobial therapy generally is continued for at least 6 weeks, and treatment for 8 weeks often is recommended. However, if an aminoglycoside is necessary in small animals, it is discontinued after 7–10 days, or sooner if any sign of renal toxicity develops. Close monitoring of the urine sediment is indicated to detect early signs of aminoglycoside nephrotoxicity. Fluid therapy is given concurrently because of the concern for aminoglycoside nephrotoxicity. Furosemide should not be administered during aminoglycoside treatment because it can exacerbate nephrotoxicity. Therefore, aminoglycoside use generally is contraindicated in patients with CHF or underlying renal disease.

It is important to seek confirmation of suspected *Bartonella* endocarditis infection because treatment could require extremely long-term antibiotic therapy (for example, up to 3 months) using at least two antimicrobial drugs with different modes of action, in an attempt to eliminate the organism. However, the most effective strategy for eliminating *Bartonella* in dogs and cats currently remains unproven.

In vitro testing and reported antibiotic minimal inhibitory concentration do not reflect efficacy against *Bartonella* in the host animal. Bacterial persistence can lead to recurrent clinical infection, especially with immunosuppression or concurrent disease. Although previous recommendations have included use of azithromycin, this drug is no longer recommended as first line therapy for *Bartonella* because of the rapid development of resistance to it (Breitschwerdt, 2010 and 2015).

For dogs with *Bartonella* endocarditis (or myocarditis), initial therapy with amikacin (15–30 mg/kg q24h IV, IM, or SC) for 7–10 days, combined with doxycycline ([5–]10 mg/kg q12h PO) has been recommended. Renal function must be closely monitored when using an aminoglycoside; this agent should not be used in certain patients (see the previous paragraphs). After amikacin is discontinued, an oral fluoroquinolone is added. Currently recommended oral therapy for *Bartonella* infection includes doxycycline (5–10 mg/kg q12h PO; or minocycline at 10 mg/kg q12h PO), combined with enrofloxacin (5–20 mg/kg q24h PO) or pradofloxacin (5–10 mg/kg q24[–12]h PO; not approved for dogs in the United States) for 28–42 days, at minimum (Breitschwerdt, 2015). In clinically stable *Bartonella* patients where initial IV therapy is not used, it is recommended to start oral treatment with one drug (for example, doxycycline at 5 mg/kg q12h), followed in 5–7 days with the addition of the second drug. However, in patients severely ill with endocarditis or myocarditis this might not be possible. This recommendation is based on the observation that when both antibiotics are begun simultaneously for *Bartonella* infection, a reaction (Jarisch-Herxheimer-like reaction) can occur within 4–7 days (or longer) which can include lethargy, fever, and vomiting (Breitschwerdt, 2015). It is thought that the reaction, which can last a few days, relates to acute bacterial injury or death and host cytokine release. Unless the patient's clinical status continues to deteriorate from this reaction, the PO antibiotic strategy should be continued as planned and supportive care given as appropriate. The addition of antiinflammatory doses of a glucocorticoid might be helpful for patients experiencing this reaction; however, the glucocorticoid should be discontinued after a few days, as those signs abate.

For cats, with cardiac *Bartonella* infection, initial therapy with amikacin (10–14 mg/kg q24h IV, IM, or SC) for 7–10 days, combined with doxycycline ([5–]10 mg/kg q12h PO) has been recommended (Breitschwerdt, 2015). Aminoglycoside precautions pertaining to patient selection and renal function monitoring are as for dogs. When the amikacin is discontinued, oral pradofloxacin (5–10 mg/kg q24[–12]h PO) can be added. Currently recommended oral therapy for *Bartonella* infection includes doxycycline (5–10 mg/kg q12h PO; or minocycline at 8.8 mg/kg q12h PO), combined with pradofloxacin (5–10 mg/kg q24[–12]h PO) for 28–42 days (at least). Because higher doses and longer treatment duration generally are needed for *Bartonella* infection and because cats are at risk for retinotoxicity when enrofloxacin is used at doses exceeding 5 mg/kg/day, this agent is no longer recommended for *Bartonella* infections in cats. Jarisch-Herxheimer-like reactions (see the previous paragraph) also can occur in cats.

Supportive care for infective endocarditis includes monitoring for and management of CHF (Chapter 22) and cardiac arrhythmias (Chapter 25), as appropriate. Complications related to the primary infection source, secondary TE, or immune responses also must be addressed. Blood pressure and renal function should be monitored, along with other parameters as indicated for the individual patient. Hypertension must be vigorously controlled (Chapter 38). Even in patients with normal blood pressure, modest additional afterload reduction with an arteriolar vasodilator can help support cardiac function, especially with advancing aortic or mitral valve regurgitation. Corticosteroids are contraindicated, except in the limited context described above for managing reactions to initial combination therapy for *Bartonella*.

A nonsteroidal anti-inflammatory drug often is administered to horses to reduce fever and signs of systemic illness; however, the same is not generally used in dogs or cats for this purpose. Resolution of fever often is an indication of effective (initial) antimicrobial therapy. The usefulness of aspirin or clopidogrel in reducing vegetative lesion growth and incidence of TE is unresolved. In people, there are conflicting data; although a number of studies have shown benefit from daily administration of aspirin or clopidogrel, others have not, and it might depend in part on comorbidities and the source of infection (for example, prosthetic devices). However, aspirin (salicylic acid) appears to reduce the virulence of *S. aureus* by downregulating fibrinogen, fibronectin and alpha-hemolysin production; such factors are important for bacterial replication in host tissues. Although aspirin use has been advocated in horses for this purpose, its efficacy is unclear. The potential adverse effects of aspirin must be considered if this drug is used in clinical cases of endocarditis. In general, anticoagulant and antiplatelet therapies are not recommended; however, an exception might be the patient with protein-losing nephropathy, DIC, or other hypercoagulable condition, or infection related to an infected device.

Follow-up and Monitoring

Follow-up for patients with initially positive blood or urine cultures ideally includes repeated culture(s) 1–2 weeks after beginning antibiotic therapy, and again 2 weeks after discontinuing the antibiotics. Animals with a positive *Bartonella* antibody titer, can be retested in 4 weeks after starting antibiotic therapy to verify that titers are decreasing. Persistently elevated titers suggest the need to alter antibiotic strategy. Patients testing positive for *Bartonella* via serologic and BAPGM enrichment blood culture techniques before antibiotic therapy is begun, should have these tests repeated at 2 and 6 weeks after therapy has been discontinued, to evaluate treatment efficacy.

Other tests or monitoring might be indicated depending on the type and severity of concurrent disease and secondary complications in the individual patient. Follow-up echocardiographic examinations are useful to assess progressive changes in vegetation size, valve function, chamber dimensions, and LV function. Rechecks at 2 and 6–8 weeks after starting antibiotic therapy, and at 2–3 weeks after its termination are suggested. Even when antibiotic therapy has been successful in clearing the infection, progressive cardiac enlargement and dysfunction are likely, depending on the severity of valve and myocardial damage. Therefore, continued cardiac monitoring is recommended. Therapy for CHF probably will be required eventually. A novel approach to managing CHF secondary to severe AR caused by endocarditis could involve palliative placement of a porcine bioprosthetic valve in the descending aorta (Arai, 2007). In the case of this report, the CHF resolved.

Prognosis Mitral or aortic valve endocarditis often confers a guarded to grave prognosis. Aortic endocarditis is associated with shorter survival compared with mitral valve infections in dogs, particularly if caused by *Bartonella* spp (MacDonald, 2004). Endocarditis is likely to be the cause of death in over half of affected dogs. Median survival time was 54 days in one survey (Sykes, 2006). CHF, sepsis, systemic embolization, arrhythmias, and renal failure are common causes of death. Negative prognostic signs include thrombocytopenia, renal dysfunction, and TE. Even with successful antimicrobial therapy in the short-term, the long-term prognosis often is guarded to poor because residual valve damage leads to progressive volume overload, cardiac remodeling, and ultimately, CHF. Nevertheless, aggressive therapy might be successful in cases without large vegetations or severe valve dysfunction.

Prognosis in cats with endocarditis likewise is guarded to grave, with median survival of about a month (Palerme, 2016). This could relate to the high prevalence of CHF by the time of diagnosis. Survival time in cats does not appear to be influenced by whether the aortic or mitral valve is affected.

Prognosis in horses with vegetative lesions on the mitral or aortic valve, with associated marked valve regurgitation, also is poor (Henderson, 2020). Horses with endocarditis usually die or are euthanatized because of persistent infection or CHF secondary to the cardiac valve damage. Vegetative lesions are only rarely cleared of bacterial colonization, although there have been some successful cases. Tricuspid endocarditis is relatively rare, but when it does occur the prognosis tends to be better than with mitral or aortic valve endocarditis. Tricuspid valve endocarditis was curable in several reported equine cases.

Antibiotic Prophylaxis Prophylactic antibiotic use is controversial. Experience in people suggests most infective endocarditis cases are not preventable; the risk of endocarditis involved with a specific (such as a dental) procedure is very low compared with the cumulative risk associated with normal daily activities. However, in view of the increased prevalence of endocarditis with certain cardiovascular malformations (especially SAS), antimicrobial prophylaxis usually is recommended for these cases prior to dental cleanings or other "dirty" procedures (including those involving the oral cavity or intestinal or urogenital systems). Antimicrobial prophylaxis also is advised for animals with an implanted pacemaker or other device, or with a history of endocarditis. Prophylaxis should be considered in immunocompromised animals, as well. Recommendations have included: high-dose ampicillin, amoxicillin, or a cephalosporin 1 hour prior to, and 6 hours after, oral or upper respiratory procedures; clindamycin prior to dental procedures; ampicillin with an aminoglycoside (given IV) 1/2 hour prior to, and 8 hours after, gastrointestinal or urogenital procedures; and ticarcillin or a first generation cephalosporin (IV) 1 hour prior to, and 6 hours after, a procedure.

Suggested Additional Reading and References

Also See Online Comprehensive Bibliography at: https://www.routledge.com/9781482246223.

Alvarez-Fernandez A, Breitschwerdt EB, Solano-Gallego L. Bartonella infections in cats and dogs including zoonotic aspects. Parasites and Vectors 2018;11:624.

Arai S, Wright BD, Miyake Y, et al. Heterotopic implantation of a porcine bioprosthetic heart valve in a dog with aortic valve endocarditis. J Am Vet Med Assoc 2007;231:727–730

Billeter SA, Breitschwerdt EB, Levy MG. Invasion of canine erythrocytes by *Bartonella vinsonii subsp. Berkhoffii*. Vet Microbiol 2012;156:213–216.

Breitschwerdt EB. Feline bartonellosis and cat scratch disease. Vet Immunol Immunopathol 2008;123:167–171.

Breitschwerdt EB. Bartonellosis of the cat and dog. Plumbstherapeuticsbrief.com, Nov 2015;18–23.

Breitschwerdt EB. Did *Bartonella henselae* contribute to the deaths of two veterinarians? Parasites and Vectors 2015;8:317.

Breitschwerdt EB, Blann KR, Stebbins ME, et al. Clinicopathological abnormalities and treatment response in 24 dogs seroreactive to Bartonella vinsonii (berkhoffii) antigens. J Am Anim Hosp Assoc 2004;40:92–101.

Breitschwerdt EB, Maggi RG, Chomel BB, et al. Bartonellosis: an emerging infectious disease of zoonotic importance to animals and human beings. J Vet Emerg Crit Care 2010;20:8–30.

Breitschwerdt EB, Suksawat J, Chomel B, et al. The immunologic response of dogs to Bartonella vinsonii subspecies berkhoffii antigens: as assessed by Western immunoblot analysis. J Vet Diagn Invest 2003;15:349–354.

Bryan LK, Clark SD, Diaz-Delgado J, et al. Rhodococcus equi infections in dogs. Vet Pathol 2017;54:159–163.

Buergelt CD, Cooley AJ, Hines SA, et al. Endocarditis in six horses. Vet Pathol 1985;22:333–337.

Caywood DD, Wilson JW, O'Leary TP. Septic polyarthritis associated with bacterial endocarditis in two dogs. J Am Vet Med Assoc 1977;171:549–552.

Cherubini GB, Rusbridge C, Singh BP, et al. Rostral cerebellar arterial infarct in two cats. J Feline Med Surg 2007;9:246–253.

Chomel BB, Kasten RW, Williams C, et al. Bartonella endocarditis: a pathology shared by animal reservoirs and patients. Ann N Y Acad Sci 2009;1166:120–126.

Cook LB, Coates JR, Dewey CW, et al. Vascular encephalopathy associated with bacterial endocarditis in four dogs. J Am Anim Hosp Assoc 2005;41:252–258.

Costa A, Lahmers S, Barry SL, et al. Fungal pericarditis and endocarditis secondary to porcupine quill migration in a dog. J Vet Cardiol 2014;16:283–290.

Davis AZ, Jaffe DA, Honadel TE, et al. Prevalence of Bartonella sp. in United States military working dogs with infectious endocarditis: a retrospective case-control study. J Vet Cardiol 2020;27:1–9.

Decloedt A. Pericardial disease, myocardial disease, and great vessel abnormalities in horses. Vet Clin North Am Equine Pract 2019;35:139–157.

Donovan TA, Balakrishnan N, Carvalho Barbosa I, et al. Bartonella spp. as a possible cause or cofactor of feline endomyocarditis-left ventricular endocardial fibrosis complex. J Comp Pathol 2018;162:29–42.

Doyle CG, Allen JW, Ettinger SJ. Foxtail-associated endocarditis in a cat. J Feline Med Surg 2011;13:116–119.

Durack DT, Lukes AS, Bright DK. New criteria for diagnosis of infective endocarditis: utilization of specific echocardiographic findings. Duke endocarditis service. Am J Med 1994;96:200–209.

Elwood CM, Cobb MA, Stepien RL. Clinical and echocardiographic findings in 10 dogs with vegetative bacterial endocarditis. J Small Anim Pract 1993, 34:420–427.

Glickman LT, Glickman NW, Moore GE, et al. Evaluation of the risk of endocarditis and other cardiovascular events on the basis of the severity of periodontal disease in dogs. J Am Vet Med Assoc 2009;234:486–494.

Guptill L. Bartonellosis. Vet Microbiol 2010;140:347–359.

Henderson B, Diaz M, Martins C, et al. Valvular endocarditis in the horse: 20 cases (1993–2020). Can Vet J 2020;61:1290–1294.

Jesty SA, Reef VB. Septicemia and cardiovascular infections in horses. Vet Clin North Am Equine Pract 2006;22:481–495, ix.

Kornreich BG, Craven M, McDonough SP, et al. Fluorescence in-situ hybridization for the identification of bacterial species in archival heart valve sections of canine bacterial endocarditis. J Comp Pathol 2012;146:298–307.

Li JS, Sexton DJ, Mick N, et al. Proposed modifications to the Duke criteria for the diagnosis of infective endocarditis. Clin Infect Dis 2000;30:633–638.

Macdonald K. Infective endocarditis in dogs: diagnosis and therapy. Vet Clin North Am Small Anim Pract 2010;40:665–684.

MacDonald KA, Chomel BB, Kittleson MD, et al. A prospective study of canine infective endocarditis in northern California (1999–2001): emergence of Bartonella as a prevalent etiologic agent. J Vet Intern Med 2004;18:56–64.

Malik R, Barrs VR, Church DB, et al. Vegetative endocarditis in six cats. J Feline Med Surg 1999;1:171–180.

Marr CM. Equine acquired valvular disease. Vet Clin North Am Equine Pract 2019;35:119–137.

Maxson AD, Reef VB. Bacterial endocarditis in horses: ten cases (1984–1995). Equine Vet J 1997;29:394–399.

Meier H, Shouse CL. Acute vegetative endocarditis in the dog and cat. J Am Vet Med Assoc 1956;129:278–289.

Meurs KM, Heaney AM, Atkins CE, et al. Comparison of polymerase chain reaction with bacterial 16s primers to blood culture to identify bacteremia in dogs with suspected bacterial endocarditis. J Vet Intern Med 2011;25:959–962.

Miller MW, Fox PR, Saunders AB. Pathologic and clinical features of infectious endocarditis. J Vet Cardiol 2004;6:35–43.

Ohad DG, Morick D, Avidor B, et al. Molecular detection of Bartonella henselae and Bartonella koehlerae from aortic valves of Boxer dogs with infective endocarditis. Vet Microbiol 2010;141:182–185.[

Palerme JS, Jones AE, Ward JL, et al. Infective endocarditis in 13 cats. J Vet Cardiol 2016;18:213–225.

Pappalardo BL, Brown TT, Tompkins M, et al. Immunopathology of Bartonella vinsonii (berkhoffii) in experimentally infected dogs. Vet Immunol Immunopathol 2001;83:125–147.

Peddle GD, Boger L, Van Winkle TJ, et al. Gerbode type defect and third degree atrioventricular block in association with bacterial endocarditis in a dog. J Vet Cardiol 2008;10:133–139.

Peddle GD, Drobatz KJ, Harvey CE, et al. Association of periodontal disease, oral procedures, and other clinical findings with bacterial endocarditis in dogs. J Am Vet Med Assoc 2009;234:100–107.

Peddle G, Sleeper MM. Canine bacterial endocarditis: a review. J Am Anim Hosp Assoc 2007;43:258–263.

Pennisi MG, Marsilio F, Hartmann K, et al. Bartonella species infection in cats: ABCD guidelines on prevention and management. J Feline Med Surg 2013;15:563–569.

Pesavento PA, Chomel BB, Kasten RW, et al. Pathology of bartonella endocarditis in six dogs. Vet Pathol 2005;42:370–373.

Porter SR, Saegerman C, van Galen G, et al. Vegetative endocarditis in equids (1994–2006). J Vet Intern Med 2008;22:1411–1416.

Ralph AG, Saunders AB, Hariu CD, et al. Spontaneous echocardiographic contrast in three dogs. J Vet Emerg Crit Care 2011;21:158–165.

Sage AM. Cardiac disease in the geriatric horse. Vet Clin North Am Equine Pract 2002;18:575–589, viii.

Schmiedt C, Kellum H, Legendre AM, et al. Cardiovascular involvement in 8 dogs with blastomyces dermatitidis infection. J Vet Intern Med 2006;20:1351–1354.

Semedo-Lemsaddek T, Tavares M, Sao Braz B, et al. Enterococcal infective endocarditis following periodontal disease in dogs. PLoS One 2016;11:e0146860.

Sisson D, Thomas WP. Endocarditis of the aortic valve in the dog. J Am Vet Med Assoc 1984;184:570–577.

Smarick SD, Jandrey KE, Chomel BB, et al. Aortic valvular endocarditis caused by Bartonella vinsonii subsp. Berkhoffii in 2 dogs presenting for fulminant pulmonary edema. J Vet Emerg Crit Care 2004;14:42–51.

Sykes JE, Kittleson MD, Chomel BB, et al. Clinicopathologic findings and outcome in dogs with infective endocarditis: 71 cases (1992–2005). J Am Vet Med Assoc 2006;228:1735–1747.

Sykes JE, Kittleson MD, Pesavento PA, et al. Evaluation of the relationship between causative organisms and clinical characteristics of infective endocarditis in dogs: 71 cases (1992–2005). J Am Vet Med Assoc 2006;228:1723–1734.

Szatmari V. Incidence of postoperative implant-related bacterial endocarditis in dogs that underwent trans-catheter embolization of a patent ductus arteriosus without intra- and post-procedural prophylactic antibiotics. Vet Microbiol 2017;207:25–28.

Travers CW, van den Berg JS. Pseudomonas spp. associated vegetative endocarditis in two horses. J S Afr Vet Assoc 1995;66:172–176.

Winter RL, Gordon SG, Zhang S, et al. Mural endocarditis caused by Corynebacterium mustelae in a dog with a VSD. J Am Anim Hosp Assoc 2014;50:366–372.

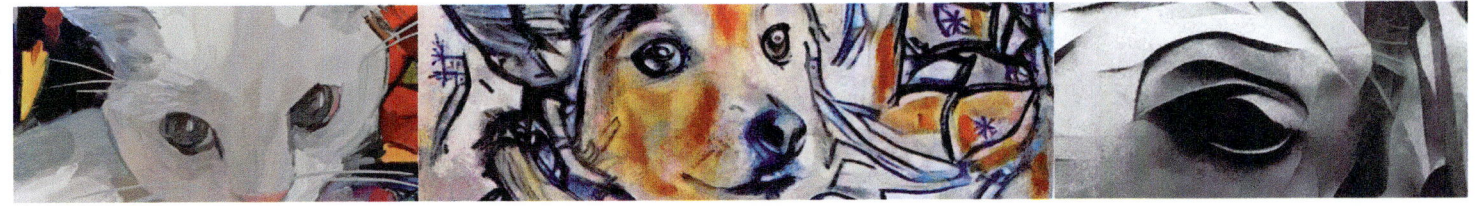

32
MYOCARDIAL DISEASES OF THE DOG

A variety of etiologies cause myocardial disease and dysfunction. From a clinical perspective, these largely can be categorized into echocardiographic (echo) phenotypes of which dilated cardiomyopathy (DCM) predominates in dogs. Other phenotypes include hypertrophic cardiomyopathy (HCM) and restrictive cardiomyopathy. Various authors use the label "dilated cardiomyopathy" somewhat differently in veterinary medicine. For some, it is limited to DCM of genetic or unknown cause (idiopathic). For others, it refers to an echo phenotype, regardless of cause. In this chapter, we will adopt the former approach, although we acknowledge that there is no consensus regarding this; for example, in people secondary causes of the DCM phenotype, such as myocarditis and doxorubicin toxicity, are labeled as "dilated cardiomyopathy" in some consensus papers (Pinto, 2016; Mathew, 2017).

Primary (idiopathic) DCM is the most important cause of heart disease in many large breed dogs. This disorder represents the end stage of abnormal cellular function and myocardial remodeling of unclear origin, although various alterations in gene structure and expression are certainly involved in multiple canine breeds. However, these alterations and related signaling abnormalities are only beginning to be understood. Secondary causes of myocardial damage and dysfunction that can lead to a DCM phenotype include chronic hemodynamic (pressure or volume) overloads (Katz, 1990), as well as persistent tachyarrhythmias (p. 630), nutritional disorders (p. 632), infectious (p. 636) and inflammatory myocarditis, and toxin- and drug-induced injuries. A generalized muscular disorder that can affect the heart is Duchenne's cardiomyopathy in Golden Retrievers. These dogs pass through a preclinical phase of ventricular dysfunction and, nearer the end of life, myocardial failure (p. 635). English Springer spaniels reportedly are prone to atrial muscular disease that can lead to silent atrium or persistent atrial standstill. Other genetic diseases that can result in a cardiomyopathic phenotype in dogs are likely to be recognized in the future.

Cardiac rhythm disturbances can be an early manifestation of myocardial disease. These often occur before ventricular dysfunction is evident by routine echocardiography. Arrhythmias are common with progressive disease and heart failure also. Sudden arrhythmic death can occur in either early or late stages of disease. Over time, most primary and secondary myocardial diseases in dogs involve progressive reduction in ventricular systolic (contractile) function. This limits cardiac output and eventually results in progressive ventricular dilation and other remodeling changes. Additional volume loading, caused by primary or secondary valvular insufficiency, exacerbates this cardiac dysfunction.

Primary HCM (p. 629) is rare in dogs, in contrast to cats. Secondary causes of myocardial hypertrophy include chronic systolic pressure overload, imposed by ventricular outflow obstruction or increased vascular resistance (systemic or pulmonary hypertension). Sporadic causes of hypertrophic myocardial disease can involve the trophic effects of chronic, excessive catecholamine, thyroid hormone or growth hormone exposure. Restrictive cardiomyopathy, characterized by extensive endomyocardial or myocardial fibrosis, is exceedingly rare in dogs and probably is a consequence of prior myocarditis.

The clinical phases of cardiomyopathies frequently are referred to as preclinical (occult) and overt or clinical. This categorization is somewhat unsatisfying because dogs with arrhythmias can fall into either group; furthermore, dogs with ventricular dysfunction and early signs of (low output) heart failure might be overlooked unless they are stressed by exercise. Regardless, this categorization is ingrained in both the veterinary and human literature and will be used in this chapter.

Idiopathic Dilated Cardiomyopathy

Idiopathic DCM is characterized by left ventricular (LV) or biventricular dilation and impaired systolic function unexplained by congenital or valvular heart disease, hypertension, or coronary disease. Although it mainly involves the left side of the heart, DCM affects both sides in many dogs, which leads to "four-chamber dilation." Congestive heart failure (CHF) and tachyarrhythmias are common; these are the usual causes of death or euthanasia. Secondary causes of myocardial failure and cardiac dilation should be excluded before making a diagnosis of idiopathic or genetic DCM. The sequence of events is not always consistent, as discussed under "Echocardiography". In early disease, some cases have impaired systolic function without dilation, while some have dilation without impaired function; some have normal echocardiograms but persistent atrial or ventricular arrhythmias. This variability is evident in people with DCM, too (Pinto, 2016).

The occurrence of DCM also varies among types of dog. A genetic basis is expected in breeds with a high prevalence or a familial occurrence. DCM is most common in large and giant breeds. It frequently is observed in spaniels; but it is comparably rare in small and toy breeds. An overview of inherited disorders within functional dog breed groups indicated that the prevalence of presumably inherited DCM ranges from almost 0.5% in the "sporting dog" group to almost 2% in the "working dog" group, especially the sighthound haplotype (Oberbauer, 2015). The working dog group includes German Shepherds, Doberman Pinschers, Portugese Water Dogs, Mastiffs, retrievers, sight hounds, and spaniels. Pedigree analysis suggests that inheritance patterns could differ among breeds or lines. Familial DCM in Doberman Pinschers, Newfoundlands, and Irish Wolfhounds shows an autosomal dominant inheritance pattern, as does arrhythmogenic right ventricular cardiomyopathy (ARVC) in Boxers (p. 624). One study of Great Danes with DCM suggested inheritance was an X-linked recessive trait; however, another showed an autosomal dominant pattern. In contrast, the rapidly fatal familial DCM affecting Portuguese Water Dog puppies has an autosomal recessive inheritance pattern. Juvenile DCM in Toy Manchester Terriers and a litter of Doberman puppies also has been described, with inheritance thought to be recessive or multigenic. Multiple genes, mostly related to various structural cardiac proteins, have been associated with familial DCM in people. Studies in dogs of different breeds with DCM have shown differential expression of many genes, and especially, down-regulation of many associated with energy metabolism and cardiac function. However, it is unclear whether any of these alterations might be primary to the pathogenesis of DCM, or a secondary consequence. A combination of multiple genetic factors could influence DCM risk in different breeds.

A mutation in the gene for pyruvate dehydrogenase kinase isozyme 4 (PDK4) on chromosome 14 is present in some Dobermans with DCM, especially in the United States. PDK4 is involved in mitochondrial energy production; myocardial ultrastructural abnormalities involving the cardiomyocyte Z-lines, T-tubules, sarcoplasmic reticulum, and mitochondria were found in these dogs (Meurs, 2012). Mitochondrial function was most severely impaired in dogs homozygous for the PDK4 mutation, with intermediate impairment in heterozygotes. As with other mutations known to affect the heart, disease penetrance is incomplete; yet the PDK4 mutation is thought to confer a ten-fold increase in risk for DCM (Stern, 2018). The PDK4 mutation appears to be uncommon in European Dobermans. However, another mutation was identified on chromosome 5 in European Dobermans (Mausberg, 2011). This mutation involves a sarcomeric gene; it has a proprietary designation. The chromosome 5 mutation appears to be most prevalent in Dobermans with ventricular tachyarrhythmias as their major disease manifestation, compared to those with marked ventricular dilation. The risk for DCM in both homozygote and heterozygote carriers of this mutation is increased by over twenty-fold. For Dobermans with both the chromosome 5 and PDK4 mutations, the risk is thought to be increased thirty-fold (Stern, 2019). A third mutation that is strongly associated with DCM in Doberman Pinschers has been identified in the United States. It is a missense variant in the titin (TTN) gene, involving the sarcomere and cardiac contraction (Meurs, 2019). Some Dobermans with DCM have both the PDK4 and TTN mutations, some have one or the other, but some have neither mutation (Meurs, 2020). Given the genetic heterogeneity of familial cardiomyopathies in general, it is likely that still other mutations, yet to be identified, are involved with DCM of Doberman Pinschers and of other breeds, as well. Additional factors also could be important in the pathogenesis of DCM.

Genome expression patterns involving abnormal levels of calstabin2 and triadin expression, among others, have been identified in Great Danes with DCM. These proteins are involved in regulating the cardiac ryanodine receptor (RyR2), which suggests that DCM pathogenesis might involve abnormal intracellular Ca^{++} fluxes in these dogs. Multiple gene loci could be involved with DCM in Irish Wolfhounds. Increased messenger ribonucleic acid (RNA) expression for enzymes involved in myocardial matrix remodeling, such as certain matrix metalloproteinases (MMPs) and tissue inhibitors of these proteinases (TIMPs), also has been identified in dogs with DCM. These might be a consequence of end-stage disease, or could play a role in disease progression. Differential expression of microRNAs (miRNAs) occurs in people with DCM; however, in the few Dobermans Pinschers evaluated, no difference was found between normal and DCM dogs. MiRNAs are short, noncoding RNAs with gene-regulating functions.

Pathophysiology

DCM as an entity probably represents the end-stage of different pathologic processes or metabolic defects involving myocardial cells or the intercellular matrix. These result in diminished cardiomyocyte contractility and increased interstitial collagen content. Underlying disease mechanisms, many presumably related to altered expression of various genes, could include abnormal Ca^{++} fluxes, biochemical or nutritional deficiencies, toxins, immunologic mechanisms, or even infectious agents, in some cases. Impaired intracellular energy homeostasis, with reduced myocardial adenosine triphosphate (ATP) has been found in Doberman Pinschers with DCM. Increased expression of a skeletal muscle sarco-endoplasmc reticulum calcium ATPase (SERCA) isoform was identified in the myocardium of German Shepherds with DCM. This could represent a response to impaired myocardial calcium handling. In addition, increased myocardial cytokine expression, found in some dogs with myocardial disease, is consistent with inflammatory system activation. The extent to which viral or bacterial pathogens might play a causal role in the development of DCM is unclear, although it has not been thought substantial. Recently, however, endomyocardial biopsy samples from a small series of dogs with unexplained myocardial and rhythm disorders (including 25 with DCM) revealed nucleic acid from various cardiotropic pathogens in 52% of the dogs with DCM (Santilli, 2019). Some of these also had lymphoplasmacytic infiltrates and interstitial fibrosis.

Nutritional causes or contributors to poor myocardial function and CHF could relate to inadequate intake of important amino acids or proteins (such as taurine, L-carnitine, or their precursors), altered bioavailability or interference with the uptake of such amino acids, other dietary deficiencies, or even toxic dietary components. DCM that occurs in dog breeds not usually associated with this condition, as well as some cases in typical breeds, could involve a nutritional cause or interaction (see p. 633).

Serotonin (5-hydroxytryptophan, 5-HT)-R2B receptors are present on endothelial and smooth muscle cells, fibroblasts, cardiomyocytes, and valve interstitial cells. In dogs with DCM, cardiac expression of messenger RNA for 5-HTR2B is significantly increased. Greater serotonin signaling within the heart correlates with increased inflammatory cytokine, MMP, and TIMP expression, and therefore, likely contributes to cardiac remodeling and functional impairment in DCM. LV dilation and increasing wall stress also might increase local serotonin production through stimulation of ventricular mechanoreceptors. By inducing inflammatory cytokines such as interleukin (IL)-1, IL-6, tumor necrosis factor (TNF)-alpha and transforming growth factor (TGF)-beta1, increased serotonin signaling is thought to promote cardiomyocyte hypertrophy, myocardial fibrosis, and increased ventricular stiffness. These changes ultimately lead to reduced cardiac systolic and diastolic function.

Regardless of the etiology and triggers, the key features identified by echocardiography involve progressive deterioration of systolic pump function followed by ventricular dilation, although this might be reversed in some cases. As cardiac output declines and leads to periods of arterial underfilling, compensatory mechanisms are activated to maintain blood pressure and expand the circulating volume (**Figures 32.1** and **32.2**, also **Figure 20.1**, p. 302). Typically, all chambers dilate, although left atrial (LA) and LV enlargement often predominate. Eccentric hypertrophy produces an

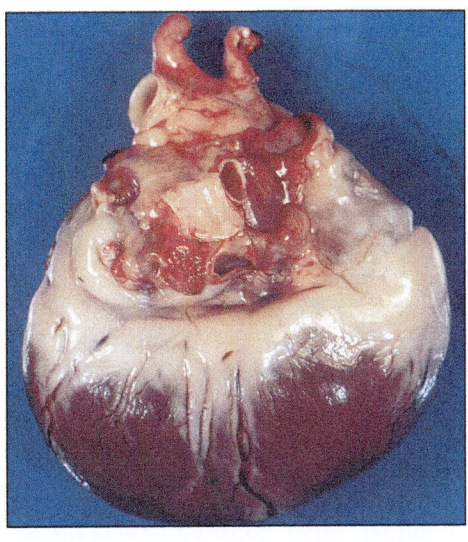

Figure 32.1 Dilated heart from a dog with end-stage dilated cardiomyopathy. View from caudal right aspect. Courtesy of Dr R Myers.

increased heart weight to body weight ratio, although LV wall thickness might appear decreased due to myocardial remodeling, especially when compared with lumen size. Flattened, atrophic papillary muscles and endocardial thickening also are evident sometimes. Atrioventricular (AV) valve thickening tends to be only mild, if present at all. Yet marked degenerative (myxomatous) changes do occur in some large-breed dogs, as they do in smaller breeds. Chamber dilation and papillary muscle dysfunction typically cause mild to moderate AV valve insufficiency by distracting the valves atypically, interfering with leaflet apposition, and stretching the valve annulus. In advanced disease, diastolic function also worsens. The increasing ventricular diastolic stiffness (along with the reduced ejection fraction, AV valve regurgitation, and cardiac arrhythmias) contributes to rising end-diastolic pressure, venous congestion, and ultimately, CHF.

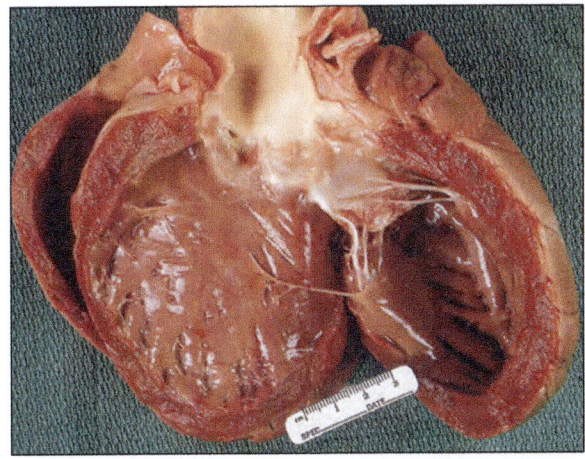

Figure 32.2 Open left ventricular (LV) outflow tract and aorta shows pronounced LV chamber dilation, with normal to slightly diminished wall thickness, in a dog with dilated cardiomyopathy. The opened right ventricular outflow tract is to the left.

Two distinct types of histopathology are described in dogs with DCM and are thought to relate to underlying disease mechanisms. One is characterized by narrowed (attenuated) myocardial cells with a wavy appearance. This type occurs commonly in many medium- to giant-breed dogs with DCM, including some Dobermans and Boxers. Attenuated wavy fibers also have been observed in some dogs predisposed to DCM (such as Newfoundlands), but without clinical or echo signs of the disease. However, some pathologists have found attenuated wavy fibers in heart diseases unrelated to idiopathic DCM, too. The other histologic type is characterized by myofiber degeneration, myocyte atrophy and lysis, fatty infiltration, and fibrosis. This fatty infiltration-degenerative type is described in Boxers and some Doberman Pinschers; it is similar to histologic findings in human ARVC. Some dogs have both types of histologic features. In contrast, other dogs with DCM might have non-specific histopathologic findings that include scattered areas of myocardial degeneration and necrosis with replacement fibrosis, especially in the left ventricle. Inflammatory cell infiltrates and myocardial hypertrophy occur inconsistently; active myocarditis is rare.

DCM appears to develop insidiously over a prolonged period in most cases. There are no clinical signs during this occult (preclinical) stage. As cardiac output decreases, sympathetic, hormonal, and renal compensatory mechanisms become activated to support arterial filling and blood pressure. These compensations help maintain cardiac function by increasing heart rate, peripheral vascular resistance, and vascular volume; however, they also are maladaptive. Chronic neurohormonal activation contributes to progressive myocardial damage, as well as the syndrome of CHF (Chapter 20). Left-sided or biventricular CHF and low-output signs are common in dogs with overt DCM. Poor forward blood flow, combined with increased ventricular diastolic pressure, also can compromise coronary perfusion, further impairing myocardial function and provoking arrhythmias. Profound myocardial dysfunction can lead to cardiogenic shock.

Atrial fibrillation (AF) and other atrial or ventricular tachyarrhythmias are common. Because atrial contraction contributes importantly to ventricular filling at faster heart rates, AF and the loss of the "atrial kick" can markedly reduce cardiac output and precipitate acute clinical decompensation. Furthermore, persistent tachycardia associated with AF or other arrhythmias can accelerate the deterioration of myocardial function (p. 630). Episodic weakness, syncope and sudden death generally are associated with tachyarrhythmias, usually of ventricular origin. However, paradoxical bradyarrhythmias (of the vasovagal type) also have caused syncope, especially in Doberman Pinschers and Boxers.

Although hypothyroidism is common in Doberman Pinchers and can mildly impair ventricular function, low thyroid levels do not appear to cause DCM progression. Nor does thyroid hormone treatment seem to prevent DCM progression or improve outcome. It can make CHF worse by increasing the demand for cardiac output; this is under-recognized. No association between growth hormone insufficiency and DCM has been found in dogs.

Clinical Features

Idiopathic DCM is most common in large and giant breeds of dog, especially Doberman Pinschers, Great Danes, and Irish Wolfhounds. Other commonly affected breeds include Saint Bernards, Scottish Deerhounds, Boxers, Newfoundlands, Afghan Hounds, Dogue de Boudeaux, and Dalmatians. Among smaller breeds, English and American Cocker Spaniels, English Bulldogs, Standard Schnauzers, and others have been affected; however, the disease is rare in dogs weighing less than 12 kg. There is some regional variation in the occurrence of DCM and some breeds or families have much higher disease prevalence. For example, cumulative disease prevalence in Dobermans is quite high; an estimated 45 to 63% of dogs across Europe and North America develop DCM (Wess, 2017). Reported disease prevalence was estimated to be up to 47% in Great Danes (Stephenson, 2012) and 43% in Irish Wolfhounds (Vollmar, 2013).

DCM is diagnosed most often in middle-aged dogs and the occurrence of overt (clinical) DCM increases with age. The median age at diagnosis for Irish Wolfhounds appears to be younger than for most other breeds. Occasionally, dogs of various breeds develop clinical signs of DCM when younger than 3 years of age. Juvenile forms of DCM in Portuguese Water Dogs and Toy Manchester Terriers affect puppies under a year old and are rapidly progressive. Their manifestations include sudden death without premonitory signs of heart disease, or an acute onset of CHF. Some reports indicate a male preponderance for DCM, especially in dogs with clinical heart failure. However, others show no clear gender predilection when dogs with occult disease are included. In Doberman Pinschers, male dogs are known to have earlier onset of echo changes. Sudden death before CHF develops is relatively common in this breed.

The preclinical phase of DCM can be prolonged and it can involve ventricular dysfunction, chamber dilation, or heart rhythm disturbances. In some dogs, either LV dilation or borderline to low ejection fraction is identified; these changes can remain static for months to years. In some families of Doberman Pinschers, ventricular (or supraventricular) tachyarrhythmias occur beginning months to several years before echo or clinical signs of DCM develop. Once LV function begins to deteriorate, progressive chamber dilation occurs and tachyarrhythmias become more likely. Sudden death from ventricular tachycardia and fibrillation is estimated to occur in up to 30% of affected Doberman Pinschers. In addition to Boxers (p. 624), Great Danes and other breeds can have increased rates of ventricular tachyarrhythmia, as well as sudden death, in the preclinical phase. Nevertheless, AF reportedly is the most common arrhythmia found in giant breed dogs with DCM. In 151 Irish Wolfhounds identified with DCM, about 81% were preclinical (stage B2 disease) at the time of initial diagnosis and about 71% of those had AF; the 19% of Wolfhounds with overt CHF (stage C) at diagnosis also had AF (Vollmar, 2019a). Although lone AF (p. 409) often precedes DCM in giant breed dogs, not all dogs with lone AF develop clinical DCM. Cardiac screening of 645 clinically normal Irish Wolfhounds revealed AF in almost 9%; over 55% of those with AF had an abnormal echocardiogram (Tyrell, 2020). Another study comparing a group of 52 Irish Wolfhounds with asymptomatic AF (and no echo evidence for DCM) with a group of normal Wolfhounds in sinus rhythm found that half of the AF dogs eventually developed DCM (Vollmar, 2019b). Most of these died from either CHF or sudden death. In contrast, only about 21% of the Wolfhounds with sinus rhythm at study entry eventually developed DCM, and only about 10% died suddenly or from CHF. For dogs with AF, compared to those in sinus rhythm, odds ratios of 3.7 for DCM development and 7.2 for cardiac-related death were reported. Yet, median survival times for the AF and sinus rhythm groups did not differ significantly.

Physical Findings The clinical history for many dogs with early preclinical DCM is unremarkable. As DCM progresses to the clinical phase, initial signs might be limited to decreased exercise stamina (representing heart failure without congestion). Weakness or collapse episodes can stem from intermittent arrhythmias, or the development of CHF. Physical exam findings during the preclinical phase often are normal. However, in some dogs, a soft murmur of mitral (MR) or tricuspid regurgitation (TR), an arrhythmia, or (occasionally) a soft S_3 gallop sound is heard on auscultation.

Some clinicians confine the diagnosis of overt (clinical) DCM to dogs with signs of CHF. Its onset can appear rather sudden, despite a protracted preclinical phase, especially in non-working dogs where early signs might be unnoticed. The duration of clinical signs prior to presentation could range from a day to several weeks. Presenting complaints include any or all of the following: tachypnea or dyspnea, exercise intolerance, cough (sometimes described as "gagging"), weakness, lethargy, anorexia, abdominal distension (ascites), syncope, and even sudden death (**Figure 32.3**). Some giant breed dogs with only mild to moderate LV dysfunction are relatively asymptomatic, even in the presence of AF. In the later stages of DCM, loss of muscle mass (cardiac cachexia) can become pronounced, especially in dogs with signs of right-sided CHF (**Figure 32.4**).

Physical findings vary with the degree of cardiac decompensation. Poor cardiac output, with high sympathetic tone and peripheral vasoconstriction, causes mucous membrane pallor, prolonged capillary refill time, and sometimes, palpably cool extremities. The femoral arterial pulse and precordial impulse often are weak and rapid. Uncontrolled AF and frequent ventricular premature complexes (VPCs) cause a rapid and irregular rhythm, with pulse deficits and variable pulse strength (**Figures 32.5** and **14.2**, p. 256). Dogs

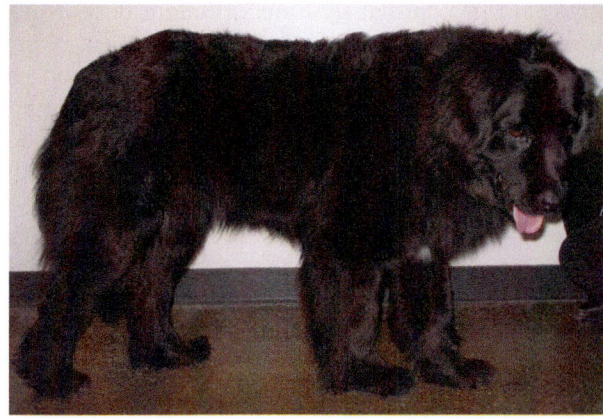

Figure 32.3 Reduced exercise tolerance, excessive panting, and a soft cough were the initial signs of congestive heart failure in this male Newfoundland with dilated cardiomyopathy.

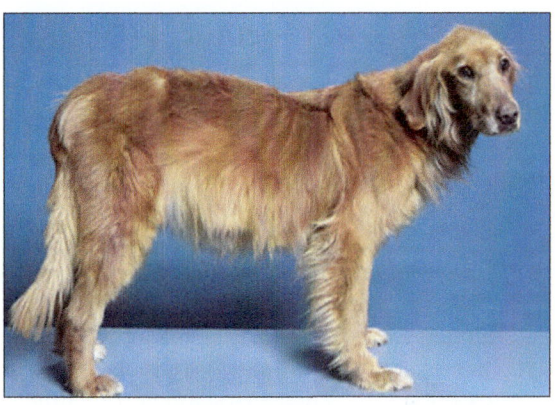

Figure 32.4 Golden Retriever with dilated cardiomyopathy, biventricular congestive failure, and cardiac cachexia. Note marked muscle mass loss along ribs and back, and abdominal distension from ascites.

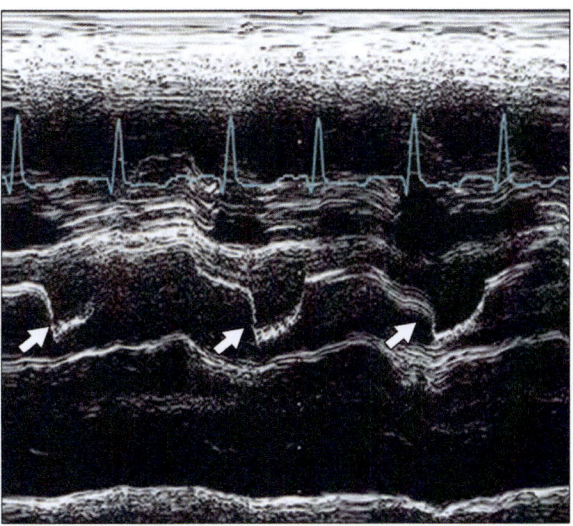

Figure 32.5 Pulse deficits in a Doberman Pinscher with dilated cardiomyopathy and atrial fibrillation (ECG near top). M-mode echocardiogram at aortic root level shows the motion of one aortic valve cusp. Left ventricular systolic pressure generation sufficient to cause aortic valve opening (arrows) and ejection only occurs with every other QRS complex.

with profound myocardial dysfunction might develop *pulsus alternans* (p. 256), related to an every-other-beat alteration in stroke volume. This is discovered only rarely on physical examination, but is easier to detect by echocardiography. Signs of CHF can include tachypnea, loud bronchial sounds, pulmonary crackles, jugular venous distension or pulsations, pleural effusion or ascites, hepatomegaly, and possible splenomegaly. Right-sided CHF manifestations are common in dogs with rapid ventricular response to AF. Heart sounds might be muffled secondary to pleural effusion or poor cardiac contractile strength. An audible third heart sound (S_3 gallop) is a classic finding in dogs with DCM, especially those with decompensated CHF, although an irregular heart rhythm can obscure this. Soft to moderately intense systolic murmurs of MR, TR, or both, are common.

Diagnostic Tests in Preclinical (Occult) DCM

The diagnosis of preclinical (occult) DCM is challenging. Many of the published criteria suggested for diagnosis, while logical, are not widely tested to the endpoint of predicting overt (clinical) DCM with CHF. A history of DCM in close relatives or genetic testing for known mutations associated with DCM can help in gauging overall risk. However, few genetic tests are available currently, and geographic differences in disease prevalence for specific breeds might influence the effectiveness of some genetic tests. Especially in the typical breeds, an arrhythmia or systolic murmur found on physical exam should raise suspicion of preclinical DCM. Elevated N-terminal probrain natriuretic peptide (NT-proBNP) and possibly cardiac troponin (cTn)I concentrations further raise suspicion. Routine electrocardiography can be useful when abnormal, but ambulatory electrocardiograms (ECGs) recorded for 24 to 48 hours are recommended to screen for arrhythmias. Thoracic radiography might show some degree of cardiomegaly; however, this is an insensitive screening tool for early DCM.

Most screening today focuses on the Holter ECG and echocardiogram. One challenge in predicting which echo and Holter ECG cutoffs are "abnormal" is that some numbers must be selected based on statistical analyses. These values have imperfect and sometimes marginal sensitivities or specificities. Moreover, results of one test often are used to validate the predictive values of other diagnostic tests, including biomarker and genetic tests. This can create a circuitous argument, or base classification on "how many VPCs/day are normal?" or, what is the "lower end of normal fractional shortening (FS) or ejection fraction (EF)?" In contrast, the phenotype of clinical DCM is straightforward, and potential abnormalities identified as predictive in preclinical disease ultimately need to be validated in canine patients with overt disease. The authors have tried to summarize available evidence related to screening dogs for DCM in the preclinical phase; but much more work is needed in all breeds.

Screening evaluations are important for breeding programs, as well as the health of individual dogs. **Table 32.1** summarizes current screening recommendations for occult DCM in Doberman Pinschers, from a panel of the European Society of Veterinary Cardiology. The principles embodied in these guidelines are reasonable and applicable to other breeds; of critical importance, however, is that the precise "cutoff" values listed cannot be extrapolated to all breeds.

Table 32.1   ESVC Cardiac Screening Guidelines for Doberman Pinschers[a]

Recommended Screening Tests, Beginning at 3(–4) Years of Age and Yearly Thereafter

- Echocardiography[b]
- Holter monitoring[c]

Echocardiographic Criteria Consistent with DCM

- LV volume determined by SMOD is the preferred test (p. 614)
  - EDVI >95 mL/m^2, or ESVI >55 mL/m^2
- Alternatively, normalized (p. 614) or breed-specific LV systolic or diastolic dimensions could be considered
  - Normalized LVIDd >1.73, or normalized LVIDs >1.14
  - LVIDd > 47(–49) mm for males and >46 mm for females, or LVIDs >36(–38) mm for either sex

Holter Criteria Consistent with DCM

- Either >300 VPCs/24 hours, or two Holter recordings within a 1-year period documenting 50–300 VPCs/24 hours

Holter Criteria Suspicious for DCM (Follow-up Holter Recommended in 3–6 Months)

- Presence of any VPC couplets, triplets or runs of ventricular tachycardia, especially with close coupling intervals (>250–260 bpm)
- Although <50 single VPCs/24 hours could be within acceptable limits, any VPCs are of concern

Ancillary Tests (Might Be Helpful, But Not Considered Diagnostic By Themselves)[d]

- Follow-up echocardiogram and Holter monitoring indicated if any of the following abnormalities
  - Cardiac troponin I >0.22 ng/mL
  - NT-proBNP >500 pmol/L
  - 5-minute resting ECG showing any VPCs or AF

[a] Adapted from European Society for Veterinary Cardiology (ESVC) Recommendations (Wess, 2017).
[b] Exam should be done by a well-trained echocardiographer.
[c] Usable recording of >23 hour duration, with analysis by trained individual.
[d] See p. 613 for additional information.

Abbreviations: AF, atrial fibrillation; DCM, dilated cardiomyopathy; ECG, electrocardiogram; EDVI, end-diastolic volume index; ESVI, end-systolic volume index; LV, left ventricular; LVIDd, LV internal dimension at end-diastole; LVIDs, LV internal dimension at end-systole; NT-proBNP, N-terminal probrain natriuretic peptide; SMOD, Simpson's method of disks; VPCs, ventricular premature complexes.

Additional longitudinal studies are needed to confirm these guidelines. In particular, a sufficient number of dogs labeled with "preclinical" DCM must advance to a definitive endpoint of overt DCM with CHF. Different echo cutoffs for DCM relate allometrically to body size, but breed also must be considered (Esser, 2020). We also have concerns about using only M-mode values for diagnosing preclinical DCM (see "Echocardiography in Preclinical DCM"). Similar to the European guidelines for Doberman Pinschers, the authors recommend that ventricular volumes be calculated from 2D imaging and that Simpson's method of discs (SMOD) be used for EF calculation, in preference to M-mode measurements only, for diagnosis of preclinical DCM. Beyond the Doberman Pinscher, echo screening, with or without Holter ECG recordings, are recommended for dogs of other breeds thought to have higher risk for developing DCM. However, different values for cardiac size and potentially, for biomarker values, must be determined.

Blood tests that screen for higher risk of heart disease are practical and do not require specialty examination. There are some data describing positive and negative predictive values or optimal cutoffs for these tests, but additional information is needed. Elevated natriuretic peptide levels have been documented in Dobermans with preclinical DCM. NT-proBNP concentrations >550 pmol/L indicated the presence of echo changes with a high degree of sensitivity and specificity in one study (Wess, 2011). However, this cutoff is well within normal limits for most dogs and this precise value should not be extrapolated to other breeds. Furthermore, in another study of NT-proBNP, many of the "healthy" Doberman Pinschers (screened by echocardiography) had much higher levels of this biomarker than 550 pmol/L (Sjöstrand, 2014). Marked breed differences also are reported, and many normal dogs exceed the all-breed upper limit of 900 pmol/L. Substantial upward trends in natriuretic peptide measurements are likely to be more useful than a single value. Still, while further clarification will be important, NT-proBNP concentration measurements should be useful in screening other dog breeds, as well.

Elevation in serum cTnI also occurs in many dogs with occult, as well as overt, DCM. Mild ("trickle") cTnI elevations in the 0.1 to 0.3 ng/mL range are common with any form of cardiomyopathy. A standard sensitivity cTnI >0.22 ng/mL had fairly good sensitivity and specificity to detect underlying DCM in one study (Wess 2017). In Doberman Pinschers with cardiac enlargement, a cTnI >0.34 was associated with increased risk for sudden death. The high-sensitivity cTnI test, at a cutoff value >0.113 ng/mL, appears better able to identify Dobermans destined for DCM before echo changes or arrhythmias are detected, compared to the conventional cTnI test (Klüser, 2019). These specific cutoffs need validation in other populations of this and other breeds. Occasionally, marked elevations of cTnI are encountered (>10× to 20× upper reference values); this finding should prompt consideration of myocarditis (p. 636), especial in younger dogs, atypical breeds, or when echocardiography shows myocardial wall thickening or speckling. In such cases, appropriate immunodiagnostic or polymerase chain reaction (PCR) tests might be indicated for an underlying vector-borne infectious disease, such as Lyme carditis, Chagas disease, or myocarditis cause by rickettsia, protozoa, or *Bartonella* spp.

Electrocardiography in Preclinical DCM Electrocardiography is one of the two main approaches used when screening for preclinical DCM. Although routine electrocardiography might reveal ectopy or possibly, changes in the amplitude, duration, or morphology of sinus complexes, it is neither sensitive nor specific enough for most situations. The 24- to 48-hour ambulatory ECG (Holter) recording is the current standard for detecting DCM-associated ventricular arrhythmias in Doberman Pinschers, Boxers (p. 627), English bulldogs, and likely other breeds at risk, such as the Great Dane. A more prolonged period of Holter monitoring (over several days to a week) probably would identify more dogs with evidence for occult DCM. Yet for other breeds, the ECG is neither sensitive nor specific enough to be used as a screening tool. In Doberman Pinschers, the occurrence of more than (50–)100 VPCs/24 hours or any couplets or triplets is likely to signal future DCM. However, dogs with <50 VPCs/24 hours on initial evaluation also have developed DCM several years later. Additionally, different authors have used different cutoffs or even changed their cutoffs over time to "recognize" or "classify" dogs as preclinical DCM. This simply emphasizes that, rather than employing binary cutoff values reported as "normal" or "preclinical DCM," it might be better to consider the relative risk of developing the disease. In reality, many healthy dogs of breeds rarely affected by DCM have no ventricular ectopy, aside from a few escape complexes, in a 24-hour Holter recording.

The frequency and complexity of ventricular arrhythmias do appear to correlate negatively with echo FS. This might indicate a true relationship of VPCs predicting LV systolic dysfunction, or might relate to tachycardia-induced cardiomyopathy (TICM, p. 630), which in humans can occur when 15 to 20% of total daily beats are premature. Sustained ventricular tachycardia undoubtedly can impair ventricular function acutely and has been associated with increased risk of sudden death. The variability in total number of VPCs among repeated Holter recordings in the same dog can be quite high. Nevertheless, in Doberman Pinschers, the occurrence of any VPCs during a 5-minute resting ECG reportedly is predictive for occult DCM, although the sensitivity of this test is too low for it to be a reliable screening tool. Analysis of heart rate variability (HRV) has not been helpful for differentiating mildly or moderately affected dogs from normal, or in predicting sudden death. However, HRV does predictably decrease with CHF, as vagal tone is withdrawn and sympathetic activity increases. Measures of heart rate turbulence also reflect autonomic changes as DCM progresses, with a decrease in parasympathetic output apparently preceding increased sympathetic activation (Harris, 2017). The technique of signal-averaged electrocardiography can identify the presence of ventricular late potentials; these have been associated with increased risk for sudden death, as shown in some Doberman Pinschers with occult DCM that died suddenly.

Echocardiography in Preclinical DCM Echocardiography is the other primary method for screening dogs at increased risk for DCM; this is also true of human DCM, although cardiac magnetic resonance imaging (MRI) also plays a prominent role. Measurable abnormalities are variable in preclinical canine DCM. In some dogs, the diagnostic criteria of ventricular enlargement or depressed systolic function are identified years before overt DCM develops. This has been reported in the Newfoundland and Doberman Pinscher (and also in humans; Mathew, 2017; Pinto, 2016). The condition of hypokinetic, non-dilated cardiomyopathy is considered part of the spectrum of DCM in humans; other people with preclinical familial DCM express only mild LV dilation with preserved or borderline LV EF (40-44% by SMOD). As suggested, some echo changes can be ambiguous and more than a few dogs fall into a grey zone; these require follow-up examinations to look for trends. Doppler studies tend to have less value in preclinical than in overt DCM, but might show MR or TR, as well as diastolic dysfunction (inconsistently) that might simply be age-related. Clinically silent valve regurgitation commonly is observed. Tissue Doppler imaging and newer modalities such as speckle tracking strain imaging hold potential for early diagnosis, but require additional investigation.

LV enlargement is a major echo finding in preclinical and overt DCM. An experienced examiner can subjectively identify moderate to severe cardiomegaly, yet detecting mild enlargement this way is difficult. When the internal LV dimensions are referenced to another internal structure, typically the aorta (Ao), the ratio of LV/Ao can be used to detect mild to moderate cardiomegaly (see Chapter 4). However, the precise method used for aortic measurement is critical, and experience suggests that LV/Ao ratios are sensitive in some breeds but less so in others. Therefore, to identify the earliest signs of DCM, measurements aimed at recognizing increased LV end-diastolic volume are needed. The LV internal dimensions at end-diastole (LVIDd) and at end-systole (LVIDs), whether measured by 2D or M-mode imaging, are simply surrogates for LV volumes. LVIDd measurements using M-mode and (long- or short-axis) 2D images are used to identify LV dilation; these are derived from a minor axis and ignore the other two axes of this three-dimensional chamber (Chapter 4). Echo software calculations of LV volume from measurements of minor axis dimension frequently are based on Teicholz modifications of the cubed formula. This method commonly overestimates LV volume, especially when the chamber is dilated; the authors recommend that such calculations be ignored. Instead, 2D length-area methods or SMOD should be performed to obtain LV volumes. This involves tracing LV internal area and length at end-diastole and systole, and then directing the echo software to calculate the volumes using one or two planes. Although the apical four-chamber view typically is used in people, and can be used in dogs, parasternal long-axis images from the right thorax often provide slightly larger volumes and better endocardial border resolution in dogs. Ideally, both long-axis and apical image planes should be measured and averaged, although this is not a true biplane approach (that involves adding the orthogonal, apical two-chamber view). In at least one study, SMOD was considered more sensitive for detecting preclinical DCM in the Doberman pinscher (Wess, 2010a).

Limited breed-specific cutoffs based on internal LV dimensions and volumes (**Table 32.1**) also have been used to detect LV dilation and identify preclinical DCM; but, ignoring body size variation even within a breed could be problematic. For example, the upper prediction limit of normal for LVIDd in the Doberman Pinscher is not consistent across all studies, and cutoff values often are based on relatively small numbers of healthy dogs (O'Grady, 2009; Kobal, 2007). These differences likely relate to methodology and potentially, to differing weights and ages of the canine samples. The preferred method for recognizing LV dilation in most canine breeds, when making linear measurements in diastole and systole, employs allometric scaling of the dimensions (that is, relative to body weight or surface area). When breed-specific cutoff values are unavailable, allometry is essential because the relationship between LV chamber size and body weight is non-linear. Arguably, allometric scaling also should be integrated into single-breed reference values when there is substantial individual size variation. This should result in tighter (more sensitive) reference intervals, in contrast to using multi-breed data. Most studies do not show sex-based differences in ventricular size, aside from its impact on body weight. The challenge of including older dogs when generating reference intervals relates to potentially higher liability for acquired heart disease; however, their inclusion should improve the quality of the sample, unless specific age intervals are desired.

The allometric approach for normalizing measurement data to body size is analogous to the situation employed in growing children (and in adults), where (heteroscedastic) Z-scores based on large databases are used to identify both cardiomegaly and progression of disease (Chubb, 2012; Pinto, 2016; Matthews, 2017). The study data (measurements and associated bodyweight) are related by the equation $Y = ax^b$, where Y = M-mode measurement; a = the constant of proportionality; x = bodyweight; and b = the scaling exponent. The coefficients "a" and "b" are derived from the study data and log transformed to generate 95% prediction intervals, more commonly referred to as reference intervals. This is now the preferred approach for many purebred and mixed breeds. Use of the normalized LV dimension represents a practical approach and it is simple to calculate, or program into a spreadsheet or echo software. Normalized LVID = LV dimension (cm)/kg bodyweight^{exp}, where "exp" represents the exponent based on the allometric scaling. Depending on the dogs sampled, body size distribution, methodology, and measured data in the sample, somewhat different exponents have been generated for dogs. The three largest multi-breed studies have reported exponents (and correlation r^2) based on M-mode values for LVIDd and LVIDs as follows: LVIDd 0.294 (r^2 = 0.874) and LVIDs 0.315 (r^2 = 0.777; Cornell, 2004); LVIDd 0.299 (r^2 = 0.894) and LVIDs 0.387 (r^2 = 0.790; Visser, 2019); and for non-sighthound dogs, LVIDd 0.322 (r^2 = 0.766) and LVIDs 0.387 (r^2 = 0.680; Esser, 2020).

In general, the upper prediction (reference) limit in a normally distributed sample falls at approximately the upper 97.5 percentile of the sample data. Generation of appropriate exponents in multi-breed studies presumes a sufficient sample size (at least 120 dogs), an unbiased distribution across breeds and body sizes, and attention to technical details of recording and measurement. Smaller sample sizes might be suitable for single breeds, provided robust confidence intervals are generated by appropriate statistical techniques, such as bootstrapping around the reference intervals (Ozarda, 2016). Very large sample sizes are likely to have higher correlation coefficients, but when data are submitted by multiple individuals, more variability in technique is likely; depending on one's perspective, such data can represent "real-life" or be considered "insensitive" for cardiomegaly. The same arguments can be made for single versus multicenter studies, where there is likely to be wider variation in the latter's design. Unfortunately, not all breeds fall neatly within the prediction limits of multi-breed studies. In the large study reported by Esser (2020), where just over 6,000 dogs were used to generate prediction intervals, LVIDd and LVIDs were overestimated for both the Newfoundland dog and the Irish Wolfhound. For other sighthounds in this study, these were underestimated, suggesting a need for breed-specific data.

For the veterinarian performing basic echocardiography, we interpret the published data as showing both substantial congruence, but also some differences that are likely to be clinically relevant. Based on these published data, *"practical cutoffs"* suggested to identify a dilated left ventricle are: *normalized LVID >1.65 to 1.7, and normalized LVIDs >1 to 1.1*. To be more conservative, an additional 5% can be added to the cutoff (as sometimes is recommended in people). As an example, for a 30 kg dog with an LVIDd of 44 mm, the normalized LVIDd = 4.4 cm/30kg$^{0.30}$ = 1.59, which is considered nondilated (<1.65). If exponents of .294 or .322 are used instead, the normalized LVIDd becomes 1.62 or 1.47, respectively. Although the differences in exponents seem relatively small, they can yield different results. Additional details of these studies are beyond the scope of this chapter; interested readers and especially those who regularly perform echocardiography are encouraged to consult these references for more details.

There are numerous technical issues to consider, as well. 2D imaging should assure optimal LV length in the long-axis or apical image to minimize foreshortening, while fine plane angulation across the LV should be done to avoid a truncated lumen. When identifying LV dilation from an M-mode study, proper cursor alignment perpendicular to the ventricular walls is critical to minimize angulation errors. One good check is to measure the LVIDd in both short- and long-axis planes. The short-axis measurement often is slightly larger, but the two values should be close if properly obtained. As an additional point, excessive heart rate can reduce apparent systolic function.

Reduced LV EF is the human standard for diagnosing systolic dysfunction in DCM. Functional criteria for canine DCM include LV EF<40%, FS <20%, and fractional area change (FAC) <35%. The LV EF = (LV diastolic volume − LV systolic volume)/(LV diastolic volume), or LV stroke volume/LV diastolic volume. The LVIDs and the LV FS, calculated as (LVIDd − LVIDs)/LVIDd, are simply minor axis surrogates for end-systolic volume and EF, respectively. Normal SMOD EF usually is >45%, and FS usually is ≥25%; but many healthy large-breed dogs have an EF of 40-44%, and FS of 20-24%, that remains stable for years. The LV short-axis FAC at the high papillary muscle level, calculated as (LV Area$_d$ − LV Area$_s$)/LV Area$_d$ (Chapter 4), incorporates numerous short-axis measurements; yet also fails to account for apical-basilar contraction. Values ≥40% are normal. When these linear and area measurements are normal and the heart subjectively appears normal, it is likely that calculated ventricular volumes will be also. However, it is possible to both underestimate cardiac size and falsely diagnose systolic dysfunction when only M-mode or FAC are used. The LVIDs and the LV volume (and end-systolic volume index) derived from one-dimensional measurements have been advanced as relatively specific indices of LV systolic function. However, other factors affect these values, including initial diastolic LV size and ventricular dyssynchrony. Dyssynchrony is common in both healthy and cardiomyopathic dogs. Normally, the ventricular septum and LV wall contract at nearly the same time, with the septum usually reaching its maximum amplitude slightly before the free wall. However, if there is a substantial time delay between these two movements, the LVIDs grossly underestimates systolic function and overestimates end-systolic volume. Even with synchronous contraction, the often quoted "normal" end-systolic volume index of 30 ml/m^2 is too low for many larger breeds, so we advise against using it. The LV FAC is somewhat less affected by dyssynchrony because multiple short axis diameters are recorded; however, measuring the short axis area is technically more difficult, especially with off angle images. Instead, a length-area technique, where volumes are calculated by SMOD, is recommended. The echo frame used for LV end-diastolic volume is timed to the onset of the QRS complex (on simultaneously recorded ECG); the end-systolic volume is obtained from the frame showing the smallest systolic volume, just prior to mitral valve opening.

Little has been published on the predictive value of strain echocardiography or tissue Doppler imaging with respect to identifying preclinical DCM that will progress to overt DCM. Most reported strain and tissue Doppler studies have validated abnormalities using conventional ejection phase indices like LV FS, or reported low values in dogs already in CHF (Chetboul, 2007). In Great Danes with preclinical DCM, speckle tracking echocardiography was not found to be a strong predictor of disease (Pedro, 2007). Yet these newer modalities have the potential to identify DCM before conventional methods can, although so far this has been shown only in isolated case reports and in Golden Retrievers with Duchenne's cardiomyopathy (Chetboul, 2004). It seems that strain imaging should be useful in dogs with idiopathic DCM, but additional study is required before clear recommendations can be made. In people, speckle tracking myocardial strain mainly is used to identify ischemia with stress or doxorubicin-related cardiomyopathy, prior to declines in EF.

There has been much focus on early identification of DCM in Dobermans. Besides the normalized LVID guidelines, M-mode LV diameter measurements sometimes are used in this breed to screen for occult DCM; for example, LVIDd > 47(–49) mm for males and >46 mm for females, or LVIDs >36(–38) mm (for both sexes) are commonly used cutoffs. However, body surface area-indexed LV volumes (volume/m²) calculated from 2D echo images (using 4-chamber right parasternal long-axis or left apical view optimized for LV size) and using SMOD were reported to be a more sensitive screening tool than M-mode-derived LV dimensions. It is recommended that volumes be obtained using both of these echo views; then the view showing the largest volumes should be used (also see **Figure 4.27**, p. 104, and related text). Recommended SMOD cutoff values for identifying preclinical DCM in Dobermans are: end diastolic volume index (EDVI) >95 mL/m² and end systolic volume index (ESVI) >55 mL/m². Other factors that appear useful for identifying early DCM in Dobermans include a mitral E-point-to-septal separation (EPSS) >6.5 mm (or >8 mm, based on more conservative earlier reports) or a FS <25%. The occurrence of any VPCs during initial exam also has been considered a "high-risk" predictor for future DCM in this breed. It is important to remember that EPSS can be spuriously increased if aortic valve insufficiency or other cause of restricted mitral valve motion is present, or if M-mode cursor positioning is suboptimal.

While previously proposed diagnostic guidelines using LV dimension, sphericity, and other criteria (ESVC Guidelines, Dukes-McEwan, 2003) can be useful for identifying dogs that warrant serial evaluation for progression to DCM, at least in Dobermans, the use of the SMOD and EPSS cutoffs listed above are more straightforward and just as effective. One major criterion of the previously proposed system is the sphericity index (SI), which is based on the observation that the left ventricle becomes more spherical in shape as it dilates. The SI = LV length at end-diastole (measured from 2D right parasternal long-axis 4-chamber view) divided by LVIDd. A SI <1.65 is considered to be abnormal. This cutoff was shown to be fairly sensitive and specific for differentiating Dobermans with DCM from normal. Nevertheless, SI and EPSS appear less sensitive than the SMOD method (and no better than M-mode measurements) for identifying early DCM in Dobermans. Dobutamine stress echocardiography, has reportedly detected early myocardial dysfunction in Doberman Pinschers, but rarely is done in clinical patients.

In Great Danes also, the 2D Simpson's ESVI can reportedly identify dogs with DCM; ESVI was more sensitive than FS or EF for detecting early DCM, with a cut-off of >44.3 mL/m² reported (only) for males (Stephenson, 2012). Normal M-mode LV dimensions were smaller in female Danes compared to males because of body size differences. Allometric scaling eliminated the gender difference and was useful for identifying occult DCM in this breed, too. In addition, suggested M-mode cutoff values for normal LV dimensions in Great Danes were reported as LVIDd of 56.1 mm (males) and 54 mm (females), and LVIDs of 42.7 mm (males) and 41.7 mm (females). Normal Great Danes had lower than expected FS, with a median FS of 27% (and 5–95% reference interval of 20–37%).

Diagnostic Tests in Overt DCM

Clinical laboratory tests in dogs with overt (stage C) DCM can be normal, although prerenal azotemia (from poor renal perfusion) or mildly increased liver enzyme activities (from passive hepatic congestion) are common. Hypoproteinemia, hyperkalemia, and hyponatremia accompany some cases of severe heart failure. Hypochloremia is common with aggressive loop diuretic therapy. Hypothyroidism with hypercholesterolemia is present in some dogs with DCM, with higher prevalence suspected in Dobermans and Great Danes. However, most dogs with DCM have normal thyroid stimulating hormone and free T_4 concentrations. Circulating natriuretic peptides and other neurohormones, such as norepinephrine (NE), aldosterone, and endothelin (ETN)-1 increase in dogs with overt DCM (also see Chapter 20). Progressive increases in circulating concentrations of NE and ETN-1 have been associated with worse prognosis. Cardiac troponin concentrations increase in some dogs with DCM and CHF; however, marked elevations are not expected with idiopathic DCM. Tests for other cardiac or systemic diseases that can depress LV function are appropriate before making a diagnosis of primary (idiopathic) DCM.

Blood taurine concentrations are normal in the vast majority of dogs tested, especially dogs with DCM of suspected genetic etiology. However, because the DCM-phenotype has been associated with certain diets in some dogs (p. 632), clinicians should consider measuring whole blood taurine concentration and obtaining a detailed diet history for dogs with DCM. This is especially important in breeds without known genetic risk, as well as in dogs eating a diet possibly associated with DCM.

Radiography in Overt DCM Generalized cardiomegaly is typical, although left heart enlargement predominates in some cases (**Figures 32.6** and **32.7**). Especially in Doberman

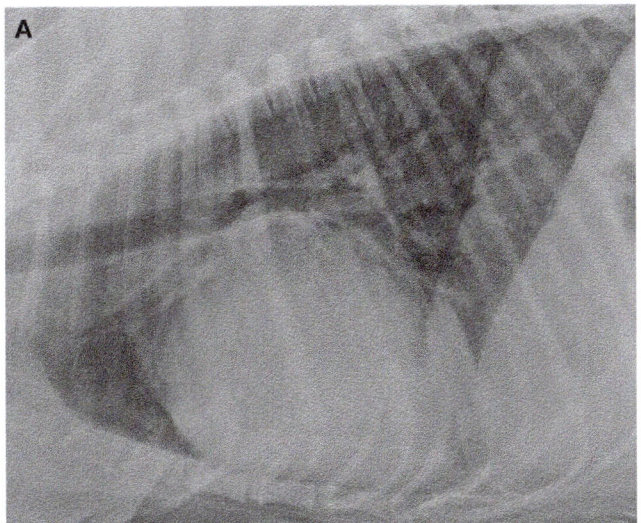
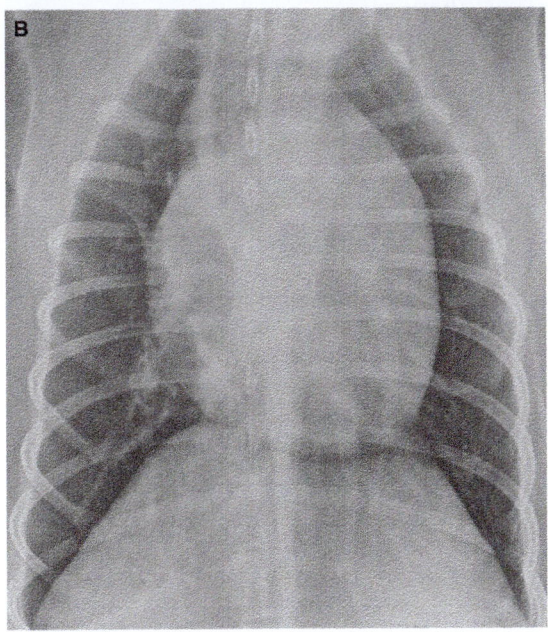

Figure 32.6 Lateral (A) and dorsoventral (B) radiographs show generalized cardiomegaly (VHS = 11.9 v) and mild pulmonary venous distension in a 6-year-old male Golden Retriever with dilated cardiomyopathy. There is no sign of pulmonary edema.

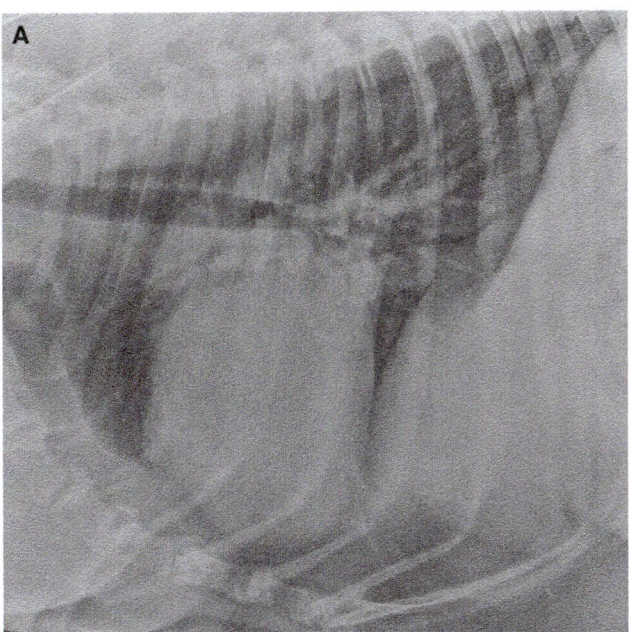
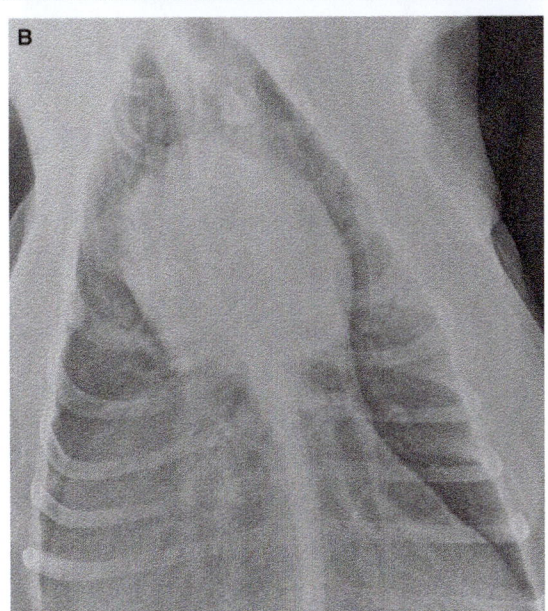

Figure 32.7 Lateral (A) and dorsoventral (B) radiographs from an 8-year-old male Doberman Pinscher being treated for stage C dilated cardiomyopathy. Pulmonary edema is now resolved and the pulmonary vasculature appears normal. Note the predominantly left atrial and ventricular enlargement (VHS = 11v) and vertical heart long-axis (A). The dog's heart was radiographically normal 2 years ago (**Figure 3.2**, p. 48).

Pinschers and Boxers, LA enlargement without marked cardiomegaly is common. Pulmonary interstitial or alveolar opacities, particularly in the hilar and dorsocaudal regions, accompany left-sided CHF. Yet, an asymmetrical or widespread distribution of pulmonary edema infiltrates is evident in some dogs (**Figures 32.8** and **32.9**). Distended pulmonary veins (**Figure 3.17D**, p. 60) are a hallmark of elevated pulmonary venous pressure, although this is not always radiographically apparent. Some dogs with severe left-sided CHF have both enlarged pulmonary lobar veins and arteries because of postcapillary pulmonary hypertension associated with fulminant pulmonary edema (**Figure 32.9**). Variable degrees of caudal vena caval distension, hepatomegaly, pleural effusion, and ascites are common and become pronounced in dogs with overt right-sided CHF signs.

Electrocardiography in Overt DCM The QRS complex voltage might be increased (consistent with LV dilation), normal, or smaller than usual. Increased QRS complex duration is common with myocardial disease, along with a sloppy R wave descent, suggesting intraventricular conduction disturbance;

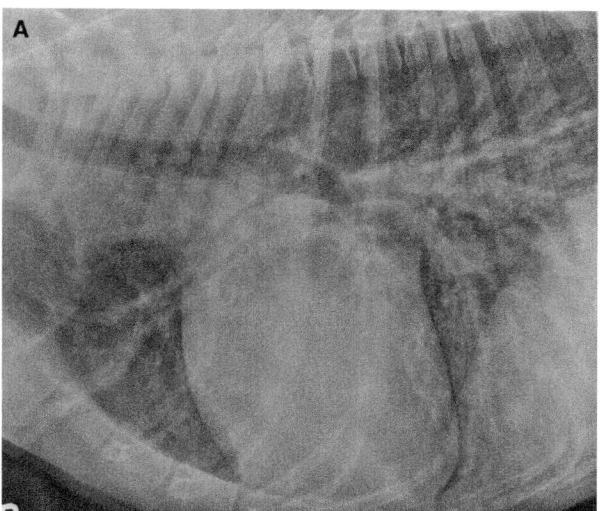

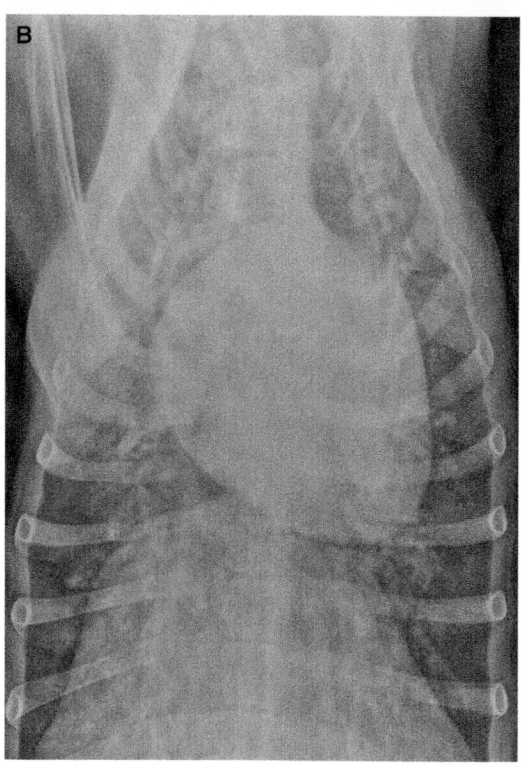

Figure 32.8 Lateral (A) and dorsoventral (B) radiographs show moderately severe pulmonary edema in a 4-year-old male Great Dane with dilated cardiomyopathy and decompensated left-sided heart failure. The dog started coughing 5 days prior, followed by progressively increasing tachypnea with mildly increased respiratory effort. Atrial fibrillation with a rapid ventricular response rate (~220 beats/min) was present on admission. Moderate left-sided to generalized cardiomegaly (VHS ~12v) is present. The diffuse, unstructured interstitial to alveolar lung pattern is most prominent in perihilar and caudodorsal lung fields, but is present throughout all lobes. Pulmonary lobar vessels are enlarged.

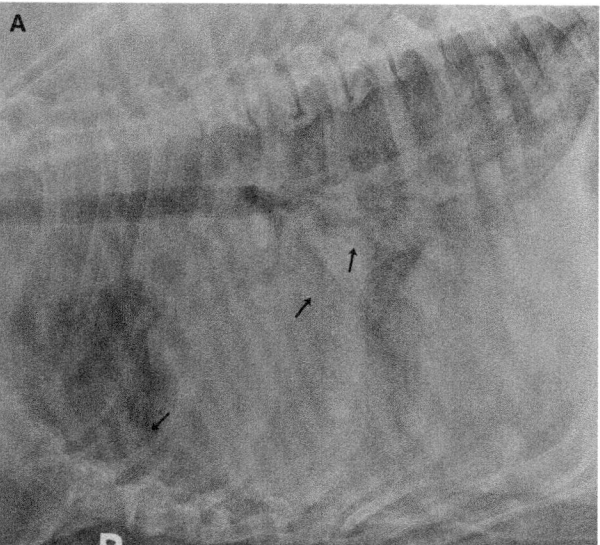

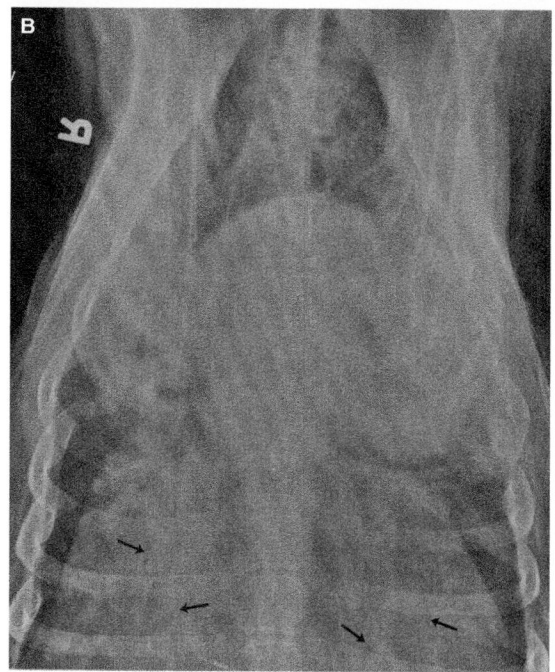

Figure 32.9 Fulminant pulmonary edema is present in this 9-year-old male Doberman Pinscher with dilated cardiomyopathy. A gagging cough was noted about a week before presentation; the owner initially thought the dog had a bone stuck in his throat. Progressive decrease in exercise tolerance and increase in respiratory effort followed. Lateral (A) and dorsoventral (B) radiographs show moderate left heart enlargement (VHS ~11 v), with diffusely increased pulmonary soft tissue-fluid opacity and air bronchograms (arrows). The cardiac silhouette, diaphragm, and pulmonary vessels are partially border-effaced. Where visible, both veins and arteries appear mildly enlarged. Spondylosis deformans also is evident in the thoracic spine.

the ST segment might be slurred (**Figure 32.10**). A bundle branch block pattern, usually left-sided, sometimes is present (**Figure 5.49**, p. 154). In dogs with sinus rhythm, widened and notched P waves suggest LA enlargement. AF is a common arrhythmia, especially in Irish Wolfhounds, Great Danes and other giant breeds (**Figure 32.11**; also **Figure 5.24**, p. 146). Uniform or multiform VPCs and paroxysmal ventricular tachycardia, with a background of sinus rhythm or AF, are

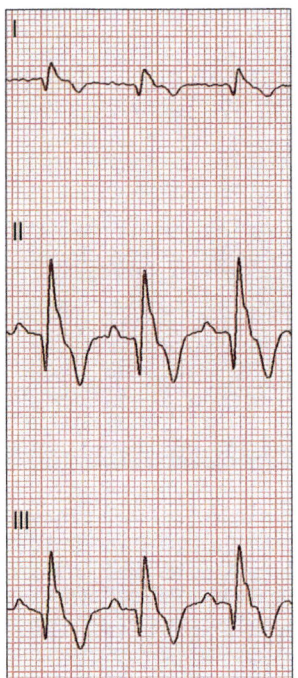

Figure 32.10 Sinus tachycardia in a 9-year-old female Doberman Pinscher with dilated cardiomyopathy and pulmonary edema. The wide P waves are consistent with left atrial enlargement; wide QRS complexes with slow and "sloppy" R wave descent suggest myocardial disease with slowed intraventricular conduction. Leads as marked; 50 mm/s, 1 cm = 1 mV.

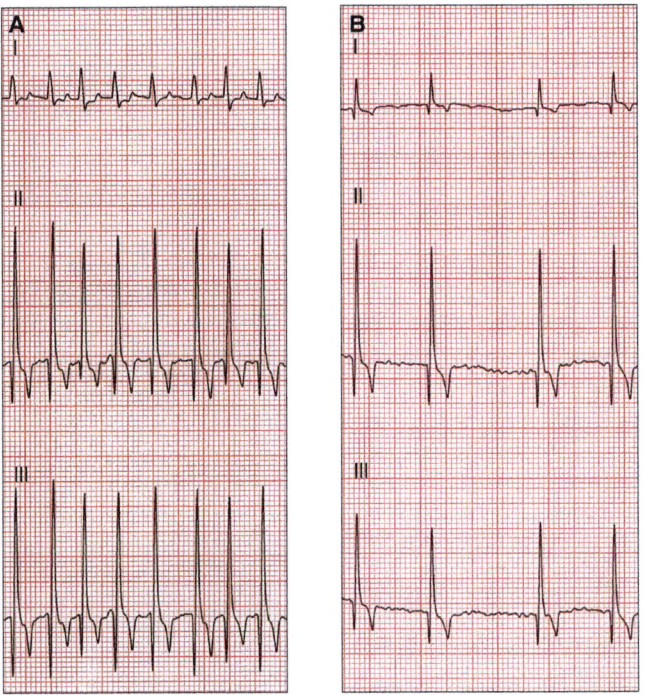

Figure 32.11 (A) Atrial fibrillation with uncontrolled ventricular response rate (~230 beats/min) in a 3-year-old male Doberman Pinscher with severe signs of heart failure from dilated cardiomyopathy. (B) Recording from the same dog following treatment, after signs of congestion had resolved. The ventricular rate is now 110 beats/min; baseline fibrillation waves are clearly evident. Leads as marked; 25 mm/s, 1 cm = 1 mV.

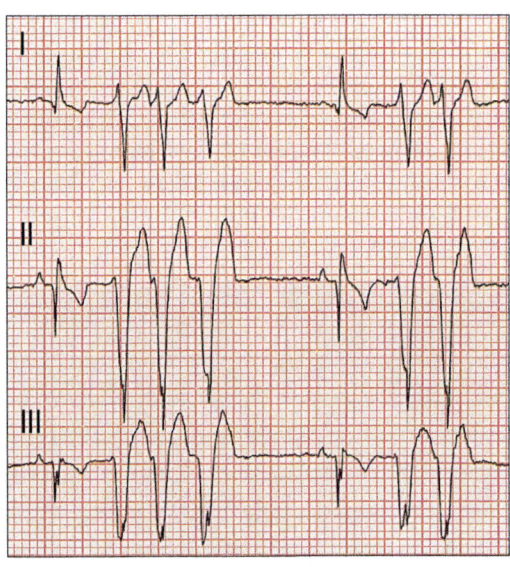

Figure 32.12 Frequent ventricular premature complexes (a triplet and pair (couplet) seen here) in a 9-year-old female Doberman Pinscher with dilated cardiomyopathy and decompensated congestive heart failure. Leads as marked; 25 mm/s, 1 cm = 1 mV.

typical in Doberman Pinschers and Boxers. Such arrhythmias often occur in other affected dogs, too (**Figures 32.12** and **32.13**; also **Figures 5.33** and **5.39**, pp. 149 & 150). Measures of heart rate variability and turbulence are decreased in dogs with overt DCM compared to normal dogs, consistent with the autonomic neural alterations that occur (reduced parasympathetic and increased sympathetic activation).

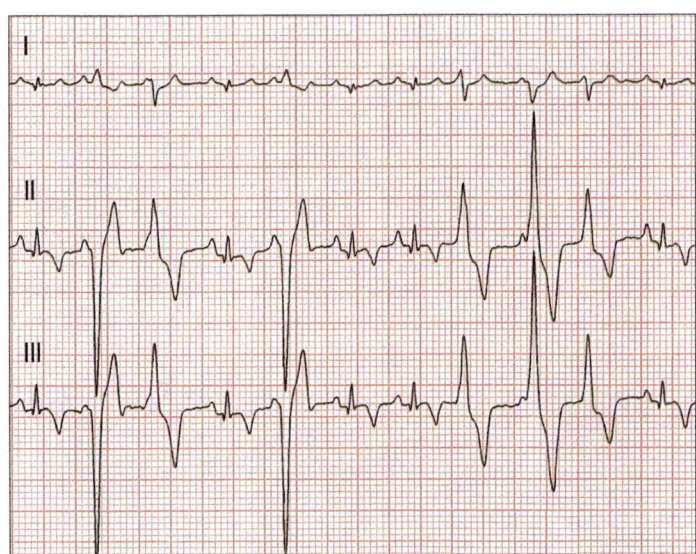

Figure 32.13 Multiform ventricular premature complexes in a 5-year-old male Labrador Retriever with dilated cardiomyopathy. The sinus QRS complex voltage is quite low; however, no effusion or other cause was found. The P waves are slightly wide. Leads as marked; 25 mm/s, 1 cm = 1 mV.

Echocardiography in Overt DCM Compared to the preclinical state, overt DCM is a straightforward diagnosis in most dogs. Dilated and rounded cardiac chambers, increased sphericity index, reduced systolic ventricular wall and septal motion, increased ESVI, reduced FS and EF, and increased mitral EPSS are characteristic findings (**Figures 32.14** and **32.15**). LV free wall and septal thicknesses are normal or decreased.

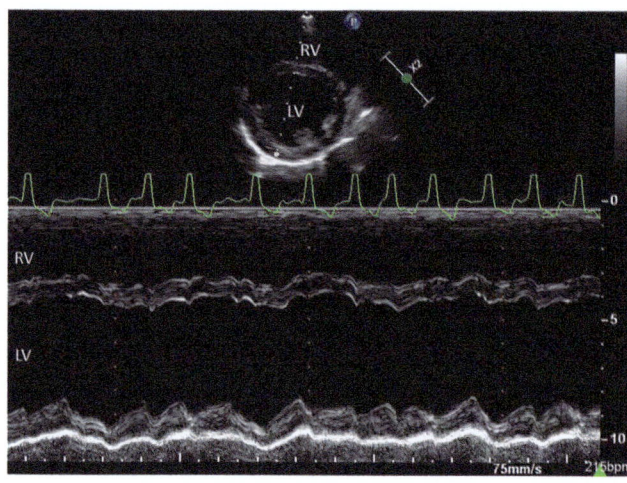

Figure 32.15 M-mode image at the ventricular level in a 7-year-old male Labrador Retriever with dilated cardiomyopathy and biventricular congestive failure. The cardiac rhythm is atrial fibrillation with an uncontrolled ventricular response rate (~215 beats/min). Ventricular dilation with chaotic, attenuated wall and septal motion (fractional shortening <12%) are evident. LV, left ventricle; RV, right ventricle.

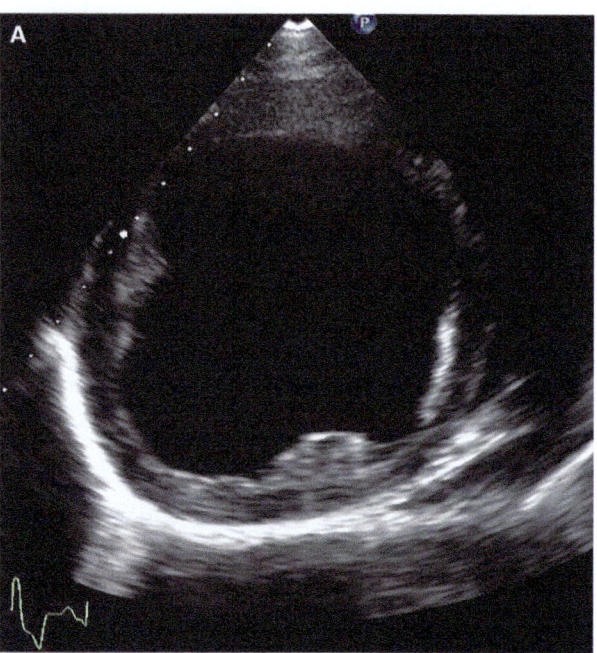

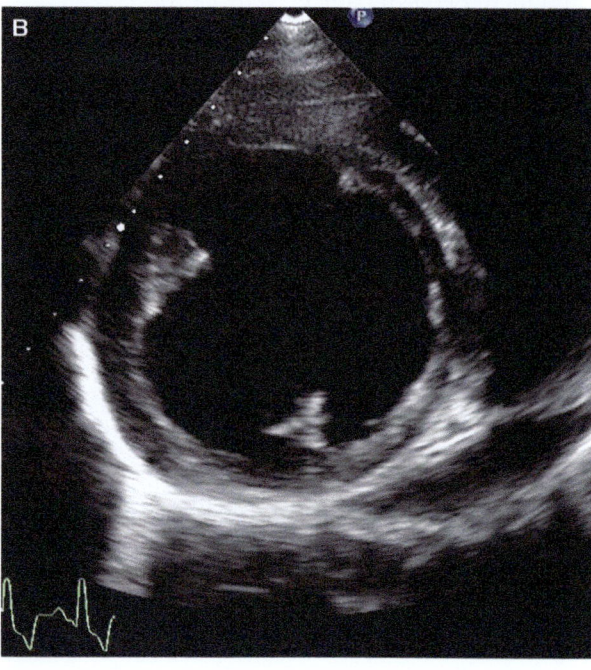

Figure 32.14 Right parasternal short-axis echocardiographic images at the ventricular level in end-diastole (A) and maximal systole (B) show marked left ventricular (LV) dilation in a 6-year-old male Great Dane with idiopathic dilated cardiomyopathy. There is minimal change in LV dimension throughout the cardiac cycle.

In some dogs with severe LV volume overload, diastolic displacement of the septum toward the right ventricle leads to exuberant septal motion, which can be confusing. However, poor LV free wall motion strongly supports the diagnosis, if the chamber is dilated. Once CHF has developed, all cardiac chambers tend to be enlarged; although right heart size can be relatively normal in some dogs, including many Dobermans and Boxers. In these two breeds, as well as Irish Wolfhounds and some other dogs with CHF, LA enlargement can be prominent while LV dilation might be only mild to moderate. Conversely, right heart enlargement can be marked in Boxers and English Bulldogs with ARVC with LV involvement (DCM-phenotype). AF can increase systemic venous pressures, leading to further right heart dilation. LV end-diastolic and end-systolic volumes, calculated using the SMOD and indexed to body surface area, or LV dimensions (from M-mode or 2D images) assessed by the allometric scaling method or compared with breed-specific normal values, should be obtained (see p. 614 and Chapter 4). Dogs with overt DCM typically have an ESVI well over 80 mL/m^2 and a SI well below normal. Increased LV sphericity is a characteristic of DCM; a SI <1.65 represents increased chamber rounding. Other signs of CHF might be evident, such as dilated pulmonary veins and caudal vena cava.

Doppler imaging provides additional information regarding myocardial and valvular function, but is not needed to establish the diagnosis in overt DCM. Mild to moderate AV valve regurgitation commonly is evident with color Doppler imaging (**Figure 32.16**). These regurgitant jets tend to be central and easily seen, even if silent to auscultation. They result from annular dilation and tethering of the AV valve apparatus to the ventricle, which distracts the co-optation points apically relative to the annular plane. This tenting of

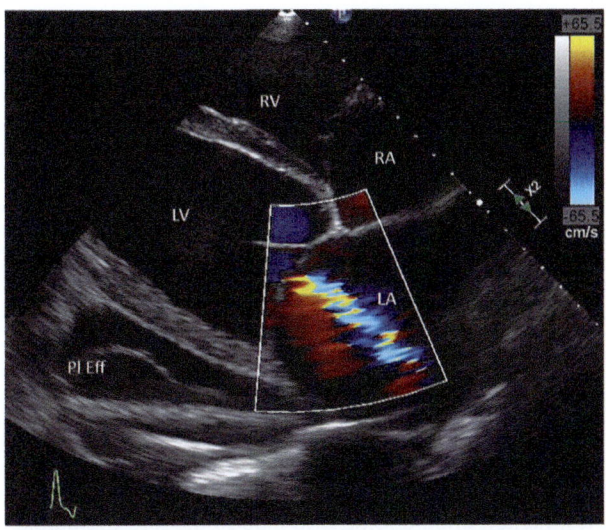

Figure 32.16 Mild to moderate mitral (and tricuspid) regurgitation develops with progressive ventricular enlargement in animals with dilated cardiomyopathy (DCM). Mild mitral regurgitation is evident in this systolic color-flow Doppler frame from a 4-year-old male Great Dane with stage C DCM. All four cardiac chambers are dilated and there is pleural effusion behind the LV. This dog also had atrial fibrillation, with a ventricular rate of 240 beats/min. LA, left atrium; LV, left ventricle; Pl Eff, pleural effusion; RA, right atrium; RV, right ventricle.

the valve differs from the prolapse seen in primary mitral valve disease; nevertheless, many dogs have some degree of myxomatous valve change. Spectral Doppler can verify the timing of regurgitation and estimate pressure differences between the ventricle and atrium. This information helps establish the presence or absence of pulmonary hypertension (or systemic hypertension), as long as atrial pressure also is taken into account (Chapter 4). Diastolic function becomes increasingly abnormal as overt DCM develops. Spectral Doppler imaging typically shows a restrictive transmitral filling pattern (p. 129), shortened mitral E wave deceleration time, shortened isovolumic relaxation time (IVRT), and increased mitral E/IVRT ratio, correlated with increased LA and LV diastolic pressures. Tissue Doppler imaging shows that the time from QRS onset to mitral annulus systolic motion is prolonged, and peak annular velocity is decreased, in dogs with DCM compared to normal. Resolution of pulmonary edema after CHF therapy usually is associated with an increase in IVRT, decrease in E/IVRT (by a mean of ~50% compared to its value during decompensated CHF), and often, improvement in diastolic functional class from restrictive to pseudonormal (p. 129).

Management of Preclinical DCM

General recommendations for stage B dogs include avoidance of strenuous exercise and instructing owners about home-monitoring of RRR, so that they can determine their dog's normal baseline RRR (p. 338 and **Table 22.1**, p. 339). Periodically checking the RRR can alert owners to a persistent increase, which provides an early indicator of CHF onset. In addition, the discovery of reduced myocardial function in a breed not typically associated with DCM, a mixed-breed dog, or a dog eating a diet associated with DCM, should prompt measurement of cTnI and blood taurine concentrations, as previously noted. Alternatively taurine supplementation can be added empirically for at least 4 months; p. 634). Feeding a well-balanced diet that is mildly or moderately reduced in salt, or at minimum avoiding high salt foods, is prudent. Cardiac reevaluation every 4–6 months will help in monitoring for disease progression and early signs of decompensation.

Several strategies have been used in attempting to slow progressive LV dysfunction and delay CHF onset in occult DCM. These variably include administration of an angiotensin converting enzyme (ACE) inhibitor, spironolactone, beta-blocker (such as carvedilol), pimobendan, and omega-3 fatty acid supplements. Several of these agents are thought to have a beneficial effect on pathologic ventricular remodeling. Although the optimal strategy in all cases is unclear, in Dobermans, pimobendan alone was found to delay CHF onset by about 9 months and increase total survival time (Summerfield, 2012). In Irish Wolfhounds with preclinical DCM (with or without AF), pimobendan markedly prolonged (by over 2 years) the time to CHF or sudden death, compared to an ACE inhibitor or methyldigoxin (Vollmar, 2016b). Another study in Dobermans that used benazepril alone, showed a delay in CHF onset of about 3 months (O'Grady, 2009). The authors' preference is to recommend beginning cardiac muscle protection with RAAS inhibition, and discussion with the owner (or a cardiology specialist) the pros and cons of up-titrating a beta-blocker at this stage of disease. We also recommend initiating pimobendan in breeds where it is been proven beneficial, or when moderate to severe decrease in systolic function is associated with LV dilation. We do not typically prescribe pimobendan for mild LV systolic dysfunction, especially if LV enlargement is only borderline. Another indication for pimobendan might be when antiarrhythmic therapy with sotalol, or other agent with negative inotropic effect, is initiated in a dog with systolic dysfunction.

The decision to use antiarrhythmic drug therapy in dogs with ventricular tachyarrhythmias is influenced by whether clinical signs (such as episodic weakness or syncope) have occurred, as well as by the arrhythmia's frequency and complexity. The best antiarrhythmic drug regimen(s) and ideal time to institute therapy are not entirely clear. Furthermore, reduction in VPC number on repeat Holter recordings does not assure protection from sudden death. In general, drugs (or combinations) that increase the ventricular fibrillation threshold, as well as reduce arrhythmia frequency and complexity, are desirable. The class III agents sotalol and amiodarone, or the combination of mexiletine with sotalol (or possibly atenolol), appear most promising (see Chapters 24 and 25).

Prognosis in Preclinical DCM In Dobermans, the presence of LV dilation or any arrhythmia on a 3-minute ECG is associated with increased risk for CHF or sudden death. Pimobendan treatment potentially could reduce heart size and improve prognosis. A greater decrease in LV function, higher heart rate on physical exam, and ≥4 VPCs on a 3-minute ECG recording were independent predictors of CHF or sudden death (Summerfield, 2012). The prognosis for Irish Wolfhounds with occult DCM appears relatively good. In a retrospective report of 151 Wolfhounds with DCM, a slight majority of dogs originally identified with stage B2 disease (with or without AF) eventually died of noncardiac causes. Median survival for those initially diagnosed with AF and occult DCM was almost 22 months; for those in sinus rhythm at initial diagnosis, median survival was about 29 months (Vollmar, 2019a). In contrast, the prognosis for Wolfhounds with overt CHF is much worse (see section "Prognosis in Overt DCM"). Wolfhounds with lone AF that do develop DCM also are likely to develop CHF over the next several years; sudden death has occurred.

Management of Overt DCM

Therapy for dogs with stage C disease is aimed at controlling congestive signs, optimizing cardiac output, managing arrhythmias, improving quality of life, and prolonging survival. Pimobendan, an ACE inhibitor, furosemide, and spironolactone form the core treatment for most dogs. The severity of CHF signs determines the aggressiveness of therapy. Additional inotropic, diuretic, vasodilator, antiarrhythmic, or other agents might be needed, especially for dogs in fulminant heart failure (**Table 32.2** and **Table 22.2**, p. 342; also see Chapter 25 for arrhythmia management and Chapters 20–22 for more information to guide heart failure management).

Frequent reevaluation is important for patients with acute heart failure because clinical status can deteriorate rapidly. Respiratory rate and character, lung sounds, pulse quality, heart rate and rhythm, peripheral perfusion, blood pressure, serum electrolyte and hydration status, renal function, body weight, rectal temperature, and mentation are important parameters. Although diuresis alleviates venous congestion and edema, the resulting preload reduction could cause an inadequate cardiac output, with hypotension. Cardiogenic shock can develop with severe DCM, especially after excessive diuresis and vasodilation, because high cardiac filling pressure often is necessary to maintain cardiac output (p. 313 and p. 347). Cautious fluid administration (either SC or IV) might be needed in some dogs, especially after aggressive diuretic therapy. Five percent dextrose in water (D_5W) with potassium chloride added (12 mEq/500 mL), or 0.45% sodium chloride and 2.5% dextrose with potassium chloride added, can be administered at conservative rates (such as 15–30 mL/kg/day). Careful monitoring is essential to avoid overhydration and recurrent pulmonary edema. As always, thoracocentesis is indicated for moderate- to large-volume pleural effusion.

Table 32.2 Treatment Outline for Dogs with Overt (Stage C) Dilated Cardiomyopathy

Mild to Moderate Signs of CHF[a]
- Furosemide
- Pimobendan
- ACE inhibitor
- Spironolactone
- Antiarrhythmic therapy, if necessary[b]
- Complete exercise restriction until signs abate
- Moderate dietary salt restriction

Severe, Acute Signs of CHF[a]
- Supplemental O_2
- Furosemide (parenteral)
- Pimobendan (initiate as soon as possible; IV, if available)
- Other inotropic support, as needed (IV dobutamine or other)
- ACE inhibitor, once edema and blood pressure are stable
- Other vasodilator only with caution (such as IV nitroprusside or PO hydralazine with topical nitroglycerine)
- Antiarrhythmic therapy, as necessary[b]
- Sedation (such as butorphanol), as needed for anxiety
- Cage rest
- Minimize patient handling & stress
- Monitor respiratory rate, heart rate and rhythm, arterial blood pressure, peripheral perfusion, urine output, renal function, serum electrolytes, etc.

For AF and Inadequate Heart Rate Control with Digoxin[b]
- Acute: cautiously add IV diltiazem or incremental PO doses of the standard preparation
- Chronic: diltiazem long-acting and digoxin, ±beta-blocker if needed

Chronic DCM Management[a]
- Pimobendan
- ACE inhibitor
- Furosemide (lowest effective dosage and frequency)
  - Or torsemide for refractory edema, pleural effusion or ascites
- Spironolactone
- Antiarrhythmic therapy as indicated
- ± Other medications for refractory CHF (p. 354)
- Client education and resting respiratory rate (and heart rate, if possible) monitoring at home
- Regular mild exercise, if tolerated, as long as signs of CHF are controlled
- Dietary salt restriction
- Routine health maintenance (including heartworm testing and prophylaxis in endemic areas)
- Manage other medical problems

[a] See text, Tables 22.2 (p. 342) and 22.3 (p. 345), and Chapters 21 and 22 for further details.
[b] See Tables 25.1 (p. 398) and 25.2 (p. 402), and Chapters 24 and 25 for further details.

When acute heart failure signs are controlled, the patient is transitioned to long-term oral therapy. This involves pimobendan, furosemide, an ACE inhibitor, reduced-sodium diet, and exercise restriction. Spironolactone usually is added for its potential cardioprotective effect at the first recheck. Although the concurrent use of an ACE inhibitor and spironolactone could potentially increase serum blood urea nitrogen (BUN), potassium, and magnesium concentrations, this usually does not occur to a clinically relevant degree. Nevertheless, it is important to monitor these parameters. Spironolactone is prescribed mostly for its antialdosterone effect, although it might support diuresis in these patients, too. Aldosterone contributes to adverse cardiac remodeling (p. 307). Inadequate aldosterone suppression (aldosterone escape or breakthrough) develops in some dogs despite ACE inhibition. The addition of spironolactone to standard heart failure therapy has improved survival in people with myocardial dysfunction, and might in dogs, as well. If pimobendan administration is not possible for some reason (including financial), digoxin could be used cautiously instead; however, it is not advised in dogs with serious ventricular ectopy, azotemia or hypokalemia (p. 327).

Some dogs benefit from an increase in dosage or frequency of pimobendan when CHF is difficult to control (p. 354). While this drug's potential for increasing the risk of ventricular tachyarrhythmias is small, it is not zero. In cases of advanced CHF, and where it is not relatively contraindicated, digoxin could be used with pimobendan for additional inotropic effect. However, besides being a less powerful inotrope, digoxin carries significant risk for toxicity so conservative dosing and monitoring of serum digoxin concentration are essential (p. 328). Digoxin toxicity occurs at relatively low dosages in some dogs. The total daily dosage generally should not exceed 0.5 mg for most large and giant breed dogs (and 0.25–0.375 mg for Doberman Pinschers). If this drug is used, serum digoxin concentration measurement is recommended at 7–10 days after initiating digoxin therapy, or after a dosage change. Serum electrolyte and creatinine or BUN concentrations also should be monitored, because hypokalemia and azotemia predispose to digoxin toxicity.

Additional medical therapy (see following paragraphs and p. 354) might also be helpful. Client education about the disease process and medications prescribed is important. Home monitoring of RRR (**Table 22.1**, p. 339), as well as heart rate if possible, is advised. The time frame for periodic reevaluation depends on the animal's status; visits once or twice a week might be needed initially.

For dogs with AF, digoxin is helpful for controlling heart rate especially in those with CHF. It usually is co-administered with diltiazem, unless otherwise contraindicated. Previously, an oral "loading" dose of twice the usual digoxin maintenance dose often was advocated; but today, diltiazem co-administration generally is preferred and is started immediately. Initial diltiazem doses can be given IV if the patient is hospitalized, or started PO with standard preparations. Because of diltiazem's negative inotropic effect, it is safest to begin with low initial doses and then up-titrate as needed (for example 0.05-0.1 mg/kg IV every 2 hours for 3 or 4 doses, or 0.5 mg/kg PO repeated every 2 hours, up to 4-6 mg/kg/day for the first 24h). A standard oral dose of digoxin can be started, as well. Heart rate control is extremely important for dogs with AF. A maximum ventricular rate of 140–150 beats/minute in the hospital (a stress-inducing setting) is the recommended target; lower heart rates (125 beats/minute or less) are expected at home, assuming the ventricular response rate is well-controlled. Because it is difficult to accurately count the heart rate by auscultation or chest palpation in dogs with AF, ECG recording is recommended. Femoral pulses never should be used to assess heart rate in the presence of AF because pulse deficits are likely. Home heart rate monitoring, using a smartphone-based ECG app (p. 242), helps with diltiazem (or beta-blocker) dosage titration to achieve a desired heart rate. It also might detect other intermittent arrhythmias.

With regard to nutritional supplements, only a small percentage of dogs have shown marked clinical improvement in response to oral L-carnitine supplementation. In the absence of myocardial deficiency, high doses of L-carnitine are unlikely to be beneficial. Carnitine supplementation should be considered optional, but might be considered particularly in Boxers for 3- to 6-months (see p. 634). Taurine deficiency or impaired bioavailability could be part of the DCM syndrome in some dogs, especially Golden Retrievers and Cocker Spaniels, or in dogs eating a BEG diet (p. 632). Whole blood (or the less desirable plasma) taurine concentration measurement can be helpful. Yet, levels are usually normal even in dogs eating atypical diets. Taurine supplementation should be provided when blood concentration is low; it might help in some other cases, too (see p. 634). Nevertheless, most dogs of breeds commonly affected with DCM have normal taurine levels and do not respond to supplementation.

The value of other nutritional supplements for most dogs is uncertain. Preliminary evidence suggests that omega-3 fatty acid supplements in the form of fish oil capsules, or enriched diets, might help reduce cytokine (including TNF) production associated with cardiac cachexia. This is probably the most often recommended supplement beyond taurine. Oxygen free-radical damage also can contribute to myocardial dysfunction. Experimental evidence in other species suggests that antioxidant vitamins might reduce oxidative stress and possibly attenuate associated myocardial and endothelial dysfunction. Whether supplementation with vitamin C or other antioxidant vitamins would have a measurable benefit in canine DCM remains to be discovered. Clients are often overwhelmed by the number of prescription medication pills and encouraging them to take supplements of marginal or unproven value is probably unwise unless they are eager to "try anything."

Long-term, low-dose beta-blocker therapy with carvedilol or metoprolol would appear to have theoretical benefit over time, if the individual can tolerate the drug. However, convincing clinical evidence in dogs is lacking; this approach has fallen out of favor and we do not recommend it presently. If a beta-blocker was used previously in the preclinical stage for cardiac muscle protection, the drug should be markedly reduced or discontinued. Despite the theoretical concern about abruptly withdrawing a beta-blocker, dogs with fulminant heart failure should not be treated with these drugs. If used, this therapy should only be given to dogs with stable DCM; it must be initiated with very low doses and titrated upward slowly (see p. 331). Perhaps the most promising use for drugs like carvedilol is as a low-dose add-on to digoxin and diltiazem in patients with AF where heart rate is difficult to control. In these cases, the beta-blocker dose is increased every 2 to 4 weeks, as needed. Caution is necessary to avoid clinical decompensation or AV block.

Resolution of CHF is associated with reduction in RRR (to the patient's normal baseline rate) and serum NT-proBNP concentration (by >20%), as well as resolution of radiographic pulmonary edema (and pleural effusion). Changes in several Doppler echo variables also accompany CHF resolution, including decreases in mitral E/IVRT and mitral E to early annular velocity (Ea) ratios.

Several surgical treatment modalities for DCM have been explored, with mixed results. At present, surgical approaches for DCM management are not advocated. Biventricular pacing (cardiac resynchronization therapy) is helpful in some people with myocardial failure, but so far there is little experience with this in dogs. Novel strategies using stem cells, gene therapy or other techniques might become available in the future.

Prognosis in Overt DCM Historically, the prognosis for dogs with overt DCM has been guarded to poor. Most Doberman Pinschers survived only 2–6 months, with only a small minority surviving more than a year after the onset of clinical CHF. For Irish Wolfhounds with overt CHF and AF at the time of diagnosis, a median survival time of about 7 months and a cardiac-related death rate of almost 90% were reported (Vollmar, 2019a). For dogs with DCM of all breeds, the probability of surviving for 2 years after CHF onset has been estimated at 7.5–28%. However, pimobendan and other treatment advances appear to be improving survival times. Some dogs live well for several years after initial decompensation. Nevertheless, CHF can be difficult to control and sudden death is common. An estimated 20–40% of affected Doberman Pinschers experience sudden death, often before clinical heart failure develops.

Initial echo estimates of myocardial function do not consistently correlate with survival, although an ESVI >140 mL/m² has been associated with reduced survival time. Young age at CHF onset, ascites, and dyspnea were independent risk factors for shorter survival in an older study where ACE inhibitors and pimobendan were not yet in common use. A survey of DCM dogs, where most received an ACE inhibitor and almost a third received pimobendan, revealed ESVI as the best prognostic indicator (Martin, 2010). Other variables associated with a negative prognosis were radiographic pulmonary edema, presence of VPCs, higher creatinine, lower plasma protein, and the Great Dane breed. Others suggest a worse prognosis with right-sided or biventricular CHF signs or concurrent AF, which itself is a risk factor for right-sided congestive signs. A restrictive transmitral flow pattern on Doppler echo could be the most important negative prognostic indicator. This supports the concept that diastolic dysfunction is an integral pathophysiologic factor in DCM. Other indicators that have been associated with reduced survival time include a QRS duration ≥60 ms, marked increase in NT-pro BNP concentration, moderate increase in cTnI concentration, and cardiac cachexia (p. 312).

Sudden cardiac death in Doberman Pinschers appears to be most strongly predicted by the degree of LV dilation, particularly an EDVI >91 mL/m², with the probability of sudden death increasing over eight-fold for every 50 mL/m² increase in EDVI (Klüser, 2016). ESVI, ejection fraction, and NT-proBNP concentration correlate closely with EDVI. Other important risk factors for sudden death include increased cTnI concentration and the occurrence of ventricular tachycardia (although not total number of VPCs), as well as heart rates exceeding 260 beats/minute during ventricular tachycardia episodes. In Dobermans with these serious (malignant) ventricular arrhythmias, antiarrhythmic therapy might improve survival time.

Arrhythmogenic Right Ventricular Cardiomyopathy

ARVC is an inherited myocardial disease, with clinical and histopathologic characteristics similar to those found in people with the analogous disease. ARVC sometimes is called "arrhythmogenic cardiomyopathy," because the associated lesions are not necessarily limited to the right ventricle. In dogs, ARVC occurs mainly in Boxers. Clinically, it is characterized by ventricular tachyarrhythmias that can cause syncope or sudden death. LV dysfunction similar to that with idiopathic DCM in other large dog breeds also develops in some cases, leading to signs of left- or right-sided CHF. Presumptive diagnosis of ARVC in Boxers is based on a combination of the patient's signalment and presence of ventricular arrhythmias without other identifiable cause. Supportive evidence includes a history of ARVC in related dogs, a positive genetic test, and typical (postmortem) myocardial histopathological findings. In theory, an MRI would show fatty replacement of myocardium and late gadolinium uptake (fibrosis). Infrequently, a high resolution echocardiogram will show areas of RV wall thinning. Similar clinical and pathological findings occasionally occur in other dog breeds (including the English Bulldog, Shetland Sheepdog, Labrador Retriever, Dalmatian, and Weimaraner) and in cats; marked right heart dilation, signs of right-sided CHF, and severe ventricular tachyarrhythmias are described in such cases.

The disease in Boxers is thought to be the same in dogs from both the United Kingdom and United States and to have originated in a small number of dogs from the latter. Three clinical forms of ARVC were originally described: (1) asymptomatic dogs with ventricular tachyarrhythmia (typically with positive QRS configuration in lead II); (2) dogs with normal heart size and LV function, but with syncope or weakness caused by paroxysmal or sustained ventricular tachycardia; (3) Boxers with poor myocardial function and ventricular dilation (the so-called DCM phenotype) and CHF, in addition to ventricular (and sometimes supraventricular) tachyarrhythmia (Harpster, 1991). The latter form carries an especially poor prognosis. These three clinical forms are thought to be manifestations of the same underlying disease. Similarly, in human patients with ARVC there is a spectrum of clinical manifestations.

ARVC in Boxers shows autosomal dominant inheritance, with incomplete penetrance and variable expression, which likely are influenced by environmental, as well as genetic, factors. The fact that some dogs develop asymptomatic arrhythmias at an older age is consistent with a low disease penetrance. Because of incomplete penetrance, breeding dogs with the causative mutation might not become clinically affected themselves, but can produce offspring that develop ARVC. In people with ARVC, several mutations in genes coding for desmosomal proteins have been identified, although these same mutations have not been found in dogs. Genome-wide association study followed by gene sequencing led to the identification of a deletion mutation in the striatin gene (on chromosome 17) which is associated with ARVC in Boxers (Meurs, 2010). However, despite a strong association with ARVC and the frequent development of the DCM phenotype in Boxers homozygous for the mutation, the likelihood that this specific striatin mutation is causative has been questioned. Some Boxers with DCM lack the mutation. A large pedigree-based evaluation of 3 descendent lines concluded that the causative mutation must be located in close proximity on the same chromosome, but was not the striatin gene itself (Cattanach, 2015). Separation of these two genes could have occurred during cell division in certain dogs, explaining why some dogs in one pedigree line developed ARVC but did not have the striatin mutation. Other mutation(s) also might be involved in some lines. While the specific causative mutation might be unidentified as yet, the striatin mutation could at minimum be considered a marker for the ARVC gene. Dogs homozygous for the striatin (and presumed underlying ARVC) mutation tend to become severely affected at an early age. Disease progression is signaled by more frequent and complex ventricular arrhythmias, syncope, and development of myocardial dysfunction. Striatin plays a role in cardiomyocyte function, so its interactions with possible other (unknown) ARVC mutation(s) could contribute to disease development, as could exercise, stress or other heart conditions.

ARVC screening recommendations for Boxers include genetic testing (regardless of whether the striatin mutation is specifically causative) and Holter monitoring (**Table 32.3**). General guidelines have been published, largely for guiding breeders regarding the degree of ventricular ectopy that

Table 32.3 Cardiac Screening Guidelines for Boxers[a]

Recommended Screening Test, Beginning at 3 Years of Age and Yearly Thereafter

- 24–hour Holter monitoring[b]
- Interpretation of Holter results:
  - 0–20 single VPCs/24 hours: within acceptable limits of normal
  - 20–100 VPCs/24 hours: indeterminate, suggest repeat Holter monitoring in 6–12 months
  - 100–300 single VPCs/24 hours: suspicious for ARVC
  - 100–300 VPCs/24 hours & increased complexity (frequent couplets, triplets, ventricular tachycardia): likely affected with ARVC
  - 300–1000 single VPCs/24 hours: likely affected with ARVC
  - >1000 VPCs/24 hours: affected with ARVC

For Dogs with, or Suspected to Have, ARVC

- Echocardiography recommended (in addition to Holter monitoring), to evaluate myocardial function
- See p. 628 for treatment considerations

[a] Adapted from Meurs, 2017. Also see text.
[b] Usable recording of >23 hour duration, with analysis by trained individual.
Abbreviations: ARVC, arrhythmogenic right ventricular cardiomyopathy; VPCs, ventricular premature complexes.

might be considered normal or suspicious for cardiomyopathy. These cutoffs should be considered as relative liabilities, and not absolute. As an example, a dog with five VPC triplets might only have 18 VPCs in 24h, but most certainly would not be considered normal. A dog with VPCs mainly of LV morphology could have a splenic tumor, for example, and not ARVC. It can be helpful to consult with a cardiologist when interpreting Holter data from dogs being screened for ARVC, so that supraventricular arrhythmias with aberrancy are not misinterpreted and ventricular escapes are not misclassified as VPCs. Echocardiography usually is optional in asymptomatic dogs, but should be performed if genetic tests or Holter ECG are abnormal. Dogs homozygous for the mutation should be restricted from breeding. Homozygous-positive dogs reportedly are more likely to develop overt ARVC, especially the DCM phenotype, and at a younger age. Heterozygous dogs have less risk for developing overt disease than homozygotes; however, avoiding prolonged strenuous exercise for these dogs is prudent. Heterozygous dogs with no signs of ARVC and possessing desirable breed-traits could be bred, but not to a dog homozygous for the striatin mutation, because of the risk of producing homozygous puppies.

Pathophysiology

Abnormalities of intercellular adhesion and electrical signaling at the intercalated disks, and the desmosomes in particular, are thought to underlie ARVC, although the mechanisms are not fully understood. Desmosomes are intercalated disk components important for anchoring adjacent cells together. Loss of desmosomal integrity reduces cell-to-cell adhesion and can promote myocyte death, ultimately impairing the heart's ability to withstand mechanical stress. In Boxers, as in people with ARVC, desmosomal integrity is abnormal. Even if the striatin gene mutation is not the specific cause for ARVC, abnormal striatin could play a role in disease pathogenesis. Striatin is a structural protein within the intercalated disk. However, the connections among abnormal desmosomal structure and function, or that of other intercalated disk components, and the development of myocardial fibro-fatty infiltration is unclear.

Abnormal localization of beta-catenin and striatin proteins occurs within the cardiomyocytes from ARVC Boxers, regardless of striatin gene mutation status. Abnormal beta-catenin trafficking could negatively affect normal adherens junctions, desmosomes, and gap junctions at the intercalated disks. The mislocalization of beta-catenin and dysfunction of beta-catenin and striatin might disrupt Wnt signaling, which is a molecular pathway important for the survival and proliferation of cells. The Wnt signaling pathway is involved in epithelial to mesenchymal cell transition as well as adipocyte proliferation. Abnormal Wnt signaling is thought to be associated with an increase in fatty and fibrous tissue. Abnormalities of a related protein (plakoglobin, or gamma-catenin) that interacts or competes with beta-catenin also might be involved in the pathogenesis of ARVC. Reduction in myocardial calstabin2 messenger RNA and protein also have been observed in AVRC Boxers compared to normal dogs. This protein is important to the normal functioning of the cardiac ryanodine receptor (RyR2). Calstabin deficiency is associated with increased RyR2 channel opening and abnormal intracellular Ca^{++} leakage, which could trigger ventricular tachyarrhythmias.

Myocardial histologic changes are more extensive in Boxers with ARVC compared to those in other dogs with DCM. These histologic features include myofiber atrophy, progressive loss of cardiomyocytes, fatty or fibrofatty infiltration, and fibrosis. Focal areas of myocytolysis, necrosis, hemorrhage, and mononuclear cell infiltration also occur. Despite the focus on the right ventricular (RV) component of this disease, fatty or fibrofatty replacement occurs in the LV and also in atrial myocardium in almost half of affected Boxers. Because of the widespread distribution of lesions within the heart, a change in name to Arrhythmogenic Cardiomyopathy has been proposed.

Ultrastructural changes in ARVC support the notion that proteins important for anchoring the cytoskeletal structure to the intercalated disks are disrupted. Reduced numbers of desmosomes, adherens junctions, and gap junctions are found at the intercalated disks of dogs with ARVC compared to normal dogs. Additional abnormalities involving Z-line and sarcomere appearance also suggest a connection between ARVC and the contractile apparatus. Intercalated disc and gap junction protein abnormalities also occur in the atrial myocardium of Boxers with ARVC and could underlie the atrial arrhythmias seen in some dogs.

ARVC disease progression appears to be exacerbated by strenuous exercise and endurance training, perhaps because of increased myocardial stress. The disease is thought to progress more slowly in sedentary dogs. Thus, the appearance of clinical disease in middle-aged or older dogs might relate to the cumulative effects of myocardial stress.

Clinical Features

ARVC occurs in both male and female Boxers at about equal rates; its prevalence has been estimated at 9%. Median age at diagnosis is between 5 and 7 years; however, clinical disease onset can occur in dogs under 3 and over 10 years of age. Geographical variation in clinical manifestations is reported. Ventricular tachyarrhythmias with normal LV contractility and chamber size could be the more common presentation in the United States, while a more classical DCM presentation with CHF predominates in Europe.

ARVC also is reported in adult to older English Bulldogs; there is sporadic occurrence in other breeds, too. Male Bulldogs appear to be affected more often than females. While probably over half of dogs have ventricular tachyarrhythmias, supraventricular tachyarrhythmias, including atrial flutter, also occur in a minority. CHF is common in these Bulldogs. Some have sudden death. Cardiac-related death occurred in about half of the Bulldogs in one report, with median survival after diagnosis at just over 8 months (Cunningham, 2018b).

A history of syncope is common in dogs with ARVC, occurring in about a third of affected Boxers (Meurs, 2014). Episodic weakness, syncope, or sudden death can be the only disease manifestation in Boxers, or other dogs, with a tachyarrhythmia and relatively well-preserved ventricular function. However, it is important to note that syncope in Boxers also can occur secondary to neurocardiogenic reflexes or other mechanisms, rather than ventricular tachycardia (Domingues, 2020). Even in dogs with VPCs, the mechanism of syncope might not be ventricular tachycardia. For dogs with neurocardiogenic syncope, empirical treatment with sotalol often exacerbates the collapse episodes. As in Doberman Pinschers with DCM, progression from "silent" ventricular tachyarrhythmia to an overt DCM-phenotype occurs in some Boxers with ARVC, unless sudden death interferes. Dogs with the DCM-phenotype can show increased respiratory rate or effort, poor appetite, weight loss, and abdominal distension (ascites).

Physical findings are normal early in the disease, although a cardiac rhythm disturbance might be detected on physical exam. While VPCs are most common, AF or atrial ectopy can occur, too. A soft systolic murmur also is a common finding in dogs with ARVC. This might relate to MR or TR in dogs with ventricular dysfunction and dilation; however, nonpathologic left-basilar flow murmurs (p. 228) are common in Boxers, as is congenital subaortic stenosis (SAS; p. 480). Other physical findings in dogs with poor ventricular contractility are similar to those described for dogs with DCM. When CHF occurs, left-sided signs predominate in most cases, although ascites and other evidence of biventricular failure also are common, especially in dogs with AF.

Diagnostic Tests

Routine clinical laboratory tests generally are not helpful for diagnosing the disease. Increased serum cTnI concentration, correlated with VPC number and arrhythmia grade, has been identified in Boxers with ARVC. However, there is too much overlap between normal and affected Boxers for cTnI to be a discriminating test. Increases in NT-proBNP concentration are expected only in dogs with the DCM-phenotype and ventricular dilation.

The characteristic *ECG finding* is ventricular ectopy, usually with a background of sinus rhythm or sinus arrhythmia. Supraventricular arrhythmias, including AF or atrial premature complexes, and other ECG abnormalities also occur with ARVC but are less common. The ventricular ectopic complexes occur singly, in pairs, short runs, or as sustained ventricular tachycardia (**Figures 32.17** and **32.18**; also **Figure 5.30**, p. 148). Typically, these VPCs have an upright configuration (left bundle branch block pattern) in leads II and aVF, which suggests a RV origin. However, some Boxers have VPCs with multiform or negative (right bundle branch block) configuration. Finding any VPCs (of suspected RV origin) in a 5-minute resting ECG recording is reportedly specific for occult cardiomyopathy in Boxers, although the sensitivity of this is too low for the 5-minute ECG to be an adequate screening tool. Even in dogs that do have VPCs on a brief ECG recording, the resting ECG generally cannot provide a broader assessment of arrhythmia frequency and complexity. QRS complexes in Boxers often are relatively small; increased voltages are

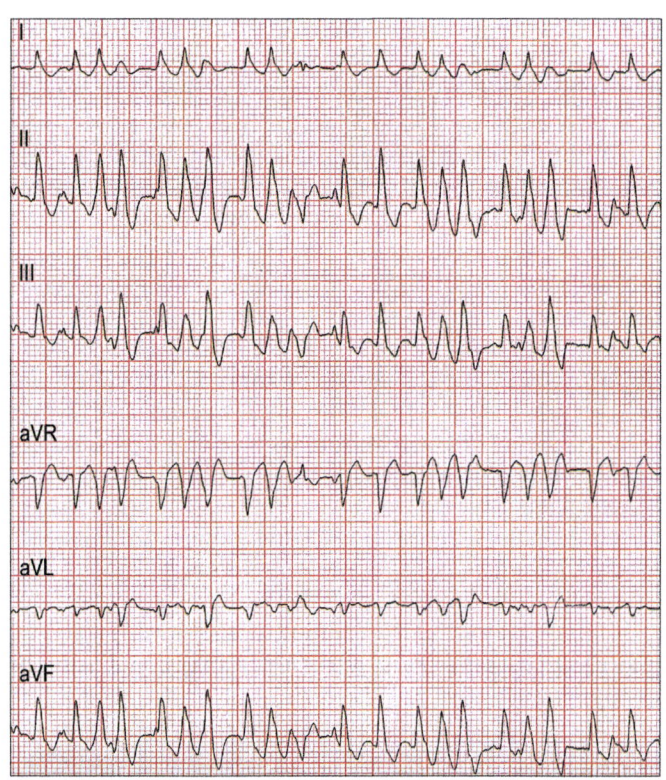

Figure 32.18 Severe, multiform ventricular tachyarrhythmia in a 3-year-old female Boxer with poor left ventricular function and congestive failure. Sudden death followed shortly. Leads as marked; 25 mm/s, 0.5 cm=1 mV.

atypical. Occasional dogs have widened QRS complexes and secondary T-wave changes.

Holter or other ambulatory monitoring is recommended whenever ARVC is suspected, based on an auscultated arrhythmia or a history of weakness or syncope (**Table 32.3**). Likewise, Holter monitoring is used to screen asymptomatic Boxers, especially those with a positive genetic test or family history of disease. For patients being treated for arrhythmias, Holter monitoring also is helpful for evaluating antiarrhythmic drug efficacy. The presence of ventricular couplets and R-on-T phenomenon (p. 422) appear to be independent predictors of ARVC (Meurs, 2014). An absolute number of VPCs/24 hours that might separate normal from abnormal dogs is not totally clear, however. Some researchers consider more than 100 VPCs/24 hours to be consistent with ARVC, while others have used the criteria of >300 VPCs/24 hours or the presence of any ventricular tachycardia runs. Many affected Boxers have well over 1000 VPCs/24 hours. Between 50 and 100 (-300) VPCs/24-hour period could present a diagnostic "grey-zone." Less than 50 isolated VPCs/24 hours is within the realm of acceptable, if not assuredly normal. The number of VPCs found with Holter monitoring can vary widely from day to day and year to year in the same dog. Spontaneous variability of >80% in the number of VPCs/day has been reported in Boxers with ARVC (and >500 VPCs/24 hours); however, the severity grade of the arrhythmia appears to be fairly consistent for individual dogs.

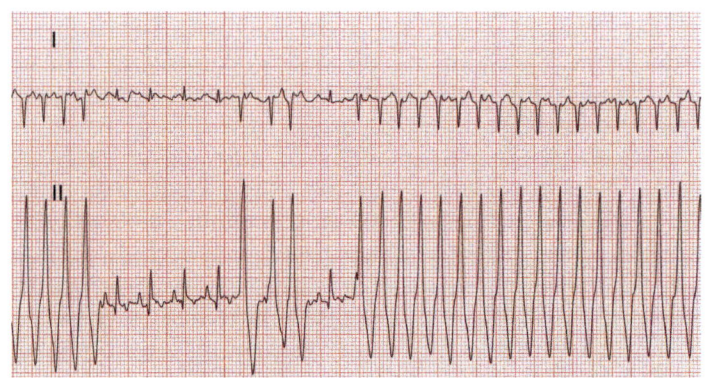

Figure 32.17 ECG from a 6-year-old male Boxer with recent collapse. Sinus activity is evident, but the predominant rhythm is a rapid ventricular tachycardia, with upright QRS configuration (left bundle branch block pattern) in lead II. This is typical for arrhythmogenic right ventricular cardiomyopathy (arrhythmogenic cardiomyopathy) in Boxers. Cardiac size and function were normal. Lidocaine suppressed the tachycardia and sotalol controlled it for at least 3 months, before the dog was lost to follow-up. Leads I & II; 25 mm/s, 1 cm=1 mV.

A Holter study in over 300 clinically normal Boxers showed that the number of VPCs/24 hours is quite low in most dogs (Stern, 2010). Arrhythmia frequency and grade increased with patient age, and the number of VPCs/24 hours was correlated with arrhythmia grade. Circadian variation in VPC frequency appears minimal, although a slight increase in VPC number might occur in mid- to late morning and early- to mid-evening.

While ventricular tachycardia probably is the most common cause for syncope in Boxers, sinus bradycardia or sinus arrest occasionally underlies the collapse episodes. These episodes of bradycardia are thought to be neurocardiogenic in nature. They usually are associated with excitement (as ventricular tachycardia also is). Some affected Boxers have concurrent ventricular tachyarrhythmias. Therefore, ambulatory ECG monitoring is important for evaluating dogs with episodic weakness or syncope. An event monitor or implantable loop recorder might be needed to document the heart rhythm during collapsing spells.

Radiographic findings are normal in dogs without ventricular dysfunction and dilation. Progressive cardiomegaly develops in those with the DCM phenotype. Infiltrates of pulmonary edema are expected with the onset of left-sided CHF; pulmonary venous enlargement often is seen, as well. Right-heart failure signs can include ascites, caudal vena caval distension, and pleural effusion. Cardiac MRI can show reduced myocardial function prior to ventricular dilation.

Echo findings vary from normal cardiac size and function to marked chamber dilation with poor contractility (**Figure 32.19**). Several echo measures can be used to evaluate myocardial function (see p. 614 and Chapter 4). RV function, as assessed using the index of myocardial performance (Tei index), could not differentiate ARVC Boxers without LV dysfunction from normal dogs. However, RV systolic function, as assessed by tricuspid annular plane systolic excursion (TAPSE; p. 94), was found to be reduced in Boxers with suspected ARVC and ≥50 VPCs/24 hr, compared to clinically normal Boxers (with <50 VPCs/24 hr; Kaye, 2015). In addition, a TAPSE <15.1 mm was associated with shorter survival time, even in dogs with normal measures of LV contractility; TAPSE was an independent predictor of time to cardiac death on multivariate analysis, with a Hazard ratio over 4.

Management

Boxers with a history of episodic weakness or syncope should undergo ambulatory ECG monitoring in an effort to identify the cardiac rhythm just prior to and during such episodes. Prior to prescribing a ventricular antiarrhythmic agent, it is important to verify that a ventricular tachyarrhythmia, rather than bradyarrhythmia, underlies the episodes. Sotalol and other drugs used to suppress ventricular ectopy could exacerbate episodic bradycardia and precipitate syncope in susceptible Boxers. In addition, echocardiography is indicated to evaluate myocardial function.

Antiarrhythmic therapy clearly is indicated in dogs with clinical signs caused by arrhythmias (see Chapters 24 and 25). Whether asymptomatic dogs should receive antiarrhythmic therapy is less clear, although dogs with complex or very frequent ventricular tachyarrhythmias typically are treated. Factors influencing the decision to treat include the severity of recorded arrhythmia, presence of ventricular dysfunction or dilation, the clinician's judgement, and owner preference. If possible, a pretreatment 24-hour Holter recording is obtained just prior to starting the antiarrhythmic drug, in order to better assess treatment efficacy. However, for dogs presented with symptomatic ventricular tachycardia, antiarrhythmic therapy should be started right away. Most cardiologists will treat dogs that have runs of ventricular tachycardia, whether sustained or not. How VPC couplets are viewed depends in part on their timing, because some are closely coupled on the prior T-wave and others clearly occur after the T-wave has been fully inscribed. The former tend be of more concern. Patterns of long-short cycle length that precipitate ventricular tachycardia also are of concern. When the number of VPCs/24h constitutes 20% or more of total heartbeats, or if the average *daily* heart rate exceeds 100 beats/minute, the potential for TICM probably is high; this might constitute another indication for therapy. Follow-up Holter monitoring is done a week or so after instituting antiarrhythmic therapy; a decrease of over 80% in VPC number and reduction in arrhythmia complexity define effective drug therapy. Sotalol and mexiletine have been shown to reduce arrhythmia severity and syncopal episode frequency. The authors typically use sotalol as the drug of first choice in ARVC. However, some Boxers respond better to a combination of both sotalol and mexiletine. Some Boxers require electrocardioversion to finally break sustained

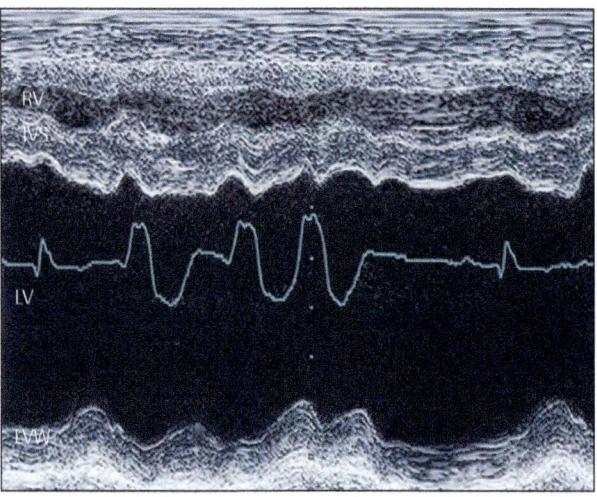

Figure 32.19 M-mode echocardiogram at the ventricular level from a 4-year-old female Boxer with arrhythmogenic cardiomyopathy and depressed left ventricular function (dilated cardiomyopathy phenotype). Fractional shortening in the dilated LV is poor. The 3 ventricular premature complexes visible here have an "upright" configuration, typical for Boxers (ECG displayed within the LV). Note the arrhythmia's effect on the motion of the IVS and LVW. IVS, interventricular septum; LV, left ventricle; LVW, left ventricular wall, RV, right ventricle.

ventricular tachycardia. In sporadic cases, amiodarone with a beta-blocker or another combination might be needed for arrhythmia control. No clear survival advantage has yet been identified among the different antiarrhythmic strategies.

For dogs with reduced myocardial function but no evidence for CHF, RAAS inhibition with an ACE inhibitor and spironolactone might be helpful. The use of pimobendan is unstudied in preclinical disease, and the previously noted recommendations for idiopathic DCM are suggested here. Therapy for dogs that have developed CHF is as for those with idiopathic DCM (p. 622, and Chapters 21 and 22). Because myocardial carnitine deficiency has been documented in a small number of Boxers with myocardial failure and CHF, a trial period of L-carnitine supplementation could be considered in Boxers with the DCM-phenotype (p. 634). However, few dogs show clinical response to this.

General recommendations for all dogs with ARVC include avoidance of strenuous exercise and excessive excitement. In addition, whether antiarrhythmic drug therapy is prescribed or not, adding a daily fish oil supplement could help reduce the number of VPCs. This was shown in a small study of Boxers with ARVC where fish oil capsules were given for 6 weeks at a dose of 2 gm (78 mg eicosapentaenoic acid and 497 mg docosahexaenoic acid) per day (Smith, 2007).

Prognosis The prognosis for dogs with ARVC is surprisingly variable. This might be due in part to misclassification of Boxers with occasional asymptomatic VPCs that faint from more benign neurocardiogenic mechanisms, but are misdiagnosed as ARVC. Despite the risk of sudden death and poor outcome in Boxers with CHF, overall prognosis for most Boxers with ARVC appears to be less dismal than previously thought. In one study, median survival age for ARVC dogs was 11 years, compared to 10 years for control dogs (Meurs, 2014). Thus, many affected Boxers have a normal life-span. Shorter survival time is associated with poor ventricular systolic function and increased frequency and complexity of ventricular tachyarrhythmia, including ventricular tachycardia and polymorphic VPCs. Even in dogs with normal LV function, reduced RV systolic function (as assessed by TAPSE) is associated with shorter survival, as noted in the paragraph on echo findings with ARVC. Older dogs are more likely to have greater arrhythmia frequency and complexity. In Boxers with normal LV function, the presence of ventricular tachycardia and older age were independent predictors of shorter survival (Motskula, 2013). There is conflicting evidence regarding whether males have worse prognosis. Likewise, reports conflict as to whether syncope is associated with worse outcome. One study found an almost five-fold increase in probability of death within a year for dogs with a history of syncope, despite the exclusion of dogs with LV dysfunction (Caro-Vadillo, 2013). Another found no association (Motskula, 2013). Results could be influenced by the age or LV function of the population studied, or whether syncope from causes other than ventricular tachycardia were included. The presence of atrial premature complexes, supraventricular tachycardia, or episodic bradycardia does not appear to influence patient outcome.

Hypertrophic Cardiomyopathy

Idiopathic HCM is rare in dogs. Although its cause is unknown, a genetic basis is suspected. As in cats, it might be that several disease processes produce similar ventricular changes. Secondary causes of LV hypertrophy must be ruled out. These include compensatory concentric hypertrophy induced by chronic systolic pressure overload (fixed or dynamic LV outflow obstruction, severe systemic hypertension), as well as trophic effects on the heart caused by excessive thyroid or growth hormone, persistent catecholamine release (as with pheochromocytoma), and chronic administration of an alpha- or beta-adrenergic agonist agent.

Dynamic LV outflow obstruction occasionally is identified in young dogs. Terrier breeds might be overrepresented. This usually is associated with mitral valve malformation and systolic anterior motion of the valve. Regression of the dynamic obstruction and LV hypertrophy over time, with or without treatment with a beta-blocker, suggests that this condition is not truly HCM.

Pathophysiology

Abnormal and excessive myocardial hypertrophy characterizes HCM. Similar to cats with HCM, increased ventricular stiffness leads to diastolic dysfunction (Chapter 33). The hypertrophy usually is symmetrical in dogs, although regional variation in wall or septal thickness can occur. Severe ventricular hypertrophy is likely to compromise coronary perfusion, which can provoke myocardial ischemia, exacerbate arrhythmias, slow ventricular active relaxation, and further impair filling. Increased LV diastolic (filling) pressure can cause pulmonary congestion and edema. These abnormalities are magnified when heart rate increases. In addition to impaired diastolic function, some dogs have dynamic LV outflow obstruction during systole. Malposition of mitral apparatus components could contribute to abnormal systolic mitral leaflet motion and dynamic outflow obstruction, as well as to MR. Asymmetrical septal hypertrophy also could contribute to outflow obstruction in some dogs. LV outflow obstruction increases ventricular wall stress and myocardial oxygen requirement. It also can further impair coronary flow and worsen ischemia. Whether dynamic LV outflow obstruction results from a congenital abnormality (of LV outflow tract or mitral apparatus structure) or is a form of primary myocardial disease can be unclear in a particular individual.

Clinical Features

Young to middle-aged, large breed dogs are more commonly diagnosed with HCM, although various breeds and a wide age distribution are affected. Males might be affected more often. Clinical signs of heart failure, episodic weakness, and syncope (presumably from ventricular ectopy) develop in some dogs. Sudden death can occur even before other signs appear. A systolic murmur of LV outflow obstruction or mitral insufficiency sometimes is heard. The ejection-type murmur of outflow obstruction becomes accentuated whenever ventricular contractility is increased (for example, with exercise or in the heartbeats following VPCs) or when systemic arterial pressure is decreased (as from a vasodilator). An atrial gallop sound (S_4) is evident in some affected dogs.

Diagnostic Tests

Thoracic radiographs could be normal or indicate LA and LV enlargement, with or without pulmonary edema. Ventricular tachyarrhythmias and conduction abnormalities, including complete heart block, 1st degree AV block, and fascicular blocks, appear to be common ECG findings. Criteria for LV enlargement are variably present. Characteristic echo findings include an abnormally thick LV wall, with or without LV outflow narrowing and asymmetrical septal hypertrophy, and LA enlargement. MR can be evident on Doppler studies. Sometimes, the RV wall is mildly to moderately thickened as well; this raises questions of whether some circulating trophic factor is involved, or if the disease has different manifestions in dogs. In these cases, volume depletion and pseudohypertrophy must be excluded. Dynamic LV outflow obstruction is associated with mitral valve systolic anterior motion (SAM) and partial mid-systolic aortic valve closure. Careful imaging of the mitral valve usually reveals leaflet thickening and possible chordal abnormalities. This thickening persists, even if the outflow obstruction improves in the future. Other causes of secondary LV hypertrophy should be excluded, including congenital SAS, systemic hypertension, thyrotoxicosis, pheochromocytoma, and a history of chronic sympathomimetic drug administration (such as phenylpropanolamine).

Management

Treatment goals are to enhance ventricular filling, control pulmonary edema, and suppress arrhythmias. A beta-blocker can help reduce HR and increase ventricular filling time, minimize LV outflow obstruction, decrease myocardial oxygen requirement, and reduce sympathetically mediated tachyarrhythmias. Resolution of dynamic LV outflow obstruction with atenolol therapy has been documented in several young dogs, although the exact cause of obstruction was unclear. Diltiazem also can reduce HR and might enhance myocardial relaxation, but would be less useful for ameliorating dynamic outflow obstruction, especially in view of its vasodilating effect. Both beta- and calcium-channel blocker drugs could worsen any AV conduction abnormality that might exist, and therefore, are relatively contraindicated in that situation. A diuretic and RAAS inhibition are suggested for congestive signs. Pimobendan could exacerbate dynamic LV outflow obstruction because of its positive inotropic and vasodilating effects. Furthermore, systolic function generally is not depressed in HCM; therefore, pimobendan probably is best avoided in these cases. An exception might be the development of chronic refractory CHF from advanced HCM; in such cases, pimobendan might help control CHF signs. Similarly, digoxin is avoided with hypertrophic heart disease because it could worsen outflow obstruction, increase myocardial oxygen requirement, and predispose to arrhythmias. Recommendations for monitoring, exercise restriction, and dietary considerations are as for other chronic heart failure patients (Chapter 22).

Secondary Myocardial Diseases

A variety of agents and conditions are known to harm the myocardium (**Table 32.4**). In this review, we classify known causes as secondary etiologies of myocardial disease or the DCM-phenotype. Acute myocardial injury can abruptly impair ventricular function, or progress more gradually to a secondary DCM. Often the initiating cause is unknown in end-stage disease. As for idiopathic DCM, arrhythmias often are a prominent feature of secondary myocardial diseases.

Tachycardia-Induced Cardiomyopathy

Rapid, incessant tachycardia causes progressive myocardial dysfunction, activation of neurohormonal compensatory mechanisms, and CHF. This is known as TICM; arrhythmia-induced cardiomyopathy and ectopy-induced cardiomyopathy are other names for this, especially in people. TICM is well-recognized in dogs with AV nodal reciprocating tachycardia associated with accessory conduction pathways that bypass the AV node (such as Wolff–Parkinson–White syndrome, p. 417). It also occurs with other sustained tachycardias and uncontrolled AF. Rapid artificial ventricular pacing (>200 beats/minute) is a common model for inducing experimental myocardial failure that simulates DCM. LV dysfunction also can result from frequent premature beats, as demonstrated by a pacing model simulating persistent ventricular bigeminy.

The ECG allows identification of the persistent tachyarrhythmia, which then guides antiarrhythmic therapy. Reentrant supraventricular tachycardia, atrial tachycardia, or AF underlies TICM most often. Nevertheless, a sustained or persistently recurrent ventricular tachyarrhythmia also can impair myocardial function. Radiographs commonly indicate cardiomegaly, with or without evidence for CHF. Echocardiography shows the extent of LV dilation and myocardial dysfunction, which is exacerbated during the tachycardia. Dogs with a concurrent congenital cardiac malformation show the associated structural abnormalities. In some cases, it is unclear whether the arrhythmia is the underlying cause of myocardial dysfunction or is a consequence of primary cardiomyopathy.

Table 32.4 Causes of Secondary Myocardial Disease and Myocarditis

Cardiac Toxins
- Anesthetic drugs
- Antineoplastic drugs (doxorubicin, p. 631; potentially also cyclophosphamide, 5-fluorouracil, interleukin-2, alpha-interferon)
- Catecholamines (endogenous, "brain–heart syndrome"; or exogenous amphetamines)
- Cobalt
- Cocaine
- Ethyl alcohol (when administered rapidly or undiluted for ethylene glycol toxicity)
- Heavy metals (arsenic, lead, mercury)
- Insect toxins (wasp or scorpion stings, spider bites)
- Ionophores (monensin)
- Other drugs (lithium, thyroid hormone)
- Plant toxins (*Taxus* species, foxglove, black locust, buttercups, lily-of-the-valley, gossypol)
- Snake venom

Infective Myocardial Diseases (p. 636)
- Bacterial (*B. burgdorferi*, *Bartonella* species, other)
- Protozoal (*T. cruzi*, *T. gondii*, *B. canis*, other)
- Rickettsial (and similar) organisms
- Viral (parvovirus, other)

Myocardial Inflammation
- Antimicrobial and diuretic drugs (hypersensitivity myocarditis documented in people)
- Immunologic responses to infectious agents
- Various systemic immune-mediated diseases (documented in people)

Myocardial Ischemia or Infarction (p. 636)
- Coronary atherosclerosis
- Coronary thromboembolic disease
- Intramural coronary arteriosclerosis

Neoplastic or Other Infiltrative Disease (p. 732)

Nutritional/metabolic deficiency (p. 632)
- Taurine
- L-carnitine
- Other diet-related issues

Other Metabolic or Endocrine Disease
- Diabetes mellitus
- Glycogen storage disease
- Hyperthyroidism
- Hypothyroidism
- Muscular dystrophies
- Pheochromocytoma

Tachycardia-Induced Cardiomyopathy (p. 630)
- Persistent tachycardia of supraventricular or ventricular origin, and atrial fibrillation with uncontrolled ventricular rate
- Frequent premature ventricular beats

Physical Injury
- Blunt or sharp trauma
- Electric shock
- Hyperthermia
- Hypothermia
- Ionizing radiation

Arrhythmia control is essential. Appropriate antiarrhythmic drug therapy should be instituted immediately (Chapters 24 and 25). Other therapy is directed at supporting myocardial function and controlling CHF, if present (Chapters 21 and 22). Cardiac electrophysiologic study with catheter ablation could successfully abolish the underlying arrhythmia in selected cases, especially those with an accessory pathway. This procedure is available at several cardiac specialty centers. Consultation with a veterinary cardiologist can help determine whether a particular patient would be a good candidate for an ablation procedure. If the arrhythmia can be controlled and heart rate normalized, the myocardial dysfunction associated with TICM usually improves greatly and sometimes resolves (Wright, 2018).

Doxorubicin Toxicity

The anthracycline antineoplastic drug doxorubicin induces both acute and chronic cardiotoxicity. Acute doxorubicin toxicity can include hypersensitivity reactions and anaphylaxis, arrhythmias, and tissue necrosis following extravasation. Histamine, secondary catecholamine release, and free-radical production appear to be involved in the pathogenesis of myocardial injury. Progressive myocardial damage and fibrosis develop with cumulative doses of over 160 mg/m^2, and sometimes as low as 100 mg/m^2. Histologic findings include myofibrillar degeneration and loss, sarcoplasmic vacuolar degeneration, and myocyte loss. Decreased myocardial function and arrhythmias result. In dogs with normal pretreatment cardiac function, clinical cardiotoxicity might not appear until the cumulative dose exceeds 240 mg/m^2, although echo evidence for reduced myocardial function can appear at <90 mg/m^2. Breeds with a higher prevalence of idiopathic DCM and dogs with underlying cardiac disease appear to have greater risk for doxorubicin-induced cardiotoxicity. In a survey of almost 500 dogs treated with doxorubicin, breeds at high risk for DCM had a 15% incidence of clinical cardiotoxicity, while low-risk breeds had a 3% incidence (Hallman, 2019). Anthracycline-induced cardiomyopathy is irreversible and can be the cause of death.

Clinical features are similar to those of idiopathic DCM. Elevated serum cTnT and cTnI concentrations have been found in dogs after doxorubicin administration. Circulating cardiac troponin concentrations might become useful in monitoring for doxorubicin-induced myocardial injury; however, specific guidelines are not clear. Elevations in NT-proBNP can become apparent as chronic cardiotoxicity develops.

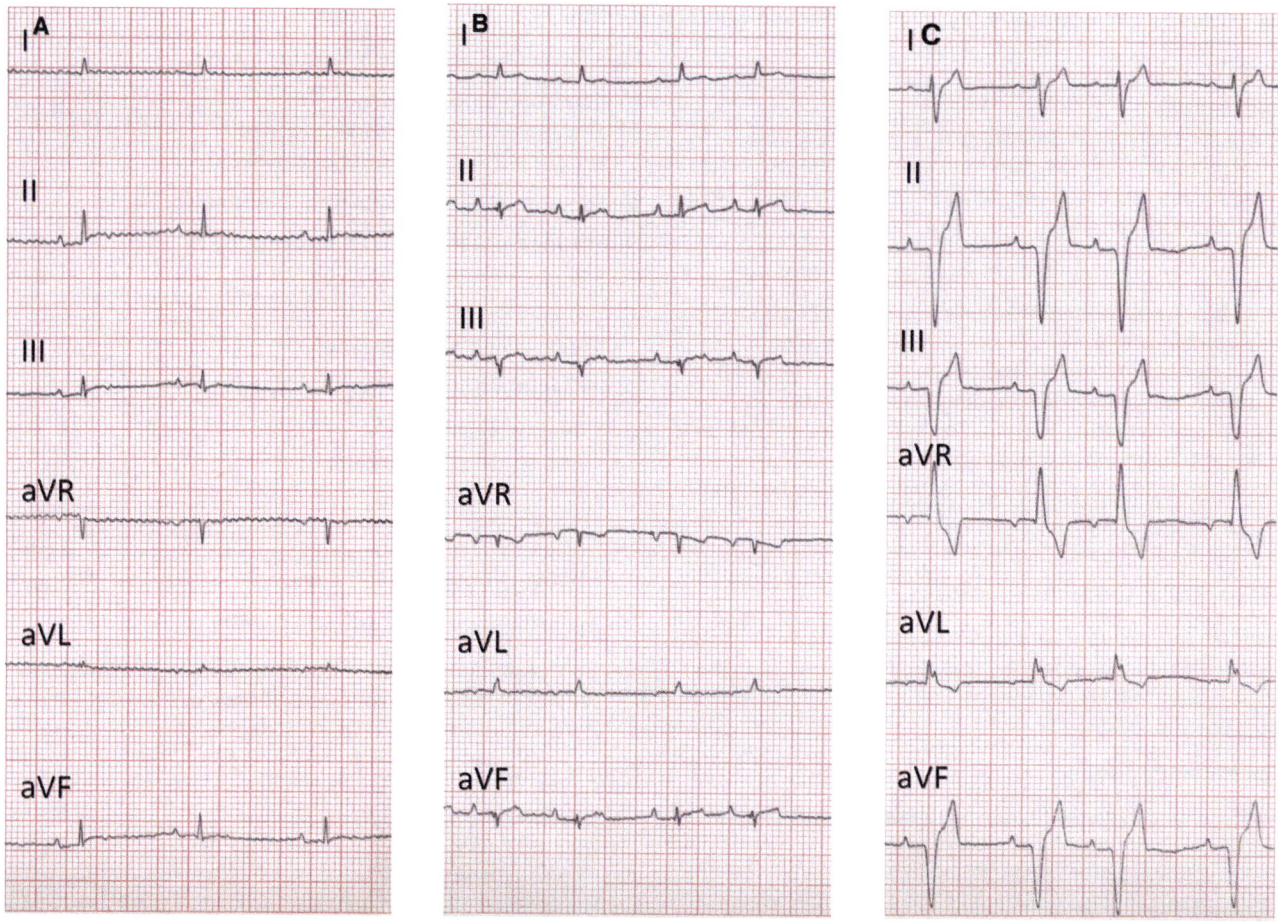

Figure 32.20 An 11-year-old female Standard Schnauzer with gastric adenocarcinoma initially was treated with doxorubicin. (A) ECG recorded about the time of the first doxorubicin dose. Although QRS complex voltages are small, the mean electrical axis is normal. There is some baseline 60 Hz artifact. (B) Four weeks later, subtle shifts in QRS morphology and a left axis deviation are evident. (C) Five weeks after the first recording (A), the ECG now shows a complete right bundle branch block pattern. Doxorubicin was discontinued and 5-fluorouracil instituted. This dog's cumulative doxorubicin dose was not excessive (exact dose unclear from available records). Leads as marked, 25 mm/s, 1 cm = 1 mV.

Ventricular and supraventricular tachyarrhythmias can occur acutely during or following drug infusion. They also can accompany chronic cardiotoxicity. Infranodal AV and bundle branch blocks sometimes develop (**Figure 32.20**). However, ECG changes do not necessarily precede clinical heart failure. Chronic cardiotoxicity produces echo changes related to reduced LV contractility and progressive ventricular dilation. These can develop at variable cumulative doxorubicin dosage. The M-mode and 2D changes are like those of other causes of DCM. Early decline in LV diastolic function, as indicated by reduced Doppler mitral E/A ratio compared to pretreatment value, reportedly occurs prior to 2D echo changes in dogs. Early evidence for chronic cardiotoxicity also was shown with tissue Doppler imaging in people.

When ventricular tachyarrhythmias are found on pretreatment ECG, doxorubicin infusion often is delayed or suspended. Echo evidence for deteriorating myocardial function is an indication to discontinue doxorubicin therapy whenever possible. Clearly, this decision depends on patient status and availability of other antineoplastic treatment options. Therapy for anthracycline-induced cardiomyopathy is similar to that for other causes of DCM.

Strategies for avoiding anthracycline-induced cardiomyopathy could include using epirubicin (49-epidoxorubicin), a related compound with lesser cardiotoxicity; co-administration of an agent such as dexrazoxane, which inhibits anthracycline free-radical induction; liposome encapsulated doxorubicin; or alternative antineoplastic agents. Attempts to provide cardioprotection using a calcium-channel or beta-adrenergic blocking drug, phosphodiesterase-5 inhibitor, ACE inhibitor, or anticytokine agent have not been effective. It is unclear whether use of certain antioxidant substances could reduce cardiotoxicity. Doxycycline infusion duration does not appear to influence the development of clinical cardiotoxicity.

Nutritional Deficiencies and Metabolic Abnormalities

DCM is associated with dietary factors in some dogs. Certain breed predispositions to deficiencies in taurine, L-carnitine, or both and the related development of a DCM phenotype were recognized years ago. These include taurine (with or without L-carnitine) deficiency in American Cocker Spaniels and L-carnitine-associated DCM in a small number of Doberman Pinschers and Boxers. However, in recent years a growing number of other cases of systolic myocardial dysfunction are suspected to be diet-related. These involve breeds not usually affected by DCM, mixed-breed dogs, as well as the more typical large breeds. Much concern is focused on the amino acid taurine, which is the main nutrient discussed in the next paragraphs. Nevertheless, abnormalities related to other nutrients or their combinations could be involved, especially because blood taurine concentration appears adequate in the majority of these cases. Problems could stem from deficiencies in the food as fed, reduced nutrient uptake, or factors related to nutrient metabolism. Various diets have been implicated, including commercial lamb meal and rice-based diets; some "boutique," exotic protein-based or grain-free (sometimes collectively referred to as "BEG") diets; low protein, high fiber, vegetarian or vegan diets; and home-made diets. Although the scientific merits of reports and retrospective studies on diet-related DCM have been criticized by members of the pet food industry (McCauley, 2020), experienced clinicians are observing more cases of partially to completely reversible DCM following dietary changes from certain BEG diets. A preliminary United States Federal Drug Administration (FDA) report noted that, in reported cases of DCM where only a single primary diet was fed, 90% of the foods involved were labelled "grain-free" or zero grain; 10% of the diets contained grains, although some were vegan or vegetarian (FDA, 2019). A large proportion of the reported diets included peas or lentils. Yet, almost all the diets appeared to have a content of crude protein, fat, fiber, starch, cysteine, methionine, and taurine comparable to the nongrain-free diets analyzed. Investigations are on-going; veterinarians are urged to obtain complete diet histories on suspected diet-related DCM cases and to report these cases to the FDA[1]. It also might be useful for the pet owner to save packaging labels and food samples for possible analysis. In addition, other dogs in the household that eat the same diet should be screened for myocardial dysfunction. Yet many dogs fed these types of diets do not develop overt DCM. Furthermore, it is possible that completely different factors underlie DCM in some of these cases.

Links between the "BEG" or other diets and DCM might involve: the use of a high percentage of pulses (such as lentils, peas, chickpeas, fava beans, and others) or potatoes as replacements for grain ingredients; other components like unusual or exotic meat proteins, flaxseed, or probiotics; imbalances of nutrients within the diet; "anti-nutritional" factors (such as trypsin or chymotrypsin inhibitors) normally present in some ingredients, but not destroyed by heat-processing; or possible inadvertent inclusion of toxic components (Freeman, 2018; Mansilla, 2019). Furthermore, even diets that might seem equivalent could have substantial differences in nutrient bioavailability. For example, some grain-free diets have been associated with more pronounced negative effects on cardiac remodeling (greater increase in LV dimensions and sphericity) compared to other grain-free diets (Adin, 2019). Longer survival after hospital release has been identified in retrospective studies of DCM in dogs switched from BEG diets to more conventional diets, although these results have been challenged. Prospective studies are needed to identify the potential cardiac issues and mechanisms associated with diets high in pulses/legumes.

Multiple factors could influence the bioavailability of taurine and its precursor amino acids (especially methionine), or other nutrients, in diets that seem to contain adequate amounts. Such factors could include effects of manufacturing processes, the particular source ingredients used, and impaired nutrient absorption related to effects of other ingredients (Mansilla, 2019). For example, diets with a high concentration of pulse ingredients or soybean meal, while apparently high in protein, can have important imbalances in amino acids, including low methionine content; intestinal protein digestibility can be lower, also. In addition, plant-based ingredients are low in taurine. Diets high in fiber, including beet pulp and legume ingredients, increase the amount of taurine or its precursors (such as methionine and cysteine) needed in the diet because of the effects of fermentation (including intestinal microbial degradation of taurine) and greater fecal excretion of taurine-conjugated bile. Physiologic or metabolic factors also could influence taurine status in some cases. For example, taurine synthesis tends to be lower in large dogs, because of their comparatively lower metabolic rate, than in small dogs. Likewise, taurine requirements might differ among breeds or morphologic body types.

Taurine Taurine serves as a mediator for various biologic processes. It comprises about 60% of the total free amino acid content in the heart. Taurine is thought to increase myofilament sensitivity to Ca^{++} and Ca^{++} reuptake into the sarcoplasmic reticulum. Reduced taurine intake or synthesis, therefore, could have negative effects on myocardial calcium handling and contractility. Unlike cats, dogs can synthesize taurine from dietary methionine and cysteine.

DCM is associated with taurine deficiency in some dogs, as well as in cats (p. 682). American Cocker Spaniels with DCM often have low plasma taurine, and sometimes carnitine, concentrations. Oral supplementation of these two amino acids has improved LV function and reduced the need for heart failure medication in this breed; supplementation with taurine only is useful in some of these dogs. Taurine deficiency has not been identified as a common cause for DCM in English Cocker Spaniels, which often have a prolonged course of DCM. Other breeds with possible predisposition to taurine deficiency are the Golden Retriever and perhaps Newfoundlands, Irish Wolfhounds, English Setters, and Saint Bernards. In Irish Wolfhounds, whole blood taurine concentrations do not appear to be correlated with DCM; low taurine levels were found in some dogs with DCM, as well as some without. It is unclear whether certain dogs have lower rates of taurine biosynthesis or increased taurine loss, which could predispose them to cardiomyopathy even when dietary taurine content is thought to be adequate. Sporadic cases of DCM accompanied by a low taurine concentration have occurred in Labrador Retrievers, Dalmatians, and others. Taurine deficiency in some dogs has been associated with low-protein, lamb meal-based, or high-fiber diets. Low blood taurine was identified in some Newfoundland dogs without clinical DCM that were eating lamb and rice diets. High-fat/low-protein diets also could lead to decreased blood and plasma taurine. Newer grain-free and other diets have been implicated in the development of DCM, as well (see previous paragraphs).

Whole blood samples are preferred for measuring taurine concentration. Most taurine is located intracellularly, including within platelets. Plasma free taurine concentrations are comparatively low and might not accurately represent taurine status. Nevertheless, whole blood might not always accurately represent taurine content in muscle tissue. Thrombocytopenic blood samples also can underestimate taurine status. Specific sample collection and submission requirements should be confirmed with the testing laboratory. Whole blood taurine concentrations <200 (or 150) nmol/mL are considered deficient. However, DCM responsive to taurine supplementation and diet change has occurred in some Golden Retrievers with whole blood taurine concentrations between 200 and 250 nmol/mL. This suggests that adequate taurine levels in this breed might be >250 nmol/mL; there could be other important breed variations, as well (Freeman, 2018). Plasma taurine concentrations <25 (to 40) nmol/mL also are considered deficient.

While some dogs with suspected diet-related DCM have reduced blood taurine levels, most do not. Taurine supplementation and a change in diet can bring improvement not only in dogs with low blood taurine, but also in some with normal taurine concentrations. Recommendations for taurine supplementation are 250 mg PO q12h for dogs weighing <10 kg; 500 mg PO q12h for dogs between 10–25 kg; and 1000 mg PO q12h for dogs >25 kg. The supplement can be mixed into the food. Supplementation for 3–6 months usually is needed to determine if echo improvement will occur. Feeding a diet made by a well-established pet food manufacturer that contains standard ingredients, or consultation with a veterinary nutritionist for other dietary recommendations, is advised. Other therapy is as for DCM in general (p. 622). The prognosis is good for dogs that respond to taurine supplementation or diet change. Gradual decrease and eventual withdrawal of heart failure therapy is possible in some dogs.

L-carnitine DCM has been associated with L-carnitine–linked defects in myocardial metabolism in some dogs. Systemic carnitine deficiency is a known cause of DCM in children and adults with primary carnitine deficiency, an autosomal recessive disorder of fatty acid metabolism. Inherited or acquired metabolic defects, rather than simple L-carnitine deficiency, are suspected in dogs, as well. L-carnitine is present in high concentrations in cardiac and skeletal muscle. It is an essential component of the mitochondrial membrane transport system for fatty acids, which are the heart's primary energy source. It also binds with and transports potentially toxic metabolites out of the mitochondria; excess production of such metabolites can result in L-carnitine depletion. L-carnitine is present mainly in foods of animal origin. Although dogs can synthesize carnitine from lysine and methionine, DCM has developed in some dogs fed strict vegetarian diets. An association between DCM and carnitine deficiency might exist in some families of Boxers, Doberman Pinschers, Cocker Spaniels, and possibly Great Danes, Irish Wolfhounds, and Newfoundlands. Clinical and echo findings are similar to those caused by idiopathic DCM. Plasma carnitine concentration is not a sensitive indicator of myocardial carnitine deficiency, although it is specific (at <8 mmol/L free carnitine). Most dogs with myocardial carnitine deficiency or abnormal esterified:free carnitine ratio confirmed on endomyocardial biopsy, have had normal or high plasma carnitine concentrations.

Management is as for DCM in general (p. 622). L-carnitine supplementation is indicated when deficiency is suspected, although the response to oral carnitine supplementation is inconsistent and few dogs have shown echo evidence of improved function since the initial reports. Supplemental L-carnitine does not suppress preexisting arrhythmias or prevent sudden death. Only the L-carnitine isomer should be used for supplementation. Dosage guidelines are 1 g (for dogs <25 kg) to 2 g (for dogs 25–40 kg) mixed with food, q8h. Up to 200 mg/kg PO q8h also has been recommended. About 1/2 teaspoonful of pure substance contains 1 g. Dogs that respond generally show improved activity within a month.

Echo improvement appears in some dogs after 2–3 months of supplementation, although a response plateau usually is reached in 6–8 months. Medication for CHF usually is still needed. The prognosis for dogs that respond to L-carnitine treatment is likely to be good, with continued supplementation. For dogs that show no echo improvement after 3 months of supplementation, L-carnitine usually is discontinued. Their outcome is likely to be similar to that with other causes of DCM.

Catecholamine-Associated Myocardial Disease Excessive sympathetic stimulation from brain or spinal cord injury causes myocardial hemorrhage, necrosis, and arrhythmias (so-called brain–heart syndrome). Catecholamine-secreting pheochromocytomas of the adrenal medulla also cause cardiac pathology, as well as severe hypertension. Catecholamines, especially norepinephrine, secreted by functional tumors can stimulate tachycardia and arrhythmias, as well as cardiac hypertrophy and other injury. Although described in only a minority of canine pheochromocytoma cases, postmortem cardiac lesions include multifocal cardiomyocyte degeneration and necrosis with contraction bands, myocardial hemorrhage, lymphohistiocytic myocarditis, and interstitial fibrosis. These findings are similar to catecholamine-induced cardiomyopathy reported in people with pheochromocytoma. Mechanisms underlying catecholamine-induced cardiomyocyte damage include coronary vasoconstriction and vasospasm, which lead to local myocardial hypoxia or infarction. High catecholamine concentrations also can increase intracellular Ca^{++} to levels which have a direct toxic effect on cardiomyocytes. The effects of systemic hypertension, persistent tachycardia, oxidation injury and other factors might be involved with pheochromocytoma, as well. Phenylpropanolamine, administered chronically or at high dosage, also can stimulate arrhythmias and myocardial hypertrophy, as well as hypertension.

Clinically evident effects of excess catecholamine stimulation can include unexplained tachycardia, agitation, and systemic hypertension. Besides a complete history and physical evaluation, blood pressure measurements, ECG, an imaging search for a possible endogenous source of excess catecholamine exposure, and echocardiogram are advised. Arrhythmias associated with pheochromocytoma in dogs have included idioventricular rhythms, premature atrial and ventricular contractions, and surprisingly, complete (3rd degree) AV block. Repolarization abnormalities and QT prolongation have been associated with pheochromocytoma in people, although these have yet to be reported in dogs. Echocardiography might show ventricular dilation or unexpected myocardial hypertrophy.

Antihypertensive therapy can include alpha- and beta-adrenergic blocking agents, an ACE inhibitor, or calcium-channel blocker (Chapter 38). Captopril, an older ACE inhibitor, might have additional benefit because of its free-radical scavenging effect. Free-radical damage is thought to contribute to the cardiac pathology of catecholamine-induced cardiomyopathy. Calcium-channel blockers might reduce vasospasm and its consequences. When possible, surgical excision of pheochromocytoma should be pursued.

Muscular Dystrophy Muscular dystrophy of the fasciohumoral type is reported in Springer Spaniels. It can result in atrial standstill (p. 416) and heart failure. Canine X-linked muscular dystrophy also has been associated with myocardial fibrosis and mineralization; this disease is analogous to Duchenne muscular dystrophy in people. Although described mainly in Golden Retrievers, the mutation has occurred in Labrador Retrievers and other breeds. The mutation causes loss of dystrophin, a cytoskeletal protein important to normal muscle structure and signaling pathways.

Lack of dystrophin leads to progressive muscle wasting and fibrosis. The associated cardiomyopathy is characterized by cardiomyocyte loss with replacement fibrosis. Affected dogs typically develop a slowly progressive skeletal myopathy and a dilated form of cardiomyopathy. In rare cases, signs suggestive of acute myocardial infarction can occur, with markedly elevated cTnI and NT-proBNP concentrations and tachyarrhythmias. LV wall motion abnormalities can be identified using tissue Doppler imaging, even before other signs of reduced contractility appear in dogs with X-linked muscular dystrophy. Other early echo changes include hyperechoic foci within the ventricular myocardium that represent fatty, fibrotic, and/or mineralized changes. Reduced global LV function and progressive chamber dilation develop with advancing cardiomyopathy. NT-proBNP concentrations also rise. Thoracic radiographic abnormalities can include diaphragmatic asymmetry, as well as progressive cardiomegaly. The ECG typically shows deep Q waves in the caudal leads, with increased ratio of Q-to-R wave amplitudes, and shortened PR interval. Various arrhythmias can occur. ACE inhibitor therapy has been tried for management prior to CHF onset with unclear effect. Experimental evidence suggests that phosphodiesterase-5 inhibition could slow the onset of dystrophic cardiomyopathy. Signs of CHF and arrhythmias are treated with standard therapy (Chapters 22 and 25).

Other Conditions Reduced myocardial function also has been associated with diseases such as hypothyroidism and diabetes mellitus; however, clinical heart failure secondary to these conditions alone is unusual in dogs. Obese dogs can have mild LV hypertrophy with mild diastolic dysfunction (as indicated by slight IVRT prolongation), as well as slightly elevated systolic blood pressure. Clinically evident consequences typically are absent.

Rarely, nonneoplastic (such as glycogen storage disease) and neoplastic (metastatic and primary) infiltrative myocardial diseases can interfere with normal myocardial function (also see p. 732). Immunologic mechanisms might play an important role in the pathogenesis of myocardial dysfunction in some dogs. Autoantibodies directed against the heart have been found in some dogs with apparent DCM. The extent to which free radical damage causes clinical myocardial injury is not clear. Evidence for increased oxidative stress occurs in dogs, as well as people, with CHF and myocardial failure. A negative correlation between disease severity and plasma vitamin E concentration has been observed in dogs with DCM.

Disease conditions that induce systemic inflammatory response, especially sepsis but also trauma, major surgery, cancer, autoimmune or other inflammatory diseases, and heatstroke can be associated with depressed myocardial function. Circulating cTnI is a marker of myocardial injury in dogs with systemic inflammatory disease. Higher cTnI concentrations are associated with poor short-term outcome. In patients that survive the underlying disease process, the myocardial depression can be reversible. Some circulating myocardial depressant factor(s) is thought to be causative, rather than hypotension alone. Various inflammatory cytokines, including TNF-alpha, might negatively affect myocardial function directly or by altering Ca^{++} homeostasis, reducing cyclic adenosine monophosphate (cAMP) production, or triggering sympathetic neural overstimulation. Activation of toll-like receptors could play a mediating role.

Ischemic Heart Disease

Acute myocardial infarction caused by coronary embolization occurs uncommonly in dogs. In most cases, there is an underlying disease associated with increased risk for thromboembolism (TE), such as bacterial endocarditis, neoplasia, severe renal disease, immune-mediated hemolytic anemia, acute pancreatitis, disseminated intravascular coagulation (DIC), or corticosteroid use. Myocardial infarction also has occurred sporadically in dogs with congenital ventricular outflow tract obstructions, patent ductus arteriosus (PDA), HCM, and degenerative mitral valve disease (DMVD). In dogs with advanced DMVD, a partial LA tear would promote localized mural thrombus formation and increase the risk for coronary and systemic arterial embolization. Atherosclerosis of major coronary arteries is rare in dogs; however, it can accompany hypercholesterolemia from severe hypothyroidism and diabetes mellitus. Occasionally, this leads to acute myocardial infarction, as well as thrombosis and infarction of other tissues.

Nonatherosclerotic narrowing of small coronary arteries might be more clinically important than previously appreciated. Hyalinization of small intramural coronary vessels and intramural myocardial infarctions occur with DMVD. These also are seen in older dogs without endocardiosis. Fibromuscular arteriosclerosis of small coronary vessels is described, too. These mural changes cause coronary luminal narrowing and could impair resting coronary blood flow and vasodilatory responses. Small myocardial infarctions, focal myocardial necrosis, and secondary fibrosis can lead to myocardial function deterioration and a variety of tachyarrhythmias and conduction disturbances. One study of dogs with histopathologically confirmed intramural coronary arteriosclerosis (with or without multiple chronic or acute infarctions) found that almost half of the cases had died from CHF (Falk, 2000). An additional 20% of cases died suddenly; most of these had hyaline arteriosclerosis without degenerative valve disease. Another 15% of cases died during or after general anesthesia. Moderately decreased myocardial contractility was evident in most cases that had an echocardiogram. The majority of dogs in this study were of larger breeds; Cocker Spaniels and Cavalier King Charles Spaniels were the most common small breeds. Myocardial necrosis also has been associated with some drugs, central nervous system (CNS) lesions, trauma, stress, pancreatitis, gastric dilatation/volvulus, viral infections, splenic masses, immune-mediated hemolytic anemia, renal disease, and neoplasia.

Acute obstruction of a major coronary artery would be likely to cause abrupt onset of arrhythmias, pulmonary edema, marked ST segment changes on ECG, and regional or widespread myocardial dysfunction evident on an echocardiogram. Various rhythm disturbances, depressed contractility, progressive ventricular enlargement, and CHF also can occur with more chronic coronary artery disease. Increased circulating cTnI and creatine kinase concentrations are expected with myocardial injury and necrosis. Evidence for TE elsewhere might also be present.

Therapy is aimed at managing arrhythmias, supporting myocardial function, and controlling signs of CHF (Chapters 22 and 25). Underlying disease conditions should be addressed as possible. Antiplatelet prophylaxis could be helpful when risk of TE is increased (Chapter 36). A beta-blocker could reduce (myocardial oxygen) demand ischemia, and possibly, arrhythmias. This is the rationale for empirical use of atenolol in dogs with severe congenital subaortic stenosis. Prognosis is affected by the underlying disease process and extent of myocardial damage. There is increased risk for sudden death, and for progressive CHF.

Infective Myocarditis

Many infectious agents can affect the myocardium, although disease manifestations in other organ systems often predominate. In a recent case series of approximately 200 dogs diagnosed with myocarditis, an infectious cause was identified in 55% (Lakhdhir, 2020). Direct invasion by an infective agent, elaborated toxins, or host immune responses can cause myocardial injury. The classic clinical presentation of acute myocarditis involves an unexplained onset of arrhythmias or heart failure after a recent episode of infective disease or drug exposure. However, findings often are nonspecific and identifying the specific etiology in a case of suspected myocarditis can be difficult. Definitive antemortem diagnosis in people is based on histologic confirmation from endomyocardial biopsy specimens. Evidence for myocardial inflammation and injury is expected on postmortem exam, although the causative agent is not always identified.

Clinical Features and Diagnostic Tests

Cardiac arrhythmias and impaired myocardial function are likely consequences of myocarditis. These can cause clinical signs of lethargy, reduced appetite, weakness, syncope, CHF, or sudden death, in addition to systemic signs of the infection. Fever and cardiac murmur also are common; some dogs show gastrointestinal (GI) signs, as well. For other signs associated with specific organisms, see sections that follow.

Elevated cTnI concentrations provide an indication of active myocardial damage, although not specific cause. Serum cTnI concentration increases within 2 hours of myocardial injury and peaks 12–24 hours after initial insult. Persistent cTnI elevation is consistent with ongoing, active myocyte damage. Dramatic increases exceeding 50 ng/mL sometimes are encountered. Other laboratory tests recommended as part of a broad database could include CBC, serum biochemical profile, urinalysis, thoracic and abdominal radiographs, an echocardiogram, and ECG. Common findings on CBC have included thrombocytopenia, neutrophilia, monocytosis, and anemia. Biochemical abnormalities might include elevated liver enzymes, hypoalbuminemia, hypocalcemia, or azotemia. In dogs with persistent fever, serial blood cultures occasionally are rewarding.

Serologic or PCR tests help identify exposure to certain infectious agents. However, inconsistent clinical presentation and lack of specific noninvasive tests often makes establishing a definitive diagnosis difficult. The diagnostic criteria for myocarditis are histologic and include inflammatory infiltrates with myocyte degeneration and necrosis. Endomyocardial biopsy specimens currently are the only means of obtaining a definitive antemortem diagnosis. While endomyocardial biopsy is available in some veterinary specialty settings, the procedure is not without risk. Furthermore, findings might not be diagnostic if the lesions are focal and representative myocardial samples are missed. In many cases, the underlying cause of myocarditis remains unknown.

The ECG might show nonspecific changes (such as an ST segment shift, T wave or QRS voltage change, or AV conduction abnormality), as well as various arrhythmias. Ventricular tachyarrhythmias are most common, and can be highly resistant to medical therapy. Supraventricular tachycardia or various bradyarrhythmias, including AV block, occur occasionally. Radiographs might indicate cardiomegaly, evidence for CHF, or other abnormalities. Echocardiography sometimes reveals areas of abnormal myocardial echogenicity, thickening, reduced regional or global ventricular wall motion, or pericardial effusion (**Figures 32.21** and **32.22**).

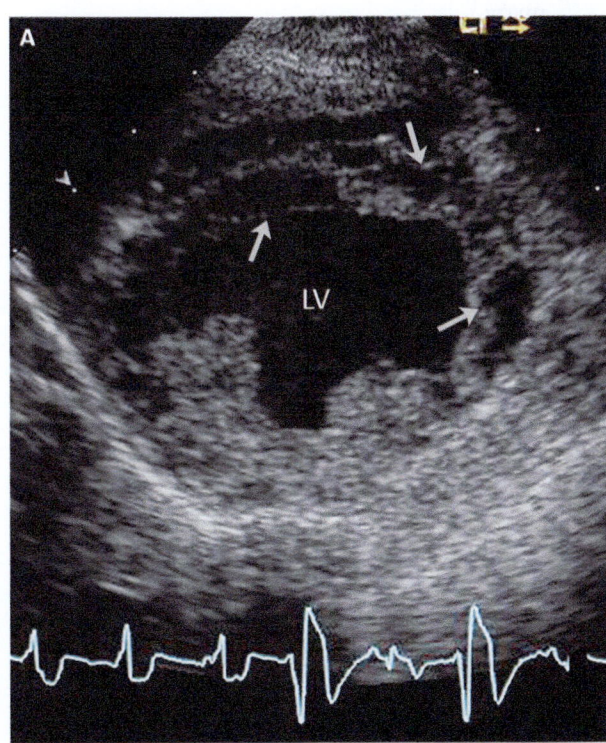
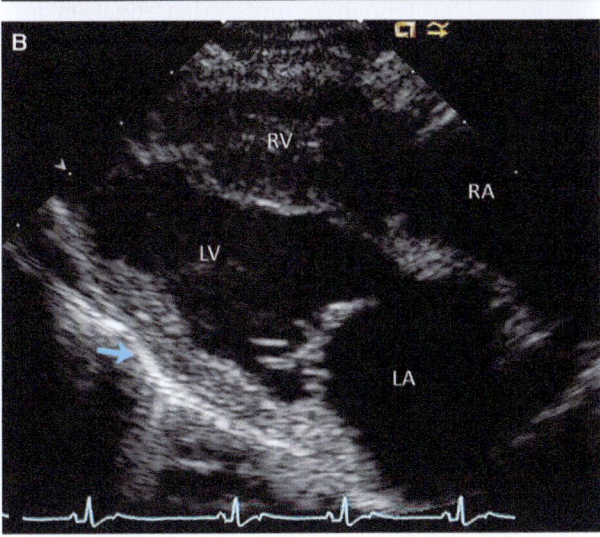
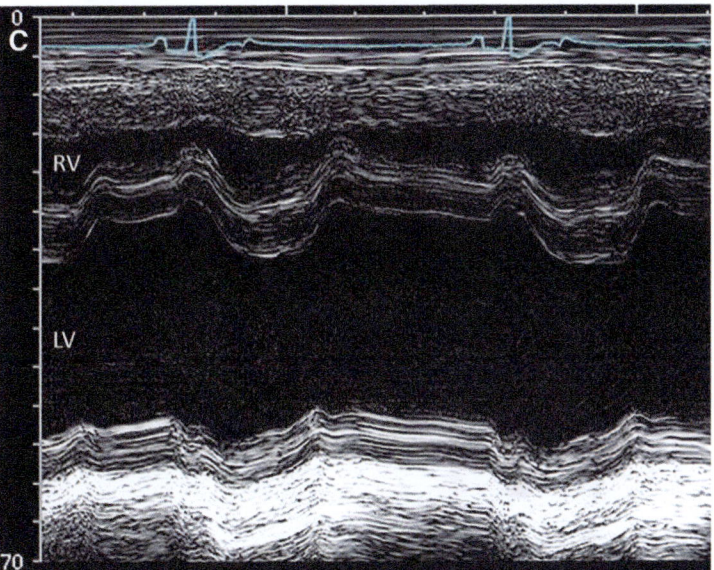

Figure 32.21 (A) Right parasternal short-axis image in diastole from a 4-year-old female Pembroke Welsh Corgi with lethargy, weakness episodes, decreased exercise tolerance, heavy breathing, and weight loss. Left ventricular size and function appeared normal at this time. However, the ventricular myocardium looked mottled, with areas of hypoechogenicity (arrows) and variable hyperechogenicity. An intermittent accelerated idioventricular rhythm, some multiform ventricular premature complexes (VPCs), and paroxysmal ventricular tachycardia occurred during the echo exam. Mild left atrial enlargement and a small volume of cellular pericardial effusion also were present (not visible here). Cardiac troponin (cTn)I was >40 ng/mL. Treatment with sotalol, enalapril, and a combination of antimicrobial drugs was begun. Test results for multiple infectious causes of myocarditis were negative. A week later, the dog was clinically improved, in sinus rhythm with only occasional VPCs, and had normal ventricular chamber size and no pericardial effusion. However, the mid-region of the left ventricular free wall showed dyskinetic motion. (B) By 5 weeks after initial presentation, the dog was clinically well and cTnI was 0.11 ng/mL. Yet the area of dyskinesis persisted and left ventricular diameter had increased. This long-axis image in systole shows outward bulging of the mid-dorsal left ventricular wall (arrow). Mitral regurgitation and thinning of apical wall and posterior papillary muscle also had developed. (C) M-mode image at mid-ventricular level shows systolic left freewall motion in the opposite direction from the vigorous septal motion. Although the etiology of the myocarditis is unknown, the dog remained clinically stable for at least 3 more years. LA, left atrium; LV, left ventricle; RA, right atrium; RV, right ventricle.

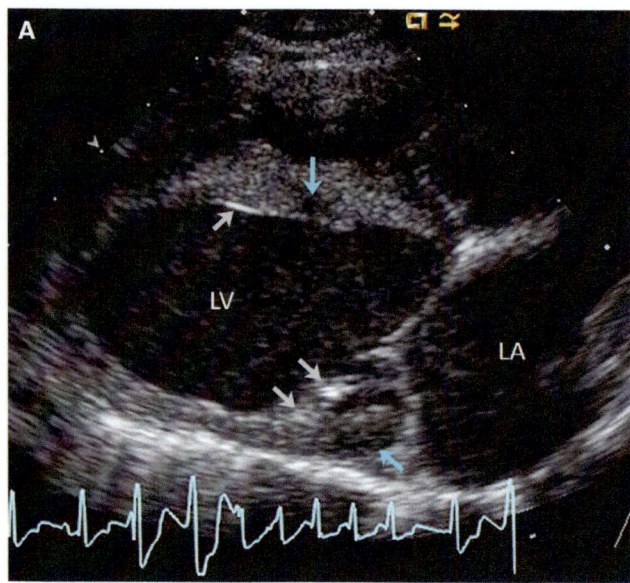
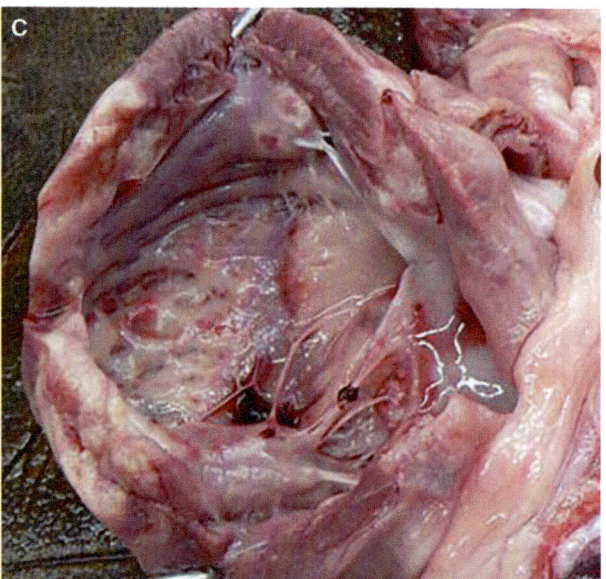
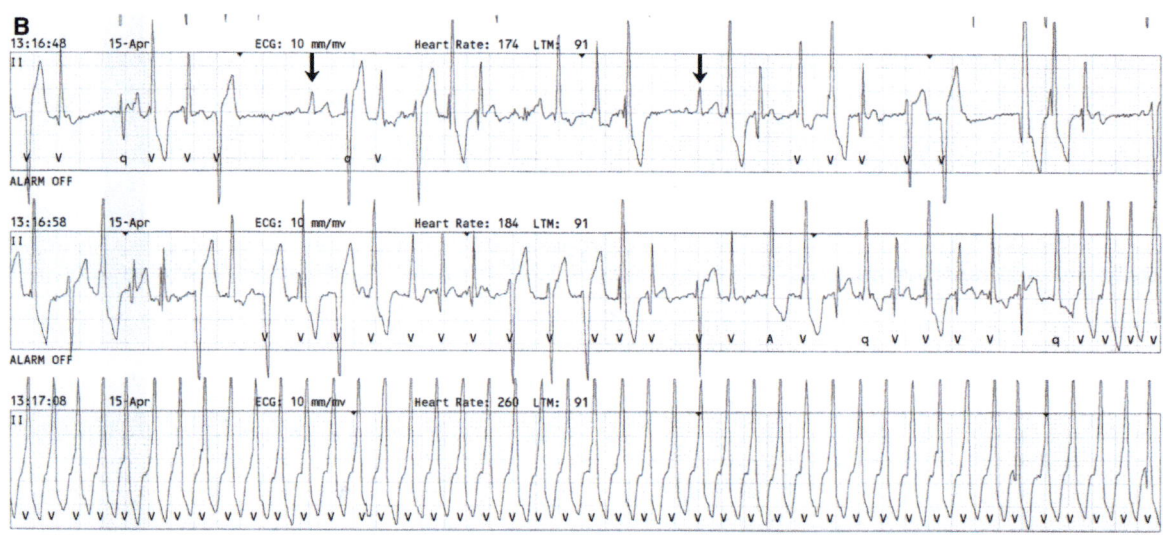

Figure 32.22 (A) The ventricular myocardium has a mottled appearance, with areas of both hyperechogenicity (grey arrows) and lucency (blue arrows), in a 4-month-old female Vizsla. Spontaneous contrast appears within the mildly dilated left ventricle (LV) and left atrium (LA). The ECG monitor lead shows a variable ventricular tachyarrhythmia. Right parasternal long-axis view, early systole. (B) Portion of a continuous lead II ECG recording from this puppy shows paroxysms of irregular, multiform ventricular tachycardia, with only occasional sinus complexes (arrows, top strip). The rhythm evolves into a rapid, monomorphic ventricular tachycardia at 260 beats/min (middle to bottom strips). (C) Postmortem image of the open LV from this pup (apex to the left); the anterior mitral leaflet has been partially incised. Large, full thickness pale regions are visible within the interventricular septum and toward the ventricular apex, along with areas of intramyocardial hemorrhage. Based on gross appearance, lymphoma was suspected; however, histopathology showed widespread suppurative to lymphohistiocytic inflammation, with areas of myocardial necrosis and fibrosis. No bacterial or protozoal agents were identified despite application of multiple special stains, and immunohistochemistry for Toxoplasma and Neospora spp. Although the specific cause was not determined, it is possible that a drug, environmental substance, cardiotropic virus or other infective agent could have triggered a hypersensitivity reaction. At least one other puppy from the same breeding was found to have similar lesions.

Management

Therapy for suspected myocarditis is largely supportive, unless the specific etiology can be identified and treated. Management strategies include: strict rest; antiarrhythmic therapy as appropriate (Chapter 25); an ACE inhibitor, with or without pimobendan, for myocardial dysfunction; furosemide and other therapy as indicated for signs of CHF (Chapter 22); antibiotic therapy for suspected bacterial myocarditis; and other supportive measures, as needed. Corticosteroids are not of proven clinical benefit in dogs with myocarditis and, considering the possible infective etiologies, they are not recommended as nonspecific therapy. Immunosuppressive therapy appears to be of little benefit in most human myocarditis cases; however, exceptions include confirmed immune-mediated disease, drug-related or eosinophilic myocarditis, and confirmed myocarditis that fails to resolve. Pericardial effusion and azotemia were associated with nonsurvival on multivariate analysis, in one case series (Lakhdhir, 2020). However, prognosis often is poor for dogs with myocarditis.

Viral Myocarditis

Acute viral infection can cause nonsuppurative or lymphocytic myocarditis. The animal's immune responses to viral, as well as nonviral, antigens provoke acute myocardial inflammation and can lead to persistent myocardial damage. If the animal survives, secondary myocardial fibrosis and remodeling eventually could lead to a DCM phenotype. Active myocarditis is uncommon in dogs with DCM, though. An association between acute (viral) myocarditis and subsequent deterioration in myocardial function to end-stage DCM has long been recognized in people. An earlier study employing postmortem myocardial PCR analysis in a small number of DCM-affected dogs suggested that viral agents were only rarely associated with canine DCM. However, in another small group of dogs with DCM, endomyocardial biopsy samples contained nucleic acid from various cardiotropic pathogens in over half of those cases (Santilli, 2019).

A syndrome of parvoviral myocarditis was widely recognized in the late 1970s. It was characterized by peracute necrotizing myocarditis and sudden death, with or without signs of acute respiratory distress, usually in 4–8-week-old puppies. Necropsy findings included cardiac dilation with pale myocardial streaks, gross evidence of congestive failure, large basophilic or amorphophilic intranuclear viral inclusion bodies, myocyte degeneration, necrosis and focal lymphocytic mononuclear cell infiltrates. Acute, subacute, and chronic parvoviral myocarditis has been described (Ford, 2017). The inflammatory response is more severe in pups 6–9 weeks old compared to younger pups, while chronic inflammatory changes are typical in pups over 3 months old. Immunohistochemistry can identify the virus. Parvovirus myocarditis is uncommon today, presumably because maternal antibody protection in pups lasts for several weeks. However, smoldering myocarditis and myocardial fibrosis in young dogs could often be unrecognized, and might not be evident unless unexpected anesthetic death occurs during spay or neutering. Cells are most susceptible to canine parvovirus infection when rapidly dividing; for the heart, this occurs in utero and during the first few weeks after birth. So puppies infected during this time often develop acute myocarditis and sudden death without showing GI signs. Because virus is not yet being shed in the stool of these puppies, fecal ELISA testing is not useful. Presumptive antemortem diagnosis in young pups of a non- or poorly vaccinated dam is based on clinical signs, chest radiographs, elevated cTnI, and echo or ECG abnormalities. Most pups in an affected litter are likely to die within the first 2 months of life. Those that survive can develop myocardial failure later, similar to DCM.

Canine distemper virus can cause myocarditis in young puppies, although multisystemic signs usually predominate. Myocardial histologic changes are mild compared with those in acute parvovirus myocarditis. Herpesvirus infection of pups *in utero* also can cause fatal necrotizing myocarditis with intranuclear inclusion bodies. Myocarditis has occurred in association with West Nile Virus, Pseudorabies, and presumably other viral infections, too.

Bacterial Myocarditis

Bacteremia and bacterial endocarditis or pericarditis sometimes cause suppurative myocardial inflammation or abscessation. Malaise, weight loss, arrhythmias and cardiac conduction abnormalities are common. An audible murmur is rare unless concurrent valvular endocarditis or another underlying cardiac defect is present. Fever is an inconsistent finding. Serial bacterial, or fungal, blood cultures might allow identification of the organism. *Bartonella vinsonii* subsp. *berkhoffii* and related species have been associated with cardiac arrhythmias (including high-grade AV block), myocarditis, endocarditis, and sudden death in dogs. Multifocal areas of myocardial inflammation also are found in some dogs with endocarditis from *B. vinsonii* subsp. *berkhoffii* (see Chapter 31 for more information). Retrospective PCR testing of histologic samples from a group of military dogs with culture-negative endo- or myocarditis revealed *Bartonella* DNA in a majority of cases (Davis, 2020). Miscellaneous other bacterial species have been identified in dogs with myocarditis, including *Citrobacter* and *Moraxella* spp.

Lyme Disease Lyme borreliosis is recognized in certain geographic areas, especially the northeastern and north central United States, as well as in Europe, Japan, and other areas. The spirochete *Borrelia burgdorferi*, or a closely related species, is transmitted to dogs by ticks, frequently of the genus *Ixodes*. Small mammals and birds serve as reservoir hosts. Histopathologic findings of myocarditis are similar to those found in human Lyme carditis, with infiltrates of plasma cells, macrophages, neutrophils, and lymphocytes, in conjunction with areas of myocardial necrosis. Lyme carditis, with rapid onset of progressive CHF, sudden death, and pyogranulomatous myocarditis has been reported in puppies. Occasionally, vegetative or cystic forms of *B. burgdorferi* could be evident on histopathology, or cardiac immunohistopathology might be positive for the organism.

Systemic signs include lymphadenopathy and arthritis. Onset of clinical signs commonly occurs in late summer or early fall. Third-degree and high-grade second-degree heart block have been identified in dogs with Lyme disease. Syncope, CHF, impaired myocardial contractility, and ventricular arrhythmias also can occur in affected dogs. Presumptive diagnosis is made on the basis of positive (or increasing) serum titers and concurrent signs of myocarditis, with or without other systemic signs. Endomyocardial biopsy, if available, could help confirm the diagnosis. Antibiotics (doxycycline, azithromycin) are used in treatment. Cardiac drugs are prescribed as necessary.

Protozoal Myocarditis

The protozoal organisms *Trypanosoma cruzi*, *Toxoplasma gondii*, *Neosporum caninum*, *Babesia canis*, *Leishmania infantum chagasi*, and *Hepatozoon canis* can affect the myocardium.

Chagas Disease American trypanosomiasis (Chagas disease) is an important cause of myocarditis and secondary DCM in people of Central and South America. In the United States, canine infections have occurred mostly in southeast Texas, but also in Louisiana, Oklahoma, Georgia, Virginia, and other southern states. The prevalence appears to be increasing; in some areas of Texas and Louisiana, infection rates could reach about 50% in some hunting dog kennels. Historically, young working dogs have been affected most often. More recently, infection has occurred in many breed groups, including nonsporting and toy breeds of dog (Meyers, 2019). There appears to be no sex or breed predilection; however, the risk of infection is substantially increased among dogs living with an infected animal.

The organism is carried by bloodsucking insects of the family *Reduviidae* ("kissing bugs") and is enzootic in wild animals of the region. Infected insects can transmit infective trypomastigotes during or after their blood meal by defecating near or in the bite wound. Dogs also can become infected by eating infected vectors or meat. *T. cruzi* can be transmitted through the placenta or during nursing, and by blood transfusion. Parasitemia can begin three days after infection, usually peaks within three weeks, then subsides by the fourth week. Acute, chronic asymptomatic (latent), and chronic symptomatic phases of Chagas myocarditis are described. Prevention of *T. cruzi* infection involves avoiding contact with vectors and reservoir hosts. Transmission to people via infected blood or tissue is possible, so care is warranted in handling samples from dogs suspected of being infected.

Acute *T. cruzi* myocarditis involves trypomastigote-induced cell damage and rupture, with subsequent inflammation. Diffuse granulomatous myocarditis, parasitic pseudocysts and minimal fibrosis are described. Chronic changes include multiple foci of interstitial mononuclear cell infiltrate, perivasculitis, and marked fibrosis. Parasitic pseudocysts are rare in the chronic stage; immunohistochemistry might be needed for definitive diagnosis. The development of progressive myocardial dysfunction and arrhythmias is thought to involve immune-mediated injury, microvascular disease, and toxic effects from the parasite. Preliminary experimental evidence suggests that statin drugs might reduce cardiac remodeling during this period by modifying immune responses; no clinical recommendations are yet available.

Signs of acute myocarditis might not be recognized, but if evident, occur around 2 weeks after infection and resolve over the following 2 weeks. Although clinical signs can be subtle, acute trypanosomiasis can cause lethargy, depression, pallor, lymphadenopathy, and other systemic or neurologic signs, as well as respiratory distress, various tachyarrhythmias, AV conduction disturbances, and sudden death in dogs. The mortality rate is high in immature dogs, especially. In the acute stage, trypomastigotes sometimes are found in thick peripheral blood smears, although they are more likely to be found by Wright- or Giemsa-stained buffy coat smears and other plasma concentrations methods. Organisms also might be identified on lymph node aspirate or abdominal fluid cytology, isolated in cell culture, or by inoculation into mice.

Survivors of the acute phase enter a chronic asymptomatic (latent) phase of variable duration. During this time, parasitemia resolves and antibodies develop against the organism, as well as components of the heart, which leads to fibrosing myocardial inflammation. Variable shedding of the organisms can occur, also. A complete cure of *T. cruzi* infection is unlikely. For dogs diagnosed in the acute stage, therapy with benznidazole (which might be available from the Centers for Disease Control in Atlanta) can reduce parasite burden (if the strain is susceptible); this could reduce myocardial damage. However, most cases of chronic Chagas disease develop cardiomyopathy.

Some dogs develop chronic symptomatic myocardial disease during the several years following infection. This is when most *T. cruzi* diagnoses are made. An index of suspicion is important for dogs that have been in an endemic area at any time. Chronic Chagas disease appears clinically as DCM, characterized by progressive right-sided or generalized cardiomegaly and arrhythmias. Clinical signs of biventricular failure are common. Severe ventricular tachyarrhythmias are most notable, although supraventricular tachyarrhythmias, right bundle branch block, and AV conduction disturbances can occur also. Some dogs experience sudden death. Ventricular dilation and myocardial dysfunction usually are evident on echocardiography. Serologic and PCR testing are useful for diagnosis in the latent and chronic stages of Chagas disease; however, *T.cruzi* antibody tests might cross-react with Leishmania antibodies. While PCR testing for *T. cruzi* DNA is highly specific, sensitivity often is low. Nevertheless, clinical signs in conjunction with positive serology appear to be the best means of diagnosis.

Therapy for chronic Chagas disease is aimed mainly at supporting myocardial function, controlling congestive signs, and managing arrhythmias. Several drugs with trypanocidal activity are being investigated, although efficacy in clinical trials has not been well-tested. *T. cruzi* shares similar sterol biosynthesis pathways with fungi; therefore, antifungal azole drugs such as itraconazole, which disrupt sterol biosynthesis, have been used in some human patients. Recently, the combination of itraconazole and the antiarrhythmic drug, amiodarone, was reported to have synergistic effects against *T. cruzi* in dogs (Madigan, 2019). Besides its antiarrhythmic action, amiodarone can disrupt calcium homeostasis and inhibit sterol production in the parasite, among other effects. Such sterols are necessary for parasite proliferation. Amiodarone also appears to promote improved myocardial function in affected dogs.

Other Protozoal Diseases Toxoplasmosis and neosporiosis occasionally cause clinical myocarditis, along with generalized systemic disease, especially in the neonatal or immuno-compromised animal. Infection can occur from eating infected meat. Vertical transmission of neosporiosis is suspected in affected neonates. After initial infection, the organism becomes encysted in the heart and various other body tissues. When these cysts rupture, expelled bradyzoites induce a hypersensitivity reaction and tissue necrosis. Other systemic signs often predominate over signs of myocarditis. Immunosuppressed dogs with chronic toxoplasmosis (or neosporiosis) could be at risk for active disease, including clinically relevant myocarditis, pneumonia, chorioretinitis, and encephalitis. Serology and PCR tests are helpful in diagnosis. Therapy with appropriate antiprotozoal agents might be successful. Immunohistochemistry testing can provide a post-mortem diagnosis.

Babesiosis sometimes has been associated with cardiac lesions in dogs, including myocardial hemorrhage, inflammation, and necrosis. Pericardial effusion and variable ECG changes are also noted in some cases. A correlation between plasma cTnI concentration and clinical severity, survival, and cardiac histologic changes was reported in dogs with babesiosis.

Dogs with Leishmania (*L. infantum chagasi*) infection commonly have cardiac lesions, even if overt clinical signs of myocarditis are absent. Lymphoplasmacytic myocarditis, myocyte necrosis and increased interstitial collagen accumulation are the most common observations. Less common changes include lepromatous-type granulomatous myocarditis, fibrinoid vascular changes and vasculitis. A higher number of parasitized cells correlates with greater inflammatory response and more granulomas.

Myocardial involvement with *H. canis* infection has been found in dogs along the Texas coast in the United States. Infection results from ingestion of the organism's definitive host, the brown dog tick (*Rhipicephalus sanguineus*). Reported clinical signs include stiffness, anorexia, fever, neutrophilia, and periosteal new bone reaction.

Miscellaneous Causes of Myocarditis

In rare instances, fungi (such as *Aspergillus, Cryptococcus, Coccidioides, Histoplasma, Blastomyces,* and *Paecilomyces* spp.), rickettsiae (*Rickettsia rickettsii, Ehrlichia canis*), algae-like organisms (*Prototheca* spp.), and nematode larval migration (*Toxocara* spp.) cause myocarditis. Affected animals usually are immunosuppressed and have systemic signs of disease. Monocytic ehrlichiosis in dogs is associated with high frequency of various arrhythmias, cTnI elevation, and decreased heart rate variability (Gianfranchesco, 2019). Rocky Mountain spotted fever (*R. rickettsii*) occasionally causes fatal ventricular arrhythmias, along with necrotizing vasculitis, myocardial thrombosis, and ischemia. *Angiostrongylus vasorum* infection (p. 870), in association with immune-mediated thrombocytopenia, rarely has caused myocarditis, thrombosing arteritis, and sudden death.

Noninfective Myocarditis

Drugs, toxins, immunologic responses, and trauma can cause myocardial inflammation. Although little clinical documentation exists for many of these in animals, many potential causes have been identified in people (**Table 32.4**). Immune-mediated diseases and pheochromocytoma can cause myocarditis. Sporadic cases of apparently noninfective myocarditis are reported in dogs with polymyositis and steroid-responsive meningitis-arteritis. Eosinophilic myocarditis has occurred with mast cell tumors. Other primary or metastatic cardiac neoplasia also could cause myocardial inflammation. An eosinophilic myocarditis of unknown cause was characterized by tachycardia, lethargy, severely increased cTnI, myocardial thickening with a mottled echo appearance, and reduced contractility. Hypersensitivity reactions to antiinfective agents and other drugs are known to cause myocarditis in people. Eosinophilic and lymphocytic infiltrates characterize drug-related myocarditis. As in cases of infective myocarditis, supraventricular and ventricular tachyarrhythmias, serious AV block, and sudden death can occur with noninfective myocarditis.

Traumatic Myocarditis

Blunt trauma to the chest and heart is more common than penetrating wounds in companion animals. Being struck by a motor vehicle is the usual cause. Besides orthopedic injuries, lung contusions and cardiac arrhythmias are common sequelae. There also are sporadic case reports of cardiac rupture or laceration resulting from blunt trauma, as well as instances of direct cardiac injury from a bullet or other projectile. Traumatic avulsion of papillary muscles, septal perforation, and laceration of the pericardium also have occurred. Acute low-output failure and shock, or rapid-onset CHF, as well as arrhythmias, can result from severe cardiac trauma. If it is nonlethal, an intracardiac bullet fragment can cause transient myocardial injury, with arrhythmias and mild pericardial hemorrhage or effusion (**Figure 32.23**). In rare cases, it could be an incidental finding (**Figure 32.24**).

Dogs that have been hit by a motor vehicle often develop posttraumatic cardiac arrhythmias, even when there is no visible thoracic trauma. Mechanisms of myocardial injury and subsequent arrhythmias could include compression or acceleration-deceleration forces, autonomic imbalance, ischemia,

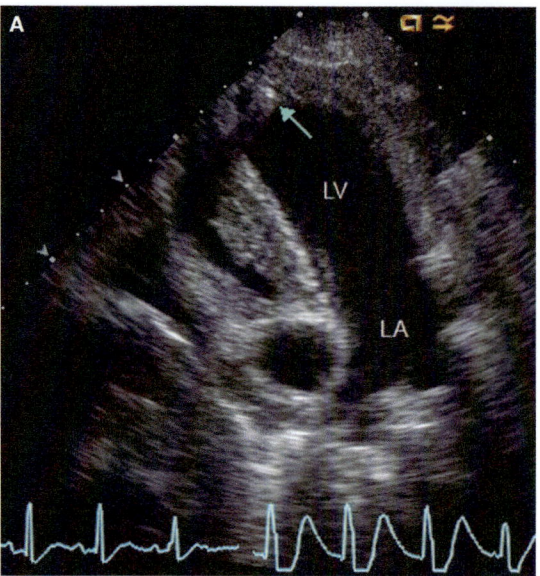
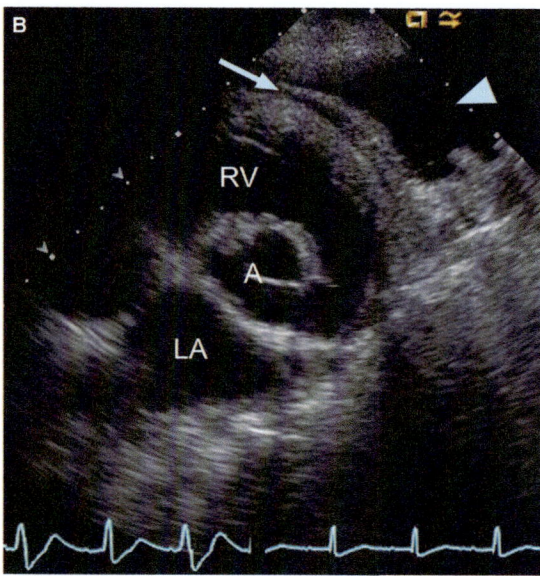

Figure 32.23 A 6-year-old male Labrador Retriever, on emergency presentation for acute-onset lethargy, weakness and heavy breathing over several hours, was found to have a small wound on the left thorax. Pallor, hypotension, and progressive decrease in hematocrit were noted. Thoracic radiographs showed mild pleural effusion and a 5 × 5 mm metal opacity within the chest. The dog's condition stabilized after treatment with O_2, IV fluid, packed red cell transfusion, cefazolin, hydromorphone, and lidocaine (after ventricular tachycardia developed). (A) The following day, echocardiography showed a metal projectile (bullet, arrow) lodged in the left ventricular apex and casting an acoustic shadow distally. Paroxysmal ventricular tachycardia is evident on the ECG monitor lead. Left apical view. (B) A small volume of pericardial effusion (arrow) and a larger volume of pleural fluid (arrowhead) are visible on this right parasternal short-axis image. The pleural (and presumably pericardial) fluid was blood. The dog made a good clinically recovery. A, aorta; LA, left atrium; LV, left ventricle; RV, right ventricle.

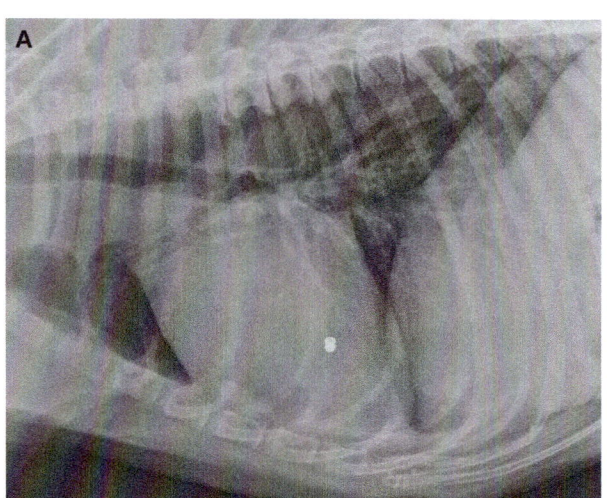
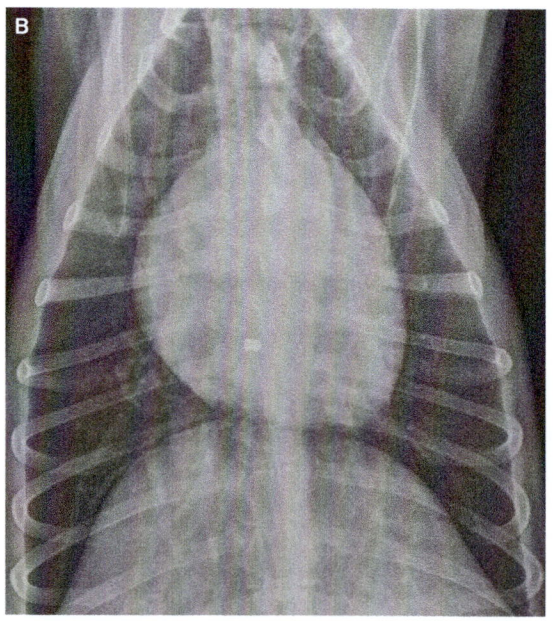
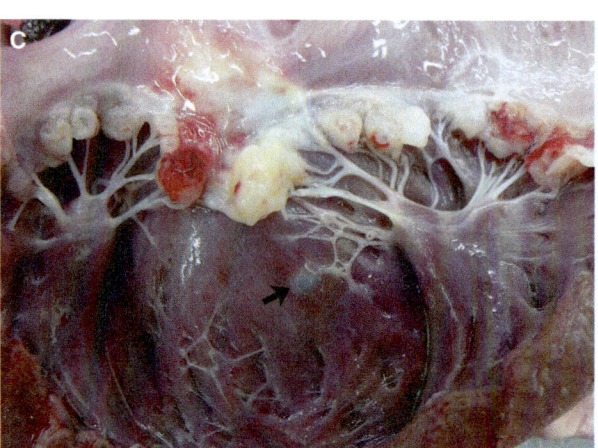

Figure 32.24 Lateral (A) and DV (B) thoracic radiographs from a 9-year-old female mixed-breed dog presented for evaluation of suspected myxomatous mitral valve disease. Except for the typical mitral regurgitant murmur, her physical exam was unremarkable. The cardiac silhouette is mildly enlarged (VHS = 10.9v). There is a metal pellet in the area of the heart. The lungs and pulmonary vessels are normal. Echocardiography showed mild left ventricular and atrial dilation, thickened mitral and tricuspid valve leaflets, moderate mitral regurgitation, and a bright highly reverberating echo (~5 mm) within the interventricular septum. Three years later, the dog died from advanced biventricular congestive heart failure. (C) Postmortem exam showed cardiac changes consistent with advanced degenerative mitral and tricuspid valve disease. Note the prominent nodular (Whitney class 4) lesions along the edges of the mitral leaflets in this image of the open left ventricle. The previously identified metal pellet (arrow) is visible as a discolored bulge beneath the septal endocardium, surrounded by fibrous tissue. Histologically, there was no inflammation surrounding the pellet nor visible damage in adjacent myocardium.

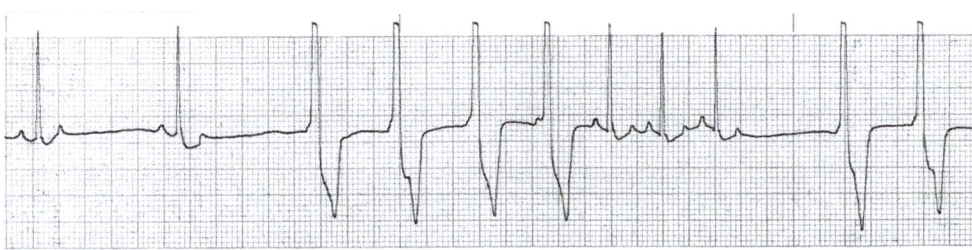

Figure 32.25 Sinus arrhythmia is interrupted by an accelerated idioventricular rhythm in an 8-year-old female Golden Retriever. The dog had been hit by a car several days prior and sustained a femoral fracture. Her left ventricular function was normal. Note that the idioventricular rhythm appears after a pause, during slower cycles of the sinus rhythm. An increase in the sinus rate suppresses the abnormal rhythm. Lead II, 25 mm/s, 1 cm = 1 mV.

reperfusion injury, or electrolyte and acid-base disturbances. Arrhythmias usually appear within 24–48 hours after trauma. Isolated VPCs, accelerated idioventricular rhythms (at 60–100 beats/minute or slightly faster), and ventricular tachycardia are more common than supraventricular tachyarrhythmias or bradyarrhythmias. The occurrence of frequent VPCs and ventricular tachycardia appears to affect only a small percentage of cases. An accelerated idioventricular rhythm often becomes evident only when the sinus rate slows (**Figure 32.25**; also **Figure 5.36**, p. 149). Accelerated idioventricular rhythms usually are benign and tend to disappear in a week or so in animals with a functionally normal heart.

ECGs, radiographs, serum biochemical tests, cTnI, and echocardiography are useful for assessing these patients, and defining preexisting cardiac disease and myocardial function. For dogs with a history of blunt trauma within the previous 24 hours, normal cTnI concentration and ECG findings at hospital admission predicted very low risk for the development of clinically important cardiac arrhythmias over the subsequent 24 hours (Biddick, 2020). Antiarrhythmic therapy for posttraumatic accelerated idioventricular rhythm usually is unnecessary, although close monitoring is warranted. If more serious arrhythmias (including faster rate or multiform configuration) or hemodynamic deterioration develops, antiarrhythmic therapy might become necessary (Chapter 25).

NOTE

1. US FDA. How to report a pet food complaint. Available at: www.fda.gov/AnimalVeterinary/SafetyHealth/ReportaProblem/ucm182403.htm.

Suggested Additional Reading and References

Also See Online Comprehensive Bibliography at: https://www.routledge.com/9781482246223.

Adin D, DeFrancesco TC, Keene BK, et al. Echocardiographic phenotype of canine dilated cardiomyopathy differs based on diet type. J Vet Cardiol 2019; 21:1–9.

Alves de Souza RC, Camacho AA. Neurohormonal, hemodynamic, and electrocardiographic evaluations of healthy dogs receiving long-term administration of doxorubicin. Am J Vet Res 2006;67:1319–1325.

Baumwart RD, Meurs KM, Atkins CE, et al. Clinical, echocardiographic, and electrocardiographic abnormalities in Boxers with cardiomyopathy and left ventricular systolic dysfunction: 48 cases (1985–2003). J Am Vet Med Assoc 2005;226:1102–1104

Baumwart RD, Orvalho J, Meurs KM. Evaluation of serum cardiac troponin I concentration in Boxers with arrhythmogenic right ventricular cardiomyopathy. Am J Vet Res 2007;68:524–528.

Beier P, Reese S, Holler PJ, et al. The role of hypothyroidism in the etiology and progression of dilated cardiomyopathy in Doberman Pinschers. J Vet Intern Med 2015;29:141–149.

Biddick AA, Bacek LM, Fan S, et al. Association between cardiac troponin I concentrations and electrocardiographic abnormalities in dogs with blunt trauma. J Vet Emerg Crit Care 2020; 30:179–186.

Bulmer BJ. Cardiovascular dysfunction in sepsis and critical illness. Vet Clin North Am Small Anim Pract 2011;41:717–726.

Caldas IS, Menezes APJ, Diniz LF, et al. Parasitaemia and parasitic load are limited targets of the aetiological treatment to control the progression of cardiac fibrosis and chronic cardiomyopathy in *Trypanosoma cruzi*-infected dogs. Acta Trop 2018;189:30–38.

Calvert CA, Jacobs G, Pickus CW, et al. Results of ambulatory electrocardiography in overtly healthy Doberman Pinschers with echocardiographic abnormalities. J Am Vet Med Assoc 2000;217:1328–1332.

Caro-Vadillo A, Garcia-Guasch L, Carreton E, et al. Arrhythmogenic right ventricular cardiomyopathy in Boxer dogs: a retrospective study of survival. Vet Rec 2013;172:268.

Cattanach BM, Dukes-McEwan J, Wotton PR, et al. A pedigree-based genetic appraisal of Boxer ARVC and the role of the Striatin mutation. Vet Rec 2015;176:492.

Chetboul V, Escriou C, Tessier D, et al. Tissue Doppler imaging detects early asymptomatic myocardial abnormalities in a dog model of Duchenne's cardiomyopathy. Eur Heart J 2004;25:1934–1939.

Chetboul V, Gouni V, Sampedrano CC, et al. Assessment of regional systolic and diastolic myocardial function using tissue Doppler and strain imaging in dogs with dilated cardiomyopathy. J Vet Intern Med 2007;21:719–730.

Chubb H, Simpson JM. The use of Z-scores in paediatric cardiology. Ann Pediatr Cardiol 2012;5:179–184.

Cornell CC, Kittleson MD, Della Torre P, et al. Allometric scaling of M-mode cardiac measurements in normal adult dogs. J Vet Intern Med 2004;18:311–321.

Cunningham SM, Aona BD, Antoon K, et al. Echocardiographic assessment of right ventricular systolic function in Boxers with arrhythmogenic right ventricular cardiomyopathy. J Vet Cardiol 2018a; 20:343–353.

Cunningham SM, Sweeney JT, MacGregor J, et al. Clinical features of English bulldogs with presumed arrhythmogenic right ventricular cardiomyopathy: 31 cases (2001–2013). J Am Anim Hosp Assoc 2018b;54:95–102.

Davis AZ, Jaffe DA, Honadel TE, et al. Prevalence of Bartonella sp. in United States military working dogs with infectious endocarditis: a retrospective case-control study. J Vet Cardiol 2020;27:1–9.

Domingues M, Brookes VJ, Oliveira P, et al. Heart rhythm during episodes of collapse in Boxers with frequent or complex ventricular ectopy. J Small Anim Pract 2020;61:127–136.

Dukes-McEwan J, Borgarelli M, Tidholm A, et al. Proposed guidelines for the diagnosis of canine idiopathic dilated cardiomyopathy. J Vet Cardiol 2003;5:7–19.

Dutton E, López-Alvarez J. An update on canine cardiomyopathies – is it all in the genes? J Small Anim Pract 2018;59:455–464.

Edmondson EF, Bright JM, Halsey CH, et al. Pathologic and cardiovascular characterization of pheochromocytoma-associated cardiomyopathy in dogs. Vet Pathol 2015;52:338–343.

Elamm C, Fairweather D, Cooper LT. Pathogenesis and diagnosis of myocarditis. Heart 2012;98:835–840.

Esser LC, Borkovec M, Bauer A, et al. Left ventricular M-mode prediction intervals in 7651 dogs: Population-wide and selected breed-specific values. J Veter Intern Med 2020;34:2242–2252.

Falk T, Jonsson L. Ischaemic heart disease in the dog: a review of 65 cases. J Small Anim Pract 2000;41:97–103.

FDA Investigation into Potential Link between Certain Diets and Canine Dilated Cardiomyopathy. Feb 19, 2019; https://www.fda.gov/AnimalVeterinary/NewsEvents/ucm630993.htm (accessed 3/12/19).

Fine DM, Shin J-H, Yue Y, et al. Age-matched comparison reveals early electrocardiography and echocardiography changes in dystrophin-deficient dogs. Neuromuscul Disord 2011;21:453–461.

Fonfara S, Hetzel U, Oyama MA, et al. The potential role of myocardial serotonin receptor 2B expression in canine dilated cardiomyopathy. Vet J 2014;199:406–412.

Fonfara S, Hetzel U, Tew SR, et al. Myocardial cytokine expression in dogs with systemic and naturally occurring cardiac diseases. Am J Vet Res 2013;74:408–416.

Fonfara S, Loureiro J, Swift S, et al. Cardiac troponin I as a marker for severity and prognosis of cardiac disease in dogs. Vet J 2010;184:334–339.

Ford J, McEndaffer L, Renshaw R, et al. Parvovirus infection is associated with myocarditis and myocardial fibrosis in young dogs. Vet Pathol 2017;54:964–971.

Freeman LM, Stern JA, Fries R, et al. Diet-associated dilated cardiomyopathy in dogs: what do we know? J Am Vet Med Assoc 2018;253:1390–1394.

Friedenberg SG, Chdid L, Keene B, et al. Use of RNA-seq to identify cardiac genes and gene pathways differentially expressed between dogs with and without dilated cardiomyopathy. Am J Vet Res 2016;77:693–699.

Gallay-Lepoutre J, Belanger MC, Nadeau ME. Prospective evaluation of Doppler echocardiography, tissue Doppler imaging and biomarkers measurement for the detection of doxorubicin-induced cardiotoxicity in dogs: a pilot study. Res Vet Sci 2016;105:153–159.

Gasparini S, Fonfara S, Kitz S, et al. Canine dilated cardiomyopathy: diffuse remodeling, focal lesions, and the involvement of macrophages and new vessel formation. Vet Pathol 2020;57:397–408.

Gianfranchesco Filippi M, de Castro Ferreira Lima M, Paes AC, et al. Evaluation of heart rate variability and behavior of electrocardiographic parameters in dogs affected by chronic *Monocytic ehrlichiosis*. PLoS One 2019;14:e0216552.

Gunasekaran T, Olivier NB, Sanders RA. Comparison of single- versus seven-day Holter analysis for the identification of dilated cardiomyopathy predictive criteria in apparently healthy Doberman Pinscher dogs. J Vet Cardiol 2020;27:78–87.

Hallman BE, Hauck ML, Williams LE, et al. Incidence and risk factors associated with development of clinical cardiotoxicity in dogs receiving doxorubicin. J Vet Intern Med 2019;33:783–791.

Hammers DW, Sleeper MM, Forbes SC, et al. Tadalafil treatment delays the onset of cardiomyopathy in dystrophin-deficient hearts. J Am Heart Assoc 2016;5.

Hanson KR, Ware WA. Myocardial hypertrophy associated with long-term phenylpropanolamine use in a dog. J Am Vet Med Assoc 2018;253:1452–1459.

Harpster N. Boxer cardiomyopathy. In, Kirk R (editor). Current Veterinary Therapy VIII. WB Saunders, Philadelphia, PA. 1983. pp. 329–337.

Harris JD, Little CJL, Dennis JM, et al. Heart rate turbulence after ventricular premature beats in healthy Doberman Pinschers and those with dilated cardiomyopathy. J Vet Cardiol 2017;19:421–432.

Holler PJ, Wess G. Sphericity index and E-point-to-septal-separation (EPSS) to diagnose dilated cardiomyopathy in Doberman Pinschers. J Vet Intern Med 2014;28:123–129.

Katz AM. Cardiomyopathy of overload. A major determinant of prognosis in congestive heart failure. N Engl J Med 1990;322:100–110.

Kaye BM, Borgeat K, Motskula PF, et al. Association of tricuspid annular plane systolic excursion with survival time in Boxer dogs with ventricular arrhythmias. J Vet Intern Med 2015;29:582–588

Kim YH, Kim JH, Park C. Evaluation of tissue Doppler ultrasonographic and strain imaging for assessment of myocardial dysfunction in dogs with type 1 diabetes mellitus. Am J Vet Res 2018;79:1035–1043.

Klüser L, Holler PJ, Simak J, et al. Predictors of sudden cardiac death in Doberman Pinschers with dilated cardiomyopathy. J Vet Intern Med 2016;30:722–732.

Klüser L, Maier ET, Wess G. Evaluation of a high-sensitivity cardiac troponin I assay compared to a first-generation cardiac troponin I assay in Doberman Pinschers with and without dilated cardiomyopathy. J Vet Intern Med 2019;33:54–63.

Ko KS, Fascetti AJ. Dietary beet pulp decreases taurine status in dogs fed low protein diet. J Anim Sci Technol 2016;58:29.

Kobal M Petric AD. Echocardiographic diastolic indices of the left ventricle in normal doberman pinschers and retrievers. Slov Vet Res 2007;44:31–40.

Kornegay JN. The golden retriever model of Duchenne muscular dystrophy. Skeletal muscle 2017;7:9.

Lakhdhir S, Viall A, Alloway E, et al. Clinical presentation, cardiovascular findings, etiology, and outcome of myocarditis in dogs: 64 cases with presumptive antemortem diagnosis (26 confirmed postmortem) and 137 cases with postmortem diagnosis only (2004–2017). J Vet Cardiol 2020;30:44–56.

Langhorn R, Oyama MA, King LG, et al. Prognostic importance of myocardial injury in critically ill dogs with systemic inflammation. J Vet Intern Med 2013;27:895–903.

Legge CH, Lopez A, Hanna P, et al. Histological characterization of dilated cardiomyopathy in the juvenile toy Manchester terrier. Vet Pathol 2013;50:1043–1052.

Madigan R, Majoy S, Ritter K, et al. Investigation of a combination of amiodarone and itraconazole for treatment of American trypanosomiasis (Chagas disease) in dogs. J Am Vet Med Assoc 2019;255:317–329.

Mansilla WD, Marinangeli CPF, Ekenstedt KJ, et al. The association between pulse ingredients and canine dilated cardiomyopathy: addressing the knowledge gaps before establishing causation. J Anim Sci 2019; 97:983–997.

Martin MW, Stafford Johnson MJ, Strehlau G, et al. Canine dilated cardiomyopathy: a retrospective study of prognostic findings in 367 clinical cases. J Small Anim Pract 2010;51:428–436.

Mathew T, Williams L, Navaratnam G, et al. Diagnosis and assessment of dilated cardiomyopathy: a guideline protocol from the British Society of Echocardiography. Echo Res Pract 2017;4:G1–G13.

Mausberg TB, Wess G, Simak J, et al. A locus on chromosome 5 is associated with dilated cardiomyopathy in Doberman Pinschers. PLoS One 2011;6:e20042.

Maxson TR, Meurs KM, Lehmkuhl LB, et al. Polymerase chain reaction analysis for viruses in paraffin-embedded myocardium from dogs with dilated cardiomyopathy or myocarditis. Am J Vet Res 2001;62:130–135.

McCauley SR, Clark SD, Quest BW, et al. Review of canine dilated cardiomyopathy in the wake of diet-associated concerns. J Anim Sci. 2020;98:skaa155. Erratum in: J Anim Sci. 2020;98: PMID: 32542359; PMCID: PMC7447921.

Meurs KM. Arrhythmogenic right ventricular cardiomyopathy in the Boxer dog: an update. Vet Clin North Am Small Anim Pract 2017;47:1103–1111.

Meurs KM, Friedenberg SG, Kolb J, et al. A missense variant in the titin gene in Doberman Pinscher dogs with familial dilated cardiomyopathy and sudden cardiac death. Hum Genet 2019; 138:515–524.

Meurs KM, Lahmers S, Keene BW, et al. A splice site mutation in a gene encoding for PDK4, a mitochondrial protein, is associated with the development of dilated cardiomyopathy in the Doberman Pinscher. Hum Genet 2012;131:1319–1325.

Meurs KM, Mauceli E, Lahmers S, et al. Genome-wide association identifies a deletion in the 3' untranslated region of striatin in a canine model of arrhythmogenic right ventricular cardiomyopathy. Hum Genet 2010;128:315–324.

Meurs KM, Stern JA, Adin D, et al. Assessment of PDK4 and TTN gene variants in 48 Doberman Pinschers with dilated cardiomyopathy. J Am Vet Med Assoc 2020;257:1041–1044.

Meurs KM, Stern JA, Reina-Doreste Y, et al. Natural history of arrhythmogenic right ventricular cardiomyopathy in the Boxer dog: a prospective study. J Vet Intern Med 2014;28:1214–1220.

Meurs KM, Stern JA, Sisson DD, et al. Association of dilated cardiomyopathy with the striatin mutation genotype in Boxer dogs. J Vet Intern Med 2013;27:1437–1440.

Meyers AC, Hamer SA, Matthews D, et al. Risk factors and select cardiac characteristics in dogs naturally infected with Trypanosoma cruzi presenting to a teaching hospital in Texas. J Vet Intern Med 2019;33:1695–1706.

Motskula PF, Linney C, Palermo V, et al. Prognostic value of 24-hour ambulatory ECG (holter) monitoring in Boxer dogs. J Vet Intern Med 2013;27:904–912.

Noszczyk-Nowak A. NT-pro-BNP and troponin I as predictors of mortality in dogs with heart failure. Pol J Vet Sci 2011;14:551–556.

Oberbauer AM, Belanger JM, Bellumori T, et al. Ten inherited disorders in purebred dogs by functional breed groupings. Canine Genet Epidemiol 2015;2:9.

O'Grady MR, O'Sullivan ML, Minors SL, et al. Efficacy of benazepril hydrochloride to delay the progression of occult dilated cardiomyopathy in Doberman Pinschers. J Vet Intern Med 2009;23:977–983.

O'Sullivan ML, O'Grady MR, Minors SL. Plasma big endothelin-1, atrial natriuretic peptide, aldosterone, and norepinephrine concentrations in normal Doberman Pinschers and Doberman Pinschers with dilated cardiomyopathy. J Vet Intern Med 2007;21:92–99.

Owczarek-Lipska M, Mausberg TB, Stephenson H, et al. A 16-bp deletion in the canine PDK4 gene is not associated with dilated cardiomyopathy in a European cohort of Doberman Pinschers. Anim Genet 2013;44:239.

Oxford EM, Danko CG, Fox PR, et al. Change in beta-catenin localization suggests involvement of the canonical Wnt pathway in Boxer dogs with arrhythmogenic right ventricular cardiomyopathy. J Vet Intern Med 2014;28:92–101.

Oxford EM, Danko CG, Kornreich BG, et al. Ultrastructural changes in cardiac myocytes from Boxer dogs with arrhythmogenic right ventricular cardiomyopathy. J Vet Cardiol 2011;13:101–113.

Ozarda Y. Reference intervals: current status, recent developments and future considerations. Biochem Med (Zagreb) 2016;26:5–16.

Palermo V, Stafford Johnson MJ, Sala E, et al. Cardiomyopathy in Boxer dogs: a retrospective study of the clinical presentation, diagnostic findings and survival. J Vet Cardiol 2011;13:45–55.

Pedro BM, Alves JV, Cripps PJ, et al. Association of QRS duration and survival in dogs with dilated cardiomyopathy: a retrospective study of 266 clinical cases. J Vet Cardiol 2011;13:243–249.

Pedro B, Stephenson H, Linney C, et al. Assessment of left ventricular function in healthy Great Danes and in Great Danes with dilated cardiomyopathy using speckle tracking echocardiography. J Vet Cardiol 2017;19:363–375.

Pinto YM, Elliott PM, Arbustini E, et al. Proposal for a revised definition of dilated cardiomyopathy, hypokinetic non-dilated cardiomyopathy, and its implications for clinical practice: a position statement of the ESC working group on myocardial and pericardial diseases. Eur Heart J 2016;37:1850–1858.

Ratterree W, Gieger T, Pariaut R, et al. Value of echocardiography and electrocardiography as screening tools prior to Doxorubicin administration. J Am Anim Hosp Assoc 2012;48:89–96.

Rosa FA, Leite JH, Braga ET, et al. Cardiac lesions in 30 dogs naturally infected with Leishmania infantum chagasi. Vet Pathol 2014;51:603–606.

Santilli RA, Grego E, Battaia S, et al. Prevalence of selected cardiotropic pathogens in the myocardium of adult dogs with unexplained myocardial and rhythm disorders or with congenital heart disease. J Am Vet Med Assoc 2019;255:1150–1160.

Santos FM, Mazzeti AL, Caldas S, et al. Chagas cardiomyopathy: the potential effect of benznidazole treatment on diastolic dysfunction and cardiac damage in dogs chronically infected with Trypanosoma cruzi. Acta Trop 2016;161:44–54.

Schober KE, Hart TM, Stern JA, et al. Effects of treatment on respiratory rate, serum natriuretic peptide concentration, and Doppler echocardiographic indices of left ventricular filling pressure in dogs with congestive heart failure secondary to degenerative mitral valve disease and dilated cardiomyopathy. J Am Vet Med Assoc 2011;239:468–479.

Simpson KE, Devine BC, Woolley R, et al. Timing of left heart base descent in dogs with dilated cardiomyopathy and normal dogs. Vet Radiol Ultrasound 2008;49:287–294.

Simpson S, Dunning MD, Brownlie S, et al. Multiple genetic associations with Irish Wolfhound dilated cardiomyopathy. Biomed Res Int 2016;2016:6374082.

Sjöstrand K, Wess G, Ljungvall I, et al. Breed differences in natriuretic peptides in healthy dogs. J Vet Intern Med 2014;28:451–457.

Smith CE, Freeman LM, Rush JE, et al. Omega-3 fatty acids in Boxer dogs with arrhythmogenic right ventricular cardiomyopathy. J Vet Intern Med 2007;21:265–273.

Spier AW, Meurs KM. Evaluation of spontaneous variability in the frequency of ventricular arrhythmias in Boxers with arrhythmogenic right ventricular cardiomyopathy. J Am Vet Med Assoc 2004;224:538–541.

Stern JA, Meurs KM, Spier AW, et al. Ambulatory electrocardiographic evaluation of clinically normal adult Boxers. J Am Vet Med Assoc 2010;236:430–433.

Stern JA, Ueda Y. Inherited cardiomyopathies in veterinary medicine. Pflugers Arch 2019;471:745–753.

Steudemann C, Bauersachs S, Weber K, et al. Detection and comparison of microRNA expression in the serum of Doberman Pinschers with dilated cardiomyopathy and healthy controls. BMC Vet Res 2013;9:12.

Stephenson HM, Fonfara S, Lopez-Alvarez J, et al. Screening for dilated cardiomyopathy in Great Danes in the United Kingdom. J Vet Intern Med 2012;26:1140–1147.

Summerfield NJ, Boswood A, O'Grady MR, et al. Efficacy of pimobendan in the prevention of congestive heart failure or sudden death in Doberman Pinschers with preclinical dilated cardiomyopathy (the PROTECT study). J Vet Intern Med 2012;26:1337–1349.

Thomason JD, Kraus MS, Surdyk KK, et al. Bradycardia-associated syncope in 7 Boxers with ventricular tachycardia (2002–2005). J Vet Intern Med 2008;22:931–936.

Thomason JD, Rapoport G, Fallaw T, et al. The influence of enalapril and spironolactone on electrolyte concentrations in Doberman Pinschers with dilated cardiomyopathy. Vet J 2014;202:573–577.

Tyrrell WD Jr., Abbott JA, Rosenthal SL, et al. Echocardiographic and electrocardiographic evaluation of North American Irish Wolfhounds. J Vet Intern Med 2020; 34:581–590.

Vila J, Pariaut R, Moise NS, et al. Structural and molecular pathology of the atrium in Boxer arrhythmogenic right ventricular cardiomyopathy. J Vet Cardiol 2017;19:57–67.

Vischer AS, Connolly DJ, Coats CJ, et al. Arrhythmogenic right ventricular cardiomyopathy in Boxer dogs: the diagnosis as a link to the human disease. Acta Myol 2017;36:135–150.

Visser LC, Ciccozzi MM, Sintov DJ, et al. Echocardiographic quantitation of left heart size and function in 122 healthy dogs: A prospective study proposing reference intervals and assessing repeatability. J Vet Intern Med 2019;33:1909–1920.

Vollmar AC, Aupperle H. Cardiac pathology in Irish wolfhounds with heart disease. J Vet Cardiol 2016a;18:57–70.

Vollmar AC, Fox PR. Long-term outcome of Irish Wolfhound dogs with preclinical cardiomyopathy, atrial fibrillation, or both treated with pimobendan, benazepril hydrochloride, or methyldigoxin monotherapy. J Vet Intern Med 2016b;30:553–559.

Vollmar AC, Fox PR, Servet E, et al. Determination of the prevalence of whole blood taurine in Irish wolfhound dogs with and without echocardiographic evidence of dilated cardiomyopathy. J Vet Cardiol 2013;15:189–196.

Vollmar C, Vollmar A, Keene BW, et al. Dilated cardiomyopathy in 151 Irish Wolfhounds: characteristic clinical findings, life expectancy and causes of death. Vet J 2019a;245:15–21.

Vollmar C, Vollmar A, Keene B, et al. Irish wolfhounds with subclinical atrial fibrillation: progression of disease and causes of death. J Vet Cardiol 2019b;24:48–57.

Wess G, Butz V, Mahling M, et al. Evaluation of N-terminal pro-B-type natriuretic peptide as a diagnostic marker of various stages of cardiomyopathy in Doberman Pinschers. Am J Vet Res 2011;72:642–649.

Wess G, Domenech O, Dukes-McEwan J, et al. European Society of Veterinary Cardiology screening guidelines for dilated cardiomyopathy in Doberman Pinschers. J Vet Cardiol 2017;19:405–415.

Wess G, Maurer J, Simak J, et al. Use of Simpson's method of disc to detect early echocardiographic changes in Doberman Pinschers with dilated cardiomyopathy. J Vet Intern Med 2010a;24:1069–1076.

Wess G, Schulze A, Butz V, et al. Prevalence of dilated cardiomyopathy in Doberman Pinschers in various age groups. J Vet Intern Med 2010b;24:533–538.

Wess G, Schulze A, Geraghty N, et al. Ability of a 5-minute electrocardiography (ECG) for predicting arrhythmias in Doberman Pinschers with cardiomyopathy in comparison with a 24-hour ambulatory ECG. J Vet Intern Med 2010c;24:367–371.

Wess G, Simak J, Mahling M, et al. Cardiac troponin I in Doberman Pinschers with cardiomyopathy. J Vet Intern Med 2010d;24:843–849.

Wright KN, Connor CE, Irvin HM, et al. Atrioventricular accessory pathways in 89 dogs: clinical features and outcome after radiofrequency catheter ablation. J Vet Intern Med 2018;32:1517–1529.

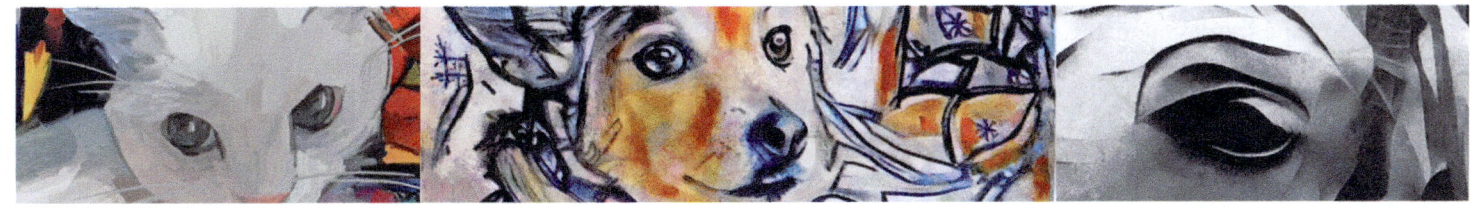

33
MYOCARDIAL DISEASES OF THE CAT

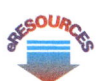

Feline myocardial diseases (cardiomyopathies) are characterized by a variety of structural and pathophysiologic abnormalities that develop in the absence of an identifiable cause. The cardiomyopathies as a group are the most common cause of heart disease in cats. Their overall estimated prevalence in the general cat population is ~15%, depending on the echocardiographic (echo) criteria used for diagnosis. The vast majority of cases express a hypertrophic form of disease. Several cardiomyopathy phenotypes are recognized in cats (**Table 33.1**; American College of Veterinary Internal Medicine, ACVIM, consensus statement; Luis Fuentes, 2020). Yet even within these recognized phenotypic categories, morphologic variation exists and features of more than one phenotype could coexist in an individual. Furthermore, cardiac remodeling over time can change an individual's phenotype.

Hypertrophic cardiomyopathy (HCM) is much more common than other forms of cardiomyopathy in cats. These include restrictive (RCM, p. 678), dilated (DCM, p. 682), and arrhythmogenic right ventricular cardiomyopathy (ARVC, also known as arrhythmogenic cardiomyopathy, p. 686). Some cats with myocardial disease have cardiac features that do not align well with these classic phenotypic categories. Such cats previously were considered to have "unclassified" cardiomyopathy. However, this name does not provide much insight into the nature of their disease. Therefore, the currently preferred term for these cats is "cardiomyopathy of non-specific phenotype" (p. 687); this identifier should be accompanied by a description of the individual cat's cardiac morphology and function. Congestive heart failure (CHF), cardiac rhythm disturbances, arterial thromboembolism (TE), and cardiac death are serious outcomes in cats with cardiomyopathies.

Several conditions are known to cause secondary myocardial disease and should be ruled out in relevant clinical settings. It is important to test for these disorders prior to making a diagnosis of idiopathic cardiomyopathy. Before such underlying conditions have been excluded in an individual suspected to have (idiopathic) cardiomyopathy, appending the modifier term "phenotype" initially is recommended. For example, hyperthyroidism and systemic hypertension can stimulate myocardial hypertrophy; therefore, before these conditions can be ruled out, cats observed to have left ventricular (LV) hypertrophy are described initially as having a "HCM phenotype." Similarly, taurine deficiency can lead to ventricular systolic failure and dilation; so until this cause is eliminated, a cat with LV dilation and failure would be identified as having a "DCM phenotype." If no explanatory disease condition subsequently is found, the cat then is diagnosed with "HCM," or "DCM," or other cardiomyopathy, as appropriate (Luis Fuentes, 2020). Other abnormalities are associated sporadically with secondary myocardial disease (p. 688) or myocarditis (p. 689).

Disease staging in cats with cardiomyopathy can be done in a similar manner as for dogs with degenerative (myxomatous) mitral valve disease (**Table 33.2**). This is helpful for assessing risk of clinical disease and, to a limited extent, guiding therapy. Cats with stage B1 disease have relatively low risk for CHF and arterial TE. Those at stage B2 are at much higher risk for developing CHF or arterial TE in the near future. Left atrial (LA) size is useful for classifying asymptomatic cats into stage B1 or B2, and as a prognostic marker. LA function, LV function, and presence of extreme hypertrophy also are important variables.

Hypertrophic Cardiomyopathy

Idiopathic (primary) HCM is by far the most common form of feline myocardial disease. It is characterized by LV hypertrophy without dilation. The hallmark pathophysiologic feature of HCM is LV diastolic dysfunction, or impaired filling. The disease has many similarities to HCM in people. Various patterns of hypertrophy occur among affected cats, ranging from symmetrical LV and septal hypertrophy to focal thickening of papillary muscles or wall segments. One common HCM

Table 33.1 Feline Cardiomyopathy Phenotypes

Cardiomyopathy Phenotype	Description
Hypertrophic cardiomyopathy	Diffusely or regionally increased LV wall thickness with nondilated LV chamber
Restrictive cardiomyopathy - endomyocardial form	Macroscopically prominent endocardial scar that usually bridges the IVS and LV free wall, and could cause fixed mid-LV obstruction; often with apical thinning or aneurysm. LA or biatrial enlargement usually present
Restrictive cardiomyopathy - myocardial form	Normal LV dimensions and wall thickness, with LA or biatrial enlargement
Dilated cardiomyopathy	LV systolic dysfunction, with progressively increasing ventricular dimensions, normal or reduced wall thickness, and atrial dilation
Arrhythmogenic (Arrhythmogenic RV) cardiomyopathy	Severe RA and RV dilation and often, RV systolic dysfunction and wall thinning. Left heart might also be affected. Arrhythmias and right-sided CHF common
Nonspecific cardiomyopathy	Cardiomyopathic phenotype not adequately described by other categories. The individual's cardiac morphology & function should be described in detail

Adapted from ACVIM consensus statement guidelines (Luis Fuentes, 2020).
Abbreviations: CHF, congestive heart failure; IVS, interventricular septum; LA, left atrial; LV, left ventricular; RA, right atrial; RV, right ventricular.

Table 33.2 Clinical Cardiomyopathy Staging in Cats

Stage	Description
A	No apparent structural disease yet, but considered predisposed or "at risk" for developing cardiomyopathy (mainly HCM).
B	Evidence for cardiomyopathy is present, but no clinical signs of heart failure have occurred.
• B1	Asymptomatic, with no or only minimal LA enlargement.
	• Considered to be at low risk, although increasing age, male gender, family history of cardiomyopathy, or a loud systolic murmur are more likely to be associated with disease progression.
• B2	Asymptomatic, but with moderate to severe LA enlargement.
	• Considered to be at higher risk, especially if severe LA enlargement with poor function, spontaneous contrast or intracardiac thrombus, extreme LV hypertrophy, decreased LV systolic function or regional dyskinesis, audible gallop sound, or arrhythmia is present.
C	Cardiomyopathy is present and signs of CHF or arterial TE have occurred, either currently or in the past (and now resolved with therapy).
D	Persistent or end-stage CHF; clinical signs difficult to control or refractory to standard therapy.

Abbreviations: CHF, congestive heart failure; HCM, hypertrophic cardiomyopathy; LA, left atrial; LV, left ventricular; TE, thromboembolism.

variation involves dynamic (systolic) LV outflow tract obstruction. This is known as hypertrophic obstructive cardiomyopathy (HOCM) because of its additional systolic abnormality. While HOCM carries a higher risk for sudden cardiac death in people, this has not been so in cats. Asymmetric ventricular septal hypertrophy is common, although not consistently present, in these cats. Similar to humans, affected cats also can have abnormal mitral or papillary muscle structure. The degree, or even presence, of dynamic LV outflow tract obstruction can vary dramatically at different times in the same cat, largely related to prevailing sympathetic tone. The dynamic obstruction also can decrease over time, often because of impaired LV systolic function.

Secondary causes of myocardial hypertrophy are especially important in middle-aged to older cats with some well-defined comorbidities. For example, LV hypertrophy from the systolic pressure overload of systemic arterial hypertension often is associated with chronic kidney disease (Chapter 38). Hyperthyroidism and acromegaly exert trophic effects on the myocardium that can stimulate hypertrophy. Most cats with acromegaly also have diabetes mellitus, and both are considered potential risk factors for LV hypertrophy and cardiomyopathy. Other abnormalities that sometimes cause myocardial thickening include myocarditis and congenital LV outflow obstructions stemming from mitral dysplasia or aortic stenosis; congenital subvalvular, valvular, and supravalvular forms of aortic stenosis are all reported in the cat. Rarely, infective endocarditis causes an acquired valvular aortic stenosis. When hypertrophic myocardial disease is identified, testing for these potential causes is indicated. Secondary myocardial hypertrophy (p. 688) is not considered to be true HCM.

Many, if not most, cases of feline HCM are thought to be familial, with autosomal dominant inheritance and variable penetrance. Phenotypic expression varies from mild to severe LV hypertrophy. Clinical consequences also range widely, from no signs of disease at all to CHF or sudden death. Disease expression is greater in older cats; but as in human teenagers, severe HCM sometimes is identified in relatively young cats, even at <1 year of age. Congenital HCM even has been reported. In people with HCM, over 1400 different mutations involving sarcomeric genes, which code for myocardial proteins, have been identified in different families. Mutations related to other cardiomyocyte structures or calcium kinetics also could be associated with HCM. Thus far, only a handful of genetic markers have been identified in the domestic cat.

Two mutations in the gene encoding the cardiac isoform of myosin binding protein C (MYBPC3) and that are associated with HCM have been identified in cats. One is in the Maine Coon breed (MYBPC3-A31P mutation; Meurs, 2005) and the other in Ragdolls (MYBPC3-R820W mutation; Meurs, 2007). Recently, a proprietary genetic test was released for the Sphynx (Sphinx) breed, although a scientific paper describing the mutation was unavailable at the time of this writing. Myosin binding protein C has structural and regulatory functions within the sarcomere. Feline HCM associated with a variant in MYH7, another sarcomeric gene that codes for the beta-myosin heavy chain protein, also has been reported (Schipper, 2019). Genetic testing can be valuable for indicating a likely risk of developing HCM, or of breeding animals passing this to their offspring.

The MYBPC3-A31P mutation is estimated to occur in 30 to slightly over 40% of all Maine Coon cats, although it could be higher in some geographic regions. Cats homozygous for this mutation have increased risk for HCM. These homozygous cats often develop more severe disease and at an earlier age than heterozygous cats that develop HCM. In other words, there is high disease penetrance in homozygous cats. However, in young heterozygous cats, disease penetrance is fairly low; furthermore, HCM usually does not develop before the age of 6 years in this population. Still, even with normal LV wall thickness, mild diastolic dysfunction might be detectable by tissue Doppler imaging (TDI) in heterozygous cats. It also is important to note that some Maine Coon cats with HCM do not have the MYBPC3-A31P mutation.

In the Ragdoll breed, prevalence of the MYBPC3-R820W mutation is estimated at 17–30%. Based on questionnaires sent to owners of over 230 Ragdoll cats, those cats homozygous for the mutation have a shorter lifespan and are more likely to die from cardiac disease, and sooner, compared to heterozygous or mutation-negative cats (Borgeat, 2014a). Conversely, Ragdolls that are heterozygous for the mutation have relatively low HCM prevalence, similar to the situation in Maine Coon cats. The mutation could be associated with slightly greater LV wall thickness, although there is much overlap with normal cats. LV wall thickness also is independently associated with body size. Yet, increased circulating levels of a type I collagen marker was identified in Ragdoll cats with the MYBPC3-R820W mutation, but without measurable LV hypertrophy. This might be an early indicator of developing hypertrophy, increased collagen turnover, and a profibrotic state in cats with the mutation, even if they appear clinically normal. Furthermore, some Ragdolls without the mutation have LV hypertrophy, suggesting other mutations or factors likely are involved, too. In some cats with the R820W mutation that have only minimal or no LV hypertrophy, subtle functional abnormalities could exist.

Testing of Maine Coon, Ragdoll, and Sphynx cats for their specific mutation is recommended, especially in animals intended for breeding, even though genetic status does not fully correlate with disease occurrence. Cats that are homozygous for the mutation should not be bred. Although breeding nonaffected cats together is optimal, selective breeding of a heterozygous cat with desired breed characteristics to a nonaffected or another heterozygous cat is reasonable, as long as the offspring are tested. Echocardiography still is needed to screen potential breeding cats because of the variable disease penetrance and the likelihood that other mutations exist.

Other single nucleotide polymorphisms of the MYBPC3 gene, A74T variants, have been identified in Maine Coon cats, Persians, Norwegian Forest cats, and several other breeds, as well as Domestic Shorthair cats. However, there appears to be no correlation between the A74T mutation and HCM. Presently unidentified mutations probably underlie other cases of HCM in cats. Variant polymorphisms in angiotensin converting enzyme (ACE) and cardiac beta-adrenergic receptor genes occur in some cats, although the significance of these is unclear. A distinct pattern of micro ribonucleic acid (RNA) expression has been observed in cats with HCM, compared to normal cats. MicroRNAs are important post-transcriptional regulators of messenger RNA expression and protein levels. They could play a role in cardiac disease development and also might eventually serve as potential biomarkers.

Pathophysiology

The pathogenesis of myocardial hypertrophy in HCM is not well-understood. Various mutations in genes coding for myocardial contractile or regulatory proteins presumably are involved, although only a limited number have been identified (see previous paragraphs). Mechanisms postulated to contribute to HCM development include increased myocardial sensitivity to, or excessive production of, catecholamines; an abnormal hypertrophic response to myocardial ischemia, fibrosis, or trophic factors; primary collagen abnormalities; and abnormal myocardial calcium-handling processes. An analogous abnormality of myofilament regulation was identified in both humans and cats with HCM, despite differences in sarcomeric gene mutations (or presumed mutations; Messer, 2017). Increased myofilament sensitivity to Ca^{++} that was not modulated by cTnI phosphorylation was found in HCM hearts, but not in normal hearts. These changes were associated with sarcomeric hypercontractility, as well as abnormalities of Ca^{++} regulation, and appeared to be the same in both humans and cats with HCM. These findings might reflect a common underlying molecular pathway, not dependent on specific gene mutations, that ultimately leads to the myocardial hypertrophy, fiber disarray, and fibrosis characteristic of HCM. Sarcomere hypercontractility probably contributes importantly to the dynamic LV outflow obstruction of HOCM. An experimental study in cats with HOCM showed that a novel small molecule (MYK-461), which decreases sarcomeric contractility by interfering with the myosin filament's ability to engage with actin, was able to abolish mitral systolic anterior motion (SAM) and markedly reduce LV outflow obstruction in a dose-dependent manner (Stern, 2016). In addition, systolic blood pressure (BP) increased slightly despite reductions in LV contractility (as estimated by fractional shortening, FS). Whether strategies aimed at directly counteracting sarcomere hypercontractility also might reduce ischemia risk or LV hypertrophy, or increase survival time, is unknown.

There are gene-nutrient interactions that might influence HCM development. Some echocardiographic and laboratory variables might be modified by diet. Preliminary evidence suggests that increased insulin-like growth factor-1 (IGF-1), larger skeletal size, and perhaps body weight, are more associated with HCM compared to normal cats. Possibly, early growth rate and nutrition might interact in some way with a genetic predisposition to HCM. Insulin, as well as inflammation, might contribute to the development of myocardial hypertrophy; higher serum insulin concentrations have been found in some cats with preclinical HCM. Cats with preclinical HCM fed a diet restricted in starch (to minimize insulin release) and supplemented with omega-3 fatty acids had reduced LV thickness measurements and IGF-1 concentration after 12 months; however, compared to a control diet group, overall differences were not significant (van Hoek, 2020). Cats with HCM have some alterations in plasma fatty acids, compared with healthy controls, although overall omega-3 fatty acid levels are not decreased in HCM cats. There could be a role for the adipokine, leptin, in the cardiac remodeling process of HCM. In people, leptin production increases in association with cardiac disease, as well as with obesity. It also is thought to enhance platelet aggregation. Compared to normal cats, increased myocardial leptin messenger RNA expression and transcription have been identified in cats with HCM, especially in atrial tissue (Fonfara, 2017). In addition, this correlated with transcription levels of some inflammatory cytokines and markers of remodeling. However, in HCM cats with an atrial thrombus, leptin expression was reduced; it is unclear what this means, although variation in gene expression related to disease stage might be a factor.

Cardiac Morphologic Abnormalities Hypertrophy of the LV free wall and/or interventricular septum (IVS) is evident grossly (**Figure 33.1**), although its extent and distribution vary. Hypertrophy might encompass the entire ventricle symmetrically or involve only certain regions. Asymmetrical septal thickening is a common pattern. In some cats, hypertrophy is limited to portions of the LV wall or papillary muscles. The LV lumen often appears small, especially in cats with severe hypertrophy; it can become virtually obliterated during systole.

Some cats with HCM also have right ventricular (RV) free wall hypertrophy, the severity of which might relate to the degree of LV hypertrophy or presence of CHF. In general, RV hypertrophy is variable, and while statistically significant

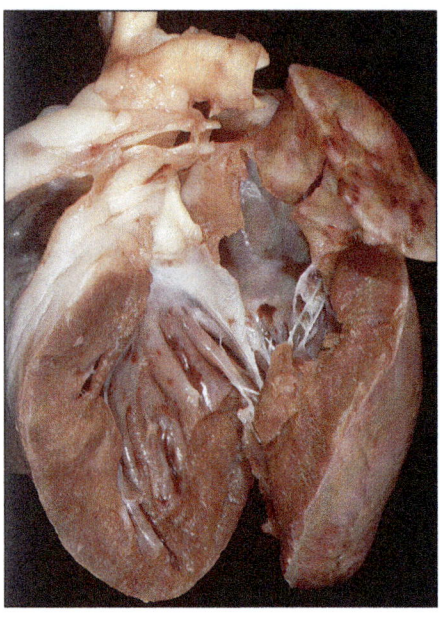

Figure 33.1 Open left ventricle & atrium from a cat with hypertrophic cardiomyopathy. Note thick ventricular wall and dilated auricle (top right).

compared to controls, usually is mild. Left apical aneurysmal dilation, with myocardial fibrosis and myocyte atrophy, occurs rarely. Secondary LA enlargement varies from mild to massive, depending largely on the severity of diastolic dysfunction. Pulmonary edema or pleural effusion from CHF might be evident on autopsy, if not clinically, in cats with advanced HCM. A thrombus sometimes is found within the left atrium, especially its appendage, or attached to the ventricular wall (**Figure 33.2**). Evidence for systemic arterial TE is common.

Except for cases of focal thickening, the heart weight to body weight ratio is increased above normal. In one postmortem study, heart weight as a percentage of body weight was 0.36 (±0.07)% in normal cats, and 0.57 (±0.17)% in cats with HCM, although some overlap was noted (Kershaw, 2012). The

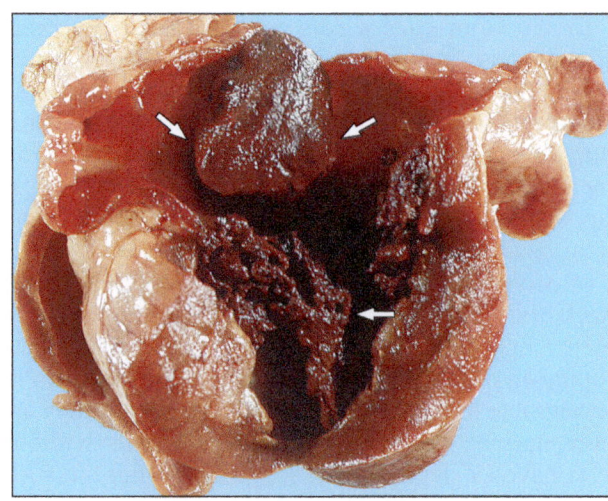

Figure 33.2 Large thrombi (arrows) present in both the left atrium (top) and ventricle in a cat with hypertrophic cardiomyopathy.

feline heart often appears thick at autopsy (even when not hypertrophied) because of muscle contracture and lack of blood volume in the chambers. Weighing the heart is a relatively quick and useful method for identifying increased myocardial mass. Most cats with HCM have a heart weight over 20 g (after removing the pericardium and retaining only the proximal segments of the aorta and pulmonary artery). Combined with the heart weight-to-body weight ratio, this measurement might help confirm a diagnosis of HCM. Another postmortem method for assessing relative heart size is to compare the heart weight (in grams) to the distance between the cat's first and eighth vertebral bodies; average distance between these vertebrae in normal and HCM cats is about 8.7–8.9 cm. Although not fully validated, values above 2.5 g/cm distance appeared to indicate increased heart weight, and clearly demarcated the two study groups; however, mild or early hypertrophy might not be detected (Kershaw, 2012). This method is somewhat analogous to the vertebral heart size (VHS) method used radiographically. It also avoids the confounding effect of body fat on total weight. Cross-sectional slices through the heart (for example, midway between the coronary groove and apex) also show increased total myocardial area in HCM. With regard to diagnostic usefulness, myocardial wall thickness (or total cross-sectional area) and relative heart weight (especially indexed to the distance between 1st and 8th vertebrae) appear superior to histologic/morphometric criteria.

Histologic findings in cats with HCM include variable cardiomyocyte hypertrophy and myocardial fiber disarray (disorganization; **Figure 33.3**). Some cats have severe, diffuse myocyte hypertrophy with much myofiber disarray. In others, the myocyte disorganization might be focal and not apparent on all sections. Some histologic morphometric evaluations comparing normal and HCM cats have shown only minimally increased cardiomyocyte diameter and cross-sectional area in HCM cats, with no increase in myocyte branching or myocardial fibrosis. Others report inconsistent amounts of interstitial fibrosis, cardiomyocyte hypertrophy and fiber disarray, as well as some arteriolar wall hypertrophy. However, the specific areas sampled or other factors could influence the histologic observations. Focal or diffuse areas of fibrosis within the endocardium, conduction system, or myocardium are common. Endomyocardial fibrosis was noted in Norwegian Forest cats with familial cardiomyopathy, and can occur in others as well. Focal areas of inflammatory cell infiltrates and increased myocardial collagen also have been observed in cats with mild preclinical HCM. Inflammatory cytokines could contribute to the increased interstitial collagen and fibrosis seen in HCM. Ultrastructural changes, observed with transmission electron microscopy in a small number of cats with HCM, involve cardiomyocyte and interstitial structural abnormalities, including myofibrillar disorganization, decreased mitochondrial numbers, and excessive intercellular matrix formation.

Arteriosclerosis and narrowing of small intramural coronary arteries are common findings in cats with HCM. This can predispose to myocardial ischemia, focal myocardial infarctions and replacement fibrosis, which are evident in some cats with HCM. A relative reduction in myocardial capillary density also occurs as hypertrophy progresses; this can contribute to the increased ischemia risk. Ischemia not only exacerbates ventricular stiffness and impaired filling, it can provoke tachyarrhythmias, which then further reduce filling time, increase filling pressure, and promote more ischemia, ultimately leading to CHF and other adverse effects. Cats with subclinical HCM and sudden unexpected death commonly have histopathologic findings of interstitial fibrosis, intramural coronary arteriosclerosis and narrowing, as well as myocardial fiber disarray. Presumably, the small vessel changes predispose to ischemia with subsequent lethal arrhythmias. Microvascular disease, as well as interstitial fibrosis, probably also facilitate progression to end-stage LV remodeling in other cats.

Myocardial Functional and Hemodynamic Abnormalities

The pathophysiology of diastolic dysfunction in HCM involves impaired myocardial active relaxation in early diastole, and abnormal ventricular wall stiffness that impedes filling during the rest of diastole. Multiple factors, many of which are unstudied in cats, could contribute to diastolic heart failure in different individuals. These include: the myocardial hypertrophy itself, myocyte injury caused by ischemia or inflammation, intercellular matrix changes, cell death, interstitial fibrosis, disordered myofiber orientation (cardiomyocyte disarray), abnormal intracellular calcium handling, and increased myocardial calcium sensitivity. Disorganized myocardial cell structure and fibrosis contribute to higher LV filling pressure

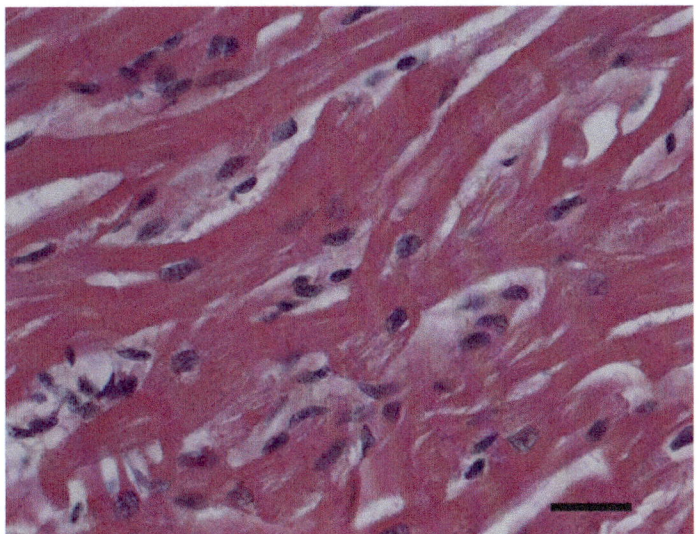

Figure 33.3 Histopathologic section from a cat with preclinical hypertrophic cardiomyopathy. Mild myocyte hypertrophy is present, along with an area of myocardial fiber disarray (bottom half of image); some cardiomyocytes are oriented at oblique angles to each other. Hematoxylin and eosin stain; bar = 60 μm. (From Khor, 2015)

during mid- and late diastole. Slowed or incomplete early (active) relaxation interferes with the normally rapid early diastolic LV pressure drop, prolongs isovolumic relaxation time (IVRT; p. 18), reduces early ventricular filling, and increases the importance of atrial contraction to cardiac filling in late diastole. Delayed relaxation can manifest as an atrial (S_4) gallop sound, especially when the heart is under sympathetic stimulation.

Myocardial ischemia (of both the supply and demand types) further impairs diastolic function. This can be labile, and might explain some cases of "flash" pulmonary edema observed often in cats (and people) with diastolic heart failure. Anatomical and pathophysiological factors likely contribute to reduced myocardial perfusion in HCM. Anatomical factors include intramural coronary artery narrowing, and reduced myocardial capillary density associated with pathologic hypertrophy. Any stress-induced tachycardia decreases coronary perfusion because it impairs active relaxation, elevates LV filling pressures, and shortens diastole and coronary filling time. High sympathetic tone also increases BP, myocardial contractility and dynamic outflow obstruction. Each of these consequences increases myocardial oxygen demand. Recurrent or chronic ischemia leads to myocardial cell necrosis and fibrosis; it also predisposes to lethal arrhythmias and perhaps even to exertional thoracic pain (angina).

Considering these adverse adrenergic effects on the hypertrophied heart, it has long been speculated that sympathomimetic surges are a cause of the sudden decompensation that can occur following stressful events in cats with HCM. This idea is one rationale used for empirically prescribing atenolol to cats with HCM. Such stressors could include veterinary hospital examinations or procedures, introduction of a new cat into the household, and even moving to a new home. Another speculation is whether cats that suffer sudden sympathetic stress to the heart might develop ischemic cardiac "stunning," or sudden changes in ventricular stiffness or function. Some cats are presented emergently in cardiogenic shock, with moderate to severe LV hypertrophy, bradycardia, normal to enhanced systolic function, and no clear proximate cause, such as an arterial thromboembolim (TE). Some of these cats recover completely. Clearly, much remains to be learned about the influence of ischemia and the sympathetic nervous system on the feline heart in this disease.

With regard to hemodynamics, increased ventricular stiffness leads to reduced ventricular filling and elevated LV filling pressure, which raises LA and pulmonary venous pressures. LV diastolic volume can be normal; however, it often is decreased in HCM. From a practical standpoint, cats with diastolic dysfunction are less able to tolerate a fluid overload, because this further increases LV filling pressure and predisposes to pulmonary congestion or overt CHF. HCM often is "revealed" after fluid therapy in cats with previously preclinical disease. Ventricular stiffness and relaxation abnormalities do not always correlate to the degree or distribution of hypertrophy; however, markedly impaired LV filling often accompanies severe LV hypertrophy. Reduced ventricular end-diastolic volume yields a lower stroke volume, although by LaPlace's law, wall thickening might compensate by decreasing peak wall stress. Cats with compensated HCM, and even many with pulmonary edema, exhibit a hyperdynamic LV with high ejection fraction, which can be appreciated by echocardiography. Yet reduced cardiac output eventually can contribute to neurohormonal activation. Compensatory increases in heart rate (HR) shorten diastolic filling time and can further reduce LV filling, and exacerbate myocardial ischemia and heart failure. Thus, advanced LV diastolic dysfunction typically leads to clinical signs of CHF, despite seemingly normal global systolic function. This is known as heart failure with preserved ejection fraction in people.

Experience indicates that cats with HCM in respiratory distress usually have either acute pulmonary edema or a moderate to large pleural effusion. While both of these situations are emergent, their pathogenesis likely differs. Cats with a large pleural effusion clearly have retained a large volume of fluid, and they often have reduced systolic function and marked LA enlargement. Cats with sudden-onset pulmonary edema also have LA enlargement, but it often is mild; after diuresis, some even have an LA size that appears normal. This suggests that other decompensating factors might be involved in a sudden worsening of LV diastolic function. In some of these cats, pulmonary edema is labile, occasionally resolving even when diuretics are discontinued.

When HCM progresses more gradually to clinical signs of CHF, moderate to severe LA dilation is anticipated. Gradual LA enlargement and a more vigorous atrial contraction initially buffer the progressive rise in LV diastolic, LA, and pulmonary venous pressures. Likewise, enhanced pulmonary lymphatic flow can mitigate the effects of increasing pulmonary capillary pressure. Over time, however, LA compliance and function decrease; this is evidenced by reduced LA fractional area change and diminished LA appendage ejection velocities. As LA pressure rises, pulmonary congestion and edema can occur. In experimental pulmonary edema (in opened-chest cats), an increase in LA pressure to ~30 mm Hg resulted in marked accumulation of lung water and alveolar flooding (Hauge, 1977). It is likely that LA pressures are higher in some cats with chronic disease, and probably lower in those with flash pulmonary edema. LV and papillary muscle geometric changes, as well as abnormal systolic mitral valve motion, can interfere with mitral valve closure. Secondary mitral regurgitation (MR), if substantial, could exacerbate the increasing LA volume and pressure. Additionally, severe LA dilation could increase that chamber's stiffness and impede RV output.

Pulmonary blood volume, and the time required to traverse the pulmonary vasculature (pulmonary transit time), are increased in HCM. The lung's capacity to hold additional blood volume is much lower than that of the systemic circulation, and increased blood volume predisposes to pulmonary congestion and edema. A larger LA to aortic root dimension ratio (LA/Ao) is associated with greater pulmonary blood volume, as well as prolonged normalized pulmonary transit times; this suggests reduced cardiac output and higher risk for CHF (because cardiac output from both ventricles must equalize over time).

The development of pulmonary edema generally is the initial manifestation of CHF in cats with HCM. Pleural (and sometimes mild pericardial) effusion also are common with CHF, especially in later stages of disease. The effusion typically is a modified transudate, although the pleural fluid often becomes chylous over time. In some cats with incipient CHF, a small pericardial effusion (observed during echo exam) is an indication to obtain thoracic radiographs and consider preemptive therapy.

As heart failure develops, activation of the renin-angiotensin-aldosterone system (RAAS), and presumably other neurohormonal mechanisms, occurs (p. 303). Circulating cardiac troponin (cTn)I and natriuretic peptide concentrations increase with moderate to severe HCM, with higher levels associated with overt CHF (p. 660). Cardiac adrenomedullin RNA expression also increases in cats with HCM. Adrenomedullin is another peptide that promotes vasorelaxation and natriuresis. The precise role of these mediators in the progression of feline myocardial disease and development of heart failure is unknown; as such, the value of RAAS inhibition therapies for feline cardiomyopathies is unresolved.

Feline HCM is considered a diastolic heart failure disorder. Yet LV systolic function is relevant. Based on FS (or other estimates of ejection fraction), global LV function is normal to hyperdynamic in most cats with HCM. However, depression of contractile function at the cellular level might occur. Based on Laplace's law, wall thickening should normalize peak LV wall tension and therefore, the peak afterload on the ventricle. Along with an increase in HR, these can compensate for a reduced preload and so maintain cardiac output. Although afterload might increase in cats with dynamic LV outflow tract obstruction, the peak pressure gradient does not develop until nearly all of the stroke volume has been ejected; thus, wall stress should be lower than for a fixed aortic stenosis. However, some cats develop regional or global LV systolic dysfunction; this is supported by the aforementioned prolongation in normalized pulmonary transit time reported in cats with progressive cardiomyopathy. Depressed contractile function likely stems from myocardial infarction or fibrosis, and perhaps is exacerbated by neurohormonal injury. End-stage ("burned out") HCM is characterized by progressive decline in segmental or global systolic function, along with increasing LA dilation. Often there is regional or global LV wall thinning in areas that previously were hypertrophied. Marked LA enlargement, a restrictive LV filling pattern on Doppler echocardiography (see p. 669, below, and **Figure 4.31B**, p. 109 and related text), and increased myocardial fibrosis indicate an advanced stage of disease. Echo findings in such cases can be confused with RCM, especially if there is little residual wall thickening or prior echo studies are unavailable for comparison. These cats might have a "normal" LV FS by echocardiography, but clearly reduced LV free wall or septal excursion. Progression to global ventricular systolic failure with LV dilation occurs in some cats with end-stage disease, and so overlaps with the DCM phenotype. Similar progressions are observed in some people with chronic HCM.

At least four types of dynamic ventricular outflow obstruction have been observed in cats with HCM: (1) mitral valve SAM; (2) midventricular obstruction, between the hypertrophied septum and papillary muscles; (3) dynamic RV outflow tract obstruction, which could be physiologic but possibly is enhanced by septal thickening; and (4) potentially, subaortic septal bulges (although these rarely cause obstruction in isolation). The classic LV outflow obstruction is SAM of the mitral valve; this is what most clinicians refer to when discussing HOCM or outflow obstruction in cats (or in humnas). The systolic mitral leaflet–septal contact of HOCM generates a mid- to late systolic flow acceleration (and pressure gradient) in the LV outlet, which is detectable by continuous wave (CW) Doppler imaging. Coinciding with this, an eccentric MR jet forms as the mitral leaflets and chords are pulled towards the septum. Several mechanisms could underlie SAM; these include: (1) septal hypertrophy that narrows the LV outlet; (2) generalized myocardial hypertrophy that reduces LV volume; (3) papillary muscle hypertrophy that alters the normal traction on the leaflet(s); (4) structural abnormalities of the mitral apparatus; and (5) a suction (Venturi) effect that pulls the mitral leaflet toward the IVS during ejection. The last mechanism is probably additive to the others. Mid-ventricular obstruction also is common, and usually related to LV cavity obliteration during systole. This obstruction can be recognized by color and spectral Doppler imaging. Dynamic RV outflow obstruction can occur, too, although it is not always associated with HOCM and tends to be mild. However, it can produce a prominent systolic murmur in some cats. Some degree of tricuspid regurgitation (TR) also is common in cats with HCM, but this does not necessarily correlate to dynamic obstruction or detectable murmurs. Pulmonary hypertension has not been a common finding in cats with HCM (Vezzosi, 2019). However, it also can be difficult to recognize, as strong TR jets are few.

The LV outflow tract gradient produced by SAM is labile, as is its accompanying murmur's intensity. Both increase with stress and excitement as higher sympathetic tone enhances contractility, shortening, and HR. Mild to moderate functional MR typically accompanies SAM (p. 669); its severity tends to parallel the degree of SAM and dynamic LV outflow obstruction. The systolic murmur detected in HOCM likely relates to MR as much as to the subaortic obstruction, although both probably contribute. Beta-blockade tends to diminish or eliminate SAM, as well as audible murmurs, in many cats. SAM can provoke endocardial scar tissue formation where the mitral leaflet repeatedly contacts the IVS during systole. This contact lesion is evident at autopsy and sometimes, with two-dimensional (2D) echocardiography. LV systolic outflow obstruction increases intraventricular pressure, at least in mid- to late systole. Thus, SAM might increase LV wall stress during a portion of systole. Theoretically, this would increase myocardial oxygen demand and induce transient subendocardial myocardial ischemia. Increased N-terminal probrain (B-type) natriuretic peptide (NT-proBNP) and cTnI concentrations have been associated independently with the presence of SAM, even in cats without LV hypertrophy or LA enlargement. Whether SAM in cats with HOCM is simply a pathophysiologic curiosity and diagnostic clue (by generating murmurs), or clinically important to the pathogenesis of this disease is uncertain. It is an independent predictor of sudden death in people, but this has not been shown in cats.

Because most cats with HCM have only mild to moderate MR, a markedly enlarged LA usually indicates long-standing and advanced diastolic (± systolic) dysfunction. The strength of LA chamber and appendage contractile force (which together generates the "atrial kick") typically declines in these cats. Pulsed wave (PW) Doppler echocardiography can demonstrate this. These factors promote blood stasis, which can trigger clot formation. Spontaneous contrast (echocontrast, "smoke"), seen on echocardiogram, is thought to represent cellular aggregates forming in poorly moving blood. It is an indication that conditions are ripe for thrombus formation within the heart, especially within a dilated, hypocontractile left auricle. If dislodged, the devastating complications of systemic TE can follow (Chapter 36). A large thromboembolus is likely to lodge in the distal aorta or another major artery, resulting in acute and severe clinical signs. Small emboli could be clinically silent, depending on their location. Renal infarcts are common. Elevations in mean fibrinogen and von Willebrand factor antigen concentrations, as indicators of hypercoagulability and endothelial injury, respectively, have been observed in cats with spontaneous echocontrast and in those with arterial TE. An increase in biomarkers of platelet activation also was observed in cats with severe HCM.

Clinical Features

The prevalence of HCM has been estimated at between 10 and 16% of the general (mixed and purebred) cat population, and over 25% in some breeds, such as the Maine Coon and Ragdoll. Besides these breeds, HCM probably is inherited in Sphynx, Norwegian Forest, American and British Shorthairs, Persian, Bengal, Birman, Chartreux, Cornish Rex, and possibly other breeds. It also occurs in families of domestic shorthair (DSH) cats. An autosomal dominant inheritance pattern has been found in the families studied, similar to the most common inheritance pattern in people. The occurrence of HCM increases with age. In a survey of 780 clinically healthy cats, HCM prevalence ranged from about 4% in cats under 1-year old to ~29% in those ≥9 years old (CATSCAN study, Payne, 2015b). When evaluating any study of HCM, one should understand the criteria used for diagnosis and the method of wall (or septal) thickness measurement (Chapter 4). The criterion for HCM in CATSCAN was a wall thickness of ≥ 6mm measured by 2D imaging at the tissue/blood interface. Values 5.5 to 5.9 mm were considered equivocal. In general, 2D measurement of wall thickness generates slightly greater values (by 1 to 3 mm) than a leading edge-to-leading edge M-mode study. However, the 6 mm criterion used in CATSCAN is conservative and relatively specific, except for very large cats and perhaps some Bengal cats. Besides age, other factors associated with HCM in this population were male gender, increased body condition score, and a moderate to loud heart murmur. HCM is reported most often in middle-aged male cats, but it can occur in young, as well as geriatric, animals. British Shorthair, Maine Coon and Sphynx cats appear to develop HCM at an earlier age than other breeds. For the Maine Coon breed, this largely is influenced by MYBPC3 status. Despite an increased prevalence of HCM in males, the mutations identified in Maine Coon and Ragdoll cats do not show a sex bias.

When considering the clinical presentation of HCM in cats, it is helpful to divide patient groups into "clinically normal" (asymptomatic cats) and cats that demonstrate signs of "clinical disease." The first group is by far the largest. Two important subgroups of healthy cats are those that are about to undergo an anesthetic procedure, and cats that will be used for breeding. HCM screening, especially for these cats, is described in the following paragraphs.

Screening for Hypertrophic Cardiomyopathy Whenever a cat without cardiovascular signs is examined by a veterinarian, it is, in a sense, undergoing a screening for HCM. This most important feline heart disease can occur at virtually any age. In healthy cats, or those without clinical signs of cardiovascular disease, clinically silent cardiomyopathy generally will be exposed only through abnormalities fortuitously uncovered by auscultation, biomarker tests, ECG, or diagnostic imaging (radiography or ultrasound). With a few exceptions (summarized in the next paragraphs), there currently are no compelling data indicating that all cats should undergo extensive cardiac testing for HCM beyond the physical examination. Routine NT-proBNP or cTnI measurement in all healthy cats with normal auscultation is discouraged. Such screening for all healthy cats undoubtedly will lead to many false positives, simply based on the lower disease prevalence in that wide population. Similarly, the use of thoracic radiography, electrocardiography, and even echocardiography as screening tools for the general feline population is not supported by data, and is too insensitive and cost-ineffective.

One major exception to the preceding statements involves HCM screening in cats to be used for breeding, especially those of a breed at known risk or positive for a genetic mutation associated with HCM. These cats should be tested for available genetic markers – something most reputable breeders do outside the veterinary practice – and by echocardiography (see "Echocardiography" section). Results of genetic testing can influence breeding recommendations; for example, cats homozygous for a breed-specific mutation should not be bred. However, genetic testing alone does not provide adequate screening for HCM. Likewise, currently available natriuretic peptide tests are not sufficiently sensitive or specific for this pre-breeding screen. Echocardiography is the most effective screening method for purebred breeding cats, and should be done prior to first breeding and every 1–2 years thereafter. The technical challenges involving in acquiring and interpreting feline echocardiograms are substantial, especially in cats with mild disease. Therefore, it is recommended that these exams be performed by a cardiology specialist. Echo evaluation includes cardiac chamber dimension and wall thickness measurements, systolic function assessment, LA size and function determination, additional subjective observations, and ideally, Doppler and TDI interrogations.

Other asymptomatic cats at potentially higher risk, if preclinical HCM were to remain undiscovered, are those undergoing general anesthesia. In addition, cats with systemic illnesses are at potentially higher risk, especially those needing large volume or recurrent fluid therapy. Requiring an echo exam for every cat prior to anesthesia probably is unwarranted, for the reasons cited previously and the need for appropriate ultrasound training. However, some veterinarians do routinely obtain a pre-procedure NT-proBNP, either using the ELISA-based point-of-care (POC) or reference laboratory tests, in an attempt stratify risk of occult HCM (see "Laboratory Tests" section). For cats with a "positive" NT-proBNP result, an echo exam usually is recommended. A POC "quick" thoracic ultrasound examination has been advocated by some to screen for underlying HCM in asymptomatic cats. A clinically normal cat's age is relevant in deciding whether or when to pursue a complete echo exam. HCM prevalence is relatively low in young cats; but it becomes much higher in those older than 9 years. Therefore, the relative importance for echo screening increases in older cats, especially those needing prolonged general anesthesia, fluid therapy, as well as long-acting (depot) corticosteroids. Results of the preanesthetic echo exam can modify the planning of anesthetic regimens (Clark, 2020). There also are some data showing that brief POC ultrasound scans conducted by trained, non-specialist individuals can identify moderate to severe heart disease prior to anesthesia. Yet rigorous cost-benefit analysis of echo or biomarker screening in these cats (that have no other signs of heart disease) has not been reported.

However, the discovery of a cardiac murmur, gallop sound or arrhythmia on routine auscultation, or the fortuitous discovery of cardiomegaly on thoracic radiographs, indicates increased relative risk for structural heart disease, especially in cats >6 months of age. These findings warrant follow-up testing, especially in middle-aged and older cats. The usual initial test in general practice is NT-proBNP; additional guidelines are summarized in **Figure 33.4**.

History Cats with mild HCM can remain asymptomatic for years and many never develop cardiac signs. The majority of cats diagnosed with preclinical HCM or HOCM have good long-term survival (p. 672). For cats that develop clinical disease, signs associated with CHF occur most commonly; those of arterial TE are next in frequency. Syncope, likely related to cardiac arrhythmias, affects some cats. Sudden death without premonitory signs occurs occasionally. Arterial TE typically produces signs of sudden and painful posterior paresis, although other manifestations can occur (p. 755).

Early signs of CHF can include withdrawal, inactivity, reduced tolerance for play or exercise, increased respiratory rate or effort, panting with exertion (although this can be normal after vigorous play), lethargy, and poor appetite. The onset of CHF might seem sudden, although pathologic changes develop gradually. Tachypnea and overt respiratory distress are the most common signs of severe acute CHF, as well as of progressive but previously tolerated CHF that was unrecognized until becoming urgent. Coughing, sometimes misinterpreted as retching or vomiting, is uncommon in cats with CHF; however, it can occur, especially with severe cardiomegaly or edema. Stress from anesthesia and surgery, fluid administration, systemic illness (such as infections with fever, anemia, or thyrotoxicosis), and even boarding or veterinary appointments can precipitate CHF in cats with occult HCM or other cardiomyopathy. Cats with stress-induced peracute pulmonary edema that resolves following emergent diuretic treatment, might not experience recurrent pulmonary edema for a prolonged time. Cats that develop signs of acute CHF are likely to be middle-aged or older.

Physical Findings - Auscultation Physical examination findings often are normal in cats with preclinical (occult) HCM. Yet in many cases, a murmur, gallop sound, or arrhythmia heard during auscultation signals the presence of disease. According to some reports, about 20% of HCM cases in a referral population have normal cardiac auscultatory findings at the time of diagnosis. Some cats have no murmur even with marked ventricular hypertrophy; these cats are unlikely to be identified unless they become symptomatic. It is important to note that a murmur is not considered specific for cardiomyopathy in otherwise healthy cats, especially those of young age (p. 226). But for cats with a murmur, the likelihood of HCM being the underlying cause increases with age, greater murmur intensity (grade 3–4/6), male sex, and possibly, larger body size. Up to 80% of cats with preclinical HCM could have a murmur; however, this figure probably is biased, because only those healthy cats with a murmur are likely to be further evaluated. An audible gallop sound generates much stronger suspicion for cardiomyopathy, particularly in younger cats, because it usually indicates increased ventricular stiffness or LA pressure. Nevertheless, gallop sounds are heard in some cats with hyperthyroidism, hypertension, or anemia, as well as in some stressed geriatric cats without apparent myocardial disease. The cause in some of these cases might be slowed ventricular relaxation associated with aging, with vigorous atrial contraction in compensation.

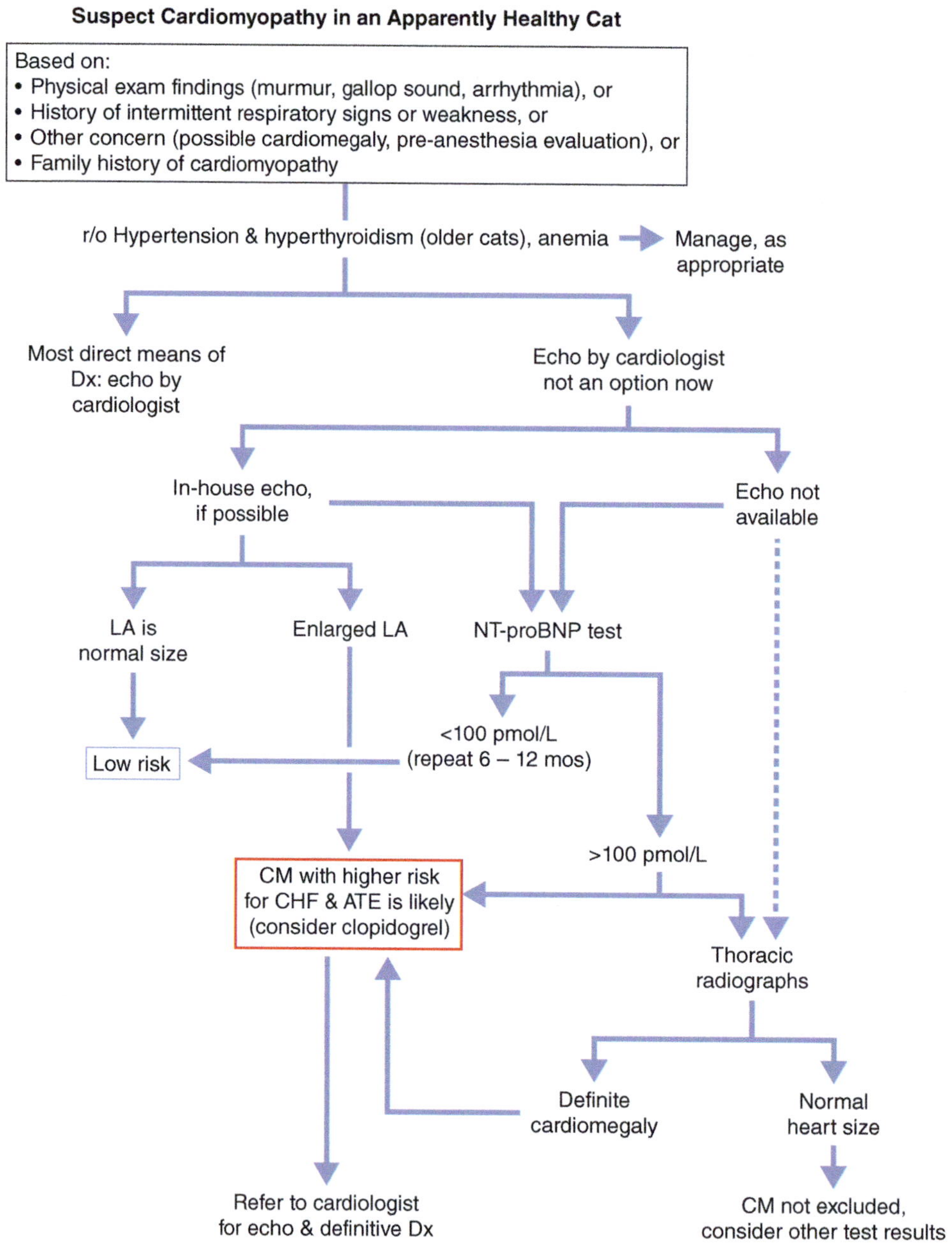

Suspect Cardiomyopathy in an Apparently Healthy Cat

Based on:
- Physical exam findings (murmur, gallop sound, arrhythmia), or
- History of intermittent respiratory signs or weakness, or
- Other concern (possible cardiomegaly, pre-anesthesia evaluation), or
- Family history of cardiomyopathy

↓

r/o Hypertension & hyperthyroidism (older cats), anemia → Manage, as appropriate

↓

- Most direct means of Dx: echo by cardiologist
- Echo by cardiologist not an option now

↓

- In-house echo, if possible
- Echo not available

↓

- LA is normal size → Low risk
- Enlarged LA
- NT-proBNP test
  - <100 pmol/L (repeat 6 – 12 mos) → Low risk
  - >100 pmol/L

↓

CM with higher risk for CHF & ATE is likely (consider clopidogrel)

↓

Thoracic radiographs
- Definite cardiomegaly → Refer to cardiologist for echo & definitive Dx
- Normal heart size → CM not excluded, consider other test results

Figure 33.4 Suggested approach for evaluating a cat suspected to have cardiomyopathy. (Derived from ACVIM consensus statement guidelines; Luis Fuentes, 2020). ATE, arterial thromboembolism; CHF, congestive heart failure; CM, cardiomyopathy; Dx, diagnosis; echo, echocardiography; LA, left atrium; NT-proBNP, N-terminal probrain natriuretic peptide; r/o, rule out.

A murmur detected in an asymptomatic cat frequently prompts referral for echocardiography. Many of these cats have HCM, but most do not. For practical purposes, a heart murmur in a cat indicates one of three general causes: (1) a functional (physiologic) murmur; (2) a congenital heart defect; or (3) a primary or secondary form of cardiomyopathy, usually associated with LV thickening. A congenital cardiac malformation should be considered when a loud murmur is heard, especially in a younger cat or one new to a veterinary practice. Functional systolic murmurs often relate to noncardiac disorders, including anemia, hyperthyroidism, systemic hypertension (p. 228), and pulmonary hypertension. Each of these conditions enhances sympathetic tone and alters peripheral vascular resistance, which can cause a functional murmur. When chronic, these diseases also are associated with secondary cardiac remodeling. Functional heart murmurs thought to arise from "stress" and associated increases in LV or RV outflow tract ejection velocity occur in many cats (Rishniw, 2002), although the pathogenesis of RV outflow tract murmurs has been challenged as iatrogenic in some cases (Ferasin, 2020). Functional murmurs commonly increase and decrease in intensity with varying sympathetic tone; however, this also is true of pathological murmurs in cats. Additionally, while louder heart murmurs are more likely to be associated with structural heart disease, some functional murmurs can be quite intense, although many are soft and localized.

Many veterinarians do not appreciate how frequently functional (nonpathologic) murmurs occur in cats. These account for the large majority of systolic murmurs in young cats and roughly half of the heart murmurs detected in mature cats. These estimates are based on reported studies, but are substantially influenced (raised or lowered) depending on the wall thickness criteria used to diagnose HCM (for example, 5.2 mm by M-mode versus 6.0 mm by 2D echo exam; see "Echocardiography" section). In the CATSCAN study (Payne, 2015b), a systolic murmur was detected in approximately 40% of the 780 healthy cats studied. Of those cats, 70% were considered functional based on echo exam, using 6 mm wall thickness as the HCM criterion). Importantly, most of these cats were auscultated more than once, and in many, murmurs were not detected at each examination. The multiple evaluations also probably account for the higher murmur prevalence in this study compared to prior studies of healthy cats, where prevalence was lower (15.5 to 33.7%). The overall negative predictive value of auscultation (that is, a cat with no murmur, gallop or arrhythmia) is high for ruling out HCM in younger cats. In older cats (with a greater prevalence of HCM), the positive predictive value of hearing a cardiac murmur becomes greater, although still relatively low. Furthermore, murmur intensity does not correlate with the severity of disease in cats.

Systolic murmurs in cats with HCM could arise from at least four types of outflow obstruction, as well MR and possibly TR, as previously noted (see "Pathophysiology"). Often more than one potential cause can be identified by Doppler echocardiography. Dynamic LV or RV outflow tract obstruction, subaortic narrowing, and midventricular cavity obliteration are all potential sources of variable systolic murmurs in HCM. It is challenging to differentiate a murmur of outflow obstruction from MR by auscultation alone, considering that the stethoscope chest piece covers a good portion of the feline heart, both murmurs can occur concurrently, and the rapid HR makes precise murmur timing difficult. Some animals with dynamic LV outflow obstruction and MR caused by mitral SAM have loud murmurs with minimal LA enlargement. Others with advanced HCM have soft (or absent) murmurs because of reduced systolic function or LV dilation, which reduces SAM and dynamic obstructions. Murmurs of MR are most prominent when mitral SAM is present. At slower HRs, this murmur's onset after the S_1 (at the time of mitral septal contact) could be discernable. In cats with LV outflow obstruction, murmur intensity varies with the degree of obstruction and concurrent mitral SAM. The murmur can be quite soft or even inaudible in the relaxed cat, especially those on beta-blocker therapy. The intensity (grade) of any of these murmurs can increase as dynamic obstruction worsens with higher sympathetic tone and its associated increases in HR, contractility, and ventricular pressures. In some cats, the only potential murmur source identified on Doppler echo exam is dynamic RV outflow obstruction. This generally is considered nonpathologic (functional), although in HCM, septal thickening that impinges on the right ventricle might provoke it.

An audible cardiac gallop sound is a manifestation of impaired LV relaxation, compliance, and filling. It reportedly is present in only a minority of cases but can be challenging to identify, especially when there also is a heart murmur. Gallop detection probably depends in part on the experience and training of the examiner. A gallop sound (usually S_4 or a summation gallop, p. 232) is more likely to become audible in cats with incipient or overt CHF, as LA pressure increases. Whether some transient sounds detected in HCM are systolic clicks is uncertain, although this was suggested by one study (Blass, 2013).

Cardiac arrhythmias also might be heard in cats with asymptomatic HCM, as well as those with clinical signs. In both groups, simple and complex ventricular and supraventricular tachyarrhythmias occur with some frequency. Premature beats often are recognized by the pause following the extrasystole, or during an echo exam. Electrocardiography is recommended to further define these. Femoral pulses usually are normal in cats with HCM, unless a tachyarrhythmia or distal aortic TE has occurred. A vigorous precordial impulse often is palpable. BP generally is normal in both preclinical HCM and overt CHF.

Physical Findings–Congestive Heart Failure Respiratory distress is reported in about a third of cats with CHF. Moderate to severe LV diastolic dysfunction typically is present in these cases. Physical exam findings in cats with CHF can include prominent bronchial sounds as well as tachypnea and, in those with severe pulmonary edema, pulmonary crackles and cyanosis. Pleural effusion is common with chronic and end-stage HCM and usually attenuates ventral lung sounds. A moderate to large pleural effusion points to more chronic CHF. Tachypnea also is a manifestation of pain in cats with arterial TE, even in those without pulmonary edema or pleural effusion. Body temperature tends to be lower in cats with clinical signs. Some cats with acute CHF or arterial TE are hypothermic, which often foreshadows a worse outcome. The triad of hypothermia, bradycardia, and systemic hypotension is common in cats with cardiogenic shock, although hypovolemic and septic shock should be excluded. Some cats in shock from heart failure have evidence of intra-abdominal disease such as pancreatitis.

Cats with CHF often have sinus rhythm with a normal or somewhat lower HR (compared to cats with preclinical disease); this is in contrast to the sinus tachycardia typically seen in dogs with CHF. Nevertheless, many cats with CHF have HRs over 200 beats/min. Besides sinus tachycardia, a rapid HR could stem from frequent premature beats, supraventricular or ventricular tachycardia, or atrial fibrillation (AF). A slower than expected HR can result from sinus bradycardia or advanced atrioventricular (AV) block. Hypothermia might underlie sinus bradycardia. While murmurs are common in cats with asymptomatic HCM, only about half of those with CHF appear to have an audible murmur. Abnormal rhythms and an audible gallop sound are more common in cats with CHF; a gallop sound is reported in about a third of cases. The type of gallop sound most often detected in cats with CHF has not been studied rigorously with phonocardiography; but based on limited recordings, it likely is an S_3 or a summation ($S_3 + S_4$) gallop. Other physical findings in cats with acute CHF include weakness, mucous membrane pallor, and weak or irregular femoral pulses. Jugular vein distension or pulsations and, rarely, ascites are most often found in cats with advanced disease and a moderate to large pleural effusion. Cardiac cachexia develops in some cats with CHF; associated findings include older age, pleural effusion, azotemia, and lower body condition score (Santiago, 2020).

Diagnostic Tests

Initial screening of cats with a cardiac murmur can involve measuring NT-proBNP concentration and if possible, LA size by focused thoracic (cardiac) ultrasound scan (see p. 665 and p. 80). NT-proBNP concentration rises in cats with moderate to severe disease (see next section); however, this test does not reliably distinguish normal cats from those with mild disease. Likewise, standard serum cTnI testing, ECG, and thoracic radiography are not sensitive enough tests to distinguish mildly affected cats from normal. While high-sensitivity cTnI test results >0.06 ng/mL have differentiated cats with HCM from normal cats with good sensitivity and specificity, echocardiography still is recommended for confirmation (Hertzsch, 2019). Echocardiography is the "gold standard" screening test; again, referral to a veterinary cardiologist for this is advised when feasible. In equivocal cases, repeated echo evaluations over time (perhaps every 6–12 months) can help identify progressive changes and separate early HCM from normal variation.

Cats suspected to have HCM should be screened for potential secondary myocardial diseases as appropriate for their age and comorbidities, such as chronic kidney disease. Secondary myocardial disease also can occur with systemic hypertension (Chapter 38), hyperthyroidism, diabetes mellitus, and acromegaly, especially in older cats. Other causes of LV wall thickening identified on echo exam, might include myocarditis, congenital aortic stenosis, mitral valve malformations with dynamic LV outflow obstruction, and lymphoma or other infiltrative neoplasia. Myocarditis can cause transient myocardial thickening (p. 688).

Laboratory Tests Routine complete blood count (CBC) and biochemical laboratory tests are not helpful for diagnosing HCM in cats with (or without) CHF. Biochemical and hematologic changes often relate to medication effects or concurrent disease. Cats with HCM and CHF can have greater variation in RBC size (increased RBC distribution width, RDW) than those with preclinical HCM or normal hearts. RDW an indicator of regenerative anemia. However, overlap among groups precludes its use as a diagnostic test. Reports conflict as to whether greater RDW on a single sample is associated with worse prognosis in cardiomyopathic cats with CHF. In people with CHF, progressively increasing RDW on serial measurements is associated with shortened survival. Elevations in symmetric dimethylarginine (SDMA) concentration consistent with early renal dysfunction, along with evidence for systemic inflammation, also have been observed in cardiomyopathic cats with CHF. Increased SDMA concentration appears to be associated with shorter survival.

Cardiac biomarkers, mainly NT-proBNP and cTnI, might identify cats with preclinical HCM or CHF. Two proprietary tests (Cardio-Pet proBNP and "SNAP" Feline proBNP; IDEXX Laboratories, Westbrook, ME) are currently available that measure NT-proBNP in the blood. The POC "SNAP" ELISA test is generally considered a binary "negative/positive" test. The reference laboratory test quantifies the amount of natriuretic peptide fragment in the blood in pmol/L. There are three general patient types where natriuretic peptide testing is most often directed. The first is the asymptomatic cat with a murmur, gallop, arrhythmia or incidental cardiomegaly. The second is the cat in respiratory distress where CHF is a possible cause. The third type of feline patient has a systemic disease that can affect the heart (systemic hypertension, hyperthyroidism, diabetes mellitus), or with a comorbidity where therapy (IV fluids, repositol corticosteroids) might destabilize underlying occult HCM. These tests should be selected, and results interpreted, with these points in mind.

The reference laboratory indicates that values of NT-proBNP >100 pmol/L are associated with increased risk of HCM in healthy, asymptomatic cats. Earlier multicenter studies showed that values between 50 and 100 pmol/L were equivocal. In general, there are more false positives than false negatives for the NT-proBNP test, in terms of predicting asymptomatic HCM. This likely stems from studies that group together "normal" and "mildly affected" cats, and because there is no uniformly agreed on gold-standard echo measurement for the diagnosis of mild HCM. Thus, some overlap between normal and affected cats should be expected. In general, natriuretic peptide concentrations should not be used to quantify the severity of LV hypertrophy, because there is too much overlap between groups. Concentrations are increased in most cats with moderate to severe LV hypertrophy and LA dilation, and especially in those with clinical signs of CHF. Other abnormalities can be associated with NT-proBNP elevation, including congenital heart disease, hyperthyroidism, azotemia, and pulmonary hypertension. Overall, NT-proBNP should be viewed as a test that denotes relative risk of heart disease. Treatment never should be initiated based only on this test.

The NT-proBNP test has been studied in a number of cats with respiratory distress. For unspecified reasons this biomarker increases in these feline patients whether the cause is cardiac failure or primary respiratory disease. A higher cutoff value must be used to identify CHF in these symptomatic patients. Based on different clinical trials, the reference laboratory recommends that values >270 pmol/L are consistent with CHF-induced pulmonary edema or pleural effusion; conversely, NT-proBNP <100 pmol/L in a dyspneic cat points away from a diagnosis of CHF. Intermediate values do not indicate a clear cause. Pleural effusion fluid (diluted 1:1 with saline to increase specificity) also can be used for NT-proBNP testing; concentrations are comparable to or higher than those in plasma. NT-proBNP in pleural effusion showed good sensitivity for diagnosis of HCM, but lower specificity (Hezzell, 2016). Similarly, median plasma atrial natriuretic peptide (ANP) concentration is higher in cardiomyopathic cats with CHF, although the test is only moderately sensitive and specific for distinguishing cardiomyopathic cats from normal. Values in cats without LA enlargement are comparable to those in normal cats. There is no commercially available ANP test validated for cats at this time.

The POC ELISA-based "SNAP" Feline proBNP test can be useful for identifying moderate to severe occult HCM and to a lesser extent, ruling out CHF as a cause of dyspnea (**Figure 19.3**, p. 292 and text). Based on the manufacturer's guidelines, the SNAP test turns "positive" at approximately 150 pmol/L in cats with moderate to severe cardiomyopathy, and a darker sample compared to reference spot on the test kit suggests an NT-proBNP of >200 pmol/L. The main use for this SNAP test is asymptomatic cats with abnormal cardiac auscultation. However, it also can be used to some benefit for cats with respiratory distress. The POC test is good at identifying the absence of moderate to severe cardiac disease (high negative predictive value) in both symptomatic and asymptomatic cats. However, its positive predictive value in a general practice population would appear only fair, although it is higher in a referral setting. A positive SNAP test in an asymptomatic cat could indicate moderate or severe occult HCM, but might not identify milder myocardial disease. Whether to pursue a follow-up echocardiogram immediately or monitor and retest the cat over time would depend on the clinical situation and the owner's wishes. A negative POC SNAP test (usually indicating <150 pmol/L) in a cat with dyspnea from pleural effusion is strong evidence for a noncardiac cause; however, a positive test (generally >200 pmol/L) is less specific, as noted above for the reference laboratory test.

Troponins are subcellular constituents of the myocardial contractile apparatus that are released into the blood with cardiomyocyte injury and necrosis. There are standard assays for this biomarker that are reasonably conserved across species, and so can be obtained from veterinary reference and human laboratories; there also are high-sensitivity tests that are in less common use and carry lower reference intervals. The cTnI is more likely to be elevated with moderate to severe myocardial disease. In such cases, it could have prognostic as well as diagnostic value. cTnI usually is increased in cats with respiratory distress caused by cardiac disease. But otherwise, there is much overlap in cTnI between cardiac and noncardiac groups that have been studied. cTnI appears less helpful than NT-proBNP for discriminating mild disease. Nevertheless, a recent study reported that a cTnI concentration >0.163 ng/mL was moderately sensitive, but highly specific, for differentiating asymptomatic HCM cats without LA enlargement from normal cats (Hori, 2018). Values >0.234 ng/mL had excellent sensitivity and good specificity for identifying cats with CHF. Some cTnI elevation also can occur with hyperthyroidism, which might reflect myocardial injury caused by increased catecholamine release or the hormone itself. Nevertheless, an elevated cTnI can help differentiate cardiac from noncardiac causes of dyspnea in cats. Earlier reports indicated that a cTnI <0.24 ng/mL was suggestive of noncardiac disease. However, variation in reported cut-off values could relate to differences in test methodology among studies. Cats with respiratory distress caused by CHF can have cTnI concentrations exceeding 0.7 ng/mL. Still, considerable overlap exists between cats with primary respiratory and cardiac causes of dyspnea. Circulating cTnI (and cTnT) concentrations are higher in cats that experience cardiac death, compared to longer-term survivors. In one study, cats with a cTnI over 0.7 ng/mL at diagnosis had shorter survival time regardless of LA size and function or presence of CHF (Borgeat, 2014b). Furthermore, cats with regional LV hypokinesis had significantly higher circulating cTnI than those without. This likely reflects myocardial damage from regional ischemia or infarction. It is unclear whether the rate of change in biomarker concentrations is correlated with prognosis, and how much day-to-day variability there might be in individual cats. Rapid POC assays are available (Biosite Triage Meter, Biosite, San Diego, CA; iStat 1 analyzer, Abbott, Abbott Park, IL). The potential utility of high-sensitivity cTnI testing in cats with myocardial disease is being explored. Because cTnI (as well as NT-proBNP) can be elevated in hyperthyroid cats, it is important to determine thyroid status in older cats.

Radiography Radiography is a fairly insensitive tool for identifying cardiomyopathy. The cardiac silhouette typically appears normal in cats with mild HCM. However, a variable degree of cardiomegaly, often with LA prominence, usually accompanies advanced cases of cardiomyopathy (**Figures 33.5–33.7**; also **Figure 3.5**, p. 52). Radiographic estimation of LA size using a modified VHS scoring system has been described (p. 50). Yet LA enlargement is not always radiographically evident, even in cats with CHF. Echocardiography is more sensitive for identifying LA enlargement.

Cats with dyspnea caused by CHF are likely to have cardiomegaly, with a VHS > 9 v (Sleeper, 2013). A VHS between 8 and 9.3 v suggests cardiac disease; however, echocardiography is needed to discriminate between cardiac and primary respiratory causes of dyspnea. The classic "valentine"-shaped appearance of the heart on DV or VD view is caused by left

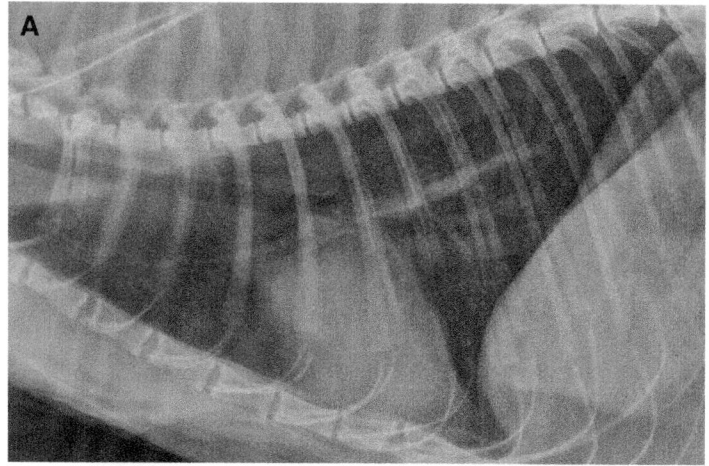
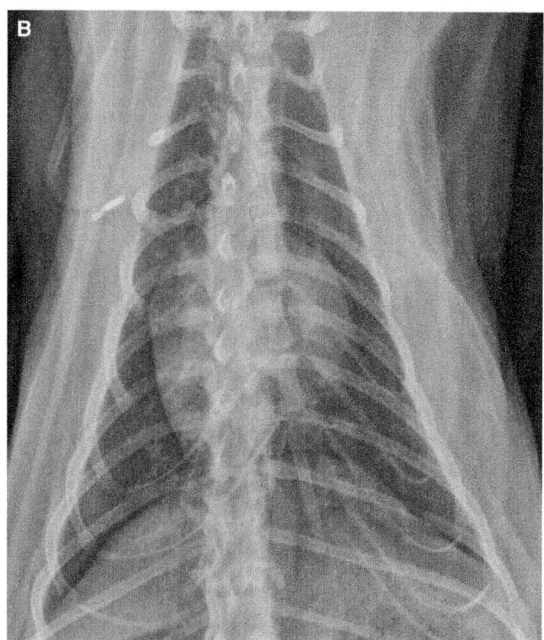

Figure 33.5 Lateral (A) and DV (B, slightly rotated) radiographs show only mild cardiomegaly (VHS ~8.2v) in a 5-year-old male cat with stage C hypertrophic cardiomyopathy. Images obtained 1 day after starting therapy for mild congestive heart failure.

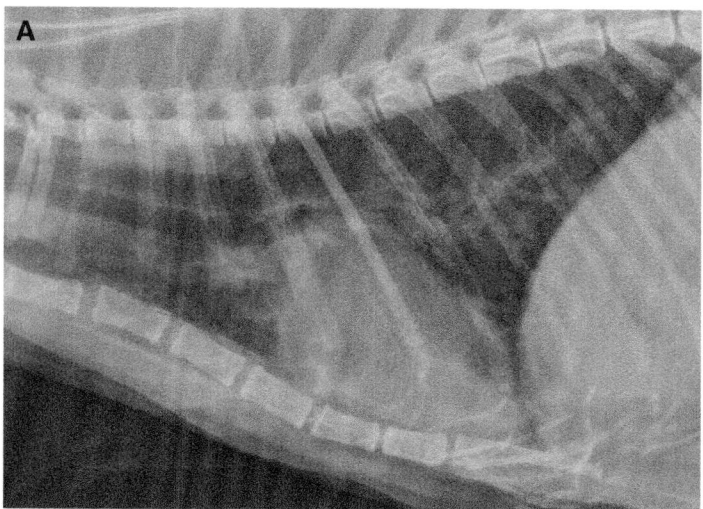
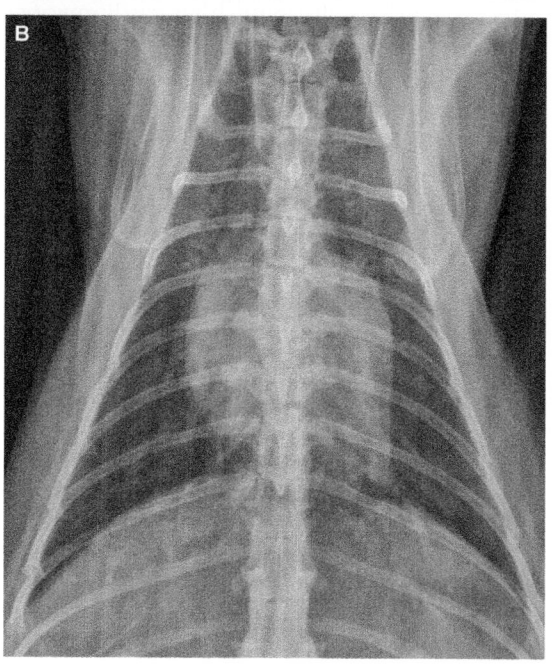

Figure 33.6 Lateral (A) and DV (B) radiographs in a 16-year-old female Domestic Shorthair cat with hypertrophic cardiomyopathy and resolving pulmonary edema. There is moderate cardiomegaly (VHS ~9v), with mild residual pulmonary opacity, especially in cranial right lung. Prominent left atrium and tortuous caudal pulmonary vein are more easily seen in (A).

auricular enlargement, apex shifting to the right, and possibly some right atrial (RA) dilation (**Figures 33.7B** and **3.14B**, p. 57), but it is not always present. Most cats with this cardiac shape do have some type of cardiomyopathy or other structural heart disease, although often not HCM with biatrial enlargement specifically. Mild to moderate pericardial effusion further increases apparent cardiomegaly in some cats with CHF. Following diuretic therapy, the heart size can decrease substantially both from reduced venous pressures and mobilization of pericardial effusion. Other causes of cardiomegaly, including congenital cardiac malformations, other types of primary and secondary cardiomyopathies, and peritoneopericardial diaphragmatic hernia must be excluded (**Figure 35.3**, p. 708).

Enlarged, tortuous pulmonary veins indicate chronically elevated LA and pulmonary venous pressures. Variable degree and distribution of unstructured interstitial or alveolar pulmonary infiltrates develop with pulmonary edema in cats (**Figure 33.8**, also **Figure 3.22**, p. 64). The distribution of these infiltrates can be nonuniform yet spread throughout the lung regions; sometimes it is uniform. Patchy, multifocal opacities occur less often; a focal area of infiltrate also could be evident. Cats with overt pulmonary edema often exhibit enlargement of lobar pulmonary veins and arteries. Arterial dilation might stem from hypoxia-induced vasoconstriction,

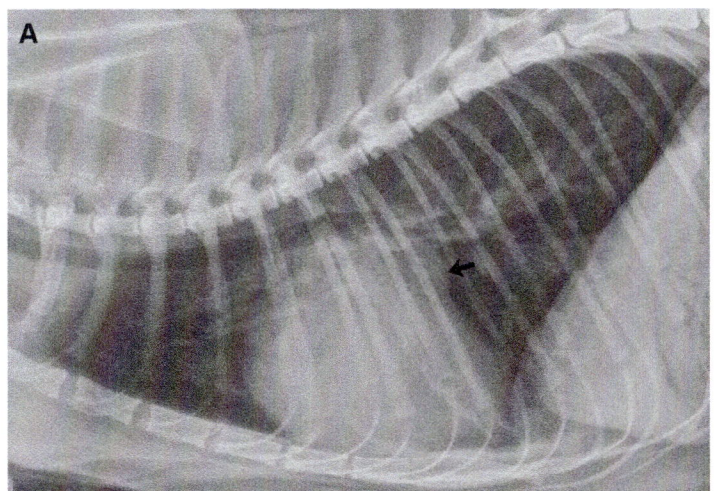
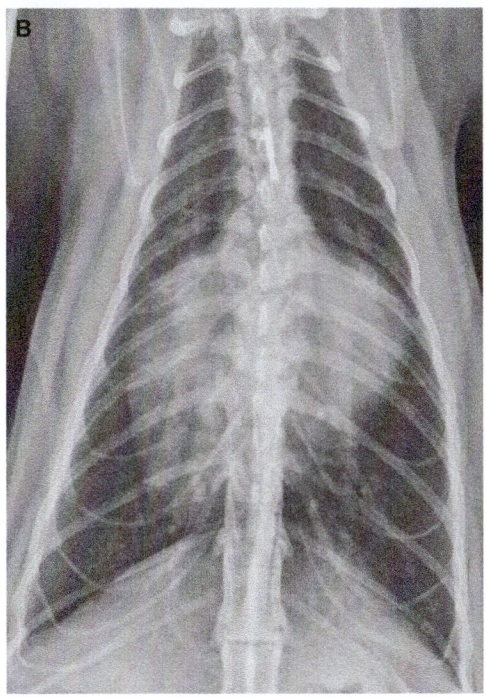

Figure 33.7 More severe left ventricular (LV) and atrial (LA) enlargement is evident in a 4-year-old Selkirk Rex with hypertrophic cardiomyopathy. (A) Note the carina's dorsal elevation and the markedly convex LA border (suggesting severe enlargement, arrow) on lateral view. The VHS is ~10.5v. (B) DV projection shows a large left auricular bulge in the 2:00–3:00 o'clock region. The LV apex point is maintained, although shifted to the right on this radiograph.

or perhaps as a protective response from sudden increases in LA pressure, shown experimentally to constrict small pulmonary arteries in cats (Shirai, 1991). From a practical standpoint, many cats in distress are radiographed in dorsoventral recumbency; the clinician should remember that this will magnify all the caudodorsal pulmonary vessels. Lobar vessel size can appear normal after diuretic therapy. Pleural effusion is common with advanced left or biventricular CHF (**Figure 3.24**, p. 65). Some cats with CHF have caudal vena caval distention, hepatomegaly, and rarely, ascites.

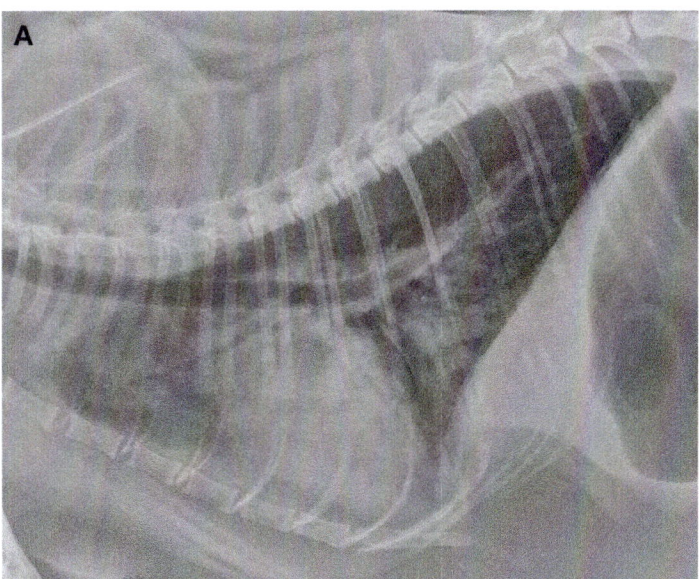
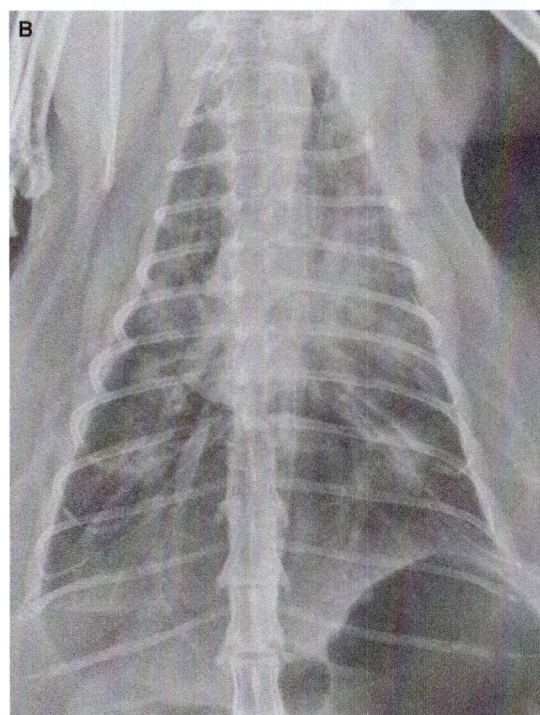

Figure 33.8 Lateral (A) and DV (B) radiographs in a 9-year-old male Domestic Shorthair cat with hypertrophic cardiomyopathy and congestive heart failure. Patchy soft tissue opacities are present in all lung regions, with air bronchograms in the cranio- and caudoventral fields. The heart is moderately enlarged (VHS 9.5v). Lobar pulmonary vessels (both veins and arteries) are distended. Air within the thoracic esophagus and stomach (aerophagia) implies respiratory distress.

Electrocardiography ECG abnormalities are common in cats with HCM, although ECG sensitivity for detecting LV hypertrophy or LA enlargement is too low for this to be an effective screening test for cardiomyopathy. The ECG is normal in many affected cats. Criteria for LA and LV enlargement, ventricular or supraventricular premature complexes, and a left axis deviation are the most common abnormalities (**Figures 33.9** and **33.10**; also **Figure 5.27**, p. 147). In a study of cats with preclinical HCM, few ectopic complexes were found on 24-hour Holter recordings in the home environment, similar to normal cats (Hanas, 2017). Yet ventricular tachyarrhythmias often occur with HCM, as well as other forms of cardiomyopathy. Another small Holter-based study found wide variation in frequency of ventricular premature complexes (VPCs) and paroxysmal tachycardia in cats with HCM (Bartoszuk, 2019). The median number of VPCs was highest in those with decompensated CHF, although median VPC number in the cats with "compensated" HCM also was significantly greater than in normal cats. This study was conducted in the hospital setting. Elevated sympathetic tone presumably caused the higher median HRs observed, even in cats without CHF (compared to the at-home Holter study), and might have provoked more arrhythmias. Plasma cTnI was highest in the CHF group, but this biomarker did not correlate with arrhythmia frequency. No association was found between arrhythmia frequency or complexity and survival in this study, although others have identified arrhythmias as a negative prognostic factor. AF develops in some cats, especially those with marked LA enlargement (**Figure 5.25**, p. 146). Supraventricular tachycardia, AV conduction delays, complete AV block, or sinus bradycardia also occur occasionally (**Figure 5.46**, p. 152). Atrial standstill is a rare cause of bradycardia in HCM and most often associated with cardiogenic shock. Sinus rhythm often resumes if the cat can be effectively resuscitated, warmed, and made normotensive. Ambulatory ECG recordings can be especially useful in cats with a history of weakness or collapse.

Echocardiography   Echocardiography is the best noninvasive means to identify HCM and differentiate it from other cardiac disorders. It is used to screen breeding cats, evaluate those with abnormal cardiac auscultation or radiographic findings, and assess cats with respiratory difficulty in urgent settings. Elective echocardiography also is used to screen cats at higher risk for structural heart disease prior to anesthesia or treatments that would expand plasma volume. Both 2D and M-mode echo imaging can be used to assess LA size and the extent and distribution of hypertrophy within ventricular walls, septum,

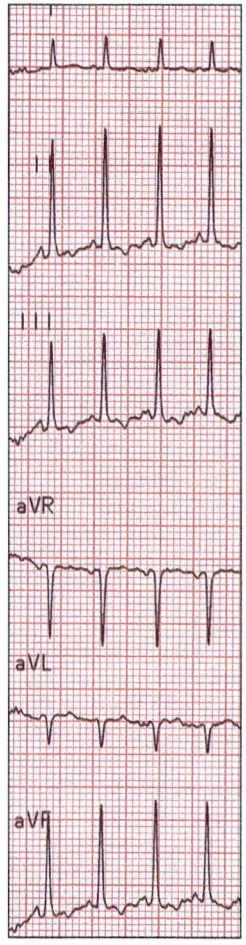

Figure 33.9   Tall and wide R waves on this ECG suggest left ventricular enlargement in a cat with cardiomyopathy. Sinus rhythm and a normal electrical axis are present. Leads as marked; 25 mm/sec; 1 cm = 1 mV.

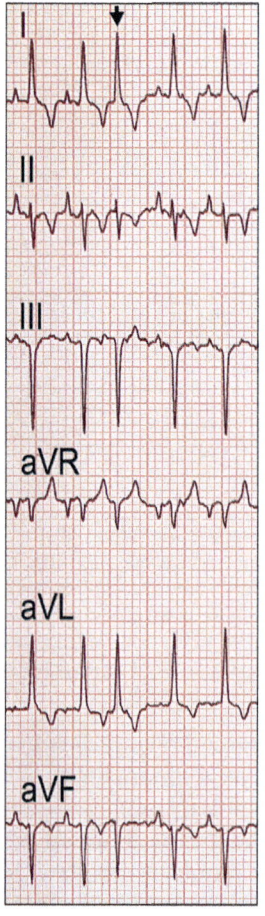

Figure 33.10   ECG from a 16-year-old Domestic Shorthair cat with hypertrophic cardiomyopathy shows sinus rhythm with an atrial premature complex (arrow). The mean electrical axis is deviated leftward. Leads as marked; 25 mm/sec, 2 cm = 1 mV.

and papillary muscles, although measurements obtained by one method are not interchangeable with the other. These and Doppler echo modalities can identify dynamic LV outflow obstruction, as well as systolic and diastolic functional abnormalities. Echocardiography can be particularly challenging in this species, and it requires higher frequency transducers for optimal imaging. Clear and accurate measurements can be difficult to obtain in cats without suitable equipment and meticulous technique; accordingly, referral to a veterinary cardiologist generally is recommended for a complete echo examination.

Nevertheless, a POC thoracic (lung) ultrasound with focused echo exam (p. 82) can inform the clinician with minimal echo training. Learning to identify LA enlargement, pulmonary infiltrates, pleural and pericardial effusions, and LV systolic dysfunction are key aspects for proficiency with this examination. Especially important for cats in respiratory distress, such information helps differentiate CHF from noncardiac disease and facilitates immediate therapeutic decisions. The POC ultrasound exam can be done quickly, with the patient in sternal or standing position and without shaving, to minimize patient stress. While not a replacement for a complete echo exam (nor for thoracic radiographs!), it can help direct acute therapy until the patient is stable enough for additional diagnostic tests. The heart base usually can be visualized in a short-axis plane from the right side of the thorax. Evidence for LA enlargement, with increased LA/Ao ratio, in a cat with respiratory distress increases the likelihood that CHF is causative. Pulmonary infiltrates cause artifacts known as "B" lines (also called lung rockets, comet tails, ring-down artifacts) on lung ultrasound scans. B lines appear as hyperechoic, nonattenuating vertical artifacts or streaks that originate from the pleural-pulmonary interface, extend down through the entire image field, and move with respiration (**Figure 33.11**). Although various pulmonary infiltrates could cause these artifacts, cardiogenic pulmonary edema in cats is strongly associated with the presence of ≥3 B lines in at least 2 of 4 standard positions on both sides of the chest, especially when LA/Ao is increased (Ward, 2018). Pleural and pericardial effusions also can be identified and differentiated on rapid thoracic ultrasound exam.

A focused cardiac ultrasound exam also could be useful as a screening tool for cardiomyopathy in asymptomatic cats, when a complete echo evaluation with Doppler is not available or cost effective. Additionally, this can identify cats that would benefit from referral to a cardiologist for more detailed evaluation. A multicenter study involving 289 cats and several nonspecialists minimally trained in echocardiography, reported that the nonspecialists and cardiology specialists were in agreement as to the presence or absence of occult cardiac disease in 62% of cats after focused echo exam (Loughran, 2019). Agreement was high for cats with moderate to severe cardiac disease. The abnormal cardiac findings identified most consistently by nonspecialists were LA enlargement and ventricular septal hypertrophy, as well as cardiac murmurs. The focused cardiac exam described in this study used the right parasternal transducer position, with short- and long-axis views optimized for the left atrium and ventricle.

LA enlargement can range from mild to severe in cats with HCM. The degree of LA enlargement generally correlates with the severity of cardiac disease, although some artifactual increase in LA size can occur in cats given a parenteral fluid overload. Conversely, aggressive diuresis or other causes of dehydration can artificially reduce LA size. Progressive LV diastolic dysfunction is the largest contributor to LA enlargement in cats with HCM, along with volume retention as heart failure develops and increases venous pressures. Moderate to severe MR also could contribute in some cases, although this rarely is a major factor. Marked LA enlargement correlates with more severe, chronic LV diastolic stiffness and impaired filling (**Figures 33.12–33.14**). The LA wall can visibly hypertrophy,

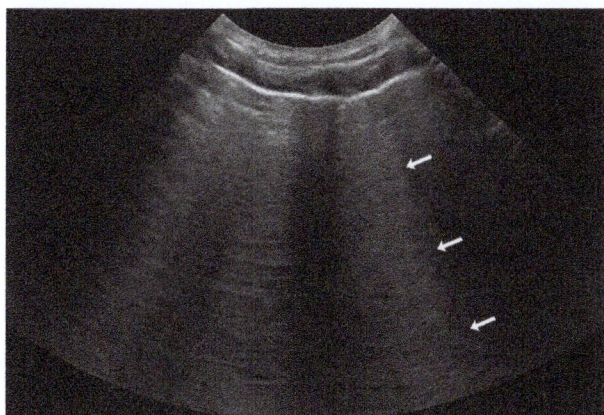

Figure 33.11 Lung ultrasound image shows several B-line artifacts (arrows), consistent with pulmonary edema, in a 7-year-old Domestic Shorthair cat with congestive heart failure caused by hypertrophic cardiomyopathy.

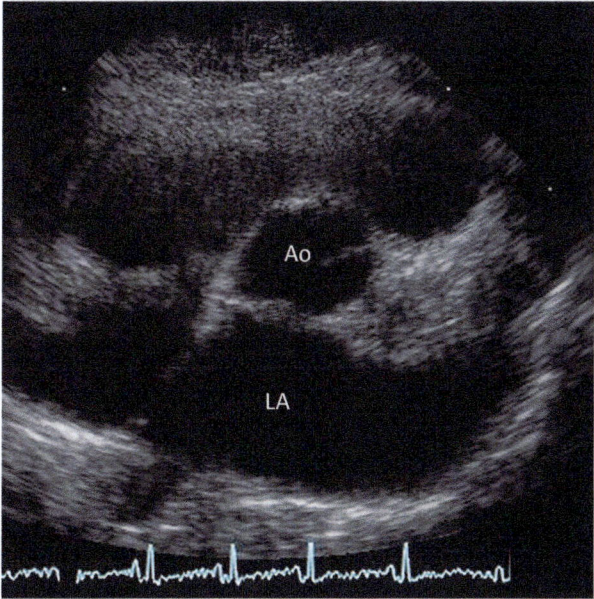

Figure 33.12 Only minimal left atrial enlargement is evident in this 10-year-old female Persian cat with early hypertrophic obstructive cardiomyopathy. Right parasternal short-axis view. Ao, aorta; LA, left atrium.

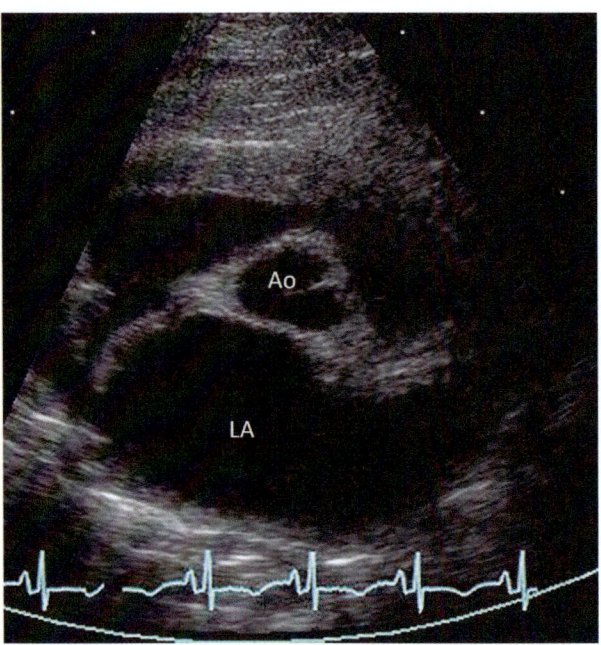

Figure 33.13 The left atrium is moderately enlarged in this 7-year-old female Sphynx cat with cardiomyopathy. No thrombus is evident, although spontaneous contrast was seen intermittently. Right parasternal short-axis view. Ao, aorta; LA, left atrium.

too. Cats with HCM and CHF have greater LA size compared to those with asymptomatic HCM and especially, normal cats. LA size is an indicator of risk for CHF, as well as arterial TE. Spontaneous echocontrast (p. 656) is visible within the

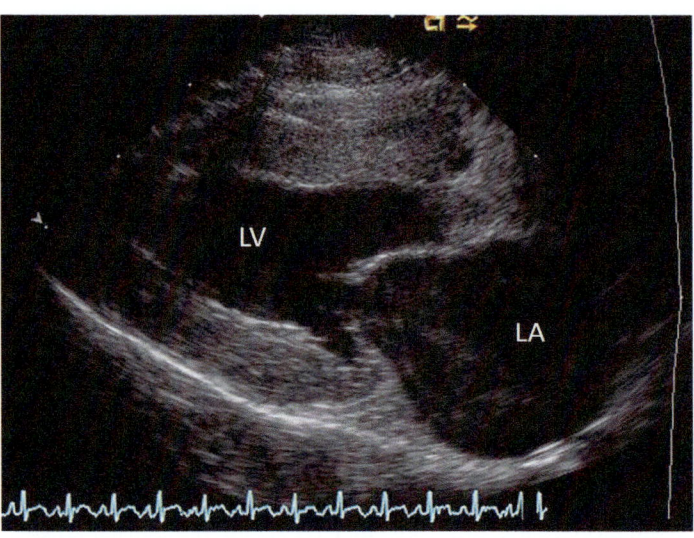

Figure 33.15 Swirls of spontaneous contrast (echo "smoke") extend from dorsocaudal LA through the open mitral valve in this image from a 6-year-old male cat with end-stage hypertrophic cardiomyopathy. Right parasternal long-axis view. LA, left atrium; LV, left ventricle.

enlarged left atrium and auricle of some cats (**Figure 33.15**) and also indicates increased risk for TE. Prophylactic antiplatelet or anticoagulant therapy is strongly recommended for these cats. A thrombus sometimes is visible within the heart, usually in the left auricle but occasionally attached to the LV wall (**Figure 33.16**, also **Figures 36.3** and **36.16**, pp. 751 & 761). It is important to image the left auricle from the left cranial and dorsal transducer position, where smoke

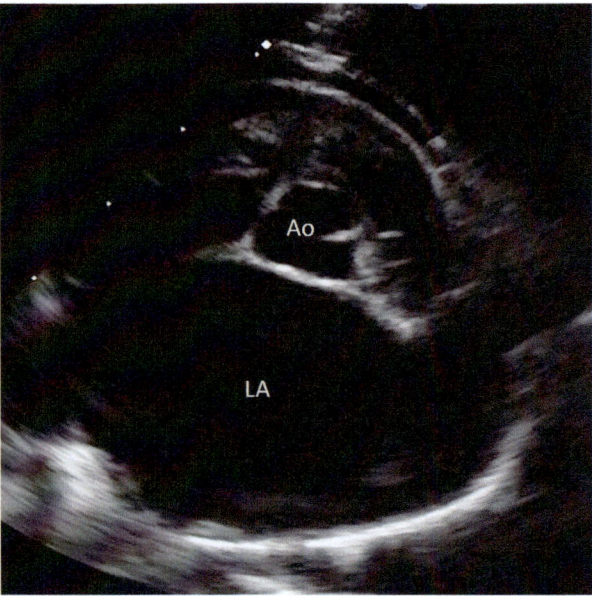

Figure 33.14 Severe left atrial enlargement is present in this 6-year-old male Domestic Shorthair cat with advanced hypertrophic cardiomyopathy and congestive heart failure. The cardiac rhythm was atrial fibrillation. A small volume of pleural effusion is present. Right parasternal short-axis view. Ao, aorta; LA, left atrium.

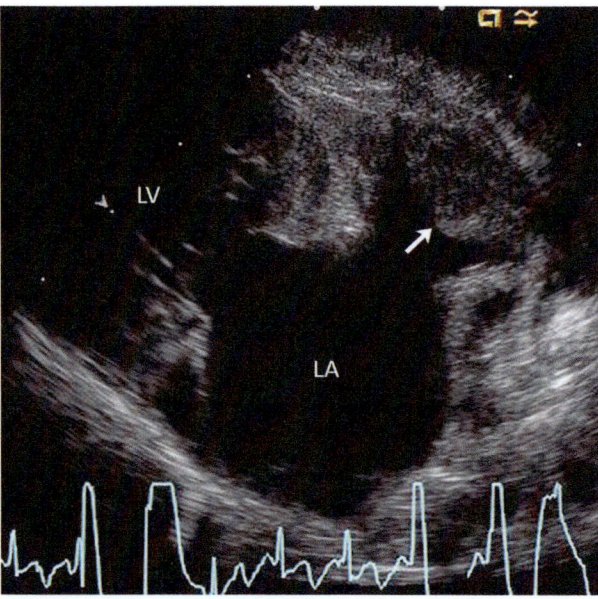

Figure 33.16 A large thrombus (~1.4 × 0.9 cm; arrow) is present within the dilated left auricle of this 8-year-old female Domestic Longhair cat with end-stage cardiomyopathy. Although not evident in this frame, spontaneous contrast also was seen during this cat's echo study. The ECG monitor lead (at bottom) contains much artifact. Left cranial view optimized for LA and auricle. LA, left atrium; LV, left ventricle.

and thrombus are more readily identified. This position also is optimal for Doppler assessment of the appendage's function.

Even when a complete, detailed echo evaluation is not possible, the LA size usually can be estimated fairly easily from either the right parasternal short-axis view of the aortic root and LA or from the right long-axis 4-chamber view optimized for the mitral inflow region (Chapter 4, p. 103). There are a number of approaches to measuring the feline left atrium. A diastolic LA/Ao root ratio >1.4–1.5 (from short-axis view) typically is considered abnormal; an LA/Ao >1.6 indicates increased risk for CHF and is anticipated in cats with overt CHF. From the long-axis 4-chamber view, the cranial-caudal maximum dimension is measured at end-systole. Average-sized, healthy cats have a maximal LA (systolic) dimension <16 mm; although, for an extremely large cat, an LA dimension up to 17 or 18 mm might be acceptable. LA long-axis dimensions between 19 and 24 mm indicate (arbitrarily) moderate LA enlargement; >24 mm indicates severe LA enlargement. Cats with respiratory distress and an LA diameter ≥17 mm most likely have CHF as the underlying cause, rather than primary respiratory disease.

Other echo measures that might help identify CHF include the ratios of pulmonary vein to pulmonary artery diameters, or pulmonary vein to aortic diameters. The ratio of measured minimum diameters for pulmonary vein/pulmonary artery appears most accurate; a proposed ratio of >0.81 was highly sensitive and specific for identifying CHF in cats (Patata, 2020). These measurements are obtained using a modified right parasternal long-axis 4-chamber view, with an M-mode cursor positioned to transect perpendicularly both the (longitudinal) pulmonary vein near its LA entry and the adjacent right pulmonary artery (in cross-section). From the M-mode recording, the minimum diameters of vein and artery are measured using the blood-tissue interface method. The timing of these differs; minimum diameter of the artery occurs at end-diastole and of the vein, slightly later. Furthermore, a ratio of minimum pulmonary vein diameter/aortic diameter (measured from 2D short-axis) of >0.3 also had good sensitivity and specificity for CHF.

LA function, estimated by LA fractional shortening or ejection fraction, is reduced in cats with HCM and CHF (p. 103). LA function often decreases as the left atrium dilates. LA contractile function also can be estimated by measuring maximal flow velocity generated when the left auricle contracts; velocities under 0.20 m/second indicate poor LA function and are associated with spontaneous echocontrast and increased TE risk. Cats with CHF that develop pleural effusion have worse LA function; they also typically have a larger RV diameter than those without pleural effusion. Cats with HCM and an RV internal diameter >3.6 mm are likely to have pleural effusion as a manifestation of CHF.

Ventricular hypertrophy commonly is widespread and diffuse; however, more asymmetrical and segmental patterns of LV hypertrophy frequently occur (**Figures 33.17** and **33.18**). Some cats show only papillary muscle or LV free wall

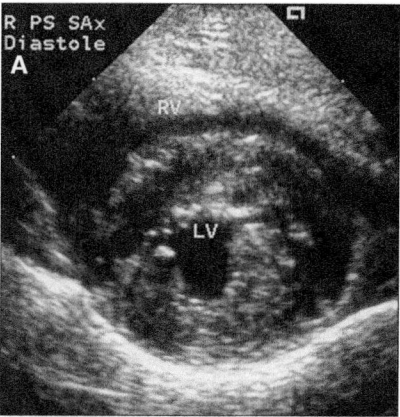

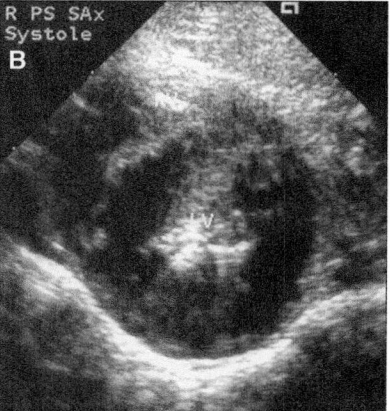

Figure 33.17 Example of symmetrical left ventricular wall and septal hypertrophy, with thick papillary muscles, in diastole (A) and systole (B). The lumen is virtually obliterated in systole. Increased subendocardial echogenicity is evident. LV, left ventricle; RV, right ventricle.

hypertrophy; others have basilar or diffuse septal hypertrophy with normal LV wall thickness. Cats with septal hypertrophy appear more likely to have dynamic LV outflow obstruction, with mitral SAM and increased LV outflow turbulence. Cats with papillary muscle or LV free wall hypertrophy commonly have MR. Mild to moderate MR usually accompanies SAM, also. LA enlargement seems to develop more often in cats with diffuse LV or free wall hypertrophy, compared to septal hypertrophy alone, and this distribution poses a higher risk for CHF.

If an M-mode cursor can be properly aligned perpendicular to areas of greatest wall and septal thickness, M-mode images can provide better temporal resolution and clearer endocardial edge visualization for measuring diastolic thicknesses (**Figure 33.19**). Use of 2D guidance helps ensure proper M-mode beam positioning. However, end-diastolic 2D image frames often are used to measure wall thickness also, especially of focally hypertrophied areas outside the standard positions and if accurate M-mode beam orientation is problematic. The leading edge-to-leading edge method typically is used for M-mode measurements; because different practices sometimes are used for 2D measurements, the method used should be specified (p. 95). The leading edge technique (with

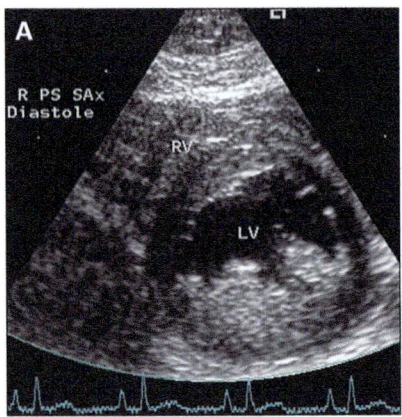 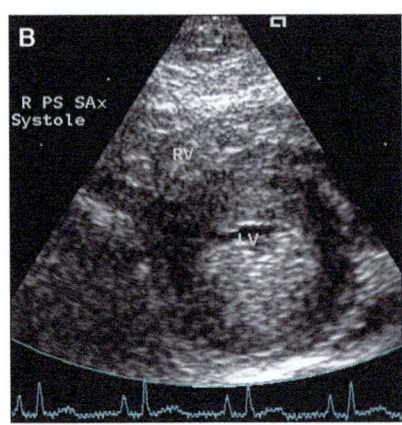 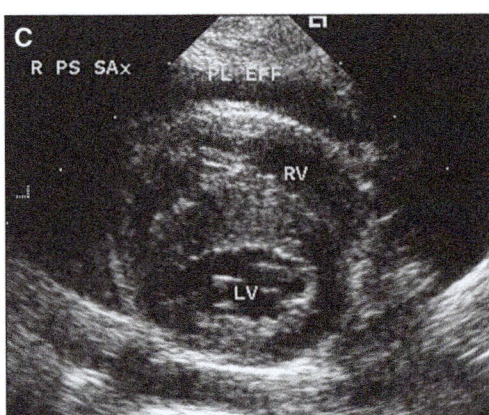

Figure 33.18 Images in diastole (A) and systole (B) from an older cat show hypertrophy localized to the left ventricular free wall and papillary muscles. Increased subendocardial and mid-myocardial echogenicity in those regions suggests chronic ischemia and fibrosis. (C) Diastolic frame from a 4-year-old cat with asymmetric septal hypertrophy. Right parasternal short-axis view. LV, left ventricle; PL EFF, pleural effusion; RV, right ventricle.

only one endocardial thickness included) is often 2-3 mm less than if 2D echo is used and diastolic measurements are made at the blood/endocardial interface. This difference might seem trivial but can literally change the "diagnosis,"

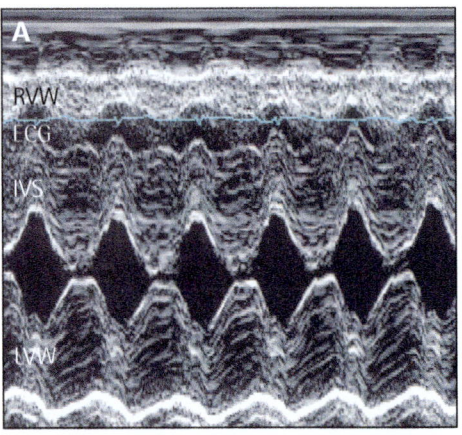

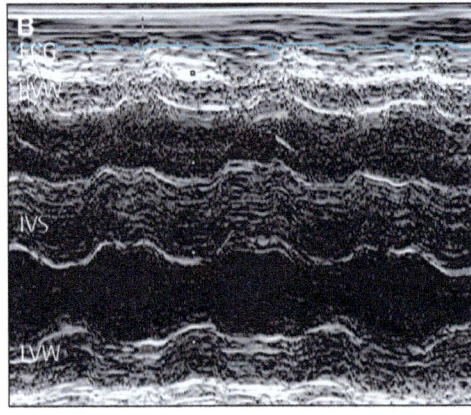

Figure 33.19 (A) M-mode image from a 16-year-old male cat with symmetrical left ventricular hypertrophy shows typical vigorous systolic motion and normal right ventricular size. ECG monitor lead superimposed over the right ventricle. (B) Marked septal hypertrophy in a 4-year-old female cat with hypertrophic obstructive cardiomyopathy. ECG, electrocardiogram; IVS, interventricular septum; LVW, left ventricular wall, RVW, right ventricular wall.

and subsequently, the life of the cat and client in terms of follow-up examinations and costs for veterinary care. As with M-mode measurements, 2D measurements should be made perpendicular to the thickest areas of the LV and septal walls. With either method, the LV lumen should be measured near the tips of the open mitral leaflets or at the chordal level, taking care to avoid including the papillary muscles. Additionally, all measurements should be averaged from at least 3 cardiac cycles and from orthogonal views. The examiner should provide a description of the distribution of hypertrophy, because maximal linear measurements do not necessarily relate to the overall severity of HCM. Falsely increased measurement values for LV wall and IVS thicknesses can result from: inadequate positioning; poor image resolution; use of image frames that are not timed to end-diastole (especially a problem in cats with tachycardia); inclusion of extraneous structures in the measurement of the LV wall (such as papillary muscle, chordal structure or false tendon) or IVS (including septal tricuspid leaflet, chordal structure or false tendon); and LV pseudohypertrophy (from dehydration).

The upper limit of normal for diastolic LV wall and septal thickness and the value that defines the presence of HCM are controversial and not definitively established. Some clinicians consider end-diastolic values of 5.0–5.5 mm as upper limits of normal, based on M-mode studies. Most normal cats, except perhaps those of exceptionally large body size or specific breeding, have measurements below these limits. Some consider an LV or septal diastolic thickness between 5.5 and 6 mm to be abnormal, while others consider this an "equivocal" zone. Again, interpretation should take into account the cat's body size, family history, and other echo findings. An end-diastolic LV wall or septal thickness ≥6 mm is considered specific, but not necessary sensitive, as a cutoff for diagnosing LV hypertrophy. Again, exceptions might be made for a very large cat or mild septal thickening in certain breeds (especially the Bengal cat). Allometric scaling or breed specific values can guide interpretation of measurements in such cats (**Table 4.6**, p. 98). Cats with severe HCM can have diastolic LV wall or septal thicknesses exceeding 8 mm. Although the degree of hypertrophy is not necessarily correlated with the severity of clinical signs, extreme LV hypertrophy generally is a negative prognostic indicator.

Compensatory concentric myocardial hypertrophy (as from systemic hypertension or congenital aortic stenosis) and other causes of myocardial hypertrophy (including hyperthyroidism in cats ≥6 years old) should be excluded before a diagnosis of idiopathic HCM is made (p. 688). Myocardial thickening also can result from infiltrative disease, including myocarditis and cardiac lymphoma; variation in myocardial echogenicity or wall irregularities might be evident in such cases. Excess moderator bands or false tendons, which could represent a congenital anomaly, appear as bright, linear echoes within the LV cavity. They can complicate accurate wall thickness measurements. Focal myocardial thickening is common at false tendon insertion sites and is normal. In middle-aged to older cats with aortic dilation and an abnormal septal-to-aortic angle, a subaortic sepal bulge is common. This sometimes is called discrete upper septal thickening ("DUST") or discrete interventricular septal hypertrophy ("DISH"); the condition might represent a growth response to flow disturbance in the area, as opposed to focal HCM. Signs of early HCM can include isolated papillary muscle hypertrophy or dynamic LV outflow obstruction with mitral SAM. However, it is unclear whether cats with SAM and normal LV wall thickness actually have early HOCM, a congenital mitral apparatus malformation, or possibly even normal structure with hyperdynamic function.

Cats with HOCM might have greater papillary muscle hypertrophy, anterior mitral leaflet length, and presence of false tendons (excess chordae) in the LV outflow tract, compared to cats with HCM but without outflow obstruction. Besides mitral SAM (**Figure 33.20**), mid-systolic partial closure of the aortic valve leaflets might be evident on M-mode scans in cats with dynamic LV outflow tract obstruction. Color Doppler imaging can reveal areas of increased turbulence associated with dynamic outflow obstruction and valvular insufficiency; this helps guide cursor placement for measurement of peak velocities by spectral (CW) Doppler. Mild MR and mid- to late systolic increase in LV outflow velocity are typical with HOCM (**Figure 33.21**). Optimal beam alignment with the outflow jet's maximal velocity can be difficult and, along with the dynamic nature of HOCM, makes accurate systolic gradient estimation challenging. Dynamic LV midventricular obstruction is an uncommon variant in cats with marked papillary muscle and mid-ventricular wall or septal hypertrophy; color and spectral Doppler modalities can document this, as well.

Marked papillary muscle hypertrophy and systolic LV cavity obliteration are observed in some cats. Increased echogenicity (brightness) of papillary muscles and LV subendocardial areas is common and thought to be a marker for chronic myocardial ischemia and subsequent fibrosis. LV diastolic size in cats with HCM is usually normal to reduced. Systolic function estimated by LV FS generally is normal to increased; however, some cats develop mild to moderate LV dilation and reduced contractility (with FS ~23–29%). Poor or regionally paradoxical wall motion can occur with myocardial infarction or replacement fibrosis. In end-stage HCM, it is common to see reduced free wall amplitude during systole, compared to the septum, and this is a sign of impaired systolic function. Mild to moderate pericardial effusion, without tamponade, often accompanies CHF in cats with advanced disease (**Figure 35.24**, p. 719). RV enlargement and pleural effusion also are common in advanced CHF.

Doppler-derived measures are important for further characterizing diastolic function. These include transmitral and pulmonary venous inflow patterns and TDI annular velocities. However, accurate images must be obtained, which is difficult in many cats. Furthermore, tachycardia often prevents separation of early (E) and late (A) LV filling waves, although a vagal maneuver (or a drop of intraocular timolol) can be effective for slowing the HR in some cats. Abnormal mitral inflow patterns occur with delayed (impaired) LV myocardial relaxation, reduced LV compliance, and increased LV filling pressure. Early change in diastolic function (impaired relaxation pattern) includes reduced maximal velocity of the mitral early filling (E) wave, slowed E wave deceleration rate, a mitral late filling (A, atrial contraction) wave peak velocity that exceeds the E wave velocity (E/A ratio <1), and prolonged IRVT (**Table 4.13**, p. 128, and **Figure 4.31**, p. 109). This pattern is common in older but healthy animals, too. Moderate diastolic dysfunction produces a "pseudonormal" mitral inflow pattern as LV stiffness causes LA pressure to rise, which then increases early filling (E) velocity and shortens IVRT, despite impaired relaxation. The pseudonormal pattern is transitional, between the impaired relaxation and restrictive patterns. TDI measurement of lateral mitral annulus motion and an abnormal pulmonary venous inflow pattern help differentiate pseudonormal from true normal mitral filling. Severe diastolic dysfunction is characterized by a restrictive filling pattern, where the mitral E wave peak velocity is increased but rapidly decelerates, the A wave velocity is blunted, E/A ratio exceeds 2, and IVRT is shortened. Greater LV stiffness and increased LV filling pressure characterize the restrictive filling pattern. LA function often is poor, as well. Mitral inflow A wave velocity is influenced by both LV compliance and LA contractility. A study evaluating Doppler echo parameters in cats with HCM showed that an E/A ratio >1.77 was sensitive and specific for the presence of CHF (Rohrbaugh, 2020). In cats with fused E and A waves, a ratio of fused EA to fused (TDI) e′a′ velocities >15 was fairly sensitive, but highly specific, for the presence of CHF; nevertheless, caution should always be exercised when measuring fused waves.

Abnormalities of right heart size and function also are a factor in HCM. Almost a third of cats with HCM have some degree of RV wall thickening. Furthermore, increases

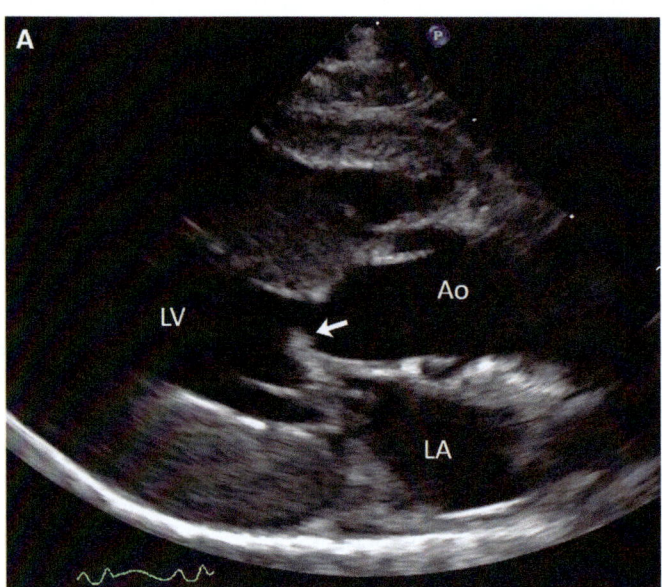
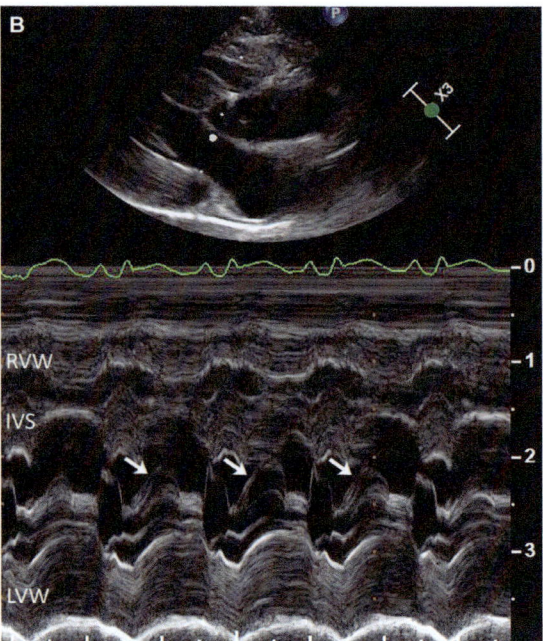
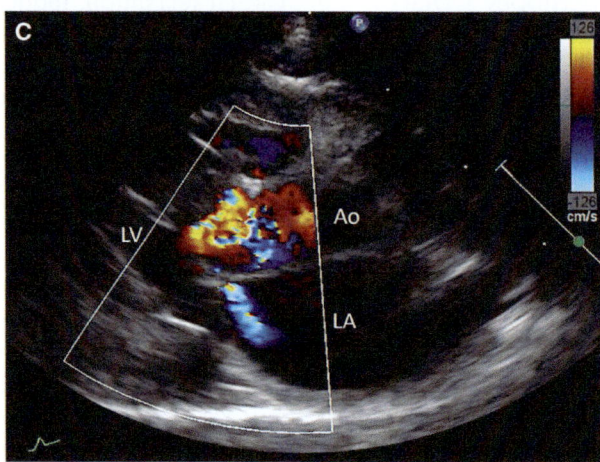

Figure 33.20 (A) Right parasternal long-axis image in systole from a 7-year-old male Domestic Shorthair cat with hypertrophic obstructive cardiomyopathy and transient neurologic signs. The interventricular septum and free wall are hypertrophied. Systolic anterior motion (SAM) of the anterior mitral leaflet (arrow), contributes to the dynamic left ventricular outflow obstruction, as the leaflet is sucked toward the outflow tract during ejection. Two open aortic valve leaflets are visible. (B) M-mode image at the mitral valve level shows the anterior leaflet motion (SAM, arrows) toward the IVS during systole. (C) Color Doppler image in systole, as in (A), shows a small caudally directed jet of mitral regurgitation, which typically accompanies mitral SAM. The dynamic outflow obstruction (from mitral SAM and septal contraction) causes mid-systolic flow acceleration and turbulence within the outflow tract. Ao, aorta; IVS, interventricular septum; LA, left atrium; LV, left ventricle; LVW, left ventricular wall; RVW, right ventricular wall.

in LV wall thickness and diastolic RV chamber dimension, as well as decreased tricuspid annular plane systolic excursion (TAPSE; p. 94), correlate independently with increased LA size (Visser, 2017). Cats with CHF caused by HCM have increased right heart size and reduced RV systolic function, compared to normal cats. Those with pleural effusion as a manifestation of CHF appear more likely to have a thicker RV free wall, larger RA diameter, and decreased TAPSE, compared to cats without pleural effusion. However, postcapillary pulmonary hypertension (Chapter 39) was detectable in a relatively small minority of cats with left-sided CHF (Vezzosi, 2019). Measurements of TAPSE and mitral annular plane systolic excursion (MAPSE) assess longitudinal ventricular systolic function; both are reduced in cats with HCM and are lowest in those with CHF (Spalla, 2018). Cats with pleural effusion, rather than pulmonary edema alone, had the lowest values, particularly of MAPSE at the septal annulus. However, these measures did not independently predict survival.

Other echocardiographic modalities used (mostly in academic settings) to evaluate myocardial function in cats with

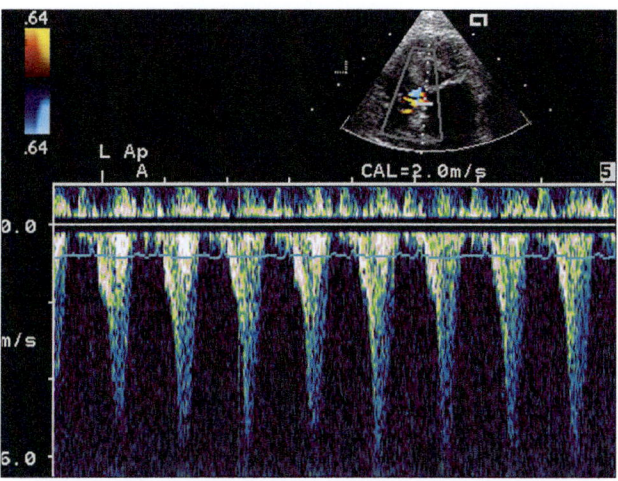

Figure 33.21 Continuous wave Doppler image of aortic flow in a 4-year-old Persian cat with dynamic left ventricular outflow obstruction shows the pattern of mid-systolic flow acceleration (as obstruction worsens) and high peak velocity (almost 6 m/sec).

HCM include LV strain (and strain rate) analysis by 2D speckle tracking or TDI. TDI studies can show reduced diastolic, and sometimes systolic, function in cats with HCM. Strain analysis appears to be more sensitive for detecting early changes in cardiac function, even in cats with minimal hypertrophy and no LA enlargement. Strain (myocardial deformation) imaging might detect early systolic dysfunction before there is any echo evidence for hypertrophy or change in systolic function. Decreased longitudinal and radial myocardial deformations have been found in cats with HCM and normal echo indices of systolic function, as well as those with preclinical HCM. Cats with advanced disease and CHF also have reduced circumferential strain, which might play a role in clinical decompensation. Measures of LV peak systolic torsional deformation (apical rotation and torsion) appear to be increased in cats with HCM, especially those with HOCM.

Management

Because the major pathophysiology of HCM relates to impaired LV filling, strategies to lower HR should allow more time for ventricular filling and coronary perfusion, as well as reduce myocardial oxygen demand and risk of ischemia. This is theoretically beneficial, even if myocardial relaxation or stiffness characteristics are not altered directly. Although a beta- or calcium channel-blocker might be used for this in selected cases (p. 676), these agents currently are not advocated in most situations now. Neither is proven to delay CHF, prolong survival, or even improve owner-assessed activity level or quality of life. Several other therapies, including those aimed at RAAS inhibition, also have theoretical benefit. Unfortunately, there still are no convincing data to indicate any therapy has long-term benefit in preventing CHF or sudden cardiac death in feline HCM. (The only assured outcome will be substantial inconvenience to most cats and their owners). Ivabradine is a newer drug that might prove helpful by moderating sinus tachycardia in HCM. Ivabradine slows HR by inhibiting the "funny" current (I_f) which is important in sinus node impulse generation and is modulated by sympathetic activity. Although ivabradine has equivalent HR effects to oral atenolol, it does not reduce dynamic outflow obstruction as effectively in cats with HOCM (p. 333). Other effects on systolic and diastolic function appear to be negligible. But clinical experience is needed to determine if ivabradine will have a positive impact on outcomes.

Currently, beyond avoidance of stressful situations and excess fluid loads, clear strategies for preventing CHF and improving survival unfortunately remain to be defined. Better data are available for arterial TE prevention. Screening for systemic hypertension and hyperthyroidism in middle-aged and older cats is important, because these treatable conditions not only can mimic HCM, but also cause greater problems for cats that concurrently have idiopathic HCM. For cats with overt CHF, furosemide and thoracocentesis (as indicated) are used to manage excess fluid accumulation. For TE prophylaxis, clopidogrel is superior to aspirin; its efficacy compared to or in combination with the newer oral anticoagulant drugs remains to be seen. Anticoagulant and antiplatelet drugs help manage acute arterial TE and future risks (p. 763). Beyond these basic tenets, optimal management for HCM largely remains a mystery.

Management of Preclinical HCM Many cats with mild LV hypertrophy or other evidence of preclinical HCM never develop signs of disease. Therefore, watchful waiting and periodic echo monitoring is a rational approach. For cats with stage B1 disease, if echo is not feasible, a biomarker and radiographic recheck every 12–18 months is suggested. More frequent rechecks could be helpful in younger cats, in case disease progression is more rapid. For cats with stage B2 disease (LA enlargement), reevaluation every 6–12 months is suggested. However, the cat's level of stress during these visits must be considered. Strategies to minimize patient fear and excitement are important and should be employed as needed. Less frequent rechecks or home administration of a sedative (for example, 50–100 mg gabapentin mixed into ~1 teaspoonful of wet food or tuna) prior to the appointment, or both, can help. Also, the cat's resting respiratory rate (and effort) periodically should be monitored at home for changes that could suggest early CHF (**Table 22.1**, p. 339). Change in activity level or appetite should be noted, too.

Again, there is little evidence that any specific treatment delays or prevents the onset of CHF or improves long-term survival in cats with preclinical HCM. Nevertheless, multiple recommendations for managing preclinical HCM have been made, although they remain theoretical. Yet for those cats with disease features that are associated with worse prognosis (see "Prognosis" section), attempting to mitigate these abnormalities with medical therapy seems reasonable, and worth a discussion with clients while emphasizing the lack of evidence, aside from the potential benefits of clopidogrel. The drugs used in cats with preclinical HCM generally are aimed at reducing the risk of arterial TE, improving LV diastolic filling, or managing tachyarrhythmias. Factors to consider when deciding whether to begin drug therapy include the cat's medical history, specific echo findings, potential adverse medication effects, costs, and ease of drug administration. Besides the expense, the level of stress for both owner and cat are likely to rise substantially with the number of drugs prescribed and the frequency of dosing. The negative impact of this on quality of life and the owner-pet relationship must be considered, especially given the unproven efficacy for most treatments. Particularly in cats that are difficult to medicate, poor treatment compliance can further confuse assessment of benefit.

Cats with moderate or severe LA enlargement, reduced LA function, or prior embolic event should benefit from antiplatelet therapy. Clopidogrel is preferred over aspirin, although they can be administered together since they have different mechanisms of action. For cats thought to have particularly high risk for arterial TE (severe LA size and function changes, spontaneous echocontrast, intracardiac thrombus, or prior embolic event), combination therapy using clopidogrel and aspirin, or clopidogrel and an oral Factor Xa inhibitor (p. 766) should be considered. Low molecular weight heparin (enoxaparin or dalteparin) can be used instead of apixaban or rivaroxaban, if affordable and acceptable to cat and client.

Cats with severe dynamic LV outflow obstruction might benefit from atenolol or other beta-blocker, because this drug can reduce obstruction as well as HR. The dosage of atenolol can be titrated by checking the HR in the exam room (with the cat in its carrier) two to three hours after administration. A target HR usually is between 120 and 160 beats/min, considering the stress of a veterinary visit. Reduction in murmur intensity is indirect evidence of diminished obstruction and mitral SAM. Alternatively, atenolol at 6.25 mg PO q12 often is recommended for most cats. A recheck echocardiogram in 3 to 6 months is advised to assess any benefit or potential adverse effect, such as increased LA size. Atenolol can depress LA function; it should be administered cautiously if there is moderate to severe LA dilation or reduced LA appendage ejection velocity. For severe LV outflow tract obstruction that responds inadequately to beta-blocker therapy, a preliminary report suggests concurrent administration of disopyramide might improve or resolve the obstruction; however, further study is needed (Hori, 2020). Nevertheless, it is uncertain how important therapy to reduce dynamic LV outflow obstruction really is, as the degree of obstruction that occurs in the home setting is unknown. Furthermore, cats with dynamic LV outflow obstruction might actually fare better than those without, possibly because their heart murmur leads to earlier diagnosis. Beta-blocker therapy (atenolol, or sotalol for malignant tachyarrhythmias) also is the drug of first choice for frequent supraventricular or ventricular tachyarrhythmias (Chapter 25). Nevertheless, atenolol does not appear to reduce NT-proBNP or cTnI concentrations in cats with preclinical HCM, even with marked LV hypertrophy. Atenolol also had no significant effect on 5 year mortality rate in preclinical HCM (Schober, 2013; Fox, 2018, REVEAL study).

Regarding other medications for preclinical disease, diltiazem generally is not used anymore. An exception might be for HR management in a cat with uncontrolled AF that does not tolerate a beta-blocker. Currently, there is no convincing evidence that RAAS inhibition with an ACE inhibitor or spironolactone will delay the onset of CHF, improve diastolic function, or reduce myocardial hypertrophy. Spironolactone is not recommended for preclinical HCM. Although theoretically it might reduce myocardial fibrosis, it did not decrease LV mass or improve diastolic function in Maine Coon cats with subclinical familial HCM (MacDonald, 2008). However, it did cause severe facial ulcerative dermatitis in almost a third of the study cats. This adverse effect likely was related to both dose and duration of treatment; lower clinical doses seem to be better tolerated when used for CHF.

Concurrent systemic diseases that increase cardiac workload or persistently increase HR, such as hyperthyroidism, systemic hypertension, and anemia should be identified and addressed. Other recommendations for cats with preclinical disease involve avoidance of excessive excitement and strenuous play. Stress associated with boarding, hospitalization, anesthesia and surgery have precipitated clinical signs in some cats. Likewise, high-dose or repositol corticosteroid use and parenteral fluid administration also have been associated with clinical decompensation.

Prognosis in Preclinical HCM The majority of cats diagnosed with preclinical HCM remain asymptomatic for a long time. A multinational survey (including >1700 cats) found that over 2/3 of the (~1000) cats with occult HCM showed no clinical evidence of disease for at least 5 years; ~10% of study cats reached 9–15 years of age (REVEAL study, Fox, 2018). During the REVEAL study period, just over 30% of HCM cats developed CHF, ATE, or both and ~28% experienced cardiac-related death. The risk for developing these outcomes increases with age. For CHF and arterial TE, the risks over time were 7.0% and 3.5%, 19.9% and 9.7%, and 23.9% and 11.3% at one, five, and ten years after entering the study. The risks for cardiac or vascular death were 6.7%, 22.8%, and 28.3% for the same periods. Cats with dynamic LV outflow obstruction but without LV hypertrophy do not appear to have worse prognosis, in contrast to the analogous situation in people. A follow-up subanalysis of the REVEAL data showed that noncardiac causes of death in cats with occult HCM occurred at the same rate (~31%) as in apparently healthy cats, and also increased with age (Fox, 2019). Nonetheless, the occurrence of cardiovascular death in the HCM cats that developed clinical disease caused all-cause mortality to be ~60% higher in this group. In a smaller study of over 280 cats with HCM (±CHF), median survival time was 5.9 years; median age at diagnosis in this report was just over 6 years (Payne, 2013).

Because HCM is such a heterogeneous disease, predicting which individuals are most likely to develop progressive disease and future clinical signs can be challenging; however, several characteristics have been associated with a worse prognosis. These include marked LA enlargement (LA/Ao >1.8), severe (≥9 mm) LV wall or septal hypertrophy, subnormal LV systolic function (FS <30%), and older age (Payne, 2013). Other indicators associated with increased risk for CHF or arterial TE include an audible gallop sound, arrhythmias, decreased LA function, presence of spontaneous echocontrast ("smoke") or intracardiac thrombus, a restrictive (Doppler) mitral inflow pattern, and regional LV thinning with hypokinesis. Low vitamin D status also has been associated with shorter survival time.

Acute Congestive Heart Failure Sudden onset or rapid worsening of respiratory distress is the usual presentation for cats with acute CHF (**Figure 33.22**). Some cats have no prior indication of underlying heart disease; others might have been diagnosed years previously and could be receiving some treatments. When respiratory distress is of uncertain cause, the following findings suggest underlying CHF: gallop sounds and pulmonary crackles on auscultation, a positive POC (or reference laboratory) NT-proBNP test (p. 291), LA enlargement and multiple B-lines at ≥2 sites on POC thoracic ultrasound exam (**Figure 33.11**), and radiographic cardiomegaly with lung opacities consistent with pulmonary edema (**Figures 33.8** and **3.22**, p. 64). As with any cause of acute dyspnea, cats with fulminant CHF are clinically fragile. It is important to avoid further stress, which can worsen their status or precipitate cardiac arrest.

When CHF is suspected, the cat should be sedated and administered oxygen followed by an initial furosemide dose (2–4 mg/kg) given IM, if immediate IV catheter placement is deemed too stressful. Continued furosemide therapy is administered IV, if possible, until brisk diuresis ensues; at this point the dose usually is reduced. For milder respiratory signs of pulmonary edema, an initial furosemide dose of 1–2 mg/kg IV might be adequate. Mild sedation is continued as needed to reduce patient anxiety (**Table 33.3** and **Table 22.2**, p. 342). Supplemental O_2 should be provided in

Table 33.3 Treatment Outline for Cats with Stage C Hypertrophic Cardiomyopathy

Acute Signs of CHF[a]

- Supplemental O_2
- Cage rest
- Minimize patient handling and stress
- Furosemide (parenteral)
- Sedation (butorphanol, or buprenorphine for greater analgesia)
- Thoracocentesis, if pleural effusion
- ± Nitroglycerin (topical; for pulmonary edema; uncommonly used)
- ±Pimobendan for cardiogenic shock, reduced LV systolic function, moderate to large pleural effusion, or insufficient response to diuretic (see text)
- ±IV Dobutamine
- For rapid tachyarrhythmia: IV esmolol (or diltiazem or other, as indicated; do not use IV propranolol)[b]
- ±Albuterol for suspected bronchospasm (1–2 puffs by inhaler/spacer/facemask)
- Monitor: urinary output, respiratory rate, HR and rhythm, arterial BP, renal function and serum electrolytes, weight, appetite.

Chronic Heart Failure Management[a]

- Furosemide as necessary (lowest effective dose and frequency)
  - Or torsemide, for refractory CHF
- Antithrombotic prophylaxis (clopidogrel ± other drug; see text)[c]
- Thoracocentesis as needed
- ±Pimobendan (indications above; see text)
- ±ACE inhibitor (see text)
- ±Spironolactone (see text)
- Manage other medical problems, as indicated (rule out hyperthyroidism, anemia, hypertension, if not done previously)
- Atenolol for severe LV outflow obstruction
- Dietary salt restriction, if accepted
- ±Additional antiarrhythmic, if indicated
- Home monitoring: resting respiratory rate and effort, activity, appetite, compliance
- Follow-up veterinary examinations:
  - Monitor renal function and electrolytes
  - Note HR and rhythm
  - Measure systolic BP
  - Focused cardiac and thoracic ultrasound
  - ±Thoracic radiographs

[a] See text, as well as **Tables 22.2** and **22.3**, pp. 342 and 345, and Chapter 22 for further details.
[b] See **Table 25.2**, p. 402, and Chapter 25 for further details.
[c] See **Table 36.2**, p. 751, and Chapter 36 for further details.

Abbreviations: ACE, angiotensin converting enzyme; BP, blood pressure; CHF, congestive heart failure; HR, heart rate; LV, left ventricular.

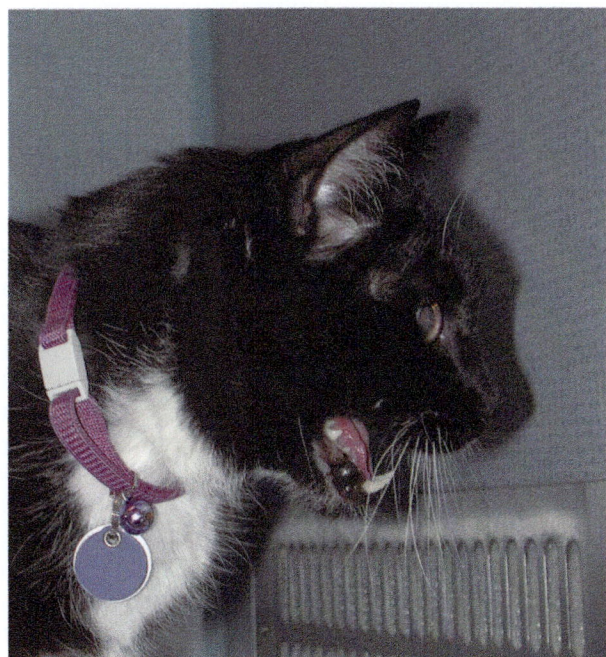

Figure 33.22 Respiratory distress with panting in a 10-year-old male Domestic Shorthair cat with a large volume of pleural effusion secondary to congestive heart failure. Thoracocentesis relieved the respiratory distress.

the least stressful way possible. A commercial temperature-controlled O_2 cage is ideal. Alternatives include flow-by O_2 via face mask or other more creative solutions (p. 217). Allowing the patient to remain sternal and avoiding restraint as much as possible helps ease ventilation.

POC thoracic ultrasound can rapidly reveal pleural and pericardial effusions, as well as LA size, with minimal patient stress prior to radiography (p. 82, and see "Suggested Additional Reading and References"). Pleural effusion also might be suspected during auscultation, if lung sounds are absent ventrally and accentuated dorsally. For those experienced in thoracic percussion, areas of dullness over the ventral thorax will be noted (p. 42). Moderate-to-large volume pleural effusion should be drained as soon as possible to improve ventilation. Although a diuretic will be coadministered, thoracocentesis has the greatest and most immediate impact. Mild sedation, with or without a local lidocaine block, helps reduce patient stress and movement during the procedure. Bilateral effusion usually can be removed from one side of the chest, because of mediastinal fenestrations. It is important to monitor for complications, including pneumothorax or hemorrhage. Pleural fluid can be used in the POC feline NT-proBNP SNAP test (p. 660), especially when serum is not immediately available. IV catheter placement, thoracic radiography and blood sampling for clinical laboratory tests should be done after the cat appears stable enough to tolerate them.

Monitoring of respiratory rate and effort is done every 30 minutes or so initially, without disturbing the cat, to help guide furosemide therapy. Additional furosemide boluses (1–2 mg/kg q1–4h, or as needed) are provided, with dose and frequency dependent on the cat's diuretic and respiratory response. For cats that do not respond adequately to 2–3 IV bolus doses, a furosemide constant rate infusion (CRI) can be tried for several hours. Caution is advised if or when furosemide dosing exceeds 12 mg/kg over a 24-hour period. Although there is no absolute maximum dose, renal function is the limiting parameter. Furthermore, resolution of alveolar flooding could take some hours to days, depending on the severity of secondary capillary injury; additional high-dose diuretics might not necessarily hasten this repair. Once the respiratory distress is alleviated, furosemide administration is continued at reduced doses q8–12h. Diuretic therapy is guided by the cat's respiratory rate and effort, as well as renal and electrolyte status.

Although topical 2% nitroglycerine ointment might promote venodilation and help redistribute blood from the pulmonary to the splanchnic circulation, this has not been proven in cats and most clinicians currently do not recommend this therapy. Nevertheless, 1/8 to 1/4 of an inch of the ointment usually is tolerated. Other strategies for fulminant pulmonary edema could include low-dose nitroprusside or nitroglycerin CRI; however, the risk of severe hypotension (especially in cats with HOCM), drug expense, and the intensive monitoring required make this impractical in nearly all cases (**Table 22.2**, p. 342). Artificial ventilation sometimes is used in emergency centers to good effect.

ACE inhibitor and other arterial vasodilator therapies generally are not used for acute CHF. RAAS inhibition might be considered after respiratory distress resolves and the cat is eating again; however, its efficacy in controlling CHF in cats is largely unstudied.

The use of pimobendan in cats with HCM is controversial at this time, and its use for acute CHF varies widely across teaching hospitals and emergency clinics. Cats with mainly left-sided CHF (pulmonary edema with small pleural effusions) usually have normal to hyperdynamic LV systolic function, unless myocardial infarction has occurred. Cats with moderate to large pleural effusions are more likely to have end-stage HCM or show some other evidence of combined diastolic and systolic heart failure. The greatest concern regarding pimobendan is for cats with HOCM, where an inodilator would conceivably worsen outflow tract obstruction and increase MR. However, pimobendan supports LA function and RV function, and these effects can be beneficial. Yet many cats with pulmonary edema respond well to just sedation, oxygen, and diuresis. Without controlled study, it is impossible to know if pimobendan would provide further benefit in this situation. Conversely, cats with moderate to large pleural effusions probably have more chronic in heart failure, and are presented only after pulmonary atelectasis has become critical. Many of these cats have no visible pulmonary edema or only a mild interstitial change following thoracocentesis. They usually have volume expansion, jugular venous distention and evidence of biventricular CHF. Although there are a number of clinical studies and reports regarding the tolerability of pimobendan in cats, all the available studies have substantial limitations and none can be considered pivotal in terms of recommending treatment.

To us, a *reasonable approach* based on current information is to identify cats that are likely to have LV dynamic obstruction; this is where pimobendan's use has been most challenged in acute CHF. Although LV outflow obstruction might be observed with POC ultrasound, it is probably more practical to auscultate the cat for a murmur. Accepting the challenges of auscultation in the dyspneic cat, the absence of a prominent systolic murmur argues against HOCM. If the cat mainly has pulmonary edema, we recommend withholding pimobendan for at least 4-6 hours and observing the cat's response to furosemide, supplemental O_2, and sedation. If the response is insufficient, then consider adding in pimobendan. For cats with a moderate to large pleural effusion, we recommend including pimobendan in the initial therapy. In addition, if hypotension or reduced systolic function is identified, oral pimobendan is recommended once the cat can tolerate PO administration. For cats with cardiogenic shock (hypothermia, hypotension with systolic BP<90, and sinus bradycardia or apparent atrial standstill), diuretic therapy (±thoracocentesis, as indicated) can treat the CHF and a dobutamine CRI is recommended to support cardiac function (**Table 22.2**). Adverse effects can include tachycardia and arrhythmias. Pimobendan PO or IV (where available) works by a different mechanism and also is administered.

Cats with severe, refractory pulmonary edema and signs of respiratory fatigue (such as slowing respirations, with hypercapnia and depressed mentation) might benefit from mechanical ventilation, if adequate intensive care monitoring, equipment, and technical expertise are available. When reactive airway disease is suspected as a contributor to the respiratory distress, a puff or two of inhaled albuterol or salbutamol, delivered by an administration mask and spacer chamber, can be tried. Sinus tachycardia or other tachyarrhythmias are potential adverse effects, so HR and rhythm should be monitored closely.

A beta-blocker usually is avoided in cats with acute CHF, although a $beta_1$ selective agent should be less likely to provoke bronchoconstriction. If the cat already is on a beta-blocker, at minimum, the dose should be reduced. While in theory beta-blocker therapy should not be terminated abruptly, this is an extrapolation from human medicine and in practice, atenolol often is stopped and then its use reassessed once the cat is stable.

Patient monitoring includes BP measurement (q4–12hr depending on the individual cat), respiratory rate and effort (q15–30 minute initially, gradually increasing to q1hr or more, depending on progress), mentation, HR and heart rhythm (either frequently or by continuous ECG). Recording of body temperature and weight, as well as estimated urine output, also is recommended. Parenteral fluid administration is almost never indicated for animals with acute CHF. An uncommon exception might be the cat whose pulmonary edema has resolved, but that has moderate to severe azotemia and refuses to drink. In such a case, a small volume (15–20 mL/kg/day) of 0.45% saline or 5% dextrose in water (D_5W), or other low-sodium fluid can be administered cautiously. If IV fluid must be given, potassium chloride should be supplemented, because diuresis is likely to reduce serum K^+ concentration in the acute setting.

For cats with uncontrolled AF or rapid supraventricular tachycardia (>250 bpm), diltiazem can be tried, either slowly IV or PO (**Table 25.2**, p. 402). Ventricular tachycardia usually is treated with low-dose lidocaine or possibly esmolol (**Table 25.2**), although the concern regarding beta-blocker use in animals with severe pulmonary edema stands. Similarly, if the cat is able to take oral medication, sotalol or atenolol are other options, if pulmonary edema is fairly well controlled. Hypokalemia and hypomagnesemia predispose to ventricular arrhythmias, so these should be corrected if identified.

When oral medication administration is possible, an antiplatelet drug is added. Clopidogrel is preferred because of its greater efficacy. However, its bitter taste causes some cats to reject it. Hiding the pill fragment in a small gelatin capsule or pill pocket might help. If this fails, aspirin (or an anti-Xa agent) might be more readily accepted.

Ideally, a serum chemistry profile was obtained before treatment began, but if not, this should be done as soon as the patient is stable. Renal function and electrolyte concentrations are measured again in 24–36 hours, or rechecked prior to hospital discharge. Some degree of azotemia is common after aggressive diuresis; it usually resolves with oral rehydration, although this should be monitored. Hypokalemia typically improves once the cat starts eating again. Although there is an increasing tendency to place a nasogastric tube in cats where this is delayed, some restraint is suggested, except in the sickest and immobile patients. Thoracic radiographs, to verify improvement in pulmonary edema and pleural effusion, can be obtained before hospital discharge or at the first recheck visit within a week or so.

When respirations become normal or at least appear comfortable and the cat is drinking water voluntarily, it generally is safe to send the patient home on chronic heart failure medications (see next section). Even if food intake is poor in the hospital, this often improves once the cat is home. An appetite stimulant, such capromorelin, can be considered if anorexia persists at home. Adverse effects are uncommon, but can include marked polydipsia and polyuria which diuretic therapy can augment, leading to volume depletion and azotemia.

An initial recheck exam is recommended within a week, or sooner if problems occur. CHF control, renal function and electrolyte status, BP, HR and rhythm, appetite, and activity level all should be assessed. The normal resting (sleeping) respiratory rate (RRR) in most cats is under 30 breaths/min. It is important to verify that the owner is able to effectively monitor the RRR, and effort, and can administer all medications consistently. Any client concerns should be addressed. The patient's clinical status influences the frequency of follow-up exams.

Chronic Heart Failure The main goals of long-term therapy are to prevent arterial TE and control excess fluid accumulation, while maintaining a cardiac output sufficient to permit good quality of life, activity, and near-normal renal function. Other treatment goals might include controlling arrhythmias, minimizing myocardial ischemia, and enhancing LV filling (**Table 33.3** and **Table 22.3**, p. 345). Most recommendations for chronic heart failure therapy still are based largely on clinical experience and theoretical speculation, because high-quality evidence-based recommendations are essentially lacking, aside from the value of clopidogrel. The heterogeneous nature of HCM and its different clinical manifestations are confounding factors also.

Furosemide is adjusted to find the lowest dosage (and longest dosing interval) that effectively controls congestive signs in the individual cat. Oral doses of 1–2 mg/kg q12–24hr might be adequate initially and can be a reasonable starting point in cats with mild CHF. Higher dosages are needed in cats with moderate to large pleural effusions to prevent or delay recurrence. Over the following weeks, some cats can be titrated to lower doses and once daily, or occasionally every other day, administration. Others require increasingly higher doses, especially as the disease advances. Careful at-home observation of RRR and effort by the owner is important for optimizing furosemide dosage. Furosemide generally is used in combination with other therapy. Renal function and electrolytes should be monitored periodically. Thoracocentesis is indicated for moderate- to large-volume pleural effusion, followed by intensified therapy to slow further fluid accumulation. Mild azotemia should be anticipated and it generally is well tolerated. A disconnection between serum urea nitrogen and creatinine concentrations often develops, probably related to the diffusability of urea nitrogen and the reduced creatinine generation in cats with cardiac cachexia. In those cases, monitoring serum urea nitrogen, in preference to creatinine, might be more useful.

As noted previously, therapy to reduce risk of arterial TE also is important, especially when LA enlargement is moderate to severe. Virtually every cat that has experienced CHF will be sent home on clopidogrel (1/4 of 75 mg tablet q24h), because this was shown to be more effective than aspirin in secondary arterial TE prevention (Hogan, 2015). Cats judged to be at high risk for initial or recurrent arterial TE can be treated with both clopidogrel and aspirin, or more aggressively, with clopidogrel and an anti-Xa agent, such as apixaban, rivaroxaban, or with a low molecular weight heparin (**Table 36.2**, p. 751).

Other long-term therapy in cats with chronic heart failure (that accept being medicated reasonably well) can include an ACE inhibitor, spironolactone, and/or pimobendan (see following paragraphs). An ACE inhibitor might be of benefit in a cat with suspected myocardial infarction; it also should moderate RAAS activation in cats receiving diuretic therapy. Enalapril or benazepril, with or without spironolactone, can be considered, especially in cats with advanced CHF and a large pleural effusion, or in cats with recurrent pulmonary edema. Unfortunately, there currently is insufficient evidence that RAAS inhibitor drugs improve survival or quality of life, beyond open-label studies or small studies that show promise but cannot be considered pivotal (James, 2018). Additionally, these drugs can negatively affect renal function or appetite in some cats. Initial dose(s) of enalapril or benazepril of 0.25 mg/kg q24h could be increased to 0.5 mg/kg q24(–12)h, as long as renal function, appetite, and BP are not adversely affected. Spironolactone usually is dosed at 1-2 mg/kg daily. Another indication for these drugs is persistent hypokalemia. In general, they should not be given with an oral potassium supplement. Enclosing these multiple pill fragments into an empty gelatin capsule, pill pocket, or compounding it into a strongly flavored (such as fish or tuna) suspension can help with owner and patient treatment compliance.

The routine addition of a beta-blocker or calcium channel blocker currently is not recommended for chronic CHF management. There is no clear evidence for benefit and possibility for negative effects. However, there might be some advantage for selected individuals. For example, in cats with severe HOCM, the ability of beta-blockers to reduce dynamic LV outflow obstruction and HR would be expected to reduce myocardial oxygen demand and could help protect from ischemia- or sympathetic-induced arrhythmias. Therefore, atenolol can be considered in cats with marked dynamic LV outflow obstruction, frequent ventricular or supraventricular tachyarrhythmias, or suspected myocardial infarction. If the cat was not previously being medicated with atenolol, therapy usually is initiated after pulmonary edema has been controlled and with a low-moderate dose (such as ¼ of a 25 mg tab q12h). Monitoring is as previously discussed for preclinical disease. Beta-blockers are relatively contraindicated if bradycardia or marked contractility failure exists.

Although diltiazem has the theoretical benefit of improving diastolic function, its clinical efficacy is unconfirmed. Potential adverse effects include inappetence, hepatotoxicity, and possible behavioral changes. The nonsustained form requires q8hr dosing and there are pharmacokinetic inconsistencies with sustained-release forms. Therefore, diltiazem (and verapamil) are not recommended, except for uncontrolled AF, or other supraventricular tachyarrhythmia, that does not respond to atenolol or sotalol.

Pimobendan often is added in the management of chronic CHF caused by HCM. The potential benefits and concerns regarding this drug have been previously noted (see "Acute Congestive Heart Failure"). Definitive evidence regarding its effect on survival and quality of life in cats with HCM and CHF currently is lacking; available data are conflicting and based only on small numbers of cats. A single-center, retrospective report suggested possible survival benefit, although many factors, including owner compliance, disease severity, and comorbidities could have influenced results (Reina-Doreste, 2014). In contrast, a randomized, double-blind, multicenter prospective trial found no benefit on outcome at 9 months, compared to placebo (Schober, 2021). However, those cats were not treated with pimobendan until after CHF was stable (a requirement of enrollment), and there was considerable case dropout over the course of the study. As the authors indicated, the study was "exploratory" and "non-pivotal." At least in a small number of cats studied, pimobendan did not appear to worsen dynamic outflow obstruction, although this finding is somewhat surprising. A relatively large number of retrospective studies in cats with heart failure have shown the drug is well-tolerated.

Pimobendan's effects as an inodilator might be less relevant in heart failure caused primarily by diastolic dysfunction with well-preserved systolic function, although the ventricular unloading effect might be useful in cats with CHF; its positive inotropic effect on LA, and probably RV, function also are likely to help. Pimobendan was shown to improve measures of LA function somewhat, and these effects appear to be greater in cats with HCM compared to healthy cats (Kochie, 2020). This might especially benefit cats with LA enlargement and poor atrial contractility. Other postulated benefits for pimobendan in cats with HCM might include possible reduced platelet aggregation, enhanced myocardial relaxation from phosphodiesterase-3 (PDE-3) inhibition, and enhanced myocardial perfusion from increased vascular endothelium-derived relaxation effects.

The authors' recommendations for using pimobendan in cats with chronic heart failure are similar to those already noted for acute CHF. It probably is unnecessary in cats that had good response to diuretic therapy. It potentially can be beneficial in cats where diuretic and RAAS inhibitor therapies are failing. It is recommended strongly in cats with moderate or large pleural effusions or any echo evidence of impaired systolic function. It should be used cautiously in cats with moderate to severe HOCM; then, we cautiously add pimobendan, carefully monitoring these patients (including with HR and BP measurements, especially after the initial dose, and on recheck exams). Cats with poor LA function and marked LA enlargement might particularly benefit from the drug. The empirical dose used typically is the same as the dog label dose, usually falling between 0.625 to 1.25 mg/per cat. Although there are pharmacokinetic differences in cats, including a longer half-life, twice daily dosing still is used.

Other cardiac drugs either are not indicated or are contraindicated. Digoxin is relatively contraindicated in HCM, because it can increase myocardial oxygen demand and worsen dynamic LV outflow obstruction. Drugs that accelerate HR are potentially detrimental, because tachycardia decreases filling time and predisposes to myocardial ischemia. In addition, arterial vasodilators could cause hypotension and reflex tachycardia because cats with HCM have little preload reserve. Hypotension also can exacerbate dynamic outflow obstruction. Although ACE inhibitors have this potential, their vasodilating effect usually is mild enough that this is not clinically apparent.

For cats with persistent or recurrent congestive signs despite progressively higher furosemide doses (such as >6 mg/kg/day), one strategy is to give one of the daily furosemide doses by SC injection (rather than PO) a number of times weekly. This has limitations in terms of compliance but can be useful if GI absorption is suboptimal, or when frequent oral dosing is becoming difficult. A more practical strategy for suspected diuretic resistance is to switch from furosemide to torsemide (starting at ~1/10 to 1/12 of the cat's furosemide dose in mg/day; **Table 22.3**, p. 345). Torsemide is a more potent loop diuretic with a longer duration of effect compared to furosemide; however, caution is needed to avoid dehydration, azotemia and electrolyte abnormalities. There is limited clinical experience with this drug in cats, compared to furosemide. Torsemide (or furosemide) therapy combined with pimobendan, spironolactone, and an ACE inhibitor is recommended for end-stage HCM. In addition, beta-blocker therapy is withdrawn unless needed for serious arrhythmia. As always, careful home monitoring and prophylaxis against arterial TE remain important.

Recurrent pleural (or occasionally, abdominal) effusion often accompanies refractory or end-stage CHF. Thoraco- (or abdomino-)centesis is performed as needed to improve ventilation. Medication doses are intensified, as possible, to reduce the rate of fluid accumulation while avoiding worsened renal function. If pimobendan and torsemide are not being administered, these should both be considered.

Ventricular and supraventricular tachyarrhythmias are common in advanced HCM. Atenolol usually is the antiarrhythmic drug of first choice for in cats (Chapters 24 and 25). However, if atenolol does not adequately suppress these arrhythmias, sotalol might be more efficacious, especially if the arrhythmia is complex or associated with syncope or weakness. Caution is advised when congestive signs are present, especially in cats with reduced systolic function. A sotalol dose of 10 mg/cat q12h usually is tried initially; some cats might need up to 20 mg/cat q12h. The negative inotropic effect of higher doses should be recognized.

Medication administration can be extremely challenging. If possible, "pilling" the cat rather than trying to hide medication in food helps assure that the dose has been taken and can reduce food avoidance associated with distasteful medicine (such as clopidogrel). Some cats accept medications more easily when put into a pill pocket, a small empty gelatin capsule, or even a small piece of cold butter. A gelatin capsule or pill pocket usually can hold all the needed pill fragments, except pimobendan. If the drug can be mixed into a suspension (with strong tuna, chicken, or other desired flavor), this can be a good alternative for some cats.

A diet moderately low in salt is desirable, as for dogs with chronic CHF. However maintaining appetite and food intake often is more challenging in cats. Adding a small amount of reduced-salt food to the cat's regular diet, then slowly increasing the proportion over time, might work with some cats. If not, it is better that the cat eat a higher-salt diet than become anorexic. Inappetence also can result from azotemia, adverse medication effects, congestion, or other causes. Managing identifiable underlying abnormalities, reducing drug dosage(s), or even providing a brief drug "holiday," if possible, might help. Offering a variety of different foods or using an appetite stimulant (such as mirtazapine or capromorelin) could help slow the development of cardiac cachexia.

Home management for cats with chronic heart failure should include periodic RRR monitoring. Most cats with normal lungs have a RRR <30 breaths/minute. However, it also is important to monitor respiratory effort, because accumulating pleural effusion might not increase breathing rate but will increase effort. As always, stress avoidance is important and making the cat's environment as stress-free as possible is advised.

Periodic recheck exams are helpful to assess CHF control. As a stress reduction tool, use of gabapentin administration prior to hospital visits should be discussed with clients. Rechecks at 2 weeks after hospital discharge and then every 2 to 4 months are appropriate for many cats; however, the individual cat's clinical status, as well as the level of stress caused by hospital visits, influence reevaluation schedules. If clients are carefully monitoring respirations at home, the cat's activity and appetite are good, and treatment compliance is acceptable, then veterinary rechecks can be relatively simple. Such examinations would include: assessment of HR, rhythm, and respiratory status; noninvasive BP measurement;

serum renal function and electrolyte panel; and usually, a brief thoracic ultrasound exam to screen for pleural effusion, pulmonary B-lines, and thrombus formation or smoke in the left atrial appendage. These are high-yield evaluations for cats with chronic CHF and might circumvent the need for radiographs. Often, these procedures can be conducted from a single examination table while the cat rests in sternal recumbency. This can minimize the stress of rechecks.

Other Complications and Prognosis The prognosis for cats with HCM is quite variable overall. Although cats with HCM have a higher rate of death from cardiac causes than normal cats, the majority of cats with preclinical HCM survive for at least two to over five years after diagnosis and some never develop clinical signs (see "Prognosis in Preclinical HCM"). Longer survival is associated with younger age and absence of clinical signs. The 5-year cumulative incidence of cardiac death for cats diagnosed with HCM (at any age) was estimated at ~23% in the REVEAL study, and for cats that developed CHF or arterial TE, mean survival time was fairly short at 1.3 (±1.7 years; Fox, 2018). CHF, arterial TE, or reduced LV systolic function present at diagnosis were associated with <2-year survival in another report also (Payne, 2015a). Many cats survive for <6–12 months following CHF onset. However, cats that develop CHF following IV fluid therapy, general anesthesia or other stress, or long-acting corticosteroid treatment might have a better prognosis than cats without such history.

Cats presented with TE and concurrent CHF generally live for <6 months; a great many die or are euthanized within days of the event. Even in cats without CHF, outcomes depend very much on client and veterinary expectations and the attendant cost of care. Yet some cats do quite well for longer, especially if congestive signs can be controlled and infarction of vital organs has not occurred. For example in the FATCAT study (Hogan, 2015), median survival in cats receiving clopidogrel was nearly one year (346 days to composite endpoint of recurrent TE or cardiac related death). Even in the aspirin-treated group, median survival (to the composite endpoint) was about four months (Hogan, 2015). Recurrent TE is common and some cats have survived several episodes (Chapter 36).

Various retrospective studies have associated different factors with an increased likelihood of cardiac death (whether from CHF, arterial TE, sudden death, or euthanasia). These are not controlled, prospective studies and do not address client motivation and resources; however, they do represent "real-life" data. Negative prognostic factors include: increased LA size and LA/Ao (>1.8, on short-axis 2D imaging); diminished LA function (peak LA appendage flow velocity <0.20 m/s, LA systolic shortening <12%); presence of spontaneous echocontrast ("smoke"); severe LV hypertrophy (≥9 mm, end-diastole); reduced LV regional or global systolic function (with FS <30%); arterial TE; arrhythmias; and older patient age. Doppler echo evidence for a restrictive LV filling pattern (with mitral inflow E/A velocity ratio >2) indicates advanced diastolic dysfunction and worse prognosis. Other factors that probably reflect a negative outcome include AF (presumably a consequence of severe LA enlargement), progressive pleural effusion, and cardiac cachexia. A high cTnI (≥0.7 ng/mL) has been associated with increased mortality, regardless of LA size. For cats presented in CHF, those with a larger percentage decrease in NT-proBNP concentration from the time of admission to hospital discharge, and without evidence for CHF at reevaluation, had longer survival time. Survival was shorter in cats that still had signs of CHF at reevaluation and in those that were difficult for owners to medicate (Pierce, 2017). Cats with a history of syncope or arrhythmias on presentation might have increased risk for sudden death.

Restrictive Cardiomyopathy

Cardiomyopathy characterized by what is considered mainly restrictive pathophysiology occurs less often than HCM, but is not uncommon. Affected cats have marked left or biatrial enlargement with relatively normal ventricular wall thickness, chamber size, and contractility. Affected cats often develop CHF, with or without arterial TE. The etiology is unknown but probably multifactorial, as there is a spectrum of pathophysiologic findings. RCM might be a sequela of endo/myocarditis (either infectious or immune mediated) or it could represent the end-stage of myocardial failure and infarction from HCM. Evidence for viral nucleic acid or endo/myocarditis was lacking in a group of cats tested, however (Kimura, 2016). A secondary form of RCM occasionally could result from neoplastic (as with lymphoma) or other infiltrative disease.

Pathophysiology

Cats with RCM can have extensive endocardial, subendocardial, or myocardial fibrosis and prominent left or biatrial enlargement, with some atrial wall hypertrophy. These are the salient features. The LV chamber size and function are more heterogeneous. Typically, LV size is normal, although it can be slightly decreased or increased. LV wall thickness usually is normal, although mild or regional hypertrophy can occur, suggesting the cat has end-stage or burned out HCM. Heart weight is greater than in normal cats.

Both endomyocardial (eRCM) and myocardial (mRCM) forms of fibrosis are seen in RCM, similar to that described in people. The myocardial form is characterized by normal LV dimension and wall thickness, with restrictive pathophysiology and prominent LA enlargement. The endomyocardial form, also known as endomyocardial fibrosis, might be most common in cats; however, not all reports agree. Extensive patchy or diffuse LV endocardial scarring and chamber deformity characterize eRCM. Rarely, the RV also is affected. Patchy areas of thickening appear more common than the diffuse form. Large trabecular or irregular broad bands of fibrous tissue might be associated with these patchy LV lesions, with multiple "false tendons" (previously known as LV moderator bands) providing a framework for the fibrous band formation. Thick bands of fibrous tissue bridging between the LV wall and septum can cause intraventricular obstruction. Excess and thickened false tendons (extending along or between the LV wall and septum) are found in some cats with RCM. However, these could represent a congenital anomaly; they have been identified in young kittens as well as older cats. It is possible that some of these are a nonspecific response to cardiac enlargement or injury. The mitral valve apparatus and papillary muscles can be distorted and fused to surrounding structures. Thrombi commonly are found within the enlarged left atrium, and sometimes in the left ventricle or systemic vasculature.

Histopathologic changes include patchy endocardial and myocardial fibrosis. Variable degrees of myocyte disarray are present in some cats. A spectrum of endocardial lesions has been observed with the endomyocardial form of RCM, which probably reflects a progressive process. One form (Type 1) is found in young cats up to 3 years of age, while more advanced (Type 2 and 3) lesions involve more fibrous tissue and tend to be seen in middle-aged and older cats, respectively. Immunohistochemistry has revealed mesenchymal cells with smooth muscle differentiation associated with areas of connective tissue, which could be involved in the development of the fibrous endocardial lesions. Histologically, false tendons appear to consist of central Purkinje fibers surrounded by collagen. Intramural coronary arteriosclerosis, with thickened vascular walls and luminal narrowing, is common. Other findings can include hypertrophied myocytes, areas of myocardial degeneration and necrosis, and, sometimes, endomyocardial cellular infiltrates. Myocyte disarray has been reported, which supports the idea that many of these cats are really end-stage HCM.

Ventricular filling is impeded (restricted) because of abnormal ventricular stiffness. Contractility is normal or only mildly reduced in most affected cats; however, contractility might decline with time as more functional myocardium is lost. Regional LV dysfunction occurs in some cats, which reduces overall systolic function. Such cases might be better categorized as cardiomyopathy of "non-specific phenotype," rather than restrictive. LA enlargement is secondary to marked LV diastolic dysfunction and the progressively increasing pressure required to fill the stiff ventricle. Arrhythmias and myocardial ischemia or infarction also can contribute to diastolic dysfunction. MR can occur, although usually it is mild and does not explain the degree of LA enlargement, which often is massive. A murmur is found only inconsistently. Progressive increase in left heart filling pressure, presumably in combination with compensatory neurohormonal and renal compensations, eventually leads to left-sided or biventricular CHF. Poor LA emptying with blood stasis predisposes to thrombus formation and TE.

Clinical Features

The mean age at diagnosis appears to be between 7 and 10 years; however, RCM can occur in cats <6 months to >18 years old. There is no apparent breed predilection. Although some reports indicate no sex predominance, in others, males account for up to 70% of cases. Clinical signs are variable; but most cats with RCM are presented initially for respiratory signs caused by pleural effusion, pulmonary edema, or both. Based on two recent surveys, 62 to >80% of cats with RCM have overt respiratory distress at presentation (Locatelli, 2018; Chetboul, 2019). Signs often are precipitated by stress or a concurrent disease that increases cardiovascular demand. Clinical signs are likely to develop or worsen suddenly. Thromboembolic events are common. Inactivity, poor appetite, vomiting, weight loss, or syncope might be part of the cat's recent history. Preclinical RCM sometimes is discovered upon finding abnormal heart sounds or radiographic evidence of cardiomegaly.

Auscultation is variable although most have some abnormality. A soft systolic murmur of MR or TR might be heard; however, many cats have no obvious murmur, which likely explains why their cardiac disease was never identified prior to presentation with clinical signs. Careful auscultation usually indicates a gallop sound in cats with CHF. As noted by Harpster (1977), who first reported this disorder calling it "intermediate cardiomyopathy," cardiac arrhythmias commonly are heard in cats with RCM. Soft heart sounds suggest either pleural or pericardial effusion, or impaired contractility. Muffled or abnormal lung sounds might be evident with pleural effusion or pulmonary edema, respectively. Femoral arterial pulses are normal or slightly weak, unless blocked by TE. Jugular vein distension and pulsation are indicative of elevated right heart filling pressures, especially in cats with pleural effusion. Ascites occasionally is present as a manifestation of right-sided CHF. Signs of arterial TE usually relate to distal aortic obstruction with hind limb paresis, although other body regions are affected in some cats (see Chapter 36). Cats with CHF often are hypothermic.

Diagnostic Tests

As for cats with HCM, clinicopathologic findings are non-specific. Cardiac biomarker concentrations are likely to be elevated, especially in cats with clinical disease. Severe cTnI elevation suggests myocarditis or possibly acute myocardial infarction. Pleural effusions usually are a modified transudate or chyle. Plasma taurine concentration occasionally is low, and should be measured if decreased LV contractility is evident.

Radiographs show LA or biatrial enlargement, with LV or generalized cardiomegaly (**Figures 33.23** and **3.14**, p. 57). Mild to moderate pericardial effusion (associated with CHF) can magnify the cardiomegaly. Proximal pulmonary veins might appear dilated and tortuous. Patchy or diffuse alveolar

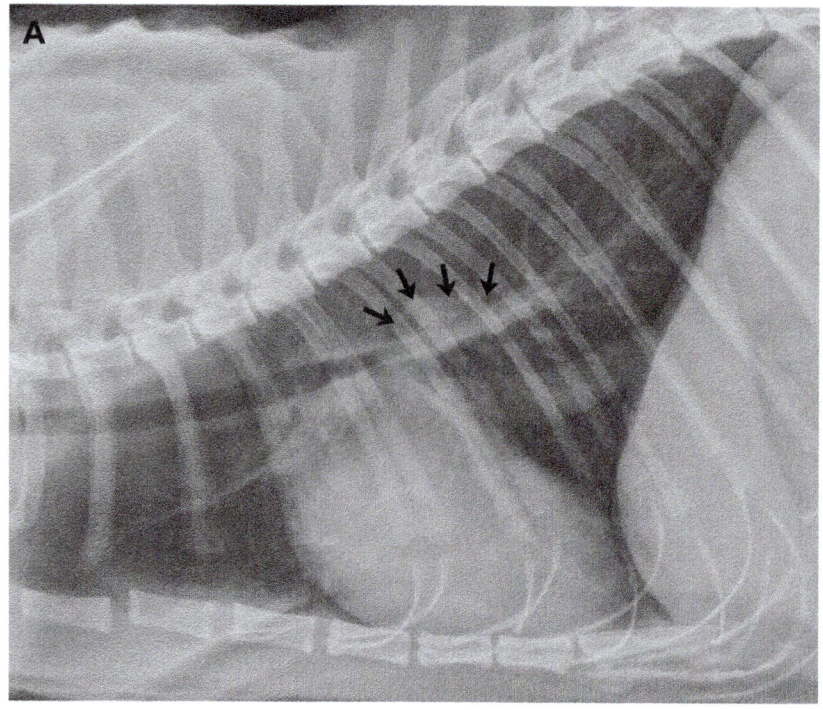
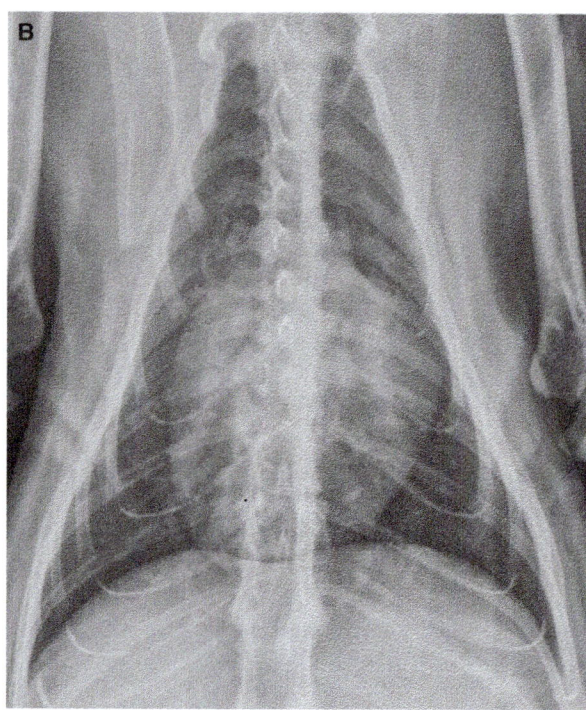

Figure 33.23 Lateral (A) and DV (B) thoracic radiographs from a 7-year-old male Domestic Shorthair cat with restrictive cardiomyopathy show left-sided cardiomegaly (VHS = 9 v). Pulmonary edema has resolved, but the indicated tortuous caudal pulmonary vein (A, arrows along dorsal border) suggests chronically elevated pulmonary venous pressure. (B) The cardiac apex has shifted into the right hemithorax. Echocardiography showed severe left atrial enlargement, with normal left ventricular dimensions, wall thickness, and systolic function. There was no pericardial effusion. Paroxysmal supraventricular tachycardia (at ~300 beats/min), identified during the echo, likely contributed to the cat's clinical decompensation.

or interstitial infiltrates of pulmonary edema, pleural effusion, and sometimes, caudal vena caval distension, hepatomegaly or ascites are seen in cats with CHF.

The ECG often is abnormal. Wide QRS complexes, tall R waves, wide P waves, and evidence of disturbed intraventricular conduction, including right bundle branch block, might be seen. Various arrhythmias also are common in cats with RCM. These include supraventricular or ventricular premature complexes and tachycardia, AF, and varying degrees of AV block (**Figures 33.24** and **33.25**).

Echo features include moderate to severe LA (with or without RA) enlargement and patchy or extensive areas of hyperechoic, thickened endocardium. RA enlargement probably depends in part on the presence of CHF, as increased systemic pressures will distend this chamber. Usually the LV wall and septal thicknesses are normal (<6 mm), although focal thickening might be evident in some cases. LV wall motion is normal to only mildly depressed; FS usually exceeds 25%, but this is quite low for most cats. Hyperechoic areas of fibrosis can appear within the LV wall or endocardial areas, although this is not prominent in all cats (**Figures 33.26** and **33.27**). In some cats, endocardial scarring can be extensive, bridging to the septum and constricting portions of the LV lumen. Mitral SAM or other evidence for dynamic LV outflow obstruction is highly unlikely in RCM. RV dilation is common in cats with CHF. An intracardiac thrombus might be present within the left atrium or occasionally, the ventricle (**Figure 33.28**). Color Doppler evaluation sometimes shows mild (to moderate) MR or TR (**Figure 33.29**). Spectral Doppler interrogation generally reveals a restrictive LV filling pattern (see **Figure 4.31B**, p. 109). However, this simply

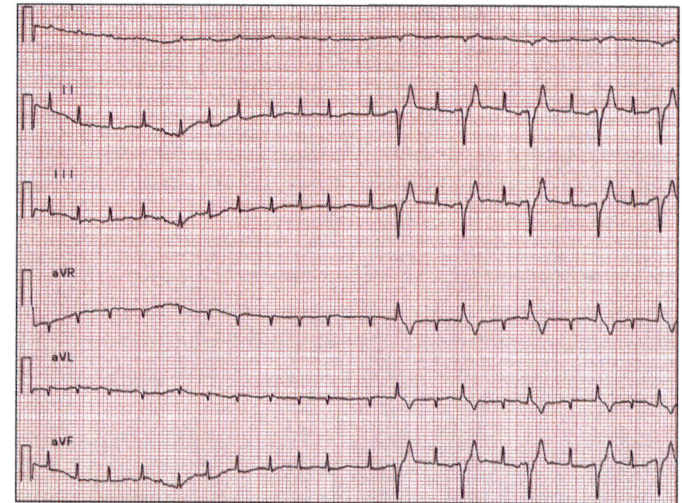

Figure 33.24 ECG from a cat with restrictive cardiomyopathy shows atrial fibrillation, suggesting marked atrial enlargement. Ventricular premature complexes occur in bigeminal pattern on the right side of the recording. Leads as marked; 25 mm/sec, 1 cm = 1 mV.

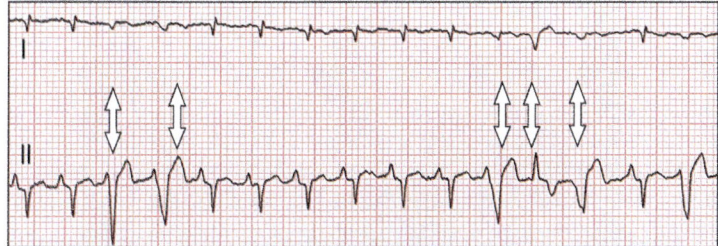

Figure 33.25 Sinus rhythm with multiform ventricular premature complexes (arrows) in a cat with restrictive cardiomyopathy. Abnormal intraventricular conduction caused a right axis shift. Leads as shown; 25 mm/sec, 1 cm=1 mV.

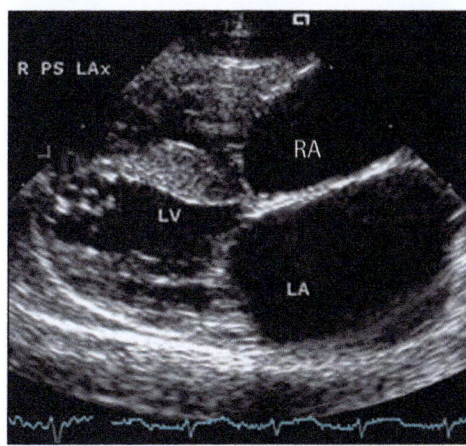

Figure 33.26 Fibrotic areas produced multiple irregular, bright echoes near the left ventricular apex in a cat with restrictive cardiomyopathy. Note the absence of significant hypertrophy and marked left atrial enlargement. The RA is moderately enlarged. Right parasternal long-axis view. LA, left atrium; LV, left ventricle; RA, right atrium.

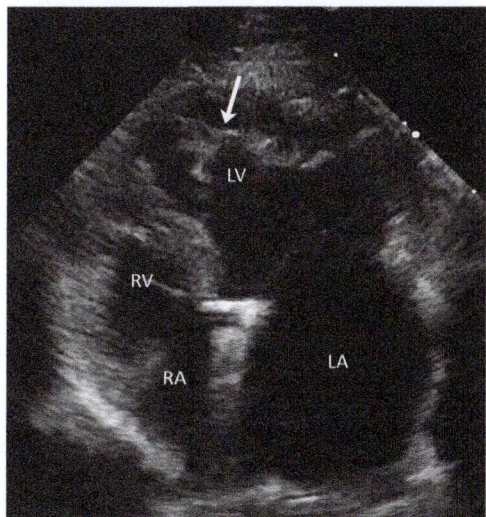

Figure 33.27 Bright fibrous bands (arrow) bridge between the interventricular septum and left ventricular free wall in the mid- to apical LV in a 9-year-old male Domestic Shorthair cat with restrictive cardiomyopathy. Increased endocardial echogenicity also was present in this region. The LA is severely enlarged. Left ventricular wall and septal thicknesses are normal. Fractional shortening was mildly reduced (24%). Left apical 4-chamber view. LA, left atrium; LV, left ventricle; RA, right atrium; RV, right ventricle.

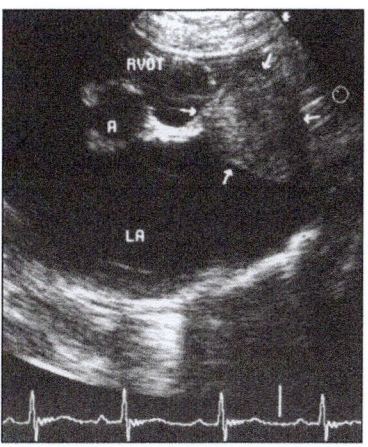

Figure 33.28 Massive enlargement of the LA with an auricular thrombus (arrows) in an older cat with restrictive cardiomyopathy. A, aorta; LA, left atrium; LV, left ventricle; RA, right atrium; RVOT, right ventricular outflow tract.

indicates high LA pressure superimposed on a stiff ventricle; it is not specific for RCM. Occasional cats have marked regional wall dysfunction (especially of LV free wall) which depresses FS and mild LV dilation. These could represent cases of myocardial infarction or cardiomyopathy of nonspecific phenotype, rather than RCM.

Management

Therapy for acute CHF is as for cats with HCM (p. 673, **Table 33.2** and **Table 22.2**, p. 342). Most cats will require thoracocentesis for stabilization. Treatment for acute TE is outlined in Chapter 36 (p. 763). Recommended long-term CHF therapy includes furosemide at the lowest effective dose, with pimobendan and RAAS inhibition (an ACE inhibitor and spironolactone). Prophylaxis against TE is important (p. 769). Dietary considerations, at-home monitoring, and reevaluation recommendations are as for cats with HCM.

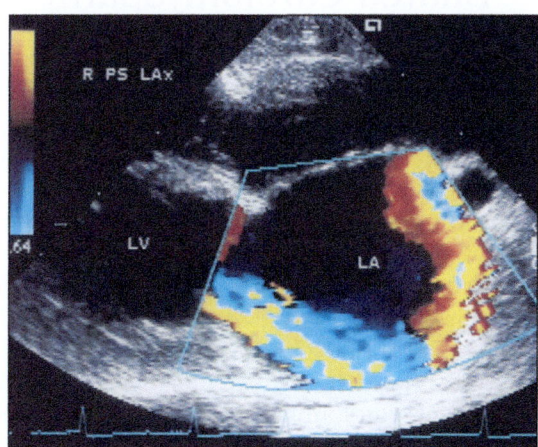

Figure 33.29 Color Doppler image in systole reveals a jet of mitral regurgitation swirling around the large LA of a 10-year-old Domestic Shorthair cat with restrictive cardiomyopathy. Right parasternal long-axis view. LA, left atrium; LV, left ventricle. (ECG in **Figure 33.24**.)

Refractory heart failure with pleural effusion is difficult to manage. Besides repeated thoracocenteses, furosemide dosage can be increased (or torsemide used instead) unless limited by worsening renal function. It might be possible to increase the dose of pimobendan or ACE inhibitor somewhat, or spironolactone can be added to the regimen if not already included. Renal function and serum electrolyte concentrations, as well as BP, must be monitored. Diuretic and/or ACE inhibitor dosages are reduced if hypotension or (more than mild) azotemia develops. Some cats with progressive azotemia require SC fluid support (such as 20–40 mL/kg/day); however, this can exacerbate congestive signs, and generally indicates that death or euthanasia is near.

A beta-blocker usually is prescribed only for tachyarrhythmias or perhaps if an acute myocardial infarction is suspected. Most chronic infarctions appear as thinned areas of LV freewall myocardium. Atenolol is likely to depress LV and LA function; sotalol, which has lesser negative inotropic effect, might be preferred as an antiarrhythmic drug. As a less desired alternative, diltiazem could be used for AF with an uncontrolled ventricular rate or for atrial tachycardia (**Table 25.2**, p. 402). Refractory ventricular tachyarrhythmias might respond to sotalol.

Prognosis The overall prognosis for cats with RCM generally is guarded to poor. Median survival time in some reports is as short as 30 days. More recently, a median survival time of slightly over 2 months was reported for cats presented in respiratory distress; although, for the small minority of cats without respiratory signs, it was over 15 months (Locatelli, 2018). However, a median survival time >21 months also has been reported for cats with mRCM (Chetboul, 2019). Cats with severe LA enlargement (LA/Ao ≥2) have the highest risk of cardiac death. CHF, arterial TE, and occasionally, sudden death are the usual causes of death. The time course of subclinical RCM is unknown.

Dilated Cardiomyopathy

LV systolic dysfunction, with progressive increase in ventricular dimensions, characterizes DCM. Atrial enlargement follows and typically is less severe than in HCM and RCM. After taurine deficiency was discovered to be a major etiology underlying feline DCM in the late 1980s, the taurine content of commercial feline diets was increased and occurrence of clinical DCM fell dramatically. Taurine-induced myocardial failure, therefore, is really a form of secondary (nutritional) myocardial disease. The few cats identified with DCM now typically are not taurine deficient, although testing is warranted to verify this. These cases might represent the end-stage of another cardiomyopathy, a myocardial metabolic abnormality, toxicity, or infection. Although myocardial toxicity from chronic doxorubicin therapy is possible in cats, this species appears fairly resistant to clinical dilated myocardial failure. Nevertheless, the drug causes characteristic myocardial histologic lesions in cats, as in dogs, and some cats have

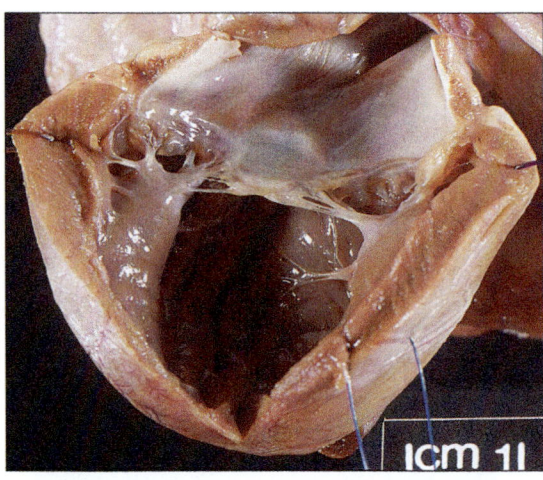

Figure 33.30 Caudal view of the open left atrium (top) and ventricle from a 9-year-old male Siamese cat with dilated cardiomyopathy and low blood taurine. Note the chamber dilation without hypertrophy.

developed echo changes consistent with DCM after receiving cumulative doxorubicin doses of 170–240 mg/m^2.

Pathophysiology

The features of DCM in cats are similar to those in dogs (p. 609). Poor myocardial contractility is the hallmark, with dilation of left heart or all four cardiac chambers (**Figure 33.30**). Mild to moderate AV valve regurgitation develops secondary to chamber enlargement and papillary muscle atrophy. Compensatory neurohormonal mechanisms should be activated as cardiac output decreases, leading to clinical manifestations of CHF. Arrhythmias and pleural effusion are common in cats with DCM. Signs of low output failure and cardiogenic shock sometimes occur.

Clinical Features

Affected cats tend to be older, although DCM can occur in cats of any age, with no breed or sex predilection. Increased respiratory rate or effort, lethargy, anorexia, dehydration, and hypothermia are common clinical findings following the onset of CHF and shock. Subtle physical evidence of poor ventricular function might be present, such as hypokinetic arterial pulses, a weak precordial impulse, and a soft first heart sound, even in the absence of pleural effusion. A gallop sound (usually S_3) and jugular venous distension are signs of heart failure. Left- or right-sided systolic murmurs (of MR or TR) are common, but often very soft. Normal sinus rhythm might be present, although various brady- or tachyarrhythmias can occur. Sinus bradycardia frequently accompanies cardiogenic shock. Increased lung sounds with pulmonary crackles are heard in some cats. Pleural effusion can muffle ventral lung sounds. Arterial TE occurs in some affected cats (Chapter 36). In the taurine deficiency era, central retinal degeneration was evident in about 1/3 of cats with taurine deficiency, and many affected cats were of young age. This rarely is seen today.

Diagnostic Tests

Prerenal azotemia, mildly increased liver enzyme activity, and a stress leukogram are common clinicopathologic findings. NT-proBNP elevation is likely. High serum muscle enzyme activities, an abnormal blood clotting profile, and disseminated intravascular coagulation (DIC) often occur with TE. Pleural fluid in cats with DCM usually is a modified transudate, although chylous effusions can develop, especially over time. Plasma or blood taurine concentration should be measured. Plasma taurine concentrations are influenced by the amount of taurine in the diet, the type of diet, and the time of sampling in relation to eating; however, a plasma taurine concentration of ≤20–30 nmol/mL in a cat with DCM is considered diagnostic for taurine deficiency. Nonanorexic cats with a plasma taurine concentration of <60(–80) nmol/mL probably should receive taurine supplementation or have their diet changed. Normal plasma taurine in cats is approximately 80–120 nmol/mL. Results are more consistent if whole blood, rather than plasma, is used for taurine determination. Normal whole blood taurine concentrations usually are in the range of 300–600 nmol/mL; <140–200 nmol/mL is considered deficient.

A typical radiographic finding is generalized cardiomegaly, with rounding of the cardiac apex. Pleural effusion can obscure the heart silhouette, and any evidence of pulmonary edema or venous congestion (**Figure 33.31**). Hepatomegaly and, infrequently, ascites might be present. ECG findings frequently include an LV enlargement pattern, AV conduction disturbance, and various arrhythmias.

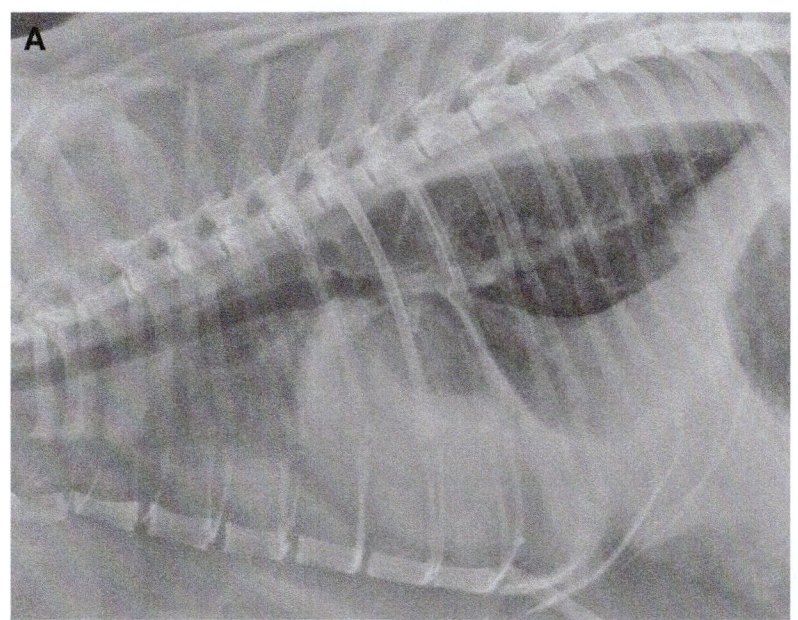
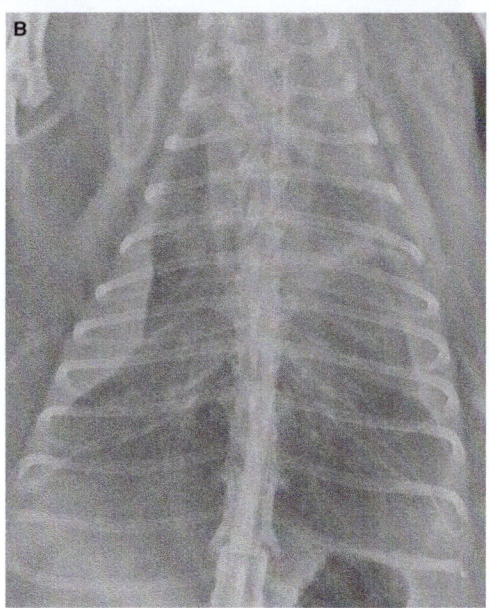
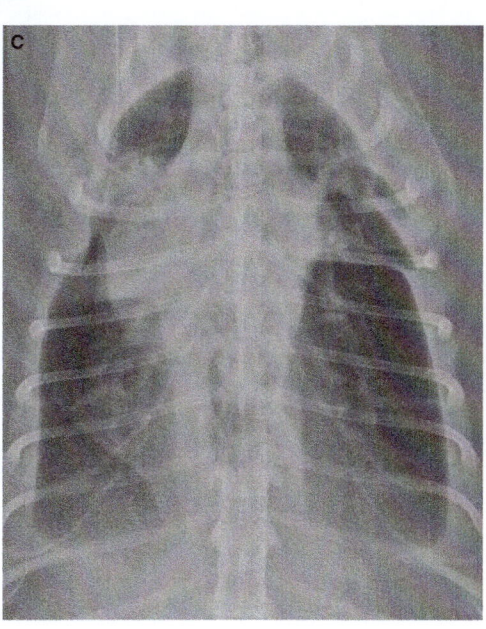

Figure 33.31 (A) Despite the presence of pleural effusion, cardiac enlargement (with tracheal elevation) is evident on this lateral radiograph from an obese, 8-year-old male Domestic Shorthair cat with congestive heart failure from dilated cardiomyopathy. (B) The effusion totally obscures the cardiac silhouette on DV view. (C) The VD view allows better appreciation of the cardiomegaly, with much of the pleural fluid pooled in the dorsal thorax. An S_3 gallop, but no murmur, was heard during auscultation of this cat.

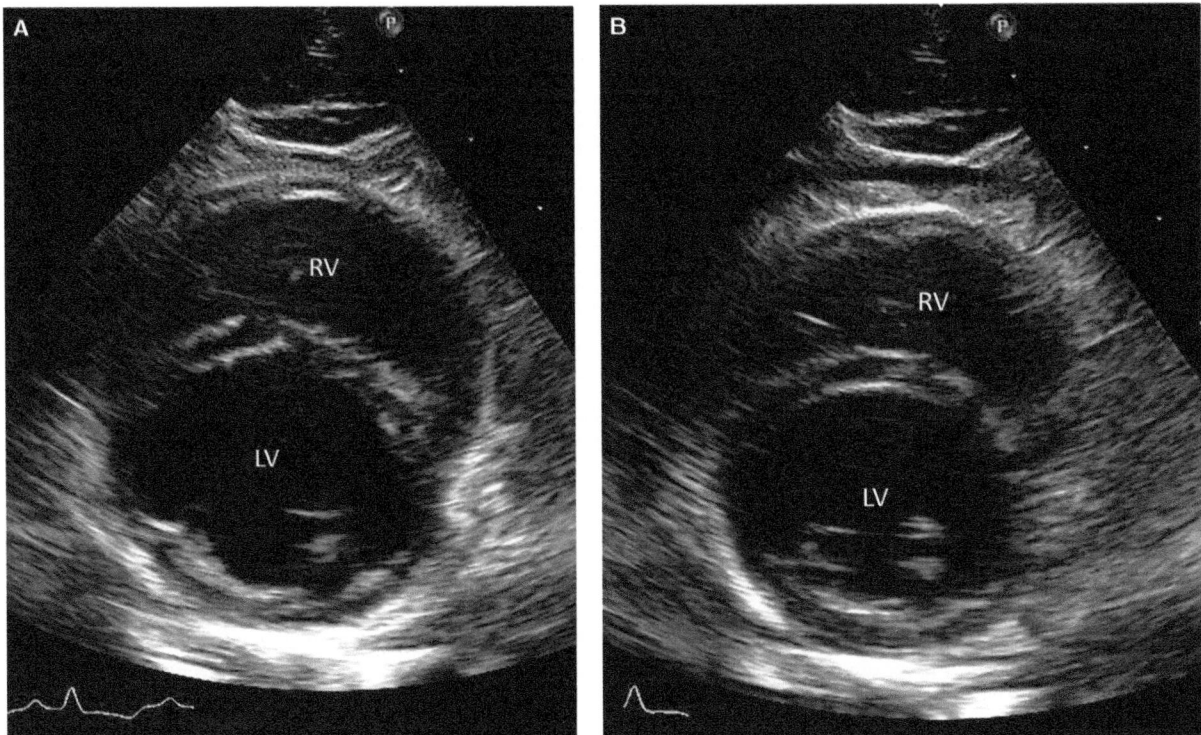

Figure 33.32 Right parasternal short-axis images at the ventricular level in end diastole (A) and systole (B) from a cat with dilated cardiomyopathy. Both ventricles are dilated. There is little change in ventricular dimensions throughout the cardiac cycle. LV, left ventricle; RV, right ventricle.

Definitive diagnosis is made using echocardiography (**Figures 33.32–33.34**). Findings can be analogous to those in dogs with DCM (p. 620), although some cats have focal areas of hypertrophy, or hypokinesis, of either the septum or LV free wall with relatively hyperdynamic motion of the opposite wall. LV systolic function indices (such as FS, ejection fraction, and LV ejection time) are reduced; the preejection period is prolonged. Diastolic

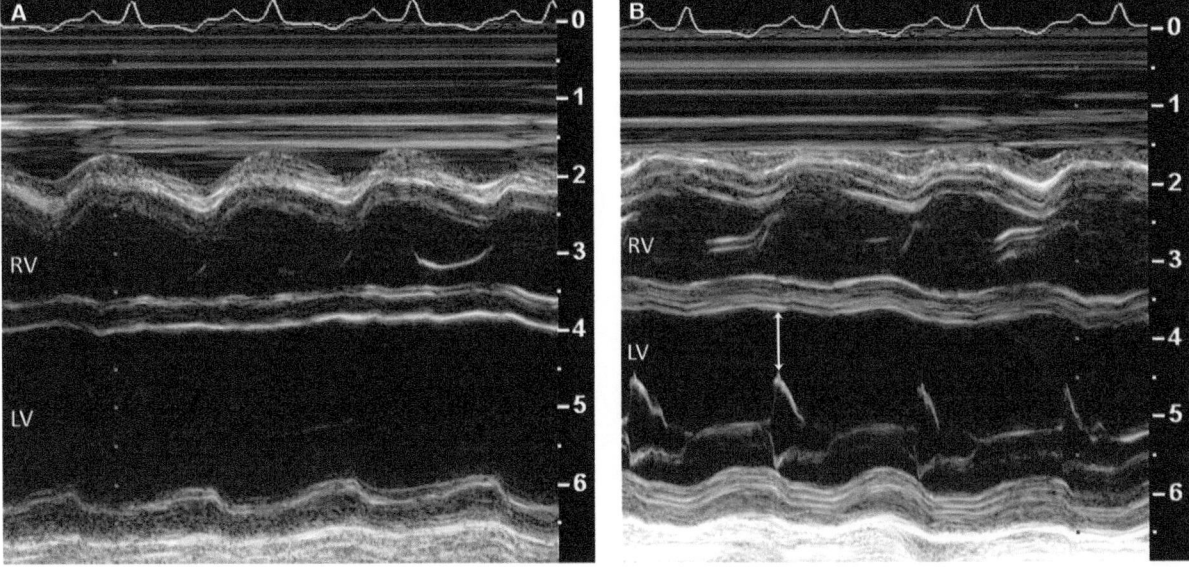

Figure 33.33 M-mode images at the ventricular (A) and mitral (B) levels from the cat in **Figure 33.31**. (A) Left ventricular free wall motion is quite poor and, septal motion is virtually nonexistent. Ventricular dilation is evident. A small volume of pleural effusion is adjacent to the right ventricular free wall. (B) The motion of both mitral leaflets is visible within the dilated LV. The E-point-septal separation (double-headed arrow) is markedly increased at 8 mm. LV, left ventricle; RV, right ventricle.

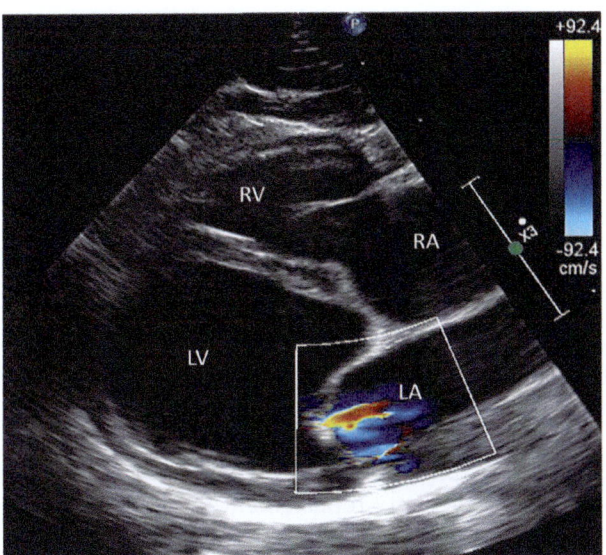

Figure 33.34 Echocardiographic image in systole shows findings typical of advanced dilated cardiomyopathy in a cat. All cardiac chambers are markedly enlarged, but not hypertrophied. Mild mitral regurgitation, secondary to valve annulus dilation, is evident within the color Doppler sector. The cat also had mild tricuspid regurgitation. Pleural effusion is visible in the near field. Right parasternal long-axis view. LA, left atrium; LV, left ventricle; RA, right atrium; RV, right ventricle.

function also is impaired. Sometimes an intracardiac thrombus is found.

Echocardiography has rendered nonselective angiocardiography unnecessary as a diagnostic test now; nevertheless, **Figure 33.35** is instructive in illustrating the characteristic generalized chamber enlargement, atrophied papillary muscles, decreased aortic diameter, and slowed circulation time of DCM. Complications of angiography, especially in cats with extremely poor myocardial function or decompensated CHF, have included vomiting with aspiration, arrhythmias, and cardiac arrest.

Management

Treatment goals essentially are the same as for dogs with DCM, with the addition of TE prophylaxis. For acute CHF, furosemide is given as for HCM; however, greater caution is needed with regard to dosing. Thoracocentesis often is needed for moderate to severe volumes of pleural effusion; this will help stabilize the patient, reducing the diuretic dosage required. Overly aggressive diuresis can markedly decrease cardiac output and BP because of the poor LV systolic function, and cardiogenic shock can develop. Supplemental O_2 should be provided, as needed.

Pimobendan is administered as soon as possible for inotropic support. However, a dobutamine or dopamine CRI (or IV pimobendan, if available) is often needed for cats that are in cardiogenic shock or too dyspneic for oral medications (p. 347 and **Table 22.2**, p. 342). Adverse effects of dobutamine can include seizures or tachycardia; if these occur, the infusion rate is decreased by 50% or discontinued. Adverse effects of dopamine, usually at higher doses, include tachycardia and increased peripheral vascular resistance (alpha-adrenergic effect).

Close monitoring of BP, hydration, renal function, electrolyte balance, and peripheral perfusion is indicated. Hypothermia occurs commonly in cats with decompensated DCM; external warming should be provided, as needed. Supportive therapy for cats with TE is described in Chapter 36 (p. 763). Once pulmonary edema is controlled, furosemide is tapered to the lowest effective dosage.

Furosemide and any vasodilating agents reduce cardiac filling and can predispose to hypotension and cardiogenic shock in cats with DCM, as they can in dogs with DCM. In cases where this is a concern, cautious fluid therapy might be needed along with IV positive inotropic therapy to support BP; for example, 0.45% saline, D_5W, or other low-sodium fluid could be administered at 15–30 mL/kg/day by CRI or in several divided doses. Potassium supplementation might be needed.

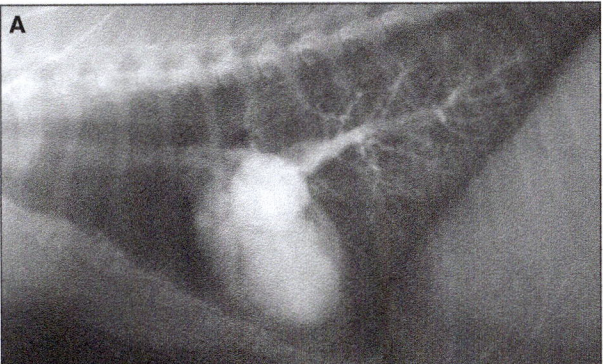
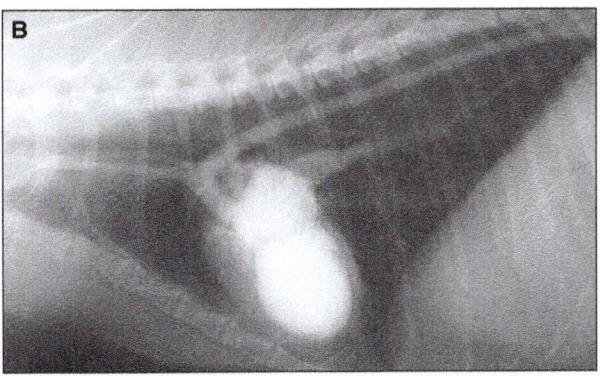

Figure 33.35 Nonselective angiocardiogram from a 13-year-old Siamese cat with dilated cardiomyopathy. (A) 3 seconds after radiopaque contrast injection, the pulmonary venous bed and dilated left heart are opacified. (B) Image taken 13 seconds postinjection. The continued presence of contrast agent within the left atrium and ventricle documents a remarkably slow circulation time in this cat. (From Ware WA. Myocardial diseases of the cat. In, Small Animal Internal Medicine (5th edition). Nelson RW & Couto GC (editors), 2014, Elsevier-Mosby, St Louis, MO, p. 156.)

Long-term therapy for DCM in cats includes PO furosemide, pimobendan, an ACE inhibitor, spironolactone, and antithrombotic prophylaxis (p. 769). Pimobendan is well-tolerated and probably improves survival time in cats with DCM. Digoxin is not recommended.

Home monitoring of RRR and effort and other parameters is as described for HCM. If not done previously, testing for taurine deficiency is indicated. Taurine supplementation (250–500 mg PO q12h) should be instituted as soon as possible in cats with low or unmeasured plasma taurine concentration. Clinical improvement, if it occurs, follows 1–2 weeks of supplementation, so supportive cardiac care is important. Echo evidence of improved systolic function develops in most taurine-deficient cats within 6 weeks of starting supplementation. Some cats can be weaned from heart failure drug therapy after 6–12 weeks, although resolution of pleural effusion and pulmonary edema should be confirmed before reducing the dosages. When LV systolic function is at or near normal, taurine supplementation can be decreased and perhaps eventually discontinued, as long as a diet known to support adequate plasma taurine concentration is fed (this generally includes the name-brand commercial cat foods). Dry diets with 1,000–1,200 mg of taurine per kilogram of dry weight and canned diets with 2,000–2,500 mg of taurine per kilogram of dry weight are thought to maintain normal plasma taurine concentrations in adult cats. Plasma taurine concentration measurement 2–4 weeks after supplement discontinuation is advised.

Prognosis Taurine deficient cats that survive more than a month after initial DCM diagnosis appear to have about a 50% chance for 1-year survival (at least). The prognosis for cats unresponsive to taurine supplementation (or not supplemented) is guarded to poor. Hypothermia and FS <20% are associated with poor prognosis. TE is a grave sign.

Arrhythmogenic Right Ventricular Cardiomyopathy

ARVC is sometimes called "arrhythmogenic cardiomyopathy" because the left side of the heart also can be involved. From an echo perspective, it might be better called "RV cardiomyopathy." It is an uncommon and idiopathic cardiomyopathy with some similarities to ARVC in English Bulldogs, probably more so than in Boxers where severe RV and RA dilation are less common (p. 624). Dilation of those right-sided chambers characterize ARVC in cats; RV systolic dysfunction, RV wall thinning, and ventricular tachyarrhythmias also occur frequently. The left heart is involved to a lesser degree. Right-sided CHF is common and sudden death occurs in some cases. There might be a family history, but this is not well defined. Other conditions that can appear similar to feline ARVC, in terms of right sided enlargement, include congenital tricuspid dysplasia, atrial septal defect, anomalous pulmonary venous drainage, and Uhl's anomaly, which is a rare congenital malformation characterized by partial or total absence of RV myocardium. These congenital malformations also can lead to marked right heart enlargement and right-sided CHF signs. Right-sided CHF caused by congenital pulmonary stenosis, pulmonary hypertension, or double-chambered right ventricle have different echocardiographic findings.

Pathophysiology

Moderate to severe dilation of the RV chamber, with either focal or diffuse RV wall thinning, is typical. The RV wall can become so thin as to appear translucent at autopsy. An RV wall aneurysm can occur as well. RA and sometimes LA dilation occurs. Histologic findings include myocardial atrophy with fatty and fibro-fatty replacement tissue. Focal myocarditis and evidence of apoptosis can be present. These histologic changes are most prominent in the RV wall. Fibrous tissue or fatty infiltration sometimes is present within the LV and LA walls.

Clinical Features

No age or breed predisposition has been identified for feline ARVC. It has occurred in Domestic Shorthair, Burmese, and Birman cats. Birmans might be overrepresented, suggesting a possible hereditary effect, although the genetics are unknown.

The clinical presentation usually relates to signs of right-sided CHF, with pleural effusion or chylothorax causing labored or rapid respirations, and less often, abdominal distension (ascites). Occasionally, syncope or sudden death is reported. The history also can include lethargy and inappetence without overt heart failure. Physical findings generally reflect right-sided CHF, with jugular venous distension or pulsation, ventrally muffled lung sounds (from pleural effusion), and hepatosplenomegaly commonly present; some cats also have ascites. Cardiac auscultation might reveal a soft systolic murmur, as well as a tachyarrhythmia.

Diagnostic Tests

Thoracic radiography suggests right heart and sometimes LA enlargement. Pericardial effusion contributes to the cardiomegaly in some cases. Pleural effusion is common. Caudal vena caval distension and ascites might be evident.

Various arrhythmias have been documented in affected cats, including VPCs, ventricular tachycardia, AF, and supraventricular tachyarrhythmias. A right bundle branch block pattern appears to be common. An AV block occurs in some cats.

Echocardiography reveals RA and RV enlargement that often is severe. Abnormal RV thinning, aneurysmal dilation, areas of dyskinesis, and paradoxical septal motion also might be seen. TR commonly is evident on color Doppler examination.

Management

Therapy for CHF includes furosemide, pimobendan, clopidogrel, and sometimes an ACE inhibitor and/or spironolactone. Additional therapy for specific arrhythmias might be needed (see Chapter 25). Recommendations for at-home monitoring and reevaluation are similar to those for other cardiomyopathies.

Prognosis Long-term prognosis usually is poor once signs of heart failure appear. Death from progressive CHF or sudden death is likely.

Cardiomyopathy of "Nonspecific Phenotype"

Previously described as "unclassified" cardiomyopathy, this designation is applied when the structural or functional characteristics of a cat's myocardial disease do not conform to those of other described cardiomyopathies. This likely reflects the wide variability in triggers, progression, and manifestations of feline myocardial disease, rather than representing a specific form of cardiomyopathy. Cats with cardiomyopathy of non-specific phenotype can have variable LV hypertrophy or mural thinning. Diastolic dysfunction is predominant in many of these cats, although varying degrees of systolic dysfunction also are common. In each case, a description of the specific morphologic and functional features present in that individual cat should accompany the designation "cardiomyopathy of nonspecific phenotype."

A rare form of myocardial disease that appears analogous to noncompaction cardiomyopathy in people was reported in a cat (Kittleson, 2017). LV noncompaction is characterized by prominent myocardial trabeculae, with deep sinusoidal recesses in between that communicate with the ventricular lumen. The subepicardial layer of myocardium is more normally structured. The excessive trabeculation of subendocardial to mid-myocardial regions creates a "moth-eaten" appearance on echo exam. LV noncompaction might represent an incomplete maturation of the ventricular wall(s). Mutations in genes coding for sarcomeric proteins have been identified in some people with the condition, suggesting a possible relationship to other forms of cardiomyopathy.

Clinical Features and Diagnostic Tests

The clinical history and physical findings in cats with a nonspecific phenotype can be like those of any other type of cardiomyopathy. Laboratory test results, ECG findings, and radiographic appearance are likely to mimic those of other cardiomyopathies. Echocardiography reveals LV structural or functional changes that defy neat categorization as HCM, RCM, or DCM (**Figure 33.36**). Some LA enlargement is expected, with or without variable right heart enlargement. There can be evidence for impaired LV filling, as well as reduced contractility.

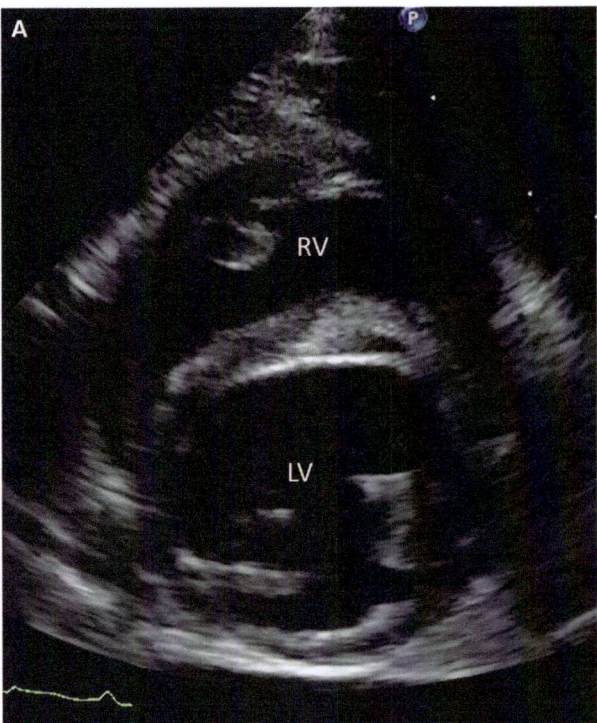

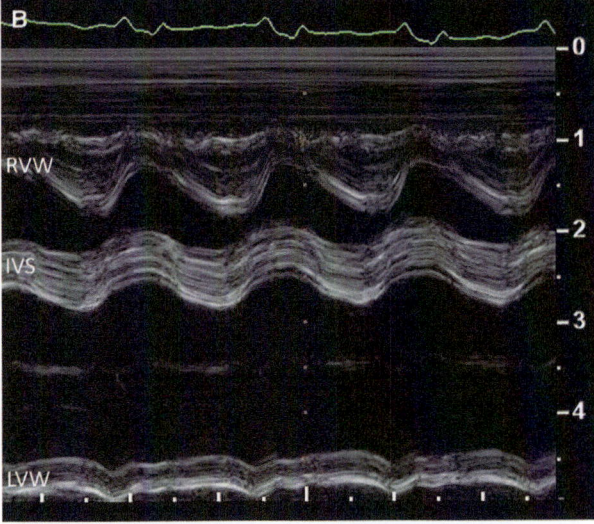

Figure 33.36 Advanced cardiomyopathy of nonspecific phenotype in an 11-year-old male cat is characterized by moderate left and right ventricular enlargement, normal septal thickness, and a thin, poorly contracting left ventricular free wall (LVW). (A) Right parasternal short-axis image in diastole shows chamber enlargement and thinned LVW. (B) Poor systolic LVW motion evident on M-mode resembles DCM, but septal thickness is disproportionate to the LVW. Severe left atrial dilation & biventricular congestive failure also were present. IVS, interventricular septum; LV, left ventricle; RV, right ventricle; RVW, right ventricular wall.

Management

Recommendations are the same as for cats with HCM and RCM. These include pimobendan, especially when LV systolic function is reduced.

Secondary Myocardial Disease

When LV hypertrophy is identified, secondary causes of wall thickening should be ruled out. Myocardial concentric hypertrophy is a compensatory response to certain stresses or disease (p. 16 and the next paragraphs). Such cases are not considered idiopathic HCM. Reduced systolic function also can be secondary to identifiable causes. Most notable is myocardial failure induced by taurine-deficiency (see "Dilated Cardiomyopathy" section). Other causes of secondary myocardial disease are mentioned in this section, as well.

There are reports of some cats with apparent HCM and CHF where both LV hypertrophy and congestive signs resolve, and no longer require therapy. This has been called "transient myocardial thickening" (Novo Matos, 2018). These cats tend to be slightly younger and are more likely to have had some kind of prior stressful event, including general anesthesia or a traumatic incident. Although various medications might have been used, only a minority received a corticosteroid. The cause of the myocardial thickening is unclear. It could involve edema or cellular infiltrate associated with catecholamine-induced or other myocarditis. Myocarditis is a likely etiology in many cats, and some cases have demonstrated extremely high cTnI concentrations. Cardiac drugs eventually can be discontinued in many of these cats.

Causes

Pressure Overload LV concentric hypertrophy is the expected compensatory response to increased ventricular systolic pressure (afterload). Systemic arterial hypertension is the most common cause (Chapter 38). BP always should be measured in cats with increased LV wall thickness. Increased LV systolic pressure load also occurs because of fixed (usually from congenital aortic stenosis, p. 480) or dynamic LV outflow tract obstruction. Congenital mitral valve dysplasia is an uncommon cause of dynamic LV outflow obstruction. Severe LV hypertrophy is more likely to result from marked LV outflow obstruction (or HCM) rather than systemic hypertension.

Hyperthyroidism Other conditions increase LV wall thickness by their trophic effects on the myocardium, and sometimes also by raising BP. Hyperthyroidism is the most common abnormality here, but other potential causes include excessive growth hormone secretion and chronic exposure to catecholamines. Testing for hyperthyroidism is indicated in cats 6 years of age and older that have myocardial hypertrophy. A cat with hyperthyroidism and concurrent LV hypertrophy is said to have hyperthyroidism with an HCM phenotype.

Thyroid hormone affects the heart directly by altering myocardial protein synthesis and stimulating contractility. Thyroid hormone also interacts with the sympathetic nervous system, which produces effects on both the heart and circulation. Increased HR and reduced peripheral vascular resistance (from thyroid-induced vascular smooth muscle relaxation and increased basal metabolic rate) further raise cardiac output. Thyroid hormone also increases blood volume (and preload), via RAAS activation in response to systemic vasodilation. Hyperthyroidism thus creates a hyperdynamic circulatory state characterized by increases in cardiac output, oxygen demand, blood volume, and HR. Concurrent systemic hypertension can further stimulate myocardial hypertrophy.

Clinical cardiovascular signs of hyperthyroidism frequently include a systolic murmur, hyperdynamic precordial and arterial impulses, tachycardia and arrhythmias. Some affected cats have an audible gallop sound. Evidence for LV enlargement or hypertrophy typically is present on ECG, thoracic radiographs, and echocardiogram (**Figure 33.37**). Some hyperthyroid cats develop CHF, usually with normal

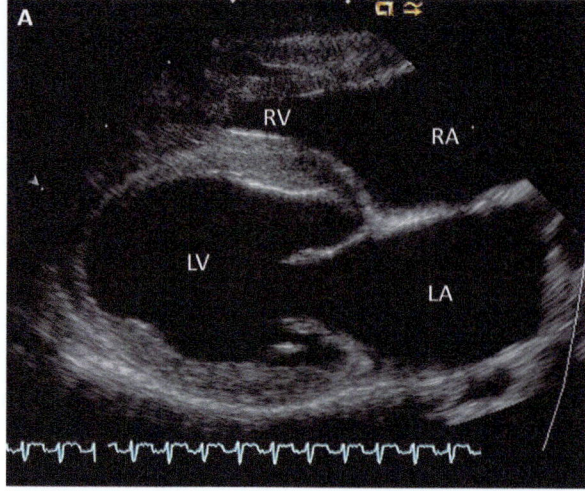 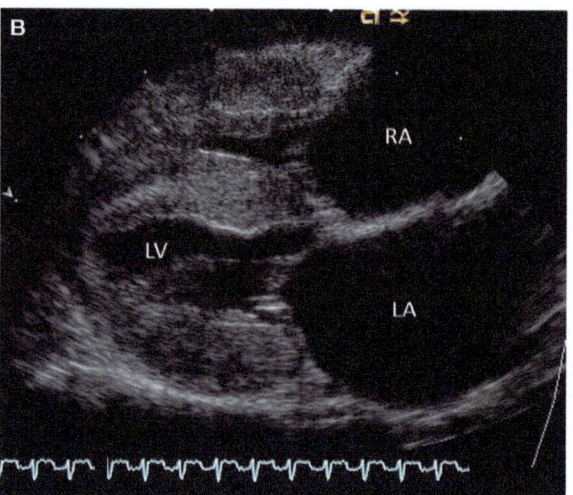

Figure 33.37 Diastolic (A) and systolic (B) 2D echo frames from a 12-year-old Domestic Shorthair cat with hyperthyroidism and hyperdynamic heart disease. Biatrial enlargement, moderate left ventricular dilation, vigorous systolic motion (fractional shortening >54%), and sinus tachycardia (250 beats/min) are evident. There is only borderline hypertrophy of the interventricular septum. A loud systolic murmur (moderate mitral and tricuspid regurgitation documented) and S_4 gallop sound were heard on auscultation. Right parasternal long-axis view. LA, left atrium; LV, left ventricle; RA, right atrium; RV, right ventricle.

to high FS, although a few have poor contractile function. In addition to antithyroid treatment, other therapy might be needed to manage cardiac complications of hyperthyroidism. A beta-blocker can temporarily control adverse cardiac effects of excess thyroid hormone, especially tachyarrhythmias. CHF signs are treated as described for HCM. The rare hypodynamic (dilated) cardiac failure is treated as for DCM. However, beta-blocker or other cardiac therapy is not a substitute for antithyroid treatment. Cardiac changes usually regress or normalize after the cat becomes euthyroid.

Miscellaneous Causes Cardiac hypertrophy develops in cats with hypersomatotropism (acromegaly), as a result of growth hormone's trophic effects on the heart. Most of these cats have diabetes mellitus as well. Myocyte hypertrophy, with minimal fiber disarray, and interstitial fibrosis are the major histopathologic findings in acromegaly. CHF occurs in some of these cats. If the causative pituitary tumor is removed and growth hormone concentrations normalize, the cardiac hypertrophy regresses.

Chronic beta- (or potentially alpha-) adrenergic stimulation also has the potential to cause myocardial hypertrophy, although this would be rare. Hyperviscosity stemming from plasma cell neoplasia has been associated sporadically with LA enlargement, increased LV wall thickness, and CHF. Additionally, increased myocardial thickness not caused by myocardial hypertrophy occasionally results from infiltrative myocardial disease (such as lymphoma).

CHF leading to death has occurred in cats with diabetes mellitus (Little, 2008). LA enlargement appears to be common, although LV hypertrophy might be only sporadic. Right-sided CHF signs (pleural effusion and occasionally, ascites) can predominate and various arrhythmias can occur. It is unclear whether hypertension, acromegaly or hyperthyroidism also plays a role. In addition, myocardial hypertrophy is known to occur with hypertrophic feline muscular dystrophy, an X-linked recessive dystrophin deficiency similar to Duchenne muscular dystrophy in people (p. 635); however, CHF is uncommon in these cats.

Moderate to severe anemia (packed cell volume <20%) is a cause of four-chamber dilation with signs of volume overload; pleural effusion can occur. A rare cause of secondary myocardial failure in cats is tachycardia-induced cardiomyopathy (TICM; p. 630). As in dogs, a persistent rapid tachyarrhythmia can lead to poor ventricular contractility with generalized chamber dilation that mimics idiopathic DCM. Finally, myocardial failure and CHF or sudden death has occurred rarely with hypocalcemia associated with primary hypoparathyroidism.

Whether viral myocarditis plays an important role in the pathogenesis of feline cardiomyopathy is unclear. A small study using formalin-fixed cardiomyopathic feline hearts, indicated that 58% showed evidence of myocarditis; panleukopenia virus DNA was found in almost 45% of those with myocarditis, in 15% of cardiomyopathic cats without myocarditis, and in none of the normal cat hearts examined (Meurs, 2000). Original reports of feline cardiomyopathy by Liu (1975) identified endomyocarditis as one form of this disease.

Corticosteroid-Associated Congestive Heart Failure In some cats, CHF signs develop subsequent to glucocorticosteroid administration, especially long-acting repositol forms. The genesis of this is unclear. Small increases in LA and LV dimensions and NT-proBNP concentration sometimes have occurred after oral steroid administration, although whether more consistent or pronounced effects occur following repositol glucocorticoisteroid administration is not known. Subclinical HCM might exist in some cases. Affected cats experience acute onset of lethargy, anorexia, tachypnea, and respiratory distress. Auscultatory abnormalities are identified in a minority of cases. The HR is not elevated in most cats, and BP might be low. Moderate cardiomegaly, moderate to severe diffuse pulmonary infiltrates, and mild to moderate pleural effusion can be seen radiographically. Reported ECG findings include sinus bradycardia, intraventricular conduction abnormalities, atrial standstill, AF, and VPCs. Echocardiographically, most cats show some increase in diastolic septal and LV wall thicknesses and in LA diameter; however, this can be minimal. AV valve insufficiency or SAM sometimes occurs. Cats that survive the initial episode of CHF seem to experience at least partial resolution of abnormal cardiac findings. Gradual withdrawal of all cardiac medications without recurrence of CHF is possible. Further use of corticosteroids, especially long-acting forms, should be avoided.

Myocarditis

Inflammation of the myocardium and adjacent structures occurs in cats, as in other species (see Chapter 32, p. 636). Various infectious agents can affect the myocardium, as well as other organs, through direct invasion, elaborated toxins, or host immune responses. Disease manifestations in other body systems are likely to predominate. Noninfective causes of myocarditis also can occur. Consequences of myocarditis include cardiac arrhythmias, CHF and sudden death. Definitive diagnosis of myocarditis and its underlying etiology is challenging.

Causes

Several viruses have been associated with myocarditis in cats. Panleukopenia viral DNA has been found in myocardial samples from some cardiomyopathic cats with histologic evidence of myocarditis. Myocarditis associated with feline immunodeficiency virus (FIV) also was identified in several young cats with HCM (Rolim, 2016). In these cats, multifocal inflammatory myocardial infiltrates of T lymphocytes and macrophages were present, and FIV antigen within the inflammatory cells was identified using immunohistochemistry. Nevertheless, the possible role of viral myocarditis in the pathogenesis of cardiomyopathy in other cats is not clear.

Bacterial myocarditis can result from sepsis or from bacterial endocarditis or pericarditis, as it does in other species. Both lymphoplasmacytic and pyogranulomatous myocarditis have been found sporadically in cats with *Bartonella* infections. Bartonella-associated myocarditis probably is often subclinical. It is unclear whether or how often natural infections have any role in the development of cardiomyopathy. However, *Bartonella* spp. DNA was identified in about half of the cardiac tissues examined from cats with endomyocarditis-LV endocardial fibrosis complex, yet in only a small minority of HCM cats and in no normal controls (Donovan, 2018). *Borrelia burgdorferi* infection (Lyme carditis) has been associated with bradyarrhythmias in cats.

Myocarditis caused by *Toxoplasma gondii* occurs occasionally, usually in immunosuppressed cats as part of a generalized disease process. *Trypanosoma cruzi* infection (p. 640) has been identified in some cats in south Texas. Other protozoal infections rarely have involved the myocardium, as well as other tissues. A migrating foreign body such as a grass awn (foxtail) is another uncommon cause of myocarditis and vegetative endocarditis.

Noninfective myocarditis secondary to thoracic trauma (p. 641) is recognized only rarely in cats (**Figure 33.38**).

Pathophysiology

Myocarditis can cause clinical disease by disrupting normal cardiac electrical function, reducing myocardial contractility, or impairing ventricular filling. Diastolic dysfunction can occur from slowed early diastolic ventricular relaxation or altered myocardial stiffness characteristics. Inflammatory infiltrates and their effects can lead to all of these cardiac alterations. The consequences of reduced ventricular filling and contractility include increased venous pressure, CHF, and in some cases, poor cardiac output. Tachy- or bradyarrhythmias associated with myocarditis and impaired cardiac function exacerbate these pathophysiologic sequelae. AV block is possible if the inflammation spreads into the atrial or ventricular septum.

Histologic findings relate to the underlying etiology. An endomyocarditis has been described, mostly in young cats, that is of unclear relation to viral infection. Histopathologic characteristics of acute endomyocarditis include focal or diffuse lymphocytic, plasmacytic, and histiocytic infiltrates with a few neutrophils. Others cases of endomyocarditis are characterized by suppurative infiltration with prominent numbers of mononuclear cells (Stalis, 1995). Degenerative and lytic changes can occur in adjacent myocytes. Chronic endomyocarditis has been associated with minimal inflammatory response, but much myocardial degeneration and fibrosis. RCM could represent the end-stage of nonfatal endomyocarditis.

Clinical Features

Clinical findings often are nonspecific. Cardiac arrhythmias and impaired myocardial function are likely consequences of myocarditis. Cats with severe or widespread myocarditis can experience clinical signs of weakness, syncope, CHF, or sudden death. An unexpected anesthetic-related death in a young cat could relate to underlying myocarditis. The

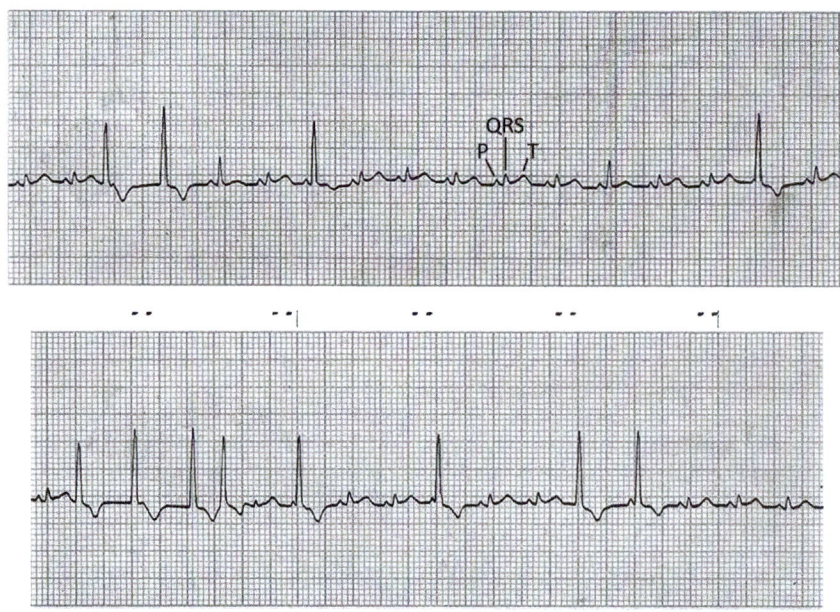

Figure 33.38 Continuous ECG strip from a 3½ month old kitten that had been attacked by a dog 4 days ago. The kitten suffered chest trauma with rib fractures. Ventricular premature complexes, most of which suggest a competing accelerated idioventricular rhythm, interrupt the sinus rhythm (waveforms indicated; 160 beats/min). This is consistent with traumatic myocarditis. Echocardiographic findings were normal. The cardiac rhythm returned to normal within a couple days without antiarrhythmic therapy. Lead II; 25 mm/sec, 1 cm = 1 mV.

endomyocardial inflammation can be extensive. Cats with focal myocardial inflammation might be asymptomatic, or have other systemic signs of infection. Acute and chronic cases of suspected viral myocarditis and pericarditis–epicarditis (as from coronavirus) have been described, although a viral cause rarely is documented. Acute death, with or without signs of pulmonary edema for a day or two, is the most common presentation reported with endomyocarditis.

Diagnostic Tests

Elevations in cTnI, and possibly NT-proBNP, are likely with ongoing myocardial damage. Radiographic findings could be nonspecific, especially in the absence of cardiomegaly or signs of CHF. The ECG might show various arrhythmias, including isolated premature ectopic complexes, rapid atrial tachycardia, multiform ventricular tachycardia, and AV or major conduction bundle blocks. Echocardiography can reveal heterogeneous echogenicity of the myocardium, reduced ventricular function, or variable chamber enlargement. Transient myocardial thickening also has been observed.

Management

Therapy for suspected myocarditis largely is supportive, unless the specific etiology can be identified and treated. In cases with myocardial thickening, appropriate serologic or immunodiagnostic tests should be performed with consideration of *Bartonella* spp., toxoplasmosis, and tick borne diseases. Strict rest, antiarrhythmic therapy as indicated (see Chapter 25), an ACE inhibitor with or without pimobendan for myocardial dysfunction, furosemide for signs of congestion or edema (see Chapter 22), and other supportive treatments are directed as needed.

Suggested Additional Reading and References

Also See Online Comprehensive Bibliography at: https://www.routledge.com/9781482246223.

Bartoszuk U, Keene BW, Baron Toaldo M, et al. Holter monitoring demonstrates that ventricular arrhythmias are common in cats with decompensated and compensated hypertrophic cardiomyopathy. Vet J 2019;243:21–25.

Blass KA, Schober KE, Bonagura JD, et al. Clinical evaluation of the 3M Littmann Electronic Stethoscope Model 3200 in 150 cats. J Feline Med Surg 2013;15:893–900.

Borgeat K, Casamian-Sorrosal D, Helps C, et al. Association of the myosin binding protein C3 mutation (MYBPC3 R820W) with cardiac death in a survey of 236 Ragdoll cats. J Vet Cardiol 2014a;16:73–80.

Borgeat K, Connolly DJ, Luis Fuentes V. Cardiac biomarkers in cats. J Vet Cardiol 2015;17(Suppl 1):S74–86.

Borgeat K, Sherwood K, Payne JR, et al. Plasma cardiac troponin I concentration and cardiac death in cats with hypertrophic cardiomyopathy. J Vet Intern Med 2014b;28:1731–1737.

Borgeat K, Stern J, Meurs KM, et al. The influence of clinical and genetic factors on left ventricular wall thickness in Ragdoll cats. J Vet Cardiol 2015;17(Suppl 1):S258–267.

Chetboul V, Passavin P, Trehiou-Sechi E, et al. Clinical, epidemiological and echocardiographic features and prognostic factors in cats with restrictive cardiomyopathy: a retrospective study of 92 cases (2001-2015). J Vet Intern Med 2019;33:1222–1231.

Chetboul V, Petit A, Gouni V, et al. Prospective echocardiographic and tissue Doppler screening of a large Sphynx cat population: reference ranges, heart disease prevalence and genetic aspects. J Vet Cardiol 2012;14:497–509.

Christiansen LB, Prats C, Hyttel P, et al. Ultrastructural myocardial changes in seven cats with spontaneous hypertrophic cardiomyopathy. J Vet Cardiol 2015;17(Suppl 1):S220–232.

Clark L, Kavanagh JA, Pang DSJ, et al. Impact of preanaesthetic echocardiography on the planned anaesthetic management of cats. Vet Anaesth Analg 2020;47:614–620.

Coleman AE, DeFrancesco TC, Griffiths EH, et al. Atenolol in cats with subclinical hypertrophic cardiomyopathy: a double-blind, placebo-controlled, randomized clinical trial of effect on quality of life, activity, and cardiac biomarkers. J Vet Cardiol 2020;30:77–91.

DeFrancesco TC. Management of cardiac emergencies in small animals. Vet Clin North Am Small Anim Pract 2013;43:817–842.

Donovan TA, Balakrishnan N, Carvalho Barbosa I, et al. Bartonella spp. as a possible cause or cofactor of feline endomyocarditis-left ventricular endocardial fibrosis complex. J Comp Pathol 2018;162:29–42.

Ferasin L, DeFrancesco T. Management of acute heart failure in cats. J Vet Cardiol 2015;17(Suppl 1):S173–189.

Ferasin L, Ferasin H, Kilkenny E. Heart murmurs in apparently healthy cats caused by iatrogenic dynamic right ventricular outflow tract obstruction. J Vet Intern Med 2020;34:1102–1107.

Ferasin L, Kilkenny E, Ferasin H. Evaluation of NT-proBNP and cTnI levels in cats with systolic anterior motion of the mitral valve (SAM) in the absence of left ventricular hypertrophy. J Vet Cardiol 2020;30:23–31.

Finn E, Freeman LM, Rush JE, et al. The relationship between body weight, body condition, and survival in cats with heart failure. J Vet Intern Med 2010; 24:1369–1374.

Fonfara S, Kitz S, Hetzel U, et al. Myocardial leptin transcription in feline hypertrophic cardiomyopathy. Res Vet Sci 2017;112:105–108.

Fox PR, Basso C, Thiene G, et al. Spontaneously occurring restrictive nonhypertrophied cardiomyopathy in domestic cats: a new animal model of human disease. Cardiovasc Pathol 2014;23:28–34.

Fox PR, Keene BW, Lamb K, et al. International collaborative study to assess cardiovascular risk and evaluate long-term health in cats with preclinical hypertrophic cardiomyopathy and apparently healthy cats: the REVEAL study. J Vet Intern Med 2018; 32:930–943.

Fox PR, Schober KA Management of asymptomatic (occult) feline cardiomyopathy: challenges and realities. J Vet Cardiol 2015;17(Suppl 1):S150–158.

Fox PR, Keene BW, Lamb K, et al. Long-term incidence and risk of noncardiovascular and all-cause mortality in apparently healthy cats and cats with preclinical hypertrophic cardiomyopathy. J Vet Intern Med 2019;33:2572–2586.

Freeman LM, Rush JE, Feugier A, et al. Relationship of body size to metabolic markers and left ventricular hypertrophy in cats. J Vet Intern Med 2015;29:150–156.

Gordon SG, Cote E. Pharmacotherapy of feline cardiomyopathy: chronic management of heart failure. J Vet Cardiol 2015;17(Suppl 1):S159–172.

Granstrom S, Godiksen MT, Christiansen M, et al. Genotype-phenotype correlation between the cardiac myosin binding protein C mutation A31P and hypertrophic cardiomyopathy in a cohort of Maine Coon cats: a longitudinal study. J Vet Cardiol 2015;17(Suppl 1):S268–281.

Häggström J, Luis Fuentes V, Wess G. Screening for hypertrophic cardiomyopathy in cats. J Vet Cardiol 2015;17(Suppl 1):S134–149.

Hanas S, Tidholm A, Holst BS. Ambulatory electrocardiogram recordings in cats with primary asymptomatic hypertrophic cardiomyopathy. J Feline Med Surg 2017;19:158–164.

Harpster NK. Feline cardiomyopathy. Vet Clin North Am 1977;7:355–371.

Harris AN, Beatty SS, Estrada AH, et al. Investigation of an N-terminal prohormone of brain natriuretic peptide point-of-care ELISA in clinically normal cats and cats with cardiac disease. J Vet Intern Med 2017;31:994–999.

Hauge A, Bo G, Aarseth P. Hydrostatic pulmonary edema in the cat. Effects on pulmonary blood and water volumes and on lung compliance. Acta Anaesthesiol Scand 1977;21:413–422.

Hertzsch S, Roos A, Wess G. Evaluation of a sensitive cardiac troponin I assay as a screening test for the diagnosis of hypertrophic cardiomyopathy in cats. J Vet Intern Med 2019;33:1242–1250.

Hezzell MJ, Rush JE, Humm K, et al. Differentiation of Cardiac from Noncardiac Pleural Effusions in Cats using Second-Generation Quantitative and Point-of-Care NT-proBNP Measurements. J Vet Intern Med 2016;30:536–542.

Hickey MC, Jandrey K, Farrell KS, et al. Concurrent diseases and conditions in cats with renal infarcts. J Vet Intern Med 2014;28:319–323.

Hogan DF, Fox PR, Jacob K, et al. Secondary prevention of cardiogenic arterial thromboembolism in the cat: the double-blind, randomized, positive-controlled feline arterial thromboembolism; Clopidogrel vs. Aspirin trial (FAT CAT). J Vet Cardiol 2015;17(Suppl 1):S306–317.

Hori Y, Fujimoto E, Nishikawa Y, et al. Left ventricular outflow tract pressure gradient changes after carvedilol-disopyramide cotherapy in a cat with hypertrophic obstructive cardiomyopathy. J Vet Cardiol 2020;29:40–46.

Hori Y, Iguchi M, Heishima Y, et al. Diagnostic utility of cardiac troponin I in cats with hypertrophic cardiomyopathy. J Vet Intern Med 2018;32:922–929.

Humm K, Hezzell M, Sargent J, et al. Differentiating between feline pleural effusions of cardiac and non-cardiac origin using pleural fluid NT-proBNP concentrations. J Small Anim Pract 2013;54:656–661.

Jackson BL, Adin DB, Lehmkuhl LB. Effect of atenolol on heart rate, arrhythmias, blood pressure, and dynamic left ventricular outflow tract obstruction in cats with subclinical hypertrophic cardiomyopathy. J Vet Cardiol 2015;17(Suppl 1):S296–305.

Jackson BL, Lehmkuhl LB, Adin DB. Heart rate and arrhythmia frequency of normal cats compared to cats with asymptomatic hypertrophic cardiomyopathy. J Vet Cardiol 2014;16:215–225.

James R, Guillot E, Garelli-Paar C, et al. The SEISICAT study: a pilot study assessing efficacy and safety of spironolactone in cats with congestive heart failure secondary to cardiomyopathy. J Vet Cardiol 2018;20:1–12.

Johns SM, Nelson OL, Gay JM. Left atrial function in cats with left-sided cardiac disease and pleural effusion or pulmonary edema. J Vet Intern Med 2012;26:1134–1139.

Jung SW, Kittleson MD. The effect of atenolol on NT-proBNP and troponin in asymptomatic cats with severe left ventricular hypertrophy because of hypertrophic cardiomyopathy: a pilot study. J Vet Intern Med 2011;25:1044–1049.

Kershaw O, Heblinski N, Lotz F, et al. Diagnostic value of morphometry in feline hypertrophic cardiomyopathy. J Comp Pathol 2012;147:73–83.

Khor KH, Campbell FE, Owen H, et al. Myocardial collagen deposition and inflammatory cell infiltration in cats with preclinical hypertrophic cardiomyopathy. Vet J 2015;203:161–168.

Kimura Y, Karakama S, Hirakawa A, et al. Pathological features and pathogenesis of the endomyocardial form of restrictive cardiomyopathy in cats. J Comp Pathol 2016;155:190–198.

Kittleson MD, Fox PR, Basso C, et al. Naturally occurring biventricular noncompaction in an adult domestic cat. J Vet Intern Med 2017;31:527–531.

Kittleson MD, Meurs KM, Harris SP. The genetic basis of hypertrophic cardiomyopathy in cats and humans. J Vet Cardiol 2015;17(Suppl 1):S53–73.

Kochie SL, Schober KE, Rhinehart J, et al. Effects of pimobendan on left atrial transport function in cats. J Vet Intern Med 2020.

Linney CJ, Dukes-McEwan J, Stephenson HM, et al. Left atrial size, atrial function and left ventricular diastolic function in cats with hypertrophic cardiomyopathy. J Small Anim Pract 2014;55:198–206.

Lisciandro GR, Fulton RM, Fosgate GT, et al. Frequency and number of B-lines using a regionally based lung ultrasound examination in cats with radiographically normal lungs compared to cats with left-sided congestive heart failure. J Vet Emerg Crit Care 2017;27:499–505.

Little CJ, Gettinby G. Heart failure is common in diabetic cats: findings from a retrospective case-controlled study in first-opinion practice. J Small Anim Pract 2008;49:17–25.

Liu SK, Tilley LP, Lord PF. Feline cardiomyopathy. Recent Adv Stud Cardiac Struct Metab 1975;10:627–64.

Locatelli C, Pradelli D, Campo G, et al. Survival and prognostic factors in cats with restrictive cardiomyopathy: a review of 90 cases. J Feline Med Surg 2018;20:1138–1143.

Luis Fuentes V, Abbott J, Chetboul V, et al. ACVIM consensus statement guidelines for the classification, diagnosis, and management of cardiomyopathies in cats. J Vet Intern Med 2020; 34:1062–1077.

MacDonald KA, Kittleson MD, Kass PH, et al. Effect of spironolactone on diastolic function and left ventricular mass in Maine Coon cats with familial hypertrophic cardiomyopathy. J Vet Intern Med 2008;22:335–341.

Machen MC, Oyama MA, Gordon SG, et al. Multi-centered investigation of a point-of-care NT-proBNP ELISA assay to detect moderate to severe occult (pre-clinical) feline heart disease in cats referred for cardiac evaluation. J Vet Cardiol 2014;16:245–255.

Maron BJ, Fox PR. Hypertrophic cardiomyopathy in man and cats. J Vet Cardiol 2015;17 (Suppl 1):S6–9.

Mary J, Chetboul V, Sampedrano CC, et al. Prevalence of the MYBPC3-A31P mutation in a large European feline population and association with hypertrophic cardiomyopathy in the Maine Coon breed. J Vet Cardiol 2010;12:155–161.

Messer AE, Chan J, Daley A, et al. Investigations into the sarcomeric protein and Ca(2+)-regulation abnormalities underlying hypertrophic cardiomyopathy in cats (Felix catus). Front Physiol 2017;8:348.

Meurs KM, Fox PR, Magnon AL, et al. Molecular screening by polymerase chain reaction detects panleukopenia virus DNA in formalin-fixed hearts from cats with idiopathic cardiomyopathy and myocarditis. Cardiovasc Pathol 2000;9:119–126.

Meurs KM, Norgard MM, Ederer MM, et al. A substitution mutation in the myosin binding protein C gene in ragdoll hypertrophic cardiomyopathy. Genomics 2007;90:261–264.

Meurs KM, Sanchez X, David RM, et al. A cardiac myosin binding protein C mutation in the Maine Coon cat with familial hypertrophic cardiomyopathy. Hum Mol Genet 2005;14:3587–3593.

Novo Matos J, Pereira N, Glaus T, et al. Transient myocardial thickening in cats associated with heart failure. J Vet Intern Med 2018;32:48–56.

Paige CF, Abbott JA, Elvinger F, et al. Prevalence of cardiomyopathy in apparently healthy cats. J Am Vet Med Assoc 2009;234:1398–1403.

Patata V, Caivano D, Porciello F, et al. Pulmonary vein to pulmonary artery ratio in healthy and cardiomyopathic cats. J Vet Cardiol 2020;27:23–33.

Payne J, Luis Fuentes V, Boswood A, et al. Population characteristics and survival in 127 referred cats with hypertrophic cardiomyopathy (1997 to 2005). J Small Anim Pract 2010;51:540–547.

Payne JR, Borgeat K, Connolly DJ, et al. Prognostic indicators in cats with hypertrophic cardiomyopathy. J Vet Intern Med 2013;27:1427–1436.

Payne JR, Borgeat K, Brodbelt DC, et al. Risk factors associated with sudden death vs. Congestive heart failure or arterial thromboembolism in cats with hypertrophic cardiomyopathy. J Vet Cardiol 2015a;17(Suppl 1):S318–328.

Payne JR, Brodbelt DC, Luis Fuentes V. Cardiomyopathy prevalence in 780 apparently healthy cats in rehoming centres (the CatScan study). J Vet Cardiol 2015b;17(Suppl 1):S244–257.

Peck CM, Nielsen LK, Quinn RL, et al. Retrospective evaluation of the incidence and prognostic significance of spontaneous echocardiographic contrast in relation to cardiac disease and congestive heart failure in cats: 725 cases (2006-2011). J Vet Emerg Crit Care 2016;26:704–712.

Pellegrino A, Daniel AG, Pereira GG, et al. Assessment of regional left ventricular systolic function by strain imaging echocardiography in phenotypically normal and abnormal Maine coon cats tested for the A31P mutation in the MYBPC3 gene. Can J Vet Res 2017;81:137–146.

Pierce KV, Rush JE, Freeman LM, et al. Association between survival time and changes in NT-proBNP in cats treated for congestive heart failure. J Vet Intern Med 2017;31:678–684.

Rishniw M, Pion PD. Is treatment of feline hypertrophic cardiomyopathy based in science or faith? A survey of cardiologists and a literature search. J Feline Med Surg 2011;13:487–497.

Rishniw M, Thomas WP. Dynamic right ventricular outflow obstruction: a new cause of systolic murmurs in cats. J Vet Intern Med 2002;16:547–552.

Roderick KV, Abelson AL, Nielsen L, et al. Evaluation of red blood cell distribution width as a prognostic indicator in cats with acquired heart disease, with and without congestive heart failure. J Feline Med Surg 2017;19:648–656.

Rohrbaugh MN, Schober KE, Rhinehart JD, et al. Detection of congestive heart failure by Doppler echocardiography in cats with hypertrophic cardiomyopathy. J Vet Intern Med 2020;34:1091–1101.

Rolim VM, Casagrande RA, Wouters AT, et al. Myocarditis caused by feline immunodeficiency virus in five cats with hypertrophic cardiomyopathy. J Comp Pathol 2016;154:3–8.

Santiago SL, Freeman LM, Rush JE. Cardiac cachexia in cats with congestive heart failure: prevalence and clinical, laboratory, and survival findings. J Vet Intern Med 2020;34:35–44.

Schipper T, Van Poucke M, Sonck L, et al. A feline orthologue of the human MYH7 c.5647G>A (p.(Glu1883Lys)) variant causes hypertrophic cardiomyopathy in a Domestic Shorthair cat. Eur J Hum Genet 2019;27:1724–1730.

Schober KE, Chetboul V. Echocardiographic evaluation of left ventricular diastolic function in cats: hemodynamic determinants and pattern recognition. J Vet Cardiol 2015;17(Suppl 1):S102–133.

Schober KE, Rush JE, Luis Fuentes V, et al. Effects of pimobendan in cats with hypertrophic cardiomyopathy and recent congestive heart failure: Results of a prospective, double-blind, randomized, nonpivotal, exploratory field study. J Vet Intern Med 2021.

Schober K, Savino S, Yildiz V. Reference intervals and allometric scaling of two-dimensional echocardiographic measurements in 150 healthy cats. J Vet Med Sci 2017;79:1764–1771.

Schober KE, Wetli E, Drost WT. Radiographic and echocardiographic assessment of left atrial size in 100 cats with acute left-sided congestive heart failure. Vet Radiol Ultrasound 2014;55:359–367.

Schober KE, Zientek J, Li X, et al. Effect of treatment with atenolol on 5-year survival in cats with preclinical (asymptomatic) hypertrophic cardiomyopathy. J Vet Cardiol 2013;15:93–104.

Seo J, Payne JR, Novo Matos J, et al. Biomarker changes with systolic anterior motion of the mitral valve in cats with hypertrophic cardiomyopathy. J Vet Intern Med 2020;34:1718–1727.

Shirai M, Ninomiya I, Sada K. Constrictor response of small pulmonary arteries to acute pulmonary hypertension during left atrial pressure elevation. Jpn J Physiol 1991;41:129–142.

Sleeper MM, Roland R, Drobatz KJ. Use of the vertebral heart scale for differentiation of cardiac and noncardiac causes of respiratory distress in cats: 67 cases (2002-2003. J Am Vet Med Assoc 2013;242:366–371.

Spalla I, Locatelli C, Riscazzi G, et al. Survival in cats with primary and secondary cardiomyopathies. J Feline Med Surg 2016;18:501–509.

Spalla I, Payne JR, Borgeat K, et al. Prognostic value of mitral annular systolic plane excursion and tricuspid annular plane systolic excursion in cats with hypertrophic cardiomyopathy. J Vet Cardiol 2018;20:154–164.

Stalis IH, Bossbaly MJ, Van Winkle TJ. Feline endomyocarditis and left ventricular endocardial fibrosis. Vet Pathol 1995;32:122–126.

Stern JA, Markova S, Ueda Y, et al. A small molecule inhibitor of sarcomere contractility acutely relieves left ventricular outflow tract obstruction in feline hypertrophic cardiomyopathy. PLoS One 2016;11:e0168407.

Streitberger A, Modler P, Häggström J. Increased normalized pulmonary transit times and pulmonary blood volumes in cardiomyopathic cats with or without congestive heart failure. J Vet Cardiol. 2015;17:25–33.

Suzuki R, Mochizuki Y, Yoshimatsu H, et al. Early detection of myocardial dysfunction using two-dimensional speckle tracking echocardiography in a young cat with hypertrophic cardiomyopathy. JFMS open reports 2018;4:1–7. doi: 10.1177/2055116918756219.

Taillefer M, Di Fruscia R. Benazepril and subclinical feline hypertrophic cardiomyopathy: a prospective, blinded, controlled study. Can Vet J 2006;47:437–445.

Tornqvist-Johnsen C, Dickson SA, Rolph K, et al. First report of Lyme borreliosis leading to cardiac bradydysrhythmia in two cats. JFMS open reports 2020;6:1–6. doi: 10.1177/2055116919898292.

Trehiou-Sechi E, Tissier R, Gouni V, et al. Comparative echocardiographic and clinical features of hypertrophic cardiomyopathy in 5 breeds of cats: a retrospective analysis of 344 cases (2001–2011). J Vet Intern Med 2012;26:532–541.

van Hoek I, Hodgkiss-Geere H, Bode EF, et al. Association of diet with left ventricular wall thickness, troponin I and IGF-1 in cats with subclinical hypertrophic cardiomyopathy. J Vet Intern Med 2020;34:2197–2210.

Vezzosi T, Schober KE. Doppler-derived echocardiographic evidence of pulmonary hypertension in cats with left-sided congestive heart failure. J Vet Cardiol 2019;23:58–68.

Visser LC, Sloan CQ, Stern JA. Echocardiographic assessment of right ventricular size and function in cats with hypertrophic cardiomyopathy. J Vet Intern Med 2017;31:668–677.

Ward JL, Kussin EZ, Tropf MA, et al. Retrospective evaluation of the safety and tolerability of pimobendan in cats with obstructive vs nonobstructive cardiomyopathy. J Vet Intern Med 2020;34:2211–2222.

Ward JL, Lisciandro GR, Ware WA, et al. Evaluation of point-of-care thoracic ultrasound and NT-proBNP for the diagnosis of congestive heart failure in cats with respiratory distress. J Vet Intern Med 2018;32:1530–1540.

Ware WA, Freeman LM, Rush JE, et al. Vitamin D status in cats with cardiomyopathy. J Vet Intern Med 2020;34:1389–1398.

Wagner T, Fuentes VL, Payne JR, et al. Comparison of auscultatory and echocardiographic findings in healthy adult cats. J Vet Cardiol. 2010;12:171–182.

Wess G, Schinner C, Weber K, et al. Association of A31P and A74T polymorphisms in the myosin binding protein C3 gene and hypertrophic cardiomyopathy in Maine Coon and other breed cats. J Vet Intern Med 2010;24:527–532.

Wilkie LJ, Smith K, Luis Fuentes V. Cardiac pathology findings in 252 cats presented for necropsy; a comparison of cats with unexpected death versus other deaths. J Vet Cardiol 2015;17(Suppl 1):S329–340.

Winter MD, Giglio RF, Berry CR, et al. Associations between "valentine" heart shape, atrial enlargement and cardiomyopathy in cats. J Feline Med Surg 2015;17:447–452

Wolf OA, Imgrund M, Wess G. Echocardiographic assessment of feline false tendons and their relationship with focal thickening of the left ventricle. J Vet Cardiol 2017;19:14–23.

Zecca IB, Hodo CL, Slack S, et al. Prevalence of Trypanosoma cruzi infection and associated histologic findings in domestic cats (Felis catus). Vet Parasitol 2020;278:109014.

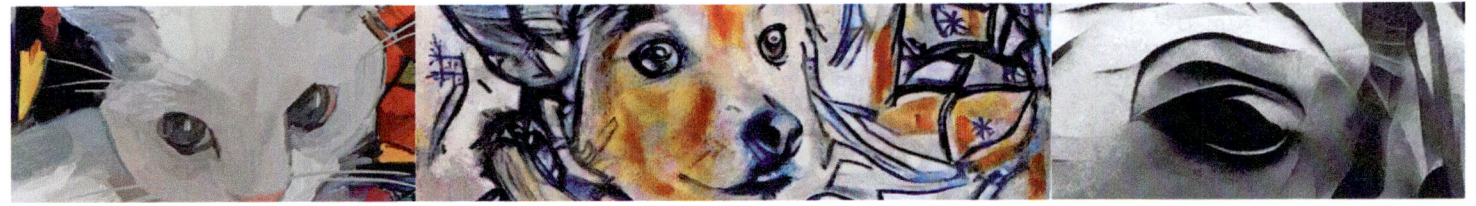

34
MYOCARDIAL DISEASES OF THE HORSE

The myocardium constitutes the bulk of the atrial and ventricular tissues. Cardiomyocytes exhibit the electrical properties of excitability and current conduction and the mechanical properties of contraction, active relaxation, passive elongation, and stiffness. The cardiomyocytes are joined by intercellular junctions and interstitial connective tissues that influence both electrical and mechanical functions of the heart. Myocardial diseases affect cardiomyocytes, cell junctions and supporting tissues. Clinical consequences can include arrhythmias, decreased contractility, and impaired myocardial relaxation and chamber distensibility. Severe myocardial disease can induce exercise intolerance, heart failure, arrhythmias, and sudden cardiac death.

Causes of Equine Myocardial Disease

Heart muscle diseases include congenital malformations of the cardiac septa. Ventricular septal defects are most common in horses; atrial septal defects and complex atrioventricular (AV) septal defects occur sporadically. The mobile tissues of the foramen ovale, a normal fetal structure, can be visualized in premature and full-term foals by two-dimensional (2D) echocardiography shortly after birth. While not considered a cardiac defect, a patent foramen ovale in the newborn can function as a conduit for right-to-left shunting in foals with pulmonary hypertension (PH), stenosis of the tricuspid or pulmonary valves, or atresia of the right ventricular (RV) inlet or outlet. See Chapter 26 for more information on congenital septal defects.

Acquired myocardial diseases include those of known etiology, idiopathic cardiomyopathies, and myocardial hypertrophy as an adaptive response to work or injury (**Table 34.1**). Despite the many potential causes, clinically impactful myocardial diseases appear of comparably low incidence in horses. The true prevalence of primary and secondary myocardial disease in this species is unknown. Recognition of subtle or occult myocardial disease is challenging (see "Diagnostic Tests").

Myocardial hypertrophy occurs as an adaptive response to a sustained increase in workload. The increased ventricular mass that develops in response to exercise training is considered physiological (an "athletic heart"); however, as in humans, extreme exercise training has been associated with increases in interstitial fibrosis, affecting both atrial and ventricular muscle. Idiopathic and genetically determined dilated and hypertrophic forms of cardiomyopathy (so often seen in dogs and cats) are not established as important disorders in the horse, although rare cases compatible with hypertrophic cardiomyopathy and arrhythmogenic right ventricular cardiomyopathy have been seen (Cullimore, 2018; Freel, 2010; Raftery, 2015). However, secondary injuries to the myocardium or increased cardiac (volume or pressure) workloads can induce adaptive increases in myocardial mass (p. 16; **Table 34.1**).

Eccentric hypertrophy is the usual response to ventricular volume overloading, typically caused by a congenital shunt or significant valvular insufficiency (see Chapters 26 and 30). Concentric and mixed (dilation plus wall thickening) ventricular hypertrophy are compensatory responses to increased ventricular systolic pressure, as occurs with systemic and pulmonary hypertension (Chapters 38 and 39), or with congenital outflow obstructions (Chapter 27). Pressure overloads related to congenital heart diseases are uncommon in horses; whereas, systemic and pulmonary hypertension likely are underdiagnosed. Pathologic ventricular hypertrophy is associated with both diastolic and systolic myocardial dysfunction, and with increased interstitial and replacement fibrosis.

Other sporadic, but well-recognized, reasons for acute or chronic myocardial injury occur. These include various toxicities, such as from ionophores, poisonous plants, and heavy metals, as well as relentless junctional or ventricular

Table 34.1 Myocardial Diseases in Horses

Congenital Myocardial Diseases

- Atrial septal defects
- Ventricular septal defects

Ventricular Eccentric Hypertrophy from Increased Workload

- Valvular regurgitation
- Congenital shunt

Ventricular Concentric or Mixed[a] Hypertrophy from Increased Workload

- Congenital outflow tract obstructions (pulmonary stenosis)
- Systemic hypertension
- Metabolic syndrome
- Pulmonary hypertension (causing right ventricular hypertrophy)
  - Left-sided heart disease
  - Pulmonary veno-occlusive disease
  - Idiopathic pulmonary fibrosis
  - Chronic airway disease (bronchitis-asthma)
- Congenital shunts (Eisenmenger's pathophysiology)

Dilated Cardiomyopathy Phenotype

- Idiopathic dilated cardiomyopathy
- Cardiomyopathy of chronic (volume) overload
- Tachycardia-induced cardiomyopathy
- Consequent to myocarditis
- Toxic myocardial injury

Myocarditis

- Infective (postviral, bacterial, parasitic, fungal)[b]

Infiltrative Myocardial Diseases

- Neoplasia (lymphoma, others)
- Amyloidosis
- Inflammatory infiltrates (myocarditis with edema)

Nutritional Deficiencies

- Vitamin E and selenium
- Copper

Myocardial Fibrosis (Consequence of Myocardial Injury)

Toxicosis

- Ionophore feed additives
- Cantharidin toxicity (blister beetles)
- Heavy metals (cobalt)
- Cardiotoxic poisonous plants (a partial list):
  - Glycoside-containing plants (*Taxus* spp.), oleander (*Nerium oleander*), foxglove (*Digitalis* spp.) summer pheasant's eye (*Adonis aestivalis*), and milkweeds,
  - Maple tree seeds (*Acer* spp.) and Marshmallow (*Malva parviflora*).
  - White snakeroot (*Ageratina altissima*) with tremetol toxicosis
  - Various plants containing grayanotoxins (including rhododendron, azalea, fetterbush, laurels, and mountain pieris)

Snake Envenomation

Trauma to the Thorax

Vascular Events

- Ischemia/reperfusion
- Infarction
- Catecholamine-induced injury
- Hypotension (hemorrhage)
- Vasculitis

[a] Mixed hypertrophy means wall thickening plus chamber dilation.
[b] See Decloedt (2019) for more details.

tachycardias, which can induce a potentially reversible, dilated cardiomyopathy (DCM) phenotype. Dissection of the ventricular septum can occur in association with a ruptured sinus of Valsalva aneurysm (p. 784); RV dissection is a rare, idiopathic lesion.

Pathophysiology

Most myocardial diseases involve the left ventricular (LV) myocardium. The underlying pathophysiology leading to clinical signs usually relates to *systolic dysfunction*, from reduced myocardial contractility (inotropy). Other pathophysiologic features of myocardial diseases often include: abnormal ventricular filling (*diastolic dysfunction*), caused by impaired relaxation or increased chamber stiffness; secondary mitral (or tricuspid) valve incompetency, resulting from annular dilation or papillary muscle dysfunction; and cardiac *arrhythmias*. Chronic left heart dysfunction can lead to the clinical syndrome of left-sided congestive heart failure (CHF), as well as "post-capillary" PH (Chapter 39) and secondary right-sided enlargement with biventricular CHF signs. Other pulmonary causes of RV hypertrophy, or cor pulmonale, include severe equine bronchial disease with asthma, idiopathic interstitial fibrosis, and pulmonary veno-occlusive disease (**Table 34.2**).

Recurrent ventricular premature complexes (VPCs) or ventricular tachycardias are common with myocardial disease. Although atrial arrhythmias more often are a primary electrical disturbance in horses, these also can develop with cardiomyopathies. While it is tempting to diagnose "myocardial disease" in the setting of any heart rhythm

Table 34.2 Clinical Manifestations of Heart Failure in the Horse[a]

History and General Observations
- Altered behavior (depression)
- Exercise intolerance
- Sweating (sympathetic activation)
- Colic-like signs
- Ventral edema
- Muscle wasting (cardiac cachexia)
- Exertional collapse or sudden death

Respiratory Signs
- Tachypnea
- Coughing
- Loud bronchial sounds
- Pulmonary crackles
- Muffled breath sounds on auscultation
- Fluid line on auscultation/percussion

Extravascular Fluid Accumulation[b]
- Subcutaneous ventral edema (right-sided CHF)
- Pulmonary edema (left-sided CHF)
  - Increased B-lines (lung rockets) on thoracic ultrasound (r/o pulmonary edema)
  - Pulmonary vascular prominence with increased lung opacities on thoracic radiographs
- Pleural effusion on thoracic ultrasound or thoracic radiography
- Ascites on abdominal ultrasound (right-sided CHF)

Physical Diagnosis—Cardiac Examination
- Observational abnormalities (see "History and General Observations")
- Resting (sinus) tachycardia
- Arterial pulse and superficial vein abnormalities
  - Hypokinetic ("thready") or irregular arterial pulse
  - Hyperkinetic pulse - widened arterial pulse pressure (r/o aortic regurgitation)
  - Jugular and superficial venous distension
  - Pathologic jugular pulsations
- Abnormal heart sounds
  - Soft first sound (S_1; r/o decreased contractility, pleural or pericardial effusion)
  - Tympanic second heart sound (S_2; r/o pulmonary hypertension)
  - Absent fourth (S_4, atrial) sound due to atrial fibrillation
  - Loud third (S_3, ventricular) sound due to high filling pressures
  - Arrhythmias
  - Murmur(s): mitral or tricuspid regurgitation (often soft in equine cardiomyopathies). Murmurs might indicate other causes of CHF, including congenital or acquired shunts and primary valvular diseases (congenital, degenerative, infective, valvulitis)[a]
- Pericardial friction rubs (pericarditis)[a]

Abnormal Electrocardiogram
- Premature atrial or ventricular beats, including tachyarrhythmias
- Atrial fibrillation
- Conduction blocks

Abnormal Diagnostic Imaging Findings
- Extravascular fluid accumulation[b] – edema or effusions (see above)
- Echocardiographic signs of structural heart disease
- Cardiomegaly on radiographs
- Systemic or pulmonary venous distension
- Dilation of the pulmonary artery

Clinical Laboratory Abnormalities
- Azotemia (nonspecific sign; from reduced cardiac output)
- Elevated concentration of:
  - Blood cardiac troponin I (cTnI)
  - Serum creatine kinase (myocardial band, CK-MB)
  - Serum aspartate aminotransferase (AST)
  - Blood natriuretic peptides
- Markers of inflammation (myocarditis, endocarditis, pericarditis)[a]

---

[a] As indicated in this table, these signs are not exclusive to myocardial disease with CHF; they also can occur with congenital, valvular, and pericardial diseases or sustained tachyarrhythmias, as well as from noncardiac diseases. Manifestations of equine myocardial disease are variable.
[b] Might be evident from inspection, auscultation, ultrasonography, or radiography.
Abbreviations: CHF, congestive heart failure; r/o, rule out.

---

disturbance, rhythm abnormalities can occur as primary electrical disturbances, without a gross anatomical substrate. This point is especially relevant to horses with electrolyte or other metabolic imbalances, excessive adrenergic stimulation, sepsis or toxemia, hypoxemia, or hypotension-ischemia-reperfusion syndromes. For example, in horses examined for sudden death at a racetrack, gross or microscopic myocardial lesions were relatively uncommon findings (Gelberg, 1985). Conceivably, some horses might have an (ion) channelopathy (genetic or acquired) that renders the heart susceptible to arrhythmias; however, none have been identified thus far. Infiltrative myocardial diseases have been associated with conduction disturbances in horses, including complete AV block.

Specific Myocardial Disorders

As outlined in **Table 34.1**, a wide variety of myocardial diseases have been reported or observed in horses. These include toxic, inflammatory, and degenerative lesions; fibrosis of undetermined etiology; and idiopathic, hypertensive, and tachycardia-induced cardiomyopathies, among other lesions. Some of the key aspects of these disorders are considered below.

Myocardial Toxicity

Toxins that can injure the myocardium include ionophore antibiotic feed additives, poisonous plants, cantharidin (blister beetle), snake venoms, and heavy metals such as cobalt. Myocardial toxins also can alter cardiac cell electrophysiology, either directly by affecting ion channels (ionophores) or by causing myocardial necrosis, inflammation or fibrosis. Toxicity should be strongly considered when multiple animals in a barn or pasture are affected, although individual susceptibility to intoxicants can vary. Whenever toxicosis is suspected, feedstuff samples should be obtained for possible analysis and a reference laboratory consulted.

Toxic myocardial injury can occur following ingestion of a variety of poisonous plants. Some plants contain cardiac glycosides, which block sodium-potassium adenosine triphosphatase (ATPase) activity; the consequent intracellular accumulation of sodium thereby indirectly affects the sodium-calcium exchanger. Glycosides induce gastrointestinal irritation and often, heart rhythm disturbances (p. 328). Myocardial injury and necrosis also have occurred following envenomation by rattlesnakes or other vipers, from systemic infections, or subsequent to blunt or penetrating thoracic trauma.

Horses are especially susceptible to injury from ionophore antibiotics, which are used as coccidiostats and growth promoters, mainly in poultry. These substances include monensin (acute oral LD50, 2–3 mg/kg), salinomycin (acute oral LD50, 0.6 mg/kg), and lasalocid (acute oral LD50, 21.5 mg/kg). Clinical signs of ionophore toxicosis also relate to skeletal muscle and neurological injury, evidence of which sometimes overshadows cardiac signs. Other signs are nonspecific and include colic, diarrhea, and excessive urination. Serum muscle enzyme and cardiac troponin concentrations rise because of rhabdomyolysis and cardiac muscle injury. Some horses recover but show evidence of residual myocardial damage, including arrhythmia and reduced ventricular function.

Myocarditis

Myocardial inflammation and necrosis can occur secondary to a variety of infective agents, either as a primary insult or perhaps as an immune-mediated response to a virus. Eosinophilic myocarditis was reported in a horse with complete AV block (Luethy, 2017). Numerous viruses can replicate in the equine myocardium, so it is likely that some unexplained cardiac arrhythmias are a consequence of infection, inflammation, and necrosis. Such lesions also can develop from other myocardial insults, such as ischemia/infarction or toxic injury. In this context, inflammation and necrosis are not caused primarily by myocarditis, but occur secondary to the initial insult. Definitive diagnosis of myocarditis is challenging

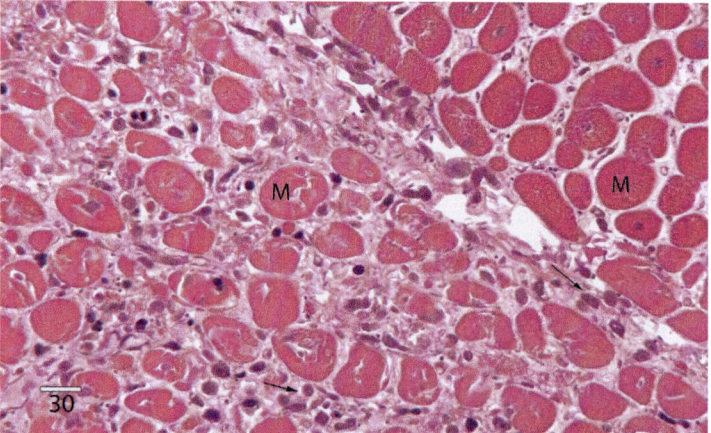

Figure 34.1 Histopathology of myocardial necrosis with inflammation. In upper right corner are more normal appearing cardiomyocytes (M) in cross section. Note the necrosis and overall loss of cardiomyocytes in center and lower left, with many inflammatory cell nuclei between cardiomyocytes (arrows). Calibration bar, 30 microns. Image courtesy of Dr T Papenfuss.

and requires histologic confirmation (**Figure 34.1**), as well as consideration of the clinical scenario. Definitive antemortem diagnosis of myocarditis might be obtained with transvenous endomyocardial biopsy (Decloedt, 2016); however, this test is rarely done.

Idiopathic Dilated Cardiomyopathy

Idiopathic DCM is relatively uncommon in horses; there is no clear genetic basis. Generalized two- or four-chamber dilation, increased ventricular sphericity, and rounding of affected chambers are classic features observed by echocardiography and at postmortem examination (**Figure 34.2**). The pathophysiology and clinical presentation are similar to those of DCM in dogs (Chapter 32) and signs of CHF are likely (**Table 34.2**). The condition is recognized by echocardiographic (echo) evidence for ventricular dilation and LV hypokinesis in the absence of congenital malformation, toxin exposure, antioxidant deficiency, persistent tachycardia, or primary valvular disease. However, some cases with a DCM phenotype are likely secondary to previously unrecognized toxic injury or myocarditis.

Idiopathic DCM must be distinguished from chronic, severe valvular disease (Chapter 30) or congenital shunts, which also can lead to ventricular dilation. Horses with DCM can develop substantial mitral regurgitation with apical distraction ("tenting") of the mitral leaflets. However, in contrast to DCM, many horses with primary mitral valve disease maintain a hyperdynamic left ventricle. Nevertheless, some horses with chronic volume overload seemingly progress to a DCM phenotype, which can create confusion about the primary disorder. The diagnosis of idiopathic DCM also can be uncertain in the setting of

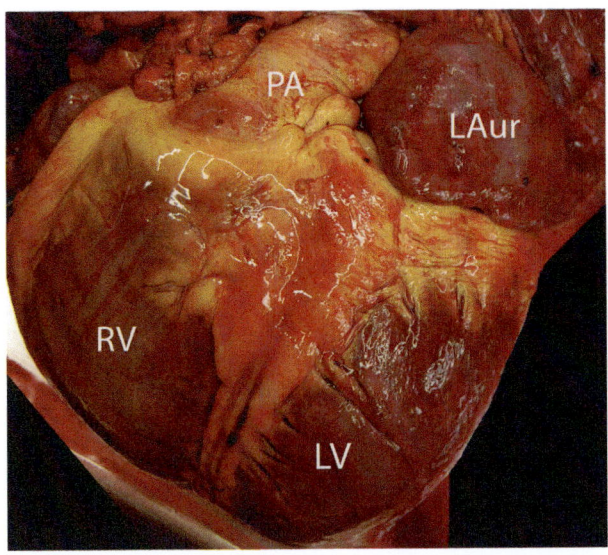

Figure 34.2 Specimen from a horse with dilated cardiomyopathy and congestive heart failure (left craniolateral aspect). Dilation of left atrial appendage (LAur) and apical regions of both right ventricle (RV) and left ventricle (LV) is evident. PA, pulmonary trunk.

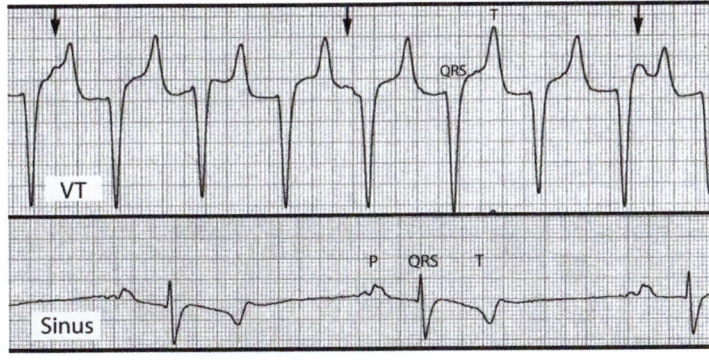

Figure 34.3 Base-apex ECGs recorded from a 15-year-old Quarterhorse gelding with tachycardia-induced cardiomyopathy. Upper strip shows ventricular tachycardia at 150 beats/min, with atrioventricular dissociation and independent P waves (arrows). Lower strip shows normal sinus rhythm after successful antiarrhythmic therapy with quinidine sulfate. The cardiomyopathy later reversed. Courtesy of Dr J Stern.

relentless tachyarrhythmia, as this can reduce ventricular function, both acutely and chronically.

Tachycardia-Induced Cardiomyopathy

Tachycardia-induced cardiomyopathy (TICM; p. 630) is a potentially reversible form of DCM caused by relentless tachycardia (Stern, 2012). The ectopic rhythm often is ventricular in origin, with heart rates >130 beats/min for many days (**Figures 34.3** and **34.4**). TICM potentially is reversible within days to weeks, so long as the rhythm (or heart rate) be controlled.

Infiltrative Cardiomyopathy

Antemortem diagnosis of infiltrative cardiomyopathy is rare in horses. Potential causes include neoplastic cells and amyloid fibrils. These can induce arrhythmias or myocardial dysfunction, although effects of extracardiac lesions can overshadow cardiac signs. The diffuse infiltration of lymphoma and hemangiosarcoma into the myocardium create a mixed echo texture (Beaumier, 2020). Diffuse, symmetrical neoplastic infiltration must be distinguished from concentric hypertrophy, myocarditis, or other myocardial infiltrates, such as from amyloidosis (**Figure 34.5**).

Ischemic Myocardial Disease

Myocardial (demand) ischemia undoubtedly occurs during maximal exercise, as evidenced by exercise ECG analysis (marked ST-T changes) and research studies (Manohar, 1994).

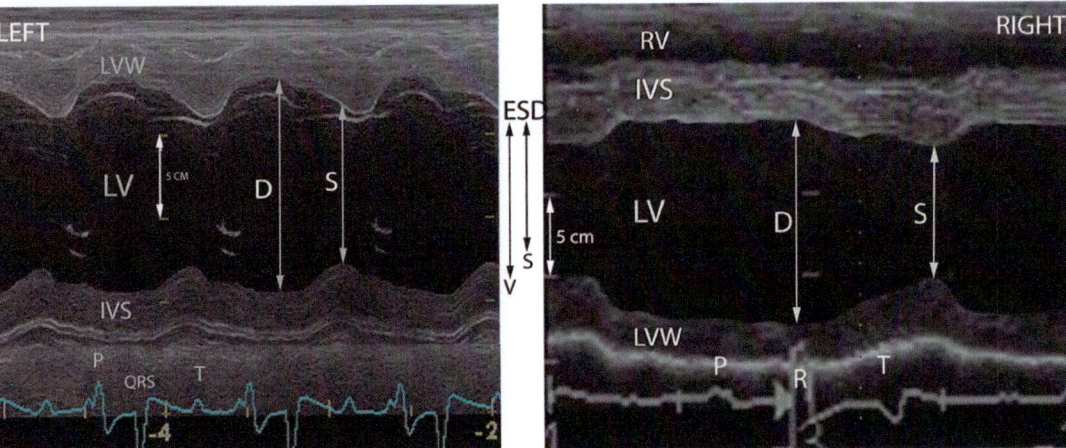

Figure 34.4 Tachycardia-induced cardiomyopathy in a 2-year-old Standardbred filly. Left: M-mode image recorded some hours after conversion to sinus rhythm with amiodarone (lidocaine & Mg salts were ineffective). The left ventricle (LV) is dilated for the breed (increased diastolic dimension, D); systolic shortening is reduced and end-systolic (S) dimension increased. Image obtained from left thorax due to severe subcutaneous edema from congestive heart failure. Right: Follow-up echo obtained weeks later (from right thorax) shows improved systolic function of LV. End-systolic dimensions (ESD) are compared in center: after conversion from ventricular tachycardia (V) and after weeks in sinus rhythm (S). ECG at bottom of images.

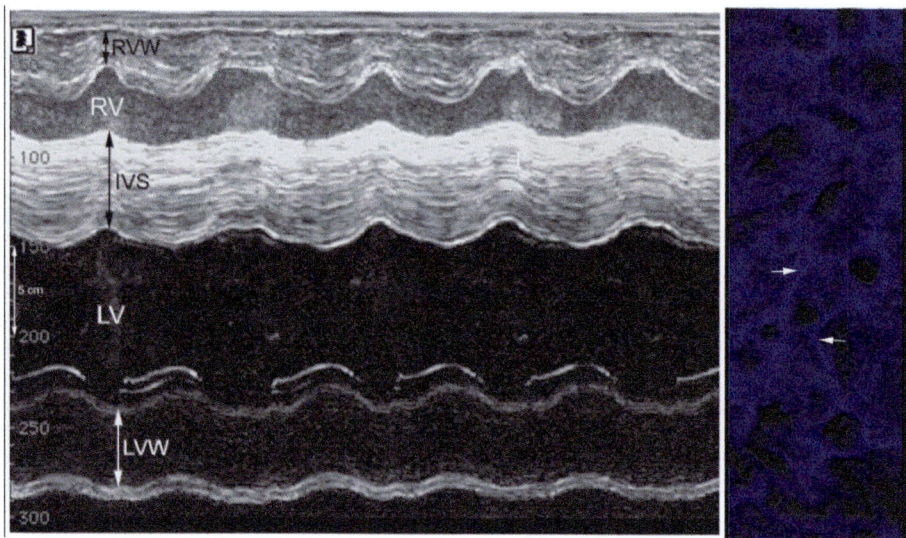

Figure 34.5 Cardiac amyloidosis in a 16-year-old Thoroughbred gelding with normal direct systemic arterial blood pressure. The M-mode image (left panel) shows marked thickening of the left ventricular free wall (LVW) and interventricular septum (IVS), with reduced systolic function of the left ventricle (LV). 2D imaging (not shown) showed hyperechogenicity throughout the myocardium. RV, right ventricle; RVW, right ventricular wall. The right panel shows pericellular amyloid deposits (arrows) under ultraviolet light (thioflavin-T staining). Histologic image courtesy of Dr T Papenfuss.

Yet, in the setting of high-intensity exercise, the boundary between physiological and pathological requires better definition. Extramural coronary disease is rare in horses. But an exercise echocardiogram that shows poor segmental wall motion suggests underlying myocardial disease; this might indicate myocardial perfusion impairment. However, stress echo exercise testing currently is not standardized sufficiently, and more importantly, has not been shown conclusively to identify myocardial dysfunction or pathologic correlation.

Hypertensive Cardiomyopathy

LV hypertrophy and dysfunction can develop secondary to systemic hypertension. This could be associated with chronic kidney disease, laminitis, chronic pain, or potentially, from hyperadrenocorticism or metabolic syndrome (Navas de Solis, 2013). Considering the few causes of LV thickening in horses, systemic blood pressure should be measured when echo exam reveals LV concentric hypertrophy or wall thickening, or when one of the disorders mentioned here is diagnosed.

Myocardial Fibrosis

Areas of myocardial fibrosis are observed regularly at gross and histopathologic postmortem examinations (Else, 1972; Moleson, 2019). The etiology for most of these lesions is unknown, although high-level training has been associated with increased microscopic fibrosis scores, compared to sedentary horses. Fibrosis can be a histopathologic finding only; visualization might require special stains, as in cases of atrial fibrosis secondary to chronic atrial fibrillation (AF). Areas of gross endocardial thickening and subepicardial and subendocardial scars also can be incidental findings, or consequent to confirmed myocardial injury (**Figures 34.6** and **34.7**). Myocardial fibrosis can develop as replacement for necrotic or apoptotic myocardium. In addition, neurohormones (including norepinephrine and aldosterone) and cytokines are known to incite more diffuse myocardial fibrosis in other species; this might be relevant in horses with

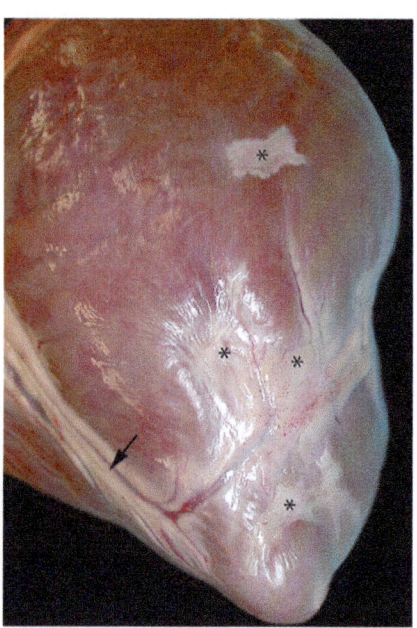

Figure 34.6 Multiple areas of superficial myocardial fibrosis (*) are evident over the left ventricular surface in this specimen from a horse. This was an incidental necropsy finding. Normal fat surrounds the left coronary artery branches within the interventricular sulcus (arrow).

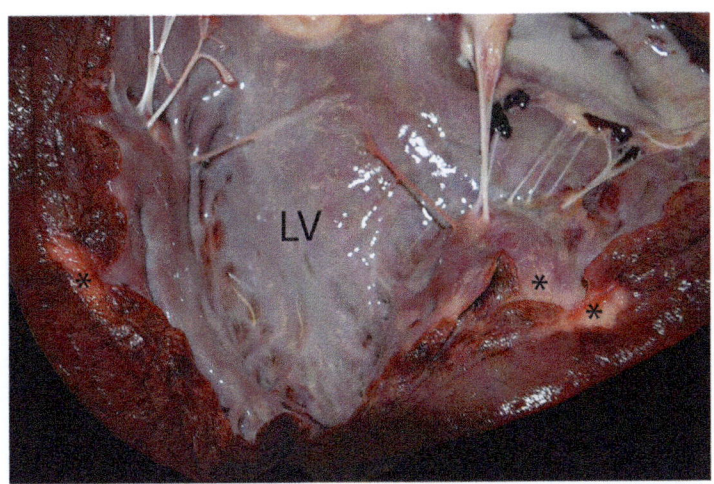

Figure 34.7 Opened left ventricle (LV) shows multiple areas of chronic myocardial scarring (*) in a young horse that also had acute myocarditis and necrosis, with various arrhythmias including rapid paroxysmal ventricular tachycardia, isolated ventricular premature complexes, 2nd-degree atrioventricular (AV) block, and accelerated idioventricular rhythm with AV dissociation. Cardiac troponin I was 17 ng/mL.

advanced valvular or congenital heart disease. Myocarditis, parasitic or toxic injuries, and ischemic necrosis are other potential causes of reactive or replacement fibrosis. Although extensive myocardial fibrosis can interfere with ventricular systolic and diastolic function, focal fibrosis is more common in horses. Yet such lesions could create conduction obstacles that facilitate re-entrant arrhythmias (p. 365).

Clinical Features

Horses that are mildly affected by a myocardial disease might show no detectable clinical signs, especially when performance expectations are low. However, exercise intolerance, hemodynamically significant arrhythmias, heart failure, and sudden cardiac death are potential consequences of myocardial diseases. The onset of clinical signs can lag from the initial insult, especially in cases of myocarditis or recurrent myocardial injury. For example, a horse that has apparently recovered from an infection or sublethal ionophore exposure might develop problems once rigorous training begins. Affected horses could take longer to cool down after a workout. In more severe cases, overt exercise intolerance, weakness, ataxia, or even collapse can occur. More severe clinical signs of systemic involvement or of CHF might be identified from the history, or during observation (**Figure 10.5**, p. 212 and **Figure 20.5**, p. 312), clinical examination, or diagnostic testing (see **Table 34.2**). Sudden death sometimes occurs without premonitory signs.

Clinical examination findings vary in horses with myocardial disease and there are no pathognomonic signs. Cardiac findings might include persistent sinus tachycardia at rest, premature atrial or ventricular beats or even more sustained cardiac arrhythmias, a systolic murmur of mitral or tricuspid valve regurgitation, or clinical signs of CHF. Manifestations of CHF are caused in part by fluid retention and elevated systemic venous pressures (Chapter 20). Postexercise examination might reveal abnormal heart rate elevation that persists after exercise ceases. Despite its value for revealing arrhythmias and other functional abnormalities, clinicians and clients should understand that exercise testing is potentially unsafe in horses with persistent resting tachycardia or myocardial dysfunction.

Diagnostic Tests

The diagnosis of myocardial disease typically requires a high level of clinical suspicion, integrated with findings from echo and ancillary tests. Yet, the variability and nonspecific nature of most findings means that the diagnosis of myocardial disease is mainly presumptive. The following paragraphs note some specific diagnostic points.

Laboratory Tests

Routine hematologic and biochemical tests are not diagnostic for myocardial diseases (**Table 34.2**). Specific circulating cardiac biomarkers are useful for identifying myocardial cell injury or necrosis, but it is important to recognize that these tests do not distinguish myocarditis from other causes of myocardial cell injury or death. A relatively specific marker for myocardial damage is serum cardiac troponin (cTn)I, or the less-often used cTnT. Troponins are regulatory constituents of myocardial sarcomeres. Unequivocal cTnI elevations point to recent cardiac muscle injury, such as that induced by inflammation, toxicosis, hypoxia, hypotension, or ischemia. Normal values are relatively low in horses (usually <0.08 ng/mL, for most of the normal sensitivity assays). Normal or borderline biomarker concentrations do not exclude myocardial disease. Persistently elevated plasma cTnI concentrations (>0.08 ng/mL) and even "trickle" elevations in the 0.08–0.1 ng/mL range, can indicate ongoing heart muscle damage, inasmuch as cTnI plasma half-life is relatively short in horses. Values exceeding 30 ng/mL have occurred in horses with active severe myocardial injury, but most results in horses with heart disease are much lower. Nevertheless, cause and effect can be challenging to determine. Primary arrhythmias and hypotension (from hemorrhage, for example) also seem to elevate troponins, at least mildly.

Serum muscle enzyme concentrations traditionally were evaluated as indicators for myocardial cell injury; these maintain some utility, considering cTnI is not part of routine serum biochemical profiles. Elevated plasma or serum creatine kinase (CK) and aspartate aminotransferase (AST) activities are compatible with myocardial cell injury, but are nonspecific. Increases in specific fractions (myocardial bands) of creatine kinase (CK-MB) or lactate dehydrogenase

(LDH) 1–2 more strongly suggest myocardial injury. However, cardiac origin of such elevations should be verified by measuring serum cTnI. These muscle enzymes also can increase with skeletal muscle injury, and secondary or combined injuries, as observed with ionophore toxicity and some other conditions.

Electrocardiography

The resting electrocardiogram (ECG) might show a normal sinus mechanism, but at a faster rate. Sinus tachycardia is a nonspecific finding. However, further investigation generally is warranted to explore the reason for elevated sympathetic tone, and compensation for cardiac disease is one consideration. An exercising ECG might document provoked arrhythmias (**Figure 34.8**) or an inappropriately high heart rate for the level of work; however, the aforementioned caution must be reemphasized.

Echocardiography

Straightforward equine cases of DCM phenotype demonstrate a dilated LV with reduced systolic function (low ejection fraction or fractional shortening) and left atrial (LA) or biatrial enlargement, findings similar to dogs with DCM (Chapter 32; and **Figure 34.4**). Dilation of all four chambers is more common when clinical CHF signs or AF also are present. Depending on the type of myocardial disease, the LV wall thickness relative to LV chamber size can be increased (as with inflammatory, infiltrative or hypertensive cardiomyopathy, **Figure 34.5**) or decreased (as with DCM, **Figure 34.9** or TICM, **Figure 34.4**). Marked increase in LV or LA spontaneous echocontrast might be observed in horses with poor myocardial function, although this is not a specific finding and can occur in healthy horses with bradycardia. Abnormal areas of myocardial echogenicity, as well as thinning or scarring have been described; however, myocardial tissue characterization by echocardiography is not well-established in

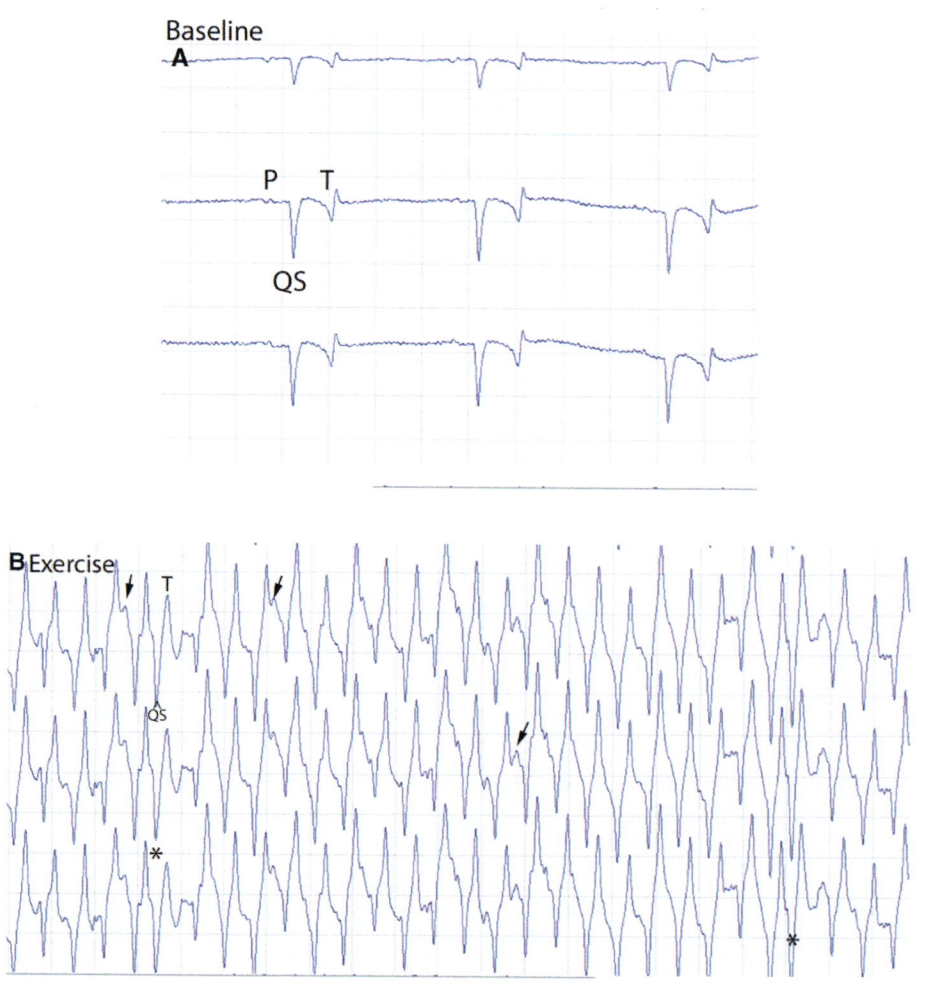

Figure 34.8 (A) Multiple lead ECG in a horse at baseline. Normal waveforms are marked. (B) ECG recorded during exercise reveals premature complexes. The challenges of interpreting an exercise ECG are evident in terms of faster rate, fusion of T and P waves (arrows indicate some P waves), motion artifact and ventilation, and the precise origin of premature complexes (*). These are thought to be supraventricular premature complexes, based on QRS morphology in multiple leads. QS, ventricular activation ("QRS"); P, atrial activation; T, ventricular repolarization.

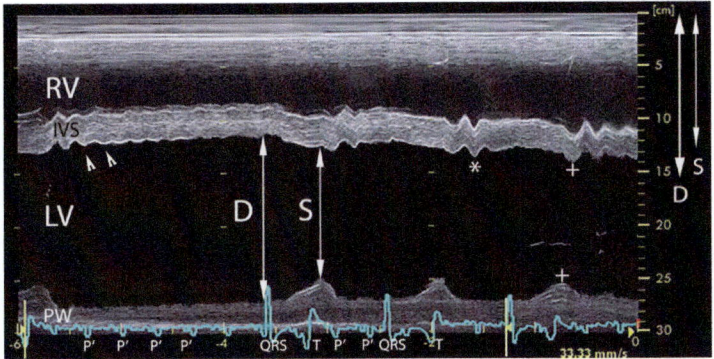

Figure 34.9 M-mode image from the right thorax in a horse with dilated cardiomyopathy (DCM) phenotype and sustained atrial tachyarrhythmia (focal atrial tachycardia or atypical atrial flutter). Diastolic minor dimension (D) and end-systolic dimension (S) are both increased, indicating a dilated left ventricle (LV; D ~15 cm) with reduced systolic function. The atrial rhythm is rapid (P′) and ventricular response rate irregular. Note small deflections (arrowheads) in interventricular septum (IVS) caused by atrial contractions. These should not be confused with the normal diastolic septal dip (*). There is ventricular dyssynchrony, with longer than normal offset between septal and left posterior wall (PW) contractions (+). This could be primary DCM with secondary atrial arrhythmia, or tachycardia-induced cardiomyopathy. Successful cardioversion and time in sinus rhythm would clarify this. RV, right ventricle.

horses and gray-scale density depends on numerous technical factors. Overtly thin or hyperechoic segments of myocardium are compatible with myocardial fibrosis. Hyperechoic regions might be observed with inflammation, ionophore injury, and amyloid. Doppler imaging, when available, commonly reveals secondary mitral or tricuspid regurgitation.

In more subtle cases, advanced echo techniques are needed to detect mild ventricular dysfunction; however, these methods (such as strain imaging) are largely investigational. The ability of postexercise, or pharmacological, stress echocardiography to detect mild myocardial disease or myocardial ischemia is controversial. However, a positive test could demonstrate a paradoxical reduction of LV shortening or regional wall motion abnormalities after exercise. It is imperative to acquire images quickly, once exercise has ceased, so that the heart rate is at least 100 beats/minute.

Management

The treatment for horses affected by myocardial disease is supportive (Chapter 22). The horse should be rested, preferably in a stall, until myocardial function, heart rhythm and cardiac troponin concentrations return to normal, or at least remain stable for several weeks. Supplementation with vitamin E and selenium might be beneficial in the odd case with suspected nutritional deficiencies. For suspected bacterial myocarditis, antibiotic treatment is indicated. If noninfective myocarditis is thought responsible for the arrhythmia or other clinical signs, anti-inflammatory corticosteroid therapy (dexamethasone) might be administered; however, while such therapy is commonly used, validation of this treatment requires controlled clinical trials.

Antiarrhythmic therapy is administered when indicated for potentially life-threatening arrhythmias (see Chapters 24 and 25). Typically, lidocaine, magnesium salts, quinidine and amiodarone are used in the management of sustained ventricular tachycardias (procainamide is relatively unavailable). Theoretically, an angiotensin converting enzyme (ACE) inhibitor such as benazepril or an aldosterone antagonist like spironolactone could limit adverse myocardial remodeling and unload the ventricles. However, the efficacy of such treatment for equine myocardial diseases is unknown. Benazepril would seem a logical therapy in definitive cases of myocardial disease with DCM phenotype or CHF.

Medical Therapy for Congestive Heart Failure

Medical therapy for CHF generally involves furosemide, an ACE inhibitor (benazepril in the United States), and digoxin. Parenteral furosemide is a mainstay for CHF treatment; initially, it is given IV. Chronic IM administration sometimes is possible. ACE inhibitors are potentially teratogenic in the first and second trimesters of pregnancy. When this is not of concern, benazepril could be used. Enalapril is ineffective in horses (p. 322). Digoxin is especially relevant in the setting of AF. However, digoxin is (relatively) contraindicated in horses with ventricular ectopy. Chronic administration should involve serum digoxin concentration monitoring (therapeutic target: 0.8 to 1.2 ng/mL at ~12 hours post-dosing). Digoxin has been safely administered in the final trimester of pregnancy. Initial IV digoxin doses (typically 1 mg for an adult horse) are administered every 12 hours; this is followed by chronic oral administration every 12–24 hours, if feasible (p. 413). Pimobendan might be useful for horses in CHF. Pimobendan has been administered to healthy horses, but it is considered investigational and treatment is quite expensive.

Prognosis

The prognosis for horses with myocardial disease depends on the underlying etiology, disease severity, and the electrical and hemodynamic consequences. When the principal manifestation of myocardial disease is electrical (arrhythmias with otherwise normal myocardial function), the prognosis is fair to good for resolution of the arrhythmias. The prognosis for horses with impaired systolic function, cardiac dilation, or CHF is guarded to poor for life and poor for future work. It is notable, however, that some horses with LV hypertrophy (or thickening) and dysfunction, and some with acute onset of CHF, have recovered completely and returned to their prior performance level. Such horses most likely suffered from acute myocarditis that resolved spontaneously, or perhaps following anti-inflammatory therapy. As noted previously, TICM potentially is reversible. Other horses might achieve incomplete recovery, yet might still stand for breeding.

Suggested Additional Reading and References

Also See Online Comprehensive Bibliography at: https://www.routledge.com/9781482246223.

Bauquier J, Stent A, Gibney J, et al. Evidence for marsh mallow (Malva parviflora) toxicosis causing myocardial disease and myopathy in four horses. Equine Vet J 2017;49:307–313.

Beaumier A, Dixon CE, Robinson N, et al. Primary cardiac hemangiosarcoma in a horse: echocardiographic and necropsy findings. J Vet Cardiol 2020;32:66–72.

Bonagura JD. Overview of equine cardiac disease. Vet Clin North Am Equine Pract. 2019;35:1–22.

Cranley JJ, McCullagh KG. Ischaemic myocardial fibrosis and aortic strongylosis in the horse. Equine Vet J. 1981;13:35–42.

Cullimore AM, Lester GD, Secombe CJ, et al. Hypertrophic cardiomyopathy in a Clydesdale gelding. Aust Vet J 2018;96:212–215.

Cushing TL. Endocardial fibroelastosis in a quarterhorse mare. J Comp Pathol. 2013;149:318–321.

Decloedt A. Pericardial disease, myocardial disease, and great vessel abnormalities in horses. Vet Clin North Am Equine Pract 2019;35:139–157.

Decloedt A, de Clercq D, Ven S, et al. Right atrial and right ventricular ultrasound-guided biopsy technique in standing horses. Equine Vet J 2016;48:346–351.

Decloedt A, Verheyen T, De Clercq D, et al. Acute and long-term cardiomyopathy and delayed neurotoxicity after accidental lasalocid poisoning in horses. J Vet Intern Med 2012;26:1005–1011.

Durando MM. Cardiovascular causes of poor performance and exercise intolerance and assessment of safety in the equine athlete. Vet Clin North Am Equine Pract. 2019;35(1):175–190.

Else RW, Holmes JR. Cardiac pathology in the horse. 2. Microscopic pathology. Equine Vet J. 1972;4(2):57–62.

Freel KM, Morrison LR, Thompson H, et al. Arrhythmogenic right ventricular cardiomyopathy as a cause of unexpected cardiac death in two horses. Vet Rec 2010;166:718–721.

Gelberg HB, Zachary JF, Everitt JI, et al. Sudden death in training and racing Thoroughbred horses. J Am Vet Med Assoc. 1985;187(12):1354–1356.

Hoffman A, Levi O, Orgad U, et al. Myocarditis following envenoming with *Vipera palaestinae* in two horses. Toxicon 1993;31:1623–1628.

Gy C, Leclere M, Bélanger MC, et al. Acute, subacute and chronic sequelae of horses accidentally exposed to monensin-contaminated feed [published online ahead of print, 2020 Mar 7]. Equine Vet J. 2020;10.1111/evj.13258. doi:10.1111/evj.13258

Jesty SA, Reef VB. Septicemia and cardiovascular infections in horses. Vet Clin North Am Equine Pract 2006; 22(2):481–495.

Luethy D, Slack J, Kraus MS, et al. Third-degree atrioventricular block and collapse associated with eosinophilic myocarditis in a horse. J Vet Intern Med 2017;31:884–889.

Manohar M, Goetz TE, Hutchens E, et al. Atrial and ventricular myocardial blood flows in horses at rest and during exercise. Am J Vet Res. 1994;55(10):1464–1469.

Molesan A, Wang M, Sun Q, et al. Cardiac pathology and genomics of sudden death in racehorses from New York and Maryland racetracks. Vet Pathol 2019;56:576–585.

Nath LC, Anderson GA, Hinchcliff KW, et al. Serum cardiac troponin I concentrations in horses with cardiac disease. Aust Vet J. 2012;90(9):351–357.

Navas de Solis C. Exercising arrhythmias and sudden cardiac death in horses: review of the literature and comparative aspects. Equine Vet J. 2016;48(4):406–413. doi:10.1111/evj.12580

Navas de Solis C, Slack J, Boston RC, et al. Hypertensive cardiomyopathy in horses: 5 cases (1995-2011). J Am Vet Med Assoc. 2013;243(1):126–130.

Nout YS, Hinchcliff KW, Bonagura JD, et al. Cardiac amyloidosis in a horse. J Vet Intern Med. 2003;17(4):588–592.

Raftery AG, Garcia NC, Thompson H, et al. Arrhythmogenic right ventricular cardiomyopathy secondary to adipose infiltration as a cause of episodic collapse in a horse. Ir Vet J 2015;68:24. Erratum in: Ir Vet J 2017;70:19.

Reef VB, Bonagura J, Buhl R, et al. Recommendations for management of equine athletes with cardiovascular abnormalities. J Vet Intern Med. 2014;28(3):749–61.

Sandersen C, Detilleux J, Art T, et al. Exercise and pharmacological stress echocardiography in healthy horses. Equine Vet J Suppl. 2006;(36):159–162.

Schwarzwald CC. Cardiovascular diseases. In, Reed SM, Bayly WM, Sellon DC (editors). Equine Internal Medicine. 4th edition. 2017. Elsevier, St. Louis, MO. pp 387–541.

Stern JA, Doreste YR, Barnett S, et al. Resolution of sustained narrow complex ventricular tachycardia and tachycardia-induced cardiomyopathy in a Quarter Horse following quinidine therapy. J Vet Cardiol 2012;14:445–451.

Traub-Dargatz JL, Schlipf JW Jr, Boon J, et al. Ventricular tachycardia and myocardial dysfunction in a horse. J Am Vet Med Assoc. 1994;205:1569–1573.

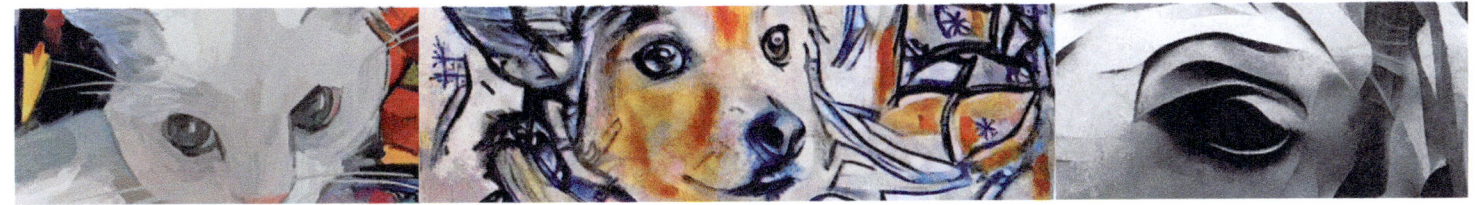

35
PERICARDIAL DISEASES AND CARDIAC TUMORS

The pericardium forms a double-layered sac around the heart; it is attached to the great vessels at the heart base (**Figure 35.1**). There is an outer fibrous layer (parietal pericardium) and an inner serous membrane, which covers the heart (visceral pericardium, or epicardium). A small volume (~0.25 mL/kg) of serous fluid between these layers serves as a lubricant. The pericardium helps balance the output of the right and left ventricles, limits acute distension of the heart, and maintains the normal cardiac position within the chest. The pericardium also provides a barrier to infection or inflammation that might occur in surrounding structures.

Diseases involving the pericardium and intrapericardial space can disrupt normal cardiac function, most often by impairing cardiac filling. Some disorders are congenital in origin, but the vast majority stem from excess or abnormal fluid accumulation in the pericardial space (pericardial effusion). Clinical evidence of this occurs most often in dogs, subsequent to the development of cardiac tamponade (p. 712). Most canine pericardial effusions are associated with cardiac (or pericardial) neoplasia or, in younger dogs, an idiopathic hemorrhagic effusion. Other causes include pericardial or cardiac infections, noninfective pericarditis, hemorrhage into the pericardial space, and congestive heart failure (CHF), among others. Pericardial effusion, usually without tamponade, is known to occur in dogs with systemic inflammatory disease. Increased cardiac troponin (cTn) concentrations and depressed myocardial function often coexist in these dogs. The condition presumably is mediated by circulating inflammatory cytokines with associated vasculitis; resolution commonly occurs with successful treatment of underlying disease (Covey, 2018). Various inflammatory conditions have been implicated, including steroid-responsive meningitis-arteritis in particular (Spence, 2019).

Pericardial effusion as a primary disorder is less common in cats and in horses, compared to dogs. In cats, it most often is associated with CHF, caused by hypertrophic or other forms of cardiomyopathy. Concurrent pleural effusion (with or without pulmonary edema) also is identified in many cases, although some cats develop a small pericardial effusion prior to the onset of obvious CHF. Regardless, when there is cardiac enlargement and pericardial effusion the presumption should be underlying myocardial disease, rather than a primary effusion with cardiac tamponade. In these cases, the pericardial effusion typically diminishes or resolves with treatment for CHF, and tamponade is rare. Other disorders that can cause pericardial effusion include feline infectious peritonitis, lymphoma and other neoplasia, systemic infections, and, rarely, renal failure. Similar to cats, primary pericardial diseases are uncommon in horses. These usually involve infective or sterile fibrinous pericarditis with effusion (p. 715), intrapericardial hemorrhage, or (rarely) direct trauma to the thorax.

Constrictive pericardial disease (p. 730) is recognized occasionally in dogs, and rarely in cats and horses. It can be a consequence of chronic pericarditis. The majority of canine cases represent what, in people, is termed constrictive–effusive pericardial disease.

Cardiac tumors (p. 732) develop more often in dogs, and uncommonly in cats and horses. Pericardial effusion accumulates with many cardiac tumors and it often causes cardiac tamponade. Mass lesions that involve the heart or heart base can obstruct venous return or impede ejection of blood from the right ventricle.

Spontaneous pneumopericardium is a rare abnormality reported sporadically in the dog and cat. Underlying or associated conditions could include pneumonia, bronchopulmonary disease, and pulmonary abscess or neoplasia. Pneumopericardium also can occur from iatrogenic (including from bone marrow biopsy in the horse) or traumatic causes. It can cause signs of dyspnea and cardiac tamponade.

Cardiovascular Disease in Companion Animals

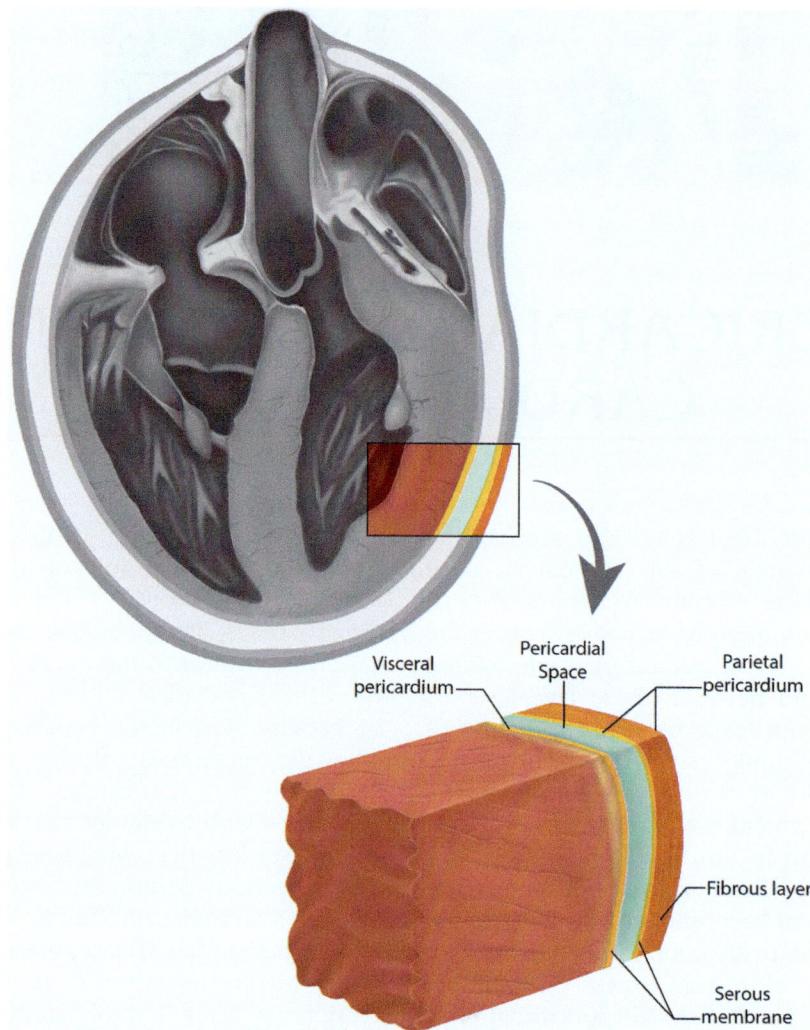

Figure 35.1 Schematic illustration of pericardial structure. The pericardium is adhered to the great vessels at the heart base. The serous visceral pericardial layer reflects back at the heart base onto the parietal pericardium, which consists of a tough fibrous layer lined by this thin serous membrane. Normally, the pericardial space is more of a virtual space, containing only a small amount of lubricating serous fluid, unless an abnormal accumulation of fluid distends it.

Congenital Pericardial Malformations

Peritoneopericardial diaphragmatic hernia (PPDH) is the most common congenital pericardial malformation in dogs and cats. It occurs sporadically in horses. Other congenital pericardial anomalies are quite rare; most are discovered on postmortem examination. Pericardial cysts are anomalies thought to originate from abnormal fetal mesenchymal tissue development or from incarcerated omental or falciform fat secondary to a small PPDH (Sisson, 1993). An expansive pericardial cyst could compress cardiac chambers and cause pathophysiology analogous to cardiac tamponade. The clinical presentation of such cases is similar to that of animals with pericardial effusion and tamponade. The cardiac silhouette could appear enlarged or deformed on radiographs. Echocardiography or other imaging modalities, including computed tomography (CT), magnetic resonance imaging (MRI), or even pneumopericardiography, can reveal the diagnosis. Drainage and surgical removal of the cyst, in conjunction with partial pericardiectomy (pericardectomy), usually has resulted in cure, although some cases are complicated by local adhesions.

Congenital defects of the pericardium itself are extremely rare. Occasional cases of partial (usually on the left side) and complete absence of the pericardium have been reported in dogs and horses. A possible complication resulting from partial absence of the pericardium is herniation of a portion of the heart, such as an atrial appendage (**Figure 35.2**). This can lead to arrhythmias, syncope, embolic disease, or sudden death. Echocardiography, CT, MRI, or angiocardiography facilitate antemortem diagnosis. A partial pericardial defect might remain clinically silent for years.

Pericardial Diseases and Cardiac Tumors

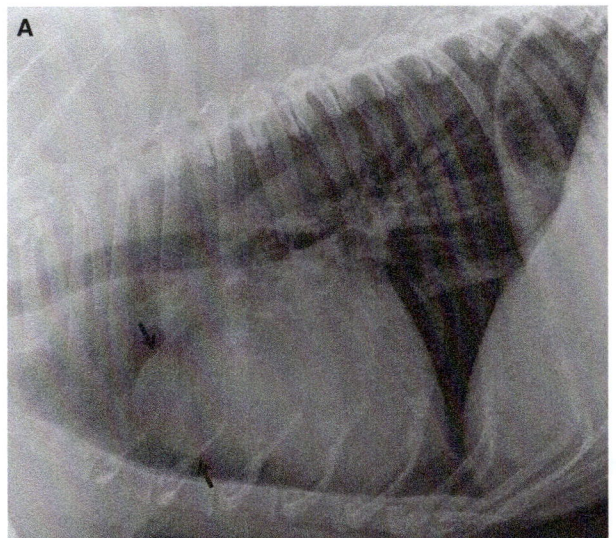
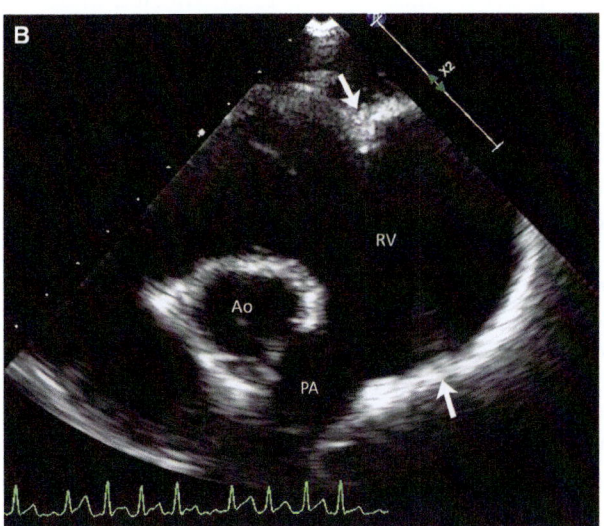
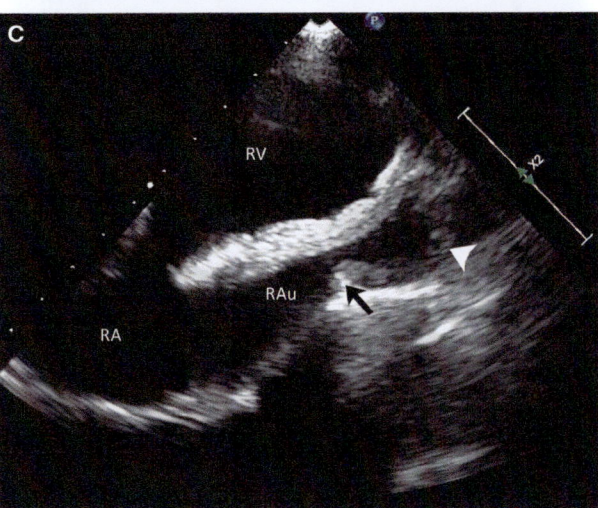

Figure 35.2 (A) Left lateral thoracic radiograph shows a bulge (arrows) at the right cranial aspect of the cardiac silhouette in an 8-year-old male German Shepherd, referred for suspected cardiac neoplasm and syncope. (The differential diagnosis for this radiograph also would include traumatic rupture of the heart into the pericardium.) Radiograph courtesy of VCS Midwest Veterinary Referral. (B) Echocardiography showed outward bulging of the cranial right ventricular wall through a pericardial defect (partial absence of the pericardium). Right parasternal short-axis view. (C) Image from the left cranial long-axis position, with medial angulation, shows a constricted area (black arrow) in the middle of the right auricle, while the auricular tip (white arrowhead) extends across the pericardial defect into the pleural space. The dog's ECG at presentation showed intermittent atrial fibrillation and ventricular premature complexes; after sotalol was prescribed, no further syncope was reported. Ao, aorta; PA, pulmonary artery; RA, right atrium; RAu, right auricle; RV, right ventricle.

Peritoneopericardial Diaphragmatic Hernia

Abnormal embryonic development, probably of the septum transversum, allows persistent communication between the pericardial and peritoneal cavities at the ventral midline. The pleural space is not involved. Other congenital defects such as umbilical hernia, sternal malformations, and cardiac anomalies might coexist. Although the peritoneal–pericardial communication is not trauma-induced, trauma can facilitate movement of abdominal contents through a preexisting defect. Hepatic lobes, falciform fat and the gall bladder are the structures most often identified within the pericardial space in cats. The herniated viscera in dogs can be as for cats, or can include multiple bowel loops, as well as small cystic lesions. The diaphragmatic defect can vary in size from small to massive; smaller defects are most evident ventrally and near the midline.

Pathophysiology A small volume of herniated content probably causes negligible effect, considering PPDH is an incidental finding in many mature animals. However, PPDH can lead to impaired cardiac function when abdominal organs (either partially or entirely) or falciform fat migrate from the cranial abdomen into the pericardial space and compress or displace the heart. Likewise, compression, torsion, or other compromise to the integrity and function of the abdominal structures within the pericardium also can cause gastrointestinal (GI) or other systemic signs. Animals with PPDH sometimes develop some degree of pericardial effusion, usually a modified transudate, presumably from altered capillary forces within the entrapped abdominal tissues. The translocated abdominal soft tissues, with or without pericardial effusion, potentially can compromise cardiac filling enough to cause signs of right-sided CHF or low cardiac output, similar to those of cardiac tamponade. Increased volume within the pericardial space also can impair pulmonary function, which probably contributes to the exertional respiratory difficulty sometimes observed. The impact of the hernia on diaphragmatic function has not yet been studied insofar as the authors can determine.

Clinical Features Males appear to be affected more often than females. Weimaraner dogs might be predisposed. The malformation is common in cats, as well; Himalayan and Domestic Longhair cats could be predisposed, and a family of affected Persian cats has been reported (Margolis, 2018). The authors and others have observed pericardial cystic lesions with small PPDH in Miniature Schnauzer dogs (Simpson, 1999). PPDH also occurred in multiple Golden Retriever puppies exposed to potentially teratogenic drugs during gestation (Kaplan, 2018).

The initial onset of clinical signs associated with PPDH can occur at any age. However, the majority of cases are discovered during the first 4 years of life, usually within the first year. Some animals with PPDH never develop clinical signs. In about half of small animal cases, the malformation might be an incidental finding on thoracic radiographs, echocardiography, or postmortem exam. Clinical signs are variable and result from the herniation of abdominal contents into the pericardial space. Signs usually relate to the GI or respiratory systems. Vomiting, diarrhea, anorexia, weight loss, abdominal pain, cough, dyspnea, and wheezing are reported most often. Shock and collapse also can occur. Physical examination can reveal muffled heart sounds on one or both sides of the chest, displacement or attenuation of the apical precordial impulse (and heart sounds), thoracic borborygmus, and, with herniation of multiple organs, an "empty" feel on abdominal palpation. Occasionally, signs of cardiac tamponade can develop, including those of right-sided CHF with chylothorax.

Diagnostic Tests Thoracic radiography often is diagnostic or highly suggestive of PPDH. Characteristic findings include enlargement of the cardiac silhouette with dorsal tracheal displacement, overlap of the diaphragmatic and caudal heart borders, and abnormal fat opacity or gas within the cardiac silhouette (**Figures 35.3** and **35.4**). The heart itself is displaced cranially and dorsally in many cases, which is indicated by the location of the tracheal carina. A pleural fold (persistent mesothelial remnant) usually is evident on lateral view, extending between the caudal aspect of the cardiac silhouette and the diaphragm ventral to the caudal vena cava (**Figure 35.3A**; Berry, 1990). Gas-filled loops of bowel extending across the diaphragm into the pericardial sac, a small liver, and few organs within the abdominal cavity also might be evident. *Pectus excavatum* or other thoracic or sternal skeletal deformity is present in some cases, as well.

ECG changes are inconsistent. Decreased QRS complex amplitude and axis deviation caused by a shift in the cardiac position sometimes occur. Echocardiography can help confirm the diagnosis (**Figure 35.5**) and ultrasound imaging is now the usual diagnostic method of choice in both general and specialty practices. A GI barium series is diagnostic if stomach or intestines are within the pericardial cavity (**Figure 35.6**); however, this usually is unnecessary today. Other older imaging studies that can be diagnostic include

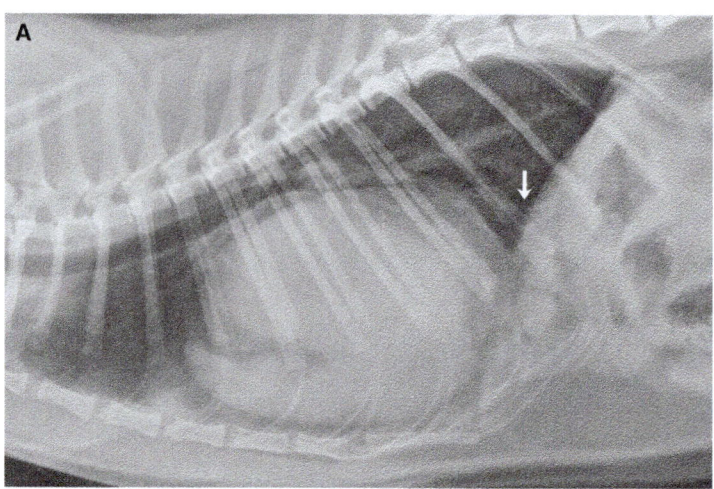

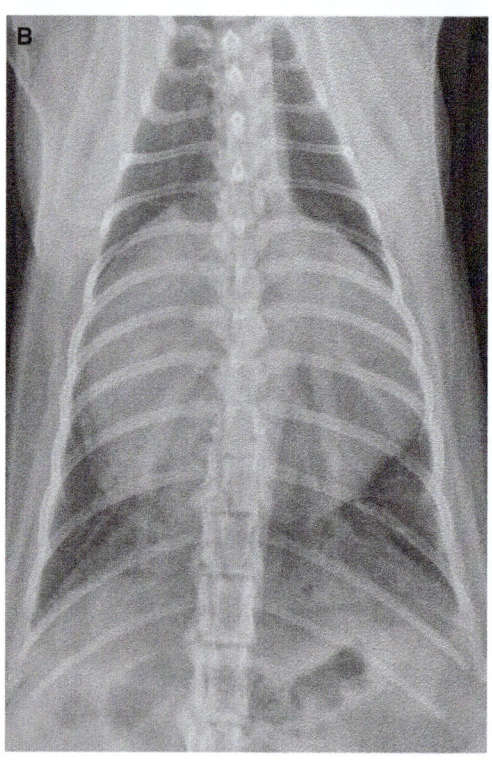

Figure 35.3 Lateral (A) and DV (B) radiographs from a 6-month-old male Domestic Longhair kitten with a history of tachypnea at rest and open-mouth breathing during play or excitement. There is no visible separation between the greatly enlarged cardiac silhouette and the diaphragm in either view because of a peritoneopericardial diaphragmatic hernia. A pleural fold (arrow) is visible extending between them on lateral view; an area of gas density also is evident in the cranial cardiac silhouette.

fluoroscopy, nonselective angiography (especially if only falciform fat or liver has herniated; **Figure 35.7**), positive contrast peritoneography, and pneumopericardiography. CT (**Figure 35.8**) or MRI studies are performed in some cases.

Management Therapy for symptomatic animals involves surgical closure of the peritoneal–pericardial defect after viable organs are returned to their normal location. Surgery usually is successful in resolving clinical signs. However, trauma

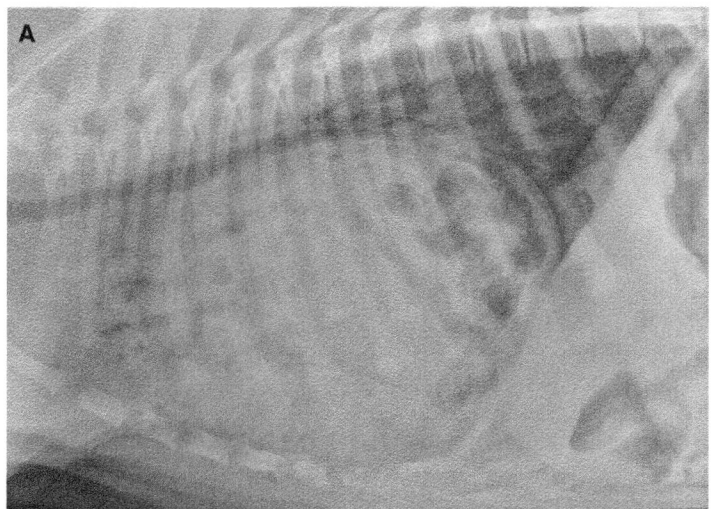

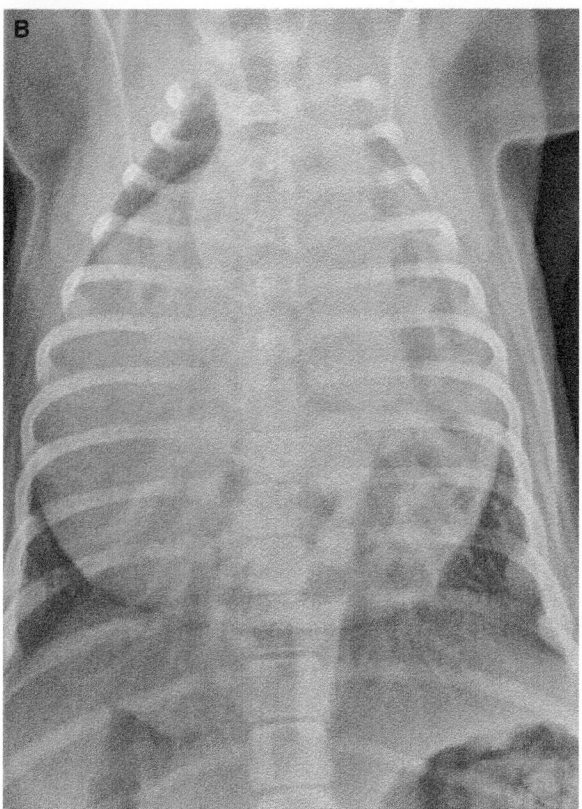

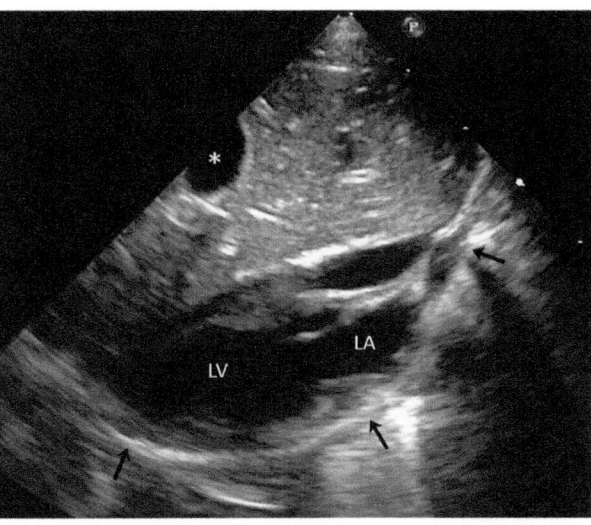

Figure 35.5 Right parasternal echocardiographic image from the cat of **Figure 35.3** shows a large portion of liver within the pericardium (black arrows) which has displaced the heart leftward and craniodorsally. Prior to the echo exam, cardiac auscultation had revealed muffled heart sounds over the right chest wall and bilaterally near the sternal border; but the heart sounds were unusually prominent over the mid-left chest wall. LA, left atrium; LV, left ventricle; *, gallbladder.

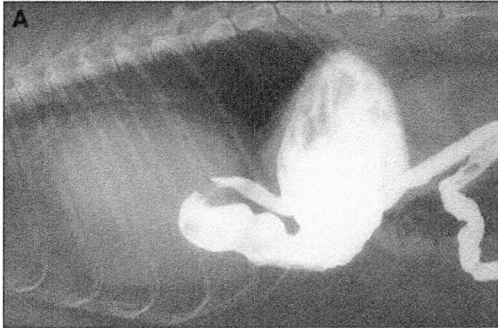

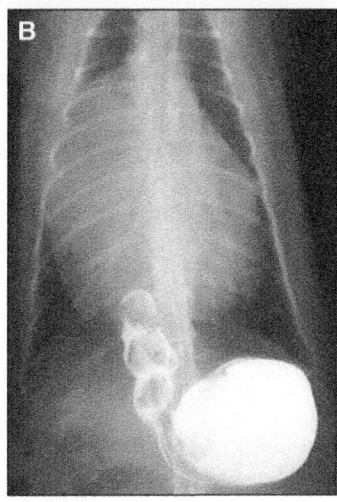

Figure 35.4 Lateral (A) and DV (B) radiographs from a 3-month-old male Labrador Retriever with peritoneopericardial diaphragmatic hernia; a cranial abdominal wall defect had been repaired earlier by the referring veterinarian. The massive cardiac silhouette contains multiple linear gas densities (intestines).

to organs chronically adhered to the heart or pericardium is of concern during attempted repositioning. Animals without clinical signs, and some with mild signs, often do well without surgery (Morgan, 2020). The presence of other congenital or acquired abnormalities and the animal's clinical signs influence the decision to operate. In uncomplicated cases, the prognosis is excellent, although minor complications from

Figure 35.6 A barium swallow can identify a peritoneopericardial diaphragmatic hernia when the stomach or intestines extend across the defect. Lateral (A) and DV (B) images from a 5-year-old male Persian cat with exercise-induced respiratory signs.

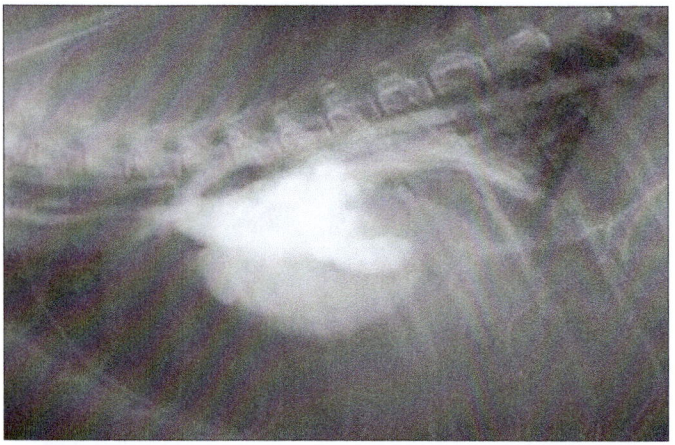

Figure 35.7 Nonselective angiocardiography can help identify peritoneopericardial diaphragmatic hernia, especially when no hollow viscera have crossed the defect, but echocardiography or computed tomography are used more commonly. This cat's normal heart is displaced dorsally by liver and omental fat.

surgery are common. Mortality associated with surgery occurs in a small percentage of cases. Rare sequelae of surgery for PPDH have included pericardial cyst formation, arrhythmias and constrictive pericardial disease. Overall, long-term survival appears to be similar between dogs and cats treated surgically compared to those not operated.

Acquired Pericardial Effusions

Most pericardial effusions in dogs are serosanguineous or sanguineous and are of neoplastic or idiopathic origin. The latter also has been described as "benign" idiopathic pericarditis, idiopathic hemorrhagic pericardial effusion, and similar terms. Transudates, modified transudates, and exudates occur occasionally in both dogs and cats. Pericardial effusion in horses often is fibrinous or serofibrinous. An infectious or immune-mediated process is likely in many if not most equine cases, although a specific etiology can be elusive. Some horses with fibrinous pericarditis have little to no effusion. Constrictive–effusive pericarditis is discussed under "Constrictive Pericardial Disease."

Types of Effusion

Transudative Effusions Pure transudates are clear, with a low cell count (usually <1,000 cells/microliter), specific gravity <1.012, and protein content <25 g/L (<2.5 g/dL). Modified transudates might appear slightly cloudy or pink-tinged. Cellularity is low (~1,000–8,000 cells/microliter) but specific gravity (1.015–1.030) and total protein concentration (25–50 g/L [2.5–5.0 g/dL]) are higher than those of a pure transudate. Transudative effusions (**Figure 35.9**) can be caused by CHF, PPDH, hypoalbuminemia, pericardial cyst, or toxemias that

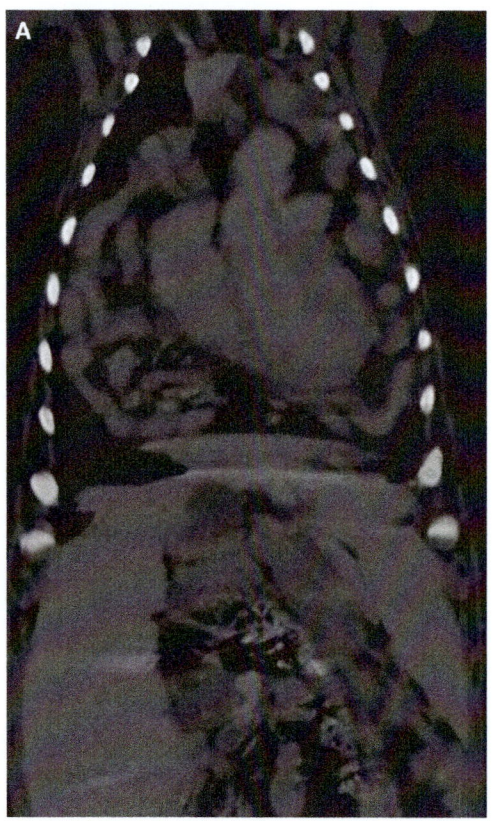
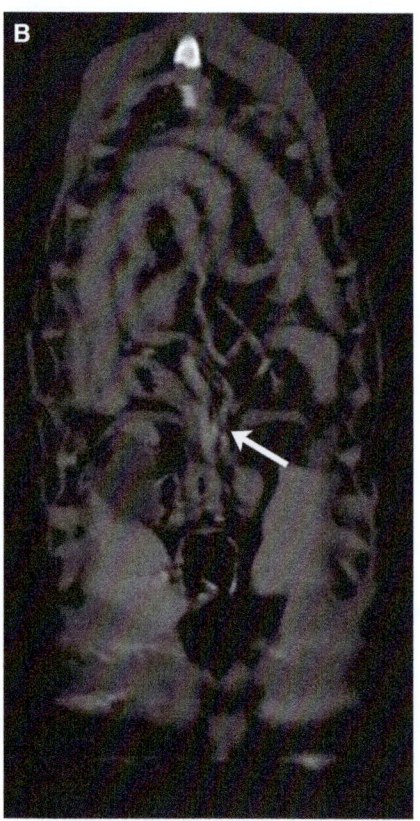

Figure 35.8 (A) Computed tomographic image in the frontal plane shows intestines surrounding the heart in a young dog with peritoneopericardial diaphragmatic hernia. (B) A more ventral slice depicts intestines extending through the diaphragmatic defect (arrow) and into the pericardial space.

hemorrhagic effusion. Hemangiosarcoma (HSA; p. 732) most commonly is responsible; however, hemorrhagic effusions also occur with other neoplasms, including heart base tumors (chemodectoma, ectopic thyroid carcinoma, and other neuroendocrine tumors) and pericardial mesothelioma. Pericardial effusion secondary to tumor metastasis develops rarely, although myocardial metastasis probably is underdiagnosed.

Idiopathic pericardial effusion occurs most often in medium- to large-breed dogs, with possible predilection for Golden Retrievers and Saint Bernards. Dogs of any age can be affected, but the median age appears to be ~6–7 years. Histologic evidence of mild inflammation with areas of hemorrhage and diffuse pericardial fibrosis, especially perivascular, has been described in cases of idiopathic pericardial effusion. Although several viruses are associated with pericarditis in people, there is little evidence to support an infective cause in dogs. Nevertheless, deoxyribonucleic acid (DNA) of various vector-borne pathogens was detected in a greater number of dogs with pericardial effusion, compared to those without, although no relation to the effusion's etiology was apparent (Tabar, 2018). Less commonly, intrapericardial hemorrhage occurs because of left atrial (LA) rupture secondary to advanced degenerative (myxomatous) mitral valve disease, coagulopathy (including rodenticide toxicity), penetrating trauma (including iatrogenic coronary artery laceration during pericardiocentesis or from a metal projectile), and severe non-penetrating chest trauma (as from a fence post). Rarely, acute hemorrhage into the pericardium with cardiac tamponade has occurred secondary to aortic dissection. In horses, intrapericardial rupture of the aorta causes acute hemopericardium and sudden death.

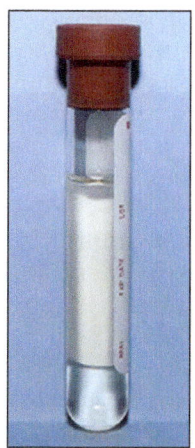

Figure 35.9 Transudative pericardial effusion from a dog with chronic degenerative mitral valve disease and congestive heart failure.

increase vascular permeability, including uremia. In addition, rare occurrence of *Dirofilaria repens* microfilariae in abdominal and pericardial fluid has been described, although any potential cause and effect relationship is undefined. Usually, only a small volume of pericardial effusion is associated with conditions causing transudative pericardial effusion. Cardiac tamponade rarely develops.

Hemorrhagic Effusions This fluid typically is dark red (**Figure 35.10**), with a packed cell volume (PCV) >7%, specific gravity >1.015, and protein concentration >30 g/L (>3 g/dL). Cytology shows mostly red blood cells (RBCs), although reactive mesothelial, neoplastic, or other cell types might be seen. The fluid does not clot unless the hemorrhage was very recent, or the heart was perforated during sampling. Older dogs are more likely to have a neoplastic

Exudative Effusions Exudates can appear cloudy to opaque, or serofibrinous to serosanguineous (**Figure 35.11**). They are characterized by a high nucleated cell count (usually well over 3,000 cells/microliter), protein concentration usually much higher than 30 g/L (3 g/dL), and specific gravity >1.015. Cytologic findings relate to the etiology. Exudative pericardial effusions are uncommon in small animals. Infectious causes usually relate to a foreign body (such as a migrating plant awn or porcupine quill), bite wounds, other penetrating wounds, systemic infection, or extension of infection in nearby structures (Aronson, 1995). Various aerobic and anaerobic bacteria, actinomycosis, disseminated tuberculosis and, rarely, other fungal or protozoal infections have been identified. In endemic regions, coccidioidomycosis is a regular cause of pericarditis in dogs (Heinritz, 2005). Immune-compromised patients, including those undergoing chemotherapy, are probably at greater risk for infectious causes. Myocarditis of various etiologies can produce some pericardial effusion. This includes infection with *Trypanosoma cruzi* (p. 640). Sterile exudative effusions have occurred with leptospirosis, canine distemper, and idiopathic pericardial effusion in dogs, and

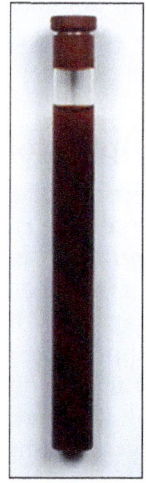

Figure 35.10 Most pericardial effusions in dogs are hemorrhagic, as is this fluid from a dog with "benign" idiopathic pericardial effusion.

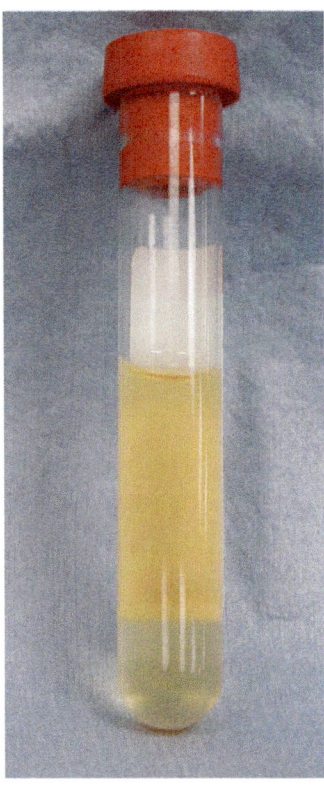

Figure 35.11 Nonseptic, exudative pericardial effusion from a 4-year-old male Domestic Shorthair cat with feline infectious peritonitis and cardiac tamponade.

with feline infectious peritonitis and toxoplasmosis in cats. Chronic uremia occasionally causes a sterile, serofibrinous or hemorrhagic effusion.

Pericarditis in Horses Bacterial infection, viral infection, or immune-mediated mechanisms are thought to underlie most cases of pericarditis in horses. An estimated one third of cases are bacterial in origin. Primary infection or extension from pleuropneumonia can occur. The most common bacteria isolated are *Actinobacillus* and *Streptococcus* species (spp.). Others have included *Escherichia coli*, *Enterococcus faecalis*, *Pseudomonas aeruginosa*, *Pasteurella* spp., *Corynebacterium* spp., and *Mycoplasma*, among others. Viruses thought to be associated with some cases of pericarditis include Equine Herpes Virus, Equine Viral Arteritis, and Equine Influenza Virus. However, a specific etiology often is not identified, so many cases are considered idiopathic. Nevertheless, it is possible that a virus or secondary immune responses could underlie idiopathic pericarditis. A history of recent respiratory disease is common in affected horses. Sporadically, pericarditis is associated with fungal, parasitic, or neoplastic disease. Rarely, thoracic trauma, a penetrating foreign body, or vascular rupture causes intrapericardial hemorrhage and inflammation.

Pericardial inflammation often causes a fibrinous response (fibrinous pericarditis) in horses. Some cases have a variable amount of pericardial effusion as well (fibrino-effusive pericarditis); other cases are primarily effusive. Cardiac tamponade can occur (see "Pathophysiology"). Constrictive pericardial disease (p. 730) appears to be an uncommon sequela of pericarditis.

Pericarditis occurs in adult horses of all ages, breeds, and sexes, although younger horses and intact males might be over-represented. Fibrino-effusive pericarditis has occurred in foals with systemic inflammatory response syndrome; the exudative pericardial effusion could be sterile, but prognosis appears poor. An outbreak of fibrino-effusive pericarditis occurred as a component of the mare reproductive loss syndrome in the early 2000s in Kentucky (United States); although other horses also were affected. This appeared to be associated with ingestion of a certain type of caterpillar (Eastern Tent Caterpillar). The specific disease mechanism is unclear, but might involve a toxin or breach of intestinal mucosal integrity caused by the stiff hairs of the caterpillar. Postmortem findings include serofibrinous pericardial fluid and fibrin tags on the pericardium (**Figure 35.12**). A thick layer of fibrinous to fibrinopurulent exudate, consisting of neutrophils and mononuclear cells mixed with proliferating fibroblasts and fibrin, can be present on the visceral pericardium; the inflammation sometimes extends into the myocardium (Bolin, 2005).

Chylous Effusions Chylous pericardial effusion sometimes develops secondary to systemic fungal disease or mesothelioma, as well as with embolization of apparently benign mesothelial cells to local lymph nodes. Sporadically, the latter also has been seen in dogs with idiopathic pericardial effusion. In cases of chylous pericardial effusion, the pericardial fluid characteristics might have evolved from hemorrhagic into chylous. Lymphatic damage secondary to inflammation of the pericardium and adjacent structures, or from lymphatic embolization, can be involved.

Pathophysiology

Pericardial effusion impairs cardiac function by restricting filling as intrapericardial pressure rises. If the effusion accumulates slowly enough, sufficient pericardial stretching and enlargement might occur to accommodate the increased pericardial fluid volume at a low intrapericardial pressure. As long as intrapericardial pressure stays below normal right heart filling pressures, cardiac filling and output remain relatively normal and clinical signs are absent. However, pericardial tissue is relatively noncompliant. Rapid pericardial fluid accumulation or a large volume of effusion will cause intrapericardial pressure to rise markedly (**Figure 35.13**). This impedes ventricular filling and creates the condition

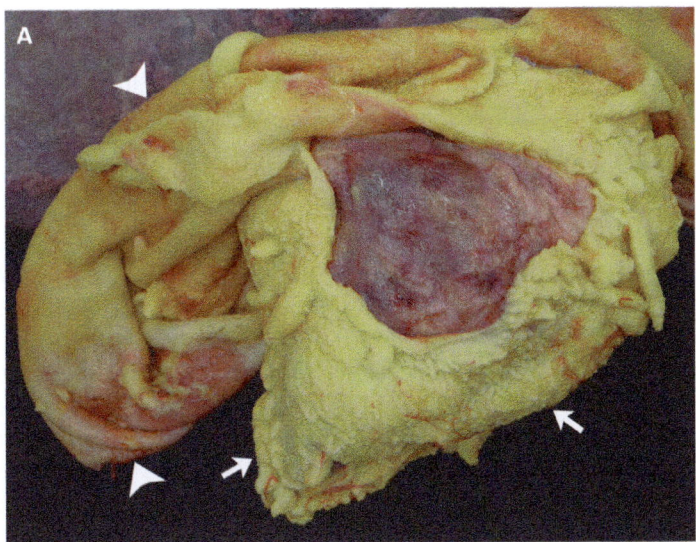 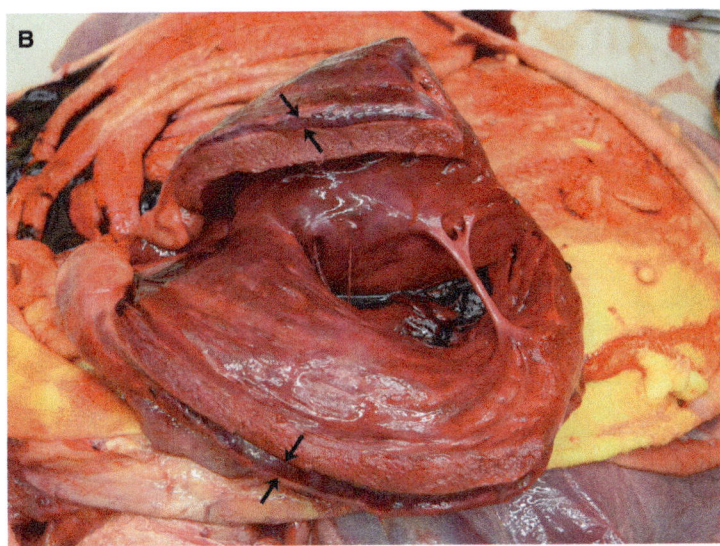

Figure 35.12 (A) Thick (to ~2 cm) yellow shaggy material (fibrin), with finger-like protrusions, covers the visceral pericardium/epicardium (arrows) of a mare with severe chronic-active fibrinous pericarditis. A small area is peeled back to expose the thick irregular cardiac surface. The thick, rough parietal pericardium (arrowheads) is pulled away from the heart. ~8 L of deeply pigmented yellow pericardial fluid was present, as well as ~2 L of pleural fluid with fibrin strands and ~20 L of ascites. (B) The opened right ventricle reveals severe epicardial-subepicardial edema (arrows).

known as *cardiac tamponade*. Pericardial fibrosis and thickening further limit the compliance of this tissue. Pericardial fibrosis and inflammatory infiltrates can occur with idiopathic, inflammatory, and neoplastic effusions.

Other pathophysiologic mechanisms also probably influence some of the observed clinical signs in animals with pericardial disease. For example, an extremely large-volume pericardial effusion might cause clinical signs by virtue of its size, even in the absence of cardiac tamponade. Displacement and compression of the lungs and major airways can cause dyspnea or cough. Esophageal compression could cause dysphagia or regurgitation. Animals with infective causes of pericarditis can have clinical signs related to systemic inflammation before cardiac tamponade develops. Similarly, multicentric or metastatic neoplasia can produce clinical signs caused by extracardiac organ involvement. The pericardial sac, especially when inflamed, can be involved in reflexes that include cough and increasing vagal tone to the heart. This might explain why sinus arrhythmia (rather than tachycardia) occurs in some cases and why larger dogs with pericardial disease might be more prone to atrial fibrillation. Additionally, at least in dogs, vomiting and cough often are reported with pericardial disease. The pericardium contains cough receptors in some species, and it is possible that phrenic nerve stimulation or sudden onset of hypotension might precipitate vomiting in dogs with pericardial effusion (Fahey, 2017).

Cardiac Tamponade Pericardial effusion with cardiac tamponade is a relatively common cardiac diagnosis in dogs; however, tamponade is uncommon in cats and horses. Tamponade develops when intrapericardial pressure rises to equal and exceed normal cardiac diastolic pressures. The rate of pericardial fluid accumulation and the distensibility of the pericardial sac determine whether, and how quickly, cardiac tamponade develops. Rapid accumulation of even a small volume (such as 50–100 mL in dogs) could markedly raise intrapericardial pressure because the pericardium can stretch only slowly. Presence of a large volume of pericardial fluid volume (sometimes >1 L in larger dogs) implies a gradual process. This external cardiac compression limits right then left heart filling. Systemic venous pressure increases while cardiac output falls. Diastolic pressures in all the cardiac chambers and

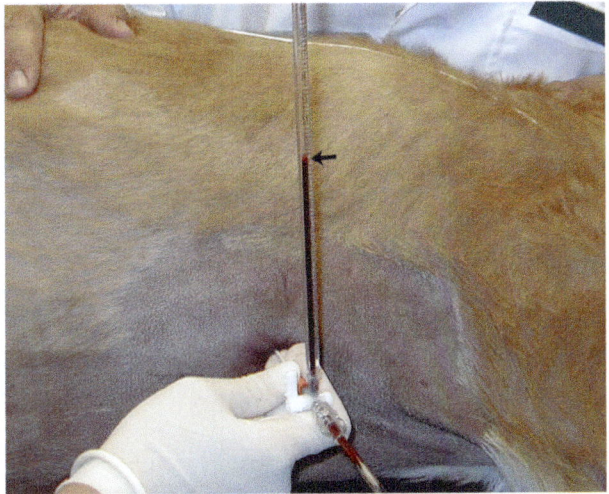

Figure 35.13 Intrapericardial pressure measurement using a water manometer in a dog with cardiac tamponade. In this case, the intrapericardial pressure was just over 12 cm H_2O (arrow). After pericardiocentesis, intrapericardial pressure dropped to ~0 mm Hg.

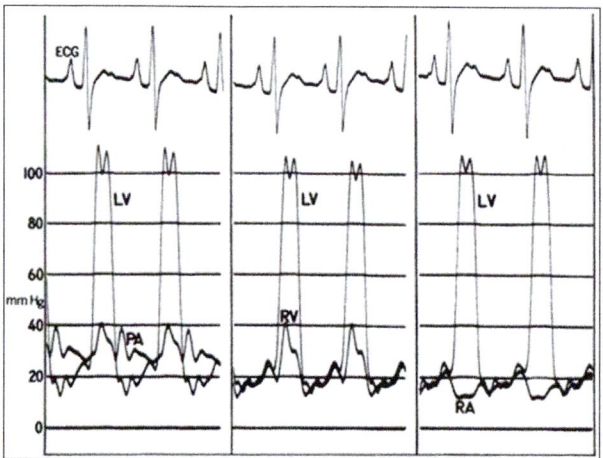

Figure 35.14 Simultaneous pressure recordings from the LV and PA, LV and RV, and LV and RA in a dog with cardiac tamponade. Note the elevated end-diastolic pressure (20–25 mm Hg), equilibrated across the heart; PA and RV systolic pressures also are mildly increased (40 mm Hg). LV, left ventricle; PA, pulmonary artery; RA, right atrium; RV, right ventricle. (From Thomas WP. Pericardial disease. In, Textbook of Veterinary Internal Medicine, 2nd edition. (Ettinger SJ, editor) 1983. WB Saunders, Philadelphia, PA, p. 1082.)

great veins eventually become equilibrated (**Figure 35.14**). Although myocardial contractility is not affected directly by pericardial effusion, reduced coronary perfusion occurs during tamponade, which can impair both systolic and diastolic function. Low cardiac output, arterial hypotension, and poor perfusion of other organs, as well as the heart, ultimately can lead to cardiogenic shock and death. The neurohormonal and renal compensatory mechanisms of heart failure become progressively activated as cardiac output falls. Given sufficient time, increases in plasma volume and systemic venous pressures produce clinical signs of systemic venous congestion and right-sided CHF. However, acute cardiac tamponade can quickly cause profound hypotension or sudden death without congestive signs.

Cardiac tamponade also causes an exaggerated respiratory variation in arterial blood pressure, called *pulsus paradoxus*. Inspiration lowers intrapericardial and right atrial (RA) pressures somewhat, which enhances right heart filling from extrathoracic veins. At the same time, left heart filling is reduced as more blood is held within the pulmonary vessels. Importantly, the interventricular septum bulges leftward from the inspiratory increase in right ventricular (RV) filling; this ventricular interdependence can be appreciated by echocardiography. Consequently, left heart output and systemic arterial pressure decrease during inspiration. Tamponade exaggerates this inspiratory reduction in cardiac output. In patients with pulsus paradoxus, arterial pressure falls by 10 mm Hg or more during inspiration (**Figure 35.15**). During exhalation, the relative differences in right versus left heart filling reverse.

Clinical Features

Beyond a possible predilection to pericardial effusion in the St. Bernard and Golden Retriever breeds, the risks of developing specific neoplasms, especially HSA and chemodectoma, are relevant. These predispositions, as well as breed popularity, clearly influence the canine breeds most often seen for pericardial effusion; some of these breed risks are enumerated in section "Cardiac Tumors." Clinical findings associated with cardiac tamponade typically reflect poor cardiac output and congestion behind the right heart (**Figure 35.16**). The two common presentations are those of collapse due to hypotension or progressive right-sided CHF signs. Although signs of biventricular failure might exist, pulmonary edema is rare. Historical findings of weakness, exercise intolerance, abdominal enlargement, tachypnea, syncope, and cough are

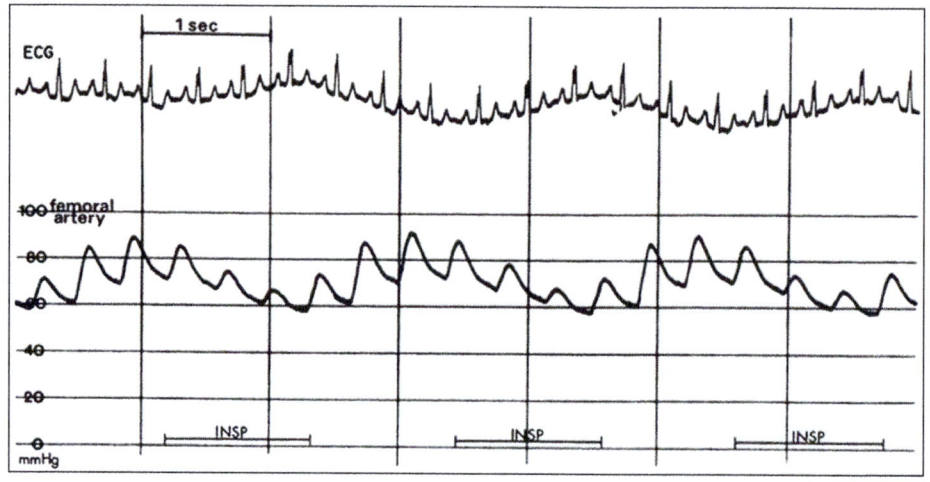

Figure 35.15 Pulsus paradoxus caused by cardiac tamponade. Directly measured femoral arterial pressure shows an exaggerated fall in mean pressure (by ~15–20 mm Hg) and markedly decreased pulse pressure during normal inspiration (INSP). (From Thomas WP. Pericardial disease. In, Textbook of Veterinary Internal Medicine, 2nd edition. (Ettinger SJ, editor) 1983. WB Saunders, Philadelphia, PA, p. 1089.)

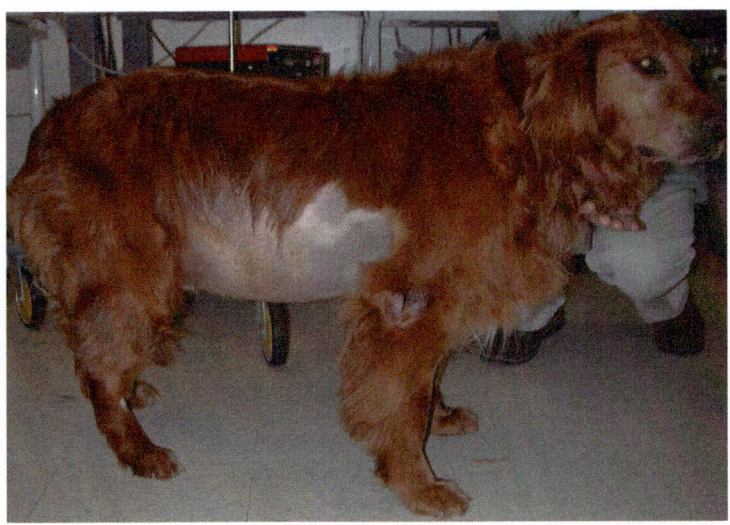

Figure 35.16 7-year-old male Golden Retriever with cardiac tamponade presented for enlarged belly (ascites), lethargy and excessive panting. Weak arterial pulses, distended jugular veins, almost imperceptible precordial impulse, and muffled heart sounds were detected. The dog had cardiac hemangiosarcoma with pulmonary metastases.

typical. Vomiting also appears to be a common historical sign (reported in about half of dogs in one report; Fahey, 2017). Nonspecific findings might occur before obvious ascites develops, including lethargy, weakness, poor exercise tolerance, inappetence, or other GI signs. Loss of lean body mass (cachexia) develops in some chronic cases (**Figure 2.1**, p. 35). Pain related to pericardial stretching, inflammation, or neoplastic processes could be present in some patients, as it is in some people with pericardial disease; however, this is not well studied in animals. Rapid pericardial fluid accumulation can cause acute tamponade, shock, and death. In such cases, jugular venous distension, hypotension, and possibly pulmonary edema could develop without evidence of pleural effusion, ascites, or marked radiographic cardiomegaly.

Physical Findings The classic features of cardiac tamponade are the (Beck's) triad of jugular vein distension, distant or muffled heart sounds, and pulsus paradoxus (paradoxicus). Collapse or right-sided CHF signs are the usual reasons for presentation. Pleural effusion is common with cardiac tamponade. Respiratory signs can be pronounced especially if there is a large pleural effusion. Detection of the jugular venous distension often requires gentle palpation over the vein, as older dogs tend to have thick skin and hair coats. A positive abdominojugular (hepatojugular) reflux (p. 37) also might be apparent. Kussmaul's sign (jugular distension during inspiration, when the right heart is overwhelmed with venous return) is challenging to detect. However, jugular distention can be absent if the patient was inappropriately treated with diuretics prior to examination. In dogs with CHF signs, hepatomegaly, ascites, labored respiration, and weakened femoral pulses are common physical examination findings. Systemic hypotension and collapse could be the predominant signs in dogs with a cardiac mass (or severely enlarged LA) that ruptures, compared to those without such conditions. Ascites suggests a more gradual development or progression of tamponade, and can be present with either non-neoplastic or neoplastic causes of pericardial effusion.

Pulsus paradoxus sometimes is discernable by femoral pulse palpation. Alternatively, pulsus paradoxus might be detected using a Doppler crystal applied to an artery (by listening for audible changes in the signal), or applied as for indirect blood pressure measurement (p. 796) with slow deflation of the cuff. The systolic sounds are heard during expiration only, if the cuff pressure is maintained at just slightly higher than systolic blood pressure during inspiration. High sympathetic tone commonly produces sinus tachycardia, pale mucous membranes, and prolonged capillary refill time; however, some dogs have a normal heart rate or even sinus arrhythmia. An association of pericardial disease with atrial fibrillation in larger breed dogs is probably under-recognized; it can occur before or after pericardiocentesis or surgery. The precordial impulse is palpably weakened when the pericardial fluid volume is large, and it can be imperceptible in some cases. However, acute tamponade with a small pericardial fluid volume is unlikely to reduce precordial impulse strength substantially.

Heart sounds similarly are muffled by a moderate- to large-volume pericardial effusion, yet might seem normal with a small effusion. Pleural effusion will cause muffled lung sounds ventral to the fluid line, and possibly could depress heart sound intensity. Although pericardial effusion does not cause a murmur, concurrent cardiac disease could do so. In dogs with LA rupture secondary to chronic degenerative valve disease, the heart murmur might be considerably softer than at the time of a previous examination. Fever might accompany infectious pericarditis and pericardial friction rubs are sometimes detectable.

Pericarditis in Horses Clinical signs in horses with pericarditis often include lethargy, respiratory signs, anorexia, fever, weight loss (**Figure 35.17**), and signs of colic. But some mares with reproductive loss syndrome show minimal clinical evidence of disease. On physical examination, tachycardia and tachypnea are common. Right-sided congestive signs (jugular venous distension or pulsation, ventral edema, pleural effusion, ascites), as well as low cardiac output signs (weakness, collapse, prerenal azotemia) are likely when cardiac tamponade or constrictive pathophysiology is present. Some cases have muffled heart sounds, especially when the volume of pericardial effusion is large.

Pericardial friction rubs often are described; these are thought to be caused by the rubbing of inflamed visceral and parietal pericardial layers. Classically, pericardial friction rubs have three components (triphasic); these are associated with atrial contraction (presystolic timing), ventricular contraction (systolic), and the end of the rapid ventricular filling phase (diastolic). However, less commonly, only two components (biphasic) might be heard (systolic and diastolic). In

Radiography Radiography depicts the cardiac silhouette enlargement caused by pericardial fluid accumulation. Massive pericardial effusion causes the "classic" globoid-shaped cardiac shadow ("basketball," or "soccer ball," heart) seen on both lateral and DV views (**Figures 35.18** and **35.19**). However, despite the fact that pericardial effusion generally creates a larger and more rounded cardiac silhouette than that seen with other cardiac diseases, radiographic vertebral heart size (VHS) or measures of sphericity are only moderately accurate for identifying pericardial effusion. These indices are neither sensitive nor specific enough to differentiate dogs with pericardial effusion and cardiac tamponade from those with other causes of right-sided CHF signs. For example, both dilated cardiomyopathy and tricuspid dysplasia can cause a similarly large and rounded cardiac silhouette, although subtle contours might be apparent. Generally, with large effusions, the caudodorsal border of the cardiac silhouette on the lateral projections appears more rounded when compared to LA enlargement seen with other causes of heart failure. Smaller volumes of pericardial fluid allow some cardiac contours to be identified, especially those of the atria. Furthermore, the appearance can change between right and left lateral views. With cardiac tamponade, pulmonary vascular markings usually appear normal to

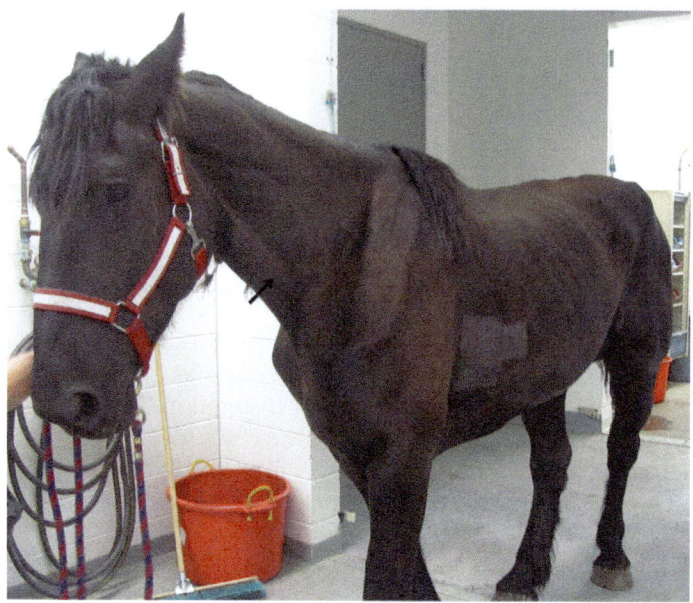

Figure 35.17 Cardiac cachexia (with weight loss of ~350# over 4 months) in a 4-year-old Percheron mare with pericarditis and cardiac tamponade. Jugular venous distension (black arrow) is evident. Other physical findings included subcutaneous edema in the cranioventral and caudoventral trunk (not seen well in photo), sinus tachycardia (HR ~70 beats/min), a weak precordial impulse, and muffled heart sounds with no murmur.

rare cases, only a single friction rub sound might be evident; this could mimic a cardiac murmur. The sounds generated by pericardial friction rubs have been compared to those caused by walking on dry snow, the creaking of a leather saddle, or sawing of wood. Concurrent pleural effusion can produce ventral thoracic dullness on percussion and auscultation. Horses with pericarditis might have concurrent pleuropneumonia or pleuritis, which contributes to pleural fluid accumulation and other clinical signs.

Diagnostic Tests

Laboratory Tests Routine serum biochemistry tests in animals with pericardial effusion and tamponade could reflect hepatic congestion and low cardiac output (prerenal azotemia), but otherwise are non-contributory. The hemogram sometimes shows a nonregenerative or poorly regenerative anemia in dogs with neoplastic, as well as benign, effusions. Occasional cases have hypoproteinemia. Serum cTnI could be useful in differentiating pericardial effusion caused by HSA from other causes, especially when a mass lesion is not obvious on echocardiogram. Based on one report, cTnI elevation suggests that cardiac HSA is more likely (Chun, 2010). HSA involving other organs does not increase serum cTnI concentration. Pericardial fluid also can be used for cTnI assay, although this does not provide improved sensitivity. Serum N-terminal probrain (B-type) natriuretic peptide (NT-proBNP) concentration is likely to be low in patients with pericardial effusion, in contrast to other cardiac diseases. It might increase slightly after pericardiocentesis.

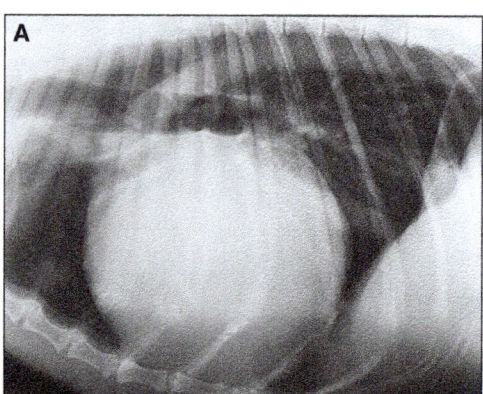
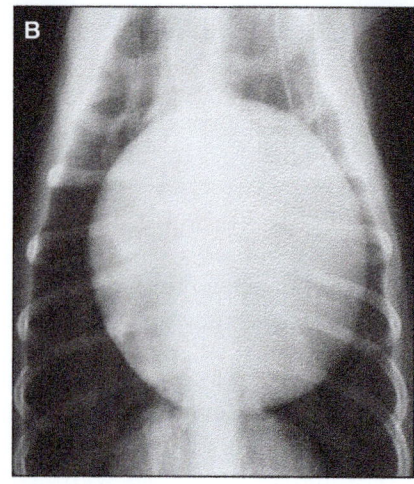

Figure 35.18 Lateral (A) and DV (B) radiographs show the classic "ball-shaped" cardiac silhouette in an Afghan Hound with large pericardial effusion. Cardiac contours are completely obscured.

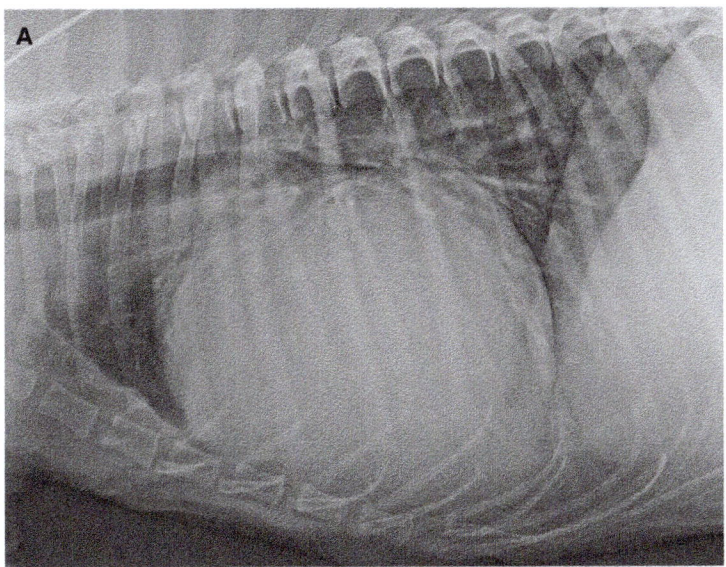
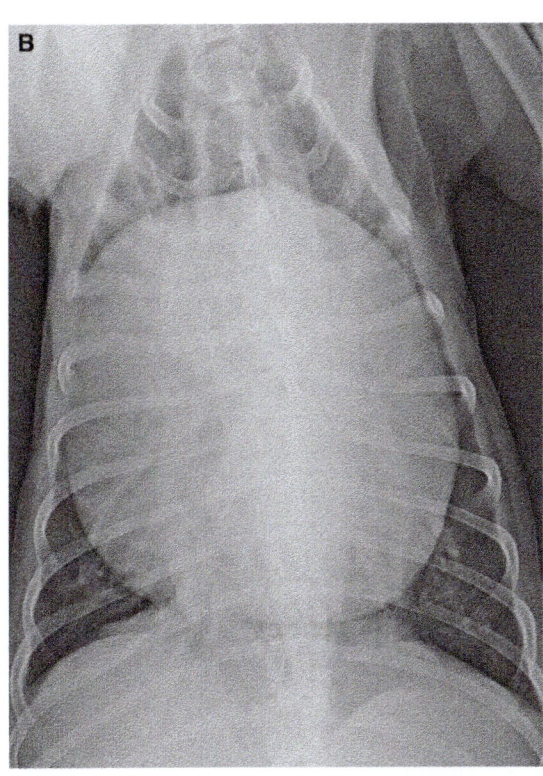

Figure 35.19 Lateral (A) and DV (B) thoracic radiographs from a 13-year-old Coonhound with massive pericardial effusion and a heart base tumor. The presenting complaint was a hacking cough. A slow process of fluid accumulation over time is necessary to generate such a large volume of pericardial effusion; >1 L of hemorrhagic fluid was removed.

diminished, in contrast to other causes of heart failure (such as dilated cardiomyopathy) where vessels often are prominent to enlarged. A large heart base tumor could cause supravalvular pulmonary stenosis, and compromise flow to certain lung lobes. Other findings associated with cardiac tamponade, as well as other causes of right-sided CHF, include pleural effusion, caudal vena caval distension, hepatomegaly, and ascites (**Figure 35.20**). In experimental pericardial disease of the dog, interstitial pulmonary edema can develop; however, pulmonary opacities of edema and distended pulmonary veins are only occasionally present. Some heart base tumors cause (leftward) deviation or elevation of the trachea, a soft tissue mass effect, or both, especially just cranial to the heart. Although these findings are strongly suggestive of a heart base mass, radiographic findings usually are not adequately sensitive for identifying such tumors. Metastatic lung lesions are common in dogs with HSA, but might only be evident by CT imaging.

Electrocardiography ECG findings can include small-amplitude QRS complexes (<1 mV in all frontal plane leads for dogs), electrical alternans, and ST segment elevation (**Figures 35.21–35.23**). Electrical alternans is a recurring, every-other-beat alteration in the size or configuration of the QRS complex and sometimes, the T wave. It is seen most often with large-volume pericardial effusions and results from the heart's rhythmic swinging back and forth within the pericardial fluid. Electrical alternans might be more evident at heart rates between 90–140 beats/min or in certain body positions (especially standing). In the absence of supraventricular tachycardia, it is relatively specific but insensitive for identifying pericardial effusion. Electrical alternans could be confused with respiratory artifact, but that also will lead to marked baseline movement. ST segment depression usually indicates myocardial ischemia. ST segment elevation is less common and usually relates to an epicardial injury current associated with pericarditis and epicardial inflammation. Sinus tachycardia often accompanies cardiac tamponade, although a normal heart rate and sinus arrhythmia can be present. Atrial or ventricular tachyarrhythmias are relatively common. Recurrent isolated atrial premature complexes might be an indication of tumor infiltration within the atrium. The combination of atrial distention, activation of vagal reflexes, and premature atrial beats could trigger atrial fibrillation. Ventricular premature complexes are quite common, whether the effusion is neoplastic or not. Iatrogenic ventricular beats also can occur during pericardiocentesis. Persistent ventricular tachycardia that is resistant to therapy should heighten suspicion for neoplastic infiltration within the ventricle.

Echocardiography Echocardiography is the diagnostic test of choice because it is highly sensitive for noninvasively detecting even small-volume pericardial effusions, and it can document the large majority of underlying mass lesions or other

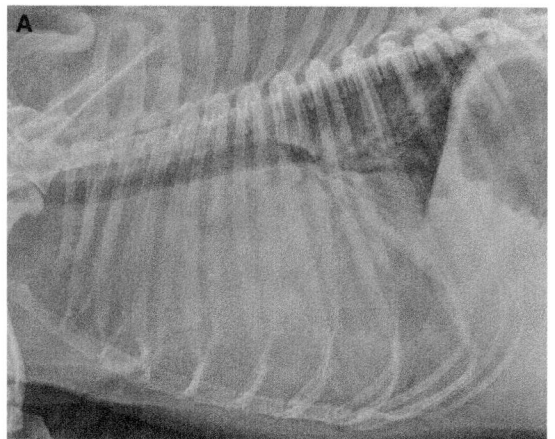
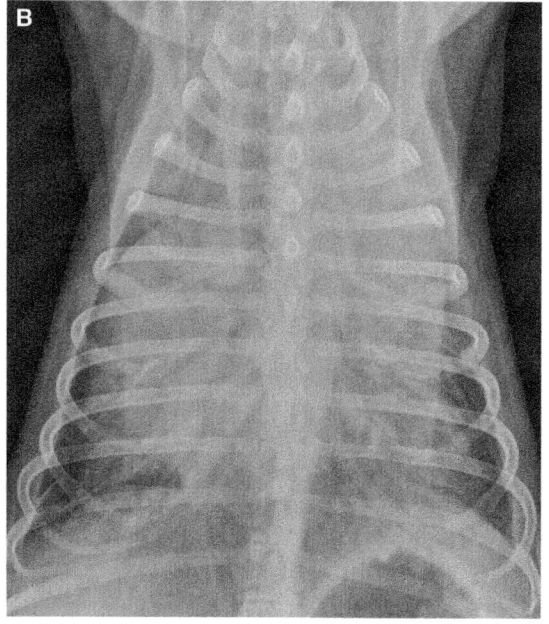
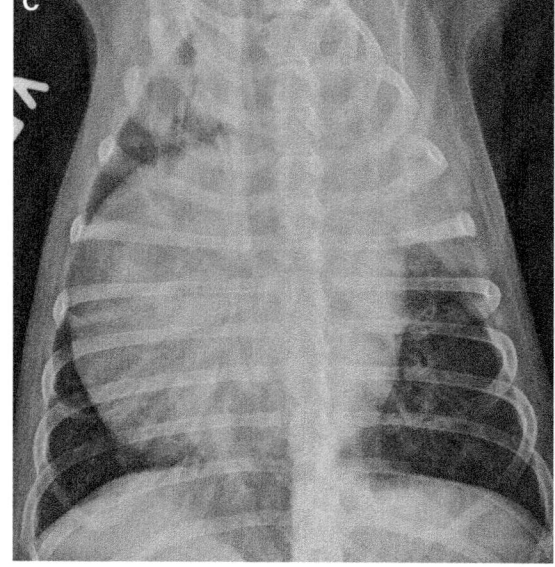

Figure 35.20 Cardiac tamponade eventually produces right-sided congestive signs, as in this 10-year-old male Cocker Spaniel, presented for inappetence, coughing and ascites. Lateral (A) and DV (B) radiographs show a modest amount of pleural effusion. Nevertheless, marked enlargement of the cardiac silhouette is still evident, especially with the dorsal tracheal displacement (A). The VD view (C) clearly reveals a globoid cardiac silhouette, as pleural fluid has collected in the gutters along the spine. A large heart base mass was identified in this case.

cardiac conditions. Clinicians with basic training in echocardiography or only the "thoracic focused assessment with sonography for trauma" (TFAST) ultrasound exam should be able to identify and differentiate pericardial and pleural effusions. Especially important in patients with collapse or respiratory distress, a TFAST exam can reveal pericardial effusion and tamponade quickly, before radiographs are obtained. The diaphragmaticohepatic view shows the pericardial effusion in most cases, although small-volume effusion might be missed; the TFAST pericardial view or serial exams can increase the sensitivity of this test. Nevertheless, after the patient has been stabilized, a more detailed echocardiographic (echo) exam is warranted to identify and define any mass lesions or other cardiac disease. This echo exam should entail all standard right- and left-sided views and might require some off-angle views. The left cranial long-axis plane, angled to visualize the RA appendage, is especially important (p. 718). This exam preferably would be done by a cardiologist, or other individual with advanced training and skill in echocardiography.

Pericardial effusion appears as an echo-free space between the bright parietal pericardium and the epicardium (**Figures 35.24–35.28**). Echocardiography also reveals abnormal cardiac wall motion and chamber shape, as well as intrapericardial or intracardiac mass lesions that might be present (**Figures 35.29–35.31**). Sometimes pleural effusion, marked LA (and auricular) enlargement, a dilated coronary sinus, or persistent left cranial vena cava might be misinterpreted as pericardial effusion, so images must be obtained and evaluated carefully (**Figure 29.25**, p. 548). Visualizing an atrial appendage surrounded by fluid, as well as identifying the parietal pericardium in relation to the echo-free fluid, helps in differentiating pleural from pericardial effusions.

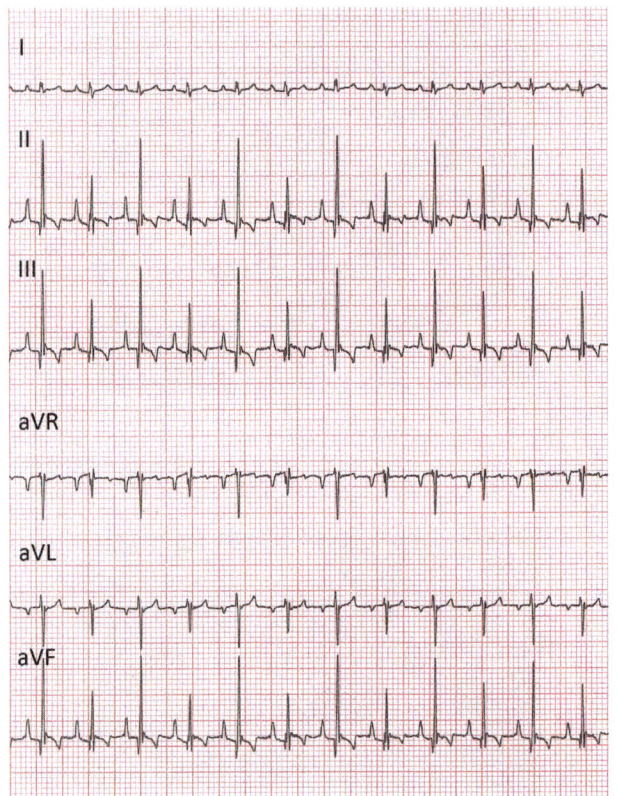

Figure 35.21 Electrical alternans is prominent in this ECG from a 13-year-old mixed-breed dog with a large pericardial effusion. Sinus rhythm. Leads as marked, 25 mm/s, 1 cm = 1 mV.

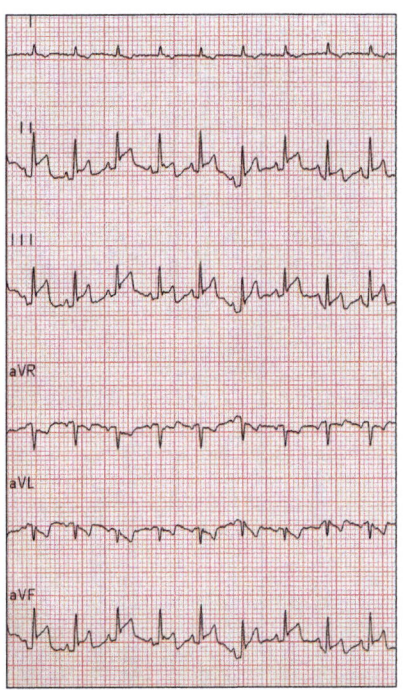

Figure 35.23 ECG from a 10-year-old dog with pericardial effusion and large tumor invading lateral right atrial and ventricular walls. Note ST-segment elevation and small QRS complexes. Sinus rhythm. Leads as marked, 25 mm/s, 1 cm = 1 mV.

The pericardium typically produces the brightest echoes, so if the operator progressively damps returning echo signals, this structure's echoes persist the longest. Furthermore, evidence of collapsed lung lobes or pleural folds usually can be seen within pleural effusion. Because pericardial fluid is subject to gravity, most appears around the ventricles. However,

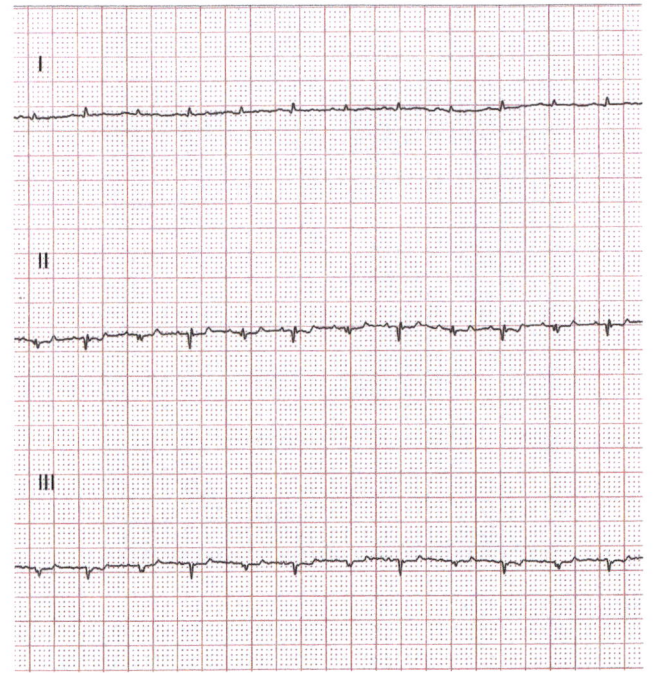

Figure 35.22 Tiny QRS complexes in an 8-year-old male Boxer with large pericardial effusion and tamponade. Low-voltage QRS complexes are common with large-volume pericardial effusion. Note the subtle electrical alternans. Sinus rhythm. Leads as marked, 25 mm/s, 1 cm = 1 mV.

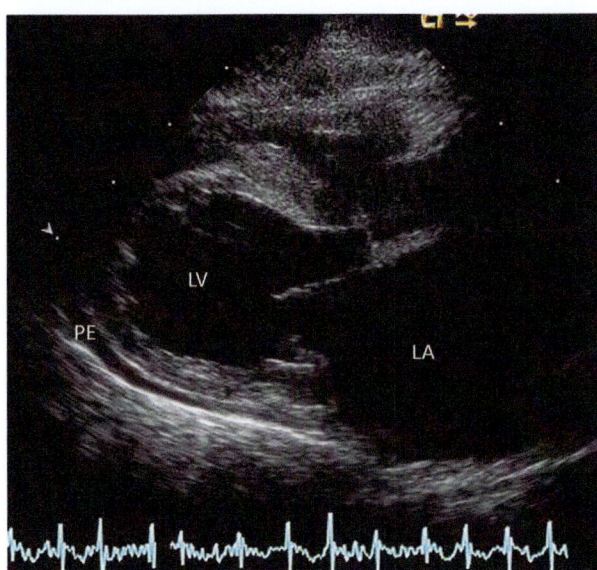

Figure 35.24 Echocardiography reveals a small rim of pericardial effusion behind the LV in this 10-year-old male Domestic Shorthair cat with restrictive cardiomyopathy. Right parasternal long-axis view. LA, left atrium; LV, left ventricle; PE, pericardial effusion.

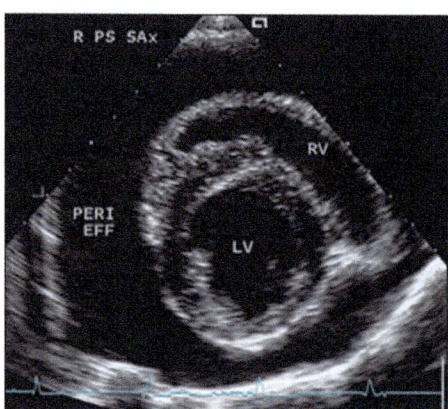

Figure 35.25 Moderately large pericardial effusion (PERI EFF) in a 2-year-old female Labrador Retriever. In this unusual case, the fluid was chylous and caused by systemic blastomycosis. Right parasternal short-axis view. LA, left atrium; LV, left ventricle.

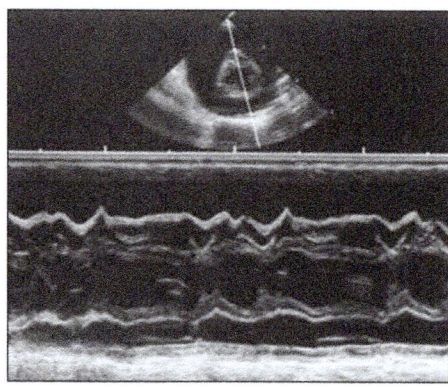

Figure 35.26 Large echolucency of pericardial effusion surrounds the heart in this duplex 2D/M-mode image at ventricular level, from a 10-year-old female Miniature Schnauzer with a heart base tumor. Cardiac tamponade caused poor ventricular filling.

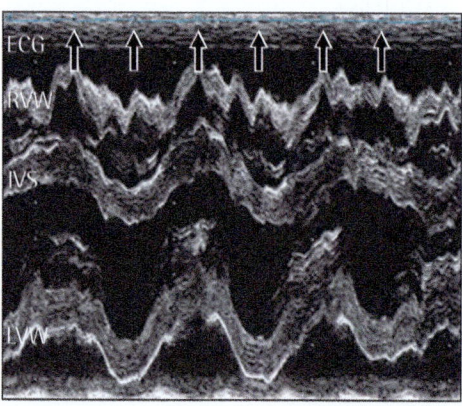

Figure 35.27 Large-volume pericardial effusion allows the heart to swing back and forth on alternating heartbeats, causing the electrical alternans seen on ECG in some dogs. This M-mode image (ventricular level) shows this motion. Note how the heart's relative position shifts with every QRS complex (arrows). ECG, electrocardiogram; IVS, interventricular septum; LVW, left ventricular wall; RVW, right ventricular wall.

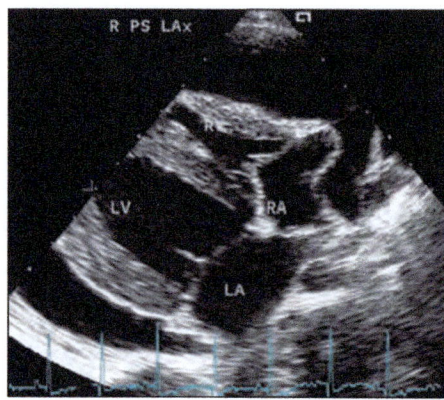

Figure 35.28 Cardiac tamponade compresses the RV and RA, causing variable mural collapse (here at onset of diastole). Right parasternal long-axis. LA, left atrium; LV, left ventricle; RA, right atrium; RV, right ventricle.

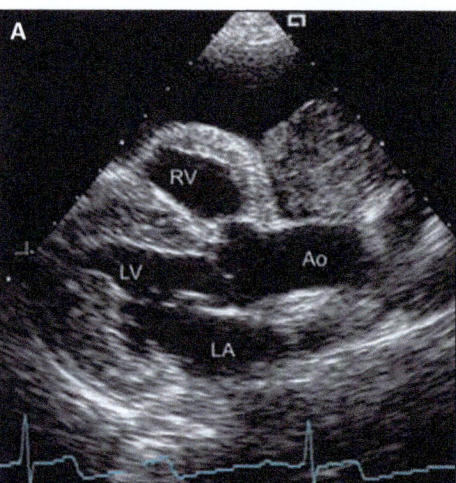

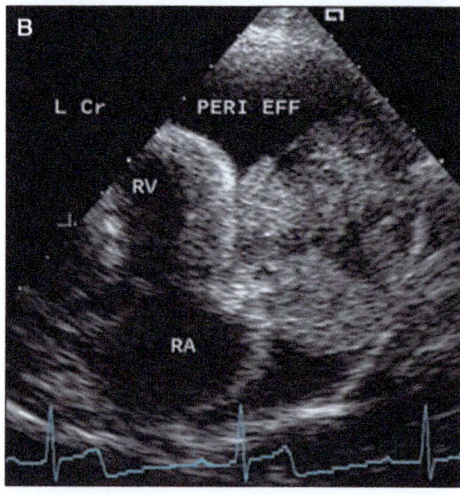

Figure 35.29 (A) A large soft tissue mass is near the right ventricular wall and ascending aorta in a 10-year-old Keeshond with cardiac tamponade. The origin of the mass is not clear from this right parasternal long-axis 2D view. (B) Left cranial long-axis view, optimized for RA and auricle. The tumor mass appears to arise from the auricular tip, as is typical for hemangiosarcoma. This is the best view for evaluating the right auricular area. Ao, aorta; LA, left atrium; LV, left ventricle; PERI EFF, pericardial effusion; RA, right atrium; RV, right ventricle.

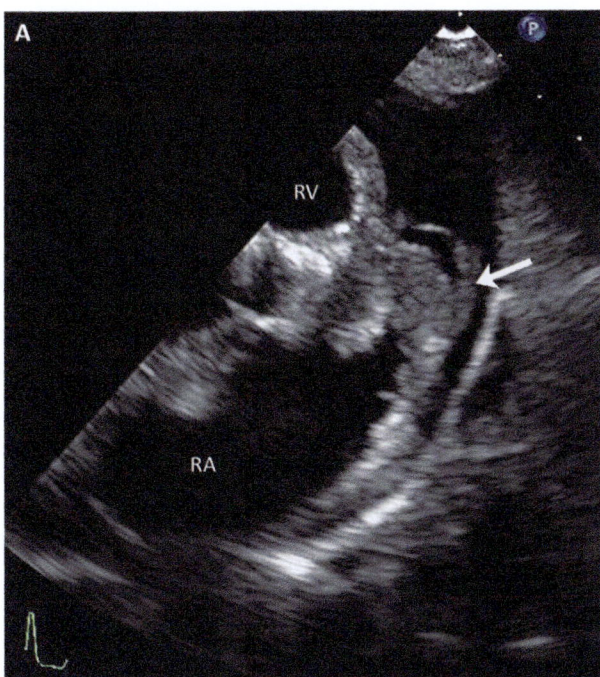

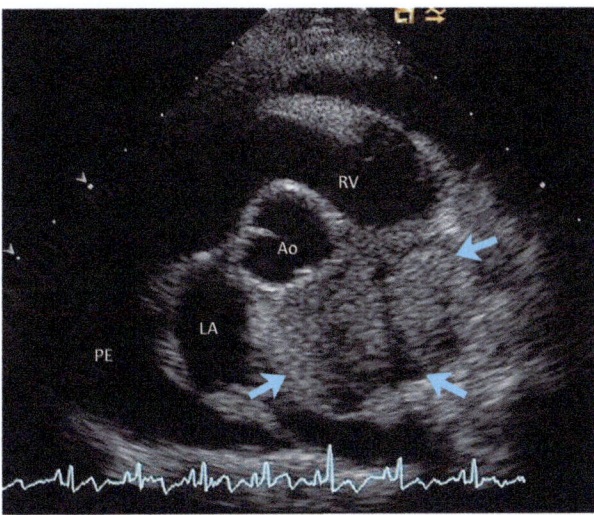

Figure 35.31 An aortic body tumor (arrows) is visible at the heart base, nestled between the aortic root, LA and origin of the main pulmonary artery in a 13-year-old female French Bulldog. Ao, aorta; LA, left atrium; PE, pericardial effusion; RV, right ventricle.

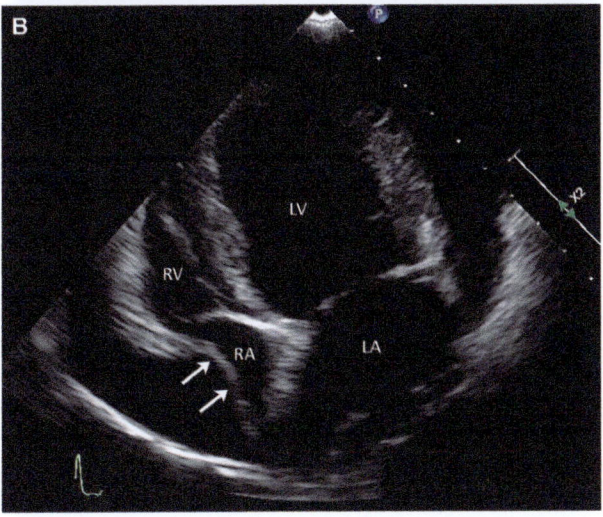

Figure 35.30 (A) A small hemangiosarcoma mass (arrow) is present at the tip of the right auricle in an 11-year-old Labrador Retriever. This left cranial long-axis imaging plane was the only view where a mass was visible. (B) Left apical 4-chamber view documents the right atrial wall collapse (arrows) associated with cardiac tamponade in this dog. LA, left atrium; LV, left ventricle; RA, right atrium; RV, right ventricle.

unlike the situation in humans, some pericardial effusion can be seen more dorsally and behind the left atrium. Subcostal imaging can be helpful, as it often shows both pleural and pericardial effusions. In addition, subcostal imaging in dogs with tamponade typically reveals vena caval and hepatic vein dilation, with loss of respiratory variation in caval diameter. Ascites can be absent or massive in pericardial disease.

Cardiac tamponade is characterized by collapse of the RA, and sometimes RV, wall (**Figures 35.28** and **35.30B**). As intrapericardial pressure rises with the accumulating effusion, compression then collapse of the RA wall signals the onset of cardiac tamponade. Initially, the RA wall collapses transiently during ventricular systole. As tamponade worsens, RA wall collapse intensifies and extends into diastole. Diastolic RV compression and collapse occur with advancing tamponade and suggest that intrapericardial and intracardiac pressures have equalized. Further rise in intrapericardial pressure exacerbates the diastolic RV collapse, compresses the left ventricle, and signals severe tamponade with its extreme hemodynamic compromise. Immediate pericardiocentesis is especially urgent in patients with this degree of cardiac tamponade and showing clinical signs of hypotension. Large pleural effusions also can cause some degree of right heart collapse; however, collapse extending over 50% of the cardiac cycle is more likely to be caused by cardiac tamponade. Furthermore, pulmonary hypertension and plasma volume status can affect the degree of right heart chamber collapse. In compensated tamponade, high systemic venous pressure opposes RA and RV collapse. Conversely, diuretic administration diminishes this compensation so RA and RV wall collapse (signaling tamponade) is more likely to occur.

The cardiac chamber size (volume) is normal to small with typical cardiac tamponade. Following pericardiocentesis, the elevated venous pressures can abruptly enlarge the chambers. However, marked atrial dilation prior to pericardiocentesis suggests a concurrent cardiac disease, such as mitral or tricuspid valvular disease, cardiomyopathy, or the uncommon constrictive-effusive pericardial disease. In cats, the heart should be evaluated comprehensively because even a moderate to large effusion can be secondary to heart failure from cardiomyopathy. Precisely why this occurs is unknown, but it might relate to the effect of increased venous pressures on lymphatic drainage from the pericardial space. In general, an enlarged left atrium in a cat predicts that the pericardial effusion stems from CHF, accepting the potential for coexistent pericardial disease and cardiomyopathy. Considering the higher risk of pericardiocentesis in this species, medical therapy for heart failure usually is initiated first (unless there is evidence for severe tamponade).

Idiopathic pericardial effusion is a diagnosis of exclusion, after neoplastic, infectious, or other causes have been ruled out. Unfortunately, some mass lesions are not easily visualized. An estimated 15-20% of HSAs and chemodectomas are probably missed at the first examination, even by skilled personnel. Furthermore, mesothelioma without a discrete mass lesion cannot be reliably distinguished by noninvasive tests. It is easier to define small masses on or near the heart when they are surrounded by anechoic fluid. So if the patient is stable enough, it is helpful to do the echocardiogram before pericardiocentesis. However, if signs of severe tamponade (such as collapse, hypotension or dyspnea) are present and especially if there would be delay in obtaining an advanced cardiology evaluation, pericardiocentesis (p. 724) should be done immediately.

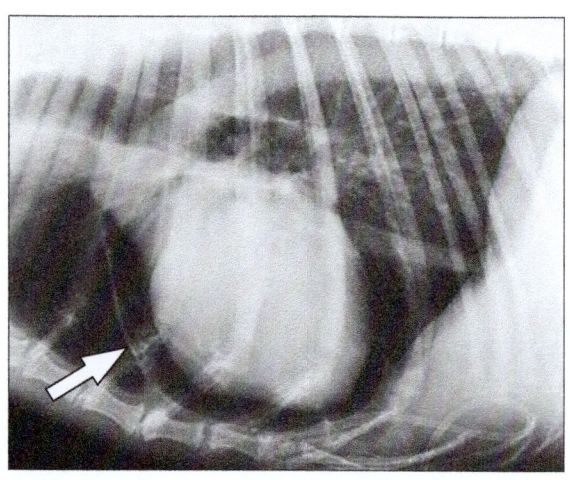

Figure 35.32 Lateral pneumopericardiogram from the dog in **Figure 35.18** shows the pericardium (arrow) distended with air and normal cardiac contours, with no evidence of a mass lesion. The intrapericardial catheter lies cranioventral to the heart.

Other Imaging CT and MRI imaging provides greater detail than plain radiographs and can better reveal pulmonary metastases and other extracardiac lesions. Yet based on limited reports, these modalities are not proven better than echocardiography for identifying pericardial effusion and associated mass lesions. Cardiac MRI could better define anatomical structures, including the location and extent of mass lesions or vascular obstructions in cases where echo findings cannot clearly define whether small mass lesions are present in the heart or pericardium. However, neither MRI nor CT necessarily detect all mass lesions. Diagnosis of cardiac masses also can be challenging if the study is not ECG-gated. As with echocardiography, misinterpretation or over-reading of mass lesions can occur, and some experience is required to find the best balance of sensitivity and specificity.

Other imaging techniques can yield diagnostic information, although echocardiography has essentially replaced them. Fluoroscopy can differentiate a large pericardial effusion from cardiomegaly, because motion of the cardiac silhouette is diminished to absent when fluid surrounds the heart. Angiocardiography, although now rarely used to diagnose pericardial effusion and cardiac neoplasia, can reveal increased endocardial-to-pericardial distance; cardiac tumors often displace normal structures and cause filling defects or angiographic vascular "blushing" (during the systemic arterial phase). Echocardiography (as well as CT and MRI) also has replaced the use of pneumopericardiography, where injection of CO_2 or air into the drained pericardial sac is used to outline the heart radiographically (**Figure 35.32**). Left lateral and DV views allow the injected gas to outline the RA and heart base areas, respectively, where tumors are most commonly located.

Central Venous Pressure and Right Heart Catheterization Central venous pressure (CVP) measurement is a potential diagnostic aid for recognizing elevated systemic pressure, although it is probably most valuable in constrictive disease, where the heart is not enlarged or effusion is absent. CVP measurement also might be helpful when the jugular veins are difficult to assess. Normally, CVP is <8 cm H_2O in dogs; a CVP >10–12 cm H_2O is common with cardiac tamponade (lower in cats; higher in horses). It might not be as elevated in the setting of volume depletion (low-pressure tamponade). Tamponade alters the RA pressure (and CVP) waveforms by markedly diminishing the y descent (which occurs during ventricular relaxation and filling) while maintaining or exaggerating the x' descent. During tamponade, ventricular diastolic expansion immediately raises intrapericardial and RV diastolic pressures, so caval flow into the right atrium is impaired then. However, blood flow into the right atrium (and x' descent) continues to occur during ventricular contraction. As noted earlier, cardiac tamponade also raises RV filling pressure, leading to diastolic pressure equilibration across the heart (**Figure 35.14**).

Pericardial Fluid Evaluation Cytologic evaluation helps characterize the fluid, although reliable differentiation of sanguineous neoplastic effusions from benign hemorrhagic pericarditis usually is not possible. Pericardial fluid cytology is nondiagnostic in most (>90%) dogs, especially those with hemorrhagic effusion (Cagle, 2014). It often is nondiagnostic in horses, as well (see next paragraphs). Even in cases where a mass lesion is visualized with echocardiography, cytology rarely provides an etiologic diagnosis. Reactive mesothelial cells within the effusion can resemble neoplastic cells. Furthermore, common tumors such as chemodectoma and HSA often do not shed cells into the effusion. Nevertheless, in a small percentage of animals with pericardial effusion, fluid cytology might reveal a neoplastic or infectious cause. The likelihood of cytologic diagnosis is higher (~20%) in effusions of low hematocrit (<10%). Pericardial fluid associated with cardiac lymphoma tends to be serous, and neoplastic lymphocytes usually are apparent on cytologic examination.

Neoplastic (and other noninflammatory) effusions tend to have a pH of 7.0 or greater; inflammatory effusions (including benign idiopathic pericarditis) tend to have lower pH values. However, there is too much overlap between these groups for pericardial fluid pH to be a reliable discriminator. However, if cytologic evaluation and fluid pH suggest an infectious or inflammatory cause, pericardial fluid culture is advised. Immunodiagnostic tests for coccidioidomycosis or Chagas disease might be helpful in endemic areas, and other immunodiagnostic tests also could be useful in some patients. Elevated cTnI, either in serum or pericardial fluid, is more suggestive of cardiac HSA, or other cause of myocardial injury. Patient diagnosis should not be based only on cTnI concentration.

Pericarditis in Horses There are no specific findings on routine clinical laboratory tests. Some cases have leukocytosis, hyperproteinemia or hyperfibrinogenemia. Horses with pericarditis associated with chronic or immune-mediated disease sometimes are anemic. Prerenal azotemia and electrolyte abnormalities can occur with cardiac tamponade or constrictive pericardial disease. Serologic testing for equine herpes viral arteritis or influenza virus titers might suggest a viral etiology. For horses with concurrent respiratory disease, tracheal wash or pleural fluid cytology and culture could be helpful.

Thoracic radiography generally is not useful for diagnosis. Echocardiography allows identification of pericardial fluid (as in small animals), as well as evidence for cardiac tamponade or constrictive pathophysiology, if present. The volume of pericardial fluid is quite large in some cases. Fibrin (fibrinous pericarditis) causes the pericardial surfaces to appear shaggy (**Figure 35.33**). The fibrin tags have variable distribution and echogenicity over the epicardial and parietal pericardial surfaces. An ECG might show electrical alternans in cases with large-volume pericardial effusion, as in dogs (**Figures 35.21** and **35.22**); the QRS complex amplitude also might be diminished.

Pericardial fluid analysis is important, although it often is nondiagnostic. Cytologic examination, bacterial culture and sensitivity testing, and virus isolation or titers might yield an etiologic diagnosis in some cases; however, findings are negative in many. In some septic exudative effusions, bacteria could be evident. Yet culture and sensitivity testing often is unrewarding, especially if antimicrobial therapy was used prior to pericardial fluid sampling. *Streptococcus* spp. historically have been the most common bacteria isolated from equine pericarditis cases. However, both Gram-positive and Gram-negative organisms could be found on cytologic examination of pericardial fluid from horses. Pericarditis associated with mare reproductive loss syndrome typically produces pericardial fluid with a low white count (mostly neutrophils) and a high protein content. Although the pericardial fluid appears to be a sterile exudate in many cases, *Actinobacillus* spp. might be isolated in some horses; *Escherichia coli* and *Enterococcus faecalis* also have been found. Neoplastic cells might be evident in cases with an underlying cardiac or pericardial tumor.

Management

In all species, it is important to differentiate cardiac tamponade from other causes of right-sided CHF signs because its treatment is so different. Diuretic and vasodilator drugs can further decrease cardiac output and exacerbate hypotension by reducing cardiac filling pressure; the compressed cardiac

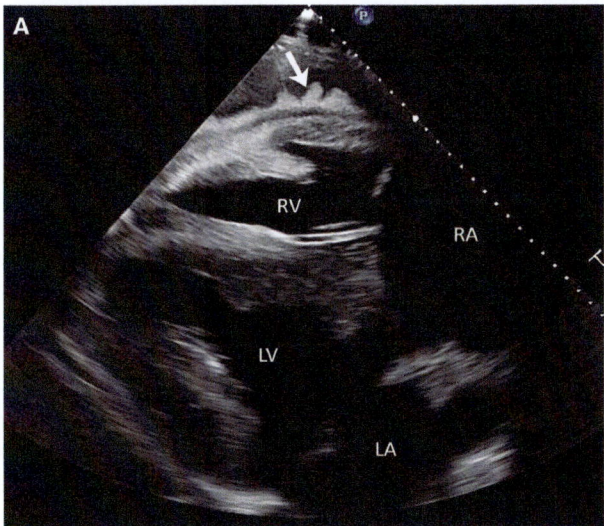 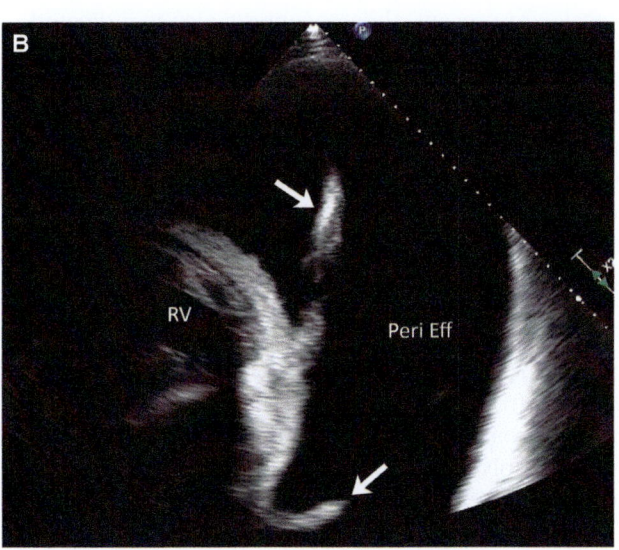

Figure 35.33 (A) Right parasternal long-axis echocardiogram from the horse of **Figure 35.12** shows the shaggy layer of fibrinous material (arrow) covering the visceral pericardium and somewhat cellular-appearing pericardial effusion in the near field. The thin line of echolucency between the shaggy material and the ventricular myocardium corresponds to the edematous epicardial-subepicardial region seen in **Figure 35.12B**. (B) An off-angle image from the same patient shows two of the large finger-like projections (arrows) that extended from the thick visceral pericardial coating into the pericardial space. LA, left atrium; LV, left ventricle; Peri eff, pericardial effusion; RA, right atrium; RV, right ventricle.

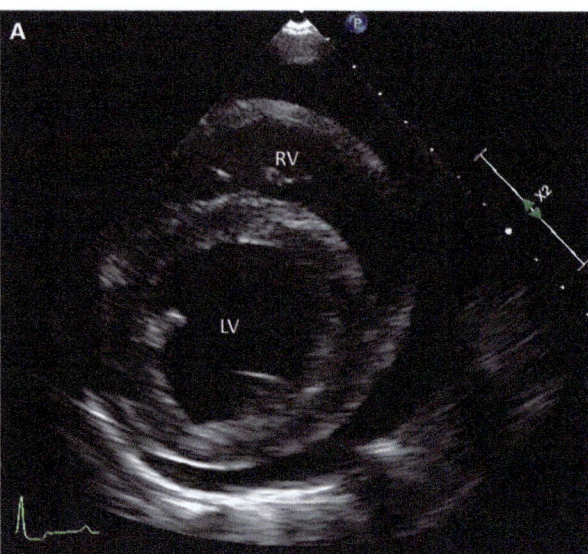 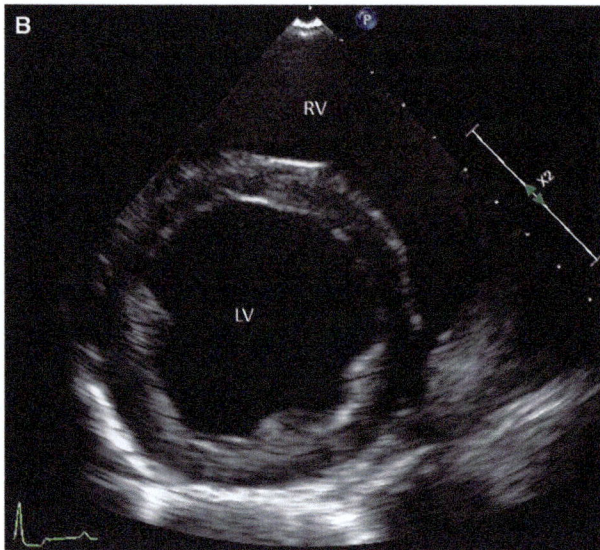

Figure 35.34 (A) End-diastolic 2D echo frame showing the compressed RV and LV in an 11-year-old Labrador Retriever with cardiac tamponade. Although the volume of effusion in this case is only modest, intrapericardial pressure had increased enough to cause tamponade. (B) End-diastolic frame after pericardiocentesis shows a marked increase in ventricular filling, once the elevated intrapericardial pressure was reduced. Right parasternal short-axis view. LV, left ventricle; RV, right ventricle.

chambers require high venous pressure in order to fill. Positive inotropic drugs do not improve cardiac output or ameliorate the signs of tamponade because the main underlying pathophysiology is impaired cardiac filling, not poor contractility. The effect of small volume resuscitation is somewhat more controversial, but in hypotensive patients with systolic pressure <100 mm Hg, a rapid bolus of crystalloid fluid (~5 to 10 ml/kg) should be considered. Although this will raise venous and intrapericardial pressures, it can increase blood pressure in most patients. When a large pleural effusion and compression atelectesis are present, thoracocentesis also is indicated.

Immediate pericardiocentesis is the initial therapeutic procedure for cardiac tamponade (**Figure 35.34**). It could also provide some diagnostic information. Signs of hypotension usually abate within minutes and those of CHF resolve soon (usually over 1-3 days) after intrapericardial pressure is reduced by fluid removal. Some animals with severe fluid retention might benefit from a modest dose or two of furosemide after pericardiocentesis, to help mobilize secondary abdominal or pleural effusions. Identification of the underlying cause for the pericardial effusion is important to guide further management. Pericardial effusion that develops secondary to CHF from other acquired or congenital cardiac disease, or to hypoalbuminemia, usually does not cause tamponade, often resolves with management of the underlying disease, and therefore, usually does not need to be drained.

Pericardiocentesis Pericardiocentesis is a relatively safe procedure when performed carefully. There is no single "best" way to perform this procedure and different operators hold various preferences for the technique. Nevertheless, some principles apply. Mild sedation (butorphanol) is helpful, depending on the clinical status, blood pressure, and temperament of the animal. Continuous ECG monitoring during the procedure is strongly recommended because needle or catheter contact with the heart commonly provokes ventricular arrhythmias. An IV catheter should be placed prior to pericardiocentesis, to provide access for sedative, antiarrhythmic, or other drug administration, as needed. Especially in hypotensive patients, as noted previously, an IV fluid bolus can help support cardiac output and blood pressure during preparations for the pericardial tap. However, the pericardiocentesis procedure should not be unduly delayed because of fluid administration.

Pericardiocentesis typically is approached from the right side of the chest to minimize the risk of trauma to the lung (by using the cardiac notch area) and coronary vessels on the left lateral cardiac surface (**Figure 35.35**). Echo-guidance is useful to identify an optimal location from which to reach the pericardial fluid, but the probe generally is removed once the procedure starts. It also is helpful to measure the distance from the superficial chest wall to the parietal pericardium and to the heart; this informs the selection of an appropriate pericardiocentesis catheter or needle. However, for compartmentalized or very small volume effusions, continual ultrasound guidance during pericardiocentesis is valuable. In this situation, the probe could be covered with a sterile sheath and sterile coupling gel used if placement within the sterile field is required.

The small animal patient generally is placed in left lateral or sternal recumbency, or in an intermediate position (left lateral, with a foam wedge under the spine), to allow more stable restraint. Alternatively, good success can be had using an elevated echocardiography table with a large cut-out; in this situation, the animal is placed in right lateral recumbency and the tap is performed from underneath (**Figure 35.36**). The

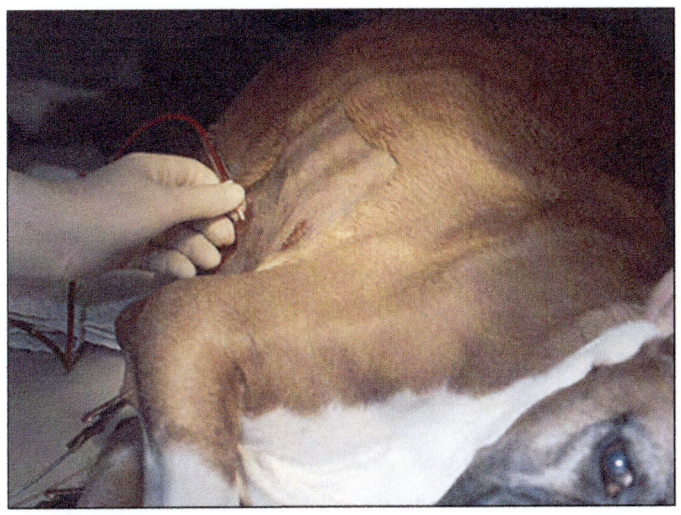

Figure 35.35 Pericardiocentesis was performed with this Boxer in left lateral recumbency. Note the (typical) hemorrhagic pericardial fluid.

advantage of this method is that gravity pulls fluid down to the right side; however, if adequate space is not available for wide sterile skin preparation or needle/catheter manipulation, this approach is not advised. Needle pericardiocentesis can be successfully performed on a standing dog, but the risk of injury is increased if the patient moves suddenly. In horses, pericardiocentesis is done with the animal standing (also see p. 729).

A variety of equipment can be used for pericardiocentesis. In an emergency situation, an appropriately long hypodermic or spinal needle attached to extension tubing could be used; for a tiny dog or cat, a butterfly needle can be effective. However, a far safer alternative is an over-the-needle catheter system. For example, an 18–20 gauge, 3.75–5.0 cm (1.5–2.0 inch) long catheter is adequate for small dogs. Larger over-the-needle catheter systems, such as a 12–16 gauge, 10–15 cm (4–6 inch) system, allow for faster fluid removal in large dogs. Another option for pericardiocentesis is to use a

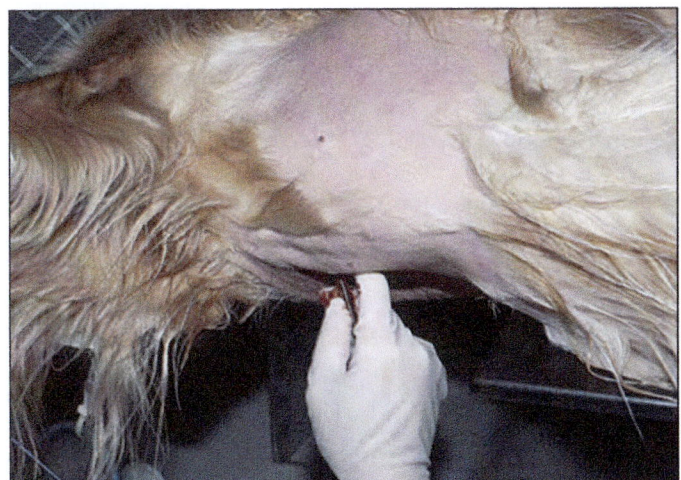

Figure 35.36 Gravity can facilitate drainage of pericardial effusion when the animal is placed in right lateral recumbency on an elevated tabletop with a large cut-out, as used for echocardiography.

hemodialysis fistula needle (Celona, 2017). If pericardiocentesis is indicated in a cat, a small-gauge butterfly needle or 20–22 g over-the-needle catheter can be used. An alternative method in larger dogs and horses is to use a drainage catheter system designed for pericardiocentesis, or other large bore catheter with end- and side holes near the tip. This catheter is introduced into the pericardial space over an exchange guide wire (see alternative method description on p. 727). Great caution is advised when contemplating this method in patients with suspected HSA (and perhaps it should be avoided), because wire or catheter contact with this friable tumor could induce bleeding. In horses, smaller gauged thoracic drains ("chest tubes") with a central trocar and over the needle fenestrated tube can be effective; these often are sutured in place.

Additional equipment should be gathered prior to beginning the procedure. This includes sterile extension tubing (except if using a butterfly needle), a 3-way stopcock, a 20–60 mL collection syringe, a 3 mL syringe and small gauge needle for local block, 2% lidocaine (without epinephrine), a small surgical blade (for stab incision when using a larger catheter), sterile gloves, sterile ethylene diamine tetraacetic acid (EDTA) and clot (red-top) tubes for fluid samples, a large fluid collection receptacle, and an ECG monitor. Personnel able to help restrain the animal and assist with fluid aspiration also are essential.

The hair is clipped and the skin surgically prepared over the puncture site, generally from about the right third to seventh intercostal spaces and from sternum to well above the costochondral junction. Before the final scrub, the putative puncture site is marked with an indelible ink pen or a needle scratch. In most cases, the point of strongest precordial impulse (typically between the 4th and 6th rib near the costochondral junction) is the best site for needle entry, but this can be verified by using the ultrasound probe prior to final skin scrub. A small volume of 2% lidocaine is infiltrated into the skin and underlying intercostal muscle to the pleura at the puncture site (alternatively, some clinicians prefer to do this later using sterile technique). Operators differ in the volume of local anesthetic used, with some selecting 0.5–1 mL for dogs and others (including one author) preferring to distribute 2.5 to 3.0 mL of lidocaine across the various layers for large dogs (such as Golden Retrievers). A sufficient volume is especially necessary when using a larger-bore catheter. In addition to humane issues, the purpose of the analgesia is to avoid sudden patient movements that might result from insufficient local block. It should be noted that the pericardium is difficult to block, and initial puncture might generate some reaction. The pericardium also can be extremely thick in certain patients, especially horses. Patient movement can be minimized by using sufficient local anesthesia along with IV sedation with butorphanol (or xylazine in a horse).

After sterile skin preparation is complete, sterile gloves are donned and the drainage catheter assembly prepared. Commercial pleurocentesis and pericardiocentesis catheters generally have multiple side holes, in addition to the end hole. If a large-gauge over-the-needle catheter is to be used, a 2-3 tiny

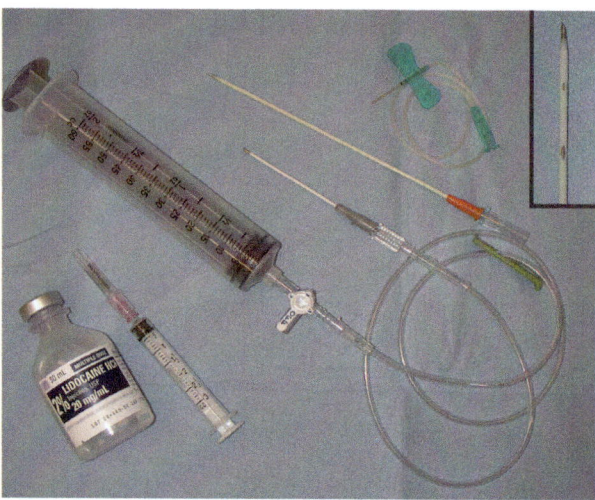

Figure 35.37 Examples of equipment for pericardiocentesis. Local anesthetic is helpful, and necessary when using a larger gauge catheter. A three-way stopcock connects the collection syringe to extension tubing (or, for a very small dog or a cat, a butterfly needle assembly). For most dogs, an over-the-needle catheter is used to access the pericardial space; the needle-stylet then is withdrawn and the extension tubing attached directly to the catheter. For faster drainage of a large-volume effusion, a few small side holes can be made near the tip of a large (12–16 g) catheter (inset) prior to placement. See text for details.

(~1 mm) side holes can be added by smoothly cutting the catheter with a sharp sterile blade or iris scissors near the catheter tip; this will facilitate fluid drainage (**Figure 35.37**). Care must be taken to offset these holes from each other and avoid making them too large, so that the catheter tip is not excessively weakened, because it could break off within the pericardial or pleural space. After carefully replacing the catheter over the needle/stylet the operator should review the procedure again with staff, insure the ECG leads and IV line are attached, and have additional lidocaine available in case of ventricular tachyarrhythmias.

Different techniques could be employed at this point. Some operators prefer to make a small skin stab incision, which certainly is needed if a large bore catheter will be placed. Most commercial catheter needles are quite sharp, and the catheter itself is slippery. If the operator pulls up and penetrates the skin first, and then re-grips the catheter with two hands, the catheter and needle usually can be advanced without any skin incision. Once the catheter is through the skin, approaches also vary. Some operators simply advance the system deliberately but without hesitation across the intercostal and pleural spaces to enter the pericardial space. At this point, (usually dark red) fluid spontaneously flows out of the needle without any need for aspiration. Once the needle tip is within the pericardial space, the system is advanced a few millimeters and the catheter gently rotated into the pericardial space as the needle is retracted from the thorax. A three way stopcock attached to extension tubing then is connected to the catheter and an assistant drains the fluid by aspirating it into the collection syringe. One advantage of this approach is that the operator is able to hold the catheter itself with both hands, can readily re-palpate the intercostal space landmarks, and can place the side of one hand against the thorax in case the patient suddenly moves. Although pneumothorax is a theoretical concern, this usually is not a practical issue. Pleural fluid uncommonly exits the catheter spontaneously, while pericardial fluid generally flows out within seconds, so confusion is unlikely.

A similar approach that also allows the operator use of both hands during needle/catheter penetration, and avoids the risk of iatrogenic pneumothorax, involves sterilely preassembling the: collection syringe to 3-way stopcock to extension tubing. The stopcock is set "off" to air and the extension tubing is attached to the needle stylet (which is within the catheter). Before inserting the needle/catheter into the chest, the collection syringe with attached stopcock is handed carefully (to maintain operator sterility) to an assistant. The operator then palpates the intercostal landmarks and inserts the needle/catheter into the skin, as described in the paragraph above, being careful to avoid the intercostal vessels which run caudal to each rib. Although a perpendicular needle/catheter orientation to the skin initially might help avoid intercostal vessels, it often is helpful to "aim" the needle tip toward the point of the patient's opposite (left) shoulder as the chest is entered. As soon as the needle has penetrated the skin, the assistant applies very slight negative pressure to the collection system as the operator advances the needle/catheter assembly toward the pericardium. If pleural effusion is present, a small amount is likely to enter the extension tubing when the pleural space is entered; this generally is a modified transudate. If the patient has a large volume of pleural fluid, an additional amount could be drained at this time to improve lung expansion. Otherwise, the needle/catheter is advanced until the pericardial space is entered and (usually hemorrhagic) pericardial fluid appears in the extension tubing. As described in the previous paragraph, the needle/catheter system is advanced a little further, then the catheter is rotated and advanced into the pericardial space while the needle stylet is withdrawn. Once the needle is fully removed from the catheter, the extension tubing is detached from the needle and reattached to the catheter, being careful to maintain sterility. The assistant then can continue draining the pericardial fluid while the operator stabilizes the catheter.

Finally, some operators prefer to place a 3 mL syringe on the needle(/catheter system) prior to inserting it into the chest and aspirate as soon as the pleural space is entered. However, pleural fluid could fill the syringe under negative pressure before the pericardium has been entered. Ensuring that the pericardium actually has been penetrated could therefore be difficult. Also, this method requires one hand to manipulate the syringe, leaving only one hand to stabilize the needle during advancement. This could lead to inadvertent and excessive needle movement within the thorax.

Regardless of the method used, it is important to hold the needle/catheter assembly steady during insertion to avoid extraneous motion of the sharp tip within the chest. The pericardium, when contacted, causes increased resistance to needle advancement and might produce a subtle scratching sensation. The needle is advanced by applying gentle pressure until it penetrates through the pericardium. A loss of resistance might be felt with needle penetration and pericardial fluid will appear in the tubing or flow from the needle/catheter. Initial pericardial fluid samples should be saved into the sterile EDTA and clot tubes for evaluation. As much fluid as possible then is aspirated. When fluid collection becomes difficult or ceases, adjusting the catheter position slightly, tilting the (small animal) patient into a slightly more sternal position, or raising the hindquarters slightly might allow retrieval of additional fluid. A small back flush into the catheter also might help clear fibrin or clot from the catheter.

If the needle or catheter contacts the heart, a scratching or tapping sensation usually is felt. In addition, the needle (catheter) tends to move with the heartbeat and ventricular premature contractions (VPCs) often are provoked – the device should be retracted slightly to avoid cardiac trauma. It is important to check the ECG monitor frequently. The operator also must be mindful that if the catheter has been directed too dorsally, RA penetration could occur and this will not result in VPCs. If it is unclear whether pericardial fluid or intracardiac blood (from inadvertent cardiac penetration) is being aspirated, a few drops can be placed on the table or into a red top tube; a sample also could be put into a hematocrit tube if someone is available to immediately spin it. Pericardial fluid does not clot (unless associated with very recent hemorrhage) because the blood becomes defibrinated soon after entering the pericardial cavity. Additionally, the PCV of pericardial fluid typically is much lower than that of the patient's peripheral blood, and the supernatant appears yellow-tinged (xanthochromic; **Figure 35.38**). As more pericardial fluid is removed, the patient's ECG complexes often increase in amplitude while tachycardia diminishes. Many animals take a deep breath and appear more comfortable at this point. Conversely, if intracardiac blood is being aspirated, the patient is likely to become more tachycardic and hypotensive. If ultrasound assistance is available, the catheter might be visible. However, a more definitive method of verifying catheter location is to rapidly inject a small bolus of sterile, agitated saline through the pericardiocentesis catheter (via the 3-way stopcock) to create an echocontrast ("bubble") study. If the catheter tip is within the pericardial space, small bright microbubbles will appear within the pericardial fluid around the heart. If the catheter tip has penetrated into a cardiac chamber, the bubbles will appear within the heart. However, if bubbles appear outside of the pericardium, the catheter was never placed properly or has retracted during the procedure.

When no additional pericardial fluid can be aspirated, the catheter is slowly withdrawn under continued but gentle negative pressure. If there is a significant pleural effusion and the catheter still is functional, this fluid can be drained, usually with the patient in sternal recumbency. A quick echo recheck should verify whether any pericardial fluid remains, tamponade has been resolved, and cardiac filling is improved (**Figure 35.34B**). If substantial fluid remains, pericardiocentesis can be repeated using a fresh catheter system and slight adjustment in the patient's position, as needed. A sample of the effusion (in the EDTA tube) should be submitted for fluid analysis and cytological evaluation; another sample should be reserved in the sterile clot tube for possible culture, pending cytology results. Further echo monitoring of the patient for acute recurrence of pericardial effusion before hospital discharge is wise, especially when HSA is suspected.

For the alternative pericardial drainage catheter method, a modified Seldinger technique is used to introduce the pericardiocentesis catheter into the pericardial space. It is important to maintain sterility during the procedure, which can be challenging because of the longer wire length and exchange process. First, an appropriately sized access needle is inserted through the skin stab incision and into the pericardial space. An exchange guide wire (that previously was verified to fit through the needle) is inserted through the needle into the pericardial space. The needle is withdrawn, leaving enough length of guide wire within the pericardium so that it does not slip out. The pericardiocentesis catheter is passed over the guide wire and into the pericardial space; a sufficient length of the catheter must be introduced into the pericardial space so that its tip does not slip out of the pericardium as the effusion is drained. A skin suture is used to secure the catheter in place during drainage. The pericardial drainage catheter could remain in place for a few hours to a few days if a need for repeated drainage is anticipated; the development of arrhythmias that might require antiarrhythmic therapy can be an adverse consequence (Cook, 2019).

Complications of Pericardiocentesis Adverse events associated with pericardiocentesis are estimated to occur in about 15% of cases within 48 hours of the procedure (Humm, 2009). VPCs commonly occur during the procedure from direct myocardial contact or puncture. These usually are self-limiting when the needle is retracted slightly; however, more

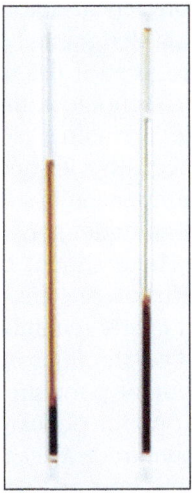

Figure 35.38 Hemorrhagic pericardial effusion (left) usually has a lower hematocrit than peripheral blood (right). Red cell break-down in the effusion produces a yellow-tinged (xanthochromic) supernatant.

serious arrhythmias develop in some cases, so having a preplaced IV catheter is prudent. Myocardial ischemia or an invasive neoplastic process also can provoke arrhythmias. When VPCs persist, IV lidocaine is administered (and possibly continued after the procedure), as needed. Other arrhythmias, including atrial fibrillation also could develop during or following pericardiocentesis; appropriate antiarrhythmic therapy should be provided, if indicated (Chapter 25). Some dogs will spontaneously convert back to sinus rhythm.

Coronary artery laceration, with myocardial infarction or further bleeding into the pericardial space, can occur although this is uncommon, especially when pericardiocentesis is approached from the right side. Rarely, death can result from arrhythmias or coronary laceration. Cardiac perforation and lung laceration leading to pneumothorax or pulmonary hemorrhage also are potential complications of the procedure. Effective patient restraint, as well as carefully holding the needle/stylet steady and advancing slowly during placement, help prevent cardiac and pulmonary trauma. In some cases, dissemination of infection or neoplastic cells into the pleural space is exacerbated.

Management After Pericardiocentesis Idiopathic pericarditis generally is treated conservatively at first, with pericardiocentesis repeated as needed. Although anti-inflammatory doses of a glucocorticoid have been given in some cases after pericardial fluid analysis rules out an infectious cause, the value of glucocorticoid or colchicine therapy in preventing recurrent idiopathic pericardial effusion is unknown and cannot be advocated without data. Some clinicians prescribe a course of broad-spectrum antibiotics, but this should be unnecessary if sterile technique was used and the effusion shows no evidence of infection. Periodic reevaluation by radiography or echocardiography is advised to detect fluid recurrence. Effusion recurs in up to 64% of idiopathic cases. Mesothelioma or HSA can underlie some recurrent effusions that initially were thought to be idiopathic. However, persistent non-neoplastic pericarditis or hemorrhage also can be a cause of recurrent effusion. If pericardial effusion recurs persistently despite conservative treatment (for example, after 2 or 3 pericardial taps), strong consideration should be given to pericardiotomy (pericardial window) or subtotal pericardiectomy (removing the pericardium ventral to the phrenic nerves); this allows drainage to the larger absorptive surface of the pleural space, thus reducing the risk of tamponade. There are pros and cons of each of these procedures and appropriate surgical specialists, cardiologists, and oncologists should be consulted when considering these approaches. Client expectations also play a large role in deciding on the follow-up course. There are no definitive prospective studies to indicate the best approach for non-neoplastic effusions or those associated with cancer.

Neoplastic effusions also are drained as needed to relieve cardiac tamponade. Pleural effusion also needs to be managed, in many cases. Recurrent effusion is expected, and with HSA, this can occur within hours of pericardiocentesis. For that reason, many patients are kept for observation for variable periods after initial centesis, and occasionally a pericardiocentesis catheter is sewn into place. Depending on the cause and situation, additional therapy might involve attempted surgical resection or surgical biopsy, partial pericardiectomy or pericardiotomy, chemotherapy, stereotaxic radiation therapy, or repeated pericardiocentesis until episodes of cardiac tamponade become unmanageable. Surgery can be associated with significant morbidity and mortality and is only palliative in most cases. Prognosis generally is poor in dogs with HSA or mesothelioma. Because heart base tumors (such as chemodectoma) tend to be slow growing, partial pericardiectomy or pericardiotomy might prolong survival for months to years.

Compared to thoracotomy, thoracoscopy provides a less invasive approach for pericardiotomy and biopsy sample acquisition for histopathologic evaluation. It can be effective for idiopathic and some cases of neoplastic pericardial effusion, especially heart base tumors. The thoracoscopic pericardial window procedure generally requires shorter procedure and hospitalization times than open thoracotomy and has low morbidity. Partial pericardiectomy is possible using thoracoscopy in some animals. A minimally invasive, transxiphoid surgical approach to the caudoventral thoracic cavity and pericardium also has been described. These procedures are best performed by surgical specialists. Subtotal pericardiectomy, at least when performed via open thoracotomy, has provided increased survival time and longer time to recurrent clinical signs compared to pericardiotomy (pericardial window) created by thoracoscopy. Whether this relates to erroneous classification of some neoplastic effusions as idiopathic, or whether a pericardial window truly is inferior to subtotal pericardiectomy for idiopathic disease is unclear. Subtotal pericardiectomy also can be accomplished successfully using a transdiaphragmatic approach. When pericardial effusion is inflammatory, subtotal pericardiectomy is strongly recommended to prevent loculated effusions.

Percutaneous balloon pericardiotomy is a minimally invasive means of providing long-term continuous pericardial drainage. It can be considered if the more preferred surgical options (thoracoscopy and thoracotomy) are unacceptable to the owner or unavailable. Premature closure of the pericardial opening is possible, especially with neoplastic disease, which could lead to recurrent tamponade in some cases. Balloon pericardiotomy in dogs is done under general anesthesia and with fluoroscopic guidance. There should be at least a moderate volume of pericardial effusion present prior to the procedure. The dog is placed in left lateral recumbency with the sternum tilted slightly downward on the fluoroscopy table. Ultrasound is used to verify the optimal puncture site. Continuous ECG monitoring is important. As for pericardiocentesis, the area is shaved and surgically prepared. After making a stab incision at the puncture site, a large-bore access needle or 16–18 gauge over-the-needle catheter is inserted into the pericardial space; a small injection of iodinated contrast material can be made to verify intrapericardial position. A guide wire (such as a 180 cm,

0.035," J- or floppy-tipped) is then inserted through the needle (or catheter) into the pericardial space under fluoroscopic guidance. The needle (or catheter) is withdrawn and a percutaneous vascular sheath introducer is advanced over the guide wire, which is left in place. A low-profile balloon (~20 mm × 4 cm) dilation catheter is inserted over the guide wire. The balloon is positioned so that it straddles the parietal pericardial wall, in order to create a hole when inflated. Fluoroscopy is used to verify proper balloon positioning; a narrowed "waist," caused by the pericardium, should be seen in the center of the balloon during its initial inflation. The waist should disappear with full balloon dilation, which is held for 3–5 minutes before deflating the balloon. It might be necessary to partially withdraw the vascular sheath from the chest so that it does not interfere with full balloon dilation. Also, it can help to position the dog into full lateral recumbency or even elevate the sternum slightly so that the heart falls away from the chest wall. Balloon dilation is repeated until the pericardium no longer creates a waist in the balloon. After the balloon catheter, wire, and vascular sheath are withdrawn, a single skin suture is used to close the incision. Complications of this procedure are similar to those of pericardiocentesis, although the risk of cardiac puncture, tumor disruption (if present) and continued hemorrhage can be greater.

The *prognosis* for animals with pericardial effusion depends on the underlying disease process. Idiopathic effusion in dogs carries a much better prognosis than neoplastic effusion. Retrospective studies show better results with surgery but these are probably related in part to client motivation to continue treatment for recurrent idiopathic hemorrhage. Median survival time for idiopathic pericardial effusion in one report ranged from 10 months to almost 3 years, while estimated median survival for dogs with neoplastic effusion was about 2 to 4 weeks, overall (Stafford-Johnson, 2004). A small study of dogs with recurrent pericardial effusion thought to be idiopathic identified a median survival time of ~1 year following thoracoscopic subtotal pericardiectomy; yet 25% of the dogs actually had a neoplastic effusion with median survival of 76 days (Michelotti, 2019). Another small report of dogs with presumptive idiopathic pericardial effusion that were managed by thoracoscopic examination followed by pericardiectomy found that half the dogs actually had small mass lesions; these dogs had a median survival time of 66 days, whereas median survival time was not reached in the dogs without identified lesions (Carvajal, 2019). For more information on prognosis in dogs with cardiac tumors, see p. 741. Cats with pericardial effusion that live longer than 24 hours after diagnosis have an estimated overall median survival between 4–5 months (Hall, 2007). Pericardial effusion associated with CHF appears to confer a worse prognosis than effusion not related to CHF in cats.

Management of Pericardial Effusion in Horses

Treatment involves rest, vigorous systemic broad-spectrum antimicrobial therapy (unless a bacterial cause appears unlikely), and pericardiocentesis to drain the pericardial effusion. IV fluid therapy can help support cardiac filling and output prior to pericardiocentesis in horses with cardiac tamponade; however, pericardiocentesis (with ECG monitoring during the procedure) should not be delayed. Diuretics should not be used in horses with cardiac tamponade, because this will further reduce cardiac output. Pericardiocentesis in the standing horse typically is approached via the right or left 5th intercostal space, dorsal to the lateral thoracic vein. A large-bore catheter, teat cannula, or chest tube can be used to drain the pericardial space. However, a chest tube is preferred for indwelling pericardial access when repeated drainage and pericardial lavage are anticipated, as for septic or idiopathic fibrinous pericarditis management.

The combination of local intrapericardial therapy with systemic antimicrobial drugs can be effective for septic pericarditis in some cases. Lavage of the pericardial space, followed by (or combined with) antimicrobial instillation, usually is done immediately following the initial pericardiocentesis. Sodium penicillin and gentamicin have been recommended as generally safe to use within the pericardial space. Indwelling catheter placement into the pericardial space at the time of initial pericardiocentesis allows for repeated pericardial drainage and lavage. Pericardial lavage helps remove fibrin, inflammatory cells, immune-complexes, bacteria, and other debris. A sterile 0.9% saline solution often is used for pericardial lavage, sometimes with the addition of an anticoagulant such as heparin. At about 12-hour intervals, as much pericardial effusion as possible is drained, then 1–2 L of lavage solution is flushed into the pericardial space and immediately drained along with any additional effusion. The chosen antibiotic can be mixed into the last half of the fluid used at each lavage, or instilled into the pericardial space following lavage. Pericardial lavages are continued for several days, or until the accumulated volume of pericardial fluid over a 12-hour period becomes minimal (<1 L), the fluid itself appears less inflammatory, and the patient's clinical status is improved. If pericardial fluid culture results are positive, antibiotic therapy can be adjusted, as needed. When excessive production of pericardial effusion appears controlled, the pericardial catheter is removed. A nonsteroidal antiinflammatory drug usually is given as well, to reduce inflammation and risk of subsequent constrictive pericardial disease. Equine pericarditis of suspected viral or immune-mediated origin sometimes is treated with a corticosteroid (such as antiinflammatory doses of dexamethasone), although this is controversial. First, there should be no evidence for bacterial infection on pericardial fluid cytology and culture. The *prognosis* for horses with bacterial pericarditis, including the fibrino-effusive pericarditis associated with mare reproductive loss syndrome, generally is guarded even with vigorous therapy. For horses with idiopathic pericarditis, prognosis might be positive if aggressive therapy can be provided without delay; however, the condition could become chronic. Constrictive pericarditis is a potential sequela, especially with inflammatory pericardial disease.

Constrictive Pericardial Disease

Constrictive pericardial disease occurs when visceral and parietal pericardial membranes are thickened, adhered, and restrict ventricular diastolic filling. Usually the entire pericardium is involved symmetrically. In true constrictive pericardial disease, fusion of the parietal and visceral pericardial layers can occur and obliterate the pericardial space. In some cases, the visceral layer (epicardium) alone is involved. Most commonly in dogs a small amount of pericardial effusion is present (constrictive–effusive pericarditis). Constrictive pericardial disease is diagnosed occasionally in dogs, but only rarely in cats and horses. Histopathologically, increased fibrous connective tissue and variable amounts of inflammatory and reactive infiltrates are present in the pericardium. Pericardial mineralization occurs rarely. The etiology of constrictive pericardial disease often is unknown. Specific associations that have been identified in some animals include recurrent idiopathic hemorrhagic effusion, infectious pericarditis (including from actinomycosis, mycobacteriosis, coccidioidomycosis), a metallic foreign body in the pericardium, mesothelioma and other neoplasia, idiopathic osseous metaplasia and fibrosis of the pericardium, and prior surgery for PPDH.

Pathophysiology

Pericardial fibrosis creates a stiff shell around the heart and increases ventricular interdependence. With constrictive disease, ventricular filling is limited to early- and possibly mid-diastole before ventricular expansion becomes curtailed and filling stops abruptly. Diastolic pressures within the atria and ventricles become equalized at this time (**Figure 35.39**). It is only with increasingly high venous and atrial pressures that any further filling occurs. The phasic variations in right and left heart filling, which occur during the respiratory cycle, are magnified in constrictive pericardial disease because of increased ventricular interdependence. During inspiration, reduced intrapleural pressure increases venous return to the right heart. However, the stiffened pericardium curtails normal RV free wall expansion, causing the septum to shift leftward; this further compromises LV filling. During exhalation, the increased intrapleural pressure reduces right heart filling but increases pulmonary venous return to the left heart, shifting the interventricular septum rightward.

The compromised cardiac filling raises CVP and reduces cardiac output. Compensatory neurohormonal and renal activations lead to the right-sided CHF signs of jugular venous distension, pleural effusion and ascites, along with tachycardia and vasoconstriction. The modified-transudate pleural effusion can become chylous over time. Radiographically, the heart might not appear enlarged; consequently, constrictive pericardial disease often is misdiagnosed as intra-abdominal disease because most canine cases present with ascites.

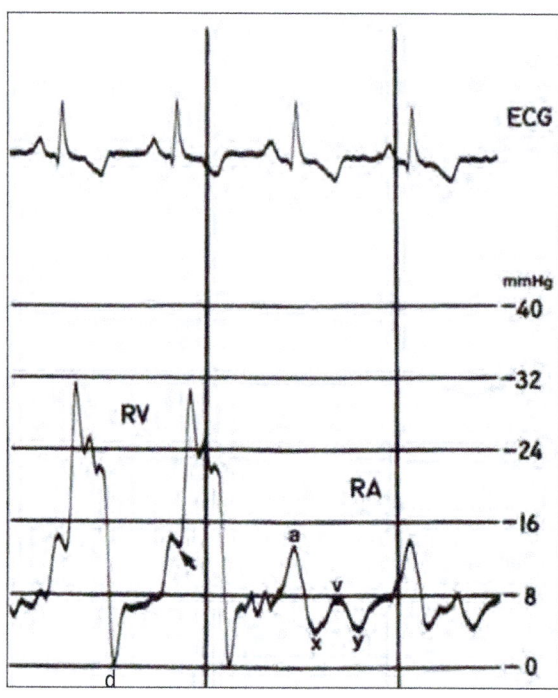

Figure 35.39 Pressure recordings from right ventricle (RV) and atrium (RA) in a dog with constrictive pericardial disease. A characteristic early diastolic dip (d; when most filling occurs), mid-diastolic plateau, and elevated end-diastolic pressure (14 mm Hg in this case; arrow) are evident in the pressure trace from the RV. The pressure waveforms from the RA show a tall a wave (corresponding to the high end-diastolic pressure in the RV), and prominent x and y descents. (From Thomas, 1984).

Clinical Features

Large to medium-sized, middle-aged dogs are affected most often; males and German Shepherd dogs might be at higher risk. Clinically, right-sided CHF signs predominate. Client complaints include abdominal distension (ascites), dyspnea or tachypnea, tiring, syncope, weakness, and weight loss. Signs can develop over a period of weeks to months. Occasionally, there is a prior history of pericardial effusion. As in cases of cardiac tamponade, ascites and jugular venous distension are the most consistent clinical findings. Weakened femoral pulses and muffled heart sounds also are detected in many cases. An audible pericardial "knock," caused by the abrupt deceleration of ventricular filling in early diastole, has been described in people, horses, and rarely, in dogs (Schwartz, 1971). A systolic murmur or click, probably caused by valvular disease unassociated with the pericardial pathology, might be heard.

Diagnostic Tests

Constrictive pericardial disease is a diagnostic challenge. Radiographic findings can include mild to moderate cardiomegaly, pleural effusion, and caudal vena caval distension. Reduced cardiac motion might be evident on fluoroscopy. ECG abnormalities have included sinus tachycardia, P wave prolongation, and small-amplitude QRS complexes.

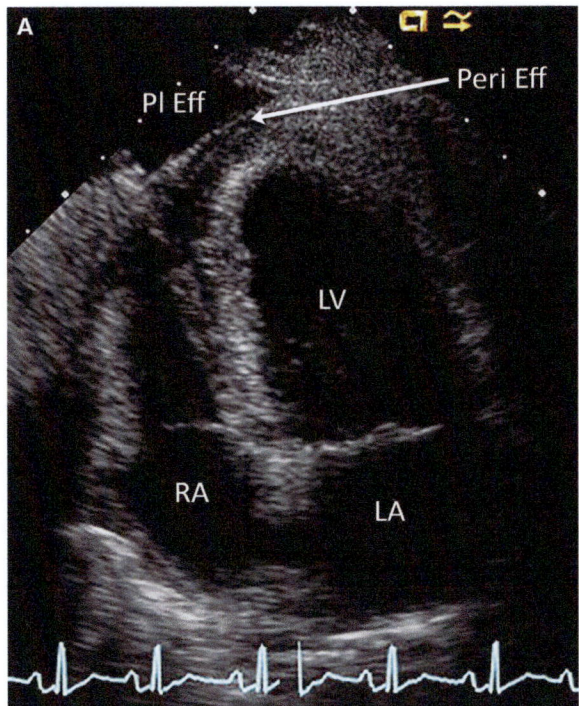
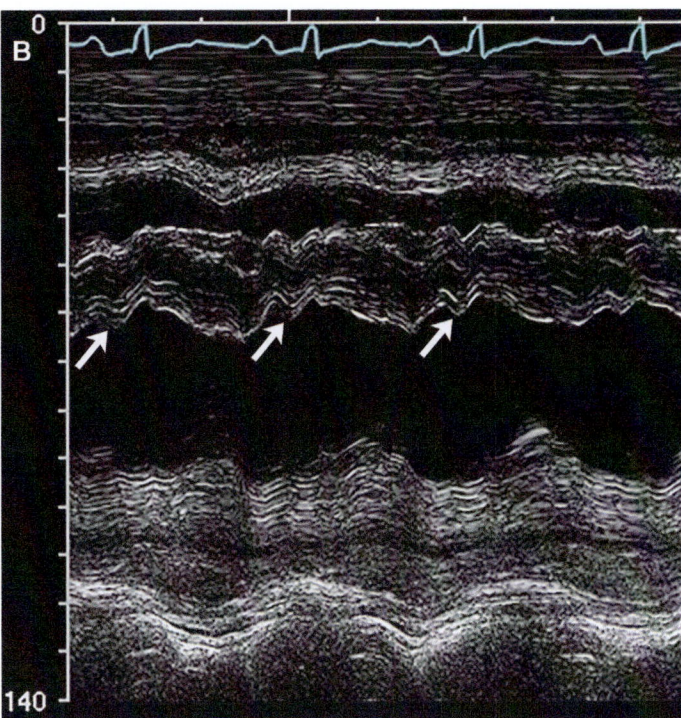

Figure 35.40 (A) Left apical 2D image in mid-systole from a 9-year-old male Labrador Retriever with pleural and abdominal effusions caused by constrictive pericardial disease. Only a tiny rim of pericardial effusion (Peri Eff, arrow) is present. The RA is mildly enlarged and the LV slightly small. Central venous pressure was 16 mm Hg. Radiographically, only equivocal cardiomegaly was present (VHS ~11.5v). LA, left atrium; LV, left ventricle; Pl Eff, pleural effusion; RA, right atrium. (B) M-mode at the ventricular level from the same dog shows a sudden leftward septal wobble ("bounce") in diastole (arrows) that reflects transiently higher pressure in the RV compared to the LV. Inspiration accentuates this motion. The subtle early "diastolic septal dip" (just after maximal freewall excursion) preceding the "bounce" is a normal finding.

Constrictive pericardial disease produces subtle but suggestive echo changes. Abnormal and abrupt septal motion in diastole (septal "bounce") reflects the ventricular interdependence of a heart surrounded by an inflexible "shell" (**Figure 35.40**). Small changes in intraventricular pressures cause septal shifts because the free walls cannot expand further. Diastolic flattening of the LV free wall also might be seen. During inspiration, greater leftward deviation of both the interventricular and atrial septa reflects the relative increase in right heart filling at the expense of left heart filling during this respiratory phase. During exhalation, the septa shift back toward the right. Ventricular chamber dimensions are likely to be reduced or normal with constrictive pericardial disease. RA collapse is not expected with constrictive disease, in contrast to pericardial effusion with tamponade; atrial dilation is possible. The pericardium might appear thickened and intensely echogenic, but differentiating this from its normal echogenicity can be difficult. Pleural effusion and vena caval dilation (with blunted respiratory fluctuation in diameter) also can be evident. Doppler findings illustrate the increased ventricular interdependence. Marked respiratory fluctuation occurs in peak flow velocities across the mitral and tricuspid valves, as well as into both atria. Transtricuspid early filling (E wave) peak velocity is greatest in early inspiration, while maximum peak transmitral E wave velocity occurs with the onset of expiration (**Figure 35.41**). In humans, 25-50% variation is considered significant; however, this is not established in dogs and is not likely to be very specific

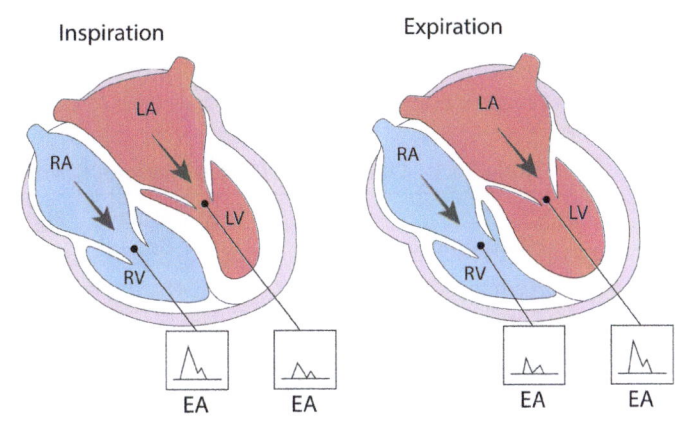

Figure 35.41 Schematic diagram of transvalvular flow velocities in constrictive pericarditis. During inspiration, the decrease in left ventricular filling causes a leftward septal shift, which allows increased flow into the RV. The opposite occurs during expiration. Note the respiratory variation in transtricuspid and transmitral early filling (E wave) velocities. A, late diastolic inflow velocity; E, early diastolic inflow velocity; LA, left atrium; LV, left ventricle; RA, right atrium; RV, right ventricle.

in this species. Additionally tissue Doppler imaging shows a normal velocity for early diastolic LV e′.

Invasive hemodynamic studies can verify the diagnosis. In the dog, a CVP >15 mm Hg and high mean atrial and diastolic ventricular pressures are expected. Constrictive pericardial disease causes a prominent y descent in the atrial pressure curve, in contrast to the diminished y descent typical of cardiac tamponade. Classically, there is an early diastolic dip in ventricular pressure, followed by a mid-diastolic plateau as filling is curtailed (see RV pressure trace in **Figure 35.39**); however, this is not found consistently in dogs with constrictive pericardial disease and might require some volume loading to identify. Angiocardiography could show atrial and vena caval enlargement with increased endocardial to pericardial distance, although images can be normal. MRI is a standard for identifying thick pericardium in humans.

Management

Pericardiectomy is necessary to improve ventricular filling. Although this might be possible using thoracoscopy in sporadic cases, creating just a pericardial window generally is ineffective. Pericardiectomy is most likely to be successful when the parietal pericardium is mainly responsible for the constrictive pathophysiology (constrictive-effusive disease). True constrictive disease or extensive visceral pericardial involvement requires epicardial stripping (decortication), which dramatically increases the difficulty and associated complications of surgery. Pulmonary thrombosis, sometimes massive, could be a relatively common postoperative complication. Tachyarrhythmias are another complication. Moderate doses of diuretic might be helpful postoperatively. The effectiveness of angiotensin converting enzyme (ACE) and aldosterone inhibition is unclear; positive inotropic and arteriolar vasodilator drugs are unstudied and not likely to be helpful. Without successful surgical intervention, disease progression and death are expected. Repeated thoracocentesis often is necessary to stabilize the patient; a pleural port, if it remains patent, might improve management options.

Cardiac Tumors

The overall prevalence of cardiac tumors in dogs was estimated at 0.19% (1383/729,265 dogs), with at least 90 breeds affected, based on a large multi-institutional database survey (Ware, 1999). Primary heart tumors are thought to be much more common than secondary (metastatic) neoplasia in dogs. Approximately 84% of heart tumors were identified as primary to the heart in this database survey, while only 16% were identified as metastatic. Of the cardiac metastatic tumors that were identified histologically, over 33% were diagnosed as HSAs (including angiosarcoma, malignant hemangioendothelioma) and about 20% as adenocarcinomas. Other metastatic tumors found in the heart have included lymphoma, various sarcomas including osteosarcoma, and mast cell tumors. In a smaller necropsy survey of dogs, cardiac metastases from extracardiac neoplasms were found in over a third of the cases (Aupperle, 2007).

Primary cardiac tumors in dogs usually are malignant; between 50 to over 65% metastasize. HSA is by far the most common cardiac tumor (**Table 35.1**). Most primary cardiac tumors in dogs involve the right side of the heart, presumably because they are likely to be HSA. Of the 66% (914/1383) of cardiac tumor cases identified histologically in the study mentioned above, HSA accounted for over two-thirds (69%). This highly malignant tumor appears to be more common in the dog than in other species. The right heart, especially the RA appendage, is one of the most common primary sites for this tumor. Sporadically, cardiac HSA also can arise in the interventricular septum or LV, or even the pericardium itself. Other common primary sites for HSA are the spleen, subcutaneous tissues, and liver. Primary cardiac HSA is likely to metastasize to other organs, including the lung and spleen. Extensive metastases often can be found in the lungs (and elsewhere)

Table 35.1 Occurrence Rate of Various Cardiac Tumors in Dogs

Histologic Diagnosis	% of Cardiac Tumor Cases[a]	Number of Cases[a] (total n = 1383)	% of Cardiac Tumor Cases[b]	Number of Cases[b] (total n = 309)
Hemangiosarcoma	46	633	61	187
Aortic body tumor	5	69	15	46
Lymphoma	2	34	4	12
Thyroid carcinoma	1	13	3	9
All other histologic types	12	165	17	55
Unknown[c]	34	469		

[a] Ware, 1999. Data source: Survey of Purdue Veterinary Medical Database.
[b] Walter, 1996. Cardiac tumor cases found from 10,090 canine autopsies; includes primary & secondary cardiac tumors.
[c] Histologic diagnosis not reported; probably most were hemangiosarcomas, with a lesser number of aortic body tumors.

on postmortem exam, even before they are radiographically apparent. Primary splenic HSA only occasionally metastasizes to the heart. In dogs with splenic HSA, the risk of developing concurrent HSA in the RA appears to be fairly low (<9%; Boston, 2011).

Tumors involving the aortic root and heart base region also are fairly common in dogs. Usually these are aortic body tumors, also known as chemodectomas or nonchromaffin paragangliomas. They are the second-most common type of cardiac tumor in dogs. Of heart tumors identified histologically in dogs, almost 8% (69/914) were aortic body tumors in one study (Ware, 1999), and ~15% in another (Walter, 1996). These neoplasms arise from chemoreceptor cells, which are sensitive to blood oxygen and carbon dioxide tensions, as well as other factors. Clusters of these cells are located near the aortic root (aortic bodies), carotid bifurcations (carotid bodies), and elsewhere; however tumors most often develop in the aortic bodies in dogs. Aortic body tumors are locally invasive, although they often do metastasize. Unless they cause symptomatic pericardial effusion or dysfunction of surrounding structures, aortic body tumors (chemodectomas) can be an incidental finding on echo or autopsy examination. It is likely that these are recognized antemortem more often today, with the higher-quality imaging available and more individuals trained in echocardiography. Other heart base tumors include thyroid, parathyroid, lymphoid, neuroendocrine, and connective tissue neoplasms.

Pericardial mesothelioma occurs less frequently in the dog and cat. This neoplasm can appear in variable forms and can be difficult to identify on echo exam. Mesothelioma might be more common in certain geographic locations; exposure to environmental asbestos or possibly other substances might be a factor, as in people. Myocardial lymphoma and sporadic cases of cardiac myxoma and various (nonhemangio-) sarcomas, as well as other neoplasms also occur in dogs (Treggiari, 2017).

Cats are less likely to be affected by cardiac tumors than dogs, with an estimated occurrence rate of <0.03% (58/210,388 cats in database). The most common cardiac tumor in cats is lymphoma, accounting for 31% of cases in a large database survey (Ware, 1995; **Table 35.2**). Lymphoma also could primarily involve the pericardium. Various carcinomas, mostly metastatic, occurred in about 19% of cases. Cardiac HSA, aortic body tumor, ectopic thyroid tumor, and fibrosarcoma are uncommon in cats.

Primary cardiac tumors are rare in horses. Occasionally, metastatic lesions are found in the heart. Sporadic reports in horses have described thoracic lymphoma, mesothelioma, and HSA, as well a case of intracardiac malignant melanoma that caused septal hemorrhage, atrioventricular (AV) node dysfunction and sudden death.

Rarely, nonneoplastic mass lesions affect the heart or pericardium in animals. These have included fungal granuloma or pyogranuloma (as from coccidioidomycosis or blastomycosis), other granulomatous or cystic inflammatory lesions, and auricular aneurysm.

Pathophysiology

Cardiac tumors cause a variety of effects, depending on their anatomic location and consequent hemodynamic or other derangements. In general, physiologic disturbances relate either to external cardiac compression which impedes filling (as with pericardial effusion and resulting cardiac tamponade; p. 713), obstruction of blood flow into or out of the heart, arrhythmias, impaired ventricular systolic or diastolic function secondary to myocardial infiltration or ischemia, or to a combination of these abnormalities. Most reports describe tumors causing pericardial effusion and cardiac tamponade; the majority of these are HSAs or aortic body tumors (chemodectomas; **Figures 35.42–35.44**). Yet, a tumor mass also could obstruct blood flow, either by externally compressing or infiltrating into the heart or an adjacent great vessel. For example, chondroid tumors in the ascending aorta have caused acquired aortic stenosis (Kohnken, 2015). Intracardiac tumors of various histologic types can cause congestive or low-output signs by obstructing blood flow and inducing arrhythmias, rather than by causing pericardial effusion with

Table 35.2 Occurrence Rate of Various Cardiac Tumors in Cats[a]

Histologic Diagnosis	% of Cardiac Tumor Cases	Number of Cases (total n = 58)
Lymphoma	31	18
Metastatic carcinomas	19	11
Hemangiosarcoma	9	5
Aortic body tumor	3	2
Other sarcomas	3	2
Unknown[b]	35	20

[a] Ware, 1995. Data source: Survey of Purdue Veterinary Medical Database (from 1982 to 1993).
[b] Histologic diagnosis not reported.

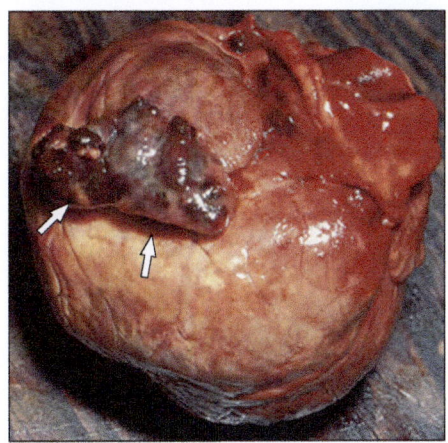

Figure 35.42 Hemangiosarcoma (arrows) originating at the right auricle. View from cranial aspect of the heart; note small left auricle visible on the right side of photo. Specimen from a German Shepherd.

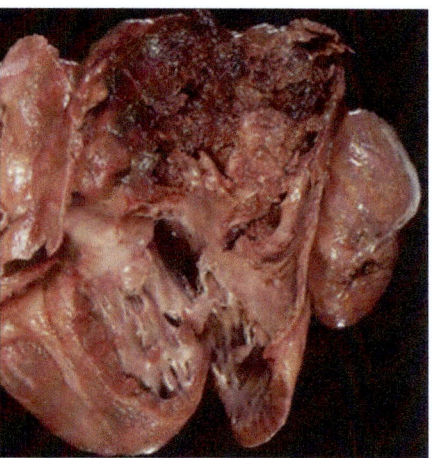

Figure 35.43 A hemangiosarcoma almost obliterates the right atrium (RA) and protrudes outside the heart (at right) in an older Beagle. View from caudal aspect of open RA (top) and right ventricle (bottom).

tamponade (**Figures 35.45–35.47**). The location and size of the tumor influence the degree of functional disruption. RV inflow obstruction is most common, although RV and, occasionally, LV outflow obstruction sometimes occurs.

Clinical Features

Cardiac tumors are more common in middle-aged to older dogs (7–15 years old). The previously mentioned database survey identified the highest occurrence rate in dogs 10–15 years of age. Surprisingly, cardiac tumor occurrence in dogs over 15 years old was low. About 55% of dogs with cardiac HSA or aortic body tumor were 10–15 years old; about 35% were 7–10 years old. Pericardial mesothelioma also occurs more often in middle-aged dogs. In contrast, lymphoma was more likely to affect dogs 7 years old and younger. Almost 28% of

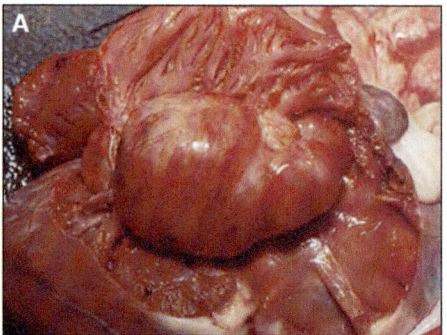

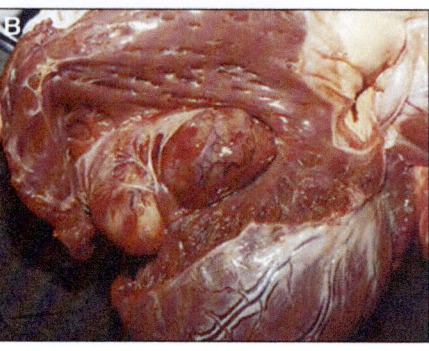

Figure 35.45 (A) An intracardiac sarcoma arising from the lateral right atrial wall occupies most of that chamber. It obstructed venous return to the heart, but did not cause pericardial effusion. View from the open right atrium. (B) This tumor bulged into the tricuspid orifice during diastole. View from the open right ventricle shows the tumor mass straddling the parietal tricuspid leaflet, chordae, and a papillary muscle.

cats with a heart tumor were 7 years old or younger, which likely reflects the greater percentage of lymphoma cases in this species. However, at least two thirds of cats with heart tumors were >7 years old in the database survey.

Although equal numbers of male and female dogs were affected, reproductive status appears to have an effect on

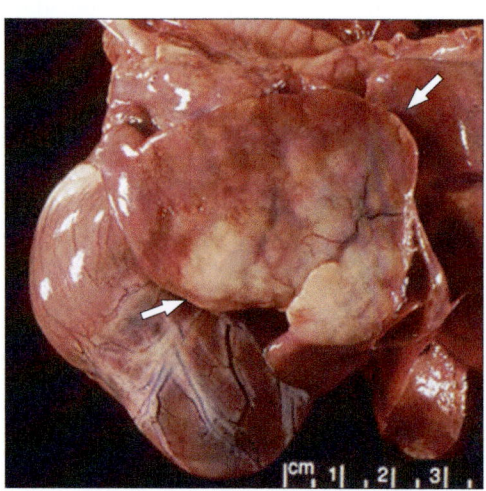

Figure 35.44 A large aortic body tumor (chemodectoma, arrows) extends from the heart base caudally and to the left in an older Schnauzer. View from left. The mass was flattened against the chest wall and also invaded the lung (pushed caudally) and left atrium.

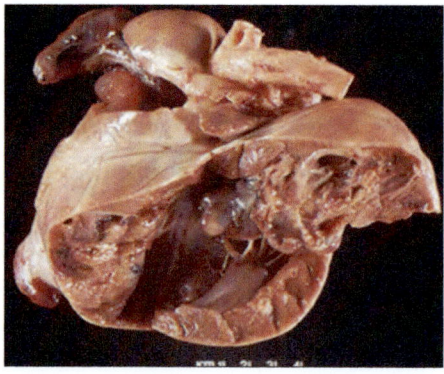

Figure 35.46 Intracardiac rhabdomyosarcoma extensively infiltrated the myocardium of both ventricles and protruded from the apex in a young female Golden Retriever, causing a systolic murmur, malignant ventricular tachyarrhythmias (**Figure 5.32**, p. 149), and syncope. There was no pericardial effusion. The tumor formed bulbous projections that obstructed outflow from both right ventricle (RV; top left in photo) and left ventricle (LV; middle of photo). View from left cranial aspect; left apex to lower left of photo, open LV in center, open RV at top.

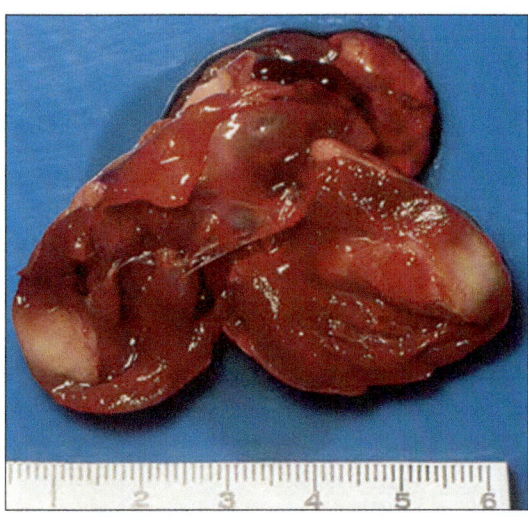

Figure 35.47 Myocardial lymphoma (focal pale areas) in the open left and right (top) ventricles of a cat. (Image courtesy of Dr JO Noxon.)

relative risk for cardiac neoplasia. Spayed females had an overall 4-fold greater risk of cardiac tumor than intact females (5-fold greater for HSA); the risk for castrated males was estimated at 1.6 times that of intact males, and for intact males was about 2.4 times greater than for intact females. The overall relative risk for cardiac tumor appears similar between spayed females and neutered males. In a similar database survey in cats, 53% of affected cats were female and 47% were male; however, the effect of reproductive status is unknown.

Breed predilections have been identified for some cardiac tumors in dogs. Breeds with higher rates of HSA, and all cardiac tumors in general, include the Afghan Hound, English Setter, German Shepherd Dog, and Golden Retriever. Other breeds that appear to have increased risk for HSA include the American Cocker Spaniel, Doberman Pinscher, Labrador Retriever, Miniature Poodle, Miniature Dachshund, and Schnauzer, among others. The majority of canine aortic body tumors reported in the literature have been in brachycephalic breeds, specifically Boxers, Boston Terriers, and Bulldogs; however, not all dogs diagnosed with aortic body tumor are of brachycephalic breeds. Conversely, some breeds appear to have a significantly lower prevalence of cardiac tumors, including the Pomeranian, Pug, Jack Russell Terrier, and others.

Physical Findings Signs of right-sided CHF are common with tumors that obstruct blood flow within the right atrium or ventricle, or that cause pericardial effusion and cardiac tamponade. These signs include ascites, pleural effusion, jugular vein distension, abnormal jugular pulsations, and occasionally, subcutaneous edema. Weakness and syncope with exertion or excitement also are common signs. These low cardiac output signs can result from cardiac tamponade, blood flow obstruction, arrhythmias, impaired myocardial function, or a combination of these factors. In addition, lethargy and collapse can occur with bleeding tumors (especially HSA) that also have invaded extracardiac locations. Abnormal heart sounds in animals with a cardiac tumor can include a murmur (caused by intracardiac blood flow obstruction or from unrelated disease, such as degenerative mitral valve disease), or unusual transient sounds (including a systolic click or snap, or diastolic gallop or tumor "plop"). Arrhythmias are common, especially with myocardial invasion, and can be intractable to manage. As noted earlier, muffled heart sounds are likely with large-volume pericardial effusion. Yet some cases have no auscultable abnormalities.

Diagnostic Tests

Median cTnI concentration was higher in dogs with cardiac HSA compared to dogs with non-cardiac HSA, dogs with other neoplasms, and dogs with pericardial effusion not caused by HSA (Chun, 2010). A plasma cTnI concentration >0.25 ng/mL reportedly was 81% sensitive and 100% specific for identifying cardiac HSA in dogs with pericardial effusion. Other routine laboratory tests rarely are useful in cardiac tumor diagnosis.

Radiographic suggestion of pericardial effusion or cardiac tamponade might be found as noted earlier (p. 716). Mass lesions within or extending through a wall of the heart also can enlarge or create an unusual contour of the chamber(s) they affect (**Figure 35.48**). Dorsal deviation of the trachea, a mass-like opacity cranial to the heart, increased perihilar opacity, or a combination of these findings occur with some heart base tumors. Large heart base masses create unusual bulges at the dorsal aspect of the cardiac silhouette, with or without the presence of pericardial effusion (**Figures 35.49** and **35.50**). Pulmonary metastases might be evident with primary or secondary (metastatic) cardiac neoplasms. Caudal vena caval distension, pleural effusion, and ascites commonly occur with marked RV inflow or outflow obstructions. Large heart base masses that obstruct the right or left pulmonary artery can result in diminished perfusion of that lobe. Pulmonary venous obstruction probably is under-recognized, and sometimes can be seen on echo exam. Such obstruction potentially could produce pulmonary infiltrates in affected lobes. Some intracardiac tumors cause no noticeable radiographic changes.

The ECG might suggest pericardial effusion (**Figures 35.21–35.23** and text, p. 717). Atrial or ventricular premature complexes and paroxysmal tachycardias can result from tumor infiltration (**Figure 35.51**). Varying degrees of bundle branch or AV block and symptomatic bradycardia can develop secondary to conduction system infiltration (**Figure 35.52**). Intracardiac tumors that obstruct RV outflow could cause a right axis shift and RV hypertrophy pattern on the ECG, secondary to the RV systolic pressure overload. Other chamber enlargement or abnormal conduction patterns could occur, depending on tumor location and hemodynamic sequelae.

Echocardiography has good sensitivity and specificity for identifying a variety of cardiac masses (**Figures 35.53–35.57**, also **Figures 35.29–35.31, 35.48, 35.50,** and **35.51**). Nevertheless, 15 to 20% of cardiac masses probably are missed on initial evaluation (MacDonald, 2009). The presence

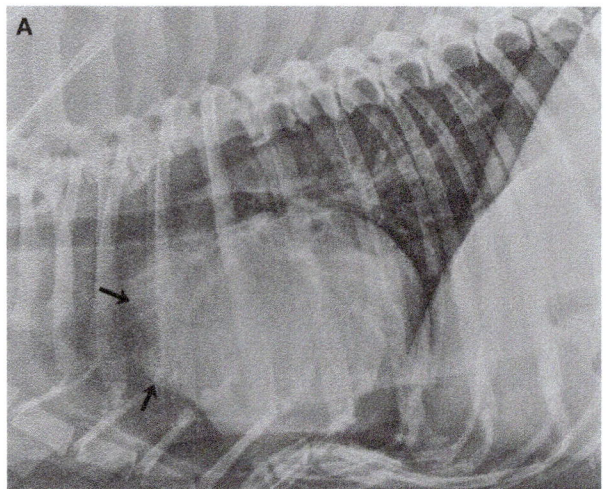
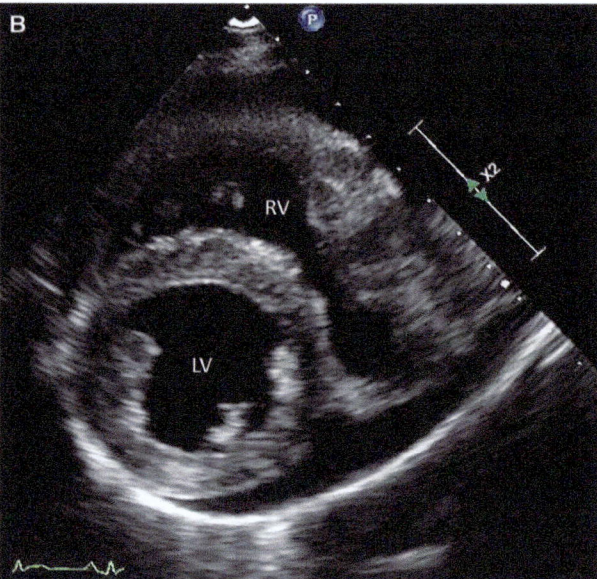
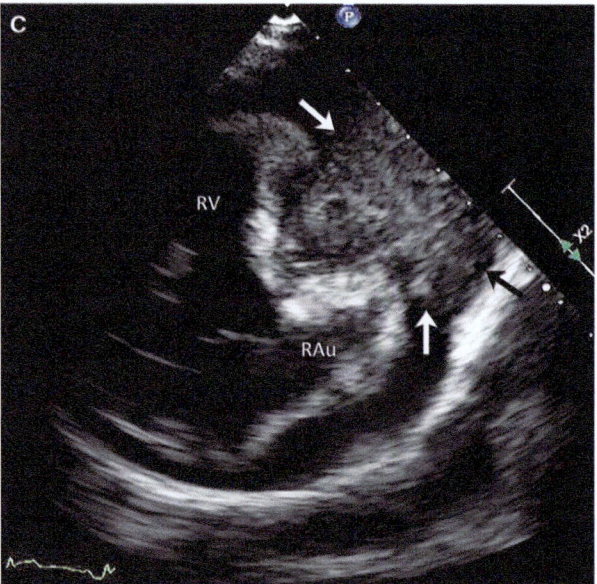

Figure 35.48 (A) Left lateral radiograph shows an unusual bulge (arrows) at the cranial aspect of the cardiac silhouette in a 9-year-old female Labrador Retriever with signs of cardiac tamponade. Spondylosis of the thoracic spine and *pectus excavatum* also are evident. (B) Right parasternal short-axis echocardiographic image at the ventricular level shows a small amount of pericardial effusion and a large, invasive soft-tissue mass. The mass involves the full thickness of the cranial right ventricular wall and extends into the lumen, as well as into the pericardial space. (C) Left cranial long-axis image optimized for the right ventricle (RV) and right auricle (RAu) shows a mass (arrows) also extending from the tip of the RAu in this dog. Based on the location of the mass(es), hemangiosarcoma was suspected; unfortunately, the dog was lost to follow-up. A, Radiograph courtesy of Jordan Creek Animal Hospital.

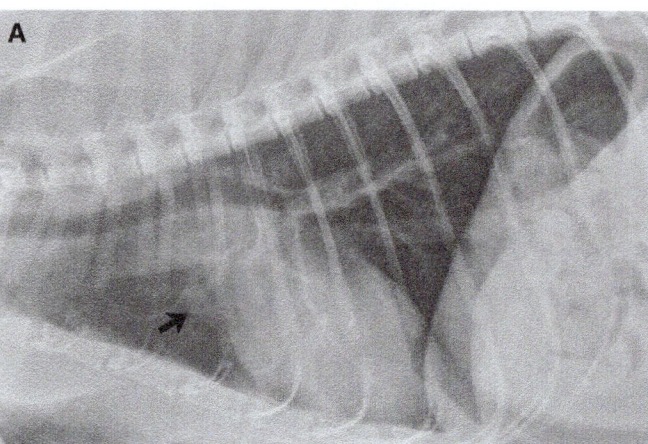
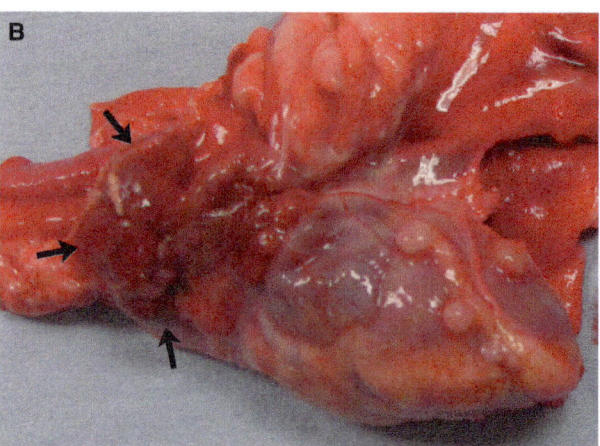

Figure 35.49 (A) Lateral thoracic radiograph from a 6-year-old male Domestic Shorthair cat shows that the distal trachea is pushed dorsally, just cranial to the cardiac silhouette. A soft tissue bulge also is evident at the dorsocranial aspect of the heart (arrow). (B) Postmortem exam (view from left) shows the cause of the radiographic abnormalities: a large aortic body tumor (arrows). The pericardium is still intact in this image.

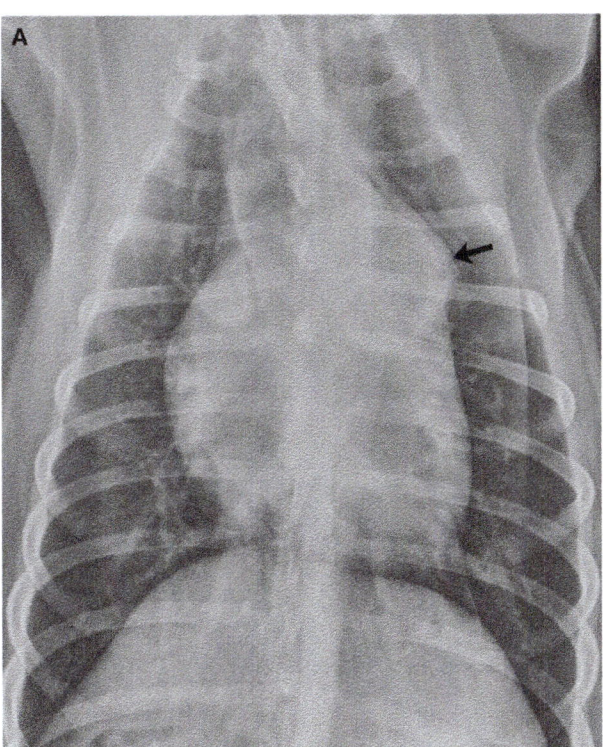 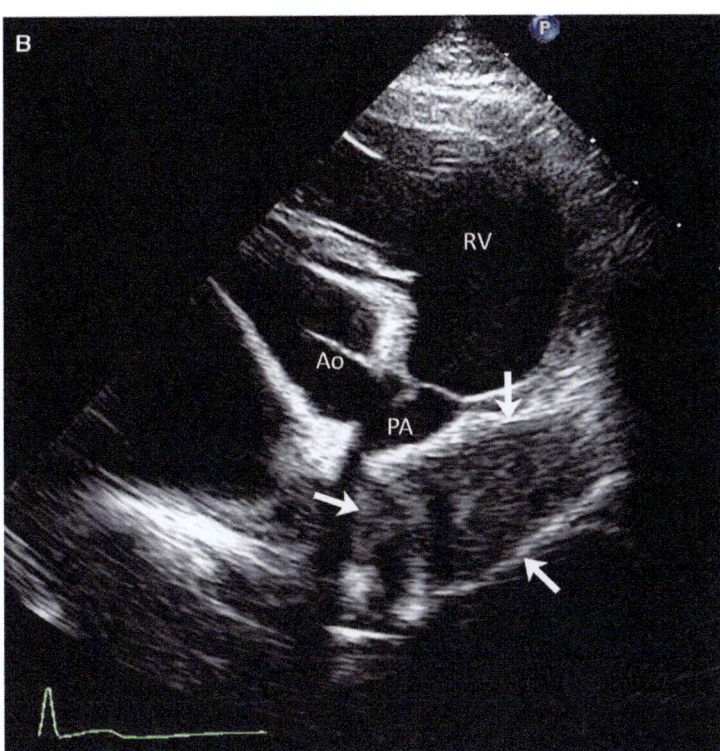

Figure 35.50 A 2-year-old female Golden Retriever presented for a 3–4 months history of making grunting sounds when lying down. (A) Based on the bulge (arrow) seen on DV radiograph, pulmonic stenosis or heartworm (HW) disease initially was suspected. However, the dog had no murmur, a HW test the month before was negative, and the dog was being given HW prophylaxis. (B) Echocardiography revealed a soft tissue mass (arrows) adjacent to (and slightly impinging on) the main pulmonary artery (PA). The aortic root and ascending aorta did not appear involved. Such masses sometimes are so obstructive as to cause right-sided CHF. Angled right parasternal short-axis view. Ao, aortic root; RV, right ventricle.

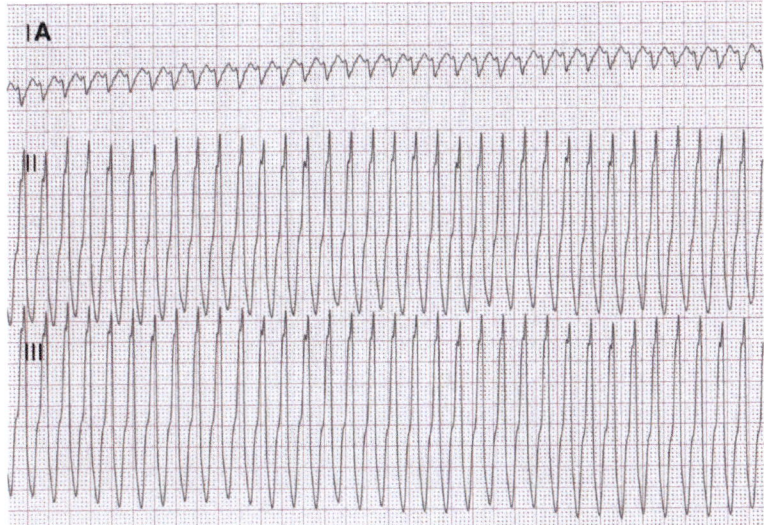 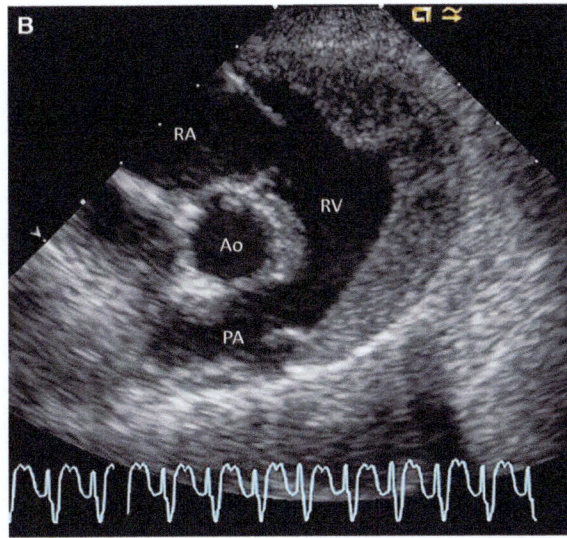

Figure 35.51 (A) Rapid sustained ventricular tachycardia (~280 beats/min) in a 4-year-old female English Cocker Spaniel with a history of inflammatory bowel disease. Leads I, II, III, 25 mm/s, 1 cm = 1 mV. (B) Echocardiography showed marked thickening and variable echogenicity of the right ventricular free wall and portions of left ventricular myocardium (not seen on this image), with no evidence for pulmonary hypertension nor right ventricular outflow obstruction. The ventricular tachycardia had become refractory to several antiarrhythmic drugs by the time of the echo exam. Myocardial lymphoma was suspected. Because of the dog's grave condition, L-asparaginase and dexamethasone were administered empirically, along with multiple antiarrhythmic drugs and other supportive care. The following day the dog was in sinus rhythm. Over the next few days, the myocardial thickening regressed dramatically; chemotherapy for lymphoma was continued.

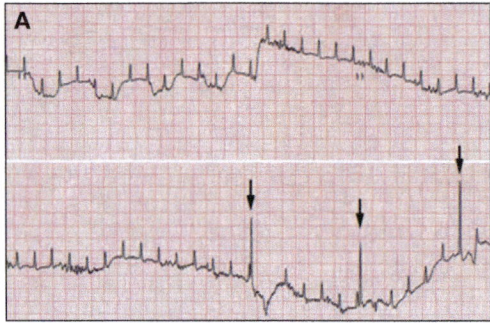

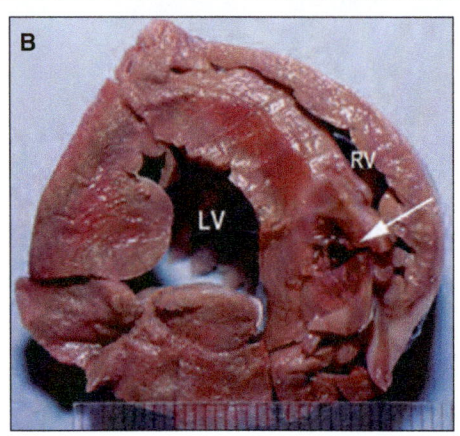

Figure 35.52 A 17-year-old female dog with recent-onset collapse episodes had variable atrioventricular (AV) block. (A) Continuous lead II ECG shows sinus tachycardia (tall P waves) and complete AV block. No ventricular activity occurs until a few ventricular escape complexes finally appear (arrows, bottom strip). (B) At postmortem, a small hemangiosarcoma (arrow) was found within the region of the AV conduction system in the basal ventricular septum. No other cardiac lesions were identified.

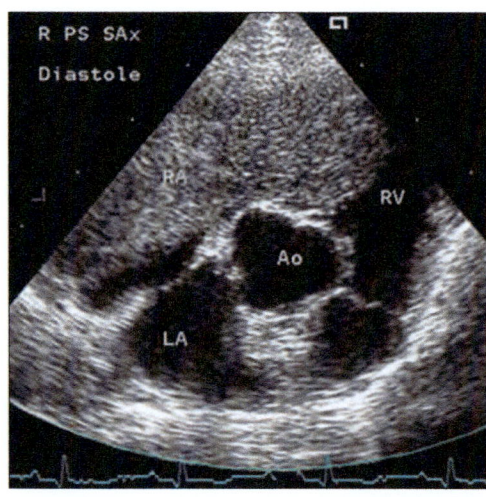

Figure 35.54 An extensive soft tissue mass is in the RA of a 16-year-old male Cockapoo with ascites and hindlimb weakness. The mass bulges through the tricuspid orifice into the RV in diastole. In systole, it would move back into the RA as the tricuspid valve closed. There is no pericardial effusion. Radiographic heart size was normal. Right parasternal short-axis. Ao, aorta; LA, left atrium; RA, right atrium; RV, right ventricle.

of pericardial effusion aids in finding, and assessing the location and extent of, heart base and other masses that extend into the pericardial space. Although most masses that appear to arise from the heart base are aortic body tumors (or less often, ectopic thyroid tumors), other neoplasia could have

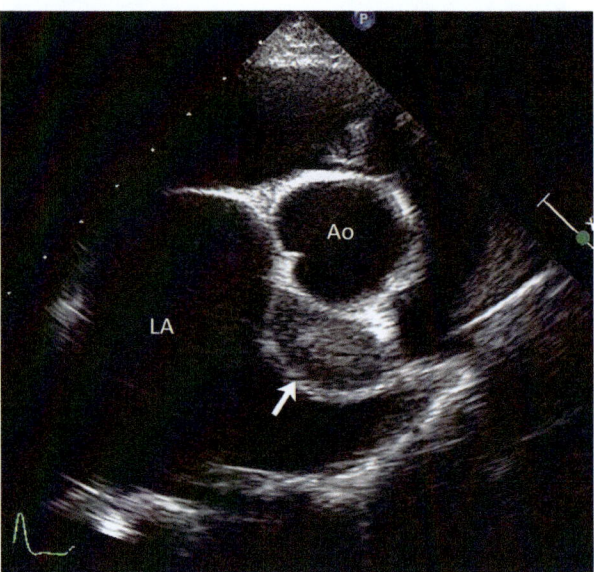

Figure 35.53 A small heart base tumor (arrow) was an incidental echocardiographic finding in a 7-year-old male mixed-breed dog with stage B2 myxomatous mitral valve disease. There was no pericardial effusion. Right parasternal short-axis view. Ao, aorta; LA, left atrium.

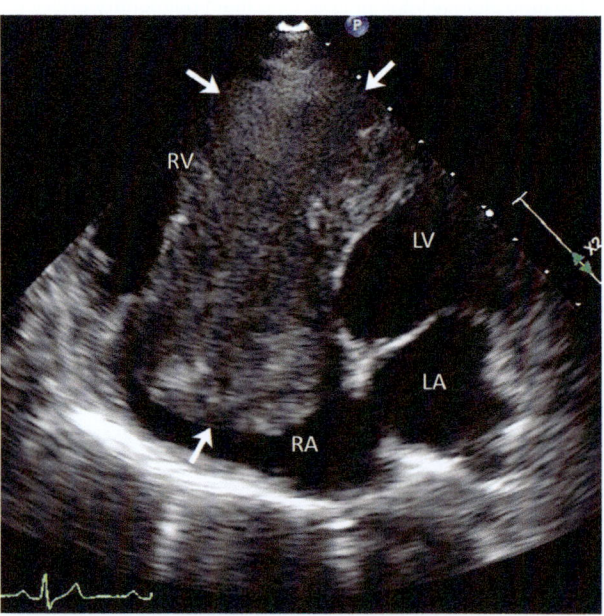

Figure 35.55 A huge soft tissue mass (arrows) extends from the cranial RA and its auricle across the tricuspid valve and into the RV, obstructing ventricular inflow. The mass almost fills the RV and reaches into its outflow tract. No pericardial effusion is present. The 9-year-old male, large mixed-breed dog had a history of decreasing exercise tolerance, weight loss, malaise, and abdominal enlargement (ascites) over the prior 3–4 weeks. Medical therapy for right-sided heart failure signs would be counterproductive in this case, as it would in a case of cardiac tamponade. LA, left atrium; LV, Left ventricle; RA, right atrium; RV, right ventricle.

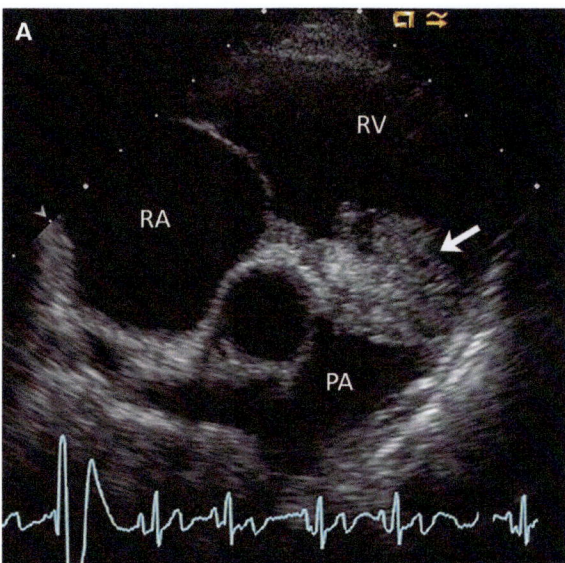

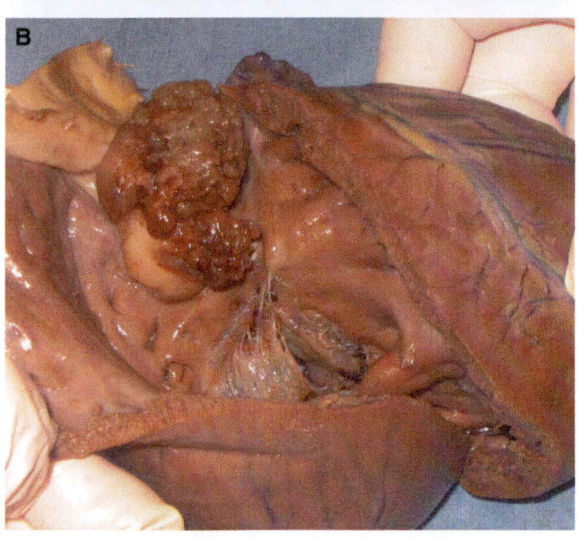

Figure 35.56 A 15-year-old female Australian Shepherd with a history of syncopal or seizure episodes, poor appetite, generalized weakness, and hyperadrenocorticism was referred for increasingly frequent collapse. Radiographically, the cardiac silhouette was normal; however, a grade 3/6 systolic murmur could be heard at the left heart base. (A) An irregular soft-tissue mass (arrow) encompassing the pulmonary valve is evident on this right parasternal short-axis echocardiogram. The mass obstructed outflow, which explained the systolic murmur and dilated RA and RV. The owner declined a surgical attempt to excise or debulk the mass. As expected, weakness and syncopal events continued with increasing frequency until the dog died suddenly about 2 weeks later. PA, pulmonary artery; RA, right atrium; RV, right ventricle. (B) Postmortem image of open right ventricular outflow region in this dog. A multilobulated mass obliterates the pulmonary valve. Histological description indicated chondroid metaplasia, possibly originating as chondroma or myxoma.

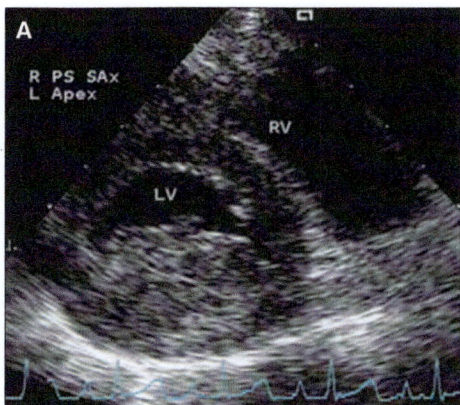

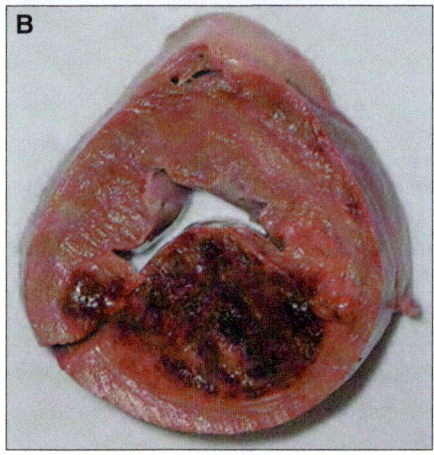

Figure 35.57 (A) A soft tissue mass involving the left ventricular apical region invades the free wall of the LV and extends into the lumen in a 17-year-old female Keeshond. There is no pericardial effusion. The dog had recent-onset weakness and acute collapse episodes. ECG showed paroxysmal ventricular tachycardia. Right parasternal short-axis. LV, left ventricle; RV right ventricle. (B) Cut section through the ventral LV from this dog shows the dark tumor mass (a hemangiosarcoma). This tumor rarely develops within the left heart.

similar anatomic location and appearance, including HSA, mesothelioma, and other neuroendocrine tumors. Likewise, despite the fact that most RA masses or those invading the right AV groove are HSA, a variety of other histologic tumor types might arise in this location, including aortic body tumor, ectopic thyroid tumor, mesothelioma, lymphoma, and various sarcomas. Furthermore, tumors that appear unusual on echocardiogram often are of a common histologic type. Therefore, prediction of cardiac tumor type based on location probably is only moderately accurate. Non-neoplastic masses occur rarely, as well. Echocardiography can depict the hemodynamic effects of various mass lesions. Secondary changes in cardiac chamber size, wall thickness, and valve motion could be evident. Even when mass lesions are not clearly apparent, abnormal chamber shape and pericardial adhesions can occur with mesothelioma (**Figure 35.58**) or rarely, a granulomatous inflammatory process. Doppler echocardiography can define intracardiac blood flow abnormalities (**Figure 35.59**). Determination of the location, size, attachment (pedunculated or broad-based), and extent (superficial or deeply invading adjacent myocardium) of the cardiac tumor(s) is of value when assessing whether surgical resection or biopsy might be possible.

CT, MRI, or other imaging techniques (including pneumopericardiography and angiocardiography, although rarely

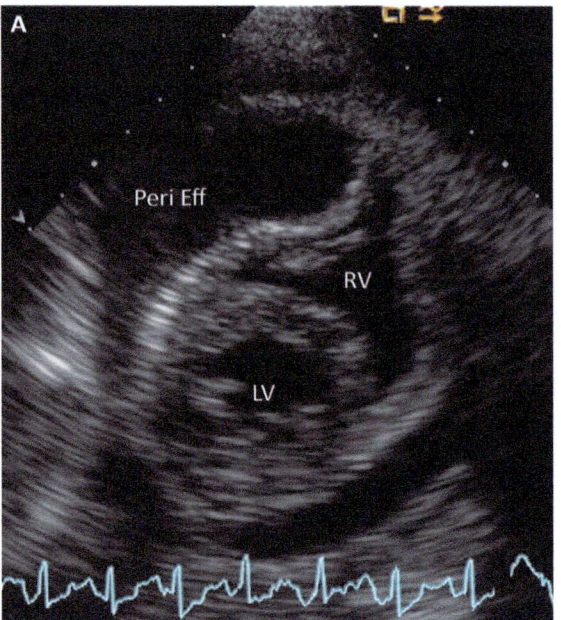
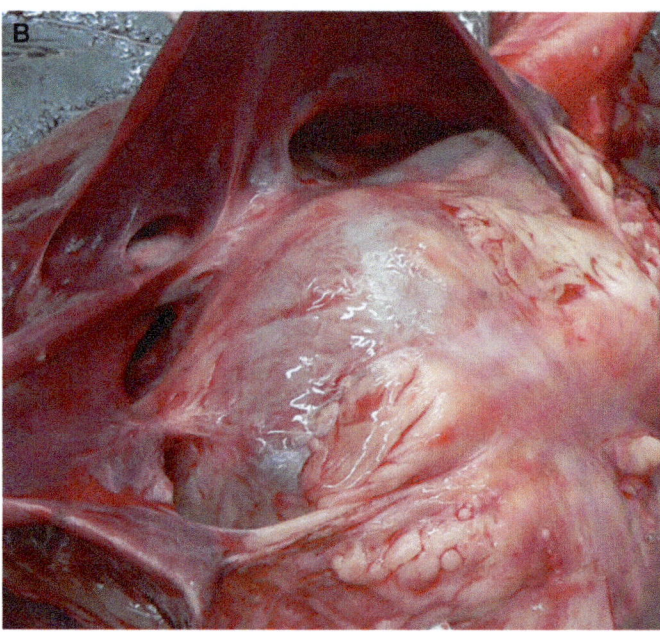

Figure 35.58 A 10-year-old male Golden Retriever developed cardiac tamponade three times over the course of about 6 months. No mass lesion was visible prior to pericardiocentesis on either of the first two echo exams. (A) Right parasternal echocardiographic image from the third presentation shows adhesions between the right ventricular free wall and pericardium. Again, no definite mass lesion was identified. Pericardial fluid was drained, but surgical exploration was declined. The dog died one month later. LV, left ventricle; Peri Eff, pericardial effusion; RV, right ventricle. (B) Postmortem image shows multiple areas of adhesion between the pericardium and epicardium. The diagnosis was mesothelioma of the pericardium, also involving portions of pleura, with multifocal dense fibrous tissue (scirrhous) reaction. Neoplastic emboli were evident within some small pericardial vessels. A large (fibrinous) pulmonary thromboembolus also was found.

used now; **Figures 35.60** and **35.61**) also can help identify cardiac tumors. Differentiation of neoplastic effusions from benign hemorrhagic pericarditis usually is not possible solely by pericardial fluid analysis (p. 722); nevertheless, lymphoma and occasionally some other tumors can be identified cytologically. Ultrasound-guided transthoracic fine needle aspiration of certain cardiac mass lesions might be possible depending on their location, which could yield cytologic diagnosis. Anesthesia or sedation alone might be adequate for this in some cases.

Management

Pericardiocentesis is indicated immediately for cardiac tamponade (p. 724). Conservative therapy, with pericardiocentesis as needed, is used in some patients until episodes of

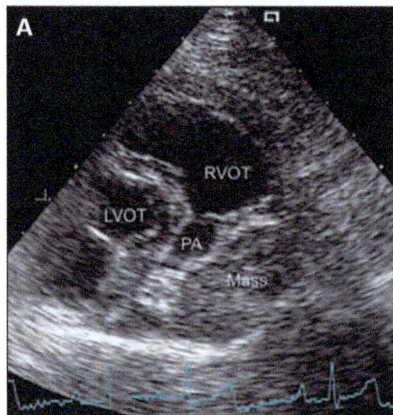
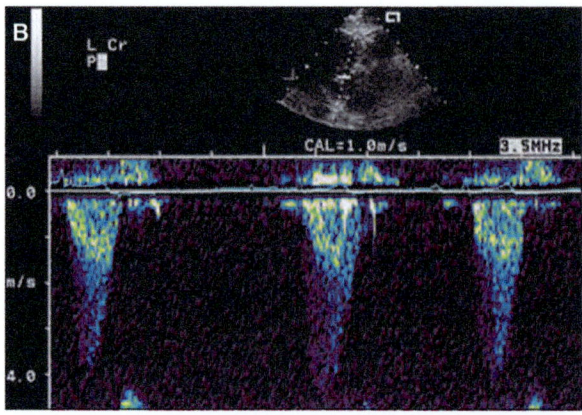

Figure 35.59 (A) A mass within the pericardium compressed the right ventricular outflow tract (RVOT) and main pulmonary artery (PA) area, without causing pericardial effusion, in a 9-year-old male Keeshond. It caused a systolic ejection murmur and compensatory right ventricular hypertrophy. Right parasternal short-axis. LVOT, left ventricular outflow tract. (B) Continuous wave Doppler shows increased pulmonary velocity to ~4 m/s (gradient ~64 mm Hg), resulting from outflow obstruction. The denser, lower velocity signal represents proximal (prestenotic) blood velocity (V_1).

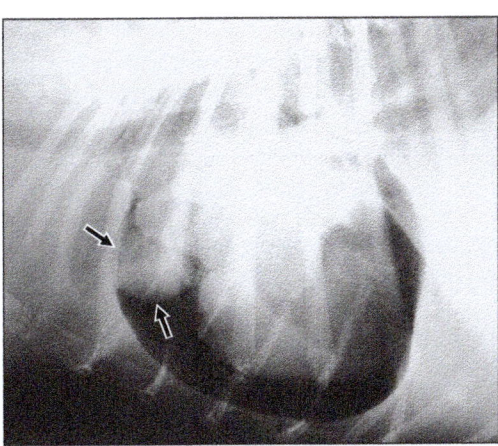

Figure 35.60 Pneumopericardiogram in an older Boxer with cardiac tamponade shows abnormal soft tissue opacity (arrows) at the cranial heart base, consistent with an aortic body tumor. Compare with the normal study in **Figure 35.32**.

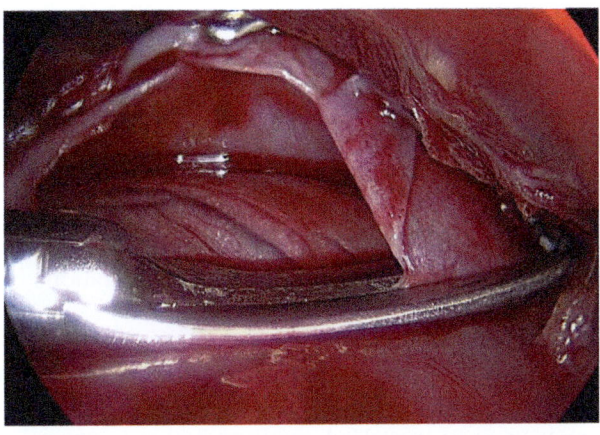

Figure 35.62 A section of pericardium is being cut away to create a pericardial window during thoracoscopic surgery in a different 9-year-old male Boston Terrier with a large heart base tumor. (Courtesy Dr J Naiman.)

cardiac tamponade become unmanageable. Whether antiinflammatory doses of a glucocorticoid are of benefit is unclear. Surgical pericardiotomy or subtotal pericardiectomy can prevent recurrent tamponade but might facilitate metastatic dissemination throughout the thoracic cavity. However, this does not appear to affect survival time with HSA or mesothelioma. Heart base tumors (such as chemodectoma) tend to be slow growing, so partial pericardiectomy could prolong survival for months to years. A thoracoscopic (**Figure 35.62**) or open surgical approach could be used. While balloon pericardiotomy (p. 728) might provide a less invasive alternative to surgery in some patients, this procedure is not advocated in most instances. Guide wire contact with a HSA during the

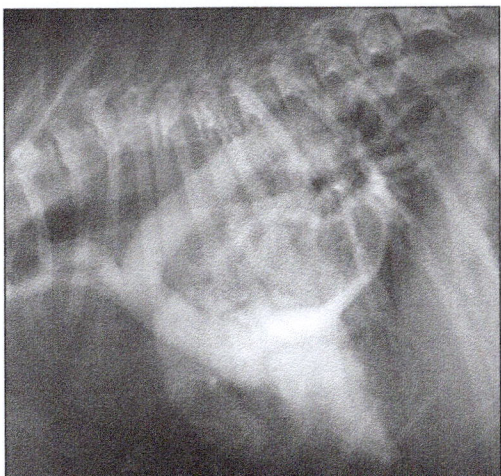

Figure 35.61 Levo-phase of a nonselective angiocardiogram shows radiopaque contrast material in the left heart and aorta (and faintly in the pulmonary artery). A large heart base mass has compressed the left atrium and pushed the carina and descending aorta dorsally. From a 9-year-old Boston Terrier. (Image courtesy of Dr E Riedesel.)

procedure could cause extensive bleeding, because this tumor is so friable. Furthermore, the pericardial opening created by balloon pericardiotomy is more likely to become occluded over time compared to a surgically created pericardial window or partial pericardiectomy.

Because heart base and some other tumors are quite locally invasive, complete surgical resection rarely is possible. Nevertheless, occasional tumors might be amenable to surgical resection, depending on their location and extent. Resection of a small mass at the tip of the right auricle has been successfully accomplished using thoracoscopy. Open thoracotomy probably is needed to attempt removal or debulking of larger right auricular masses; this might also require pericardial patch grafting. Surgical biopsy of a nonresectable mass could be helpful if chemotherapy is contemplated. In cases where the tumor has externally compressed a major vessel, stent placement might provide some palliation (Bussadori, 2020).

In general, dogs with a heart base tumor have much longer median survival time than those with an RA mass (historically, ~5 months vs less than 1 week, respectively). One study of dogs with a heart base mass found that successful pericardiectomy improved median survival time to about 2 years, compared to dogs with no surgery, where median survival was just over 1 month (Ehrhart, 2002). While many cardiac tumors are unresponsive to conventional therapies, some are treated with short-term success. Stereotaxic radiation therapy combined with elective pericardial window resulted in a median survival of about 400 days in a study of 28 dogs with chemodectoma; most dogs had at least partial response, with low rate of adverse radiation effects (Kruckman-Gatesy, 2020). Caval obstruction, regional lymph node enlargement, tachyarrhythmias, and clinical signs were negatively associated with survival in that study. In a retrospective study of toceranib (Palladia®), 27 dogs with heart base tumors had an overall median survival time of 823 days, with a wide range of survival (Lew, 2019). This study indicates that dogs affected by this tumor can have prolonged survival. Nevertheless, the retrospective nature of that study and the need for stringent disease staging and treatment blinding demands prospective assessment of toceranib for treating these neoplasms. Until that is available, an oncologist should be consulted regarding treatment options for chemodectoma. Because chemodectoma often is an incidental finding, clinical status and tumor staging at the time of diagnosis are considerations when assessing potential survival times.

Management of canine HSA is less successful, in part because of the high rate of metastasis, as well as multicentric localization in some cases. Doxorubicin and carboplatin have been used to treat HSA, with or without surgical mass resection. Overall, the results of chemotherapy alone or with surgery are dismal to poor. Even with surgery and adjunctive chemotherapy, median survival times of <6 months are anticipated, although occasional dogs live longer. For dogs with presumptive cardiac HSA, radiation therapy appears to be well-tolerated and can reduce the frequency of pericardiocentesis required to manage recurrent tamponade; median survival time was 79 days in one study (Nolan, 2017). With regard to delaying the recurrence of tamponade or prolonging survival in dogs with presumptive HSA, no benefit was shown for treatment with Yunnan Baiyao (either alone or in combination with the plasminogen activation inhibitor, epsilon aminocaproic acid) compared with pericardiocentesis only. Yunnan Baiyao is a Chinese herbal remedy with hemostatic properties. Immunotherapy might become a viable option for some tumors. Consultation with an oncologist, as well as current sources for antineoplastic drug protocols and other tumor treatment modalities, is recommended. At present, the long-term prognosis for animals with cardiac tumors is generally guarded to poor.

Suggested Additional Reading and References

Also See Online Comprehensive Bibliography at: https://www.routledge.com/9781482246223.

Alleman AR. Abdominal, thoracic, and pericardial effusions. Vet Clin North Am Small Anim Pract 2003;33:89–118.

Amati M, Venco L, Roccabianca P, et al. Pericardial lymphoma in seven cats. J Feline Med Surg 2014;16:507–512.

Armstrong SK, Raidal SL, Hughes KJ. Fibrinous pericarditis and pericardial effusion in three neonatal foals. Aust Vet J 2014;92:392–399.

Aronson LR, Gregory CR. Infectious pericardial effusion in five dogs. Vet Surg 1995;24:402–407.

Atencia S, Doyle RS, Whitley NT. Thoracoscopic pericardial window for management of pericardial effusion in 15 dogs. J Small Anim Pract 2013;54:564–569.

Aupperle H, Marz I, Ellenberger C, et al. Primary and secondary heart tumours in dogs and cats. J Comp Pathol 2007;136:18–26.

Barbur LA, Rawlings CA, Radlinsky MG. Epicardial exposure provided by a novel thoracoscopic pericardectomy technique compared to standard pericardial window. Vet Surg 2018;47:146–152.

Baumwart RD, Hanzlicek AS, Lyon SD, et al. Plasma N-terminal pro-brain natriuretic peptide concentrations before and after pericardiocentesis in dogs with cardiac tamponade secondary to spontaneous pericardial effusion. J Vet Cardiol 2017;19:416–420.

Beaumier A, Dixon CE, Robinson N, et al. Primary cardiac hemangiosarcoma in a horse: echocardiographic and necropsy findings. J Vet Cardiol 2020;32:66–72.

Berry CR, Koblik PD, Ticer JW. Dorsal peritoneopericardial mesothelial remnant as an aid to the diagnosis of feline congenital peritoneopericardial diaphragmatic hernia. Vet Radiol US 1990;31:239–245.

Boddy KN, Sleeper MM, Sammarco CD, et al. Cardiac magnetic resonance in the differentiation of neoplastic and nonneoplastic pericardial effusion. J Vet Intern Med 2011;25:1003–1009.

Bolin DC, Donahue JM, Vickers ML, et al. Microbiologic and pathologic findings in an epidemic of equine pericarditis. J Vet Diagn Invest 2005;17:38–44.

Boston SE, Higginson G, Monteith G. Concurrent splenic and right atrial mass at presentation in dogs with HSA: a retrospective study. J Am Anim Hosp Assoc 2011;47:336–341.

Burns CG, Bergh MS, McLoughlin MA. Surgical and nonsurgical treatment of peritoneopericardial diaphragmatic hernia in dogs and cats: 58 cases (1999–2008). J Am Vet Med Assoc 2013;242:643–650.

Bussadori CM, Claretti M, Borgonovo S, et al. Branch pulmonary artery stent placement in a dog with heart base neoplasia. J Vet Cardiol 2020;30:17–22.

Cagle LA, Epstein SE, Owens SD, et al. Diagnostic yield of cytologic analysis of pericardial effusion in dogs. J Vet Intern Med 2014;28:66–71.

Carvajal JL, Case JB, Mayhew PD, et al. Outcome in dogs with presumptive idiopathic pericardial effusion after thoracoscopic pericardectomy and pericardioscopy. Vet Surg 2019;48:O105–O111.

Case JB. Advances in video-assisted thoracic surgery, thoracoscopy. Vet Clin North Am Small Anim Pract 2016;46:147–169.

Case JB, Maxwell M, Aman A, et al. Outcome evaluation of a thoracoscopic pericardial window procedure or subtotal pericardectomy via thoracotomy for the treatment of pericardial effusion in dogs. J Am Vet Med Assoc 2013;242:493–498.

Celona B, Crino C, Giudice E, et al. Evaluation of pericardial effusion in dogs and successful treatment using a hemodialysis fistula needle: a retrospective study. Top Companion Anim Med 2017;32:72–75.

Chun R, Kellihan HB, Henik RA, et al. Comparison of plasma cardiac troponin I concentrations among dogs with cardiac hemangiosarcoma, noncardiac hemangiosarcoma, other neoplasms, and pericardial effusion of nonhemangiosarcoma origin. J Am Vet Med Assoc 2010;237:806–811.

Cook S, Cortellini S, Humm K. Retrospective evaluation of pericardial catheter placement in the management of pericardial effusion in dogs (2007–2015):18 cases. J Vet Emerg Crit Care 2019;29:413–417.

Cote E, Schwarz LA, Sithole F. Thoracic radiographic findings for dogs with cardiac tamponade attributable to pericardial effusion. J Am Vet Med Assoc 2013;243:232–235.

Covey HL, Connolly DJ. Pericardial effusion associated with systemic inflammatory disease in seven dogs (January 2006–January 2012). J Vet Cardiol 2018;20:123–128.

Davidson BJ, Paling AC, Lahmers SL, et al. Disease association and clinical assessment of feline pericardial effusion. J Am Anim Hosp Assoc 2008;44:5–9.

De Ridder M, Kitshoff A, Devriendt N, et al. Transdiaphragmatic pericardiectomy in dogs. Vet Rec 2017;180:95.

Decloedt A. Pericardial disease, myocardial disease, and great vessel abnormalities in horses. Vet Clin North Am Equine Pract 2019;35:139–157.

DeFrancesco TC. Management of cardiac emergencies in small animals. Vet Clin North Am Small Anim Pract 2013;43:817–842.

Ehrhart N, Ehrhart EJ, Willis J, et al. Analysis of factors affecting survival in dogs with aortic body tumors. Vet Surg 2002;31:44–48.

Fahey R, Rozanski E, Paul A, et al. Prevalence of vomiting in dogs with pericardial effusion. J Vet Emerg Crit Care 2017;27:250–252.

Fine DM, Tobias AH, Jacob KA. Use of pericardial fluid pH to distinguish between idiopathic and neoplastic effusions. J Vet Intern Med 2003;17:525–529.

Ghaffari S, Pelio DC, Lange AJ, et al. A retrospective evaluation of doxorubicin-based chemotherapy for dogs with right atrial masses and pericardial effusion. J Small Anim Pract 2014;55:254–257.

Guglielmini C, Baron Toaldo M, Quinci M, et al. Sensitivity, specificity, and interobserver variability of survey thoracic radiography for the detection of heart base masses in dogs. J Am Vet Med Assoc 2016;248:1391–1398.

Guglielmini C, Diana A, Santarelli G, et al. Accuracy of radiographic vertebral heart score and sphericity index in the detection of pericardial effusion in dogs. J Am Vet Med Assoc 2012;241:1048–1055.

Hall DJ, Shofer F, Meier CK, et al. Pericardial effusion in cats: a retrospective study of clinical findings and outcome in 146 cats. J Vet Intern Med 2007;21:1002–1007.

Heinritz CK, Gilson SD, Soderstrom MJ, et al. Subtotal pericardectomy and epicardial excision for treatment of coccidioidomycosis-induced effusive-constrictive pericarditis in dogs: 17 cases (1999-2003). J Am Vet Med Assoc 2005;227:435–440.

Holak P, Szalecki P, Adamiak Z, et al. Thoracoscopic creation of a pericardial window in dogs. Pol J Vet Sci 2009;12:419–421.

Humm KR, Keenaghan-Clark EA, Boag AK. Adverse events associated with pericardiocentesis in dogs: 85 cases (1999-2006). J Vet Emerg Crit Care 2009;19:352–356.

Jesty SA, Reef VB. Septicemia and cardiovascular infections in horses. Vet Clin North Am Equine Pract 2006;22:481–495, ix.

Kaplan JL, Gunther-Harrington CT, Sutton JS, et al. Multiple midline defects identified in a litter of golden retrievers following gestational administration of prednisone and doxycycline: a case series. BMC Vet Res 2018;14:86.

Kohnken R, Durham JA, Premanandan C, et al. Aortic chondroid neoplasia in two Labrador Retriever dogs. J Vet Cardiol 2015;17:314–320.

Kruckman-Gatesy CR, Ames MK, Griffin LR, et al. A retrospective analysis of stereotactic body radiation therapy for canine heart base tumors: 26 cases. J Vet Cardiol 2020;27:62–77.

Kurt S, Kovacevic A. Atrial rupture and pericardial effusion as a complication of chronic mitral valve endocardiosis. Schweiz Arch Tierheilkd 2012;154:397–401.

Lew FH, McQuown B, Borrego J, et al. Retrospective evaluation of canine heart base tumours treated with toceranib phosphate (Palladia): 2011–2018. Vet Comp Oncol 2019;17:465–471.

Linde A, Summerfield NJ, Sleeper MM, et al. Pilot study on cardiac troponin I levels in dogs with pericardial effusion. J Vet Cardiol 2006;8:19–23.

Lisciandro GR. Abdominal and thoracic focused assessment with sonography for trauma, triage, and monitoring in small animals. J Vet Emerg Crit Care 2011;21:104–122.

Lisciandro GR. The use of the diaphragmatico-hepatic (DH) views of the abdominal and thoracic focused assessment with sonography for triage (AFAST/TFAST) examinations for the detection of pericardial effusion in 24 dogs (2011–2012). J Vet Emerg Crit Care 2016;26:125–131.

MacDonald KA, Cagney O, Magne ML. Echocardiographic and clinicopathologic characterization of pericardial effusion in dogs: 107 cases (1985–2006). J Am Vet Med Assoc 2009;235:1456–1461.

MacGregor JM, Faria ML, Moore AS, et al. Cardiac lymphoma and pericardial effusion in dogs: 12 cases (1994–2004). J Am Vet Med Assoc 2005;227:1449–1453.

Margolis C, Zakosek Pipan M, Demchur J, et al. Congenital peritoneopericardial diaphragmatic hernia in a family of Persian cats. JFMS Open Reports 2018;4:2055116918804305.

Mayhew KN, Mayhew PD, Sorrell-Raschi L, et al. Thoracoscopic subphrenic pericardectomy using double-lumen endobronchial intubation for alternating one-lung ventilation. Vet Surg 2009;38:961–966.

Mayhew PD, Dunn M, Berent A. Surgical views: thoracoscopy: common techniques in small animals. Compend Contin Educ Vet 2013;35:E1.

Michelotti KP, Youk A, Payne JT, et al. Outcomes of dogs with recurrent idiopathic pericardial effusion treated with a 3-port right-sided thoracoscopic subtotal pericardiectomy. Vet Surg 2019;48:1032–1041.

Monnet E. Interventional thoracoscopy in small animals. Vet Clin North Am Small Anim Pract 2009;39:965–975.

Morgan KRS, Singh A, Giuffrida MA, et al. Outcome after surgical and conservative treatments of canine peritoneopericardial diaphragmatic hernia: A multi-institutional study of 128 dogs. Vet Surg 2020;49:138–145.

Murphy LA, Panek CM, Bianco D, et al. Use of Yunnan Baiyao and epsilon aminocaproic acid in dogs with right atrial masses and pericardial effusion. J Vet Emerg Crit Care 2017;27:121–126.

Murphy LA, Russell NJ, Dulake MI, et al. Constrictive pericarditis following surgical repair of a peritoneopericardial diaphragmatic hernia in a cat. J Feline Med Surg 2014;16:708–712.

Nelson DA, Miller MW, Gordon SG, et al. Minimally invasive transxiphoid approach to the cardiac apex and caudoventral intrathoracic space. Vet Surg 2012;41:915–917.

Nolan MW, Arkans MM, LaVine D, et al. Pilot study to determine the feasibility of radiation therapy for dogs with right atrial masses and hemorrhagic pericardial effusion. J Vet Cardiol 2017;19:132–143.

Oricco S, Perego M, Poggi M, et al. Aortic dissection in four cats: clinicopathological correlations. J Vet Cardiol 2019;25:52–60.

Pazdzior-Czapula K, Otrocka-Domagala I, Myrdek P, et al. Dirofilaria repens-an etiological factor or an incidental finding in cytologic and histopathologic biopsies from dogs. Vet Clin Pathol 2018;47:307–311.

Pedro B, Linney C, Navarro-Cubas X, et al. Cytological diagnosis of cardiac masses with ultrasound guided fine needle aspirates. J Vet Cardiol 2016;18:47–56.

Ployart S, Libermann S, Doran I, et al. Thoracoscopic resection of right auricular masses in dogs: 9 cases (2003-2011). J Am Vet Med Assoc 2013;242:237–241.

Rajagopalan V, Jesty SA, Craig LE, et al. Comparison of presumptive echocardiographic and definitive diagnoses of cardiac tumors in dogs. J Vet Intern Med 2013;27:1092–1096.

Reimer SB, Kyles AE, Filipowicz DE, et al. Long-term outcome of cats treated conservatively or surgically for peritoneopericardial diaphragmatic hernia: 66 cases (1987-2002). J Am Vet Med Assoc 2004;224:728–732.

Rivera PA, Borgarelli M. Cardiovascular images: constrictive pericarditis and tricavitary effusion in a dog with pericardial mesothelioma. J Vet Cardiol 2020;32:55–59.

Rush JE, Keene BK, Fox PR. Pericardial disease in the cat: a retrospective evaluation of 66 cases. J Am Anim Hosp Assoc 1990;26:39–46.

Scollan KF, Bottorff B, Stieger-Vanegas S, et al. Use of multidetector computed tomography in the assessment of dogs with pericardial effusion. J Vet Intern Med 2015;29:79–87.

Schwartz A, Wilson GP, Hamlin RL, et al. Constrictive pericarditis in two dogs. J Am Vet Med Assoc 1971;159:763–776.

Schwarzwald CC. Disorders of the cardiovascular system. In, Reed SM, Bayle WM, Sellon DC (editors), Equine Internal Medicine, 4th edition. 2018. Elsevier, St. Louis. pp. 387–541.

Sebastian MM, Bernard WV, Riddle TW, et al. Review paper: mare reproductive loss syndrome. Vet Pathol 2008;45:710–722.

Shaw SP, Rozanski EA, Rush JE. Cardiac troponins I and T in dogs with pericardial effusion. J Vet Intern Med 2004;18:322–324.

Sidley JA, Atkins CE, Keene BW, et al. Percutaneous balloon pericardiotomy as a treatment for recurrent pericardial effusion in 6 dogs. J Vet Intern Med 2002;16:541–546.

Simpson DJ, Hunt GB, Church DB, et al. Benign masses in the pericardium of two dogs. Aust Vet J 1999;77:225–229.

Sisson D, Thomas WP, Reed J, et al. Intrapericardial cysts in the dog. J Vet Intern Med 1993;7:364–369.

Spence S, French A, Penferis J, et al. The occurrence of cardiac abnormalities in canine steroid-responsive meningitis arteritis. J Small Anim Pract 2019.

Stafford Johnson M, Martin M, Binns S, et al. A retrospective study of clinical findings, treatment and outcome in 143 dogs with pericardial effusion. J Small Anim Pract 2004;45:546–552.

Stepien RL, Whitley NT, Dubielzig RR. Idiopathic or mesothelioma-related pericardial effusion: clinical findings and survival in 17 dogs studied retrospectively. J Small Anim Pract 2000;41:342–347.

Tabar MD, Movilla R, Serrano L, et al. PCR evaluation of selected vector-borne pathogens in dogs with pericardial effusion. J Small Anim Pract 2018;59:248–252.

Thomas WP, Reed JR, Bauer TG, et al. Constrictive pericardial disease in the dog. J Am Vet Med Assoc 1984;184:546–553.

Treggiari E, Pedro B, Dukes-McEwan J, et al. A descriptive review of cardiac tumours in dogs and cats. Vet Comp Oncol 2017;15:273–288.

Tse YC, Rush JE, Cunningham SM, et al. Evaluation of a training course in focused echocardiography for noncardiology house officers. J Vet Emerg Crit Care 2013;23:268–273.

Vicari ED, Brown DC, Holt DE, et al. Survival times of and prognostic indicators for dogs with heart base masses: 25 cases (1986-1999). J Am Vet Med Assoc 2001;219:485–487.

Walter JH, Rudolph R. Systemic, metastatic, eu- and heterotope tumours of the heart in necropsied dogs. Zentralbl Veterinarmed A. 1996;43:31–45.

Ware WA, Hopper DL. Cardiac tumors in dogs: 1982-1995. J Vet Intern Med 1999;13:95–103.

Ware WA. Cardiac neoplasia. In, Bonagura JD (editor). Kirk's Current Veterinary Therapy XII. WB Saunders, Philadelphia, PA. 1995. pp. 873–876.

Zini E, Glaus TM, Bussadori C, et al. Evaluation of the presence of selected viral and bacterial nucleic acids in pericardial samples from dogs with or without idiopathic pericardial effusion. Vet J 2009;179:225–229.

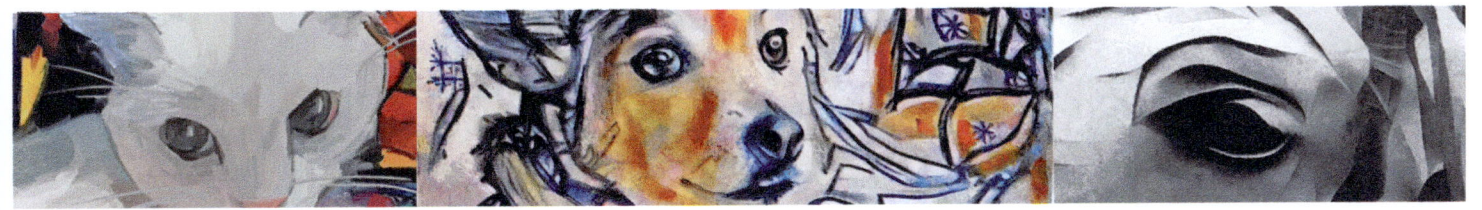

36
THROMBOEMBOLIC DISEASE

Coauthored by Brian A. Scansen

Thromboembolic (TE) disease can result when normal hemostatic mechanisms are disturbed. A thrombus is a locally formed (*in situ*) clot or aggregation of platelets and other blood elements that partially or completely obstructs blood flow either in a vessel or in the heart. An embolus is a clot or other aggregate (such as a foreign body or tumor) that breaks away from its origination site and is carried by blood flow until it lodges in a smaller vessel. Any part of the body can be affected, but most clinically recognized TE events involve the distal aorta, pulmonary arteries, heart, and cranial vena cava. Thrombi and emboli both can occur concurrently in some individuals.

Tissue injury, inflammation, and other situations can disturb the normal balance among factors that promote or inhibit clot formation and break-down. In general, conditions that cause cardiovascular (CV) endothelial damage, blood stasis, or hypercoagulability (including impaired fibrinolysis) promote TE disease. The clinical sequelae of thromboemboli depend mainly on their size and location, which determine the degree of organ or tissue compromise. Thromboemboli can cause acute and profound clinical signs or subclinical tissue damage that ultimately leads to varying degrees of pathology. TE disease sometimes is suspected antemortem; however, in other cases it is discovered only at necropsy (or not at all). This chapter focuses on principles of thromboembolism, related pathophysiology, and clinical TE disorders that mainly affect cats and dogs. Although a number of vascular disorders affect the horse (see Chapter 37), clinical syndromes of TE disease seem relatively uncommon or under-recognized in this species. In some situations, the pathogenesis of a systemic or pulmonary artery thrombosis is ill-defined and might represent either a TE event or localized thrombosis.

Normal Hemostasis

Normal hemostasis depends on the interplay among several different factors that promote coagulation, inhibit coagulation, and promote fibrinolysis. A proper balance of these factors maintains blood fluidity and minimizes loss when vessels are damaged. Hemostasis involves the vascular endothelium, platelets, proteins of the coagulation cascade, and the fibrinolytic system. Injury to the vascular endothelium quickly induces several reactions that cause vasoconstriction, hemostatic plug formation, and attempts at vascular repair. These are the normal hemostatic mechanisms used by the body to prevent blood loss. When a thrombus forms, the fibrinolytic system immediately begins to break it down. Normally, contraction and complete dissolution of the thrombus soon follow, although if hemostatic and fibrinolytic processes are disrupted, the thrombus might persist and become more extensive. Over time, persistent thrombi usually organize and eventually recanalize.

Intact vascular endothelial cells secrete substances that help prevent inappropriate thrombosis and participate in vasoregulation. Damaged endothelial cells promote thrombus formation. While this reduces blood loss in the event of vascular laceration, in other settings TE disease can result. Endothelial damage can contribute to thrombus formation in several ways. Injured endothelial cells release endothelin, which promotes vasoconstriction and decreases local blood flow. Exposed subendothelial collagen and other substances stimulate platelet adherence, activation and aggregation. Injured endothelial and other cells also release tissue factor (thromboplastin), which initiates coagulation and contributes to further platelet activation (**Figure 36.1**).

The hemostatic process has been described in several ways; for example, primary vs. secondary, or cell-based model vs. coagulation cascade. The currently accepted model

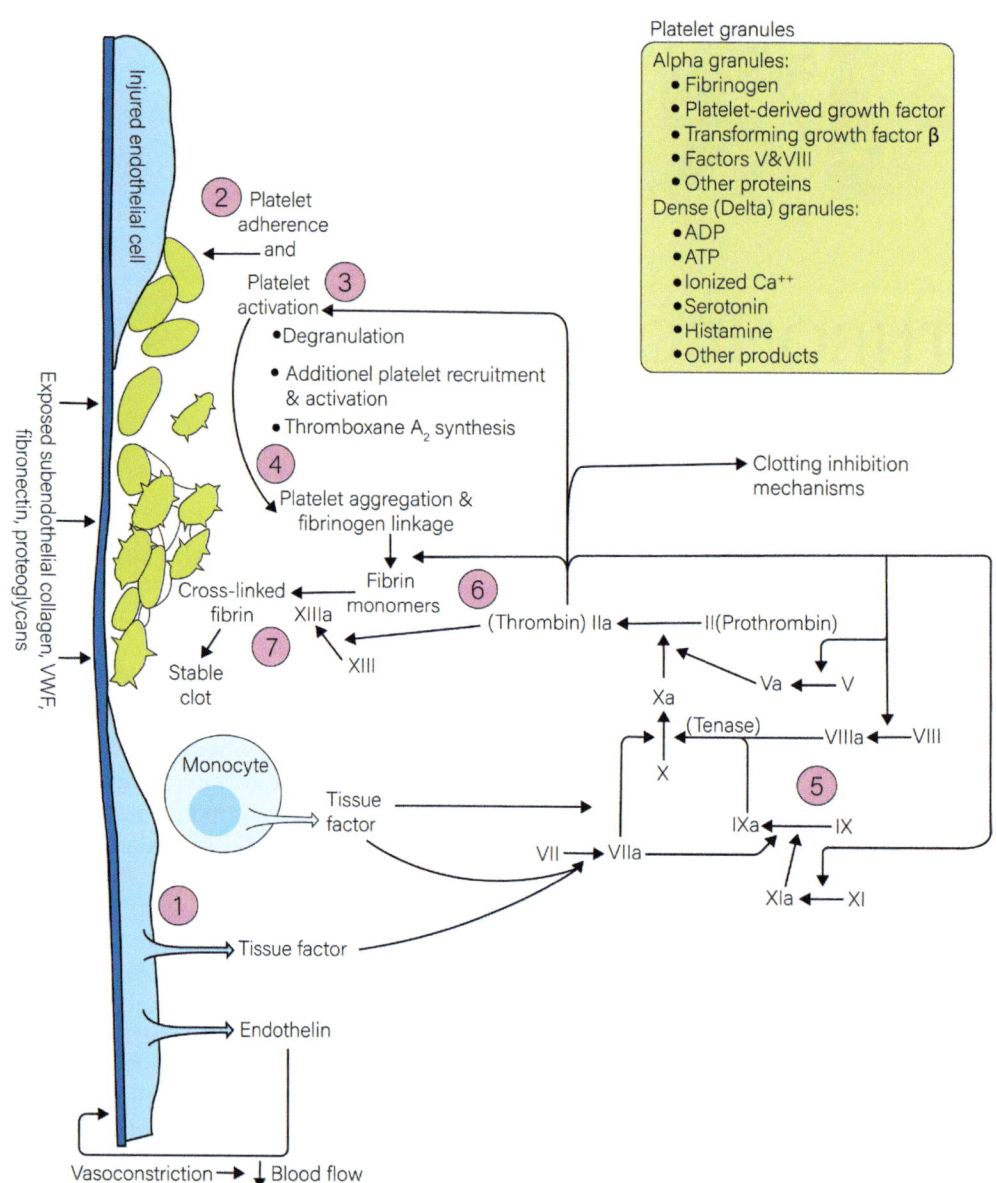

Figure 36.1 Schematic diagram summarizing major events in the hemostatic process. (1) Endothelial injury initiates clotting by (a) exposing collagen and other substances that promote platelet adherence, (b) releasing tissue factor which activates the coagulation cascade and thrombin production, and (c) stimulating vasoconstriction via endothelin release. Coagulation initiation also can occur in the absence of endothelial damage via expression of active tissue factor from various cells or circulating microparticles (see text). Active tissue factor triggers the generation of thrombin, which promotes platelet activation and degranulation, and which ultimately leads to fibrin formation. (2) Platelets adhere to the injured area. (3) Platelets become activated to release their granule contents. Platelet degranulation amplifies the coagulation process by recruiting and activating more platelets, as well as contributing to platelet interactions. Platelets also secrete thromboxane A_2, which fosters interplatelet signaling and aggregation. (4) Platelet aggregation increases (via linkage with fibrinogen). (5) Activated coagulation factors coalesce around the activated platelets; factors IXa and VIIIa (bound together as the tenase complex) activate more factor Xa. On platelet surfaces, factor Xa complexes with factor Va, which generates a burst of additional thrombin. (6) Thrombin also activates more factors VIIIa and Va, which further stimulate thrombin generation. Thrombin production stimulated by the coagulation cascade further promotes platelet aggregation and helps stabilize the clot by cleaving fibrinogen to fibrin. Thrombin also stimulates clot-inhibiting mechanisms. (7) Final clot stabilization occurs as thrombin-activated factor XIIIa catalyzes cross-linkage of fibrin monomers into insoluble fibrin. Activated clotting factors are designated by "a" following the Roman numeral. ADP, adenosine diphosphate, vWF, von Willebrand's factor.

of coagulation is the cell-based model, in which coagulation occurs in overlapping steps: initiation, amplification, and propagation. The initiation phase can begin in a couple of ways. One is by the exposure of subendothelial collagen caused by vascular trauma; this triggers the accumulation and activation of platelets at the site. Activated platelets adhere to collagen of the injured vessel wall and release contents of their granules. Interactions of platelet glycoproteins with exposed vascular collagen and collagen-bound von Willebrand factor (vWF) are important to the process of platelet adhesion and subsequent activation when subendothelial collagen exposure is an initiating factor. Another means of initiating thrombus formation is through the expression of active tissue factor, without requiring collagen exposure or vWF. Tissue factor can be released from cells in the vessel wall, or from fibroblasts, monocytes, other cells, and circulating microparticles. Tissue factor contained in circulating microparticles could be activated when the particles are recruited to a vascular injury site or, under pathological conditions, while in the circulation. Activated platelets, as well as endothelial cells, are thought capable of catalyzing the activation of latent tissue factor in the blood.

Active tissue factor is the initiator of thrombin generation and ultimately, fibrin formation. Tissue factor complexes with activated factor VII (VIIa), which promotes the activation of factor X (either directly or via factor IXa). Factor Xa (the activated form of factor X) localizes to the surface of the tissue factor-bearing cell and catalyzes the generation of thrombin (factor IIa) from prothrombin (factor II) at this site. Initially, just a small amount of thrombin is formed. Thrombin binds to thrombin receptors on the surface of platelets, which promotes platelet activation and stimulates the release of platelet (alpha and dense) granule contents (including adenosine diphosphate, ADP; serotonin; thromboxane A2; and other products). Platelet degranulation products further amplify the process by activating still more platelets and contributing to thrombus formation. Activation of platelet integrin alpha$_{IIb}$beta$_3$ mediates the recruitment of additional platelets and interplatelet interactions. During the amplification and propagation processes, thrombin promotes the activation of factors VIIIa and Va, which then facilitate additional factor Xa and thrombin generation that can continue without additional tissue factor.

During the propagation phase, platelet-platelet interactions and aggregation increase. Coagulation factors, activated during thrombus initiation and amplification, coalesce around the activated platelets. Factor IXa bound with factor VIIIa (the tenase complex) activates more factor Xa. On platelet surfaces, factor Xa complexes with factor Va (prothrombinase) and promotes a burst of additional thrombin generation. Thrombin converts fibrinogen into fibrin monomers. These polymerize to soluble fibrin, which then becomes cross-linked by the action of thrombin-activated factor XIIIa to form insoluble fibrin. The now-insoluble fibrin stabilizes the clot. Besides stimulating further platelet aggregation and fibrin formation, thrombin also contributes to negative feedback inhibition of clotting by interacting with thrombomodulin, proteins C and S, and antithrombin.

The above description differs somewhat from the traditional view of hemostasis as a primary platelet plug followed by the coagulation cascade. Conceptually, the coagulation cascade with its two arms (intrinsic and extrinsic pathways) that feed into the common pathway to produce thrombin remains useful for understanding the factors involved (**Figure 36.2**). However, this system only partially explains the hemostatic process in vivo.

Fibrinolysis

Once a thrombus forms, several mechanisms limit the extent of the clot and promote its breakdown. Thrombolysis requires

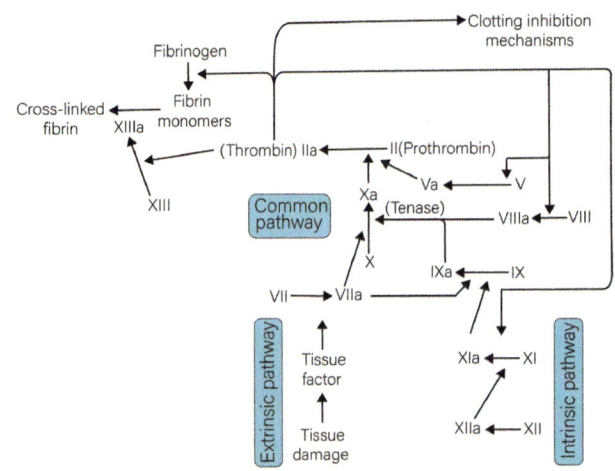

Figure 36.2 Traditional coagulation cascade concept, with intrinsic and extrinsic pathways that feed into a common pathway, leading to thrombin production. "a" designates activated factor. See text.

plasmin. Its inactive precursor, plasminogen, is converted to plasmin by tissue plasminogen activator (t-PA) when fibrin is present. During coagulation, endothelial cells simultaneously release t-PA. Other substances also act as plasminogen activators, including urokinase, bradykinen, kallikrein, and factor VII. Plasmin degrades fibrinogen and soluble (noncrosslinked) fibrin to yield fibrinogen/fibrin degradation products (FDPs). Plasmin also cleaves cross-linked fibrin within stabilized clots into large fragments (x-oligomers), which are further broken down into D-dimers and other fragments. D-dimers are produced only with active coagulation and subsequent fibrinolysis. There also are negative feedback constraints on fibrinolysis (such as plasminogen activator inhibitors, alpha$_2$-antiplasmin, thrombin-activated fibrinolytic factor). Defective fibrinolysis is thought to play a role in pathologic thrombosis.

Mechanisms Opposing Thrombosis

Inhibition of platelet adherence and activation is important in preventing the amplification process. In addition, there are three main mechanisms that limit thrombus formation: antithrombin, protein C, and the fibrinolytic system. Malfunction of one or more of these systems promotes thrombosis.

Intact endothelium normally produces factors that have antiplatelet, anticoagulant, or fibrinolytic effects. Antiplatelet substances include nitric oxide, prostacyclin, and adenosine diphosphatase (ADPase). Nitric oxide inhibits platelet activation and promotes local vasodilation. Prostacyclin also inhibits platelet activation and aggregation, while mediating vascular smooth muscle relaxation. Endothelial prostacyclin synthesis is stimulated by thrombin, bradykinin, and histamine. ADPase, on the endothelial surface, degrades ADP released from activated platelets, preventing ADP-induced platelet aggregation. Anticoagulant substances synthesized by intact endothelium include thrombomodulin, protein S, heparan sulfate, and tissue factor pathway inhibitor (TFPI).

Thrombomodulin binds thrombin at the cell surface, which inhibits its procoagulant effect; after the thrombin is degraded, thrombomodulin is recycled within the cell. Thrombomodulin also binds factor Xa, which inhibits prothrombin activation, and enhances protein C activation by thrombin (see below). Endothelial-produced protein S enhances the action of protein C. Heparan sulfate acts as a cofactor to antithrombin to inactivate several coagulation factors (IXa, Xa, XIa, XIIa). TFPI, a protease inhibitor, is synthesized mainly by the liver but also by endothelial cells, especially in the presence of inflammation. TFPI, combined with factor Xa, inhibits the tissue factor-factor VIIa complex, which limits coagulation. The endothelium contributes to fibrinolysis by producing t-PA.

Antithrombin is a small (up to 65,000 daltons) alpha$_2$-globulin that is produced by the liver. It is responsible for most of the anticoagulant effect of plasma. Antithrombin binds to and inactivates thrombin; factors IXa, Xa, XIa and XIIa; and kallikrein. Cofactors (such as heparan sulfate and heparin) accelerate this process.

Protein C is a vitamin K-dependent glycoprotein involved in countering thrombosis. Thrombin converts it to its active form. Activation is accelerated on vascular surfaces by the cofactor thrombomodulin. Protein S, another vitamin K-dependent protein, also acts as a cofactor. When activated by the thrombin–thrombomodulin complex, protein C, along with protein S, acts as an anticoagulant and profibrinolytic. It inhibits thrombin generation (by inactivating factors Va and VIIIa) and stimulates fibrinolysis (by inhibiting plasminogen activator inhibitor type 1, PAI-1). Deficiency of protein C could occur with neoplastic, infectious or other disease processes, although this is not yet clear in companion animals.

Pathophysiology

Mechanisms of Pathologic Thrombosis

TE disease is more likely to occur when changes in normal hemostatic processes create conditions that favor clot formation or impair thrombolysis. Three general situations, the so-called Virchow's triad, promote pathologic thrombosis: abnormal endothelial structure or function; slowed or static blood flow; and a hypercoagulable state, either from increased procoagulant substances or decreased anticoagulant or fibrinolytic substances. A number of common diseases can produce such conditions (see following paragraphs and **Table 36.1**). Several mechanisms could be involved to a variable degree in pathologic thrombus formation, depending on the vascular site affected and underlying disease process(es). Arterial thromboemboli, formed in areas of high-velocity flow, including cardiac valves, are more likely to contain many platelets because of shear stress-induced platelet activation. Venous thrombi tend to have greater fibrin content because coagulation occurs under low-velocity conditions. These differences have some influence on therapeutic approach, as discussed later.

Table 36.1 Thrombosis Risk Assessment

Considered at High Risk for Thrombosis—Antithrombotic Therapy is Recommended

- Dogs with immune-mediated hemolytic anemia
- Dogs with protein-losing enteropathy
- Cats with cardiomyopathy and LA enlargement, spontaneous echocontrast, decreased LA function, or prior TE event
- Animals with 2 or more other disease conditions associated with thrombosis, including:
    - Systemic inflammatory disease
    - Immune-mediated disease
    - Neoplasia (including adenocarcinoma and lymphoma, among others)
    - Vegetative endocarditis
    - Sepsis
    - Severe pancreatitis
    - Heartworm disease (pulmonary arteries)
    - Vascular trauma (iatrogenic or other injury, or from increased turbulence)
    - Prolonged indwelling catheter presence
    - Arteritis
- Postischemic injury
- Primary vascular disease (Cavalier King Charles Spaniels?)
- Poor blood flow or areas of blood stasis (including from prolonged recumbency, circulatory shock, cardiac disease)
- Conditions associated with antithrombin loss, reduced synthesis, or increased consumption (DIC)
- Endocrine diseases such as hyperadrenocorticism or diabetes mellitus
- Exogenous corticosteroid administration (dogs primarily)
- Shock
- Severe hepatopathy
- Heatstroke
- Atherosclerosis (dogs)
- Vascular obstruction
- Aortic dissection
- Chronic intersititial nephritis (dogs)
- Gastric dilatation-volvulus (dogs)
- Hypereosinophilic syndrome (dogs)
- After cardiopulmonary bypass procedure
- Prosthetic heart valve or other CV implant

Considered at Low to Moderate Risk for Thrombosis

- Animals with a single risk factor or disease condition
- Animals with disease condition(s) associated with risk for thrombosis, but that are expected to resolve within days to weeks, with treatment

Abbreviations: CV, cardiovascular; DIC, disseminated intravascular coagulation; LA, left atrial; TE, thromboembolic.

Vascular endothelial integrity is highly important. Diseases that induce severe or widespread endothelial injury also promote the loss of normal endothelial antiplatelet, anticoagulant and fibrinolytic functions while exposing tissue factor. In addition, injured endothelium produces antifibrinolytic factors such as PAI-1. Subendothelial tissue, exposed because of endothelial cell damage, promotes thrombosis by acting as a substrate for clot formation and stimulating platelet adherence and aggregation. Increased coagulability and platelet activation favor pathologic thrombosis. Systemic release of inflammatory cytokines (including tumor necrosis factor, various interleukins, platelet activating factor, and nitric oxide) can cause widespread endothelial injury. This occurs with sepsis and probably with other systemic inflammatory conditions as well. Neoplastic invasion, vascular disruption from other disease, and postischemic injury also induce endothelial damage. Primary vascular disease as an underlying cause is suggested in Cavalier King Charles Spaniels by a genetic predisposition to femoral artery and pulmonary artery (PA) thrombosis. Mechanical trauma to the vascular endothelium (as can occur with catheterization) also can precipitate thromboembolism, especially when other predisposing conditions exist. Pulmonary arterial endothelial injury caused by heartworm disease (HWD) is well known (Chapter 40). The inflammatory reaction to dead worms and worm fragments exacerbates the endothelial damage and prothrombotic conditions.

Stagnant blood flow promotes thrombosis by impeding the dilution and clearance of coagulation factors. There normally is a low background level of systemic coagulation factor activation; however, adequate blood flow rapidly disperses the activated factors. This dilution, along with hepatic clearance of activated factors and normal anticoagulation mechanisms, usually prevents thrombus formation. Blood stasis negates such protections against thrombosis. Poor blood flow also can promote local tissue hypoxia and endothelial injury. In addition, abnormal turbulence has been associated with thrombus formation. Turbulence can mechanically injure the endothelial surface. Heart diseases that cause low intracardiac blood flow velocity or increased turbulence can create prothrombotic conditions. Other diseases that produce localized blood stasis could similarly create conditions favorable for thrombosis. These include circulatory shock and prolonged recumbency. Hyperviscosity syndromes increase resistance to blood flow and so can reduce flow velocity.

Hypercoagulability develops secondary to various systemic diseases. Multiple mechanisms probably are involved; however, thrombus formation in these animals might also require altered endothelial integrity or blood flow characteristics. Antithrombin deficiency is the most common cause of hypercoagulability. Inadequate antithrombin can be secondary to decreased synthesis (possibly congenital), increased consumption (as with disseminated intravascular coagulation, DIC), accelerated loss from the intravascular compartment (such as with nephrotic syndrome), or increased protein catabolism (as with hyperadrenocorticism). An inadequate amount or function of proteins C and S could occur in animals with hypercoagulability associated with malignancy, DIC, and other conditions, as it does in some people. Reduced protein C and antithrombin activities, as well as evidence for DIC, have been shown in dogs with sepsis. Excessive platelet activation and aggregability can contribute to a prothrombotic state. Increased platelet aggregability has been associated with neoplasia, some heart diseases, diabetes mellitus, and nephrotic syndrome in some animals. However, thrombocytosis alone, without an increase in platelet aggregability, is not thought to create greater risk for thrombosis.

Defective fibrinolysis can promote pathologic thrombosis by preventing efficient breakdown of physiologic clots. Reduced levels of fibrinolytic substances (such as t-PA, plasminogen, and urokinase) or increased amounts of plasminogen activator inhibitors (which reduce conversion of plasminogen to plasmin) are implicated. The major inhibitor of the fibrinolytic system is PAI-1, which is produced mainly by macrophages. Systemic inflammation stimulates its synthesis (as well as that of alpha$_2$-antiplasmin and thrombin-activated fibrinolytic factor) through the effects of various cytokines.

Thromboembolism and Common Disease Conditions

Several diseases are known to increase risk for TE disease (**Table 36.1**). Dogs with immune-mediated hemolytic anemia (IMHA), protein-losing nephropathy, or a combination of multiple risk factors are considered to be at high risk for thrombosis (deLaForcade, 2019). Similarly, cats with cardiomyopathy and left atrial (LA) enlargement or hypocontractility, as well as cats with a combination of disease factors conveying higher risk, are prone to thrombosis. Conversely, for dogs and cats with just a single risk factor that is less-commonly associated with TE complications, or with a disease condition likely to resolve within days to a few weeks with treatment, the risk for thrombosis is considered to be low or perhaps only moderate. Although much remains to be clarified about TE disease in these situations, animals at high risk are likely to benefit from antithrombotic prophylaxis.

Conditions that induce a systemic inflammatory response promote TE disease in multiple ways. Thrombosis also promotes further inflammation. Various proinflammatory cytokines, such as tumor necrosis factor and interleukins, cause endothelial damage, induce tissue factor expression on monocytes and endothelial cells, inhibit anticoagulant mechanisms (including protein C, TFPI, and antithrombin), and limit fibrinolysis. Acute necrotizing pancreatitis, shock, trauma, sepsis, neoplasia, severe hepatopathy, heatstroke, immune-mediated disease, and other conditions can lead to gross thrombosis, as well as DIC. DIC involves massive activation of thrombin and plasmin, with generalized consumption of coagulation factors and platelets. DIC produces extensive thrombosis, as well as hemorrhage, in the microcirculation and results in widespread tissue ischemia and multiorgan failure.

IMHA in dogs frequently is complicated by thrombosis. Its genesis probably is multifactorial, with the systemic inflammatory (immune-mediated) response playing a large role (Kidd, 2013). Increased tissue factor expression, platelet activation, and procoagulant microparticles are implicated in causing a hypercoagulable state. In addition, thrombocytopenia, elevated bilirubin, and hypoalbuminemia have been identified as risk factors for thromboembolism. These might reflect the severity of disease or could contribute to hypercoagulability or increased platelet aggregability. DIC is common with IMHA. Free hemoglobin, released by hemolysis, serves as a scavenger of nitric oxide; when coupled with inflammatory cytokines and activated monocytes, this might induce endothelial cell expression of tissue factor and initiate thrombosis. The potential role of high-dose corticosteroid therapy in pathologic thrombosis is unclear. Although most often considered idiopathic, IMHA can develop secondary to systemic lupus erythematosis, neoplasia, and blood parasites. These diseases exacerbate conditions that favor thrombosis. Pulmonary thromboembolism (PTE) or thrombosis appears to be most common with IMHA; however, multiple systemic arterial sites also can be affected. Common postmortem findings include macro- and microthrombosis, fibrin deposition, and hemorrhage, as well as pulmonary thromboemboli and splenic, renal and cardiac infarction (McManus, 2001). Antithrombotic therapy is recommended for dogs with IMHA (CURATIVE guidelines, Goggs, 2019).

Protein-losing nephropathy also is strongly associated with TE disease in dogs. Its causes include glomerulonephritis, renal amyloid deposition, or hypertensive injury. Hypercoagulability and marked antithrombin deficiency occur. Because of its small size, antithrombin is lost through damaged glomeruli more easily than most procoagulant proteins. This predisposes to thrombosis. Although protein-losing enteropathies also cause antithrombin deficiency, concurrent loss of larger proteins often tends to maintain balance between procoagulant and anticoagulant factors. Other factors that might contribute to TE disease in animals with protein-losing nephropathy include increased thromboxane and fibrinogen concentrations, as well as enhanced platelet aggregability associated with hypoalbuminemia and hypercholesterolemia. Thrombosis also has been associated with chronic interstitial nephritis and acute tubular necrosis. The mechanism might relate to endothelial damage caused by uremic toxins or possibly to altered coagulability, although this is unclear. Other predisposing conditions could be involved. As with IMHA, PTE appears to occur most commonly, although systemic arterial TE events and venous thrombosis also occur. Antithrombotic therapy is recommended for dogs with protein-losing nephropathy (Goggs, 2019).

Exogenous corticosteroid administration is thought to promote a hypercoagulable state in dogs; in some, TE events have occurred. In healthy dogs, such treatment can increase coagulation factors, platelet aggregation, fibrinogen and thrombin generation, while reducing antithrombin, but the actual risk of thromboembolism is not known. Nevertheless, especially in patients with another risk factor for thrombosis, corticosteroid use could foster thromboembolism. It is unclear if corticosteroid therapy promotes thrombosis in cats.

TE disease has occurred in a minority of dogs with spontaneous hyperadrenocorticism. Although some have identified decreased fibrinolysis (from increased PAI activity) and elevated levels of several coagulation factors associated with this endocrinopathy, others have not shown evidence for a hypercoagulable state. Renal glomerular damage, associated with hypertension in some cases, could promote antithrombin loss. Other predisposing factors might be present, as well. However, at this time, prophylactic antithrombotic therapy is not advocated for dogs with hyperadrenocorticism, unless other risk factors are present concurrently (deLaForcade, 2019). Diabetes mellitus occasionally is associated with TE disease in dogs. Platelet hyperaggregability and possibly hypofibrinolysis might be involved.

Cats with myocardial disease (Chapter 33) are at risk for intracardiac thrombus formation and subsequent arterial embolization. A thrombus sometimes is found within the left heart (especially the left atrium or its auricle) during echocardiography or at necropsy in cats with cardiomyopathy. Increased LA size, and especially reduced LA function, increase risk for intracardiac thrombosis and an arterial TE event in cats with cardiomyopathy. Spontaneous echocontrast (p. 656) is evident in many of these cats. Mechanisms involved probably relate to poor intracardiac flow, especially within the LA appendage, altered blood coagulability, local tissue or blood vessel injury, or a combination. Increased platelet reactivity occurs in some of these cats. DIC can accompany thromboembolism in these patients. Some cats with TE disease have decreased plasma arginine and vitamin B_6 and B_{12} concentrations; hyperhomocysteinemia might be a factor in some. Hyperhomocysteinemia and low plasma vitamin B are risk factors for thromboembolism in people. It is not known if hypercoagulability induced by a genetic abnormality exists in some cats, as occurs in people. Antithrombotic therapy is recommended for cats with cardiomyopathy, especially those with increased LA size or reduced LA function, or if other risk factors coexist. In contrast, dogs with cardiac disease have not been shown to have increased risk for thrombosis, except those with a valve prosthesis or perhaps another implanted CV device.

Systemic Arterial Thromboembolic Disease

The systemic arterial system is a high-shear environment. Platelet activation and clumping are integral to the formation and expansion of thromboemboli here. Therapeutic strategies that impair platelet activation, aggregability, and adherence are likely to be most effective. Therefore, antiplatelet therapy generally is advocated for patients at high risk for arterial TE disease, although anticoagulant therapy might be a useful adjunct (see paragraphs that follow and **Table 36.2**).

The most common cause for arterial TE disease in cats is cardiomyopathy, of any form, including myocarditis (Chapter 33), although initial thrombus formation is likely to occur in the low-flow left atrium. Thrombi that form in the left heart can become quite large (**Figure 36.3**, also **Figure 33.2**, p. 652). While some remain in the heart (usually in the left auricle), others embolize to the distal aorta or less often, other

Table 36.2 Suggested Dosages for Antithrombotic Drugs

Antiplatelet Drugs

- Clopidogrel (preferred)
  - Dogs: 1.1–3 mg/kg PO q24h for arterial thromboembolism prophylaxis (up to 4 mg/kg q24h); can give single loading dose of 4–10 mg/kg PO to more rapidly reach therapeutic plasma concentration
  - Cats: 18.75 mg/cat (~3–6 mg/kg) PO q24h for arterial thromboembolism prophylaxis; to obtain rapid therapeutic plasma concentration, can give a single loading dose of 37.5 mg/cat
- Aspirin
  - Dogs: 0.5–1 mg/kg PO q24h
  - Cats: 10–25 mg/kg (or 20–81 mg/cat) PO q72h (or 2–3 times/week); low-dose, 5 mg/cat q72h

Anticoagulant Drugs

- Unfractionated heparin
  - Dogs: IV dosing—one 100 U/kg IV bolus is suggested, followed by 480–900 U/kg q24h CRI (20–37.5, or up to 50, U/kg/h); or, SC doses of 150–300 U/kg q6h. Optimal dosage probably varies among individuals. Administration PO or by inhalation not recommended. Base individual dosage adjustments on anti-Xa monitoring (p. 765)
  - Cats: 250 U/kg SC q6h. Can use anti-Xa monitoring for dosage adjustments, although optimal target not established (p. 765)
  - Horses: 40–100 IU/kg SC q6h
- Dalteparin
  - Dogs: 100–175 U/kg SC q8h
  - Cats: 75 U/kg SC q6h initial dose; up to 150 U/kg SC q6h
  - Horses: 50–100 IU/kg SC q24h
- Enoxaparin
  - Dogs: 0.8-1 mg/kg SC q6-12h
  - Cats: 0.75–1 mg/kg SC q6(–12)h
- Fondaparinux
  - Cats: (?) 0.06 or 0.2 mg/kg SC q12h (low dose for prophylaxis; high dose for thrombosis treatment)
- Rivaroxaban
  - Dogs: 1–2 mg/kg PO q24h
  - Cats: 0.5–1 mg/kg PO q24h (or 2.5 mg/cat q24h)
- Apixaban
  - Dogs: 0.25-0.5 mg/kg PO q8-12h
  - Cats: 0.625 mg/cat PO q12h
- Warfarin (p. 770)

Fibrinolytic Drugs

- rt-PA (p. 766)
- Streptokinase (p. 767)

Abbreviation: CRI, continuous rate infusion.

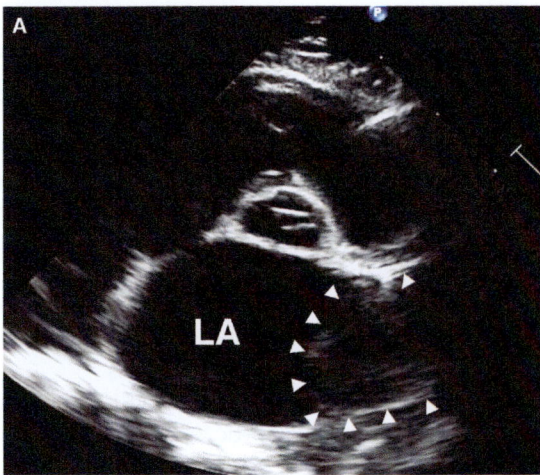 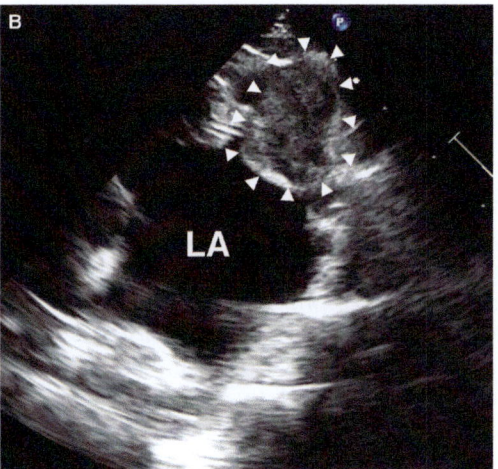

Figure 36.3 Transthoracic echocardiographic images from right parasternal short-axis (A) and left cranial (B) views in a cat with hypertrophic cardiomyopathy and congestive heart failure. A large mass of mixed echogenicity (thrombus, arrowheads) extends from the left auricle into the body of the left atrium (LA).

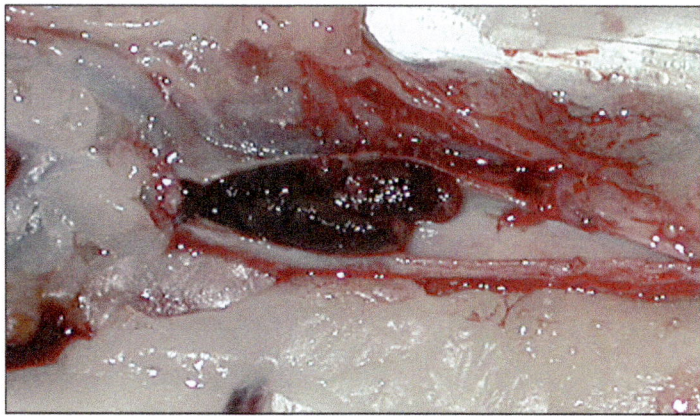

Figure 36.4 A thromboembolus is visible within the opened distal aorta in this postmortem image from a male cat (cranial is to the right). This cat had left atrial enlargement and congestive heart failure secondary to congenital mitral valve dysplasia and subaortic stenosis.

sites (**Figure 36.4**). Hyperthyroidism might be a risk factor for thromboembolism in cats independent of its cardiac effects. Arterial thromboembolism has been observed in cats with congenital heart diseases, especially mitral stenosis or supravalvular mitral ring. Neoplasia, particularly pulmonary carcinoma, and systemic inflammatory disease occasionally underlie systemic TE disease in cats. Infective endocarditis of aortic and mitral valve leaflets is uncommon in cats, but arterial thromboembolism can occur, including embolization to the distal aorta. In some cases, no precipitating cause is identified.

Arterial TE disease is relatively uncommon in dogs compared with cats. Nevertheless, it has been associated with many conditions, including protein-losing nephropathy, hyperadrenocorticism, neoplasia, chronic interstitial nephritis, dirofilariasis, hypothyroidism, gastric dilatation-volvulus, pancreatitis, hypereosinophilic syndrome, and occasionally, CV disease, among others (**Figure 36.5**). Often, more than one potential association exists concurrently. Kidney disease is present in a large proportion of cases. In-situ thrombosis, rather than an acute TE event, is likely in many canine cases. Perhaps the most common canine CV disease associated with systemic thromboembolism is vegetative endocarditis (Chapter 31). Other CV associations include patent ductus arteriosus (PDA; from surgical occlusion site), myocardial infarction, arteritis, aortic intimal fibrosis, atherosclerosis, aortic dissection, mitral valve myxosarcoma, granulomatous inflammatory erosion into the LA, a prosthetic heart valve, intracardiac surgery, other thrombi in the left heart, and occasionally, dilated cardiomyopathy. TE disease, as a rare complication of arteriovenous (A-V) fistulae, could develop secondary to venous stasis related to distal venous hypertension. Atherosclerosis is an important risk factor for arterial thromboembolism in people. Although atherosclerosis is uncommon in dogs, it has been associated with TE disease in this species, as well. Endothelial disruption in areas of atherosclerotic plaque, hypercholesterolemia, increased PAI-1,

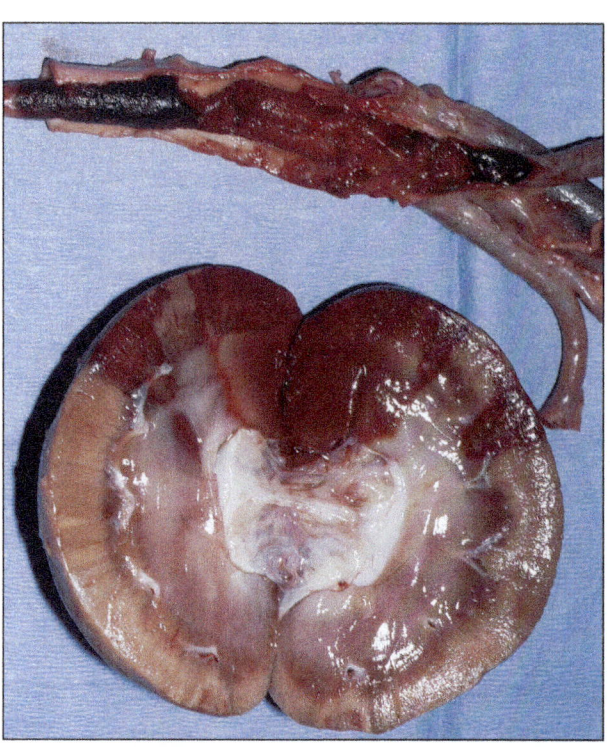

Figure 36.5 Specimens from a dog that had multiple thromboembolic events. A long thromboembolus fills this section of caudal aorta and iliac arteries (top; cranial is to the left). The opened left kidney has a large infarcted (dark) area. A mycotic infection of the hilar lymph node(s) had eroded into the dorsal left atrium, creating an inflammatory nidus for intraatrial thrombus formation and subsequent arterial thromboembolic events.

and possibly other mechanisms are thought to be involved in thrombus formation. Some canine cases of apparent arterial thrombosis or TE disease appear similar to a form of aortoiliac occlusive disease observed in people (Leriche's syndrome) and in horses; these dogs actually might develop local thrombosis rather than an embolic event (**Figure 36.6**). Atherosclerosis can develop with profound hypothyroidism, hypercholesterolemia, and hyperlipidemia, as perhaps rarely caused by disorders of lipid metabolism (**Figures 37.5** and **37.6**, pp. 779 and 780). The aorta, as well as coronary and other medium to large arteries, can be affected. Myocardial and cerebral infarctions occur in some cases. There also is a high rate of interstitial myocardial fibrosis in affected dogs. Vasculitis related to infectious, inflammatory, immune-mediated, or toxic disease occasionally can underlie TE events. Arteritis of immune-mediated pathogenesis has occurred in some young Beagles and other dogs. Inflammation and necrosis affect small to medium-sized arteries and are associated with thrombosis in these cases.

Larger systemic arterial emboli (originating in the heart) usually lodge at the aortic trifurcation (the so-called "saddle thrombus"), although coronary, iliac, femoral, renal, brachial, and other arteries can be affected by an embolus, depending on its size and flow path. Some small emboli are clinically "silent", in that they cause no obvious effects. Emboli

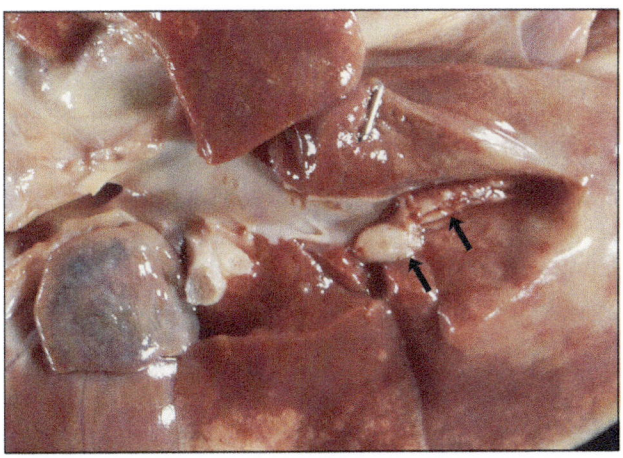

Figure 36.7 Postmortem image of opened left pulmonary artery, obstructed by a thromboembolus (arrows), from a 5-year-old male Dachshund with immune-mediated hemolytic anemia. Pulmonary trunk is to the left; left auricle and dorsal left ventricle are visible at lower left corner.

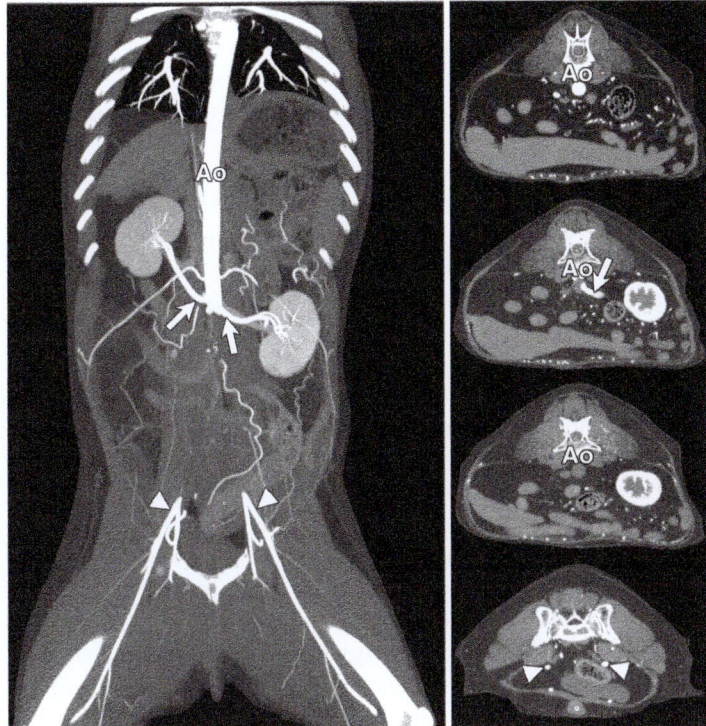

Figure 36.6 Dorsal maximum intensity projection reformat (left) and transverse sections (right) from a computed tomography angiography scan on a 13-year-old Labrador Retriever with rear limb weakness. Aortoiliac thrombosis is present. In the left image, the contrast column within the descending aorta (Ao) ends abruptly, just distal to the renal arteries (arrows). Patency returns at the femoral arterial level (arrowheads). The transverse images on the right show progression from cranial (top) to caudal (bottom): a patent aortic lumen, partial obstruction at the level of the left renal artery (arrow), complete aortoiliac obstruction, and recanalization of the femoral arteries (arrowheads).

can originate from within the heart or an upstream vascular site; they can consist only of blood elements or could contain neoplastic cells or infectious organisms. Emboli also can form from fat, tissue fragments, gas, or parasites. Pulmonary thromboemboli and intracardiac or venous thrombi can exist concurrently with arterial thromboemboli. In-situ thrombosis causes arterial occlusion in some cases.

Besides obstructing arterial flow, thromboemboli release vasoactive substances (such as thromboxane A_2 and serotonin) that induce vasoconstriction and compromise the development of collateral flow around the obstructed vessel. The resulting tissue ischemia causes further damage and inflammation. An ischemic neuromyopathy occurs in the affected limb(s), with peripheral nerve dysfunction and degeneration, as well as pathologic changes in associated muscle tissue.

Coronary artery thromboembolism or thrombosis can cause myocardial ischemia and infarction. Reported causes include infective endocarditis, neoplasia that involves the heart directly or via neoplastic emboli, coronary atherosclerosis, dilated cardiomyopathy, degenerative (myxomatous) mitral valve disease with congestive heart failure, LA tear, and coronary vasculitis. In some dogs, coronary TE events have occurred in association with severe renal disease, IMHA, exogenous corticosteroids or hyperadrenocorticism, or acute pancreatic necrosis. Such cases often have TE lesions in other locations, too. Coronary thromboembolism with myocardial necrosis has occurred in cats with cardiac disease, especially severe hypertrophic cardiomyopathy or infective endocarditis, as well as from carcinoma emboli.

Pulmonary Arterial Thromboembolic Disease

Pulmonary thromboemboli in dogs can develop with HWD, other heart diseases, IMHA, neoplasia, DIC, sepsis, hyperadrenocorticism, nephrotic syndrome, pancreatitis, trauma, hypothyroidism, gastrointestinal (GI) disease, and right atrial thrombosis (**Figures 36.7** and **36.8**). Deep vein thrombosis, the main cause of PTE in people, is not a recognized clinical problem in dogs and cats. Massive pulmonary thrombi

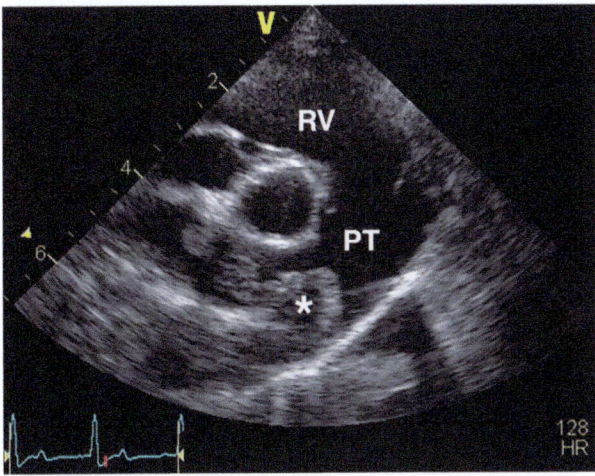

Figure 36.8 Transthoracic right parasternal short-axis image from a Cavalier King Charles Spaniel shows a large thrombus (*) at the bifurcation of the dilated main pulmonary trunk (PT). RV, right ventricle.

also can occur in-situ; this has been described in the Cavalier King Charles Spaniel. PTE also occurs in cats with a variety of systemic and inflammatory disorders. These have included neoplasia, HWD, anemia (probably immune-mediated), pancreatitis, glomerulonephritis, encephalitis, pneumonia, heart disease, sepsis, glucocorticoid administration, protein-losing enteropathy, and hepatic lipidosis. Nevertheless, PTE appears to be rare in cats compared to dogs, except in those with HWD. Almost half of cats with necropsy-confirmed pulmonary thromboemboli had multiple predisposing disorders. Diagnosis usually has been made at postmortem, although most affected cats had respiratory signs before death or euthanasia.

TE obstruction within the pulmonary circulation generally must be extensive before pathophysiologic manifestations are observed at rest. These include increased pulmonary vascular resistance and impaired gas exchange. Sudden onset of pulmonary hypertension (PH) places acute strain on the right ventricle and in severe cases can impair cardiac output. When thromboemboli completely obstruct blood flow to a pulmonary region, functional gas exchange ceases there; this creates physiologic dead space and decreases the total area available for gas diffusion. Another potential consequence is an increase in blood flow velocity in well-perfused lung regions; accelerated red cell capillary transit time reduces the time available for gas exchange, although this normally occurs extremely quickly. Nevertheless, these mechanisms together could reduce pulmonary gas exchange via diffusion impairment and increase the alveolar-arterial (A-a) pO_2 gradient (p. 220). Severe PH caused by massive PTE can lead to right-to-left shunting in patients with a patent foramen ovale or other pulmonary-to-systemic communication, which exacerbates systemic hypoxemia.

Venous Thrombosis

In contrast to the platelet-rich thromboemboli that characterize arterial TE disease, venous thrombosis occurs in a low shear stress environment. These clots are rich in fibrin and less dependent on platelet number and activation for their development. The rationale for an anticoagulant as first-choice drug for venous thrombosis is based on these features. Nevertheless, antiplatelet therapy probably is important, as well.

Thrombosis in large veins is more likely to be clinically evident than small vessel thrombosis (**Figure 36.9**). Cranial vena caval thrombosis has occurred with IMHA, immune-mediated thrombocytopenia, sepsis, neoplasia, protein-losing nephropathy, mycotic disease, heart disease, presence of a transvenous pacemaker lead, and glucocorticoid therapy in dogs (especially with systemic inflammatory disease), as well as after cardiopulmonary bypass procedures. Most cases have more than one predisposing factor. An indwelling jugular venous catheter increases the risk for cranial vena caval thrombosis, probably by causing vascular endothelial damage or laminar flow disruption, or by acting as a nidus for thrombus formation. Caudal vena caval thrombosis also can occur with neoplasia, especially adrenal tumors. Thrombosis can develop around a redundant transvenous pacemaker lead here, as well.

Portal vein thrombosis (**Figure 36.10**) in dogs is associated with hepatic disease, distant or local neoplasia, immune disorders, infectious disease, hyperadrenocorticism, protein-losing enteropathy, pancreatitis, and exogenous glucocorticoid administration. Portal vein thrombosis can be acute or chronic. Circulatory shock or DIC can result.

Thrombophlebitis can occur secondary to local vascular trauma associated with IV catheterization or injections. This is a common cause of jugular and other peripheral venous thrombosis in horses and other animals (**Figure 37.12**, p. 783). Factors that increase the risk for catheter-associated thrombophlebitis include suboptimal catheterization technique, prolonged indwelling catheter duration, poor catheter hygiene, systemic inflammatory disease or infection, hypoproteinemia, and other conditions that increase coagulability. Some degree of thrombophlebitis is estimated to occur in almost a third of ill horses with a long-term indwelling venous catheter (Geraghty, 2009). Although the venous thrombus might be sterile, invasion by blood-borne

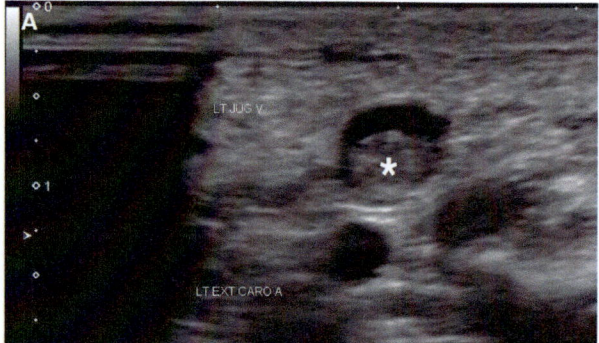
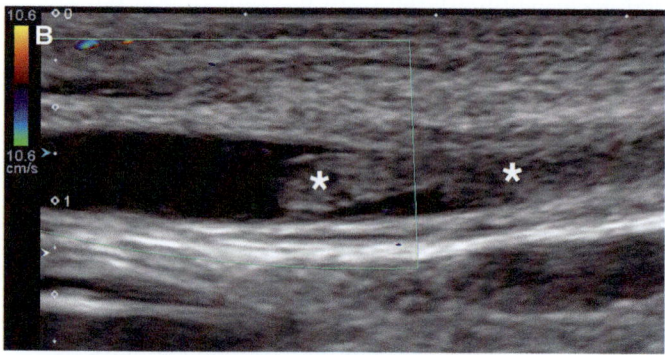

Figure 36.9 Vascular ultrasound images of the left external jugular vein (LT JUG V) from a dog with pleural effusion and central venous thrombosis. (A) Short-axis view shows a mixed echogenic thrombus (*) within the lumen of the vein. The lumen of the left external carotid artery (LT EXT CARO A) is visible below and slightly leftward. (B) Long-axis image of the vein toward the thoracic inlet shows the extensive thrombus (*).

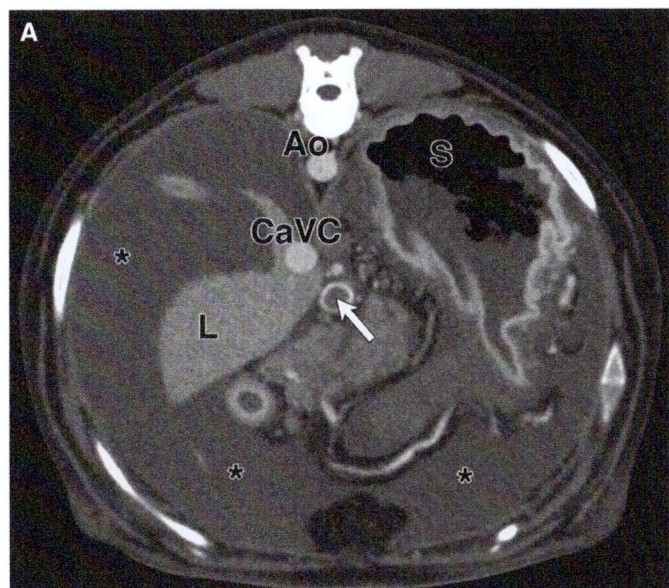

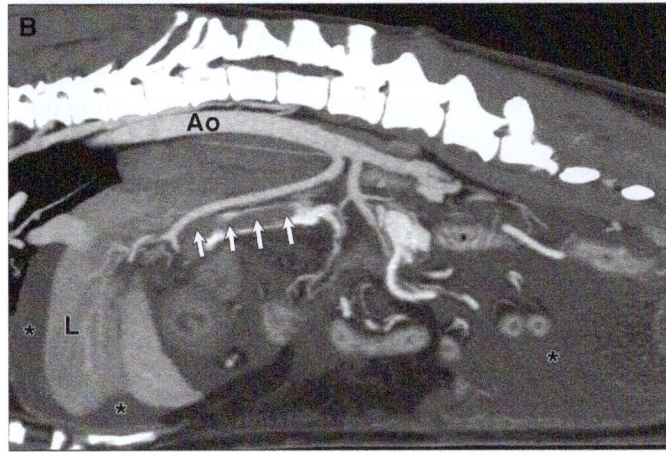

Figure 36.10 Axial (A) and sagittal (B) computed tomography angiography images from a dog with portal venous thrombosis and ascites (*). Contrast material is visible around a central hypoattenuating thrombus (arrows: A&B). Ao, aorta; CaVC, caudal vena cava; L, liver; S, stomach.

organisms or skin contaminants often causes infective thrombophlebitis, with attendant signs of infection and inflammation locally and possibly, systemically.

Clinical Features

Clinical manifestations of TE disease depend on the type, number, and location of vessels affected, the duration and degree of vascular obstruction, the extent of tissue damage, and any related complications. Most reported cases involve thrombi in the distal aorta, heart, brachial or other large systemic artery, the pulmonary arteries, cranial vena cava, or portal vein. Multiple sites are affected in some animals. An index of suspicion for TE disease is important for ante-mortem diagnosis. This is based on the patient's history, physical findings, and concurrent disease(s).

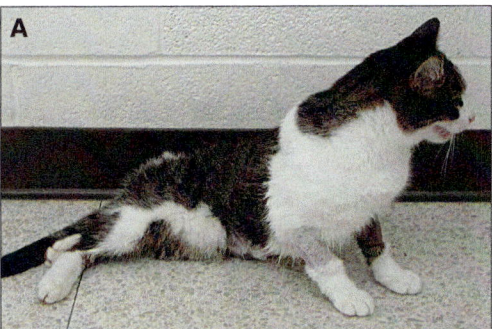

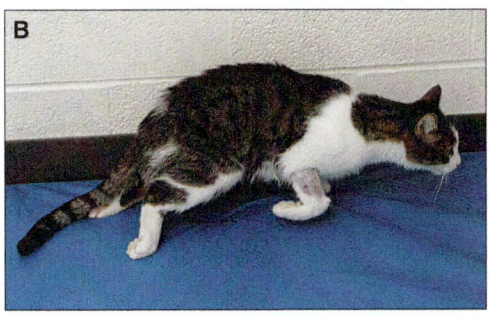

Figure 36.11 Acute caudal aortic thromboembolism caused respiratory distress and panting (A), as well as posterior paresis (B), in this 4-year-old male Domestic Shorthair cat with restrictive cardiomyopathy. The cat could ambulate with difficulty by shifting his weight to the forelimbs and dragging the hindlimbs and tail.

Arterial Thromboembolism

Arterial Thromboembolism in Cats Arterial TE disease in cats usually causes acute and dramatic clinical signs secondary to tissue ischemia and its vascular, musculoskeletal, neurologic, and metabolic consequences. Male cats are at higher risk for thromboembolism, although this gender bias appears related to the prevalence of hypertrophic cardiomyopathy (HCM). Cats that previously suffered an arterial TE event or that have reduced LA function have an increased risk of dying from arterial thromboembolism (Payne, 2015). Distal aortic embolization occurs in most cases (**Figures 36.11** and **36.12**).

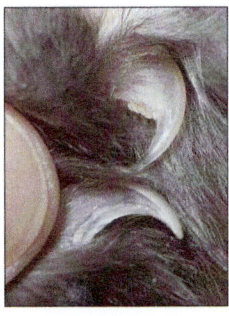

Figure 36.12 A cyanotic hindlimb nail bed (lower) from another cat with caudal aortic thromboembolism, shown next to the pink nail bed (upper) of a forelimb.

Acute hindlimb paresis without palpable femoral pulses is most typical. Common clinical findings are summarized in **Table 36.3**). Signs of pain and poor systemic perfusion usually are present. Sensation to the lower limbs is reduced. One side might show greater deficits than the other. The distal portions of affected limbs exhibit the most severe neurologic deficits; return of function progresses from proximal to distal. Emboli sometimes are small enough to lodge more distally in only one limb, which causes paresis of the lower limb alone. Embolization of a brachial artery produces forelimb monoparesis. Intermittent claudication (see next section, in dogs) occurs rarely. Thromboemboli within the renal, mesenteric, or pulmonary arterial circulation can result in failure of these organs and death; cats suffering from mesenteric thrombi often are presented in intractable pain. Emboli to the brain could induce seizures or various neurologic deficits. Hypothermia and azotemia are common, even when a site other than the distal aorta is affected.

A cardiac murmur, gallop sound, or arrhythmia often is noted; however, these signs might not be evident even with underlying heart disease (Chapter 33). Clinical signs of heart disease prior to the TE event often are absent. About 10% of cats experience vomiting in association with the onset of arterial TE signs. Tachypnea and open-mouth breathing frequently occur with acute arterial embolization, despite the absence of overt CHF in many cats. This might represent a pain response, although it could relate to increased pulmonary venous pressure. It is important to determine if CHF underlies the acute respiratory signs. A rapid lung ultrasound scan at presentation can be helpful, although thoracic radiographs are recommended once the cat is stabilized. Motor function in the lower limbs is minimal to absent in most cases, although the cat usually is able to flex and extend the hips.

Table 36.3 Common Signs of Acute Arterial Thromboembolic Disease in Cats

Acute Limb Paresis
- Posterior (hind limb) paresis
- Monoparesis
- ±Intermittent claudication (rare, p. 756)

Characteristics of Affected Limb(s)
- Painful
- Cool distal limb
- Pale footpads
- Cyanotic nailbeds
- Absent arterial pulse
- Contracture of affected muscles, especially gastrocnemius and cranial tibial (with caudal aortic thromboembolus)

Other Systemic Signs
- Tachypnea or respiratory distress (rule out pain, CHF, or other cause)
- Vocalization (pain and distress)
- Hypothermia
- ±Vomiting

Signs of Heart Disease (Not Always Present)
- Systolic murmur or gallop sound
- Arrhythmia
- Cardiomegaly
- Anorexia
- Lethargy/weakness

Signs of CHF (Not Always Present)
- Pulmonary edema
- Pleural effusion

Common Hematologic and Biochemical Abnormalities
- Azotemia
- Increased activity of:
  - Creatine kinase
  - Aspartate aminotransferase
  - Alanine aminotransferase
  - Lactate dehydrogenase
- Metabolic acidosis or mixed acidosis (respiratory) alkalosis
- Increased blood lactate
- Hyperglycemia (stress response)
- Lymphopenia (stress response)
- Disseminated intravascular coagulation

Abbreviation: CHF, congestive heart failure

Arterial Thromboembolism and Thrombosis in Dogs

Arterial thrombosis in dogs has no clear age, breed, or sex predilections, although Greyhounds appear to be affected relatively often. Most dogs with arterial (usually distal aortic) thrombosis display some clinical signs between one and eight weeks before presentation, which might suggest an embolic event, although this is not well established. Less than a quarter of cases have peracute paralysis without prior signs of lameness, as usually occurs in cats. Most dogs are presented for signs related to the thrombosis or thromboembolism. These include pain, hindlimb paresis, lameness or weakness (which might be progressive or intermittent), and chewing or hypersensitivity of the affected limb(s) or lumbar area. Dogs might develop sudden paralysis, although some studies suggest the majority of dogs remain ambulatory. *Intermittent claudication*, which is common in people with peripheral occlusive vascular disease, can be a manifestation of distal aortic TE disease in dogs (and horses as well). Intermittent claudication involves pain, weakness, and lameness that develop during exercise. These signs intensify until walking becomes impossible, and then they resolve with rest. Inadequate perfusion during exercise leads to lactic acid accumulation and cramping. Physical findings in dogs with aortic thromboembolism are similar to those in cats, including absent or weak femoral pulses, cool extremities, hindlimb pain, loss of sensation in the digits, hyperesthesia, cyanotic nailbeds, and neuromuscular dysfunction. Occasionally, a brachial or other artery is embolized (**Figure 36.13**). TE disease involving an abdominal organ

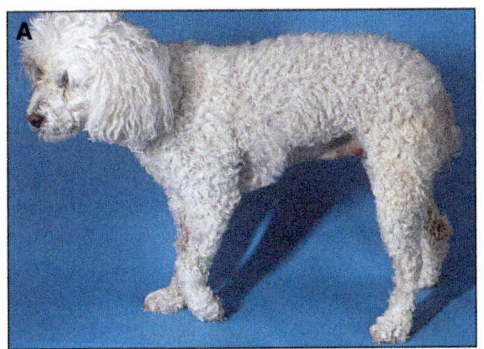
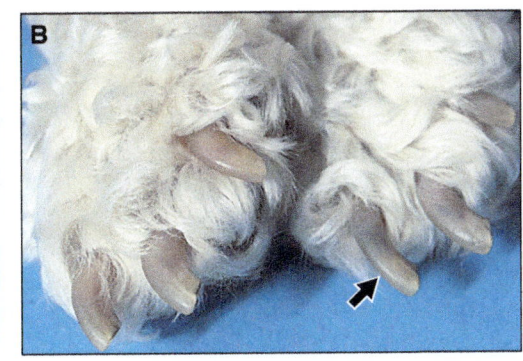

Figure 36.13 (A) This 6-year-old female Poodle developed acute paresis of the left forelimb because of a thromboembolic event soon after surgery for cystotomy. The dog recovered normal function following supportive therapy. (B) Cyanosis of the left forepaw is seen best on the nail of the 3rd digit (arrow); the normal pink right forepaw is to the left in the image.

causes visceral pain, along with clinical and laboratory evidence of damage to the affected organ(s).

Coronary Thromboembolism Coronary artery thromboembolism or thrombosis is likely to be associated with arrhythmias, as well as ST segment and T wave changes on ECG. Ventricular or other tachyarrhythmias are common. Conduction block can develop if atrioventricular (AV) nodal tissue is injured. Clinical signs of acute myocardial infarction and necrosis mimic those of severe pulmonary TE disease; these include weakness, tachypnea or respiratory distress, and collapse. The respiratory signs might develop from preexisting pulmonary pathology, left-sided heart failure, and/or cardiac pain (angina), depending on the underlying disease and degree of myocardial ischemia and dysfunction. Other findings in animals with myocardial necrosis can include tachycardia, weak pulses, increased lung sounds or crackles, cough, cardiac murmur, hyperthermia or hypothermia, GI signs (uncommonly), and sudden death. Signs of other systemic disease can be concurrent. Radiographically evident pulmonary infiltrates are present in some animals with respiratory distress. However, in others, an absence of pulmonary infiltrate could relate to acute increases in pulmonary venous pressure (from acute myocardial dysfunction) prior to the accumulation of overt edema, to concurrent pulmonary emboli, or to pain. Acute myocardial ischemic injury that causes sudden death might not be detectable on routine histopathology.

Pulmonary Thromboembolism Pulmonary TE disease (also see Chapter 39) shows no apparent age or sex predilection in dogs or cats. Classically, PTE causes dyspnea or tachypnea, although this is not evident in all cases. Increased lung sounds, a cardiac murmur, and hepatosplenomegaly also are reported in many affected dogs. Chest pain and hemoptysis are typical signs in people, but not usually recognized in animals.

Venous Thrombosis Systemic venous thrombosis produces signs related to increased venous pressure upstream from the obstruction. Thrombosis of the cranial vena cava leads to the cranial caval syndrome (p. 277 and **Figures 17.5A** and **17.6**). Pleural effusion occurs commonly. This effusion often is chylous because lymph flow from the thoracic duct into the cranial vena cava also is impaired. Palpable thrombosis can extend into the jugular veins in some cases (**Figure 36.9**). Portal vein thrombosis can cause ascites, with elevated liver enzyme activities and hemostatic abnormalities consistent with DIC. Because vena caval obstruction reduces pulmonary blood flow and left heart filling, signs of poor cardiac output are common. Infective thrombophlebitis, involving the jugular or other peripheral veins, can cause local swelling, redness, pain over the site, and possibly, fever and other signs of systemic infection. Conversely, a sterile venous thrombus might not cause any signs of inflammation and if the vessel is not completely obstructed, obvious clinical signs might be absent. Complete venous obstruction typically causes upstream venous distension and often, subcutaneous edema near or ventral to the obstruction. As with cranial vena caval obstruction, bilateral jugular vein thrombosis is likely to cause edema of the head and ventral neck.

Diagnostic Tests

Laboratory Tests

Results of routine clinical laboratory tests depend largely on the disease process underlying the TE event(s). Systemic arterial TE disease elevates muscle enzyme concentrations secondary to skeletal muscle ischemia and necrosis. Aspartate aminotransferase (AST) and alanine aminotransferase (ALT) activities rise soon after the TE event. Widespread muscle injury also causes increased lactate dehydrogenase and creatine kinase (CK) activities. In cases of transient ischemia with functional limb recovery, as occasionally occurs with forelimb arterial thromboembolism, elevation in these muscle enzymes 24 hours later can be a clue to a previous vascular event. Azotemia is common with arterial thromboembolism, especially in cats. This can be prerenal from poor systemic perfusion or dehydration, primary renal from embolization of the renal arteries or preexisting kidney disease, or a combination of both. Metabolic acidosis, increased blood lactate, DIC, electrolyte abnormalities (especially low serum Na^+, Ca^{++}, and K^+ and elevated phosphorus) are common in cats, as is stress hyperglycemia. Hyperkalemia can develop secondary to ischemic muscle damage and reperfusion. Comparison of lactate and glucose concentrations between affected and unaffected limbs in patients with suspected systemic arterial thromboembolism can support vascular obstruction as the cause of clinical signs, although this rarely is needed. Lower glucose and higher lactate concentrations in the affected limb compared to an unaffected limb or central value often are found.

Myocardial damage from coronary artery embolization increases circulating cardiac troponin (cTn) concentrations, although this could also relate to underlying heart disease. Increased AST activity also has been reported with myocardial necrosis. Total CK and ALT increase variably within a few hours of injury. Elevation in the cardiac-specific isoenzyme of CK (CK-MB) is expected, although not usually measured in animals anymore. Values peak in 6–12 hours then return to normal within 1–2 days. Continued increase indicates ongoing injury. Other laboratory parameters reflect underlying disease, as is the case with pulmonary TE disease and venous thrombosis. Leukocytosis and increased liver enzymes appear to be common in patients with PTE; thrombocytopenia is common with cranial caval thrombosis.

Routine coagulation test results are variable with TE disease. Levels of FDPs can be increased; however, this can occur with inflammatory disease and is not specific for a TE event or DIC. Cats with arterial TE disease usually have a normal coagulation profile. Coagulation test results are more variable in dogs with systemic arterial (including coronary) and pulmonary TE disease. Prolonged coagulation times and thrombocytopenia consistent with DIC are reported in many cases, although results are normal in some dogs. Many conditions that underlie TE disease also are associated with DIC themselves. Coagulation profile results frequently are normal with cranial vena caval thrombosis. However, shortened coagulation (prothrombin, activated partial thromboplastin, and thrombin) times might indicate a hypercoagulable state and increased risk for thrombosis (Song, 2016). Plasma antithrombin concentration could be low in dogs with arterial TE events, particularly if protein-losing nephropathy is present.

D-dimer assays provide a more specific indicator of clot breakdown than FDPs. A number of assays have been developed to measure D-dimers in dogs. D-dimers are degradation products specific to cross-linked fibrin. FDP assays do not discriminate between the breakdown of fibrinogen and stable clots, and are not sensitive enough to detect thromboemboli. D-dimer concentrations rise with TE disease; higher concentrations are more specific for thromboemboli. A small clinical study in dogs found significantly higher D-dimer concentrations in the cases with shortened coagulation times, compared to those with normal coagulation times; more thrombus formation and suspected PTE occurred in the dogs with abbreviated coagulation times, too (Song, 2016). Modestly increased D-dimer concentrations can occur with other conditions such as neoplasia, liver disease, and IMHA. This could reflect subclinical TE disease or another clot activation mechanism, because these conditions are associated with a procoagulant state. Body cavity hemorrhage also causes a rise in D-dimers. Because this condition is associated with increased fibrin formation, elevated D-dimers might not indicate TE disease in these cases. The specificity of D-dimer testing for pathologic thromboembolism is less at lower D-dimer concentrations; but there is high sensitivity at lower concentrations, which provides an important screening tool. D-dimer testing appears to be as specific for DIC as FDP measurement. However, it is important to interpret D-dimer results in the context of other clinical and laboratory findings. The applicability of D-dimer testing in cats and horses is not yet clear.

Assays for circulating antithrombin and proteins C and S also are available for dogs and cats. Deficiencies of these proteins are associated with increased risk for thrombosis. Factor Xa activity and anti-Xa activity also can be measured, which can be especially useful for monitoring heparin therapy. A number of methods are described to test for antithrombin activity. Sample submission instructions and normal reference values should be obtained from the laboratory performing the testing.

Measures of platelet function are available and variably used in veterinary medicine. Such tests provide more information than quantitative platelet counts. Many diseases associated with thromboembolism can impair platelet function. Most tests are measures of platelet aggregometry or the time to cessation of blood flow under high shear conditions.

Thromboelastography (TEG) is a viscoelastic test of coagulation that assesses initial clot formation, clot strength, and fibrinolysis (**Figure 36.14**). Although animal studies are ongoing, TEG could provide a broader overview of hemostasis than other testing modalities. It might be more representative of the patient's clinical state (hypo-, normo-, or hypercoagulable). However, results have been within normal limits in some animals (particularly sight hounds) with aortic thrombosis. Nevertheless, TEG could be helpful in monitoring response to anticoagulant therapy. Individual lab variation appears to exist with TEG, so lab-specific reference values should be consulted.

Arterial blood gas analysis is helpful when respiratory signs are severe or persistent (p. 220). Animals with PTE often have hypoxemia, hypocapnia, and an increased A-a gradient. The hypoxemia usually improves with supplemental O_2, perhaps because of improved ventilation in areas of low ventilation-to-perfusion (V/Q) or improved diffusion from higher partial pressure of alveolar oxygen in areas with greater perfusion. Progressive decrease in PaO_2 despite O_2 therapy suggests intrapulmonary shunting. Cranial vena caval thrombosis that causes complete caval obstruction also leads

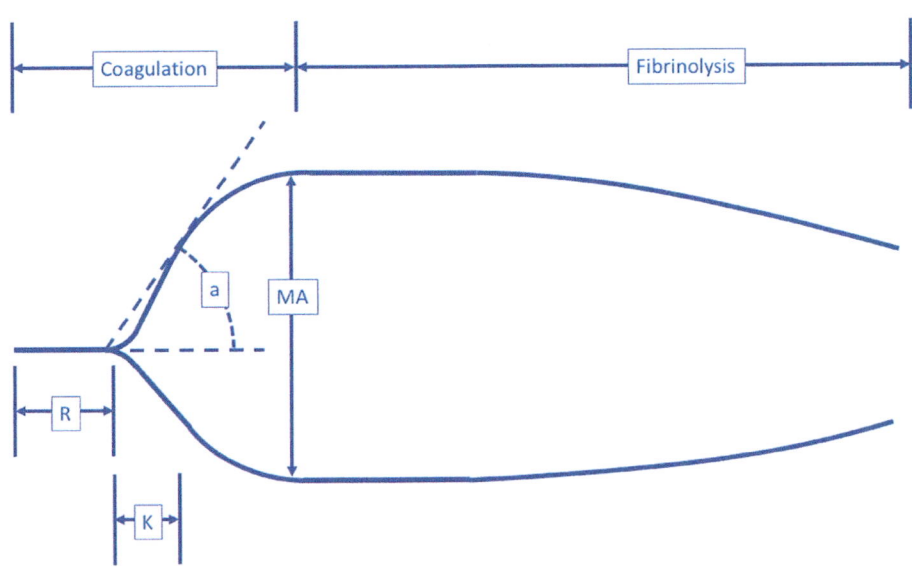

Figure 36.14 Diagram of thromboelastography tracing. For this test, blood is placed into a small container; then a wire moving through the sample monitors changes in viscoelastic properties and thereby, clot formation and strength. Assessed variables include: reaction time (R, a measure of initial clot formation); clotting time (K, the time from the end of R to a predetermined clot strength); angle (a, the rate of clot build-up); and maximum amplitude (MA, the peak strength of the clot). Fibrinolysis is represented by the rate of clot strength dissolution. A measure of the fibrinolysis rate is the amplitude at 30 minutes after MA is reached (A30; not depicted here).

to hypocapnia and hypoxemia. Respiratory alkalosis (from hyperventilation) and metabolic acidosis (possibly from poor tissue oxygenation induced by hypoxemia and low cardiac output) can occur. Partial improvement with O_2 therapy indicates some degree of V/Q mismatch.

Radiography

Thoracic radiography is used to screen for cardiac abnormalities, especially in animals with systemic arterial TE disease, and for pulmonary changes in animals suspected to have pulmonary thromboemboli. Evidence for CHF or other pulmonary disease associated with thromboemboli (such as pulmonary carcinoma or another neoplasm, HWD, or other infections) also might be found. Most cats with arterial TE disease have some degree of cardiomegaly (especially LA enlargement) when cardiomyopathy is underlying (**Figures 3.14** and **3.22**, pp. 57 and 64; **Figures 33.6–33.8** and **33.23**, pp. 662 and 680, and Chapter 33). A minority of affected cats have no radiographic evidence of cardiomegaly. Signs of CHF (including dilated pulmonary veins, pulmonary edema, or pleural effusion) might or might not be present. PTE produces variable radiographic findings (**Figure 36.15**). Pleural effusion, truncated lobar pulmonary arteries, alveolar infiltrates, hyperlucent lungs and areas of relative oligemia (suggesting reduced pulmonary blood flow), pulmonary trunk enlargement, and sometimes, lung atelectasis are described in dogs. However, any radiographic pattern is possible in the setting of PTE. Cats with PTE also can develop pleural effusion, alveolar opacification, peribronchial and interstitial markings, or pulmonary vascular congestion similar to dogs. Radiographs sometimes are unremarkable, even with clinical signs of respiratory compromise.

Echocardiography

A complete echocardiographic examination is important to define whether, and what type of, heart disease might be present. Thrombi within the left or right heart chambers and proximal great vessels can be readily identified with two-dimensional (2D) echocardiography provided sufficient right- and left-sided images are obtained (**Figures 36.3**, **36.8**, and **36.16**; also **Figure 33.16**, p. 666). The most common intracardiac site for thrombosis is the LA appendage. A small auricular thrombus is seen best from a left craniodorsal transducer position. Doppler modalities help define abnormal (or absent) blood flow in affected regions, and often indicate depressed active LA appendage ejection velocities (<20 cm/s). Cats with arterial TE disease associated with cardiomyopathy usually have some degree of LA enlargement and often, reduced LA shortening fraction or fractional area change. An LA dimension over 20 mm (measured from the 2D long-axis 4-chamber view) increases the risk for TE disease, although over half of aortic thromboembolism cases had a smaller LA size in one study (Smith, 2003). Increasing LA size and depressed LA function (regardless of how these are measured) increase the liability for arterial thromboembolism in cats. Spontaneous echogenic contrast ("smoke") indicates a clear risk for thrombosis.

PTE severe enough to cause PH variably produces right ventricular (RV) enlargement and hypertrophy, interventricular

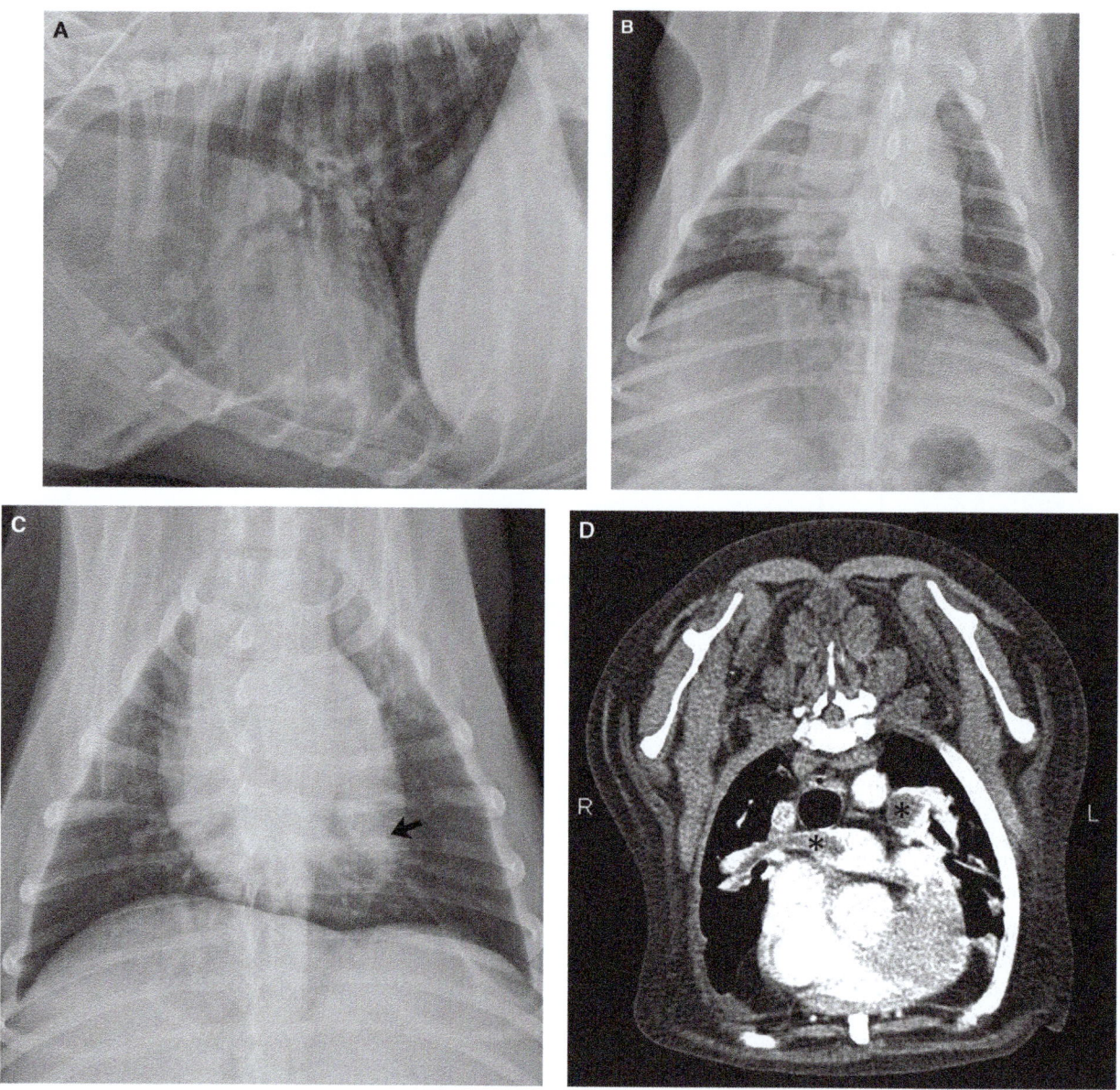

Figure 36.15 Right lateral (A), DV (B), and VD (C) radiographs from a 9-year-old female Dalmatian presented for lethargy, anorexia, and tachypnea. Tachycardia, harsh lung sounds, weak peripheral pulses, and hypoxemia were noted on exam. Two months prior, the dog had normal thoracic radiographs. These images show a multifocal alveolar infiltrate with an indistinct nodular pattern near the right cranial lobar vessels and bronchus (A). The right (B) and left (C, arrow) caudal lobar arteries are somewhat dilated. (D) Transverse computed tomography image after contrast administration shows intraluminal filling defects (*) in both left (seen in cross-section) and right primary pulmonary arteries, consistent with extensive pulmonary thromboembolism. L, left; R, right. Images courtesy of Dr E Hawkins.

septal flattening, and a high tricuspid regurgitation jet velocity (p. 828 and **Figures 39.12** and **39.13**, pp. 829 and 830). An experimental study of chronic embolic PH in dogs showed that the ratios of PA/aorta dimensions and PA flow acceleration time (AT)/ejection time (ET) had the highest sensitivity and specificity for predicting PH in this model (Akabane, 2019). The right PA distensibility index (RPADI), normalized RV internal diameter in diastole, and normalized tricuspid annular plane systolic excursion (TAPSE) also correlated with directly measured PA pressures.

Sometimes, thrombosis is visible within the main PA or right atrium (RA; **Figures 36.8** and **39.6C**, p. 822). Likewise, vena caval thrombosis might be visible sonographically, especially when the clot extends into the RA (**Figure 36.17**). In animals with coronary TE disease, the echo examination might indicate reduced myocardial contractility, with or without regional dysfunction. Areas of myocardial fibrosis secondary to chronic ischemia or infarction appear hyperechoic, hypokinetic or akinetic, and often thinner compared with the surrounding myocardium.

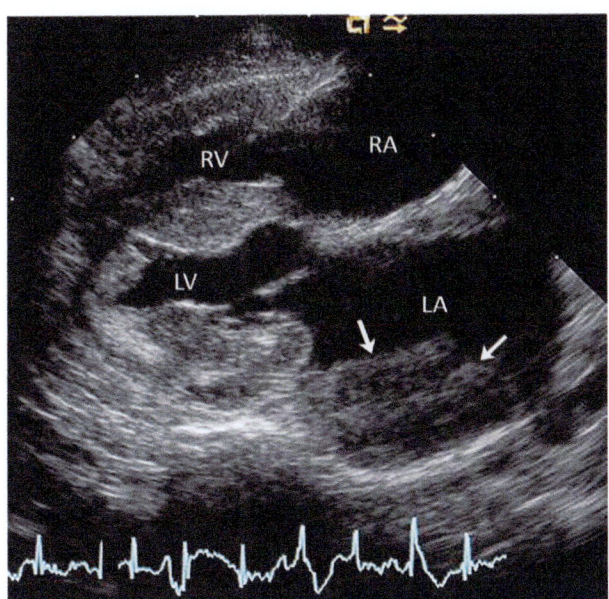

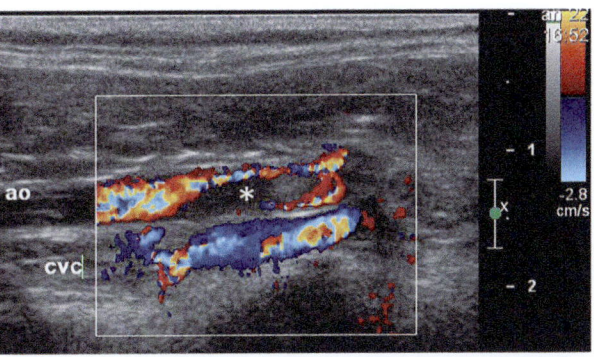

Figure 36.18 Color Doppler ultrasound image of the distal aorta (ao) and caudal vena cava (cvc) from a 9-year-old male Domestic Shorthair cat with hypertrophic cardiomyopathy and acute posterior paresis. The aortic flow signal is disturbed by an elongated soft tissue mass (thromboembolus, *). The lower-velocity, unobstructed caval flow is coded mostly blue. This cat had 4 occurrences of acute aortic thromboembolism over a period of 3 years. Image courtesy of Dr D L'Heureux.

Figure 36.16 A large thrombus (arrows) is present along the free wall of the massively dilated LA of this 10-year-old male Domestic Shorthair cat with end-stage cardiomyopathy and congestive heart failure. The thrombus extended into the left auricle. LA, left atrium; LV, left ventricle; RA, right atrium; RV, right ventricle.

Other Diagnostic Imaging

Ultrasonography can reveal the presence of a thromboembolus in the distal aorta or other large artery, as well as thrombosis of the portal vein and vena cava (**Figures 36.9, 36.18,** and **36.19**). Angiography can document vascular occlusion when ultrasonography is inconclusive or unavailable (**Figure 36.20**). It also can show the extent of collateral circulation. The choice of selective or nonselective technique depends on patient size and the suspected location of the obstruction. Especially in cats, if echocardiography is unavailable, nonselective angiocardiography can help define the nature of underlying cardiac disease and determine the location and extent of the thromboembolus. Pulmonary angiography can identify major obstructions to

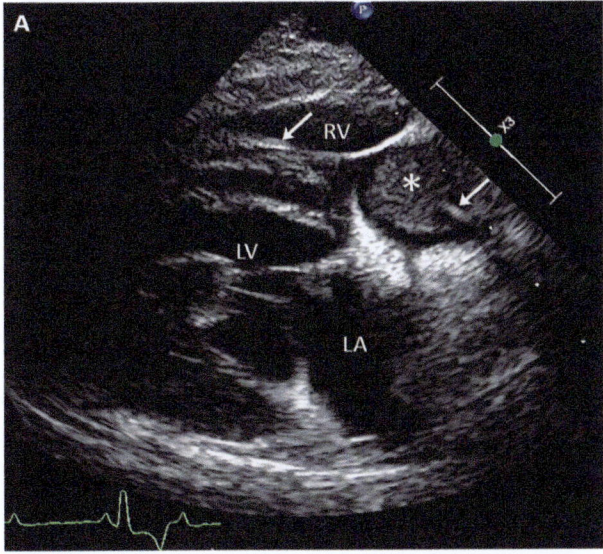
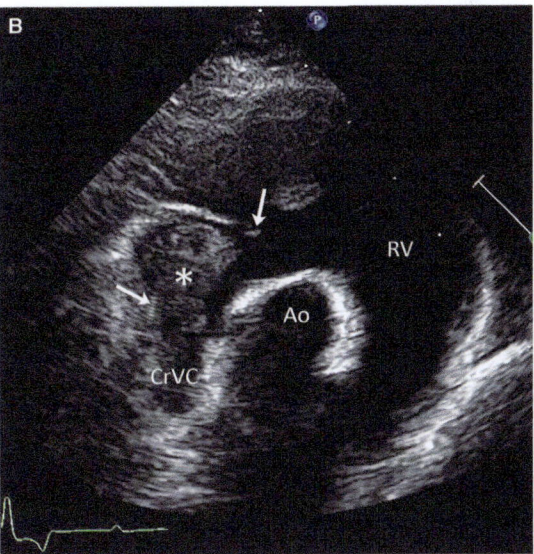

Figure 36.17 A few weeks after a transvenous pacing system was implanted in a 6-year-old Brussels Griffon with 3rd degree heart block, the dog developed ventral cervical and cranial thoracic subcutaneous edema. A large thrombus had formed around the pacing lead wire, obstructing right atrial inflow. The dog also had protein-losing nephropathy. (A) Right parasternal 4-chamber image recorded ~2½ weeks after initiation of antithrombotic therapy; subcutaneous edema had resolved and the thrombus had diminished in size. Thrombus (*) is evident within the right atrium and surrounds the lead wire (arrows). ECG (at bottom left) shows 1 paced QRS complex and 3 nonconducted P waves. (B) Angled short-axis view shows the thrombus (*) extending into the CrVC. Only small segments of the lead wire (arrows) are visible in this frame. Ao, aorta; CrVC, cranial vena cava; LA, left atrium; LV, left ventricle; RV, right ventricle.

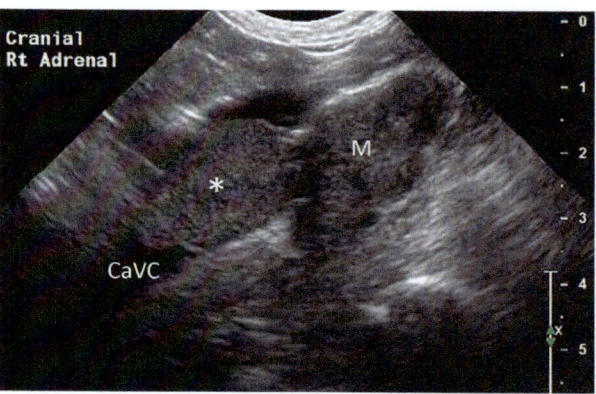

Figure 36.19 A 5-year-old female German Shorthair Pointer was being rechecked for stage B2 myxomatous mitral valve disease. The owner mentioned that the dog had shown right rear limb weakness over the previous 3–4 weeks, which prompted additional testing. This abdominal ultrasound image shows the dog's right adrenal gland, obliterated by a hypoechoic mass lesion (M, most likely pheochromocytoma or adrenal carcinoma) that eroded into the caudal vena cava (CaVC). A thrombus (*), possibly including an extension of the mass, lies within and partially occludes the CaVC. Image courtesy of Dr K Miles.

pulmonary flow (**Figure 36.21**). Angiography traditionally has been done using fluoroscopic imaging. However, cross-sectional imaging (computed tomography, CT; or magnetic resonance imaging, MRI) also can be used; these modalities require only peripheral venous access for contrast material injection, rather than selective central catheterization. Furthermore, the ability to generate 3-dimensional models from high-resolution CT angiography studies has allowed a level of anatomic understanding not previously available (**Figure 36.22**). To perform CT angiography, a bolus of contrast material is injected into a cephalic (or other peripheral) vein, then the CT scan is initiated as the contrast reaches the vascular structure of interest. Multiple phases are obtained to

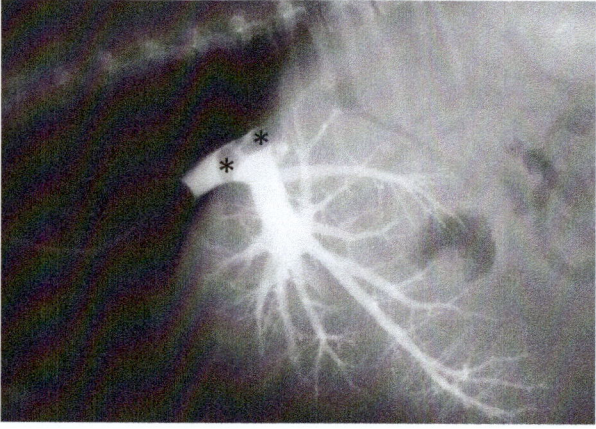

Figure 36.20 Caudal vena caval angiogram from an older male Dachshund with massive ascites. A multilobed thrombus (*) is obstructing flow caudal to the hepatic vein. An inflated balloon at the tip of the injection catheter prevents dye from flowing into the heart during the injection. A pheochromocytoma had invaded into the caudal vena cava.

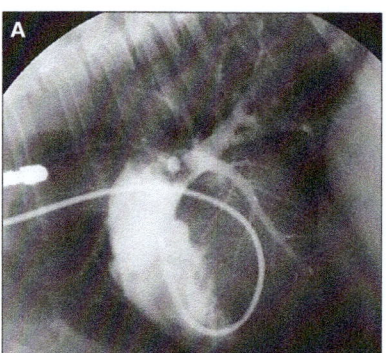

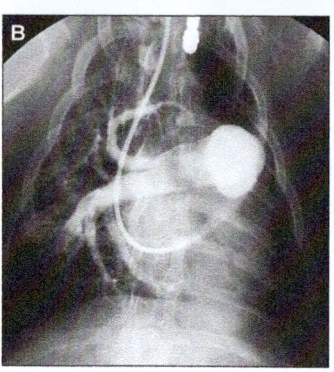

Figure 36.21 Lateral (A) and DV (B) pulmonary angiograms from a dog with hypothyroidism, exercise intolerance, and postexercise cyanosis. A large thromboembolus (TE) obstructed flow into the left pulmonary artery and its branches. Although arteries serving the right cranial and ventral lung regions are perfused, another TE blocked flow to the right caudodorsal lung region. Images courtesy of Dr E Riedesel.

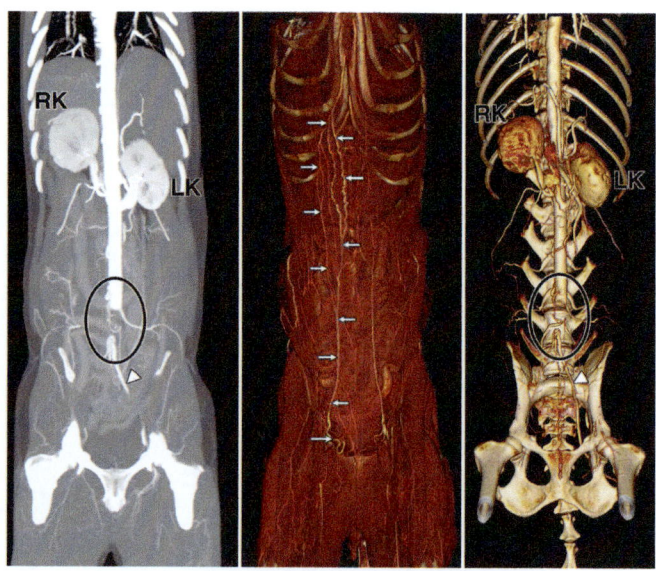

Figure 36.22 Computed tomography angiography reformats from a Whippet with aortic thrombosis. Left: dorsal maximum intensity projection reformat shows absent aortic filling proximal to iliac trifurcation (circle). Middle: 3D reformat highlights prominent superficial epigastric collateral vessels (arrows indicate right-sided arteries) on the dog's ventrum that bypass the caudal aortic obstruction. Right: volume-rendered 3D reformat shows the aortic filling defect (circle). Surfaces of left kidney (LK) and right kidney (RK) have multifocal depressions, consistent with embolic infarctions.

highlight both arterial and venous anatomy; a delayed phase also is commonly recorded, roughly 90 seconds to 3 minutes after the arterial and venous phases. Various protocols for contrast timing can be used, with test scan or bolus-tracking being the two primary methods.

Thermography, to evaluate surface infrared radiation, presents another tool for detecting arterial thromboembolism. In patients with PTE, ventilation/perfusion scintigraphy might show unperfused lung regions. Nuclear scintigraphy can help evaluate perfusion in other obstructed regions as well.

Management of Thromboembolic Disease

General Therapeutic Principles

The goals of therapy are to: (1) stabilize the patient by supportive treatment as needed; (2) prevent extension of the thrombus and additional TE events; and (3) reduce the size of existing thrombi and restore perfusion, when possible. Management strategies used for TE disease are outlined in **Table 36.4**). Supportive care also is provided to help improve tissue perfusion, minimize further endothelial damage and blood stasis, optimize organ function, and allow time for collateral circulation development. Antiplatelet and anticoagulant drugs form the foundation of antithrombotic therapy. These therapies are aimed at reducing platelet aggregation and growth of existing thrombi. They essentially are a component of supportive care, in anticipation of thrombus dissolution by the animal's endogenous fibrinolytic system. Although direct fibrinolytic therapy could be used in some cases, dosage uncertainties, the need for intensive care, and the potential for serious complications limit its application. In addition, it is important to manage underlying disease condition(s), as far as is possible.

Fluid therapy, depending on individual patient needs, can help expand vascular volume, support blood pressure, and correct electrolyte and acid/base abnormalities. However, this usually is not appropriate for animals with overt CHF (p. 348), and for those with subclinical heart disease, must be used only with great caution. Cardiac-specific therapy is provided if indicated. In patients with acute respiratory signs, it is important to determine whether CHF, pain, PTE, or other abnormality is responsible. In animals without CHF, diuretic or vasodilator therapy could worsen perfusion.

Acute arterial embolization is particularly painful and analgesic therapy is indicated, especially for the first 24–36 hours. However, chronic in-situ aortic thrombosis, which is more likely in dogs, appears to be less painful; analgesic therapy might be less urgent. For IV drug administration in animals with caudal aortic obstruction, cranial venous access is advised; the lumbar musculature can be used for IM injection. A strong mu agonist is likely to provide analgesia that is more effective, and so is recommended for initial pain

Table 36.4 Management Outline for Thromboembolic Disease

General Supportive Care

- Fluid therapy to improve tissue perfusion, support blood pressure, and correct electrolyte or acid/base imbalances, as indicated (except if CHF present, see text)
- Supplemental O_2, as needed
- Analgesia for acute arterial thromboembolism, especially during initial 24–36 hours (see p. 763). Options include:
  - Fentanyl citrate
    - Dog: 0.002–0.005 mg/kg IV bolus, then 0.002–0.005 mg/kg/h CRI
    - Cat: same
  - or Hydromorphone
    - Dog: 0.05–0.2 mg/kg IM, IV, SC q4–6h
    - Cat: same
  - or Oxymorphone
    - Dog: 0.05–0.2 mg/kg IM, IV, SC q2–4h
    - Cat: same
  - or Morphine
    - Dog: 0.2–0.4 mg/kg IM, IV, SC q4–6h
    - Cat: 0.1 mg/kg IM, IV, SC q4–6h
  - or Methadone
    - Dog: 0.5-1.0 mg/kg IV q3-4h
    - Cat: 0.1 (-0.2) mg/kg IV q3-4h
  - or Buprenorphine
    - Dog: 0.01–0.03 mg/kg IM, IV, SC q6–8h
    - Cat: same; or PO, for transmucosal absorption

Prevent thrombus extension and additional TE events

- Antiplatelet therapy (see **Table 36.2** and associated text)
  - Clopidogrel preferred over aspirin in dogs and cats
- Anticoagulant therapy (see **Table 36.2** and associated text)
  - UFH typically used initially for acute thromboembolism, although LMWH could be used instead
  - LMWH or direct Xa inhibitor for chronic use
- ± Consider fibrinolytic or other therapy (see p. 766)
  - (Intensive care setting, with continuous ECG and frequent renal and electrolyte monitoring needed for fibrinolytic therapy)

Monitoring and Follow-Up Care

- Monitor body temperature, respiratory status, renal function, electrolytes, blood pressure, and other parameters, as appropriate
  - Provide external warming, if hypothermic
- Evaluate for underlying or concurrent disease (echocardiography and other tests, as indicated)
  - Manage underlying disease, including CHF (see Chapter 22, and chapters on specific diseases), if present
- For nonambulatory patients: periodically rotate body position, provide postural support and physical therapy (when stable)

Abbreviations: CHF, congestive heart failure; LMWH, low molecular weight heparin; TE, thromboembolic; UFH, unfractionated heparin.

management, especially in cats (**Table 36.4**). Depending on the type of practice and level of monitoring, a number of opioids can be effective. These include an IV bolus followed by CRI of fentanyl, as well as parenteral administration of methadone, hydromorphone, oxymorphone, or morphine. Buprenorphine is a mixed mu agonist/antagonist; it usually is reserved for follow up analgesia. Potential adverse effects of opioids include respiratory depression, reduced GI motility, and in cats, dysphoria and temperature dysregulation. A fentanyl patch (such as 25 mcg/hour size for cats, applied to shaved skin) could be used for analgesia lasting up to 3 days; however, because of the delayed onset of effect, another analgesic must be given concurrently for the initial 12 hours.

Hypothermia is addressed by providing gentle external warming. Renal function and serum electrolyte concentrations should be monitored daily, or more frequently if fibrinolytic therapy is used. Continuous ECG monitoring during the first several days can help the clinician detect acute hyperkalemia associated with reperfusion (p. 160). For nonambulatory patients, periodic rotation of body position and postural support during urination and defecation (or bladder expression) should be provided, as needed. Loosely bandaging the affected limb(s) to prevent self-mutilation might be necessary in some animals with arterial TE disease. Physical therapy can be helpful after the animal is stabilized. Nutritional support becomes important if anorexia persists after the initial treatment period. Supplemental O_2 improves hypoxemia related to V/Q mismatch and alveolar hypoventilation. Oxygen therapy is especially important with PTE and could be helpful with other TE disease. The use of tissue plasminogen activator is not established for treatment but has been used (see below).

For horses with thrombophlebitis, heparin or dalteparin have been used to reduce thrombus extension. Local infusion of a fibrinolytic agent, especially for jugular thrombosis, might be considered also, although the efficacy of this is unclear. When infective thrombophlebitis is suspected, broad-spectrum antibiotic therapy is used pending results of catheter-tip or aspirate culture and sensitivity testing. Flunixin meglumine (1 mg/kg q12h) could help reduce inflammation.

Antiplatelet Therapy

Antithrombotic therapy is used to prevent thrombosis in cases at high risk or as secondary prevention when a thrombotic event has already occurred. A drug to block platelet activation and aggregation is recommended, especially with arterial TE disease. Clopidogrel, a second-generation thienopyridine, has greater antiplatelet effects than, and now is preferred over, aspirin (acetylsalicylic acid) for cats. These two drugs also can be administered concurrently, especially for secondary prevention or in patients at the highest risk for arterial thromboembolism. Clopidogrel can be co-administered with heparin(s) or with a factor Xa-inhibitor, such as apixaban or rivaroxaban. This combination is used most often for secondary prevention in patients with preexisting or prior embolic events. Clopidogrel probably is more efficacious in dogs also, although there currently is less evidence to support this. The current cost of some anticoagulants render them impractical for the majority of veterinary patients, although the smaller size of the cat provides greater opportunities for combination antithrombotic therapy.

Clopidogrel Clopidogrel (at 18.75 mg/cat PO q24h) significantly reduced the recurrence of thromboembolism in the high-risk population of cats that had a prior arterial TE event (FATCAT study, Hogan, 2015). In addition, for cats that did have another TE event, clopidogrel more than doubled the median time to TE recurrence (to over 440 days), compared to aspirin. As a platelet membrane $P2Y_{12}$ receptor antagonist, clopidogrel inhibits ADP binding, which subsequently decreases platelet binding to fibrinogen and vWF and leads to reduced ADP-mediated platelet aggregation. Clopidogrel also reduces platelet release of serotonin, ADP, and other factors that promote platelet aggregation and vasoconstriction. The drug requires hepatic bioconversion to an active metabolite for its effects. Genetic differences in individual ability to biotransform clopidogrel could exist in cats, as in people, with questionable drug efficacy in poor metabolizers. Clopidogrel's antiplatelet effect peaks within 72 hours of dosing and dissipates in about a week after administration ceases. A loading dose (**Table 36.2**), given as soon as possible after an acute arterial TE event, can achieve therapeutic plasma concentrations within 1½ hours, appears to be well-tolerated, and might have a positive effect on collateral blood flow. The generic clopidogrel formulation appears to yield comparable levels of active metabolite as the original branded form in cats. In horses, oral clopidogrel causes variable and competitive, rather than irreversible, platelet inhibition and its terminal half-life is less than 2 hours (Norris, 2019). Therefore, more frequent administration is likely to be needed in horses than in other species.

Clopidogrel could cause GI ulceration or other GI signs, but is much less likely to do so compared to aspirin. When given in conjunction with aspirin, a reduced aspirin dosage is recommended (such as 5 mg/cat q72h). Some cats experience vomiting; icterus has occurred rarely. Clopidogrel tablets have a bitter taste when split, causing excess salivation and intolerance in some cats. This can make administration to some cats unacceptable. Coating the tablet fragment in butter or placing it in a gel capsule or pill pocket might improve compliance in some patients. A related drug, ticlodipine, caused a high rate of anorexia and vomiting at the effective antiplatelet dose in a preliminary study in cats.

Aspirin Aspirin irreversibly inhibits cyclooxygenase, which reduces prostaglandin and thromboxane A_2 synthesis and, therefore, subsequent platelet aggregation, serotonin release, and vasoconstriction. Because platelets cannot synthesize additional cyclooxygenase, the reduction of procoagulant prostaglandins and thromboxane persists for the platelet's lifespan (7–10 days). Endothelial prostacyclin production (also via the cyclooxygenase pathway) is reduced by aspirin, although only transiently because endothelial cells synthesize additional cyclooxygenase. Aspirin's benefit might relate more to in-situ thrombus formation; efficacy in acute arterial thromboembolism is unknown. The optimal aspirin dose is unclear. Cats lack the enzyme glucaronyl transferase, which is needed to metabolize aspirin; therefore, less frequent dosing is required compared with dogs. Doses of 10–25 mg/kg (1.25 grains/cat) given PO once every (2–)3 days inhibit platelet aggregation in-vitro and appeared to improved collateral circulation when given prior to experimental aortic thrombosis in cats. Clinical outcomes in cats with arterial TE disease were comparable when either low-dose aspirin (5 mg/cat q72h) or more typical doses (40–81 mg/cat q72h) were used. However, fewer GI side-effects occurred with the lower dose. In general, the adverse effects of aspirin tend to be mild and uncommon. However, adverse GI effects (including vomiting, inappetence with weight loss, ulceration, hematemesis) occur in some animals, especially with higher or more frequent doses; a buffered formulation or aspirin-Maalox combination product might help minimize this. Although aspirin's antiplatelet efficacy is inferior to that of clopidogrel, the FATCAT trial (Hogan, 2015) demonstrated a likely benefit of treatment and aspirin could be useful in animals that do not tolerate clopidogrel. Aspirin might also be used in combination with clopidogrel for a high-risk patient with adequate platelet count, although the use of a low molecular weight heparin (LMWH) or anti-Xa anticoagulant drug as adjunct to clopidogrel would appear to be of greater advantage.

Other Antiplatelet Drugs Some drugs block platelet glycoprotein IIb/IIIa receptors (alpha$_{IIb}$beta$_3$ integrin inhibitors) and thereby interfere with platelet binding to fibrinogen. Abciximab is one of these agents. In a preliminary study, pretreatment with abciximab plus aspirin was more effective than aspirin alone in reducing platelet aggregation and in-vivo thrombosis in cats, although there was much inter-cat variability, as well as prolongation of mucosal bleeding time; the potential clinical utility of this drug for veterinary patients is unknown (Bright, 2003). However, a similar drug (eptifibatide) caused unpredictable CV collapse and death in an experimental cat study. Newer antiplatelet drugs include other P2Y$_{12}$ platelet inhibitors, such as prasugrel (a third-generation thienopyridine) and ticagrelor (a nonthienopyridine), although their potential for veterinary use is unexplored.

Anticoagulant Therapy

Heparin is used in animals with acute thromboembolism to limit extension of existing thrombi and prevent further TE episodes. It does not promote thrombolysis. Unfractionated heparin (UFH) and a number of LMWH products are available and can be used for thrombosis management. In addition, LMWHs and several oral anticoagulant drugs are becoming more widely used for longer-term and prophylactic therapy. Warfarin (p. 770) is not used for acute thrombosis management and currently has very little, if any, role in long-term anticoagulant treatment.

Unfractionated Heparin Heparin's main anticoagulant effect is produced by complexing with antithrombin, which in turn inhibits factors IXa, Xa, XIa, XIIa, and IIa (thrombin). This prevents fibrin formation and reduces thrombin-induced activation of platelets and factors V, VIII, and XI. UFH binds thrombin, as well as antithrombin. Heparin also stimulates the release of tissue factor inhibitor from vascular sites, which helps reduce thrombus initiation. Optimal dosing protocols for animals are undefined. UFH usually is given as an initial IV bolus followed by SC injections or constant infusion in dogs (**Table 36.2**). IM administration is avoided because of the risk for hemorrhage at the injection site. Heparin doses (from 75–500 U/kg) have been used with uncertain efficacy. Anti-Xa activity measurement is recommended for monitoring UFH therapy (the Cornell Comparative Coagulation laboratory, http://ahdc.vet.cornell.edu/Sects/Coag/ can provide this test for dogs and cats). An anti-Xa target of 0.35–0.7 U/mL is used in dogs, although minor hemorrhage could still occur at this level. The same anti-Xa target range could be used in cats, although additional study to support this is needed. Other methods (such as monitoring activated partial thromboplastin time, activated clotting time, or thromboelastography) continue to be used despite lack of adequate evidence to support their use. Monitoring activated partial thromboplastin time (with a goal of prolongation to 1.5–2.5 times baseline) does not consistently predict serum heparin concentrations. Likewise, activated clotting time is not recommended for monitoring heparin therapy, although it might be useful intraoperatively or during a catheter-based procedure. Hemorrhage is the major complication of UFH, which has complex pharmacodynamics. Heparin-induced bleeding might be counteracted by use of protamine sulfate, although overdose of this agent can itself cause hemorrhage and other life-threatening adverse effects. Fresh frozen plasma might be needed to replenish antithrombin. Heparin treatment typically is continued until the patient is stable and has been transitioned to oral antithrombotic medication(s).

Low Molecular Weight Heparin LMWH products are a diverse group of depolymerized heparins that vary in size, structure, and pharmacokinetics. LMWHs bind to antithrombin and accelerate its inactivation of factor Xa. Their smaller size prevents simultaneous binding to thrombin and antithrombin. LMWHs have minimal ability to inhibit thrombin, so they are less likely to cause bleeding. Thus, they are safer than heparin, especially for longer-term use. LMWHs have greater bioavailability and a longer half-life than UFH when given SC because of lesser binding to plasma proteins, as well as endothelial cells and macrophages. LMWHs do not markedly affect coagulation times. Their effect can be monitored indirectly by anti-Xa activity, although the necessity for routine monitoring is not firmly established. In dogs, dosage adjustments could be considered based on anti-Xa activity 2–4 hours postdosing, using a target level of 0.5–1.0 IU/mL. Dalteparin sodium and enoxaparin are the LMWHs used most commonly in dogs and cats, although the most efficacious dosing is not entirely clear. Predicted feline doses to maintain anti-Xa activity within therapeutic range for people

(0.3–1.0 IU/mL) have been suggested as 150 IU/kg SC q4h for dalteparin, and 1.5 mg/kg SC q6h for enoxaparin. However, such doses might not be necessary for antithrombotic activity. Enoxaparin (at 1 mg/kg SC q12h) had significant antithrombotic effect for at least 12 hours, with no correlation between plasma anti-Xa activity and thrombus formation in a feline venous thrombosis model. Whether efficacy is similar in cardiomyopathic cats with arterial TE is not clear, but this regimen is recommended most often in clinical practice.

Newer Anticoagulant Agents Novel anticoagulant drugs now available have a relatively predictable pharmacodynamic profile, with demonstrated superiority over chronic warfarin therapy in limiting cardiogenic TE disease in people. Most are administered orally. These agents include the direct factor Xa inhibitors rivaroxaban (Xarelto), apixaban (Eliquis) and fondaparinux (Arixtra), as well as the direct thrombin inhibitor, dabigatran. The direct factor Xa inhibitors enhance antithrombin's effects without affecting thrombin or platelet function. Anti-Xa activity could be used to monitor their effect; routine coagulation tests are affected by these agents at peak concentrations, but optimal monitoring strategies are not established.

Rivaroxaban has good oral bioavailability in dogs. Peak anti-Xa activity occurs at between 1.5–3 hours postdose; feeding can delay absorption. The magnitude of anti-Xa effect varies among individuals. Duration of effect is thought to be <12 hours; however, it is unclear whether more than once daily dosing is clinically advantageous. Rivaroxaban is excreted through the kidney and in bile. A small study in normal dogs found good correlations between the drug's anti-Xa activity and the ratio of peak (3-hour) time value-to-baseline value for both PT and R value in TEG (using a tissue factor or RapidTEG as an activator; Bae, 2019). Prolongation of either the PT or TEG-R ratio by 1.5–1.9 times its baseline value was calculated to produce anti-Xa concentrations of 140–260 ng/mL, or within the human therapeutic range. Recommended clinical dosage for dogs is 1–2 mg/kg PO q24h (Blais, 2019). In healthy cats, rivaroxaban's peak anti-Xa activity occurs at about 3 hours following administration. A clinical dosage of 0.5–1 mg/kg q24h has been suggested (Blais, 2019). Doses of 1.25 mg q12h and 2.5 mg q24h have been tolerated adequately in healthy cats. Based on antifactor Xa activity, twice daily dosing might be preferable although this is unclear.

Apixaban, in healthy cats, reduces factor Xa activity following oral and IV dosing (0.2 mg/kg), although chronic oral dosing studies are not available. There appears to be high bioavailability, fairly brief half-life, and much intercat variability. Clinically, doses of 0.625 mg/cat once daily have been tried. Fondaparinux (at 0.06 or 0.2 mg/kg SC injection q12h) produced presumed therapeutic anti-Xa activity in a small number of healthy cats. Studies in dogs suggest higher dosing might be needed; early safety studies describe 0.25-0.5 mg/kg PO q8-12h.

The clinical efficacy and optimal dosing of these direct factor Xa inhibitors for preventing or managing arterial thromboembolism remain to be more fully documented. Use of dabigatran in clinical veterinary patients is not yet reported.

Andexanet Alfa is a modified recombinant, inactive form of human factor Xa developed as a reversal agent for factor Xa inhibitors; its potential for clinical use in animals is unexplored.

Fibrinolytic Therapy

Drugs used to promote lysis of thrombi have included human recombinant tissue plasminogen activator (rt-PA), streptokinase, and urokinase. These agents increase conversion of plasminogen to plasmin to facilitate fibrinolysis. Although they can break down thrombi, frequent complications and high mortality related to reperfusion injury and hemorrhage, as well as the costly intensive care typically required, uncertain dosing protocols, and lack of clear survival advantage have prevented their widespread use. If pursued, this therapy is probably best instituted within 3–4 hours of vascular occlusion; nevertheless, beneficial effects might be possible up to a week after thrombosis. An intensive care setting, including continuous serum potassium concentration (or ECG) monitoring to detect reperfusion-induced hyperkalemia, is recommended during fibrinolytic therapy. The consequences of reperfusion injury present serious and sometimes fatal complications. Attempts to mitigate these using the iron chelator deferoxamine mesylate (to reduce oxidative damage from free radicals involving iron) or allopurinol have been met with uncertain results.

Tissue Plasminogen Activator rt-PA is a single-chain polypeptide serine protease with a higher specificity for fibrin within thrombi and a low affinity for circulating plasminogen. Although the risk of hemorrhage is less than with streptokinase, there is potential for serious bleeding as well as other side effects. rt-PA also is potentially antigenic in animals because it is a human protein. rt-PA induces platelet dysfunction but not hyperaggregability. Optimal dosing in animals is not known. Ten cats with distal aortic TE disease that received rt-PA were reported initially, although the data were never published in a peer-reviewed format. Doses used were 0.25–1 mg/kg/hour IV continuous rate infusion (CRI) for a total of 1–10 mg/kg. A prospective study of 11 cats with arterial TE disease evaluated two different rt-PA protocols: 5 mg of rt-PA given over 1.5 hours or 4 hours (Welch, 2010). Although there was evidence for reperfusion, serious complications and high mortality occurred. Cause of death in most cats was attributed to reperfusion injury (hyperkalemia, metabolic acidosis) or hemorrhage; CHF, neurologic signs, and arrhythmias also occurred. In another retrospective report (Guillaumin, 2019), 16 cats with arterial TE disease that received rt-PA (most at a dose of 1 mg/kg infused over one hour) along with standard supportive care were compared to 38 similarly affected cats that received the current standard care. Statistically, there were no differences in complication rates (reperfusion injury, acute kidney injury), clinical improvement, or short-term survival between the treatment groups. A prospective study of rt-PA compared to conventional therapy in cats with acute arterial thromboembolism is currently undergoing analysis.

In dogs, the half-life of rt-PA is about 2–3 minutes, although effects persist longer because of binding to fibrin. rt-PA has been given as IV boluses (1 mg/kg q1h) for 10 doses, with IV fluid, other supportive therapy, and close monitoring. It also has been used in 2 mg aliquots infused into dialysis catheters to restore catheter patency. For venous thrombosis, one author (BAS) has administered rt-PA locally via an indwelling infusion catheter using a bolus of 2 to 4 mg followed by CRI at 0.5 mg/hour for 24 hours (**Figure 36.23**).

Other Fibrinolytic Agents Streptokinase and urokinase no longer are marketed in the United States, although they still might be available elsewhere. These drugs are nonspecific plasminogen activators that promote the breakdown of fibrin as well as fibrinogen. This leads to the degradation of fibrin within thrombi and clot lysis, but also potentially leads to systemic fibrinolysis, coagulopathy, and bleeding. Streptokinase also degrades factor V, factor VIII, and prothrombin. Although the half-life of streptokinase is about 30 minutes, fibrinogen depletion continues for much longer. Streptokinase has been used with variable success in a small number of dogs with arterial thromboembolism. The reported protocol for dogs and cats is 90,000 IU of streptokinase infused IV over 20–30 minutes, then at a rate of 45,000 IU/hour for 3 hours (up to 8–12, in dogs). For cats, dilution of 250,000 IU into 5 mL saline, then into 50 mL to yield 5,000 IU/mL for infusion with a syringe pump has been suggested. However, no survival benefit was shown for streptokinase compared with combination aspirin and heparin treatment in cats. In a series of 46 cats with arterial TE disease, about 33% of those that received streptokinase infusion survived, which was roughly equivalent to the conventional therapy group. Local infusion of streptokinase into a femoral arterial thrombus was effective in one dog that had not improved with IV streptokinase. Local infusion of urokinase for distal aortic thromboembolism in a cat also was effective when intravenous therapy had failed. Although adverse effects were minor in some cases and bleeding might respond to discontinuation of streptokinase, there is potential for serious hemorrhage and high mortality. Acute hyperkalemia secondary to thrombolysis and reperfusion injury, metabolic acidosis, bleeding, and other complications can lead to death. Streptokinase can increase platelet aggregability and induce platelet dysfunction. Streptokinase used with heparin therapy can increase the risk of hemorrhage, especially

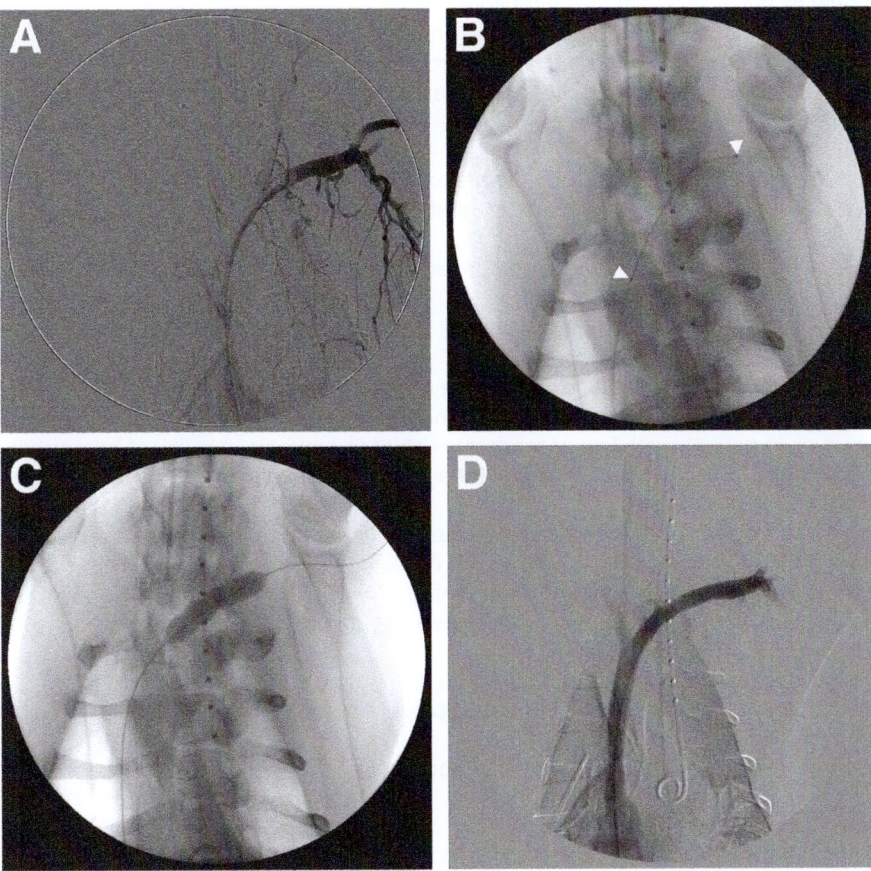

Figure 36.23 Images obtained during transcatheter intervention in a dog with central venous thrombosis that caused swelling of the head and pleural effusion. (A) Digitally subtracted angiogram with contrast injection into the left subclavian vein shows filling defects (thrombi) within the brachiocephalic vein, as well as poor filling of the cranial vena cava and prominent collaterals along the left lateral thorax. (B) An infusion catheter is placed throughout the thrombosed area in preparation for recombinant tissue plasminogen activator (rt-PA) infusion; the infusion site is denoted by radiopaque marks (arrowheads). (C) After rt-PA infusion, balloon angioplasty of the thrombus is performed throughout the brachiocephalic vein and cranial vena cava. (D) Final digitally subtracted angiogram shows normal venous return has been restored; flow is not seen in the previously noted collateral vessels.

when coagulation times are increased. Streptokinase is potentially antigenic, because it is produced by beta-hemolytic streptococci.

Other Considerations

Surgical removal of a thromboembolus generally is not advised in cats. The surgical risk is high and substantial neuromuscular ischemic injury is likely to have already occurred by the time of surgery. Nevertheless, successful surgical embolectomy for acute thromboembolism at the aortic trifurcation has been reported. Thrombus removal using an embolectomy catheter has not been effective in cats, but might be more successful in dogs of larger size. Rheolytic thrombectomy produced successful revascularization in 5 of 6 cats, although survival was comparable to medical therapy alone. Interventional transcatheter options for treating thrombotic and TE disease also could include local delivery of a fibrinolytic drug, angioplasty, and intravascular stent implantation (**Figure 36.23**). Transcatheter therapies for TE disease have not been evaluated rigorously against conventional medical therapies in animals. However, these alternative approaches might benefit select cases.

Some patients should remain on antithrombotic therapy indefinitely. Others might be safely weaned from treatment after a period of time. Decisions related to how long antithrombotic therapy should be continued in a particular patient can be challenging. Likewise, it can be difficult to decide whether therapy should be suspended prior to a surgical procedure or not. **Table 36.5** provides

Table 36.5 Considerations for Continuing or Stopping Antithrombotic Therapy

High Risk Patients (see Table 36.1)

- Recommend continuing antithrombotic therapy indefinitely.
  - Even after *in-situ* arterial or venous thrombus resolution, antithrombotic therapy should be continued indefinitely because of increased risk for recurrent thromboembolism.
- Presurgical considerations
  - Antiplatelet therapy should be continued using a single agent.
    - If 2 antiplatelet drugs are being administered, discontinue one.
  - Anticoagulant therapy should be continued prior to invasive procedures.
    - Continue heparin (UFH or LMWH) therapy; ideally, surgery should occur at the nadir of anticoagulant effect (for example, ~6–8 hours after SC injection).
- Surgical and postsurgical considerations
  - Because of increased risk for bleeding, close attention to hemostasis is important.
  - If antithrombotic therapy was discontinued prior to surgery, institute therapy as soon as possible, as long as there is no evidence of ongoing bleeding.
  - Antithrombotic therapy should be initiated immediately in patients that develop thrombosis postoperatively.

Low to Moderate Risk Patients

- Following resolution of *in-situ* arterial or venous thrombus
  - If underlying causative conditions have resolved, antithrombotic therapy can be discontinued after thrombus resolution.
  - If underlying conditions are unknown, or known conditions cannot be cured or resolved, recommend continuing antithrombotic therapy indefinitely. However, in patients with low or moderate risk of thrombosis, the risk of hemorrhage, as well as ability of the animal to tolerate antithrombotic therapy, should be weighed against the risk of recurrence of the prothrombotic condition.
- Guidelines for discontinuing anticoagulant therapy
  - If UFH is being given as an IV infusion, the dose should be tapered (weaned) rather than abruptly discontinued.
  - If UFH is being administered SC, consider weaning down the dosage.
  - If a LMWH is being used, it can be discontinued without weaning.
  - If a direct factor Xa inhibitor is being administered, consider weaning before discontinuing.
- Presurgical considerations
  - Recommend discontinuing antiplatelet therapy within 5(–7) days prior to elective procedures.
  - Possibly discontinue anticoagulation therapy prior to invasive procedures, especially where bleeding might be catastrophic or difficult to control.
    - Consider tapering (UFH) or stopping (LMWH) therapy 24 hours prior to procedure. Must balance thrombosis risks versus bleeding risks.
- Surgical and postsurgical considerations
  - Suggest restarting antithrombotic therapy once there is no evidence of ongoing bleeding.
  - Antithrombotic therapy should be started immediately in patients that develop thrombosis postoperatively.

Abbreviations: LMWH, low molecular weight heparin; UFH, unfractionated heparin.
(Adapted from Goggs R, Blais MC, Brainard BM, et al. American College of Veterinary Emergency and Critical Care (ACVECC) Consensus on the Rational Use of Antithrombotics in Veterinary Critical Care (CURATIVE) guidelines: Small animal. J Vet Emerg Crit Care (San Antonio) 2019;29:12–36.)

some considerations for making these decisions, based on current consensus guidelines (CURATIVE guidelines, Goggs, 2019).

Prognosis The prognosis generally is poor for cats with arterial TE disease. Historically, only a third survive the initial TE episode. However, survival statistics improve when cats that were euthanized without any or only limited therapy are excluded, or when only cases from recent years are analyzed. Significant embolization of the kidneys, intestines, or other organs carries a grave prognosis. Survival is better when only one limb is involved and if some motor function is preserved. Hypothermia and CHF at presentation both are associated with poor survival in cats. Rectal temperature at admission of 37.2°C (98.9°F) predicted a 50% probability of survival in one study (Smith, 2003). Other negative factors could include: hyperphosphatemia, progressive hyperkalemia or azotemia, progressive limb injury (continued muscle contracture after 2–3 days, necrosis), severe LA enlargement or LA dysfunction, presence of intracardiac thrombi or spontaneous echogenic contrast ("smoke"; **Figure 33.15**, p. 666) on echocardiogram, DIC, and a history of thromboembolism (Payne, 2015).

Barring complications, limb function in cats that survive the initial event should begin to return within 1–2 weeks. Some cats become clinically normal within 1–2 months, although residual deficits can persist for a variable time, particularly distal proprioceptive defects. In some cats, tissue necrosis might require wound management, skin grafting, or even amputation (**Figure 36.24**). Permanent limb deformity develops in some cats (**Figure 36.25**). Repeated TE events occur in at least a quarter of surviving cats.

The prognosis in most dogs with aortic thrombosis appears to be mixed; many cases have a more insidious onset, with less acute disease, so overall prognosis is unclear. Approximately 50% to 60% of reported cases leave the hospital alive. For these dogs, return of rear limb function is likely to take two weeks or longer, although some show improvement within several days of beginning antithrombotic therapy. Prognosis for dogs that are still ambulatory upon presentation and have had chronic clinical signs is more favorable than for dogs with acute-onset signs or that are unable to walk at presentation.

Thromboembolic Disease Prophylaxis

Antiplatelet and Anticoagulant Strategies

An antiplatelet or anticoagulant drug is recommended for animals thought to be at high risk for thrombosis (**Table 36.1**). Antiplatelet therapy is thought to be better for reducing arterial TE disease, while an anticoagulant drug might be better for reducing venous thrombosis or PTE (including that associated with HWD in dogs). However, the efficacy of

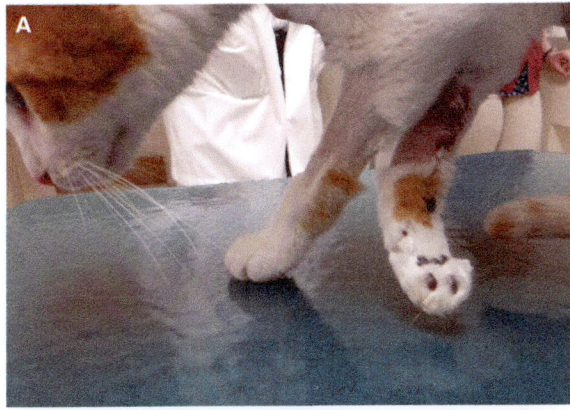

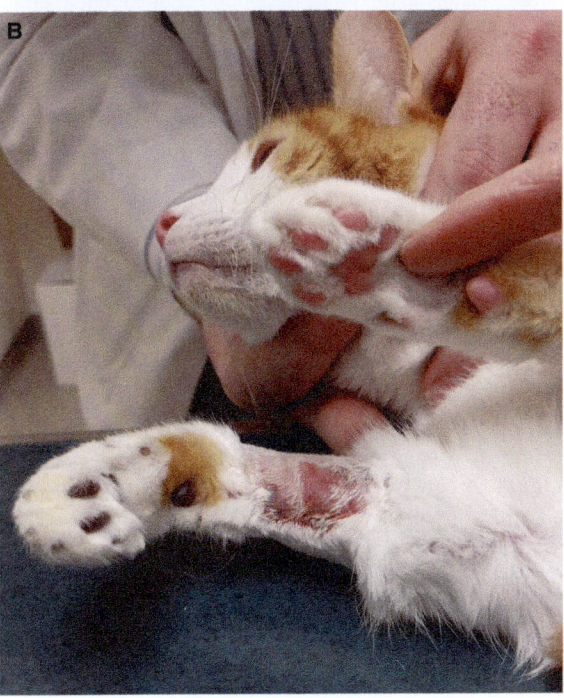

Figure 36.24 (A) This 3-year-old male Domestic Shorthair cat had been receiving medical therapy for an acute arterial thromboembolism to the right forelimb that occurred 10 days prior. Anorexia, a malodorous oozing lesion on the right antebrachium, and inability to use the right forelimb prompted the owner to return to the clinic. The leg was severely infected and gangrenous, with nonviable tissues distal to the carpus. (B) The right paw (with previously pink pads) was dark, shrunken, and hard (compare to the normal left forepaw). Following amputation of the right forelimb, supportive care and a few weeks of convalescence, the cat recovered. However, he died following another thromboembolic event a couple months later. The underlying diagnosis was restrictive cardiomyopathy with atrial fibrillation.

prophylaxis for TE disease is unknown and a strategy that consistently prevents thromboembolism is not yet clear.

In cats, clopidogrel is superior to aspirin for reducing recurrent arterial thromboembolism (Hogan, 2015) and probably first events, too. At-risk cats treated with aspirin alone, have a high rate of arterial thromboembolism recurrence. Any benefit to combining clopidogrel with aspirin, or adding an anticoagulant to either, is unclear. Nevertheless, for cats at

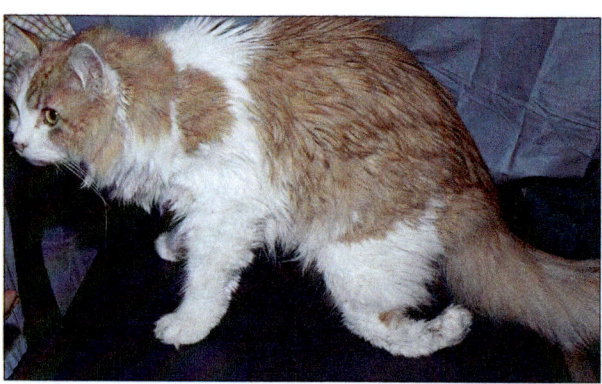

Figure 36.25 Hindlimb deformity developed subsequent to an episode of caudal aortic thromboembolism in this cat with restrictive cardiomyopathy, severe left atrial enlargement, and atrial fibrillation. The cat was able to ambulate well, despite weight-bearing on the dorsal aspect of the left metatarsus.

extremely high risk for arterial thromboembolism, the combination of clopidogrel with a LMWH or direct factor Xa inhibitor might provide better protection. For owners not motivated to give daily SC injections of LMWH, rivaroxaban or apixaban could be attractive alternatives. In cats without thrombocytopenia, concurrent aspirin (or clopidogrel) use could be considered. The risk of bleeding must be balanced against the likely risk for thrombosis, however.

For dogs at risk for arterial thromboembolism, clopidogrel probably is better than aspirin, although there is no strong evidence supporting one over the other. Dogs at high risk for arterial TE disease might benefit from the combination of an antiplatelet drug with a LMWH or direct factor Xa inhibitor (rivaroxaban or apixaban). Nevertheless, there is currently no strong evidence to support this either.

The preferred options for long-term anticoagulant drug therapy include LMWHs and the oral direct factor Xa inhibitor agents. In people, the oral Xa inhibitors rivaroxaban and apixaban have comparable or better efficacy than warfarin (coumadin), with less risk for hemorrhage. They require less monitoring and are more convenient to use.

Warfarin Although warfarin has been used for thromboprophylaxis in the past, it generally is not recommended now because of its complicated dosing, risk for hemorrhage, and the frequent monitoring required. Warfarin is considered only a last-choice alternative for larger dogs. The information related to warfarin is included only for this context, when use of a LMWH or direct anti-Xa anticoagulant is cost-prohibitive. Warfarin is not recommended for use in cats. It has been associated with a higher rate of fatal hemorrhage and no survival benefit compared to aspirin in this species. Furthermore, recurrent thromboembolism has occurred in almost half of cats treated with warfarin.

Warfarin inhibits vitamin K epoxide reductase which activates the vitamin-K dependent factors (II, VII, IX, and X), and proteins C and S. Warfarin initially causes transient hypercoagulability because anticoagulant proteins have a shorter half-life than most procoagulant factors; therefore, UFH or LMWH is given concurrently for 2–4 days after warfarin initiation. There is wide variability in dose response and potential for serious bleeding, even with close monitoring. The drug is highly protein-bound. Changes in serum protein content, as well as presence of other protein-bound drugs, can influence its anticoagulant effect.

In dogs, LMWH or a direct factor Xa inhibitor is recommended instead of warfarin as an anticoagulant. However, if warfarin is used, a baseline coagulation profile, platelet count, and international normalization ratio (INR) should be obtained, and antiplatelet drugs discontinued, before beginning treatment. There can be uneven distribution of drug within warfarin tablets, so compounding rather than use of tablet fragments is advised, if necessary to achieve appropriate dosing. Drug administration and blood sampling times should be consistent. An initial dose between 0.05 to 0.2 mg/kg PO q24h has been used in dogs. Dosage adjustments are based on the INR or prothrombin time (PT). The INR method is recommended because of variation in commercial PT assays. The INR is calculated by dividing the animal's PT by the control PT and raising the quotient to the power of the international sensitivity index (ISI) of the thromboplastin used in the assay; that is, INR = (animal PT/control PT)^{ISI}. An INR of 2–3 is thought to be as effective as higher values, with less chance for bleeding. The INR is rechecked at 1–3 days after beginning warfarin therapy, and then at progressively increasing intervals as needed to achieve a stable INR within the target range of 2–3. Warfarin dose adjustments are made by increasing or decreasing the total dose per week by 5–20%, depending on the measured INR. Heparin overlap is recommended until the INR is >2. If PT is used to monitor warfarin therapy (not advised), the goal is 1.25–1.5 (to 2) times pre-treatment PT at 8–10 hours after dosing. PT is checked several hours after initial dosing, then at progressively increasing time intervals (such as daily, then, twice weekly, then once weekly, then every 1–2 months) as long as the animal's condition appears stable. Warfarin overdose is treated by discontinuing the drug and administering vitamin K_1 (1–2 mg/kg/day PO or SC) until the patient's hematocrit is stable and PT is normal. Transfusion (fresh frozen plasma, packed red blood cells, or fresh whole blood) might be needed.

Suggested Additional Reading and References

Also See Online Comprehensive Bibliography at: https://www.routledge.com/9781482246223.

Akabane R, Shimano S, Sakatani A, et al. Relationship between right heart echocardiographic parameters and invasive pulmonary artery pressures in canine models of chronic embolic pulmonary hypertension. J Vet Med Sci 2019;81:1485–1491.

Alwood AJ, Downend AB, Brooks MB, et al. Anticoagulant effects of low-molecular-weight heparins in healthy cats. J Vet Intern Med 2007;21:378–387.

Bae J, Kim H, Kim W, et al. Therapeutic monitoring of rivaroxaban in dogs using thromboelastography and prothrombin time. J Vet Intern Med 2019;33:1322–1330.

Barrera JS, Bernard F, Ehrhart EJ, et al. Evaltion of risk factors for outcome associated with adrenal gland tumors with or without invasion of the caudal vena cava and treated via adrenalectomy in dogs: 86 cases (1993–2009). J Am Vet Med Assoc 2013;242:1715–1721.

Birkbeck R, Humm K, Cortellini S. A review of hyperfibrinolysis in cats and dogs. J Small Anim Pract 2019;60:641–655.

Blois S. Hyper- and hypocoagulable states. In, Ettinger SJ, Feldman EC, Cote E, (editors). Textbook of Veterinary Internal Medicine. 8th edition. Elsevier, St. Louis, MO. 2017. pp. 822–829.

Borgeat K, Wright J, Garrod O, et al. Arterial thromboembolism in 250 cats in general practice: 2004-2012. J Vet Intern Med 2014;28:102–108.

Bright JM, Dowers K, Hellyer P. In vitro anti-aggregatory effects of the GP IIb/IIIa antagonist eptifibatide on feline platelets. J Vet Intern Med 2002;16:v.

Bright JM, Dowers K, Powers BE. Effects of the glycoprotein IIb/IIIa, antagonist abciximab on thrombus formation and platelet function in cats with arterial injury. Vet Therapeutics 2003;4:35–46.

Carr AP, Panciera DL, Kidd L. Prognostic factors for mortality and thromboembolism in canine immune-mediated hemolytic anemia: a retrospective study of 72 dogs. J Vet Intern Med 2002;16:504–509.

Cook AK, Cowgill LD. Clinical and pathological features of protein-losing glomerular disease in the dog: a review of 137 cases (1985–1992). J Am Anim Hosp Assoc 1996;32:313–322.

Conversy B, Blais MC, Dunn M, et al. Anticoagulant activity of oral rivaroxaban in healthy dogs. Vet J 2017;223:5–11.

Cunningham SM, Ames MK, Rush JE, et al. Successful treatment of pacemaker-induced stricture and thrombosis of the cranial vena cava in two dogs by use of anticoagulants and balloon venoplasty. J Am Vet Med Assoc 2009;235:1467–1473.

deLaforcade A, Bacek L, Blais MC, et al. Consensus on the rational use of antithrombotics in veterinary critical care (CURATIVE): domain 1-defining populations at risk. J Vet Emerg Crit Care (San Antonio) 2019;29:37–48.

de Laforcade AA, Freeman LA, Shaw SP, et al. Hemostatic changes in dogs with naturally occurring sepsis. J Vet Intern Med 2003;17:674–679.

Dixon-Jimenez AC, Brainard BM, Brooks MB, et al. Pharmacokinetic and pharmacodynamic evaluation of oral rivaroxaban in healthy adult cats. J Vet Emerg Crit Care (San Antonio) 2016;26:619–629.

Drees R, Frydrychowicz A, Keuler NS, et al. Pulmonary angiography with 64-multidetector-row computed tomography in normal dogs. Vet RadiolUltrasound 2011;52:362–367.

Driehuys S, Van Winkle TJ, Sammarco CD, et al. Myocardial infarction in dogs and cats: 37 cases (1985–1994). J Am Vet Med Assoc 1998;213:1444–1448.

Dunn ME. Thrombectomy and thrombolysis: the interventional radiology approach. J Vet Emerg Crit Care 2011;21:144–150.

Falk T, Jonsson L. Ischaemic heart disease in the dog: a review of 65 cases. J Small Anim Pract 2000;41:97–103.

Furie B, Furie BC. Mechanisms of thrombus formation. N Engl J Med 2008;359:938–949.

Gant P, McBride D, Humm K. Abnormal platelet activity in dogs and cats - impact and measurement. J Small Anim Pract 2020;61:3–18.

Gara-Boivin C, de Castillo JRE, Dunn ME, et al. Effect of dalteparin administration on thrombin generation kinetics in healthy dogs. Vet Clin Pathol 2017;46:269–277.

Geraghty TE, Love S, Taylor DJ, et al. Assessment of subclinical venous catheter-related diseases in horses and associated risk factors. Vet Rec. 2009;164:227–231.

Goggs R, Blais MC, Brainard BM, et al. American College of veterinary emergency and critical care (ACVECC) consensus on the rational use of antithrombotics in veterinary critical care (CURATIVE) guidelines: small animal. J Vet Emerg Crit Care (San Antonio) 2019;29:12–36.

Good LI, Manning AM. Thromboembolic disease: physiology of hemostasis and pathophysiology of thrombosis. Compend Cont Educ Pract Vet 2003;25:650–659.

Good LI, Manning AM. Thromboembolic disease: predispositions and clinical management. Compend Cont Educ Pract Vet 2003;25:660-.

Guillaumin J, Gibson RM, Goy-Thollot I, et al. Thrombolysis with tissue plasminogen activator (TPA) in feline acute aortic thromboembolism: a retrospective study of 16 cases. J Feline Med Surg 2019;21:340–346.

Guillaumin J, Hmelo S, Farrell K, et al. Canine aortic thromboembolism (2005–2011): a retrospective study of 50 cases. J Vet Emerg Crit Care 2012;22:S6.

Habing A, Coelho JC, Nelson N, et al. Pulmonary angiography using 16 slice multidetector computed tomography in normal dogs. Vet Radiol Ultrasound 2011;52:173–178.

Hoffman M. Remodeling the blood coagulation cascade. J Thromb Thrombolysis 2003;16:17–20.

Hogan DF. Feline cardiogenic arterial thromboembolism: prevention and therapy. Vet Clin North Am Small Anim Pract 2017;47:1065–1082.

Hogan DF, Andrews DA, Green HW, et al. Antiplatelet effects and pharmacodynamics of clopidogrel in cats. J Am Vet Med Assoc 2004;225:1406–1411.

Hogan DF, Andrews DA, Talbott KK, et al. Evaluation of antiplatelet effects of ticlopidine in cats. Am J Vet Res 2004;65:327–332.

Hogan DF, Fox PR, Jacob K, et al. Secondary prevention of cardiogenic arterial thromboembolism in the cat: the double-blind, randomized, positive-controlled feline arterial thromboembolism; Clopidogrel vs. Aspirin trial (FAT CAT). J Vet Cardiol 2015;17 Suppl 1:S306–317.

Jung J, Chang J, Oh S, et al. Computed tomography angiography for evaluation of pulmonary embolism in an experimental model and heartworm infested dogs. Vet Radiol Ultrasound 2010;51:288–293.

Kidd L, Mackman N. Prothrombotic mechanisms and anticoagulant therapy in dogs with immune-mediated hemolytic anemia. J Vet Emerg Crit Care (San Antonio) 2013;23:3–13.

Kidd L, Stepien RL, Amrheiw DP. Clinical findings and coronary artery disease in dogs and cats with acute and subacute myocardial necrosis: 28 cases. J Am Anim Hosp Assoc 2000;36:199–208.

Klainbart S, Kelmer E, Vidmayer B, et al. Peripheral and Central venous blood glucose concentrations in dogs and cats with acute arterial thromboembolism. J Vet Intern Med 2014;28:1513–1519.

Langston C, Eatroff A, Poeppel K. Use of tissue plasminogen activator in catheters used for extracorporeal renal replacement therapy. J Vet Intern Med 2014;28:270–276.

Laste NJ, Harpster NK. A retrospective study of 100 cases of feline distal aortic thromboembolism: 1977-1993. J Am Anim Hosp Assoc 1995;31:492–500.

Levi M, van der Poll T. Inflammation and coagulation. Crit Care Med 2010;38:S26–34.

Li RH, Stern JA, Ho V, et al. Platelet activation and clopidogrel effects on ADP-induced platelet activation in cats with or without the A31P mutation in MYBPC3. J Vet Intern Med 2016;30:1619–1629.

Lozada Miranda B, Walton R, LeVine DN, et al. Use of rivaroxaban for treatment of cranial vena cava syndrome secondary to transvenous pacemaker lead thrombosis in a dog. J Vet Cardiol 2019;25:7–13.

Lynch AM, deLaforcade AM, Sharp CR. Clinical experience of anti-Xa monitoring in critically ill dogs receiving dalteparin. J Vet Emerg Crit Care (San Antonio) 2014;24:421–428.

Malkawi M, Woolcock AD, Lee PM, et al. Comparison of metabolomics and platelet aggregometry between Plavix and generic clopidogrel in cats: a pilot study. J Feline Med Surg 2019;21:951–958.

McManus PM, Craig LE. Correlation between leukocytosis and necropsy findings in dogs with immune-mediated hemolytic anemia: 34 cases (1994–1999). J Am Vet Med Assoc. 2001;218:1308–1313.

McMichael MA, Freeman LM, Selhub J, et al. Plasma homocysteine, B vitamins, and amino acid concentrations in cats with cardiomyopathy and arterial thromboembolism. J Vet Intern Med 2000;14:507–512.

Mischke RH, Schuttert C, Grebe SI. Anticoagulant effects of repeated subcutaneous injections of high doses of unfractionated heparin in healthy dogs. Am J Vet Res 2001;62:1887–1891.

Morassi A, Bianco D, Park E, et al. Evaluation of the safety and tolerability of rivaroxaban in dogs with presumed primary immune-mediated hemolytic anemia. J Vet Emerg Crit Care (San Antonio) 2016;26:488–494.

Murray JD, O'Sullivan ML, Hawkes KC. Cranial vena caval thrombosis associated with endocardial pacing leads in three dogs. J Am Anim Hosp Assoc 2010;46:186–192.

Myers JA, Wittenburg LA, Olver CS, et al. Pharmacokinetics and pharmacodynamics of the factor Xa inhibitor apixaban after oral and intravenous administration to cats. Am J Vet Res 2015;76:732–738.

Nelson OL, Andreasen C. The utility of plasma D-dimer to identify thromboembolic disease in dogs. J Vet Intern Med 2003;17:830–834.

Norris CR, Griffey SM, Samii VF. Pulmonary thromboembolism in cats: 29 cases (1987–1997). J Am Vet Med Assoc 1999;215:1650–1654.

Norris JW, Watson JL, Tablin F, et al. Pharmacokinetics and competitive pharmacodynamics of ADP-induced platelet activation after oral administration of clopidogrel to horses. Am J Vet Res 2019;80:505–512.

Olsen LH, Kristensen AT, Haggstrom J, et al. Increased platelet aggregation response in cavalier king charles spaniels with mitral valve prolapse. J Vet Intern Med 2001;15:209–216.

Panek CM, Nakamura RK, Bianco D Use of enoxaparin in dogs with primary immune-mediated hemolytic anemia: 21 cases. J Vet Emerg Crit Care (San Antonio) 2015;25:273–277.

Payne JR, Borgeat K, Brodbelt DC, et al. Risk factors associated with sudden death vs. Congestive heart failure or arterial thromboembolism in cats with hypertrophic cardiomyopathy. J Vet Cardiol 2015;17:S318–S328.

Reimer SB, Kittleson MD, Kyles AE. Use of rheolytic thrombectomy in the treatment of feline distal aortic thromboembolism. J Vet Intern Med 2006;20:290–296.

Respess M, O'Toole TE, Taeymans O, et al. Portal vein thrombosis in 33 dogs: 1998-2011. J Vet Intern Med 2012;26:230–237.

Schermerhorn T, Pembleton-Corbett JR, Kornreich B. Pulmonary thromboembolism in cats. J Vet Intern Med 2004;18:533–535.

Schober KE, Maerz I. Assessment of left atrial appendage flow velocity and its relation to spontaneous echocardiographic contrast in 89 cats with myocardial disease. J Vet Intern Med 2006;20:120–130.

Schoeman JP. Feline distal aortic thromboembolism: a review of 44 cases (1990–1998). J Feline Med Surg 1999;1:221–231.

Scott KC, Hansen BD, DeFrancesco TC. Coagulation effects of low molecular weight heparin compared with heparin in dogs considered to be at risk for clinically significant venous thrombosis. J Vet Emerg Crit Care 2009;19:74–80.

Smith CE, Rozanski EA, Freeman LM, et al. Use of low molecular weight heparin in cats: 57 cases (1999–2003). J Am Vet Med Assoc 2004;225:1237–1241.

Smith SA, McMichael M. Coagulation testing. In, Ettinger SJ, Feldman EC, Cote E (editors). Textbook of Veterinary Internal Medicine. 9th edition. Elsevier, St. Louis, MO. 2017. pp. 818–822.

Smith SA, Tobias AH, Jacob KA, et al. Arterial thromboembolism in cats: acute crisis in 127 cases (1992–2001) and long-term management with low-dose aspirin in 24 cases. J Vet Intern Med 2003;17:73–83.

Song J, Drobatz KJ, Silverstein DC. Retrospective evaluation of shortened prothrombin time or activated partial thromboplastin time for the diagnosis of hypercoagulability in dogs: 25 cases (2006–2011). J Vet Emerg Crit Care 2016;26:398–405.

Stokol T, Brooks MB, Erb HN, et al. D-dimer concentrations in healthy dogs and dogs with disseminated intravascular coagulation. Am J Vet Res 2000;61:393–398.

Stokol T, Brooks M, Rush JE, et al. Hypercoagulability in cats with cardiomyopathy J Vet Intern Med 2008;22:546–552.

Thompson MF, Scott-Moncrieff JC, Hogan DF. Thrombolytic therapy in dogs and cats. J Vet Emerg Crit Care 2001;11:111–121.

Van De Wiele CM, Hogan DF, Green HW, et al. Antithrombotic effect of enoxaparin in clinically healthy cats: a venous stasis model. J Vet Intern Med 2010;24:185–191.

Van Winkle TJ, Liu SM, Hackner SG. Clinical and pathological features of aortic thromboembolism in 36 dogs. J Vet Emerg Crit Care 1993;3:13–21.

Welch KM, Rozanski EA, Freeman LM, et al. Prospective evaluation of tissue plasminogen activator in 11 cats with arterial thromboembolism. J Feline Med Surg 2010;12:122–128.

West JB, Luks AM. Vascular diseases. West's Pulmonary Pathophysiology: The Essentials. 9th edition. Wolters Kluwer, Philadelphia, PA. 2017. pp. 119–145.

Winter RL, Sedacca CD, Adams A, et al. Aortic thrombosis in dogs: presentation, therapy, and outcome in 26 cases. J Vet Cardiol 2012;14:333–342.

Yang VK, Cunningham SM, Rush JE, et al. The use of rivaroxaban for the treatment of thrombotic complications in four dogs. J Vet Emerg Crit Care (San Antonio) 2016;26:729–736.

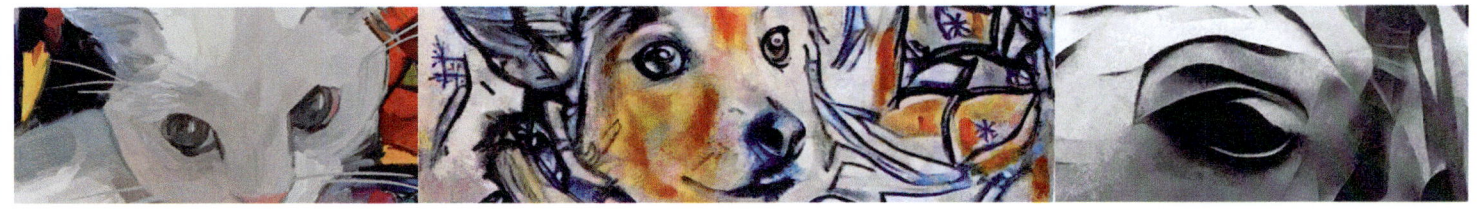

37
VASCULAR DISEASES

Companion animals are affected by multiple vascular diseases. These can be congenital (Chapter 28) or acquired in origin, can affect arteries and veins of varying size, and incite clinical signs ranging from mild to life threatening. Diseases of lymphatic vessels cause clinical signs that are similar to those induced by vasculitis or phlebitis. This chapter summarizes some of the more important vascular and lymphatic disorders affecting dogs, cats, and horses. Systemic and pulmonary hypertension, as well as systemic and pulmonary arterial thromboembolism (TE), are addressed more fully in Chapters 38, 39, and 36, respectively.

Pathophysiology

Arteries and veins are organized structurally into three layers: intima, media, and adventitia (**Figure 1.25**, p. 24). These histologic layers, along with the vascular lumen they surround, represent the anatomic targets for most vascular diseases. **Table 37.1** summarizes general types of vascular disease. The pathophysiology of various vascular diseases can be understood by considering how the disease disrupts normal vascular functions (**Table 37.2**). Three major clinical outcomes of vascular diseases include signs related to *ischemia*, *edema*, and *hemorrhage* (**Figure 37.1**).

Vascular diseases often cause organ dysfunction and tissue injury secondary to loss of blood flow or ischemia. Arterial obstruction results in downstream tissue hypoxia with attendant loss of cell and organ function. Without suitable collateral circulation, tissue necrosis (infarction) and eventually replacement fibrosis occur. Clinical consequences of ischemia depend on the location of the obstructed vascular territory and the presence (or adequacy) of collateral circulation. A notable example is the acute neuromuscular injury that follows distal aortic TE or a "saddle thrombus" in cats with cardiomyopathy (p. 755 and **Figures 36.24** and **36.25**, pp. 769 and 770). Another is mesenteric arteritis in the horse, which causes bowel ischemia and severe abdominal pain (colic).

Tissue edema is a common pathologic and clinical feature of vascular diseases. When edema occurs with arterial obstruction or infection, it usually is a consequence of secondary inflammation within infarcted or inflamed tissues. An example is hind-limb rhabdomyolysis from aortic TE (**Figure 37.1A**). In contrast, localized venous obstruction causes edema secondary to the increased hydrostatic pressure within capillary beds drained by the obstructed vein. Edema also can stem from physical, infective, or immunologic injuries to small vessels that increase vascular permeability or disrupt the vascular wall. This leads to leakage of protein-rich fluid into the surrounding interstitial tissues. Examples include numerous causes of systemic vasculitis, pulmonary injury from smoke inhalation and sepsis, and anaphylaxis, where edema can be localized or widespread. Clinical consequences of edema depend on the site of formation. In the lung for instance, a high-protein, noncardiogenic pulmonary edema increases lung stiffness, impairs ventilation, and induces arterial hypoxemia.

Profound hemorrhage can result from traumatic injury or spontaneous rupture of an artery, large vein, or an arteriovenous (A-V) communication, even in the absence of a coagulopathy. The clinical consequences of hemorrhage often are explained by hypotension, hypovolemic shock, or space-occupation. There are many causes of severe bleeding that can lead to acute hypotension or shock (**Table 37.2**). These often occur secondary to trauma or spontaneous rupture of vascular tumors, as with acute bleeding from splenic or right atrial hemangiosarcoma. Fatal bleeding also occurs sometimes from idiopathic thymic hemorrhage in young dogs or rupture of the uterine artery or intrapericardial aorta in horses. Confined hemorrhage can have severe consequences when it places pressure on adjacent vessels, peripheral nerves,

Table 37.1 Clinically Important Vascular Diseases of Companion Animals

Arteriovenous Fistula
- Congenital
- Acquired

Arteriosclerosis (including intimal thickening and medial hypertrophy)
- Atherosclerosis
- Intramural arterial sclerosis (myocardial)
- Medial hypertrophy of pulmonary arteries
- Associated with pulmonary hypertension
  - Congenital shunts (atrial septal defect, ventricular septal defect, patent ductus arteriosus)
  - Chronic lung diseases
  - Parasitic diseases
  - Idiopathic

Vascular Mineralization

Thrombosis and Embolism
- From arteritis (see next section)
- From phlebitis/thrombophlebitis (due to irritating drugs, chemicals, catheters, pacing leads, infections)
- Systemic diseases causing hypercoagulability
- Systemic arterial (thrombo)embolism
- Pulmonary thromboembolism
  - Parasitic infection (heartworm disease)
  - Hematologic disorders (such as immune-mediated hemolytic anemia)
- Neoplastic diseases invading veins or causing tumor thrombi

Vasculitis | Arteritis
- Associated with infectious diseases (numerous)
- Associated with parasitic diseases (such as *Dirofilaria immitis*, *Strongylus vulgaris, Angiostrongylus vasorum*, *Spirocera lupi/sanguinolenta*)
- Associated with toxicosis (such as insect and snake bites)
- Immune-mediated
- Drug-induced (itraconazole, carbimazole, among others)
- Idiopathic
  - Meningitis arteritis syndrome
  - Cutaneous and renal glomerular vasculopathy syndrome

Other Vascular Diseases
- Vascular Disruption or physical obstruction of blood vessels
  - Preexisting vascular disease (including parasitic, neoplastic)
  - Traumatic injury to vessels
  - Neoplasms of vascular and nonvascular tissues
  - Iatrogenic (including surgery and catheterization)
  - Client related: constricting bands, collars or restraints
  - Dissection of an artery or vein
  - Rupture secondary to a preexisting vascular lesion or systemic hypertension
  - Torsion with obstruction of the vascular pedicle (spleen, liver, stomach, lung)
- Aortopathy (dilation) or idiopathic aneurysm
  - Older cats with aortoannular ectasia
  - Aortic rupture in horses
  - Connective tissue disorders (Ehlers-Danlos, Marfan's-like elastin dysplasia)
- Parasitic diseases
- Hamartoma (developmental within various tissues and organs)
- Neoplasms of blood vessel elements
- Varicosities (venous)
- Pulmonary veno-occlusive disease

This is a partial listing and does not include many systemic vasculitides associated with infections, drugs, or immunological reaction. Some categories overlap, for example: parasitic infections can cause arteritis, thrombosis, aneurysm, or rupture of the involved blood vessel.

or organs such as the brain, eyes, heart, and lungs. Even focal hemorrhage can be devastating in certain locations, for example when causing hemorrhagic stroke (**Figure 37.1B**) or retinal hemorrhage secondary to systemic hypertension (**Figure 38.1**, p. 793).

Lymphatic vessels also are integral to microcirculatory function. Impaired lymphatic drainage leads to formation of *lymphedema* (the accumulation of interstitial fluid in tissues) or effusions within serous body cavities. Lymphangitis from infections can alter lymphatic function and increase permeability or obstruct lymphatic flow. Metastatic invasion of lymphatic vessels by carcinomas or neoplastic transformation (lymphangiosarcoma) are other causes for lymphedema. The resulting clinical signs can include subcutaneous edema and peritoneal, pleural, and pericardial effusions, depending on the location of the lymphatic disease. Idiopathic (congenital) lymphedema occurs sporadically in dogs and causes nonpainful, subcutaneous edema (**Figure 37.2**). The pelvic limbs are affected more often, although edema can be generalized (**Figure 17.7**, p. 278). Lymph nodes in the affected areas usually are smaller than normal, or completely absent, in young dogs. Affected limbs are more prone to infection. Consultation with a specialist regarding diagnosis and possible treatments can be helpful. Some cases improve spontaneously, especially when hind limbs are affected.

Arteriovenous Fistula

An A-V fistula is a congenital or acquired communication between an artery and vein. Congenital A-V fistulae can involve single or multiple malformations; these are described further in Chapter 28 (p. 523). Acquired cases are traumatic in origin, with patency between an artery and its satellite vein established during the healing process. Etiologies include missiles (bullets), fractures, and surgical procedures, including inexpert feline declawing. The pathophysiology of A-V fistulae involves the transmission of high arterial blood pressure directly to the low-pressure venous system. This increases hydrostatic pressure at the venous side of the associated capillaries, which results in vascular congestion and edema formation within the affected region. Rare congenital forms of A-V fistula involve the limbs, head, or internal organs such as the liver. Multiple, small, acquired A-V fistulae can develop with neoplasms, as observed with thyroid adenocarcinoma in the dog.

Clinical Features

Typical clinical findings with a peripheral A-V fistula include nonpainful swellings, anatomically adjacent or distal to the fistula. In some cases, the swelling represents an abnormal plexus of vessels or dilated vascular channels (**Figure 37.3**).

Table 37.2 Pathophysiologic Mechanisms and Clinical Consequences of Vascular Disease

General Mechanism	Clinical Consequences
Increased systemic vascular resistance	Systemic hypertension with target organ damage to brain, eyes, heart, kidneys, and small arteries
Increased pulmonary vascular resistance	Pulmonary arterial hypertension with signs of cor pulmonale and right heart dysfunction or failure
Ischemia and impaired tissue perfusion	Tissue hypoxia, impaired organ function, cell death (infarction and replacement fibrosis)
Hemorrhage	Space occupying effect Impaired tissue function Hypotension, shock or sudden death
Vascular tumors and hamartomas	Space occupying lesions and disruption of normal organ function
Impaired venous drainage (from organs and regional circulations)	Increased capillary hydrostatic pressures leading to tissue congestion, edema, and impaired metabolism and wound healing
Impaired venous return to the heart	Hypotension and (obstructive) shock Cavity effusions Subcutaneous edema
Redistribution of blood flow	"Steal" phenomenon (causing ischemia) Increased venous return (shunt) Space occupying vascular lesion
Increased vascular permeability (from immune-mediated or infectious diseases, and other injuries to the vessel)	Tissue edema and hemorrhage Cavity effusions

When the swelling is caused by interstitial edema, subsequent tissue hypoxia, dysfunction, and secondary infections can occur and lead to clinical signs of lameness or localized discomfort. Large fistulae can compress adjacent organs. A superficial A-V fistula, if traumatized, can hemorrhage profusely. Congenital hepatic A-V fistulae can increase intra-sinusoidal (hepatic capillary) pressure and cause ascites.

A typical peripheral A-V fistula produces continuous, high-velocity flow from the arterial to the venous circulation. Auscultation directly over a large fistula might reveal a continuous murmur or "bruit." Theoretically, transient shunt closure (by applying pressure) could reflexively slow the heart rate (the "Branham reflex"). This is similar to what occurs when a large patent ductus arteriosus is suddenly closed.

Diagnostic Tests

Definitive diagnosis of an A-V fistula often is established from the history, physical examination, and noninvasive imaging studies. Ultrasound imaging, complemented by color and

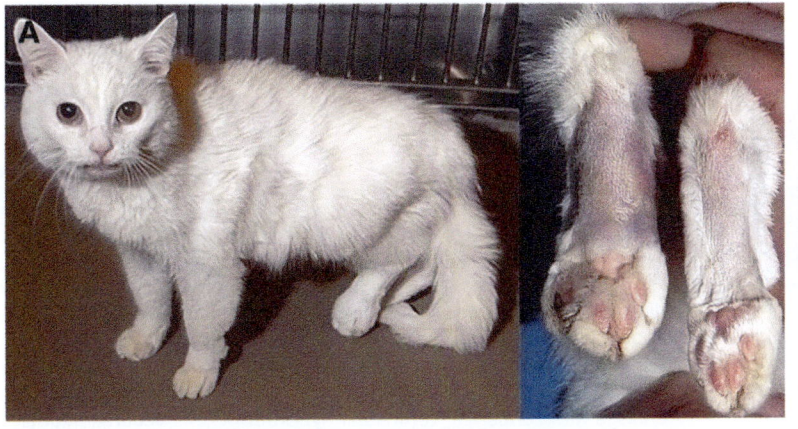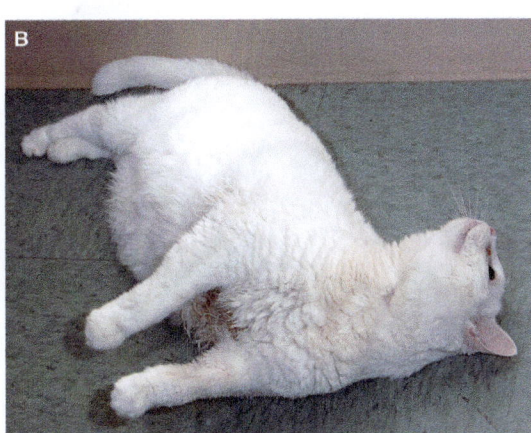

Figure 37.1 Clinical consequences of vascular disease. (A) Severe tissue edema secondary to ischemia in a cat recovering from aortic thromboembolism. The right panel shows tissue edema and discoloration from rhabdomyolysis-induced hemorrhage and inflammation. (B) Decerebration-type posture, secondary to hemorrhagic stroke associated with systemic hypertension, in a different cat.

spectral Doppler studies, is especially helpful for identifying abnormal vascular communications and flow patterns. In some cases, advanced vascular imaging is required for diagnosis. This could include traditional angiography or carefully timed computed tomography (CT) angiography over the affected area.

Management

Typical therapy for an A-V fistula involves surgical ligation of the communication or occlusion of the feeding artery or arteries. These procedures are challenging and are best referred to a surgical specialist. Minimally invasive techniques that include coil embolization or delivery of thrombogenic materials to occlude the arterial feeder sometimes are feasible. However, these treatments are confined to specialized centers.

Arteriosclerosis

Arteriosclerosis ("hardening" of arteries) refers to a degenerative or hypertrophic arterial disease that causes vascular wall thickening and luminal narrowing of affected vessels. In most cases, lesions of arteriosclerosis involve microscopic changes in small arteries. However, larger vessels can be involved, with macroscopic lesions evident. Morphologic changes can localize to the subintimal or medial layers, or involve multiple mural layers of the artery. Lesions can be characterized by cellular infiltration, vascular reaction, smooth muscle proliferation, or by the incorporation of largely acellular materials such as glycosaminoglycans (acid-staining mucopolysaccharides) or lipid (**Figure 37.4**).

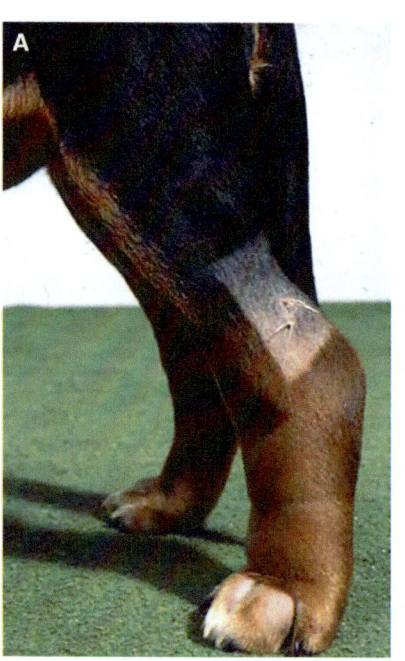
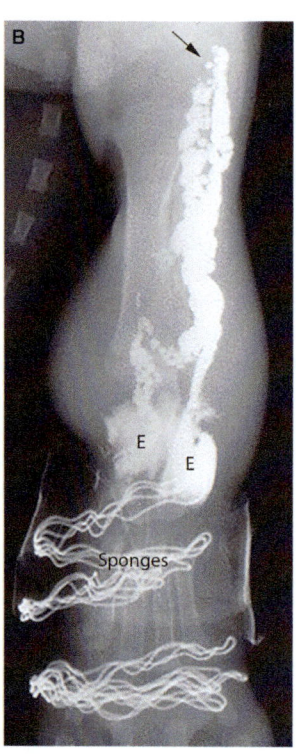

Figure 37.2 (A) Pelvic limb edema in a puppy with congenital lymphatic dysplasia. (B) Dilated, tortuous and blindly ending (arrow) lymphatic vessels are evident following injection of oily contrast media into a peripheral lymphatic vessel. Extravasation (E) of contrast is present above radiopaque surgical sponges. While this lymphangiogram demonstrates the pathology well, newer contrast methods, including computerized tomography angiography and scintigraphy, can be used to confirm the diagnosis today.

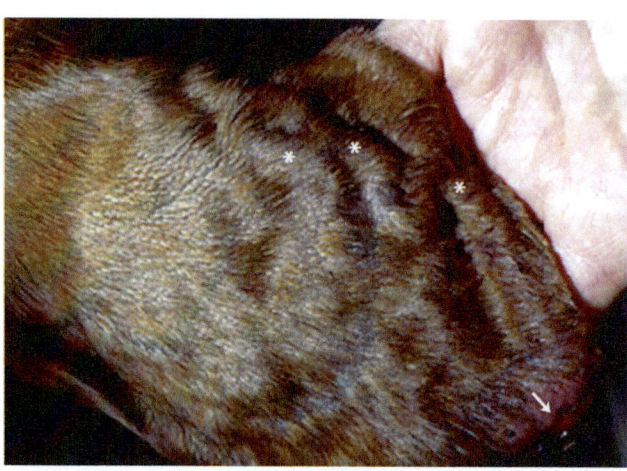

Figure 37.3 Arteriovenous fistula in the ear pinna of a hunting dog. The ear was traumatized and the walls of an artery and a vein fused during the healing process. The result is direct transmission of high arterial pressure into the venous system, which caused marked distention of superficial auricular veins (*). Trauma to one of the vessels resulted in profuse hemorrhage from a relatively small focus (arrow, lower right) just after this picture was obtained.

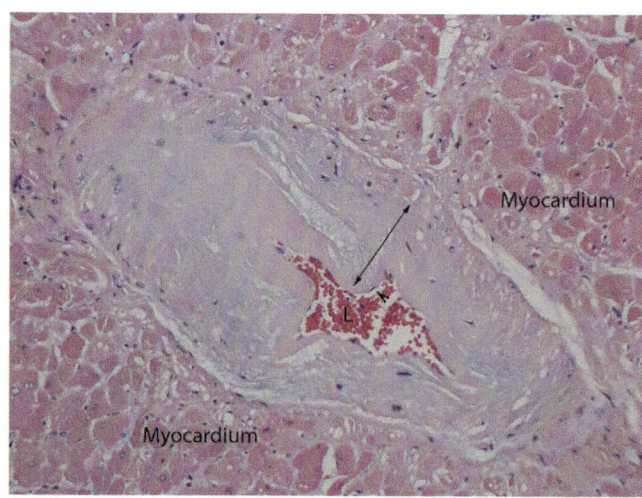

Figure 37.4 Fibrinoid change with arteriosclerosis in a cat with cardiomyopathy. Cross-section through an intramyocardial coronary artery shows subintimal tissue expansion (arrow) with relatively acellular material. This usually represents either fibrinoid necrosis, as can occur with hypertension, or glycosaminoglycan deposition, a common degenerative change with concentric ventricular hypertrophy; this occurs in aged dog hearts, too. Endothelial cells line the intima (at this low-power only the nuclei are evident; arrowhead). The vascular lumen (L), containing red blood cells, is small. Courtesy of Drs R Kohnken and R Cianciolo.

Arteriosclerosis stiffens and narrows the artery, which increases vascular resistance and reduces downstream tissue perfusion. These changes create risk for organ ischemia, tissue hypoxia, and infarction. With intimal layer involvement, there is added potential for localized thrombosis, or embolization of thrombotic material or plaque. Several arteriosclerotic disorders of varying histological character are known to occur in companion animals. Some have obvious clinical significance, although that is not always the case.

Atherosclerosis

Atherosclerosis is a specific form of arteriosclerosis characterized by lipid deposition in the vessel walls (**Figure 37.5**). In typical canine cases, the lipid accumulates within the vascular media as opposed to the subendothelial intimal layer, as is usually seen in humans. However, there are exceptions and diffuse subintimal atherosclerosis has occurred in dogs (**Figure 37.6**). The most recognized cause of canine atherosclerosis is hypothyroidism with severe hypercholesterolemia (generally >700 mg/dL). It is likely that familial dyslipidemias

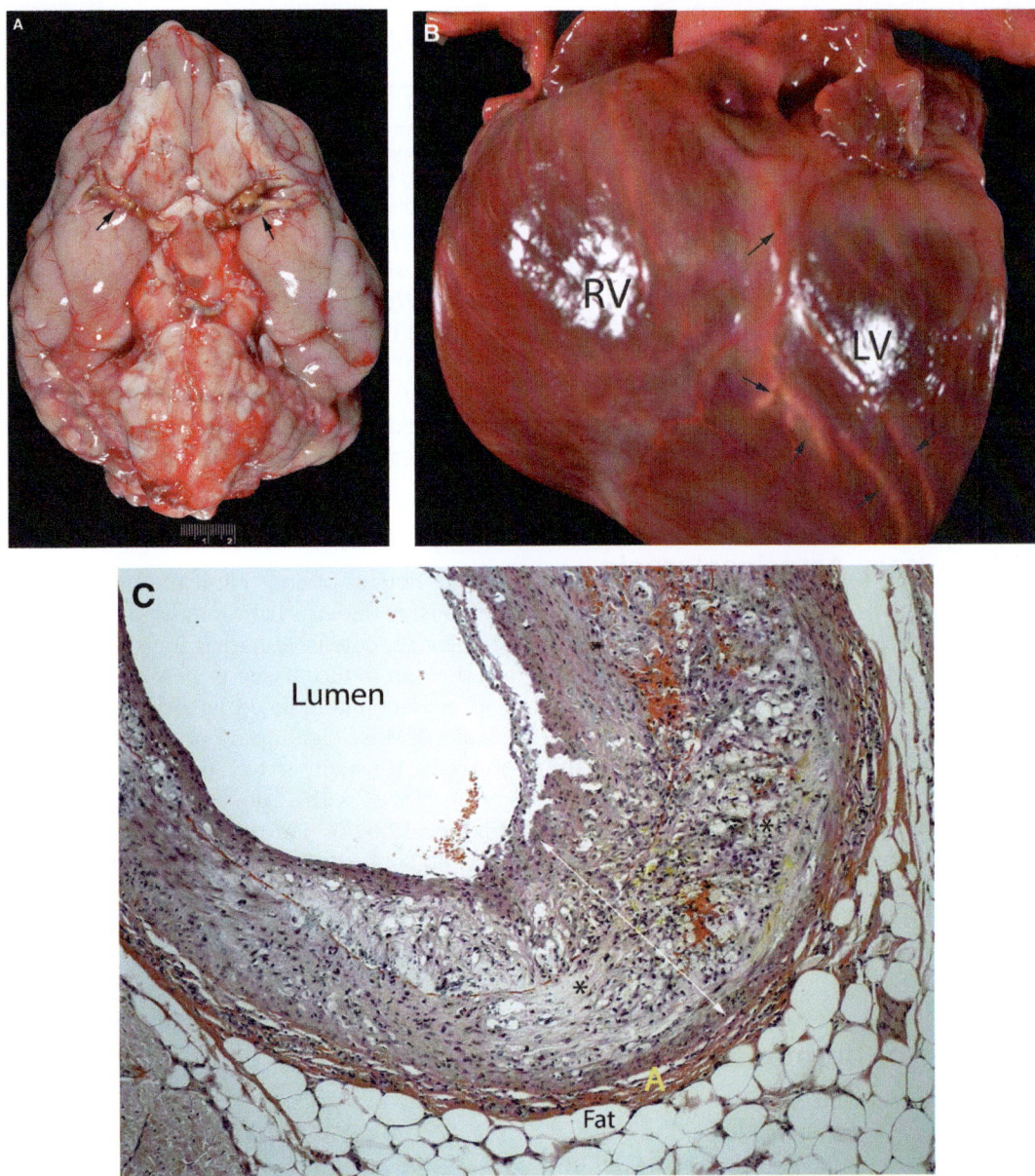

Figure 37.5 Grossly evident atherosclerosis (arrows) in canine cerebral (A) and extramural coronary (B) arteries. (C) Cross-section of atherosclerotic canine coronary artery shows typical histological changes. Note marked lipid accumulation within the media (white arrow). Fat cells also surround this extramural coronary artery. A, vascular adventitia; LV, left ventricle; RV, right ventricle. Courtesy of Drs. Charles C Capen, R Duncan, R Kohnken, and R Cianciolo.

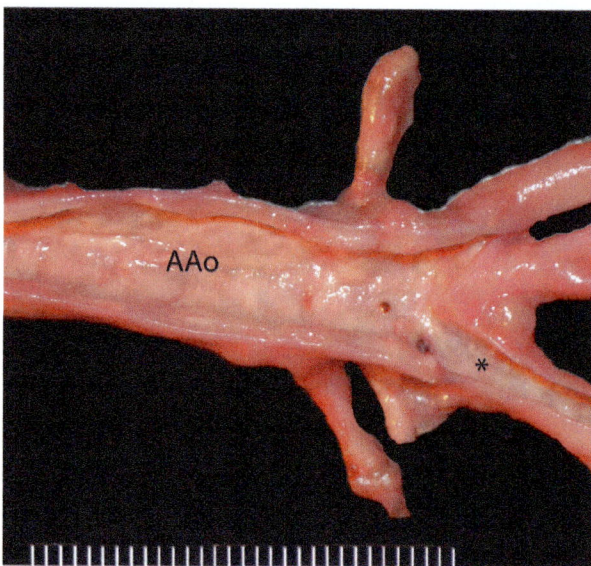

Figure 37.6 Severe intimal atherosclerotic change in a dog with a congenital dyslipidemia. The abdominal aorta (AAo), opened at autopsy, reveals an irregular intimal surface that extends into branch vessels such as the opened right external iliac artery (*). Lipid is grossly evident as a yellow discoloration to the vessel lining. In this case, lipid is located atypically for dogs, within the vessel's subintimal and intimal layers. Blood flow to the limbs and numerous organs was reduced in this dog.

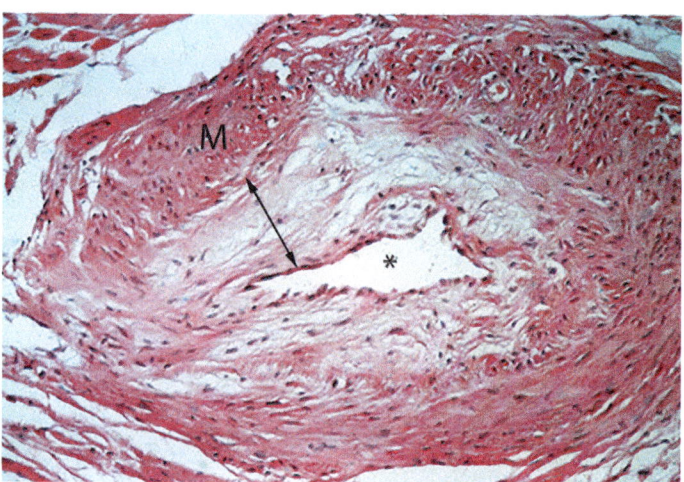

Figure 37.7 Tangential cross-section of an intramyocardial coronary artery shows arteriosclerosis in an older dog with degenerative mitral valve disease. Relatively acellular, lightly eosinophilic material within the subintima (arrow) also extends into the media (M) and narrows the vessel lumen (*). Nuclei of intimal endothelial cells lining the vascular lumen are evident.

that cause atherosclerosis are underrecognized in dogs (Scaglione, 2018). Atherosclerosis can affect coronary vessels in dogs, as well as those in the brain, where it has been associated with stroke and other neurological signs.

Intramural Coronary Arteriosclerosis

This relatively common lesion is observed in the small, intramyocardial vessels of dogs and cats with various heart diseases (Falk, 2000). It is frequently found in older dogs with degenerative (myxomatous) valvular disease. Subintimal or medial deposition of acellular glycosaminoglycans, and in some cases, proliferation of vascular smooth muscle cells, characterize the lesion (**Figure 37.7**). Similar lesions affecting coronary arteries in dogs with aortic stenosis and pulmonary stenosis, and in cats with hypertrophic and restrictive forms of cardiomyopathy, have been reported. Areas of adjacent myocardial replacement fibrosis or scar sometimes are present, suggesting this lesion might be clinically relevant in some dogs and cats, although this point is unresolved.

Medial Hypertrophy of Pulmonary Arteries

This arterial change, which is characterized by expansion of the vascular smooth muscle, often is an incidental histological finding in cats. Medial hypertrophy also occurs with pulmonary vascular injury stemming from heartworm disease and in pulmonary hypertension associated with congenital left-to-right shunts and other lung pathologies (see related Chapters). Medial hypertrophy can develop in conjunction with other arterial lesions, including intimal proliferation and plexiform lesions (**Figures 39.3** and **39.4**, p. 818). The consequence of extensive medial hypertrophy, especially when accompanied by intimal thickening, is an increase in pulmonary vascular resistance. This can lead to pulmonary arterial hypertension and related clinical signs, such as syncope or right-sided congestive heart failure (see Chapter 39).

Clinical Features of Arteriosclerosis

Arteriosclerosis often is clinically silent. However, as described previously under "Pathophysiology," **Table 37.2**, and in Chapter 36, extensive narrowing or obstruction of distributing arteries can induce tissue ischemia, and lead to organ dysfunction or ischemia-induced lameness and associated pain (claudication). Muscle cramping or weakness secondary to vascular obstruction usually is worse with activity as observed in dogs and in horses with various forms of aorto-iliac arteriosclerosis (**Figure 37.6**). When the heart is affected, myocardial infarction and subsequent fibrosis, if extensive, can impair ventricular systolic function, increase ventricular diastolic stiffness, and serve as a substrate for reentrant arrhythmias. It is likely that some of the apparent scars and regional ventricular wall abnormalities observed by echocardiography in cats with cardiomyopathy are related to coronary vascular lesions and secondary infarctions (**Figure 37.8**).

Vascular Mineralization

Calcification of blood vessels can be idiopathic or a consequence of vasculitis or a high blood calcium-phosphorus product. Vascular calcification usually is a histologic lesion. However, in occasional cases, mineral deposition in the

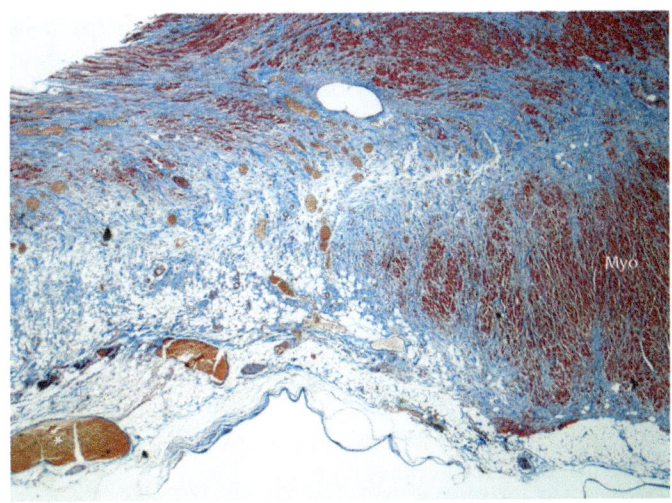

Figure 37.8 Trichrome stain of myocardium from a cat with ischemic cardiac injury. There is widespread loss of myocardium (Myo) with fibrous connective tissue replacement (blue-staining). Larger coronary vessels (*, lower left) that likely represent neovascularization also are evident. Courtesy of Drs R Kohnken, R Cianciolo, and D Russell.

intimal layer is evident grossly at autopsy or identified during imaging studies. For example, diffuse calcification of the feline aorta has been observed on thoracic radiographs.

Vasculitis (Arteritis)

Vasculitis generally refers to inflammation of arteries. It often is associated with systemic infectious or immune-mediated diseases but can be focal, especially when associated with a parasitic infection such as *Spirocera lupi* in dogs or *Strongylus vulgaris* in horses (**Figure 37.9**). There are numerous other examples in companion animals, including the feline infectious peritonitis virus in cats, rickettsial infections (such as *Ehrlichia canis* and *Rickettsia rickettsii*, Rocky Mountain spotted fever) in dogs, and mycotic (guttural pouch) arteritis in horses. Clinical signs vary with the location and distribution of vascular involvement. Tissue edema (**Figure 17.4A**, p. 276), hemorrhage (**Figure 37.10**), or thrombosis associated with vasculitis can lead to central nervous system (CNS) signs, organ dysfunction, disseminated coagulopathies, or signs of severe ischemia, such as colic. Therapy generally is supportive, unless a specific microorganism or parasite can be identified and addressed. Immunosuppressive therapies are used in some patients with suspected vasculitis; however, consultation with a specialist is advised when vasculitis is suspected, and potential underlying infectious causes sought.

A notable vascular lesion in the horse is fungal infection of the guttural pouches, which can be caused by a number of mycotic agents. Invasion of the carotid or maxillary artery can result in arteritis, mural erosion, and profuse hemorrhage that can be fatal (**Figure 37.11**). Severe epistaxis is the clinical sign that should alert the clinician to this consideration.

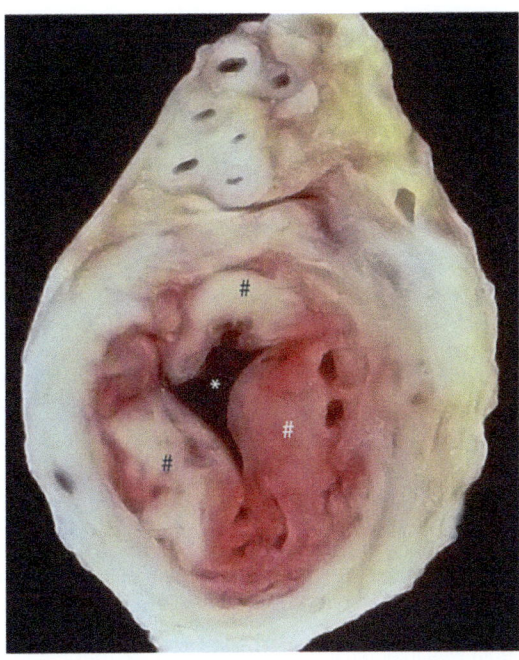

Figure 37.9 Severe narrowing of the cranial mesenteric artery in a horse, secondary to infection with the parasite *Strongylus vulgaris*. The vascular lumen (*) is narrowed by a thrombotic arterial reaction seen in various stages of organization and scarring (#). This reduces arterial flow to the gut resulting in ischemia and abdominal pain or colic.

The diagnosis is made by endoscopy, and can be verified by angiography at the time of treatment. Therapy involves either ligation of the feeding vessels (such as the carotid artery, with risk of ocular or CNS injury) or more often today, catheter-delivered embolization coils or plugs placed into the affected vessels under fluoroscopic or endoscopic guidance.

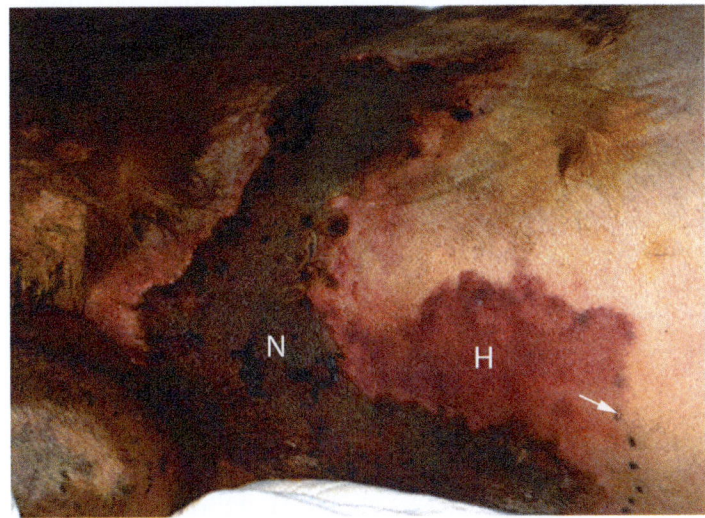

Figure 37.10 Subcutaneous edema, dermal hemorrhage (H) and tissue necrosis (N) in a dog with histologically confirmed vasculitis of unknown cause. The dog also developed severe pancreatitis. The small black dots (arrow) delineate the extent of tissue damage at time of admission. The dog recovered with immunosuppressive and supportive care.

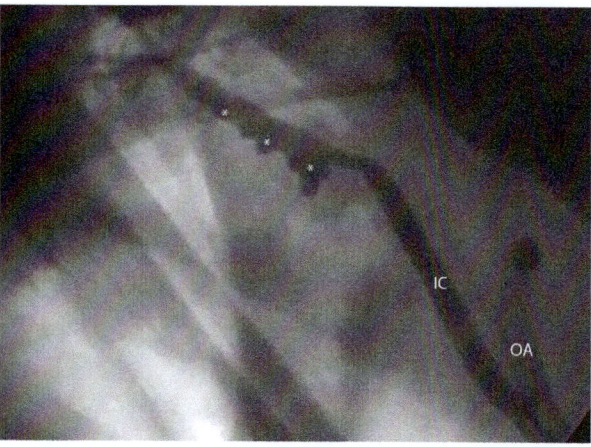

Figure 37.11 Mycotic arteritis in a horse secondary to fungal invasion of the vessel wall. Angiography reveals marked irregularity of the internal carotid artery, especially along its ventral surface (*), as it courses through the guttural pouch. Compare this to the proximal segments of the internal carotid (IC) and occipital arteries (OA). Erosion of the artery typically leads to severe hemorrhage and epistaxis that can be fatal. Contrast media was injected in the common carotid artery.

Various clinical syndromes relate to arterial disease and associated systemic and immunologic disorders, such as abortion in equine viral arteritis. Another example is the cutaneous and renal glomerular vasculopathy ("Alabama rot") that causes ulcerative dermatitis and kidney failure in dogs (Holm, 2020). Histopathology in these cases demonstrates a microscopic, thrombotic angiopathy in renal tissues.

Thrombosis and Embolism

Thrombosis represents pathological antemortem blood clotting predisposed by Virchow's triad of (1) damaged vascular intima or endocardium, (2) stagnant blood flow, and (3) a prothrombotic state. The best-known syndrome in cats is left auricular thrombosis associated with cardiomyopathy (p. 755). TE defines the pathological and clinical consequences of a thrombus formed at one location and carried by blood flow to another. Other biological or foreign material also can embolize, including fat, tumor cells, parasites, foreign bodies, and air. More information about thromboembolic disease and its treatment is in Chapter 36.

Thrombotic Diseases

Arterial thrombosis forms in-situ. For example, aortic thrombosis affecting the terminal aorta and iliac trifurcation of horses and dogs (p. 756 and **Figure 36.22**, p. 762) is thought to form locally, in contrast to the common situation in cats where the left atrium is the source of the aortic thrombus (thromboembolus). The etiology of distal aortic thrombosis in horses is unknown, and while *S. vulgaris* larval migration is suspected, it rarely is proven. Similarly, in dogs with aortic thrombosis the cause often appears idiopathic, except in situations of protein-losing disorders with demonstrable hypercoagulability (as with renal amyloidosis).

Acute coronary artery occlusions ("heart attacks") do occur in dogs and cats, are considered relatively rare, but probably are underdiagnosed. In dogs, the most common clinical association is systemic illness and hypercoagulability. In cats, coronary thrombosis has been associated with cardiomyopathy; it might represent localized thrombosis or a small embolus originating from the left auricle. These are challenging to detect in feline coronary vessels by histopathology. Infrequently, thrombotic (or thromboembolic) stroke is diagnosed in animals, but it also is likely underrecognized. Clinical signs relate to the location of the thrombus, vascular territory affected, and collateral circulation.

Thrombosis in the pulmonary arteries can develop locally or result from thromboembolic disease originating in systemic veins, typically vessels within the abdomen. Large thromboses within the main branches of the pulmonary artery have been observed with protein losing nephropathies, surrounding adult heartworms, and as an idiopathic disorder in Cavalier King Charles Spaniels (**Figures 36.15D**, **36.21**, and **39.6C**, pp. 760, 762 and 822). Pulmonary arterial thrombosis also is reported with canine hyperadrenocorticism.

The clinical signs of thrombotic disease depend on the vascular localization, severity of obstruction, and collateral circulation around the obstructed vessel. Many cases of distal aortic thrombosis in dogs and horses are chronic; the diagnosis can be elusive. Narrowing or occlusion of the distal aorta causes exercise-induced lameness or cramping (claudication), with physical signs of insufficient pelvic limb circulation. Arterial pulses can be normal, weak, or absent. The limb might feel cold. In horses, there is poor saphenous venous return. Ultrasound examination of the distal aorta and external iliac system reveals thromboses with varying degrees of blood flow.

Therapy for TE involves identifying and addressing the underlying disorder when possible. Treatment can involve antiplatelet drugs, especially for sources of arterial embolism, but drugs that inhibit coagulation usually are more effective, especially for venous sources of thrombosis. These include heparins, warfarin or factor Xa inhibitors, such as apixaban or rivaroxaban, although the costs for some of these treatments can be a challenge. The administration of tissue plasminogen activator is a consideration if the thrombosis is known to be of very recent onset. Interventional catheterization procedures such as balloon catheter embolectomy or stenting open of obstructed vessels have been applied to dogs, cats, and horses with varying success (p. 763; **Figure 36.23**, p. 767). Localized thrombophlebitis is addressed first by removing any physical cause such as a catheter and culturing the device. Antimicrobials are often administered empirically and local therapies provided, such as hot compresses and DMSO (in horses).

Arterial Embolic Disease

Embolism occurs when the material occluding a blood vessel travels from one source to another via the arterial or venous circulation. Embolized material often is thrombus, although there are other types of thromboembolic disease. As mentioned, acute TE from the left auricle to the terminal aorta or a brachial artery in cats with cardiomyopathy is the most common example in small animals. Sudden and complete occlusion leads to predictable signs of vascular incompetency (cold, pale, pulseless limbs lacking blood flow by Doppler flow detection); peripheral neuropathy (paresis, loss of reflexes and proprioception); and ischemic skeletal muscle injury (cramping, severe pain, markedly elevated muscle enzymes, and rhabdomyolysis; **Figure 37.1** and **Table 36.3**, p. 756). A less well-recognized cause of arterial TE in cats is a primary lung tumor, where presumably, local invasion of pulmonary vein(s) leads to transit of a thrombus through the left heart and into the systemic arterial circulation.

Infective (bacterial) endocarditis (Chapter 31) is another cause of systemic arterial TE in domesticated animals. Thrombi can be bland (sterile) or septic (infected) and lead to metastatic infection downstream from the infected valve. For example, meningitis is a common sequela in dogs with aortic or mitral valve endocarditis. Cats also can develop arterial TE secondary to infective endocarditis. Any downstream organ system can be affected, including the heart, brain, or kidneys.

Relatively rare clinical causes of TE include tumor emboli, air emboli (from catheters or diagnostic radiologic procedures), embolization of heartworm larvae or adults into the systemic circulation, and fat emboli (from fractures or bone surgery). These are probably common events, but when signs are subclinical or subtle they go unrecognized. Pulmonary arterial thrombosis is common in canine and feline heartworm disease (Chapter 40).

Venous Embolic Disease

Systemic venous emboli occur secondary to local injury or inflammation (*phlebitis*) of a systemic vein, or to systemic disease that leads to pathological clotting. Pulmonary TE occurs when systemic venous thrombi travel through the vascular system and right heart to eventually lodge in one or more pulmonary arteries (see Chapters 36 and 39 for additional information). These emboli can be large enough to occlude a branch of the pulmonary trunk, or small and numerous, causing diffuse or localized pulmonary disease. The pelvic limbs are the main source of pulmonary TE in humans; however, the spleen or another abdominal organ is likely to be the dominant source in animals (Johnson, 1999; Specchi, 2020).

A state of hypercoagulability predisposes to venous thrombosis. This often is related to systemic infections, immune-mediated hemolytic anemia, pancreatitis, and some neoplastic disorders. Neoplastic invasion of veins can result in localized venous occlusion, as well as tumor-laden or bland thrombotic emboli; an example is caudal vena caval invasion by a pheochromocytoma (**Figures 36.19** and **36.20**, p. 762). Complete obstruction has caused obstructive shock.

Phlebitis is another potential source of localized thrombosis and pulmonary thromboembolism. This frequently results from intravenous injection of irritating drugs or chemicals (**Figure 37.12**). Phlebitis also stems from physical injury to veins during IV catheterization, or infection in or around an intravenous catheter. Transvenous pacemaker leads occasionally serve as a nidus for vena caval or cardiac thrombosis, especially in cases that have protein losing nephropathy or stagnant flow due to dilated cardiomyopathy.

Clinical consequences of venous thrombosis and TE include local and pulmonary findings. Locally, obstruction of venous return and elevated capillary hydrostatic pressure lead to congestion and edema of tissues drained by that venous system (**Figure 17.6**, p. 277). Any thrombosis obstructing the cranial vena cava is likely to lead to the cranial vena caval syndrome (characterized by subcutaneous edema of the face, neck, and brisket; p. 277), or to pleural effusion including chylothorax. Obstruction of the caudal vena cava can cause a Budd-Chiari type of pathophysiology with marked ascites.

Pulmonary TE that obstructs one or more pulmonary arteries can lead to otherwise unexplained tachypnea or respiratory distress. Thoracic radiographs might indicate peripheral pulmonary infiltration or a subtle variation in pulmonary circulation, with redistribution of flow away from the obstructed lobes (often missed on thoracic radiographs). Clinical laboratory tests might be useful, but are not as helpful as in humans. These can include measurement of D-dimers (if these are low, pulmonary TE is unlikely) and thromboelastography (**Figure 36.14**, p. 759). Definitive diagnosis

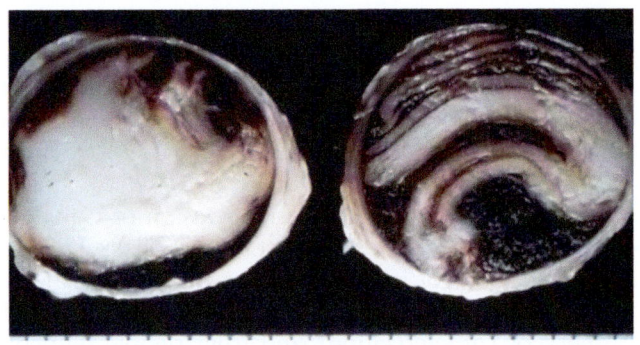

Figure 37.12 Cut surfaces across the jugular vein of a horse. Chronic thrombophlebitis has nearly occluded the vessel. Sections show organized thrombus with fibrosis (white areas) interspersed with areas of postmortem (dark red) clotting within the remaining vascular channels. Notice the layered appearance to the thrombosis within the segment at the upper right. In most cases, this is iatrogenic and caused by inexpert injections or extravasation of tissue-irritating drugs or chemicals.

generally involves CT angiography (**Figure 36.15D**, p. 760); however, this often requires general anesthesia and is not routinely performed in the seriously ill patient. Pulmonary arteriography is another imaging option (**Figure 36.21**, p. 762), although this procedure is rarely pursued. A large TE located in the pulmonary trunk or its bifurcation usually can be identified echocardiographically (**Figure 39.6C**, p. 822). Complete thrombosis or acute embolization of a large pulmonary artery (or the vena caval vessel) can lead to shock from blood flow obstruction. Chronic pulmonary TE can be associated with increased pulmonary vascular resistance and pulmonary arterial hypertension (Chapter 39). Potential consequences include signs of low cardiac output such as exercise intolerance, exertional collapse or syncope, and possible progression to right-sided congestive heart failure.

Other Vascular Diseases

A number of other vascular conditions are reported in dogs, cats, and horses (**Table 37.1**); a brief listing follows. Hamartomas are thought to be developmental malformations that resemble focal neoplasms and are composed of different cellular elements related to the site of origin. Hamartomas often include prominent vascular elements; these masses can be prone to bleeding or function as a space-occupying lesion. Examples include some cutaneous hemangiomas, renal hamartomas, and rare hamartoma formations in cardiac valves, cardiac chambers, and great vessels. These should not be confused with valvular hematocysts, which are common and usually benign developmental abnormalities located mainly on the tricuspid valves in many species.

Tumors of vascular and nonvascular origin can affect blood vessels. For example, hemangiosarcoma and chemodectoma (aortic body tumor) are important causes of pericardial effusion in older dogs (Chapter 35). Large heart base tumors can obstruct the branch pulmonary artery (usually the right) causing supravalvular pulmonary stenosis. The caudal vena cava or pulmonary veins often are displaced, and occasionally obstructed, by a chemodectoma. Chondrosarcoma has occurred rarely in the ascending aorta and can obstruct aortic outflow. Nonvascular tumors of any type can obstruct arteries or veins, resulting in shock, organ dysfunction, localized swellings, or limb edema. Neoplastic invasion of veins could produce localized thrombosis or distant embolism.

Beyond emboli or local thrombosis, physical obstruction of blood vessels can stem from trauma, iatrogenic injury (during surgery or catheterization), and from people who place tight-fitting bands, collars, or other restraints on animals. Torsion of the vascular pedicle of an intra-abdominal organ such as the spleen, liver, or stomach exerts profound vascular and systemic effects. Lung lobe torsion commonly leads to pulmonary hemorrhage, as well as pleural effusion.

Dissection or aneurysm with rupture of a great vessel occurs sporadically; some are probably associated with connective tissue disorders (**Table 37.2**). Associated signs are too varied to address here, but can range from a murmur to sudden death. Pulmonary artery dissection can develop in association with surgical or catheter-device closure of patent ductus arteriosus. Dissection of the aorta is rare whether blood pressure is normal or elevated (**Figure 37.13**).

Rupture of the aorta, usually involving a sinus of Valsalva with acquired aortic to cardiac fistula, is of clinical importance in horses (**Figure 37.14**); it also occurs rarely in other species with infective endocarditis. This fistula often causes systolic and diastolic murmurs, as blood shunts continuously from the aorta into the right atrium, right ventricle, or ventricular septum. Although affected horses can be asymptomatic and appear normal aside from a heart murmur, dissection of the ventricular septum can occur, with associated ventricular arrhythmias. Rupture of the aorta into the pericardial space can lead to acute cardiac tamponade, hypotension, and sudden cardiac death; anecdotally, this is most common in aged stallions.

Friesian horses are prone to a more distal rupture of the aorta with fistulation into the pulmonary artery, near the level of the ductus arteriosus (Ploeg, 2013). Diagnosis in these cases can be confirmed by echocardiography or ultrasound examination. The cause of the aortic rupture and pulmonary fistulation is uncertain. Reported clinical signs include coughing, false colic, sustained tachycardia, and subcutaneous edema from CHF. Aortic dissection has been observed, and associated, with a form of supravalvular aortic stenosis. Prognosis is variable. In equine cases, an expert should be consulted regarding use of the horse and safety issues.

Dilation of the great vessels actually is quite common, although rarely of clinical consequence (beyond yet unstudied effects on ventricular-to-arterial coupling and blood pressure). Dilation downstream from aortic or pulmonic stenosis is common and, in some cases, probably represents an aortopathy or pulmonary arteriopathy, as opposed to turbulence-induced post-stenotic dilation (Chapter 28). Isolated aortopathies (dilatation of the aortic root, ascending aorta, and arch) are recognized most often in Leonberger dogs and other large breeds prone to subaortic stenosis (including Rottweiler, Newfoundland and Golden Retriever, even in the absence of outflow obstruction). These can be confused with heart base tumors radiographically. Idiopathic aortic dilation (aortoannular ectasia) also is common in mature cats and can be dramatic, with "redundancy" of the ascending aorta and aortic arch (**Figures 38.7** and **38.8**, pp. 800 and 801). Some of these cats have systemic hypertension; however, many do not. This finding often is associated with a systolic heart murmur and focal, dorsal ventricular septal hypertrophy. Aortic regurgitation (silent to auscultation) is a common Doppler echocardiographic finding (**Figure 38.13**, p. 802).

Venous abnormalities can include varicosities; these might involve long segments of systemic veins. As in humans, "varicose veins" are associated with venous valve

Vascular Diseases 785

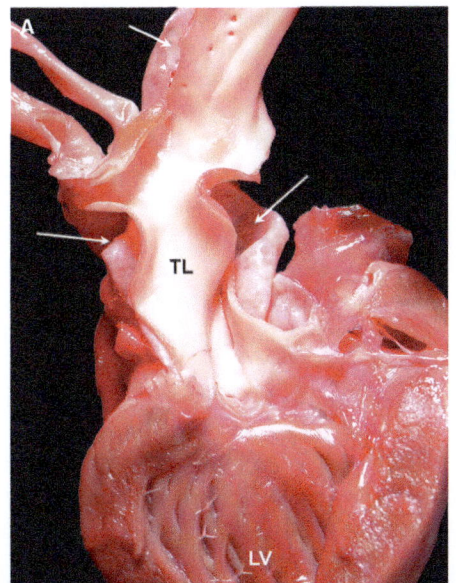

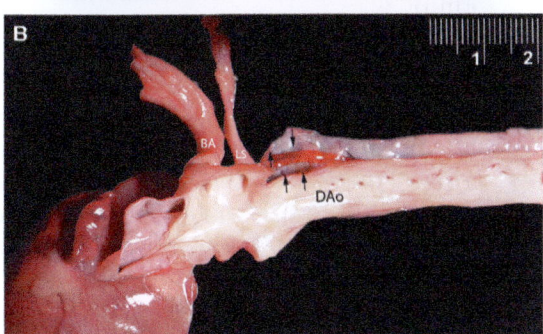

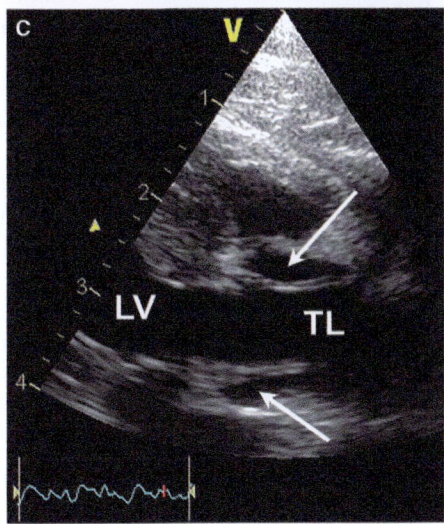

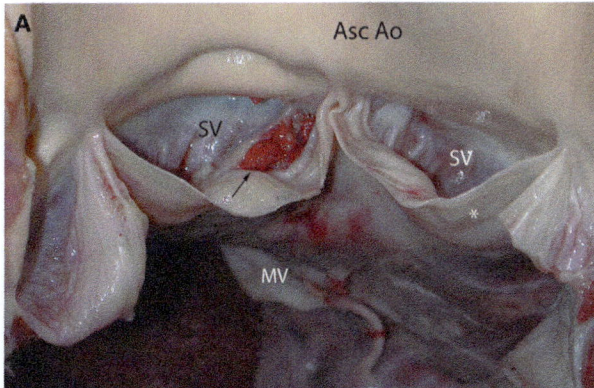

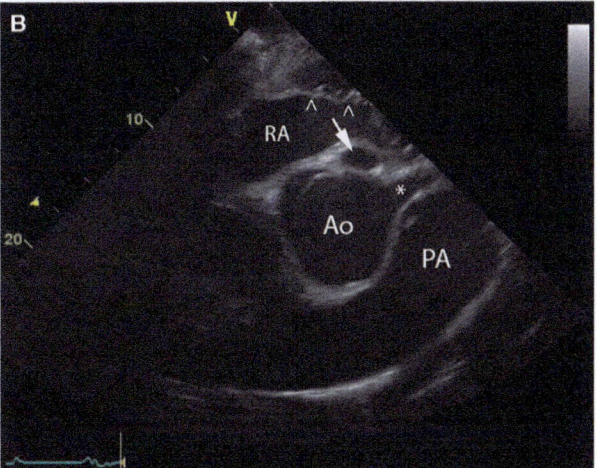

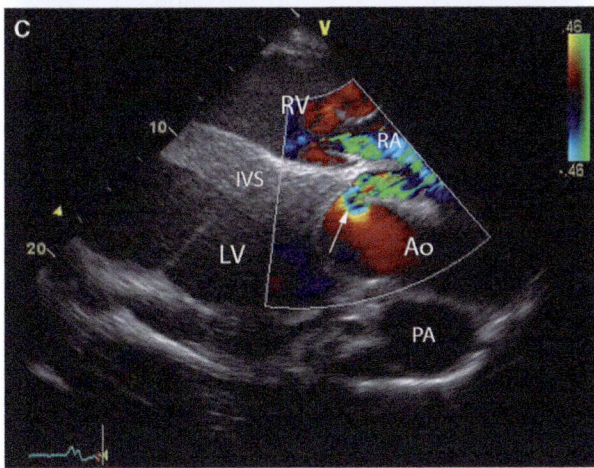

Figure 37.13 Postmortem (A&B) and 2D echocardiographic (C) images from a 16-year-old cat with dissection of the aorta. This lesion most often is associated with systemic hypertension in this species, which was the cause in this case. Note, in (A) and (C), the separation of the aortic layers into a true lumen (TL) and false lumen (arrows). (B) The opened descending aorta (DAo) distal to the brachiocephalic artery (BA) and left subclavian artery (LS) shows the edges of the false lumen (upward arrows) and thrombus formation throughout the extent of the false lumen (downward arrow). LV, left ventricle. Images courtesy of Dr BA Scansen.

Figure 37.14 Ruptured aortic sinus of Valsalva in two horses. (A) Postmortem specimen shows a thrombus within the tear in the right aortic sinus (arrow). Compare this to the normal sinus of Valsalva (SV) adjacent to the left coronary cusp of the aortic valve (*). The dissection extended subendocardially down toward the ventral left aspect of the ventricular septum in this horse. (B) 2D echocardiogram from another horse with a tear in the right sinus of Valsalva, which led to communication (arrow) with the RA. (C) Color Doppler image from the horse in (B) shows shunting (arrow) from Ao into the RA, which caused the RV and PA to dilate; angled, right parasternal long-axis view. Ao, aorta; Asc Ao, ascending aorta; IVS, interventricular septum; LV, left ventricle; MV, anterior mitral valve leaflet; PA, pulmonary artery; RA, right atrium; RV, right ventricle; ^^, parietal tricuspid valve leaflet;* (B), right coronary artery.

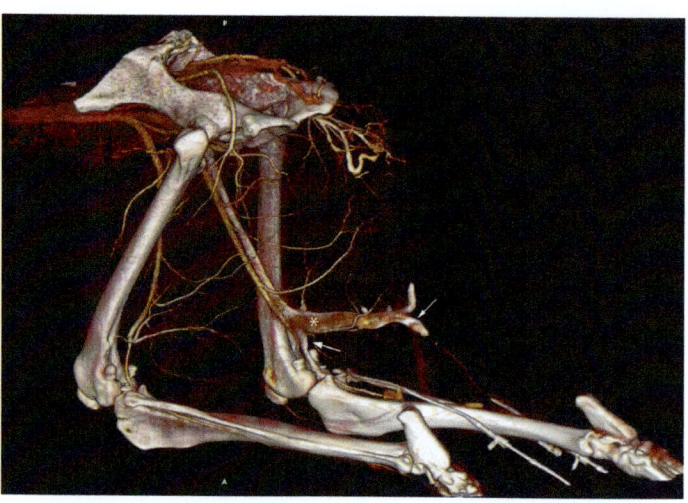

Figure 37.15 3D reconstruction of computed tomography angiogram from a mature Greyhound with edema and cutaneous ulcers of the distal pelvic limb. The rotated image shows severe dilation (varicosities) within the saphenous venous system (*). Note transition from normal to abnormal veins (arrows). The cause was unknown, but prior trauma is a possibility. Venous insufficiency, from loss of normal venous valve and vascular functions, can cause impaired training, elevated capillary pressure and edema. Secondary skin lesions (stasis dermatitis) occurred here.

insufficiency, pooling of blood (especially in long-legged dogs), and the potential for subcutaneous edema and stasis dermatitis (**Figure 37.15**). Diagnosis generally is by clinical suspicion and advanced imaging, including duplex Doppler imaging of peripheral blood vessels and noninvasive CT angiography. Definitive (angiographic) diagnosis and possible catheter-based treatments require catheterization of the vessels.

Suggested Additional Reading and References

Also See Online Comprehensive Bibliography at: https://www.routledge.com/9781482246223.

Decloedt A. Pericardial disease, myocardial disease, and great vessel abnormalities in horses. Vet Clin N Am Equine Pract 2019;35:139–157.

Dias DP, de Lacerda Neto JC. Jugular thrombophlebitis in horses: a review of fibrinolysis, thrombus formation, and clinical management. Can Vet J. 2013;54:65–71.

Falk T, Jönsson L. Ischaemic heart disease in the dog: a review of 65 cases. J Small Anim Pract 2000;41(3):97–103.

Giacchi A, Marcatili M, Withers J, et al. An atypical presentation of leiomyosarcoma causing extremity compartment syndrome of the crural region in a Dutch Warmblood mare: a case report. J Vet Sci. 2020;21:e3.

Holm LP, Stevens KB, Walker DJ. Pathology and epidemiology of cutaneous and renal glomerular vasculopathy in dogs. J Comp Pathol 2020;176:156–161.

Johnson LR, Lappin MR, Baker DC. Pulmonary thromboembolism in 29 dogs: 1985–1995. J Vet Intern Med 1999;13(4):338–345.

Oricco S, Perego M, Poggi M, et al. Aortic dissection in four cats: clinicopathological correlations. J Vet Cardiol. 2019;25:52–60.

Marr CM, Reef VB, Brazil TJ, et al. Aorto-cardiac fistulas in seven horses. Vet Radiol Ultrasound. 1998;39(1):22–31.

Ploeg M, Saey V, de Bruijn CM, et al. Aortic rupture and aorto-pulmonary fistulation in the Friesian horse: characterisation of the clinical and gross post mortem findings in 24 cases. Equine Vet J. 2013;45(1):101–106.

Scaglione J, Diaz SF, Bonagura JD, et al. Ischemic necrosis of the digits and hyperlipidemia associated with atherosclerosis in a miniature American shepherd. J Am Vet Med Assoc 2018;253(2):209–214.

Scansen BA, Bonagura JD. Venous and lymphatic disorders. In, Ettinger SJ, Feldman EC, Cote E (editors). Textbook of Veterinary Internal Medicine, 8th edition. 2017. pp. 1349–1362.

Scansen BA, Simpson EM, López-Alvarez J, et al. Pulmonary artery dissection in eight dogs with patent ductus arteriosus. J Vet Cardiol. 2015;17(2):107–119.

Specchi S, Bertolini G. CT angiography identifies collaterals in dogs with splenic vein obstruction and presumed regional splenic vein hypertension. Vet Radiol Ultrasound 2020;61:636–640.

Walker D, Holm L, Hawkins I, et al. Suspected idiopathic cutaneous and renal glomerular vasculopathy in dogs. Vet Rec. 2014;174(5):124.

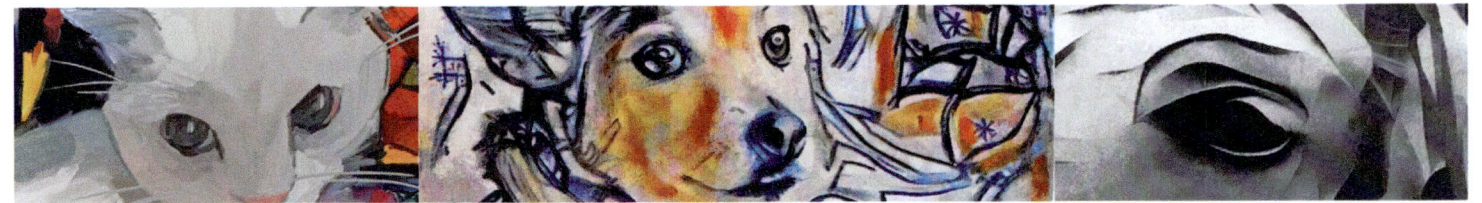

38

SYSTEMIC HYPERTENSION

Persistently elevated systemic arterial blood pressure (BP) defines systemic hypertension (HT). HT can have serious consequences in animals, as it can in people. Progressive damage to the vasculature and so-called "target organs" (or "end organs") is likely when perfusion pressure is excessively high (see section "Pathologic Effects of Hypertension"). The eye, kidney, heart, and brain are particularly vulnerable to damage from chronic HT and its associated vascular changes. Some animals experience acute and dramatic clinical signs. Target organ damage can become manifest as sudden blindness from retinal detachment or ocular hemorrhage, rapidly worsening renal dysfunction, neurologic signs of encephalopathy or stroke, left ventricular (LV) hypertrophy (seen on echocardiogram), and other signs.

Most animals with systemic HT also have an associated disease condition and therefore, are considered to have secondary HT. Chronic kidney disease or an endocrinopathy are involved most often; HT also is common with acute kidney injury (see "Predisposing Conditions" and "Pathophysiology" sections). In some cases, HT develops after administration of certain drugs. The prevalence of HT increases with age. As most commonly associated diseases tend to develop during or after middle-age this is not surprising, although age-related vascular changes also could contribute.

Systemic HT is considered to be idiopathic (primary or "essential") if no underlying or predisposing disease can be identified. This is a diagnosis of exclusion. Idiopathic HT is uncommon in companion animals, yet it has been documented sporadically in dogs and possibly in up to 20% of cats with HT. However, some cases probably are secondary to subclinical kidney disease, in which azotemia might not be evident. Anxiety induced increase in BP could mimic idiopathic HT in some cases, also.

It is well known that patient anxiety can increase BP (the so-called "white-coat" effect in human medicine). Veterinary clinic visits often provoke BP elevation. Systolic BP can exceed 180 mm Hg in some stressed, normal animals, and increases in systolic pressure of 80 mm Hg have been recorded in some cats during simulated clinic visits. This could result in a false diagnosis of HT. Therefore, the importance of maintaining a quiet, calm environment and allowing time for patient acclimatization before measuring BP cannot be overemphasized. It also is important to verify elevated BP readings by repeating the measurement process at different times. Other factors that might influence BP include the patient's age, breed, body condition, underlying disease, and prescribed medications.

Blood Pressure in Normal Animals

BP typically is reported as systolic/diastolic pressures (mm Hg) when both measurements are available. Several studies have aimed to define normal BP levels in different veterinary populations. While direct intra-arterial pressure measurement is likely to be most accurate, and was used initially to identify HT in dogs and cats at risk (Littman, 1994), it generally is impractical as a screening tool for small animal practice. Available indirect BP methods also have limitations. Factors related to measurement equipment and technique, as well as the individual animal, can influence the BP readings achieved. Importantly, no study has shown indirect BP measurements to meet human standards of accuracy and most studies show clinically relevant differences between noninvasive methodologies (Cerna, 2021). There probably also are differences in the accuracy of BP measurements obtained from animals with HT compared to normotensive or hypotensive animals.

In normal dogs, reported average direct (intraarterial) systolic BP measurements have ranged from 144 to 154 mm Hg, with diastolic pressures of 81–96 mm Hg and mean BP of 102–115 mm Hg. Indirect BP measurement studies, using the oscillometric method, report normal median systolic BP values from 131 to 150 mm Hg, with diastolic values of 74–91 mm Hg and mean BP of 97–110 mm Hg. Reported median systolic BP, assessed by Doppler ultrasonography, is approximately 145–150 mm Hg in most normal dogs. Some breed-related variation in BP is reported. Sight hounds (such as Greyhounds, Deerhounds) typically have BPs approximately 10–20 mm Hg higher than mixed breed dogs. Almost a third of retired racing greyhounds appear to have a systolic BP over 160 mm Hg (Surman, 2012). Minor variation in normal BP could occur in other breeds as well. Whether the higher BP observed in sight hounds is a functional adaptation or pathologic is unclear. Recent studies in Greyhounds suggest increased risk for target organ damage. Average values for systolic, diastolic, and mean BP in large and giant breed dogs (except the sight hounds) generally appear lower than those in small breed dogs (such as Beagles). Minor effects on BP related to age have been observed, along with a substantially lower BP and responsiveness in puppies <8 weeks old. Sex and reproductive status, as well as body size, have been variably reported to affect BP in normal dogs. Some canine studies found a small BP increase with age, while others demonstrated no age effect. Male dogs might have a small (<10 mm Hg) increase in BP compared to females. Obesity has been associated with only slightly higher BP in dogs.

In normal cats, average direct (intraarterial radiotelemetric) measurements for systolic BP are about 125–126 mm Hg, with diastolic values of 89–91 mm Hg and mean BP of 105–106 mm Hg. Indirect BP measurements, using the oscillometric technique, indicate normal median systolic BP values ranging from 115 to 139 mm Hg, with diastolic values of 74–77 mm Hg and mean BP of 96–99 mm Hg. Median systolic BP, assessed by Doppler ultrasonography, in a large study of clinically normal cats was approximately 120 mm Hg (110–132, interquartile range; Payne, 2017). Other studies using the Doppler technique report mean systolic BP between 118 and 139 mm Hg in normal cats, although a mean systolic BP of 162 mm Hg was found in one older study. The varying results likely reflect different recording conditions, equipment, and populations. Some studies report slightly higher systolic BP related to age in cats, while others do not. Likewise, a minor increase in median systolic BP in male compared to female cats is reported inconsistently. The large normal cat survey (noted earlier) found higher median systolic BPs in neutered compared to sexually intact animals; there also was a weak positive correlation between body weight and systolic BP. As expected, a cat's demeanor can significantly influence BP results, even within the normal range. Calm cats have lower median systolic BP than cooperative but anxious cats, which have lower median BP than excited or aggressive cats. No breed differences in BP have been reported for cats, although there might be some diurnal effect.

Average values obtained for BP (±standard deviation) in normal standing adult horses, using noninvasive monitoring at the tail base (corrected for vertical distance above the heart, see p. 798), are approximately 135 ±15 mm Hg, systolic; 90 ±15 mm Hg, diastolic; and 110 ±15 mm Hg, mean (Schwarzwald, 2018). Foals less than a month old have lower BPs. Some breed variation in BP has been reported. For example, higher BP was observed in Thoroughbreds compared to Standardbreds, and in Friesians compared to Warmbloods (Vera, 2020). Draft breeds tend to have lower BP than racehorses. Changes in head position can have an influence on BP measurements made from the coccygeal artery in standing horses and variations of about 20 mm Hg have been reported; raising the head increases BP, while lowering it decreases BP. This emphasizes the importance of maintaining consistency of patient positioning, in addition to other recording conditions, when measuring BP. During exercise or other conditions where cardiac output markedly increases, systolic BP can exceed 200 mm Hg.

Risk for Target Organ Disease

Abnormally elevated BP usually is categorized according to its severity and the perceived risk for target organ disease (**Table 38.1**; American College of Veterinary Internal Medicine, ACVIM, consensus statement, Acierno, 2018; International Society of Feline Medicine consensus statement, Taylor, 2017; International Renal Interest Society, IRIS). Most animals with evidence for target organ damage have a systolic BP exceeding 160 mmHg. Animals with repeatable systolic BP less than 140 mm Hg are considered normotensive. Animals with BPs under 150 mm Hg, systolic, and under 95 mm Hg, diastolic, are considered to have minimal risk for target organ damage. A BP of 150–159 mm Hg, systolic, and 95–99 mm Hg, diastolic, that is repeatable on at least 3 occasions is considered to imply relatively low risk for target organ disease. The repeated BP measurements can occur over a 4–8-week period without unduly increasing patient risk. A designation of "prehypertensive" sometimes is used to describe systolic BPs between 140 and 159 mm Hg, (although this designation is no longer used in humans). Systolic BPs higher than 160 mm Hg are likely to cause some renal damage, even when azotemia is absent. Animals with a BP between 160 and 179 mm Hg, systolic, and 100 to 119 mm Hg, diastolic, are thought to have moderately increased risk for target organ

Table 38.1 Classification of Hypertension[a]

Description	Blood Pressure, Systolic (/Approximate Diastolic)	Comment
Normotensive	<140(/<85) mm Hg	Minimal risk for TOD[b]
Prehypertensive	140–159(/85–99) mm Hg	Low risk for TOD
Hypertensive	160–179(/100–119) mm Hg	Moderate risk for TOD
Severely Hypertensive	≥180(/≥120) mm Hg	High/severe risk for TOD

[a] Categorizations based on ACVIM Consensus Guidelines (Acierno, 2018). ISFM Guidelines define systolic blood pressure <150 mm Hg as "Normotensive" and the range of 150–159 mm Hg as "Borderline Hypertensive" (Taylor, 2017).

[b] TOD, target organ damage.

disease; however, BP measurements to confirm this generally can occur over a 4–8-week period, also. Animals with repeatable systolic BPs of 180 mm Hg and higher (and diastolic ≥120 mm Hg) are at severe risk for target organ damage. In these cases, repeated BP measurements should be completed within a 1–2-week period, except for patients showing evidence for acute target organ damage, which are given antihypertensive therapy immediately. An additional 10–20 mm Hg allowance for these categories typically is used for sight hounds. An animal's actual BP can vary in different situations. The duration, as well as degree, of HT likely influences subsequent target organ damage.

Some dogs and cats clearly have HT-induced clinical disease. Yet many with elevated BP show no evidence of related pathology, although subclinical injury might exist. In general, unless there are acute signs of target organ damage, BP measurements are repeated over several occasions before HT is definitively diagnosed. Underlying, predisposing disease should be identified and managed as possible. Animals with mild HT might not require specific antihypertensive therapy. Most animals with moderate (risk of) HT (also previously known as Risk Category III) could benefit from antihypertensive therapy. Treatment definitely is indicated when there is evidence for target organ disease. Similarly, animals with any degree of HT and more than trivial mitral or aortic valve insufficiency (for example, dogs with degenerative mitral valve disease or animals with infective endocarditis) should be treated to normalize BP and reduce LV afterload. Animals with severe HT should be treated to reduce target organ damage. Some animals require emergency antihypertensive therapy (see p. 805).

Predisposing Conditions

Secondary, rather than idiopathic, HT usually is identified in companion animals (**Table 38.2**). Chronic kidney disease is the condition most commonly associated in both dogs and cats. The prevalence of HT in animals with chronic kidney disease could be as high as 75%. HT also is associated with several endocrinopathies, especially hyperadrenocorticism in dogs (Ortega, 1996) and hyperthyroidism in cats. Less commonly, primary hyperaldosteronism or pheochromocytoma underlies HT. Occasionally, HT is identified in dogs with diabetes mellitus. In horses, HT is recognized only infrequently; however, it has been associated with laminitis, other painful conditions, chronic renal disease, equine metabolic syndrome, pheochromocytoma, and multiple endocrine neoplasia. HT discovered during a routine examination could be an early marker of previously unrecognized underlying disease.

Because of the increased risk for HT in patients with these associated diseases, BP measurement is indicated at the time of diagnosis and periodically thereafter. This is especially urgent if evidence of target organ disease exists. In addition to these predisposing conditions, several drugs can increase BP, at least transiently. These include phenylpropanolamine,

Table 38.2 Secondary Hypertension Associations

- Kidney disease (chronic or acute; especially glomerular)
- Hyperadrenocorticism
- Hyperthyroidism
- Pheochromocytoma
- Hyperaldosteronism
- Diabetes mellitus (dog)
- Metabolic syndrome (horses)
- Laminitis (horses)
- Chronic anemia (cats)
- Intracranial lesions (↑ intracranial pressure)
- Brachycephalic sleep apnea?

Certain drugs and toxins (observed mainly in dogs; p. 792):

- Phenylpropanolamine
- Alpha-2 adrenergic agonist agents (dexmedetomidine, others)
- Phenylephrine; ephedrine; pseudoephedrine
- Glucocorticoids
- Mineralocorticoids
- Erythropoietin
- Toceranib phosphate
- Cocaine
- Methamphetamine; amphetamine
- 5-hydroxytryptophan
- Garlic toxicity; other toxins

Other conditions associated with hypertension in people:

- Acromegaly
- Inappropriate antidiuretic hormone secretion
- Hyperviscosity/erythrocytosis (polycythemia)
- Renin-secreting tumors
- Hypercalcemia
- Hypothyroidism with atherosclerosis
- Hyperestrogenism
- Coarctation (narrowing) of the aorta
- Pregnancy
- Central nervous system disease

glucocorticoids, mineralocorticoids, erythropoietin, nonsteroidal antiinflammatory agents, sodium chloride, and even topical ocular phenylephrine. Primary cardiac disease, including hypertrophic cardiomyopathy, does not cause systemic HT.

Pathophysiology

BP is a function of cardiac output and peripheral vascular resistance. There is continuous interplay between these variables and the factors that influence them. Conditions that raise cardiac output (such as increased heart rate, stroke volume, or blood volume) or that increase vascular resistance tend to raise BP. Normally, arterial pressure is maintained within narrow limits by the actions of the autonomic nervous system (including arterial baroreceptor feedback), as well as hormones (including angiotensins, aldosterone, vasopressin/antidiuretic hormone, and natriuretic peptides), endothelial signaling mechanisms, vasodilatory prostaglandins, pressure natriuresis, and ultimately blood volume regulation by the kidney (p. 25). Persistently high systemic BP suggests some type of dysfunction in the neurohormonal or renal mechanisms responsible for arterial BP regulation.

Secondary HT sometimes is subclassified into renal and endocrine HT, although HT can result from multiple mechanisms that might exist concurrently. These could involve the renin-angiotensin-aldosterone system (RAAS), sympathetic nervous system, endothelial (dys)function, vascular remodeling, and progressive renal (especially glomerular) disease. RAAS activation, with subsequent salt and water retention and vasoconstriction, can result from enhanced angiotensinogen production (for example, with hyperadrenocorticism) and diseases that increase sympathetic nervous activity (as with hyperthyroidism), as well as from compromised renal perfusion (as with renal artery obstruction). Other conditions also could cause or facilitate the development of HT. Reduced endothelial function could contribute to HT in older animals. The cause of minor BP increases sometimes found in obese dogs and cats is unclear. Sympathetic nervous system and RAAS activation, or perhaps other hormonal mechanisms, could be involved. BP can become abnormally high when sympathetic nervous activity or responsiveness is enhanced (such as with hyperthyroidism or hyperadrenocorticism), or catecholamine production is increased (as with pheochromocytoma). The role of central sympathetic controls on BP including during stress is a focus of active investigation. Volume expansion secondary to sodium retention that might occur from renal failure, hyperaldosteronism, acromegaly, or hyperadrenocorticism also could raise BP.

Kidney Disease

The reported prevalence of HT in dogs with renal disease has ranged widely from under 20% to well over 75%. Some degree of proteinuria generally is present in these cases, although there appears to be no direct association among BP, urine protein/creatinine ratio and fractional excretion of electrolytes. Studies in dogs have shown that loss of functional renal tissue leads to increases in BP, plasma renin activity, and angiotensin (Ang)I, AngII, and aldosterone (ALD) concentrations, in addition to azotemia. Angiotensin converting enzyme (ACE) inhibitor administration reduces BP, as well as AngII and ALD concentrations. Dogs with chronic kidney disease and systemic HT reportedly have higher urinary protein (albumin)/creatinine ratios than those without HT. Marked proteinuria with HT is a negative prognostic sign. Macroalbuminuria usually is evident when urine protein/creatinine ratio exceeds 1. For dogs with renal disease, HT and a urine protein/creatinine ratio of 1 or less, testing for microalbuminuria is useful, in the absence of overt proteinuria.

HT can occur at any stage of chronic kidney disease or with acute kidney injury, such as from a toxic, infectious or ischemic insult. In dogs, an inverse correlation between exogenous creatinine plasma clearance and systolic BP, as well as a weak but significant positive correlation between urine protein/creatinine ratio and systolic BP, have been reported; some studies report no direct relation between serum creatinine concentration and BP. HT associated with chronic renal disease could develop by a number of mechanisms. For example, BP could rise if decreased glomerular filtration rate (GFR) and reduced sodium excretion increase blood volume, or if poor renal blood flow or localized renal ischemia activates the RAAS cascade, or if production of vasodilator substances (such as prostaglandins and kallikreins) decreases. Effects related to secondary hyperparathyroidism might be involved, also. High BP has been associated with low serum potassium concentration in animals with renal disease; this could relate to effects of ALD, or other mechanisms.

In dogs with renal disease, RAAS activation is thought to be an important mechanism underlying HT. Endothelin (ETN)-1 also could play a role in the pathogenesis of both inflammation and HT associated with kidney disease, although it might merely be associated with renal disease severity. Serum levels of homocysteine and big ETN-1 often are elevated in dogs with renal disease, especially those with proteinuria. Correlation between serum homocysteine and creatinine concentrations has been reported, but not with the degree of HT. Serum big ETN-1 concentration typically is elevated in dogs with advanced (IRIS stage IV) renal disease, compared to normal dogs. Correlations between serum ETN-1 and serum creatinine, proteinuria (urine protein/creatinine ratio), systolic BP, and increased C-reactive protein levels have been found. Reduced GFR and HT also are associated with mild increase in plasma N-terminal prohormone B-type (brain) natriuretic peptide (NT-proBNP) concentration.

Between 19 and 65% of cats with chronic kidney disease have HT, or develop it within a few months of initial renal disease diagnosis. Cats with chronic kidney disease are more likely to develop HT as they age, compared to healthy cats, especially if their BP was in the upper-normal range at initial evaluation. Creatinine concentration is an independent risk factor for HT in cats. Up to 75% of cats with HT have some elevation in serum creatinine. However, HT severity does not appear correlated to renal disease severity. Cats with HT at the time of chronic kidney disease diagnosis also are highly likely to have evidence of target organ damage.

The mechanism of HT in cats with chronic renal disease is incompletely understood, although it could involve RAAS activation as well as fluid retention. The limited changes in ALD concentrations, plasma renin activity, and BP in response to ACE inhibitor therapy suggest RAAS activation is not a major mechanism in cats. Nevertheless, elevated ALD could play a role in some cats. Increased ALD concentrations have been identified in older cats with azotemia and HT, compared to normotensive cats. Changes in plasma renin activity do not appear to affect ALD concentrations in these cats, which suggests possible autonomous ALD production or Ang-ALD activation not related to renin activity. Local tissue-specific Ang and ALD production (rather than systemic RAAS activation) could be responsible. Other mechanisms for HT in cats with kidney disease could include sodium retention, increased sympathetic stimulation, or other abnormalities. Increased vascular tone (vasoconstriction) appears to play an important mechanistic role, based on the positive therapeutic response to amlodipine in most cats with HT.

Endocrine Disease

Endocrinopathies as a group rank closely behind renal disease as a cause of secondary HT. An estimated 10–23% of cats diagnosed with hyperthyroidism have HT, although concurrent renal disease is the likely etiology of HT in some cases. Furthermore, perhaps up to one fourth of hyperthyroid cats that are normotensive at diagnosis develop HT later, even after becoming euthyroid. Similar to cats with hyperthyroidism, some dogs with a functional thyroid adenocarcinoma develop HT. Barring metastatic disease, their HT is likely to resolve after successful thyroidectomy assuming the sole cause is excess thyroid hormone. The mechanism of HT associated with hyperthyroidism is not fully understood. Increased sensitivity to circulating catecholamines or direct cardiac effects probably are important. RAAS activation does not appear to be the main cause of HT in hyperthyroid cats, although some cats with hyperthyroidism might develop RAAS upregulation or dysfunction. Plasma renin activity appears to be similar among hyperthyroid cats with and without HT, and in those that develop HT after antithyroid therapy; it decreases in all groups after treatment. In hyperthyroid cats that develop HT after antithyroid treatment, however, a discordance between plasma renin activity and ALD concentrations suggests that RAAS dysfunction might contribute to HT in these cats.

Hyperadrenocorticism commonly is associated with HT, which can be severe. Between 47 and 86% of affected dogs have HT. The rate of HT occurrence reportedly is greater in dogs with adrenal-dependent hyperadrenocorticism, compared to those with pituitary-dependent disease. Hyperadrenocorticism, either pituitary-dependent or caused by an adrenal tumor, also can be associated with severe HT in cats. Glucocorticoids enhance production of angiotensinogen by the liver, which increases RAAS activation. Other hormones besides cortisol could contribute to HT, such as ALD, and gluco- or mineralocorticoid precursors. Albuminuria and increased urine protein/creatinine ratio are common in dogs with hyperadrenocorticism. The presence of albuminuria does not seem directly correlated with systolic BP. Nevertheless, pressure-induced glomerular basement membrane damage could promote albuminuria. Systolic BP has shown weak correlation with urine protein/creatinine ratio. BP elevation and cardiac hypertrophy appear to be more common with adrenal-dependent, compared to pituitary-dependent, disease although hypertrophy has not been correlated specifically with BP. Mild LV and septal hypertrophy, and slightly reduced systolic function, have been seen in dogs with hyperadrenocorticism, even in the absence of HT. Perhaps in addition to HT, stimulation of the RAAS, as well as myocyte mineralocorticoid and glucocorticoid receptors, might promote cardiac hypertrophy and myocardial fibrosis development, as in people.

Exogenous glucocorticoid administration can increase BP over time, although not necessarily to a higher risk level. Administration of antiinflammatory doses of prednisone have increased systolic BP by an average of almost 20 mm Hg in dogs, although not all studies show significant change from baseline BP. Albuminuria and urine protein/creatinine ratio also increase with chronic glucocorticoid administration. These changes usually are reversible after the drug is discontinued

HT can be associated with an adrenal cortical tumor (carcinoma or adenoma) causing excessive secretion of ALD or an ALD-like substance that mimics the effects of mineralocorticoid excess. Functional adrenal neoplasia also can produce excessive estradiol and progesterone. Although primary hyperaldosteronism caused by an adrenal tumor is uncommon, it should be considered, especially in middle-aged and older age cats with HT and hypokalemic polymyopathy. Between 40 and 60% of cats with primary hyperaldosteronism have HT, which can be severe. Other mechanisms besides sodium retention and volume expansion that might contribute to HT include vascular remodeling and increased responsiveness to sympathetic stimulation.

A functional pheochromocytoma is another cause for HT. Increased secretion of catecholamines by the tumor sometimes leads to severe HT. Other causes of increased sympathetic nervous system activity, as well as exogenous adrenergic agonists, also can raise BP to pathological levels.

Diabetes mellitus has been associated with BP elevation in over 50% of affected dogs; diastolic hypertension appears more common than systolic. In most cases, the HT is only mild; however, moderate to severe HT develops sporadically. Microalbuminuria and increased urine protein/creatinine are common, although no significant association among BP, urine albumin concentration, urine protein/creatinine ratio, and occurrence of retinopathy have been identified. Mild increases in BP have been found in cats with diabetes mellitus, but severe HT is uncommon. Experimentally, diabetes mellitus has been associated with vascular complications including nephropathy and retinopathy, as well as HT.

Insulin resistance is known to be related to HT and impaired vasodilation in people, and insulin administration can lower BP. Decreases in systolic, mean and diastolic BPs after insulin administration also were demonstrated in healthy horses. Horses with normal insulin sensitivity have greater systolic and mean BP reduction than those with insulin resistance. In ponies prone to laminitis, higher BP, as well as insulin resistance and other metabolic responses (including elevated plasma triglycerides and uric acid), were observed after they grazed on summer pasture, but not when on winter pasture. These metabolic changes are described as a prelaminitic phenotype. Intra-abdominal fat accumulation in horses is associated with reduced insulin sensitivity (hyperinsulinemia), glucose intolerance, dyslipidemia, HT, and insidious-onset laminitis.

Other Associations

Obesity, by itself, has not been clearly identified as a risk factor for HT in dogs. While mean systolic BP was shown to be mildly increased in obese compared to lean dogs, it was still within normal limits and the BP ranges of obese and lean groups did not differ. In obese hypertensive dogs and horses, another abnormality, such as kidney or endocrine disease, probably underlies the HT. Nevertheless, obesity has been associated with RAAS activation, increased sympathetic nervous activity, insulin resistance, renal glomerular hypertrophy (from high caloric intake and renal blood flow), and increased cortisol concentrations. Some LV hypertrophy also can occur in obese animals. Although HT has not been attributed to obesity in cats, lipoprotein changes similar to those in obese people have been observed.

Certain drugs can increase BP. Alpha-agonist agents stimulate vasoconstriction and raise BP. Even phenylephrine eyedrops can raise BP to some degree. Alpha$_2$-agonist agents (xylazine, detomidine, medetomidine, and dexmedetomidine) are known to increase BP acutely, often leading to reflex bradycardia and in some cases, atrioventricular (AV) block. Overdose of phenylpropanolamine can cause potentially severe HT, as well as tachyarrhythmias and other clinical signs. Cocaine and methamphetamine toxicoses likewise can produce HT and tachycardia, as well as neurologic and other disturbances. Erythropoietin has been associated with HT, also. Tyrosine kinase inhibitor therapy is associated with HT and proteinuria in people; in normotensive dogs, toceranib phosphate sometimes increases systolic BP to over 160 mm Hg. Ingestion of 5-hydroxytryptophan (5-HTP; serotonin) supplements can lead to serotonin syndrome, with tachycardia, HT, tachypnea, and hyperthermia. It is important to remember that animals with a failing ventricle or severe mitral (or aortic) regurgitation are likely to be less tolerant of commonly used drugs that raise BP. These include the sedative dexmedetomidine and phenylpropanolamine used to treat urinary incontinence.

Impaired cerebral perfusion can provoke bradycardia, HT, and apnea too. A reflex central nervous system (CNS) ischemic response probably is responsible. This could occur with cerebral or subarachnoid hemorrhage, an intracranial mass lesion, or during cisternal myelography.

Chronic magnesium deficiency with intracellular depletion has been associated with systemic HT. The antihypertensive effects of magnesium likely relate to its calcium channel blocking effect and ability to reduce arterial stiffness. There appears to be a connection between magnesium depletion and hypercapnia from obstructive sleep apnea. This could be an underlying mechanism in Bulldogs, and other dogs with brachycephalic conformation, and HT. Hypercapnia is thought to promote magnesium deficiency, which in turn promotes pharyngeal muscle weakness and further airway collapse, hypoxemia and hypercapnia. Nocturnal hypoxemia, and HT, can worsen with age. Other potential mechanisms involved with brachycephalic conformation and the associated HT could include increased sympathetic activity, endothelial damage, decreased nitric oxide production, and excessively negative intrathoracic pressures. In people with obstructive sleep apnea, mechanisms of HT are thought to include RAAS activation, arterial wall stiffening, oxidative damage, endothelial dysfunction, and systemic inflammation. Hypoxemia and hypercapnia stimulate aortic and carotid chemoreceptors. The resulting brainstem reflexes promote increased ventilatory rate and sympathetic enhancement of vascular tone. Increases in heart rate accompanying these changes can outweigh chemoreceptor-stimulation of vagal tone.

Greyhounds often have elevated BP or overt HT and proteinuria. They also appear to have a higher prevalence of stroke compared to other dog breeds. Increased production of arachidonic acid metabolites in this breed could promote vascular dysfunction and contribute to higher BP and albuminuria. While HT is common, coagulation abnormalities do not appear to underlie ischemic stroke in greyhounds.

In people, there is an inverse association between vitamin D status (as assessed by serum 25-hydroxyvitamin D concentration) and HT, among other cardiovascular abnormalities. Whether this is a causative mechanism or an epiphenomenon, or whether the same association is present in dogs and cats is unknown. However, vitamin D can affect the cardiovascular system through several pathways, including the RAAS, parathyroid hormone, vascular endothelial growth, and the immune system.

Various toxins can cause HT, including garlic toxicity, chronic cadmium exposure, and black widow spider envenomation. Garlic ingestion can lead to intravascular hemolysis and methemoglobinemia (p. 249). Postulated mechanisms of methemoglobinemia-induced HT include vasoconstriction secondary to endothelial damage and nitric oxide dysregulation, hypoxia-induced sympathetic nervous system activation, and activation of the RAAS. Chronic exposure to the heavy metal cadmium could underlie HT. Higher urinary cadmium excretion has been found in cats with HT. In dogs, experimental low-level cadmium exposure was associated with HT, although acute high doses were not. Postulated mechanisms include cadmium-induced renal injury and effects on vascular endothelial or smooth muscle function. Higher cadmium concentrations were observed in the kidneys of geriatric cats, compared to young adult and middle-aged cats, and also in older horses. Because cadmium has a long half-life in the body, years of chronic accumulation could produce signs of toxicity. Passive exposure to cigarette smoke can increase cadmium levels in the body.

Pathologic Effects of Hypertension

High perfusion pressure can damage the smallest arteries and capillary beds. Normally, increases in arterial BP invoke autoregulatory arteriolar vasoconstriction in most tissues. This vascular autoregulation protects capillaries from large pressure fluctuations and maintains constant blood flow, at least when arterial BP is in the range of about 60–160 mm Hg. However, underlying organ disease can interfere with normal autoregulation. In addition, prolonged arteriolar constriction secondary to chronic HT leads to medial hypertrophy and other vascular remodeling, which can further increase vascular resistance. Vascular structural changes and spasm can cause local hypoxia, tissue damage, hemorrhage, and infarction. Variable signs of organ dysfunction can result. In cats, arteriopathy of the small vessels that supply the walls of larger vessels (the *vasa vasorum*) was found to correlate strongly with hypertensive status, as well as degree of renal arteriosclerosis and degenerative aortic wall lesions.

In the kidney, autoregulation is important for maintaining GFR, as well as renal perfusion. Glomerular capillary pressure normally is maintained at 60–65 mm Hg by autoregulatory vasoconstriction or dilation of afferent arterioles. Changes in efferent arteriolar resistance also help maintain glomerular capillary pressure and promote optimal GFR. If vascular autoregulation is impaired by renal disease, glomerular pressure is likely to rise or fall directly with systemic BP. Glomerular hypertension causes hyperfiltration, which over time leads to glomerulosclerosis, atrophy, and proliferative glomerulitis. Although not necessarily pathognomonic for HT, increased prevalence of glomerulosclerosis and arteriosclerosis has been observed in cats with higher BP. Vascular damage from chronic HT also leads to renal tubular degeneration and interstitial fibrosis, which contribute to proteinuria, deteriorating renal function and increasing vascular resistance. Proteinuria, an important manifestation of renal damage, has been associated experimentally with severity of HT in cats and dogs. Chronic HT, therefore, tends to perpetuate itself, exacerbate renal disease and potentially, reduce survival.

Ocular lesions are common in patients with HT. Positive correlations between BP and degree of ocular fundic changes and age have been demonstrated in cats. Hypertensive damage can develop at systolic BPs under 170 mm Hg, although risk increases substantially as BP exceeds 180 mm Hg. Breakdown of vascular autoregulation in precapillary arterioles causes dilation and leakage, especially in the retina and choroid. Retinal edema (either focal or generalized), papilledema, focal perivascular transudate, arteriolar sclerosis, vascular tortuosity or narrowing, focal retinal arteriolar dilations (macroaneurysms), retinal hemorrhages, and ischemic lesions can occur with hypertensive disease (**Figures 38.1** and **38.2**). Focal bullous retinal detachment is a common manifestation of hypertensive retinopathy. Total retinal detachment occurs

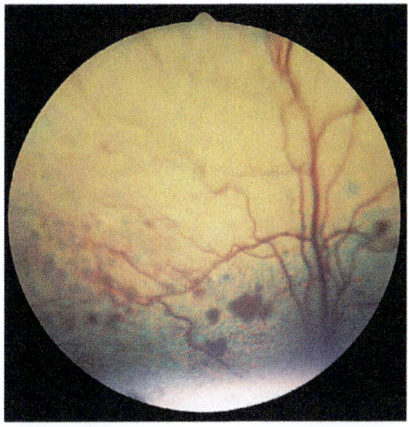

Figure 38.1 Fundic image from a dog with hypertension shows multiple retinal hemorrhages (associated with blood vessels) in the bottom (ventral) half of the image. Some vascular tortuosity is present. Small dark spots (in 8–9 o'clock position) are thought to be subretinal hemorrhage. Light artifact is at bottom edge. (Image courtesy of Dr D Betts.)

less commonly. Vitreal hemorrhage, hyphema, secondary glaucoma, and uveitis also can occur, as can hypertensive optic neuropathy secondary to ischemia and edema. The reported prevalence of ocular lesions varies widely, which probably relates to how early the HT was diagnosed. For example, lesions have been reported in 41–100% of hypertensive cats; however, most of these cases had advanced disease when diagnosed. In the general population of middle-aged to geriatric cats, the prevalence of hypertensive ocular lesions appears to be well under 20%, including many preclinical lesions. Retinopathy or choroidopathy also is common in hypertensive dogs. Most retrospective reports describe severe ocular damage, such as retinal detachment and hyphema, presumably because a visual disturbance or obvious ocular hemorrhage prompted the examination. Sudden blindness is more likely to occur with severe HT.

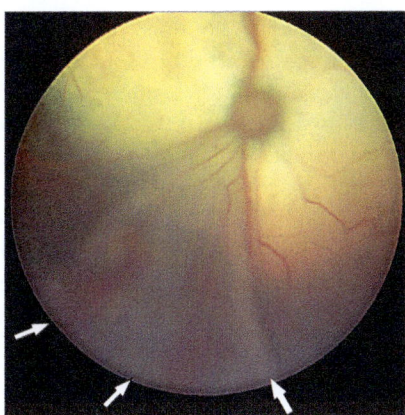

Figure 38.2 Fundic image from an older, mixed breed cat with systolic blood pressure >300 mm Hg. Partial retinal detachment is evident ventrally (arrows), with areas of hemorrhage on the detached segment. There is nonuniform retinal edema dorsally and around the optic disk. (Image courtesy of Dr D Betts.)

Cerebral blood flow also is influenced by autoregulation in response to changes in perfusion pressure. In addition, increased $PaCO_2$ and perivascular acidosis cause vasodilation and increase blood flow locally. Disease can interfere with normal cerebral vascular autoregulation. Cerebral blood flow could increase when BP rises above 160 mm Hg, depending on several factors. Conditions that increase intravascular pressure within the brain include HT, vascular obstruction, and abnormal cerebral autoregulation. Elevated vascular pressure can promote edema formation and increase intracranial pressure, which can lead to hemorrhage in and around the brain. Conversely, elevated systemic BP can develop secondary to intracranial pathology that raises intracranial pressure, as a reflex mechanism to maintain cerebral blood flow (Cushing's reflex). Therefore, HT can cause neurologic signs or be a secondary manifestation of elevated intracranial pressure.

Neurologic signs occur in 15–46% of hypertensive cats. Hypertensive encephalopathy is more likely when BP rises acutely and/or exceeds 180 mm Hg. Lesions associated with hypertensive encephalopathy include cerebral arteriosclerosis, vasogenic brain edema, and intracranial hemorrhage. Clinical abnormalities can include disorientation or other mentation change, especially depression. Other signs, including ataxia, vestibular signs or other focal neurologic deficits, seizures, recumbency, or blindness can occur (**Figure 37.1B**, p. 777). Neurologic signs might improve after BP normalization. Owners of hypertensive cats often remark that their pet is more active after normal BP has been restored. Exercise-induced neurologic signs, including ataxia and central vestibular signs, have been associated with HT. These could represent transient ischemic attacks, which are episodes of focal brain dysfunction caused by vascular disease. Transient ischemic attacks generally resolve within 24 hours and often are recurrent; HT is a common preexisting condition. Stroke is cerebrovascular disease caused by an intracranial vascular event and characterized by sudden onset of focal neurologic deficits that usually last at least 24 hours. In people, HT is the most common risk factor for ischemic, as well as hemorrhagic, stroke. HT is associated with stroke in dogs, too; although stroke also can occur with other conditions, such as neoplasia, sepsis, hypothyroidism, parasitic disease, vascular malformation, and coagulopathy. Nevertheless, in one report, almost a third of dogs with brain infarction had HT (Garosi, 2005). Greyhounds could be at increased risk for stroke compared to other breeds. Spinal infarction also has occurred in patients with HT.

The heart is another target organ of HT. Secondary cardiac remodeling can result from chronic HT. High systolic BP increases LV afterload and wall stress, activates myocardial mechanoreceptors, and stimulates the development of LV concentric hypertrophy. Cats with higher BPs are more likely to have measurable LV hypertrophy; HT should be ruled out before making a diagnosis of hypertrophic cardiomyopathy (p. 649). However, the degree of LV concentric hypertrophy in most companion animals with systemic HT usually is only modest. Just under half of hypertensive dogs had measurable concentric LV hypertrophy in one case series (Misbach, 2011), although the reference values in use at the time now are considered somewhat insensitive for the diagnosis of LV thickening. Notably, dogs with HT had thicker walls and evidence of diastolic dysfunction compared to controls. Although HT could decrease cardiac output, hypertensive heart disease usually does not progress to CHF in companion animals unless there is preexisting myocardial or valvular disease; this is in contrast to the situation in people. The difference might relate to the effects of underlying disease on lifespan in companion animals. Nevertheless, LV hypertrophy can increase ventricular stiffness and impair diastolic function. This could explain the occurrence of gallop sounds or unexpected congestive signs that sometimes develop following fluid therapy in older, hypertensive cats.

Coronary artery disease generally is not a clinical problem in companion animals with HT, in contrast to people. Yet, as with other diseases causing LV hypertrophy, medial hypertrophy of intramural coronary arteries has occurred in hypertensive cats. Chronic systemic HT is a risk factor for aortic dilation, as well as aneurysm, in people. Aortic dilation is observed commonly in cats and dogs with HT, and many have silent aortic regurgitation evident on color Doppler examination. However, aortic aneurysm and aortic dissection have been described only sporadically in dogs and cats (**Figure 37.13**, p. 785), and HT was not documented in all cases. Aortic rupture in horses typically occurs more often during periods of excitement and presumably, elevated BP, such as during racing or in stallions when breeding (p. 784). Another uncommon manifestation of hypertensive vascular damage is epistaxis, caused by rupture of nasal mucosal vessels. In dogs, this has been reported mainly with pheochromocytoma.

Clinical Features

The prevalence of HT in apparently healthy dogs has been estimated at 0.5–10%. The situation in apparently normal cats could be similar, with an estimated 2% prevalence suggested. Many animals show no overt signs of HT, so unless BP is measured, HT could be markedly underdiagnosed. The prevalence of HT in apparently healthy horses is unknown. Clinical HT is more common in middle-aged and older animals. These are populations with greater prevalence of the associated diseases. In cats, the median age at HT diagnosis is estimated to be 13–15 years, although HT has been found in cats as young as 5–7 years.

Clinical signs often relate to the underlying or associated disease process. Presenting signs in dogs can include polyuria and polydipsia, weight loss, anorexia, lethargy, ocular signs, vomiting, seizures, ataxia or other neurologic signs, and syncope. Signs of target organ damage can predominate when HT is severe or sustained. Overt clinical manifestations of HT often involve ocular signs. Sudden blindness caused by acute retinal hemorrhage or detachment, or hyphema are most visible to the owner and likely to prompt veterinary attention. Polyuria and polydipsia are common complaints; these signs probably are caused by renal disease, hyperadrenocorticism (in dogs and possibly horses), or hyperthyroidism (mainly in cats). Although pressure diuresis is one of the major compensations for HT, its contribution to polyuria is mainly speculative and this mechanism likely is overwhelmed once chronic BP elevation becomes established. Hypertensive encephalopathy can cause mentation changes, seizures, paresis, ataxia, collapse, vocalization, or other neurologic deficits. These might be short-lived manifestations of a transient ischemic attack, or the result of cerebrovascular accident (stroke) caused by hypertensive arteriolar spasm and occlusion or hemorrhage. Other nonspecific signs might include wimpering, inappetence, or behavioral changes, including marked depression. Epistaxis, caused by HT-induced nasal mucosal bleeding, occurs occasionally. Rarely, severe AV block and syncope are associated with severe HT and reflex vagal responses.

Physical Findings

Abnormal heart sounds often are heard in hypertensive animals, although they do not appear to correlate with the degree of LV hypertrophy. Soft systolic murmurs usually relate to abnormal LV flow dynamics or valve function. Two-thirds of hypertensive dogs are estimated to have a systolic murmur; however, degenerative mitral valve disease is likely to be the main contributor in older dogs. A gallop sound might be heard in hypertensive cats, likely reflecting increased ventricular stiffness. The heart rate usually is normal, although tachycardia or arrhythmias occur in some hypertensive animals. Clinical signs of heart failure from HT are uncommon in cats, and unreported in dogs. Fundic examination in hypertensive animals often reveals retinal hemorrhages; other signs can include bullous to complete effusive retinal detachment, subretinal edema, vascular tortuosity, hyperreflective scars, retinal atrophy, papilledema, and perivasculitis (**Figures 38.1** and **38.2**). Vitreal or anterior chamber hemorrhage, closed-angle glaucoma, and corneal ulceration also can occur (p. 793). Rarely, another complication could be retrobulbar thrombus. Over 60% of dogs with HT reportedly have some type of ocular lesion. Abnormal neurologic exam findings occur in some cases.

Blood Pressure Measurement

BP measurement beginning in young adulthood could help establish individual baseline values. Rechecks every 2–3 years through middle-age, and then yearly for older to geriatric animals, have been recommended in order to detect HT at an early stage (Taylor, 2017). Others suggest screening should begin in dogs and cats at about 9 years of age, unless circumstances warrant BP measurement earlier (Acierno, 2018). For animals that develop signs suggestive of target organ damage, BP should be measured right away (**Figure 38.3**). BP

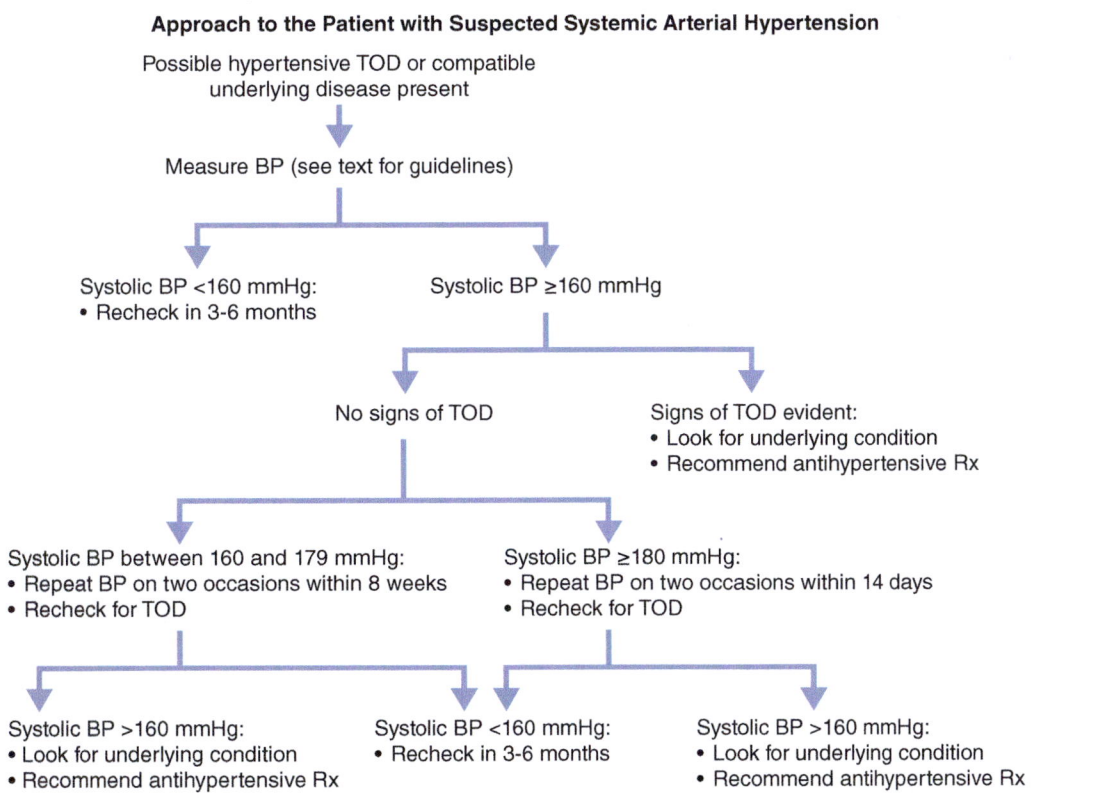

Figure 38.3 An approach to the patient with suspected systemic arterial hypertension. (Adapted from ACVIM consensus statement guidelines; Acierno, 2018.) BP, blood pressure; Rx, therapy; TOD, target organ damage.

measurement also is indicated whenever a disease commonly associated with HT is diagnosed, with additional follow-up measurements every 3–6 months, if normal. It is important to confirm suspected HT by obtaining BP measurements more than once, ideally on different days, unless emergency treatment is indicated (p. 805). Several methods can be used to measure systemic arterial BP. Variation in measured BP can relate to the technique used (direct and various noninvasive methods), as well as to patient factors, especially anxiety.

Direct Measurement

BP measurement through a needle or catheter placed directly into an artery is considered the gold standard. However, besides the greater technical expertise required, the physical restraint and discomfort associated with arterial puncture in awake animals can falsely increase BP. Nevertheless, when sustained arterial pressure monitoring is needed, an indwelling arterial catheter is the best approach. The dorsal metatarsal artery often is used for this. An electronic pressure monitor will provide continuous measurement of systolic and diastolic pressures and calculated mean pressure. With fluid-filled systems, the pressure transducer should be positioned at the same horizontal level as the patient's right atrium, to avoid false increases or decreases in measured pressure caused by gravitational effects on the fluid within the connecting tubing. In addition, under- and overdamping of the pressure waveform can cause erroneous BP measurements. For intermittent direct BP measurement, a small-gauge needle attached directly to a pressure transducer can be used to puncture the dorsal metatarsal or femoral artery. After removing the catheter or needle, pressure should be applied to the arterial puncture site for several minutes to prevent hematoma formation. Direct arterial pressure measurement is more accurate than indirect methods in hypotensive animals. Direct measurement occasionally is needed to accurately determine BP, if indirect readings between sites are markedly disparate; this sometimes is observed between fore- and rearlimb measurements in dogs (as in Dalmatians and some others).

Indirect Measurement

Noninvasive BP measurement is used for most clinical situations. Methods available include Doppler ultrasonic flow detection, oscillometry, and photoplethysmography. The latter occasionally is employed in small dogs (<10 kg) and cats for continuous BP estimation, although it most often is used in people. Photoplethysmography uses infrared light transmission to measure arterial volume changes, usually on a (human) finger.

Doppler and oscillometric methods are used most commonly in companion animals and are the recommended techniques (**Figure 38.4**). Ideally, the device selected has been validated for use in the particular species, although this often is not the case; standards for validating indirect BP devices in

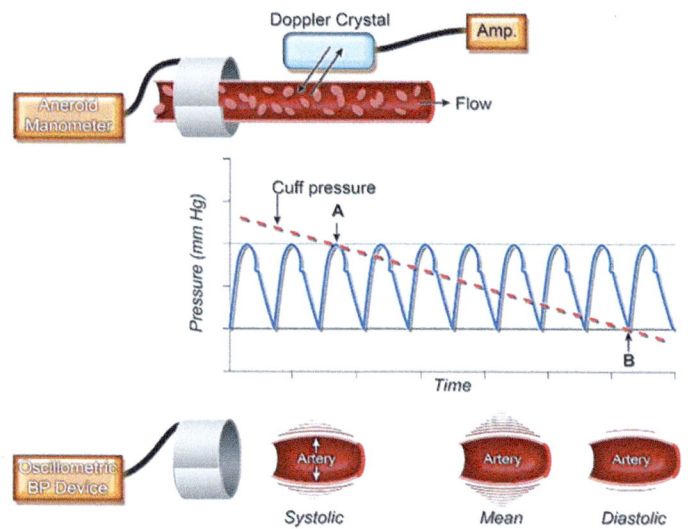

Figure 38.4 Schematic of commonly used noninvasive blood pressure (BP) measurement methods. Doppler method (top) uses the frequency shift between emitted and reflected ultrasound signals to detect return of arterial flow when compression from the occluding cuff falls to the level of systolic (A) BP. Oscillometric systems (bottom) use an automated method to detect characteristic oscillations in cuff pressure which originate from arterial wall oscillations that begin at systolic BP, are maximal at mean BP, and return to baseline at diastolic BP. During occluding cuff deflation, the system's microprocessor measures and averages arterial BP oscillations over several cardiac cycles. Some devices record the three separately; others measure mean arterial BP, then calculate systolic (A) and diastolic (B) pressures from this value using proprietary algorithms. In general, mean arterial BP – the average over the entire cardiac cycle – is most accurate with this method. At normal heart rates, mean arterial BP is about ~(1/3 × pulse pressure) + diastolic pressure.

awake dogs and cats are available (Brown, 2007). However, as noted previously, no devices have achieved an accuracy or reliability standard that would be acceptable for human BP determination. Moreover, differences in recorded BP in the same subject often occur between different technologies or instruments. Indirect BP methods use an inflatable cuff, placed around a limb or the tail, to occlude blood flow through the brachial, radial, saphenous, or the median caudal (or coccygeal) artery (**Figure 38.5**). Controlled release of cuff pressure is monitored to detect the return of flow through the artery. In the case of Doppler technology, the amplified audible Doppler shifts, caused by blood moving through the previously occluded artery, are recorded at the onset of systolic BP. With oscillometric methods, vibrations in the blood vessel wall (which vary at systolic, mean, and diastolic pressures) are detected by the microprocessor. Both techniques can yield measurements fairly well correlated with direct BP measurement, although different devices can produce different BP readings; yet even with reasonable correlations, there often is a wide bias (± deviation) from direct measurements. Indirect methods generally are more reliable in normotensive and hypertensive animals, and trends certainly are useful if methods are applied consistently. In conscious cats, greater correlation with direct BP measurement has been found using

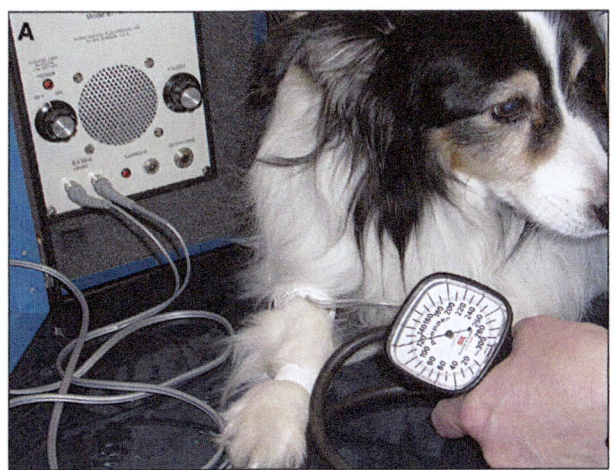
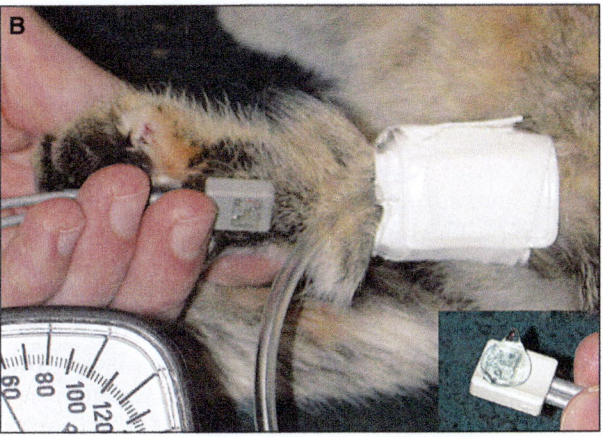
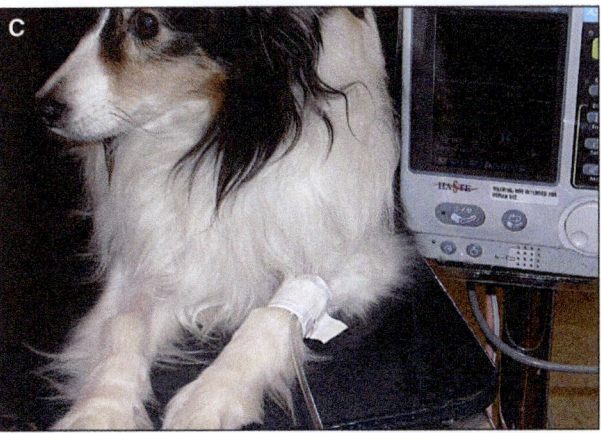

Figure 38.5 (A) Doppler method of indirect systolic blood pressure (BP) measurement in a dog. The ultrasonic probe is positioned over the palmer common digital artery so that a clear flow signal can be heard, then taped in place. The cuff (on the forearm over the radial artery) is inflated to occlude arterial flow, then slowly deflated to detect the pressure at which systolic flow recurs. (B) The Doppler flow probe can be held gently in position during BP measurement, as in this cat. It is important to shave the hair over the target artery and use sufficient ultrasonic coupling gel (inset) to achieve an air-free interface between the Doppler probe and skin. (C) Oscillometric method of indirect BP measurement using the radial artery in a dog.

the Doppler method for systolic BP, rather than the traditional oscillometric method, which tends to underestimate BP at higher levels. It sometimes is difficult or impossible to obtain BP measurements in cats with traditional oscillometric equipment. However, high definition oscillometry equipment can provide better results in cats. Only systolic BP values are thought to have acceptable accuracy, though (Taylor, 2017).

Other methods (such as auscultation and arterial palpation) are not recommended for BP estimation. The auscultatory method (used to detect Korotkoff sounds in people) is not technically feasible in dogs and cats, mainly because of limb conformation. Direct arterial palpation is not a reliable or accurate method to estimate BP, especially in hypertensive patients. This is because the perceived pulse strength depends on the pulse pressure (defined as systolic minus diastolic arterial pressure), not the absolute level of systolic or mean pressure. Pulse strength also is influenced by body conformation and other factors.

The most common causes of spurious BP readings are operator inexperience or technical error and patient anxiety. Consistent technique is important to minimize variability in BP measurements. Because surges in endogenous catecholamine release can rapidly raise BP, it is important to maintain a quiet and distraction-free environment away from other animals and clinic activity. It is important to allow time (at least 5–10 minutes) for patient acclimation and to use the least restraint possible. Sometimes it is helpful to have the owner present. The same trained person should obtain the measurements whenever possible. Allowing additional time for the patient to relax after cuff placement might help further reduce patient anxiety. Erroneously low BP readings also can occur; these could result from technical error during measurement, dehydration, or other factors.

The animal should be restrained gently and comfortably. Lateral (or sternal) recumbency often is used for dogs, so the cuff is close to right atrial level. For lateral recumbency, the nondependent limb is used for BP measurements. A sitting position also is used sometimes, but can produce poor repeatability and systematic overestimation of BP. For cats, using minimal restraint and allowing the animal to assume its position of choice can work well. Placing the cat on a towel or bedding from home, if available, can help reduce anxiety. The radial and coccygeal arteries commonly are used for BP measurement in cats. Many cats tolerate a cuff on the tail better than on either a fore- or rear limb. Systolic BP measurements from the tail might be slightly higher than from the limbs.

The technical skill and experience of the individual who obtains the BP measurements are integral to achieving consistent results. With indirect BP methods especially, the specific measurement protocol used can affect results. Whenever possible, and as a standard procedure, the same limb should be used to obtain BP measurements from animal to animal. It is especially important to use the same limb (or tail) and protocol for repeated measurements in the same patient.

Poor correlation between forelimb and hindlimb BP values has been shown for repeated within-dog BP measurements (Scansen, 2014). In a large cat study (Payne, 2017), although body position during BP recording did not affect results, the use of the right forelimb produced higher median BP readings than the left forelimb. The limb (artery) used, cuff size, and patient's body position all should be noted in the medical record so that the same conditions can be used for repeated measures. Heart rate is relevant, too; ideally, BP should be remeasured if tachycardia is present initially. It also is helpful to record the patient's demeanor during BP recording (for example: calm, anxious, uncooperative, aggressive, etc.).

The size of the occlusion cuff is important for accurate indirect BP measurement. The width of the inflatable balloon (bladder) within the cuff should be about 40% of the circumference of the extremity it encircles in dogs, 30–40% in cats, and 40(–60)% of the tail base in horses. The length of the balloon should cover at least 60% of this circumference. Some of the cuff inflation pressure goes toward tissue compression. Measurements using cuffs that are too narrow are more affected by this and produce falsely increased pressure readings. Cuffs that are too wide can cause BP underestimation. Human pediatric and infant size cuffs can be used in dogs and cats. It is important to note that the printed cuff "size" is not necessarily the cuff's width in cm. The cuff should encircle the limb snugly, but not be excessively tight. Common cuff locations are: midway between the elbow and carpus, in the tibial region, or at the base of the tail; skeletal prominences are avoided. Tape (not just velcro on the cuff) can be used to secure the cuff in position. This often is done to permit multiple uses of the cuff; however, cuff slippage during inflation should prompt replacement of what are (by design) disposable cuffs.

Cuff location in relation to the heart also is important. The cuff should be positioned at (or close to) the same height above the table or floor as the patient's right atrium, with the cuff bladder centered over the target artery. For oscillometric devices, the cuff area nearest the connector tubes often has an arrow or mark that should be centered over the artery for optimal system sensitivity. For animals in lateral recumbency, the sternum can be used to approximate right atrial (RA) level. For cats in sitting or sternal position, a distance of about 40% of the total length from sternum to dorsal spinous processes along the caudal edge of the scapula can be used to estimate RA level. In the standing horse, the vertical distance from the cuff at the tail head (coccygeal artery) down to RA level introduces greater error from hydrostatic effect than in small animals (**Figure 38.6**). Therefore, correction is made by measuring the vertical distance between RA level and the tail cuff in cm, multiplying this distance by a factor of 0.75 (to 0.77), and adding the resulting number (in mm Hg) to the measured BP.

Multiple BP measurements should be taken. The first measurement generally is discarded; then the average of at least 3 (ideally 5–7) consecutive measurements is used to increase accuracy. When readings differ widely from each other (by >20%), the cuff's placement should be readjusted and measurements repeated. If the BP readings are progressively declining during the measurement session, measures should be repeated until a plateau is achieved followed by 5–7 consistent and consecutive readings. On the other hand, if BP readings begin to increase during the measurement session, results must be interpreted within the specific patient's clinical context. Because patient anxiety can falsely increase BP, before definitively diagnosing HT high readings should be confirmed by repeated measurement at a later time, either on the same day or on separate occasions. The exception to this guideline occurs when there are clinical signs of target organ disease thought to be caused by HT. In these cases, antihypertensive therapy should be started immediately (p. 803).

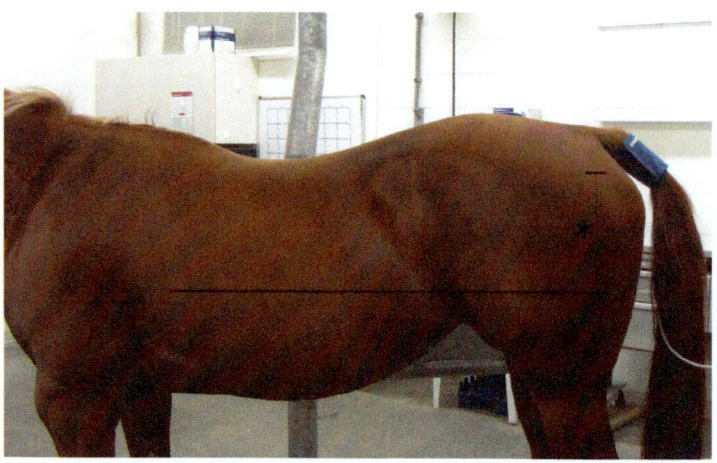

Figure 38.6 Indirect blood pressure (BP) measurement in the standing horse. The vertical distance (*) between right atrium and tail cuff is measured, multiplied by a correction factor, and the product added to the measured BP, to account for the hydrostatic effect of gravity (see text).

Several indirect BP measurement devices are available. Different devices and techniques can give disparate results, even in the same animal at the same measurement session. Because of this, BP measurement values obtained using different devices cannot be reliably compared. Therefore, consistency in the device, as well as measurement protocol, used is recommended, especially for repeated measurements in the same patient.

Doppler Method The Doppler method uses the change in frequency between emitted ultrasound and echoes reflected back from moving blood cells, or vessel wall, to detect blood flow in a superficial artery. This frequency change (the "Doppler shift") is in kilohertz and therefore within the audible range. The shifts are converted into an audible signal and amplified. Effective locations for pressure measurement include the palmer common digital (forelimb), median caudal (tail), and dorsal metatarsal arteries. One of the most commonly employed Doppler systems in animals (Ultrasonic Doppler Flow Detector, Parks Medical Electronics Inc.) has been used for over 4 decades in veterinary practice, but other vendors make similar devices. Some manufacturers have different sized ultrasound crystals; the smaller ones should be used in cats and small to medium dogs. The probe is placed over the artery, distal to the occluding cuff. If necessary, a small area of hair is shaved or wetted down where the probe is to be placed to optimize skin contact; clipping should be done if the signal acquisition is poor. Ultrasonic coupling gel (as opposed to alcohol) is applied to the flat Doppler flow probe to achieve an air-free interface with the skin. The probe is positioned so that a clear flow signal can be heard. The probe should be perpendicular to the target artery and not held so tightly as to occlude flow. The probe must be held still to minimize noise; it can be taped in place, especially for prolonged or repeated monitoring. A low volume setting on the Doppler unit helps minimize patient disturbance; alternatively, the operator can use headphones (which is especially useful for cats and horses). The flow-occluding cuff is attached to an aneroid sphygmomanometer and inflated to a pressure 20–30 mm Hg above where arterial flow stops and no audible signals can be heard. As the cuff is deflated slowly, by a few mm Hg/second, the return of blood cell motion produces characteristic flow signals during systole. The pressure at which pulsatile blood flow first recurs, indicated by brief "taps" or short "swishing" sounds, is the systolic pressure. The cuff should be completely deflated between measurements. Sometimes, a change in the flow sound from short and pulsatile to a longer, more continuous "swishing" can be detected as cuff pressure declines. The pressure at which this occurs approximates diastolic pressure; however, diastolic BP measurement is less accurate with this system because its determination is subjective. This change in flow sound might not be detectable, especially with small or stiff vessels. Although only systolic pressure is estimated reliably with the Doppler method, most animals with HT are thought to have elevated systolic BP, as opposed to isolated diastolic HT. It can be difficult to measure BP in small or hypotensive animals; Doppler methods might better approximate mean arterial BP in that setting. Patient movement also interferes with measurement.

Oscillometric Method The oscillometric method uses an automated system for detecting and processing oscillations in cuff pressure signals. Generally, oscillometric devices measure mean arterial pressure most accurately and some will calculate systolic and diastolic pressures from algorithms. Other devices might directly measure the changes in oscillations occurring from systolic through mean to diastolic BP. Accurate results depend on carefully following the instructions for use and holding the animal still. Studies in both dogs and horses indicate that oscillometric measurements track acceptably with direct (invasive) BP measurements, although they tend to slightly underestimate direct measurements. Mean arterial pressure readings correlate more precisely with direct measurements. Most correlative studies involve anesthetized or sedated animals and are not necessarily transferrable to all clinical situations, where greater differences between invasive and noninvasive techniques might be anticipated over the wide range of BPs and technical challenges. Experience suggests there is variability among devices from different manufacturers.

The flow occlusion cuff must be applied snugly so that oscillations are accurately detected. The cuff is inflated to a pressure above systolic pressure, then slowly deflated. The system's microprocessor measures, and averages over several heartbeats, the resulting pressure oscillations characteristic of systolic, diastolic, and/or mean pressures (depending on the system). The limb used to obtain BP readings should not be bearing weight, because muscle contraction can produce oscillations. At least 5 readings are obtained, the lowest and highest are discarded, and the remaining measurements are averaged. Effective use of the oscillometric method might be difficult in small dogs and cats, and underestimation of systolic BP is common. In horses, oscillometric BP measurements, especially mean pressure, usually approximate direct BP measurements closely. This assumes cuff placement at the tail base (cuff bladder width 40% of circumference), with the cuff bladder centered over the middle coccygeal artery. Hypotension produces larger discordance, however. Oscillometric BP readings are less likely to be accurate at slow heart rates, if arrhythmias are present, and when mean arterial pressure is less than 60 mm Hg. Again, correction should be made for the hydrostatic effect caused by difference in vertical distance between cuff and RA levels (p. 798).

Other Diagnostic Tests

Besides BP measurements, other tests are indicated to screen patients with suspected or confirmed HT for predisposing disease, as well as target organ damage. A thorough physical examination is important, including neurologic, cardiac, and ophthalmologic (with indirect ophthalmoscopy) evaluations.

Laboratory Tests

A routine hemogram, serum biochemical profile, and urinalysis with urine protein/creatinine ratio provide an initial laboratory database. Because hypertensive animals without overt azotemia or proteinuria still could have microalbuminuria, symmetric dimethylarginine (SDMA) testing can help identify early glomerular disease. Microalbuminuria was found in a majority of retired racing Greyhounds with systolic BP over 160 mm Hg, although serum biochemical tests were normal. Depending on the patient's physical findings and initial laboratory results, other tests that might be useful include endocrine function tests (especially T_4 measurement in older cats), radiography, abdominal ultrasonography, echocardiography, measurement of serum and urine ALD or catecholamine concentrations, measurement of GFR, electrocardiography (ECG), computed tomography (CT) or magnetic resonance imaging, or others.

Increases in certain biomarkers can occur with HT. Serum NT-proBNP concentration increases in cats with HT, especially when target organ disease is evident (Bijsmans, 2017). NT-proBNP usually decreases with antihypertensive therapy. Cardiac troponin I (cTnI), and vascular endothelial growth factor, also increase with HT. Elevated cTnI concentrations were identified in 70% of dogs and cats with renal failure, as well as in 70% of dogs with various systemic noncardiac disease (Porciello, 2008). However, cTnI was not specifically correlated with the degree of azotemia or HT, or type of noncardiac disease. Nevertheless, this suggests subclinical myocardial injury, although altered cTnI elimination cannot be excluded. In dogs with ischemic stroke, elevations in cTnI were noted, which also were associated with creatinine concentrations (Goncalves, 2020).

Radiography and Electrocardiography

Thoracic radiographs often indicate some degree of cardiomegaly in dogs and cats with chronic HT. Other findings reported in cats include a prominent aortic arch and an undulant (wavy) thoracic aorta (**Figures 38.7** and **38.8**). Aortic undulation was positively correlated with systolic BP, but not age in one feline study (Nelson, 2002). Nevertheless, although aortic dilation also is evident in some patients with HT, others with aortic dilation are normotensive; some of these findings might relate to geriatric variation or aortopathy. An interesting but unstudied point in companion animals is the impact of any aortic dilation on characteristic input impedance and compliance. Physiologically, a "stiffer" aorta augments systolic and reduces diastolic blood pressures. Increasing input impedance and reducing aortic compliance in canine models results in increased LV afterload and hypertrophy (Yamashita, 2019).

The ECG sometimes shows changes consistent with left atrial (LA) or LV enlargement in animals with HT, including left cranial axis deviation suggestive of concentric hypertrophy. However, this is not consistent. Arrhythmias are uncommon and could reflect underlying disease, rather than HT itself.

Echocardiography

Echocardiography might reveal mild to moderate LV hypertrophy (**Figures 38.9** and **38.10**). Severe LV thickening occurs uncommonly. The prediction limits for wall thicknesses in dogs and cats of different body sizes are quite wide, even within a specified weight. This likely leads to under-diagnosis of LV hypertrophy. Consequently, wall measurements are often within the normal range and the degree of hypertrophy does not correlate to individual BP measurements. Therefore, normal LV wall thickness does not rule out HT. Slightly over half of spontaneously hypertensive dogs had no overt LV hypertrophy in one study, although the dogs generally had LV wall thickness measurements somewhat above expected

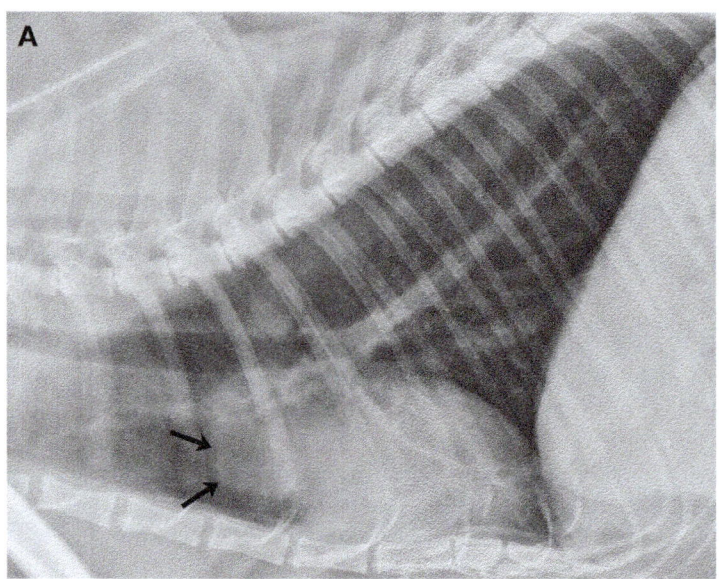

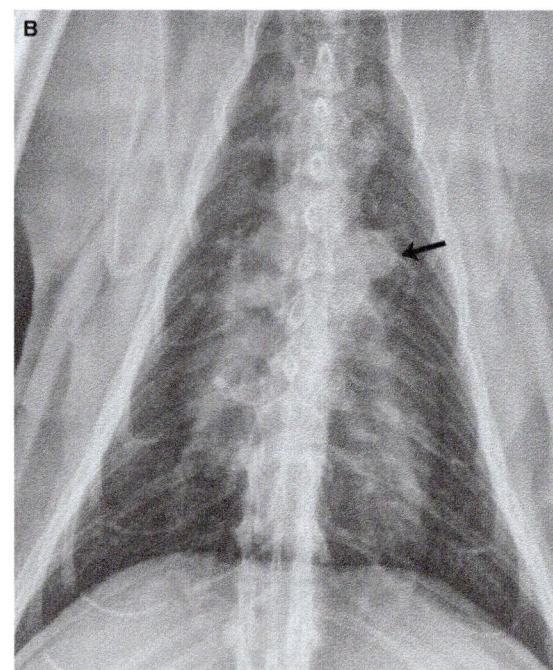

Figure 38.7 Thoracic radiographs from an 11-year-old female Domestic Shorthair cat with hypertension and a soft systolic murmur. (A) Lateral view shows a horizontal cardiac orientation, with a prominent bulge in the area of the ascending and arch aorta (arrows). There is mild cardiomegaly (VHS = 8.2v). (B) The aortic arch forms a knob-like projection (arrow) on DV view. A mild bronchial pattern also is present.

mean values, based on allometric scaling (Misbach, 2011). In addition, group means for LV wall and septal thicknesses were greater in hypertensive, compared to normal, dogs. In hypertensive dogs with LV concentric hypertrophy, a symmetrical pattern is most typical, although a few cases have septal thickness greater than LV free wall thickness. In hypertensive cats, LV wall and septal hypertrophy can appear symmetric or asymmetric, with variable patterns. Some degree

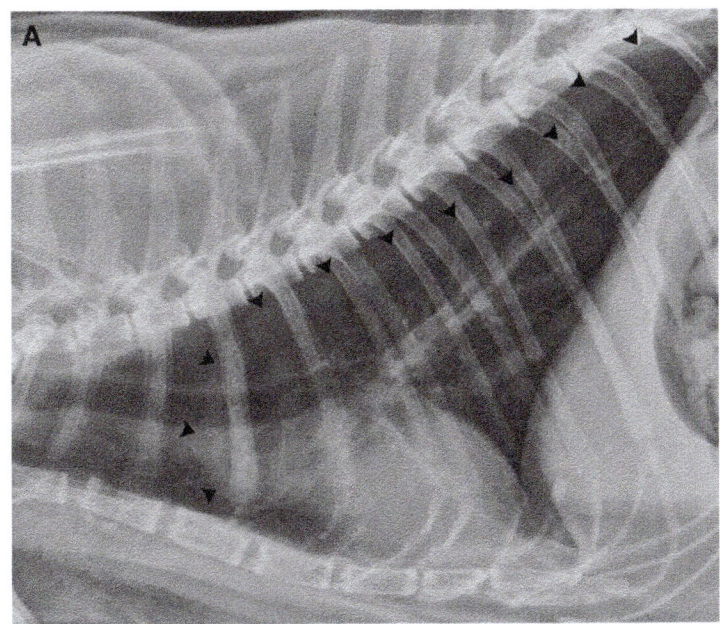

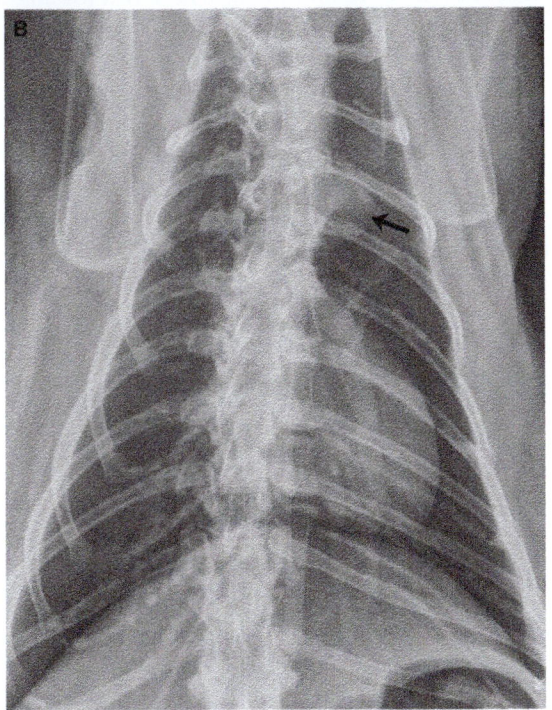

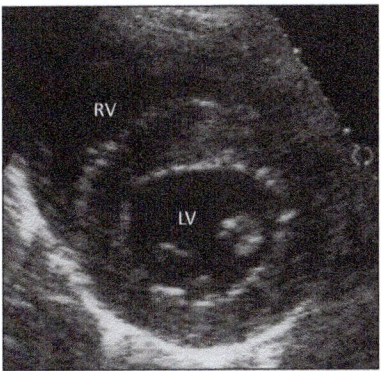

Figure 38.9 This 2D echo image in diastole from a 16-year-old female Domestic Shorthair cat with severe hypertension (BP >240 mm Hg) shows mild-moderate hypertrophy of the interventricular septum (7 mm) and left ventricular wall (6–7 mm). Right parasternal short-axis view. LV, left ventricle; RV, right ventricle.

LV chamber diameter typically is normal, although reduced lumen size is present in some hypertensive animals. Mild LA enlargement, sometimes associated with mitral regurgitation, has occurred in cats. In dogs, LA enlargement appears to be uncommon with HT. Aortic valve annulus diameter usually is normal, although the ascending aorta might be dilated (**Figures 38.11–38.13**). Correlation between ascending aortic diameter and systolic BP, but not age, is reported in cats, as it is in people. The ratio of proximal ascending aortic diameter to aortic valve annulus diameter is equal to or greater than 1.25 in most hypertensive cats, but not in healthy older cats (Nelson, 2002). Trivial or mild aortic insufficiency is more common in dogs than in cats; about a third of hypertensive dogs have some degree of aortic regurgitation. Hypertensive dogs with a systolic murmur usually have some degree of mitral regurgitation.

Subclinical reductions in LV systolic and diastolic function have been found with Doppler tissue imaging in hypertensive dogs and cats, with or without measurable LV hypertrophy. Abnormalities in diastolic function (Chapter 4) must

Figure 38.8 Lateral (A) and DV (B) thoracic radiographs from a 17-year-old male Siamese cat with chronic kidney disease, severe hypertension, and bilateral retinal detachment. The thoracic aorta is wavy (undulant). The cardiac silhouette has a horizontal orientation (A), but is of normal size; arrowheads indicate the dorsal border of the aorta. The aortic arch forms a prominent knob (arrow) on DV view (B). A gallop sound, but no cardiac murmur, was heard in this cat.

of LV wall and septal hypertrophy also is reported in horses with chronic hypertension. Dehydration can increase wall thickness (pseudohypertrophy) and is relevant to some of the causes of HT. This usually involves both ventricles and resolves with sufficient hydration.

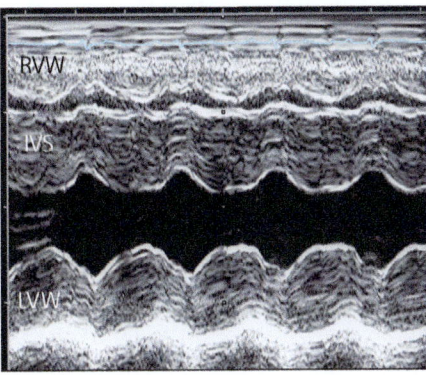

Figure 38.10 M-mode image at the ventricular level from a different 17-year-old cat with chronic hypertension shows mild hypertrophy of the LVW (6.5 mm) and IVS (6 mm). IVS, interventricular septum; LVW, left ventricular wall; RVW, right ventricular wall.

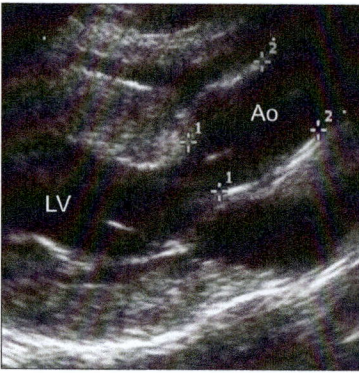

Figure 38.11 Right parasternal long-axis 2D image in diastole from a hypertensive cat shows widening of the ascending aorta (between measurement markers #2), compared with the aortic valve annulus (measurement markers #1). Moderate left ventricular hypertrophy also is present. Ao, aorta; LV, left ventricle. (Image courtesy of Dr OL Nelson.)

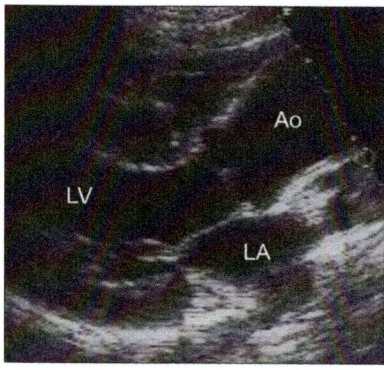

Figure 38.12 Marked dilation of the ascending aorta is evident in this echo image from the cat in **Figure 38.9**. Right parasternal long-axis, in diastole. Ao, aorta; LA, left atrium; LV, left ventricle.

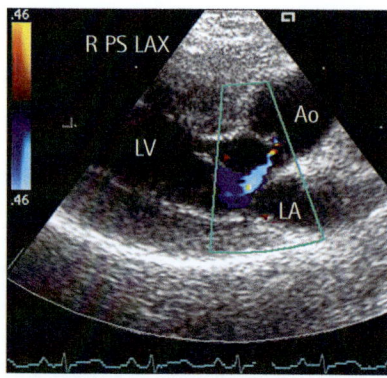

Figure 38.13 Mild aortic valve regurgitation is visible on color Doppler exam in the cat of **Figure 38.10**. Ao, aorta; LA, left atrium; LV, left ventricle.

be added to the estimated LA pressure (often ~8 mm Hg) to predict systolic aortic pressure. However, multiple confounding factors can affect the accuracy of this method and it is not considered a reliable means of BP determination (Tou, 2006).

Abdominal ultrasonography can be used to compare the diameter of the abdominal aorta with that of the caudal vena cava. Mean abdominal aorta/caudal vena cava ratio was about 1.52 in a group of 128 dogs with confirmed systemic HT; in contrast, the ratio was 1.03 in a comparison group of 18 normotensive dogs (Holland, 2020). In this study, the vessels were imaged longitudinally, cranial to the aortic trifurcation, and measured from outer (mural) border to outer border.

Management

The goal of antihypertensive therapy is to reduce the risk of further vascular and target organ damage. Ideally, successful medical therapy will decrease systolic BP to below 140 (–150) mm Hg (and diastolic BP to <95 mm Hg), where risk for target organ damage is minimal. To be considered "adequate," therapy should produce systolic BPs of no more than 159 mm Hg on recheck exams. Antihypertensive therapy should be intensified if systolic BP is over 160 mm Hg on recheck exam. However, if systolic BPs are under 120 mm Hg, accompanied by clinical signs of weakness, syncope or tachycardia, the antihypertensive drug dose(s) should be reduced as needed to normalize BP and relieve hypotension. Management of underlying or concurrent disease is important for all patients, and sometimes is sufficient to normalize BP. However, many cases also need antihypertensive drug therapy (**Figure 38.14**).

Decision to Treat

Animals with confirmed severe HT (previously called Risk Category IV), and those with clinical signs presumed to be caused by HT, clearly should be treated right away. BP often is over 200/110 mm Hg in these patients. Hypertensive emergencies (malignant HT), including sudden loss of vision, should be treated immediately and optimally, with intensive monitoring (p. 805). However, most hypertensive animals can be managed relatively conservatively. Gradual BP reduction over a period of weeks is thought to be safer for most animals with chronic HT. Vascular adaptations in cerebral autoregulatory mechanisms occur in response to sustained high BP; consequently, sudden BP reduction could adversely affect cerebral perfusion.

Whether all animals with mild or even moderate HT (systolic BP 160–179 mm Hg) derive clinical benefit from antihypertensive treatment is not necessarily clear. However, if there is evidence for target organ disease possibly caused by HT, treatment is initiated. Elevated BP in dogs with degenerative (myxomatous) mitral valve disease, or any animal with clinically relevant mitral or aortic valve insufficiency, generally should be treated to reduce LV afterload. This should help

be distinguished from age-related changes. Theoretically, spectral Doppler-derived peak mitral regurgitation velocity could be used to estimate systolic arterial BP by means of the Bernoulli relationship (pressure gradient = 4 × peak velocity^2); the calculated LV to LA pressure gradient would

Stepwise Approach to Antihypertensive Therapy

```
Establish need for antihypertensive treatment
                │
                ▼
     Institute first-line therapy
                │
                ▼
   Recheck BP in 7-10 days  ◄──────────────┐
   (or 1-3 days, if TOD present)           │
        │         │         │              │
        ▼         ▼         ▼              │
  Systolic BP  Systolic BP  Systolic BP    │
  <160 mmHg    <120 mmHg &  >160 mmHg      │
  (minimal     signs of                    │
  goal)        hypotension                 │
  <140 mmHg                                │
  (optimal                                 │
  goal)                                    │
    │            │            │            │
    ▼            ▼            ▼            │
  Continue     ↓Medication  ↑Medication    │
  therapy;     dosage       dosage or      │
  Recheck in                add another    │
  (1-)4 (or 6)              drug           │
  months,                                  │
  depending on                             │
  patient                                  │
  stability                                │
               └────────────┴──────────────┘
```

Figure 38.14 Guidelines for monitoring and adjusting antihypertensive therapy. (Adapted from ACVIM consensus statement guidelines; Acierno, 2018.) BP, blood pressure; TOD, target organ damage.

decrease the degree of valvular regurgitation. The decision to institute antihypertensive therapy for other animals with mildly to moderately elevated BP is based on the individual's clinical situation. Treatment decisions for individual patients also might be influenced by the ability to accurately measure BP, an owner's willingness or ability to commit to adequate follow-up and medication recommendations, or other factors. **Table 38.3** contains general guidelines for initiating antihypertensive therapy, based on both ACVIM and ISFM consensus guidelines (Taylor, 2017; Acierno, 2018).

Antihypertensive Strategies

Several drugs have been used as antihypertensive agents in dogs and cats (**Table 38.4**). Usually, one drug is prescribed at a time, starting at a low or moderate initial dose, depending on the severity of pressure elevation. The drugs most commonly used as antihypertensives are the ACE inhibitors, amlodipine, and angiotensin receptor blockers (ARBs). A beta-adrenergic blocker sometimes is used as adjunct therapy; alone it usually does not provide adequate BP control. Other drugs also might be indicated. More information about specific drugs is located below. One useful way to think of these drugs is as first-line, second-line, and third-line agents. The latter group is used uncommonly, either for refractory HT or for special situations such as pheochromocytoma or hyperthyroidism.

The initial agent of choice for dogs usually is an ACE inhibitor, typically enalapril or benazepril, although an ARB such as telmisartan could be considered instead. In dogs, amlodipine generally is not used as the sole antihypertensive

Table 38.3 Guidelines for Initiating Antihypertensive Therapy[a]

Immediate (Emergency) Antihypertensive Therapy Is Indicated When

- Acute or worsening TOD (especially ocular or neurologic, p. 793) is evident and systolic BP is ≥170–180 mm Hg, on even a single measurement session (p. 805 and **Table 38.5**).

Antihypertensive Therapy Is Indicated When

- Systolic BP is ≥170–180 mm Hg, measured on at least 2 separate occasions within a 1–2-week period (and "white coat"/situational hypertension is thought unlikely). Search for possible associated condition (**Table 38.2**) and institute plan for monitoring and reevaluation.
- Systolic BP is 160–170 mm Hg, measured on at least 2 separate occasions within a 4–8-week period, especially with evidence for TOD (p. 793). Search for possible associated condition and institute plan for monitoring and reevaluation.

Consider Antihypertensive Therapy Trial If

- Systolic BP is 140–159 mm Hg, measured on at least 2 separate occasions within a 4–8-week period, AND clear evidence of ocular or neurologic TOD is present. (However, if clinical signs do not respond to antihypertensive therapy as expected and systolic BP is <160 mm Hg, reassess the presumption of underlying HT and need for continued therapy by antihypertensive drug withdrawal, with repeated monitoring of BP and clinical signs.) Note: prehypertension generally is not treated, although increased BP monitoring frequency is recommended.

[a] Base decision to treat on carefully obtained BP measurements, as well as the individual patient's clinical situation.

Abbreviations: BP, blood pressure; HT, hypertension; TOD, target organ damage.

Table 38.4 Oral Antihypertensive Drugs[a]

Angiotensin Converting Enzyme Inhibitors
(also see Chapter 21)

- Enalapril
  - Dog: 0.5 mg/kg PO q12(–24)h
  - Cat: 0.5 mg/kg PO q(12–)24h
- Benazepril
  - Dog: 0.5 mg/kg PO q12–24h
  - Cat: 0.5 mg/kg PO q12–24h
  - Horse: 0.5 mg/kg PO q12-24h

Angiotensin Receptor Blockers

- Telmisartan
  - Dog: 1(–2?) mg/kg PO q24h
  - Cat: 1.5 mg/kg PO q12h for 14 days, then 2 mg/kg PO q24h; (if necessary, decrease dose by 0.5 mg/kg increments to minimum of 0.5 mg/kg q24h)
- Losartan
  - Dog: 0.5 mg/kg(?) PO q24h
- Irbesartan
  - Dog: 5 mg/kg(?) PO q24h

Calcium Channel-blocker

- Amlodipine
  - Dog: 0.1–0.25 (to 0.5) mg/kg PO q24(–12)h
  - Cat: 0.1–0.25(to 0.5) mg/kg PO q24h, or 0.625(–1.25) mg/cat q24(–12)h

Beta-adrenergic blockers (also see Chapter 24)

- Atenolol
  - Dog: 0.2–1.0 mg/kg PO q12h (start low)
  - Cat: 1–2 mg/kg PO q12h, or 6.25–12.5 mg/cat PO q12h
- Propranolol
  - Dog: 0.2–1.0 mg/kg PO q8(–12)h (start low)
  - Cat: 0.2–1.0 mg/kg PO q8–12h, or 2.5–5 mg/cat PO q8h

Alpha$_1$-adrenergic Blockers

- Phenoxybenzamine
  - Dog: 0.25 mg/kg PO q(8–)12h, or 0.5 mg/kg PO q24h
  - Cat: 0.25mg/kg or 2.5 mg/cat PO q(8–)12h, or 0.5 mg/kg PO q24h
- Prazosin
  - Dog: 0.05–0.2 mg/kg PO q8–12h, or 0.5–4 mg/dog PO q8-12h
  - Cat: 0.25–0.5 mg/cat PO q12–24h
  - Horse: Start at 5-10 mg per horse PO q12h (optimal dose unknown)

Direct Arteriolar Vasodilator

- Hydralazine (not usually for long-term therapy)
  - Dog: 0.25–2 (to 4) mg/kg PO q12h (start low)
  - Cat: 0.25–2 mg/kg PO q12h, or 2.5 mg/cat PO q12–24h

Aldosterone Antagonist

- Spironolactone
  - Dog: 1–2 mg/kg PO q12(–24h)
  - Cat: 1–2 mg/kg PO q(12–)24h

[a] See text for further information.

agent for mild to moderate HT, because it preferentially dilates the renal afferent arterioles and so can expose the glomerular capillaries to excessive pressure. It also could provoke RAAS activation. Amlodipine can be added to ACE inhibitor (or ARB) therapy, if needed; the combined effect should minimally affect glomerular capillary hydrostatic pressure. For dogs with severe HT (systolic BP >200 mm Hg), using the combination of a RAAS inhibitor (ACE inhibitor or ARB) with amlodipine is appropriate for initial therapy. Caution is advised in dogs that are dehydrated, because antihypertensive drug administration (especially RAAS inhibitors) could dramatically reduce GFR. Unless rapidly progressive target organ damage is evident, these animals should be rehydrated then reevaluated before antihypertensive therapy is administered.

For cats, the recommended first-line antihypertensive agent historically has been amlodipine. Telmisartan often is an effective alternative; however, telmisartan's efficacy against severe HT is uncertain, because so far it has been evaluated only in cats with mildly to moderately elevated BP (<190 to 200 mm Hg). Therapy with an ACE inhibitor alone tends to be less effective for BP control in cats, although drugs in this class (or an ARB) can be helpful as adjunct therapy with amlodipine to manage HT. In dehydrated cats, initiation of ACE inhibitor or ARB therapy could markedly decrease GFR, so such agent should be delayed until the animal is rehydrated and BP rechecked. When hyperthyroidism is the underlying cause of HT, atenolol (or another beta-blocker) can help reduce tachycardia or arrhythmias provoked by excessive thyroid hormone. This will lower BP; however, beta-blockers are third-line drugs and monotherapy with atenolol is less effective than amlodipine for controlling BP in hyperthyroid cats. Atenolol should probably be reserved as co-therapy with amlodipine or telmisartan for initial control of extreme sinus tachycardia or supraventricular tachyarrhythmias in this disease. It can be considered for longer-term co-therapy in cats unable to undergo radioactive iodine treatment and that do not tolerate methimazole or related compounds. Systemic HT in cats with hyperthyroidism and proteinuric renal disease could be treated first with an ARB or ACE inhibitor.

Other treatment approaches to HT might be employed for particular conditions. For example, spironolactone, as an ALD antagonist, would be appropriate for a cat with hyperaldosteronism. Nevertheless, another antihypertensive agent often is needed concurrently to control BP in these cases. Potassium supplementation should be given, as appropriate, and adrenalectomy pursued, if possible. For HT caused by pheochromocytoma, an alpha-adrenergic antagonist is used, with a beta-blocker added secondarily if needed for tachyarrhythmias. However, an additional antihypertensive agent also might be necessary to control BP. Horses with HT associated with hyperadrenocorticism (Cushing's disease) or metabolic syndrome should have their underlying disorder managed, as possible. Benazepril, if not contraindicated, can be used as antihypertensive therapy and if needed, prazosin can be considered for BP control. Management strategies for hypertensive emergencies are described below.

Adverse effects of antihypertensive therapy usually relate to hypotension. This generally is manifested by periods of lethargy, weakness, or ataxia. Reduced appetite might be another adverse effect. Additional adverse effects have been associated with specific agents (see below). If antihypertensive therapy should become unnecessary, the dosage should be gradually tapered before the drug is withdrawn. Rebound HT from sudden drug discontinuation is a concern, especially with beta- or alpha$_2$-blockers.

Several ancillary strategies have been used in conjunction with antihypertensive drug therapy. High-salt foods should be avoided. A diet moderately reduced in salt (for example, 0.22–0.25% sodium on a dry matter basis) sometimes is recommended; however, this alone is not expected to normalize BP. Neurohormonal activation and potassium excretion appear to increase in cats with renal dysfunction that are fed a low-sodium diet. Although in some cats, a high-salt diet might be involved in the development of HT, dietary salt intake generally does not affect BP in normal cats. Weight reduction typically is recommended for obese animals, yet this probably has minimal effect on BP. Drugs that can potentiate vasoconstriction (such as phenylpropanolamine, or other alpha$_1$- and alpha$_2$-adrenergic agonists) should be avoided. Glucocorticoids and progesterone derivatives also are to be avoided when possible, because steroid hormones can increase BP.

Monitoring Therapy The ability to monitor BP accurately is important when prescribing antihypertensive medications. Serial measurements are crucial for establishing effective therapy and avoiding hypotension. In nonemergency cases, outpatient BP monitoring can be done every 7 to 10 days to assess treatment efficacy (**Figure 38.14**). The dosage of the initial antihypertensive agent is increased within recommended guidelines if adequate BP control has not been achieved, or reduced if systolic BP is below 120 (especially if <110) mm Hg. It can take 2 or more weeks before a satisfactory BP is established. If the first agent is not sufficiently effective by itself, a second drug can be added. When control has been achieved, BP monitoring is repeated every 1–4 months, depending on patient stability. Recheck intervals could be extended to every 6 months for stable patients. Other tests are done as needed to monitor target organ status. It is important that owners understand the necessity of repeated monitoring and long-term medication. For hospitalized patients, especially those receiving fluid therapy or medications with cardiac or vascular effects, daily BP measurement is advised.

Some animals become refractory to therapy that initially was effective. An increased dosage, adjunctive therapy, or a change of antihypertensive drug can be tried. Continued attention to the underlying disease process also is important. Routine hemogram, serum biochemistry profile, urinalysis, and urine protein/creatinine ratio usually are recommended every 6 months. Other tests are done as appropriate for the individual patient. If proteinuria persists after BP is controlled, the addition (or increased dose) of an ACE inhibitor or ARB should be considered in the hope that further RAAS inhibition will reduce proteinuria. Decreasing severity of proteinuria is considered a positive sign.

Management of Hypertensive Emergencies Emergency antihypertensive therapy is indicated for animals with new or progressive signs caused by markedly high BP (**Table 38.5**). These include acute retinal detachment and ocular hemorrhage, encephalopathy or other evidence of intracranial hemorrhage, acute renal or heart failure, or aortic aneurysm. Treatment in a hospital with 24-hour critical care monitoring is advised. Based on recommendations for people, BP reduction should occur over a period of several (up to about 6) hours, with a systolic BP goal of 160 mm Hg. BP should be rechecked every 1–3 hours. During the first hour of emergency antihypertensive therapy, a decline in BP of about 10% is the goal; this is followed by an additional decrease of about 15% over the next few hours, and then a gradual return to normal BP (Acierno, 2018). BP should not be allowed to fall by over 20–25% during the first hour or two of treatment. Because of HT-induced autoregulatory adaptation, rapid and marked BP decreases could provoke ischemia in target organs.

A parenteral antihypertensive drug that can be titrated to effect provides better control for incrementally reducing BP. One choice, if available, is fenoldopam; this drug is a selective dopamine-1 receptor agonist that is used for human hypertensive emergencies. Fenoldopam increases renal vasodilation, natriuresis, and GFR in normal dogs. Although it has not been studied in acute hypertensive crisis in dogs or cats, it appears safe in animals with acute kidney injury. Fenoldopam has a short half-life in dogs and cats; effects dissipate within several minutes of drug discontinuation. Alternatively, other parenteral drugs that could be used IV for hypertensive emergency include the beta-blocker labetalol, or hydralazine or nitroprusside; although these three agents do not induce renal vasodilation like fenoldopam does (Acierno, 2018). Again, the capacity to provide accurate continuous IV infusion and BP monitoring, as well as intensive supportive care, is crucial. Hypotension can be a significant adverse effect. Other agents that have been used successfully in a hypertensive crisis include enalaprilat, other IV beta-blockers (such as esmolol or propranolol), and acepromazine. A parenteral drug could be used in combination with oral amlodipine or hydralazine, if BP has not been sufficiently reduced within 12 hours. After BP control has been achieved for 12–24 hours, oral antihypertensive therapy is begun (or continued) as the parenteral drug is titrated down, then discontinued.

Alternatively, oral antihypertensive drugs such as amlodipine or hydralazine could be effective for expedient BP reduction in a hypertensive emergency, with less risk of hypotension than with parenteral agents (**Table 38.5**). Oral therapy is especially appropriate for patients with BP classified as severely hypertensive, but without evidence for acute target organ disease, or when parenteral agents or appropriate

Table 38.5 Management Options for Hypertensive Crisis[a]

Parenteral Therapy Options[b]

- Fenoldopam
  - Dog: 0.1 mcg/kg/min IV CRI, to start; uptitrate q15 min, as needed based on systolic BP, by increments of 0.1 mcg/kg/min to maximum of 1.6 mcg/kg/min
  - Cat: Same?
- Labetolol
  - Dog: 0.25 mg/kg IV over 2 min (can repeat to total dose of 3.75 mg/kg, based on BP); follow with 25 mcg/kg/min CRI
  - Cat: Same?
- Esmolol
  - Dog: 25–75 (to 200) mcg/kg/min IV CRI
  - Cat: Same
- Propranolol
  - Dog: 0.02 (initial)–0.1 mg/kg slow IV q8–12h
  - Cat: 0.02 (initial)–0.06 mg/kg slow IV q8–12h
- Hydralazine
  - Dog: 0.1 mg/kg IV over 2 min, followed by 1.5–5 mcg/kg/min CRI; or can try 0.1–0.2 mg/kg IV or IM, repeat q2h as needed based on BP
  - Cat: 0.5 mg/cat SC, repeat after 15–30 min, to total dose of up to 2.5 mg, if necessary
- Nitroprusside
  - Dog: 1 mcg/kg/minute CRI (initial); increase q15 to 30 min, up to maximum of 15 mcg/kg/min IV CRI, if needed based on systolic BP
  - Cat: Same initial dose, up to 3 mcg/kg/min IV CRI
- Phentolamine (alpha-adrenergic blocker for pheochromocytoma-induced HT)
  - Dog: 0.1 mg/kg IV to start, followed by 1–2 mcg/kg/min CRI, as needed
  - Cat: Same?
- Enalaprilat
  - Dog: 0.2 mg/kg IV, repeated q1–2h as needed; or 0.1–1.0 mg/dog IV q6h, as needed
- Acepromazine
  - Dog: 0.05–0.1 mg/kg (up to 3 mg/kg total) IV
  - Cat: 0.01–0.05 (to 0.1) mg/cat IV or SC
- Nicardipine
  - Dog: 0.5–5 mcg/kg/min IV CRI
  - Cat:?

Intensive Oral Therapy Options

- Amlodipine (can dissolve in water and administer rectally, if PO not possible)
  - Dog: 0.25 mg/kg PO initial dose; repeat as needed q1–3h until systolic BP is 140–160 mm Hg, up to total dose of 1 mg/kg/day (see text, p. 806). OR, 0.2–0.4 (up to 0.6) mg/kg PO q24h
  - Cat: 0.1–0.25 mg/kg PO, can repeat after 4–8 hours if needed, up to total of 0.6(–1) mg/cat within first 24 hours. OR, 0.2–0.4 (up to 0.6) mg/kg PO q24h
- Hydralazine
  - Dog: 0.5–2 mg/kg PO q12h, titrate up to effect
  - Cat: 0.25–2 mg/kg PO q12h, titrate up to effect
- Prazosin (see **Table 38.4**)
- Acepromazine
  - Dog & Cat: 0.5–2 mg/kg PO q8h

[a] See text for further information.
[b] Continuous BP monitoring (ideally by arterial catheterization) strongly recommended with use of parenteral antihypertensive medication.
Abbreviations: BP, blood pressure; CRI, constant rate infusion; HT, hypertension.

monitoring are not available. An amlodipine protocol that could effectively reduce BP within several hours in dogs with severe HT was reported (Geigy, 2011). This uses an initial amlodipine dose of 0.25 mg/kg, which is repeated every 1–3 hours until systolic BP is between 140 and 160 mm Hg, or to a maximum dose of 1 mg/kg/day. However, if systolic BP falls by 20 mm Hg or more between doses, the next dose should be postponed for 2 hours. The 24-hour cumulative dose needed for initial control and the patient's BP response guide subsequent therapy. Although amlodipine is an oral drug, for patients with persistent vomiting, the same doses can be dissolved in water and administered rectally. Some dogs require a second antihypertensive drug; in these cases, combination with an ACE inhibitor or ARB is suggested. For cats, oral amlodipine might be preferable to parenteral therapy because the risk of hypotension is less. Whether telmisartan might be effective for acute treatment of severe HT is uncertain; studies in cats with systolic BP >200 mm Hg are needed. Oral hydralazine also could be effective in dogs, as an alternative to amlodipine (**Table 38.5**, and p. 323). In addition, hydralazine has been administered SC in cats for acute HT. Following initial BP stabilization, long-term oral therapy can be started. Frequent BP monitoring is important, especially in animals with rapidly progressive signs. Horses with high BP can respond to incremental doses of the alpha-1 antagonist, prazosin. This drug has been used for urine retention in this species. The authors have limited experience with it in horses with HT related to hyperadrenocorticism.

For hypertensive crisis caused by catecholamine excess (as with pheochromocytoma), the alpha-adrenergic blocker phentolamine can be given by initial IV bolus, followed by an infusion titrated to effect (**Table 38.5**). A beta-blocker also might be indicated for pheochromocytoma-induced tachyarrhythmias. However, it should not be used alone or before a nonselective or selective alpha$_1$-blocker is administered, to avoid exacerbation of hypertension by unopposed alpha$_1$-receptors. Selective alpha$_2$-blockers (such as clonidine) are contraindicated. Antihypertensive treatment for 2–3 weeks prior to surgery for pheochromocytoma excision is recommended. For inoperable pheochromocytoma, long-term antihypertensive therapy is advised to avoid hypertensive emergencies.

Prognosis Because most cases of HT are associated with severe and progressive underlying disease, the long-term prognosis often is guarded despite apparent response to antihypertensive drugs. Even when underlying disease has been well-managed, HT can persist, especially in dogs with hyperadrenocorticism and cats with hyperthyroidism. However, proactive BP monitoring and attention to management goals are likely to reduce HT-associated damage. Some primary disease treatments can exacerbate HT, including fluid therapy, corticosteroids, and erythropoietin. High BP has been associated with shorter survival time in animals with chronic kidney disease. The severity of proteinuria is a negative prognostic indicator. Cats with the most severe HT are likely to have the greatest degree of proteinuria. A median survival time of about 15 months was noted for cats without proteinuria at diagnosis; however, it was less than 6 months for cats with proteinuria (Jepson, 2007). Telmisartan is more likely to reduce proteinuria than amlodipine. The degree of BP control itself does not seem to be correlated with survival in cats. In dogs with chronic renal failure, HT and marked proteinuria also are associated with shorter survival time (Wehner, 2008).

Antihypertensive Agents

Angiotensin Converting Enzyme Inhibitors

The ACE inhibitors (enalapril, benazepril, and others) diminish AngII production, thereby reducing RAAS-related systemic vascular resistance and volume retention (p. 320 and **Figure 21.2**, p. 321). Concurrent increase in bradykinin levels are thought to contribute, as well. These agents have been more effective in hypertensive dogs, although their effect would be dependent on the degree of RAAS activation. The effectiveness of these drugs is greater in animals with increased RAAS activation and with proteinuric renal disease (glomerular hypertension). Otherwise, they have relatively weak vasodilating effect. For optimal RAAS suppression in dogs, every 12 hour dosing is recommended; once daily dosing is thought adequate in cats. If BP control is not adequate at 0.5 mg/kg PO q12h in dogs, (q24h in cats), further dosage increase probably will not increase effectiveness. In these cases, amlodipine usually is added.

ACE inhibitors generally are well-tolerated. However, some animals develop gastrointestinal (GI) upset, electrolyte disturbances or hypotension. Animals with chronic kidney disease could experience worsening azotemia related to reduced GFR caused by drug-induced efferent arteriolar dilation. Rarely, a dry cough might occur; although this is not well-documented in animals, it is a known adverse effect in people and thought to be induced by bradykinin.

Hypertensive cats with chronic renal failure typically are inadequately responsive to ACE inhibitors, either long-term or initially, although benazepril can reduce BP in some. Reduced renin activity has been shown in some cats with end-stage renal disease. Nevertheless, an ACE inhibitor might help protect against hypertensive renal damage; however, the ARB, telmisartan, appears more efficacious (see next section). Because AngII preferentially constricts renal efferent arterioles, ACE inhibitors (and ARBs) tend to produce greater dilation of efferent rather than afferent arterioles. As long as adequate GFR is maintained, the reduction in glomerular hypertension can especially benefit animals with renal disease. This benefit might be realized even without substantial reduction in systemic BP. ACE inhibitors can reduce proteinuria and slow the progression of renal disease. ACE inhibitors might also inhibit growth factors associated with intrarenal Ang formation that promote glomerular hypertrophy and sclerosis.

There is little information about use of ACE inhibitors for HT in horses. In normal horses, oral benazepril (at 0.5 mg/kg) reduced serum ACE activity by over 70%, and minimized exercise-induced rise in systolic and diastolic BP at about 1.5 hours postdose (Munoz, 2016). In contrast, enalapril had minimal effect on ACE activity and exercise-induced BP increases. The effects of ramipril and quinapril were intermediate.

Angiotensin Receptor Blockers

The ARB drugs block Ang type-1 receptors (Ang1R), displacing AngII and thereby blocking its effects of vasoconstriction, sympathetic activation, ALD release, and renal sodium retention. An increase in ACE2 activity and Ang1-7 formation also could augment ARB efficacy (p. 305). Like ACE inhibitors, ARBs preferentially dilate glomerular efferent arterioles and thereby decrease intraglomerular pressure. Although this reduces proteinuria, it also could decrease GFR and exacerbate azotemia. ARBs can decrease peripheral vascular resistance in a dose-dependent manner without substantial change in heart rate or cardiac output.

Veterinary clinical experience with ARBs is growing. Losartan, telmisartan, and irbesartan have been used in dogs. In healthy Beagles, irbesartan produced a significant reduction in systolic BP at 5 mg/kg; there was no direct correlation between BP and plasma concentration. Telmisartan also has reduced BP in dogs with proteinuric kidney disease. Telmisartan is increasingly being used in hypertensive cats. The drug is licensed for this purpose in the United States and Europe (Semintra, Boehringer-Ingelheim Vetmedica).

Telmisartan In normal cats, telmisartan (at 3 mg/kg) provided an antihypertensive effect against AngI challenge more effectively than irbesartan and benazepril, even at

24 hours post dose; however, losartan did not (Jenkins, 2015). In another study involving healthy cats, telmisartan, at a total daily dose of 1–3 mg/kg (either as single dose, or split into two equal doses q12h), was shown to be well-tolerated and to produce BP reduction for up to 2 days following the last dose (Coleman, 2019b). In normal fasted cats, peak plasma concentration is reached in about 30 min; terminal elimination half-life is about 8 hours. Telmisartan is metabolized by hepatic glucaronidation in both cats and dogs. Some cats experience hypersalivation shortly after telmisartan administration. Other potential adverse effects could include vomiting, diarrhea, reduced appetite, weight loss, and lethargy.

A prospective multicenter placebo-controlled study in cats showed telmisartan (2 mg/kg/day) reduced systolic BP at 2 and 4 weeks by about 20 mm Hg; over half of the treated cats reached the target BP of <150 mm Hg by 4 weeks, although cats with severe HT (BP >200 mm Hg) or overt ocular or neurologic signs were excluded from study (Glaus, 2019). Another prospective, double-blind study in cats with systolic BPs between 160 and 200 mm Hg also showed that telmisartan (1.5 mg/kg PO q12h for 2 weeks, then at 2 mg/kg PO q24h) produced a clinically relevant (mean ~23 mm Hg) decrease in systolic BP after 2 weeks of treatment (Coleman, 2019a). The decrease was sustained at 1 and 6 months, during an extended trial period. Over half of the telmisartan-treated cats "responded", with systolic BPs decreasing to below 150 mm Hg, or by at least 15% of baseline. Additionally, cats with the highest BPs (~180–200 mm Hg) at study entry experienced a greater decrease in BP with telmisartan, compared to cats with a lower entry BP (~160–179 mm Hg). This suggests the drug might be more efficacious in cats with even higher BPs. Telmisartan was well-tolerated in these (mostly) geriatric cats, including those with chronic kidney disease (IRIS stages 1–3). However, about 20% of the telmisartan-treated cats did not respond adequately by the 2 week recheck and needed other antihypertensive therapy because of persistent HT (BP >180 mm Hg). About 13% of the cats required a reduction in the telmisartan study dose because of a systolic BP below 120 mm Hg; a few developed hypotension and were removed from the study.

RAAS activation has been identified in some hypertensive cats with kidney disease or hyperthyroidism, and some with idiopathic HT. However, the relative importance of RAAS activation in feline HT appears inconsistent. The effectiveness of telmisartan in the majority of cats in this study supports a mechanism of RAAS involvement in at least some cats with HT. Drugs that oppose RAAS activation can have a protective effect on the kidneys by their ability to reduce intraglomerular pressure and proteinuria. By directly blocking Ang1R, telmisartan leaves Ang2R unopposed, as well as circumventing the effects of AngII produced by ACE-independent pathways. This could explain why it has efficacy in feline HT, when benazepril monotherapy generally does not. Telmisartan also reduces proteinuria to a greater degree than benazepril in cats with renal dysfunction (Sent, 2015). The concurrent use of an ACE and an ARB is not advised. Combined therapy of telmisartan (or an ACE inhibitor) with amlodipine appears to be well tolerated in the few cats where it was studied.

Amlodipine

Calcium channel blocking drugs, as a group, decrease free Ca^{++} concentration in arteriolar and cardiac muscle cells, resulting in vasodilation and reduced cardiac output (p. 324 and p. 384). Amlodipine besylate is a long-acting dihydropyridine blocker of L-type calcium channels in vascular smooth muscle. It has vasodilating effects, without appreciable cardiac effects. Amlodipine dilates the glomerular afferent arterioles and can thereby act synergistically with an ACE inhibitor or ARB to reduce glomerular hypertension. The drug's gradual onset and offset of action relate to relatively slow binding and dissociation from its receptors. Amlodipine plasma concentration correlates directly to the dose administered. Amlodipine tablets are difficult to split evenly; however, the drug can be compounded. Transdermal amlodipine delivery appears less effective than oral, although improvements in formulation or dosing might be developed.

Adverse events, including systemic hypotension, are uncommon; however, BP monitoring is recommended. Gingival hyperplasia has occurred in dogs (**Figure 38.15**), and sporadically in cats, treated with amlodipine over several months. This adverse effect also is well-recognized in people; its pathogenesis is unclear. The hyperplasia usually recedes after drug discontinuation, although surgical removal of the overgrown tissue might be needed. Diffuse peripheral edema is another rare adverse reaction to amlodipine reported in dogs.

Amlodipine is effective as a single agent in the majority of hypertensive cats, with BP reductions of about 30–70 mm Hg reported. Peak serum concentrations of amlodipine occur in 3–6 hours, with maximal effect after a single oral dose in

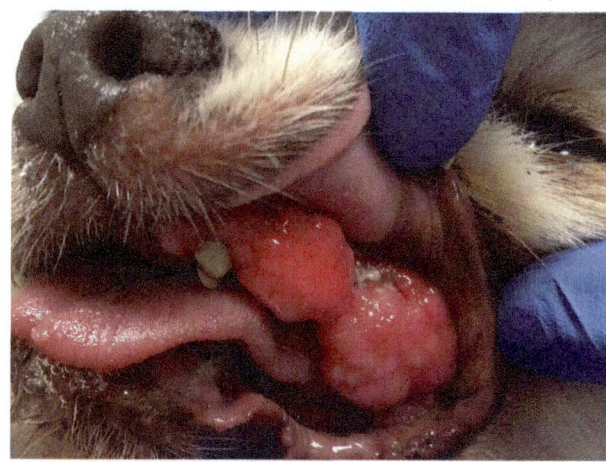

Figure 38.15 Severe gingival hyperplasia developed after ~2½ years of amlodipine therapy in a 12-year-old male Pomeranian-mix with well-managed systemic arterial hypertension and stage B2 myxomatous mitral valve disease. Amlodipine was prescribed because enalapril monotherapy did not provide adequate blood pressure control.

4–6 hours. Amlodipine's effect on BP lasts up to 30 hours, so once daily dosing is adequate in most cats (**Table 38.4**). It can be given with or without food. Intercat differences in amlodipine pharmacokinetics do not appear to influence the antihypertensive response. The drug generally does not affect serum creatinine concentration in cats with chronic renal failure. Mild reductions in serum K^+ concentration respond to oral potassium supplementation. RAAS activation with amlodipine could occur in cats, although this has not been fully studied in this species. The usual starting dose in cats is 0.625 mg/cat (~0.125 mg/kg) q24h. If adequate BP control is not achieved within 3 weeks, the dose can be doubled. However, BP reduction appears to be dose related, so for severely hypertensive cats (systolic BP >200 mm Hg) an initial amlodipine dose of 1.25 mg/cat (~0.25 mg/kg) q24h could be more effective. Rarely, an even higher dose might be needed (2.5 mg/cat q24h). However, it is especially important to carefully minimize patient anxiety while rechecking BP and verify medication compliance before any dosage increase. If HT cannot be controlled adequately with amlodipine alone, an ACE inhibitor or telmisartan can be added; alternatively, telmisartan alone might be effective. Amlodipine has reduced proteinuria in hypertensive cats with kidney disease.

In dogs, amlodipine is a useful adjunct if ACE inhibitor (or ARB) therapy does not sufficiently control BP. Amlodipine is added at a low initial dose and titrated upward, as needed. The combined effect of these agents produces both afferent and efferent renal arteriolar dilation, which helps balance glomerular pressure and GFR. The half-life of amlodipine is about 30 hours in dogs; maximal effect is not reached until 4–7 days after starting therapy. Amlodipine's bioavailability is high. Plasma concentrations peak in 3–8 hours postdose and increase with chronic therapy, because of the long half-life. The drug is metabolized in the liver. Caution is warranted when liver function is poor. First-pass elimination is not extensive. The drug is excreted through the urine and feces.

Concerns about using amlodipine alone for chronic HT treatment in dogs relate to its propensity to cause RAAS activation. Also, kidney damage could possibly be accelerated because amlodipine's preferential afferent arteriolar dilation could cause glomerular hypertension, although reduction in systemic BP might protect against this. On the other hand, at least in dogs with acute kidney injury, there also are concerns about using ACE inhibitors alone because their efferent arteriolar dilation could reduce GFR. Combination therapy with amlodipine and an ACE inhibitor, therefore, would appear to provide a balanced effect on glomerular pressure and GFR. Nevertheless, amlodipine can be useful for in-hospital treatment of severe HT in dogs (p. 805 and **Table 38.5**).

Other Drugs

A beta-blocker might be useful for adjunctive antihypertensive therapy by reducing heart rate, cardiac output, and renal renin release. Atenolol and propranolol have been used most often (p. 379). Yet, atenolol does not significantly decrease BP in normotensive cats and beta-blocker monotherapy generally is ineffective for treating HT in cats with renal disease. For cats with hyperthyroidism, a beta-adrenergic blocker (particularly atenolol) often is recommended to manage tachycardia and HT. Increased sympathetic nervous activity or responsiveness could contribute to HT in this disease. Also, beta-blockers can inhibit peripheral conversion of T_4 to active T_3. Nevertheless, while atenolol monotherapy (at 1–2 mg/kg q12h) does significantly reduce both systolic BP and heart rate in hyperthyroid cats with HT, it appears to reduce BP by only about 15 mm Hg. Therefore, most of these cats require an additional drug to adequately control HT.

A diuretic (thiazide or furosemide; p. 317) theoretically might help by reducing blood volume and sodium content; however, a diuretic alone rarely is effective for reducing HT in companion animals. In azotemic patients, diuretics should be avoided, or used only with great caution. It is important to monitor serum potassium concentration, especially in cats with chronic renal disease.

Spironolactone (p. 319), as an ALD antagonist, could help control HT in animals with hyperaldosteronism. Not only does ALD regulate sodium and potassium balance, it also has proinflammatory and profibrotic effects that contribute to vasoconstriction, vascular remodeling, and endothelial dysfunction. Spironolactone's efficacy is questionable with other causes of HT.

$Alpha_1$-adrenergic antagonists reduce peripheral vascular resistance by opposing the vasoconstrictive effects mediated by these adrenergic receptors. These agents are used primarily to treat HT caused by pheochromocytoma. Phenoxybenzamine is a noncompetitive $alpha_1$- and $alpha_2$-receptor blocker used for pheochromocytoma-induced HT (**Table 38.4**). Initially, a low dose is administered, with upward titration as necessary. Prazosin is another oral $alpha_1$-blocker that could be used for pheochromocytoma when another alpha-blocker is unavailable. A beta-blocker can be added as adjunctive therapy to help control tachycardia and arrhythmias after the $alpha_1$-blocker is initiated. However, with pheochromocytoma, a beta-blocker should not be used alone or prior to alpha-blockade, because leaving $alpha_1$-receptors unopposed is likely to exacerbate HT. Prazosin also could be used as a 3rd- or 4th-line drug for refractory HT in small animals. In horses with systemic HT related to equine Cushing's like syndrome, prazosin has been observed to exert an antihypertensive effect. The potential effects of this drug on BP also should be considered when it is prescribed to reduce urethral sphincter tone.

Hydralazine (p. 323) is an arteriolar dilator that acts by increasing endothelial nitric oxide synthesis. It can be effective in hypertensive crisis; however, it generally is not used for chronic therapy, especially in patients with kidney disease. Hydralazine can provoke reflex tachycardia, sodium retention, and marked hypotension; other side effects can include GI upset. Sodium nitroprusside (p. 324) is a powerful arteriolar and venodilator that sometimes is used for hypertensive crisis (**Table 38.5**). Nitroprusside stimulates nitric oxide release, which leads to cyclic guanine monophosphate-mediated inhibition of calcium influx and results in vascular smooth muscle relaxation. Because it can cause severe hypotension, nitroprusside should only be used with close BP monitoring. Prolonged infusion of nitroprusside, especially in patients with renal or hepatic insufficiency, could potentially cause cyanide toxicity. Other injectable agents that occasionally are used for hypertensive crisis include enalaprilat (an ACE inhibitor), nicardipine (a calcium channel blocker), and fenoldopam (a dopamine type-1 receptor agonist).

Suggested Additional Reading and References

Also See Online Comprehensive Bibliography at: https://www.routledge.com/9781482246223.

Acierno MJ, Brown S, Coleman AE, et al. ACVIM consensus statement: guidelines for the identification, evaluation, and management of systemic hypertension in dogs and cats. J Vet Intern Med 2018; 32:1803–1822.

Bailey SR, Habershon-Butcher JL, Ransom KJ, et al. Hypertension and insulin resistance in a mixed-breed population of ponies predisposed to laminitis. Am J Vet Res 2008;69:122–129.

Bijsmans ES, Doig M, Jepson RE, et al. Factors influencing the relationship between the dose of amlodipine required for blood pressure control and change in blood pressure in hypertensive cats. J Vet Intern Med 2016;30:1630–1636.

Bijsmans ES, Jepson RE, Chang YM, et al. Changes in systolic blood pressure over time in healthy cats and cats with chronic kidney disease. J Vet Intern Med 2015;29:855–861.

Bijsmans ES, Jepson RE, Wheeler C, et al. Plasma N-terminal pro-brain natriuretic peptide, vascular endothelial growth factor, and cardiac troponin I as novel biomarkers of hypertensive disease and target organ damage in cats. J Vet Intern Med 2017;31:650–660.

Brown S, Atkins C, Bagley R, et al. Guidelines for the identification, evaluation, and management of systemic hypertension in dogs and cats. J Vet Intern Med 2007;21:542–558.

Buranakarl C, Ankanaporn K, Thammacharoen S, et al. Relationships between degree of azotaemia and blood pressure, urinary protein:creatinine ratio and fractional excretion of electrolytes in dogs with renal azotaemia. Vet Res Commun 2007;31:245–257.

Cannon MJ, Brett J. Comparison of how well conscious cats tolerate blood pressure measurement from the radial and coccygeal arteries. J Feline Med Surg 2012;14:906–909.

Carlucci L, Song KH, Yun HI, et al. Pharmacokinetics and pharmacodynamics (PK/PD) of irbesartan in Beagle dogs after oral administration at two dose rates. Pol J Vet Sci 2013;16:555–561.

Carter J. Hypertensive ocular disease in cats: a guide to fundic lesions to facilitate early diagnosis. J Feline Med Surg 2019;21:35–45.

Carter JM, Irving AC, Bridges JP, et al. The prevalence of ocular lesions associated with hypertension in a population of geriatric cats in Auckland, New Zealand. N Z Vet J 2014;62:21–29.

Cerna P, Archontakis PE, Cheuk HO, et al. Comparison of Doppler ultrasonic and oscillometric devices (with or without proprietary optimisations) for non-invasive blood pressure measurement in conscious cats. J Feline Med Surg 2021;23:121–130.

Cole LP, Jepson R, Dawson C, et al. Hypertension, retinopathy, and acute kidney injury in dogs: A prospective study. J Vet Intern Med 2020;34:1940–1947.

Cole L, Jepson R, Humm K. Systemic hypertension in cats with acute kidney injury. J Small Anim Pract 2017;58:577–581.

Coleman AE, Brown SA, Traas AM, et al. Safety and efficacy of orally administered telmisartan for the treatment of systemic hypertension in cats: results of a double-blind, placebo-controlled, randomized clinical trial. J Vet Intern Med 2019a; 33:478–488.

Coleman AE, Brown SA, Stark M, et al. Evaluation of orally administered telmisartan for the reduction of indirect systolic arterial blood pressure in awake, clinically normal cats. J Feline Med Surg 2019b;21:109–114.

Conroy M, Chang YM, Brodbelt D, et al. Survival after diagnosis of hypertension in cats attending primary care practice in the United Kingdom. J Vet Intern Med 2018;32:1846–1855.

Cortadellas O, del Palacio MJ, Bayon A, et al. Systemic hypertension in dogs with leishmaniasis: prevalence and clinical consequences. J Vet Intern Med 2006;20:941–947.

Daniel G, Mahony OM, Markovich JE, et al. Clinical findings, diagnostics and outcome in 33 cats with adrenal neoplasia (2002–2013). J Feline Med Surg 2016;18:77–84.

Djajadiningrat-Laanen S, Galac S, Kooistra H. Primary hyperaldosteronism: expanding the diagnostic net. J Feline Med Surg 2011;13:641–650.

Ebner T, Schanzle G, Weber W, et al. In vitro glucuronidation of the angiotensin II receptor antagonist telmisartan in the cat: a comparison with other species. J Vet Pharmacol Ther 2013;36:154–160.

Elliott J, Barber PJ, Syme HM, et al. Feline hypertension: clinical findings and response to antihypertensive treatment in 30 cases. J Small Anim Pract 2001;42:122–129.

Finch NC, Syme HM, Elliott J. Association of urinary cadmium excretion with feline hypertension. Vet Rec 2012;170:125.

Garosi L, McConnell JE, Platt SR, et al. Results of diagnostic investigations and long-term outcome of 33 dogs with brain infarction (2000–2004). J Vet Intern Med 2005;19:725–731.

Geigy CA, Schweighauser A, Doherr M, et al. Occurrence of systemic hypertension in dogs with acute kidney injury and treatment with amlodipine besylate. J Small Anim Pract 2011;52:340–346.

Glaus TM, Elliott J, Herberich E, et al. Efficacy of long-term oral telmisartan treatment in cats with hypertension: results of a prospective European clinical trial. J Vet Intern Med 2019;33:413–422.

Goncalves R, Sanchez-Masian D, Maddox TW, et al. Preliminary investigation of serum cardiac troponin I in dogs with acute ischaemic stroke. J Small Anim Pract 2020;61:93–100.

Green BA, Frank EL Comparison of plasma free metanephrines between healthy dogs and 3 dogs with pheochromocytoma. Vet Clin Pathol 2013;42:499–503.

Guyenet PG. The sympathetic control of blood pressure. Nat Rev Neurosci 2006;7:335–346.

Heliczer N, Lorello O, Casoni D, et al. Accuracy and precision of noninvasive blood pressure in normo-, hyper-, and hypotensive standing and anesthetized adult horses. J Vet Intern Med 2016;30:866–872.

Helms SR. Treatment of feline hypertension with transdermal amlodipine: a pilot study. J Am Anim Hosp Assoc 2007;43:149–156.

Herring IP, Panciera DL, Werre SR. Longitudinal prevalence of hypertension, proteinuria, and retinopathy in dogs with spontaneous diabetes mellitus. J Vet Intern Med 2014;28:488–495.

Hoareau GL, Jourdan G, Mellema M, et al. Evaluation of arterial blood gases and arterial blood pressures in brachycephalic dogs. J Vet Intern Med 2012;26:897–904.

Holland M, Hudson J, Bao Y, et al. Aortic to caudal vena cava ratio measurements using abdominal ultrasound are increased in dogs with confirmed systemic hypertension. Veterinary Radiology & Ultrasound 2020;61:206–214.

Hori Y, Heishima Y, Yamashita Y, et al. Relationship between indirect blood pressure and various stages of chronic kidney disease in cats. J Vet Med Sci 2018;80:447–452.

Huhtinen M, Derre G, Renoldi HJ, et al. Randomized placebo-controlled clinical trial of a chewable formulation of amlodipine for the treatment of hypertension in client-owned cats. J Vet Intern Med 2015;29:786–793.

Jenkins TL, Coleman AE, Schmiedt CW, et al. Attenuation of the pressor response to exogenous angiotensin by angiotensin receptor blockers and benazepril hydrochloride in clinically normal cats. Am J Vet Res 2015;76:807–813.

Jepson RE, Elliott J, Brodbelt D, et al. Effect of control of systolic blood pressure on survival in cats with systemic hypertension. J Vet Intern Med 2007;21:402–409.

Jepson RE, Syme HM, Elliott J. Plasma renin activity and aldosterone concentrations in hypertensive cats with and without azotemia and in response to treatment with amlodipine besylate. J Vet Intern Med 2014; 28:144–153.

Johnson PJ. The equine metabolic syndrome peripheral Cushing's syndrome. Vet Clin North Am Equine Pract 2002;18:271–293.

Kang MH, Park HM. Hypertension after ingestion of baked garlic (Allium sativum) in a dog. J Vet Med Sci 2010;72:515–518.

Karck J, von Spiessen L, Rohn K, et al. [Interrelation between the degree of a chronic renal insufficiency and/or systemic hypertension and ocular changes in cats]. Tierarztl Prax Ausg K Kleintiere Heimtiere 2013;41:37–45.

Kent M, Glass EN, Haley AC, et al. Ischemic stroke in Greyhounds: 21 cases (2007–2013). J Am Vet Med Assoc 2014;245:113–117.

Kohnken R, Scansen BA, Premanandan C. Vasa vasorum arteriopathy: relationship with systemic arterial hypertension and other vascular lesions in cats. Vet Pathol 2017;54:475–483.

Lalor SM, Connolly DJ, Elliott J, et al. Plasma concentrations of natriuretic peptides in normal cats and normotensive and hypertensive cats with chronic kidney disease. J Vet Cardiol 2009;11 Suppl 1:S71–79.

Leblanc NL, Stepien RL, Bentley E. Ocular lesions associated with systemic hypertension in dogs: 65 cases (2005–2007). J Am Vet Med Assoc 2011;238:915–921.

Lee SK, Park S, Cheon B, et al. Body weight, blood pressure, and systemic changes following low-dosage prednisolone administration in dogs. Am J Vet Res 2017;78:1091–1097.

Lien YH, Hsiang TY, Huang HP. Associations among systemic blood pressure, microalbuminuria and albuminuria in dogs affected with pituitary- and adrenal-dependent hyperadrenocorticism. Acta Vet Scand 2010;52:61.

Lin CH, Yan CJ, Lien YH, et al. Systolic blood pressure of clinically normal and conscious cats determined by an indirect Doppler method in a clinical setting. J Vet Med Sci 2006;68:827–832.

Littman MP. Spontaneous systemic hypertension in 24 cats. J Vet Intern Med 1994;8:79–86.

Lo AJ, Holt DE, Brown DC, et al. Treatment of aldosterone-secreting adrenocortical tumors in cats by unilateral adrenalectomy: 10 cases (2002–2012). J Vet Intern Med 2014;28:137–143.

Maggio F, DeFrancesco TC, Atkins CE, et al. Ocular lesions associated with systemic hypertension in cats: 69 cases (1985–1998). J Am Vet Med Assoc 2000;217:695–702.

Marsh PS. Approach to equine critical care: monitoring arterial blood pressure. In, Reed SM, Bayly WM, Sellon DC (editors). Equine Internal Medicine. 3rd edition. Saunders, St. Louis, MO. 2010. pp. 254–256.

Martinez JT, Rogers LK, Kellogg C, et al. Plasma vasoprotective eicosanoid concentrations in healthy greyhounds and non-greyhound dogs. J Vet Intern Med 2016;30:583–590.

Martin-Flores M, Mercure-McKenzie TM, Campoy L, et al. Controlled retrospective study of the effects of eyedrops containing phenylephrine hydrochloride and scopolamine hydrobromide on mean arterial blood pressure in anesthetized dogs. Am J Vet Res 2010;71:1407–1412.

Masters AK, Berger DJ, Ware WA, et al. Effects of anti-inflammatory glucocorticoids on clinicopathologic, echocardiographic, and hemodynamic variables in clinically healthy dogs. Am J Vet Res 2018;79:411–423.

Mehlman E, Bright JM, Jeckel K, et al. Echocardiographic evidence of left ventricular hypertrophy in obese dogs. J Vet Intern Med 2013;27:62–68.

Misbach C, Gouni V, Tissier R, et al. Echocardiographic and tissue Doppler imaging alterations associated with spontaneous canine systemic hypertension. J Vet Intern Med 2011;25:1025–1035.

Miyagawa Y, Tominaga Y, Toda N, et al. Relationship between glomerular filtration rate and plasma N-terminal pro B-type natriuretic peptide concentrations in dogs with chronic kidney disease. Vet J 2013;197:445–450.

Munoz-Durango N, Fuentes CA, Castillo AE, et al. Role of the renin-angiotensin-aldosterone system beyond blood pressure regulation: molecular and cellular mechanisms involved in end-organ damage during arterial hypertension. Int J Mol Sci 2016;17.

Navas de Solis C, Slack J, Boston RC, et al. Hypertensive cardiomyopathy in horses: 5 cases (1995–2011). J Am Vet Med Assoc 2013;243:126–130.

Nelson L, Reidesel E, Ware WA, et al. Echocardiographic and radiographic changes associated with systemic hypertension in cats. J Vet Intern Med 2002;16:418–425.

Nostell KE, Lindase SS, Brojer JT. Blood pressure in Warmblood horses before and during a euglycemic-hyperinsulinemic clamp. Acta Vet Scand 2016;58:65.

Olsen E, Pedersen TL, Robinson R, et al. Accuracy and precision of oscillometric blood pressure in standing conscious horses. J Vet Emerg Crit Care 2016;26:85–92.

O'Neill J, Kent M, Glass EN, et al. Clinicopathologic and MRI characteristics of presumptive hypertensive encephalopathy in two cats and two dogs. J Am Anim Hosp Assoc 2013;49:412–420.

Ortega TM, Feldman EC, Nelson RW, et al. Systemic arterial blood pressure and urine protein/creatinine ratio in dogs with hyperadrenocorticism. J Am Vet Med Assoc 1996;209:1724–1729.

Payne JR, Brodbelt DC, Luis Fuentes V. Blood pressure measurements in 780 apparently healthy cats. J Vet Intern Med 2017;31:15–21.

Perez-Sanchez AP, Del-Angel-Caraza J, Quijano-Hernandez IA, et al. Obesity-hypertension and its relation to other diseases in dogs. Vet Res Commun 2015;39:45–51.

Peterson KL, Lee JA, Hovda LR. Phenylpropanolamine toxicosis in dogs: 170 cases (2004–2009). J Am Vet Med Assoc 2011;239:1463–1469.

Peterson ME. Black widow spider envenomation. Clin Tech Small Anim Pract 2006;21:187–190.

Porciello F, Rishniw M, Herndon WE, et al. Cardiac troponin I is elevated in dogs and cats with azotaemia renal failure and in dogs with non-cardiac systemic disease. Aust Vet J 2008;86:390–394.

Rattez EP, Reynolds BS, Concordet D, et al. Within-day and between-day variability of blood pressure measurement in healthy conscious Beagle dogs using a new oscillometric device. J Vet Cardiol 2010;12:35–40.

Rossi G, Giordano A, Breda S, et al. Big-endothelin 1 (big ET-1) and homocysteine in the serum of dogs with chronic kidney disease. Vet J 2013;198:109–115.

Scansen BA, Vitt J, Chew DJ, et al. Comparison of forelimb and hindlimb systolic blood pressures and proteinuria in healthy Shetland Sheepdogs. J Vet Intern Med 2014;28:277–283.

Schwarzwald CC. Disorders of the cardiovascular system. In, Reed SM, Bayly WM, Sellon DC (editors). Equine Internal Medicine, 4th edition. 2018. Elsevier, St. Louis, MO. pp. 387–541.

Sent U, Gossl R, Elliott J, et al. Comparison of efficacy of long-term oral treatment with Telmisartan and Benazepril in cats with chronic kidney disease. J Vet Intern Med 2015;29:1479–1487.

Surman S, Couto CG, Dibartola SP, et al. Arterial blood pressure, proteinuria, and renal histopathology in clinically healthy retired racing greyhounds. J Vet Intern Med 2012;26:1320–1329.

Syme H. Hypertension in small animal kidney disease. Vet Clin North Am Small Anim Pract 2011;41:63–89.

Taylor SS, Sparkes AH, Briscoe K, et al. ISFM consensus guidelines on the diagnosis and management of hypertension in cats. J Feline Med Surg 2017; 19: 288–303.

Theobald A, Volk HA, Dennis R, et al. Clinical outcome in 19 cats with clinical and magnetic resonance imaging diagnosis of ischaemic myelopathy (2000–2011). J Feline Med Surg 2013;15:132–141.

Thomas EK, Drobatz KJ, Mandell DC. Presumptive cocaine toxicosis in 19 dogs: 2004–2012. J Vet Emerg Crit Care 2014;24:201–207.

Tjostheim SS, Stepien RL, Markovic LE, et al. Effects of toceranib phosphate on systolic blood pressure and proteinuria in dogs. J Vet Intern Med 2016;30:951–957.

Tou SP, Adin DB, Estrada AH. Echocardiographic estimation of systemic systolic blood pressure in dogs with mild mitral regurgitation. J Vet Intern Med 2006;20:1127–1131.

Tropf M, Nelson OL, Lee PM, et al. Cardiac and metabolic variables in obese dogs. J Vet Intern Med 2017;31:1000–1007.

Tsugawa N. Cardiovascular diseases and fat soluble vitamins: vitamin D and vitamin K. J Nutr Sci Vitaminol (Tokyo) 2015;61 Suppl:S170–172.

Valverde A. Alpha-2 agonists as pain therapy in horses. Vet Clin North Am Equine Pract 2010;26:515–532.

Vera L, De Clercq D, Van Steenkiste G, et al. Differences in ultrasound-derived arterial wall stiffness parameters and noninvasive blood pressure between Friesian horses and Warmblood horses. J Vet Intern Med 2020; 34:893–901.

Violette NP, Ledbetter EC Punctate retinal hemorrhage and its relation to ocular and systemic disease in dogs: 83 cases. Vet Ophthalmol 2018;21:233–239.

Wehner A, Hartmann K, Hirschberger J. Associations between proteinuria, systemic hypertension and glomerular filtration rate in dogs with renal and non-renal diseases. Vet Rec 2008;162:141–147.

Wernick MB, Hopfner RM, Francey T, et al. Comparison of arterial blood pressure measurements and hypertension scores obtained by use of three indirect measurement devices in hospitalized dogs. J Am Vet Med Assoc 2012;240:962–968.

Wessmann A, Chandler K, Garosi L. Ischaemic and haemorrhagic stroke in the dog. Vet J 2009;180:290–303.

Willi B, Kook PH, Quante S, et al. [Primary hyperaldosteronism in cats]. Schweiz Arch Tierheilkd 2012;154:529–537.

Williams TL, Elliott J, Syme HM. Renin-angiotensin-aldosterone system activity in hyperthyroid cats with and without concurrent hypertension. J Vet Intern Med 2013;27:522–529.

Yamashita Y, Oishi Y, Motomatsu Y, et al. Thoracic endografting increases cardiac afterload and leads to left ventricular hypertrophy in dogs. Eur J Cardiothorac Surg 2019;55:618–625.

Young WM, Zheng C, Davidson MG, et al. Visual outcome in cats with hypertensive chorioretinopathy. Veterinary Ophthalmol 2019;22:161–167.

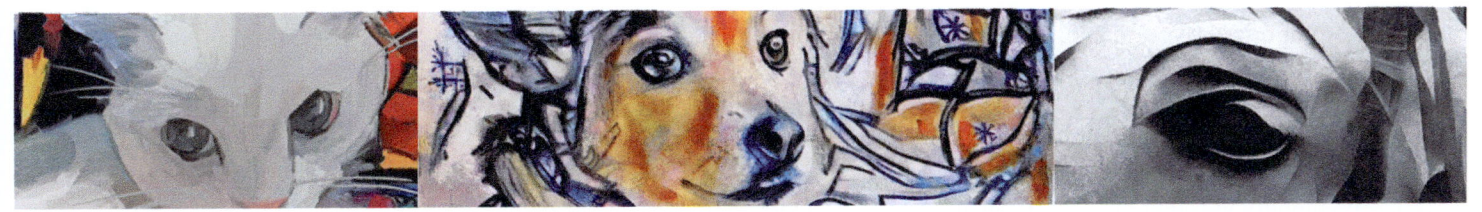

39
PULMONARY HYPERTENSION

The pulmonary and systemic circulations connect in series and pump the same cardiac output (CO), but are functionally and structurally different. Compared to the systemic circulation, the pulmonary circulation has a much lower pressure, vascular resistance, and venous capacitance. However, it has a substantial flow reserve and can accommodate marked increases in CO with little change in pressure. Vascular resistance across the pulmonary circulation relates not only to the pulmonary arterioles, but also to left atrial (LA) pressure and the pulmonary capillary circulation. Resistance and flow across the pulmonary capillary beds are altered by expansion or collapse of alveoli and by gravity. The pulmonary circulation resides within the negative pressure pleural space, while receiving venous return from largely extrathoracic systemic veins.

Normal pulmonary arterial (PA) pressures in resting dogs are approximately 25 mm Hg, systolic; 8 mm Hg, diastolic; and 12–15 mm Hg, mean. PA pressures in anesthetized cats are slightly lower than for dogs. In standing horses with a normal resting heart rate, systolic PA pressure is approximately 40 to 45 mm Hg. Low PA pressures minimize right ventricular (RV) work (the area under the pressure-volume loop), thereby accommodating the relatively thin walls of that chamber and maintaining optimal RV myocardial blood flow. In the absence of any RV outflow stenosis, peak RV systolic pressure equals the PA systolic pressure within a few mm of Hg. At rest, the normal PA end-diastolic pressure just exceeds, or equilibrates with, the LA (or pulmonary arterial wedge) pressure. Exercise-induced increases in pulmonary blood flow can be accepted with only mild elevation in PA pressures unless the exertion is extreme. This accommodation relates to the thin-walled and highly distensible pulmonary vasculature, recruitment of underperfused pulmonary vessels, and a large pulmonary capillary surface area. One notable exception occurs in the exercising horse, where PA and right-heart pressures increase relatively more than in exercising dogs. Transient, but severe, increases in PA pressures develop during maximal exercise in horses. Systolic PA pressures can reach 120 mm Hg during maximal exercise and this often is associated with transient or persistent pulmonary hypertension (PH), as discussed later in this chapter.

PH is a pathophysiologic state involving high PA pressures, rather than a specific disease. PH in dogs and in cats generally is defined as a systolic PA pressure >30 or 35 mm Hg, diastolic PA pressure >19 mm Hg, and mean PA pressure ≥25 mm Hg at rest. Somewhat higher systolic PA pressures can occur in athletic, geriatric, and obese people without clinical consequence; whether the same occurs in small animals is unknown. Pulmonary compliance and airway resistance also influence PA pressure because of pulmonary parenchymal and vascular interdependence. Specific values indicating PH in horses depend in part on the study, but are somewhat higher than those used in dogs. PH likely is present in a resting horse with mean PA pressure >30 to 35 mm Hg.

Pulmonary reserves for maintaining gas exchange and vascular resistance are high, and therefore, PH and its causes can remain subclinical for quite some time. For example, in a dog with normal lungs, up to 60% of the pulmonary vascular bed can be destroyed before PH develops. Many cases of PH associated with primary lung disease are not identified until later in the course of the disease, once clinical signs become overt. Multiple disorders, including those summarized for dogs in **Table 39.1**, can lead to PH. The general etiologic groupings in that table, as well as many of the listed causes, also are relevant to cats and to horses. Overall, PH is less common in cats, although a congenital cardiac shunt, pulmonary thromboembolism (PTE), or other pulmonary pathology could underlie it. Aside from the "physiological" PH of exercise, chronic bronchitis/asthma (also called reactive airway disease and previously, chronic obstructive pulmonary disease) is probably the most common reason for PH in horses. In one study of horses undergoing right heart catheterization at sea level, acute reactive airway disease (asthma, or chronic obstructive pulmonary disease) roughly doubled the resting

Table 39.1   Pulmonary Hypertension Disease Classification Scheme for Dogs[a,b]

Group 1: Pulmonary Arterial Hypertension

- Conditions characterized by pulmonary arteriopathy induced by known or unknown stimuli in susceptible individuals.
- Includes idiopathic (1a) & heritable PH (1b, mainly in people);
- Includes PH associated with large congenital cardiovascular shunts (1d1); drugs or toxins (1c); as well as pulmonary vasculitis (1d2), pulmonary vascular amyloid deposition (1d3), connective tissue & other diseases (such as scleroderma), portal hypertension, and also persistent PH in the newborn (people).
- Pulmonary veno-occlusive disease & pulmonary capillary hemangiomatosis also are considered a subcategory of pulmonary arterial hypertension (group 1′).

Group 2: Pulmonary Hypertension Secondary to Left Heart Disease

- Caused by left-sided congestive heart failure and other causes of chronic pulmonary venous hypertension.
- Includes acquired (2b1) and congenital (2c1) diseases of the mitral or aortic valve (degenerative, congenital malformation, infective endocarditis);
- Includes left ventricular dysfunction (2a) from cardiomyopathy (dilated, hypertrophic, restrictive) or myocarditis; as well as other congenital or acquired left heart inflow or outflow obstruction/stenosis (2c1) or causes of left ventricular dysfunction; also pulmonary venous inflow obstruction (rare).

Group 3: Pulmonary Hypertension Secondary to Respiratory Disease, Hypoxia, or Both

- Caused by primary lung or airway diseases and chronic hypoxia.
- Includes chronic obstructive airway diseases (3a), such as tracheal or mainstem bronchial collapse (3a1) and bronchomalacia (3a2).
- Includes interstitial lung diseases (3b1) such as fibrotic lung disease (3b1a), cryptogenic organizing pneumonia (3b1b), pulmonary alveolar proteinosis (3b1c), unclassified interstitial lung disease (3b1d), and eosinophilic pneumonia/bronchopneumopathy (3b1e); infectious pneumonias (3b2); diffuse pulmonary neoplasia (3b3);
- Also includes obstructive sleep apnea/sleep-disordered breathing (3c), alveolar hypoventilation, chronic high-altitude exposure (3d), developmental lung disease (3e); and miscellaneous conditions (3f) such as bronchiolar disorders, bronchiectasis, emphysema, pneumonectomy.

Group 4: Pulmonary Hypertension Secondary to Pulmonary Thromboembolic Disease

- Caused by massive acute (4a) or chronic (4b) pulmonary embolism, thrombosis, or thromboembolism.
- Could be associated with immune-mediated hemolytic anemia, protein-losing nephropathy or enteropathy, neoplasia, sepsis, hyperadrenocorticism or long-term exogenous glucocorticoids, cardiac disease, pancreatitis, disseminated intravascular coagulation, or other disease.

Group 5: Pulmonary Hypertension Secondary to Parasitic Disease

- Caused by *Dirofilaria immitis* or *Angiostrongylus vasorum* (dogs)

Group 6: Pulmonary Hypertension Associated with Multifactorial or Unclear Causes

- Includes cases with two or more concurrent disease conditions from groups 1–5 that both contribute to PH (6a);
- Includes mass lesions that compress the pulmonary arteries (6b); and other disorders with unclear mechanisms (6c). In people, this includes myeloproliferative disease, systemic disorders (sarcoidosis, pulmonary histiocytosis, lymphangioleiomyomatosis), metabolic disorders (glycogen storage disease, thyroid disorders), and others (neoplastic obstruction, fibrosing mediastinitis, chronic renal failure, segmental PH).

[a] Canine classification adapted from human PH classification guidelines (Simonneau, 2013) and the ACVIM consensus statement guidelines for the diagnosis, classification, treatment, and monitoring of pulmonary hypertension in dogs (Reinero, 2020); subclassification designations from the latter are in parentheses. Further study and documentation of diseases causing PH in animals could lead to changes in these classifications.

[b] Diseases in groups 1 and 3–5 are considered precapillary causes of PH, those in group 2 are postcapillary causes; group 6 could have either pre- or combined pre- and postcapillary causes.

Abbreviation: PH, pulmonary hypertension.

PA pressures from a systolic (mean) pressure of 34 (24) mm Hg to 66 (45) mm Hg (Dixon, 1978). However, there was marked individual variation in the degree of PH; this could not be explained solely by alveolar hypoxia because mean PA pressure decreased only ~5 mm Hg after oxygen supplementation. Equine interstitial lung diseases and chronic left heart disease probably are under-recognized causes of PH in this species. Group 1 etiologies of PH are rarely reported in horses.

Classification of PH is based on its pathological and hemodynamic features in people (Simonneau, 2013). A similar classification scheme is proposed for dogs (**Table 39.1**; and American College of Veterinary Internal Medicine, ACVIM, consensus guidelines, Reinero, 2020). PH also is categorized into precapillary and postcapillary causes, according to underlying pathophysiology; some conditions have elements of both (so-called combined PH). Precapillary PH results from injury at the

PA or arteriolar level that produces increased pulmonary vascular resistance (PVR). Most classification systems also include primary pulmonary diseases in this category. Hemodynamic characteristics of precapillary PH in people (based on right heart catheterization data) include a mean PA pressure ≥25 mm Hg and a pulmonary capillary wedge pressure (PCWP) ≤15 mm Hg. Causes of precapillary PH include heartworm disease (HWD; Chapter 40), cardiovascular shunts (Chapter 26), vascular occlusive disease, chronic hypoxemia from various pulmonary diseases, and idiopathic PA hypertension. Postcapillary PH results from increased pulmonary venous pressure and congestion, originating downstream from the pulmonary capillary bed. In almost all cases, postcapillary PH occurs secondary to left-sided heart failure. The most common etiology in dogs is degenerative (myxomatous) mitral valve disease (DMVD). Hemodynamic characteristics of postcapillary PH, as described in people, include a mean PA pressure ≥25 mm Hg and a PCWP >15 mm Hg. Because PVR is fairly normal in patients with isolated postcapillary PH, the difference between diastolic PA pressure and PCWP is small (<7 mm Hg). However, with combined pre- and postcapillary PH, PVR is elevated and the gradient between diastolic PA pressure and PCWP is ≥7 mm Hg (human guidelines). LA enlargement is typical with postcapillary PH, whereas this is not a feature of precapillary PH. The clinical presentation and response to treatment can differ between pre- and postcapillary PH. Although the exact values quoted for human patients are not transferrable to animals, the concepts do hold and are relevant to understanding the causes and therapy of PH in dogs, cats and horses.

PH exacerbates the clinical manifestations and mortality associated with the underlying disease process(es). Hypoxic pulmonary disease and pulmonary vascular obstructive disease probably account for almost half of the PH cases in dogs. Chronically elevated pulmonary venous pressure is estimated to account for almost one quarter of canine PH cases. In dogs with DMVD, development of PH relates to the severity of valvular disease and regurgitation. Most of these cases develop mild to moderate PH, although PH can be severe in some (presumably reflecting combined pre- and postcapillary PH). PTE, as another potential cause of PH, can occur with multiple clinical conditions (Chapter 36).

Pathophysiology

Increased PVR raises PA pressure according to the relationship: pressure = cardiac output × resistance (or, CO = pressure/resistance; see p. 22). Increases in pulmonary flow are well-accommodated, unless extreme, provided PVR remains normal. For example, a left-to-right shunting patent ductus arteriosus (PDA) can double or triple pulmonary flow; yet, PH is uncommon (except at high altitudes). However, when an increase in PVR preexists, increased CO through the lungs can significantly raise PA pressures. Pulmonary arteriolar vasoconstriction increases PVR in response to hypoxia and other stimuli; however, the development of severe PH also involves angioproliferative changes that permanently reduce vascular compliance and lumen size. PVR is inversely related to the total cross-sectional area of pulmonary resistance vessels. When enough of these vessels become narrowed or destroyed, and when their capacity to dilate is impaired by disease, even a normal CO generates increased PA pressure.

Pulmonary vasoconstriction is a normal response to alveolar hypoxia, although response magnitude varies among species. Usually this helps optimize ventilation/perfusion (V/Q) balance by preferentially shifting blood flow to better-ventilated lung regions. Hypoxia-induced pulmonary vasoconstriction can occur with hypoventilation, low inspired O_2 concentrations (as with high altitude), and a variety of respiratory diseases. Examples include major airway collapse or obstruction, chronic bronchitis and asthma, lung lobe torsion, interstitial lung diseases such as pulmonary fibrosis, and pneumonias. The prevalence of clinically important PH with these conditions is unknown, however, especially near sea level. Normal dogs exposed to lower inspired O_2 concentration at high altitude typically show only mild pulmonary vasoconstriction, although it can be more prominent when a concurrent reason for PH exists, such as a left-to-right shunt. With most primary respiratory diseases, the associated PH is mild or mild-to-moderate; in many cases, it appears to be clinically unimportant and without erythrocytosis. Vasoconstriction associated with transient hypoxia usually is reversible; however, chronic hypoxia can lead to morphologic changes in the small pulmonary arteries and arterioles. Such hypoxia can cause or contribute to reactive PH in people and might be a factor in some dogs, as well. Increases in erythropoietin, endothelin (ETN), and vascular endothelial growth factor concentrations have been identified in dogs living at high altitude, despite the absence of erythrocytosis.

Severe pulmonary parenchymal disease or fibrosis can destroy normal pulmonary vascular structure, as well as stimulate regional hypoxic vasoconstriction, thereby further increasing PVR. In patients with chronic lung disease, the development of PH could relate to hypoxia, inflammation, and increased sheer stress in vessels; all of these factors promote pulmonary vascular morphologic changes. Restrictive pulmonary diseases (including chronic interstitial pulmonary disease and fibrosis) decrease dynamic lung compliance and can contribute to PH because of abnormal pulmonary mechanics. Animals with multiple underlying mechanisms for PH sometimes have more severe elevations in PA pressure.

Abnormal endothelial function contributes to the pathogenesis of vascular changes associated with PH. These include smooth muscle hypertrophy, intimal proliferation and fibrosis, and increased extracellular matrix deposition. Chronic vasoconstriction can provoke such vascular remodeling, perhaps related to persistent pulmonary inflammation with exuberant expression of growth factors and increased release of vasoactive mediators. Individual genetic predisposition likely plays an important role in cases of severe PH. Endothelial cells normally modulate vascular smooth muscle cell activity through production of substances with vasodilator/antimitotic (such as prostacyclin and nitric oxide, NO) and vasoconstrictor/mitogenic (including thromboxane A_2 and ETN) activities. With PH, the balance between vasodilation and vasoconstriction is upset. Increased circulating levels of thromboxane and ETN have been found in animals with PH. Thromboxane A_2 causes platelet activation and vasoconstriction and contributes to cell proliferation.

NO is important to normal pulmonary vascular function. NO is synthesized from L-arginine and oxygen by the enzyme nitric oxide synthetase (NOS). Variable decrease in NOS expression or inhibition of NOS function can occur with PH. NO directly promotes vascular smooth muscle relaxation via increased intracellular cyclic guanosine monophosphate (cGMP) production. cGMP also inhibits smooth muscle proliferation, as well as platelet aggregation. However, cGMP is inactivated rapidly by phosphodiesterase (PDE) isoenzymes, especially PDE-5. Prostacyclin, produced from arachidonic acid, induces smooth muscle relaxation via cyclic adenosine monophosphate (cAMP) production. This leads to reduced intracellular Ca^{++} availability in vascular smooth muscle, and vasorelaxation. Prostacyclin also inhibits growth of smooth muscle cells and inhibits platelet aggregation.

Excessive vasoconstrictor production, with relative vasodilator deficiency, leads to abnormal endothelial–smooth muscle interactions, which promote pulmonary vasoconstriction and vascular remodeling. ETN induces vascular remodeling in various disease conditions associated with PH, including PTE and HWD. Increased ETN-1 serum concentrations have been correlated with the severity of PH. Besides vasoconstriction, ETN stimulates smooth muscle proliferation, collagen production, and platelet aggregation; it also has proinflammatory actions. Other mediators include serotonin, which is known to be a potent vasoconstrictor and can stimulate platelet aggregation, as well as pulmonary smooth muscle proliferation.

Activation of the renin-angiotensin-aldosterone system (RAAS) also is thought to contribute to the development and severity of PH (Hu, 2015). It is known that the RAAS can induce endothelial dysfunction, promote vascular remodeling, and cause pulmonary vasoconstriction. Experimentally, aldosterone inhibition with spironolactone has reduced PA pressure and PVR without causing systemic hypotension. In another experimental model, angiotensin receptor blockade also decreased PA pressure and vascular remodeling. Furthermore, in people with PH, renal sympathetic denervation diminishes RAAS activation, improves cardiac function, and reduces ventricular dyssynergy. Thus, RAAS modulation might be a useful adjunct to other therapeutic strategies for PH management, although this has not been demonstrated in veterinary clinical trials. Traditionally, medical strategies in humans have been aimed at antagonizing the effects of ETN (as with bosentan), providing prostacyclin analogs (such as epoprostanol), and inhibiting PDE-5 (with sildenafil, tadalafil and related drugs; Brown, 2010).

Exercise intolerance is a prominent consequence of PH. During exercise, there is a need for increased pulmonary blood flow. In order to accommodate increased flow without a marked increase in pressure, pulmonary vasodilation and recruitment of pulmonary capillaries must occur. However, because pulmonary vascular compliance is abnormal in patients with PH, increased flow leads to further increases in PA pressures and RV afterload stress. Depending on the underlying cause of PH, hypoxemia and pulmonary infiltration or edema also might contribute to reduced exercise capacity, hyperventilation and respiratory distress. Other factors that could contribute to exercise intolerance include abnormal respiratory muscle function and skeletal muscle deconditioning.

Cor Pulmonale

Cor pulmonale is the term used to describe the cardiac changes caused by moderate to severe PH. Progressively worsening PH increases afterload on the right ventricle. This systolic pressure overload stimulates the development of RV hypertrophy, which helps reduce myocardial wall stress. The nature of ventricular remodeling depends in part on the time course of PH. In neonates or young animals with PH caused by congenital shunts, concentric RV hypertrophy is more likely. In acute PH, as with a massive pulmonary embolus, simple RV dilation would be found (this is rarely observed). Most often, acquired PH leads to a mixed form of hypertrophy with increased RV wall thickness and myocardial mass, but with varying degrees of RV dilation (**Figures 39.1** and **39.2**). Tricuspid regurgitation (TR) sometimes develops or worsens as RV dilation progresses. Although TR is variable in PH, and may not be evident even with severe PH, when present it adds a volume load to the existing pressure overload. Severe TR further reduces forward CO. Again, the degree of myocardial hypertrophy that develops is variable; marked RV wall thickening is most common in young animals with Eisenmenger's (patho)physiology or in older ones with pulmonary arterial hypertension (Group 1). Eisenmenger's (patho)physiology is the term used to describe severe PH caused by systemic to pulmonary arterial overcirculation, which then leads to right-to-left or bi-directional shunting (p. 438). RV diastolic (filling) pressure also rises as RV stiffness increases and function deteriorates. Forward CO progressively declines as the right ventricle fails, a situation that initially can present as heart failure without overt congestion. When sufficient neurohormonal and renal compensations develop, elevated systemic venous pressures can lead to signs of right-sided congestive heart failure (CHF; Chapter 20).

Severe PH is characterized in many cases by low output signs of heart failure. Although RV stroke volume might be adequate at rest, circulatory needs during exertion often cannot be met, which leads to exertional tachypnea or distress, fatigue, weakness, and exertional collapse or syncope. The latter, especially, is a sign of severe disease. Syncope implies that RV output cannot increase sufficiently to maintain blood pressure and perfusion in the face of exercise-induced systemic vasodilation. RV contractility that is unable

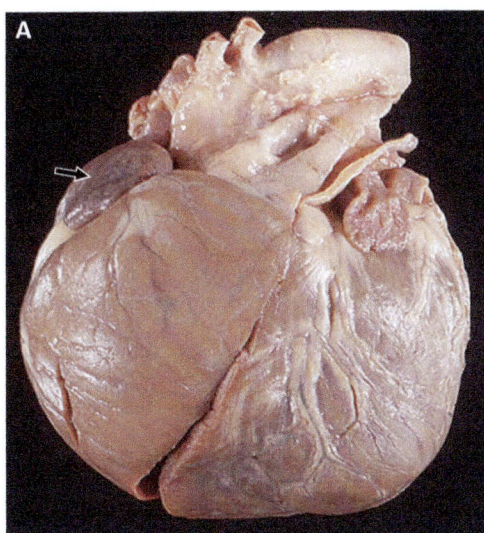
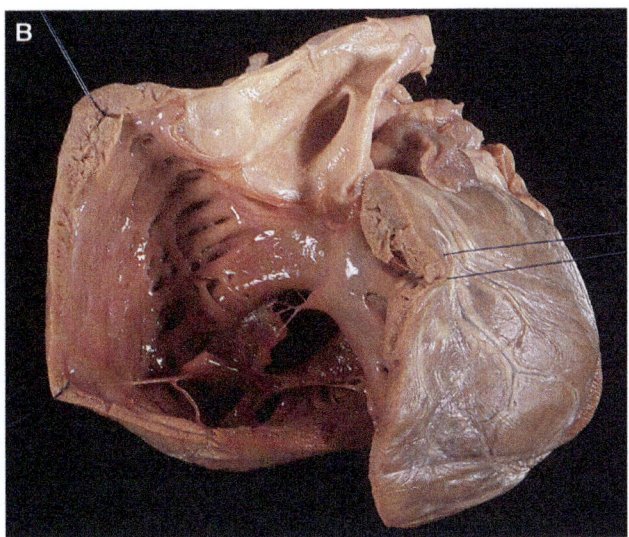

Figure 39.1 (A) Photo showing the cranial left aspect of the heart from a dog with severe pulmonary hypertension and tricuspid insufficiency. Enlargement of the right ventricle (RV) and right auricle (arrow) is evident. (B) Opened outflow tract and main pulmonary artery from the same dog shows marked dilation of the RV and pulmonary trunk; ventricular wall thickening is minimal in this dog. The left ventricular apex is toward the lower right of the image.

to overcome the high afterload (known as ventriculoarterial uncoupling) is a consequence of RV dysfunction (Tran, 2018). The few published studies of humans with exertional collapse from PH show that reduced systemic blood pressure, as opposed to arrhythmias or reflex mediated syncope, is most likely responsible; this is compatible with an inability of the right ventricle to maintain sufficient CO with exercise. Similar studies are not reported in animals. Furthermore, people with severe PH often have exertional angina secondary to RV ischemia, especially during systole. It is unclear if the same occurs in animals, but it is certainly possible.

Pulmonary Arterial Hypertension

Pulmonary arteriopathy refers to vascular disease processes that lead to irreversible narrowing and obliteration of the arterial lumen. A spectrum of pathologic features can accompany pulmonary vascular disease, including PA myointimal proliferation, vascular occlusion, fibrosis, inflammation and necrosis (**Figure 39.3**). Advanced pulmonary arteriopathy causes severely increased PVR, PH, and often, right-sided CHF, unless there is a shunt that can serve as a pressure "pop-off valve". These findings are characteristic of idiopathic PH (usually referred to as primary PH in humans), although multiple causes are known to underlie precapillary PH characterized by pulmonary arteriopathy (**Table 39.1**, group 1). Histologic characteristics of idiopathic pulmonary arteriopathy, as described in people, also are observed in dogs. These include various combinations of PA intimal thickening, medial hypertrophy, plexiform lesions, and isolated arteritis (**Figure 39.4**). Other lesions might include exudative alveolitis, which, along with complex vascular lesions, appears to be associated with worse outcome. Most group 1 causes of precapillary PH share the findings of diffuse vascular narrowing caused by proliferative PA wall remodeling and complex plexiform arterial lesions. The human histopathological classification (Heath-Edwards) scheme, which uses a scale of I to VI to describe

Figure 39.2 Heart specimen from a 10-year-old, female Miniature Schnauzer presented for a month-long history of collapse episodes during activity shows right ventricular dilation and moderate to severe hypertrophy or wall thickening (at bottom), as well as septal compression toward the left ventricle. Severe pulmonary hypertension was secondary to proliferative pulmonary arteriopathy.

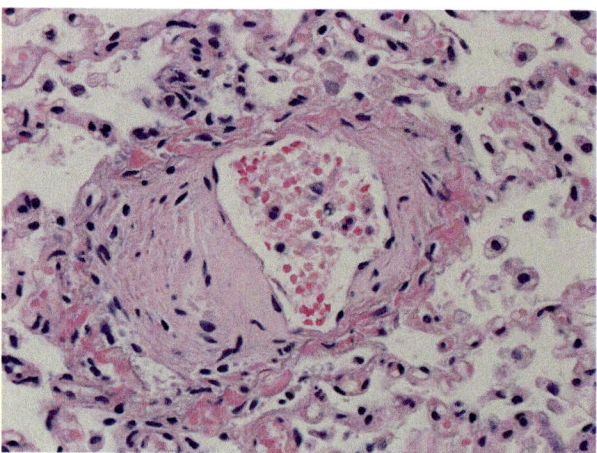

Figure 39.3 An accumulation of fibrocytes and collagenous matrix within the wall of a small pulmonary artery narrows the vessel lumen. Histologic image from the dog of **Figure 39.2**. Hematoxylin & eosin; 100X magnification. (Courtesy of Dr J Smith.)

progressive pulmonary vasculopathy changes, sometimes is applied to animals. Although HWD could fit into group 1 PH based on the pulmonary arteriopathy it causes, it instead has been classified in the veterinary scheme into group 5 because multiple factors contribute to PH in this disease (see section "Parasitic Disease").

Pulmonary overcirculation, caused by an initially left-to-right congenital cardiovascular shunt, can provoke arterial remodeling and eventually lead to increased PVR and PH. Greatly increased blood flow can induce vascular damage and raises perfusion pressure in the lungs. Excessively high pulmonary flow can disrupt normal pulmonary vasorelaxation

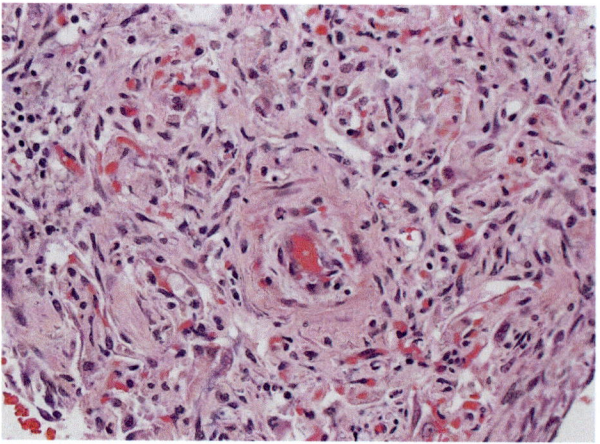

Figure 39.4 Histologic image of a plexiform pulmonary arterial lesion from a 6-year-old, female Welsh Corgi with marked pulmonary hypertension and secondary cor pulmonale. These complex proliferative lesions include irregular intimal thickening and clusters of irregular branching arterioles and fibrous tissue surrounding small pulmonary arteries. An idiopathic pulmonary arteriopathy was presumed, as neither a (reversed) cardiac shunt nor heartworm disease was present. Hematoxylin & eosin; 100X magnification. (Courtesy of Dr R Myers.)

mechanisms and increase ETN release. Shunt location and size, as well as species and individual susceptibility, influence the development and severity of PH. For example, the burden of an unrestrictive PDA or ventricular septal defect is likely to induce PH more rapidly than a large atrial septal defect, where PA flow is increased but direct transmission of high pressure from the systemic circulation is not. The development of pulmonary vascular disease associated with shunt lesions seems to be more gradual in cats when compared to dogs. The arterial changes include medial hypertrophy, intimal proliferation and fibrosis, occlusion of small vessels, and eventually, plexiform lesions similar to those of human idiopathic PH. Erythrocytosis and hyperviscosity that develop secondary to systemic hypoxemia could exacerbate the increased PVR. Generally, animals with PH and right-to-left shunting do not show signs of CHF, because the shunt acts as a "pop-off valve" which mitigates the degree of PA pressure increase and lends some protection to the right ventricle. However, in sporadic cases, right-sided CHF signs do develop with severe PH caused by a reversed shunt.

Human heritable or idiopathic PH is a primary pulmonary vascular disease. Mutation of the bone morphogenic protein receptor type-2 gene, a member of the transforming growth factor (TGF)-beta super family, is found in most affected people. PH also has been associated with use of certain drugs in people, especially appetite suppressants (including fenfluramine, phenylpropanolamine) and other amphetamines. Liver disease with portal hypertension, human immunodeficiency virus infection, and connective tissue diseases sometimes are accompanied by PH, also. People with severe PH associated with another disease tend to have marked pulmonary vascular changes, similar to those found in idiopathic PH. The pathobiology appears to be similar in animals. Yet, while primary (idiopathic or familial) PH is well known in people, documentation for this in animals is rare. Endothelial dysfunction and vascular structural changes, not just pulmonary vasoconstriction, underlie the greatly increased PVR of severe PH. Individual predisposition is probably important in these severe PH cases, too. Thrombosis in-situ also can be a factor.

Aside from HWD and severe pulmonary overcirculation, the underlying cause for many cases of pulmonary arterial hypertension in companion animals is unknown and the label "idiopathic PH" seems appropriate. It is likely that a number of canine cases (especially some rescued dogs) are secondary to longstanding heartworm infection where viable filarial worms are no longer present. Regardless of the cause, chronic arteritis or inflammation can produce progressive intimal thickening, mural hypertrophy, and irreversible fibrosis in affected vessels, leading to PH. The severity of PH ultimately is proportional to the reduction in total cross-sectional area of the pulmonary vasculature.

Acute necrotizing pulmonary vasculitis of small to moderate-size pulmonary arteries is a rare condition that causes PH in dogs. Although most often associated with congenital cardiovascular malformations, such as PDA, it has occurred in isolation. Manifestations can include acute lethargy, anorexia, coughing, respiratory distress, weakness, and cyanosis. The necrotizing pulmonary vasculitis is associated with circumferential myointimal thickening and fibrinoid necrosis affecting small to moderately sized pulmonary arteries. This can be accompanied by an acute fibrinous pneumonia with macrophage infiltration and fibrinous alveolar exudate. The resulting PH is severe and leads to progressive right-sided CHF and death, assuming the initial pulmonary insult was survived.

Pulmonary veno-occlusive disease (PVOD) is another rare cause of primary PH in people. Similar histologic features are described in small case reports in dogs and horses with severe PH of unexplained cause and associated respiratory distress (den Toomb, 2018; Williams, 2008). So far, neither the pathogenesis nor prevalence of PVOD in dogs, horses, or other species is known. Lung histopathologic characteristics include pulmonary venous and arterial occlusive remodeling that involves endothelial and smooth muscle cells, and sometimes, fibrous connective tissue. Segmental congestion of alveolar capillaries results from downstream venous occlusion. Focal vascular lesions that resemble pulmonary capillary hemangiomatosis (PCH) in people also can occur in these canine cases (Reinero, 2019). PCH is a rare vasoproliferative disorder that is reported sporadically in dogs and cats. It involves multifocal pathologic alveolar capillary proliferation, which often extends into adjacent pulmonary veins, arteries and bronchioles. Type II pneumocyte hyperplasia, alveolar hemorrhage, and multifocal pulmonary arterial thrombosis also can occur. Although PVOD and PCH mainly affect pulmonary veins and capillaries, the associated pulmonary arterial lesions of intimal fibrosis and medial hypertrophy place these conditions into the group 1 PH category. Clinically, based on an acute onset of respiratory distress, radiographic pulmonary infiltrates that can resemble those of pulmonary edema, as well as evidence for PH, these conditions can be mistaken for left-sided CHF. However, there usually is no evidence of clinically relevant left heart disease. PVOD and PCH also mimic idiopathic PH in people. Unfortunately, the typical vasodilator (including PDE-5 inhibitor) therapy for PH can provoke fatal pulmonary edema. Definitive diagnosis might require special staining (Verhoeff-Van Gieson) of lung tissue to histologically differentiate pulmonary arteries and veins. Treatment in people involves lung transplantation. One could speculate that judicious diuretic doses plus pimobendan might be useful in controlling pulmonary edema and supporting right heart function, but at the risk of volume depletion and hypotension.

Pulmonary Venous Hypertension

Postcapillary PH is caused by chronically elevated pulmonary venous pressure (**Table 39.1**, group 2). Left-sided CHF associated with valvular or myocardial disease, whether acquired or congenital, is the usual cause. The overall prevalence of PH in dogs with (stages B2 and C) DMVD is estimated at just under 40%, although more stage C dogs are affected (Borgarelli, 2015). Moderate to severe PH is associated with worse outcome in dogs with DMVD (p. 561). Postcapillary PH also occurs in some cats with left heart failure, although its prevalence is probably less than half that in dogs. PH can be a complication in horses with severe mitral or aortic valve regurgitation, as well.

In some cases, concurrent precapillary increase in PVR is likely, either from acute hypoxia-induced pulmonary vasoconstriction associated with cardiogenic pulmonary edema, or from reactive pulmonary vascular remodeling and narrowing secondary to chronic hypoxia, induced either by underlying pulmonary disease or chronic pulmonary venous hypertension. Chronically elevated pulmonary venous pressure can induce structural changes in pulmonary capillaries and increase the muscularity of resistance arterioles. In addition, pulmonary congestion and edema caused by high venous pressure could contribute to the increasing PVR by reducing lung compliance and increasing resistance to air flow.

Persistent neurohormonal activation, including increased ETN production and reduced endothelium-dependent vasodilation contribute to PH in animals with left-sided CHF, as well as those with other pulmonary disease. Compared to normal dogs, increased serum big ETN-1 concentrations were found in those with cardiopulmonary disease regardless of PH status; however, levels were higher in dogs with PH (Fukumoto, 2014). Natriuretic peptides normally contribute to cGMP-mediated vasodilation. However, with heart failure, sensitivity to natriuretic peptides and other endogenous vasodilators can be blunted within the pulmonary vasculature. Increased stiffness of the pulmonary (and also the systemic) vasculature occurs, as well. Decreased cGMP synthesis and enhanced degradation by PDE-5 are mechanisms thought to be involved in PH associated with heart failure.

Unusual causes of postcapillary PH have included congenital intra-LA or pulmonary venous obstructive lesions. Congenital valvular or supravalvular mitral stenosis, cor triatriatum sinister, and double-outlet right atrium (pp. 500, 512, and 466, respectively) are rare malformations that cause postcapillary PH. Stenotic lesions above the mitral valve are reported more often in cats, with PH accompanying about half of reported cases. Respiratory signs of pulmonary edema usually develop within the first few years of life in affected cats, although some become symptomatic later, especially when pulmonary hypertension develops. Arterial thromboembolism (Chapter 36) can be a complication.

Pulmonary Disease and Hypoxia

Primary pulmonary diseases also cause precapillary PH (**Table 39.1**, group 3). Alveolar hypoxia, as well as vasoactive and mitogenic substances produced by pulmonary endothelial and vascular smooth muscle cells, cause arterial vasoconstriction and vascular remodeling. These changes progressively increase PVR. Pulmonary fibrosis is a progressive interstitial lung disease that is thought to represent the healing phase of lung injury. Although there are well-defined causes in people, most veterinary cases are idiopathic. There is a genetic predisposition to (idiopathic) pulmonary fibrosis in West Highland White Terriers (Clercx, 2018). Pulmonary fibrosis occasionally has been linked to use of certain drugs, including nitrosoureas (cats, people), amiodarone (people, dogs?), and bleomycin (rodent models). Besides pulmonary fibrosis, histopathologic findings can include type II pneumocyte hyperplasia, smooth muscle hypertrophy, and sometimes, epithelial metaplasia. Pulmonary fibrosis is associated with loss of functional alveoli, as well as increased deposition of abnormal collagen. It leads to restrictive pulmonary pathophysiology, often accompanied by varying degrees of PH. Exercise intolerance, tachypnea, variable coughing, and eventually, respiratory distress are common historical signs; coarse pulmonary crackles are characteristic findings on auscultation. Radiographically, these changes can produce a variety of lung patterns ranging from subtle to severe and in horses can include pulmonary nodularity. Most canine cases are associated with an increase in unstructured interstitial opacity, which is best appreciated by computed tomography (CT) imaging. Varying degrees of bronchial involvement are common and likely to be associated with coughing. Radiographic, CT, and echocardiographic (echo) abnormalities associated with elevated PA pressure are identifiable in some cases, as well as cor pulmonale. Other interstitial lung disease, without clear histopathologic classification, also can underlie PH.

Some dogs with severe PH develop what appears to be a form of noncardiogenic pulmonary edema, with patchy to diffuse alveolar opacities distributed throughout the lungs (Kellihan, 2015; **Figure 39.5**). This disorder seems most common in small breed dogs (such as the Shih Tzu); many of these have concurrent mitral regurgitation but no evidence of significant left heart enlargement. The precise pathogenesis of this disorder and the optimal treatment approaches require further definition. Clearly, there must be some degree of "acute on chronic" pulmonary injury. The magnitude of PH in these cases is so severe that if it were only of acute onset, the RV afterload would be intolerable. Additionally, these dogs generally show evidence of cor pulmonale with a mixed pattern of compensatory RV hypertrophy. Although the source of lung injury is uncertain, pulmonary crackles persist long after stabilization and likely represent fibrosis, which predisposes to PH. However, the initial insult responsible for alveolar injury is unknown. One proposed mechanism involves nonuniform pulmonary capillary overperfusion, resulting from variability in pulmonary vasoconstrictive responses to hypoxia across the lung. This is similar to the mechanism described for people suffering from acute high-altitude pulmonary edema: pulmonary capillary beds served by arterioles with a less robust hypoxic vasoconstrictive response are subjected to high hydrostatic pressure and flow. Damage to alveolar capillary membrane integrity in those areas leads to formation of pulmonary edema with high protein and red cell content. The distribution of this edema is patchy because not all capillary beds are overperfused. This type of pulmonary edema should improve or resolve with reduction of PA pressure (as with PDE-5 inhibitor and O_2 therapy). Clinically, it can be confused with cardiogenic pulmonary edema or pneumonia. However, excessive diuretic therapy only worsens CO and perfusion.

Pneumonia caused by *Pneumocystis carinii* is a rare condition that has been associated with PH in dogs (Schiborra, 2018). It has been reported mainly in Cavalier King Charles Spaniels and Miniature Dachshunds, although other breeds can be affected. An underlying immunodeficiency is suspected as a predisposing condition. The pathogenesis involves inflammation and thickening of alveolar walls from an inflammatory infiltrate, with subsequent interstitial involvement. Lesions can have a diffuse or multifocal distribution.

Airway obstruction is another potential cause of PH. Horses with severe asthma (recurrent lower airway obstructive disease) can experience reversible PH of variable severity during acute attacks of airway inflammation triggered by allergens in dust and moldy hay (Decloedt, 2017). The greatest increases in PA pressure typically occur in horses with the most severe clinical signs and marked hypoxemia. More pronounced pulmonary vasoconstriction, and greater PVR, would be expected in these animals. Alveolar hypoxia is associated with reduced NO and increased ETN-1 levels; this promotes vasoconstriction and inhibits vasodilation. However, O_2 administration during asthmatic episodes in these horses does not completely normalize PA pressure, so other mechanisms are likely, too. Such mechanisms might involve inflammatory mediator-induced vasoconstriction, and pulmonary capillary compression or destruction associated with pulmonary emphysema. Focal myocardial neutrophilic infiltrate also is evident histologically in some animals. During asthma attacks, echo changes associated with PH can develop, including PA dilation, abnormal interventricular septal motion, and reduced left ventricular (LV) size. Other manifestations of *cor pulmonale* include RV hypertrophy and dilation with mildly reduced ventricular systolic and diastolic function. However, the cardiac changes secondary to acute airway obstruction in horses often are largely reversible. Even severely asthmatic horses might only occasionally show signs of cor pulmonale, presumably because of intermittent and reversible episodes of PH. Cardiac structure and function could be echocardiographically normal during the intervals between acute asthma episodes in asthmatic horses (Johansson, 2007). Nevertheless, some degree of persistent RV hypertrophy is likely in severely affected horses. Besides secondary RV hypertrophy, increased risk for arrhythmias can occur.

Chronic upper airway obstruction sometimes produces marked hypoxemia and hypercarbia. This could be another cause of PH and cor pulmonale. PH induced by upper airway obstruction is well-documented in people and has occurred with feline upper airway inflammatory polyps.

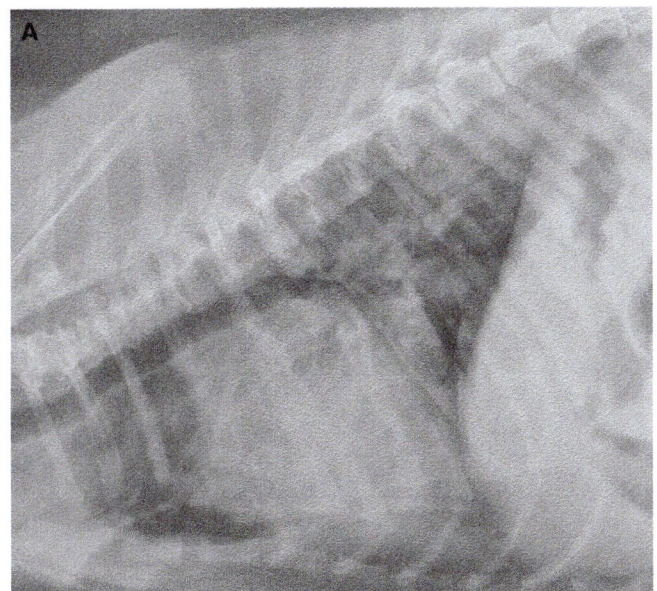
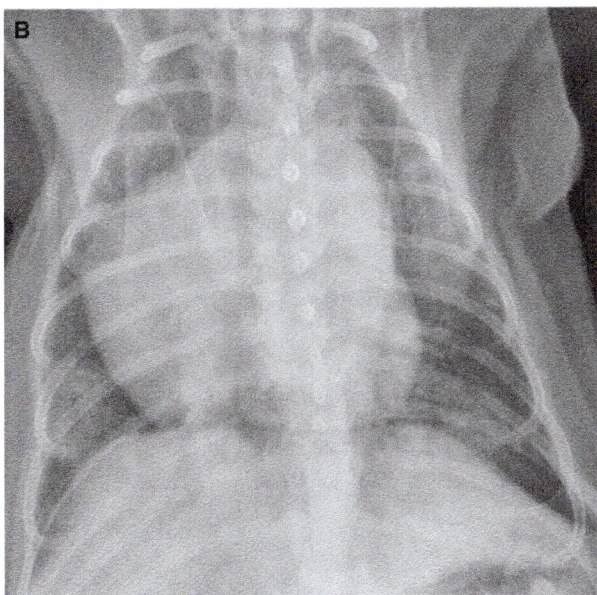
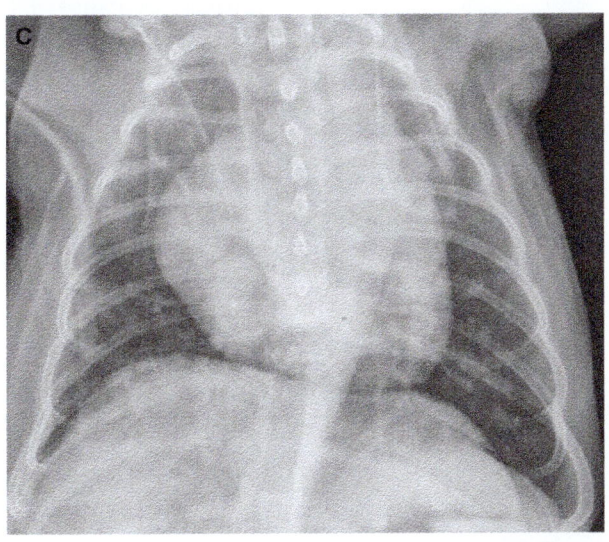

Figure 39.5 Right lateral (A) and DV (B) radiographs from a 13-year-old, female Chihuahua presented for acute respiratory distress and inappetance. Clinical findings included bilateral pulmonary crackles, muddy oral membranes, and a moderately loud systolic murmur over the tricuspid region. The respiratory distress improved following supplemental O_2 and furosemide administration. These initial radiographs show right heart enlargement with bilateral pulmonary infiltrates, especially in the right caudodorsal region (B). Although left-sided congestive heart failure was suspected at hospital admission, the ventral angulation of the main bronchi distal to the carina (A) does not support left atrial enlargement (or heart failure caused by mitral regurgitation). Furthermore, the prominent right heart enlargement and caudal vena caval distension (B), as well as the murmur consistent with tricuspid regurgitation, suggest the presence of severe PH. Echocardiography confirmed normal left atrial size, with minimal mitral regurgitation; moderate right atrial and ventricular dilation; moderate tricuspid regurgitation (TR); and severe pulmonary hypertension (PH; estimated TR pressure gradient >92 mm Hg). Sildenafil was prescribed and furosemide discontinued, because chronic lung pathology was thought to underlie the PH (and episode of presumed noncardiogenic pulmonary edema). The following day, radiographs (C, DV view) showed marked reduction of pulmonary infiltrates, as well as right heart size. At recheck exam a week later, the dog was breathing comfortably and had a normal appetite. The TR murmur was softer and Doppler exam showed modest decrease in peak TR velocity.

Pulmonary Thromboembolism

A pulmonary (thrombo)embolus large enough to obstruct one or more major vessel(s) can cause PH (**Figure 39.6**; also **Figure 36.8**, p. 753). Alternatively, numerous small emboli could block many small arteries and arterioles. PTE can occur in situations of hypercoagulability, endothelial damage, or blood stasis (Chapter 36). Besides PTE, pulmonary vascular obstructive disease (obliterative pulmonary arterial hypertension) can result from in-situ pulmonary thrombosis, as well as HWD.

Vascular obstruction reduces total cross-sectional pulmonary vascular area, not only by mechanically occluding

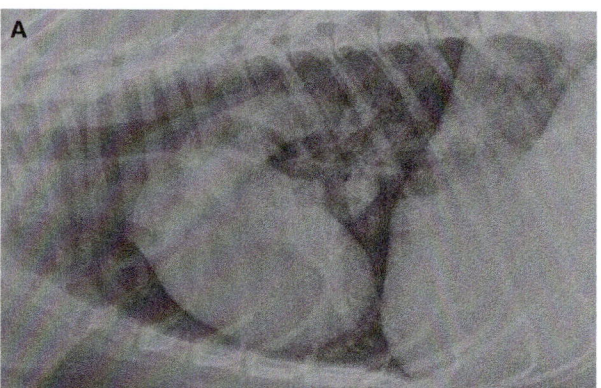
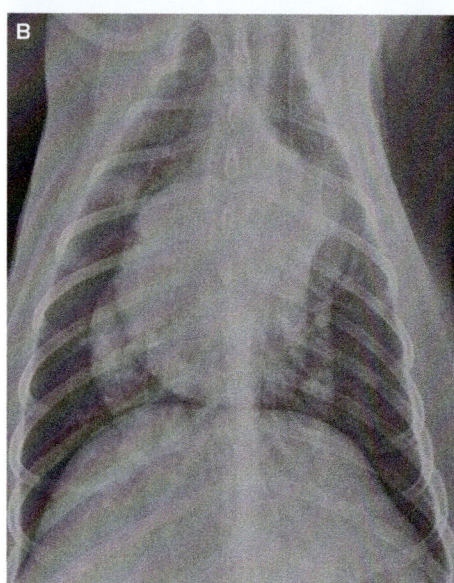
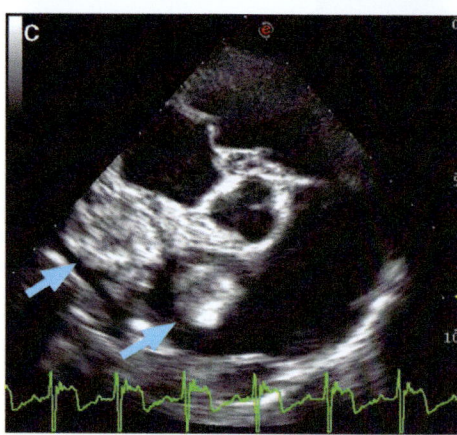

Figure 39.6 Right lateral (A) and DV (B) radiographs from a 10-year-old female English Setter with progressive exercise intolerance and recent onset of collapse after minimal exertion. Physical exam revealed pale mucous membranes, jugular venous pulsation, weak femoral pulses, a murmur of tricuspid regurgitation, and a snapping S_2 sound. There is severe enlargement of the right ventricle and the pulmonary trunk and its major branches. Note the cardiac apex elevation from the sternum (A), and reverse "D" configuration of the cardiac silhouette, with prominent pulmonary trunk bulge (B). The peripheral pulmonary arteries are markedly truncated. (C) Echocardiography revealed large in-situ pulmonary thrombi (arrows) within the markedly dilated right pulmonary artery. (Images courtesy of Dr OL Nelson.)

vessels, but also by provoking local hypoxic pulmonary vasoconstriction. In addition, neurogenic stimulation and release of vasoconstrictor substances contribute to pulmonary arteriolar vasoconstriction. Abnormal pulmonary blood flow and endothelial dysfunction promote platelet aggregation, activation of the clotting cascade, and elaboration of vasoconstrictor substances such as ETN, thromboxane A_2, and serotonin. NO production is decreased, impairing endothelial-mediated vasodilation. These factors exacerbate the vascular obstruction. Additionally, a PA wall baroreflex might contribute to vasoconstriction as pulmonary pressure increases. Associated pulmonary parenchymal disease could exacerbate the reduction in vascular area.

Acute PH caused by PTE has been identified in cats and dogs. The majority of cases are presumed emboli from abdominal veins, but the source of the thrombus often is uncertain. One well-appreciated cause of a major embolus with related thrombosis is spontaneous heartworm death in cats or after adulticidal therapy in dogs (Chapter 40). Regardless of cause, PTE can provoke respiratory distress with signs of RV dilation and, if truly acute, hypotension. Acute on chronic PTE potentially can lead to cor pulmonale and right-sided CHF. Sometimes, clinical signs are reversible with anticoagulant therapy, supplemental O_2 and supportive care. Reduction in active pulmonary arteriolar vasoconstriction by direct or indirect activation of the NO-cGMP pathway is helpful in PTE. In dogs and in cats, that means treatment with sildenafil or tadalafil, along with support of RV function with pimobendan. In people, sudden, massive PTE is the most common cause of acute precapillary PH. Acute PTE has been known to resolve spontaneously in some cases; it might even be subclinical in others. However, incomplete resolution, recurrent PTE, or in-situ thrombosis can cause chronic disease. Acute clinical signs of painful breathing are thought to relate to pleuritis in some cases. This can only be inferred in animals. Many affected animals have tachypnea, probably stemming from pulmonary infiltrates related to the PTE; these can be severe with heartworm embolism. Exercise-induced dyspnea in people with PH from chronic PTE is thought to involve not only impaired CO because of the elevated PVR, but also increased ventilatory drive caused by V/Q mismatch. Progressive vascular remodeling associated with chronic PTE can lead to worsening PH, RV failure, and ultimately, death. Prognosis is negatively correlated with PA pressure in people.

Parasitic Disease

This category (**Table 39.1**, group 5) deviates from the human PH classification scheme and was added by the ACVIM consensus panel on canine PH to encompass HWD caused by *Dirofilaria immitis*, as well as PH associated with *Angiostrongylus vasorum* infection (Chapter 40). Multiple mechanisms underlie PH in HWD. Proliferative intimal lesions within the pulmonary arteries (a group 1 lesion), luminal obstruction by dead worms and thrombi (a group 4 lesion), and inflammation of surrounding parenchyma (a group 3 lesion) all damage the pulmonary vasculature and lead to sustained PH. Besides *D. immitis*, other pulmonary parasitic diseases occasionally cause PH. An estimated 15% of dogs infected with *A. vasorum* have PH, and underlying severe pulmonary parenchymal and vascular injury can lead to marked hypoxemia (Borgeat, 2015; also see p. 871). These cases generally have pronounced hyperglobulinemia consistent with longstanding infection, and shorter survival time than infected dogs without PH. In cats, sporadic cases of *Aelurostrongylus abstrusus* and *Troglostrongylus brevior* have caused PH. Pulmonary vasculitis can occur with other infectious diseases, too, which should be considered in endemic areas. These have included leishmaniasis, ehrlichiosis, Rocky Mountain spotted fever, bartonellosis, borreliosis, hepatozoonosis, and sepsis.

Other Causes of Pulmonary Hypertension

PH of unclear or multifactorial mechanisms is assigned to group 6 (in people, this is group 5). This group includes patients with various comorbidities that contribute importantly, but by different mechanisms, to the development of PH. An example would be a small-breed dog with CHF caused by advanced DMVD (group 2 PH) that also has severe interstitial lung disease (group 3 PH). Another would be inflammatory lung diseases of uncertain etiology in cats and in horses. Animals with PH of multiple underlying mechanisms will likely need therapy aimed at each cause.

Another veterinary example that might be considered in PH group 6 is recurrent exercise-induced pulmonary hemorrhage (EIPH) in horses (Manohar, 1999; DeCloedt, 2017). While not considered a cardiovascular disease per se, EIPH occurs following rupture of pulmonary capillaries secondary to development of high pressures in the left atrium, pulmonary veins, and pulmonary arteries during maximal exertion. EIPH is particularly common in Thoroughbred horses used for racing. Maximal systolic PA pressures can exceed 120 mm Hg with extreme exercise and EIPH has been reported to occur once mean PA pressure exceeds 75 mm Hg (Poole, 2016, Birks 1985). This is not specifically an issue of PH because the dramatic increases in CO literally overwhelm the pulmonary circulation and left side of the heart. Dramatic increases in LV diastolic, LA, and pulmonary venous and capillary pressures occur. Inasmuch as LA pressure can exceed 65 mm Hg, there is a prominent post-capillary component to this transient PH. Mitral regurgitation, if present, could contribute by increasing pulmonary venous pressure, although EIPH is not specifically associated with AV valve regurgitation, age or body weight. Horses with chronic EIPH also exhibit structural lesions in pulmonary veins, along with abnormalities in pulmonary arterioles and capillaries. While these lesions are not as severe as those associated with PVOD and PCH (and stem from a different cause), they still might contribute to chronic increases in PVR. The increase in RV dimensions found in horses with more pronounced EIPH, apart from age or weight effects, is consistent with PH and associated RV remodeling.

Clinical Features

Clinical signs reflect the level of functional impairment in animals with PH. While these signs might relate directly to PH itself, they also could be manifestations of the underlying disease process(es). When evaluating a patient with suspected PH, a newer perspective is to consider relevant clinical findings from the standpoint of whether they are "strongly" or "possibly" suggestive of PH.

Clinical signs in patients with PH can be subtle and nonspecific. Persistent respiratory difficulty, fatigue, or exercise intolerance without apparent cause should raise suspicion for PH. Animals thought to have only a mild to moderate degree of PH might be asymptomatic. However, the severity of clinical signs has not necessarily correlated with the estimated severity of PH (Paradies, 2014). Middle-aged to geriatric dogs are affected most often; however, PH can develop in dogs, cats and horses of any age as a complication of underlying disease. There is no apparent sex predilection. The dog breeds affected often are those in which airway or pulmonary disease and DMVD are common. Younger animals with PH are more likely to have congenital cardiac disease or pneumonia. HWD must be ruled out in dogs. A small minority of dogs with PH have a history of previously treated HWD. Other infectious causes should be considered in endemic regions.

The most commonly reported presenting complaints in dogs with PH include exercise intolerance, cough, respiratory difficulty, and exertional syncope. The PH itself, independent of underlying pulmonary or cardiac disease, can cause tachypnea at rest, respiratory distress, exercise intolerance, syncope, and signs of right-sided CHF. The mechanism for syncope could relate to the underlying disease process, as well as an inability to increase CO in response to peripheral vasodilation during exercise. Cough, when present, is likely to indicate underlying respiratory disease. In addition to the above signs, PH in people has caused rare but potentially fatal hemoptysis. Hoarseness (related to recurrent laryngeal nerve compression caused by pulmonary artery enlargement) is unlikely in companion animals, but is another sign in people. Rupture of the pulmonary artery is a rare consequence in horses.

The clinical signs of PTE can be difficult to differentiate from those of other cardiopulmonary diseases. An index of suspicion is needed, especially when a predisposing cause such as canine hyperadrenocorticism, hemolytic anemia, or protein losing nephropathy is recognized. In cats, heartworm related pulmonary embolism is a consideration in endemic areas. Acute-onset respiratory difficulty is a classic manifestation of PTE, although it does not always occur. Other signs reported with PTE in dogs include tachycardia, lethargy, altered mentation, and, occasionally, vomiting or coughing. In cats with PTE, lethargy, anorexia, weight loss, and difficult breathing are common signs; vomiting, coughing, dehydration, hypothermia, and icterus occur occasionally. A history that includes indwelling venous catheter placement is common, although PTE might relate more to the seriousness of underlying disease. Dry cough, especially with exertion, and hemoptysis are other signs that occasionally occur in people with chronic PTE-induced PH. The typical presentation of the rarely identified PVOD involves an older dog with a short (few days) history of respiratory signs, which rapidly progress to respiratory distress.

Physical Findings

Physical examination findings in animals with PH can include signs of right-sided CHF, which can relate to cor pulmonale, as well as underlying primary cardiac disease (**Figure 39.7**). Ascites is reported in over one fourth of dogs with PH, although this figure likely relates to the type of patients referred for more severe signs. Other signs of CHF include jugular venous distension and possibly, subcutaneous edema, which is especially common in horses. Even without right-sided CHF, physical signs of marked PH can include jugular vein pulsation, a precordial impulse stronger on the right hemithorax (compared to the left), and cardiac auscultatory abnormalities (see next paragraph). Pulmonary crackles or wheezes are common in animals with underlying pulmonary or airway disease. Increased respiratory effort (inspiratory, expiratory or both, depending on the underlying disease process) could be evident. Animals with a right-to-left shunt, severe pulmonary disease, or asthma might have obvious cyanosis at rest, or with mild exertion.

A systolic heart murmur is audible in many animals with PH. This often relates to TR; increased murmur intensity typically signals a greater likelihood of PH, although there are exceptions especially when TR jets are eccentric (Ohad, 2013). The combination of stronger right precordial impulse, history of syncope, and a TR murmur is strongly indicative of PH in dogs (and presumably other species, as well). Similarly, the presence of ascites with a loud right apical (TR) murmur in a mature dog is highly suggestive of PH as the primary or secondary cause of heart disease. Mitral regurgitation murmurs also are common in animals with PH, particularly dogs with DMVD. A systolic murmur louder at the right apical region compared to the left in a dog with DMVD, suggests concurrent and clinically significant PH. A soft systolic ejection murmur localized over the pulmonary artery is detected in some cases. With severe PH especially, another common auscultatory abnormality is a loud, snapping or split S_2; this often can be heard even when a murmur is not. Uncommonly, a diastolic murmur of pulmonary regurgitation is audible.

Diagnostic Tests

The diagnostic process involves identifying that PH most likely exists and defining the underlying or associated conditions. When PH (or a condition often associated with PH) is suspected based on history and physical findings, thoracic radiographs can help support this suspicion and screen for pulmonary and cardiac diseases. Although direct measurement of PA pressures by right heart catheterization provides definitive diagnosis, echocardiography is the best noninvasive way to identify the probable presence of PH and assess its severity. It provides additional detailed information about cardiac structure and function, too. Therefore, echocardiography should be pursued early in the diagnostic process when PH is suspected based on clinical or radiographic findings. Other imaging modalities that might also be useful for individual cases include CT, pulmonary angiography (**Figures 36.15D** and **36.21**, pp. 760 and 762) and pulmonary nuclear perfusion scintigraphy (to identify PTE), and fluoroscopy (to document dynamic airway collapse). Heartworm status should be verified in dogs (and cats) with suspected PH (Chapter 40). Screening for other pulmonary parasites (including *A. vasorum*) or infectious diseases is indicated in endemic areas, as well. Arterial blood gas analysis or pulse oximetry, routine blood and urine analyses, tracheal or bronchoalveolar washings, and D-dimer assay or other tests of coagulation or immune

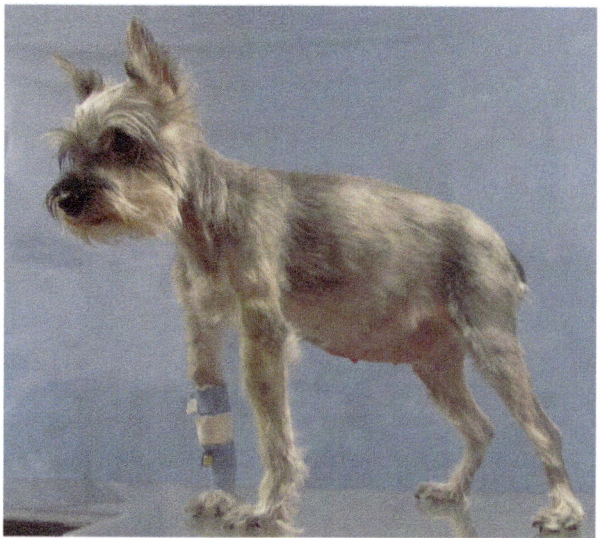

Figure 39.7 Pulmonary hypertension in an 11-year-old, female Miniature Schnauzer with advanced degenerative mitral valve disease and recent syncopal episodes. Ascites, jugular vein distension, sinus arrhythmia, and loud left and right apical systolic murmurs were present. Echocardiography showed severe left heart enlargement, moderate right heart and pulmonary artery dilation, and tricuspid regurgitation to 4.65 m/s (estimated gradient, 86 mm Hg).

system function can be helpful in some cases. Pulmonary function testing, although not widely available, might help characterize underlying disease.

Laboratory Tests

Routine clinical laboratory findings reflect abnormalities associated with the underlying disease process, rather than PH per se. Hypoxemia occurs commonly with many underlying causes of PH. Nucleated red blood cells (RBCs) often are seen with chronic hypoxemia and have been noted in over one quarter of dogs with PH. A similar percentage of dogs with PH, and most dogs with PTE, appear to have mild leukocytosis. Arterial blood gas analysis can provide information about pulmonary function, oxygenation and ventilation. Alternatively, pulse oximetry could indicate abnormal hemoglobin O_2 saturation (Chapter 10).

An association between RBC distribution width (RDW) and PH is reported in dogs; those with (either pre- or postcapillary) PH, had increased median RDW compared to healthy dogs (Mazzotta, 2016). RDW is a measure of anisocytosis. The increase in RDW might relate to underlying pathophysiologic processes associated with PH, rather than the severity of the PH itself. There are conflicting reports as to whether RDW correlates with echo indicators of PH severity, but no correlation was found with survival. Several biomarkers increase in patients with PH. However, in dogs and cats with dyspnea, currently available point-of-care tests cannot reliably differentiate between animals with PH, or CHF and concurrent PH, versus CHF alone. Elevations in circulating N-terminal prohormone B-type (brain) natriuretic peptide (NT-proBNP) occur with both pre- and postcapillary causes of PH. Thus, interpretation of NT-proBNP elevation can be problematic in animals with cardiopulmonary signs. Median NT-proBNP is higher in dogs with precapillary PH compared with dogs that have respiratory disease without PH (Kellihan, 2011). The degree of NT-proBNP elevation increases with PH severity, as estimated by peak TR gradient. Yet, in a dog model of PTE, although NT-proBNP was increased when PH was severe, it was not when PH was mild (Hori, 2012). NT-proBNP elevation also occurs in dogs without CHF but with severe arrhythmias, sepsis, or PTE, among other causes of precapillary PH. NT-proBNP concentrations between 500 and 900 pmol/L have been associated with moderately increased cardiac load, and >900 pmol/L with severe cardiac load, but there are breed variations and false positives. C-terminal BNP concentrations also rise in dogs with CHF and PH. Increases in atrial natriuretic peptide (ANP) or precursor concentrations appear to be more variable. While ANP increased with severe PH from experimental PTE, another study showed no increase in NT-proANP and cardiac troponin (cTn)I in dogs with precapillary PH.

Circulating cTnI concentration usually increases in dogs with precapillary PH compared to healthy dogs, as well as in dogs with DMVD of different stages. With DMVD, a significant increase in median cTnI accompanies decompensated left-sided CHF with postcapillary PH, although this does not appear to be the case with compensated DMVD, regardless of PH presence. Much overlap in cTnI concentrations is observed between these groups, however.

Circulating concentrations of ETNs rise with increasing severity of heart failure and pulmonary disease and are positively correlated with the severity of PH (Tessier-Vetzel, 2006). ETN-1 plasma concentration has been correlated with outcome in dogs with respiratory disease. Yet differentiating dogs with heart disease from those with primary respiratory disease using ETN-1 is problematic. Similarly, serum big ETN-1 is a potential marker for cardiopulmonary, as well as neoplastic, diseases in dogs. Although big ETN-1 levels correlate better than NT-proBNP with PH severity, big ETN probably cannot differentiate dogs with cardiopulmonary disease from those with neoplasia.

Radiography

Radiographic findings that suggest severe PH include enlargement of the right heart and main or lobar pulmonary arteries (Adams, 2017; **Figures 39.5, 39.6, and 39.8–39.10**). Evidence for primary heart disease as a cause for PH, either from a congenital shunt or secondary to left-sided CHF, should be sought. However, radiographic signs can be inconsistent, especially with lesser degrees or recent onset of PH. Additionally, a dilated main pulmonary artery is not commonly visualized in post-capillary PH. In cats, the main pulmonary artery rarely extends to the edge of the cardiac silhouette, even in feline HWD. Inspection of pulmonary lobar vessels could be more useful. For example, caudal lobar pulmonary artery diameter (at the tracheal bifurcation) divided by body surface area was evaluated as a possible tool to identify PH (Lee, 2016). Although the ratio on average is larger in dogs with PH compared to those without, the diagnostic accuracy for detecting PH was only moderate. Unfortunately, thoracic radiographs do not reliably identify PH or differentiate its severity. Radiographic findings can be unremarkable in mild to moderate PH.

Signs of right-sided CHF (including pleural effusion, caudal vena caval distension, hepatomegaly, and ascites) are visible in some advanced cases of PH. Pulmonary venous distension indicates venous congestion in dogs with underlying left-sided CHF; however, this is not always evident, especially after diuretic therapy.

For small-breed dogs (≤15 kg) with DMVD, the cardiac size on a lateral radiograph suggests PH when the cardiac short-axis dimension (as measured during vertebral heart size, VHS, assessment, p. 47) exceeds 5.2 v and the length of sternal contact exceeds 3.3 v (Mikawa, 2015). In this situation, PH with a peak TR velocity ≥3.1 m/s (or pulmonary regurgitation velocity ≥2.8 m/s) is predicted with moderate accuracy. However, the extent of sternal contact can be influenced by LV, as well as RV, enlargement. Furthermore, the criterion of

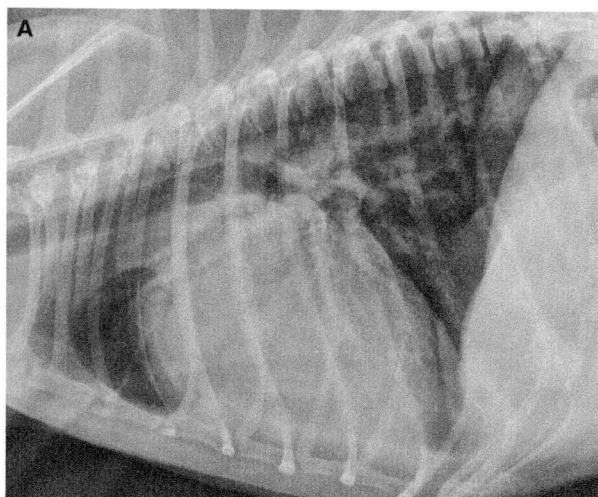
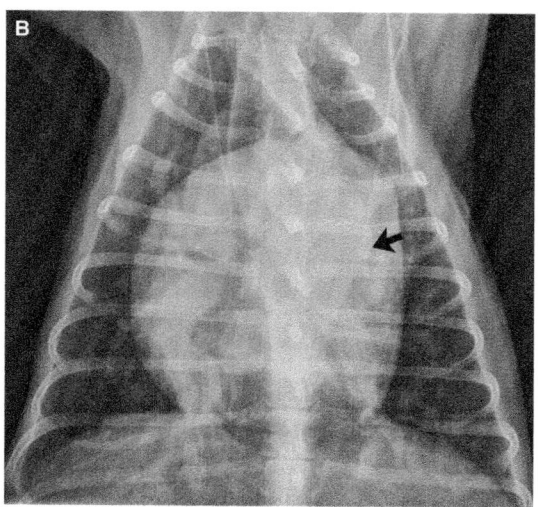

Figure 39.8 Right lateral (A) and DV (B) radiographs from an 11-year-old, female Maltese-Poodle mix with collapse episodes during the prior 3 weeks, jugular pulsation, and a soft right apical systolic murmur. Generalized cardiomegaly is evident, with enlarged and mildly tortuous caudal pulmonary arteries. There is a bulge in the descending aorta (arrow; B). Echocardiography documented right ventricular enlargement and hypertrophy, right atrial dilation, severe pulmonary trunk enlargement, tricuspid regurgitation (TR; peak velocity >4.9 m/s), and a diminutive left ventricle - all consistent with severe pulmonary hypertension. Therapy with sildenafil produced only modest reduction in TR peak velocity. However, this was sufficient for a grade 1/6 continuous left basilar murmur and small continuous Doppler flow signal within the pulmonary trunk to appear, confirming a previously undiagnosed patent ductus arteriosus.

sternal contact is unlikely to be valid in larger, deep-chested dogs because of their different chest conformation.

The pulmonary parenchymal appearance in animals with PH generally reflects underlying disease; however, this is widely variable. Pulmonary infiltrates associated with pulmonary fibrosis most often involve a bronchointerstitial pattern in dogs. In horses, nodularity might be seen by ultrasound along the lung edge. When acute lung injury or edema occurs, an alveolar pattern or a pulmonary mass effect might be evident. Sometimes dogs with inspiratory crackles typical of pulmonary fibrosis have no appreciable radiographic abnormality at all, although CT imaging will reveal abnormalities.

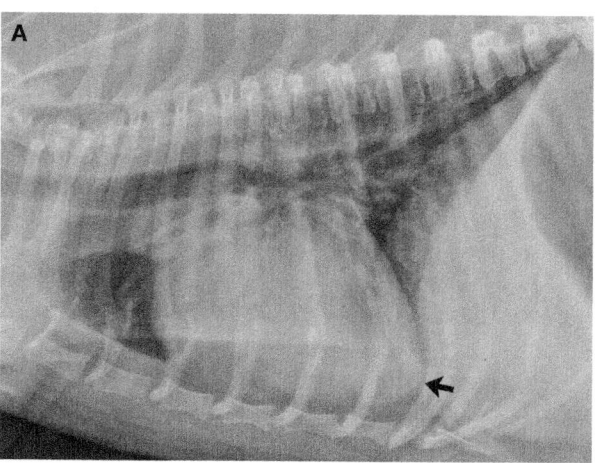
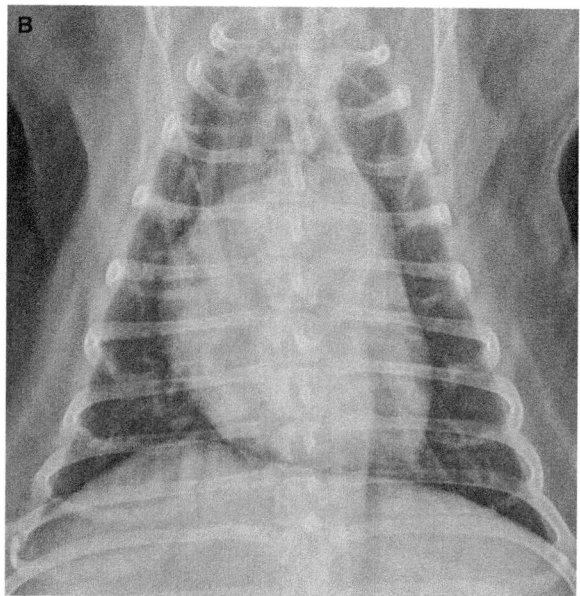

Figure 39.9 Right lateral (A) and VD (B) radiographs from a 13-year-old, female Shih Tzu with chronic pulmonary disease and severe pulmonary hypertension. Auscultation revealed coarse pulmonary crackles over all lung fields and a loud tricuspid regurgitation (TR) murmur. Although the VHS is within normal limits (10.2v; A), the widened cardiac silhouette and elevated cardiac apex (arrow) suggest right heart enlargement. Right ventricular (RV) prominence gives the cardiac silhouette a reverse "D" appearance (B); yet, pulmonary trunk dilation appears minimal. Enlarged lobar pulmonary arteries are obscured somewhat by the bronchointerstitial pattern. Echocardiography documented RV dilation and hypertrophy, pulmonary trunk dilation, moderate TR (peak velocity 4.83 m/s; gradient, 93.4 mm Hg), only trace mitral regurgitation, and normal to small left heart size.

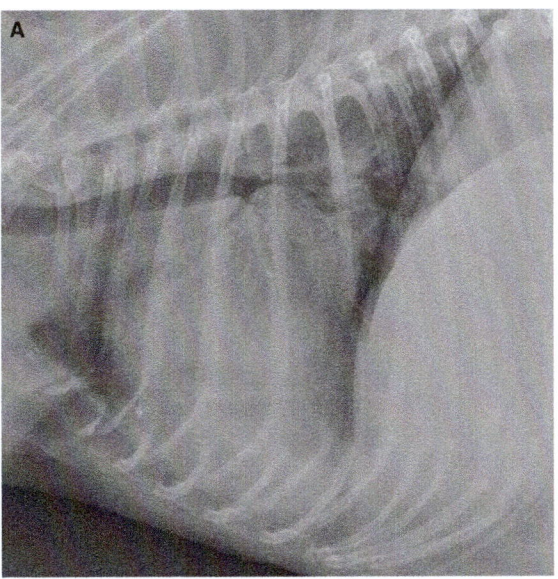 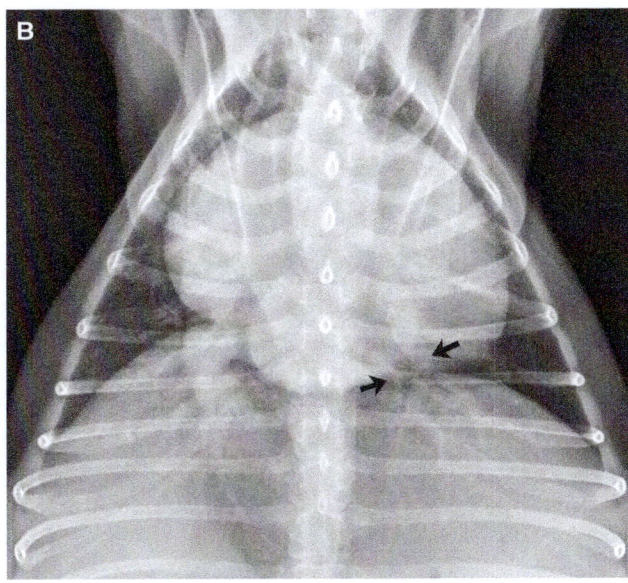

Figure 39.10 (A) Right lateral radiograph from the dog of **Figure 39.7** shows marked left atrial and ventricular enlargement (secondary to the chronic mitral regurgitation); there also is some suggestion of right heart enlargement. (B) On DV view, the enlarged right ventricle laterally displaces the left apex. The left caudal lobar pulmonary vessels best reveal the pulmonary arterial dilation (arrow on right), compared to the smaller, accompanying vein (arrow on left); also note the prominent caudal vena cava, which obscures the right caudal lobar artery.

Radiographic abnormalities in patients with PTE can include peripheral noncircumscribed consolidations, uneven pulmonary vascular diameter (and blood flow distribution) among lung lobes, proximal PA dilation with abrupt tapering, and pleural effusion. Yet radiographs sometimes appear normal (p. 759). Some dogs with moderate or severe PH caused by pulmonary fibrosis or other interstitial disease show evidence of noncardiogenic pulmonary edema, including diffuse patchy alveolar infiltrates (**Figure 39.5**). These signs could be confused with left-sided CHF, especially in dogs with DMVD, or with pneumonia. This noncardiogenic form of pulmonary edema probably relates to high perfusion pressure-induced alveolar capillary damage occurring nonuniformly within the lung. It often causes acute respiratory distress or syncope and appears to improve with sildenafil therapy. Radiographic findings with PVOD include right heart enlargement, with patchy or diffuse interstitial, and sometimes alveolar, infiltrates. Cases of PVOD and PCH usually show no radiographic evidence to support left-sided CHF as the cause for respiratory signs.

CT measurement of main PA diameter-to-aortic root (Ao) diameter might be helpful in identifying pulmonary trunk enlargement caused by PH. In normal dogs, this ratio is about 1.1 (similar to the upper normal limit (of 1.04) reported with echocardiography). However, the ratio is influenced by the phase of respiration during CT image acquisition. Expiratory scans yield a lower main PA/Ao ratio than inspiratory scans. Nevertheless, moderate correlation between this ratio and PH severity has been shown, with mean main PA/Ao ratio significantly higher in dogs with moderate and severe PH, compared to normal dogs (Sutherland-Smith, 2018). This ratio could not differentiate dogs with mild PH from normal, however. A patient suspected to have PH based on this CT finding should be followed-up with Doppler echocardiography. CT imaging also can be useful for evaluating pulmonary parenchymal lesions. Contrast studies (CT angiography) might highlight areas of neoplastic or inflammatory infiltration, or reveal PTE. Lung CT images in cases of PVOD are likely to show diffuse, perivascular nodular ground-glass opacities, as well as the PA enlargement consistent with PH.

Electrocardiography

The ECG might show evidence of right atrial (RA) or RV enlargement (p. 156) in patients with marked PH, although this is inconsistent. Arrhythmias develop in some cases. These have included atrial fibrillation and other atrial or ventricular tachyarrhythmias. Occasionally, bradycardia or slowed AV conduction occurs. Changes in the T wave or ST segment might occur in some cases, especially with marked hypoxemia or RV hypertrophy (**Figure 39.11**).

Echocardiography

Echocardiography provides the best noninvasive means of determining the probability that PH exists and estimating its severity, especially when TR is present. Imaging of pulmonary parenchyma might also reveal evidence of interstitial-alveolar syndrome in some dogs with multiple B-line ("lung rockets") suggestive of increased lung water or cellular infiltration. However, as always, pulmonary ultrasound findings should be substantiated by radiography in small animals, and echo findings interpreted within the context of the historical

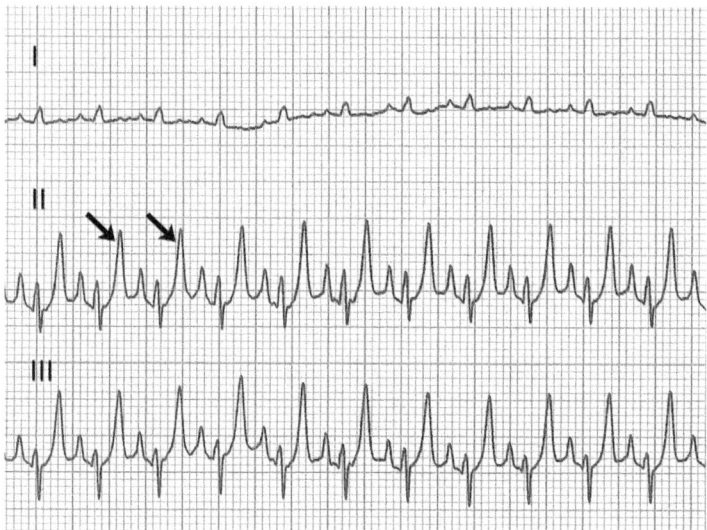

Figure 39.11 ECG from a 12-year-old, female Labrador Retriever with exercise intolerance, persistent cough, hypoxemia (PaO$_2$ 41 mm Hg; SpO$_2$ 78-82%), and marked pulmonary hypertension. The large T waves (arrows) are consistent with hypoxemia, but also could be secondary to abnormal ventricular depolarization (indeterminate electrical axis, with cranial left terminal forces). Leads as marked; 25 mm/s, 1 cm = 1 mV.

and clinical findings. It has been recommended that PH in dogs be defined as "an intermediate or high probability of PH" when characteristic echo findings are identified in animals with compatible clinical signs (Reinero, 2020; and **Table 39.2**). For dogs (and presumably cats and horses), this includes a TR peak velocity >3.4 m/s in cases with measurable TR and without RV outflow obstruction. Typical 2D and M-mode echo findings consistent with PH include: RV chamber dilation, some degree of RV hypertrophy (wall thickening), abnormal septal motion, and PA dilation (**Figures 39.12–39.14**). Impaired RV function, RA enlargement and caudal vena caval distension also might be found. In one series of dogs with PH, about half had normal RV size and wall thickness and less than a third had severe RV dilation; RV hypertrophy was considered moderate in <25% of cases, and severe in only 10% (Johnson, 1999). Severe RV concentric hypertrophy is most likely to occur in young animals, usually in association with congenital defects (**Figures 26.25**, **26.35**, and **26.41**, pp. 452, 461, and 465).

PH causes the interventricular septum to appear flattened toward the left ventricle whenever RV pressure exceeds LV pressure. This can occur in diastole, systole, or both (**Figure 39.12A** and **B**). In some cases, paradoxical septal motion is seen on M-mode exam if there is significant RV volume overload, but more often septal motion is flatter than normal (**Table 4.2**, p. 91). A small LV chamber size, with LV pseudohypertrophy (**Figure 39.12**), can signal RV failure and impaired output caused by severe PH. This is often a poor prognostic sign. Sporadically, PH (and other causes of RV pressure overload) can provoke hyperdynamic LV motion, with abnormal mitral leaflet systolic anterior motion; this probably relates to reduced pulmonary venous return combined with sympathetic activation. When PH develops secondary to left heart disease and elevated pulmonary venous pressure (postcapillary PH), moderate to severe LA enlargement is expected. LA enlargement is an indicator of clinically significant valvular regurgitation in DMVD and often of chronically increased LV filling pressure (and PCWP). However, an exception to this finding is when acute chordae tendineae rupture occurs prior to marked LA remodeling. Echo evidence for mitral or aortic valve disease or LV dysfunction also is expected in animals with postcapillary (or combined pre- and postcapillary) PH. Experience indicates that end-systolic LA pressure in dogs with severe mitral regurgitation can approach 60 mm Hg; therefore, postcapillary PH could reach the moderate to severe range, even without contribution from reflex pulmonary artery vasoconstriction. This is relevant therapeutically because most cardiologists first manage severe left-sided CHF before initiating a drug (such as sildenafil) to dilate pulmonary arteries specifically, especially when moderate to severe left heart enlargement is present. Conversely, with moderate to severe precapillary PH, left heart size often is small. After PDE-5 inhibitor therapy is begun in such cases, an increase in LV diastolic area and diameter provides a useful echo indicator of increased transpulmonary flow.

Moderate to severe PH causes distension of the RV outflow region, pulmonary valve annulus, pulmonary trunk, and branch pulmonary arteries. Consequently, the ratio of pulmonary annulus (and main PA)-to-Ao diameter generally increases. In most normal animals, this ratio is ≤1. Values >1.04 are highly sensitive, although only moderately specific, for moderate to severe PH (with a TR pressure gradient >50 mm Hg). Heartworms or a large pulmonary thrombus might be visualized in the proximal pulmonary artery of patients with such underlying conditions (**Figure 39.6C**; also **Figures 36.8**, p. 753, and **40.13**, p. 852). If a patent foramen ovale (or other intracardiac communication) exists, right-to-left shunting will occur whenever pressure on the right side exceeds that on the left. Color Doppler or an echo-bubble study can document this (**Figure 26.36A**, p. 461, and **Figures 26.40B** and **26.41B**, pp. 464 and 465). The exception is when PH is postcapillary, in which case the shunting will be from left-to-right as observed with splitting of the atrial septum.

PA pressure can be estimated noninvasively using continuous wave (CW) Doppler echocardiography when TR or pulmonary valve regurgitation (PR) is present and when pulmonic stenosis (or other RV outflow obstruction) is absent. Color Doppler imaging guides CW Doppler cursor placement, and might identify a measurable tricuspid (or pulmonary) regurgitant jet when an audible murmur is absent. Injection of agitated saline can sometimes improve the signal strength of the regurgitant jet. With TR, the modified Bernoulli relationship is used to estimate the systolic pressure gradient between the right ventricle and its atrium, based on the highest TR jet

Table 39.2 Guidelines for Estimating Probability of Pulmonary Hypertension in Dogs[a]

Probability of PH

- Low
  - Peak TR velocity ≤3.0 m/s (or not measurable), with no supportive echo evidence for PH; OR, with such evidence in only 1 anatomic site (see descriptions, below)
- Intermediate
  - Peak TR velocity ≤3.0 m/s (or not measurable) WITH supportive echo evidence for PH in 2 different anatomic sites; OR,
  - Peak TR velocity 3.0–3.4 m/s WITH supportive echo evidence for PH in only 1 (or no) anatomic site; OR,
  - Peak TR velocity >3.4 m/s even without anatomic echo evidence for PH
- High
  - Peak TR velocity ≤3.0 m/s (or not measurable) WITH supportive echo evidence for PH in 3 different anatomic sites; OR,
  - Peak TR velocity 3.0–3.4 m/s WITH supportive echo evidence for PH in ≥2 anatomic sites; OR,
  - Peak TR velocity >3.4 m/s WITH supportive echo evidence for PH in ≥1 anatomic site

Supportive Echocardiographic Evidence by Anatomic Site Includes

- Anatomic site 1 (ventricles)
  - Interventricular septal flattening (especially in systole)
  - Small (underfilled) left ventricle[b]
  - RV wall hypertrophy and/or chamber dilation
  - RV systolic dysfunction
- Anatomic site 2 (pulmonary artery)
  - PA enlargement (PA/Ao >1.0)
  - Doppler peak (early diastolic) PR >2.5 m/s
  - Right PA distensibility index <30%
  - RV outflow (Doppler) acceleration time <52–58 ms, or acceleration time/ejection time ratio <0.30
  - Systolic notching of Doppler RV outflow profile (note: false positives possible)
- Anatomic site 3 (right atrium and caudal vena cava)
  - Right atrial enlargement
  - Caudal vena caval dilation

[a] Note: these guidelines assume the absence of pulmonary valve stenosis or other cause of RV outflow obstruction. Adapted from the ACVIM consensus statement guidelines for the diagnosis, classification, treatment, and monitoring of pulmonary hypertension in dogs (Reinero, 2020).
[b] Criterion not applicable to animals with postcapillary PH because of LV remodeling from left heart disease.
Abbreviations: Ao, aorta; echo, echocardiographic; PA, pulmonary arterial; PH, pulmonary hypertension; PR, pulmonary regurgitation; RV, right ventricular; TR, tricuspid regurgitation.

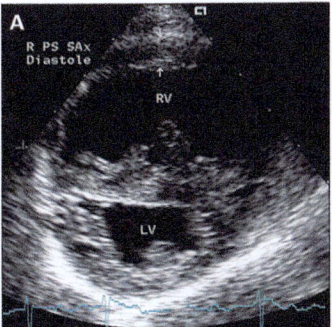
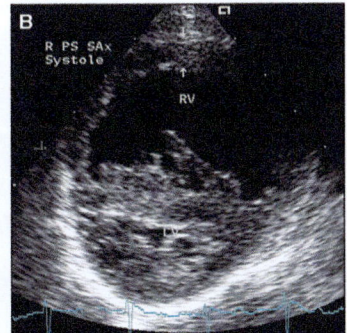
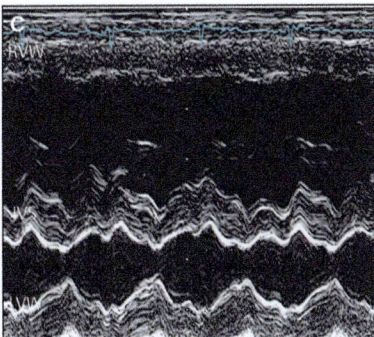
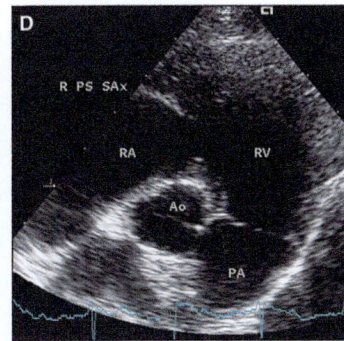

Figure 39.12 Diastolic (A) and systolic (B) 2D echo frames from a 3-year-old, female Cocker Spaniel with severe thromboembolic pulmonary hypertension (PH). The RV is hypertrophied (arrows) and dilated; high right ventricular pressures in both diastole and systole flatten the IVS toward the LV. The small left ventricular lumen size and relatively thickened walls (pseudohypertrophy) reflect poor left heart filling. (C) M-mode echocardiography depicts the right ventricular dilation and hypertrophy in this dog, with better endocardial definition. (D) 2D image at the heart base shows the right ventricular outflow and pulmonary annulus dilation caused by PH. The RA also is dilated. Right parasternal short-axis views. Ao, aorta; IVS, interventricular septum; LV, left ventricle; LVW, left ventricular wall; PA, pulmonary artery; RA, right atrium; RV, right ventricle; RVW, right ventricular wall.

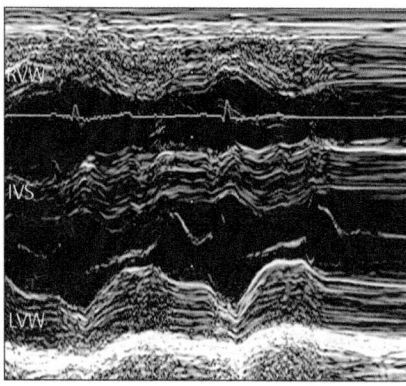

Figure 39.13 M-mode echo image at the ventricular level from a 13-year-old, male Yorkshire Terrier with severe pulmonary hypertension, diabetes mellitus, and protein-losing nephropathy. In this case, there is moderate hypertrophy of the RVW, but only modest chamber dilation. Mitral valve echoes are visible within the left ventricle. Peak tricuspid regurgitation velocity was 5.45 m/s (gradient, 120 mm Hg). IVS, interventricular septum; LVW, left ventricular wall; RVW, right ventricular wall.

velocity that can be recorded (p. 126; **Figure 39.15**; also **Figure 40.15**, p. 853). This gradient is then added to the estimated RA pressure. In the absence of right-sided CHF and when the caudal vena cava shows normal respiratory variation in size, the RA pressure often is ignored. However, in cases with elevated vena caval or jugular venous pressure, an estimate of ~5 to 10 mm Hg might be used for RA pressure. In the setting of right-sided CHF, the RA pressure probably should be added to the TR pressure gradient. This RA pressure is probably in the range of 10–15 mm Hg in most small animals prior to diuretic therapy (but much higher in the standing horse, often 30 mm Hg or more). Alternatively, central venous pressure (CVP) can be measured in order to approximate RA systolic pressure. Overall, echo estimates of RA pressure can be erroneous and produce inaccurate estimation of PA systolic pressure. Therefore, use of TR peak velocity itself (or just the calculated pressure gradient) is recommended for estimating the probability of PH. Peak TR velocities ≥3.0 m/s or peak (early) PR velocities >2.5 m/s usually suggest PH, especially when other supportive evidence exists. Based on Doppler RV-to-RA systolic pressure gradients, PH severity previously has been categorized as mild (gradient ~35–50 mm Hg; TR maximum velocity 2.9–3.5 m/s), moderate (~51–75 mm Hg; TR maximum velocity 3.6–4.3 m/s), and severe (>75 mm Hg; TR maximum velocity >4.3 m/s). However, these divisions are somewhat arbitrary and currently their use is discouraged (Reinero, 2020). End-diastolic PR jet velocity can be used similarly to estimate PA diastolic pressure: calculated PA-to-RV pressure gradient plus estimated RV diastolic pressure. The maximal (early diastolic) PR jet velocity is thought to approximate mean PA pressure. While all of this makes arithmetical sense, numerous human studies have demonstrated poor correlation between invasively measured and Doppler estimated PA pressures. Inaccuracy is especially likely when suboptimal Doppler technique is used or the regurgitant jet is small, highly eccentric, or weak.

With regard to repeatability, PH estimation using peak TR velocity is better than other echo methods. Nevertheless, several situations can confound accurate TR peak velocity measurement. Cursor malalignment with true peak TR jet velocity is a common cause of velocity underestimation. All views where TR is evident, including off-angle views, should

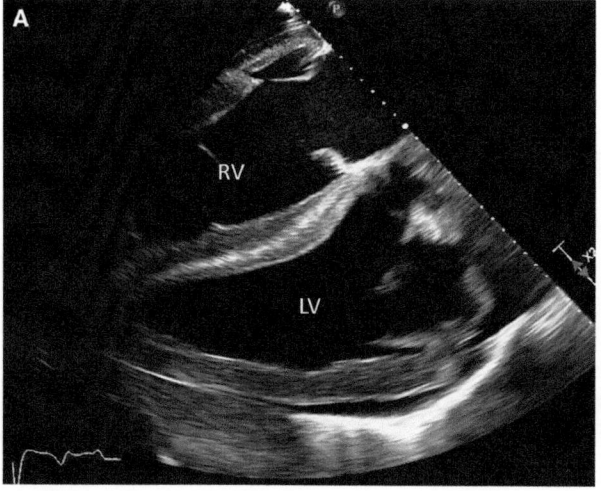
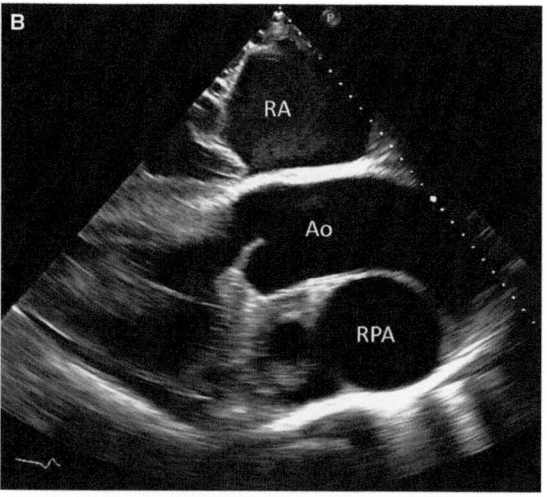

Figure 39.14 A 10-year-old Quarterhorse mare in late gestation had a 3-week history of cough and progressively increasing respiratory effort. During initial physical exam, the mare was markedly tachypneic, with jugular distension and pulsations, prominent pulmonary crackles and wheezes, and a heart rate of 80 beats/min. Arterial pO_2 was approximately 55 mm Hg. (A) Long-axis 2D echo image in late diastole shows moderate right ventricular enlargement, with leftward septal shift. A trivial amount of pericardial effusion also is present. (B) The diameter of the dilated right pulmonary artery (seen in cross-section) exceeds that of the normal aortic root. Doppler study documented peak tricuspid regurgitation velocity over 4.5 m/s (gradient, 82 mm Hg). Therapy with sildenafil and dexamethasone improved her clinical status, allowing successful foaling. Right parasternal views. Ao, aorta; LV, left ventricle; RA, right atrium; RPA, right pulmonary artery; RV, right ventricle.

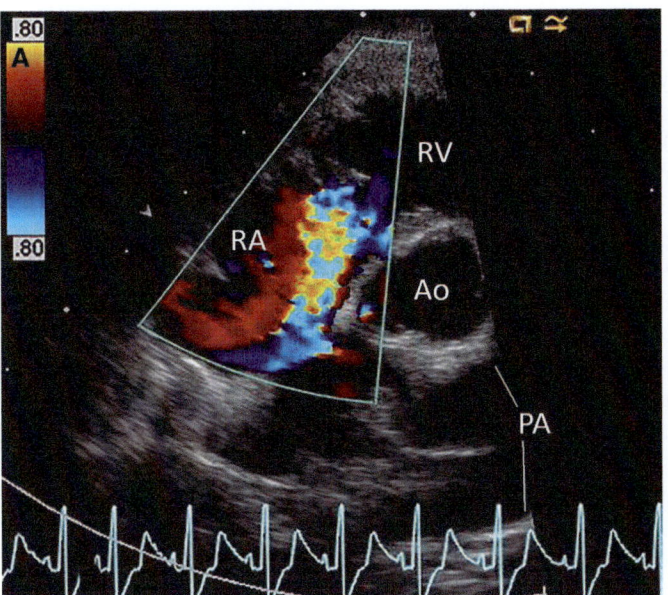
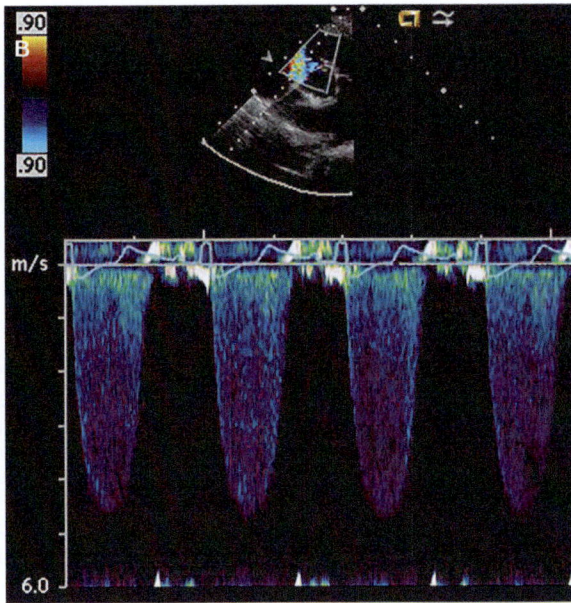

Figure 39.15 (A) Color Doppler image in systole from the dog in **Figure 39.8** shows a strongly turbulent tricuspid regurgitation (TR) jet, with indication of right ventricular dilation and hypertrophy; pulmonary arterial dilation also is evident (area of bifurcation indicated by white lines). (B) Continuous wave Doppler image shows a peak TR velocity of approximately 4.93 m/s (gradient, 97 mm Hg). Right parasternal short-axis position. Ao, aorta; PA, pulmonary artery; RA, right atrium; RV, right ventricle.

be interrogated in the search for maximal TR velocity. Other sources of error include the presence of only a tiny TR jet, an uncooperative patient, labored respiration, impaired RV contractility, pericardial constraint, and marked alteration in preload. On serial echo exams that employ consistent technique, changes in a patient's peak TR velocity of over 0.3 m/s most likely represent real differences in PA systolic pressure (Abbott, 2017). In dogs with DMVD, neither body position nor 6-minute walk test had a significant effect on TR peak velocity. However, sedation increased TR peak velocity in a majority of dogs, sometimes by over 0.4 m/s (Rhinehart, 2017). This might be an effect of slowed heart rate. In any case, it potentially could alter the clinical assessment of PH severity. An estimated (RV-to-RA) pressure gradient over 55 mm Hg has been identified as a negative predictor of survival in dogs with DMVD.

Especially when TR (or PR) is not evident, several other echo findings also help support identification of PH. These include the PA annulus/Ao ratio, alterations in the Doppler PA velocity profile (next paragraph) and associated systolic time intervals, the right pulmonary artery distensibility index (RPADI), pulmonary vein-to-right pulmonary artery ratio, and others. Nevertheless, all have potential technical limitations and are based on relatively small studies. There also are substantial differences in diagnostic cut-off points depending on the pre- or postcapillary nature of the PH.

High PA pressure alters the pulsed wave (PW) Doppler pulmonary velocity profile in characteristic ways. As PH severity increases, systolic flow acceleration becomes faster because of the increased arterial stiffness; consequently, the pulmonary flow profile becomes more like that of the aorta (**Figure 39.16**; also **Figures 40.15C**, p. 853 and **4.33**, p. 110). This shortens the pulmonary flow acceleration time (AT), prolongs ejection time (ET), and decreases the ratio of AT to ET. An AT/ET <0.30 is considered specific, although not highly sensitive, for moderate to severe PH (TR pressure

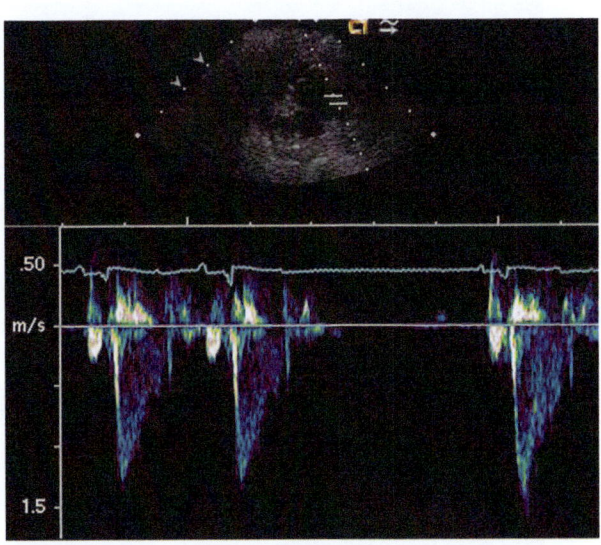

Figure 39.16 Pulsed wave Doppler recording of pulmonary arterial flow from a 5-year-old, female Yorkshire Terrier with protein-losing enteropathy, pulmonary hypertension (PH), and signs of right heart failure. Rapid systolic flow acceleration and slight notching during deceleration are evident. The acceleration time-to-ejection time ratio is 0.19 (see text). This is suggestive of precapillary PH.

gradient >50 mm Hg). Some studies have used the ratio of AT to pulmonary deceleration time (DT), with similar results. For example, in dogs with DVMD, a median pulmonary AT/DT of 0.59 was strongly correlated with an estimated systolic PA pressure >55 mm Hg (based on TR gradient), while in dogs with pressure gradients <55 mm Hg, median AT/DT was 0.84 (Tidholm, 2015). Although PA AT/ET (or AT/DT) usually is decreased by PH, this ratio can be affected by cursor position, respiration, RV systolic function, TR severity, and heart rate. In addition, abnormalities of arterial wave propagation and impedance in the pulmonary vasculature associated with marked pre-capillary PH can cause midsystolic notching of the PA velocity profile, related to prominent systolic reflection waves (**Figures 39.16**; also **4.33**, p. 110, and **40.15C**, p. 853). This finding is atypical in postcapillary PH.

In dogs with DMVD, increased TR pressure gradient is strongly associated with an increased (body) weight-normalized RV diastolic dimension. Although RV dimension can be influenced by the degree of TR, as well as PH, dogs with a TR pressure gradient >55 mm Hg had a median corrected RV diastolic dimension of 0.35, compared to 0.24 for those with lower estimated PA pressure. The weight-normalized LV diastolic dimension has a more parabolic relationship with TR pressure gradient in that severe PH is associated with both small and large LV sizes. A small LV size likely relates to poor forward flow from a failing RV secondary to severe PH, which leads to reduced LV filling. A large LV size results from the progressively increasing LV volume overload associated with severe MR and secondary PH. In these dogs, PH severity is correlated with MR severity and degree of LA dilation (LA/Ao ratio). With postcapillary PH, transmitral E wave velocities usually exceed 1 m/s.

The RPADI is the calculated percent change in diameter of this artery from systole to diastole; that is, (systolic − diastolic)/systolic × 100. The severity of PH influences this index because the increase in PA stiffness (associated with PH) reduces the change in vessel diameter that normally occurs from systole to diastole (that is, its distensibility). Measurements for the RPADI are obtained using the right parasternal short-axis view optimized for the pulmonary trunk and its right branch, as it courses toward the right lung, across the region of the left atrium; the vessel's diameter is measured from inner edge to inner edge (**Figure 39.17**). It is important to optimize the image so that both edges of the vessel are clear and translational motion throughout the cardiac cycle is minimized. The RPADI correlates strongly with calculated pressure gradients based on TR maximal velocity (Vmax), especially those >50 mm Hg. In dogs, RPADI values <29.5% predict more severe PH (similar to a TR pressure gradient of over 50 mm Hg) with 95% specificity and 84% sensitivity (Visser, 2016). Values <34.6% were shown to predict PH with a TR pressure gradient >36 mm Hg with a specificity of 91%, but sensitivity of only 74%. Others report that RPADI values ≤22% are associated with even more severe PH (estimated PA pressure >79 mm Hg), while values between 23 and 27% indicated moderate PH (56–79 mm Hg; Serrano-Parreno, 2017). Mild PH was associated with RPADI values between 28% and 35% (30–55 mm Hg). An RPADI ≥36% correlates with normal PA pressure.

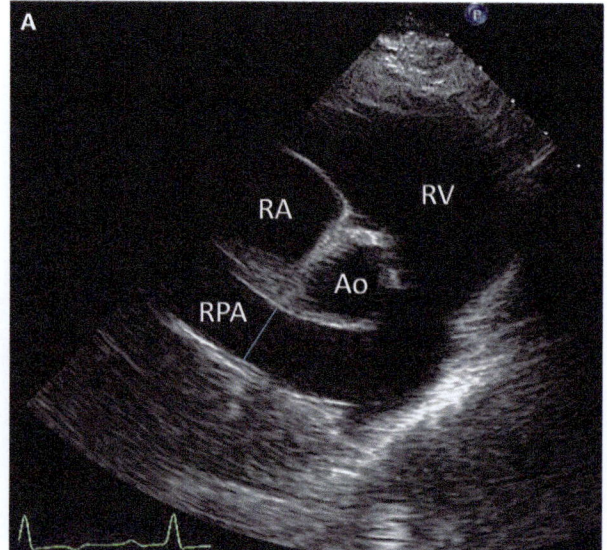 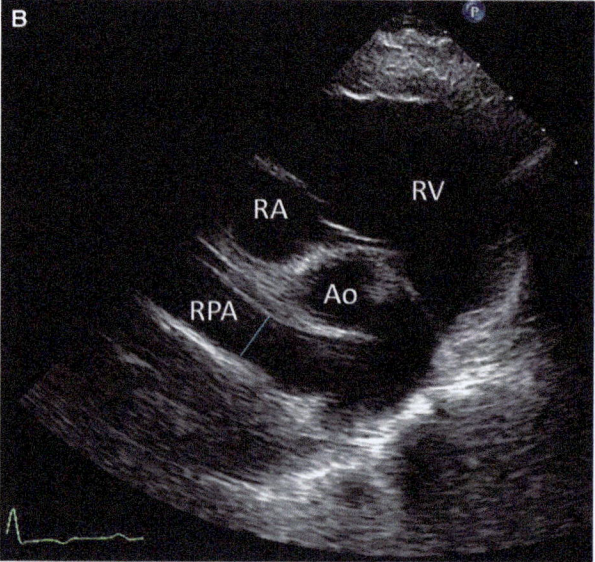

Figure 39.17 Right parasternal short-axis images from a 5-year-old mixed breed dog with pulmonary hypertension (tricuspid gradient, 62 mm Hg). The RPA distensibility index (RPADI) is calculated from diameter measurements of the RPA in systole (A) and diastole (B). This dog's RPADI is approximately 19.7%, consistent with pulmonary hypertension of at least moderate severity; see text for more information. Ao, aorta; RA, right atrium; RPA, right pulmonary artery; RV, right ventricle.

Another index described is the ratio of pulmonary vein-to-right pulmonary artery diameter, obtained using the right parasternal long-axis view. A ratio <0.7 had high sensitivity and good specificity for moderate PH (defined as TR pressure gradient >50 mm Hg) in dogs with precapillary PH (Roels, 2019). Most of these figures pertain to single center studies and specific patient types; while the principles for these indices are likely to hold true, additional studies are needed to evaluate the generalizability of these specific ratios and cutoffs.

RV systolic function can be assessed by measuring the tricuspid annular plane excursion (TAPSE; see p. 94), because RV contraction occurs mostly along the longitudinal plane. Dogs with severe PH are more likely to have a TAPSE below reference range for their body weight. Yet, TAPSE often is normal in dogs with mild or moderate PH, especially those with postcapillary PH (that is, left heart disease), where it might be increased (hyperdynamic) because of septal tethering to the left side. For dogs with DMVD, there was no difference in TAPSE between those with PH and those without (Poser, 2017). This suggests either that RV function is not decreased, or more likely, that the hyperdynamic left ventricle falsely increases TAPSE. Falsely increased TAPSE also can occur with severe TR. Ratios of TAPSE/Ao or adjusted TAPSE/Ao, and weight-adjusted TAPSE could serve as a body weight-independent means to identify severe PH, as well as to assess RV function, even in dogs with DMVD (Caivano, 2018a). Occasionally, the Tei index of myocardial performance is used as a measure of global RV function (Paradies, 2014). Positive correlation exists between the Tei index and PH severity, but this index is difficult to obtain on the right side without dual sample-volume pulsed wave Doppler systems.

RA area, indexed to body surface area, can be used to estimate RA size. RA area has prognostic value in people with PH. In dogs with moderate or severe PH, the RA area index is increased, compared to dogs with mild or no PH (Vezzosi, 2018). It also is increased in dogs with PH and right-sided CHF. A RA area index cut-off value of >12.3 cm^2/m^2 was 100% sensitive and almost 90% specific for CHF in this study. It was suggested that RA area index not only evaluates RA size but also might be a more effective predictor of CHF than TR peak velocity in dogs with PH. The severity of TR appears to be the main determinant of increased RA area index.

Tissue Doppler imaging (TDI) of the basilar RV free wall myocardium might help identify PH in animals without measurable TR or PR. A combined systolic and diastolic RV TDI index (comprised of the RV myocardial systolic velocity × the RV myocardial e'/a' velocity ratio) of <11.3 cm/s was sensitive and specific for differentiating dogs with estimated PA pressures >30 mm Hg from normal dogs (Serres, 2007). In most dogs with PH, the RV myocardial e'/a' ratio is <1. However, accurate RV TDI measurements are angle dependent, and might not be obtainable in all animals.

Cardiac Catheterization

Cardiac catheterization allows for direct PA pressure measurement, as well as selective pulmonary angiography (**Figure 36.21**, p. 762), although it rarely is done now for diagnosis of PH in clinical veterinary medicine. Measurement of PCWP can differentiate precapillary from postcapillary PH. A Swan–Ganz type or similar catheter (with end hole and inflatable balloon near its tip) is used to measure pressures within the right heart and pulmonary trunk. PCWP is obtained by inflating the balloon when the catheter tip is in the pulmonary trunk and allowing the catheter to advance passively until it (temporarily) obstructs (wedges in) a smaller PA branch. The pressure recorded here reflects downstream pressure in the pulmonary capillaries and beyond. PCWP approximates LA pressure, assuming no pulmonary venous obstruction exists. If PH is secondary to high pulmonary venous pressures (left-sided CHF; postcapillary cause), PCWP is elevated. When PH is caused by pulmonary vascular, bronchopulmonary, or other disease (with precapillary pulmonary vascular remodeling), PCWP is substantially lower than measured PA diastolic pressure. Right heart catheterization also allows evaluation of acute pulmonary vasoreactivity in response to vasodilator drugs. In people, responsiveness is defined as a decrease in mean PA pressure of at least 10 mm Hg, to a level of 40 mm Hg or lower.

Other Tests

Bronchoalveolar lavage cytology might provide diagnostic information in cases of pulmonary and airway inflammatory or neoplastic infiltration. Laryngoscopy and bronchoscopy could indicate large airway obstruction. For cases where the underlying diagnosis still is not evident, lung biopsy can be informative. This is the only way to definitively diagnose some pulmonary interstitial diseases, PVOD, and PCH; however, the potential risks involved with obtaining lung biopsy samples must be considered.

Management

There currently is no cure and few treatment options for severe PH. Medical management is aimed at addressing the underlying disease process(es) as possible, restricting exercise, attempting to reduce PH severity, and minimizing complications. Horses with PH should not be worked and are considered unsafe to ride. Routine preventative measures against infectious respiratory diseases are recommended, including vaccination and heartworm prophylaxis, as indicated. High-altitude environments, as well as airline travel, should be avoided. Likewise, elective medical or surgical procedures requiring general anesthesia are best avoided in patients with marked PH. Pregnancy also is not advised.

HWD or angiostrongylosis, when present, should be treated appropriately (Chapter 40). Animals with a right-to-left shunting congenital defect that have developed erythrocytosis are managed with maintenance of hydration (including gentle salting of the food and free access to water); periodic phlebotomy; or, if necessary, treatment with hydroxyurea (p. 454). A PDE-5 inhibitor is administered to reduce PVR. For animals with a large bidirectional shunt that becomes substantially left-to-right with PDE-5 inhibitor therapy, shunt occlusion is recommended. Therapy for animals with left heart disease that develop (postcapillary) PH is focused on delaying or controlling CHF signs and thereby, reducing pulmonary venous pressure (Chapter 22 and other relevant chapters in this text). Animals with underlying respiratory disease complicated by PH are managed as possible to mitigate inflammation, infection, airway collapse, coughing, and hypoxia. This includes avoidance of environmental irritants and excessive heat or cold, as well as patient excitement and anxiety. Current reference sources related to specific respiratory diseases should be consulted, as needed, for treatment recommendations. Obese patients might benefit from weight loss, by improvement in ventilatory mechanics. When PH is secondary to PTE or in-situ thrombosis, antithrombotic therapy is indicated (p. 763). Other medical or surgical treatment also might be indicated for individual cases. High PVR usually relates to vascular morphologic changes, which limit the capacity for pulmonary vasodilation. Supplemental O_2 administration is recommended in acute care settings. Its benefits can include a degree of pulmonary vasodilation in actively constricted vessels, reduced acidosis and ischemia, and improved right heart function. Whether at-home O_2 supplementation is of any long-term benefit is unknown. However, this could be considered in cases that show in-hospital improvement with O_2 therapy.

PDE-5 inhibitors are helpful, and especially indicated for dogs with clinical evidence for precapillary PH (see next section). Their additive value, above aggressive CHF therapy, in postcapillary PH requires more study. In contrast to sildenafil and tadalafil, other (non-PDE-5 inhibitor) vasodilator drugs such as amlodipine often produce greater systemic arterial dilation; therefore, they are of little benefit and possibly detrimental for patients with (precapillary) PH. In the case of postcapillary PH, it is reemphasized that a PDE-5 inhibitor should not be used as first-line therapy; initial management in these patients is aimed at reducing LV filling pressure and optimizing forward CO. In the rare case of PVOD or PCH, administration of a PDE-5 inhibitor is likely to precipitate acute pulmonary edema. Pimobendan usually is administered to patients with symptomatic PH also (p. 835).

The type and frequency of follow-up monitoring and recheck visits largely depend on the patient's clinical status and underlying pathology. In general, initial reevaluation for clinically stable patients could be done about 2 weeks after initiating therapy; rechecks thereafter might occur every 3–6 months, unless clinical deterioration dictates more frequent examination. The client's perception of change in the animal's tolerance for activity, respiratory signs, appetite, and other clinical parameters can be useful. An activity monitor, or exercise tolerance test (such as a 6-minute walk test) could provide more quantitative data. In addition, assessment for changes in radiographic or echo findings or in oxygenation (using pulse oximetry or arterial blood gas measurement) might help inform therapy.

Phosphodiesterase-5 Inhibitors

Selective PDE-5 inhibitors, such as sildenafil, tadalafil and similar agents increase pulmonary vascular cGMP concentrations and bolster the effect of endogenous NO. By promoting NO-mediated pulmonary vasodilation, these drugs reduce PVR and PH. PDE-5 inhibition with sildenafil has been shown to increase cGMP release and restore sensitivity of the pulmonary vasculature to cGMP-mediated vasodilation in people with heart failure and PH. In addition, sildenafil has some antioxidant effects, which might increase NO availability. In people with coronary artery disease, sildenafil also was shown to dilate epicardial coronary arteries, improve endothelial dysfunction, and inhibit platelet activity. It might have a cardioprotective effect in ischemia-reperfusion injury, too.

Sildenafil improves clinical signs and quality of life in a majority of dogs with symptomatic PH, as it does in people. In an experimental canine model of hypoxic pulmonary vasoconstriction, sildenafil significantly reduced the PA pressure increase (Mondritzki, 2017). Although decreases in Doppler-estimated PA pressure are found only inconsistently in canine patients, this might relate to study timing, PA flow events, or other factors, such as increased CO that improves clinical signs even if PA pressure reduction is only mild.

Some clinicians administer supplemental L-arginine (~100–500 mg/kg) to dogs treated with sildenafil (or another PDE-5 inhibitor) for PH, with the aim of increasing NO availability. The amino acid L-arginine is a substrate for NO-synthase. However, it is unclear whether the combination of L-arginine and sildenafil provides any greater effect, although it is unlikely to be harmful. In a model of acute PTE, use of both L-arginine and sildenafil together did not provide an advantage over sildenafil alone. In normal dogs, oral L-arginine dosed at 100 mg/kg q8h doubled plasma L-arginine concentration; however, production of L-citrulline was extremely variable (Flynn, 2017). As a byproduct of NO production from L-arginine, plasma L-citrulline concentration sometimes is used as a surrogate indicator of NO synthesis.

Oral sildenafil doses of 0.5 to 2(–3) mg/kg q12h or q8h generally are well-tolerated and have produced clinical improvement in a majority of PH dogs evaluated. These doses also reduced Doppler-estimated PA pressure in some dogs. Most clinicians reserve this therapy for cases of severe PH or those symptomatic for moderate to severe precapillary PH. Therapy should be started with lower dose(s), ideally in hospital, and resting respiratory rate monitored because in some cases, increased PA flow could precipitate pulmonary edema (see next paragraph). Sildenafil has a short half-life of 3–5 hours, so q8h dosing is likely to be more effective. Lower initial doses, with gradual up-titration, are suggested. Sildenafil can be compounded for easier dosing in small animals. Rectal administration of sildenafil (orally disintegrating film tablet form) produces lower maximum serum concentration compared to oral administration, but could be used for patients unable to take the drug orally (Yang, 2018). There are anecdotal reports of inferior potency from use of "generic" sildenafil citrate prior to the drug's release from patent. It is unclear if problems with drug equivalency persist.

Complications with sildenafil are uncommon, but have included cutaneous flushing, nasal congestion, and gastrointestinal (GI) signs. Headache, dizziness, visual disturbances, priapism, myalgia, and back pain occur in people; short-term behavioral changes have been seen in dogs. The potential for concurrent systemic vasodilation and significant hypotension must be considered, especially when non-PDE-5 inhibitor vasodilator drugs are used concurrently. For example, nitrate is a substrate that can be reduced to NO during hypoxia and tissue acidosis, so it can have beneficial effects in acute PTE and possibly other mechanisms of PH. Yet, while the combination of both sildenafil and a nitrate can produce additive effects in reducing PA pressure, it also can provoke transient systemic hypotension. Therefore, concurrent use of sildenafil (and other PDE-5 inhibitors) with a nitrate is not advised. Furthermore, sildenafil and other PDE-5 inhibitors should be used cautiously in animals with left-sided CHF or with a large congenital cardiac shunt. Reduction in pulmonary arteriolar resistance could markedly increase pulmonary venous flow and promote acute pulmonary edema in such cases.

Tadalafil and vardenafil are longer-acting PDE-5 inhibitors. Tadalafil has a half-life of about 17.5 hours in people. It has greater affinity for PDE-5 than other PDE-5 inhibitors. In an experimental dog model of vasoconstrictive PH, tadalafil produced a dose-dependent decrease in PA pressure when given by either IV infusion (100–200 mcg/kg/hr) or PO (1, 2, 4 mg/kg), although minimal effect occurred with 1 mg/kg (Hori, 2014). Tadalafil's effect is seen in about an hour and lasts at least 6 hours. Similar to sildenafil, tadalafil has improved clinical status and owner-perceived quality of life in dogs with moderate to severe PH when used at 1–2 mg/kg q24h, sometimes in combination with other therapy (including an angiotensin converting enzyme inhibitor, furosemide, spironolactone, dexamethasone, O_2). Signs of weakness or tremors might occur after initial tadalafil administration, which could reflect transient systemic hypotension. Mild decreases in systemic blood pressure have been observed during the first 48 hours of tadalafil therapy. Other adverse effects noted in a small number of dogs treated with tadalafil include decreased appetite, hindlimb weakness, and rarely, increased sexual behavior (in intact males). In people, systemic hypotension is the most common side effect of tadalafil, as well as other PDE-5 inhibitors; headache, facial flushing, nasal congestion, GI upset, and transient visual impairment also are common side effects.

Additional Medical Therapy

Pimobendan, an inodilator with PDE-3 inhibitory and calcium-sensitizing properties (p. 325), seems to have some pulmonary vasodilator effect in dogs with postcapillary PH, based on reductions in TR jet velocity that appear to be maintained long term. However, such effect on vascular tone is difficult to parse relative to its other effects; it is likely that the major clinical benefit relates to its inotropic effect. In a model of PH, pimobendan did improve CO and RV function, although it was largely ineffective in reducing PA pressures (Morita, 2020). For patients showing clinical signs of low CO or CHF stemming from PH, most cardiologists consider pimobendan, in conjunction with a PDE-5 inhibitor, as standard of care. However, one retrospective study in dogs with severe PH secondary to respiratory disease showed that combination therapy with pimobendan and sildenafil did not provide a survival benefit compared to sildenafil alone (Murphy, 2017). Digoxin, as another inotropic drug, is not indicated for PH; it is potentially proarrhythmic in the setting of hypoxia, acidosis, or cor pulmonale.

As ancillary therapy, a methyxanthine bronchodilator (if available) might help some animals with PH, although supportive studies are lacking. Theophylline and related drugs have mild positive inotropic effects on the heart, and can improve diaphragmatic contractility and reduce respiratory muscle fatigue. In addition, bronchodilation and improved intrathoracic pressure gradients might reduce the tendency for airway collapse in patients with bronchiectasis or tracheal collapse. Sustained release theophylline can be used in dogs (10 mg/kg q12h), although some dogs show adverse sympathomimetic effects at this dose. Beta$_2$-agonist bronchodilators (such as terbutaline) might also improve pulmonary hemodynamics, although this is not well studied. Terbutaline has been used in dogs (1.25–5 mg/kg q8–12h) and cats (1.25 mg/kg q12h).

Diuretics (Chapter 21) are useful for reducing blood volume in animals with CHF; however, extensive diuresis can worsen CO in patients with poor RV function. While initial diuretic therapy is appropriate for animals with respiratory distress and pulmonary infiltrates thought to be caused by CHF, if repeated diuretic doses are not improving patient status, the presumptive diagnosis of CHF should be questioned. Especially in small and mid-sized breeds of dog without a characteristic mitral regurgitation murmur or evidence for LA enlargement, such respiratory distress often relates to PH and underlying respiratory disease. Continued diuretic dosing in these cases can worsen patient status. If chronic obstructive pulmonary disease underlies PH, diuretics can further impair gas exchange by drying airway secretions and promoting mucous plug formation within bronchi. On the other hand, patients that are experiencing acute, noncardiogenic pulmonary edema secondary to severe PH could benefit from initial modest dose(s) of furosemide; however, PDE-5 inhibitor therapy is fundamental to their continued improvement.

Other Considerations

Besides PDE-5 inhibitors, prostacyclin analogues and ETN receptor antagonists are other agents used to manage PH in people. These have vasodilatory and antiproliferative properties. The rationale for prostacyclin analogues is based on the increased production of vasoconstrictors, including thromboxane A_2, and a relative deficiency of prostacyclin in patients with PH. Prostacyclin analogues (such as iloprost, epoprostenol, treprostinil) also might decrease ETN release. Improvements in exercise capacity, hemodynamics, and survival time have been shown in people. Yet, expense, the need for delivery by infusion or inhalation with some drugs, and limited duration of effect are obstacles. Beraprost is an oral prostacyclin analogue that showed relative selectivity for pulmonary vasodilation in canine experimental vasoconstrictive PH; however, its availability and efficacy appear limited, and there is little clinical experience with it. ETN-receptor antagonists (including bosentan, sitaxentan, ambrisentan) also are used for chronic PH in people. Bosentan, an oral dual ETN_A- and ETN_B-receptor antagonist, improves exercise capacity and hemodynamic status in people, but can be hepatotoxic. There are no consensus recommendations on the use of these medications.

Pentoxifylline (and similar drugs) is a xanthine-derivative PDE inhibitor with bronchodilatory effects that also increases RBC flexibility and reduces viscosity. It might also have some vasodilatory effect. Although there is anecdotal evidence of clinical improvement in patients with Eisenmenger's syndrome, the potential usefulness for acquired PH, as well as PH secondary to large cardiac shunts, is unclear and it generally is not recommended.

Tyrosine kinase inhibitors (including imatinib and toceranib) can produce PA vasodilation by inhibiting platelet-derived growth factor activation and thus, the pulmonary vascular smooth muscle proliferation that this factor stimulates. Preliminary experience with low doses of imatinib mesylate (3 mg/kg q24h PO for 30 days), was reported in dogs with PH and CHF caused by HWD (Arita, 2013). Some improvements in estimated PA systolic pressure, echo LA/Ao ratio, cardiac function indices, circulating NT-proBNP concentration, and clinical signs were observed. In people, certain tyrosine kinase inhibitors can improve refractory PH; however, serious side effects are common. Some tyrosine kinase inhibitors have caused PH in people.

Prognosis The prognosis for most patients with severe and symptomatic PH generally is poor. However, those with PH caused by HWD or *A. vasorum* (Chapter 40), or other parasitic or infectious diseases, could improve or resolve with appropriate therapy. Animals with PH from other causes might respond to medical therapy for a time. Many patients die or are euthanized within days to a few months of diagnosis. Nevertheless, others might survive for 1–2 years, and some with Eisenmenger's pathophysiology can survive beyond five years with optimal care and some luck. Factors that have been correlated with survival time in people with idiopathic PH include exercise capacity, acute pulmonary vasoreactivity, RV function, and plasma concentrations of biomarkers such as NT-proBNP, ETN-1 and cardiac troponins. A retrospective study of dogs with PH (excluding those with HWD or congenital cardiac disease) revealed shorter survival time to be independently associated with clinical right heart failure and echo variables of RA area >1.2 $cm^2/kg^{0.71}$ and TAPSE <3.23 $mm/kg^{0.284}$ (Visser, 2020). The prognosis for patients with PVOD and PCH is grave; attempted management of PH with vasodilators in these conditions is likely to provoke severe, fatal pulmonary edema.

Suggested Additional Reading and References

Also See Online Comprehensive Bibliography at: https://www.routledge.com/9781482246223.

Abbott JA, Gentile-Solomon JM. Measurement variation and repeatability of echocardiographic variables used to estimate pulmonary artery pressure in dogs. J Vet Intern Med 2017;31:1622–1628.

Adams DS, Marolf AJ, Valdes-Martinez A, et al. Associations between thoracic radiographic changes and severity of pulmonary arterial hypertension diagnosed in 60 dogs via Doppler echocardiography: a retrospective study. Vet Radiol Ultrasound 2017;58:454–462.

Aoki T, Sugimoto K, Sunahara H, et al. Patent ductus arteriosus ligation in two young cats with pulmonary hypertension. J Vet Med Sci 2013;75:199–202.

Arita S, Arita N, Hikasa Y. Therapeutic effect of low-dose imatinib on pulmonary arterial hypertension in dogs. Can Vet J 2013;54:255–261.

Atkinson KJ, Fine DM, Thombs LA, et al. Evaluation of pimobendan and N-terminal probrain natriuretic peptide in the treatment of pulmonary hypertension secondary to degenerative mitral valve disease in dogs. J Vet Intern Med 2009;23:1190–1196.

Bach JF, Rozanski EA, MacGregor J, et al. Retrospective evaluation of sildenafil citrate as a therapy for pulmonary hypertension in dogs. J Vet Intern Med 2006;20:1132–1135.

Baron Toaldo M, Guglielmini C, Diana A, et al. Reversible pulmonary hypertension in a cat. J Small Anim Pract 2011;52:271–277.

Birks EK, Mathieu-Costello O, Fu Z, et al. Very high pressures are required to cause stress failure of pulmonary capillaries in thoroughbred racehorses. J Appl Physiol 1997;82:1584–1592.

Bonagura JD. Overview of equine cardiac disease. Vet Clin North Am Equine Pract 2019;35:1–22.

Borgarelli M, Abbott J, Braz-Ruivo L, et al. Prevalence and prognostic importance of pulmonary hypertension in dogs with myxomatous mitral valve disease. J Vet Intern Med 2015;29: 569–574.

Borgeat K, Sudunagunta S, Kaye B, et al. Retrospective evaluation of moderate-to-severe pulmonary hypertension in dogs naturally infected with Angiostrongylus vasorum. J Small Anim Pract 2015;56:196–202.

Brown AJ, Davison E, Sleeper MM. Clinical efficacy of sildenafil in treatment of pulmonary arterial hypertension in dogs. J Vet Intern Med 2010;24:850–854.

Caivano D, Dickson D, Pariaut R, et al. Tricuspid annular plane systolic excursion-to-aortic ratio provides a bodyweight-independent measure of right ventricular systolic function in dogs. J Vet Cardiol 2018a;20:79–91.

Caivano D, Rishniw M, Birettoni F, et al. Right ventricular outflow tract fractional shortening: an echocardiographic index of right ventricular systolic function in dogs with pulmonary hypertension. J Vet Cardiol 2018b;20:354–363.

Campbell FE. Cardiac effects of pulmonary disease. Vet Clin North Am Small Anim Pract 2007;37:949–962, vii.

Clercx C, Fastres A, Roels E. Idiopathic pulmonary fibrosis in West Highland white terriers: an update. Vet J 2018;242:53–58.

Decloedt A, Borowicz H, Slowikowska M, et al. Right ventricular function during acute exacerbation of severe equine asthma. Equine Vet J 2017.

Decloedt A, De Clercq D, Ven S, et al. Right ventricular function during pharmacological and exercise stress testing in horses. Vet J 2017;227:8–14.

den Toom ML, Grinwis G, van Suylen RJ, et al. Pulmonary veno-occlusive disease as a cause of severe pulmonary hypertension in a dog. Acta Vet Scand 2018;60:78.

Dixon PM. Pulmonary artery pressures in normal horses and in horses affected with chronic obstructive pulmonary disease. Equine Vet J 1978;10:195–198.

Evola MG, Edmondson EF, Reichle JK, et al. Radiographic and histopathologic characteristics of pulmonary fibrosis in nine cats. Vet Radiol Ultrasound 2014;55:133–140.

Flynn KM, Kellihan HB, Trepanier LA Plasma l-citrulline concentrations in l-arginine-supplemented healthy dogs. J Vet Cardiol 2017;19:376–383.

Fukumoto S, Hanazono K, Miyasho T, et al. Serum big endothelin-1 as a clinical marker for cardiopulmonary and neoplastic diseases in dogs. Life Sci 2014;118:329–332.

Glaus TM, Tomsa K, Hassig M, et al. Echocardiographic changes induced by moderate to marked hypobaric hypoxia in dogs. Vet Radiol Ultrasound 2004;45:233–237.

Granger LA, Pariaut R, Vila J, et al. Computed tomographic measurement of the main pulmonary artery to aortic diameter ratio in healthy dogs: a comparison to echocardiographically derived ratios. Vet Radiol Ultrasound 2016;57:376–386.

Guglielmini C, Civitella C, Diana A, et al. Serum cardiac troponin I concentration in dogs with precapillary and postcapillary pulmonary hypertension. J Vet Intern Med 2010;24: 145–152.

Hori Y, Kondo C, Matsui M, et al. Effect of the phosphodiesterase type 5 inhibitor tadalafil on pulmonary hemodynamics in a canine model of pulmonary hypertension. Vet J 2014;202:334–339.

Hori Y, Uchide T, Saitoh R, et al. Diagnostic utility of NT-proBNP and ANP in a canine model of chronic embolic pulmonary hypertension. Vet J 2012;194:215–221.

Hu W, Yu SB, Chen L, et al. Renal sympathetic denervation prevents the development of pulmonary arterial hypertension and cardiac dysfunction in dogs. Kaohsiung J Med Sci 2015;31:405–412.

Jaffey JA, Leach SB, Kong LR, et al. Clinical efficacy of tadalafil compared to sildenafil in treatment of moderate to severe canine pulmonary hypertension: a pilot study. J Vet Cardiol 2019;24:7–19.

Jaffey JA, Williams KJ, Masseau I, et al. Vasoproliferative process resembling pulmonary capillary hemangiomatosis in a cat. BMC Vet Res 2017;13:72.

Jenkins TL, Jennings RN. Pulmonary capillary hemangiomatosis and hypertrophic cardiomyopathy in a Persian cat. J Vet Diagn Invest 2017;29:900–903.

Johansson AM, Gardner SY, Atkins CE, et al. Cardiovascular effects of acute pulmonary obstruction in horses with recurrent airway obstruction. J Vet Intern Med 2007;21:302–307.

Johnson L, Boon J, Orton EC. Clinical characteristics of 53 dogs with Doppler-derived evidence of pulmonary hypertension: 1992-1996. J Vet Intern Med 1999;13:440–447.

Johnson LR, Stern JA. Clinical features and outcome in 25 dogs with respiratory-associated pulmonary hypertension treated with sildenafil. J Vet Intern Med 2020;34:65–73.

Kellihan HB, Mackie BA, Stepien RL. NT-proBNP, NT-proANP and cTnI concentrations in dogs with pre-capillary pulmonary hypertension. J Vet Cardiol 2011;13:171–182.

Kellihan HB, Stepien RL. Pulmonary hypertension in dogs: diagnosis and therapy. Vet Clin North Am Small Anim Pract 2010;40:623–641.

Kellihan HB, Stepien RL. Pulmonary hypertension in canine degenerative mitral valve disease. J Vet Cardiol 2012;14:149–164.

Kellihan HB, Waller KR, Pinkos A, et al. Acute resolution of pulmonary alveolar infiltrates in 10 dogs with pulmonary hypertension treated with sildenafil citrate: 2005–2014. J Vet Cardiol 2015;17:182–191.

Lee Y, Choi W, Lee D, et al. Correlation between caudal pulmonary artery diameter to body surface area ratio and echocardiography-estimated systolic pulmonary arterial pressure in dogs. J Vet Sci 2016;17:243–251.

MacPhail CM, Innocenti CM, Kudnig ST, et al. Atypical manifestations of feline inflammatory polyps in three cats. J Feline Med Surg 2007;9:219–225.

Manohar M, Goetz TE. Pulmonary vascular resistance of horses decreases with moderate exercise and remains unchanged as workload is increased to maximal exercise. Equine Vet J Suppl 1999:117–121.

Mazzotta E, Guglielmini C, Menciotti G, et al. Red blood cell distribution width, hematology, and serum biochemistry in dogs with echocardiographically estimated precapillary and postcapillary pulmonary arterial hypertension. J Vet Intern Med 2016;30:1806–1815.

Mikawa S, Miyagawa Y, Toda N, et al. Predictive model for the detection of pulmonary hypertension in dogs with myxomatous mitral valve disease. J Vet Med Sci 2015;77:7–13.

Mondritzki T, Boehme P, Schramm L, et al. New pulmonary hypertension model in conscious dogs to investigate pulmonary-selectivity of acute pharmacological interventions. Eur J Appl Physiol 2018;118:195–203.

Morita T, Nakamura K, Osuga T, et al. Acute effects of intravenous pimobendan administration in dog models of chronic precapillary pulmonary hypertension. J Vet Cardiol 2020;32:16–27.

Murphy LA, Russell N, Bianco D, et al. Retrospective evaluation of pimobendan and sildenafil therapy for severe pulmonary hypertension due to lung disease and hypoxia in 28 dogs (2007–2013). Vet Med Sci 2017;3:99–106.

Ohad DG, Lenchner I, Bdolah-Abram T, et al. A loud right-apical systolic murmur is associated with the diagnosis of secondary pulmonary arterial hypertension: retrospective analysis of data from 201 consecutive client-owned dogs (2006–2007). Vet J 2013;198:690–695.

Paradies P, Spagnolo PP, Amato ME, et al. Doppler echocardiographic evidence of pulmonary hypertension in dogs: a retrospective clinical investigation. Vet Res Commun 2014;38:63–71.

Pariaut R, Saelinger C, Strickland KN, et al. Tricuspid annular plane systolic excursion (TAPSE) in dogs: reference values and impact of pulmonary hypertension. J Vet Intern Med 2012;26:1148–1154.

Poole DC, Erickson HH. Exercise-induced pulmonary hemorrhage: where are we now? Vet Med (Auckl) 2016;7:133–148.

Poser H, Berlanda M, Monacolli M, et al. Tricuspid annular plane systolic excursion in dogs with myxomatous mitral valve disease with and without pulmonary hypertension. J Vet Cardiol 2017;19:228–239.

Reef VB, Bonagura J, Buhl R, et al. Recommendations for management of equine athletes with cardiovascular abnormalities. J Vet Intern Med 2014;28:749–761.

Reinero CR, Jutkowitz LA, Nelson N, et al. Clinical features of canine pulmonary veno-occlusive disease and pulmonary capillary hemangiomatosis. J Vet Intern Med 2019;33:114–123.

Reinero C, Visser LC, Kellihan HB, et al. ACVIM consensus statement guidelines for the diagnosis, classification, treatment, and monitoring of pulmonary hypertension in dogs. J Vet Intern Med 2020; 34:549–573.

Rhinehart JD, Schober KE, Scansen BA, et al. Effect of body position, exercise, and sedation on estimation of pulmonary artery pressure in dogs with degenerative atrioventricular valve disease. J Vet Intern Med 2017.

Roels E, Merveille AC, Moyse E, et al. Diagnostic value of the pulmonary vein-to-right pulmonary artery ratio in dogs with pulmonary hypertension of precapillary origin. J Vet Cardiol 2019;24:85–94.

Russell NJ, Irwin PJ, Hopper BJ, et al. Acute necrotising pulmonary vasculitis and pulmonary hypertension in a juvenile dog. J Small Anim Pract 2008;49:349–355.

Schiborra F, Scudder CJ, Littler RM, et al. CT findings in Pneumocystis carinii pneumonia in five dogs. J Small Anim Pract 2018; 59: 508–513.

Schober KE, Baade H. Doppler echocardiographic prediction of pulmonary hypertension in West Highland white terriers with chronic pulmonary disease. J Vet Intern Med 2006;20: 912–920.

Schwarzwald CC, Stewart AJ, Morrison CD, Bonagura JD. Cor pulmonale in a horse with granulomatous pneumonia. Equine Vet Educ 2006;18(4):182–7.

Serrano-Parreno B, Carreton E, Caro-Vadillo A, et al. Evaluation of pulmonary hypertension and clinical status in dogs with heartworm by right pulmonary artery distensibility index and other echocardiographic parameters. Parasites & vectors 2017;10:106.

Serres F, Chetboul V, Gouni V, et al. Diagnostic value of echo-Doppler and tissue Doppler imaging in dogs with pulmonary arterial hypertension. J Vet Intern Med 2007;21:1280–1289.

Serres FJ, Chetboul V, Tissier R, et al. Doppler echocardiography-derived evidence of pulmonary arterial hypertension in dogs with degenerative mitral valve disease: 86 cases (2001–2005). J Am Vet Med Assoc 2006;229:1772–1778.

Serres F, Nicolle AP, Tissier R, et al. Efficacy of oral tadalafil, a new long-acting phosphodiesterase-5 inhibitor, for the short-term treatment of pulmonary arterial hypertension in a dog. J Vet Med A Physiol Pathol Clin Med 2006;53:129–133.

Simonneau G, Gatzoulis MA, Adatia I, et al. Updated clinical classification of pulmonary hypertension. J Am Coll Cardiol 2013;62:D34–41.

Stepien RL. Pulmonary arterial hypertension secondary to chronic left-sided cardiac dysfunction in dogs. J Small Anim Pract 2009;50 Suppl 1:34–43.

Sutherland-Smith J, Hankin EJ, Cunningham SM, et al. Comparison of a computed tomographic pulmonary trunk to aorta diameter ratio with echocardiographic indices of pulmonary hypertension in dogs. Vet Radiol Ultrasound 2018;59:18–26.

Swann JW, Sudunagunta S, Covey HL, et al. Evaluation of red cell distribution width in dogs with pulmonary hypertension. J Vet Cardiol 2014;16:227–235.

Tessier-Vetzel D, Tissier R, Chetboul V, et al. Diagnostic and prognostic value of endothelin-1 plasma concentrations in dogs with heart and respiratory disorders. Vet Rec 2006;158:783–788.

Tidholm A, Hoglund K, Häggström J, et al. Diagnostic value of selected echocardiographic variables to identify pulmonary hypertension in dogs with myxomatous mitral valve disease. J Vet Intern Med 2015;29:1510–1517.

Tran DL, Lau EMT, Celermajer DS, et al. Pathophysiology of exercise intolerance in pulmonary arterial hypertension. Respirology 2018;23:148–159.

Venco L, Mihaylova L, Boon JA. Right pulmonary artery distensibility index (RPAD index). A field study of an echocardiographic method to detect early development of pulmonary hypertension and its severity even in the absence of regurgitant jets for Doppler evaluation in heartworm-infected dogs. Vet Parasitol 2014;206:60–66.

Vezzosi T, Domenech O, Iacona M, et al. Echocardiographic evaluation of the right atrial area index in dogs with pulmonary hypertension. J Vet Intern Med 2018;32:42–47.

Vezzosi T, Schober KE. Doppler-derived echocardiographic evidence of pulmonary hypertension in cats with left-sided congestive heart failure. J Vet Cardiol 2019;23:58–68.

Visser LC, Im MK, Johnson LR, et al. Diagnostic value of right pulmonary artery distensibility index in dogs with pulmonary hypertension: comparison with Doppler echocardiographic estimates of pulmonary arterial pressure. J Vet Intern Med 2016;30:543–552.

Visser LC, Wood JE, Johnson LR. Survival characteristics and prognostic importance of echocardiographic measurements of right heart size and function in dogs with pulmonary hypertension. J Vet Intern Med 2020;34:1379–1388.

Williams KJ, Derksen FJ, de Feijter-Rupp H, et al. Regional pulmonary veno-occlusion: a newly identified lesion of equine exercise-induced pulmonary hemorrhage. Vet Pathol 2008;45:316–326.

Wung D. Treatment of canine pulmonary arterial hypertension: is tadalafil an appropriate alternative to sildenafil? Internat J Pharmaceut Comp 2013;17:24–27.

Yang HJ, Oh YI, Jeong JW, et al. Comparative single-dose pharmacokinetics of sildenafil after oral and rectal administration in healthy beagle dogs. BMC Vet Res 2018;14:291.

Young LE, Helwegen MM, Rogers K, et al. Associations between exercise-induced pulmonary haemorrhage, right ventricular dimensions and atrioventricular valve regurgitation in conditioned national hunt racehorses. Equine Vet J Suppl 2006:193–197.

Zabka TS, Campbell FE, Wilson DW. Pulmonary arteriopathy and idiopathic pulmonary arterial hypertension in six dogs. Veterinary pathology 2006;43:510–522.

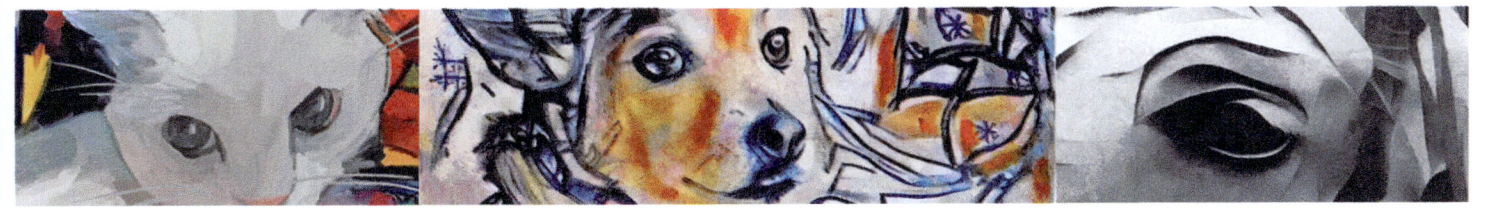

40
HEARTWORM DISEASE

Dirofilaria immitis

The nematode *Dirofilaria immitis* causes heartworm disease (HWD). Various species of mosquitoes throughout the world can serve as obligate intermediate hosts and transmit the parasite. Dogs and other canids are the preferred host species and main infection reservoir. *D. immitis* is the most prevalent nematode that affects the cardiopulmonary system of dogs and cats. Yet, other parasites can mimic some features of HWD. Depending on the geographic region, these include *Angiostrongylus vasorum* (p. 870), as well as other pulmonary parasites such as *Crenosoma vulpis*, *Filaroides* spp., *Eucoleus* (*Capillaria*) spp., and *Aelurostrongylus* spp. Circulating microfilariae (MF) of *Acanthocheilonema* (formerly *Dipetalonema*) *reconditum* could be mistaken for those of *D. immitis* (p. 849). *D. immitis* uncommonly infects people; typically, it just produces a solitary pulmonary nodule in this dead-end host.

Heartworm Transmission

HW infection in dogs occurs world-wide, including in all of the 50 United States. Although HW transmission is limited by climatic conditions, the geographic range of the parasite continues to expand aided by changing weather patterns, land development projects that increase availability of standing water (potential breeding sites), the spread of infected wild canids, and the translocation of microfilaremic dogs. In the United States, there has been significant increase in the occurrence of HW infections over the past several years, especially in southeastern states. Multiple mosquito species have the potential to spread HWD. Requirements for transmission include a climate with temperature and humidity that can support a mosquito population and sustain enough heat so that ingested MF mature into infective third stage larvae (L3) within the mosquito host. In colder regions, focal areas (such as urban "heat islands" or "microclimates") might provide favorable conditions for HWD transmission even in winter. Furthermore, some mosquito species can live and breed, or even hibernate, for several months. The time from MF ingestion to infective L3 development in mosquitoes depends on temperature. An average daily temperature over 64° F (18° C) for about a month generally is required for the parasite to mature to the infective stage within the mosquito intermediate host. Yet at about 80.6° F (27° C) and a relative humidity of 80%, it only takes 10–14 days for MF to develop into infective stage larvae. Cooler temperatures slow the process, and larval maturation stops at temperatures below 57° F (14° C); however, subsequent rewarming could resume it. In temperate latitudes of the Northern Hemisphere, HW transmission peaks in July and August. Multiple factors related to temperature fluctuation, microclimates, mosquito adaptations, and variable larval maturation time can allow for longer periods during which transmission is possible. Year-round transmission should be expected in tropical and subtropical regions. Additional information about relevant mosquito species and HW transmission can be found on the American Heartworm Society (AHS) website (www.heartwormsociety.org).

Heartworm Life Cycle   The *D. immitis* life cycle encompasses about 7–9 months. It is perpetuated when a (female) mosquito ingests MF during a blood meal from an infected dog or other host animal. As the normal definitive hosts, dogs and some wild canids have relatively long periods of microfilaremia. This promotes further spread of HWD. However, MF passed from dog to dog by blood transfusion or across the placenta do not develop into adult worms because the parasite life cycle requires the mosquito intermediate host.

Once ingested, MF develop into first stage larvae (L1) within the mosquito's malpighian tubules. The L1 moult into second stage larvae (L2), then into the infective L3, which migrate to the mosquito's head and mouthparts. The mosquito transmits the L3 to the new host during a subsequent blood meal; L3 within the mosquito's hemolymph drip onto the new host's skin and enter via the insect's puncture wound. The L3 travel subcutaneously and between muscle fibers within the new host for a few days before moulting (within 3–12 days) into fourth stage larvae (L4), which continue to migrate through the body. Between 50-70 days after infection, the L4 moult into juvenile (immature adult) worms. These enter the venous system and reach the small pulmonary arteries as early as 67 days after transmission, but typically by 90–120 days; the worms are about 1–1.5" long at this time. Juvenile worms are swept into small, distal pulmonary arteries initially; as they grow, they extend proximally into progressively larger segments of pulmonary arteries. Their eventual location is influenced by the size of the host and the worm burden. Small numbers of worms typically localize in the lobar arteries and main pulmonary artery. Increasing worm numbers, along with elevated pulmonary artery pressures and impaired right ventricular (RV) function, also increase the likelihood that some worms will migrate back into the heart (**Figure 40.1**). A burden of more than 40 worms is associated with higher risk for caval syndrome (p. 863) in dogs.

HWs reach sexual maturity at about 120 days postinfection in the canine host. Infection can become patent as early as 6 months (but usually 7-9 months) postinfection. Adult female worms grow to an average length of 10–12 inches (22–26 cm) and can live for 5–7 years; male worms are smaller. Although infected dogs might have 14–20 HWs on average, a worm burden of over 50 adult worms is not uncommon.

Cats are an imperfect host, so this species is more resistant to infection with adult HWs than dogs. The overall prevalence of HWD in cats is probably only 5–20% of that in unprotected dogs in the same geographic area. Reported prevalence in cats has ranged from 0% to over 16%, but the true infection rate is unknown. The diagnostic challenges in this species pose impediments to accurately assessing feline HWD prevalence; in addition, some infected cats display only transient clinical signs, while others die from HWD that remains undiagnosed. A large study of HW antigen (Ag) seroprevalence in cats found positive samples from 35 states within the United States, with an overall estimated seroprevalence of 0.4% (Levy, 2017). As expected, the greatest prevalence was in the southern states. Although indoor cats also are at risk of infection, the rate of seropositivity was three times greater in cats with outdoor access. Concurrent oral disease, abcesses, respiratory disease, or retrovirus infection was associated with increased risk of infection. No samples from Canada were positive for HW Ag in this study.

Infected cats generally have far fewer adult HWs than infected dogs. Worms mature more slowly in cats and fewer infective larvae mature into adults. Juvenile worms appear to have a particularly high death rate as they reach the lungs, 3–4 months after infection. The worms that survive to maturity (at around 7–8 months postinfection) are smaller than in dogs, and are about 8–9 inches (18–20 cm) long. The lifespan of adult worms in cats is only up to 2–4 years. Infected cats generally have less than 6, and usually only 1 or 2, adult worms. However, because of the small feline body size, the effects of even 1 or 2 worms can be severe and lead to death (**Figure 40.2**). Most cats have no, or only a brief period of, microfilaremia. When present, MF appear at about 195 days, and rarely persist longer than 228 days, postinfection. Host immune responses are thought responsible for clearing MF; suppression of MF production also might occur. An estimated one-third of feline cases are

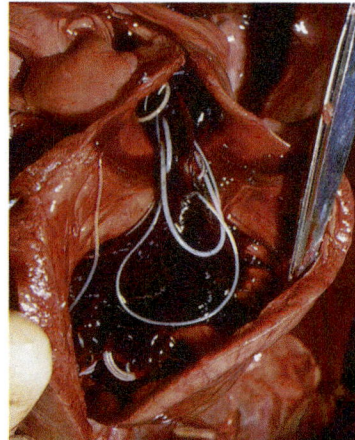

Figure 40.1 Adult heartworms within the right ventricle and pulmonary trunk of a dog with high worm burden. Open right ventricular (RV) outflow tract into pulmonary trunk, from cranial left aspect of heart. A postmortem clot partially obscures more worms in the RV inflow region.

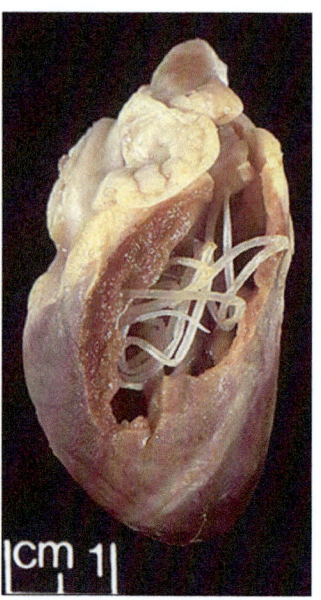

Figure 40.2 Opened right ventricular outflow region from an outdoor cat that died unexpectedly. Two heartworms were present in the heart.

unisex infections. Aberrant worm migration also is more common in cats than in dogs and this complicates necropsy confirmation of infection. Aberrant sites have included body cavities, the central nervous system (CNS), systemic arteries, and subcutaneous nodules.

Pathophysiology

Dogs HWD is an important cause of pulmonary hypertension (PH) in endemic regions. Adult worms within the pulmonary arteries incite the development of reactive vascular lesions, which precipitate PH. Pathologic changes begin within days after young adults arrive in the pulmonary arteries. Although severe disease often is associated with a large worm burden, it appears that the host–parasite interaction is more important than worm number alone in the development of HWD pathology and clinical signs. In dogs, little to no correlation has been found between pulmonary vascular resistance (PVR) and the number of worms present. On the other hand, physical activity, with its associated increase in pulmonary blood flow, exacerbates pulmonary vascular disease and PH. Sedentary dogs with a higher worm burden often develop less severe pulmonary arterial (PA) disease than dogs with far fewer worms, but that undergo moderate exercise. Thus, when cardiac output is high, even a low worm burden can lead to greater lung injury and higher PVR.

The immune response to HWs appears to be modulated largely by intracellular endosymbiont bacteria (genus *Wolbachia*) harbored by the worms. These obligate, gram-negative bacteria are integral to HW development, reproduction, and survival. *Wolbachia* bacteria possess a major surface protein and possibly other antigens that induce a strong proinflammatory response in the *D. immitis* host. They are a major contributor to the pulmonary pathology, as well as inflammation within the kidney and other areas, which occurs in the host animal following HW death. When *Wolbachia* are eliminated by doxycycline treatment, prior to HW adulticide therapy, subsequent pulmonary lesions and clinical signs associated with HW death are much less severe. Doxycycline leads to the death of L3 and L4, and in dogs with adult HWs, it gradually reduces microfilaremia. Furthermore, MF from doxycycline-treated dogs appear to develop into L3 that are unable to mature into adults.

Live worms cause endarteritis and stimulate medial hypertrophy in the pulmonary arteries, mainly in caudal lung regions. The characteristic lesion of infected pulmonary arteries is villous myointimal proliferation (**Figure 40.3**). The HW-induced changes begin with endothelial cell swelling, widening of intercellular junctions and increased endothelial permeability, which leads to periarterial edema accumulation. Endothelial sloughing stimulates adhesion of activated white blood cells and platelets. Smooth muscle cells migrate and proliferate within the media and into the intima under the influence of various trophic factors. Intimal villous proliferation develops by 3–4 weeks after the arrival of adult

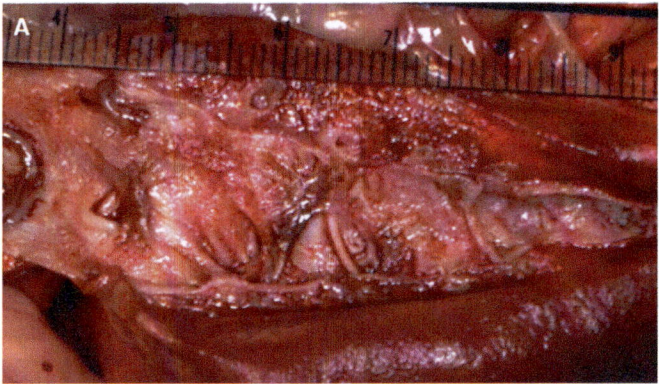

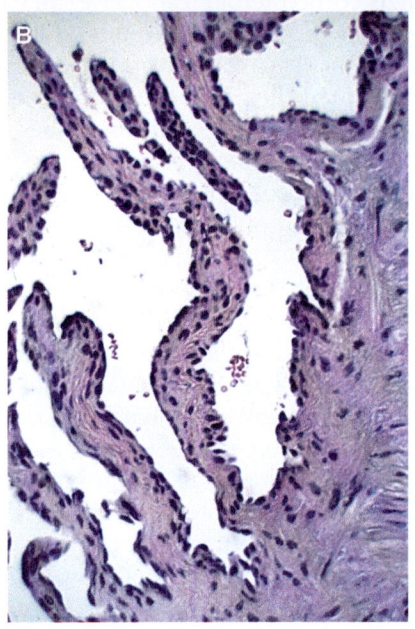

Figure 40.3 (A) Cut section of lung with longitudinally opened pulmonary artery, from a dog with severe heartworm disease. The marked intimal proliferative lesions create a roughened, rugous appearance. Ruler indicates cm scale. (B) Histological section from the same dog illustrates the exuberant intimal villous proliferation. Hematoxylin & eosin stain. (Images courtesy of Dr CE Atkins.)

worms. The villous projections, consisting of smooth muscle and collagen with an endothelium-like covering, narrow the lumen of the smaller pulmonary arteries, increase vascular resistance, and lead to further endothelial damage and proliferation. Endothelial damage promotes thrombosis and perivascular tissue reaction. Periarterial edema could be severe and partial lung consolidation develops in some animals.

Villous proliferation (and worm distribution) is most severe in the caudal and accessory lobar arteries. Affected pulmonary arteries lose their normally tapered peripheral branching and appear blunted or pruned distally. Aneurysmal dilation and peripheral occlusion can occur. The vessels dilate proximally and become tortuous as the increased PVR demands higher perfusion pressures.

Cor pulmonale, the RV dilation and hypertrophy induced by the high systolic pressure load, develops as it does with other causes of PH. The myocardial damage includes intercellular collagen loss, which might relate to HW-secreted substances or HW-host interactions that affect fibrinolytic processes. Chronic severe PH often leads to secondary tricuspid valve insufficiency and RV myocardial failure, with neurohormonal activation and clinical signs of right-sided congestive heart failure (CHF).

Dying and dead worms incite a more intense host response than healthy worms. These worsen the pulmonary disease, and can induce shock and coagulopathy. Decomposing worm fragments and thrombi stimulate further reaction. PA embolization and infarction, fibrosis, and hypersensitivity pneumonitis (that usually is corticosteroid responsive) all can contribute to the development of parenchymal lung lesions, as well as PH. Pulmonary fibrosis will not respond to any treatment. The rise in PVR intensifies in the diseased, narrowed vessels. Reduced perfusion of affected lung lobes, elevated PA pressures, increased right heart workload, and greater risk for CHF are consequences. Alveolar hypoxia, with hypoxic vasoconstriction, in consolidated lung regions exacerbates the high pulmonary resistance. Intrapulmonary hemorrhage can result in hemosiderosis of the lung, which also might be evident at autopsy.

As noted, the location of mature HWs varies with worm burden and host animal size. In dogs with a smaller HW burden, worms typically localize in lobar and main pulmonary arteries, especially the more caudal vessels. As the worm burden increases, some HWs migrate toward and into the right heart (**Figure 40.1**). Worms present in the venae cavae are associated with heavy HW burden (for example, >40 worms). Mechanical occlusion of the RV outflow tract, tricuspid valve, venae cavae, or pulmonary arteries sometimes occurs with a massive number of worms (caval syndrome; p. 863). Tricuspid regurgitation (TR) usually results from both PH and the presence of worms within the tricuspid orifice. The RV flow obstruction caused by the mass of worms, combined with TR and preexisting PH, leads to signs of low output heart failure, as well as hepatic congestion and right-sided CHF. Red blood cell fragmentation often occurs with caval syndrome, with subsequent hemolytic anemia and hemoglobinuria.

Chronic hepatic congestion secondary to HW disease can cause permanent liver damage and cirrhosis. Renal glomerular injury is associated with circulating immune complex deposition and possibly, microfilarial antigens. HW-induced glomerulopathy tends to worsen with the chronicity of infection; immature worms, as well as MF and perhaps adults, could contribute to the pathology. Renal amyloidosis also has been associated with HWD in dogs, but is rare. Impaired coagulation can accompany *D. immitis* infection. Increased fibrinolysis can occur from effects of HW-derived antigens that bind to plasminogen, which can increase plasmin levels. The HWs might release a plasminogen activator substance, also. Occasionally, aberrant worms cause embolization of the brain, eye, or other systemic arteries.

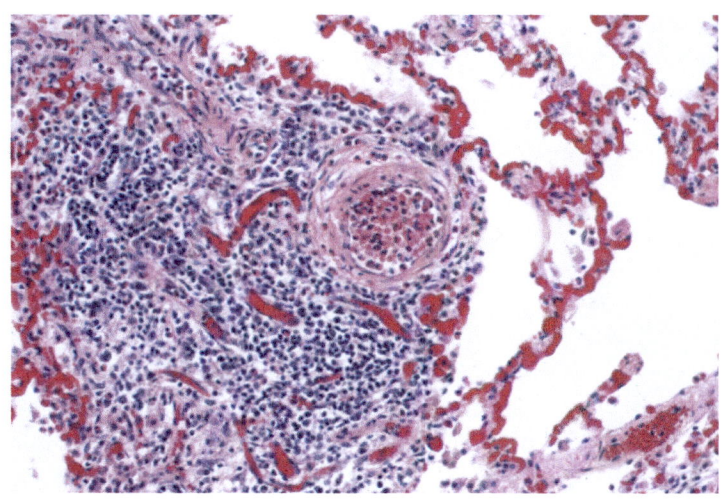

Figure 40.4 Pulmonary histologic image from a cat with heartworm infection. A transected small pulmonary artery (center) shows mild medial hypertrophy. Surrounding it, and extending to the left side of the image, is an intense inflammatory (eosinophilic) infiltrate in the adjacent lung tissue. Hematoxylin & eosin stain. Courtesy of Dr CE Atkins.

Cats HWs that reach the pulmonary arteries in cats are most likely to cause clinical signs either (1) when they initially arrive as immature (L5) worms, or (2) when adult worms die. Arrival of the juvenile worms at 3–4 months (or as early as 70–90 days) postinfection triggers an intense inflammatory response within the pulmonary arteries and arterioles where worms are located and in adjacent lung parenchyma. The immature worms stimulate activation of pulmonary intravascular macrophages. These are specialized phagocytic cells located in the pulmonary capillary beds of cats, but not dogs. These macrophages provoke acute inflammation in the pulmonary arteries and lung tissue. While interstitial lung disease occurs as in dogs, cats have more extensive alveolar type 2 (surfactant-producing) cell hyperplasia, which can interfere with alveolar O_2 exchange. The adventitial, peribronchial and perivascular inflammatory cell infiltrates consist mainly of eosinophils and neutrophils (**Figure 40.4**). This host response kills most of the young worms. The pulmonary inflammatory response can produce clinical signs similar to those of allergic bronchitis (asthma). However, it represents the syndrome known as HW-associated respiratory disease (HARD; also sometimes referred to as pulmonary larval dirofilariosis). This develops in many cats at 4–9 months after infection (even before a positive HW test or echocardiogram might be achieved). While some cats show no clinical signs during this period of acute inflammation, others develop sudden-onset and sometimes fatal respiratory distress. In cats that survive, pulmonary inflammation gradually subsides over time (up to 8 or more months); any remaining worms mature and stimulate progressive PA and parenchymal changes.

Medial hypertrophy of small pulmonary arteries is a characteristic histopathologic lesion in cats with HARD, as well as those with adult HWD. The thickening of the vascular walls compromises luminal diameter (occlusive medial

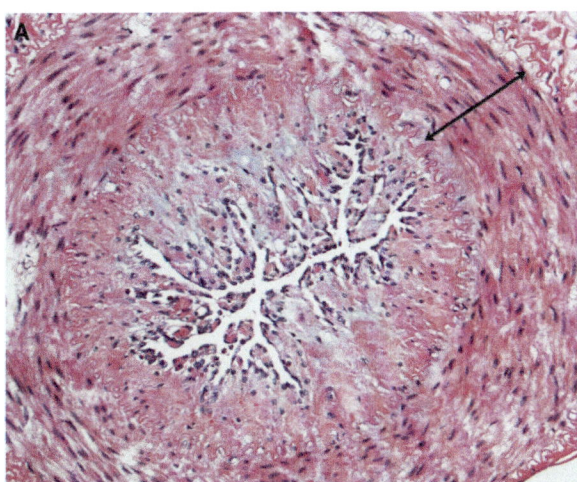
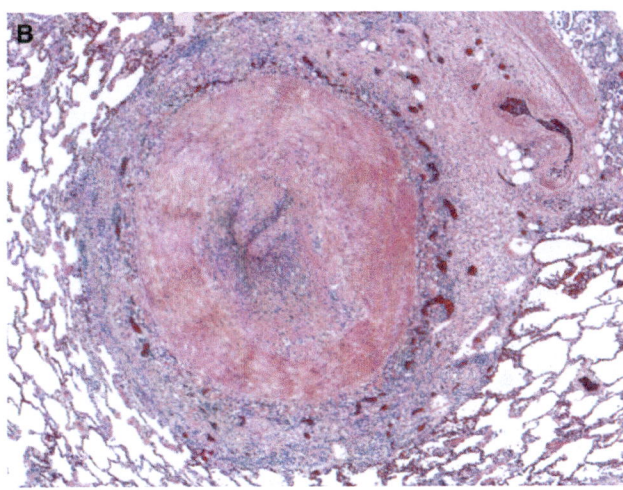

Figure 40.5 (A) Cross section of a small pulmonary artery from an 8-year-old cat that died of heartworm disease (HWD) shows marked villous proliferation of the intimal layer, which nearly occludes the vessel lumen. Hypertrophy of the tunica media is indicated by the double-headed arrow (damage to this layer on the left is artifact of fixation). Grossly, the cat's lungs were firm and appeared mottled. Moderately severe interstitial eosinophilic and lymphoplasmacytic infiltrates, some perivascular edema, and focal alveolar hemorrhage also were present. Hematoxylin & eosin stain. (B) Cross section through a larger pulmonary artery from a different cat with adult worms. Severe HW-induced medial hypertrophy and myointimal proliferation caused complete luminal obstruction. A periarterial infiltrate with eosinophils also is present. Hematoxylin & eosin stain. (B) Courtesy of Dr CE Atkins.

hypertrophy), although not all vessels are affected. Other lesions can involve the bronchi, bronchioles and alveoli. These include thickened bronchiolar walls and peribronchial inflammatory infiltrates, although there appears to be no increase in bronchial constrictive responsiveness. Similar PA and interstitial changes develop from *Toxocara cati* larval migration, although this parasite induces milder peribronchial inflammation than *D. immitis*. Nevertheless, these parasites can produce similar radiographic changes.

Cats that survive the initial HARD show progressive clinical improvement beginning at 6 to 8 months postinfection, but they are likely to have some persistent histologic lesions (including interstitial myofibrocyte proliferation) for the next 18 months, at least. HW antibody (Ab) tests become negative in about 50% of HARD cats by 8 months after infection, and all are likely to be negative by 18 months. Even cats with normal radiographs but positive HW Ab test can have mild, focal histologic pulmonary and arterial lesions.

Surviving adult worms appear to suppress the host immune response. Infected cats are likely to be asymptomatic during this stage even though adult worms provoke focal pulmonary arteritis. Vascular myointimal proliferation, eosinophilic endarteritis, intimal fibrosis, and medial hypertrophy progressively worsen in affected pulmonary arteries of cats, similar to dogs (**Figure 40.5**). These changes can be severe, causing marked obstruction within small pulmonary arteries. This occlusive hypertrophy occurs to a greater degree than in cats with HARD. In one study, over 40% of small pulmonary arteries of cats with adult HWs were affected (Browne, 2005). These lesions can be focal. Some markedly dilated areas might occur in the muscular pulmonary arteries, suggesting elevated pulmonary pressure there. However clinically relevant PH is uncommon; RV hypertrophy and right-sided CHF usually are not identified in cats. It is thought that growth of pulmonary collateral vessels protects cats from severe PH. Despite the absence of marked RV hypertrophy, reduced RV myocardial collagen content also occurs in cats and correlates with the severity of pulmonary parenchymal and arterial pathology.

Adult worms themselves are more likely to obstruct arteries in cats than in dogs because of their relative size (**Figure 40.6**). The death and degeneration of mature worms again trigger pulmonary inflammation, as well as pulmonary thromboembolism (PTE). Disease is most severe in the caudal lung lobes. Villous proliferation, thrombi, or dead HWs can cause caudal lobar arterial obstruction. However, the

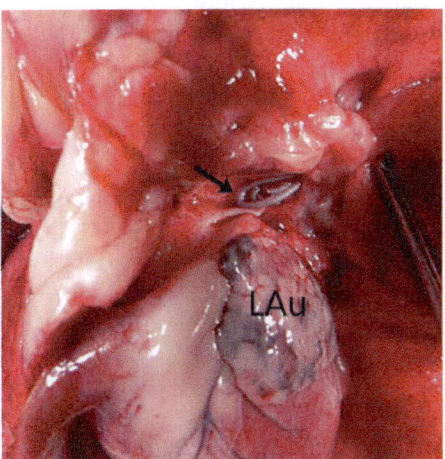

Figure 40.6 Two adult heartworms (arrow) in the pulmonary artery of the cat from **Figure 40.5A**. HWD was diagnosed 1 month earlier. A course of prednisone resolved the respiratory signs; but soon after the drug was stopped, the cat began coughing. Respiratory distress recurred 3 days later; the cat died en route to hospital. View from left dorsocranial. LAu, left auricle.

bronchopulmonary circulation in cats likely prevents pulmonary infarction. Nevertheless, the acute lung injury at this stage can trigger a high-protein pulmonary edema and respiratory distress syndrome that often is fatal for the cat. This can occur with just one adult worm present.

Sporadic vomiting occurs frequently in HW-infected cats. The underlying mechanism could relate to chemoreceptor trigger zone stimulation by inflammatory mediators, as low dose prednisone usually alleviates the vomiting. Caval syndrome occurs only rarely in cats. Nevertheless, even when just a couple of adult HWs are present, worms (or portions thereof) can be located within the heart.

Clinical Features

Dogs HWD has no specific age or breed predilection. Most affected dogs are between 4 and 8 years old, although infection in other age groups (older than 6 months) is common. Male dogs appear to be affected 2–4 times more often than females. Large-breed dogs and those primarily living outdoors are at greater risk of HW infection than small-breed or indoor dogs. Nevertheless, indoor dogs can develop HWD, too. The length of the haircoat does not appear to influence the risk of infection. The history and physical examination are important in helping determine the stage of disease and overall prognosis. Generally, a dog with no, or only minimal, clinical signs and physical examination abnormalities is likely to have a better prognosis, especially if thoracic radiographs reveal no severe changes.

Many dogs are diagnosed by a positive routine screening test, before clinical signs develop. Cough is the most common initial clinical sign. As HWD progresses, the cough becomes more severe and other signs occur, including exertional dyspnea, fatigue, syncope, weight loss, shortness of breath, and occasionally, hemoptysis. Signs of right-sided CHF (**Table 20.1**, p. 300) can develop in advanced cases. Death occurs in some. A change in or loss of a dog's bark has been reported sporadically in association with HWD. Aberrant worm migration is another uncommon occurrence; sites affected have included the CNS, eye, femoral arteries, subcutis, peritoneal cavity, and other areas. Subsequent clinical signs relate to the aberrant worm's location. Rare sequelae of microfilaremia could include keratitis caused by microfilarial infiltration of the cornea, uveitis, and MF discovered within abdominal fluid and urine.

Physical examination findings can be normal in early or mild disease. However, with severe disease, poor body condition, tachypnea or dyspnea, jugular vein distension or pulsations, ascites, or other evidence of right-sided CHF often develop. Harsh or abnormal lung sounds (wheezes and crackles), a loud and often split second heart sound (caused by PH), an ejection click or murmur at the left base, a murmur of tricuspid insufficiency, or cardiac arrhythmias might be heard on auscultation. Severe PA disease and PTE can be associated with epistaxis, disseminated intravascular coagulation (DIC), thrombocytopenia, and, possibly, hemoglobinuria. Hemoglobinuria also is a sign of caval syndrome.

Cats Cats of any age are susceptible. Strictly indoor housing is not protective. Male cats are overrepresented in some studies, but not in others. No sex predilection has been demonstrated in naturally exposed cats that test positive for HW Ab. Some studies have reported more cases diagnosed in fall and winter, presumably after infection in the spring, while others have noted fewer cases in the last quarter of the year.

Clinical signs in cats are variable and can be transient or nonspecific. The infection is self-limiting in some cats. Sometimes there is no clinical evidence of infection. The appearance of clinical signs usually is associated with the arrival of immature HWs in the lungs, and again with death of adult HWs. Respiratory signs occur in well over half of symptomatic cats, especially paroxysmal cough, wheezing, tachypnea, or increased respiratory effort. This can mimic feline asthma, especially early in HW infection. Vomiting also is common and can be the only sign in some cats; the vomiting typically is unrelated to eating. Other presenting complaints could include lethargy, anorexia, syncope, neurologic signs, hemoptysis, weight loss, and sudden death. Neurologic signs are common during aberrant worm migration; these have included seizures, dementia, apparent blindness, ataxia, circling, mydriasis, and hypersalivation. Cardiopulmonary and neurologic signs rarely coexist. Peracute respiratory distress, ataxia, collapse, seizures, and death can occur especially with the death of even one adult worm. Sudden death is more likely in cats than in dogs, and usually is related to HW death, PTE and acute respiratory distress. Serous pleural effusion, from right-sided CHF, and syncope occur much less commonly in cats than in dogs. Chylothorax, ascites, and rarely, pneumothorax also have been associated with HWD in cats. Caval syndrome develops uncommonly.

Pulmonary crackles, muffled lung sounds (from pulmonary consolidation or pleural effusion), and tachycardia might be found on thoracic auscultation. Abnormal cardiac sounds can include a gallop sound or systolic murmur, especially when a worm physically interferes with tricuspid valve function.

Heartworm Testing

In *dogs*, yearly testing for both adult HW Ag and MF are recommended for HW screening, as well as for verifying a suspected case of HWD (AHS Current Canine Guidelines, www.heartwormsociety.org, 2020). Identification and treatment of HW positive dogs is important, both for the individual animal's health and to reduce the reservoir population. When noncompliance or a break in preventative therapy has occurred, both HW serology and MF testing are recommended. A positive test indicates preexisting infection. Repeated testing in 6 months and again after another 6 months is advised. If tests are still positive, it is likely that infection occurred prior to starting, or resuming, preventative therapy. Annual retesting for both Ag and MF is recommended in these dogs.

Diagnosis of HWD is more challenging in *cats* than in dogs (AHS Current Feline Guidelines, www.heartwormsociety.org, 2020). Most infected cats do not have microfilaremia. In those that do, the MF appear later than in canine infections and rarely persist longer than 228 days postinfection. When MF are present, a MF concentration test is more likely to detect them. A combination of HW serologic testing, thoracic radiographs, and echocardiography provides the best means of clinical diagnosis in cats (**Figure 40.7**).

Serologic Tests Commercially available Ag tests detect a protein secreted mainly by the adult female HW reproductive tract. Enzyme-linked immunosorbent assay (ELISA) and immunochromatographic test methods are available. Circulating Ag is detectable no earlier than about 5 months after infection; however, antigenemia might not appear until after MF develop (at about 6 months postinfection). Macrocyclic lactone preventative drugs can suppress antigenemia until around 9 months postinfection. There is no reason to test puppies younger than 7 months for either Ag or MF. In addition, testing of adults should be done about 7 months after the end of the preceding HW transmission period. Depending on climate, this might require that monthly preventive drug treatment be started, or continued, prior to testing for possible infection during the preceding season.

These HW Ag tests are nearly 100% specific and have excellent sensitivity when the manufacturer's directions are followed carefully. They identify most occult HW infections

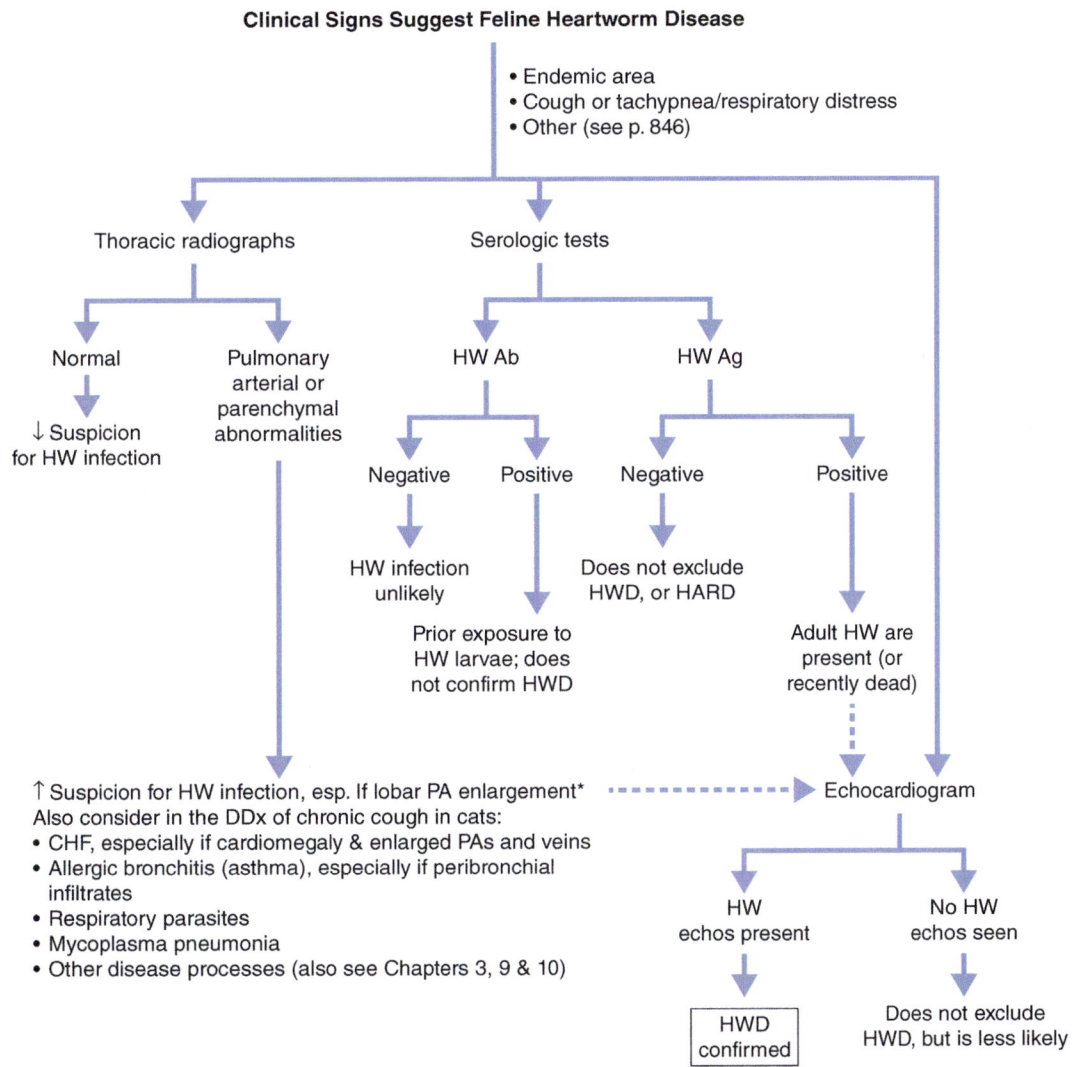

Figure 40.7 Considerations for interpreting test results in cats suspected of having HWD. *The pulmonary trunk in cats with HWD usually does not extend past the cardiac silhouette, but lobar arteries (especially right caudal) often are dilated. Ab, antibody; Ag, antigen; CHF, congestive heart failure; DDx, differential diagnosis; esp., especially; HARD, HW-associated respiratory disease; HW, heartworm; HWD, HW disease; PA, pulmonary artery. (Adapted from AHS guidelines; www.heartwormsociety.org).

(those with no detectable MF) with at least one adult female worm. A positive Ag test indicates the presence of HW-specific Ag. The circulating Ag concentration is related to the number of mature female HWs. Yet a positive Ag test's color intensity is not well-correlated with total worm number. Tests with only weakly positive or ambiguous results should be repeated. Follow-up testing by a commercial reference laboratory is helpful when results are still unclear. Sporadic false positive results are possible. Although these usually stem from technical error, several other nematode species, including *Angiostrongylus vasorum* (p. 870), might produce false positive results on a HW Ag test (Little, 2018). In any case, all positive results should be confirmed prior to administering adulticide therapy. Confirmation could be by identification of MF, positive results on a repeat test (from a different manufacturer or a reference laboratory), or visualizing HWs on an echocardiogram. Echocardiography is far more valuable for diagnosis in cats than in dogs, however. Radiographic signs consistent with HWD also are supportive.

False negative Ag test results are most likely to occur when only one or two worms, or only male or immature female worms, are present. A cold test kit or failure to follow test instructions precisely also could yield false negative results. Additionally, the formation of Ag-Ab complexes that interfere with Ag test function is another cause for false negative results in some dogs. In endemic areas, at least 5% of dogs without detectable HW Ag could test positive after serum heat treatment to destroy blocking Ab. Dogs with either microfilaremia or a history of intermittent HW preventative treatment could be more likely to have blocking Ab. Over 39% of HW-positive shelter dogs in this study had no detectable HW Ag prior to heat treatment (DiGangi, 2017). Heat treatment appears to allow earlier detection of HW infection, by about a month. However, dogs treated consistently with HW preventative medication are unlikely to develop blocking Ab. A study of canine necropsy-confirmed HW infections showed that heat treatment significantly improved HW Ag test sensitivity, not only for female unisex infections, but also overall (both including and excluding immature worms) and for male unisex infections (Gruntmeir, 2020).

Because of the potential for false negative results from HW Ag-Ab complexes, the AHS recommends that test results be reported as either "Positive" or "No Antigen Detected", rather than "Negative". This presents another reason for recommending routine MF testing, because many cases with suspected blocking Ab have circulating MF. Nevertheless, a HW-infected dog still might have neither detectable Ag nor MF. When Ag-Ab complex interference is suspected, heating the serum sample can dissociate Ag-Ab complexes, allowing free Ag to be detectable. Reference laboratories can provide heat treatment (or other nonheat methods) to release blocked HW Ag in serum samples prior to Ag testing. As a point of information, a reported method of heat treatment involves placing the serum sample in a heat block at 104°C for 10 minutes, centrifuging the sample, then collecting the resulting supernatant for HW Ag testing (Carmichael, 2017). However, it must be emphasized that routine heating of serum samples for Ag testing is not recommended and conflicts with instructions for commonly used in-house tests. Such treatment could interfere with the accuracy of combination tests for other infectious agents, as well as HW. As another consideration, confounding results could occur in dogs without active HWD if residual HW Ag (remaining after adult worm death or possibly from aberrant worms) is detectable after heat treatment, or if a non-HW Ag (denatured during heat treatment) is detected. A trichloroacetic acid method of inducing immune complex dissociation appears to be as effective as the heat-treatment method (Starkey, 2020).

In cats, serologic HW tests are useful to: (1) support an etiologic diagnosis in individuals with clinical evidence suggesting HW infection; (2) monitor the clinical course of cats diagnosed with HWD; and (3) provide a baseline reference before beginning HW preventative therapy. False-negative Ag test results are more likely in cats than dogs because of lower worm burden and greater probability of male unisex infection. An estimated 30–50% of cats with HWD have no female worms. Likewise, Ag tests do not detect infection with immature female worms. Therefore, HW Ag tests are not considered reliable for HW screening in cats. Ag test results in cats are negative during the first 5 months after infection and can be variably positive at 6–7 months; infections with mature female worms should be detectable after 7–8 months postinfection. As in dogs, circulating Ag-Ab complexes can result in no detectable Ag (false-negative) on HW Ag tests. Studies with experimentally and naturally infected cats show an increase in Ag-positive tests after heat treatment of the serum, and better concordance with samples positive for HW antibodies. However, as for dogs, routine heat treatment is not recommended.

HW Ab ELISA tests are available for cats; these use either recombinant Ag or HW Ag extract. Serum Ab to both immature and adult worms is detectable as early as 60 days postinfection. The feline Ab tests provide greater sensitivity than Ag tests regarding HW exposure, because HW larvae of either sex can provoke a host immune response. Yet, especially in cats, many immature HW larvae never develop into adults. Therefore, a positive Ab test indicates exposure to migrating larvae and adults, not the presence of adult HWs specifically. A positive Ab test should be supported by other evidence (such as a positive HW Ag test, or typical radiographic and echocardiographic, echo, findings) before a diagnosis of HWD is made. The sensitivity of feline Ab test methods to different HW developmental stages varies among the available tests. This could lead to false negatives and discordant results when different test methods are used. Ab concentration does not appear to correlate well with the number of worms present. HW Ab concentration is thought to decline over time as the worm(s) mature. Cats with clinical signs appear more likely to have a positive Ab test than asymptomatic infected cats, although some report little relation between Ab concentration and severity of radiographic or clinical signs of HWD. High Ab titers often are associated with HW death and also with heavy infection. It is unclear how long circulating Ab remains after HW infection is eliminated. False-negative Ab tests could occur in 14% to possibly 50% of cats with HWD.

Necropsy studies of naturally infected cats have shown a correlation between HW Ab production and the histopathologic finding of occlusive medial hypertrophy in many small pulmonary arterioles (**Figure 40.5B**). The majority of cats with confirmed adult HW infection, and about half of cats without adult worms but with a positive Ab test, have this prominent PA pathology. It is notable that such significant pulmonary disease can develop even in cats without adult HWs. Cats infected experimentally with many L3 and then treated with a macrocyclic lactone become negative for HW Ab within 8–16 months. However, they still develop pulmonary histologic and radiographic evidence of HARD. Pulmonary pathology is greatly diminished when HW preventative therapy is begun prior to L3 infection.

A negative HW Ab test, therefore, suggests either: (1) no HW infection, (2) infection of less than 60 days duration, or (3) a concentration of immunoglobulin-G Ab against the test Ag that is too low to be detected. If a cat's clinical findings suggest HWD despite a negative Ab test, further testing using a different Ab test and a HW Ag test is recommended. If the cat does harbor adult female worms, the HW Ag test should be positive. Chest radiographs and echocardiography also are recommended. In addition, Ab (and Ag) testing can be repeated in a few months.

Serologic testing in cats is important in several situations. One is to help establish a diagnosis in cats suspected to have HW infection; clinical signs as well as radiographic and echo findings strongly contribute here, too. Serologic testing also is used to monitor clinical progress in cats with HWD. Finally, serologic testing provides baseline information on status before beginning HW preventative therapy.

Detection of Microfilariae Testing for circulating MF is recommended for all dogs. A positive MF test confirms positive serology results, identifies dogs that are reservoirs of infection, and signals HWD in dogs with Ag-Ab complex interference on serologic testing. MF testing also can reveal the presence of high numbers of MF, which could precipitate an adverse microfilaricide reaction. The macrocyclic lactone preventive drugs eventually eliminate microfilaremia by impairing female, and possibly also male, worm reproductive function. Most dogs receiving these drugs become amicrofilaremic after 6 months. An estimated 75–90% of HW-positive dogs not treated with a monthly preventative drug (or longer-acting injectable preventative agent) have microfilaremia. Absence of circulating MF ("occult" infection) in the remaining cases can result from immunologic MF destruction within the lung, unisex or sterile adult HWs, or prepatent infection. Occult infection can lead to severe signs of disease. Other causes of false-negative MF test results include low numbers

Table 40.1 Modified Knott Test Method

- Put 1 ml blood (collected into an EDTA tube) and 9 ml of 2% formalin[a] into a centrifuge tube
- Mix well, by inverting the tube several times, to lyse the red blood cells
- Place tube into a centrifuge
- Spin at 1100–1500 rpm for 5–8 minutes
- Pour off the liquid, leaving the sediment
- Add a drop of methylene blue to the sediment
- Place stained sediment onto a glass slide
- Apply a cover slip on top
- Examine slide using low power (100X) for presence of microfilariae
- To better observe microfilariae morphology, use high-dry power (400X)

[a] Acetic acid could replace formalin; however, this will reduce microfilarial length (see p. 850).

of MF and diurnal variation in the number of peripherally circulating microfilariae.

Cats with HWD uncommonly have circulating MF and if present, the number of MF usually is small; therefore, MF tests typically are negative in this species. Nevertheless, about half of infected cats develop microfilaremia for a month or two at approximately 6.5–7 months after infection. In those cats with circulating MF, a concentration test improves the chances of detection.

MF concentration tests provide more accurate assessment of microfilaremia than nonconcentration methods. They require at least 1 ml of peripheral blood. Especially in cats, a larger volume (3–5 ml) of blood increases the probability of a positive result when MF are present. Concentration tests are done using either a millipore filter or by centrifugation with the modified Knott technique (**Table 40.1**). Both tests lyse the RBCs, and fix and stain microfilariae. The modified Knott test is preferred for measuring body dimensions and evaluating morphology to differentiate *D. immitis* from nonpathogenic filarial species, such as *Acanthocheilonema* (formerly *Dipetalonema*) *reconditum* (**Table 40.2**). Acetic acid could be used as an alternative reagent (instead of formalin) in the modified Knott test. However, this will measurably shorten the

Table 40.2 Morphologic Differentiation of Circulating Microfilariae

Smear Type	D. immitis	A. reconditum
Fresh smear	Undulate in one place	Move across field
Stained smear[a]	Straight body	Possibly curved body
	Straight tail	Curved tail (possible "hook" shape)
	Tapered head	Blunt head
	295–325 µm long	250–288 µm long
	>6 µm wide	<6 µm wide

[a] Size criteria for modified Knott test (lysate prepared using 2% formalin); microfilariae tend to be smaller with lysate of filter tests. Width and morphology are the best discriminating factors.

MF compared to when formalin is the reagent (~273 vs ~316 microns, respectively; Evans, 2019). Acetic acid also causes less hemolysis than formalin.

Nonconcentration MF tests include examination of a fresh wet blood smear or the buffy coat-plasma interface of a spun hematocrit tube. There is greater likelihood of missing low numbers of MF (under 100 MF/ml); however, these methods allow assessment of microfilarial motility. *D. immitis* MF have a stationary rather than a migratory movement pattern. A false-positive MF test could result when MF are present in the absence of live adult worms.

Other Diagnostic Tests

Many dogs in rescue shelters are HW positive, especially dogs in HW-endemic areas or transported from endemic areas to other shelters for adoption. Owners of other HW-positive dogs might be unable or unwilling to provide HW preventive medication for various reasons. Accordingly, consideration of costs associated with diagnostic testing (and therapy) is important. This section provides an overview of numerous diagnostic studies. The clinician must decide which are the most important and cost-effective for managing individual cases. Generally, the medical history, physical examination, thoracic radiographs, and heartworm tests are essential for staging. Hematocrit or PCV measurement should be done when blood is obtained for HW antigen and microfilarial testing. If possible, routine clinical laboratory tests certainly are desirable, especially in older dogs and cats, and those in poor general health or body condition. More comprehensive laboratory studies and advanced imaging (echocardiography, CT angiography) can be used in specific situations.

Dogs Eosinophilia, basophilia, and monocytosis are inconsistent hematologic findings in HWD (**Figure 40.8**). Less than 50% of dogs with HWD have eosinophilia. Mild regenerative

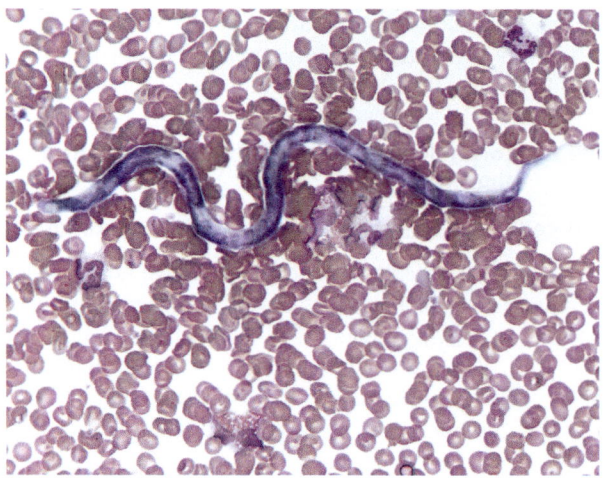

Figure 40.8 A *D. immitis* microfilaria is present in this peripheral blood smear, which also shows several eosinophils. However, concentration tests are more likely to identify microfilariae. (Courtesy of Dr M Wellman.)

anemia, likely from hemolysis, is present in <30% of cases. More severe anemia, with intravascular hemolysis, hemoglobinuria, and possible increase in bilirubin is likely in dogs with caval syndrome. Thrombocytopenia can occur secondary to platelet consumption in the pulmonary arteries, especially after adulticide treatment. DIC also can develop with advanced disease. Immune response to the HWs produces a polyclonal gammopathy. Mild to moderate elevation in liver enzyme activity and azotemia can occur. Proteinuria is found in 20–30% of affected dogs, especially those with advanced disease. Hypoalbuminemia can develop in severely affected animals. Some dogs might have other parasitic infections or comorbidities resulting from marginal preventive care, which also could alter hematologic and serum chemistry values.

Elevations in cardiac troponin I, D-dimer, and inflammatory response indicator (such as C-reactive protein, interleukin-6, haptoglobin) concentrations occur in dogs with clinically evident HWD. Higher levels are most likely in dogs with more severe clinical signs and PH. The fibrin degeneration product, D-dimer, also increases with adulticide therapy, consistent with thrombosis or PTE. Following successful treatment, elevations of these biomarkers generally resolve.

Thoracic radiographs help the clinician assess the extent of HW-induced cardiopulmonary changes. Radiographs can appear normal with mild disease; however, changes develop rapidly in dogs with a heavy worm burden. Characteristic findings with moderate to severe HWD include centrally enlarged lobar pulmonary arteries with peripheral blunting, a pulmonary trunk bulge, and RV enlargement (**Figures 40.9–40.11**). Lobar arteries often appear tortuous. The caudal lobar arteries usually are affected most severely and are seen best on DV view. The width of these vessels normally is no larger than the 9th rib, at its intersection with the vessels. On lateral view, the width of the cranial right lobar artery at its intersection with the 4th rib is no larger than the most narrow diameter of that rib in normal dogs. Enlargement of lobar pulmonary arteries, without concurrent venous distension, is strongly suggestive of HWD or other cause of PH (Chapter 39). Caudal vena caval enlargement might be seen, also; the reported normal maximal caval width is 0.75 ±0.03 times the length of the 5th thoracic vertebra (Litster, 2005). In addition, patchy pulmonary interstitial or alveolar infiltrates of variable severity are common. These suggest infarction, pneumonitis, noncardiogenic edema, pneumonia, or fibrosis. Pulmonary opacities might be mainly perivascular. Radiographic evidence of severe PA disease, as well as right heart enlargement, is present when HWD causes right-sided CHF.

The ECG usually is normal, although advanced disease can cause right axis deviation or an arrhythmia, including atrial flutter in larger dogs with right atrial dilation. Dogs with HW-induced CHF typically have ECG criteria for RV enlargement. Tall P waves, suggesting right atrial enlargement or delayed intra-atrial conduction, occur in occasional cases. Some have widened P waves, although P wave duration also relates to body size.

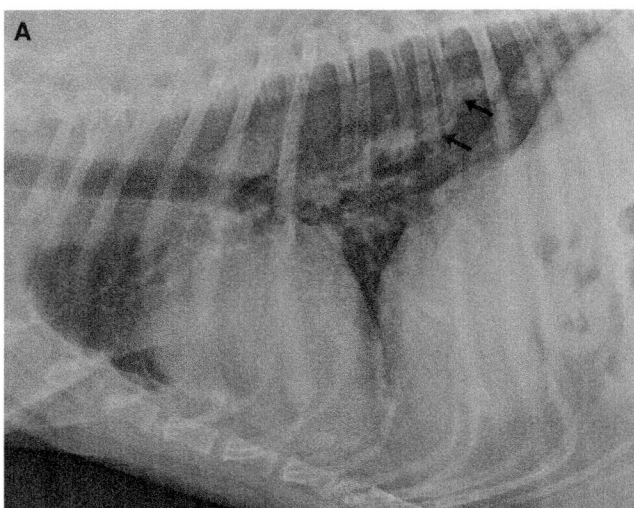
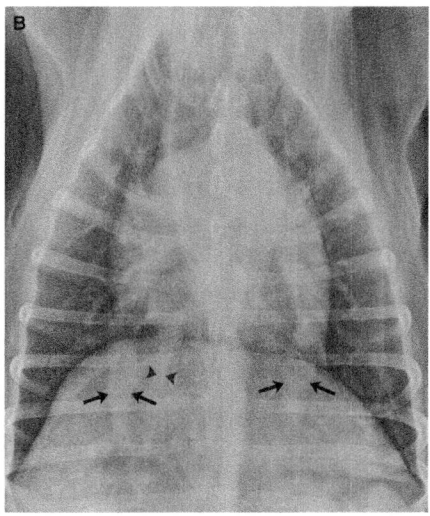

Figure 40.9 Right lateral (A) and DV (B) radiographs from a 5-year-old female Labrador Retriever diagnosed with heartworm disease by routine heartworm testing. (A) Although the cranial lobar pulmonary arteries appear normal, one or both caudal arteries are distended and tortuous (arrows). (B) Marked distension and slight tortuosity of both caudal pulmonary arteries (black arrows) are evident; grey arrowheads mark the width of the caudal right pulmonary vein. The cardiac silhouette and pulmonary parenchyma appear normal in this dog.

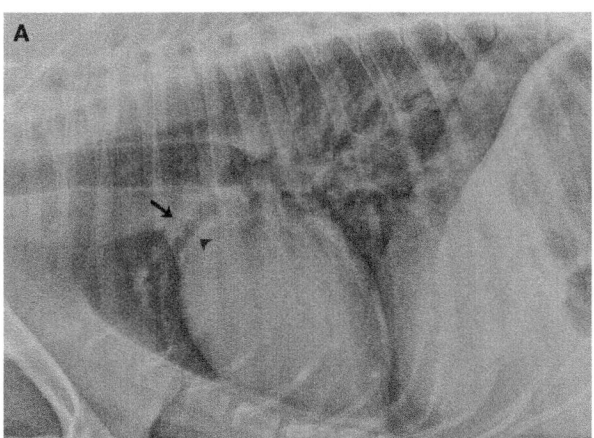
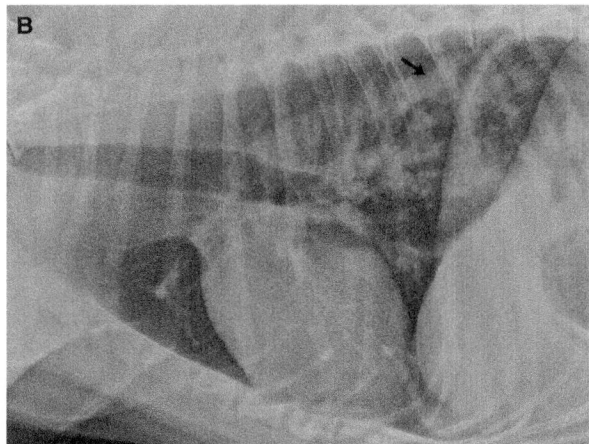
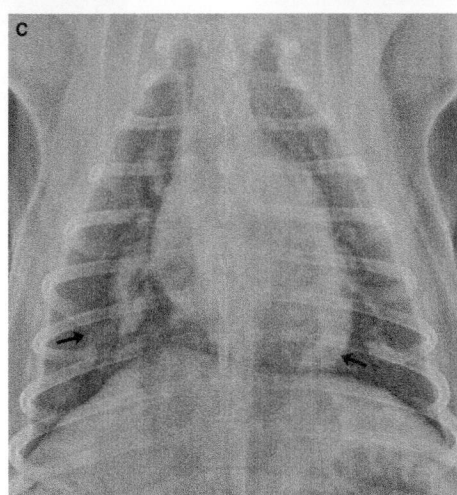

Figure 40.10 Right (A) and left (B) lateral and DV (C) radiographs from a 7-year-old male mixed breed dog with a 3 month history of coughing (partially responsive to prednisone). Occult heartworm disease was diagnosed. Moderately dilated and tortuous cranial (A, arrow; arrowhead marks accompanying lobar vein) and caudal (B & C, arrows) lobar pulmonary arteries are present. There also is a mild unstructured interstitial pulmonary pattern.

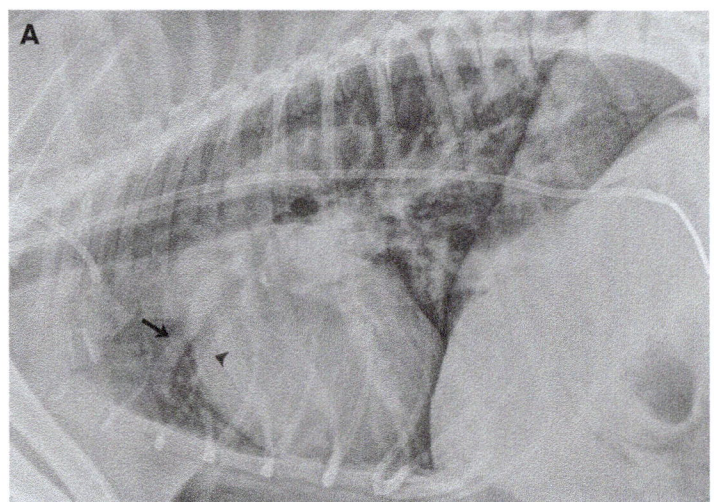

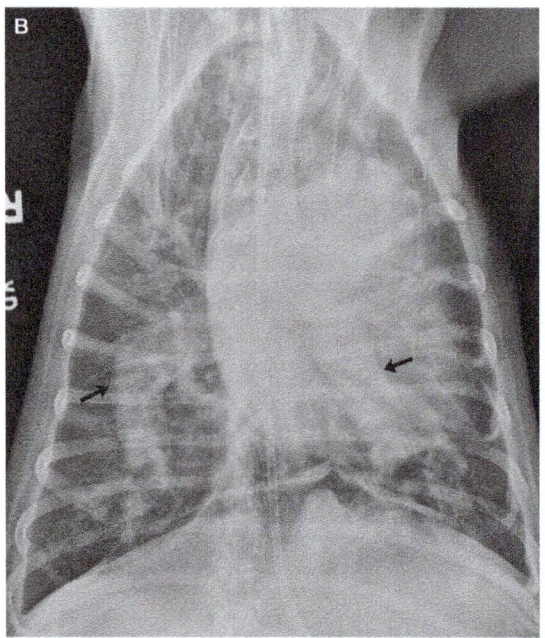

Figure 40.11 Radiographs from a mixed-breed dog presented with caval syndrome, obtained one day after worm extraction. Right ventricular enlargement, severely dilated and tortuous pulmonary arteries (arrows), and an interstitial infiltrate are evident on left lateral (A; arrowhead at cranial lobar vein) and VD (B) projections. Courtesy of Drs J Ward and S Murphy.

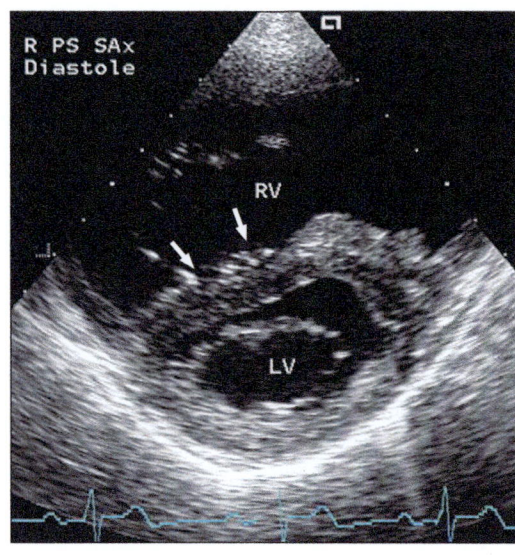

Figure 40.12 2D echo image at end-diastole from a 6-year-old male mixed breed dog with severe heartworm disease. There is right ventricular hypertrophy with marked dilation. High right ventricular pressure flattens the septum toward the left (arrows). Echos from the open mitral and tricuspid valves are present within their respective ventricles. Right parasternal short-axis view. LV, left ventricle; RV, right ventricle.

An *echocardiogram* is not part of standard care for HWD, but there are situations where an echocardiogram with Doppler will be useful. Specifically, these are in dogs with clinical signs of caval syndrome or severe PH (exertional collapse, syncope, right-sided CHF), or when radiographs indicate severe PH. Echocardiography also is useful in dogs that are likely to have concurrent cardiac disease, such as a congenital malformation, degenerative mitral valve disease, dilated cardiomyopathy, or pericardial effusion.

Echo findings in dogs with advanced HWD, as with other causes of PH (Chapter 39), are variable. These depend on PH severity, adaptive responses of the right ventricle, and presence of TR. Common echo findings include pulmonary trunk and branch pulmonary artery dilation, RV and right atrial dilation, (mixed) RV hypertrophy with increased wall thickness and chamber dilation, paradoxical to flat septal motion, and sometimes, a small left heart (**Figures 40.12 and 40.13**). HWs within the right heart, proximal pulmonary artery, or vena cava appear as bright parallel linear

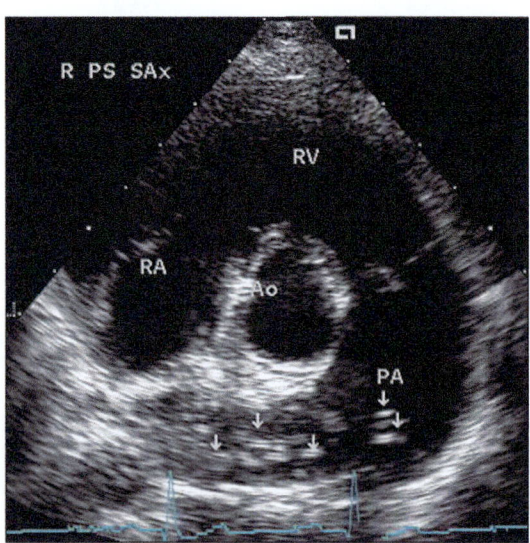

Figure 40.13 2D echo image from the 7-year-old dam of the dog in **Figure 40.12**. Heartworm-induced pulmonary hypertension caused right ventricular outflow tract and PA dilation. Portions of heartworms transected by the echo beam appear as bright parallel echoes within the main PA and its right branch (arrows). Right parasternal short-axis view. Ao, aorta; PA, pulmonary artery; RA, right atrium; RV, right ventricle.

echoes with anechoic centers, which are reflected from the parasite's body wall (**Figures 40.13** and **40.14**). Multiple variably short parallel echoes are typical because the ultrasound beam transects (at variable angles) different areas along the length of the worms. Echocardiography cannot accurately quantify adult HW number because visualized HW echos can come from multiple areas of the same worm or from several worms. Moreover, most adult worms localize to more peripheral regions of the pulmonary arteries. Therefore, HWs are not always visible on echo exam, especially in dogs with a low worm burden, large dogs, and those with only peripheral worm locations. Conversely, suspected caval syndrome can be confirmed quickly by echocardiography (p. 864). Any pleural, pericardial, or abdominal effusion also can be detected. Doppler modalities help in assessing abnormal valve function and in the diagnosis and quantitation of PH (p. 828 and **Figure 40.15**).

The right pulmonary artery distensibility index (RPADI) provides a way to screen for abnormal pulmonary artery stiffness related to PH. The RPADI is derived from the percentage change between the systolic and diastolic diameter of

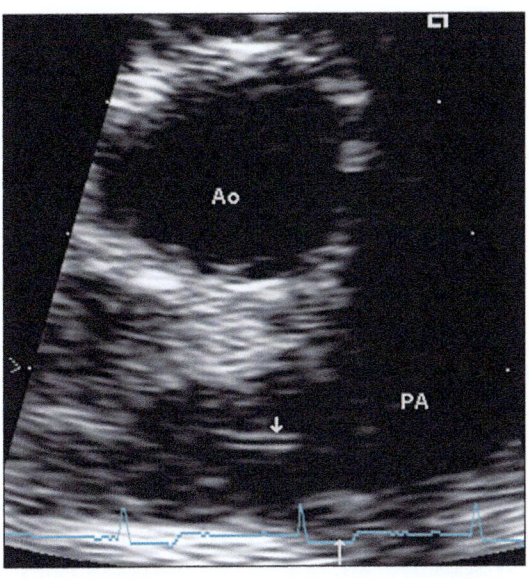

Figure 40.14 A longer heartworm segment (arrow) in the PA of another dog. Note the parallel hyperechoic walls around an anechoic center. Right parasternal short-axis. Ao, aorta; PA, pulmonary artery.

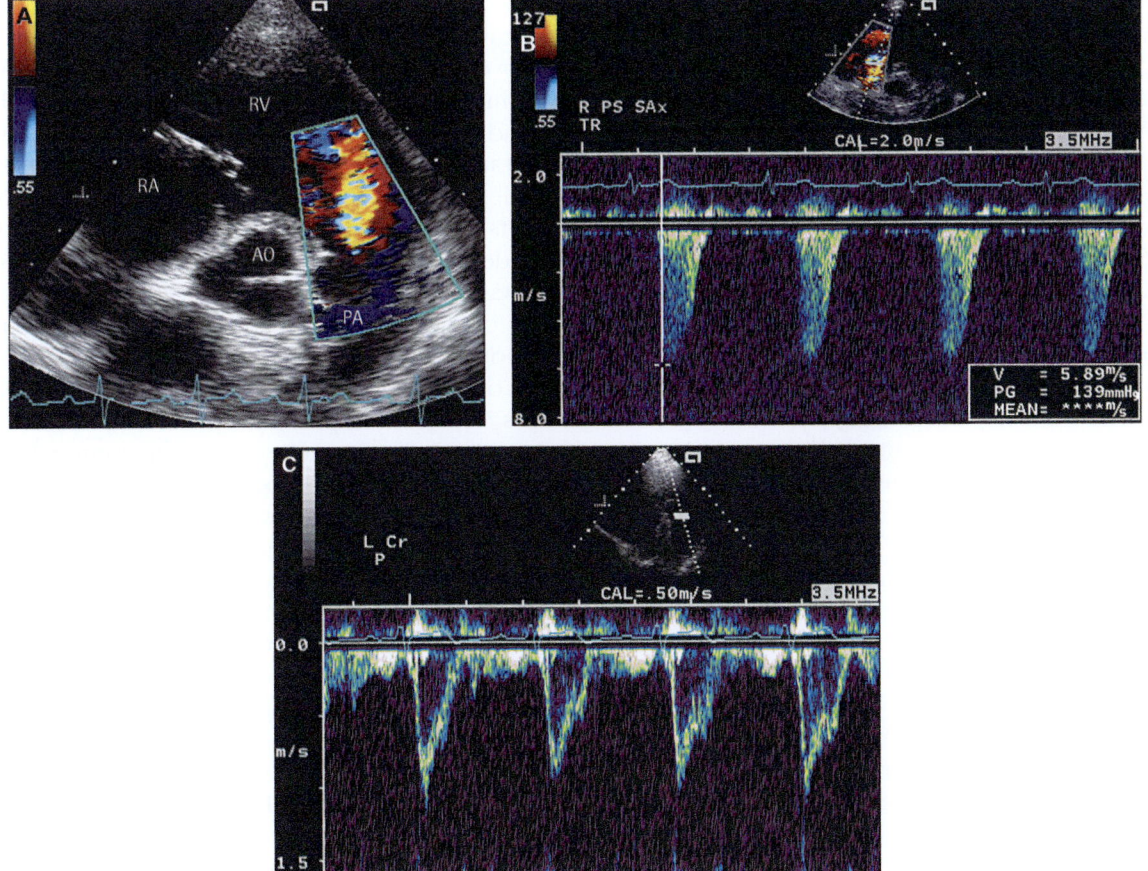

Figure 40.15 (A) Color Doppler image in diastole indicates prominent pulmonary valve regurgitation associated with heartworm-induced pulmonary hypertension (PH) in the dog of **Figure 40.12**. Right atrial and ventricular enlargement also are evident. (B) Continuous wave Doppler recording from the same dog shows high-velocity tricuspid valve regurgitation (TR, to almost 5.9 m/s; estimated RV-to-RA pressure gradient 139 mm Hg). (C) Pulsed wave Doppler pulmonary (P) flow profile shows rapid acceleration with mild mid-systolic notching, consistent with the severe PH in this dog. Images from right parasternal short-axis (A & B) and left cranial short-axis (C) views. Ao, aortic root; PA, pulmonary artery; RA, right atrium; RV, right ventricle.

the right pulmonary artery (**Figure 39.17**, p. 832 and text). Normally, the pulmonary artery expands easily during systole to accept the RV stroke volume. However, pulmonary artery elasticity becomes impaired with PH, to an extent inversely related to PH severity. Dogs with PH caused by HWD have a reduced RPADI. Nevertheless, many dogs with mild to moderate HWD-induced PH (as indicated by RPADI and pulmonary artery/aortic ratio) might not necessarily show clinical signs of disease. While the RPADI does not relate directly to HW burden or MF status, dogs with clinical signs caused by HWD generally have a lower RPADI, indicating worse pulmonary artery distensibility.

Cats HWD usually is more difficult to diagnose in cats than in dogs. Serologic testing, thoracic radiographs, echocardiography, and occasionally, MF testing are helpful, although not uniformly definitive (**Figure 40.7**). Feline HW Ab tests, while fairly sensitive, are not specific for adult HWs (p. 848). The ELISA-based Ag tests are highly specific for adult HW infection, yet their sensitivity depends on the age, sex, and number of worms. Serologic test results might be negative early in the disease process, even when clinical signs exist. Severe clinical signs and acute death from HWD can occur in Ag-negative cats. Furthermore, postmortem diagnosis can be difficult if the worms are located in distal pulmonary arteries or aberrant sites. When no worms are discovered on necropsy in a HW Ag-positive cat, considerations include spontaneous worm death, ectopic infection, or that the worms were missed during pulmonary evaluation.

Peripheral eosinophilia occurs in only in 1/3 to 2/3 of infected cats, usually between 4 and 7 months after infection. The eosinophil count is normal in many cases. Basophilia is uncommon. About one third of cases have mild nonregenerative anemia. Advanced PA disease and PTE can be accompanied by neutrophilia (sometimes with a left shift), monocytosis, thrombocytopenia, and DIC. Hyperglobulinemia is the most common biochemical abnormality, although it occurs inconsistently. The prevalence of HW-associated glomerulopathy does not appear to be high in cats with HWD.

Tracheal wash or bronchoalveolar lavage cytology could reveal an eosinophilic or mixed eosinophilic-neutrophilic inflammation consistent with allergic or parasitic disease, similar to that found with feline asthma or pulmonary parasitic infection. Experimentally, this occurs between 4 and 8 months after infection. Later in the disease, tracheal wash cytology shows nonspecific chronic inflammation or is unremarkable. Pleural fluid from cats with HWD-associated CHF generally is a modified transudate, although chylothorax can occur.

Radiographic findings can provide supportive evidence for HWD in some cats. However, radiography cannot definitively distinguish between cats currently infected with HWs and those with previous aborted infection and HARD. Radiographic findings similar to those in dogs with HWD include enlarged lobar pulmonary arteries (with or without visible tortuosity and pruning) and diffuse or focal pulmonary bronchointerstitial infiltrates (**Figure 40.16**). PA and right heart changes typically are more subtle in cats than in dogs. The main pulmonary artery segment usually is not visible radiographically, because it is located more medially in cats compared to dogs. The caudal lobar arteries appear abnormal most often (especially on the right, where worms typically are found); these are best evaluated on DV view. Although the right caudal lobar artery might be more prominent, a left caudal pulmonary artery ≥1.6 times the width of the 9th rib at the 9th intercostal space reportedly is the most discriminating radiographic finding in HW-infected, compared to noninfected, cats; unfortunately this finding might be absent in almost half of feline cases. Experimentally, the pulmonary arteries enlarge within a few weeks to 7 months of adult worm transplantation. PA enlargement tends to regress later in the disease process. Marked right-sided cardiomegaly is rare, although it is more likely when signs of right-sided CHF are evident. Reactive pneumonitis, as well as PTE, cause pulmonary infiltrates. Focal perivascular or peribronchial and interstitial changes are more common than diffuse infiltrates. The pulmonary infiltrates might spontaneously resolve over a few months. Lobar consolidation, pleural effusion, or pneumothorax are uncommon findings. Pulmonary hyperinflation sometimes is evident and, when accompanied by a bronchointerstitial infiltrate, can mimic feline allergic bronchial lung disease. Besides HW infection, other infective disease considerations in cats with similar radiographic pulmonary changes could include *Aelurostrongylus* spp. or *Toxocara cati*. Ascites occurs in some cats with HWD; it is rare in cats with CHF from cardiomyopathy. Radiographs are normal in a small minority of HW-infected cats.

Computed tomography (CT) *angiography* can show tortuous and blunted pulmonary arteries, as well as a multifocal ground-glass opacity and perivascular lung infiltrates. Although rarely done now, nonselective pulmonary arteriography might confirm a suspected diagnosis of HWD in a cat with false-negative Ag test and normal echocardiogram. Radioopaque dye injected via a large-bore jugular vein catheter outlines the morphologic changes in the pulmonary arteries. Adult worms appear as linear filling defects (**Figure 40.17**).

The ECG often is normal and, in the absence of an arrhythmia, generally is not recorded. However, cats that develop right-sided CHF usually have QRS changes suggesting RV enlargement (**Table 5.5**, p. 153). Other considerations for such criteria include congenital heart disease or a right bundle branch block, with or in the absence of cardiomyopathy. Arrhythmias appear to be uncommon, although they are more likely with advanced PA disease and CHF.

Echocardiography reveals the presence of adult HWs in an estimated 40–78% of positive cats. As the ultrasound beam transects a worm, echoes reflect from both the near and far

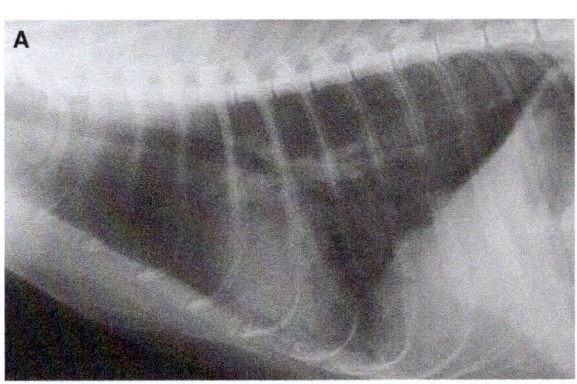
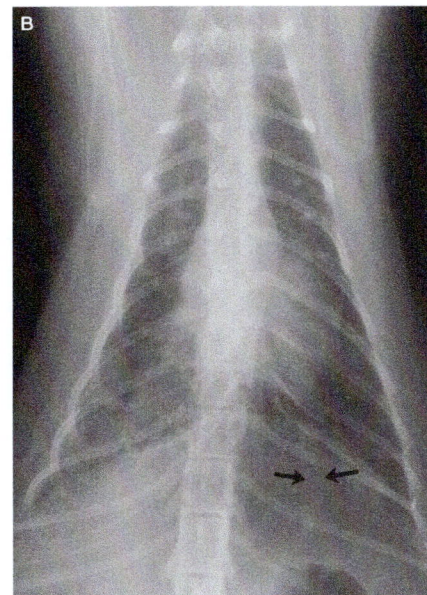
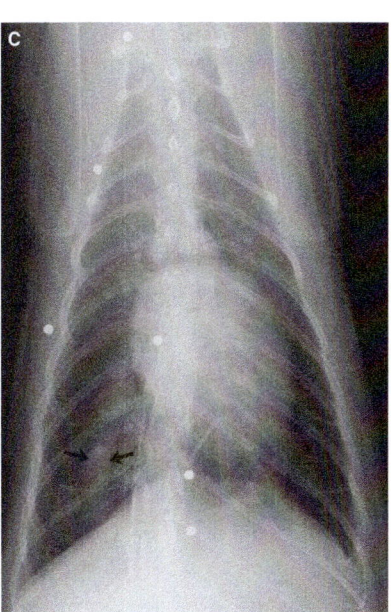

Figure 40.16 Right lateral (A) and DV (B) radiographs from an 8-year-old male cat with respiratory difficulty secondary to heartworm disease (HWD). Interstitial pulmonary infiltrates are extensive in the right caudal lobe. Lobar pulmonary arteries, especially the left caudal (B, arrows), are dilated. (C) DV radiograph from a different cat with HWD and cough history. Note the distended right caudal pulmonary artery (arrows), as well as mild pulmonary hyperinflation and slight, diffuse interstitial infiltrate that is more prominent in the right caudal lung. There is mild cardiomegaly also (VHS ~8.4v). Image (C) courtesy of Dr CE Atkins.

body wall, appearing as bright parallel line segments. The length of these parallel echoes depends on the alignment between ultrasound beam and the long axis of the worm (**Figure 40.18**). Nevertheless, echo findings can be normal unless worms extend into the heart, pulmonary trunk, or proximal right or left pulmonary arteries. It is important to inspect carefully, and to the fullest extent possible, the pulmonary trunk and especially the extended right pulmonary artery segment, which can be visualized as it crosses over the left atrium. Greater worm numbers increase the chance of echo identification. However, even with few adult worms, there is a good chance that part of a worm will extend into the proximal pulmonary artery because of the relatively large size of adult HWs compared to the cat. The number of worms present cannot be accurately gauged by echocardiography. Artifacts from pulmonary artery walls sometimes can be confusing, and therefore, higher frequency transducers are recommended to better delineate the adult parasite's

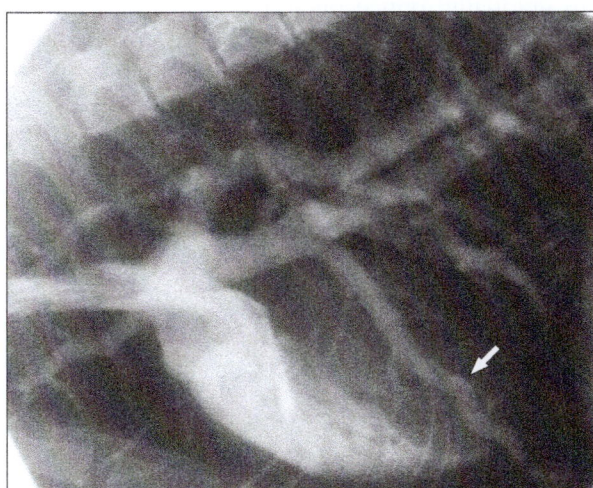

Figure 40.17 Nonselective angiogram from a cat with heartworm disease shows tortuous and dilated lobar pulmonary arteries. A linear filling defect (caused by an adult worm) is present in the middle lobar artery (arrow).

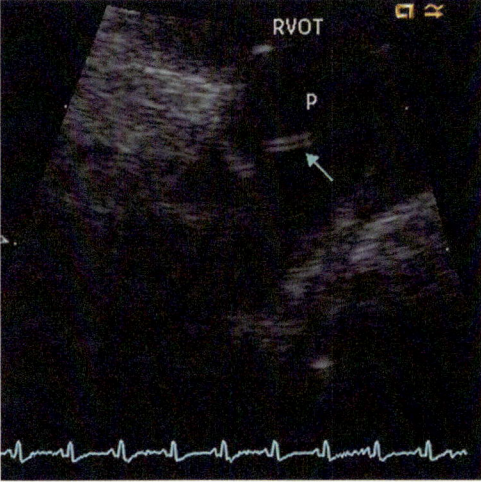

Figure 40.18 Magnified 2D echo image showing an adult heartworm (arrow) in the pulmonary trunk (P) of a cat. Note the worm's relatively large size in comparison to the artery. Right parasternal short-axis view. RVOT, right ventricular outflow tract.

morphology. Artifacts usually directly parallel, and move with, the walls of the pulmonary artery or some near field reflector; these spurious echoes relate to reverberation artifacts. Ultrasonography of other regions might allow an aberrant worm's location to be discovered, also.

Necropsy examination is important when HWD is suspected but not confirmed, as in cats with unexpected sudden death (**Figure 40.2**). Single worms easily can be overlooked, so it is important to carefully examine the right heart, venae cavae and proximal, as well as distal, pulmonary artery segments. Immature, dead and fragmented worms in the small distal pulmonary arteries are particularly easy to miss. Ectopic sites, such as body cavities, systemic arteries, and CNS might harbor worms, too.

Management of Heartworm Disease in Dogs

The recommended treatment regimen for HW-infected dogs involves an initial course of doxycycline (for 4 weeks) and a macrocyclic lactone, before administration of the adulticide, melarsomine, using the 3-dose protocol (**Table 40.3** and below). The AHS recommends this therapeutic approach for both asymptomatic and symptomatic dogs (**Table 40.4**; www.heartwormsociety.org), except for dogs with caval syndrome. This treatment protocol diminishes the severity of PA lesions and markedly reduces PTE. However, if melarsomine administration is deemed contraindicated or otherwise not suitable, an alternative approach can be considered which employs moxidectin (or ivermectin) combined with doxycycline (p. 860). It is important to note that the use of a macrocyclic lactone alone, as a so-called "slow-kill" method, is not recommended.

Dogs showing clinical signs of HWD should be stabilized prior to adulticide administration. Depending on patient status, this might include glucocorticoid therapy or management for CHF and PH (p. 860). Exercise restriction is essential in all cases! Treatment for HWD in dogs exhibiting no, or only mild, clinical signs usually proceeds well if exercise is restricted. Dogs with moderate or severe HWD signs, or with concurrent disease, often have a more challenging course. Dogs with caval syndrome should not undergo the adulticide treatment protocol until after worms have been physically extracted and the patient stabilized. Caval syndrome is an emergency that requires rapid diagnosis and immediate surgical removal of the HWs causing intracardiac blood flow obstruction (p. 863).

Elective surgical procedures in HW-positive dogs with no or only mild clinical signs do not appear to increase the rate of perioperative complications. However, for dogs with moderate to severe signs of HWD, it is advisable to avoid elective surgical and dental procedures. These dogs should be treated with the recommended 3-dose adulticide protocol (**Table 40.3**); then, if adequate recovery has occurred, the surgery can be pursued six months later.

Pretreatment Assessment The extent of preadulticide testing can vary depending on the patient's clinical status. There is no clearly defined protocol for all cases. Many dogs are treated successfully even when financial constraints have prevented ancillary testing. Postadulticide complications, although often likely, are not predictable. Even if other tests cannot be done, it usually is better to treat the HWD because HW-induced damage generally worsens over time. Nevertheless, pretreatment thoracic radiographs help the clinician assess the severity of PA disease and parenchymal reaction. A greater degree of abnormality is thought to indicate increased risk for complications. When possible, other recommended preadulticide tests include a hemogram, serum biochemistry profile, and urinalysis. A platelet count is especially important when PA disease is severe. Mild to moderate increase in liver enzyme activity can result from hepatic congestion related to HWD, although this does not preclude adulticide therapy. Liver enzyme activity usually returns to normal within 1–2 months of HW treatment. Azotemia, severe proteinuria, or both develop in some dogs with HWD. Prerenal azotemia should be corrected with fluid therapy before beginning adulticide treatment. A urine protein–creatinine ratio or quantification of urine protein loss can be useful in dogs with hypoalbuminemia or proteinuria. Severe glomerular disease can be associated with marked hypoproteinemia, nephrotic syndrome, or renal tubular damage. Loss of antithrombin III, as well as other proteins, can increase the risk for PTE in such animals. An exaggerated immune response to dead and dying HWs might also occur.

Initial Doxycycline and Macrocyclic Lactone Therapy Doxycycline is used to reduce the number of obligate endosymbiont *Wolbachia* bacteria within the HWs. Doxycycline (and minocycline) bind to the bacterial 30S ribosomal subunit and inhibit protein synthesis. This can kill L3 and L4 stages or impair their ability to develop into adult worms. Doxycycline also can gradually reduce microfilaremia. In addition, when doxycycline pretreatment is used before melarsomine therapy, lung pathology associated with HW death is less severe. Respiratory complications and mortality after adulticide treatment are reduced in dogs with naturally acquired infection. Therefore, doxycycline treatment (**Table 40.3**) is recommended prior to melarsomine to reduce *Wolbachia* bacteria with their metabolites before the worms die. The one month wait period between doxycycline treatment completion and the initial dose of melarsomine is important; this allows time for adult HWs to weaken, as well as for *Wolbachia* surface proteins and other metabolites to decrease. *Wolbachia* numbers are thought to remain low for at least a year after doxycycline therapy. The recommended doxycycline dose for HWD is 10 mg/kg q12h for 4 weeks. A lower dose (5 mg/kg q12h) might be effective, although this generally has not been recommended because of concerns that the drug's high protein binding (~92% in dogs) could interfere with its efficacy. However, some evidence suggests that the lower dose significantly diminishes patient Ab levels against *Wolbachia* surface

Table 40.3 Heartworm Adulticide Therapy Guidelines for Dogs[a]

Day 0

- Dog diagnosed and verified as HW positive:
  - Positive HW Ag test verified with MF test
  - If no MF are detected, confirm with 2nd HW Ag test from a different manufacturer
- Begin exercise restriction.
  - The more pronounced the signs, the stricter the exercise restriction
- If the dog is symptomatic:
  - Stabilize with appropriate therapy and nursing care
  - Prednisone prescribed at 0.5 mg/kg q12h for 1st week, 0.5 mg/kg q24h for 2nd week, 0.5 mg/kg q48h for 3rd and 4th weeks

Day 1

- Administer appropriate HW preventive.
  - If MF are detected, the AHS recommends antihistamine & glucocorticoid pretreatment to reduce anaphylaxis risk
  - Observe for at least 8 hours for signs of reaction

Days 1–28

- Administer doxycycline at 10 mg/kg q12h for 4 weeks (to reduce pathology associated with dead HWs and disrupt HW transmission; see p. 856)

Day 30

- Administer appropriate HW preventive
- Apply an EPA-registered canine topical product to repel and kill mosquitoes

Days 31–60

- A one month wait period following doxycycline treatment is currently recommended before administering melarsomine; this is thought to allow time for *Wolbachia* surface proteins and other metabolites to dissipate before adult HWs are killed. The delay also allows more time for the HWs to wither after elimination of the *Wolbachia* endosymbionts.

Day 61

- Administer appropriate HW preventive
- Administer 1st melarsomine injection, 2.5 mg/kg IM (follow manufacturer's instructions closely)
- Prescribe prednisone 0.5 mg/kg q12h for 1st week, then 0.5 mg/kg q24h for 2nd week, and 0.5 mg/kg q48h for 3rd and 4th weeks
- Decrease activity level even further
  - Cage restriction; on leash when using yard

Day 90

- Administer appropriate HW preventive
- Administer 2nd melarsomine injection, 2.5 mg/kg IM
- Prescribe prednisone 0.5 mg/kg q12h for 1st week, then 0.5 mg/kg q24h for 2nd week, and 0.5 mg/kg q48h for 3rd and 4th weeks

Day 91

- Administer 3rd melarsomine injection, 2.5 mg/kg IM (use opposite side from that used on day 90)
- Continue exercise restriction for 6–8 weeks following last melarsomine injection

Day 120

- Test for presence of MF
  - If positive, treat with a microfilaricide and retest in 4 weeks
- Continue a year-round HW prevention program based on risk assessment

Day 365

- HW Ag test 9 months after last melarsomine injection; screen for MF
- If still Ag positive, retreat with doxycycline, followed by two doses of melarsomine, 24 hours apart

[a] From 2020 Canine guidelines for the prevention, diagnosis, and management of heartworm (*Dirofilaria immitis*) infection in dogs. American Heartworm Society (AHS; www.heartwormsociety.org).
See text for additional information.
Abbreviations: Ag, antigen; EPA, Environmental Protection Agency; HW, heartworm; IM, intramuscular; MF, microfilariae.

Table 40.4 AHA Classification of Heartworm Disease Severity in Dogs

Disease Severity	Typical Clinical Signs
Mild	Asymptomatic, or cough
Moderate	Cough, exercise intolerance, abnormal lung sounds
Severe	Cough, exercise intolerance, dyspnea, abnormal heart & lung sounds, hepatomegaly, syncope, ascites, death
Caval syndrome	Sudden onset of severe lethargy & weakness with hemoglobinemia & hemoglobinuria

From 2020 Canine Guidelines. American Heartworm Society (www.heartwormsociety.org). The authors alternatively suggest the perspective of: 1) no or equivocal signs; 2) pulmonary signs requiring stabilization with prednisone; 3) cor pulmonale (including CHF) requiring cardiac medications and sildenafil; and 4) HWD complicated by hemolysis or caval syndrome (see text for details).

protein within 4 months, as does the standard 20 mg/kg/day. Doxycycline's oral absorption is about 60%. The half-life is widely variable (reportedly from <1 hour to >12 hour, and 6–29 hour). In a small clinical study of dogs with HWD, treatment with doxycycline or minocycline at 10 mg/kg doses was associated with more severe gastrointestinal (GI) side-effects than 5 mg/kg doses. Such side effects could lead to reduced owner compliance in medicating the dog. However, the higher doxycycline dose was more effective than the 5 mg/kg dose, and both minocycline doses, for eliminating the presence of *Wolbachia* deoxyribonucleic acid (DNA) after 28 days of treatment (Savadelis, 2018a). When possible, doxycycline should be used at 10 mg/kg, with reduction to the lower dose only if severe GI signs develop. Administering with food (except milk products) could reduce GI upset.

If doxycycline is unavailable, minocycline is an alternative. The optimal canine dose for minocycline is unclear, although a predicted dose of 5 mg/kg q12 hour was suggested based on *in vitro* and mouse studies, which demonstrated greater anti-*Wolbachia* activity with minocycline than with doxycycline (Papich, 2017). However, as noted above, a dog trial suggested the opposite. Therefore the suggested minocycline dose is (5–)10 mg/kg every 12 hours for 4 weeks. Higher minocycline doses are more likely to produce vomiting. Minocycline's oral absorption is ~50%; feeding impairs absorption. There is less protein binding (~50%) compared to doxycycline. Minocycline is more lipophilic, which should facilitate the drug's intracellular distribution. The drug has a larger volume of distribution than doxycycline. Terminal half-life is about 5 hours. Doxycycline and minocycline, like other tetracycline drugs, have activity against multiple agents besides *Wolbachia*, including some gram-positive and gram-negative bacteria, Rickettsiae, and Ehrlichiae. Other drugs are being evaluated that might have greater anti-*Wolbachia* efficacy with shorter treatment course (Turner, 2020)

A macrocyclic lactone is an integral component of HW therapy. Infected dogs could harbor adult HWs of widely varying age (from 1 month to ~7 years). Melarsomine is incompletely effective against young adult worms, so it is likely that these could survive to continue the infection. A macrocyclic lactone, administered for 2 months before the initial melarsomine injection, prevents new infection, kills susceptible larvae already in the host, and allows time for juvenile worms to mature, which will increase melarsomine's efficacy against them. However, repeated monthly treatment with a milbemycin oxime product also kills 3-month old HWs. So, another perspective is that, with current drug use, there might be no "susceptibility gap" and no increase in efficacy gained by delaying the initial dose of melarsomine. Concurrent doxycycline administration for the first month further potentiates this protective effect, thus reducing or eliminating any so-called "susceptibility gap". Concurrent ivermectin and doxycycline use kills adult worms more quickly than ivermectin alone and reduces *Wolbachia* more effectively than doxycycline alone. Both ivermectin and moxidectin, when administered with doxycycline, suppress embryogenesis and have adulticidal activity (p. 860).

Infected *dogs with a large number of circulating MF* could experience an adverse reaction following a dose of some macrocyclic lactones because of rapid MF death. In dogs with a high MF count, pretreatment with an antihistamine (diphenhydramine, 2 mg/kg PO or IM) and glucocorticoid (such as dexamethasone, 0.2 mg/kg IV) can reduce the severity of potential reactions. However, concurrent use of a glucocorticoid with a nonsteroidal antiinflammatory agent is not recommended. MF-positive dogs should be observed in the hospital after their first ivermectin dose (p. 862). Topical moxidectin has not been associated with such reactions, however. Specific microfilaricide therapy is not necessary before adulticide treatment. Concurrent macrocyclic lactone use reduces HW Ag mass by decreasing or eliminating circulating MF and tissue migrating larvae, stunts immature worm growth, and damages the adult female reproductive system.

Aspirin is not recommended as a routine preadulticide treatment; convincing evidence for beneficial antithrombotic effect is lacking. An oral anticoagulant (such as rivaroxaban or apixaban) might be more effective in preventing thrombosis in low-shear flow situations, such as the pulmonary artery in dogs with HWD, however more study is needed regarding this.

Melarsomine Treatment Melarsomine dihydrochloride is the recommended adulticide drug for dogs, except those with caval syndrome. As noted above, it should be used within the context of a multimodal treatment strategy over several months rather than by itself (**Table 40.3**). Dogs with no or only mild signs of HWD (**Table 40.4**) are considered to have lower risk for embolic complications. Most of these cases successfully undergo adulticide therapy. Although the original 2-dose melarsomine regime (2.5 mg/kg IM 24 hours apart) has been used in mild cases, the more conservative 3-dose approach is safer, more effective, and strongly recommended for all dogs (www.heartwormsociety.org). Dogs with clinical signs of moderate or severe HWD (class 2 or 3 disease) should be stabilized before adulticide administration (using the 3-dose protocol).

A single IM injection of melarsomine (2.5 mg/kg) is effective against essentially all 2-month-old HWs and over 80% of 4-month-old worms; however, efficacy against older adult HWs is less certain. Male worms appear to be more susceptible. The 3-dose melarsomine protocol is designed to partially reduce the worm burden with one initial injection, followed by the standard adulticide regimen 4–6 weeks later. The risk of fatal PTE from an initially heavy worm kill is reduced with this protocol. The overall worm kill rate is affected by the protocol used. The two-injection melarsomine protocol kills about 90% of adult worms. The more conservative three-injection protocol reportedly kills about 98% of worms and has a lower complication rate. With this latter protocol, some worms die from the initial dose while others presumably are weakened; the two injections that follow a month later kill most of the remaining worms.

Melarsomine should be given by deep IM injection into belly of the epaxial lumbar muscles, at the level of the 3rd to 5th lumbar vertebrae, exactly as recommended by the manufacturer. The drug causes mild injection site swelling and soreness, which is clinically noticeable in about a third of treated dogs. To help reduce this, after drawing the melarsomine dose into the syringe, change to a fresh needle of appropriate size for the dog's size and body condition. Also, the injection site should be gently compressed afterwards to prevent drug leakage. A nonsteroidal antiinflammatory drug given for a few days helps reduce the acute muscle soreness; however, this is contraindicated if the dog is being treated with a corticosteroid. An alternative to a nonsteroidal antiinflammatory drug is tramadol (3–5 mg/kg PO q8h) and gabapentin (10–20 mg/kg PO q8h), administered at the time of melarsomine injection, and continued for several days, as needed. The lumbar muscle site provides good vascularity and lymphatic drainage, with minimal fascial planes. Gravity also might help prevent drug leakage into subcutaneous tissues, where it can cause more irritation.

Melarsomine is absorbed quickly from the IM injection site. Unchanged drug and a major metabolite are eliminated rapidly in the feces; a minor metabolite is excreted in the urine. Posttreatment coughing and (less often) dyspnea could relate to the HWD itself, although pulmonary congestion is a toxic effect of overdosing. Adverse effects in dogs receiving recommended doses generally are mild. These typically are either behavioral (such as tremors, lethargy, unsteadiness and ataxia, restlessness), respiratory (panting, shallow breathing, coughing, labored respirations, crackles), or injection site related (edema, redness, tenderness, vocalization, increased aspartate aminotransferase, AST, and creatine kinase, CK, activities). Injection site reactions usually are of mild to moderate intensity and heal within 4(–12) weeks, although firm nodules might persist indefinitely at the sites. General signs of lethargy, depression, and anorexia develop in about 15% or fewer dogs; other adverse effects, including fever, vomiting, and diarrhea, occur occasionally. In most cases, symptomatic therapy is sufficient. However, more severe reactions can occur, rarely. These have included local, and sometimes progressive, neurologic signs. Suspected hypersensitivity reactions are treated as for those associated with rapid MF death (p. 863). For severe respiratory distress, hypotension, and other signs of shock, epinephrine also could be used (for example, 0.008–0.01 mg/kg IM q 5–15 minute, to effect; or 0.05 mcg/kg/minute CRI to effect).

Melarsomine has a low margin of safety. Overdose can cause fatal pulmonary inflammation and edema. Collapse, severe salivation, vomiting, respiratory distress, stupor, and death have occurred at triple the recommended dose in some dogs. Some clinical reversal of melarsomine toxicity could be achieved with dimercaprol (British Anti-Lewisite) administered at 3 mg/kg IM. This also will decrease adulticide activity.

Complications and outcomes after melarsomine treatment can differ depending on worm burden, host inflammatory reaction to dead and dying worms, and the effects of varying exercise restriction. Mortality in dogs with severe HWD given melarsomine has been estimated at ~10% overall; (for historical comparison, severe cases treated with thiacetarsamide under similar conditions had ~53% survival rate).

Strict rest must be enforced for at least 4–6 weeks after adulticide therapy to reduce the sequelae of adult worm death and PTE. The rest period for working dogs probably should be 8 weeks or longer, because exercise-induced increases in pulmonary blood flow exacerbate pulmonary capillary damage and subsequent fibrosis. The risk of postadulticide PTE is higher in dogs with severe pulmonary vascular disease, and especially in those with right-sided CHF or a high worm burden. Nevertheless, accurately predicting which cases will develop complications is difficult. Clearly, exercise incurs additional risk and failure to restrict physical activity is an important contributor to postadulticide complications. Owners might need reminders of this, as well as encouragement, during the period of exercise restriction. Suggestions for reducing the confined dog's boredom include use of long-lasting chew toys and puzzle feeders, and also spending quiet time in companionship with the owner (see link to "Battling Boredom: Tips for Surviving Cage Rest" in Canine Guidelines; www.heartwormsociety.org).

Assessing Adulticide Efficacy HW Ag testing is the best means to gauge the success of adulticide therapy. HW Ag should be undetectable by 6 months after all adult female worms are killed. Testing at this time is recommended, although ~80% or more of dogs with mild to moderate HWD are HW Ag negative by 4 months after melarsomine administration. Nevertheless, some larval or juvenile HWs could be present, especially if preventative medication was not given concurrently. The decision to repeat treatment in a dog with persistent antigenemia is guided by the animal's overall health, performance expectations, and age. Seroconversion approaches 100% with repeated treatment. However, complete worm kill probably is unnecessary and might not yield further clinical improvement.

Although some adult female worms might survive adulticide therapy, circulating MF disappear within 6–9 months even without microfilaricide treatment. Doxycycline in combination with a macrocyclic lactone preventative contribute to the resolution of microfilaremia. Therefore, absence of circulating MF does not verify adulticide efficacy. Microfilaremia discovered 6 months or more after adulticide therapy could result from persistence of some adult worms, maturation of immature worms (if a macrocyclic lactone was not given during adulticide treatment), or new HW infection.

It appears that the prevalence of PH (based on RPADI assessment) is not increased, but neither is it decreased, by one month after the last melarsomine dose. This suggests that regression of pulmonary vascular pathology and PH must occur over a longer period of time.

Alternatives to Melarsomine Adulticide Therapy As noted above, the AHS currently recommends the 3-dose melarsomine adulticide protocol for dogs with HWD whenever possible. However, if melarsomine treatment is not feasible or is contraindicated, an alternative approach is to use monthly topical (or oral) moxidectin, or oral ivermectin, along with a 4-week course of doxycycline (10 mg/kg q 12h). Strict exercise restriction must be enforced throughout the entire treatment period, which might last over 9–12 months. Some evidence suggests that moxidectin might be a more effective macrocyclic lactone than ivermectin for this strategy. Studies of HW positive dogs treated with monthly topical moxidectin (2.5%, with 10% imidacloprid), and with doxycycline (10 mg/kg q12 PO) for the first month, showed that circulating MF were eliminated within a month and some of the dogs tested negative for HW Ag by 4 months after treatment initiation (Genchi, 2019; Paterson, 2020). By 9 months, over 70% of these dogs had a negative HW Ag test. A small comparison group treated with melarsomine (1 dose at enrollment and 2 doses a month later) were HW Ag negative by 5 months after treatment began. Another study used moxidectin/imidacloprid twice per month for the first 3 months, followed by monthly administration, combined with a median doxycline dosage of 12.6 mg/kg/day but for only 15 days (Ames, 2020b). In this study, 21 of 22 dogs eventually converted to "no antigen dectected" status; however, this did not occur for over a year in two cases. There is growing interest in the use of this moxidectin and doxycycline strategy (nicknamed "doxymectin" or "MOXY") in HW positive dogs, because there potentially could be fewer concerns about adverse events and toxicity. However, exercise restriction is crucial. Without exercise restriction, the rate of coughing during the treatment period appears to greatly exceed that associated with the recommended HW treatment protocol. Other concerns with this alternative protocol are that HW-associated radiographic changes progress similarly to untreated dogs and evidence for PTE seems worse, even though the protocol appears over 95% effective in eliminating adult worms within 10 months (Savadelis, 2017). Signs of HW-associated PTE or pneumonitis can occur at unpredictable times. HW Ag testing should be done every 6 months. After two consecutive tests (6 months apart) have shown no detectable Ag, the dog can be considered cleared of HW. If the HW Ag test still is positive after a year, another 4-week course of doxycycline is recommended. With regard to other macrocyclic lactones, the adulticidal effectiveness of selamectin is less than that of ivermectin, and appears least for milbemycin oxime.

So-called "slow-kill" methods that employ only the monthly prophylactic doses of a macrocyclic lactone continuously throughout the year(s) are *not* recommended. It can take >2 years of continuous monthly treatment to see the adulticidal effect of these drugs (against about 95% of adult worms). Juvenile worms are more susceptible to the macrocyclic lactones; however, older adult worms are likely to persist much longer and can cause clinical disease. PA pathology and its sequelae continue to progress when worms are present. Other systemic consequences, including glomerulonephritis, also progress and could contribute to future medical complications. Exercise exacerbates the pulmonary pathology and active dogs are more likely to develop clinical signs, even with a low worm burden. Yet restrictions on physical activity are unlikely to be continuously maintained for 2 or more years. Another growing concern relates to the issue of HW drug resistance. It is possible that macrocyclic lactone monotherapy in HW-positive dogs might foster the emergence of drug-resistant HW subpopulations. Immune-complex development, leading to false-negative HW Ag test results, is more likely to occur with "slow kill" methods. Additionally, no herbal or "natural" therapies have been proven effective to prevent or treat HWD.

Treatment of Dogs with Complicated Heartworm Disease Heartworm pneumonitis occurs in some dogs with HWD. Manifestations of HW pneumonitis include a progressively worsening cough, tachypnea or dyspnea, pulmonary crackles on auscultation, and in some cases, cyanosis, weight loss, and anorexia. Eosinophilia, basophilia, and hyperglobulinemia are inconsistent findings. Serologic tests for adult HWs usually are positive. Diffuse interstitial and alveolar infiltrates typically are present on chest radiographs, especially in the caudal lobes. These might resemble infiltrates caused by pulmonary edema or blastomycosis. Cardiomegaly or lobar pulmonary artery enlargement frequently is absent. Tracheal wash often yields a sterile eosinophilic exudate with variable numbers of well-preserved neutrophils and macrophages. Glucocorticoid therapy (for example, prednisone at 1–2 mg/kg/day PO initially) usually produces rapid improvement. Prednisone, in gradually tapered doses (to 0.5 mg/kg every other day), can be continued as needed and does not appear to adversely affect the adulticide efficacy of melarsomine. For dogs with respiratory distress, IV dexamethasone (0.2 mg/kg q24h), supplemental O_2, and cage rest are recommended initially; transition to oral, tapering, corticosteroid therapy and home rest can follow.

Pulmonary eosinophilic granulomatosis is a rare syndrome that can be associated with HWD, although some affected dogs have negative HW tests. A hypersensitivity reaction to HW Ags, immune complexes, or both is thought to contribute to its pathogenesis. Pulmonary granulomas consist of a mixed population of mononuclear and neutrophilic cells, with many eosinophils and macrophages. Bronchial smooth muscle proliferation within granulomas and abundant alveolar cells in the surrounding area are common; lymphocytic and eosinophilic perivascular infiltration also might occur. Eosinophilic granulomas might concurrently involve lymph nodes, trachea, tonsils, spleen, GI tract, and the liver or kidneys. Clinical signs of pulmonary eosinophilic granulomatosis are similar to those of eosinophilic pneumonitis. Variable clinicopathologic findings can include leukocytosis, neutrophilia, eosinophilia, basophilia, monocytosis, and hyperglobulinemia. An exudative, mainly eosinophilic, pleural effusion occasionally develops. Radiographic findings include multiple pulmonary nodules of varying size and distribution, with mixed alveolar and interstitial pulmonary infiltrates. Hilar and mediastinal lymphadenopathy might be evident. Eosinophilic granulomatosis associated with HWD is treated initially with prednisone (1–2 mg/kg q12h); however, additional cytotoxic therapy sometimes is needed, as well. Incomplete response and relapse are common, especially after therapy is reduced or discontinued. HW adulticide treatment is provided after the pulmonary disease abates.

Severe PA disease is likely in dogs with long-standing HW infection and a heavy worm burden, as well as in physically active HW-infected dogs. Clinical signs can relate to pneumonitis, PTE, PH, and cor pulmonale and variably include cough, exercise intolerance, tachypnea or dyspnea, episodic weakness, syncope, weight loss, heart failure, and sudden death. Hemoptysis is noted in some cases. Radiographic evidence of marked pulmonary artery enlargement, tortuosity and blunting is common and implies the presence of PH (**Figures 40.10** and **40.11**). Pulmonary parenchymal infiltrates, which can lead to hypoxemia, are treated with prednisone (as for eosinophilic pneumonitis) until resolved. Alternate day, low-dose prednisone (0.5 mg/kg PO) should have beneficial antiinflammatory effects, but chronic high-dose corticosteroid therapy could reduce pulmonary blood flow, enhance the risk of PTE, and inhibit vascular disease resolution. Thrombocytopenia (from platelet consumption) and hemolysis can occur in dogs with severe PA disease and PTE; therefore, the packed cell volume and platelet count should be monitored. DIC develops in some dogs. Conservative therapy with oxygen, prednisone, and a bronchodilator (such as theophylline) helps improve oxygenation and decrease pulmonary artery pressures (see below). Sildenafil (or tadalafil; p. 834) could help reduce pulmonary vascular resistance in dogs with moderate to severe PH. Enforced rest is important for these cases. Clopidogrel might decrease thromboembolic risk (p. 764), although this has not been well studied in HWD and bleeding could be enhanced, especially in dogs with thrombocytopenia. After the dog's condition has been stabilized, the 3-dose melarsomine protocol is used.

Right-sided CHF develops in some dogs with severe PA disease and PH. Typical signs include jugular venous distension or pulsation, ascites, syncope, exercise intolerance, and arrhythmias. Pleural or pericardial effusion also can develop. Other signs associated with PA and parenchymal pathology might be present. Treatment is as described for dogs with severe PA disease (including sildenafil and enforced rest) with the addition of furosemide, pimobendan, and a reduced-salt diet (Chapter 22). Pimobendan is used mainly to support RV function, although this has not been well-studied in HWD. In experimental canine PH, pimobendan improved cardiac function although PA pressures were unchanged. With the reduction in pulmonary vascular resistance induced by sildenafil (or tadalafil), many dogs improve markedly. Some clinicians also prescribe an angiotensin converting enzyme (ACE) inhibitor and spironolactone; others only prescribe spironolactone, as the merits of ACE inhibition in right heart failure are uncertain. Digoxin generally is not advised for HW-induced CHF. Large-volume cavity effusions should be drained, as needed. Older studies have indicated that cage rest by itself can mobilize ascites, so exercise restriction also could be helpful for this. Adulticide therapy should be delayed until after the dog has been clinically stable for at least several weeks, although treatment with doxycycline and a macrocyclic lactone preventive can be started much sooner. After successful adulticide therapy, tapering and eventual discontinuation of sildenafil and heart failure drugs might be possible.

In a small number of *dogs with intracardiac HWs* (identified on echo exam) but without clinical signs of caval syndrome, treatment with sildenafil and pimobendan was followed by HW migration back into the pulmonary arteries within a few days (Tjostheim, 2019). The usual multimodal adulticide regime subsequently was used without complications in these dogs.

Postadulticide Pulmonary Thromboembolism Strict exercise restriction during the 4–6 weeks (or longer) following adulticide therapy is critical to reducing complications from PTE. PA disease worsens from 5–30 days after adulticide therapy and is especially severe in dogs that were symptomatic for HWD before adulticide treatment. Dead and dying worms cause thrombosis and pulmonary artery obstruction, with exacerbation of platelet adhesion, myointimal proliferation, villous hypertrophy, granulomatous arteritis, perivascular edema, and hemorrhage. Obstructed pulmonary flow and high PVR further increase RV strain. Poor cardiac output can lead to hypotension and myocardial ischemia. Poor lung perfusion, hypoxic vasoconstriction and bronchoconstriction, pulmonary inflammation, and fluid accumulation can cause serious ventilation–perfusion mismatch. As expected, the caudal and accessory lung lobes are most commonly and severely affected.

The worst signs of PTE usually develop between 5 and 10 days after adulticide therapy, although they can occur anytime within the month following. Clinical signs include lethargy, low-grade fever, cough, tachycardia, tachypnea or dyspnea, hemoptysis, and signs of right-sided CHF. Some animals experience collapse or death. Pulmonary crackles, heard on auscultation, result from lung inflammation and fluid accumulation. Focal lung consolidation can cause regionally-muffled lung sounds. A CBC might reveal thrombocytopenia or a regenerative left shift. Thoracic radiographs might show patchy alveolar infiltrates with air bronchograms, especially near the caudal lobar arteries (**Figure 40.19**). These could represent embolic pneumonia or noncardiogenic pulmonary edema. Inflammatory pulmonary infiltrates typically improve markedly with corticosteroid therapy. Persistent interstitial infiltrates that do not resolve over time suggest pulmonary scarring and fibrosis.

Symptomatic PTE is managed with strict rest (cage confinement) and glucocorticoid therapy to reduce pulmonary inflammation (for example, prednisone at 0.5 mg/kg q12h for 7 days, then q24h for another 7 days, then decreasing to 0.5 mg/kg q48h for another 1–2 weeks). Supplemental O_2 is recommended to reduce hypoxia-mediated pulmonary vasoconstriction. Likewise, sildenafil could be helpful, although this is unstudied unless there is moderate to severe PH (p. 834). The addition of pimobendan is reasonable when signs of CHF are present, as noted previously. A bronchodilator (such as aminophylline, 10 mg/kg PO, IM, or IV q8h; or theophylline, 9 mg/kg PO q6–8h), judicious fluid therapy (if there is evidence of cardiovascular shock), and a cough suppressant also might be useful on a case-by-case basis.

Antithrombotic therapy with a direct-acting oral anticoagulant (such as rivaroxaban) might be helpful for severe cases of PTE (p. 766). Other antithrombotic strategies have included low molecular weight heparin or unfractionated heparin, although excessive bleeding could be a serious adverse effect, especially with the latter agent. Aspirin is not recommended; there is no convincing evidence of a beneficial antithrombotic effect or reduced pulmonary arteritis, and possible findings of adverse effect. It is not known if clopidogrel might have any adjunct benefit in this context; bleeding could be enhanced, especially in dogs with thrombocytopenia. Because of the potential for devitalized pulmonary tissue and secondary bacterial infection in dogs with PTE, antibiotics have sometimes been prescribed empirically; however, their benefit is questionable unless concurrent bacterial infection is evident. Use of nonphosphodiesterase-5 inhibitor vasodilators brings risk of systemic hypotension. In dogs that survive, endothelial changes

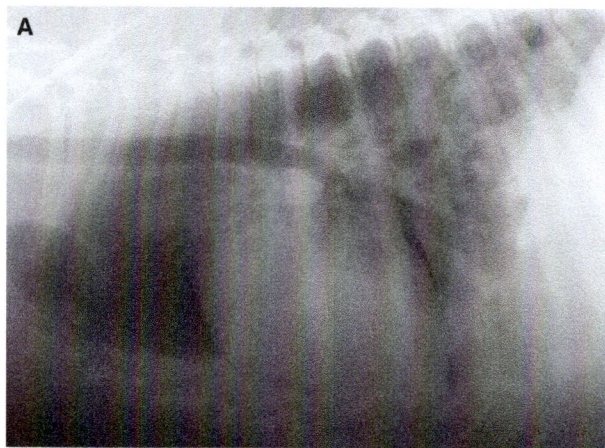

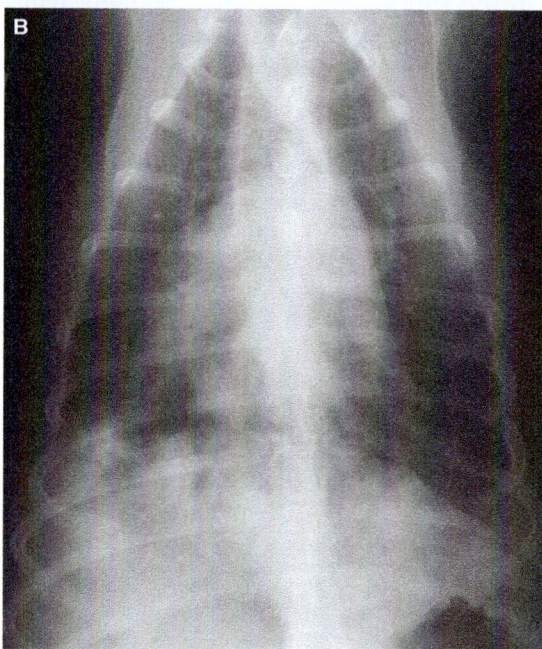

Figure 40.19 Lateral (A) and DV (B) radiographs from a 7-year-old male Golden Retriever one week after heartworm adulticide treatment. Patchy, caudal lobar interstitial infiltrates are most prominent on the right and are consistent with postadulticide pulmonary thromboembolism.

regress within 4–6 weeks. PH and radiographic signs of arterial disease begin to resolve over the next several months.

Microfilaricide Therapy Specific treatment to kill MF typically is unnecessary when the recommended adulticide protocol using doxycycline and regular preventative macrocyclic lactone doses is employed (**Table 40.3**). Microfilarial elimination should be confirmed by 6 months after adulticide treatment. Previous recommendations included giving microfilaricidal therapy 3–4 weeks after adulticide therapy; this could be done, if necessary.

Topical moxidectin will eliminate MF and has not been associated with adverse reactions. Ivermectin's microfilaricidal dose (50 mcg/kg PO) is higher than that needed for HW prevention; this preventative dose also is safe for Collies. Selamectin is known to be microfilaricidal, as well. Milbemycin oxime is (incompletely) microfilaricidal at the standard HW preventive dose (0.5–1.0 mg/kg). Other drugs previously used as microfilaricides (including levamisole and fenthion) are not recommended because of their low efficacy and frequent adverse effects.

The rapid death of many MF within 3–8 (and occasionally 12) hours of dosing could cause an acute hypersensitivity reaction. Systemic signs can include lethargy, inappetence, salivation, tachypnea, tachycardia, retching, vomiting, defecation, and pallor. Therefore, pretreatment with an antihistamine and glucocorticoid is advised for dogs with high MF numbers (see p. 858), although the concurrent use of glucocorticoid with nonsteroidal antiinflammatory agent is not recommended. These animals also should be observed closely for 8–12 hours after initial microfilaricide treatment, especially if milbemycin or ivermectin is used. Mild or moderately severe adverse effects associated with rapid microfilarial death often respond to diphenhydramine (2 mg/kg, IM), dexamethasone (0.2 mg/kg, IV) and IV fluid support. Sporadically, however, an acute hypersensitivity reaction in a dog with high numbers of circulating MF leads to circulatory collapse. Immediate treatment with shock glucocorticoid (for example, prednisolone sodium succinate, 10 mg/kg IV; or dexamethasone, 1 mg/kg IV) and IV fluid therapy (such as 80 ml/kg over 2 hours) can be successful.

Caval Syndrome The acute, shock-like condition known as the (vena) caval syndrome occurs in heavily infected dogs when a mass of worms obstructs venous inflow to the heart and interferes with tricuspid valve function (**Figure 40.20**). This condition also has been called postcaval syndrome, acute hepatic syndrome, liver failure syndrome, dirofilarial hemoglobinuria, and vena cava embolism. Although adult HWs usually locate within the pulmonary arteries, as the number of worms increases, adult worms migrate upstream in rising numbers into the right atrium (RA), caudal vena cava, and sometimes the cranial vena cava. Factors other than worm burden alone also could be involved in the development of caval syndrome. Experimentally, in dogs with equal

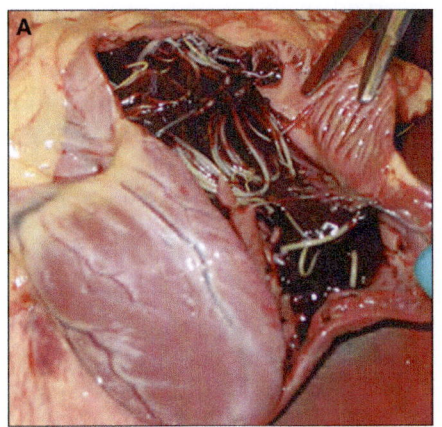
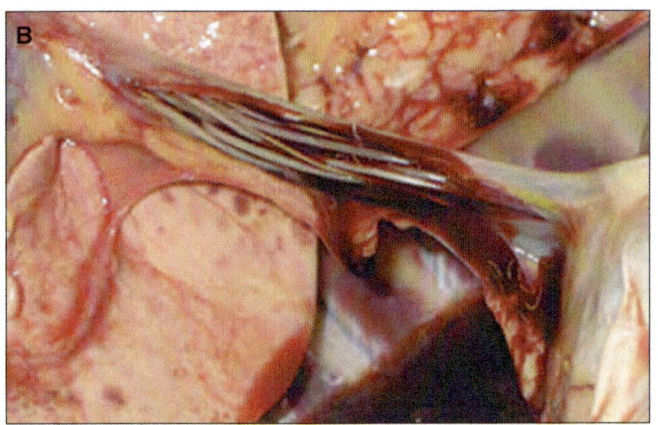
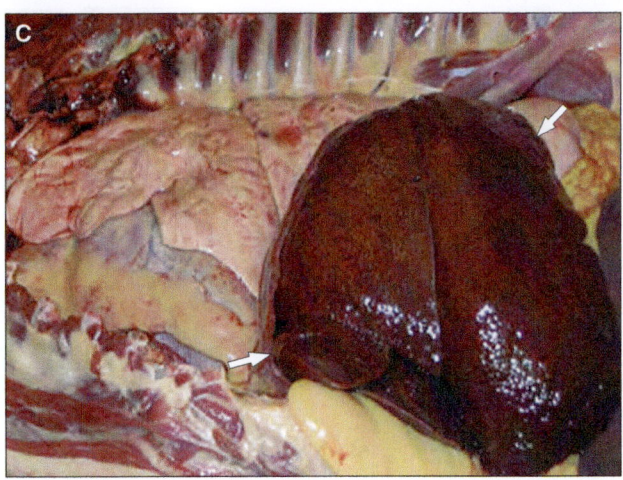

Figure 40.20 (A) Open right atrium (above) and ventricle (below) from a 9-year-old male dog presented for a suspected abdominal mass, but instead had heartworm (HW) caval syndrome. Numerous HWs are visible within the intracardiac blood pool. (B) HWs pack the caudal vena cava; the heart is to the left, diaphragm on the right. (C) The caval obstruction caused pronounced hepatic congestion (arrows); no abdominal mass was found.

worm burdens, pulmonary artery pressures were higher in those that developed caval syndrome compared with those that did not. The syndrome also has been created experimentally using a beta-blocker in heavily infected dogs, probably through reduction of cardiac output.

Caval syndrome occurs more often in geographic areas where HWD is highly endemic. Many affected dogs have no history of typical HW-related signs. The typical underlying features are a large worm burden, severe PH, cor pulmonale, and RV dysfunction. TR occurs often and can be secondary to retrograde worm migration into the valve orifice. Caval syndrome typically causes death within a couple days if surgical extraction of HWs is not accomplished right away.

Partial RV inflow occlusion caused by the mass of HWs, in conjunction with PH and TR, lead to severe hepatic congestion. Not all dogs have right-sided CHF signs (ascites), but some do. Signs of low cardiac output are typical and acute collapse or weakness is the most common presenting complaint. Other signs include tachypnea or dyspnea, pallor, hemoglobinuria and hemoglobinemia, icterus, and bilirubinuria (**Figure 40.21**). Coughing or hemoptysis occurs sometimes. Common physical findings, in addition to evidence for ascites and poor cardiac output, include jugular vein distension and pulsations, weak femoral pulses, a coarse systolic murmur of TR over the right thorax, and a loud and possibly split S_2. A cardiac gallop sound also might be heard.

Clinicopathologic findings can include Coombs-negative hemolytic anemia (from red blood cell trauma), azotemia, abnormal liver function with increased liver enzyme activity, and often, DIC. Microfilaremia is present in some cases. Intravascular hemolysis causes the hemoglobinemia and hemoglobinuria. Right heart and pulmonary artery enlargement are evident on thoracic radiographs (**Figure 40.22**). *The ECG* usually suggests RV enlargement. Ventricular and supraventricular premature complexes often occur.

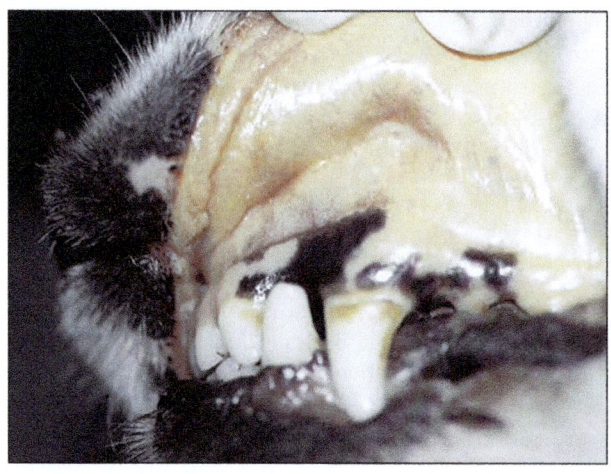

Figure 40.21 Pallor and icterus in an 8-year-old female mixed breed dog with hemolysis secondary to heartworm caval syndrome.

Echocardiography provides rapid, definitive diagnosis by showing a mass of worms entangled at the tricuspid valve and within the RA; the worm mass typically moves back into the RA in systole and into the RV inlet during diastole. Parasites often are observed in the venae cavae, too, and sometimes within hepatic veins (**Figures 40.23** and **40.24**). RV dilation and hypertrophy, paradoxical septal motion, and a small left ventricle also are features. Unless treated immediately, most dogs die within 24–72 hours from cardiogenic shock complicated by metabolic acidosis, DIC, anemia, and multiorgan failure. However, "chronic" caval syndrome occasionally is recognized, and some dogs have compatible signs that have lasted over several weeks.

The most effective and recommended *treatment* is the physical removal of worms from the RA and vena cava as soon as possible; although, a small number of dogs have shown surprising response to medical therapy (see following

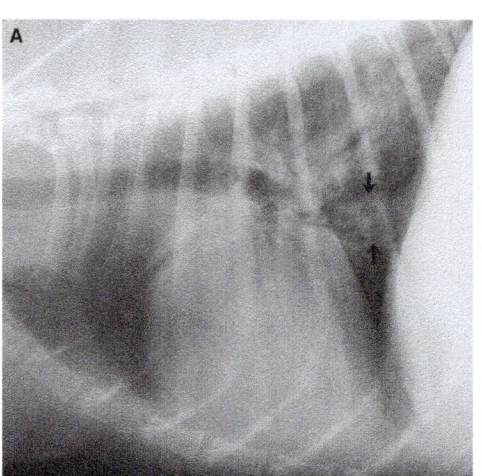
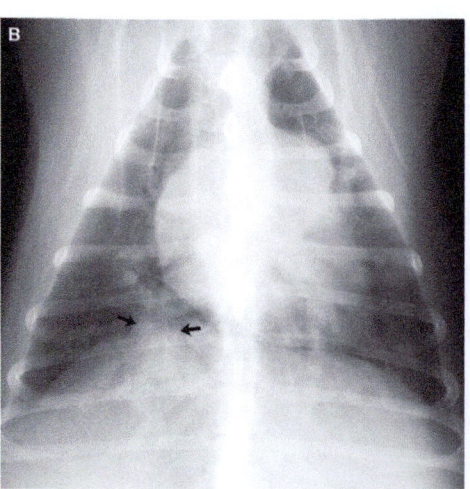
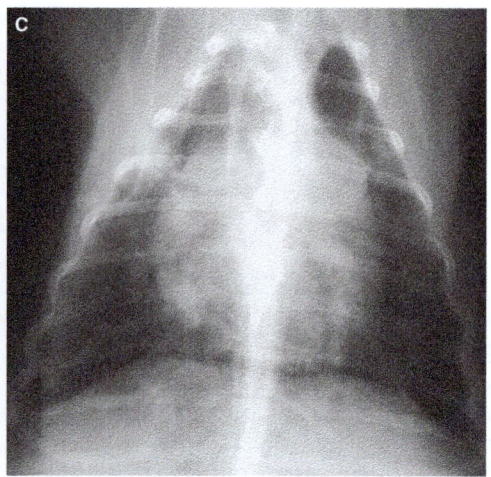

Figure 40.22 Lateral (A) and DV (B) radiographs from the dog in **Figure 40.21** at initial presentation. The caudal vena cava is markedly distended (arrows, A & B). A main pulmonary artery bulge (B), large and tortuous caudal right pulmonary artery, and patchy pulmonary infiltrates also are present. C) DV image, taken a short time after 10 adult heartworms had been extracted via jugular venotomy, shows marked increase in right heart filling.

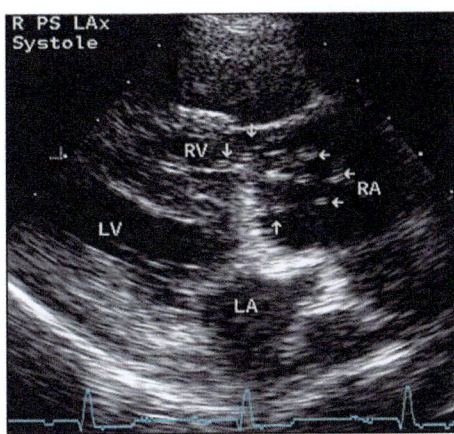

Figure 40.23 Long-axis 2D image in systole from the dog in **Figure 40.21** shows a mass of heartworms (arrows) in the right atrium (RA); they would shift into the ventricle (RV) during diastole. LA, left atrium; LV, left ventricle.

paragraphs). IV fluid, supplemental O_2, sildenafil, and possibly pimobendan could help stabilize the dog during preparations for worm removal. Also, pretreatment with an antihistamine and glucocorticoid might reduce hypersensitivity reactions caused by damage to the HW cuticle. Anesthesia is critical and a common contibutor to procedural death. Dogs with caval syndrome are fragile; standard anesthetic regimens usually depress cardiovascular function excessively. IV techniques, copious local anesthesia, and intensive monitoring often are required. Ideally, an anesthesiologist should be available or consulted.

Worm extraction is approached via right jugular venotomy, with the animal in left lateral recumbency (**Figure 40.25**); the right jugular approach provides a straighter path into the RA compared to the left jugular approach. Local anesthesia is used for markedly depressed patients, with light sedation as necessary; general anesthesia might be required in others. After the jugular vein is exposed, silk suture or umbilical tape loops are placed around the vessel cranial and caudal to the planned venotomy site to assist with vessel manipulation and hemostasis. Imaging guidance is preferred, if available. Fluoroscopy is used most often, although transesophageal echocardiography could be another option (but requires anesthesia). Various extraction devices can be used to grasp and withdraw the HWs through the jugular vein incision, including HW-specific (Ishihara) retrieval forceps, an endoscopic basket retrieval instrument, nitinol gooseneck or other intravascular retrieval snare, long alligator forceps, or a horsehair brush device. Alternatively, a flexible alligator forceps retrieval device can be used and could provide the advantage of also reaching worms in the pulmonary trunk. The instrument must be passed gently down the vein into the RA; some repositioning of the animal's neck or manipulation of the retrieval device might be needed to pass the instrument beyond the thoracic inlet. Resistance during withdrawal can occur if too many worms at one time, or a cardiovascular structure, are grasped. The retrieval device is passed repeatedly to remove as many HWs as possible. Care should be taken to avoid breaking the worms. Efforts to extract HWs are continued until 5 or 6 consecutive attempts have been unsuccessful; if available, echocardiography can verify intracardiac

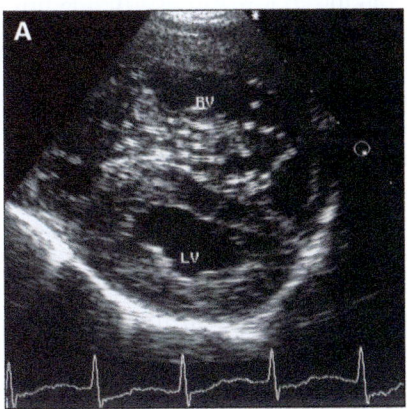

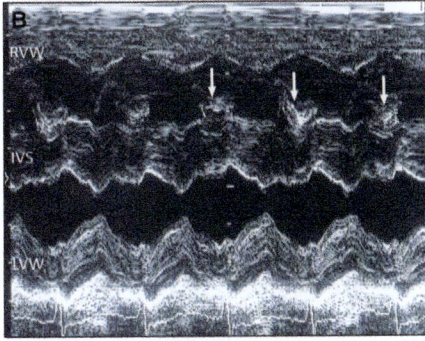

Figure 40.24 (A) Short-axis 2D image at the ventricular level from a male, mixed breed dog with caval syndrome. Within the RV are characteristic short, parallel echos from a mass of heartworms (HWs) surrounding the tricuspid valve. Right ventricular hypertrophy, dilation, and septal flattening also are evident. B) M-mode image from the same dog shows bright, irregular echos (arrows) within the RV during diastole, which are reflected from HWs entangled in the tricuspid valve. Right parasternal position; IVS, interventricular septum; LV, left ventricle; LVW, left ventricular wall; RV, right ventricle; RVW, right ventricular wall.

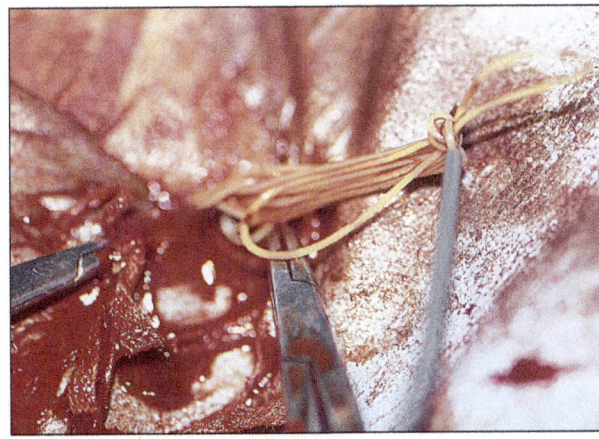

Figure 40.25 Heartworms being extracted via right jugular venotomy, using an endoscopic basket retrieval device, from the right atrium of a dog with caval syndrome.

HW removal. The jugular vein then is ligated, or repaired, and the skin incision closed. After worm extraction, the patient's murmur usually becomes much softer or disappears. Survival rates of ~50–80% have been reported for dogs undergoing this procedure. However, appropriate postprocedure intensive care is important. Right auricular cannulation performed via a thoracotomy also has been described to remove worms in very small dogs.

Cautious IV fluid administration, as well as other supportive care, is provided during and after worm extraction. Central venous pressure monitoring can help in assessing the effectiveness of worm extraction and fluid therapy. Treatment with sodium bicarbonate usually is not necessary. However, a broad-spectrum antibiotic is recommended. Anemia, thrombocytopenia, DIC, azotemia, and major organ dysfunction are likely complications, so close monitoring is important. Hemoglobinuria should resolve within 12–24 hours after successful worm extraction. Severe PTE and renal or hepatic failure are associated with poor outcome. Dogs that survive acute caval syndrome are likely to have worms remaining within the pulmonary arteries. After stabilization, these dogs can be treated with the 3-dose adulticide protocol (**Table 40.3**) to eliminate remaining worms.

A small number of dogs with caval syndrome have experienced spontaneous HW migration back into the pulmonary arteries following treatment with sildenafil, IV fluid, and O_2, with or without pimobendan, which had been administered prior to planned HW extraction procedure (Pariaut, 2020). This occurred within 2 hours to several days after the treatment was begun, and was not anticipated. A small number of dogs without caval syndrome but with intracardiac HWs also showed a similar worm migration pattern over 2(–14) days, after sildenafil and pimobendan treatment (p. 861). Nevertheless, at this time medical therapy is not recommended as a substitute for HW extraction in animals with caval syndrome.

The use of flexible alligator forceps with fluoroscopic or transesophageal echo guidance also has been employed in heavily infected dogs without caval syndrome to reduce the number of worms within the pulmonary arteries prior to adulticide therapy. Echo verification that worms are in accessible locations and appropriate technical facilities are needed for this procedure. Overall survival and recovery rate for dogs at high risk for postadulticide PTE reportedly are improved by prior physical worm removal.

Management of Heartworm Disease in Cats

Cats thought to have HWD based on radiographic or other test results are managed conservatively whenever possible (www.heartwormsociety.org). Monthly HW preventive therapy should be instituted and continued. Ivermectin (24 mcg/kg) administered monthly for 2 years reportedly reduces worm burden by 65% in cats (Guerrero, 2002). Adulticide therapy with melarsomine is *not* recommended for cats. Early clinical experience indicated frequent and severe complications in this species. Although some cats might tolerate the drug, melarsomine appears to be toxic to cats at relatively low doses (perhaps about 3.5 mg/kg).

Cats without clinical signs should be observed over time. Cats with mild to moderate respiratory signs, or radiographic evidence of pulmonary interstitial disease, are treated with a tapering course of prednisone (for example, 1 mg/kg q12h for a few days, then tapering over the next 2 weeks down to 0.5 mg/kg q48h, which then is continued for another 2 weeks before discontinuing the drug). The clinical response should be assessed after the course of prednisone therapy. Radiographs repeated at this time are useful for evaluating pulmonary parenchymal changes. Prednisone treatment can be repeated, if respiratory signs recur. While waiting for eventual natural resolution of the infection, repeated radiographs and serologic tests (for HW Ag and Ab) are recommended every 6–12 months to monitor for progression (or regression) of disease. If radiographic abnormalities resolve and a previously positive Ag test seroconverts to negative, a spontaneous cure is likely and implies markedly reduced risk for serious complications. Ag-positive cats usually become negative within 4–5 months of worm death. It is unclear how long Ab tests remain positive.

Severe respiratory distress and death can occur at any time in a HW-infected cat, especially as worms die and degenerate. The death of even one worm could trigger an anaphylactic-type reaction, as well as cause significant PTE. Cats that develop acute clinical signs require urgent treatment. Acute PTE is more likely to be fatal in cats than in dogs. Clinical signs of PTE include fever, cough, dyspnea, hemoptysis, pallor, pulmonary crackles, tachycardia, and hypotension. Radiographic findings include poorly defined, rounded, or wedge-shaped areas of interstitial (with or without alveolar) opacities that obscure associated pulmonary vessels. Depending on the situation, supportive care for acutely ill cats can include supplemental O_2, an IV glucocorticoid (such as 100–250 mg prednisone sodium succinate; or 1 mg/kg dexamethasone IV or IM), a bronchodilator, and possibly fluid therapy. Diuretics are not indicated. Aspirin or other nonsteroidal antiinflammatory drugs also are not recommended in this situation; they are without known benefit and might exacerbate pulmonary disease. However, in asymptomatic cats not being treated with a glucocorticoid drug, some clinicians have used aspirin (40–80 mg/cat PO q72h) or clopidogrel (17.5 mg/cat PO q24h) in an effort to reduce thromboembolic risk.

The contributions of *Wolbachia* bacteria to *D. immitis* viability and host disease pathogenesis also are of concern in cats, as in dogs. *Wolbachia* endotoxins and host reaction to *Wolbachia* major surface protein likely contribute to pulmonary and renal inflammation in cats, too. The potential clinical usefulness of doxycycline treatment in cats with adult HWs has not been fully investigated. But its use is suggested, because cats generally tolerate this drug and some probably are coinfected with *Mycoplasma* spp.; typical precautions should be taken to prevent erosive esophagitis when prescribing doxycycline.

Right-sided CHF develops in a small percentage of cats with severe PA disease. In these cats, respiratory distress could result from pleural effusion, as well as from pulmonary parenchymal disease or PTE. Other clinical findings can include cough, jugular venous distension or pulsation, and occasionally, ascites. Radiographic and ECG findings might suggest RV enlargement. Therapy for CHF signs includes thoracocentesis as needed, cage confinement, and conservative furosemide therapy (for example, 1 mg/kg q12–24h). Pimobendan should be helpful via its positive inotropic effects, although studies in this clinical context are not available. Sildenafil and spironolactone should be considered in cats with right-sided CHF and echo findings consistent with PH. Of course, other causes of pleural effusion, including cardiomyopathy, should first be excluded. The value of other heart failure drugs, including ACE inhibitors, is unknown. Whether apixaban or other direct anticoagulant agent would be useful also is unknown. Other supportive care is guided by the cat's clinical progress and clinicopathologic abnormalities.

Surgical or transvenous removal of adult HWs is an alternative strategy to the "wait and watch" approach, as long as the worms are in an accessible location. This must be verified echocardiographically prior to the procedure. Although technically challenging, several means could be used to extract adult HWs from cats. Worms located in the RA and venae cavae can be reached via right jugular venotomy using a loop snare, endoscopic grasping or basket retrieval forceps, small alligator forceps, or possibly other devices. Worms in the pulmonary artery have been extracted using alligator forceps via left thoracotomy and RV purse-string incision or pulmonary arteriotomy. A right thoracotomy and atriotomy approach also has been successful. Care must be taken to extract the worms gently, because traumatic worm injury or breakage during surgical removal could precipitate a potentially fatal anaphylactic reaction, with circulatory collapse and death of the cat. For this reason, pretreatment with a glucocorticoid and antihistamine might be helpful. Nevertheless, surgical worm removal could be a good alternative to conservative therapy in cats with heavy infection or persistent clinical signs, even if all adult HWs cannot be retrieved. The caval syndrome occurs rarely in cats; successful adult HW removal through a jugular venotomy has been reported. Surgical removal of aberrant worm(s) from other locations also might be possible.

As described for cats managed conservatively, repeated serologic testing is useful for *monitoring the course of infection*. Cats with a positive HW Ag test should test negative within 4–5 months of adult (female) HW elimination. After a cat has become clinically normal, with no detectable HW Ag, testing for HW Ab can cease. It is unclear how long HW Ab persists after infection has been cleared. Furthermore, repeated exposure to HW infection can result in a positive HW Ab test even in cats on preventative therapy. Thoracic radiographs and echocardiography can be useful when monitoring infected cats that have had HW-induced radiographic abnormalities and visualized worms, respectively.

Heartworm Prevention in Dogs

Until such time that an effective HW vaccine becomes available, a HW preventative drug is indicated for all dogs in endemic areas (that is, just about everywhere). Puppies should be started on HW preventative therapy by 6–8 weeks of age. Year-round chemoprophylaxis is recommended by the AHS, even in temperate regions. Besides HW chemoprophylaxis, use of a mosquito repellent/ectoparaciticide and reduction of outdoor exposure time during periods of greatest mosquito activity are recommended. Environmental control of mosquito populations and breeding environments also helps reduce exposure to HWD.

Although the time of year when infection is possible is limited in many geographic areas, continuous HW prevention is likely to increase compliance and the overall level of protection for susceptible populations. Continuous HW chemoprophylaxis is particularly important in locations with sustained warm and moist conditions, where risk for HW transmission is high during more than half the year. Especially in highly-endemic areas, even one missed or delayed preventative dose could lead to HW infection. However, in addition to the use of the macrocyclic lactones, a multimodal HW prevention strategy is thought necessary to effectively combat this disease, especially in highly endemic areas (see the next paragraphs).

In cases where a HW preventative drug was not given consistently, or when a switch to another preventative product is made, it is recommended to determine the HW status of the dog. Both HW Ag and MF tests should be negative before restarting or changing the preventative agent. Repeating these tests 6 months later also is advised. If positive, the dog likely was infected before resuming or changing preventative therapy; although rarely, a false negative test because of immature HWs or a low worm burden could miss prior infection. Both the Ag and MF tests are recommended again one year after the initial testing, and then yearly after that.

Macrocyclic Lactones Several macrocyclic lactone drugs are approved for preventing HWD: the avermectins (ivermectin, selamectin) and the milbemycins (milbemycin oxime, moxidectin). These drugs prevent maturation of infective larvae within the host and probably work with the host's immune system to kill susceptible larvae. They are administered monthly (oral or topical agents) or by semiannual or annual injection (slow-release moxidectin formulations). Macrocyclic lactones affect MF, L3, L4, and sometimes, juvenile and adult HWs when used continuously. Drug efficacy diminishes at an unpredictable rate beyond 30 days following administration of the oral and topical agents, especially against L4 and older worms. Therefore, the recommendation is that oral and topical HW preventative drugs be administered every 30 days throughout the year.

The avermectins and milbemycins induce neuromuscular paralysis and death in nematode (and arthropod) parasites by interacting with membrane chloride channels. They are almost 100% effective and exceptionally safe when used as directed, even in sensitive Collies and other P-glycoprotein-deficient dogs. Toxicosis from overdose of a macrocyclic lactone usually has been related to dosage miscalculation when a concentrated livestock preparation was used, or when combined with other P-glycoprotein-inhibiting drugs. Use of a livestock preparation in small animals is not recommended.

The drugs used for monthly oral administration are ivermectin (6–12 mcg/kg) and milbemycin oxime (0.5–1.0 mg/kg); an oral moxidectin formulation (at 24 mcg/kg) also is available. Ivermectin combined with pyrantel is available for treating roundworms and hookworms, as well as preventing HWD; products that also include praziquantel control tapeworms, too. A combination of milbemycin oxime with praziquantel is available, for protection against HWs, roundworms, hookworms, whipworms, and tapeworms. Milbemycin oxime combined with lufenuron also is available for dogs, for protection against HWs, roundworms, hookworms, and whipworms, and assistance with flea control. Other combinations might be commercially available, too. As with other medications, the potency of compounded HW preventatives (for example, milbemycin oxime) might be less than that of the original product, especially after a period of storage; because this could impact clinical efficacy, their use is not recommended.

Drugs available for topical application are moxidectin (2.5 mg/kg) and selamectin (6–12 mg/kg). These generally are applied at the base of the neck between the shoulder blades. Efficacy reportedly is unaffected by bathing or swimming at 2 hours or longer after application. Moxidectin helps control hookworms, roundworms, and whipworms, as well. A combination of moxidectin with imidacloprid also kills adult fleas. Selamectin effectively prevents HWD, kills adult fleas and prevents flea eggs from hatching, and controls ear mites in both dogs and cats. This drug also controls American dog tick infestation, as well as feline hookworm and roundworm infections.

These drugs are packaged in monthly dose units according to body weight ranges. Packaged dose units appropriate for the dog's weight range should be used. Again, dosing continuously throughout the year is recommended. However, if this is not done, administration should begin at least 1 month before the start of the HW transmission season. Treatment should continue for at least 1 month, and usually longer, after the transmission season ends. Individual product labels should be reviewed for specific recommendations.

Preventive therapy with oral and topical agents typically can begin at 6–8 weeks of age. Before administration, however, the specific product label should be consulted to verify usage guidelines in young animals. Before chemoprophylaxis is started for the first time in dogs 7 months of age and older, tests for circulating HW Ag and MF should be done. Repeat HW testing 6 months after starting preventative therapy is advised for all dogs, but especially for dogs started on preventative when older than 8 weeks of age or that are housed outdoors in heavily endemic areas. Subsequently, annual HW testing is recommended.

Sustained-release moxidectin is available as a suspension of drug-impregnated organic polymer microspheres for subcutaneous injection. Formulations are available for administration either every 6-months (0.17 mg moxidectin/kg; for dogs 6 months of age and older) or every 12-months (0.5 mg moxidectin/kg; for dogs 12 months of age and older). These sustained-release products should be administered only by personnel who have completed the manufacturer's on-line training and certification. Anaphylactic-like reactions and other adverse events have occurred in some dogs following injection (either alone or with vaccines), especially with the 12-month formulation. Some of these cases have resulted in death.

Lack of Efficacy Concerns Lack of efficacy for a HW prophylaxis product is evidenced by a dog that tests positive for HW despite consistent administration at appropriate dosage. The great majority of suspected lack of efficacy cases, however, have a root cause of inadequate medication compliance, as opposed to product failure. Besides situations where the preventative drug simply was not purchased or administered, apparent lack of efficacy can occur when too low a preventative dosage was used, the dosing interval was too long, the dog did not actually swallow the (oral) drug, or a topical agent was improperly applied or immediately washed off. These factors are of particularly urgent concern in highly endemic locations, where warm and moist conditions as well as a large population of infected animals often are present. Compliance failure can originate at any level from veterinary clinic to client to pet. Especially in highly-endemic areas, infection is possible after delay or omission of just one preventative dose.

Nevertheless, there are situations where biological variation in drug metabolism or host immune responses, or in parasite susceptibility, could impair efficacy. Some genetic polymorphism exists in populations of HWs; one or more alleles that confer decreased susceptibility or resistance to macrocyclic lactones is likely, although not yet well-defined. More than one gene might be involved. Other factors that could contribute to possible parasite resistance include genetic variations in *Wolbachia* endosymbionts, biological characteristics of the parasite itself, relative fitness of resistant and drug-susceptible genotypes, chemoprophylactic dosage used, number of dogs treated, and the size of nearby untreated HW-infected reservoir populations. HW preventatives used under certain off-label conditions could select for worms with relative resistance. This eventually could lead to the evolution of resistant HW subpopulations.

Studies to assess the efficacy of commercially available oral and topical HW preventatives against various L3 isolates suspected to be resistant have shown less than complete efficacy in preventing infection after single drug doses. While some isolates are killed by a single dose of topical (or oral) moxidectin, efficacy is incomplete for other isolates. However, three monthly doses of oral moxidectin (at least 24 mcg/kg) was highly effective against the three resistant isolates tested (McTier, 2019b). Other macrocyclic lactone strategies might also improve efficacy against resistant HW strains over time.

It is possible that a higher burden of exposure to infective L3 might magnify the effect of parasite drug resistance and contribute to possible lack of efficacy in highly endemic areas, such as the lower Mississippi River valley. The presence of other resistant HW subpopulations, and transmission of that resistance, also was found in studies using MF obtained from dogs with HWD that had been treated with microfilaricidal doses of macrocyclic lactones. Infective L3 that developed from those MF were injected into dogs, which subsequently were treated with different preventative medications. In at least one experimental trial, all of the preventative drugs (oral, topical, and parenteral formulations) failed to provide complete protection, although product differences could influence failure rate.

Additionally, interaction of macrocyclic lactones with the host's immune response to the parasite also might influence drug efficacy, or lack thereof. As an example, ivermectin interferes with the ability of *D. immitis* MF and larvae to evade recognition and destruction by the host's immune system. However, much remains to be learned about the issues involved with lack of efficacy. At this time, the macrocyclic lactones remain the best drugs available for HWD prevention. It is important that they be used as effectively and widely as possible.

No definitive test for resistance is available yet, although the predictive ability of certain single nucleotide polymorphisms to detect resistance is being studied. For now, the *microfilarial suppression test* can help in evaluating a dog with suspected resistance. This involves first performing a Knott test (**Table 40.1**) on a sample of the dog's blood and counting the number of MF present. Then administer a microfilaricidal dose of ivermectin or milbemycin oxime to the dog. After one week, repeat the Knott test and MF count. If there is less than a 75% decrease in the number of MF, resistance is highly possible. In such cases, treatment with doxycycline (along with completion of the 3-dose adulticide protocol; **Table 40.3**) is advised. Mosquito avoidance and repellent strategies also should be considered to reduce possible transmission of these MF.

Vector Control This can include efforts to reduce mosquito populations (such as eliminating standing water, treating potential mosquito breeding habitats, and other mosquito control methods), avoiding known mosquito habitats, confining pets inside (as possible) when local mosquito populations are most likely to be active (dusk and dawn), and using a mosquito repellent/insecticide (for example, containing dinotefuran-permethrin-pyriproxyfen or afoxolaner or similar agents). The latter strategy could prevent ingestion of MF by mosquitoes, as well as their maturation to infective larvae in the few mosquitoes that do feed on dogs treated with such repellent.

Minimizing Heartworm Transmission Associated with Relocated Dogs Guidelines for reducing HW transmission related to the relocation of infected dogs are summarized in **Figure 40.26**. Additional information is available from the AHS (www.heartwormsociety.org).

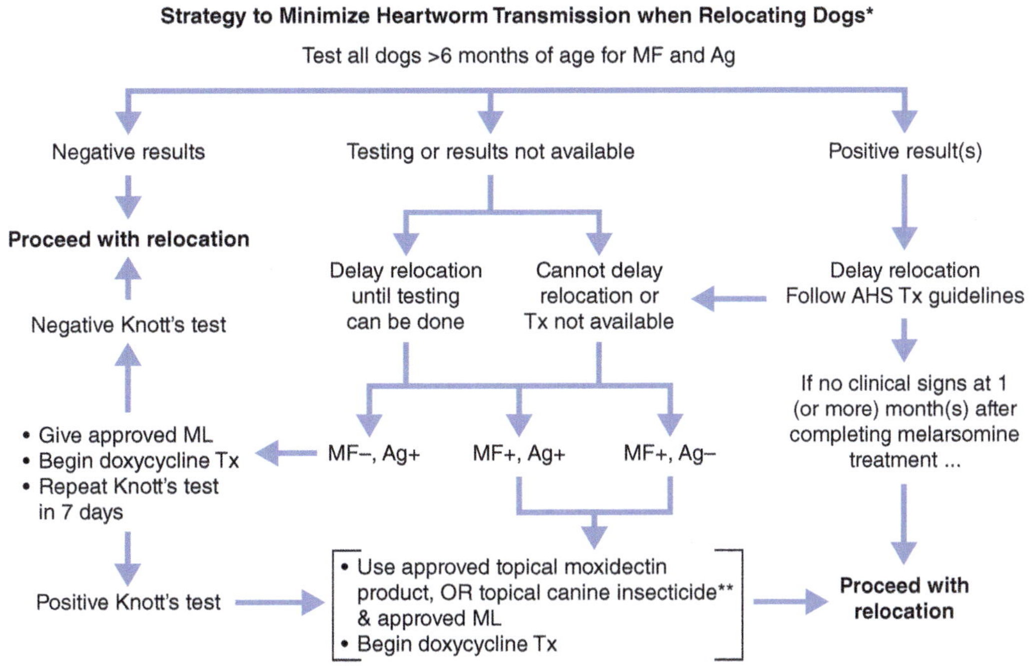

Figure 40.26 Strategy to minimize heartworm transmission during dog relocation. *Based on 2020 American Heartworm Society (AHS) Transport Guidelines. **Containing permethrin & dinotefuran & pyriproxyfen. Ag, (heartworm) antigen; MF, microfilaria; ML, macrocyclic lactone; Tx, treatment.

Heartworm Prevention in Cats

Monthly HW preventive therapy is recommended for cats in endemic areas. This includes "indoor-only" cats, because they also could be exposed to infective mosquitoes. About 25% of cats with adult HWs reportedly lived indoors, in a retrospective survey (Atkins, 2000). When preventative therapy is used, at minimum its administration should begin within 1 month of the onset of the estimated HW transmission season and continue until 30 days following this. Year-round monthly HW preventive therapy can be helpful as a means to increase compliance, as well as for the protection provided by some products against other parasites. As for dogs, it is important to consult the specific product label.

Drugs marketed for HW prevention in cats include oral ivermectin and milbemycin oxime, as well as topical selamectin, moxidectin, and eprinomectin. Some agents are combined with another drug having ecto- or endoparasiticide activity. Ivermectin is given PO at 24 mcg/kg monthly, which is four times the dose used in dogs. Milbemycin oxime's minimum recommended dose is 2 mg/kg, also higher than the dose for dogs. Selamectin is used at the same dose as for dogs (6 mg/kg, topically); the moxidectin dose is 1 mg/kg, and eprinomectin's minimum dose is approximately 0.5 mg/kg. All are safe in kittens (6–)8 weeks and older. These drugs can be administered regardless of HW Ag and Ab test results. HW Ag testing prior to starting chemoprophylaxis could be helpful in cats exposed to infection at least 8 months earlier. HW Ab testing provides a means of documenting exposure. A positive Ab test prior to HW preventative therapy suggests the cat is at increased risk for developing HARD and further justifies use of chemoprophylaxis. However, when a macrocyclic lactone is being administered, HW Ab testing does not reflect drug efficacy because an antibody response can occur from precardiac HW larval death caused by the preventative drug. MF testing is not necessary before beginning preventative therapy in cats.

Angiostrongylus Vasorum

Angiostrongylus vasorum is a metastrongyloid nematode that infects dogs and a variety of wild carnivores. Rarely, it can infect cats. This parasite, sometimes referred to as the French HW, is endemic in parts of Europe, the United Kingdom, and Africa. It occurs sporadically in other parts of the world, including the maritime provinces of Canada, and its prevalence appears to be spreading. Foxes are highly susceptible and can be a persistent source of larval shedding into the environment. Sometimes, infection by *A. vasorum* is mistaken for that of *D. immitis*. In regions where *Crenosoma vulpis* or *Eucoleus aerophilus* infection occurs (in Europe, for example), these other causes of chronic respiratory signs can be mistaken for or coexist with *A. vasorum* infection.

Similar to *D. immitis*, the adult *A. vasorum* worms live in the pulmonary arteries, and sometimes the right heart, of infected dogs and wild canids. Clinical signs can be nonspecific and the disease course, prolonged. Adult worms are about 13–21 mm in length. *A. vasorum* eggs are ovoid, thin-walled, and about 50–60 microns in diameter. Eggs are carried into the pulmonary capillaries, where they hatch. Larvae are about 320–380 microns × 18 microns in size, with a wavy or kinked tail and a cephalic button. A dorsal spine also has been noted on the tail. The L1 migrate through the alveolar epithelium into the airways. Then they are coughed up, swallowed, and passed in the feces. Maturation of L1 into the infective L3 occurs within a molluscan (slug or snail) intermediate host. Frogs and other amphibians act as paratenic hosts, as can chickens that ingest an infected snail or slug. When a dog or other host eats the intermediate (or paratenic) host, the L3 migrate from the small intestine through abdominal lymph nodes and liver to the heart and pulmonary arteries, where they mature. Larvae can be detected in the definitive host's feces after a prepatent period of about 6 weeks. Respiratory signs begin about 6–7 weeks postinfection, at the time of patency. These worsen over several weeks. Signs tend to improve by approximately 3–4 months after infection, unless there is recurrent infection. Clinical signs can relate to (verminous) pneumonia, coagulopathy and bleeding, neurologic abnormalities, or sometimes, PH. Ectopic worm migration also has been reported, including sporadic cases of ocular, hepatic and dermatologic angiostrongylosis.

The prevalence of *A. vasorum* varies across geographic regions. Seasonal variation in *A. vasorum* prevalence, as well as that of other lungworms, also has been shown in slug intermediate host populations in northern Europe. Although the risk for infection in definitive hosts is highest in summer, infection could occur throughout the year. There appears to be a fair amount of genetic diversity in *A. vasorum* populations within fox reservoir species. Other species of *Angiostrongylus* nematodes also are known to cause disease in people and other animals in different parts of the world.

Pathophysiology

The host's immune response to egg and larval antigens of *A. vasorum* provokes the development of pulmonary lesions when the infection becomes patent. Lung injury occurring during L1 migration is likely to induce clinical respiratory signs. Pathologic features in *A. vasorum*-infected dogs include pleural thickening and fibrosis, pulmonary lymphadenopathy, and multifocal pulmonary hemorrhagic and granulomatous lesions, especially in peripheral lung areas. The nematode's eggs and larvae can be found within these lesions. Pulmonary interstitial inflammation with infiltrates of lymphocytes, some eosinophils and plasma cells also occurs. Larvae (L1) might be present within dilated alveoli, as well as in tracheobronchial lymph nodes. Diffuse alveolar edema can occur. Adult worms cause PA intimal proliferation and thrombosis. Pulmonary interstitial fibrosis of varying severity can develop over time in response to the inflammatory reactions. However, most histopathologic changes appear to be largely reversible following appropriate anthelmintic therapy.

Clinically relevant PH appears to be relatively uncommon despite the sometimes severe pulmonary pathology. One retrospective survey found evidence for moderate to severe PH in only ~15% of cases (Borgeat, 2015). Infected dogs with PH had significantly greater risk of dying within 6 months compared to those without PH; although for dogs alive after this period, survival times appeared similar. This might relate to resolution of PH after anthelmintic and supportive therapy, or greater individual tolerance to PH. The prevalence of mild PH in infected dogs is unknown. Signs of acute right-sided CHF, presumably secondary to PH, occur sporadically.

A. vasorum is associated with a bleeding diathesis in some dogs. Hyperfibrinolysis and hypofibrinogenemia are common in these dogs and could contribute to hypocoagulability. Hyperfibrinolysis is present in about 2/3 of cases with clinical evidence for bleeding; this is suspected to be an important underlying mechanism in the bleeding diathesis associated with *A. vasorum* infection. The rapid degradation of cross-linked fibrin associated with hyperfibrinolysis can lead to overt bleeding. Fibrin degradation increases the circulating concentrations of fibrin degradation products (FDPs) and D-dimers, and depletes fibrinogen levels. Hyperfibrinolysis does not necessarily require prior coagulation cascade activation; it could occur when plasmin formation exceeds that of antiplasmins. The cause of hyperfibrinolysis is unclear; however, endothelial injury induced by the parasite could play a role. The coagulopathy might involve mostly pulmonary vessels, rather than systemic coagulation cascade activation. The antifibrinolytic drug, tranexamic acid, has improved hyperfibrinolysis in some cases. Plasma transfusion can mitigate hypofibrinogenemia. Although DIC might occur in some dogs, this appears to be an unlikely cause in cases with a normal platelet count and coagulation profile. Rarely, multiple hemorrhagic cerebral lesions can occur in patients with *A. vasorum* infection, with associated eosinophilic pleocytosis in cerebrospinal fluid samples. In contrast, hypercoagulability is evident in some dogs infected with *A. vasorum*.

Clinical Features

There appears to be no sex predilection for *A. vasorum* infection. It is unclear whether German Shepherd or possibly other purebred dogs might be at greater risk. Cavalier King Charles Spaniels might be more susceptible to severe clinical manifestations from *A. vasorum* infection. The clinical manifestations of infection are variable. Some infected dogs show minimal or no evidence of the disease. However, respiratory signs, such as recent-onset of a hacking cough and increased respiratory rate and effort are common; these typically are related to inflammation triggered by parasite eggs or migrating larvae. In some cases, severe and potentially fatal clinical signs develop rapidly. Lethargy, exercise intolerance, syncope, vomiting, and diarrhea can occur. Hemorrhagic diathesis also is frequently described (see above). Neurologic signs can be associated with intracranial hemorrhage. Ocular pathology caused by *A. vasorum* occurs in rare cases, also.

Physical Findings Physical exam findings could be nonspecific, although increased pulmonary sounds and tachypnea are common. About half of cases are estimated to have coughing and respiratory difficulty or tachypnea. Low-grade fever, pulmonary crackles, and a cardiac murmur have been observed in some cases. Evidence of bleeding probably occurs in about a third to half of infected dogs. PH associated with *A. vasorum* is likely to cause dyspnea and exercise intolerance, although overt signs of right-sided CHF appear uncommonly. Hypoxemia can be profound. Hemoptysis occurs in approximately 2/3 of dogs with PH; in other cases, hemoptysis occurs more sporadically. About a quarter of infected dogs show neurologic signs. Depending on the clinical presentation, *A. vasorum* infection might be mistaken for pulmonary neoplasia or other pulmonary disease, HWD, a coagulopathy, or various neurological diseases. Simultaneous infection with *D. immitis* and *A. vasorum* has occurred in endemic areas.

Diagnostic Tests

Laboratory Tests Laboratory tests might show mild eosinophilia, neutrophilia or other white blood cell abnormality, mild to moderate regenerative anemia, and/or mild to moderate hyperglobulinemia. Hypercalcemia occurs in some cases. Thrombocytopenia is common in dogs with, as well as without, signs of bleeding. Severe thrombocytopenia as the sole cause of spontaneous bleeding is uncommon, however. Coagulation times might be prolonged or can be normal. Abnormal activities of several coagulation factors have been observed. Most dogs with bleeding have evidence for hypocoagulability. Hypofibrinogenemia is present in about half of cases. Hyperfibrinolysis was reported in about 2/3 of dogs with bleeding and was associated with hypofibrinogenemia (Sigrist, 2017).

Fecal examination using the Baermann technique is diagnostic when larvae are being shed. However, larval shedding can occur irregularly. Performing a Baermann test on three consecutive fecal samples could increase the chances of finding larvae. Although examination of direct fecal smears might reveal larvae, this typically is too insensitive a test to be useful.

ELISA tests for circulating *A. vasorum* Ag and Ab have been developed. In addition, a point-of-care (POC) "SNAP" test (IDEXX AngioDetect Test, Idexx), which uses either serum or plasma, can detect *A. vasorum* Ag with fairly good sensitivity and excellent specificity. Positive results can occur as early as 9 weeks after infection. After treatment, Ag can persist for at least 3–9 weeks. The ELISA Ab test reportedly has greater sensitivity for detecting infection compared to either Ag test. *A vasorum* antigens also might cross-react with some HW Ag test kits.

Imaging Bronchoscopy can demonstrate mucosal edema and congestion in patients with *A. vasorum* infection. There also might be hemorrhagic secretions in the main bronchi. Airway washings could reveal neutrophilic or mixed neutrophilic/eosinophilic inflammation. Larvae are more likely to be found when inflammation is present, especially early in the infection (**Figure 40.27**). Quantitative polymerase chain reaction (PCR) testing of bronchoalveolar lavage (BAL) fluid also can yield the diagnosis. In a small study, quantitative PCR on BAL samples had excellent sensitivity for detecting *A. vasorum* infection, as did the ELISA Ab blood test (Canonne, 2018). In contrast, the POC Ag test, Baermann fecal analysis, and ELISA Ag test had relative sensitivities under 50% in these dogs.

Thoracic radiographs typically show signs of disease by about 2 months after infection. Bronchial thickening and patchy alveolar and interstitial infiltrates with a peripheral or multifocal (including caudodorsal) distribution commonly are seen (**Figure 40.28**). Pulmonary alveolar infiltrates become most severe at about 7–9 weeks, associated with infection patency. Later, the interstitial pattern becomes predominant, as alveolar infiltrates regress. Mild to moderate pleural effusion also is common during the time of initial patency. Hilar lymphadenopathy might be evident. The radiographic changes are likely to develop sooner and be more severe in

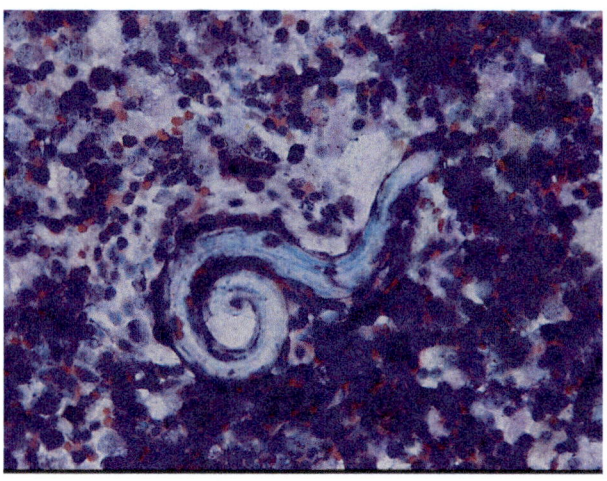

Figure 40.27 *Angiostrongylus vasorum* larva found on cytologic examination of bronchoalveolar lavage fluid, from a Labrador Retriever with progressive respiratory signs. The sample also contained multiple hemosiderin-containing macrophages, as well as neutrophils, small numbers of eosinophils, and several other larvae. Courtesy of Drs L Ferasin and O Garrdod.

dogs with greater worm burden. Although some degree of PA enlargement might be seen, cardiac changes and documented PH are uncommon. Nevertheless, right heart enlargement has been observed in occasional cases.

Thoracic CT imaging can show increased lung attenuation from ill-defined ground-glass opacity or consolidation (**Figure 40.29**). Regional mosaic attenuation, associated with peripheral bronchiectasis, and variably sized nodules with poorly

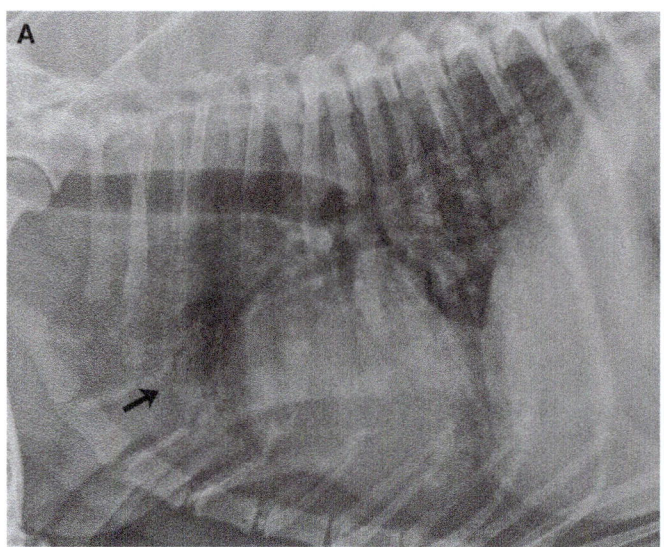
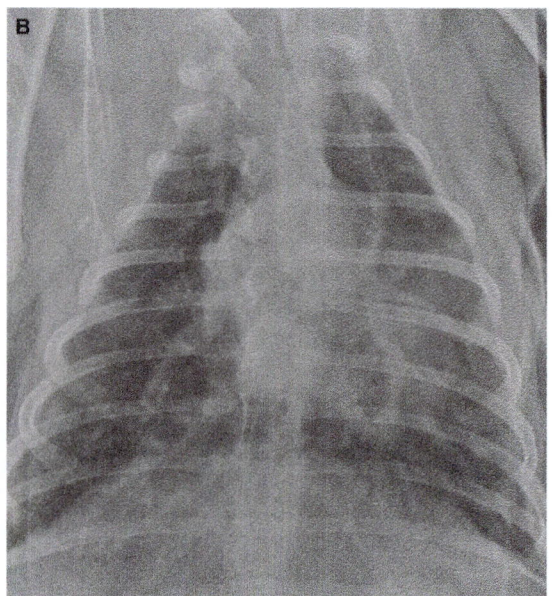

Figure 40.28 Lateral (A) and DV (B) radiographs from a 6-year-old Labrador Retriever with *Angiostrongylus vasorum* infection. Pulmonary interstitial and alveolar (A, arrow) infiltrates are most prominent in the peripheral cranioventral regions, but also are evident caudodorsally. The dog had a 3-week history of cough with progressive exercise intolerance. Pulmonary crackles were audible bilaterally. Courtesy of Drs L Ferasin and O Garrdod.

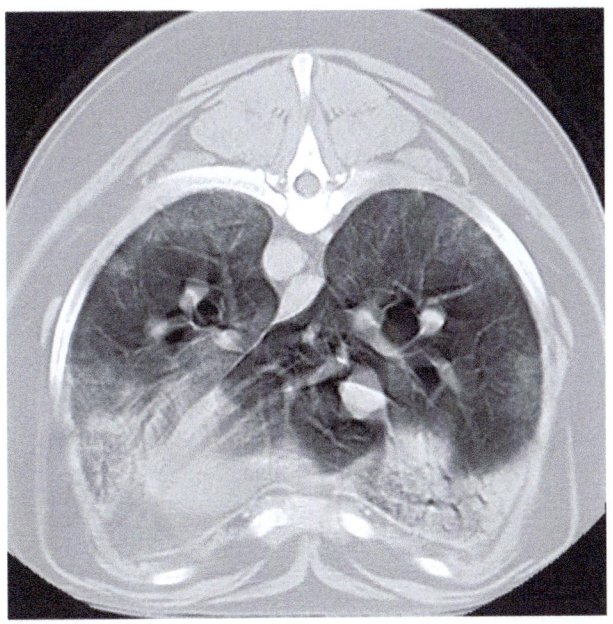

Figure 40.29 Transverse computed tomography image from the dog in Figure 40.28. Pulmonary infiltrates are most intense in the ventral lung regions, but also are evident in other peripheral locations. Courtesy of Drs L Ferasin and O Garrdod.

defined margins also are reported. Peripheral (pleural and subpleural) lung regions are affected most prominently, as opposed to peribronchial or perivascular areas. Tracheobronchial lymphadenopathy can be evident, as well.

Echo changes consistent with PH occur only in a minority of cases. Cardiac findings are unremarkable in most affected dogs.

Management

Treatment with topical moxidectin (2.5%) has been effective. One dose appears sufficient in most cases; however, if *A.vasorum* test results are still positive a month later, a second treatment can be administered. Oral moxidectin, at a minimum dose of 24 mcg/kg provided in the combination product with sarolaner and pyrantel, also is effective against immature adult *A. vasorum*; monthly use can prevent angiostrongylosis, as well as flea and tick infestation. Other parasiticide treatments that have been used include milbemycin oxime (0.5 mg/kg/week PO for 4 weeks) or fenbendazole (50 mg/kg/day PO for 10–14 days, or longer). Supportive therapy might be needed, including supplemental O_2 and antiinflammatory doses of a glucocorticoid (such as prednisolone, 0.5 mg/kg q24h for a few days, then tapered). Fresh frozen plasma can be helpful in dogs with active bleeding. For dogs with marked PH, sildenafil or other phosphodiesterase-5 inhibitor could be used (p. 834). It is unclear if this provides a survival benefit, though. Anthelmintic therapy usually leads to rapid clinical and echo improvement in a majority of dogs with PH.

Prognosis Most cases respond well to parasiticide treatment. Nevertheless, the infection can be fatal for dogs with severe respiratory signs. In one study, only about 2/3 of cases survived (Sigrist, 2017). Survival was similar between dogs with bleeding and those without. The presence of PH conveys a worse prognosis during the initial 6 months of disease; after this time, the survival rate appears similar in dogs with or without PH. Progressive neurologic signs appear to be a common cause of death.

Prevention

Monthly treatment with either moxidectin or milbemycin oxime is highly effective in preventing *A. vasorum* infection.

Suggested Additional Reading and References

Also See Online Comprehensive Bibliography at: https://www.routledge.com/9781482246223.

Dirofilaria immitis

American Heartworm Society. Current feline guidelines for the prevention, diagnosis, and management of heartworm (*Dirofilaria immitis*) infection in cats. www.heartwormsociety.org, accessed March, 2020.

American Heartworm Society. Current canine guidelines for the prevention, diagnosis, and management of heartworm (*Dirofilaria immitis*) infection in dogs. www.heartwormsociety.org, accessed March, 2020.

Ames MK, Atkins CE. Treatment of dogs with severe heartworm disease. Vet Parasit 2020a; 283:109131.

Ames MK, VanVranken P, Evans C, et al. Non-arsenical heartworm adulticidal therapy using topical moxidectin-imidacloprid and doxycycline: a prospective case series. Vet Parasitol 2020b;282:109099.

Atkins CE, DeFrancesco TC, Coats JR, et al. Heartworm infection in cats: 50 cases (1985–1997). J Am Vet Med Assoc 2000;217:355–358.

Ballesteros C, Pulaski CN, Bourguinat C, et al. Clinical validation of molecular markers of macrocyclic lactone resistance in Dirofilaria immitis. Int J Parasitol Drugs Drug Resist 2018; 8:596–606.

Bowman DD, Drake J. Examination of the "susceptibility gap" in the treatment of canine heartworm infection. Parasit Vectors 2017;10:513.

Carmichael J, McCall S, DiCosty U, et al. Evaluation of Dirofilaria immitis antigen detection comparing heated and unheated serum in dogs with experimental heartworm infections. Parasit Vectors 2017;10:486.

Carreton E, Falcon-Cordon Y, Falcon-Cordon S, et al. Variation of the adulticide protocol for the treatment of Canine heartworm infection: can it be shorter? Vet Parasitol 2019;271:54–56.

Carreton E, Morchon R, Falcon-Cordon Y, et al. Evaluation of different dosages of doxycycline during the adulticide treatment of heartworm (Dirofilaria immitis) in dogs. Vet Parasitol 2020;283:109141.

Carreton E, Morchon R, Montoya-Alonso JA. Cardiopulmonary and inflammatory biomarkers in heartworm disease. Parasit Vectors 2017;10:534.

Cochrane ZN, Berger DJ, Viall AK, et al. Evaluation of compounded aqueous milbemycin oxime: issues with formulation potency and reproducibility. J Small Anim Pract 2019;60:27–31.

DiGangi BA, Dworkin C, Stull JW, et al. Impact of heat treatment on dirofilaria immitis antigen detection in shelter dogs. Parasit Vectors 2017;10:483.

Dillon AR, Blagburn BL, Tillson M, et al. Heartworm-associated respiratory disease (HARD) induced by immature adult Dirofilaria immitis in cats. Parasit Vectors 2017;10:514.

Dillon AR, Blagburn BL, Tillson M, et al. The progression of heartworm associated respiratory disease (HARD) in SPF cats 18 months after Dirofilaria immitis infection. Parasit Vectors 2017;10:533.

Drake J, Gruntmeir J, Merritt H, et al. False negative antigen tests in dogs infected with heartworm and placed on macrocyclic lactone preventives. Parasit Vectors 2015;8:68.

Drake J, Wiseman S. Increasing incidence of Dirofilaria immitis in dogs in USA with focus on the southeast region 2013–2016. Parasit Vectors 2018;11:39.

Evans CC, Bradner JL, Savadelis MD, et al. Acetic acid as an alternative reagent in the modified Knott test. Vet Parasitol 2019;276:108975.

Falcon-Cordon Y, Montoya-Alonso JA, Caro-Vadillo A, et al. Persistence of pulmonary endarteritis in canine heartworm infection 10 months after the eradication of adult parasites of Dirofilaria immitis. Vet Parasitol 2019;273:1–4.

Genchi M, Vismarra A, Lucchetti C, et al. Efficacy of imidacloprid 10%/moxidectin 2.5% spot on (advocate(R), advantage multi(R)) and doxycycline for the treatment of natural Dirofilaria immitis infections in dogs. Vet Parasitol 2019;273:11–16.

Gonzalez-Miguel J, Morchon R, Carreton E, et al. Can the activation of plasminogen/plasmin system of the host by metabolic products of Dirofilaria immitis participate in heartworm disease endarteritis? Parasit Vectors 2015;8:194.

Grant T, Wiseman S, Snyder DE. Effects of milbemycin oxime, combined with spinosad, when administered orally to microfilaremic dogs infected with adult heartworms (Dirofilaria immitis). J Am Vet Med Assoc 2018;252:1084–1089.

Gruntmeir JM, Adolph CB, Thomas JE, et al. Increased detection of Dirofilaria immitis antigen in cats after heat pretreatment of samples. J Feline Med Surg 2017;19:1013–1016.

Gruntmeir JM, Long MT, Blagburn BL, et al. Canine heartworm and heat treatment: An evaluation using a well based enzyme-linked immunosorbent assay (ELISA) and canine sera with confirmed heartworm infection status. Vet Parasitol 2020;283:109169.

Guerrero J, McCall JW, Genchi C. The use of macrocyclic lactones in the control and prevention of heartworm and other parasites in dogs and cats. In, Vercruysse J, Rew RS (editors). Macrocyclic Lactones in Antiparasitic Therapy. CABI Publishing, Wallingford, UK. 2002. pp. 353–369.

Henry LG, Brunson KJ, Walden HS, et al. Comparison of six commercial antigen kits for detection of Dirofilaria immitis infections in canines with necropsy-confirmed heartworm status. Vet Parasitol 2018;254:178–182.

Kramer L, Crosara S, Gnudi G, et al. Wolbachia, doxycycline and macrocyclic lactones: New prospects in the treatment of canine heartworm disease. Vet Parasitol 2018;254:95–97.

Krautmann MJ, Mahabir S, Fielder A, et al. Safety of an extended-release injectable moxidectin suspension formulation (ProHeart((R)) 12) in dogs. Parasit Vectors 2019;12:433.

Levy JK, Burling AN, Crandall MM, et al. Seroprevalence of heartworm infection, risk factors for seropositivity, and frequency of prescribing heartworm preventives for cats in the United States and Canada. J Am Vet Med Assoc 2017;250:873–880.

Liebenberg J, Fourie J, Lebon W, et al. Assessment of the insecticidal activity of afoxolaner against Aedes aegypti in dogs treated with NexGard((R)). Parasite 2017;24:39.

Litster A, Atkins C, Atwell R, et al. Radiographic cardiac size in cats and dogs with heartworm disease compared with reference values using the vertebral heart scale method: 53 cases. J Vet Cardiol 2005;7:33–40.

Little S, Saleh M, Wohltjen M, et al. Prime detection of Dirofilaria immitis: understanding the influence of blocked antigen on heartworm test performance. Parasit Vectors 2018;11:186.

McCall JW, Hodgkins E, Varloud M, et al. Blocking the transmission of heartworm (Dirofilaria immitis) to mosquitoes (Aedes aegypti) by weekly exposure for one month to microfilaremic dogs treated once topically with dinotefuran-permethrin-pyriproxyfen. Parasit Vectors 2017;10:511.

McCall JW, Varloud M, Hodgkins E, et al. Shifting the paradigm in Dirofilaria immitis prevention: blocking transmission from mosquitoes to dogs using repellents/insecticides and macrocyclic lactone prevention as part of a multimodal approach. Parasit Vectors 2017;10:525.

McGill E, Berke O, Weese JS, et al. Heartworm infection in domestic dogs in Canada, 1977-2016: prevalence, time trend, and efficacy of prophylaxis. Can Vet J 2019;60:605–612.

McTier TL, Pullins A, Chapin S, et al. The efficacy of a novel topical formulation of selamectin plus sarolaner (revolution((R)) plus/Stronghold((R)) plus) in preventing the development of Dirofilaria immitis in cats. Vet Parasitol 2019a;270:56–62.

McTier TL, Six RH, Pullins A, et al. Preventive efficacy of oral moxidectin at various doses and dosage regimens against macrocyclic lactone-resistant heartworm (Dirofilaria immitis) strains in dogs. Parasit Vectors 2019b;12:444.

Moorhead AR, Evans CC, Kaplan RM. A diagnostic algorithm for evaluating cases of potential macrocyclic lactone-resistant heartworm. Parasites & vectors 2017;10:479.

Morales A, Perlmann E, Abelha ANV, et al. Keratitis due to microfilariae in dogs: a newly recognized disease. Vet Ophthalmol 2018;21:305–311.

Nelson CT, Myrick ES, Nelson TA Clinical benefits of incorporating doxycycline into a canine heartworm treatment protocol. Parasit Vectors 2017;10:515.

Papich MG. Considerations for using minocycline vs doxycycline for treatment of canine heartworm disease. Parasit Vectors 2017;10:493.

Pariaut R, Jung SW, Vila J, et al. Resolution of caval syndrome during initial hemodynamic stabilization in dogs with heartworm disease. J Vet Emerg Crit Care 2020;30:295–301.

Paterson T, Fernandez C, Burnett PJ, et al. Heartworm control in Grenada, West Indies: Results of a field study using imidacloprid 10% + moxidectin 2.5% and doxycycline for naturally-acquired Dirofilaria immitis infections. Vet Parasitol 2020;284:109194.

Pullins A, McTier TL, Mahabir S, et al. The efficacy of a topical formulation of selamectin plus sarolaner in preventing the development of a macrocyclic lactone-resistant strain of Dirofilaria immitis in cats. Vet Parasitol 2020;282:109122.

Savadelis MD, Day KM, Bradner JL, et al. Efficacy and side effects of doxycycline versus minocycline in the three-dose melarsomine canine adulticidal heartworm treatment protocol. Parasit Vectors 2018a;11:671.

Savadelis MD, Roveto JL, Ohmes CM, et al. Evaluation of heat-treating heartworm-positive canine serum samples during treatment with advantage multi((R)) for dogs and doxycycline. Parasit Vectors 2018b;11:98.

Savadelis MD, Ohmes CM, Hostetler JA, et al. Assessment of parasitological findings in heartworm-infected beagles treated with Advantage Multi® for dogs (10% imidacloprid + 2.5% moxidectin) and doxycycline. Parasit Vectors 2017;10:245.

Self SW, Pulaski CN, McMahan CS, et al. Regional and local temporal trends in the prevalence of canine heartworm infection in the contiguous United States: 2012–2018. Parasit Vectors 2019;12:380.

Serrano-Parreno B, Carreton E, Caro-Vadillo A, et al. Pulmonary hypertension in dogs with Heartworm before and after the adulticide protocol recommended by the American Heartworm Society. Vet Parasitol 2017;236:34–37.

Serrano-Parreno B, Carreton E, Caro-Vadillo A, et al. Evaluation of pulmonary hypertension and clinical status in dogs with heartworm by Right Pulmonary Artery Distensibility Index and other echocardiographic parameters. Parasit Vectors 2017;10:106.

Shin PT, Baptista RP, O'Neill CM, et al. Comparative sequences of the Wolbachia genomes of drug-sensitive and resistant isolates of Dirofilaria immitis. Vet Parasitol 2020;286:109225.

Starkey LA, Bowles JV, Blagburn BL. Comparison of acid- versus heat-treatment for immune complex dissociation and detection of Dirofilaria immitis antigen in canine plasma. Vet Parasitol 2020;282:109134.

Tjostheim SS, Kellihan HB, Grint KA, et al. Effect of sildenafil and pimobendan on intracardiac heartworm infections in four dogs. J Vet Cardiol 2019;23:96–103.

Turner JD, Marriott AE, Hong D, et al. Novel anti-Wolbachia drugs, a new approach in the treatment and prevention of veterinary filariasis? Vet Parasitol 2020;279:109057.

Venco L, Mihaylova L, Boon JA. Right Pulmonary Artery Distensibility Index (RPAD Index). A field study of an echocardiographic method to detect early development of pulmonary hypertension and its severity even in the absence of regurgitant jets for Doppler evaluation in heartworm-infected dogs. Vet Parasitol 2014;206:60–66.

Winter RL, Ray Dillon A, Cattley RC, et al. Effect of heartworm disease and heartworm-associated respiratory disease (HARD) on the right ventricle of cats. Parasit Vectors 2017;10:492.

Angiostrongylus vasorum:

Becskei C, Thys M, Doherty P, et al. Efficacy of orally administered combination of moxidectin, sarolaner and pyrantel (Simparica Trio) for the prevention of experimental Angiostrongylus vasorum infection in dogs. Parasit Vectors 2020;13:64.

Bird LE, Bilbrough G, Fitzgerald R, et al. Determining resolution of Angiostrongylus vasorum in dogs following anthelmintic treatment with an imidacloprid 10 per cent/moxidectin 2.5 per cent spot-on. Vet Rec Open 2018;5:e000215.

Boag AK, Lamb CR, Chapman PS, et al. Radiographic findings in 16 dogs infected with Angiostrongylus vasorum. Vet Rec 2004;154:426–430.

Borgeat K, Sudunagunta S, Kaye B, et al. Retrospective evaluation of moderate-to-severe pulmonary hypertension in dogs naturally infected with Angiostrongylus vasorum. J Small Anim Pract 2015;56:196–202.

Canonne AM, Billen F, Losson B, et al. Angiostrongylosis in dogs with negative fecal and in-clinic rapid serological tests: 7 cases (2013–2017). J Vet Intern Med 2018;32:951–955.

Canonne AM, Roels E, Caron Y, et al. Detection of Angiostrongylus vasorum by quantitative PCR in bronchoalveolar lavage fluid in Belgian dogs. J Small Anim Pract 2016;57:130–134.

Chapman PS, Boag AK, Guitian J, et al. Angiostrongylus vasorum infection in 23 dogs (1999–2002). J Small Anim Pract 2004;45:435–440.

Coia ME, Hammond G, Chan D, et al. Retrospective evaluation of thoracic computed tomography findings in dogs naturally infected by Angiostrongylus vasorum. Vet Radiol Ultrasound 2017;58:524–534.

Conboy G. Natural infections of Crenosoma vulpis and Angiostrongylus vasorum in dogs in Atlantic Canada and their treatment with milbemycin oxime. Vet Rec 2004;155:16–18.

Corda A, Carta S, Varcasia A, et al. Pulmonary arterial response to Angiostrongylus vasorum in naturally infected dogs: echocardiographic findings in two cases. Parasit Vectors 2019;12:286.

Di Cesare A, Traversa D, Manzocchi S, et al. Elusive Angiostrongylus vasorum infections. Parasit Vectors 2015;8:438.

Gillis-Germitsch N, Schnyder M. Impact of heat treatment on antigen detection in sera of Angiostrongylus vasorum infected dogs. Parasit Vectors 2017;10:421.

Glaus T, Schnyder M, Dennler M, et al. Natural infection with Angiostrongylus vasorum: characterisation of 3 dogs with pulmonary hypertension. Schweiz Arch Tierheilkd 2010;152:331–338.

Koller B, Hegglin D, Schnyder M. A grid-cell based fecal sampling scheme reveals: land-use and altitude affect prevalence rates of Angiostrongylus vasorum and other parasites of red foxes (Vulpes Vulpes). Parasitol Res 2019.

Kranjc A, Schnyder M, Dennler M, et al. Pulmonary artery thrombosis in experimental Angiostrongylus vasorum infection does not result in pulmonary hypertension and echocardiographic right ventricular changes. J Vet Intern Med 2010;24:855–862.

Lebon W, Tielemans E, Rehbein S, et al. Monthly administrations of milbemycin oxime plus afoxolaner chewable tablets to prevent Angiostrongylus vasorum infection in dogs. Parasit Vectors 2016;9:485.

Olivieri E, Zanzani SA, Gazzonis AL, et al. Angiostrongylus vasorum infection in dogs from a cardiopulmonary dirofilariosis endemic area of Northwestern Italy: a case study and a retrospective data analysis. BMC Vet Res 2017;13:165.

Penagos-Tabares F, Lange MK, Chaparro-Gutierrez JJ, et al. Angiostrongylus vasorum and Aelurostrongylus abstrusus: neglected and underestimated parasites in South America. Parasit Vectors 2018;11:208.

Priest JM, Stewart DT, Boudreau M, et al. First report of Angiostrongylus vasorum in coyotes in mainland North America. Vet Rec 2018;183:747.

Schnyder M, Stebler K, Naucke TJ, et al. Evaluation of a rapid device for serological in-clinic diagnosis of canine angiostrongylosis. Parasit Vectors 2014;7:72.

Sigrist NE, Hofer-Inteeworn N, Jud Schefer R, et al. Hyperfibrinolysis and hypofibrinogenemia diagnosed with rotational thromboelastometry in dogs naturally infected with Angiostrongylus vasorum. J Vet Intern Med 2017;31:1091–1099.

SUMMARY DRUG TABLE FOR DOGS

Drug	Indications	Common Dosages	Formulations	Comments	See Chapter
Acepromazine (PromAce, other)	Sedation for echo exam or respiratory distress; Or occasionally for hypertensive crisis (alpha-blocking effect)	*Sedation for echo exam*: 0.025–0.03 mg/kg IM or IV. *Sedation for respiratory distress*: 0.025–0.05 mg/kg IV or IM. *For hypertensive crisis*: 0.05–0.1 mg/kg (up to 3 mg/kg total) IV; Or, 0.5–2 mg/kg PO q8h	5-, 10-, & 25-mg tablets; 10-mg/mL injection	*Sedation for echo exam*: mixed with buprenorphine or butorphanol. *Sedation for respiratory distress*: butorphanol preferred. *For hypertensive crisis*: monitor arterial BP; Table 38.5	4 10, 22 38
Amikacin (Amiglyde-V)	Antimicrobial	For *Bartonella*: 15–30 mg/kg q24h IV, IM, or SC, for 7–10 days. ±For other endocarditis: 7–10 mg/kg IV q12h (or 20 mg/kg q24h]), for 5-10 days	50- & 250-mg/mL injection	Initial therapy, combined with doxycycline, for *Bartonella* endo/myocarditis (p. 603). Also see Table 31.3	31
Aminophylline (various generic)	Bronchodilator	10-11 mg/kg PO (or IM, IV) q8h	100-, & 200-mg tablets; 25 mg/mL injection	Table 9.3	9
Amiodarone (Cordarone, Pacerone; Nexterone injectable)	Class III antiarrhythmic	*PO Loading*: 8(–15) mg/kg PO q12h for 4(–7) days, then give same dose q24h for 7 days; then decrease to maintenance dose; *PO Maintenance*: 4–7.5(-10) mg/kg PO q24h. *IV (use Nexterone, 1.5 mg/mL)*: 2–5 mg/kg slowly IV over 15-60 min. *If effective*: 0.05 mg/kg/min CRI, if needed.	(100-), 200- & 400-mg tablets; Nexterone (amiodarone without preservative): 150 mg (1.5-mg/mL) & 360 mg (1.8 mg/mL) premixed bags for injection.	For IV injection - do not use standard older injectable formulation; and monitor BP. Alternatively, Nexterone CRI has been given at 0.8 mg/kg/hr for 6 hours, then decreased to 0.4 mg/kg/hr for 18 hours. Table 25.2	24, 25

Cardiovascular Disease in Companion Animals

Drug	Indications	Common Dosages	Formulations	Comments	See Chapter
Amlodipine (Norvasc)	Arteriolar dilator; afterload reducer & antihypertensive	*Initial*: 0.05–0.1 mg/kg PO q24h, *Up to*: 0.3(-0.5) mg/kg PO q24(–12)h *For hypertensive crisis*: 0.25 mg/kg PO initial dose; repeat as needed q1–3h until systolic BP is 140–160 mm Hg, up to total of 1 mg/kg/day (see p. 806). *Or*: 0.2–0.4 (up to 0.6) mg/kg PO q24h	2.5-, 5-, & 10-mg tablets	Monitor arterial BP. Can dissolve tablet(s) in water and administer rectally, if PO administration not possible. Tables 22.2, 22.3, 38.4 & 38.5	21, 22, 29, 38
Amoxicillin & clavulanate (Clavamox)	Antimicrobial	20–25 mg/kg PO q8h	62.5-, 125-, 250-, & 375-mg tablets; 62.5-mg/mL suspension	Table 31.3	31
Ampicillin (Omnipen, others)	Antimicrobial	22–40 mg/kg IV q6–8h	125-, 250-, & 500-mg vials (ampicillin sodium)	Table 31.3	31
Apixaban (Eliquis)	Anticoagulant	0.25 - 0.5 mg/kg PO q8 to q12h	2.5- & 5-mg tablets	Table 36.2	36
Arginine (see L-Arginine)	Amino acid				
Aspirin (various generic)	Antiplatelet	0.5–1 mg/kg PO q24h	81-, & 325-mg tablets	Table 36.2	36
Atenolol (Tenormin, others)	Beta-adrenergic blocker	0.2–1 mg/kg PO q12(–24)h	25-, 50-, & 100-mg tablets; 25-mg/mL oral suspension; 0.5-mg/mL injection (ampule)	Start with low dose. Tables 25.2 & 38.4	24, 25, 38
Atipamezole (Antisedan)	Alpha$_2$-agonist reversal	0.1 mg/kg IV or IO	5-mg/mL injection	For use during CPR Table 25.5	25
Atropine (various generic)	Anticholinergic	0.02–0.04 mg/kg IV, IM, SC; Or, 0.04 mg/kg PO q6–8h	0.05-, 0.1-, 0.4-, & 1-mg/mL injection, & others	See p. 387 for atropine response (challenge) test. Can give IT for CPR. Table 25.2	24, 25
Benazepril (Lotensin)	Angiotensin converting enzyme inhibitor	0.25–0.5 mg/kg PO q(12–)24h	5-, 10-, 20-, & 40-mg tablets	Tables 22.3 & 38.4	21, 22, 29, 32, 38
Buprenorphine (Temgesic, Vetergesic)	Sedation for echo exam; or as analgesic, opioid (mu) agonist-antagonist	*Sedation for echo exam*: 0.005–0.01 mg/kg IM or IV. *Analgesia*: 0.01–0.03 mg/kg IM, IV, SC q6–8h.	0.3 mg/mL injection	*Sedation for echo exam*: mixed with acepromazine. *As analgesic*: for follow-up analgesia in arterial thromboembolism; Table 36.4	4 36
Butorphanol (Torbutrol, Torbugesic)	Antitussive; or as sedative for echo exam or respiratory distress	*Antitussive*: 0.5–1 mg/kg PO q6–12h. *Sedation for echo exam*: 0.2–0.25 mg/kg IM or IV; (or 0.3 up to 0.5 mg/kg IM, if not using acepromazine). *Sedation for respiratory distress*: 0.1-0.3 mg/kg IM, IV	1-, 5-, & 10-mg tablets; 2- & 10-mg/mL injection	*Antitussive*: Table 9.3. *Sedation for echo exam*: mixed with acepromazine for echo sedation. *Sedation for respiratory distress*: can repeat in 30–60 min if needed.	9 4 10, 22

Drug	Indications	Common Dosages	Formulations	Comments	See Chapter
Capromorelin (Entyce)	Appetite stimulant for dogs	3 mg/kg PO q24h	30-mg/mL oral solution		22
Captopril (Capoten)	Angiotensin converting enzyme inhibitor	0.5–2.0 mg/kg PO q8–12h	25-mg tablet	Table 22.3	21, 22
Carnitine (see L-Carnitine)	Amino acid				
Carvedilol (Coreg)	Beta-adrenergic blocker	*Initial*: 0.05–0.1 mg/kg q24h. *Target*: 0.2–0.3 mg/kg q12h, if tolerated.	3.125-, 6.25-, 12.5-, & 25-mg tablets	Cardioprotection: gradually increase dosage over 1-2 months to target, as possible	21
Cefazolin sodium (Ancef, Kefzol, other)	Antimicrobial	22–33 mg/kg IV q8h	50- & 100-mg/50mL injection	Table 31.3	31
Ceftriaxone (Rocephin)	Antimicrobial	20 mg/kg IV q12h	250-, & 500-mg, & 1-, & 2-gm vials; reconstitute to 100-mg/mL for IV injection	Table 31.3	31
Chlorothiazide (Diuril)	Diuretic	10–40 mg/kg PO q12–48h (start qod with low dose)	250- & 500-mg tablets; 50-mg/mL oral suspension	Start with low dose every other (or 3rd) day Table 22.3	21, 22
Clopidogrel (Plavix)	Antiplatelet	1.1–3 (up to 4) mg/kg PO q24h. Can give 1 *initial loading dose*: 4–10 mg/kg PO	75-mg tablets	Table 36.2	36
Dalteparin (Fragmin)	Low molecular weight heparin anticoagulant	100–175 U/kg SC q8h	10,000 IU/mL (& other) for injection	Table 36.2	36
Dexamethasone (Azium, Dexaject SP, others)	Glucocorticosteroid	*Antiinflammatory*: 0.2 mg/kg IV *Shock dose*: 1 mg/kg IV	2-mg/mL injection; or Sodium phosphate form: 3.33-mg/mL injection	Anti-inflammatory; (with diphenhydramine) to prevent or treat acute hypersensitivity reaction to rapid HW microfilariae death. Shock dose for circulatory collapse	40
Dextromethorphan (Benylin, others)	Antitussive	1–2 mg/kg PO q6–8h	Multiple syrup, capsule & tablet forms	Table 9.3	9
Digoxin (Lanoxin, other)	Positive inotrope	*Maintenance*: 0.003–0.005 mg/kg PO q12h; (Or, for dogs <22 kg, 0.005–0.008 mg/kg PO q12h; for dogs >22 kg, 0.22 mg/m^2.) *Maximum*: 0.5 mg/day or 0.375 mg/day for Doberman Pinchers *Loading PO*: 1 or 2 doses at twice calculated maintenance; *Loading IV* (generally avoided): calculate 0.01–0.02 mg/kg – give 1/4 of total dose in slow boluses over 2–4 hours, to effect	0.125-, & 0.25-mg tablets; 0.05- & 0.15-mg/mL elixir; 0.1-, & 0.25-mg/1-mL injection	See text for indications. Decrease dose by 10% for elixir. Tables 22.3 & 25.2	21, 22, 24, 25, 29, 32,

Drug	Indications	Common Dosages	Formulations	Comments	See Chapter
Diltiazem (Cardizem, Dilacor)	Class IV antiarrhythmic	*Acute IV for rapid rate control of AF*: 0.05–0.15 mg/kg IV over 2–5 min, can repeat if needed. *Acute IV for SVT*: 0.1–0.2 mg/kg over 2–5 min IV, can repeat to cumulative IV dose of 0.3–0.4(–0.7?) mg/kg; monitor BP. *If effective*: 0.002–0.006 mg/kg/min CRI (or 0.12–0.36 mg/kg/h), as needed. *PO loading dose*: 0.5 mg/kg followed by 0.25 mg/kg PO q1h (or 0.5 mg/kg repeated q2h), up to total of 1.5(–2.0) mg/kg or conversion; or maximum 4-6 mg/kg over 1st 24h. *PO maintenance*: initial 0.5–1 mg/kg (up to 2–3 mg/kg) PO q8h. *Extended release* (diltiazem ER): 1–4 (up to 6) mg/kg PO q 12h.	30-, 60-, 90-, & 120-mg tablets; 5-mg/mL injection; Diltiazem ER: 60-, 120-, 180-, & 240-mg capsules (240-mg capsule contains four 60-mg tablets) Cardizem-CD: 120-, 180-, 240-mg capsules	Monitor BP, especially when using IV. Table 25.2	24, 25
Diphenhydramine (Benadryl)	Antihistamine	2 mg/kg PO or IM	25- & 50-mg tablets & capsule; 2.5-mg/mL elixir; 50-mg/mL injection	Pretreatment (with dexamethasone) before macrocyclic lactone in dogs with high number of HW microfilariae; or after, for acute hypersensitivity reaction	40
Dobutamine (Dobutrex)	Positive inotrope (catecholamine)	*Initial*: 1 mcg/kg/min CRI, *Up to*: 20 mcg/kg/min	250-mg/20-mL (12.5 mg/mL) vial for injection	Titrate upward to effect q15–30min, as needed, for 24–48 hours then wean off. See Table 22.2 for dilution & other details. Also Tables 22.3 & 25.2	21, 22, 25
Dopamine (Intropin)	Positive inotrope (catecholamine)	*Initial*: 1 mcg/kg/min initial CRI, *Up to*: 10 mcg/kg/min	40-mg/mL (also 80-, & 160-mg/mL) injection	Titrate upward to effect q15–30min, as needed, for 24–48 hours then wean off. See Table 22.2 for dilution & other details. Also Table 22.3	21, 22
Doxycycline (Vibramycin, others)	Antimicrobial	(5–)10 mg/kg q12h PO (x 4 weeks for HW disease)	50- & 100-mg tablets & capsules; 10-mg/mL oral suspension	Used for *Bartonella* endo/myocarditis (see p. 603) and HW disease (see p. 856). Table 40.3	31, 40

Drug	Indications	Common Dosages	Formulations	Comments	See Chapter
Edrophonium (Tensilon)	Short-acting cholinesterase inhibitor	0.05 to 0.1 mg/kg IV	10-mg/mL injection	Rarely used (for acute supraventricular tachycardias, p. 388). Have atropine and endotracheal tube available. Table 25.2	24, 25
Enalapril (Vasotec, others)	Angiotensin converting enzyme inhibitor	0.5 mg/kg PO q12–24h	2.5-, 5-, 10-, & 20-mg tablets	Tables 22.2, 22.3, & 38.4	21, 22, 29, 32, 38
Enalaprilat (Vasotec IV)	Angiotensin converting enzyme inhibitor, for hypertensive crisis	0.2 mg/kg IV, repeated q1–2h as needed; Or, 0.1–1.0 mg/dog IV q6h, as needed	1.25-mg/mL	Monitor arterial BP closely. Table 38.5	38
Enoxaparin (Lovenox)	Low molecular weight heparin anticoagulant	0.8 mg/kg SC q6h	100-mg/mL; in 0.3, 0.4, 0.6, 0.8, & 1 mL prefilled syringes for injection	Table 36.2	36
Enrofloxacin (Baytril)	Antimicrobial	5–20 mg/kg PO q24h, Or, 5–10 mg/kg IV q12h	5.7-, 22.7-, & 68-mg tablets; 22.7-mg/mL injection	Used for *Bartonella* (see p. 603), or other endo/myocarditis Table 31.3	31
Epinephrine (Adrenaline)	Alpha- & beta-adrenergic agonist	*Low dose*: 0.01 mg/kg IV or IO (or IT at 0.02 mg/kg) using the 1:1000 (1 mg/mL) dilution. *High dose*: 0.1 mg/kg IV or IO (or IT at 0.2 mg/kg)	1-mg/mL (1:1000) injection	For CPR: can repeat at 4-min intervals a couple times. Sometimes used at high dose for protracted CPR. Table 25.5	24, 25
Esmolol (Brevibloc)	Beta-adrenergic blocker	*Initial*: 50–100 mcg/kg (0.05–0.1 mg/kg) IV bolus; *Or, loading dose*: repeat initial dose up to total of 500 mcg/kg (0.5 mg/kg) over 5 min; *If effective*: 25–50 (up to 200) mcg/kg/min (0.025–0.05 [up to 0.2] mg/kg/min) CRI, as needed.	10-mg/mL injection	Use low doses if myocardial failure. For hypertensive crisis management, use CRI. Tables 25.2 & 38.5	24, 25, 38
Fenbendazole (Panacur, others)	parasiticide	50 mg/kg/day PO for at least 10–14 days	100-mg/mL oral liquid; 22.2% (222-mg/gm) granule form	*A. vasorum* treatment	40
Fenoldopam (Corlopam)	dopamine type-1 receptor agonist, for hypertensive crisis	*Initial*: 0.1 mcg/kg/min IV CRI; *Uptitration*: in 0.1 mcg/kg/min increments. See Comments. *Maximum*: 1.6 mcg/kg/min	10-mg/1-mL injection	Uptitrate q15 min, as needed based on systolic BP. Table 38.5	38
Fentanyl citrate (Sublimaze, other)	Opioid analgesic	*Initial*: 0.002–0.005 mg/kg IV bolus; *Follow with*: 0.002–0.005 mg/kg/h CRI	50-mcg/mL injection	For acute arterial thromboembolism. Table 36.4	36
Flecainide (Tambocor)	Class Ic antiarrhythmic	1–2 (to 3?) mg/kg PO q(8–)12h	50-, 100-, & 150-mg tablets; 200-mg extended release capsule	Start with low dose. Not advised with CHF or impaired ventricular function. Table 25.2	24, 25

Drug	Indications	Common Dosages	Formulations	Comments	See Chapter
Flumazenil (Romazicon)	Benzodiazepine reversal, during CPR	0.01 mg/kg IV or IO	100-mcg/mL (0.1-mg/mL) injection	Table 25.5	25
Fosinopril (Monopril)	Angiotensin converting enzyme inhibitor	0.25–0.5 mg/kg PO q24h	10-, 20-, & 40-mg tablets	Table 22.3	21, 22
Furosemide; frusemide (Salix, Lasix, other)	Loop diuretic	*Acute CHF*: Initial bolus, 2 mg/kg IV, IM, or SC. Repeat at 1–4 mg/kg q1–4h until RR ↓, then q6–12h; Or, 0.66–1 mg/kg/h CRI for 6(-12)h. *Maintenance*: (0.5–)1–3+ mg/kg PO q8-24h	12.5-, 50-mg tablets (veterinary); 20-, 40-, & 80- mg tablets (human); 10-mg/mL oral solution; 50-mg/mL injection	Reduce dosage as RR decreases in acute CHF. Titrate to lowest effective dosage for chronic therapy. See Chapter 22 & Tables 22.2 & 22.3 for more details. Also Table 38.4	21, 22, 29, 32, 38
Gabapentin (Neurontin)	Analgesic, for neuropathic pain	10–20 mg/kg PO q8h	100-, 300-, 400-mg tablets & capsules; 50-mg/mL oral solution	Might provide some pain relief after melarsamine injection	40
Glycopyrrolate (Robinul-V)	Anticholinergic	0.005–0.01 mg/kg IV or IM; Or, 0.01–0.02 mg/kg SC	0.2-mg/mL injection	Table 25.2	24, 25
Heparin, unfractionated	Anticoagulant	*IV dosing*: one 100 U/kg IV bolus suggested, follow with 480–900 U/kg q24h CRI (20–37.5, or up to 50, U/kg/h). *Or, SC dosing*: 150–300 U/kg SC q6h	1,000- & 10,000-U/mL injection	See Chapter 36 and Table 36.2 for more details	36
Hydralazine (Apresoline)	Arteriolar dilator for afterload reduction in CHF; or for acute control of systemic hypertension	*For CHF*: 0.5(–1.0) mg/kg PO q12h initial, can increase to 2 (up to 3) mg/kg PO q12h, as needed for maintenance. (Or for acute CHF: 0.05–0.1 mg/kg IV bolus, repeat q1–2h if needed). *For hypertensive crisis*: 0.25–2 (to 4) mg/kg PO q12h; Or, 0.1 mg/kg IV over 2 min, followed by 1.5–5 mcg/kg/min CRI; Or, 0.1–0.2 mg/kg IV or IM, repeat q2h as needed, based on BP	10-, 25-, & 50-mg tablet; 20-mg/mL injection	*For acute CHF*: can repeat initial PO dose in 2–3 hours until systolic BP is 90–110 mm Hg. Tables 22.2 & 22.3. *For hypertensive crisis*: Start with low dose, titrate up to effect. Monitor arterial BP. Tables 38.4 & 38.5	21, 22 38
Hydrochlorothiazide (Hydrodiuril, other)	Diuretic	0.5–4 mg/kg PO q12–48h	25-, & 50-mg tablets; 10- & 100-mg/mL oral solution	Start with low dose every other (or 3rd) day Tables 22.3 & 38.4	21, 22, 29, 32, 38
Hydrocodone bitartrate (Hycodan)	Antitussive	0.25 mg/kg PO q6–12h	5-mg tablet; 1-mg/mL syrup	Could dosage increase over time, if needed; Table 9.3	9
Hydromorphone (Dilaudid, Hydrostat, others)	Opioid analgesic	0.05–0.2 mg/kg IM, IV, SC q4–6h	1-, 2-, 4-, & 10-mg/mL injection	For acute arterial thromboembolism. Table 36.4	36

Drug	Indications	Common Dosages	Formulations	Comments	See Chapter
Hydroxyurea (Hydrea)	Chemotherapeutic agent, for erythrocytosis	40–50 mg/kg by mouth q48h or three times/week. (see Comments)	500-mg capsule	Depending on patient's response & tolerance: can divide dose q12h on treatment days, or administer only two times/week, or decrease dose to <40 mg/kg.	26
Hyoscyamine (Donnatal, other)	Anticholinergic	0.003–0.006 mg/kg PO q8h; Or (for large dogs), Extended release tablets, 0.01mg/kg PO q12h	Multiple forms	Table 25.2	24, 25
Imidapril	Angiotensin converting enzyme inhibitor	0.25 mg/kg PO q24h		Table 22.3	21, 22
Irbesartan (Avapro)	Angiotensin receptor blocker, antihypertensive	5 mg/kg(?) PO q24h	75-, 150-, & 300-mg tablets	Table 38.4	38
Isoproterenol (Isuprel)	Beta-adrenergic agonist	0.04–0.08 mcg/kg/min CRI	0.2-mg/mL ampules for injection	Monitor BP. Table 25.2	24, 25
Isosorbide dinitrate (Isordil, Isorbid, others)	Nitrate venodilator	0.5–2 mg/kg PO q(8–)12h	2.5-, 5-, 10-, 20-, 30-, & 40-mg tablets; 40-mg capsules	Table 22.3	21, 22
Isosorbide mononitrate (Monoket)	Nitrate venodilator	0.25–2 mg/kg PO q12h	10- & 20-mg tablets	Table 22.3	21, 22
Ivabradine (Corlanor)	I_f (HCN) channel blocker	(?) 1 mg/kg PO q12h	5- & 7.5-mg tablets; 5-mg/5-mL oral solution	Heart rate reduction in dogs with stage B DMVD	21
Ivermectin (Heartgard, others)	Macrocyclic lactone	*Heartworm prevention*: 6–12 mcg/kg PO q1month; *Microfilaricide*: 50 mcg/kg PO once	See specific product	HW prevention; microfilaricide	40
L-Arginine	Amino acid supplement	100 mg/kg PO q24h; Or, 250-500 mg PO q8h		Optimal dose unknown	22, 39
L-Carnitine	Amino acid supplement	1 g PO q8h for dogs <25 kg; 2 g PO q8h for dogs 25-40 kg. Or, 50–100 mg/kg PO q 8–12h; Or, 200 mg/kg PO q8h	250- & 500-mg capsules & tablets; also pure powder	Optimal dose unclear, if deficiency is present. Mix with food. ½ teaspoon pure L-carnitine powder = 1 g. See p. 352 or 633	22, 32
Labetalol (Normodyne, Trandate)	Beta-blocker, for hypertensive crisis	*Initial*: 0.25 mg/kg IV over 2 min (can repeat to total dose of 3.75 mg/kg, based on BP); *Follow with*: 25 mcg/kg/min CRI	5-mg/1-mL	Closely monitor systolic BP. Table 38.5	38
Lidocaine (Xylocaine, other)	Class Ib antiarrhythmic; local anesthetic	*Initial*: 2 mg/kg slowly IV (over 2 min), can repeat up to 8 mg/kg IV (over ≥10 min); *Or*, 0.8 mg/kg/min rapid IV infusion; *If effective*: 25–80 mcg/kg/ min CRI	20-mg/mL (2%) injection (also others)	Discontinue if vomiting or tremors occur. Can give IT for CPR. Table 25.2.	24, 25

Drug	Indications	Common Dosages	Formulations	Comments	See Chapter
Lisinopril (Prinivil, Zestril)	Angiotensin converting enzyme inhibitor	0.25–0.5 mg/kg PO q(12–)24h	2.5-, 5-, 10-, 20-, & 40-mg tablets	Table 22.3	21, 22
Losartan (Cozaar)	Angiotensin receptor blocker, antihypertensive	0.5 mg/kg(?) PO q24h	25-, 50-, & 100-mg tablets	Table 38.4	38
Magnesium sulfate ($MgSO_4$)	Electrolyte supplement (antiarrhythmic)	25–40 mg/kg (diluted in D_5W) slow IV bolus, followed by same dose infused over a 12–24h period.	use 100-mg/mL (10%) or 200-mg/mL (20%) solution for injection (dilute as needed)	Table 25.2	24, 25
Melarsomine (immiticide)	Heartworm adulticide	2.5 mg/kg, deep IM; see p. 858 & Table 40.3	25-mg/mL injection	Table 40.3	40
Methadone (Methadose, other)	Opioid analgesic	0.5-1.0 mg/kg IV q3-4h	10- & 20-mg/mL injection; also 5-, 10-, & 40-mg tablets; 2-mg/mL oral solution	For acute arterial thromboembolism. Table 36.4	36
Metoprolol (Lopressor)	Beta-adrenergic blocker	*Initial*: 0.1–0.2 mg/kg PO q24h. *Up to*: 1(–2) mg/kg q8(–12)h	50- & 100-mg tablets; 1-mg/mL injection	Cardioprotection: gradually increase from initial dosage over 1-2 months, as possible; *Target*: 1 mg/kg/day, if tolerated. Table 25.2	21, 24, 25
Mexiletine (Mexitil)	Class Ib antiarrhythmic	4–6 (–8) mg/kg PO q8h	150-, 200-, & 250-mg capsules	Table 25.2	24, 25
Milbemycin oxime (Interceptor, other)	Macrocyclic lactone	*D. immitis prophylaxis*: 0.5–1.0 mg/kg PO q1month; *A. vasorum parasiticide*: 0.5 mg/kg/week PO for 4 weeks	2.3-, 5.75-, 11.5-, & 23-mg tablets; or see specific product	HW prevention; parasiticide for *A. vasorum*	40
Milrinone (Primacor)	Positive inotrope (phosphodiesterase inhibitor)	*Initial*: 50 mcg/kg IV over 10 min; *Then* 0.375–0.75 mcg/kg/min CRI	1-mg/1-mL injection	For acute CHF. Human dose listed. Table 22.2	21, 22
Minocycline (Minocin)	Antimicrobial	(5-)10 mg/kg q12h PO	50-, 75-, & 100-mg tablets or capsules; 10-mg/mL oral suspension	Used for *Bartonella* endo/myocarditis (see p. 603) and sometimes for HW disease (see p. 856)	31, 40
Morphine (various generic)	Sedation for respiratory distress; or for opioid analgesia	*Sedation for respiratory distress*: 0.025–0.1 mg/kg IV; *or*, 0.1–0.5 mg/kg IM, SC, single dose. *For analgesia*: 0.2–0.4 mg/kg IM, IV, SC q4–6h	1- & 15-mg/mL injection	*Sedation for respiratory distress*: can give IV dose q2–3min to effect. *Analgesia*: for acute arterial thromboembolism. Table 36.4	22, 36
Moxidectin (Cydectin, Advantage Multi for Dogs, Trio, other)	Macrocyclic lactone	*Oral*: 24 mcg/kg PO q1month; *Topical*: 2.5 mg/kg applied to skin at base of neck, between the shoulder blades, q1month; *Injectable (sustained-release)*: 0.17 mg/kg SC q6months, or 0.5 mg/kg SC q12months	10% imidicloprid & 2.5% moxidectin; or see specific product	HW prevention; microfilaricide; Treatment & preventative for *A. vasorum*	40

Summary Drug Table for DOGS

Drug	Indications	Common Dosages	Formulations	Comments	See Chapter
Naloxone (Narcan)	Opioid reversal, during CPR	0.04 mg/kg IV or IO	20- & 400-mcg/mL injection	Table 25.5	25
Nicardipine (Cardene IV)	Calcium channel blocker, for hypertensive crisis	0.5–5 mcg/kg/min IV CRI	2.5-mg/mL (dilute before infusion); also, premixed 0.1-mg/mL & 0.2-mg/mL solutions	Closely monitor arterial BP. Table 38.5	38
Nitroglycerin ointment (2%) (Nitrol, Nitro-Bid, other)	Nitrate venodilator	~0.25-1.5" (0.6–3.8 cm) cutaneously	15-mg/inch	Apply for 8 to 12 hours, wipe off, and reapply 8 to 12h later. Or q4–6h for 24–48 hours. Can use with hydralazine or amlodipine. Tables 22.2 & 22.3	21, 22
Nitroglycerin (intravenous)	Nitrate arterio/venodilator	*Initial:* 0.5–1 mcg/kg/min CRI in D_5W. *Up to:* 6(-10) mcg/kg/min	0.5-, 0.8-, 1-, 5-, & 10-mg/mL injection	Must closely monitor blood pressure. Uptitrate slowly, to effect. Do not give for more than 24h. See Tables 22.2 & 22.3 for details.	21, 22
Na^+ Nitroprusside (Nipride, Nitropress)	Nitrate arterio/venodilator	*For Acute CHF:* 0.5–1 mcg/kg/min, initial CRI in D_5W; up to 5(–15) mcg/kg/min, as needed. *For hypertensive crisis:* 1 mcg/kg/min, initial CRI in D_5W; up to 15 mcg/kg/min, as needed.	50-mg/2-mL vial (must dilute). Protect from light.	Must closely monitor arterial BP. Uptitrate slowly, to effect. Do not give for more than 24h. See Tables 22.2 & 38.5 for details.	21, 22, 38
Norepinephrine (Levophed)	Alpha-adrenergic agonist; vasopressor agent	0.05–1 mcg/kg/min CRI, to effect	1-mg/1-mL injection	For CPR Table 25.5	25
Oxtriphylline elixir (Choledyl-SA)	Bronchodilator	14 mg/kg PO q8h	400- & 600-mg tablets; ± oral solutions	Table 9.3	9
Oxymorphone (Numorphan)	Opioid analgesic	0.05–0.2 mg/kg IM, IV, SC q2–4h	1- & 1.5-mg/mL injection	For acute arterial thromboembolism. Table 36.4	36
Phenoxybenzamine (Dibenzyline)	Alpha-adrenergic blocker	0.25 mg/kg PO q(8–)12h; *Or,* 0.5 mg/kg PO q24h	10-mg capsule	Mainly used for pheochromocytoma-induced hypertension. Monitor arterial BP. Table 38.4	38
Phentolamine (Regitine, Rogitine)	Alpha-adrenergic blocker	*Initial:* 0.1 mg/kg IV; *Follow with:* 1–2 mcg/kg/min CRI, as needed.	5-mg vial (lyophilized) reconstitute just before administration	For pheochromocytoma-induced hypertensive crisis. Closely monitor arterial BP. Table 38.5	38
Phenylephrine (Neo-Synephrine)	Alpha-adrenergic agonist; vasopressor agent	0.004 to 0.01 mg/kg IV	10-mg/mL injection	Table 25.2	24, 25

Drug	Indications	Common Dosages	Formulations	Comments	See Chapter
Phenytoin (Dilantin)	Class Ib antiarrhythmic	10 mg/kg slowly IV; Or, 20–50 mg/kg PO q8h	50-mg/mL injection; 30- & 100-mg capsules; 30- & 125-mg/mL oral suspension	For digoxin-induced ventricular tachycardia not responding to lidocaine. Table 25.2	24, 25
Pimobendan (Vetmedin)	Positive inotrope/ inodilator	0.2–0.3 (up to 0.5) mg/kg PO q12(-8)h. Initial for acute CHF: 0.15 mg/kg IV, if available.	1.25-, 2.5-, 5-, & 10-mg chewable tablets. In some countries: 1.5-, 2.5- & 5-mg capsules; & injectable	Tables 22.2 & 22.3	21, 22, 29, 32
Potassium Cl (KCl)	Electrolyte supplement	*Maintenance*: 0.05–0.1 mEq/kg/h CRI; *Up to*: 0.4–0.5 mEq/kg/h CRI for severe deficiency	2-mEq/mL injection; others	See p. 349 or Table 25.4 (p. 414) for details.	22
Prazosin (Minipress)	Alpha-adrenergic blocker	0.05–0.2 mg/kg PO q8–12h; Or, 0.5–4 mg/dog PO q8-12h	1-, 2-, & 5-mg capsules	Rarely used. Table 38.4	38
Prednisolone sodium succinate (Solu-Delta-Cortef)	Glucocorticosteroid	*Shock dose*: 10 mg/kg IV	10- & 50-mg/mL injection	Shock dose for acute hypersensitivity reaction with circulatory collapse, following rapid HW microfilariae death	40
Prednisone (various generic)	Glucocorticosteroid	0.5 mg/kg PO q12h for 1st week, 0.5 mg/kg PO q24h for 2nd week, 0.5 mg/kg PO q48h for 3rd and 4th weeks	1-, 2.5-, 5-, 10-, 20-, 25-, & 50-mg tablets; 1-mg/mL oral solutions	Anti-inflammatory therapy for HW pneumonitis, pulmonary thrombosis & thromboembolism Table 40.3	40
Procainamide (Pronestyl, other)	Class Ia antiarrhythmic	*Initial*: 2 mg/kg IV over 2 min; repeat if needed, *Up to*: cumulative 20 mg/kg; *If effective*: 10–50 mcg/kg/min CRI; Or, 6–20 (to 30) mg/kg IM q4–6h	100- & 500-mg/mL injection	Caution if heart failure. (If available, 10–20 mg/kg PO q8–12h, sustained-release) Table 25.2	24, 25
Propafenone (Rythmol, other)	Class Ic antiarrhythmic	4–5 (up to 8) mg/kg PO q8h	150-, 225-, & 300-mg tablets	Start with low dose. Table 25.2	24, 25
Propantheline (Pro-Banthine	Anticholinergic	0.25–0.5 mg/kg PO q8–12h; Or, 3.73–7.5 mg/dog PO q8–12h	7.5- & 15-mg tablets	Some clinicians have used up to 3 mg/kg PO q8h. Table 25.2	24, 25
Propranolol (Inderal, other)	Beta-adrenergic blocker	*Initial IV*: 0.02 mg/kg slow bolus; *Up to*: 0.1 mg/kg IV max. *Initial PO*: 0.1–0.2 mg/kg PO q8h, *Up to*: 1 mg/kg PO q8(-12)h	10-, 20-, 40-, 68-, 80-, & 90-mg tablets; 4- & 8-mg/mL oral solution; 1-mg/mL injection	Start with low dose. Monitor systolic BP; for hypertensive crisis, administer IV q8-12h, as needed. Tables 25.2, 38.4 & 38.5	24, 25, 38
Quinidine gluconate (Quinaglute, other)	Class Ia antiarrhythmic	6–20 mg/kg IM q6h; or, *Loading*: 14–20 mg/kg IM; Or, 6–20 mg/kg PO q6-8h	324-mg tablet; 80-mg/mL injection	Table 25.2	24, 25

Drug	Indications	Common Dosages	Formulations	Comments	See Chapter
Quinidine sulfate (Cin-Quin, other)	Class Ia antiarrhythmic	6–20 mg/kg IM q6h; or, Loading: 14–20 mg/kg IM; Or, 6–20 mg/kg PO q6-8h	100-, 200-, & 300-mg tablets; 200- & 300-mg capsules; 20-mg/mL injection	Table 25.2	24, 25
Quinidine polygalacturonate (Cardioquin)	Class Ia antiarrhythmic	6–20 mg/kg PO q6(-8)h	275-mg tablet	Table 25.2	24, 25
Ramipril (Altace)	Angiotensin converting enzyme inhibitor	0.125–0.25 mg/kg PO q24h	1.25-, 2.5-, 5-, & 10-mg capsules	Table 22.3	21, 22
Rivaroxaban (Xarelto)	Anticoagulant	1–2 mg/kg PO q(12-)24h	2.5-, 10-, 15-, & 20-mg tablets	Table 36.2	36
Sacubitril/Valsartan (Entresto)	Neprilisyn inhibitor & angiotensin receptor blocker	5-10 mg/kg q24(-12)h (?)	Tablets (sacubitril-valsartan): 24-26 mg; 49-51 mg; 97-103 mg	Discontinue ACE inhibitor 2 days before starting this drug	21, 22
Selamectin (Revolution, others)	Macrocyclic lactone	Topical: 6–12 mg/kg, applied to skin at base of neck, between the shoulder blades, q1month	See specific product	HW prevention; microfilaricide	40
Sildenafil (Viagra, Revatio, other)	Phosphodiesterase-5 inhibitor	0.5–2 (to 3) mg/kg PO q8-12h	20-, 25-, 50-, & 100-mg tablets	For palliation of pulmonary hypertension	26, 29, 39, 40
Sotalol (Betapace, other)	Class III antiarrhythmic	1–2.5 (– 5?) mg/kg PO q12h	80-, 120-, 160-, & 240-mg tablets	Table 25.2	24, 25, 32
Spironolactone (Aldactone, other)	Aldosterone antagonist, diuretic	0.5–2 mg/kg PO q24h (or divided, q12h); Target: 2 mg/kg/day	25-, 50-, & 100-mg tablets	Tables 22.3 & 38.4	21, 22, 38
Tadalafil (Cialis, Adcirca)	Phosphodiesterase-5 inhibitor	1–2 mg/kg PO q24h	2.5-, 5-, 10-, & 20-mg tablets	For palliation of pulmonary hypertension.	26, 39, 40
Taurine	Amino acid supplement	0.25 g PO q12h for dogs <10 kg; 0.5 g PO q12h for dogs 10-25 kg; 1 g PO q12h for dogs >25 kg. Or, 0.5-1 g PO q8h for dogs <25 kg; 1-2 g q8-12h for dogs 25-40 kg. Or, 0.5-1 g PO q24h	250-, 500-, 1000-mg tablets & capsules; also various powder strengths	Optimal dose unclear, if deficiency is present	22, 32
Telmisartan (Semintra, Micardis, other)	Angiotensin receptor blocker, antihypertensive	1(–2) mg/kg PO q24h	10-mg/mL feline oral suspension (4-mg/mL in Canada & Europe); also 20-, 40-, & 80-mg tablets	Table 38.4	21, 38
Terbutaline (Brethine, Bricanyl)	Bronchodilator	1.25–5 mg/dog PO q8–12h; Or, 0.14 mg/kg PO q8–12h	2.5- & 5-mg tablets; (1-mg/mL injection)	Tables 9.3 & 25.2	9, 24, 25
Theophylline (long-acting) (various generic)	Bronchodilator	10 mg/kg PO q12h	100-, 200-mg & other tablets & capsules	Tables 9.3 & 25.2	9, 24, 25, 39
Ticarcillin/ clavulanate (Timentin)	Antimicrobial	50 mg/kg IV q6h	3.1 g vial; reconstitutes to 200-mg/mL ticarcillin & 6.7-mg/mL clavulanic acid for injection	Table 31.3	31

Drug	Indications	Common Dosages	Formulations	Comments	See Chapter
Tissue plasminogen activator (Alteplase, Activase)	Fibrinolytic	See p. 766	50-mg vial lyophilized powder; reconstitute as directed		36
Torsemide; torasemide (Demadex, other)	Loop diuretic	Calculate 1/8 to 1/12 of patient's total daily furosemide dose & give as 2 divided doses	5-, 10-, 20-, & 100-mg tablets	Titrate to lowest effective dosage for chronic therapy. Table 22.3	21, 22
Tramadol (Ultram, other)	Analgesic	3–5 mg/kg PO q8h	50-mg tablet	Pain relief after melarsamine injection	40
Trazodone (Desyrel, other)	Sedation-anxiolytic, prior to echo exam	2–5 mg/kg PO (given before leaving home)	50-, 100-, 150- & 300-mg tablets	If planning to use acepromazine also, decrease its dose by 50%	4
Vasopressin (Pitressin, other)	Vasopressor agent	0.8 U/kg IV (or IO or IT) q4min	20-U/1-mL injection	Can use in place of (or sometimes with) epinephrine during CPR. Table 25.5	24, 25
Verapamil (Calan, Isoptan)	Class IV antiarrhythmic	*Initial*: 0.02–0.05 mg/kg slowly IV, can repeat q5min up to total of 0.15(–0.2) mg/kg; *Or*, 0.5–2 mg/kg PO q8h (diltiazem much preferred)	40-, 80-mg tablets; 2.5-mg/mL injection	Verapamil is *not recommended*, particularly if myocardial function is reduced; diltiazem should be used instead. Table 25.2	24, 25
Warfarin (Coumadin, other)	Anticoagulant	See p. 770	1-, 2-, 2.5-, 4-, 5-mg (& other) tablets	Other anticoagulant and/or antiplatelet strategies much preferred over warfarin for antithrombotic prophylaxis	36
Yohimbine (Yobine)	Alpha$_2$-adrenergic agonist reversal agent	0.1 mg/kg IV or IO	2-mg/mL injection	For use during CPR Table 25.5	25

Some trade names noted in parentheses; other brands as well as generic products also might be available.

Abbreviations: ACE, angiotensin converting enzyme; AF, atrial fibrillation; BP, blood pressure; CHF, congestive heart failure; CPR, cardiopulmonary resuscitation; CRI, constant rate infusion; D$_5$W, 5% dextrose in water; DMVD, degenerative mitral valve disease; echo, echocardiography; HW, heartworm; IM, intramuscularly; IO, intraosseous administration; IT, intratracheal administration (via a long catheter); IV, intravenous; PO, orally; RR, respiratory rate; SC, subcutaneously; SVT, supraventricular tachycardia.

SUMMARY DRUG TABLE FOR CATS

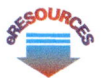

Drug	Indications	Common Dosages	Formulations	Comments	See Chapter
Acepromazine (PromAce, other)	Sedation for echo exam or respiratory distress; Or occasionally for hypertensive crisis (alpha-blocking effect)	*Sedation for echo exam*: 0.1 mg/kg IM (or 0.05 mg/kg IV). *Sedation for respiratory distress*: 0.025–0.1 mg/kg IV or IM; Or, 0.05-0.1 mg/kg SC. *For hypertensive crisis*: 0.01–0.05 (to 0.1) mg/cat IV or SC; Or, 0.5–2 mg/kg PO q8h.	5-, 10-, & 25-mg tablets; 10-mg/mL injection	*Sedation for echo exam*: mix with butorphanol. *Sedation for respiratory distress*: can use 0.05–0.1 mg/kg IM with butorphanol. *For hypertensive crisis*: monitor arterial BP; Table 38.5	4 10, 22 38
Albuterol (Proventil, other)	Bronchospasm in CHF	1–2 puffs by inhaler/spacer/facemask	90-mcg per actuation	Table 33.3	33
Alfaxalone (Alfaxan)	Sedation, echo exam	1–2 mg/kg IM	10-mg/mL injection	Either following acepromazine & butorphanol, if needed; or for heavier sedation to start, mix with butorphanol, IM	4
Amikacin (Amiglyde-V)	Antimicrobial	10–14 mg/kg q24h IV, IM, or SC, for 7–10 days	50- & 250-mg/mL injection	Initial therapy, combined with doxycycline, for *Bartonella* endo/myocarditis	31
Aminophylline (various generic)	Bronchodilator	5 mg/kg PO q12h	100-, & 200-mg tablets; 25 mg/mL injection	Table 9.3	9
Amlodipine (Norvasc)	Arteriolar dilator; antihypertensive	0.3125–0.625(–1.25) mg/cat PO q24(–12)h; Or, 0.1–0.25(to 0.5) mg/kg PO q24h. *For hypertensive crisis*: can repeat dose after 4-8 hours, if needed, up to total of 0.6(–1) mg/cat within first 24 hours. Or: 0.2–0.4 (up to 0.6) mg/kg PO q24h	2.5-, 5-, & 10-mg tablets	Monitor arterial BP. Can dissolve tablet(s) in water and administer rectally, if PO administration not possible. Tables 22.3, 38.4 & 38.5	21, 38

Cardiovascular Disease in Companion Animals 889

Drug	Indications	Common Dosages	Formulations	Comments	See Chapter
Amoxicillin & clavulanate (Clavamox)	Antimicrobial	20–25 mg/kg PO q8h	62.5-, 125-, 250-, & 375-mg tablets; 62.5-mg/mL suspension	Table 31.3	31
Ampicillin (Omnipen, others)	Antimicrobial	22–40 mg/kg IV q6–8h	125-, 250-, & 500-mg vials (ampicillin sodium)	Table 31.3	31
Apixaban (Eliquis)	Anticoagulant	0.625(-1.25) mg/cat PO q12h	2.5- & 5-mg tablets	Table 36.2	36
Aspirin (various generic)	Antiplatelet	10–25 mg/kg (or 20–81 mg/cat) PO q72h (or 2–3 times/week); Or, Low-dose: 5 mg/cat q72h	81-, & 325-mg tablets	When using with clopidogrel, use low dose; Table 36.2	36
Atenolol (Tenormin, others)	Beta-adrenergic blocker	0.2–1(–2) mg/kg PO q12h; Or, 6.25(–12.5) mg/cat PO q12(–24)h	25-, 50-, & 100-mg tablets; 25-mg/mL oral suspension; 0.5-mg/mL injection (ampule)	Start with low dose. Tables 25.2 & 38.4	24, 25, 33, 38
Atropine (various generic)	Anticholinergic	0.02–0.04 mg/kg IV, IM, SC; Or, 0.04 mg/kg PO q6–8h	0.05-, 0.1-, 0.4-, & 1-mg/mL injection, & others	Can give intratracheally for CPR. Table 25.2	24, 25
Benazepril (Lotensin)	Angiotensin converting enzyme inhibitor	0.25–0.5 mg/kg PO q24(–12)h	5-, 10-, 20-, & 40-mg tablets	Tables 22.3 & 38.4	21, 22, 33, 38
Buprenorphine (Temgesic, Vetergesic)	Opioid (mu) agonist-antagonist analgesic	0.01–0.03 mg/kg IM, IV, SC q6–8h, (or PO, for transmucosal absorption)	0.3 mg/mL injection	For follow-up analgesia in arterial thromboembolism. Table 36.4	36
Butorphanol (Torbutrol, Torbugesic)	Sedation for echo exam or respiratory distress	Sedation for echo exam: 0.2–0.25 mg/kg IM. Sedation for respiratory distress: 0.1-0.2 mg/kg IM, IV	2- & 10-mg/mL injection	Sedation for echo exam: either mixed with acepromazine; or for heavier sedation to start, use 0.2 mg/kg mixed with alfaxalone (1.5-2 mg/kg IM). Sedation for respiratory distress: or up to 0.3 mg/kg IM	4 10, 22
Capromorelin (Elura)	Appetite stimulant for cats	2 mg/kg (0.1 mL/kg) PO q24h	20-mg/mL oral solution		22
Captopril (Capoten)	Angiotensin converting enzyme inhibitor	0.5–1.25 mg/kg PO q12–24h	25-mg tablet	Table 22.3	21, 22
Cefazolin sodium (Ancef, Kefzol, other)	Antimicrobial	22–33 mg/kg IV q8h	50- & 100-mg/50mL injection	Table 31.3	31
Ceftriaxone (Rocephin)	Antimicrobial	20 mg/kg IV q12h	250-, & 500-mg, & 1-, & 2-gm vials; reconstitute to 100-mg/mL for IV injection	Table 31.3	31
Chlorothiazide (Diuril)	Diuretic	10–40 mg/kg PO q12–48h (start qod with low dose)	250- & 500-mg tablets; 50-mg/mL oral suspension	Start with low dose every other (or 3rd) day Table 22.3	21, 22

Drug	Indications	Common Dosages	Formulations	Comments	See Chapter
Clopidogrel (Plavix)	Antiplatelet	18.75 mg/cat (~3–6 mg/kg) PO q24h. Can give 1 *initial loading dose*: 37.5 mg/cat PO	75-mg tablets	Table 36.2	33, 36
Cyproheptadine (Periactin)	Appetite stimulant	2 mg/cat PO	4-mg tablet; 2-mg/5-mL oral solution		22
Dalteparin (Fragmin)	Low molecular weight heparin anticoagulant	*Initial*: 75 U/kg SC q6h; *Up to*: 150 U/kg SC q6h	10,000 IU/mL (& other) for injection	Table 36.2	36
Dexamethasone (Azium, Dexaject SP, others)	Glucocorticosteroid	1 mg/kg IV, IM	2-mg/mL injection; or Sodium phosphate form: 3.33-mg/mL injection	For acute respiratory distress from HW-associated disease	40
Digoxin (Lanoxin, other)	Positive inotrope	0.007 mg/kg (or 1/4 of 0.125 mg tab) PO q48h.	0.0625-, 0.125-, &0.25-mg tablets; 0.05- & 0.15-mg/mL elixir	Digoxin usually not recommended for cats. Table 22.3	21, 22, 25
Diltiazem (Cardizem, Dilacor)	Class IV antiarrhythmic	*Acute IV for uncontrolled AF or rapid SVT*: 0.05–0.1 mg/kg slowly IV, can repeat up to 0.25 mg/kg total. *PO maintenance*: regular diltiazem, 1.5–2.5 mg/kg (or 7.5–10 mg/cat) PO q8h; *Or extended release forms*: Diltiazem ER, 30 mg/cat q24h, up to 60 mg q24h, if necessary; *Or*, Cardizem-CD, 10 mg/kg (or 45 mg/cat) q24h	30-, 60-, 90-, & 120-mg tablets; 5-mg/mL injection; Diltiazem ER: 60-, 120-, 180-, & 240-mg capsules (240-mg capsule contains four 60-mg tablets) Cardizem-CD: 120-, 180-, 240-mg capsules	Diltiazem ER: can use ½ (up to 1) of a 60 mg controlled-release tablet within the 240 mg gelatin capsule. Table 25.2	24, 25, 33
Dobutamine (Dobutrex)	Positive inotrope (catecholamine)	*Initial*: 1 mcg/kg/min CRI, *Up to*: 10 mcg/kg/min	250-mg/20-mL (12.5 mg/mL) vial for injection	Titrate upward to effect q15–30min, as needed, for 24–48 hours then wean off. See Table 22.2 for dilution & other details. Also Tables 22.3 & 25.2	21, 22, 25
Dopamine (Intropin)	Positive inotrope (catecholamine)	*Initial*: 1 mcg/kg/min CRI, *Up to*: 5 mcg/kg/min	40-mg/mL (also 80-, & 160-mg/mL) injection	Titrate upward to effect q15–30min, as needed, for 24–48 hours then wean off. See Table 22.2 for dilution & other details. Also Table 22.3	21, 22
Doxycycline (Vibramycin, others)	Antimicrobial	(5–)10 mg/kg q12h PO	50- & 100-mg tablets & capsules; 10-mg/mL oral suspension	Used for *Bartonella* endo/myocarditis (see p. 603), also HW disease (see p. 866)	31, 40
Enalapril (Vasotec, others)	Angiotensin converting enzyme inhibitor	0.25-0.5 mg/kg PO q24(–12)h	2.5-, 5-, 10-, & 20-mg tablets	Tables 22.2, 22.3, & 38.4	21, 22, 33, 38

Drug	Indications	Common Dosages	Formulations	Comments	See Chapter
Enoxaparin (Lovenox)	Low molecular weight heparin anticoagulant	0.75–1 mg/kg SC q6–12h	100-mg/mL; in 0.3, 0.4, 0.6, 0.8, & 1 mL prefilled syringes for injection	Table 36.2	36
Enrofloxacin (Baytril)	Antimicrobial	*Initial therapy*: 5–10 mg/kg IV q12h. *Continuation*: 2.5–5 mg/kg PO q12h	5.7-, 22.7-, & 68-mg tablets; 22.7-mg/mL injection	Risk for retinotoxicity in cats. Table 31.3	31
Epinephrine (Adrenaline)	Alpha- & beta-adrenergic agonist	*Low dose*: 0.01 mg/kg IV or IO (or IT at 0.02 mg/kg) using the 1:1000 (1 mg/mL) dilution. *High dose*: 0.1 mg/kg IV or IO (or IT at 0.2 mg/kg)	1-mg/mL (1:1000) injection	For CPR: can repeat at 4-minute intervals. Sometimes used at high dose for protracted CPR. Table 25.5	24, 25
Eprinomectin (Centragard)	Macrocyclic lactone	0.5 mg/kg topical, applied to skin at base of neck, between the shoulder blades, q1month	0.3- & 0.9-mL applicators; see product weight ranges	HW prevention;	40
Esmolol (Brevibloc)	Beta-adrenergic blocker	*Initial*: 50–100 mcg/kg (0.05–0.1 mg/kg) IV; *Or, loading dose*: repeat initial dose up to total of 500 mcg/kg (0.5 mg/kg) over 5 min; *If effective*: 25–50 (up to 200) mcg/kg/min (0.025–0.05 [up to 0.2] mg/kg/min) CRI, as needed.	10-mg/mL injection	Use low doses if myocardial failure. For hypertensive crisis management, use CRI. Tables 25.2 & 38.5	24, 25, 38
Fenoldopam (Corlopam)	dopamine type-1 receptor agonist, for hypertensive crisis	*Initial*: 0.1 mcg/kg/min IV CRI; *Uptitration*: in 0.1 mcg/kg/min increments. See Comments. *Maximum*: (?)1.6 mcg/kg/min	10-mg/1-mL injection	Uptitrate q15 min, as needed based on systolic BP. Dosage uncertain, monitor closely. Table 38.5	38
Fentanyl citrate (Sublimaze, other) Fentanyl transdermal (Duragesic)	Opioid analgesic	*Initial*: 0.002–0.005 mg/kg IV bolus; *Follow with*: 0.002–0.005 mg/kg/h CRI	50-mcg/mL injection; 25-, 50-, 75-, & 100-mcg/hr patch	For acute arterial thromboembolism. Also could consider fentanyl patch (see p. 764). Table 36.4	36
Fondaparinux (Arixtra)	Anticoagulant	(?)0.06 or 0.2 mg/kg SC q12h	2.5-mg/0.5-mL (also 5-mg/0.4-mL & other) prefilled syringes for injection	Low dose for prophylaxis; high dose for thrombosis treatment. Table 36.2	36
Furosemide; frusemide (Salix, Lasix, other)	Loop diuretic	*Acute CHF*: Initial bolus, 1–2 mg/kg IV, IM or SC. Repeat at 1–2 mg/kg q1–4h until RR ↓, then q6–12h; *Or*, 0.33–0.66 mg/kg/h CRI for 6(-12)h. *Maintenance*: (0.5–)1–2 (to 3) mg/kg PO q8–12(–24)h	12.5-, 50-mg tablets (veterinary); 20-, 40-, & 80- mg tablets (human); 10-mg/mL oral solution; 50-mg/mL injection	Reduce dosage as RR decreases in acute CHF. Titrate to lowest effective dosage for chronic therapy. See Chapter 22 & Tables 22.2 & 22.3 for more details. Also Table 38.4	21, 22, 33, 38

Drug	Indications	Common Dosages	Formulations	Comments	See Chapter
Gabapentin (Neurontin)	Sedation, prior to echo exam	50-100 mg PO, for most cats (mix with ~1 teaspoon wet food & give before leaving home)	100-, 300-, 400-mg tablets & capsules; 50-mg/mL oral solution	Give 2 hours prior to scheduled echo exam	4
Glycopyrrolate (Robinul-V)	Anticholinergic	0.005–0.01 mg/kg IV or IM; Or, 0.01–0.02 mg/kg SC	0.2-mg/mL injection	Table 25.2	24, 25
Heparin, unfractionated	Anticoagulant	250 U/kg SC q6h	1,000-, 5000- & 10,000-U/mL injection	See Chapter 36 and Table 36.2 for more details	36
Hydralazine (Apresoline)	Arteriolar dilator	0.25–2 mg/kg PO q12h; Or, 2.5 (up to 10) mg/cat PO q12-24h. *For hypertensive crisis*: 0.5 mg/cat SC, repeat after 15–30 min, to max. total dose of 2.5 mg, if necessary	10-mg tablet; 20-mg/mL injection	Start with low dose, titrate up to effect. Monitor arterial BP Tables 22.3, 38.4, & 38.5	21, 38
Hydrochlorothiazide (Hydrodiuril, other)	Diuretic	0.5–2 mg/kg PO q12–48h	25- & 50-mg tablets; 10- & 100-mg/mL oral solution	Start with low dose every other (or 3rd) day Tables 22.3 & 38.4	21, 22, 38
Hydromorphone (Dilaudid, Hydrostat, others)	Opioid analgesic	0.05–0.2 mg/kg IM, IV, SC q4–6h	1-, 2-, 4-, & 10-mg/mL injection	For acute arterial thromboembolism. Table 36.4	36
Hydroxyurea (Hydrea)	Chemotherapeutic agent, for erythrocytosis	25 mg/kg by mouth q48h or three times/week; (rarely used)	500-mg capsule	Depending on patient's response & tolerance: can divide dose q12h on treatment days, or decrease dose or frequency	26
Hyoscyamine (Donnatal, other)	Anticholinergic	0.003–0.005 mg/kg PO q8h	Multiple forms	Table 25.2	24, 25
Isoproterenol (Isuprel)	Beta-adrenergic agonist	0.04–0.08 mcg/kg/min CRI	0.2-mg/mL ampules for injection	Monitor BP. Table 25.2	24, 25
Ivabradine (Corlanor)	I_f (HCN) channel blocker	(?) 0.3 mg/kg PO q8h	5- & 7.5-mg tablets; 5-mg/5-mL oral solution	Heart rate reduction in cardiomyopathy (?)	21
Ivermectin (Heartgard, others)	Macrocyclic lactone	24 mcg/kg PO q1month;	See specific product	HW prevention;	40
Ketamine (Ketavet, Vetalar, other)	Sedation, echo exam	2 mg/kg IV	100-mg/mL injection	Can give following acepromazine & butorphanol, if needed.	4
Labetalol (Normodyne, Trandate)	Beta-adrenergic blocker, for hypertensive crisis	*Initial*: 0.25 mg/kg IV over 2 min (can repeat to total dose of 3.75 mg/kg, based on BP); *Follow with*: 25 mcg/kg/min CRI	5-mg/1-mL	Dosage uncertain, closely monitor systolic BP. Table 38.5	38
Lidocaine (Xylocaine, other)	Class Ib antiarrhythmic; local anesthetic	*Initial*: 0.2–0.5 mg/kg slowly IV (over 2 min); *Can repeat at*: 0.15–0.25 mg/kg, up to total of 2(–4) mg/kg unless adverse effects; *If effective*: 10–40 mcg/kg/min CRI	20-mg/mL (2%) injection (also others)	Discontinue if vomiting, tremors, or other adverse effects occur. Table 25.2	24, 25

Drug	Indications	Common Dosages	Formulations	Comments	See Chapter
Lisinopril (Prinivil, Zestril)	Angiotensin converting enzyme inhibitor	0.25–0.5 mg/kg PO q24h	2.5-, 5-, 10-, 20-, & 40-mg tablets	Table 22.3	21, 22
Magnesium sulfate ($MgSO_4$)	Electrolyte supplement (antiarrhythmic)	(?) 25–40 mg/kg (diluted in D_5W) slow IV bolus, followed by same dose infused over a 12–24h period.	use 100-mg/mL (10%) for injection (dilute as needed)	Optimal dose uncertain. Table 25.2	24, 25
Methadone (Methadose, other)	Opioid analgesic	0.1 (-0.2) mg/kg IV q3-4h	10- & 20-mg/mL injection; also 5-, 10-, & 40-mg tablets; 2-mg/mL oral solution	For acute arterial thromboembolism. Table 36.4	36
Metoprolol (Lopressor)	Beta-adrenergic blocker	2 (to 15) mg/cat PO q 8(–12)h	50- & 100-mg tablets; 1-mg/mL injection	Start with low dose. Table 25.2	24, 25
Milbemycin oxime (Interceptor, other)	Macrocyclic lactone	2 mg/kg PO q1month;	See specific product	HW prevention;	40
Minocycline (Minocin)	Antimicrobial	8.8 mg/kg q12h PO	50-, 75-, & 100-mg tablets or capsules; 10-mg/mL oral suspension	Used for *Bartonella* endo/myocarditis (see p. 603) and sometimes for HW disease (see p. 856)	31, 40
Mirtazapine (Miritaz, other)	Appetite stimulant	1.25–4 mg/cat PO q72h; Or, 1.5" (~2 mg/cat) ointment applied to inner ear pinna	7.5-, 15-, 30-, & 45-mg tablets; Topical: 2% ointment	Wear gloves when using topical ointment	22
Morphine (various generic)	Opioid analgesic	0.1 mg/kg IM, IV, SC q4–6h	1- & 15-mg/mL injection	For acute arterial thromboembolism. Table 36.4	36
Moxidectin (Advantage Multi for Cats, other)	Macrocyclic lactone	1 mg/kg topical, applied to skin at base of neck, between the shoulder blades, q1month	10% imidicloprid & 1% moxidectin; or see specific product	HW prevention;	40
Nitroglycerin ointment (2%) (Nitrol, Nitro-Bid, other)	Nitrate venodilator	~1/8–1/4 (up to 1/2)" (0.3–0.6[-1.3] cm) cutaneously. Apply for 8 to 12 hours, wipe off, and reapply 8 to 12h later. Or q4–8h for 24–48 hours?	15-mg/inch	Apply for 8 to 12 hours, wipe off, and reapply 8 to 12h later. Tables 22.2 & 22.3	21, 22
Na^+ Nitroprusside (Nipride, Nitropress)	Nitrate arterio/venodilator	*For Acute CHF (rarely used)*: 0.5–1 mcg/kg/min initial CRI in D_5W (dilute to 100–300 mcg/mL); up to 2 mcg/kg/min, as needed. *For hypertensive crisis*: (0.5-) 1 mcg/kg/min, initial CRI in D_5W; up to 3 mcg/kg/min, as needed.	50-mg/2-mL vial (must dilute). Protect from light.	Must closely monitor arterial BP. Uptitrate slowly, to effect. Do not give for more than 24h. See Tables 22.2 & 38.5 for details.	21, 22, 38
Oxymorphone (Numorphan)	Opioid analgesic	0.05–0.2 mg/kg IM, IV, SC q2–4h	1- & 1.5-mg/mL injection	For acute arterial thromboembolism. Table 36.4	36

Drug	Indications	Common Dosages	Formulations	Comments	See Chapter
Phenoxybenzamine (Dibenzyline)	Alpha-adrenergic blocker	0.25 mg/kg PO q(8–)12h; Or, 2.5 mg/cat PO q(8–)12h; Or, 0.5 mg/kg PO q24h	10-mg capsule	Mainly used for pheochromocytoma-induced hypertension. Monitor arterial BP. Table 38.4	38
Phentolamine (Regitine, Rogitine)	Alpha-adrenergic blocker	*Initial*: 0.1 (?) mg/kg IV; *Follow with*: 1–2 (?) mcg/kg/min CRI, as needed.	5-mg vial (lyophilized) reconstitute just before administration	For pheochromocytoma-induced hypertensive crisis. Closely monitor arterial BP. Table 38.5	38
Phenylephrine (Neo-Synephrine)	Alpha-adrenergic agonist; vasopressor agent	(?) 0.004 to 0.01 mg/kg IV	10-mg/mL injection	Table 25.2	24, 25
Pimobendan (Vetmedin)	Positive inotrope-inodilator	0.2–0.3 mg/kg PO q12h; Or, 0.625-1.25 mg/cat q12h	1.25-, 2.5-, 5-, & 10-mg chewable tablets. In some countries: 1.5-, 2.5- & 5-mg capsules; & injectable	Caution if CHF from hypertrophic obstructive cardiomyopathy. Table 22.2	21, 22, 33
Pradofloxacin (Veraflox)	Antimicrobial	5–10 mg/kg q24(-12)h PO	25-mg/mL oral suspension for cats	Used for *Bartonella* endo/myocarditis (see p. 603)	31
Prazosin (Minipress)	Alpha-adrenergic blocker	0.25–0.5 mg/cat PO q12–24h	1-, 2-, & 5-mg capsules	Rarely used. Table 38.4	38
Prednisolone sodium succinate (Solu-Delta-Cortef)	Glucocorticoid	100-250 mg/cat IV	10- & 50-mg/mL injection	For acute respiratory distress from HW-associated disease	40
Prednisone (various generic)	Glucocorticoid	1 mg/kg PO q12h for 2-3 days, then taper over the next 2 weeks down to 0.5 mg/kg PO q48h, & continue this dose for another 2 weeks	1-, 2.5-, 5-, 10-, 20-, 25-, & 50-mg tablets; 1-mg/mL oral liquids	Anti-inflammatory therapy for HW pneumonitis, pulmonary thrombosis & thromboembolism	40
Procainamide (Pronestyl, other)	Class Ia antiarrhythmic	*Initial*: 1-2 mg/kg IV over 2 min; repeat if needed, *Up to*: cumulative 10 mg/kg; *If effective*: 10–20 mcg/kg/min CRI; Or, 7.5–20 mg/kg IM q(6–)8h	100- & 500-mg/mL injection	Table 25.2	24, 25
Propranolol (Inderal, other)	Beta-adrenergic blocker	*Initial IV*: 0.02 mg/kg slow bolus; *Up to*: 0.06-0.1 mg/kg IV max. Or, 2.5 (up to 10) mg/cat PO q8–12h; Or, 0.2–1.0 mg/kg PO q8–12h	10-, 20-, 40-, 68-, 80-, & 90-mg tablets; 4- & 8-mg/mL oral solution; 1-mg/mL injection	Start with low dose. Monitor systolic BP; for hypertensive crisis, administer IV q8-12h, as needed. Tables 25.2, 38.4 & 38.5	24, 25, 33, 38
Quinidine gluconate (Quinaglute, other)	Class Ia antiarrhythmic	6–16 mg/kg IM or PO q8h	324-mg tablet; 80-mg/mL injection	Table 25.2	24, 25

Drug	Indications	Common Dosages	Formulations	Comments	See Chapter
Quinidine sulfate (Cin-Quin, other)	Class Ia antiarrhythmic	6–16 mg/kg IM or PO q8h	100-, 200-, & 300-mg tablets; 200- & 300-mg capsules; 20-mg/mL injection	Table 25.2	24, 25
Rivaroxaban (Xarelto)	Anticoagulant	0.5–1 mg/kg PO q24h; *Or*, 2.5 mg/cat PO q24h (or 1.25 mg/cat PO q12h)	2.5-, 10-, 15-, & 20-mg tablets	Table 36.2	36
Selamectin (Revolution, others)	Macrocyclic lactone	6–12 mg/kg, topical, applied to skin at base of neck, between the shoulder blades, q1month	See specific product	HW prevention	40
Sildenafil (Viagra, Revatio, other)	Phosphodiesterase-5 inhibitor	0.5–2 (to 3) mg/kg PO q8-12h	20-, 25-, 50-, & 100-mg tablets	For palliation of pulmonary hypertension	26, 39
Sotalol (Betapace, other)	Class III antiarrhythmic	10(–20) mg/cat PO q12h; *Or*, 2(–4) mg/kg PO q12h	80-, 120-, 160-, & 240-mg tablets	Table 25.2	24, 25, 33
Spironolactone (Aldactone, other)	Aldosterone antagonist, diuretic	(0.5-)1–2 mg/kg PO q24h (or divided, q12h)	25-, 50-, & 100-mg tablets	Tables 22.3 & 38.4	21, 22, 33, 38
Taurine	Amino acid supplement	250–500 mg/cat PO q12h	250-, 500-, 1000-mg tablets & capsules; also various powder strengths		22, 33
Telmisartan (Semintra, Micardis, other)	Angiotensin receptor blocker, antihypertensive	*Initial*: 1.5 mg/kg PO q12h for 14 days; *Follow with*: 2 mg/kg PO q24h. If needed, ↓ dose in 0.5 mg/kg increments, to minimum 0.5 mg/kg q24h.	10-mg/mL oral suspension (4-mg/mL in Canada & Europe); also 20-, 40-, & 80-mg tablets	Monitor arterial BP. Tables 38.4 & 38.5	21, 38
Terbutaline (Brethine, Bricanyl)	Bronchodilator	1/8–1/4 (up to 1/2) of 2.5-mg tablet/cat PO q12h; *Or*, 0.1–0.2 mg/kg PO q12h; *Or*, 0.01 mg/kg SC, repeat once in 5–10 min, if needed.	2.5- & 5-mg tablets; 1-mg/mL injection	Tables 9.3 & 25.2	9, 24, 25, 39
Theophylline (long-acting) (various generic)	Bronchodilator	10-15 (up to 25) mg/kg PO q24(-48)h (in evening)	100-, 200-mg & other tablets & capsules	Tables 9.3 & 25.2	9, 24, 25
Ticarcillin/ clavulanate (Timentin)	Antimicrobial	50 mg/kg IV q6h	3.1 g vial; reconstitutes to 200-mg/mL ticarcillin & 6.7-mg/mL clavulanic acid for injection	Table 31.3	31
Tissue plasminogen activator (Alteplase, Activase)	Fibrinolytic	See p. 766	50-mg vial lyophilized powder; reconstitute as directed		36

Drug	Indications	Common Dosages	Formulations	Comments	See Chapter
Torsemide; torasemide (Demadex, other)	Loop diuretic	Calculate (1/8-) 1/10 to 1/12 of patient's total daily furosemide dose & give as 2 divided doses, Or, 0.1–0.3 mg/kg PO q12h	5-, 10-, & 20-mg tablets	Titrate to lowest effective dosage for chronic therapy. Table 22.3	21, 22
Verapamil (Calan, Isoptan)	Class IV antiarrhythmic	*Initial*: 0.025 mg/kg slowly IV, can repeat q5min up to total of 0.15(–0.2) mg/kg; Or, 0.5–1 mg/kg PO q8h (diltiazem much preferred)	40-, 80-mg tablets; 2.5-mg/mL injection	Verapamil is *not* recommended, particularly if myocardial function is reduced; diltiazem should be used instead. Table 25.2	24, 25
Warfarin (Coumadin, other)	Anticoagulant	See p. 770	1-, 2-, 2.5-, 4-, 5-mg (& other) tablets	Other anticoagulant and/or antiplatelet strategies much preferred over warfarin for antithrombotic prophylaxis	36

Some trade names noted in parentheses; other brands as well as generic products also might be available.

Abbreviations: AF, atrial fibrillation; BP, blood pressure; CHF, congestive heart failure; CPR, cardiopulmonary resuscitation; CRI, constant rate infusion; D_5W, 5% dextrose in water; echo, echocardiography; HW, heartworm; IM, intramuscularly; IO, intraosseous administration; IT, intratracheal administration (via a long catheter); IV, intravenous; PO, orally; RR, respiratory rate; SC, subcutaneously; SVT, supraventricular tachycardia.

SUMMARY DRUG TABLE FOR HORSES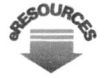

Drug	Indications	Common Dosages	Formulations	Comments	See Chapter
Acepromazine (PromAce, other)	Sedative/vasodilator	0.01–0.06 mg/kg IM q6–8h; Or, 0.1–1.0 mg/kg PO q8–12h	10- & 25-mg tablets; 10-mg/mL injection	Dose to effect & monitor BP Table 22.3	22
Amiodarone (Cordarone, Pacerone, other)	Class III antiarrhythmic	*IV loading*: 5(–6.5) mg/kg infused IV over 1h, then *IV maintenance*: 0.83(–1.1) mg/kg/h for 23 h (prior to DC cardioversion for AF); or for converting AF, continue at 1.9 mg/kg/h for 30h or to effect. *PO dosing*: 10 mg/kg q24h has been used (efficacy unclear)	Standard (older) amiodarone: 50-mg/mL injection; 200- & 400-mg tablets	Table 25.2	24, 25
Atenolol (Tenormin, others)	Beta-adrenergic blocker	0.5–1.5 mg/kg PO q12h	25-, 50-, & 100-mg tablets	Start with low dose. Table 25.2	24, 25
Atropine (various generic)	Anticholinergic	0.01–0.02 mg/kg IV, IM, SC	0.05-, 0.1-, 0.4-, & 1-mg/mL injection, & others	Table 25.2	24, 25
Benazepril (Lotensin)	Angiotensin converting enzyme inhibitor	0.5–1 mg/kg PO q24(–12)h	5-, 10-, 20-, & 40-mg tablets	Tables 22.3, 38.4	21, 22, 30, 34, 38
Dalteparin (Fragmin)	Low molecular weight heparin anticoagulant	50–100 IU/kg SC q24h	10,000 IU/mL, 95,000 IU/3.8 mL (& other) for injection	Table 36.2	36
Detomidine HCl (Dormosedan)	Sedation, echo exam	20 or 40 mcg/kg (0.2 or 0.4 mL Dormosedan/100 kg body weight) IV or IM	10-mg/mL	If needed, following xylazine	4
Digoxin (Lanoxin, other)	Positive inotrope	1 mg by slow IV push; Or, Loading: 0.0022 mg/kg IV q12 for two doses; then Maintenance: 0.0022 mg/kg IV q24h; Or, 0.011 mg/kg PO q12h	0.1-, & 0.25-mg/1-mL injection; 0.125-, & 0.25-mg tablets;	Table 22.3	21, 22, 25, 30, 34

Drug	Indications	Common Dosages	Formulations	Comments	See Chapter
Diltiazem (Cardizem)	Class IV antiarrhythmic	*Initial*: 0.125 mg/kg slowly IV over 2 min; *Can repeat* q10min to effect, up to 1.25 mg/kg total dose	5-mg/mL injection	Table 25.2	24, 25
Dobutamine (Dobutrex)	Positive inotrope (catecholamine)	*Initial*: 1 mcg/kg/min CRI, *Up to*: 5 mcg/kg/min CRI	250-mg/20-mL (12.5 mg/mL) vial for injection	Titrate upward to effect q15–30min, as needed (unless adverse signs) for 24–48 hours then wean off. Tables 22.3 & 25.2	21, 22, 24, 25
Epinephrine (Adrenaline)	Alpha- & beta-adrenergic agonist	*Low dose*: 0.01-0.05 mg/kg IV (or 0.1-0.5 mg/kg IT) using the 1:1000 (1 mg/mL) dilution.	1-mg/mL (1:1000) injection	For CPR: can repeat at 4-minute intervals. Table 25.5	24, 25
Esmolol (Brevibloc)	Beta-adrenergic blocker	*Loading dose*: 200–500 mcg/kg (0.2–0.5 mg/kg) IV over 2–5 min; *If effective*: 25–100 mcg/kg/min (0.025–0.1 mg/kg/min) CRI, titrate to effect.	10-mg/mL injection	Use low doses if myocardial failure. Table 25.2	24, 25
Flecainide (Tambocor)	Class Ic antiarrhythmic	0.2 mg/kg/min IV, up to total dose of 1–2 mg/kg/day; Or, 3–4(–6) mg/kg PO by NG tube q(4??–)24h for up to 4 days.	Injectable form not commercially available in US. 50-, 100-, & 150-mg tablets; 200-mg extended release capsule	Start with low dose. Can cause sudden death, use only with caution & consider combining with a beta-blocker. Not advised with CHF or impaired ventricular function. Table 25.2	24, 25
Flunixin meglumine (Banamine, other)	Nonsteroidal anti-inflammatory drug	1 mg/kg IV, IM q(12-)24h; (1 mg/kg PO paste q24h)	50-mg/mL injection; (also 1500-mg/syringe oral paste)	Reduce inflammation from thrombophlebitis.	36
Furosemide; frusemide (Salix, Lasix, other)	Loop diuretic	*Acute CHF*: 1–3 mg/kg IV or IM (or SC?) q6–8(–12)h to effect; Or, 1–2 mg/kg IV loading, then 0.12 mg/kg/h CRI. *Maintenance*: 1–2 mg/kg IV or IM q6–24h, as needed	12.5-, 50-mg tablets (veterinary); 20-, 40-, & 80- mg tablets (human); 10-mg/mL oral solution; 50-mg/mL injection	Table 22.3	21, 22
Gentamicin	Antimicrobial	6.6 mg/kg IV q24h	40-mg/mL injection	Table 31.3	31
Glycopyrrolate (Robinul-V)	Anticholinergic	0.005–0.01 mg/kg IV	0.2-mg/mL injection	Table 25.2	24, 25
Heparin, unfractionated	Anticoagulant	40–100 IU/kg SC q6h	1,000- & 10,000-U/mL injection	See Chapter 36 and Table 36.2 for more details	36
Hydralazine (Apresoline)	Arteriolar dilator	0.5–1.5 mg/kg PO q12h; Or, Up to 0.5 mg/kg IV q(4–)12h	10-, 25-, & 50-mg tablet; 20-mg/mL injection	Monitor BP Table 22.3	21, 22

Drug	Indications	Common Dosages	Formulations	Comments	See Chapter
Lidocaine (Xylocaine, other)	Class Ib antiarrhythmic; local anesthetic	*Initial*: 0.25–0.5 mg/kg slowly IV (over 2 min); can repeat in 5-10 min; *Up to*: total of 1.5(–2) mg/kg, unless adverse effects; *If effective*: 30–50 mcg/kg/min (0.03–0.05 mg/kg/min) CRI	20-mg/mL (2%) injection (also others)	Discontinue if tremors or other adverse effects occur. Table 25.2	24, 25
Magnesium sulfate (MgSO$_4$)	Electrolyte supplement (antiarrhythmic)	2–6 mg/kg/min CRI q2min to effect, or max. total dose of 55(–100) mg/kg	use 100-mg/mL (10%) or 200-mg/mL (20%) solution for injection (dilute as needed)	Table 25.2	24, 25
Metoprolol (Lopressor)	Beta-adrenergic blocker	0.1–0.3 mg/kg PO q12h (up to 1 mg/kg)	50- & 100-mg tablets; 1-mg/mL injection	Caution in heart failure. Table 25.2	24, 25
Milrinone (Primacor)	Positive inotrope (phosphodiesterase inhibitor)	*Initial*: 0.2 mcg/kg IV bolus; *Then* 5–10 mcg/kg/min CRI	1-mg/1-mL injection	For acute CHF; Table 22.2	21, 22
Nitroglycerin (for IV use)	Nitrate arterio/venodilator	*Acute CHF*: 5 mcg/kg/min initial CRI; *Up to*: 20 mcg/kg/min, as needed	0.5-, 0.8-, 1-, 5-, & 10-mg/mL injection	Must closely monitor blood pressure. Uptitrate slowly, to effect. Do not give for more than 24h. Table 22.3	
Penicillin G sodium	Antimicrobial	50,000 iu/kg q8 IV (or 22,000 iu/kg q6h IV)	5,000,000 iu vial (dry powder); reconstitute with either 3-mL (for 1,000,000 iu/mL) or 8-mL (for 500,000 iu/mL) of diluent for injection	Table 31.3	31
Phenylephrine (Neo-Synephrine)	Alpha-adrenergic agonist	0.1–0.2 mcg/kg/min CRI, start low & titrate to effect or max. total dose of 0.01 mg/kg	10-mg/mL injection	Table 25.2	24, 25
Phenytoin (Dilantin)	Class Ib antiarrhythmic	*Initial IV*: 7.5 (or 5–10) mg/kg IV; can follow with 1–5 mg/kg IM (or PO maintenance dose) q12h. *PO Loading*: 20 mg/kg PO q12h, for 3-4 doses, can follow with PO maintenance; *PO Maintenance*: 10–15 mg/kg PO q12h	50-mg/mL injection; 30- & 100-mg capsules; 30- & 125-mg/mL oral suspension	For digoxin-induced ventricular tachycardia not responding to lidocaine. Table 25.2	24, 25
Pimobendan (Vetmedin)	Positive inotrope/inodilator	0.25 mg/kg IV q12h (if available); PO bioavailability not established	1.25-, 2.5-, 5-, & 10-mg chewable tablets. In some countries: 1.5-, 2.5- & 5-mg capsules; & injectable	Table 22.3	21, 22, 30, 34

Drug	Indications	Common Dosages	Formulations	Comments	See Chapter
Prazosin (Minipress)	Alpha-adrenergic blocker	Start at 5-10 mg per horse PO q12h (optimal dose unknown)	1-, 2-, & 5-mg capsules	Table 38.4	38
Procainamide (Pronestyl, other)	Class Ia antiarrhythmic	1 mg/kg/min IV, up to max. total dose of 20 mg/kg	100- & 500-mg/mL injection	Monitor BP and ECG QRS & QT intervals; max dose might not be tolerated. Table 25.2	24, 25
Propafenone (Rythmol, other)	Class Ic antiarrhythmic	*Initial*: 0.5–2 mg/kg IV (in D_5W) slowly IV over 5–15 min *Follow by*: 0.07 mg/kg/min CRI for up to 2 h; *Or*, 2 mg/kg PO q8h	Injectable form not commercially available in US. 150-, 225-, & 300-mg tablets	Start with low dose. Table 25.2	24, 25
Propranolol (Inderal, other)	Beta-adrenergic blocker	0.03–0.16 mg/kg IV; PO dosing unlikely to be effective in horses (although 0.38–0.78 mg/kg PO q8h has been used)	1-mg/mL injection; (10-, 20-, 40-, 68-, 80-, & 90-mg tablets)	Start with low dose. Table 25.2	24, 25
Quinidine sulfate	Class Ia antiarrhythmic	*PO dosing (quinidine sulfate)*: 22 mg/kg, in 3–4L water, PO by NG tube q2h for up to 4(–6) doses;	100-, 200-, & 300-mg tablets; or as bulk powder	See p. 413 for more details for atrial fibrillation conversion	24, 25
Quinapril	Angiotensin converting enzyme inhibitor	0.125–0.5 mg/kg PO q24h	5-, 10-, 20-, & 40-mg tablets	Table 22.3	21, 22
Ramipril (Altace)	Angiotensin converting enzyme inhibitor	0.05–0.2 mg/kg PO q24h	1.25-, 2.5-, 5-, & 10-mg capsules	Table 22.3	21, 22
Scopolamine	Anticholinergic	0.1–0.2 mg/kg IV	0.4- & 1-mg/mL injection	Table 25.2	24, 25
Sildenafil (Viagra, Revatio, other)	Phosphodiesterase-5 inhibitor	?0.5–2 (to 3) mg/kg PO q8-12h	20-, 25-, 50-, & 100-mg tablets	For palliation of pulmonary hypertension	26, 39
Sodium bicarbonate ($NaHCO_3$)	Alkalinizing agent	1 mEq/kg IV	1 mEq/mL (& other concentrations)	If needed for quinidine toxicity signs	25
Sotalol (Betapace, other)	Class III antiarrhythmic	*Initial*: 1 mg/kg PO q12h for 2 doses, then *Maintenance*: 2–3 mg/kg PO q12h	80-, 120-, 160-, & 240-mg tablets	Table 25.2	24, 25
Spironolactone (Aldactone, other)	Aldosterone antagonist, diuretic	2–4 mg/kg PO q24h	25-, 50-, & 100-mg tablets	Table 22.3	21, 22
Torsemide; torasemide (Demadex, other)	Loop diuretic	0.5 – 1 (up to 2?) mg/kg PO q12h (?)	5-, 10-, 20-, & 100-mg tablets	Titrate to lowest effective dosage for chronic therapy. Table 22.3	21, 22

Drug	Indications	Common Dosages	Formulations	Comments	See Chapter
Vasopressin (Pitressin, other)	Vasopressor agent	0.8 U/kg IV (or IO or IT) q4min	20-U/1-mL injection	Can use in place of (or sometimes with) epinephrine during CPR.	24
Verapamil (Calan, Isoptan)	Class IV antiarrhythmic	0.025–0.05 mg/kg IV q30min, up to 0.2 mg/kg total dose (diltiazem preferred)	2.5-mg/mL injection	Verapamil is *not recommended*, particularly if myocardial function is reduced; diltiazem should be used instead. Table 25.2	24, 25
Xylazine	Sedation, echo exam	200 mg IV for typical adult horse	100-mg/mL	Often used with detomidine	4

Some trade names noted in parentheses; other brands as well as generic products also might be available.

Abbreviations: AF, atrial fibrillation; BP, blood pressure; CHF, congestive heart failure; CPR, cardiopulmonary resuscitation; CRI, constant rate infusion; ECG, electrocardiogram; IM, intramuscularly; IO, intraosseous administration; IT, intratracheal administration (via a long catheter); IV, intravenous; PO, orally; SC, subcutaneously; US, United States.

INDEX

Note: Locators in *italics* represent figures and **bold** indicate tables in the text.

A

Abciximab, 765
Abdominal distension
    approach to patient, *271*
        diagnostic testing, 271–272
        muffled heart sounds, 270
        radiographs, 271
        ultrasonography, 271
    causes, **268**, 270
    effusions
        ascites, 267, 269–270
        feline infectious peritonitis, 270
        peritoneal effusion, 267, 270
Abdominojugular (hepatojugular) reflux test, 37, 264, 539, 715
Aberrant (retroesophageal) subclavian arteries, 517–518, *518*
Abnormal blood flow
    patterns, 120
    velocity, 120–121
Abnormal cardiac conduction, *see* Cardiac conduction, abnormal
Abnormal cardiac rhythms; *see also* Cardiac rhythm, *and* individual arrhythmias
    accelerated idioventricular rhythm, 149, *149*
    atrial fibrillation (AF), *146*, 146–147, *147*
    atrial flutter, 145–146, *146*
    atrial tachycardia, 145, *145*
    atrioventricular reentrant tachycardia, 147
    escape complexes and rhythms, 150–151, *151*
    isorhythmic atrioventricular dissociation, 150, *150*
    supraventricular premature complexes, 143–145
    ventricular fibrillation (VF), 150, *150*
    ventricular parasystole, 149–150
    ventricular premature complexes (VPCs), 147–148, *148*
    ventricular tachycardia, 148–149, *149*
Abnormal endothelial structure, 748
Abnormal flow pattern, pulmonary hypertension, 831, *853*
Abnormal fluid accumulation, 4, 42, *42*, 219
Abnormal heart rate; *see also* Heart rate
    approach to patient, *243*
        atropine challenge test, 244
        sinus bradycardia, 244
        smartphone ECG recording, 242, *244*
    arrhythmias
        rapid heart rate, 240–241
        slow heart rate, 241–242
    conduction disturbance, 239
    differential diagnoses, **238**
    impulse formation, 238–239
    sinoatrial block, 238
    sinus bradycardia and tachycardia causes, **238**
    VPCs, 240
ABP, *see* Arterial blood pressure
ABV, *see* Aortic balloon valvuloplasty
Accelerated idioventricular rhythm, 149, *149*, 423–424
ACDO, *see* Amplatz® Canine Duct Occluder
Acetylsalicylic acid, 764
Acoustic enhancement, 75
Acquired pericardial effusions, *see* Pericardial effusions
Actinomycosis, 711
Activated platelets, 746
Acute arterial embolization, 763
Acute arterial thromboembolic disease in cats, **756**
Acute CHF
    dogs and cats
        diastolic dysfunction, 347–348
        diuretic therapy, 341, 344
        inotropic support, 346–347
        management, **342–343**
        monitoring and initial follow-up, 348–349
        other therapies, 346
        oxygen supplementation and ventilation, 341
        vasodilator therapy, 344, **345–346**
    horses, 358–359
Acute coronary artery occlusions, 782
Acute hyperkalemia, 767
Acute hypoxia-induced, 819
Acute myocardial infarction, 313
Acute necrotizing pancreatitis, 749
Acute necrotizing pulmonary vasculitis, 818–819
Acute-onset respiratory difficulty, 823–824
Acute respiratory distress and inappetance, *821*
Adenosine, 386
Adenosine diphosphatase (ADPase), 747
ADPase, 747
ADP-induced platelet aggregation, 747
Adrenal-dependent hyperadrenocorticism, 791
Adrenergic drive, 225
Adrenergic receptors, 20, *20*, 26
Adrenomedullin, 308–309, 536
Advanced image analysis, 72, 130
Aelurostrongylus abstrusus, 823
Aerophagia, 270
Afferent arteriolar vasodilation, 310
Afterload, 16, 21, 80, 254–255, 303
Alabama rot, 782
Alanine aminotransferase (ALT), 757
Allometric scaling, 95–96, **97–98**

Alpha$_1$-adrenergic antagonists, 809
Alpha$_2$-antiplasmin, 747
Alveolar
  edema, 205–206
  hemorrhage, 819
  hypoventilation, 214, 220
  hypoxia, 820
Ambulatory ECG
  cardiac event recording, 162–163
  exercise, horses, 164–165
  Holter monitoring, 162, *163*
  smartphone and other wireless recording, 163–164
American and European Colleges of Veterinary Internal Medicine (ACVIM/ECVIM), 581
American College of Veterinary Internal Medicine (ACVIM) staging system, **311**, 313–314
Amiodarone, 382–383, 400, **403**, 407, 408, *408*, 409, *409*, 411, 412, 414, **414**, 415, 418, 424, *425*, *426*, 427, 428, 621, 629, 641
Amlodipine, *323*, 324, **342**, 344, **345**, 349, 350, 355, **355**, 356, 384, **804**, 805–809
Amplatz® Canine Duct Occluder (ACDO), 179–180, *180*, 181, *446*, 446–447
Anemia, 564–565
Angiocardiography, 722
  equipment and supplies
    contrast agents, 174–175
    power injector, 174
  nonselective *vs.* selective injection, 174
Angiostrongylus vasorum, 841, 848, 870
  clinical features, 871
  diagnostic tests, 871–873
  infection, 822–823
  larvae, 290
  management, 873
  pathophysiology, 870–871
  prevention, 873
  prognosis, 873
Angiotensins (Ang), 26, *26*, 29, *304*, 305, *305*, 306, *307*, 309
  converting enzyme inhibitors, *see* Angiotensin converting enzyme (ACE) inhibitors
  receptor blockers, *see* Angiotensin receptor blockers
Angiotensin converting enzyme (ACE) inhibitors, 29, *29*, 289, *304*, 305–306, **345**, 534, **555**, 556–562, 564, 621, **622**, 672, 674, 677, 682, 686–687, 703, 790, 803–807
  adverse effects, 321–322
  in heart failure treatment, 320–323, **345**, 349–350, 353, 359, **555**, 558–562, 563, 589, **622**, **673**, 674, 677, 682, 686–687, 703

  benazepril, 322
  captopril, 322–323
  enalapril, 322
  imidapril, 323
  lisinopril, 323
  lowering BP, 321
  ramipril, 323
  vasodilation, 321
  in systemic hypertension, 790, 803–807
  polymorphism, 321
Angiotensin receptor blockers (ARBs); *see also* Telmisartan, Valsartan
  cats, cardiomyopathy, 306
  in heart failure treatment, 332–333
  in systemic hypertension
    telmisartan, 803–804, **804**, 806–809
Angiotensin type 1 receptors (Ang1Rs), 29, 306–307, 321, *321*, *323*, 807
Anomalous coronary anatomy, 179, *490*, 491, *491*
ANP, *see* Atrial/A-type natriuretic peptide
Antiarrhythmic drugs; *see also* Individual drug listings
  adenosine, 386
  anticholinergics, *see* Anticholinergic drugs
  cardioversion, *see* Cardioversion
  class I
    cardiac Na+ channels, 374–375
    class Ic agents, 378–379
    lidocaine, 375–376
    mexiletine, 378
    phenytoin, 378
    procainamide, 376
    quinidine, 376–378
  classification
    modernized, 375, **375**
    traditional, 373, **374**
  class II
    atenolol, 380
    beta-receptor blockers, 379–380
    carvedilol, 331, 332, 334, **374**, 379, 381, 412, 621, 623, 624
    esmolol, 381
    metoprolol, 331, 332, **374**, 379, 380–381, **402**, 623
    propranolol, **374**, 376, 379, 380, 381, 382, 388, **402**, 408, *408*, **414**, *425*, 426, *426*, 472, **673**, **804**, 805, **806**, 809
    timolol, 381, 669
  class III
    amiodarone, 382–383
    dofetilide, 383–384
    dronedarone, 383
    ibutilide fumarate, 383
    sotalol, 381–382
    vernakalant, 384
  class IV

    dihydropyridine calcium channel-blockers, 384
    diltiazem, 384–385
    verapamil, 385
  defibrillation, 393
  digoxin, 385
  edrophonium, 388
  effects of, 373, *374*
  fish oil supplements, 386
  ivabradine, 385–386
  magnesium sulfate, 386
  pacing, *see* Pacing therapy
  phenylephrine, 388
  sympathomimetic drugs, *see* Sympathomimetic drugs
  vagal maneuver, 388, 399, 407, 408, 417, 418, 669
Antiarrhythmic drug therapy, 162, 201, 242, 397, 628; *see also* Individual drugs and arrhythmias
Anticholinergic drugs
  atropine response test, 387, 402, *404*, 405
  atropine and glycopyrrolate, 386–387, **403**
  hyoscyamine, 201, 387, **403**
  propantheline, 387, **403**
  scopalamine, 387, **403**
Anticoagulant drugs
  apixaban, 107, 356, 672, 676, **751**, 764, 766, 770, 782, 858, 867
  dalteparin, 672, **751**, 764, 765, 766
  enoxaparin, 672, **751**, 765, 766
  fondaparinux, **751**, 766
  heparin, 171, **221**, 530, 729, 748, 758, 764, 765, 767, 770, 782
  low molecular weight heparin, 672, 676, **763**, 765–766, **768**, 770, 862
  rivaroxaban, 107, 356, 672, 676, **751**, 764, 766, 770, 782, 858, 862
  unfractionated heparin, **751**, **763**, 765, **768**, 862
  warfarin, 379, **751**, 765, 766, 770, 782
Antidromic AVRT, 417
Antihypertensive agents, **804**, **806**, 809–810
  amlodipine, **804**, 808–809
  angiotensin converting enzyme inhibitors, **804**, 807
  angiotensin receptor blockers, **804**, 807–808
Antimicrobial therapy for endocarditis, 602
Antiplatelet and anticoagulant strategies, TE disease prophylaxis, 769–770
Antiplatelet substances, 747
Antiplatelet therapy, **763**, 764–765, **768**, 769
  aspirin, 454, 672, 764–765
  clopidogrel, 454, 672, 764
  other agents, 765
Antithrombin, 748–749

Antithrombotic drugs, **751**
Antithrombotic therapy, 763
  cats with cardiomyopathy, 356, 750
Antitussive therapy, 207, **208**
Aorta
  coarctation, 521, *523*
  dilation, 58, **58**, *59*
  enlargement, 84
  interruption, 521
  rupture of, 784
  tubular hypoplasia, 521
Aortic arch
  anomalies
    coarctation, 521, *523*
    interruption, aorta, 521
    truncus arteriosus communis, 520–521, *521–522*
    tubular hypoplasia, 521
  embryology and anatomy, 515
Aortic balloon valvuloplasty (ABV)
  HPB catheter sizing, 183
  left ventriculography, 182, *183*
  pigtail catheter, 182
  positioning, 182
  SAS, 181
Aortic dilation, 283, 784, 794
  aortocardiac and aortopulmonary fistulae, 522
  Marfan syndrome, 521
  severe aortic aneurysm, 521, *523*
Aortic regurgitation (AR), 591, 784
  horses, 586
  hyperkinetic pulses, 255
  murmurs, 230
Aortic stenosis (AS), 16, 95, 104, 113, 122
  clinical features, *478*, 481–482
  coronary perfusion, 481
  diagnostic tests
    aortic dilation, *485*
    aorto-septal angle, *486*, *486*
    cardiac catheterization and angiocardiography, 488, *488–489*
    color and spectral Doppler echo, *486*, 486–487, *487*
    grade 1 lesions, 484
    left ventricular and atrial enlargement, 482, *483*
    left ventricular (LV) hypertrophy, *484*
    M-mode imaging, 484, *485*
    muscle hyperechogenicity, 484, *485*
    post-stenotic dilation, ascending aorta, 482, *483*
    radiographic abnormalities, 482, **482**
    sinus rhythm, 482, *484*
    stroke volume, 487
    subaortic ridge, *485*
    ventricular tachyarrhythmias, 482, *484*
  fixed/anatomic obstruction, 480
  grades, 481
  management
    beta-adrenergic blockers, 489
    exercise restriction, 488
    prognosis, 489
    transcatheter balloon dilation, 489
  subvalvular narrowing, 480
  syncope and sudden death, 481
  valvular, 480
Aortic valve, 8
  afterload, 16
  degenerative disease, 230
  Doppler examination, 113
  endocarditis, 591, *593*, 593–601, *602*, 604
  HPB catheter sizing, 183
  M-mode echocardiography, **91**, 92
  regurgitation, 8, 228
  semilunar leaflets, 8
Aortocardiac and aortopulmonary fistulae, 522
Aortoiliac thrombosis, 191, 782
APCs, *see* Atrial premature complexes
Apixaban, 672, 676, **751**, 764, 766, 770, 858
Arginine vasopressin (AVP), 307–308, 310
Arrhythmias, 10–11, 706, 710
  cardiac and hemodynamic consequences
    atrioventricular synchrony, loss of, 369
    heart rate, effects of, 368
    ineffective atrial contraction, 368
    sustained ventricular tachycardia, *368*
    ventricular dyssynchrony, 369
  clinical causes and associations
    accelerated idioventricular rhythms, 370
    autonomic imbalance, 369
    familial ventricular arrhythmia, 371
    heart rhythm disturbances, 369
    lethal arrhythmia, 370, *371*
    predisposing factors, **370**
  electrophysiologic mechanism
    abnormalities, electrical impulse formation/conduction, 363-4, *364*
    bradyarrhythmia, 364
    enhanced and abnormal automaticity, 364
    preexcitation, 364
    reentry, 365–368
    triggered activity, 365, *365–366*
  heart sound alterations, 40
  norepinephrine (NE), 304
  rapid HR, 240–241
  slow HR, 241–242
  syncope associated, 167
  tachyarrhythmias, 562
Arrhythmogenic cardiomyopathy, 624, 686
Arrhythmogenic right ventricular cardiomyopathy (ARVC), 293, 374, 624–625
  cat
    clinical features, 686
    diagnostic tests, 686
    management, 687
    pathophysiology, 686
  dog
    clinical features, 626–627
    diagnostic tests, 627–628
    Holter monitoring, **625**
    management, 628–629
    pathophysiology, 625–626
Arterial baroreceptors (pressor receptors), 20, 28, *28*, 303, 305
Arterial blood gas analysis, 220, **220**
Arterial blood pressure (ABP), 23–24
Arterial embolic disease, 783
Arterial pulse
  abnormalities
    aortic input impedance, 254
    approach to patient, 257, *258*
    and associations, **254**
    asymmetrical/absent pulses, 257
    biventricular pulsus alternans, 257
    hyperkinetic pulses, 255
    hypokinetic pulses, 254–255
    premature beat, 256
    pulse deficits, 256, *256*
    pulsus paradoxus, 257
    right ventricular pulsus alternans, 257
    systemic arterial pulsus alternans, 257
    ventricular filling, 253
  evaluation of, 36, *36*
Arterial TE disease, 752
Arterial thromboemboli, 748
Arterial thromboembolism, 5, 119, 249, 752, 755, 770
  in cats, 755–756
  coronary thromboembolism, 757
  pulmonary thromboembolism, 757
  and thrombosis in dogs, 756–757
  venous thrombosis, 757
Arteriosclerosis
  atherosclerosis, 779, 779–780
  clinical features of, 780
  congenital dyslipidemia, 780
  in dogs, 779
  fibrinoid change with, 778
  intramural coronary arteriosclerosis, 780, 780
  medial hypertrophy of pulmonary arteries, 780
Arteriovenous (A-V)
  fistula, 88, 276, 278, 284
  malformations, 523, *524*
  shunts, 88, 214, 231
Arteriovenous fistula, 776
  clinical features, 776–777

diagnostic tests, 777–778
management, 778
pathophysiologic mechanisms and
clinical consequences, **777**, 777
pelvic limb edema, 778
Arthrocentesis, 596
ARVC, see Arrhythmogenic right ventricular
cardiomyopathy
AS, see Aortic stenosis
Ascites, 267, 269–270, 511, *512*, 715, 824
hepatic, 269
posthepatic, 269
prehepatic, 269–270
ASD, see Atrial septal defect
Ashman's phenomenon, 147
Aspartate aminotransferase (AST), 757
Aspirin, 356, 357, 439, 603, 671, 672, 675,
676, **751**, **763**, 764–765, 767,
769–770, 858, 862, 866
Asymmetrical/absent pulses, 257
Atenolol, 181, 289, 331, 332, 334, 347, 357,
374, **375**, 379, 380, 385, **402**, 407,
413, **414**, *425*, *426*, 427, 472, 489,
497, 498, *502*, 621, 630, 636, 654,
671, 672, **673**, 675, 676, 677, 682,
804, 804, 809
Atherosclerosis, 752, *779*, 779–780
Atrial appendage, 706
Atrial/A-type natriuretic peptide (ANP), 29,
291, 309
Atrial enlargement, 84
ECG, **157**
patterns, 156
Atrial fibrillation (AF), 283, 610
Ashman's phenomenon, 147
atrial enlargement, 241
cats, 410, 412–413
cat with cardiomyopathy, 146, *146*
components, 410
dogs, 410
Holter monitoring, 411
management, 411–412
horses, 147, 409–410, 413–416
management
cats, 410, 412–413
dogs, 411–412
horses, 413–416
paroxysmal, 410
Atrial flutter, 145–146, *146*, 409
Atrial hemangiosarcoma, 775
Atrial natriuretic peptide (ANP), 825
Atrial premature complexes (APCs), 407
Atrial/presystolic gallop, 232
Atrial rhythm disturbances
APCs, 407
atrial fibrillation management
cats, 412–413
dogs, 411–412
horses, 413–416
atrial flutter, 409

atrial standstill, *416*, 416–417
atrial tachycardia
paroxysmal (nonsustained), 407
sustained, 407–409
Atrial septal defect (ASD)
clinical features, **436**, 462
diagnostic tests, 462–464
foramen ovale, 461
fossa ovalis, 461
ostium primum, 461
ostium secundum, 462, *462*
septum primum, 461
septum secundum, 461
Atrial standstill, *416*, 416–417
Atrial tachyarrhythmia, 537
Atrial tachycardia, 145, *145*
paroxysmal (nonsustained), 407
sustained, 407–409
Atrioventricular (AV) block
1st and 2nd degree, *420*, 421
3rd degree, 152, *152*, 262,
420, 421, *421*
causes, 419
first-degree, 151, *151*
high-grade, 421–422
idiopathic, 242, 419
physiologic, 142
P-to-QRS interval, 153
second-degree, 151–152, *152*, 256
ventricular escape rhythm, 152, *152*
ventriculophasic sinus arrhythmia, 153
Atrioventricular conduction disturbances
first-degree AV block, 151, *151*
P-to-QRS interval, 153
second-degree AV block, 151–152, *152*
third-degree AV block, 152, *152*
ventricular escape rhythm, 152, *152*
ventriculophasic sinus arrhythmia, 153
Atrioventricular reentrant (reciprocating)
tachycardia (AVRT)
ablation, 418
antidromic, 417
intracardiac electrical mapping, 418, *418*
orthodromic, 417, *418*
vagal maneuver, 418
Atrioventricular septal defect (AVSD)
clinical features, 466–467
diagnostic tests, 467, *467*–*468*
management, 467
Atrioventricular synchrony, 369
Atrioventricular valve
mitral valve, 118
PW Doppler imaging, **115–116**, 118
regurgitation, 480
stenosis, 480
tricuspid valve, 118
Atropine challenge (response) test, 244,
387, 405
Atropine sulfate and glycopyrrolate,
386–387, **403**

Auscultation, 37–40, 657–659; see also
Respiratory auscultation
in cats, *39*, 39–40
congenital CV shunts, 233
in horses, 40, *40*
murmurs, 38–39
occlusion, nostril, 38, *39*
pericardial friction rubs, 233
sound alterations, 40
splitting, 233
stethoscope, 38, *38*
valve area location, 38, *39*
Auscultatory abnormality, 225–235, 824
Autonomic control, heart, 20–21
Autoregulation, 26
AV junctional rhythms
atrioventricular blocks, 419–422
digoxin toxicity, 419
isorhythmic AV dissociation, 419
"nodal" tachycardia, 419
AVRT, see Atrioventricular reentrant
(reciprocating) tachycardia
AVSD, see Atrioventricular septal defect
Azotemia, 289, 564, 757–758

B

Bacteremia, 591
Bacterial myocarditis, 639–640
Balloon catheter embolectomy, 782
Balloon dilation catheters, 177
Balloon pulmonary valvuloplasty (BPV), see
Pulmonary balloon valvuloplasty
(PBV)
Bartonella alpha Proteobacteria growth
medium (BAPGM), 598
Bartonella infection, 594–596
Base-apex lead, 138, *138*
Basketball-shaped cardiac silhouette, 716
Benazepril, 306, 319, 321, 322, 323, 333,
339, 340, **345**, 349, 356, 358, 359,
413, 534, 557, 558, 589, 621, 676,
703, 803, 804, **804**, 807, 808
Benign idiopathic pericarditis, 710, *711*, 723
Bernoulli relationship
clinical applications, 122, **123**
pulmonary and systemic hypertension,
126
shunts, 126–127
valve stenosis, gradients, and pressure
half-time, 124–125
valvular regurgitation, 125–126
Beta-adrenergic blockers, 379–381
in CHF, 331–332, *338*, 340, 350–351,
353–354, **355**, 357, 621–624,
629–630, 676
carvedilol, 332
metoprolol and atenolol, 332
sinus tachycardia, 401
Bilateral jugular thrombosis, 261

Bilateral jugular vein thrombosis, 757
Biventricular pulsus alternans, 257
Black widow spider envenomation, HT, 792
Bland emboli, 593
Blood flow velocity, 23, 113, 228
Blood pressure measurement, systemic hypertension
  direct measurement, 796
  Doppler method, 798–799
  indirect measurement, 796–799
  in normal animals, 787–788
  oscillometric method, 799
Blood urea nitrogen (BUN), 289
BNP, *see* B-type/brain natriuretic peptide
Boxers
  cardiac screening guidelines, **625**
  ECG, **627**
  M-mode echocardiogram, **628**
  multiform ventricular tachyarrhythmia, **627**
Bradyarrhythmias, 103, 197, 241, 244
Bradycardia, 140
  Holter monitoring, 162, *163*, 201
  ventricular enlargement, 284
Bradycardia–tachycardia syndrome, 241, *241*
Bradykinen, plasminogen activators, 747
Brain–heart syndrome, 634
Branham reflex, 777
Bronchial sounds, 41
Bronchiectasis, 61–62, 66, 203
Bronchoalveolar lavage cytology, pulmonary hypertension, 833
Bronchodilator drugs, 387
Bronchomalacia, 204, 206, 211
Bronchoscopy, pulmonary hypertension, 833
B-type/brain natriuretic peptide (BNP), 29–30, 291
Bubble study, 88
Butorphanol, 346

C

Canine distemper, 711–712
Canine heart
  cardiac apex, 47
  cardiac silhouette, 46, *47*
  narrow-chested and deep-chested dogs, 46, *48*
  VHS, 47–50
Canine hyperadrenocorticism, 823–824
Capillary refill time (CRT), 35–36
Captopril, 322–323, **345**, 635
Carboxyhemoglobinemia, 287
Cardiac amyloidosis, *700*
Cardiac anomalies, 707
Cardiac arrhythmias, 10–11, 40
  atrial rhythm disturbances, *see* Atrial rhythm disturbances

AV junctional rhythms
  atrioventricular blocks, 419–422
  digoxin toxicity, 419
  isorhythmic AV dissociation, 419
  "nodal" tachycardia, 419
AVRT, *see* Atrioventricular reentrant (reciprocating) tachycardia
  decision to treat, 399–400
  intermittent, 162
  jugular pulse waves, 262
  patient assessment, 397–398, **398**
  rhythm diagnosis, 398–399, *399*
  sinus rhythm disturbances
    sinus bradycardia, 401–402, **402–404**, *404*
    sinus node dysfunction, 405–406
    sinus tachycardia, 401
  supportive measures, 400–401
  ventricular rhythm disturbances, *see* Ventricular rhythm disturbances
Cardiac biomarkers
  natriuretic peptides, 291–293
  troponins, 290–291
Cardiac cachexia, *35*, 312, *312*, 565–566, *611*, 716
Cardiac catheterization; *see also* Angiocardiography; Interventional procedures
  equipment
    hemodynamic monitoring, 169–170
    imaging, 168–169
    needles, sheaths, catheters, and wires, 170–172
  laboratory, *168*
  patient preparation, 172
  preparation and planning, 167–168
  vascular access, 172–173
Cardiac chamber measurement
  cats, 95
  enlargement, *see* Chamber enlargement
  issues, 95
  methods, 95
Cardiac conduction, abnormal
  atrioventricular, 151–153
  intraatrial, 153
  intraventricular, 153
  ventricular preexcitation, 153–155
Cardiac electrophysiology
  arrhythmias, 10–11
  depolarization, 10
  fast-response action potential, 11–12
  resting membrane potential, 11
  slow-response action potential, 12
Cardiac energy supply, 21
Cardiac hemangiosarcoma, *715*
Cardiac lesions
  echocardiography, 82, 84
  pathophysiologic abnormalities, 300
Cardiac murmurs, 596, 756; *see also* Murmurs

Cardiac output (CO), 15
Cardiac pacing
  complications, 177
  lead positioning and placement, 175–176
  lead tips, 175, *175*
  passive and active fixation, 175, *175*
  temporary, 176–177
Cardiac radiography
  additional assessment methods, 50
  additional imaging modalities, 66–67
  canine heart, 46–50
  cardiomegaly, 51–52
  chamber enlargement patterns, 52–57
  equine thoracic radiography, 66, *66–67*
  feline heart, 50–51
  intrathoracic blood vessels
    aorta, 58
    lobar pulmonary arteries and veins, 58–61
    main pulmonary artery, 58
    vena cava, 61
  patient positioning, 46
  pleural space
    pleural effusion, 64–66
    pneumothorax, 66
  pulmonary parenchyma
    patterns, 61–62
    pulmonary edema, 62–64
  small cardiac silhouette, 52
  systematic evaluation, 46
  technique considerations, 46
Cardiac resynchronization therapy, 334
Cardiac rhythm; *see also* Abnormal cardiac rhythms
  sinus arrhythmia, 143, *143*
  sinus pause/arrest, 143, *143*
  sinus rhythm and variations, 142–143, *143*
Cardiac silhouette, 706, 708
Cardiac-specific isoenzyme of CK (CK-MB), 758
Cardiac sphericity index, 50
Cardiac tamponade, 705, 708, 713, *715*, 716, *724*, *740*
  cardiac chamber size, 721
  characterized, 721
  right-sided congestive signs, *718*
Cardiac troponins (cTns), 290–291, 535–536, 578, 661, 705, 758
Cardiac tumors, 705
  clinical features, 734–735
  diagnostic tests, 735–740, *735–741*
  in dogs, **732**
  management, 740–742
  occurrence rate, **733**
  pathophysiology, 733–734, *733–735*
Cardiogenic pulmonary edema, *see also* Congestive heart failure *and relevant diseases*
  coughing, 203, 205

cats, 64, *64*
dogs, 62, *62*
horses, *67*
pulmonary veins and arteries enlargement, 61
Cardiogenic shock
  acute myocardial infarction, 313
  definition, 313
Cardiomegaly, 51–52, 826
  aorta dilation, 106
  aortic/pulmonary artery dilation, 283
  approach to patient, 284, *285*
  chamber enlargement, 282–283
  chronic hyperthyroidism, *283*
  eccentric hypertrophy, 283
  endocrinopathies, 283
  precordial impulse, 37
  valvular regurgitation, 283
Cardiomyopathy, 7, 283, 750; *see also* Arrhythmogenic right
Cardiomyopathy of nonspecific phenotype, 687
Cardiopulmonary baroreceptors, 28–29
Cardiopulmonary resuscitation, 428, **429**
Cardiorenal syndrome, 310, 564
Cardiovascular (CV) examination
  heart disease and failure, clinical signs, 33, 35, **35**
  medical history, 33, **34**
  observation, patient, 35
  physical examination
    abnormal fluid accumulation, 42, *42*
    arterial pulses, 36, *36*
    cardiac auscultation, 37–40
    jugular veins, 36–37, *37*
    mucous membrane, 35–36, *36*
    precordial palpation, 37
    respiratory auscultation, 40–42
Cardiovascular malformations; *see also* specific other congenital malformations
  aortic arch anomalies
    coarctation, 521, *523*
    interruption, aorta, 521
    truncus arteriosus communis, 520–521, *521–522*
    tubular hypoplasia, 521
  aortic dilation
    aortocardiac and aortopulmonary fistulae, 522
    Marfan syndrome, 521
    severe aortic aneurysm, 521, *523*
  arteriovenous, 523, *524*
  cor triatriatum sinister
    clinical features, 512
    diagnostic tests, 514
    embryological origin, 512
    management, 514
  CTD, *see* Cor triatriatum dexter
  endocardial fibroelastosis, 515
  portosystemic vascular anomalies, 523–524
  vascular developmental considerations
    aortic arch embryology and anatomy, 515
    venous embryology and anatomy, 515–516
  vascular ring, *see* Vascular ring anomalies
  venous, *see* Venous malformations
Cardiovascular–renal axis disorders (CvRDs), 310
Cardiovascular responses, stress and exercise, 30
Cardiovascular (CV) system
  cardiac electrophysiology, 10–12
  cardiac energy supply, 21
  circulation, 22–30
  conduction system, 9–10
  heart
    autonomic control, 20–21
    external features, 3–6
    internal features, 6–9
    as pump, 14–20
  myocardial contraction, 12–14
  responses, stress and exercise, 30
Cardioversion
  direct current (DC) shock, 391
  horses, 392, *392*
  intracardiac electrical mapping and catheter ablation, 392–393
Carotid arterial access, 173
Carvedilol, 332, 381
Cat
  arterial thromboembolism in, 755–756
  ARVC
    clinical features, 686
    diagnostic tests, 686
    management, 687
    pathophysiology, 686
  DCM
    clinical features, 682
    diagnostic tests, 683–685
    echocardiographic image, *685*
    management, 685–686
    M-mode images, *684*
    nonselective angiocardiogram, *685*
    pathophysiology, 682
    ventricular dimensions, *684*
  Dirofilaria immitis, 866–867
  HCM, 649–651
    acute congestive heart failure, 673–675
    auscultation, 657–659
    cardiac morphologic abnormalities, 652–653
    chronic heart failure, 675–678
    clinical cardiomyopathy, **650**
    clinical features, 656–660
    congestive heart failure, 659–660
    diagnostic tests, 660–671
    echocardiography, 664–671
    electrocardiography, 663–664
    histopathologic section, *653*
    history, 657
    laboratory tests, 660–661
    large thrombi, *652*
    lung ultrasound image, *665*
    management, 671–678
    myocardial functional/hemodynamic abnormalities, 653–656
    open left ventricle, *652*
    pathogenesis, 651–653
    POC thoracic ultrasound, 674
    preclinical disease, 671–672
    prognosis, 672–673
    radiography, 661–663
    refractory pulmonary edema, 675
    respiratory distress, *673*
    screening, 656–657
    septal hypertrophy, *667*
    sinus rhythm, *664*
    suspect cardiomyopathy, *658*
    treatment, **673**
  with myocardial disease, 750
  myocarditis, 689–691, *690*
  secondary myocardial diseases
    anemia, 689
    cardiac hypertrophy, 689
    causes, 688–689
    corticosteroid-associated congestive heart failure, 689
    hyperthyroidism, *688*, 688–689
    pressure overload, 688
Catecholamine-associated myocardial disease, 634–635
Catecholamines, heart failure treatment
  dobutamine, 330
  dopamine, 330
Catheter-based procedure, 765
Catheters, 170–171, *171*, 172
Caudal lobar vessels, 60
Caudal vena cava, 119
  anomalies, 526, *526*
  thrombosis, 754
Caval syndrome, 846
  Dirofilaria immitis, 863–866
Caval thrombosis, 277, *277*
Cavity effusions, echocardiography, 82
CDI, *see* Color Doppler imaging
Central cyanosis, 215, 249
Central venous pressure (CVP), 25
  and cardiac output, 261
  measurement, 264–265, *266*
Central venous pressure and right heart catheterization, 722
Cerebral blood flow and BP, 794

Chagas disease, 723
Chamber enlargement
    allometric scaling, 95–96, **97–98**
    atrial, 156
    canine breed-specific M-mode measurements, **100–101**
    canine echocardiographic left atrial and ventricular dimensions, **97**
    clinical associations, **157**
    equine echocardiographic measurements, **99**
    feline echocardiographic measurements, **98**
    feline M-mode and 2D echocardiographic measurements, **101–102**
    left atrial and left ventricular to aortic ratios, 95, **96**
    ventricular, 156
Chemodectoma, 711, 784
Chest percussion, 42, *42*, 219
Chest trauma, 711
CHF, *see* Congestive heart failure
CHF management
    acute decompensated CHF, *see* Acute CHF
    approach, 337, *338*
    cats
        ACE inhibitors, 356
        clopidogrel, 356
        diastolic dysfunction, 357
        dietary and other recommendations, 357
        monitoring and follow-up, 357–358
        pimobendan, 356–357
        refractory CHF, 358
    dogs
        diastolic dysfunction, 353
        dietary considerations, 351–352
        drug therapy, 350–351
        exercise, 352–353
        monitoring and follow-up, **353**, 353–354
        pimobendan, 349
        quad therapy, 349
        RAAS inhibition, 349
        refractory CHF, 354–356
    horses
        acute CHF, 358–359
        ongoing therapy, 359
    preclinical heart disease
        ACE inhibitor therapy, 340
        beta-blocker therapy, 339
        cats, 340
        horses, 340
        initial signs, CHF, 340
        pimobendan, 339
        routine health maintenance regimen, 337
    RRR monitoring, 338, **339**
Chlorothiazide, 320, **345**
Chordal rupture, 562
Chronically elevated pulmonary venous pressure, 819
Chronic bronchitis, *204*, 206
Chronic cadmium exposure, HT, 792
Chronic interstitial pulmonary fibrosis, 564
Chronic thrombophlebitis, *783*
Chronic upper airway obstruction, 820
Chronic uremia, *712*
Chylous abdominal effusion, 270
Chylous pericardial effusion, 712
Circulation
    control
        hormonal (humoral) factors, 29–30
        local (intrinsic) control, 26–27
        neurohormonal (extrinsic) control, 27
        vascular receptors, 27–28
        vascular reflexes, 28–29
    hemodynamic concepts, 22–23
    vasculature, 23–25
Circumcaval ureter, 526, *526*
Clindamycin, 602
Clinical laboratory abnormalities
    approach to patient, 293–294
    cardiac biomarkers
        natriuretic peptides, 291–293, 535–536, 541, 612, 613, 616, 655, 656, 660, 661, **697**, 716, 789, 790, 819, 825
        troponins, 290–291, 535, 541, 612, 616, 631, 637, 655, 697, 701, 703, 705, 800, 825, 836
    CBC, 287–289
    CV system, **288**
    D-dimer tests, 293, 758
    endocrine testing, 293
    serum biochemistries, 289–290
    tests for parasites, 290
    urinalysis, 290
Clopidogrel, 107, 671–672, **673**, *751*, 764–765, 769–770, 675–678
Clotting factors, 745
Coagulation cascade, 745–746, *747*
Coagulopathy, 711
Coarctation, aorta, 521, *523*
Coccidioidomycosis, 711, 723
Collagen-bound von Willebrand factor (vWF), 746
Color (flow) Doppler imaging (CDI)
    CW Doppler imaging, 112, 177
    TDI, 112–113
Color flow mapping, *see* Color Doppler imaging
Common arterial trunk, *see* Truncus arteriosus communis
Complete (third-degree) AV block, 284, 421–422
Complete blood count (CBC), 660
    anemia, 287
    eosinophils, 288, *288*
    erythrocytosis, 287–288, *288*
    leukocytosis, 288
    neutrophilia, 288
    RDW, 288
    thombocytopenia, 289
Computed tomography (CT) imaging, 66–67
Concentric hypertrophy, 17, 56, 104, 156, 301
Conduction system, 9–10, *10*
Congenital cardiac shunts
    ASD, *see* Atrial septal defect
    AVSD, *see* Atrioventricular septal defect
    breed predispositions, 435, **436**
    cats, 436
    CV shunts, 233
    murmur intensity (loudness), 436
    patent foramen ovale, 465–466
    pathophysiology
        left-to-right shunting, 437, *437*
        right-to-left shunting, 437–439
    PDA
        classification, 439–440
        clinical features, 441–442
        diagnostic tests, 442–444, *445*
        ductus diverticulum, 439, *440*
        management, 444, 446–449
    rASD, *see* Reversed ASD
    rPDA, *see* Reversed PDA
    rVSD, *see* Reversed ventricular septal defect
    tetralogy of Fallot, 467–472
    VSD, *see* Ventricular septal defect
Congenital dyslipidemia, *780*
Congenital pericardial malformations, 706, *707*
Congenital valvular malformations
    AS, *see* Aortic stenosis
    breed predispositions, **478**
    mitral dysplasia, *see* Mitral valve dysplasia
    pathophysiology
        atrioventricular valve regurgitation, 480
        atrioventricular valve stenosis, 480
        semilunar valve regurgitation, 479, *479*
        ventricular outflow obstruction, 478–479
    PS, *see* Pulmonic stenosis
    tricuspid dysplasia, 504–508
Congestive heart failure (CHF), 705; *see also* Heart failure
    acute, *see* Acute CHF
    consequences, 33
    dog, 591, 608
    drugs, *see* Drugs, heart failure treatment
    FAST scans, 82
    and gallop sound, 232
    horse, 703

initial signs, 340
management, *see* CHF management
presenting signs, 312–313
ring-down artifacts, 80
and subcutaneous edema, 276
VHS, 50
Conotruncal defects, 467
Constant rate infusion (CRI), 602
Constrictive pericardial disease, 710
clinical features, 730
diagnostic tests, 730–732
Labrador Retriever with, *731*
management, 732
pathophysiology, 730
Continuity relationship
blood flow velocity, 23
LVOT stenosis estimation, 124
and stenosis, 122
Continuous (machinery) murmurs, 231, 442
Continuous wave (CW) Doppler imaging, *111*, 112
Contractility/myocardial failure, 15, 300
Contrast 2D echocardiography, 88
Convulsive syncope, 195
Coronary artery disease, HT, 794
Coronary artery thromboembolism, 753
Coronary blood flow, 21, 127
Coronary thromboembolism, 757
Cor pulmonale, 816–817, 820, 824
Corticosteroids, 603, 750
Cor triatriatum, 511
Cor triatriatum dexter (CTD), 480
clinical features
distended abdominal veins, 511, *512*
persistent ascites, 511, *512*
diagnostic tests
ascites, 511, *512*
caudal vena caval angiocardiogram, *513*
dilated caudal right atrial chamber and caudal vena, *513*
Doppler studies, 511, *513*
right-to-left shunting, 511–512
management, 512, *514*
Cor triatriatum sinister, 480
clinical features, 512
diagnostic tests, 514
embryological origin, 512
management, 514
Corynebacterium spp., 712
Cough
approach to patient
alveolar edema, 205–206
antitussive therapy, 207, **208**
determination, **206**, *207*
fulminant pulmonary edema, 206
gagging/retching, 205
laryngeal paresis, 206
thoracic radiographs, 206–207
cats, 205

causes, 203, **204**
chronic bronchitis, *204*
hemoptysis, 203
horses, 205
inflammation, 203, *204*
nonproductive/dry, 203
syncope, 199
Crackles, 41
Cranial caval syndrome, 277, *277*
Cranial lobar vessels, 59
Cranial mediastinal lymphoma, 277
Cranial mesenteric artery, *781*
Cranial vena cava (CaVC), 61, *61*
Cranial vena caval thrombosis, 754, 758
Creatine kinase (CK) activities, 757
CRT, *see* Capillary refill time
CTD, *see* Cor triatriatum dexter
Cutaneous hemangiomas, 784
Cutting balloon (CB) procedure, 181–183
CVP, *see* Central venous pressure
Cyanosis
categories, 249
central, 215
differential, 249, 252
hemoglobin oxygen saturation, 247
peripheral, 215, 249
Cytokines and inflammation, 308

D

DADs, *see* Delayed afterdepolarizations
Dalteparin, **751**, 764–766
DCM, *see* Dilated cardiomyopathy
DCRV, *see* Double chambered right ventricle
D-dimers, 747
assays, 758
tests, 293
Defibrillation, 393
Defective fibrinolysis, 749
Degenerative mitral valve disease (DMVD)
in dogs, 107, 203–204, 287, 289, 301, 592, 636, 815
characteristics, 529
CHF onset (stage C management)
end-stage, 561
guidelines, **555**
heart failure therapy monitoring, 561
mild to moderate signs, 559–560
severe signs, 560
transition to home care, 560–561
clinical features
complicating factors, 540, **540**
genome-wide association studies, 538
MR murmur, 537–538
physical findings, 538–540
clinical signs
gallop sounds, 539
MR murmur, 537–538
systolic click, 539, *539*

complicating factors, 540, **540**
complications and comorbid conditions
abnormal blood pressure, 564
arrhythmias, 562
chronic respiratory disease, 563–564
left atrial tears, 562–563
pulmonary hypertension, 561–562
renal dysfunction, 564–565
ruptured chordae tendineae, 562
diagnostic tests
clinical laboratory tests, 540–541
echocardiography, 545–546
electrocardiography, 545, *545*
left heart evaluation, 546–554
radiography, 541–545
right heart evaluation, 554
systemic vascular function, 554
diagnostic tests, left heart evaluation
color-flow Doppler imaging, 549–550, *550–551*
CW Doppler, *551*, 551–552
dilated LV, *549*
echocardiography, 546–547
EROA, 551
flail chorda tendinea, *547*
LVIDdN, 548
minimal left atrial enlargement, *547*
mitral prolapse, 546, *546*
M-mode echocardiogram, *549*
PISA method, 551
PW Doppler, 552, *552–553*
severe left atrial enlargement, *548*
smooth thickening, 546
stage C, DMVD, *547*, *551*
strain (deformation) imaging, 549
dogs
ACE inhibitors, 339
pimobendan, 339
histologic grading system, 533, **533**
management
guidelines, **555–556**
stage B1, 554, **555**, 556
stage B2, **555**, 556–558
mitral valve repair and interventions, 561
normal mitral valve, 529–530, *530*
pathophysiology
diastolic function, 535
exosomal miRNA expression levels, 531
LA enlargement, 536, *536*
management guidelines, **555–556**
miRNAs dysregulation, 531
myocardial and chamber remodeling, 534–537
myxomatous valvular degeneration, 530
papillary muscle fibrosis, 536
post-capillary PH, 537
proteomic studies, 531

pulmonary arterial pressure, 537
reduced gene expression, 531
valvular changes, 531–534
vascular endothelial function and
vasodilatory responses, 537
preclinical (stage B management)
stage B1, 554, **555**, 556
stage B2, **555**, 556–558
prognosis, 565–566
Delayed afterdepolarizations (DADs), 365, *365*
Device-associated infection, 591
Diabetes mellitus, 791
Diastolic dysfunction, 127, 301
grade 1, **128**, 129
grade 2, **128**, 129
grade 3, **128**, 129
grade 4, **128**, 129
heart failure, dogs and cats, 347–348
management
cats, 357
dogs, 353
Diastolic heart failure, 17
Diastolic murmurs, 230–231, 579, *579*
Diastolic pressure, 23–24
DIC, see Disseminated intravascular coagulation
Dietary considerations, CHF management
cats, 357
dogs, 351–352
Differential cyanosis, 249, 252
Digital subtraction angiography, 174, *174*
Digoxin, **343**, **346**, 347, 348, 349, 350, **353**, 354, **355**, 356, 358, **370**, 373, **374**, **375**, 376, 377, 378, 384, 401, **404**, 406, 407, 408, *409*, 411–413, **414**, 418, 419, 422, 424, 426
antiarrhythmic effect, 385
DMVD, dogs, 559
heart failure treatment
management, toxicity, 328, 330
serum digoxin concentration, 328
toxicity, 327–328, *329*
Dihydropyridine calcium channel-blockers, 384
Dilated bronchi (bronchiectasis), abnormally, 61
Dilated cardiomyopathy (DCM), 104, 107, *189*, 283, *302*, 607, 716
cat
clinical features, 682
diagnostic tests, 683–685
echocardiographic image, *685*
management, 685–686
M-mode images, *684*
nonselective angiocardiogram, *685*
pathophysiology, 682
ventricular dimensions, *684*
dog
diagnostic tests

echocardiography in preclinical DCM, 614–616
electrocardiography in preclinical DCM, 613–614
histopathology, 610
overt (clinical) DCM, 616–621
preclinical (occult), 612
management
overt (clinical) DCM, 622–624
preclinical (occult), 621–622
prognosis in overt DCM, 624
Diltiazem, 357, **374**, **375**, 384–385, **403**, 406, 407, 408, *408*, *409*, 411–412, *418*, **622**, 623, 624, 630, 672, **673**, 675, 676, 682
Dirofilaria immitis, 822; see also Heartworm
adult heartworms, 842
alveolar hypoxia, 844
caval syndrome, *852*
chronic hepatic congestion, 844
classification, severity in dogs, **858**
clinical features
cats, 846
dogs, 846
diagnostic tests, 850–856
heartworm-induced pulmonary hypertension, *852*
HW-associated respiratory disease (HARD), 844
infected pulmonary arteries, 843, *843*
interstitial pulmonary infiltrates, *855*
life cycle, 841–842
management
alternatives to melarsomine adulticide therapy, 860
in cats, 866–867
caval syndrome, 863–866
complicated heartworm disease in dogs, 860–861
doxycycline and macrocyclic lactone therapy, 856–858
exercise restriction, 856
melarsomine treatment, 858–859
microfilaricide therapy, 862–863
postadulticide pulmonary thromboembolism, 861–862
pretreatment assessment, 856
microfilariae, **849**, 850
Modified Knott Test Method, **849**
occult heartworm disease, *851*
opened right ventricular outflow region, *842*
pathophysiology, 843–846
prevention
in cats, 870
in dogs, 867–869
testing, 846–850, *847*, *851*
transmission, 841–843
tricuspid regurgitation (TR), 844

tunica media, hypertrophy, *845*
villous proliferation, 843–844
Wolbachia bacteria, 843
Dirofilaria immitis microfilariae, 290
Dirofilaria repens, 711
Dirty procedures, 591
Discrete interventricular septal hypertrophy (DISH), 669
Discrete upper septal thickening (DUST), 669
DISH, see Discrete interventricular septal hypertrophy
Disseminated intravascular coagulation (DIC), 289, 597, 749
Distal aortic embolization, 755
Distal aortic thromboembolism, 767
Diuretics, 835–836
furosemide
dosage, 317–318
RAAS activation, 318–319
torsemide, 319
spironolactone, 319–320
thiazides, 320
Diuretic therapy, 289–290
DMVD, see Degenerative mitral valve disease
Doberman Pinschers
atrial fibrillation, *611*
DCM, 608
ESVC cardiac screening guidelines, **612**
pulmonary edema, *617–618*
Dobutamine, 330, 334, **343**, **346**, 347, 358, 380, 384, 401, **403**, **404**, 411, 422, 487, **555**, 560, 616, **622**, **673**, 674, 685
Dofetilide, 383–384
Dogs
arterial thromboembolism and thrombosis in, 756–757
arteriosclerosis in, *779*
ARVC
clinical features, 626–627
diagnostic tests, 627–628
Holter monitoring, **625**
pathophysiology, 625–626
atrial fibrillation (AF), 410–412
atrial rhythm disturbances, 411–412
cardiac tumors in, **732**
cardiogenic pulmonary edema, 62, *62*
complicated heartworm disease in, 860–861
congestive heart failure (CHF), 349–353, 591, 608
degenerative mitral valve disease (DMVD), 339
diagnostic tests, DCM, 612–621
echocardiography in preclinical DCM, 614–616
electrocardiography in preclinical DCM, 613–614

histopathology, 610
overt (clinical) DCM, 616-621
diastolic dysfunction, 353
dilated cardiomyopathy (DCM), 610-621
Dirofilaria immitis, 846, 867-869
drug therapy, 350-351
HCM, 629
    clinical features, 629-630
    diagnostic tests, 630
    management, 630
    pathophysiology, 629
herniated viscera in, 707
hyperthyroidism, 564-565
hypertrophic cardiomyopathy (HCM), 629-630
idiopathic pericardial effusion in, 711-712
management, DCM
    overt (clinical) DCM, 622-624
    preclinical (occult), 621-622
    prognosis in overt DCM, 624
myocardial disease, 607-615
myocarditis, 603
nonpathologic murmurs, 228
refractory CHF, 354-356
retinopathy, hypertensive, 793
secondary myocardial diseases
    causes, **631**
    doxorubicin toxicity, 631-632, *632*
    hypothyroidism, 635
    metabolic abnormalities, 632-636
    nonneoplastic, 635
    nutritional deficiencies, 632-636
    tachycardia-induced cardiomyopathy, 630-631
Domestic Longhair cats, 708
Domestic Shorthair cat, *662-664, 666, 668, 670, 673*
    atrial enlargement, *666*
    cardiac enlargement, *683*
    ECG, *664*
    echocardiographic images, *668*
    lung ultrasound image, *665*
    mitral leaflets, *666*
    parasternal long-axis image, *670*
    respiratory distress, *673*
    restrictive cardiomyopathy, *681*
    septal hypertrophy, *668*
    thoracic radiographs, *662-663, 680*
Dopamine, 330, **343, 346**, 347, 380, 384, *404*, 417, 422, **555**, 685
Doppler echocardiography; *see also* Color Doppler imaging
assessment
    ventricular diastolic function, 127, **128**, 129
    ventricular systolic function, 127
atrial function, 119
Bernoulli relationship, 122-127
blood flow observations, 114
diagnosis principles
    abnormal blood flow patterns, 120
    abnormal blood flow velocity, 120-121
examination, 113-114
hepatic veins and caudal vena cava, 119
jet/turbulence, 122
modalities
    PW Doppler, 112
    signal alias, 112
PISA, 121-122
presentation formats, 113
principles
    Doppler equation, 108
    Doppler shifts, 108
    spectral Doppler echocardiography, 108, *109-111*
pulmonary venous flow, 118-119
PW Doppler variables, 114, **115-116**
semilunar valves, 114, 117
TDI, *see* Tissue Doppler imaging
vena contracta, 122
Doppler equation, 108
Doppler method, systemic hypertension, 798-799
Double aortic arch, 516, *517*
Double chambered right ventricle (DCRV), *491*, 491-492
Doxorubicin, 607, 631-632, *632*
Doxycycline, 603
    Dirofilaria immitis, 856-858
    and macrocyclic lactone therapy, 856-858
Dronedarone, 383
Drug effects, ECG, **159**
    hyperkalemia, 160-161
    hypokalemia, 161
    hypomagnesemia, 159
Drugs, heart failure treatment
    ACE inhibitors, *see* Angiotensin converting enzyme
    angiotensin receptor blockade and natriuretic peptide potentiation, 332-334
    beta-blockers, 331-332
    diuretics
        furosemide, 317-319
        spironolactone, 319-320
        thiazides, 320
    positive inotropic agents
        catecholamines, 330
        digoxin, 327-330
        phosphodiesterase-3 inhibitors, 330-331
        pimobendan, 325-327
    sildenafil, 331
    vasodilators
        amlodipine, *323*, 324
        hydralazine, 323-324
        nitrates, 324-325
        prazosin, 324
Duchenne's cardiomyopathy, 607
Ductal occlusion, PDA
    ACDO, *446*, 446-447
    changes and prognosis, 448-449
    complications, 447
    surgical, 447-448
    transcatheter, 446-447
DUST, *see* Discrete upper septal thickening
Dyspnea, 211, 705

E

EADs, *see* Early afterdepolarizations
Early afterdepolarizations (EADs), 365, *366*
Eccentric hypertrophy, 16, 104, 283, 695
ECG, *see* Electrocardiography
Echocardiography; *see also* Doppler echocardiography; M-mode echocardiography; Two-dimensional (2D) echocardiography
acquired pericardial effusions, 717-722, *719-721*
cardiac chamber
    measurement, 95-102
    size and clinical decision-making, 107
cardiac lesions, 82, 84
cardiac size and function measurement, 93-95
in cat, HCM, 664-671
cavity effusions, 82
contrast 2D, 88
degenerative valvular disease, dog, 545-547
Doppler, *see* Doppler echocardiography
equine myocardial disease, 702-703, *703*
equine valvular disease, 581-586
examination, *see* Echo examination
great vessels, 106-107
guidelines and pitfalls, 74-75
hypertrophic cardiomyopathy (HCM), 664-671
image artifacts, 79-80
image planes and display, 75-79
image properties, 75
imaging technique, 81-82
infective endocarditis, *599-602*
left atrium, M-mode, 92
left ventricular size and function, 104-106
M-mode, *see* M-mode echocardiography
M-mode, aortic valve, **91**, 92
myocardial disease, *609*
patent ductus arteriosus (PDA), 444, *444-446*
patient preparation, 80
physics and terminology, 72-73, *73*
in preclinical dilated cardiomyopathy (DCM), 614-616

pulmonary balloon valvuloplasty (PBV), 177
pulmonary hypertension, 827–833
reversed PDA (rPDA), 451, *452*
right atrial and ventricular size and function, 106
sedation, 80–81
syncope, 201
systemic hypertension, 800–802, *801–802*
TEE, 129–130
transducer characteristics, 73–74
transthoracic, 177
two-dimensional, *see* Two-dimensional (2D) echocardiography
ventricular septal defect (VSD), 457, *457–459*
Echo examination
 cardiac lesions, 82, 84
 cardiac size and function, 84
 pulmonary imaging and cavity effusions, 82
 questions, 82, **83**
Echogenicity, 75
Ectopic tachycardia, 239
Ectopic thyroid carcinoma, 711
Edema, 775
 and cutaneous ulcers, *786*
Edrophonium, 388, **404**, 408
Effective regurgitant orifice area (EROA), 548, 551
Ehrlichia canis, 781
Eisenmenger's (patho)physiology, 816
Ejection fraction (EF), 612
Ejection sounds, 232
Electrical–mechanical coupling, 13–14
Electrocardiography (ECG)
 abnormalities and considerations
  drugs and electrolyte, effect of, **159**, 159–161
  electrical alternans, 157
  QT interval, **158**, 158–159
  small-voltage QRS complexes, 157
  ST-T abnormalities, 157–158
 ambulatory, *see* Ambulatory ECG
 artifacts, 161, *161–162*
 cardiac chamber enlargement
  atrial, 156
  clinical associations, **157**
  ventricular, 156
 cardiac rhythm assessment
  abnormal cardiac conduction, 151–155
  abnormal cardiac rhythms, 143–151
  sinus rhythm and variations, 142–143
 interpretation, **140**
  heart rhythm, 140–142
  HR, 139–140
 lead systems, **136**, 136–138
 MEA, 155, *156*
 measurements, 142
 normal waveforms, **136**
 in preclinical DCM, 613–614
 pulmonary hypertension, 827
 QRS complex, 135
 recording
  base-apex, 139
  electrode placement, 138, *139*
  patient positioning, 138, *138*
Electrolyte abnormalities, 723
Electrolytes, 289–290
Embolic disease, 706
Enalapril, 322, 323, *329*, **342**, **345**, 349, 359, *409*, *442*, 557, 558, 676, 703, 803, **804**, 807, *808*
Endocardial fibroelastosis, 515
Endocarditis, 290, 591
Endocrine testing, 293
Endocrinopathies, 193, 791
Endothelial-mediated regulation, 27
Endothelial-produced protein S, 748
Endothelial prostacyclin synthesis, 747
Endothelin (ETN), 293, 308, 790
End-systolic volume index (ESVI), 549
Enlargement, aorta, 84
Enoxaparin, **751**, 765–766
Enrofloxacin, 603
Enterococcus faecalis, 712
Entrance block, 149
Epinephrine, 387–388
Episodic weakness, 199
E-point to septal separation (EPSS), 90, *92*
Equine Herpes Virus, 712
Equine Influenza Virus, 712
Equine myocardial disease
 causes, 695–696, **696**
 clinical manifestations, **697**
 echocardiography, 702–703, *703*
 electrocardiography, 702, *702*
 idiopathic dilated cardiomyopathy, 698–699, *699*
 infiltrative cardiomyopathy, 699
 ischemic myocardial disease, 699–700
 management, 703
 myocardial necrosis, *698*
 myocardial toxicity, 698, *698*
 pathophysiology, 696–697
 TICM, 699, *699*
Equine thoracic radiography, 66, *66–67*
Equine valvular disease
 cardiac murmurs, **576**
  diastolic, 579, *579*
  intensity, 578
  phonocardiograms, *579*
  systolic, 579, *579*
 causes, 573, **574**
  aortic valve prolapse, *575*
  cardiac murmurs, 573, **576**
  degenerative valve disease, 573, *575*
  ill-defined noninfective valvulitis, 573, *576*
  infective endocarditis, *575–576*
  valvar stenosis, 573
 clinical findings
  arterial and jugular pulses examination, 579
  cardiac rhythm disturbances, 579–560
  CHF, 580, *580*
  chordae tendineae rupture, 580, *580*
  infective endocarditis, 579
 clinical outcomes and risk assessment, 581, **581**, *582*
 ECG monitoring, 588
 echocardiography
  aortic regurgitation, 586
  Doppler echo imaging, 581
  focal lesions, vegetative endocarditis, 581, *585*
  left heart chambers, assessment of, 586–588
  mitral regurgitation, 582–583, 585–586
  tricuspid regurgitation, 588
  valvular thickening, 581, *583*
  variables, echo assessment, 582, **584**
 management, 588–589
 thoracic radiographs, 588
 valvular regurgitation pathophysiology
  cardiac remodeling, *577–578*
  hemodynamic features, 574, *577*
  hyperdynamic systolic function, 578, *578*
  hypertrophy, 575
  left heart enlargement, *577*
  LV end diastolic pressure, 575
  ventricular ectopy, 578
Equine Viral Arteritis, 712
EROA, *see* Effective regurgitant orifice area
Erythrocytosis (polycythemia), 36, 214, 247, *248*, 249, 287–288, *288*
 and hyperviscosity, 818
Escape complexes and rhythms, 150–151
Escherichia coli, 712
Esmolol, **374**, 381, 388, 401, **403**, 408, *408*, 411, **414**, 418, *425*, 426, *426*, **673**, 675, 805, **806**
ESVI, *see* End-systolic volume index
Ethylene diamine tetraacetic acid (EDTA), 598
ETN receptor antagonists, pulmonary hypertension, 836
Examination
 abnormal fluid accumulation, 42, *42*
 arterial pulses, 36, *36*
 cardiac auscultation, 37–40
 jugular veins, 36–37, *37*
 mucous membrane, 35–36, *36*
 precordial palpation, 37
 respiratory auscultation, 40–42
Excitation–contraction coupling, 13–14
Excitement-induced syncope, *198*

Exercise
    capacity, 311–312
    dogs, CHF management, 352–353
    ECG, horses, 164–165
    intolerance, 816
        abnormal peripheral circulation, 191
        causes, **189–190**
        dilated cardiomyopathy, *189*
        inadequate oxygen delivery, 191
        intermittent tachy-/brady-arrhythmias, *191*
        low BP, 191
        patient evaluation, *192*, 192–193
        reduced forward cardiac output (CO), 191
        reversed patent ductus arteriosus, 191
Exercise-induced lameness or cramping, 782
Exercise-induced pulmonary hemorrhage (EIPH), 30, 205, 823
Exogenous corticosteroids, 750
Exogenous glucocorticoid administration, BP, 791
External cardiac event monitors, 162–163
Exudates in dogs and cats, 710
Exudative effusions, 711–712
Exudative pericardial effusion, 711–712, *712*

F

Factor VII, plasminogen activators, 747
Falciform fat, 707
Familial aneurysm, 106
Familial ventricular arrhythmia, 371
Fast-response action potential, 11–12
Feline cardiomyopathy, **650**
Feline heart
    cardiac apex, 50
    lateral view, 50, *51*
    VHS, 50–51, *52*
Feline infectious peritonitis, 270
Femoral artery and pulmonary artery (PA) thrombosis, 749
Fibrin, 723
Fibrino-effusive pericarditis, 712
Fibrinoid change with arteriosclerosis, *778*
Fibrinolysis, 747
Fibrinolytic substances, 748
Fibronectin, 592
First-pass radionuclide angiocardiography, 67
Fish oil supplements, 386
Fluid therapy, 602
Fluid therapy, thromboembolic disease, 763
Flunixin meglumine, 764
Fluoroscopic systems, 168–169
Focal atrial tachycardia (FAT), 145, *145*
Focal bullous retinal detachment, 793
Focal heart lesions, 84

Focused Assessment with Sonography in Trauma (FAST) scans, 82
Fondaparinux, **751**, 766
Fractional shortening (FS), 94
Frank–Starling relationship, 302–303
Friesian horses, 784
Fulminant pulmonary edema, 206, 539
Functional/outflow obstruction murmurs, 39–40
Functional pheochromocytoma, 791
Furosemide (frusemide), heart failure treatment, *338*, 340, 341, **342**, **343**, 344, **345**, 347, 348, 349, 350, 353–355, **355**, 356–357, 358
    dosage, 317–318
    RAAS activation, 318–319
    torsemide, 319, **345**, 349, 350, 355, **355**, 358, 359

G

Gagging/retching, 205
Gallop sounds, 232
Garlic toxicity, HT, 792
Gastric adenocarcinoma, *632*
German Shepherd, aortic valve endocarditis, *593*
Glucocorticoids, 791
Golden Retriever, *611*
    cardiac cachexia, *611*
    pulmonary venous distension, *617*
    puppies, PPDH in, 708
    sinus arrhythmia, *642*
Grass awn, 592
Great Danes, 610
    DCM, *621*
    pulmonary edema, *618*, *620*
Great imitator, 591
Great vessels
    echocardiography, 106–107
    enlargement, **94**
Guide wires, *171*, 171–172

H

Hamartomas, 784
HCM, *see* Hypertrophic cardiomyopathy
Heart
    autonomic control
        parasympathetic (vagal) stimulation, 21
        sympathetic stimulation, effects of, 20–21
    block, 151
    disease
        assessment, **311**
        clinical signs, 33, 35, **35**
    external features
        canine heart, 4, *4–5*
        equine heart, *5*
        left and right coronary arteries, 4–5
        pericardium, 4
        pulmonary venous return, 5
        RAu, 6
    internal features
        left heart, 6–8
        right heart, 8–9
    as pump
        afterload, 16
        cardiac cycle and generation of heart sounds, 18–19
        cardiac output, 15
        contractility, 15
        preload, 15–16
        pressure–volume loops, 19–20
        response to pressure/volume loading, 16–17
        stroke volume (SV), 14
        systolic function, 15
        ventricular compliance, 14–15
        ventricular function assessment, 17–18
    rhythm
        bradycardia, 140
        ectopic complexes, 140, *140*, 142
        tachycardia, 140, 142
    size, 30
    sounds, generation of, 18–19
Heart failure; *see also* Drugs, heart failure treatment
    cardiac responses, 302–303
    clinical associations, 301–302
    clinical signs, 33, 35, **35**, **300**
    definition, 299
    diagnosis, 312
    exercise capacity, 311–312
    functional classification systems, 314
    management, *see* CHF management
    neurohormonal mechanisms
        AVP, 307–308
        baroreceptor function, 305
        cytokines and inflammation, 308
        endogenous vasodilatory substances, 308–309
        ETN-1, 308
        microRNAs, 309
        natriuretic peptides, 308–309
        RAAS, 305–307
        SNS stimulation, 303–305
        systemic vasoconstriction, 303
        vitamin D, 309
    pathophysiologic abnormalities
        contractility failure, 300
        diastolic dysfunction, 301
        increased workload, 300–301
    presenting signs, 312–313
    renal responses, 310–311
    staging, 313–314
    vascular system subdivisions, 299

Heart rate (HR); see also Abnormal heart
        rate
    calculation, 139
    sinus rhythms, 140, **141**
Heart rate variability (HRV), 613
Heart sounds, abnormal; see also Murmurs
    approach to patient, 233–234, *234*, **235**
    auscultation, 233
    systolic clicks and ejection sounds, 232
    transient sounds
        gallop sounds, 232
        heart sounds, altered intensity, **231**
        split sounds, 231
Heartworm disease (HWD), 197, 749, 815
    Angiostrongylus vasorum, 870–873
    Dirofilaria immitis, 841–870
Heatstroke, 749
Heinz body anemia, 250
Hemangiosarcoma, 711, *733–734*, 784
Hemoabdomen, 267, 270
Hemodynamics, *169*, 169–170
    blood flow velocity, 23
    flow, pressure, resistance relationships, 22
    laminar and turbulent flow, 23
    resistance, 22–23
    viscosity, 23
Hemoglobinuria, 846
Hemolytic anemia, 823–824
Hemoptysis, 203
Hemorrhage, 775
Hemorrhagic effusions, 711
Hemorrhagic pericardial effusion, *727*
Hemostasis, 745–747
Hemostatic process, 745–747, *746*
Heparan sulfate, 747–748
Heparin, **751**, **763**, 764–765, **768**; see also Low molecular weight heparin
Hepatic lobes, 707
Hepatic veins, 119
Hepatojugular reflux, 37
Hepatomegaly, 42
Hepatopathy, 749
Herniated viscera in dogs, 707
Heterometric autoregulation, 15
High-pressure balloon (HPB) valvuloplasty, 181, 183
Hind-limb rhabdomyolysis, 775
Histologically confirmed vasculitis, *781*
HOCM, see Hypertrophic obstructive cardiomyopathy
Holter monitoring, 162, *163*, 201
Horse; see also Equine
    CHF, 703
    infective endocarditis
        aortic valve cusps, *593*
        chorda tendinea, *593*
        fulminant pulmonary edema, *597*
    myocarditis, 698
HPB, see High-pressure balloon

HR, see Heart rate
HW-associated respiratory disease (HARD), 844
HWD, see Heartworm disease
Hybrid catheterization, 184, *184*
Hydralazine, 323–324, **804**, 805–806, **806**, 809
Hydrochlorothiazide, 320, **345**
3-Hydroxy-3-methylglutaryl coenzyme A reductase inhibitors, 334
Hyoscyamine sulfate, 387, **403**
Hyperadrenocorticism, 193, 749–750, 789, 791
Hypercapnia, 792
Hypercoagulability, 749
Hyperechoic tissue, 75
Hyperfibrinogenemia, 723
Hyperfibrinolysis, 871
Hyperhomocysteinemia, 750
Hyperkalemia, 758, 766
    ECG changes, *160*, 160–161
    renal perfusion, 290
    slow HR, 242
Hyperkinetic pulses, 255
Hyperpnea, 211, 219
Hyperproteinemia, 723
Hypersomatotropism, 293
Hypertensive cardiomyopathy, 700
    clinical features, 701
    diagnostic tests, 701
    laboratory tests, 701–702
    myocardial fibrosis, *700*, 700–701
Hypertensive emergency, management of, 805–807, **806**
Hypertensive encephalopathy, 794
Hyperthyroidism, 564–565, 752
Hypertrophic cardiomyopathy (HCM), 92, 104, 107, 607, 755, 794
    cat, 649–651
        acute congestive heart failure, 673–675
        auscultation, 657–659
        cardiac morphologic abnormalities, 652–653
        chronic heart failure, 675–678
        clinical cardiomyopathy, **650**
        clinical features, 656–660
        congestive heart failure, 659–660
        diagnostic tests, 660–671
        echocardiography, 664–671
        electrocardiography, 663–664
        histopathologic section, *653*
        history, 657
        laboratory tests, 660–661
        large thrombi, *652*
        lung ultrasound image, *665*
        management, 671–678
        myocardial functional/hemodynamic abnormalities, 653–656
        open left ventricle, *652*

        pathogenesis, 651–653
        POC thoracic ultrasound, 674
        preclinical disease, 671–672
        prognosis, 672–673
        radiography, 661–663
        refractory pulmonary edema, 675
        respiratory distress, *673*
        screening, 656–657
        septal hypertrophy, 667
        sinus rhythm, *664*
        suspect cardiomyopathy, *658*
        treatment, **673**
    dog, 629
        clinical features, 629–630
        diagnostic tests, 630
        management, 630
        pathophysiology, 629
    pathophysiology, 629
Hypertrophic obstructive cardiomyopathy (HOCM), 650
Hypertrophic osteopathy, 596
Hyperviscosity syndromes, 749
Hypoalbuminemia, 270
Hypocalcemia, 290
Hypochloremia, 564
Hypoechoic tissue, 75
Hypoglycemia, 196, 198
Hypokalemia, 161
Hypokinetic pulses, 254–255
Hypomagnesemia, 159, 290
Hyponatremia, 290
Hypotension, 199
Hypothermia, 764
Hypothyroidism, 193, 564–565
Hypoventilation, 214
Hypoxemia, 247, 825
    assessment of, **220**
    causes, **214**
    diffusion impairmen, 214
    hypoventilation, 214
    signs, **212**
    V/Q mismatch, 214
Hypoxia-induced pulmonary vasoconstriction, 815

I

Ibutilide fumarate, 383
Icterus/jaundice, 247
Idiopathic hemorrhagic pericardial effusion, 710
Idiopathic pericardial effusion, 711, 722
    in dogs, 711–712
Idiopathic PH, 818
Idioventricular tachycardia, 149
Image artifacts
    clinical utility, 80
    echo dropout, 79
    mirror image artifacts, 79
    reverberation artifacts, 79

IMHA, *see* Immune-mediated hemolytic anemia
Imidapril, 323
Immediate pericardiocentesis, 724
Immune-mediated disease, 749
Immune-mediated hemolytic anemia (IMHA), 749
Immunodiagnostic tests, 290
Impaired cerebral perfusion, 792
Impaired lymphatic drainage, 277
Impedance, defined, 16
Impulse gradients, 114
Inadequate blood oxygen, *see* Hypoxemia
Indirect measurement, systemic hypertension, 796–799
Infective endocarditis
   antibiotic prophylaxis, 604
   aortic valve endocarditis, German Shepherd, *593*
   blood cultures, 597–598
   cardiac consequences, 593–594
   causative organisms, 594–596
   clinical features, 596
   diagnosis, 597, **598**
   echocardiography
      cardiac auscultation, *602*
      diastolic flutter, *601*
      Flat Coated Retriever, *601*
      Minature Schnauzer, *600*
      Pomeranian, *600*
      Rottweiler, *599*
      Tibetan Terrier, *601*
   electrocardiography, 599
   empirical antimicrobial therapy, **602**
   follow-up, 603–604
   horse
      aortic valve cusps, *593*
      chorda tendinea, *593*
      fulminant pulmonary edema, *597*
   management, 600, 602–603
   mitral valve, *592*
   molecular testing, 598–599
   monitoring, 603–604
   pathophysiology, 592–593
   physical findings, 596–597
   potential sequelae, **595**
   predisposing factors, 591–592
   prognosis, 604
   radiography, 599
   serologic testing, 598–599
   systemic consequences, 594
   vegetative lesions, *592*
Infective myocarditis, 636
   clinical features, 636–638
   diagnostic tests, 636–638
   management, 638–639
Insidious-onset laminitis, 792
Insulin resistance, HT, 791–792
Intermittent claudication, 756
Intermittent collapse, *see* Syncope

International normalization ratio (INR), 770
International sensitivity index (ISI), 770
International Small Animal Cardiac Health Council (ISACHC) criteria, 314
Interventional catheterization, 782
Interventional procedures
   via left heart catheterization
      ABV, 181–183
      PDA, 179–181
   via right heart catheterization
      cardiac pacing, 175–177
      PBV, 177–179
Intra-abdominal fat accumulation, insulin sensitivity, 792
Intracardiac sarcoma, *734*
Intramural coronary arteriosclerosis, 780, *780*
Intrarenal vasodilatory prostaglandins (prostacyclin), 309
Intrathoracic blood vessels
   abnormal, **58**
   aorta, 58
   lobar pulmonary arteries and veins, 58–61
   main pulmonary artery, 58
   vena cava, 61
Irbesartan, **804**, 807
Ischemia, 775
Ischemic heart disease, 636
Isoproterenol, **375**, 387, 401, **403**, *404*, 425, 422, 428
Isorhythmic atrioventricular dissociation, 150, *150*, 419
Isovolumic (isovolumetric) contraction, 19
Isovolumic relaxation time (IVRT), *621*
Ivabradine, 333–334, **374**, **375**, 385–386, 557

J

Jarisch-Herxheimer-like reaction, 603
Jet in the receiving chamber, 122
Jugular thrombosis, 764
Jugular vein distension/pulsation
   approach to patient, *265*
      abdominojugular (hepatojugular) reflux test, 264
      position, 263
   cannon a waves, 262
   carotid pulse transmission, 261
   causes, **262**
   cranial lung lobe tumor, 261, *263*
   CVP measurement
      bore jugular catheter, 264
      and cardiac output, 261
      sterile water manometer, 265, *266*
   right atrial pressure (RAP), 262, *263*
   right-sided/biventricular CHF, 261, *262*
   tricuspid regurgitation (TR), *263*
Jugular veins, evaluation of, 36–37, *37*

K

Kallikrein, plasminogen activators, 747
K-dependent protein, 748

L

Labrador Retriever
   acute-onset lethargy, *642*
   echocardiogram, *620*
   pulmonary edema, *619*
Lactic acidosis, 250
LAFB, *see* Left anterior fascicular block
Lameness, 596
Laminar and turbulent blood flow, 23
Laryngeal paralysis, 193
Laryngeal paresis, 206
Laryngoscopy, pulmonary hypertension, 833
LBBB, *see* Left bundle branch block
L-carnitine, 634
Lead axis, 137
Lead systems, ECG, **136**
   base-apex lead, 138, *138*
   deflection, 137
   lead axis, 137
   precordial leads, 138, *138*
   standard limb leads, 137, *137*
Left anterior fascicular block (LAFB), 153
Left atrial (LA) dilation, 283
   atrial cycle functions, 103–104
   suggested approach, 103
Left atrial tears, 562–563
Left atrium, M-mode echocardiography, 92
Left auricle (LAu), 5–6
Left azygous vein, 525, *525*
Left bundle branch block (LBBB), 153
Left-to-right shunts, 283
Left ventricle (LV)
   dilation, 283
   M-mode echocardiography, 90
   size and function
      allometric scaling, 105
      concentric hypertrophy, 104
      eccentric hypertrophy, 104
      suggested approach, 105
      ventricular hypertrophy, 104
Leptospirosis, 711–712
Leukocytosis, 288, 723
Lidocaine, 375–376, **402**, 408, *408*, **411**, 412, 413, **414**, 414, *415*, 418, 419, *423*, 424, *425*, 426, *426*, 427, 485, *627*, *642*, 674, 675, *699*, 703, 705
Lisinopril, 323, **345**, 321, 323
Liver and pancreatic enzymes, 289
Lobar arteries and veins
   caudal lobar vessels, 60
   left cranial lobar vessels, 59
   pulmonary vascular patterns, 58, **58**
   right cranial lobar vessels, 59

Local (intrinsic) control, 26–27
Localized thrombophlebitis, 782
Local vasodilation, 747
Losartan, **804**, 807–808
Low blood pressure, 191
Low molecular weight heparin (LMWH), **763**, 765–766, **768**, 770
    dalteparin, **751**, 764–766
    enoxaparin, **751**, 765–766
Lung ultrasound, 80, 217, 340, 665, *665*
Lung sounds, abnormal, 41
LV internal dimensions at end-diastole (LVIDd), 614
LV moderator bands, 679
Lyme disease, 639–640
Lymphangiosarcoma, 776
Lymphedema, 776
    causes, 278
    congenital, *278*
    primary, 278
    secondary, 278

M

Macroalbuminuria, 790
Macro-entrant atrial tachycardia, 145–146, *146*
Magnesium deficiency, systemic HT, 792
Magnesium sulfate, 377, 378, 386, **404**, *415*
Magnetic resonance imaging (MRI), 67
Main pulmonary artery dilation, 58
Management
    Angiostrongylus vasorum, 873
    anticoagulant therapy, 765–766
    antiplatelet therapy, 764–765
    antithrombotic therapy, **768**
    aortic stenosis (AS), 489
    atrioventricular septal defect (AVSD), 467
    cardiac tumors, 740–742
    cardiovascular malformations, 514
    congenital cardiac shunts, 444, 446–449, 460–461, 467
    constrictive pericardial disease, 732
    cor triatriatum dexter (CTD), 512, *514*
    cor triatriatum sinister, 514
    diastolic dysfunction, 353, 357
    dilated cardiomyopathy (DCM), 621–624, 685–686
    Dirofilaria immitis
        adulticide therapy, 859–860
        alternatives to melarsomine adulticide therapy, 860
        in cats, 866–867
        caval syndrome, 863–866
        complicated heartworm disease in dogs, 860–861
        exercise restriction, 856
        initial doxycycline and macrocyclic lactone therapy, 856–858
        melarsomine treatment, 858–859
        microfilaricide therapy, 862–863
        postadulticide pulmonary thromboembolism, 861–862
        pretreatment assessment, 856
    equine myocardial disease, 703
    equine valvular disease, 588–589
    fibrinolytic therapy, 766–768
    general therapeutic principles, 763–764
    HCM, 630
    infective endocarditis, 600, 602–603
    infective myocarditis, 638–639
    mitral valve dysplasia (MVD), 504
    patent ductus arteriosus (PDA), 444–449
    pericardiocentesis, 728–729
    peritoneopericardial diaphragmatic hernia (PPDH), 708–710
    pulmonary hypertension, 833–834
    pulmonic stenosis (PS), 497–500
    respiratory distress, 219–220, **220–221**
    restrictive cardiomyopathy, 681–682
    reversed ASD (rASD), 465
    reversed PDA (rPDA), 452–454
    reversed ventricular septal defect (rVSD), 460–461
    sinus bradycardia, *404*
    subaortic stenosis (SAS), 488–489
    systemic hypertension, 803–807
    tetralogy of Fallot (T of F), 471–472
    thromboembolic (TE) disease, **763**, 763–768
    tricuspid dysplasia, 506–507
    vascular diseases, 778
    vascular ring anomalies, 520
    ventricular septal defect (VSD), 458, 460
Manubrium heart scores (MHSs), 50
MAPSE, *see* Mitral annular plane systolic excursion
Marfan syndrome, 521
Matrix metalloproteinases (MMPs), 608
MEA, *see* Mean electrical axis
Mean arterial pressure (MAP), 24
Mean electrical axis (MEA), 155, *156*
Mechanical valve trauma, 591
Medial hypertrophy, pulmonary arteries, 844–845
Medial hypertrophy of pulmonary arteries, 780
Melarsomine treatment
    adulticide therapy alternatives, 860
    Dirofilaria immitis, 858–859
Mesenteric arteritis, 775
Metabolic acidosis, 758, 766
Methemoglobinemia, 249–250, *250*
Methyxanthine bronchodilator, 835
Metoprolol, 332, 380–381, **402**, 623
Metronidazole, 602
Mexiletine, 378, **402**, 411, **414**, 418, *425*, 427, 621, 628
MHSs, *see* Manubrium heart scores
Microalbuminuria, 790
Microcatheters, 171
Microcirculation and lymphatics, 24–25
Microfilaricide therapy, *Dirofilaria immitis*, 862–863
Micro-ribonucleic acids (miRNAs) dysregulation, 531
Milrinone, 330, 331, **343**, **346**, 347, 380, 385
Miniature Schnauzer dogs, PPDH in, 708
Minocycline, 603, 858
Mirror image artifacts, 79
Mitral annular plane systolic excursion (MAPSE), 670
Mitral regurgitation (MR), 206, 592; *see also* Degenerative mitral valve disease (DMVD) in dogs
    horses, 582–583, 585–586
    murmurs, 229
Mitral stenosis, 184, 480, 500, *503*,
Mitral valve, 6–8, 529–530
    disease, 711
    M-mode echocardiography, 90, **91**, 92, *92*
    PW Doppler imaging, **115–116**
    tricuspid insufficiency, 283
Mitral valve dysplasia (MVD)
    clinical features, **478**, 500
    diagnostic tests
        angiocardiography, 504, *504*
        cardiac catheterization, 501
        double-headed papillary muscle, *501*
        left heart dilation, 501, *502*
        papillary muscle-chordal malformation, *501–502*
        sinus rhythm, *503*
        valve regurgitation, *501*
        valve stenosis, *503*
    management, 504
    valvular regurgitation, 500
M-mode echocardiography
    2D image, 88, *89*
    limitations, 90
    one-dimensional view, 88, *89*
    patterns
        aortic valve and left atrium, 92
        clinical utility, 92–93
        features, 90, **91**
        image planes, 90
        left ventricle, 90
        mitral valve, 90, **91**, 92, *92*
Modified Knott Test Method, **849**
Modified Seldinger technique, 727
Modified transudates, 710
Monocytic ehrlichiosis, 641
MR, *see* Mitral regurgitation
Mucous membrane, evaluation of, 35–36, *36*
Mucous membrane color, abnormal, **248**
    approach to patient, *251*
    differential cyanosis, 252

increased HR, 250
  rear limb weakness, 252
  tests, 252
 cyanosis, 247, 249
 icterus/jaundice, 247
 methemoglobinemia, 249–250, *250*
 pale mucous membranes, 247, *248*
 pallor, 247
 severe anemia, *248*
Multifocal pulmonary arterial thrombosis, 819
Murmurs
 adrenergic drive, 225
 approach to patient, 233–234, *234*, **235**
 both systole and diastole, 231
 cardiomegaly, 284
 characteristics
  intensity, 226, **227**
  PMI, 226–227
  shape and quality, *227*, 227–228
  timing, 226, *226*
 definition, 225
 diastolic, 230–231
 horses, 573, **576**
  diastolic, 579, *579*
  intensity, 578
  phonocardiograms, *579*
  systolic, 579, *579*
 nonpathologic, 228
 pathologic causes, 226
 systolic
  MR, 229
  TR, 229
  ventricular outflow obstructions, 230
  VSD, 230
 turbulence, 38
Muscle enzymes, 290
Muscular dystrophy, 635–636
MVD, *see* Mitral valve dysplasia
Mycoplasma, 712
Mycotic arteritis, *782*
Myocardial contraction
 electrical–mechanical coupling, 13–14
 gap junctions, 12–13
 myocardial relaxation, 14
 sarcomeres, 13
Myocardial diseases, 283, 758
 cat, HCM, *see* Hypertrophic cardiomyopathy
 dog
  2D imaging, 615
  dilated heart, *609*
  echocardiography, *609*
  Great Danes, 610
  HCM, *see* Hypertrophic cardiomyopathy
  idiopathic DCM, 607–608
  LVIDs, 614–616
  overt (stage C), **622**
  pathophysiology, 608–610

 physical findings, 611, *611*
 horse, *see* Equine myocardial disease
Myocardial fibrillation, 142
Myocardial hypertrophy, 816
Myocardial ischemia, 302, 654
Myocardial lymphoma, *735*
Myocardial relaxation, 14
Myocardial speckle-tracking, 94
Myocarditis, 290, 711
 cat, 689–691, *690*
 dog, 603, 607
 horse, 698
Myosin binding protein C (MYBPC3), 651

N

Natriuretic peptide receptors (NPRs), 309
Natriuretic peptides, 291–293
  adrenomedullin, 309
  blood volume and pressure, 309
  neutral endopeptidase, 309
Necrosis, 302
Neoplasia, 749, 752
Neoplastic effusions, 723
Neoplastic invasion, 749
Nephrotic syndrome, 749
Neurocardiogenic/reflex syncope, 198, 201
Neuroendocrine tumors, 711
Neurogenic pulmonary edema, 215
Neurohormonal (extrinsic) control, 27
Neurohormonal mechanisms, heart failure
 AVP, 307–308
 baroreceptor function, 305
 cytokines and inflammation, 308
 endogenous vasodilatory substances, 308–309
 ETN-1, 308
 microRNAs, 309
 natriuretic peptides, 308–309
 RAAS, 305–307
 SNS stimulation, 303–305
 systemic vasoconstriction, 303
 vitamin D, 309
Neutrophilia, 288
Newfoundlands, 610
New York Heart Association (NYHA) classification scheme, 314
Nitric oxide (NO), 747, 816
Nitric oxide synthetase (NOS), 816
Nitroglycerin, 323, 324, 325, **342**, **343**, 344, **345**, 347, **555**, 560, 622, **673**, 674
Nitroprusside, 323, 324–325, **342**, **343**, 344, **345**, **555**, 560, **622**, 674, 805, **806**, 810
Nocturnal dyspnea, 205
Nocturnal hypoxemia, 792
Nonbacterial thrombotic endocarditis, 593
Noncardiogenic pulmonary edema, 64
Noninfective myocarditis, 641
Nonpathologic murmurs

 cats, 228
 dogs, 228
 horses, 228
Nonselective angiography, 174
Nonseptic emboli, 593
Nonsteroidal anti-inflammatory drug (NSAID), 565
Norepinephrine (NE), 304
NPRs, *see* Natriuretic peptide receptors
N-terminal prohormone of B-type natriuretic peptide (NT-proBNP), 825
NT-proBNP test, 234
Nuclear imaging studies, 67

O

Obesity, 62
Obstipation, 270
Ocular lesions, HT, 793
Oral antithrombotic medication, 765
Organomegaly, 270
Orthodromic AVRT, 417, *418*
Orthopnea, 211–212
Oscillometric method, systemic hypertension, 799
Osler–Weber–Rendu syndrome, 523
Osteoarthritis, 565
Over-the-needle (OTN) catheter, 170, *170*, 172

P

Pacing therapy
 biventricular, 390–391
 cats, 390
 complications, 391
 dual chamber pacing system, 390, *390*
 epicardial and permanent transvenous pacing, *390*
 isolated RA pacing, 389
 pacemakers, 389–390
 permanent implantation, 389–390
 revised pacemaker nomenclature, 390, **391**
 single chamber pacing, 390
 temporary pacing, 389
 transthoracic external pacing, 389
Packed cell volume (PCV), 711
Pallor, 247, 250
Paradoxical breathing, 212
Parasitic disease, pulmonary hypertension, 822–823
Parasympathetic (cholinergic) nervous system (PNS), 27
Paroxysmal ventricular tachycardia, 197
Pasteurella spp., 712
Patent ductus arteriosus (PDA), 255, 591, 636
 aberrant A-V shunts, 441

clinical features, **436**, 441–442, *442*
closure, ductus, 439; *see also* Ductal occlusion, PDA
diagnostic tests
    cardiac catheterization, 444
    cardiomegaly, 442, *443*
    Doppler echocardiographic studies, 444, *444–446*
    LV enlargement, 442, *442*
    QRS complexes, 443, *444*
    radiographic findings, **442**
ductus arteriosus, 439
ductus diverticulum, 439, *440*
echocardiography, 444, *444–446*
hyperkinetic arterial pulse quality, 440
jet lesions, 440–441, *441*
left ventricular angiocardiogram, 439–440
management
    changes and prognosis, 448–449
    CHF, 444
    surgical ductal ligation, 447–448
    transcatheter ductal occlusion, *446*, 446–447, *447*
morphologic classification, 439–440, *440*
murmurs, 231
occlusion; *see also* Ductal occlusion, PDA
    ACDO, 179–180, *180*
    nondetachable coils, 181
    procedure, 179–181
    prognosis, 181
    transarterial coil delivery, 181
    transcatheter therapy, 179, *180*
    transvenous coil delivery, 181
reversed, *see* Reversed PDA
Patent foramen ovale (PFO), 465–466
Pathologic thrombosis, mechanisms, 748–749
Pathophysiology
    acquired pericardial effusions, 712–714, *713*
    Angiostrongylus vasorum, 870–871
    arrhythmogenic right ventricular cardiomyopathy (ARVC), 625–626, 686
    cardiac tumors, 733–734, *733–735*
    congenital cardiac shunts, 437, *437*, 437–439
    congenital valvular malformations, 479–480
    constrictive pericardial disease, 730
    degenerative mitral valve disease (DMVD), 531–537
    degenerative valvular disease, dog, 530–537
    dilated cardiomyopathy (DCM), 682
    Dirofilaria immitis, 843–846
    equine myocardial disease, 696–697

hypertrophic cardiomyopathy (HCM), 629
infective endocarditis, 592–593
myocardial diseases, 608–610
peritoneopericardial diaphragmatic hernia (PPDH), 707
restrictive cardiomyopathy, 678–679
systemic hypertension, 789–793
    dyslipidemia, 792
    endocrine disease, 791–792
    hypertension, pathologic effects of, 793–794
    kidney disease, 790–791
    other associations, 792–793
thromboembolic (TE) disease, 748–755
vascular diseases, 775–776
Patient
    positioning
        cardiac radiography, 46
        ECG, 138, *138*
    preparation
        catheterization, 172
        echocardiography, 80
        radiography, 46
PBV, *see* Pulmonary balloon valvuloplasty
PCH, *see* Pulmonary capillary hemangiomatosis
PDA, *see* Patent ductus arteriosus
PDE-5 inhibitors, pulmonary hypertension, 836
Pectus excavatum, 708
Pelvic limb edema, 778
Pembroke Welsh Corgi, VPC, *637*
Pentoxifylline, 334, 836
Pericardial cysts, 706, 708, 710
Pericardial effusions, 705
    chylous effusions, 712
    clinical features
        pericarditis in horses, 715–716
        physical findings, 715
    diagnostic tests
        central venous pressure and right heart catheterization, 722
        echocardiography, 717–722, *719–721*
        laboratory tests, 716
        pericardial fluid evaluation, 722–723
        pericarditis in horses, 723
        radiography, *716*, 716–717, *717*
    exudative effusions, 711–712
    hemorrhagic effusions, 711
    in horses, management of, 729
    management, 723–727
    pathophysiology, 712–714, *713*
    pericardiocentesis
        complications of, 727–728
        management after, 728–729
    pericarditis in horses, 712
    and tamponade, 706
    transudative effusions, 710–711
Pericardial fibrosis, 713

Pericardial fluid analysis, 723
Pericardial friction rubs, 233, 715
Pericardial inflammation, 712
Pericardial mesothelioma, 734
Pericardial structure, illustration, *706*
Pericardiocentesis, 721, 724, 728–729
    complications of, 727–728
    management after, 728–729
Pericarditis in horses, 712, 715–716, 723
Pericardium, congenital defects, 706
Perioperative antibiotics, 175
Peripheral arteriovenous (A-V) fistula, 276
Peripheral cyanosis, 215, 249
Peritoneopericardial diaphragmatic hernia (PPDH), 706, *709–710*
    after barium administration, *709*
    clinical features, 708
    diagnostic tests, 708, *708–709*
    management, 708–710
    nonselective angiocardiography, *710*
    pathophysiology, 707
Peritonitis, 270
Persian cat, *665*, 671
Persistent left cranial vena cava (PLCVC)
    megaesophagus, 524
    right heart catheterization, 524–525
    size, 524
    thoracotomy, 524, *525*
Persistent right aortic arch (PRAA), 516, *516–517*
PFO, *see* Patent foramen ovale
Phenoxybenzamine, **804**, 809
Phenylephrine, 388, **404**, 408, 413, 414, **429**, **789**, 792
Phenylpropanolamine, 792
Phenytoin, 378, **402**, 426
Pheochromocytoma-induced tachyarrhythmias, 806–807
Phlebitis, 783
Phosphatidylinositol-binding clathrin assembly protein (PICALM) gene, 481
Phosphodiesterase-3 inhibitors, heart failure treatment
    amrinone, 330
    milrinone, 330–331
Phosphodiesterase-5 inhibitors, pulmonary hypertension, 834–835
Phosphodiesterase (PDE) isoenzymes, 816
Pimobendan, **555**, 556–560, 562, 564, 621–624, 674, 676–677, 681–682, 685–687, 703, 835
PISA, *see* Proximal isovelocity surface area
Pitting edema, 275–276, *276*
Plasminogen, 747
Plasminogen activator inhibitors, 747
Plasminogen activators, 747
Platelet adherence, 745, 747
Platelet aggregability, 749
Platelet degranulation products, 747

Platelet-platelet interactions, 747
Pleural effusion, 82, 216, **216**, 277, 715
    fissure lines, 64, *65*
    hypertrophic cardiomyopathy, 64, *65*
    pleural fibrosis, 66
Pleural fibrosis, 66
Pleural space
    pleural effusion, 64–66
    pneumothorax, 66
P mitrale, 156
Pneumocystis carinii, 820
Pneumonia, 820
Pneumopericardiogram, *741*
Pneumopericardium, 705
Pneumoperitoneum, 267
Pneumothorax, 66
Point-of-care (POC) NT-proBNP test, 292, *292*, 293
Polymerase chain reaction (PCR) tests, 596, 613
Porcupine quill, 592
Portal vein thrombosis, 754, *755*
Portosystemic vascular anomalies, 523–524
Positive inotropic agents, heart failure treatment
    catecholamines, 330
    digoxin, 327–330
    phosphodiesterase-3 inhibitors, 330–331
    pimobendan, 325–327
Postadulticide pulmonary thromboembolism, *Dirofilaria immitis*, 861–862
PPDH, see Peritoneopericardial diaphragmatic hernia
P pulmonale, 156
PRAA, see Persistent right aortic arch
Pradofloxacin, 603
Prasugrel, 765
Prazosin, **804**, 804, **806**, 806, 809
Precordial leads, 138, *138*
Precordial palpation, 37
Precordial thrill, 37
Preexcitation syndrome, 417
Preload, 15–16
Premature beat, 256
Prerenal azotemia, 723
Presyncope, 195
Prevention, *Dirofilaria immitis*
    in cats, 870
    in dogs, 867–869
Primary (idiopathic) DCM, 607
Procainamide, 376, **402**, 407, *408*, 409, 411, 412, **414**, 414, 415, 418, 419, 426, *426*, 427, 703
Procoagulant substances, 748
Propantheline bromide, 387, **403**
Propranolol, 380, **402**, 408, *408*, **414**, *425*, 426, *426*, 472, **673**, **804**, 805, **806**, 809
Prostacyclin, 747

Prostacyclin analogues, pulmonary hypertension, 836
Protein C, 748
Protein-losing nephropathy, 749–750
Proteins, 290
Protein S, 747–748
Proteinuria with HT, 790
Prothrombin, 747
Protozoal myocarditis, 640–641
Proximal isovelocity surface area (PISA), 121–122, 550–551
Pseudomonas aeruginosa, 712
Pseudonormal filling, 129
PTE, see Pulmonary thromboembolism
Pulmonary and systemic hypertension, 126; see also Pulmonary hypertension, Systemic hypertension
Pulmonary arterial flow, pulsed wave Doppler recording, 114, **115**, 117
Pulmonary arterial hypertension, 60, 61, 107, 197
    pulmonary hypertension, 817–819
Pulmonary arterial thromboembolic disease, 753–754
Pulmonary arteries, 60, 61
Pulmonary atresia, 492
Pulmonary balloon valvuloplasty (PBV), 177–179, 183, 471, 479, 489, 491, *493*, 497–499, *499*
    anomalous coronary anatomy, 179, 499
    ideal balloon, 177
    procedure, 177–178, *178–179*
    R2A coronary anomaly, 490, *490*, 491, *491*
    re-sterilization process, 177
    transthoracic echocardiography, Doppler, 177
Pulmonary capillary hemangiomatosis (PCH), 819
Pulmonary congestion, 859
Pulmonary crackles, 219, 846
Pulmonary disease and hypoxia, pulmonary hypertension, 819–820, *821*
Pulmonary edema, 41
    cardiogenic, 62, *62*
    Doberman Pinschers, *617–619*
    Great Dane, *618*, *620*
    increased pulmonary capillary hydrostatic pressure, 215
    Labrador Retriever, *619*
    neurogenic, 215
    noncardiogenic, 64
    patchy, 62, *63*
    progression stages, 215
    recurrent, 64, *64*
    severe, *63*
Pulmonary embolism, 823–824
Pulmonary eosinophilic granulomatosis, 861
Pulmonary fibrosis, 819–820

Pulmonary hypertension, 283, 561–562
    classification scheme for dogs, **814**
    clinical features, 823–824
    diagnostic tests, 824–825
        bronchoalveolar lavage cytology, 833
        bronchoscopy, 833
        echocardiography, 827–833
        electrocardiography, 827
        ETN receptor antagonists, 836
        laboratory tests, 825
        laryngoscopy, 833
        radiography, 825–827
    management, 833–834
    medical therapy, 835–836
        PDE-5 inhibitors, 836
        pentoxifylline, 836
        phosphodiesterase-5 inhibitors, 834–835
        prostacyclin analogues, 836
        tyrosine kinase inhibitors, 836
    prognosis, 836
    pathophysiology, 815–816
        cor pulmonale, 816–817
        exercise-induced pulmonary hemorrhage (EIPH) in horses, 823
        parasitic disease, 822–823
        pulmonary arterial hypertension, 817–819
        pulmonary disease and hypoxia, 819–820, *821*
        pulmonary thromboembolism, 821–822, *822*
        pulmonary venous hypertension, 819
    physical findings, 824
    and tricuspid insufficiency, *817*
Pulmonary metastases, *715*
Pulmonary overcirculation pattern, *60*, 60–61, 818
Pulmonary parenchyma
    patterns, 61–62
    pulmonary edema, 62–64
Pulmonary parenchymal disease, 815
Pulmonary stenosis, 301
Pulmonary thromboembolism (PTE), 216–217, 750, 757, 821–822, *822*
Pulmonary undercirculation pattern, 60, *60*
Pulmonary valve, 9
Pulmonary valve stenosis, see also Pulmonic stenosis (PS), 177
Pulmonary vascular resistance (PVR), 815
Pulmonary vasoconstriction, 815
Pulmonary veins, *60*, 61
Pulmonary veno-occlusive disease (PVOD), 819
Pulmonary venous hypertension, 33, 819
Pulmonary venous velocities, 118–119
Pulmonic stenosis (PS)
    Beagle dogs, 490, *490*
    canine PS, classification, 490

clinical features, **478**, 492, *492*
DCRV, *491*, 491–492
diagnostic tests
  angiocardiography, 497, *498*
  cardiac catheterization, 497, *497*
  caudal vena caval dilation, 494
  Doppler evaluation, *496*, 497
  dysplastic valve leaflets, 495, *496*
  pulmonary to aortic (PA/Ao) VTI ratio, 497
  pulmonary trunk bulge, 494
  radiographic features, **482**, 492, *493–494*
  right ventricular pressure overload, 495
  RV hypertrophy and enlargement, 494, *494–495*
  systolic doming, pulmonary valve, 495, *496*
management
  balloon valvuloplasty, 499
  beta-blocker (atenolol), 498
  cardiopulmonary bypass, 499
  CT angiography, 499
  palliative valvuloplasty, 498
  periodic reevaluation and echo, 497
  prognosis, 499–500
  primary infundibular stenosis, 491
  pulmonary atresia, 492
  R2A type, coronary anomaly, *490, 491, 491*
  shunting, 492
  systolic pressure overload, 490
  valvular stenosis, 490
Pulse deficits, 36, 256, *256*
Pulsed wave (PW) Doppler imaging, 112, **115–116**, 552–553, 656
Pulse oximetry, 220, **220**
Pulse pressure
  definition, 253
  HR, 254
  variations, 253
Pulsus alternans, 256
Pulsus paradoxus, 257, 714, *714*
Pulsus parvus et tardus, 255
PVOD, *see* Pulmonary veno-occlusive disease
PVR, *see* Pulmonary vascular resistance
Pyruvate dehydrogenase kinase isozyme 4 (PDK4), 608

Q

QT abnormalities, **158**, 158–159
"Quad-therapy," 320
Quinidine, 376–378, **402**, 407, *408*, 409, 410, 412–414, **414**, 415, *415*, 418, 426, 427

R

RAAS, *see* Renin–angiotensin–aldosterone system
Radiography
  canine heart, 46–50
  cardiomegaly, 51–52
  chamber enlargement patterns, 52–57
  equine thoracic radiography, 66, *66–67*
  feline heart, 50–51
  intrathoracic blood vessels
    aorta, 58
    lobar pulmonary arteries and veins, 58–61
    main pulmonary artery, 58
    vena cava, 61
  patient positioning, 46
  pleural space
    pleural effusion, 64–66
    pneumothorax, 66
  pulmonary hypertension, 825–827
  pulmonary parenchyma
    patterns, 61–62
    pulmonary edema, 62–64
  small cardiac silhouette, 52
  systematic evaluation, 46
  technique considerations, 46
Ramipril, 323, **345**
Rapid heart rate
  AF, 240–241
  sinus tachycardia, 240
  supraventricular tachyarrhythmias, 241
  ventricular tachyarrhythmias, 241
Rapid pericardial fluid accumulation, 715
rASD, *see* Reversed ASD
RBC distribution width (RDW), 288, 825
RDW, *see* RBC distribution width
Recombinant tissue plasminogen activator (rt-PA), 766
Refractory CHF
  cats, 358
  dogs, 354–356
Relaxation abnormality, 129
Renal amyloidosis, 844
Renal and endocrine HT, 789
Renal dysfunction, 564–565
Renal function tests, 289
Renal hamartomas, 784
Renin-angiotensin-aldosterone system (RAAS), 655, 789, 816
  arterial blood pressure, 290
  circadian variation, 306
  components and effects of, 29, *29*
  renal fluid retention, 281–282
  systemic activation, 305–306
Reperfusion-induced hyperkalemia, 766
Respiratory alkalosis, 759
Respiratory auscultation, 40–42
Respiratory distress
  approach to patient

breathing patterns, 218–219
clinical examination, 219
clinical testing and management, 219–220, **220–221**
O_2 administration, 217, *218*
point-of-care thoracic/lung ultrasound exam, 80, 217, 340, 665, *665*
respiratory signs, disease localization, **218**
causes, 212, **213**, 214
dyspnea, 211
hyperpnea, 211
hypoxemia, 214–215
orthopnea, 211–212
paradoxical breathing, 211–212
pleural effusion, 216, **216**
PTE, 216–217
pulmonary edema, 215, *216*
tachypnea, 211
Resting membrane potential, 11
Resting respiratory rate (RRR), 313
Restrictive cardiomyopathy, 678
  clinical features, 679
  diagnostic tests, 679–681
  management, 681–682
  pathophysiology, 678–679
Restrictive filling, 129
Retinal edema, HT, 793
Retinopathy, hypertensive dogs, 793
Retrocaval ureter, 526, *526*
Reverberation (repetition) artifacts, 79
Reversed ASD (rASD)
  clinical features and diagnostic tests, 464, *464–465*
  management, 465
  systemic embolization, venous thrombi, 464
Reversed PDA (rPDA), 191, 249
  bidirectional shunting, 449
  clinical features
    cyanosis, 450
    hindlimb weakness, 450, *450*
    S_2 sound, 450, *450*
  diagnostic tests
    cardiac catheterization, 452
    echocardiography, 451, *452*
    echocontrast studies, 451–452, *453*
    high-velocity pulmonary regurgitation, 451
    sinus rhythm, *451*
    thoracic radiographs, 450, *451*
  differential cyanosis, 450, *450*
  management
    ductal closure, 452–453
    exercise restriction, 453
    hydroxyurea, 454
    parenteral fluid therapy, 453
    PDE-5 inhibitors, 453–454
    periodic hirudotherapy, 454
    prognosis, 454

Reversed ventricular septal defect (rVSD)
  clinical features, 460
  diagnostic tests, 460, *461*
  management, 460–461
Rhonchus, 41
Rickettsia rickettsii, 781
Right atrial (RA)
  dilation, 283
  and ventricular size and function, 106
Right atrial appendage/auricle (RAu), 6
Right ductus arteriosus, 516–517
Right-to-left shunts, 283; *see also* individual Reversed shunt defects
Right ventricular (RV)
  dilation, 283
  dysfunction, 35
  pulsus alternans, 257
Rivaroxaban, **751**, 764, 766, 770, 858
Rocky Mountain spotted fever, 781
RPA distensibility index (RPADI), *832*, 832–833
RRR, *see* Resting respiratory rate
rVSD, *see* Reversed ventricular septal defect

S

S₃ gallop, 232
S₄ gallop, 232
SA block, 153
Saddle thrombus, 752, 775
Sarcoendoplasmc reticulum calcium ATPase (SERCA), 14, 609
SAS, *see* Subaortic stenosis
Scopolamine, 387, **403**
Secondary (idiopathic) DCM, 607
Secondary hypertension associations, **789**
Secondary myocardial diseases, 630
  cat
    anemia, 689
    cardiac hypertrophy, 689
    causes, 688–689
    corticosteroid-associated congestive heart failure, 689
    hyperthyroidism, *688*, 688–689
    pressure overload, 688
  dog
    causes, **631**
    doxorubicin toxicity, 631–632, *632*
    hypothyroidism, 635
    metabolic abnormalities, 632–636
    nonneoplastic, 635
    nutritional deficiencies, 632–636
    tachycardia-induced cardiomyopathy, 630–631
Sedation, echocardiography, 80–81
Selkirk Rex cat, *663*
Semilunar valves
  left ventricular outflow, 117
  maximal instantaneous velocity, 114

mean ejection velocity, 114
  regurgitation, 479, *479*
  right ventricular outflow, 117
Sepsis, 749
SERCA, *see* Sarcoendoplasmc reticulum calcium ATPase
Seroreactivity, 598–599
Serum biochemistries
  electrolytes, 289–290
  liver and pancreatic enzymes, 289
  muscle enzymes, 290
  proteins, 290
  renal function tests, 289
Serum symmetric dimethylarginine (SDMA) concentration measurement, 289
Shock, 749
"Shockable" rhythms, 393
Shunts, 126–127
Siamese cat, *682*
Sibilant rhonchi, 41
Sick sinus syndrome (SSS), 405–406
Signal aliasing, 112, 117
Sildenafil, 822, 834–835, 861–862, 866–867, 873
  in DMVD, dogs, **556**, 557, 559, 561–562
  in heart failure treatment, 331, 349, 352, **355**, 356
Silent atrium, *see* Atrial standstill
Simpson's method of discs (SMOD), 104–105, *104*, **612**, 613–616, 620
Sinoventricular rhythm, 160
Sinus arrhythmia, 21
  Holter monitoring, 162
  HRs, 238
  wandering pacemaker, 143, *143*
Sinus bradycardia, 197
  antiarrhythmic drug dosage, **402–404**
  atropine response test, 402
  causes, **238**
  clinical signs, 402
  excessive vagal tone, 401
  HR, 244
  hypotension, 401
  management, 404
Sinus node
  dysfunction, 405–406
  reentry, 143
Sinus pause/arrest, 143, *143*
Sinus rhythm
  disturbances
    sinus bradycardia, 401–402, **402–404**, *404*
    sinus node dysfunction, 405–406
    sinus tachycardia, 401
  intermittent ventricular preexcitation, 154, *155*
  LBBB, *154*
  RBBB, *154*
  and variations, 142–143, *143*
  ventricular preexcitation, *154*

Sinus tachycardia, *198*, **238**, 401
Skeletal muscle ischemia, 290
Slow heart rate
  AV block, 242
  bradycardia–tachycardia syndrome, 241, *241*
  hyperkalemia, 242
Slow-response action potential, 12
Snoring/snorting sounds, 41
Sonorous rhonchi, 41
Sotalol, 381–382, **403**, 407, 408, *408*, 409, *409*, 411, 412, **414**, 415, 416, 418, 419, 424, *425*, *426*, 427, 621, 626, *627*, 628, *637*, 672, 675, 676, 677, 682, *707*
Spectral dispersion, 113
Spectral Doppler echocardiography, 108, *109–111*
Sphynx cat, cardiomyopathy, *666*
Spirocera lupi, 781
Spironolactone, 318, *318*, 319–320, 322, 328, *338*, 339, 340, **345**, 349, 350, 353, 354, **355**, 356, 357, 358, 558–559, 809
Splenomegaly, 270
Split sounds, 233
Spontaneous pneumopericardium, 705
Sporting dog, 608
SSS, *see* Sick sinus syndrome
Standard Schnauzer, gastric adenocarcinoma, *632*
Starling's law of the heart, 15
Stenosis and continuity relationship, 122
Sterile exudative effusions, 711–712
Sternal malformations, 707
Stertor, 41
Streptococcal endocarditis, 594
Streptokinase, 766–768
Stridor, 41
Stroke, 794; *see also* Heart
Stroke distance, 127
Stroke volume (SV), 14
Strongylus vulgaris, 781, *781*
ST-T abnormalities, *157*, 157–158, **158**
Subaortic stenosis (SAS), 591; *see also* Aortic stenosis
  clinical features, 481–482
  diagnostic tests, 482–488
  management, 488–489
  murmur, 226
  radiographic abnormalities, **482**
  syncope, 196
Subcutaneous edema, 757, *781*
  approach to patient, 278–279, *279*
  causes, **277**
  cranial caval syndrome, 277
  lymphedema, 278, *278*
  myxedema, 278
  pitting edema, 275–276, *276*
  submandibular, 275, *275*

vasculitis, 276, *276*
ventral thorax and rear limbs, *275*
Subendothelial collagen, 745–746
Supplemental O_2, 341
Supravalvular pulmonary stenosis, 784
Supraventricular premature complexes, 143–145
Supraventricular tachyarrhythmias, 241
Supraventricular tachycardia (SVT), 147, 197, 262
Symmetric dimethylarginine assay (SDMA) testing, 799
Sympathetic nervous system (SNS), 27, 303–305
Sympathetic stimulation, 20–21
Sympathomimetic drugs
   bronchodilator drugs, 387
   epinephrine, 387–388
   isoproterenol, 387
Syncope, 706
   approach to patient
      ECG, 200–201
      echocardiography, 201
      endocrine tests, 200
      Holter monitoring, 201
      medical strategies, 201–202
      thoracic radiographs, 200–201
   causes, **196**
      arrhythmic, 199
      cerebral blood flow, 196
      coughing, 199
      episodic weakness, 199
      hypoglycemia, 196, 198
      neurocardiogenic reflex mechanisms, 198
      orthostatic hypotension, 198–199
      reduced cardiac output, 196
      sinus bradycardia, 197
      tachyarrhythmias, 197
      ventricular asystole, *197*
      ventricular tachycardia, 197, *197*
   convulsive syncope, 195
   definition, 195
   excitement-induced, *198*
   lateral recumbency, 195, *195*
   presyncope, 195
Systemic arterial hypertension, 289, 564
Systemic arterial hypoxemia, 249
Systemic arterial pulsus alternans, 257
Systemic arterial thromboembolic disease, 750–753
Systemic hypertension
   alpha1-adrenergic antagonists, 809
   antihypertensive agents, **803**, *803*
      amlodipine, 808–809
      angiotensin converting enzyme inhibitors, 807
      angiotensin receptor blockers, 807–808
      oral antihypertensive drugs, **804**

blood pressure in normal animals, 787–788
blood pressure measurement
   direct measurement, 796
   Doppler method, 798–799
   indirect measurement, 796–799
   oscillometric method, 799
classification, **788**
clinical features, 794–795
echocardiography, 800–802, *801–802*
hydralazine, 810–811
laboratory tests, 799–800
management
   antihypertensive strategies, 803–807
   decision to treat, 802–803
   hypertensive crisis, management options for, **806**
   hypertensive emergencies, 805–807
   monitoring therapy, 805
nitroprusside, 810
pathophysiology, 789
   endocrine disease, 791–792
   hypertension, pathologic effects of, 793–794
   kidney disease, 790–791
   other associations, 792–793
patient with suspected, **795**
radiography and electrocardiography, 800
secondary hypertension associations, **789**
spironolactone, 809
target organ disease, risk for, 788–789
Systemic hypotension, 253
Systemic veins, 25
Systolic clicks, 232, 539, *539*
Systolic heart failure, 17
Systolic heart murmur, 824
Systolic murmurs
   horses, 579, *579*
   MR, 229
   TR, 229
   ventricular outflow obstructions, 230
   VSD, 230
Systolic pressure, 23

T

Tachyarrhythmias, 197, 594, 757
Tachycardia, 140, 142
Tachycardia-induced cardiomyopathy (TICM), 630–631, 699, *699*
Tachypnea, 211, 219
Tadalafil, 822, 834–835, 861
TAPSE, *see* Tricuspid annular plane systolic excursion
Target organ disease, risk for, 788–789
Taurine, 351–352, 633–634, 682–683, 686
TDI, *see* Tissue Doppler imaging
TE, *see* Thromboembolism

TEE, *see* Transesophageal echocardiography
Telmisartan, 321, 324, 332, 564, 803, **804**, 804, 806–809
Tetralogy of Fallot (T of F)
   clinical features, **436**
      auscultation, 470
      cyanosis, *469*, 469–470
      conotruncal defects, 467
   diagnostic tests
      arterial hypoxemia, 470
      caudal caval distension, 470, *471*
      Doppler studies, 471, *472*
      infundibular hypertrophy, 469
   management
      beta-adrenergic blocker, 472
      periodic phlebotomy, 471
      prognosis, 472
   pseudotruncus arteriosus, 468
   pulmonary atresia, 469
   VSD, 468–469
Thermography, 763
Thiazide diuretics, heart failure treatment, 320
Third-degree/complete AV block, 152
Thombocytopenia, 289
Thoracic auscultation, 846
Thoracic focused assessment with sonography for trauma (TFAST) ultrasound, 718
Thoracic radiographs, 200–201, 206–207, 234, 708
Thoracic trauma, 712
Thrombin, 747
Thrombin-activated fibrinolytic factor, 747
Thrombin–thrombomodulin complex, 748
Thrombocytopenia, 758, 850
Thromboelastography (TEG), 758, *759*
Thromboembolic (TE) disease, 745
   arterial thromboembolism
      in cats, 755–756
      coronary thromboembolism, 757
      pulmonary thromboembolism, 757
      and thrombosis in dogs, 756–757
      venous thrombosis, 757
   clinical features, 755
   diagnostic tests
      angiography, 761–762
      echocardiography, 759–760
      laboratory tests, 757–759
      radiography, 759
      thermography, 763
      ultrasonography, 761–762
   fibrinolysis, 747
   management, **763**
      anticoagulant therapy, 765–766
      antiplatelet therapy, 764–765
      antithrombotic therapy, **768**
      fibrinolytic therapy, 766–768

general therapeutic principles, 763–764
mechanisms opposing thrombosis, 747–748
normal hemostasis, 745–747
pathophysiology
pathologic thrombosis, mechanisms, 748–749
pulmonary arterial thromboembolic disease, 753–754
systemic arterial thromboembolic disease, 750–753
thromboembolisim and disease conditions, 749–750
venous thrombosis, 754–755
prophylaxis, antiplatelet and anticoagulant strategies, 769–770
Thromboembolism (TE), 591, 636, 749–750, 758
Thrombomodulin, 747–748
Thrombophlebitis, 754, 764
Thrombosis
in dogs, 756–757
in pulmonary arteries, 782
Thrombosis and embolism
arterial embolic disease, 783
thrombotic diseases, 782
venous embolic disease, 783–784
Thrombosis in dogs, 756–757
Thrombotic diseases, 782
Thyrotoxicosis, 564
Ticagrelor, 765
TICM, *see* Tachycardia-induced cardiomyopathy
Timolol, 381
Tissue Doppler imaging (TDI), 112–113, 651, 833
Tissue edema, 775
Tissue inhibitors of these proteinases (TIMPs), 608
Tissue plasminogen activator (t-PA), 747, 764
T of F, *see* Tetralogy of Fallot
Tolvaptan, 333
Torsemide 319, 345, 349, 350, 355, 355, 358, 359
TR, *see* Tricuspid regurgitation
Trabeculae carneae, 6
Tracheal carina, 708
Tramlines, 61
Transcatheter therapy, 179–181
Transducers, 73–74
Transesophageal echocardiography (TEE), 129–130, *130,* 167, 169, 180–181, 599
Transforming growth factor (TGF), 609
Transient myocardial thickening, 104, 688
Transient sounds
gallop sounds, 232
heart sounds, altered intensity, **231**
split sounds, 231

Transthoracic echocardiography, 177
Transudates, 710
Transudative effusions, acquired pericardial effusions, 710–711
Traube's pulse, 256
Trauma, 749
Traumatic myocarditis, 641–643
Tricuspid annular plane systolic excursion (TAPSE), 94, 760
Tricuspid dysplasia, 716
clinical features, 505
cyanosis and metabolic acidosis, 505
diagnostic tests
QRS complexes, 506, *506*
right heart dilation, 505, *505–508*
supraventricular tachycardia, 506, *506*
malformations, tricuspid valve, 504, *504*
management
balloon valvuloplasty for stenosis, 507
prognosis, 507
thoracic duct ligation, 506
Tricuspid regurgitation (TR), 113, 118, 125–126, 655, 816, 844
horses, 588
murmurs, 229
Tricuspid valve, 8–9, *9*
PW Doppler imaging, **115–116,** 118
TR jet velocity, 830
Troglostrongylus brevior, 823
Troponins, *see* Cardiac troponins
Truncus arteriosus communis, 520–521, *521–522*
Trypanosoma cruzi, 290, 640–641, 711
Tuberculosis, disseminated, 711
Tubular hypoplasia, aorta, 521
Tumor necrosis factor (TNF), 609
Tumors of vascular and nonvascular origin, 784
Tunica media, hypertrophy, *845*
Turbulence, endothelial surface, 749
Turbulence-induced post-stenotic dilation, 784
Two-dimensional (2D) echocardiography
apical images, *78*
clinical utility, 88
four-chamber, 87
limitations, 86
RV inlet, 87, *87*
contrast, 88
cranial images, *78–79,* 88
long-axis image planes, *75–76,* 84–86
short-axis images, *76–77,* 86, *87*
temporal resolution, 84
Type II pneumocyte hyperplasia, 819
Tyrosine kinase inhibitors, 836
pulmonary hypertension, 836
Tyrosine kinase inhibitor therapy, HT, 792

U

Umbilical hernia, 707
Unclassified cardiomyopathy, 687, *687*
Unfractionated heparin (UFH), 765
Urinalysis, 290, 597
Urinary bladder
dilation, 270
rupture, 267
Urine protein/creatinine ratio, 791
Urokinase, 766–767
Urokinase, plasminogen activators, 747

V

Vagal maneuver, 388
Vagal stimulation, 21
Valsalva, ruptured aortic sinus of, *785*
Valsartan, 309, 312, 332–333, 558, 559, 561
Valve stenosis, 125
Valvular aortic stenosis, 183
Valvular heart disease (VHD), horse, *see* Equine valvular disease
Valvular regurgitation, 125–126, 283
Vascular calcification, 780–781
Vascular diseases
aortic regurgitation, 784
arteriosclerosis
atherosclerosis, 779, 779–780
clinical features of, 780
congenital dyslipidemia, *780*
in dogs, 779
fibrinoid change with, *778*
intramural coronary arteriosclerosis, 780, *780*
medial hypertrophy of pulmonary arteries, 780
arteriovenous fistula, 776
clinical features, 776–777
diagnostic tests, 777–778
management, 778
pathophysiologic mechanisms and clinical consequences, **777,** 777
pelvic limb edema, *778*
clinical consequences, 777
cranial mesenteric artery, *781*
edema and cutaneous ulcers, *786*
Friesian horses, 784
hamartomas, 784
histologically confirmed vasculitis, *781*
mycotic arteritis, *782*
pathophysiology, 775–776
thrombosis and embolism
arterial embolic disease, 783
thrombotic diseases, 782
venous embolic disease, 783–784
tumors of vascular and nonvascular origin, 784
turbulence-induced post-stenotic dilation, 784

Valsalva, ruptured aortic sinus of, *785*
vascular mineralization, 780–781
vasculitis (arteritis), 781–782, *782*
venous abnormalities, 784–785
Vascular encephalopathy, 596
Vascular endothelial integrity, 748
Vascular receptors, 27–28
Vascular reflexes, 28–29
Vascular resistance, 22–23
Vascular ring anomalies
    aberrant (retroesophageal) subclavian arteries, 517–518, *518*
    clinical features, *518*, 518–519
    diagnostic tests
        angiography, 519
        computed tomography angiography studies, 519–520, *520*
        esophageal dilation, 519, *519*
        thoracic radiographs, 519, *519*
    double aortic arch, 516, *517*
    management, 520
    PRAA, 516, *516–517*
    regurgitation, 516
    right ductus arteriosus, 516–517
Vasculature
    arterial blood pressure, 23–24
    arterial system, 23
    microcirculation and lymphatics, 24–25
    venous system, 25
Vasculitis, 276, *276*, 752, 781–782, *782*
Vasoconstriction, 26
Vasodilators; *see also* Antihypertensive agents
    acute CHF management, **345–346**
        hydralazine, 344
        sodium nitroprusside, 344
        topical nitroglycerin, 344
    heart failure treatment
        amlodipine, *323*, 324
        hydralazine, 323–324
        nitrates, 324–325
        prazosin, 324
Vaughan Williams antiarrhythmic drug classification, 373–385, **374**
Vena cava, 61, *61*
Vena contracta, 122
Venous abnormalities, 784–785
Venous aneurysms, 526
Venous embolic disease, 783–784
Venous embryology and anatomy, 515–516
Venous malformations
    caudal vena cava anomalies, 526, *526*
    left azygous vein, 525, *525*
    PLCVC, *see* Persistent left cranial vena cava
    retrocaval ureter, 526, *526*
    venous aneurysms, 526
Venous system vasculature, 25
Venous thrombosis, 754–755, 757

Ventral cervical and cranial thoracic subcutaneous edema, *761*
Ventral edema, 715
Ventricular arrhythmia
    chronic therapy, 426–428
    in-hospital therapy
        cats, *425*
        dogs, *425*
        electrocardioversion, 426, *426*
        horse, *426*
        lidocaine, 424
        phenytoin, 426
Ventricular diastolic function assessment, 127, **128**, 129
Ventricular dyssynchrony, 369
Ventricular enlargement; *see also* specific cardiac diseases
    left ventricle, **153**, *154*, **157**
    right ventricle, **153**, *154*, 156
Ventricular fibrillation (VF), 150, *150*, 428
Ventricular flutter, 150, *150*, 428
Ventricular function assessment, 17–18
Ventricular gallop, 232
Ventricular hypertrophy, 37, 104–105
Ventricular outflow obstruction
    concentric hypertrophy, *478*, 478–479
    high intraventricular pressure, 479
    murmurs, 230
    NT-proBNP concentration, 479
Ventricular parasystole, 149–150
Ventricular preexcitation, 153–155
Ventricular premature complexes (VPCs), 240, 422–423, 611, 627
    Holter monitoring, 162
    intermittent, 147, *147–148*
    interpolated, 148, *148*
    multiform, 148
Ventricular rhythm disturbances
    accelerated idioventricular rhythm, 423–424
    lethal arrhythmias and cardiopulmonary arrest
        cardiopulmonary resuscitation, 428, **429**
        unresponsive patient, 428
    therapy, ventricular arrhythmia
        chronic, 426–428
        in-hospital, 424–426
    ventricular flutter and fibrillation, 428
    ventricular tachycardia
        nonsustained (paroxysmal), 424
        sustained, 424
    VPCs, 422–423
Ventricular septal defect (VSD), 184, *184*
    classification, 454
    clinical features, **436**, 456
    diagnostic tests
        angiography, 458, *460*
        color Doppler, 458, *459*
        echocardiography, 457, *457–459*

        perimembranous defects, 457, *457*
        radiographic findings, **442**, 456, *457*
    interventricular septal formation, 454
    location, 454–455, *455*
    management, 458, 460
    murmurs, 230
    persistent truncus arteriosus, 455
    pulmonary vascular injury, 456
    shunt volume, 455–456
    supraventricular crest, 454
Ventricular systolic function assessment, 127
Ventricular tachyarrhythmias, 241
Ventricular tachycardia, 262
    capture beat, 148
    and CO, 197, *197*
    interpolated VPCs, 148, *148*
    nonsustained (paroxysmal), 424
    sustained, 424
Ventriculoarterial uncoupling, 817
Verapamil, 327, **374**, 384, 385, **403**, 411, 676
Vernakalant, 384
Vertebral heart size (VHS), 716
    canine, 47–50
    feline, 50–51, *52*
VHS, *see* Vertebral heart size
Viral myocarditis, 639
Virchow's triad, 748
Viscosity of blood, 23
Vitamin D, 310
Vitamin D and cardiovascular system, 792
Vizsla
    ECG, *638*
    ventricular myocardium, *638*
Von Willebrand factor (vWF), 746–747
VPCs, *see* Ventricular premature complexes
VSD, *see* Ventricular septal defect

W

Warfarin, 770
Waterhammer pulse, 255
Weimaraner dogs, 708
Wheezes, 41
White-coat effect in human medicine, 787
Whitney classification, mitral valve lesions, 533, **533**, *533*
Wolbachia bacteria, 843
Wolff-Parkinson-White (WPW) syndrome, 154, 417, *418*, 504, 630
Workload, heart failure, 300–301

X

Xarelto, 766
Xylazine, 80

Z

Z disk (Z line), *12*, 13, *13*, 608, 626
Z-scores, 614